MW00973806

Cancer Rehabilitation

Cancer Rehabilitation

Principles and Practice

EDITED BY

Michael D. Stubblefield, MD
Assistant Attending Physiatrist
Rehabilitation Medicine Service
Department of Neurology
Memorial Sloan-Kettering Cancer Center
Assistant Professor of Rehabilitation Medicine
Weill Cornell Medical College of Cornell University
New York, New York

Michael W. O'Dell, MD
Chief of Clinical Services
Department of Rehabilitation Medicine
New York-Presbyterian Hospital
Weill Cornell Medical Center
Professor of Clinical Rehabilitation Medicine
Weill Cornell Medical College of Cornell University
New York, New York

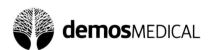

New York

Acquisitions Editor: Richard Winters and Beth Barry
Cover Design: Steve Pisano
Copyediting, Indexing, and Composition: Newgen Publishing and Data Services
Printer: Bang Printing

Visit our website at www.demosmedpub.com

Medicine is an ever-changing science. Research and clinical experience are continually expanding our knowledge, in particular our understanding of proper treatment and drug therapy. The authors, editors, and publisher have made every effort to ensure that all information in this book is in accordance with the state of knowledge at the time of production of the book. Nevertheless, the authors, editors, and publisher are not responsible for errors or omissions or for any consequences from application of the information in this book and make no warranty, express or implied, with respect to the contents of the publication. Every reader should examine carefully the package inserts accompanying each drug and should carefully check whether the dosage schedules mentioned therein or the contraindications stated by the manufacturer differ from the statements made in this book. Such examination is particularly important with drugs that are either rarely used or have been newly released on the market.

Library of Congress Cataloging-in-Publication Data

Cancer rehabilitation principles and practice / edited by Michael D. Stubblefield and Michael W. O'Dell.
    p. ; cm.
Includes bibliographical references and index.
ISBN–13: 978–1–933864–33–4 (hardcover : alk. paper)
ISBN–10: 1–933864–33–8 (hardcover : alk. paper)
1. Cancer—Patients—Rehabilitation. I. Stubblefield, Michael D. II. O'Dell, Michael W.
[DNLM: 1. Neoplasms—therapy. 2. Neoplasms—complications. 3. Neoplasms—diagnosis.
4. Pain—therapy. QZ 266 C217142 2009]
RC262.C3624   2009
616.99'405—dc22   2008048000

Special discounts on bulk quantities of Demos Medical Publishing books are available to corporations, professional associations, pharmaceutical companies, health care organizations, and other qualifying groups. For details, please contact:

Special Sales Department
Demos Medical Publishing
386 Park Avenue South, Suite 301
New York, NY 10016
Phone: 800–532–8663 or 212–683–0072
Fax: 212–683–0118
Email: orderdept@demosmedpub.com

Made in the United States of America

09 10 11 12   5 4 3 2 1

Dedication

This book is dedicated to the love of my life, Elyn. You are not only my wife, but my companion, partner, and most importantly my best friend. Without your love, encouragement, support, and patience this project would never have been possible.

—MDS

To Evelyn Brandman O'Dell my mentor, my role model, my closest friend, and my mother. Her endless optimism never ceases to inspire me. Everything I have been, everything I am, and everything I hope to be can be traced to this single, absolutely remarkable woman.

—MWO

Contents

II   INTRODUCTION TO EVALUATION AND TREATMENT OF MALIGNANCY

VII   GENERAL TOPICS IN CANCER REHABILITATION

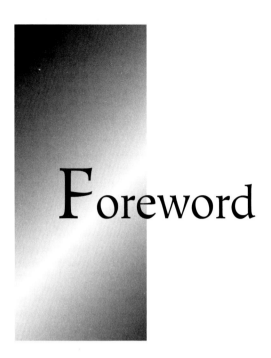

Foreword

This textbook represents a milestone.

—*Lynn H. Gerber, MD*

Dr. Howard Rusk, founder of the Rusk Institute of Rehabilitation Medicine, suggested that we needed a "service station" for cancer patients when he spoke at the first Cancer Conference on Rehabilitation Medicine in 1965 (1). In other words, a place where the multiple needs of cancer patients might be met. I credit him with the recognition that the cancer patient is a significant challenge to the health care establishment and would likely best be served in a comprehensive service organization. Others suggested that interdisciplinary efforts from the medical community, the patients, and the public sector would be needed to "reverse the defeatist attitude toward cancer and provide total continuity of care for the patient and for his family and community as well" (2).

Progress toward realizing Dr. Rusk's recommendations has been very slow. I would offer that we are still not fully there.

Several elements are needed to achieve optimal care for cancer patients. These include their rehabilitation, which makes this textbook an important contribution to the lives of cancer survivors. Cancer survivors and their families are just beginning to articulate their concerns and several priorities have been identified: the need to provide continuity of care, recognizing that care requires a team approach; the importance of quality of life as a desired outcome of treatment; and the

recognition that independence in daily function is a high priority for many cancer survivors.

The field of rehabilitation of the cancer patient received a tremendous boost from the work of Dr. J. Herbert Dietz, Jr., who worked at the Institute of Rehabilitation Medicine, New York University Hospital, and Memorial Hospital for Cancer and Allied Diseases. Dr. Dietz published the first text on rehabilitation for the cancer patient, *Rehabilitation Oncology*, in 1981 (3). This text was organized with the rehabilitation model in mind, including evaluations of impairments, disability, and societal integration (handicap). He approached the patient from the perspective of treatment goals, including extensive patient and family education (preventive, restorative, supportive, and palliative), and the phase of cancer (preoperative, postoperative, convalescence, and posthospital). He recommended the application of solid methodology in evaluating patients and assessing efficacy of treatment. The aim of treatment was goal-oriented and often vocational. The impact of Dietz's book on the next generation of oncological rehabilitation specialists was significant. In fact, in my own professional experience, it became clear to me that even without being conscious of it, Dr. Dietz's approach guided my approach to treating patients. He also offered an evaluation tool, the Dietz Scale, which became a commonly used evaluation tool for use with cancer patients.

Lehmann and colleagues (4) published a remarkable manuscript identifying the needs of patients with cancer diagnoses. They demonstrated that cancer patients had problems with self-care, mobility, and so on, and were likely to have psychological dysfunction and needed psychological support. They described the kinds of services required and valued by this population and demonstrated that when comprehensive rehabilitation was provided, there was significant clinical improvement. The authors concluded that patients with cancer need comprehensive rehabilitation, that if problems were properly identified and appropriate referrals were made, they did well. This approach presented a rationale for provision of rehabilitation services and a suggestion about which services were most needed for cancer patients. Additional studies supported the usefulness and appropriateness of inpatient rehabilitation (5–8). In fact, patients with brain tumors did as well functionally and had shorter length of hospital stay than those with stroke (9).

An important component of providing appropriate, quality care for cancer patients is good investigational work. Natural history studies, identifying the kinds of problems associated with cancer diagnoses, and clinical trials demonstrating which interventions are effective in reducing or preventing disability are critical resources for meeting the needs of these patients. Specifically, the work of Winningham and colleagues (10,11) demonstrated efficacy of aerobic training in reducing symptoms of cancer fatigue and improving functional outcomes. Dimeo demonstrated that in terms of symptoms, stamina and performance were better in bone marrow transplant recipients who received aerobic training than in those who did not (12). He further demonstrated that those who received a bicycle ergometer in the treatment room during their acute hospitalization for transplant, had improved levels of hemoglobin and white blood cell counts compared with those who did not receive in-room ergometry (13). This helped to establish the usefulness of an aerobic training program for cancer patients, and provided data to support the contention that exercise was safe during cancer treatment and had objective (eg, hematological) as well as subjective benefits.

This textbook reflects what has been learned from many of these studies. It includes results of studies of the natural history of cancer survivorship, from which we have identified problems that patients face and are of interest to them (eg, chemotherapy toxicities, impact of loss of limb, pain management, functional complications of bone marrow transplantation, etc.). It also includes important topics about rehabilitation interventions and effective treatments. For example, we have made great strides in understanding the value of exercise for cancer survivors, and, to some degree, how it works. This has enabled us to provide specific exercise prescriptions.

Cancer rehabilitation specialists have not agreed on standard core sets of evaluations or outcome measures for the cancer patient. Recent progress has been made in using new technologies to reduce the burden of data, such as item response theory, and in the quality of the psychometric properties of patient self-reports. The combination of standard objective measures of strength, range of motion, and other impairments; the use of more sensitive instruments for diagnosis and management (eg, infrared scanning for limb volume, EMG for diagnosis of neuropathy); and the widespread use of measures of symptoms, function, and quality of life, have helped define the necessary components for a comprehensive "metric" for the field. We now need to develop consensus and use these tools. These issues are discussed in this textbook, and several chapters make specific recommendations for the selection of appropriate and useful outcome measures.

Happily, cancer is no longer an acute, lethal illness. In my opinion, it is best thought of as a complex, chronic, and common disorder (14). Conceptually, the model of chronic illness best fits it. Cancers are likely to increase in prevalence as the population ages and the number of survivors increases. It will remain a challenge to treat. The biology of tumors varies considerably. Treatments for the tumor (radiation, surgery, chemotherapy, biologics) and the individual's response to them vary among patients. The impact of cancer on an individual's life is often dependent on phenomena not related to the tumor or its treatment, but rather to the individual's life needs and values. These factors present the health care professional with opportunities for collaborations and continued challenges for which the oncological and rehabilitation communities must coordinate efforts.

These observations have been known to the rehabilitation oncology community and cancer survivors for decades; but only recently has rehabilitation been acknowledged as an important contributor to the health and well-being of cancer patients and survivors. Heretofore, we were called to treat problems that were often at very late stages, such as frozen shoulder or severe lymphedema; or a problem of mobility or transfer needing adaptive equipment. This was made clear to me by the omission of the need for integrating rehabilitation services into the first National Cancer Policy Board report, "Ensuring Quality Cancer Care" (15). Rehabilitation interventions were not part of its recommendations for quality, comprehensive cancer evaluation, and treatment. The board's second report, "From Cancer Patient to Cancer Survivor: Lost in Transition," does address these concerns (16). Including rehabilitation interventions in the second report acknowledges the increasingly important role that rehabilitation plays in the lives of cancer survivors, and cites the evidence establishing efficacy of some rehabilitation treatment.

This textbook represents a milestone. It demonstrates the breadth of topics relevant to rehabilitation of the cancer patient. It also demonstrates that there is much that can be done for the cancer patient and survivor. The comprehensive nature of the content addresses the impairment, disability, and societal integration needs of this population of people. The publication of this text is likely to raise awareness of the advances in our field, the practical approach we offer for evaluating and solving problems of function, and the treatments we can offer our patients.

However, we have only just begun. Much work needs to be done to develop instruments to measure function and reconcile concerns about objective and self-reported measures. We still need to agree which are the best and most appropriate measures to use. Applying the rehabilitation model of impairment, disability, and handicap or the alternative International Classification of Disability, Functioning and Health will provide a consistent framework around which we can evaluate needs and response to treatment.

Efficacy of exercise in relieving some symptoms and improving function in the cancer survivor population has been demonstrated. Other rehabilitation interventions, such as bracing and manual therapy techniques, the use of modalities, complementary and alternative interventions have been used but would benefit from proper clinical trials.

We will need to devise interventions for all domains of the rehabilitation model. Models for delivery of care across the continuum of the phases of cancer and the life stages of survivors from infants to the very old should be evaluated for efficacy and efficiency. That is, we should evaluate the efficacy and accessibility of home health, outpatient, inpatient, and coordinated care services.

More clinical trials should be undertaken to further our goal of providing the best possible outcomes for cancer survivors. We believe the contributions of rehabilitation professionals can help improve and restore function, reduce the burden of disability, and help prevent functional decline; but more evidence is needed to demonstrate this. Achieving these outcomes will enable people who have survived cancer to attain their unique goals and enhance their quality of life. An important step in reaching these goals is to provide quality educational materials and improve access to the scope of rehabilitation practice in this population of patients. This textbook provides a comprehensive approach to the practice and the knowledge base on which the practice has been constructed. It is our hope that readers will benefit from this and enhance the nature of their practice and, ultimately, improve the lives of cancer patients.

Lynn H. Gerber, MD
Professor, Rehabilitation Science
Director, Center for the Study of
Chronic Illness and Disability
College of Health and Human Services
George Mason University
Fairfax, Virginia

REFERENCES

1. Switzer ME. Clinical Conference on Cancer, In: *Rehabilitation of the Cancer Patient*. Clark RL, Moreton RD, Healey JC, et al., eds. Chicago: Year Book Medical Publishers, Inc.; 1972.
2. Clark RL. Introduction. In: Clark RL, Moreton RD, Healey JC, et al., eds. *Rehabilitation of the Cancer Patient*. Chicago: Year Book Medical Publishers, Inc.; 1972.
3. Deitz, JH, Jr. *Rehabilitation Oncology*. New York: Wiley & Sons; 1981.
4. Lehmann JF, DeLisa JA, Warren CG, et al. Cancer rehabilitation: assessment of need, development and evaluation of a model of care. *Arch Phys Med Rehabil.* 1978;59:410–419.
5. Marciniak CM, Sliwa JA, Spill G, et al. Functional outcome following rehabilitation of the cancer patient. *Arch Phys Med Rehabil.* 1996;77:54–57.
6. Huang ME, Wartella JE, Kreutzer JS. Functional outcomes and quality of life in patients with brain tumors: a preliminary report. *Arch Phys Med Rehabil.* 2001;82:1540–1546.
7. Cole RP, Scialla SJ, Bednarz L. Functional recovery in cancer rehabilitation. *Arch Phys Med Rehabil.* 2000; 81:623–627.
8. O'Dell MW, Barr K, Spanier D, et al. Functional outcomes of inpatient rehabilitation in persons with brain tumor. *Arch Phys Med Rehabil.* 1998;79:1530–1534.
9. Huang ME, Cifu DX, Keeper–Marcus L. Functional outcomes after brain tumor and acute stroke: a comparative analysis. *Arch Phys Med Rehabil.* 1998;79:1286–1290.
10. Winningham ML, Nail LM, Burke MD, et al. Fatigue and the cancer experience. *Oncol Nurs Forum.* 1994;21:23–36.
11. MacVicar MG, Winningham ML, Nickel JL. Effects of aerobic interval training of cancer patients' functional capacity. *Nursing Res.* 1989;38:348–351.
12. Dimeo F, Rumberger BG, Keul J. Aerobic exercise training for cancer fatigue. *Med Sci Sports Exer.* 1998;4:475–478.
13. Dimeo FC, Tilmann MH, Bertz H, et al. Aerobic exercise in the rehabilitation of cancer patients after high dose chemotherapy and autologous peripheral stem cell transplant. *Cancer.* 1997;79:1717–1722.
14. Gerber LH. Cancer rehabilitation into the future. *Cancer.* 2001;92(4Suppl):975–979.
15. Hewitt, M, Simone,. *Ensuring Quality Cancer Care*. Washington DC: National Cancer Policy Board, 1999.
16. Hewitt, M. *From Cancer Patient to Cancer Survivor: Lost in Transition*. Washington DC: National Cancer Policy Board, 2005.

Preface

As of June 2008, the Centers for Disease Control (CDC) estimated that there were approximately 11 million persons in the United States living with a previously diagnosed cancer (1). This compares with fewer than 300,000 survivors of spinal cord injury and represents a threefold increase from the estimated 3 million persons who were living with cancer in 1971 (2,3). Approximately 65% of persons diagnosed with cancer today can expect to live at least five years after diagnosis compared with only 35% in the 1950s (4). This increase in cancer survivorship, largely attributable to advances in early detection and treatment, has led to a paradigm shift in how the diagnosis of cancer is perceived. Patients are increasingly described as "cancer survivors" as opposed to "cancer victims" (2). The cost of cancer survivorship is high. Patients diagnosed with cancer may look forward to various combinations of disfiguring surgery, toxic chemotherapy, and the insidiously fibrotic effects of radiotherapy. All of these potentially life-saving or prolonging modalities can result in marked impairments in every aspect of their life and function.

This textbook is intended to provide a state-of-the-art overview of the principles and practice of restoring function and quality of life to cancer survivors. The intended audience includes rehabilitation physicians, physical therapists, occupational therapists, nurses, oncologists, surgeons, and any other health care professionals with an interest in cancer rehabilitation. The successful rehabilitation of cancer patients requires a working understanding of the various types of cancer and their treatments. To this end, the section on principles, authored by some of the world's top cancer experts from wide-ranging disciplines including oncology, radiation oncology, neurosurgery, orthopedic surgery, and radiology, provides primer level overviews of the various cancer types, their evaluation, and treatment. The practice section of this text, authored by an even more diverse group of cancer rehabilitation and other specialists from a multitude of disciplines, details the identification, evaluation, and treatment of specific impairments and disabilities that result from cancer and the treatment of cancer.

The field of cancer rehabilitation has grown and changed dramatically since the pioneering work of Dietz more than a quarter century ago (5). Advances in our understanding of disease pathophysiology, improvements in imaging and electrodiagnostic testing, and enhanced treatment options including more effective medications and targeted procedures have uniquely positioned the physiatrist to benefit cancer survivors. At the Memorial Sloan-Kettering Cancer Center, the cancer rehabilitation specialist has moved into diagnostic and treatment planning roles. The rehabilitation team does not only evaluate and treat the neuromuscular and musculoskeletal pain and functional disorders associated with cancer and its treatment, but also works closely with the oncologist to determine the potential morbidity and effectiveness of a given treatment. This partnership has evolved not only due to improved patient survival but as a result of a new emphasis on maintaining or improving the cancer patient's function and quality of life. Many of the principles of cancer rehabilitation described in the text are borrowed from other rehabilitation specialties. For a variety of reasons, including to some degree fear and lack of knowledge about treating cancer patients, these principles have not been previously applied in the cancer setting. It is our intention that this work should be transformational for the discipline of cancer rehabilitation and lay the groundwork for this emerging specialty to take a leading role in cancer survivorship.

REFERENCES

1. Centers for Disease Control (CDC). Notice to readers: cancer survivorship. June 2008. MMWR 2008;57:605–606.
2. CDC. Cancer survivorship: United States, 1971–2001. MMWR 2004;53:526–529.
3. The National SCI Statistical Center. Spinal Cord Injury Facts and Figures at a Glance 2008. Available at http://www.spinalcord.uab.edu/show.asp?durki=116979.
4. Ries LAG, Melbert D, Krapcho M, Stinchcomb DG, Howlader N, Horner MJ, et al. (eds). SEER Cancer Statistics Review, 1975–2005. National Cancer Institute. Bethesda, MD. Available at http://seer.cancer.gov/csr/1975_2005/, based on November 2007 SEER data submission, posted to the SEER web site, 2008.
5. Deitz, JH, Jr. *Rehabilitation Oncology*. New York: Wiley & Sons; 1981.

Acknowledgments

Our gratitude to Theresa W. Fitzpatrick, PT, MBA and Christian M. Custodio, MD for their invaluable assistance in formulating the scope and content of this textbook.

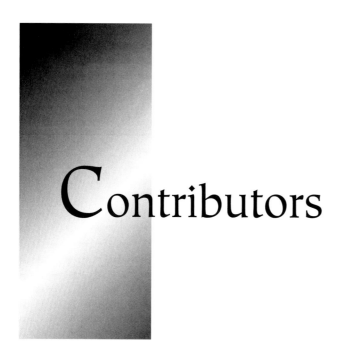

Contributors

Laura Andima, MD
Staff Anesthesiologist
VA Boston Healthcare System
Instructor
Anesthesiology
Harvard Medical School
Cambridge, Massachusetts

Edward K. Avila, DO
Assistant Attending Neurologist
Department of Neurology
Memorial Sloan-Kettering Cancer Center
New York, New York

Matthew N. Bartels, MD, MPH
John E. Dewey Associate Professor of Clinical
   Rehabilitation Medicine
Department of Rehabilitation Medicine
Columbia College of Physicians and Surgeons
Columbia University
New York, New York

Mark H. Bilsky, MD
Associate Attending Surgeon
Department of Neurosurgery
Memorial Sloan-Kettering Cancer Center
Associate Professor
Department of Neurological Surgery
Weill Cornell Medical College
New York, New York

Victoria Blinder, MD, MSc
Department of Epidemiology and Biostatistics
Health Outcomes Research Group
Department of Medicine
Breast Cancer Medicine Service
Memorial Sloan-Kettering Cancer Center
New York, New York

Patrick J. Boland, MD
Attending Orthopaedic Surgeon
Orthopaedic Service
Department of Surgery
Memorial Sloan-Kettering Medical Center
New York, New York

Julia F. Boysen, PT
Assistant Supervisor PM&R
Rochester Methodist Hospital
Rochester, Minnesota

Thomas H. Brannagan, III, MD
Associate Professor of Clinical Neurology
Director, Peripheral Neuropathy Center
Columbia University College of Physicians
   and Surgeons
Co-director, EMG Laboratory
New York-Presbyterian Hospital
New York, New York

Claudine Levy Campbell, OTR/L
Chief of Occupational Therapy
Rehabilitation Medicine Service
Department of Neurology
Memorial Sloan-Kettering Medical Center
New York, New York

Kristen E. Cardamone, DO
Fellow, Orthopedic Sports and Spine Rehabilitation
Beth Israel Medical Center
Continuum Center for Health and
    Healing/Spine Institute of New York
New York, New York

Barrie R. Cassileth, MS, PhD
Chief, Integrative Medicine Service
Department of Medicine
Memorial Sloan-Kettering Cancer Center
New York, New York

Melissa M. Center, MPH
Epidemiologist
Surveillance and Health Policy Research
American Cancer Society
Atlanta, Georgia

Leighton Chan, MD, PhD
Chief, Rehabilitation Medicine Department
National Institutes of Health
Bethesda, Maryland

Andrea L. Cheville, MD, MSCE
Associate Professor of Physical Medicine and
    Rehabilitation
Mayo Clinic
Rochester, Minnesota

Dennis S. Chi, MD
Gynecology Service
Department of Surgery
Memorial Sloan-Kettering Cancer Center
New York, New York

Kenneth Cubert, MD
Associate Attending Anesthesiologist
Pain Service
Department of Anesthesiology
    and Critical Care Medicine
Memorial Sloan-Kettering Cancer Center
New York, New York

Edward J. Cupler, MD
Associate Professor
Department of Neurology
Director, Neuromuscular Disease Center
Oregon Health and Science University
Portland, Oregon

Christian M. Custodio, MD
Assistant Attending Physiatrist
Rehabilitation Medicine Service
Department of Neurology
Memorial Sloan-Kettering Cancer Center
New York, New York

Lisa M. DeAngelis, MD
Chair
Department of Neurology
Memorial Sloan-Kettering Cancer Center
New York, New York

Robert W. DePompolo, MD
Director
Cancer Rehabilitation Program
Mayo Clinic
Rochester, Minnesota

Tim Dillingham, MD
Professor and Chairman
Physical Medicine and Rehabilitation
Medical College of Wisconsin
Milwaukee, Wisconsin

Joseph J. Disa, MD
Associate Attending Surgeon
Plastic and Reconstructive Surgery Service
Memorial Sloan-Kettering Cancer Center
New York, New York

Don S. Dizon, MD, FACP
Assistant Professor
Department of Obstetrics/Gynecology
    and Medicine
Warren Alpert Medical School
Brown University
Director, Medical Oncology and
    Integrative Care
Co-Director, Center for Sexuality, Intimacy
    and Fertility
Program in Women's Oncology
Women and Infants Hospital
Providence, Rhode Island

Edward J. Dropcho, MD
Professor, Department of Neurology
Director, Neuro-Oncology Program
Indiana University Medical Center
Indianapolis, Indiana

Austin Duffy, MD
Clinical Fellow
Medical Oncology Branch
National Cancer Institute
Bethesda, Maryland

Erin Embry, MS CCC-SLP
Instructor, Clinical Supervisor, Graduate Advisor
Department of Speech-Language Pathology
   and Audiology
New York University
New York, New York

Noel G. Espiritu, DPT
Chief Physical Therapist
Rehabilitation Medicine Service
Department of Neurology
Memorial Sloan-Kettering Cancer Center
New York, New York

Mill Etienne, MD
Fellow, Division of Epileptology
Department of Neurology
Columbia University
New York, New York

Azeez Farooki, MD
Assistant Attending Physician
Endocrinology Service
Department of Medicine
Memorial Sloan-Kettering Cancer Center
New York, New York

Mark A. Ferrante MD
Associate Professor
Co-Director, Neuromuscular Division
Director, EMG Laboratory
Department of Neurology
University of Texas Health Science Center
San Antonio, Texas

Teresa W. Fitzpatrick, PT, MBA
Rehabilitation Manager
Rehabilitation Medicine Service
Department of Neurology
Memorial Sloan-Kettering Cancer Center
New York, New York

Kevin Fox, MD
Marianne T. and Robert J. MacDonald Professor
   in Breast Cancer Care Excellence
Department of Medicine
Hospital of the University of Pennsylvania
Philadelphia, Pennsylvania

Debora Julie Franklin, PhD, MD
Director Cancer Rehabilitation
Assistant Professor
Department of Rehabilitation Medicine
Thomas Jefferson University
Philadelphia, Pennsylvania

Stacey Franz, DO, MSPT
Fellow, Musculoskeletal Medicine, Interventional
   Spine Care, Sports Medicine & Pain Management
Kessler Institute for Rehabilitation
University of Medicine and Dentistry of New Jersey
Newark, New Jersey

Mark A. Frattini, Md, PhD
Assistant Member
Department of Medicine
Memorial Sloan-Kettering Medical Center
New York, New York

Megan L. Freeland, PT, DPT
Physical Therapist
Rehabilitation Medicine Service
Department of Neurology
Memorial Sloan-Kettering Cancer Center
New York, New York

Gail Louise Gamble, MD
Medical Director
Cancer Rehabilitation
Rehabilitation Institute of Chicago
Chicago, Illinois

Sandy B. Ganz, PT, DSc, GCS
Director of Rehabiliation
Amsterdam Nursing Home
New York, New York

Susan V. Garstang, MD
Assistant Professor
Department of Physical Medicine and
   Rehabilitation
University of Medicine and Dentistry
   of New Jersey
Newark, New Jersey

Lynn H. Gerber, MD
Director, Center for Chronic Illness and
   Disability
Department of Global and Community Health
College of Health and Human Services
George Mason University
Fairfax, Virginia

Jorge E. Gomez, MD
Assistant Professor of Medicine
UM Sylvester Comprehensive Cancer Center
Miller School of Medicine
University of Miami
Miami, Florida

Clifton L. Gooch, MD
Professor and Chairman
Department of Neurology
University of South Florida College of Medicine
Tampa, Florida

Eric Graf
Senior Research Assistant
Neuromuscular Disease Center
Oregon Health and Sciences University
Portland, Oregon

Sean A. Grimm, MD
Assistant Professor of Neurology
Feinberg School of Medicine
Northwestern University
Chicago, Illinois

Jyothirmai Gubili, MS
Assistant Editor
Integrative Medicine Service
Memorial Sloan-Kettering Cancer Center
New York, New York

Amitabh Gulati, MD
Assistant Attending Anesthesiologist
Pain Service
Department of Anesthesiology and Critical Care
    Medicine
Memorial Sloan-Kettering Cancer Center
New York, New York

Sakir Humayun Gultekin
Assistant Professor
Department of Pathology
Director, Neuromuscular Pathology Laboratory
Oregon Health and Science University
Portland, Oregon

Georgi Guruli, MD, PhD
Associate Professor
Director of Urologic Oncology
Department of Surgery
Virginia Commonwealth University School
    of Medicine
Richmond, Virginia

James Han, MD
Resident Physician
Department of Physical Medicine and
    Rehabilitation
Hospital of the University of Pennsylvania
Philadelphia, Pennsylvania

Maryann Herklotz, PT
Assistant Chief Physical Therapist
Rehabilitation Medicine Service
Department of Neurology
Memorial Sloan-Kettering Cancer Center
New York, New York

Robin C. Hindery, MS
Medical Writer
Integrative Medicine Service
Department of Medicine
Memorial Sloan-Kettering Cancer Center
New York, New York

Margaret L. Ho, MA, CCC-SLP
Supervisor, Speech and Swallowing Services
Head and Neck Service
Department of Surgery
Memorial Sloan-Kettering Cancer Center
New York, New York

Jimmie C. Holland, MD
Wayne E. Chapman Chair in Psychiatric Oncology
Attending Psychiatrist
Department of Psychiatry and Behavioral Sciences
Memorial Sloan-Kettering Cancer Center
New York, New York

Dory Hottensen, LCSW
Senior Social Worker, Palliative Care
Department of Social Work
New York-Presbyterian Hospital
Weill Cornell Medical Center
New York, New York

Clifford A. Hudis, MD
Chief, Breast Cancer Medicine Service
Department of Medicine
Memorial Sloan-Kettering Cancer Center
New York, New York

Ahmedin Jemal, DVM, PhD
Department of Epidemiology and Surveillance
    Research
American Cancer Society
Atlanta, Georgia

Juan Miguel Jimenez-Andrade, PhD
Research Assistant Professor
Department of Pharmacology
University of Arizona
Tucson, Arizona

C. George Kevorkian, MD
Associate Professor and Vice Chair
Department of Physical Medicine and Rehabilitation
Baylor College of Medicine
Chief of Service
Department of Physical Medicine and Rehabilitation
St. Luke's Episcopal Hospital
Houston, Texas

Juliana Khowong, MD
Clinical Instructor
Department of Rehabilitation Medicine
Columbia University College of Physicians and
    Surgeons
New York, New York

Elizabeth M. Kilgore, MD, MS, FAAPM&R
Assistant Professor of Clinical Rehabilitation
    Medicine
Georgetown University Medical Center
Director, Cancer Rehabilitation Program
National Rehabilitation Hospital
Washington, DC

Tari A. King, MD
Assistant Attending Surgeon
Breast Service
Department of Surgery
Jeanne A. Petnek Junior Faculty Chair
Memorial Sloan-Kettering Cancer Center
New York, New York

Guenther Koehne, MD, PhD
Attending Physician
Allogeneic Bone Marrow Transplantation Service
Department of Medicine
Memorial Sloan-Kettering Cancer Center
Assistant Professor
Weill Cornell Medical College of Cornell University
New York, New York

George Krol, MD
Attending Neuroradiologist
Department of Radiology
Neuroradiology Service
Memorial Sloan-Kettering Cancer Center
Professor of Clinical Radiology
Weill Cornell Medical College of Cornell University
New York, New York

Michael Krychman, MD, FACOG
Medical Director
The Sexual Medicine Center at Hoag
Executive Director
The Southern California Center for Sexual Health
    and Survivorship Medicine
Newport Beach, California
Associate Clinical Professor
University of Southern California
Los Angeles, California

Heather J. Landau, MD
Assistant Attending
Hematology Service
Department of Medicine
Memorial Sloan-Kettering Cancer Center
New York, New York

Christine Laviano, OTR/L
Head Occupational Therapist
Acute Care
Rehabilitation Medicine Service
Department of Neurology
NewYork-Presbyterian Hospital
Columbia University Medical Center
New York, New York

Rebecca Leboeuf, MD
Assistant Professor of Medicine
Assistant Attending Physician
Endocrinology Service
Department of Medicine
Memorial Sloan-Kettering Cancer Center
New York, New York

Taryn Y. Lee, MD
Assistant Professor of Medicine
Division of Geriatrics and Gerontology
Weill Cornell Medical College of
    Cornell University
Assistant Attending Physician
New York-Presbyterian Hospital
New York, New York

Marsha Leight, PT
Senior Physical Therapist
Rehabilitation Medicine Service
Department of Neurology
Memorial Sloan-Kettering Cancer Center
New York, New York

Jon Lewis, MD
Neuroradiology Fellow
Department of Radiology
Neuroradiology Service
New York-Presbyterian Medical Center
Memorial Sloan-Kettering Cancer Center
New York, New York

Su Hsien Lim, MD
Medical Oncology and Hematology, PC
Yale-New Haven Shoreline Medical Center
Guilford, Connecticut

C. David Lin, MD
Ida and Theo Rossi Di Montelera
    Assistant Professor of Rehabilitation Medicine
Department of Rehabilitation
Weill Cornell Medical College of
    Cornell University
Assistant Attending
New York-Presbyterian Hospital
Weill Cornell Medical Center
New York, New York

Julie Lin, MD
Assistant Attending Physiatrist
Physiatry Department
Hospital for Special Surgery
Assistant Professor
Department of Rehabilitation Medicine
New York-Presbyterian Hospital
New York, New York

Todd A. Linsenmeyer, MD
Director of Urology
Kessler Institute for Rehabilitation
West Orange, New Jersey
Professor
Department of Surgery
Professor
Department of Physical Medicine and Rehabilitation
University of Medicine and Dentistry of New Jersey
Newark, New Jersey

Eric Lis, MD
Associate Attending Neuroradiologist
Director of Neurointerventional Radiology
Department of Radiology
Neuroradiology Service
Memorial Sloan-Kettering Cancer Center
New York, New York

Laura Locati, MD
Instituto Nazionale Tumori
Department of Medical Oncology
Milan, Italy

Paul Magda, DO
Clinical Assistant Professor of Neurology
Department of Neurology
St. Vincent's Catholic Medical Center-Manhattan
New York, New York

Robert G. Maki, MD, PhD
Associate Member and Co-Director
Adult Sarcoma Program
Department of Medicine
Memorial Sloan-Kettering Cancer Center
New York, New York

Vicky Makker
Assistant Member
Gynecologic Medical Oncology Service
Department of Medicine
Memorial Sloan-Kettering Cancer Center
New York, New York

Patrick W. Mantyh, PhD
Professor
Department of Pharmacology
University of Arizona
Tucson, Arizona

Enrica Marchi, MD
Herbert Irving Comprehensive Cancer Center
New York, New York

Madhu Mazumdar, PhD, MA, MS
Professor of Biostatistics in Public Health
Chief, Division of Biostatistics and Epidemiology
Department of Public Health
Weill Cornell Medical College of Cornell University
New York, New York

Christopher Mazzone
Neuroradiology Research Assistant
Department of Radiology
Neuroradiology Service
Memorial Sloan-Kettering Cancer Center
New York, New York

Heather L. McArthur, MD, MPH
Clinical Research Fellow
Breast Cancer Medicine Service
Department of Medicine
Memorial Sloan-Kettering Cancer Center
New York, New York

Colleen M. McCarthy, MD, MS
Assistant Attending Surgeon
Plastic and Reconstructive Service
Department of Surgery
Memorial Sloan-Kettering Cancer Center
New York, New York

William McKinley, MD
Director, Spinal Cord Injury Medicine
Professor of Physical Medicine and
    Rehabilitation
Virginia Commonwealth University
    Medical Center
Richmond, Virginia

Sarah A. McLaughlin, MD
Assistant Professor of Surgery
Department of Surgery
Mayo Clinic
Jacksonville, Florida

Veronica McLymont, MD, RD, CDN
Director
Food and Nutrition Services
Memorial Sloan-Kettering Cancer Center
New York, New York

Amit B. Mehta, MD
Anesthesiologist and Interventional
    Pain Physician
Premier Pain Specialists Co-founder
Co-director of the Division of Pain Management
    at MacNeal Hospital
Chicago, Berwyn, and Schaumburg, Illinois

Neel Mehta, MD
Resident
Department of Anesthesiology
Weill Cornell Medical College
    of Cornell University
New York, New York

Christina A. Meyers, PhD, ABPP
Professor and Chief
Section of Neurophysiology
M.D. Anderson Cancer Center
Houston, Texas

Amanda Molnar, MSPT
Senior Physical Therapist
Rehabilitation Medicine Service
Department of Neurology
Memorial Sloan-Kettering Cancer Center
New York, New York

Alexei Morozov, MD, PhD
Fellow, Hermatology-Oncology
Department of Medicine
Memorial Sloan-Kettering Cancer Center
New York, New York

Carol D. Morris, MD, MS
Associate Attending Surgeon
Orthopedic Surgery Service
Department of Surgery
Memorial Sloan-Kettering Cancer Center
New York, New York

Natalie Moryl, MD
Assistant Attending
Pain and Palliative Care Service
Department of Medicine
Memorial Sloan-Kettering Cancer Center
New York, New York

Rajaram Nagarajan, MD, MS
Assistant Professor of Pediatrics
Department of Pediatrics
Cincinnati Children's Hospital Medical Center
University of Cincinnati College of Medicine
Cincinnati, Ohio

Stephen D. Nimer, MD
Chief, Hematology Service
Vice Chair, Faculty Development
Department of Medicine
Alfred Sloan Chair
Memorial Sloan-Kettering Cancer Center
New York, New York

Owen A. O'Connor, MD, PhD
Director
Lymphoid Development and Malignancy Program
Herbert Irving Comprehensive Cancer Center
Chief, Lymphoma Service
College of Physicians and Surgeons
New York-Presbyterian Hospital
Columbia University
New York, New York

Michael W. O'Dell, MD
Chief of Clinical Services
Department of Rehabilitation Medicine
New York-Presbyterian Hospital
Weill Cornell Medical Center
Professor of Clinical Rehabilitation Medicine
Weill Cornell Medical College
    of Cornell University
New York, New York

Kristen M. O'Dwyer, MD
Leukemia Service
Department of Medicine
Memorial Sloan-Kettering Cancer Center
New York, New York

Kevin C. Oeffinger, MD
Attending and Member
Director
Adult Long Term Follow Up Program
Departments of Pediatrics and Medicine
Memorial Sloan-Kettering Cancer Center
New York, New York

Gary C. O'Toole, BSc, MCh, FRCS
Consultant, Orthopaedic Surgeon
St. Vincent's University Hospital
Cappagh National Orthopaedic Hospital
Dublin, Ireland

Lora Packel, MS, PT, CCS
Assistant Professor
Department of Physical Therapy
University of the Sciences
Philadelphia, Pennsylvania

Meena J. Palayekar, MD
Department of Obstetrics and Gynecology
Saint Peter's University Hospital
New Brunswick, New Jersey

Desiree A. Pardi, MD, PhD
Assistant Professor of Medicine
Division of Geriatrics and Gerontology
Weill Cornell Medical College
  of Cornell University
Director, Palliative Care Service
New York-Presbyterian Hospital
New York, New York

Rebecca A. Parks, MS, OTR/L, BCP, FAOTA
U.S. Public Health Service
National Institutes of Health
Bethesda, Maryland

Snehal Patel, MD
Attending Surgeon
Head and Neck Service
Department of Surgery
Memorial Sloan-Kettering Cancer Center
New York, New York

Mackenzi Pergolotti, MS, OTR/L
Assistant Chief of Occupational Therapy
Rehabilitation Medicine Service
Department of Neurology
Memorial Sloan-Kettering Cancer Center
New York, New York

Lucinda Pfalzer, PhD, PT, FACSM
Department of Physical Therapy
University of Michigan-Flint
Flint, Michigan

David G. Pfister, MD
Member and Attending Physician
Chief, Head and Neck Medical Oncology
Co-leader, Head and Neck Cancer Disease
  Management Team
Memorial Sloan-Kettering Cancer Center
New York, New York

Cynthia G. Pineda, MD, FAAPM&R
Assistant Profesor of Clinical Rehabilitation
  Medicine
Georgetown University Medical Center
Staff Physiatrist
National Rehabilitation Hospital
Washington, DC

Tara Post, OTR/L, ATP
Supervisor, Occupational Therapy
Department of Rehabilitation Medicine
New York-Presbyterian Hospital
Weill Cornell Medical Center
New York, New York

David William Pruitt, MD
Assistant Professor, Clinical Pediatrics
  and Clinical PMSR
Department of Pediatrics
Cincinnati Children's Hospital Medical Center
University of Cincinnati College of Medicine
Cincinnati, Ohio

Hanna Chua Rimner, BScPT
Senior Physical Therapist
Rehabilitation Medicine Service
Department of Neurology
Memorial Sloan-Kettering Cancer Center
New York, New York

Justin C. Riutta, MD, FAAPMR
Director of Lymphedema and Breast Cancer
  Rehabilitation
William Beaumont Hospital
Royal Oak, Michigan

Corey Rothrock, MD
Clinical Instructor, Orthopedic Surgery
Musculoskeletal Oncology
Norton Cancer Institute
University of Louisville
Louisville, Kentucky

Yvonne Saenger, MD
Assistant Professor
Department of Medicine, Hematology and
  Medical Oncology
Mount Sinai School of Medicine
New York, New York

Leonard B. Saltz, MD
Attending Oncologist
Gastrointestinal Oncology Service
Department of Medicine
Memorial Sloan-Kettering Cancer Center
Professor of Medicine
Weill Cornell Medical College of Cornell University
New York, New York

Sonia K. Sandhu, DO
Assistant Professor
Co-Director, Intraoperative Neurophysiologic
  Monitoring
Department of Neurology and Neuroscience
Weill Cornell Medical College of Cornell University
New York-Presbyterian Hospital
New York, New York

Annelise Savodnik, PT, MPT, CLT
Senior Physical Therapist
Rehabilitation Medicine Service
Department of Neurology
Memorial Sloan-Kettering Cancer Center
New York, New York

Oksana Sayko, MD
Assistant Professor
Department of Physical Medicine and Rehabilitation
Medical College of Wisconsin
Milwaukee, Wisconsin

Elizabeth Schack, RN, GNP, CNS
Nurse Practitioner
Palliative Care Service
New York-Presbyterian Hospital
Weill Cornell Medical Center
New York, New York

Mary J. Scherbring, CNS, RN
Prior Clinical Nurse Specialist on Cancer
and Adaptation Team
Mayo Clinic
Rochester, Minnesota

Eric Schwabe, PT, MS
Supervisor, Physical Therapy
The Sue and John L. Weinberg Inpatient
  Rehabilitation Center
Department of Rehabilitation
New York-Presbyterian Hospital
Weill Cornell Medical Center
New York, New York

Julie K. Silver, MD
Assistant Professor
Harvard Medical School
Chief Editor of Books
Harvard Health Publications
Countway Library
Boston, Massachusetts

Susan F. Slovin, MD, PhD
Associate Attending Oncologist
Genitourinary Oncology Service
Department of Medicine
Memorial Sloan-Kettering Cancer Center
New York, New York

Rebecca G. Smith, MD, MS
Assistant Professor and Chief, Division of Cancer
  Rehabilitation
Department of Physical Medicine and Rehabilitation
Hospital of the University of Pennsylvania
Philadelphia, Pennsylvania

Beth Solomon, MS, CCC-SLP
Chief, Speech Language Pathology Section
Rehabilitation Medicine Department
National Institutes of Health
Bethesda, Maryland

David Spriggs, MD
Head, Division of Solid Tumor Oncology
Winthrop Rockefeller Chair in Medical Oncology
Memorial Sloan-Kettering Cancer Center
New York, New York

Argyrios Stampas, MD
Resident Physician
Department of Physical Medicine and Rehabilitation
Hospital of the University of Pennsylvania
Philadelphia, Pennsylvania

Michelle Stern, MD
Assistant Clinical Professor
Columbia University College of Physicians
  and Surgeons
New York-Presbyterian Hospital
New York, New York

Jessica Stiles, MD
Department of Psychiatry and Behavioral Sciences
Memorial Sloan Kettering Cancer Center
New York, New York

David Martin Strick, PhD, PT
Senior Lymphedema Therapist
Mayo Clinic
Rochester, Minnesota

Michael D. Stubblefield, MD
Assistant Attending Physiatrist
Rehabilitation Medicine Service
Department of Neurology
Memorial Sloan-Kettering Cancer Center
Assistant Professor of Rehabilitation Medicine
Weill Cornell Medical College of Cornell University
New York, New York

Ping Sun, DPT
Senior Physical Therapist
Rehabilitation Medicine Service
Department of Neurology
Memorial Sloan-Kettering Cancer Center
New York, New York

Sharlynn M. Tuohy, PT, MBA
Assistant Chief Physical Therapist
Rehabilitation Medicine Service
Department of Neurology
Memorial Sloan-Kettering Cancer Center
New York, New York

Robert Michael Tuttle, MD
Professor of Medicine
Attending Physician
Endocrinology Service
Department of Medicine
Memorial Sloan-Kettering Cancer Center
New York, New York

Tracy L. Veramonti, PhD
Neuropsychologist
The Institute for Rehabilitation and Research
Memorial Hermann Hospital
Clinical Assistant Professor
Department of Physical Medicine and Rehabilitation
Baylor College of Medicine
Houston, Texas

Louis H. Weimer, MD
Associate Clinical Professor of Neurology
Director, EMG laboratory
Co-director, Columbia Neuropathy Research Center
Columbia University College of Physicians and
    Surgeons
New York, New York

Talia R. Weiss, MD
Department of Psychiatry and Behavioral Sciences
Memorial Sloan-Kettering Cancer Center
New York, New York

Golda B. Widawski, PT, MPT
Senior Physical Therapist
Department of Rehabilitation Medicine
New York-Presbyterian Hospital
Weill Cornell Medical Center
New York, New York

Jill R. Wing, PT, DPT
Assistant Chief Physical Therapist
Rehabilitation Medicine Service
Department of Neurology
Memorial Sloan-Kettering Cancer Center
New York, New York

Jedd D. Wolchok, MD, PhD
Associate Attending
Melanoma and Sarcoma Service
Department of Medicine
Memorial Sloan-Kettering Cancer Center
New York, New York

Yoshiya Yamada, MD, FRCPC
Assistant Attending Radiation Oncologist
Department of Radiation Oncology
Memorial Sloan-Kettering Cancer Center
New York, New York

David S. Younger, MD
Chief of Neuromuscular Diseases
Associate Clinical Professor
Department of Neurology
New York University School of Medicine
New York, New York

Jasmine Zain, MD
Assistant Clinical Professor
Columbia University Medical Center
New York, New York

Cancer Rehabilitation

I

PRINCIPLES OF CANCER
AND CANCER TREATMENT

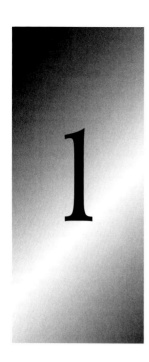

The History of Cancer Rehabilitation

C. George Kevorkian

Soon after I accepted the editors' flattering invitation to write this chapter on the history of cancer rehabilitation, I ventured into the voluminous library of the Texas Medical Center. My aim was to start research on the early years of cancer rehabilitation. Using the key words of "rehabilitation, cancer, and oncology" in a computer search, I was able to find only one volume that was published prior to 1980. This tome, entitled *Cancer Rehabilitation: An Introduction for Physiotherapists and the Allied Professions* was written by Patricia A. Downie, FCST, and published in London in 1978 (1). A meticulous and informative work, this book seems to have been written by and for physiotherapists (physical therapists). (I was later loaned a book entitled *Rehabilitation of the Cancer Patient* [1972] courtesy of Dr. Ky Shin.)

In an attempt to find resources with more of a physician orientation, I proceeded to a section on physical medicine and rehabilitation. I began my search by perusing the first (1965) and second (1971) editions of the venerable *Handbook of Physical Medicine and Rehabilitation* by Krusen, Kottke, and Ellwood (2). To my dismay, and some surprise, neither of these two first editions had a chapter, or even a paragraph, on "cancer rehabilitation." In both volumes the word cancer was only mentioned in regard to the skin cancer being caused by light, in particular, ultraviolet therapy. The word tumor appeared when discussing intramedullary spinal cord tumors in a chapter on electromyography. Malignancy and oncology were not mentioned at all.

The book entitled *Physical Medicine and Rehabilitation for the Clinician*, edited by Frank H. Krusen and published in 1951, similarly made no mention of cancer rehabilitation (3). The first, second, and third *Proceedings of the International Congress of Physical Medicine* similarly made no mention of cancer rehabilitation. Drs. Bierman and Licht edited multiple volumes of *Physical Medicine in General Practice*, where again no mention was made of cancer rehabilitation. But in one chapter, on surgical diathermy, a mention was made of electrocoagulation of malignant tissue. These volumes span the 1940s and early 1950s (4). With my search essentially revealing no information of use, I came to understand very quickly the meaning of the word *obscure* (obscure has many definitions, which include "not clear or distinct," "faint or undefined," "in an inconspicuous position," "not well known," etc.).

Finally, further desperate searching yielded "pearls." I came upon the volumes edited and/or written by a pioneer in physical medicine and rehabilitation, Dr. Howard Rusk. The volume, which he co-edited with Dr. Taylor, entitled *New Hope for the Handicapped*, which had multiple editions published in the late 1940s, actually mentioned cancer as a "special rehabilitation" problem within a chapter on rehabilitation of surgical patients (5). His first volume of the seminal work, *Rehabilitation Medicine*, had a full chapter on cancer rehabilitation in the initial 1958 edition, as well as the second and the third editions. By the fourth edition in 1977, Dr. Rusk had literally tripled the size of the chapter

KEY POINTS

- Over the last two decades, there has been a steady improvement in the survival statistics for nearly all cancers, due in large part to earlier detection and advances in surgery, radiation, and chemotherapy.
- Longer survival of patients with cancer has led to an increase in the chronic long-term toxicities associated with chemotherapy.
- Anthracycline-induced cardiovascular complications can arise acutely (during administration), early (several days to months following administration), or years to decades following exposure.
- Bleomycin therapy can result in life-threatening interstitial pulmonary fibrosis in up to 10% of patients.
- Cisplatin is used to treat testicular, ovarian, bladder, esophageal, and head and neck cancers, as well as non-small cell lung cancer, small cell lung cancer, non-Hodgkin lymphoma, and trophoblastic disease, and is commonly associated with peripheral neuropathy and ototoxicity.
- Lhermitte sign is a shocklike, nonpainful, sensation of paresthesias radiating from the back to the feet during neck flexion, which can develop in patients receiving cisplatin, and typically occurs after weeks or months of treatment.
- Taxane-induced motor and sensory neuropathies are cumulative and dose and schedule dependent.
- A peripheral neuropathy develops in approximately 75% of patients who receive prolonged thalidomide treatment.
- Almost any chemotherapeutic agent can result in postchemotherapy rheumatism, and this is a fairly common clinical phenomenon.

to now be quite inclusive (6). His wonderful 1972 volume, *A World to Care For*, not only reviewed specific medical issues and problems of the cancer patient, but also detailed specific government legislation, speculated on why there was very little cancer rehabilitation being performed in the United States, and, finally, shared with the readers his initial efforts in setting up a cancer rehabilitation program in the 1960s (7).

Armed with this information from Dr. Rusk and with added inspiration, I finally had the emotional and tangible wherewithal to commence my journey into the beginnings of cancer rehabilitation.

LEGISLATION

In the mid-1960s, President Lyndon Johnson recommended a special presidential commission to investigate and recommend ways to reduce the incidence of heart disease, cancer, and stroke, the grave killer diseases that affected millions of Americans each year (7–9). Dr. Michael DeBakey, the renowned vascular surgeon, was appointed chair of this commission, which included 25 specialists in various fields. The main purpose of the group was to work out a master plan to attack these three serious diseases. Dr. Rusk was a member of this group and effectively argued for rehabilitation, both philosophically and as a process.

Ultimately, Dr. Rusk was authorized by Dr. DeBakey to create and chair a subcommittee on rehabilitation needs and programs. Joining Dr. Rusk on this subcommittee

were several rehabilitation specialists, including William Spencer, Henry Betts, William Erdman, Arthur Abramson, Paul Elwood, and others. The commission report was the basis for the enactment and passage of Public Law 98–239, the Heart, Cancer and Stroke Act. The program was enacted in 1965 and established regional medical programs for the diagnosis, treatment, and rehabilitation of people with these three diseases.

It was determined that this mission could best be accomplished through regionalization in cooperative arrangements among a region's medical resources. It was thought that such an arrangement would enable the medical profession and its institutions to make available to all citizens the latest advances in diagnosis and treatment of these diseases. Because of the voluntary nature of American medical institutions, the legislation allowed for a flexible framework in the implementation of a regional approach. Programs were also to do research and to train professionals to deal with the diseases. Programs were to be centered in medical schools and teaching hospitals, and rehabilitation was to be a focus of all programs (9).

According to Klieger, the intent of the act toward accomplishment of this goal was to build upon and encourage the following:

1. Utilization of existing institutions and manpower resources
2. Participation of practicing physicians
3. Regional initiative, planning, and implementation under conditions that encourage innovative approaches and programs

4. Cooperation among elements of the health resources in a region
5. Effective linkages between research advances and improved patient care
6. A continuing process of education throughout the career of a physician in bringing the benefits of new knowledge to the patient (9)

The regional medical programs were to serve as instruments of synthesis within each region to reinforce the various groups seeking the latest advances in the diagnosis and treatment of these diseases. The importance of rehabilitation in the regional medical programs was outlined by the subcommittee under the chairmanship of Dr. Rusk. The subcommittee emphasized the necessity of rehabilitation as an integral part of the total rehabilitation of individuals with these diseases. It was observed, however, that despite efforts by public, professional, and voluntary agencies, the potential of rehabilitation, its concepts, and its methods were not well understood. The report pointed out that physicians must realize that rehabilitation existed as a service program for them and their patients afflicted with cancer; that programs must be designed to help the physician meet the retraining needs of patients who have been disabled as the result of surgery or radiotherapy for cancer; that comprehensive regional programs must be included as a service in every stroke center or station to accommodate patients with physical disabilities and those with communication disabilities resulting from aphasia; and that continuing education for physicians is an important contribution to the more effective utilization of rehabilitation concepts and methods in services for patients with heart disease, cancer, and stroke (9). Theoretically, this act began the special programs in stroke, cancer, and cardiac rehabilitation and lasted into the 1970s.

Other important legislation enacted by Congress in the 1960s and affecting rehabilitation medicine were the amendments to the Rehabilitation Act signed into law by President Johnson in late 1965. The act created a new facility construction program, dramatically expanded the funding for federal, state, and vocational rehabilitation services by raising the federal share of these services to 75% of total funding (10). Before Medicare, the Rehabilitation Act was the only federal health care funding for rehabilitation medicine to adult civilians who were not veterans. Again, Dr. Howard Rusk was the champion of the legislation. However, it seems that little was accomplished in the cancer rehabilitation area. Harvey notes that in 1971 only 1,000 of 260,000 clients served by the vocational rehabilitation program were cancer patients (11).

In 1971, the National Cancer Act was passed, and funds became more readily available for the development of training, demonstration, and research projects in rehabilitation and were administered through the Division of Cancer Control and Rehabilitation, National Cancer Institute (NCI) of the National Institutes of Health (NIH) (11,12). NCI contracts and grants were to be awarded to address a variety of topics, such as development of model rehabilitation programs, hospice care, pain-management programs, and interventions to reduce psychosocial morbidity. According to Mayer, these contracts and grants did not produce the desired effect. Interest and support waned and shifted to more cure-oriented areas (12). Grabois adds that " . . . the passing of this act had little impact on the rehabilitation of patients with cancer. These efforts failed due to a lack of a specific implementation plan, a lack of trained personnel, and failure to educate referring health care professionals (13)."

In 1973, legislation was promulgated that indirectly protected cancer patients from discrimination. This was the National Rehabilitation Act of 1973 and included a number of civil rights protections for people with "handicaps." Section 504 of this title prohibited discrimination against people with "handicaps," now defined as disabilities, by any federal department or agency that entered into a contract in excess of $2,500 (14,15). This included almost all educational institutions, hospitals, and most public bodies. In such institutions, affirmative action was mandated to be taken to employ, advance, or preserve the benefits of any "qualified handicapped" individuals. A violation could be filed as a grievance with the Department of Labor. This act in essence was a precursor of the Americans with Disabilities Act, which extended the prohibitions against job discrimination to all employers.

PROGRAMS AND PEOPLE

The early history of cancer rehabilitation certainly would not be complete without a review of some of the pioneer rehabilitation programs. Although the political legislation of the 1960s and 1970s was lofty and admirable, seemingly very little tangible benefit accrued to cancer patients and indeed most cancer rehabilitation programs. Nonetheless, two early programs are worth review: those at the University of Texas M.D. Anderson Cancer Center (MDACC) and a cooperative program started by Drs. Rusk and Dietz in New York City (16). It would be of benefit in understanding cancer rehabilitation history to now review those programs.

From approximately 1960 until 1973, the MDACC at the burgeoning Texas Medical Center, employed a physiatrist from a rehabilitation consultation service that had electrodiagnostic capabilities. In addition, physical and occupational therapy departments were in existence. The program was not closely aligned with any particular teaching program, as Dr. Martin Grabois has pointed out. For five years following 1973, not only was a physiatrist present at the cancer center there were also rotating residents. This rotation apparently was given favorable reviews by the rotating residents. Unfortunately, for the following decade, this program experienced quite a bit of negative turbulence. There was no longer a physiatrist, and the residency rotation ceased to exist. The Occupational Therapy Department was also discontinued and a nonphysiatrist headed the program. Finally, in 1989, the cancer center approached the Department of Physical Medicine and Rehabilitation at Baylor College of Medicine to develop a meaningful cancer rehabilitation program. According to Grabois, initial attempts at forming such a program were unsuccessful for a variety of reasons which relate to the physiatrists employed, the lack of follow-through in educating referring physicians, and insufficient clinical and office space. In the early to mid-1990s, further efforts were made to rejuvenate the program. The MDACC joined with the Department of Physical Medicine and Rehabilitation at Baylor College of Medicine in developing a program that has become quite significant (13).

Dr. Ky Shin, current head of the section, reports that there are four full-time physiatrists present, with the need for a fifth. These specialists in physical medicine and rehabilitation exclusively practice cancer rehabilitation and are in the Section of Physical Medicine and Rehabilitation in the Department of Palliative and Rehabilitation Medicine within the Division of Cancer Medicine. In addition to an inpatient rehabilitation unit and an inpatient consultation service, there is a large outpatient and electrodiagnostic practice. In recent years, the bulk of the outpatients seen have had the following diagnoses: lymphedema, pain, disability evaluations, general deconditioning, gait abnormality, fatigue and spasticity. More than 400 inpatients have been admitted yearly to the rehabilitation unit, with an average length of stay of approximately 10 days. Slightly more than half of the patients have been male and the mean age was 61 years. Twenty-eight percent of the patients were brain or spine tumor patients with up to 14% being hemorrhagic tumors. Other solid tumors included genitourinary, lung, bone, gastrointestinal, breast, head, and neck.

Approximately three-quarters of the inpatients were able to be discharged home. However, one in five of the patients, required transfer back to their acute services secondary to illness or an inability to continue participation in rehabilitation. The emphasis for admission to the MDACC rehabilitation unit has been to take patients with multiple impairments and more comorbidities or diseases. Thus, despite a variety of past tribulations and uncertainty, the cancer rehabilitation program at MDACC is now thriving.

In New York City, the seminal cancer rehabilitation program was started in the mid-1960s. Dr. Howard Rusk in *A World to Care For* details a patient with bladder cancer who required a hemicorporectomy at New York City's Memorial Hospital (7). After being transferred to the Institute of Rehabilitation Medicine, the patient ultimately was able to return home to his family. This success provided Dr. Rusk with encouragement in the rehabilitation of cancer patients. He partnered with Memorial Hospital's Dr. Herbert Dietz, a surgeon from upstate New York who came to New York City and spent two years studying rehabilitation, especially of cancer patients. Thus, a joint undertaking with Memorial Hospital and the Institute of Rehabilitation Medicine took place, and a cancer rehabilitation program developed in New York City (7). After Dr. Dietz's retirement, there were difficulties within the program. Throughout the 1980s and 1990s, there were often periods with no physiatrist and lack of a very organized program.

The current director was named in 2001. For at least one year before then there had not been a physiatrist. Similarly, there was not an outpatient therapy program for more than a year. According to Dr. Michael D. Stubblefield, Rehabilitation Medicine at Memorial Sloan Kettering Cancer Center (MSKCC) is currently a service of the Department of Neurology. It consists of 2 full-time physiatrists, 27 physical therapists, 7 occupational therapists, 3 therapy aides, and a full-time administrator. In 2006, over 2,200 outpatients were seen by the physiatrists and hundreds of EMGs and injection procedures were performed. The focus of the physiatrists in the MSKCC program has shifted from a traditional emphasis on the management of lymphedema. It is now centered on the evaluation of management of neuromuscular and musculoskeletal complications of cancer and cancer treatment. The service pioneered the use of botulinum toxin and other injections in the cancer setting to relive pain and improve function. The MSKCC rehabilitation service has become involved in a number of research trials, including collaboration with other services throughout the center. This historic program now seems to be in a strong growth phase with energetic leadership.

A review of the two historic programs detailed previously highlights the difficulties and cycles that the programs in cancer rehabilitation have endured over the past four decades. Nonetheless, both of these programs have survived and are now successful.

A recent survey of cancer rehabilitation programs and professionals has not been performed. The excellent survey by Harvey and associates was done 25 years ago (11). Anecdotal comments from professionals that I have interviewed are unanimous in emphasizing that there are only a very few centers in the United States and Canada where comprehensive rehabilitation programs exist and these are usually at larger cancer hospitals/centers. It is not known exactly how and by what means the majority of cancer patients elsewhere are treated and what attention is given to their rehabilitation needs. Logically, the rehabilitation problems of cancer patients could be addressed by their hospitals' or communities' general rehabilitation program(s).

On a professional level, more than two decades ago the Cancer Rehabilitation Special Interest Group (SIG) was formed within the American Academy of Physical Medicine and Rehabilitation. It continued until the dissolution of the SIG structure occurred in 2008.

NEED

Historically, the recognition that cancer patients had many rehabilitation needs was often clouded by common "perceptions" about the hopelessness of their condition and their acute medical needs. As early as 1969, the wonderful pioneer Mary Switzer, in a lecture given in 1970 in Houston, Texas, reported that of 260,000 people rehabilitated through the Public Vocational Rehabilitation Program in 1969, only about 1,000 were the victims of cancer (17). Fortunately, since that time, quite a few excellent papers have shed lighton the rehabilitation needs and problems of cancer patients.

In 1978, Lehman and his co-workers, provided an extremely informative and certainly convincing review of the needs of cancer patients. Surveying more than 800 patients from several hospitals, they identified many needs (Figure 1.1), including those involving activities of daily living (ADL), ambulation, family support, psychological distress, pain, and weakness. A mode of care was then organized based on the findings of the needs assessment. Ultimately, after the formation of a clinical oncology team, the number of referrals and therapy treatments greatly increased (18).

DePompolo reported the experience of the cancer rehabilitation program at the Mayo Clinic. Again, his findings certainly buoy the concept that cancer patients have many needs for rehabilitation. He outlined many of these, which included psychological issues of emotional support and assistance, pain and impairments in activities of daily living, and mobility (19). Sabers

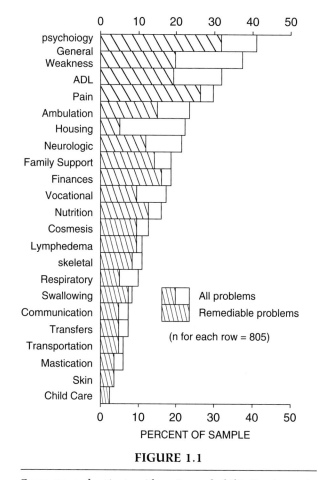

FIGURE 1.1

Percentage of patients with various rehabilitation issues in Lehman's seminal work. (From Ref. 18, with permission.)

and coworkers, also from the Mayo Clinic, reviewed the rehabilitation needs of 189 patients referred to the Cancer Adaptation Team over an eight-month period. Pain was identified as a significant need in almost three-quarters of the patients. Other findings revealed that almost the same number had difficulty rising from a chair and more than three-quarters had problems getting on and off a toilet, getting in and out of a bathtub, walking, and climbing stairs (20).

Whelan reviewed the symptoms and problems of cancer patients, which they themselves identified. Paramount among these included issues concerning sleep, pain, fatigue, and worry. These cancer patients revealed that they needed more education, more help with activities of daily living and help with social support (21). Winningham, in many scholarly works, has continued to prove that fatigue and pain are major concerns of cancer patients (22,23).

Van Harten in the Netherlands performed a comprehensive review of the literature regarding the needs of cancer patients. A wide array of psychological impairments and emotional issues was identified as well. In his own survey of 147 cancer patients, more than one-quarter felt the need for professional care and, of these, 17% indicated problems in more than one area. Their problems included not only physical function but also psychological and cognitive functions (24). Stafford and Cyr, in a review of 9,745 elderly community-based Medicare patients sampled in the 1991 Medicare Current Beneficiary Survey, found that more than 1,600 had been reported as having a diagnosis of a malignancy that was not skin cancer. These individuals reported poor health, more limitations with activities of daily living and greater health care utilization. Some of their common concerns included gait difficulty and difficulty getting out of a chair, while many had trouble completing housework and shopping (25).

Clearly, the needs of cancer patients relating to rehabilitation are multifold and complex. It is of interest that over the past 15 years, in particular, the reports of cancer rehabilitation therapy have broadened in scope. The early, pre-1980 descriptions were clearly associated with common anatomical sites of malignancy and the more obvious side effects of the tumor and the treatment. Recently documented successful efforts have gone beyond just a single anatomical site and have focused as well on more holistic issues affecting the cancer patient such as fatigue, pains and lack of social support.

EFFICACY

Dr. J. Herbert Dietz, in the 1960s, first provided some evidence as to the efficacy and worth of cancer rehabilitation. He classified his patient rehabilitation goals as:

· Restoration
· Support
· Palliation

He described 1,237 inpatients seen during the initial three years of the Cooperative Rehabilitation Program at Memorial Hospital. His ultimate conclusion was that "80% of patients treated have shown measurable benefits appropriate to the goal set for them (26)."

Unfortunately, almost a quarter of a century elapsed until further convincing evidence became available. Some of the more significant reports will be detailed. In 1991, O'Toole and Golden reviewed the progress and outcomes of patients with cancer in a freestanding rehabilitation hospital. The majority of the 70 subjects made dramatic improvement in mobility and bladder continence. Ninety days after discharge, many had maintained or improved their functional level (27).

The previously mentioned work of Sabers and coauthors reported on the efforts of a consultation-based inpatient rehabilitation team in the treatment of hospitalized cancer patients. Functional status of the patients at enrollment and discharge was evaluated with the Barthel Mobility Index and the Karnofsky Performance Status Scale (Table 1.1). Significant gains were made in both indices by the 189 patients studied (20).

Yoshioka, in Japan, reviewed more than 300 terminally ill cancer patients in an inpatient hospice setting. A variety of therapeutic interventions was performed by therapists. The Barthel Mobility Index increased from 12.4 to 19.9 ($P < 0.0001$) in those with ADL deficits. The families of these patients almost unanimously were appreciative of the care and rehabilitation efforts (28).

Phillip and coauthors surveyed the functional outcome after rehabilitation efforts of 30 children, aged three and older, who were treated for primary brain tumors. Using the Wee-Functional Independence Measure (FIM) as a functional independence measure, their study clearly documented positive effects of an interdisciplinary rehabilitation program on these pediatric patients with residual disabilities (29).

Marciniak and others at the Rehabilitation Institute of Chicago summarized the progress of 159 patients over a two-year period undergoing inpatient rehabilitation secondary to functional impairments from cancer or its treatment. All cancer subgroups made significant functional gains between admission and discharge. Also, neither the presence of metastatic disease nor the delivery of radiation treatment influenced the functional outcome (30).

TABLE 1.1 *Karnofsky Performance Scale*	
RATING (%)	**DEFINITION**
100	No evidence of disease
90	Normal activity with minor signs of disease
80	Normal activity with effort; signs of disease
70	Cannot do normal activity but cares for self
60	Requires occasional assistance
50	Requires considerable assistance; frequent medical care
40	Disabled, requires special care
30	Severely disabled; hospitalization may be indicated
20	Very sick; hospitalization necessary for supportive treatment
10	Moribund
0	Death

Kirshblum and O'Dell, in 2001, further summarized the outcomes of three prior studies of patients with brain tumors receiving inpatient rehabilitation. Although the methodology of the studies varied, it could safely be concluded that these patients with brain tumors "undergoing inpatient rehabilitation appear to make functional gains in line with those seen in similar patients with traumatic brain injury or stroke (31)." Winningham, in many excellent recent works, has reviewed the evidence, possible etiologies and theoretical models of fatigue in cancer patients. She then very clearly describes the usefulness and benefits of a variety of programs, including exercise and other effective rehabilitation interventions (22,23). Clearly, at present, the efficacy and worth of rehabilitation efforts are proven and undoubted.

CANCER REHABILITATION: FROM PAST TO FUTURE

The American Cancer Society has estimated that up to 1.4 million Americans were newly diagnosed with cancer in 2006. As our population ages, the incidence and prevalence of cancer will only increase. Dr. Richard Robbins, chair of the Department of Medicine at The Methodist Hospital in Houston, Texas, reports that the probability of a man getting cancer (not counting skin cancer) is now 1 in 2, while for women it is 1 in 3. Gerber and many others have reported that the five-year survival for many cancer sites now exceeds 50% (32). Certainly, the modern-day cancer patient has a longer lifespan and may very well be thought to have a chronic illness, not just an acute deadly malady.

Although critics may state, perhaps rightfully, that the progress made in rehabilitating cancer patients and developing cancer rehabilitation programs has been slow, the labors and persistence of our cancer rehabilitation pioneers have certainly yielded some positive fruits. Clearly, the cancer population needs, and should demand, the services of rehabilitation professionals. Supported by the convincing pioneer works of their predecessors, the modern day cancer rehabilitation specialist is empowered by evidence, inspiration and experience to march forward and provide the expertise and support for this deserving population.

References

1. Downie PA. *Cancer Rehabilitation: An Introduction for Physiotherapists and the Allied Professions.* London: Faber and Faber Ltd.; 1978.
2. Krusen FH, Kottke FJ, Ellwood PM. *Handbook of Physical Medicine and Rehabilitation.* Philadelphia, PA: WB Saunders Co.; 1965, 1971.
3. Krusen FH. *Physical Medicine and Rehabilitation for the Clinician.* Philadelphia, PA: WB Saunders Co.; 1951.
4. Bierman W, Licht S (eds). *Physical Medicine in General Practice.* New York, NY: Paul B. Hoeber, Inc.; 1944, 1947, 1952.
5. Rusk HA, Taylor EJ, eds. *New Hope for the Handicapped.* New York, NY: Harper and Brothers; 1946, 1947, 1948, 1949.
6. Rusk HA. *Rehabilitation Medicine.* St. Louis, MO: CV Mosley; 1958, 1964, 1977.
7. Rusk HA. *A World to Care For.* New York, NY: Random House; 1972:256–261.
8. Clark RL. Heath Memorial Award presentation. In: Clinical Conference on Cancer, Anderson Hospital, ed. res 8, 9, 17 *Rehabilitation of the Cancer Patient.* Chicago, IL: Year Book Medical Publishers, Inc.; 1972:5–6.
9. Klieger PA. The regional medical programs. In: *Rehabilitation of the Cancer Patient* Clinical Conference on Cancer, Anderson Hospital, ed. res 8, 9, 17. Chicago, IL: Year Book Medical Publishers, Inc.; 1972:287–290.
10. Walker ML. Beyond bureaucracy: Mary Elizabeth Switzer and rehabilitation. Blue Ridge Summit, PA: University Press of America; 1985:211–217.
11. Harvey RF, Jellinek HM, Habeck RV. Cancer rehabilitation: An analysis of 36 program approaches. *JAMA.* 1982;247:2127–2131.
12. Mayer DK. The healthcare implications of cancer rehabilitation in the twenty-first century. *Oncol Nurs Forum.* 1992;19:23–27.
13. Grabois M. Integrating cancer rehabilitation into medical care at a cancer hospital. *Cancer.* 2001;92:1055–1057.
14. Tross S, Holland JC. Psychological sequelae in cancer survivors. In: Holland JC, Rowland JH, eds. *Handbook of Psychooncology.* New York, NY: Oxford University Press; 1989:110–111.
15. Sigel CJ. Legal recourse for the cancer patient-returnee: The Rehabilitation Act of 1973. *Am J Law Med.* 1984;10:309–321.
16. Dietz JH. Introduction. In: Dietz JH, ed. *Rehabilitation Oncology.* New York, NY: John Wiley & Sons; 1981:1–2.
17. Switzer ME. The Heath Memorial Lecture: rehabilitation – an act of faith. In: Clinical conference on Cancer, Anderson Hospital, ed. res 8, 9, 17 *Rehabilitation of the Cancer Patient.* Chicago, IL. Year Book Medical Publishers, Inc.; 1972:10–11.
18. Lehmann JF, DeLisa JA, Warren CG, deLateur BJ, Bryant PLS, Nicholson CG. Cancer rehabilitation: Assessment of need, development, and evaluation of a model of care. *Arch Phys Med Rehabil.* 1978;59:410–419.
19. DePompolo RW. Development and administration of a cancer rehabilitation program. In Schwab CE, ed. *Physical Medicine and Rehabilitation: State of the Art Reviews.* Philadelphia, PA: Hanley and Belfus, Inc.; 1994:413–423.
20. Sabers SR, Kokal JE, Girardi JC et al. Evaluation of consultation-based rehabilitation for hospitalized cancer patients with functional impairment. *Mayo Clin Proc.* 1999;74:855–861.
21. Whelan TJ, Mohide EA, Willan AR, Arnold A, Tew M, Sellick S, et al. The supportive care needs of newly diagnosed cancer patients attending a regional cancer center. *Cancer.* 1997;80:1518–1524.
22. Winningham ML, Nail LM, Burke MB, Brophy L, Cimprich B, Jones LS, et al. Fatigue and the cancer experience: The state of the knowledge. *Oncol Nurs Forum.* 1994;21:23–33.
23. Winningham ML. Strategies for managing cancer-related fatigue syndrome: A rehabilitation approach. *Cancer.* 2001;92:988–997.
24. Van Harten WH, Van Noort O, Warmerdam R, Hendricks H, Seidel E. Assessment of rehabilitation needs in cancer patients. *Int J Rehabil Res.* 1998;21:247–257.
25. Stafford RS, Cyr PL. The impact of cancer on the physical function of the elderly and their utilization of health care. *Cancer.* 1997;80:1973–1980.
26. Dietz JH. Rehabilitation of the cancer patient. *Med Clin N Am.* 1969;53:621–623.
27. O'Toole DM, Golden AM. Evaluating cancer patients for rehabilitation potential. *West J Med.* 1991;155:384–387.

28. Yoshioka H. Rehabilitation for the terminal cancer patient. *Am J Phys Med Rehabil*. 1994;73:199–206.

29. Philip PA, Ayyangar R, Vanderbilt J, Gaebler-Spira DJ. Rehabilitation outcome in children after treatment of primary brain tumor. *Arch Phys Med Rehabil*. 1994;75:36–38.

30. Marciniak CM, Sliwa JA, Spill G, Heinemann AW, Semik PE. Functional outcome following rehabilitation of the cancer patient. *Arch Phys Med Rehabil*. 1996;77:54–57.

31. Kirshblum S, O'Dell MW, Ho C, Barr K. Rehabilitation of persons with central nervous system tumors. *Cancer*. 2001;92:1029–1038.

32. Gerber L. Cancer rehabilitation into the future. *Cancer*. 2001;92:975–979.

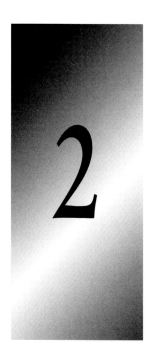

Principles of Neoplasia

Kristen M. O'Dwyer
Mark G. Frattini

Decades of cancer research have revealed that human cancer is a multistep process involving acquired genetic mutations, each of which imparts a particular type of growth advantage to the cell and ultimately leads to the development of the malignant phenotype. The consequences of the mutations in the tumor cells include alterations in cell signaling pathways that result in uncontrolled cellular proliferation, insensitivity to growth inhibition signals, resistance to apoptosis, development of cellular immortality, angiogenesis, and tissue invasion and metastasis (1). Here we address the fundamental principles of cancer genetics, cell cycle control, and invasion and metastasis. Due to limitations in space and given the complexity of the subject matter and the many excellent textbooks and review articles that are available for each topic, we will highlight the most important principles. A list of historical and current references will be provided for the interested reader.

CANCER GENETICS

The idea that human cancer is a result of multiple mutations in the deoxyribonucleic acid (DNA) sequence of a cell has developed during the past 30 years. A mutation is any change in the primary nucleotide sequence of DNA, and the mutation may or may not have a functional consequence. The field of cancer genetics emerged to study the different types of mutations, as well as the consequences of the mutations in tumor cells. Bert Vogelstein and Ken Kinzler provide the most thoroughly studied example of a human cancer that illustrates this multistep process. Their research of families with rare inherited colon cancer syndromes demonstrated that multiple somatic mutation events (5 to 10) are required for the progression from normal colonic epithelium to the development of carcinoma in situ. The mechanisms through which the mutations in the DNA occur are varied and include imprecise DNA repair processes, random replication errors, splicing errors, messenger ribonucleic acid (mRNA) processing errors, exposure to carcinogens such as radiation or chemotherapy, or incorporation of exogenous DNA into the genome such as viral DNA or RNA (2).

CLASSES OF CANCER GENES— ONCOGENES, TUMOR SUPRESSOR GENES, AND GATEKEEPER GENES

The specific genes that are mutated in the cancer cell have been described as falling into two general functional classes. The first class of genes directly regulates the processes of cell growth and includes the oncogenes and tumor suppressor genes. The second class of genes that are mutated in the cancer cell is the so-called "caretaker" genes. These genes are involved in processes of maintaining the integrity of the genome.

KEY POINTS

- Cancer is a multistep process involving acquired genetic mutations, each of which imparts a particular type of growth advantage to the cell and ultimately leads to the development of the malignant phenotype.
- The specific genes that are mutated in the cancer cell have been described as falling into two general functional classes. The first class of genes directly regulates the processes of cell growth and includes the oncogenes and tumor suppressor genes. The second class of genes that are mutated in the cancer cell is the so-called "caretaker" genes. These genes are involved in processes of maintaining the integrity of the genome.
- While the majority of cancers develop as a result of acquired somatic mutations in the genome, a small percentage (5%–10%) of cancer syndromes develop as a result of inherited mutations.

- Certain viruses are true etiologic agents of human cancers, including human papillomavirus (cervical carcinoma), hepatitis B and C viruses (hepatocellular carcinoma), Epstein-Barr virus (Burkitt lymphoma), and human T-cell leukemia virus type I (T-cell leukemia).
- Cancer metastasis is a complex multistep process and requires multiple genetic changes in the tumor cell in order for it to acquire all of the capabilities necessary to colonize a distant organ.
- It is important to realize that the single cells that form the tumor metastasis can grow fast and take over the organ quickly; in other cases, the metastatic tumors remain small and dormant for months to years. This latency is referred to as metastatic dormancy.
- Metastatic cancer of any origin is generally not curable, and complications from metastasis account for 90% of deaths from solid tumors.

Oncogenes

The study of human retroviruses in the 1970s and the discovery of reverse transcriptase (3,4) led to the finding of the first human oncogenes (5). Oncogenes are mutated forms of normal cellular genes called proto-oncogenes. Proto-oncogenes include several classes of genes involved in mitogenic signaling and growth control, typically encoding proteins such as extracellular cytokines and growth factors, transmembrane growth factor receptors, transcription factors, and proteins that control DNA replication. Importantly, all of the proteins encoded by proto-oncogenes control critical steps in intracellular signaling pathways of the cell cycle, cell division, and cellular differentiation. To date, more than 75 different proto-oncogenes have been identified (6).

In human cancer, the mutation event in the proto-oncogene typically occurs in a single allele of the gene and imitates an autosomal dominant mode of inheritance (ie, mutations in a single allele are sufficient to cause disease), producing a gain-of-function phenotype. The mutations that activate the proto-oncogene to the oncogene include point mutations, DNA amplification, and chromosomal rearrangements.

Examples of point mutations are found in three major Ras family members of proteins (HRAS, KRAS, NRAS). Briefly, Ras proteins are membrane-associated guanine nucleotide exchange proteins. Their downstream targets control diverse processes such as cell proliferation, cellular differentiation, and apoptosis. The activating mutations in the RAS genes involve

codons 12, 13, and 61 and result in an amino acid substitution in the phosphate binding domain of the protein. The functional consequence is a Ras protein that is "locked" in an active guanosine triphosphate (GTP) bound state, resulting in a constitutively active Ras-signaling pathway that now can impart a growth advantage to the cell via uncontrolled cellular proliferation and evasion of apoptosis (7).

The activating mutations in the Ras proteins have been identified in 30% of human tumors (8), though certain tumor types have a particularly high incidence of RAS mutations and include 95% of pancreatic cancers, 50% of colorectal cancers, and 30% of lung carcinomas. While Ras proteins are ubiquitously expressed in human cells, it is unclear why certain tumor types have a higher incidence of mutations.

DNA amplification is the second mechanism of activation of a proto-oncogene. Though the exact mechanism is unknown, DNA amplification results in an increase in DNA copy number of the cellular proto-oncogene. The increase in gene copy number can lead to characteristic chromosomal changes that can be identified with traditional cytogenetic studies used to asses the karyotype. These include extrachromosomal double-minute chromatin bodies (dmins) and homogeneously staining regions in which the amplified sequences are integrated into the chromosomes. The functional result is an increase in the gene expression levels and the corresponding RNA and protein levels.

The first proto-oncogene found to be amplified in a human cancer was MYC when it was identified in the HL-60 human promyelocytic leukemia cell line (9,10). MYC is a member of the basic helix-loop-helix leucine zipper family of transcription factors and regulates multiple cellular processes, including cell growth and differentiation, cell-cycle progression, apoptosis, and cell motility (11,12). MYC is frequently amplified in solid tumors, including small cell lung carcinoma (18%–31%), neuroblastoma (25%), and sarcomas, and the increased gene copy number results in concordant increases in the Myc protein level, leading to unregulated cell growth and division. An important clinical correlation is that in childhood neuroblastoma, an MYC family member, N-MYC, is amplified in approximately 40% of advanced pediatric neuroblastomas and has prognostic significance. Children with neuroblastoma and minimal or no N-MYC amplification have a very good prognosis, while children with >10 copies of N-MYC have a significantly poorer prognosis and shorter survival (13).

Another important gene that is commonly amplified in human cancer, specifically breast, ovarian, and lung cancers, is the c-erbB2/HER-2 gene. The c-erbB2/HER-2 gene encodes a transmembrane receptor of the epidermal growth factor receptor (EGFR) family with associated tyrosine-kinase activity (14,15). The signal transduction pathways that are activated control epithelial cell growth and differentiation. Amplification of the c-erbB2/HER-2 gene is correlated with an increased expression of the Her2 protein. It is estimated that HER2 is amplified in 18%–20% of breast tumors and it, too, carries prognostic value. Slamon et al. demonstrated that DNA amplification of more than five copies of HER2 per cancer cell were found to correlate with a decreased survival in patients with breast cancer (16).

Chromosomal rearrangement is the third mechanism of activation of a proto-oncogene. The mechanism of the rearrangements can be gain and loss of chromosomes that are usually seen in human solid tumors, as well as chromosome translocations, such as those seen in human leukemias, lymphomas, and sarcomas. Because proto-oncogenes are often located at or near chromosomal breakpoints, they are susceptible to mutation. The result is a structural rearrangement that juxtaposes two different chromosomal regions and typically produces a chimeric gene that encodes a fusion protein (17,18).

One of the most studied chromosomal translocations in human cancer came from the study of leukemia cells by Peter Nowell, David Hungerford, and Janet Rowley. In 1960, Hungerford observed a characteristic small chromosome in the leukemia cells of two patients with chronic myelogenous leukemia (CML) (19). At that time, the technology was such that the specific chromosome could not be identified, and so it was designated the Philadelphia chromosome (Ph), as both Hungerford and Nowell resided in Philadelphia. The development of cytogenetic banding in the 1970s was the technologic breakthrough that ultimately led Janet Rowley to identify the Philadelphia chromosome and that, in fact, the Philadelphia chromosome resulted from a translocation of a small portion of chromosome 22 being displaced to chromosome 9 (20). The next advance in this field came in 1984 when Gerard Grosveld and his colleagues cloned the 9;22 translocation and identified the Abelson leukemia (ABL) gene on chromosome 9 and the breakpoint cluster region (BCR) gene on chromosome 22, the two genes that, when joined, expressed an in-frame fusion protein and resulted in a constitutively active ABL tyrosine kinase (21). It is the unregulated BCR-ABL tyrosine-kinase activity that is the transforming event leading to the development of CML. In 2001, Brian Drucker and colleagues published the first report of a specific inhibitor of the BCR-ABL tyrosine kinase, imatinib mesylate, that is active in patients with CML (22). Imatinib mesylate is currently the first-line treatment for all patients with CML and represents one of the first examples of molecularly targeted therapy.

The identification of the Philadelphia chromosome popularized the concept that specific chromosomal rearrangements were linked to cancer. Prior to her studies in CML, Janet Rowley and colleagues had discovered the first reciprocal chromosome rearrangement between chromosomes 8 and 21 in patients with acute myeloid leukemia (AML) (23,24). In this subtype of AML, the AML1 gene (also called CBFα2 for core binding factor or PEBP2αB) on the distal long arm of chromosome 21 becomes fused to the ETO gene (eight, twenty-one gene) on chromosome 8 (24). The consequence of expression of the AML1-ETO gene rearrangement is a new fusion protein that interferes with normal transcription of a number of genes critical for hematopoietic cell development, function, and differentiation (25).

In 1977, Janet Rowley and her colleagues also discovered the 15;17 translocation that characterizes acute promyelocytic leukemia (APL) (26). In this subtype of acute leukemia, a portion of the promyelocytic leukemia (PML) gene on chromosome 15 is fused with a portion of the retinoic acid receptor alpha (RARα) gene on chromosome 17. The resulting PML-RARα fusion protein inhibits differentiation of the myeloid cell, leading to arrested differentiation in the promyelocyte stage. Additionally, the PML-RARα fusion protein acquires antiapoptotic activity that allows the malignant clone to survive under conditions of growth-factor deprivation. In the past, this type of AML was among the most fatal due to the associated coagulopathic state in patients with APL, but with the use of all-trans-retinoic acid (ATRA) and arsenic trioxide in combination with standard chemotherapy, it is now curable in the majority of patients (27), as the use of ATRA and arsenic trioxide allow for differentiation and subsequent apoptotic cell death of the malignant clone.

Tumor Suppressor Genes

Tumor suppressor genes regulate diverse cellular processes in normal cells, including cell-cycle checkpoint responses, DNA repair, protein ubiquitination and degradation, mitogenic signaling, cell specification, differentiation and migration, and tumor angiogenesis.

In human cancers, the mutation event in a tumor suppressor gene in sporadic cancers must occur in both alleles, ie, "two-hit hypothesis" to inactivate the function of the gene, producing a recessive loss-of-function phenotype (28,29). In contrast to the familial cancer syndromes, a germline inheritance of a mutant allele of a tumor suppressor gene requires only one somatic mutation to inactivate the wild-type allele, and the development of the cancer phenotype is thereby greatly accelerated. Also, the tumor suppressor gene identified in a familial syndrome must be found to be mutated in sporadic cancer in order for it to be classified as a tumor suppressor.

There are different types of mutations that inactivate tumor suppressor genes. A point mutation can lead to an amino acid substitution if it occurs in the coding region, or it can introduce a premature stop codon and, therefore, result in a truncated protein. Large deletions of nucleotide sequence of DNA may affect a portion of a gene or the entire arm of a chromosome, causing loss of heterozygosity (LOH) in the tumor DNA. The retinoblastoma gene (RB) is mutated by this mechanism and results in a large deletion in chromosome 13q14 (30).

There are epigenetic mechanisms that can inactivate tumor suppressor genes and contribute to the development of malignancy. The term *epigenetic* refers to the inheritance of genetic information on the basis of gene expression levels, and these changes are employed by mechanisms other than mutations in the primary nucleotide sequence of the DNA. The epigenetic mechanisms that modify gene expression levels include methylation of clusters of cytosine and guanine residues, known as CpG-islands, in the promoter regions of genes, histone modification, and chromatin remodeling (31,32). As the molecular evidence emerged that DNA methylation was a powerful mechanism for inactivating tumor suppressor genes and that it was a potentially reversible process, there has been significant clinical interest in developing inhibitors of DNA methylation as novel therapeutic agents. Recently, with regard to the myelodysplastic syndromes (MDS), the U.S. Food and Drug Administration approved azacitidine as the first in a new class of drugs, the demethylating agents, for the treatment of MDS, and a recent large randomized clinical trial shows improved survival (33).

To date, more than 20 tumor suppressor genes have been identified (6). The first tumor suppressor gene to be identified was the retinoblastoma (RB1) tumor suppressor gene (34). The RB1 gene, together with p107 and p130, corepress transcription of genes that regulate signal transduction pathways that govern cell-cycle progression, apoptosis, and differentiation (35). The RB1 gene product (pRb) utilizes a complex array of protein interactions to govern these processes. More than 100 proteins have been reported to interact with pRb, though the most-studied protein partners have been the E2F transcription factors and various viral oncoproteins, including the Large T antigen of simian virus 40 (SV40) and the E7 protein encoded by the oncogenic human papillomaviruses (36). Germline inactivation of RB1 causes the familial pediatric cancer retinoblastoma, and somatic loss of RB1 is common in many types of human cancer, including breast cancer and sarcomas (37–39). In addition, work from a number of laboratories has demonstrated that the key proteins in the pRb regulatory pathway may be mutated in almost 100% of human tumors (40–43). The p53 tumor suppressor gene will be discussed in the cell cycle portion of this chapter.

Caretaker Genes

The caretaker genes are involved in preserving DNA repair mechanisms and thereby protecting the genome from the various environmental and chemical compounds that cause damage to the nucleotide bases, sugars, and phosphate groups of the DNA. When the caretaker genes are mutated, all of the genes in the cell have an increased rate of mutation, including the proto-oncogenes and tumor suppressor genes. Hereditary nonpolyposis colorectal cancer (HNPCC) is an autosomal-dominant colon cancer syndrome. The mutation event in HNPCC is an inactivating germline mutation in one of the DNA mismatch repair (MMR) genes. Patients who inherit the germline mutation are at increased risk for colorectal cancers, uterine and ovarian cancers, gastric cancers, urinary tract cancers, and some brain tumors (44). Other examples of human disorders that involve a mutation in a caretaker gene and result in instability of the genome are Fanconi anemia, ataxia telangiectasia, Bloom syndrome, and xeroderma pigmentosum.

TABLE 2.1
*Common Familial Cancer Syndromes
and the Inherited Affected Gene*

INHERITED GENE	FAMILIAL SYNDROME
Rb1	Retinoblastoma and osteosarcoma
TP53	Li-Fraumeni syndrome
WT1	Wilms tumor
VHL	Von-Hippel Lindau syndrome—renal cell carcinoma
BRCA1 and BRCA2	Breast cancer and ovarian cancer
APC	Familial adenomatous polyposis; colorectal tumors
MMR	Hereditary nonpolyposis-colorectal cancer
NF1	Von Recklinghausen disease; neurofibromatosis type1; schwannoma and glioma
NF2	Neurofibromatosis type 2; acoustic neuroma and meningiomas

FAMILIAL CANCER SYNDROMES

While the majority of cancers develop as a result of acquired somatic mutations in the genome, a small percentage (5%–10%) of cancer syndromes develop as a result of inherited mutations. Typically, a specific organ is affected, and the patient develops the cancer at a much younger age than the general population. Some of the common familial cancer syndromes are listed in Table 2.1 with the corresponding affected gene.

RNA AND DNA TUMOR VIRUSES

DNA and RNA viruses were studied extensively in the 1970s, as they were thought to be the key agents that caused cancer (45,46). Ultimately, research revealed that only a minority of cancers is caused by viruses; however, the study of RNA and DNA viruses exposed the machinations of cellular growth control pathways and led to the current concepts of the genetic basis of cancer. Though the mechanism of action of these various viruses are different in regard to how they infect a human cell and integrate into the genome, the end result is either activation of a growth-promoting pathway or inhibition of a tumor suppressor. We know now that certain viruses are true etiologic agents of human cancers, including human papillomavirus (cervical carcinoma), hepatitis B and C viruses (hepatocellular carcinoma), Epstein-Barr virus (Burkitt lymphoma), and human T-cell leukemia virus type I (T-cell leukemia).

GENOMIC TECHNOLOGY TO STUDY HUMAN CANCER

High-density complementary DNA (cDNA) microarrays for "profiling" gene expression allow for the simultaneous analysis of thousands of known human genes from a biologic specimen in a single experiment (47–49). In fact, with the present technology, the gene expression levels of the entire human genome can be represented in a single experiment. This technology has been utilized by nearly all fields of cancer research, as it has provided a more comprehensive analysis of the genetic changes that occur in cancer cells and identified novel disease genes for many cancer types and cancer mechanisms. In addition, this technology has been used to classify several common cancer types at the molecular level. Current studies in many laboratories around the world are using these novel classification models to predict clinical outcomes and to propose new molecular targets for therapy (50–58). The first randomized clinical trials [The Trial Assigning IndividuaLized Options for Treatment (TAILORx) and Microarray In Node-negative Disease may Avoid ChemoTherapy (MINDACT)] using the gene expression data to make treatment decisions for patients with breast cancer are underway in the United States, Canada, and Europe (59,60).

Gene expression profiling using cDNA microarray technology is one method to obtain a more comprehensive view of the consequences of genetic changes in the cancer cell. Currently, many other microarray platforms have been developed, including oligonucleotide microarrays (61,62), microarrays of bacterial artificial chromosome (BAC) clones (63), comparative genomic hybridization (CGH) to examine high-resolution DNA copy number, and oligonucleotide single-nucleotide polymorphism (SNP) arrays that report both copy number and genotype in the same hybridization (64–66), but the principle for all of these types of microarrays is essentially the same.

A brief description of gene expression profiling is described next and is illustrated in Figure 2.1, as it is the most utilized of the genomic technologies. Gene expression profiling uses RNA from a sample of interest (tumor specimen) and a common reference source of RNA. The RNA is differentially labeled using a single round of reverse transcription and incorporating fluorescently labeled nucleotides. The fluorescently labeled reference cDNA and tumor cDNA is pooled and hybridized to the clones, or probes, on the microarray (the glass slide—Fig. 2.1A). Each clone is derived from a specific sequence of an individual human gene and located at a unique position on the array surface. The glass slide is scanned with a confocal laser microscope

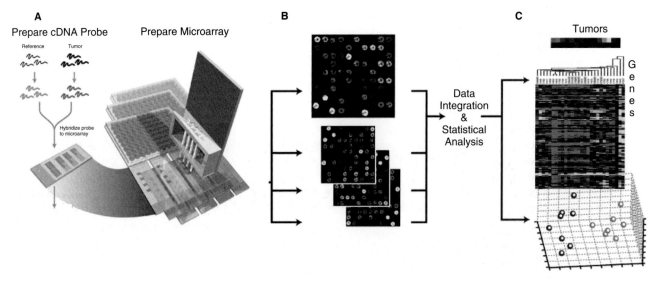

FIGURE 2.1

Gene expression profiling technology. A: Total RNA from the reference source and the tumor is fluorescently labeled with either Cye-3 or Cye-5-dUTP using a single round of reverse transcription. The fluorescently labeled cDNAs are pooled and allowed to hybridize to the clones on the array. B: The slide is then scanned with a confocal laser–scanning microscope to measure the fluorescence pattern, monochrome images from the scanner are imported into specialized software, and the images are colored and merged for each hybridization with RNA from the tumor and reference cells. C: Several statistical methods are used to visualize the expression patterns between tumor samples. (*See color insert following page 736*)

to measure the fluorescence ratio of each gene. The data from a single hybridization experiment represents the abundance of each specific gene transcript, and is viewed as a normalized ratio of each gene in each sample enumerated as either a ratio to a reference sample or as an absolute intensity value. Normalization is required for proper data analysis because differences exist in labeling and detection efficiencies of the fluorescent labels and differences exist in the quantity of RNA from the various samples. Once the ratios have been normalized, the experiment can be examined for differential gene expression. The data is then imported into statistical software programs, and the information that comes from the array is exhibited as a pseudocolor image (Fig. 2.1B). Typically, genes overexpressed in the tumor are shown in red and genes with decreased expression in the tumor are shown in green. Visualization tools are common methods used to represent the data generated from microarray experiments. Because many genes with many different expression patterns are being assayed in each experiment, these visualization tools are helpful for representing the data in a format that can produce biologic input. Two-dimensional hierarchical clustering dendograms are a frequently used method for viewing gene expression data (Fig. 2.1C). In general, the dendogram is a two-dimensional matrix where the tumor samples constitute the columns and the genes constitute the rows. The matrix makes it possible to quickly recognize the areas where

highly correlated expression sets of genes differentiate the sample types.

CELL CYCLE CONTROL

Cell division is tightly controlled through the complex interaction of multiple proteins to ensure the faithful reproduction of each component of the cell cycle—cell growth, chromosome replication, and mitosis. To guarantee the fidelity of the process, safeguards exist to prevent errors or to correct them when they occur. Genetic mutations that modify proteins that control cell-cycle regulation can weaken the safeguards, and, over time, as mutations accumulate, can result in genomic instability and ultimately lead to malignant transformation and unrestrained cell growth.

The cell cycle is separated into four phases: G_1 (gap 1), S (synthetic), G_2 (gap 2), and M (mitotic) or mitosis (67). During S phase, DNA synthesis occurs, and in M phase, the mother cell is divided into two daughter cells. The intervening gap phases, G_1 and G_2, allow for cell growth and regulatory inputs. Specifically, these gap phases of the cell cycle integrate complex signals in order to determine whether the cell should proceed into S phase and M phase, respectively, allowing the cell to make a decision to stop within the gap phases and therefore not interrupt chromosome replication and/or chromosome segregation.

Work from a number of laboratories utilizing various experimental model systems has significantly advanced our understanding of cell-cycle control by identifying many of the genes and signaling pathways that regulate the cell cycle (68,69). Exploiting the budding yeast *Saccharomyces cerevisiae* as a model system and creating conditional mutations (termed *cell division cycle*, or cdc mutations) that impaired specific phases of the cell cycle, Lee Hartwell and colleagues discovered the majority of genes that were required for regulating cell-cycle progression (68). The significance of this finding was that it demonstrated for the first time that the cell cycle is organized through a series of dependent reactions, and in order for its accurate execution, the completion of one event is required for the beginning of the next. A key finding extending from these studies was the discovery of the Cdc2 protein kinase by Nurse and colleagues (70,71). This kinase was first identified in the fission yeast *Schizosaccharomyces pombe* and later in budding yeast and was found to be the key regulator of the G_1/S and G_2/M phase transition points (72–76). This work provided the cornerstone for an entire field of molecular biology and genetics, and highlighted the role of Cdc2 in each of the major cell-cycle transitions. The next breakthrough in cell-cycle biology came with the discovery of a family of proteins in metazoans that were homologous to the yeast Cdc2, the cyclin-dependent kinases (Cdk) (77). Like Cdc2, the primary function of the Cdks is to provide information to the cell, allowing for successful passage through the cell cycle, ie, the G_1/S-phase transition, as well as the G_2/M transition (78). In fact, each phase of the cell cycle has a corresponding unique pattern of Cdk activity. The Cdks consist of a catalytic subunit (the Cdk) and a regulatory activating subunit (the cyclin). The catalytic Cdk subunit is without intrinsic enzymatic activity and thus requires the binding of the cyclin subunit in a heterodimeric conformation for full activation of the protein kinase domain. The kinase activity of the Cdk is further regulated through phosphorylation and dephosphorylation of conserved amino acid residues (usually serine or threonine) and through the binding of specific inhibitory proteins (Cdk-inhibitory proteins), specifically the INK4 proteins (p15, p16, p18, p19) and Cip/Kip proteins (p21, p27, p57).

As mentioned, safeguard mechanisms exist to regulate the timing of the cell cycle, specifically at the transition points, and to suspend progression of the cell cycle in order to remove and repair DNA damage when it occurs in order to eliminate genetic mutations during cell division and preserve genomic integrity. These biochemical regulatory pathways are termed *cell-cycle checkpoints* (79–81). Disabling the checkpoint pathways through mutations in key genes is thought to bring about the genomic instability seen in cancer cells.

The enzymes that mediate DNA replication and the segregation of chromosomes during mitosis are mostly responsible for the accurate transmission of genetic information. Though these enzymes work with great precision, they have an intrinsic error rate and cause genetic mistakes. Additionally, metabolic byproducts or exogenous exposure to certain chemicals or radiation can lead to DNA damage. Depending on the phase of the cell cycle that DNA damage occurs and is sensed, cell-cycle progression can be blocked at multiple points: prior to S-phase (G_1 DNA damage checkpoint response), during S-phase (intra-S phase DNA damage checkpoint response or DNA replication checkpoint), and prior to M-phase entry (G_2 DNA damage checkpoint response or the mitotic spindle integrity checkpoint). Otherwise, unrepaired DNA damage causes physical barriers (ie, chemical adducts and/or double-stranded breaks) to DNA replication forks, leading to replication that is predisposed to errors and followed by segregation of abnormal chromosomes during mitosis.

Though the precise molecular mechanisms for all of the checkpoint pathways are not completely understood, the G_1 DNA damage checkpoint is the best studied. Several mammalian genes regulate the DNA damage checkpoint: mutated in ataxia telangiectasia (ATM), ataxia telangiectasia and Rad-3 related (ATR), TP53, and p21. Of these, the tumor suppressor gene, TP53, is the most thoroughly studied, as well as the most commonly mutated gene in sporadically occurring human tumors (82). The human TP53 gene is located on the short arm of human chromosome 17 band 13, and the gene expressed encodes a transcription factor that is activated in response to DNA damage, such as nucleotide mismatches and double-stranded breaks. Specifically, accumulation of the p53 protein causes the cells to undergo G_1 arrest and prevents cells from entering S-phase and replicating a damaged chromosome (83). TP53 also mediates apoptosis and regulates the cellular response to DNA damage caused by ultraviolet irradiation, g-irradiation, and some chemotherapeutic agents. As mentioned, inactivating mutations of the TP53 gene have been observed in most human tumors, including osteosarcomas, soft-tissue sarcomas, rhabdomyosarcomas, leukemias, brain tumors, and lung and breast carcinomas. Germline mutations of the TP53 gene account for the majority of cases of the autosomal dominant disorder the Li-Fraumeni syndrome.

THE BIOLOGY OF HUMAN CANCER METASTASIS

Cancer metastasis is a complex multistep process and requires multiple genetic changes in the tumor cell in order for it to acquire all of the capabilities necessary to colonize a distant organ (84,85). In addition, new data is emerging that identifies genetic changes in the tumor stroma that assists in the survival of the invading tumor cell and helps to ensure stability in the distant organ (86). Though the exact genetic mutations that are necessary for the metastatic phenotype are mostly unknown, the general pathways that are involved have been studied intensely (87).

The traditional model of cancer metastasis involves the following basic steps: The cancer cell in the epithelium detaches from its neighboring cells, usually through the loss of E-cadherin, a member of the cadherin family of cell-cell adhesion molecules (88), and acquires motility to cross the basal lamina, typically by activating the signal transduction pathways that are mediated by the integrins (89). At this point, the tumor cell must also recruit new blood vessel formation, the process of angiogenesis (90). The tumor cells accomplish angiogenesis by producing powerful angiogenic factors, such as fibroblast growth factor (FGF) and vascular endothelial growth factor (VEGF). Angiogenesis creates a vascular system around the tumor and allows the tumor to grow to a larger size. The newly formed vascular system also provides a way for tumor cells to migrate into the bloodstream and subsequently to penetrate through them, a process termed intravasation. Intravasation is thought to be mediated by the microenvironment of the bloodstream, such as oxygen tension, blood pH, or a chemotactic gradient, and possibly augmented by the transcription factor Twist (91). The tumor cells circulating in the bloodstream must evade immune surveillance. Eventually the circulating tumor cells then arrest in the capillary bed and are able to grow intravascularly. The presence of the tumor cells in the blood vessels are thought to cause a physical disruption of the vessels and lead to penetration of the tumor cells out of the vessels and into the organ parenchyma, a process referred to as extravasation (92). Recently, some molecular mechanisms of extravasation have been uncovered (93–98). Lastly, there is colonization of the distant organ. This step alone is a complex process and involves not only the genetic transformation of the cancer cell, but it is thought that the cancer cell also sets in motion specific adaptations of the distant tissue stroma that will come to house the metastatic tumor cells.

This distant coordination of the stroma by the primary tumor cell may help to explain the clinical observation that certain tumor types have a preference for specific metastatic target organs. For example, in breast cancer, the bone is a significant site for metastasis and causes osteolytic lesions. The preference of breast cancer cells to metastasize to the bone is thought to be mediated by specific factors (parathyroid hormone-related protein, TNF-α, IL-1, IL6, IL8, and IL11) secreted by the tumor cells that activate osteoclasts and degrade the bone matrix. Then, once the invading tumor cells degrade the bone matrix, growth factors, such as transforming growth factor-β (TGF-β), are secreted from the bone matrix and further stimulate proliferation of the tumor cells (99–101). Similarly, prostate cancer has a tendency towards bone metastasis, though in this case, the cancer cells result in osteoblastic bone lesions. Though the precise genes that regulate prostate cancer metastasis are unknown, the proposed mechanism of regulation is similar to that described for breast cancer metastasis: The prostate tumor cells secrete paracrine factors that stimulate the osteoblasts to proliferate and cause bone remodeling, and the osteoblasts make factors that further fuel the growth of prostate tumor cells (102).

The lung, liver, and brain are other common target organs of metastasis for many solid tumors. Though extensive animal models have been developed, the mechanisms for the organ-selective metastasis are not yet thoroughly understood at the molecular level. Recent data from gene expression analysis is beginning to identify novel genes that are thought to be responsible for organ-selective metastasis in breast cancer (103,104).

It is important to realize that the single cells that form the tumor metastasis can grow fast and take over the organ quickly; in other cases, the metastatic tumors remain small and dormant for months to years. This latency is referred to as *metastatic dormancy*. Eventually, however, the metastatic tumor will expand and cause the death of the patient. In fact, metastatic cancer of any origin is generally not curable and complications from metastasis account for 90% of deaths from solid tumors. More importantly, however, the metastatic cascade offers multiple targets for therapeutic attack. For example, the angiogenesis inhibitor bevacizumab, a recombinant monoclonal antibody that targets the activity of the VEGF, when used in combination with standard chemotherapy in patients with metastatic colon cancer, has improved overall survival (105). At the root of the complexity of the metastatic cascade lies the interplay between the unique tumor microenvironment and genetic predisposition. Current research by many investigators in the field of metastasis involves developing a new paradigm that would reconcile the traditional model with recent genetic data (98).

References

1. Hanahan D, Weinberg RA. The hallmarks of cancer. *Cell.* 2000;100(1):57–70.
2. Vogelstein B, Kinzler KW. The multistep nature of cancer. *Trends Genet.* 1993;9(4):138–141.

3. Temin HM, Mizutani S. RNA-dependent DNA polymerase in virions of Rous sarcoma virus. *Nature.* 1970;226(5252):1211–1213.

4. Baltimore D. RNA-dependent DNA polymerase in virions of RNA tumour viruses. *Nature.* 1970;226(5252):1209–1211.

5. Stehelin D, Varmus HE, Bishop JM, Vogt PK. DNA related to the transforming gene(s) of avian sarcoma viruses is present in normal avian DNA. *Nature.* 1976;260(5547):170–173.

6. Hesketh. *The Oncogene and Tumor Suppressor Gene Facts Book,* 2nd ed. San Diego: Academic Press; 1997.

7. Downward J. Targeting RAS signalling pathways in cancer therapy. *Nature Rev.* 2003;3(1):11–22.

8. Bos JL. Ras oncogenes in human cancer: a review. *Cancer Res.* 1989;49(17):4682–4689.

9. Collins S, Groudine M. Amplification of endogenous myc-related DNA sequences in a human myeloid leukaemia cell line. *Nature.* 1982;298(5875):679–681.

10. Dalla-Favera R, Wong-Staal F, Gallo RC. Onc gene amplification in promyelocytic leukaemia cell line HL-60 and primary leukaemic cells of the same patient. *Nature.* 1982;299(5878):61–63.

11. Cole MD. The myc oncogene: its role in transformation and differentiation. *Annu Rev Genet.* 1986;20:361–384.

12. Henriksson M, Luscher B. Proteins of the Myc network: essential regulators of cell growth and differentiation. *Adv Cancer Res.* 1996;68:109–182.

13. Schmidt ML, Lukens JN, Seeger RC, et al. Biologic factors determine prognosis in infants with stage IV neuroblastoma: a prospective Children's Cancer Group study. *J Clin Oncol.* 2000;18(6):1260–1268.

14. Yang-Feng TL, Schechter AL, Weinberg RA, Francke U. Oncogene from rat neuro/glioblastomas (human gene symbol NGL) is located on the proximal long arm of human chromosome 17 and EGFR is confirmed at 7p13-q11.2 (Abstract). *Cytogenet Cell Genet.* 1985;40:784.

15. Coussens L, Yang-Feng TL, Liao YC, et al. Tyrosine kinase receptor with extensive homology to EGF receptor shares chromosomal location with neu oncogene. *Science.* 1985;230(4730):1132–1139.

16. Slamon DJ, Clark GM, Wong SG, Levin WJ, Ullrich A, McGuire WL. Human breast cancer: correlation of relapse and survival with amplification of the HER-2/neu oncogene. *Science.* 1987;235(4785):177–182.

17. Rowley JD. The critical role of chromosome translocations in human leukemias. *Annu Rev Genet.* 1998;32:495–519.

18. Rabbitts TH. Perspective: chromosomal translocations can affect genes controlling gene expression and differentiation—why are these functions targeted? *J Path.* 1999;187(1):39–42.

19. Nowell PC, Hungerford D. A minute chromosome in human chronic granulocytic leukemia [abstract]. *Science.* 1960;132:1497.

20. Rowley JD. Letter: a new consistent chromosomal abnormality in chronic myelogenous leukaemia identified by quinacrine fluorescence and Giemsa staining. *Nature.* 1973;243(5405):290–293.

21. Heisterkamp N, Stephenson JR, Groffen J, et al. Localization of the c-abl oncogene adjacent to a translocation break point in chronic myelocytic leukaemia. *Nature.* 1983;306(5940):239–242.

22. Druker BJ, Talpaz M, Resta DJ, et al. Efficacy and safety of a specific inhibitor of the BCR-ABL tyrosine kinase in chronic myeloid leukemia. *New Eng J Med.* 2001;344(14):1031–1037.

23. Rowley JD. Identification of a translocation with quinacrine fluorescence in a patient with acute leukemia. *Annales de genetique.* 1973;16(2):109–112.

24. Nucifora G, Rowley JD. AML1 and the 8;21 and 3;21 translocations in acute and chronic myeloid leukemia. *Blood.* 1995;86(1):1–14.

25. Tenen DG, Hromas R, Licht JD, Zhang DE. Transcription factors, normal myeloid development, and leukemia. *Blood.* 1997;90(2):489–519.

26. Rowley JD, Golomb HM, Dougherty C. 15/17 translocation, a consistent chromosomal change in acute promyelocytic leukaemia. *Lancet.* 1977;1(8010):549–550.

27. Warrell RP, Jr., Frankel SR, Miller WH, Jr., et al. Differentiation therapy of acute promyelocytic leukemia with tretinoin (all-trans-retinoic acid). *N Engl J Med.* 1991;324(20):1385–1393.

28. Knudson AG, Jr. Mutation and cancer: statistical study of retinoblastoma. *Proc Natl Acad Sci USA.* 1971;68(4):820–823.

29. Comings DE. A general theory of carcinogenesis. *Proc Natl Acad Sci USA.* 1973;70(12):3324–3328.

30. Dryja TP, Rapaport JM, Joyce JM, Petersen RA. Molecular detection of deletions involving band q14 of chromosome 13 in retinoblastomas. *Proc Natl Acad Sci USA.* 1986;83(19):7391–7394.

31. Feinberg AP. Epigenetics at the epicenter of modern medicine. *JAMA.* 2008;299(11):1345–1350.

32. Gal-Yam EN, Saito Y, Egger G, Jones PA. Cancer epigenetics: modifications, screening, and therapy. *Annu Rev Med.* 2008;59:267–280.

33. Kaminskas E, Farrell A, Abraham S, et al. Approval summary: azacitidine for treatment of myelodysplastic syndrome subtypes. *Clin Cancer Res.* 2005;11(10):3604–3608.

34. Whyte P, Buchkovich KJ, Horowitz JM, et al. Association between an oncogene and an anti-oncogene: the adenovirus E1A proteins bind to the retinoblastoma gene product. *Nature.* 1988;334(6178):124–129.

35. Weinberg RA. The retinoblastoma protein and cell cycle control. *Cell.* 1995;81(3):323–330.

36. Morris EJ, Dyson NJ. Retinoblastoma protein partners. *Adv Cancer Res.* 2001;82:1–54.

37. Friend SH, Bernards R, Rogelj S, et al. A human DNA segment with properties of the gene that predisposes to retinoblastoma and osteosarcoma. *Nature.* 1986;323(6089):643–646.

38. Friend SH, Horowitz JM, Gerber MR, et al. Deletions of a DNA sequence in retinoblastomas and mesenchymal tumors: organization of the sequence and its encoded protein. *Proc Natl Acad Sci USA.* 1987;84(24):9059–9063.

39. Horowitz JM, Park SH, Bogenmann E, et al. Frequent inactivation of the retinoblastoma anti-oncogene is restricted to a subset of human tumor cells. *Proc Natl Acad Sci USA.* 1990;87(7):2775–2779.

40. Jiang W, Zhang YJ, Kahn SM, et al. Altered expression of the cyclin D1 and retinoblastoma genes in human esophageal cancer. *Proc Natl Acad Sci USA.* 1993;90(19):9026–9030.

41. Lee EY, To H, Shew JY, Bookstein R, Scully P, Lee WH. Inactivation of the retinoblastoma susceptibility gene in human breast cancers. *Science (New York, NY).* 1988;241(4862):218–221.

42. Mori T, Miura K, Aoki T, Nishihira T, Mori S, Nakamura Y. Frequent somatic mutation of the MTS1/CDK4I (multiple tumor suppressor/cyclin-dependent kinase 4 inhibitor) gene in esophageal squamous cell carcinoma. *Cancer Res.* 1994;54(13):3396–3397.

43. Kamb A, Gruis NA, Weaver-Feldhaus J, et al. A cell cycle regulator potentially involved in genesis of many tumor types. *Science (New York, NY).* 1994;264(5157):436–440.

44. Vogelstein B, Kinzler KW. *The Genetic Basis of Human Cancer,* 2nd ed. New York. McGraw Hill Companies, Inc; 2002.

45. Ellermann V, Bang O. Experimentelle Leukaamie bei Huhnern. *Zentralb Bakteriol.* 1908;46:595–609.

46. Rous P. A transmissible avian neoplasm: sarcoma of the common fowl. *J Exp Med.* 1910;12:696–705.

47. Augenlicht LH, Wahrman MZ, Halsey H, Anderson L, Taylor J, Lipkin M. Expression of cloned sequences in biopsies of human colonic tissue and in colonic carcinoma cells induced to differentiate in vitro. *Cancer Res.* 1987;47(22):6017–6021.

48. Schena M, Shalon D, Davis RW, Brown PO. Quantitative monitoring of gene expression patterns with a complementary DNA microarray. *Science (New York, NY).* 1995;270(5235):467–470.

49. DeRisi J, Penland L, Brown PO, et al. Use of a cDNA microarray to analyse gene expression patterns in human cancer. *Nat Genet.* 1996;14(4):457–460.

50. Alizadeh AA, Eisen MB, Davis RE, et al. Distinct types of diffuse large B-cell lymphoma identified by gene expression profiling. *Nature.* 2000;403(6769):503–511.

51. Dhanasekaran SM, Barrette TR, Ghosh D, et al. Delineation of prognostic biomarkers in prostate cancer. *Nature.* 2001;412(6849):822–826.

52. Khan J, Wei JS, Ringner M, et al. Classification and diagnostic prediction of cancers using gene expression profiling and artificial neural networks. *Nat Med.* 2001;7(6):673–679.

53. MacDonald TJ, Brown KM, LaFleur B, et al. Expression profiling of medulloblastoma: PDGFRA and the RAS/MAPK pathway as therapeutic targets for metastatic disease. *Nat Genet.* 2001;29(2):143–152.

54. Rosenwald A, Wright G, Chan WC, et al. The use of molecular profiling to predict survival after chemotherapy for diffuse large-B-cell lymphoma. *N Engl J Med.* 2002;346(25):1937–1947.

55. Shipp MA, Ross KN, Tamayo P, et al. Diffuse large B-cell lymphoma outcome prediction by gene-expression profiling and supervised machine learning. *Nat Med.* 2002;8(1):68–74.

56. Sorlie T, Perou CM, Tibshirani R, et al. Gene expression patterns of breast carcinomas distinguish tumor subclasses with clinical implications. *Proc Natl Acad Sci USA.* 2001;98(19):10869–10874.

57. van 't Veer LJ, Dai H, van de Vijver MJ, et al. Gene expression profiling predicts clinical outcome of breast cancer. *Nature.* 2002;415(6871):530–536.

58. van de Vijver MJ, He YD, van't Veer LJ, et al. A gene-expression signature as a predictor of survival in breast cancer. *N Engl J Med.* 2002;347(25):1999–2009.

59. TAILORx. http://www.cancer.gov/clinicaltrials/digestpage/TAILORx.

60. MINDACT. http://www.eortc.be/services/unit/mindact/MINDACT_websiteii.asp.

61. Lucito R, Healy J, Alexander J, et al. Representational oligonucleotide microarray analysis: a high-resolution method to detect genome copy number variation. *Genome Res.* 2003;13(10):2291–2305.

62. Carvalho B, Ouwerkerk E, Meijer GA, Ylstra B. High resolution microarray comparative genomic hybridisation analysis using spotted oligonucleotides. *J Clin Pathol.* 2004;57(6):644–646.

63. Pinkel D, Segraves R, Sudar D, et al. High resolution analysis of DNA copy number variation using comparative genomic hybridization to microarrays. *Nat Genet.* 1998;20(2):207–211.

64. Bignell GR, Huang J, Greshock J, et al. High-resolution analysis of DNA copy number using oligonucleotide microarrays. *Genome Res.* 2004;14(2):287–295.

65. Huang J, Wei W, Zhang J, et al. Whole genome DNA copy number changes identified by high density oligonucleotide arrays. *Hum Genomics.* 2004;1(4):287–299.

66. Zhao X, Li C, Paez JG, et al. An integrated view of copy number and allelic alterations in the cancer genome using single nucleotide polymorphism arrays. *Cancer Res.* 2004;64(9):3060–3071.

67. Howard A, Pelc SR. Nuclear incorporation of p32 as demonstrated by autoradiographs. *Exp Cell Res.* 1951;2(2):178–187.

68. Hartwell LH, Mortimer RK, Culotti J, Culotti M. Genetic control of the cell division cycle in yeast: V. Genetic Analysis of cdc Mutants. *Genetics.* 1973;74(2):267–286.

69. Nurse P. Universal control mechanism regulating onset of M-phase. *Nature.* 1990;344(6266):503–508.

70. Lee MG, Nurse P. Complementation used to clone a human homologue of the fission yeast cell cycle control gene cdc2. *Nature.* 1987;327(6117):31–35.

71. Nurse P, Bissett Y. Gene required in G1 for commitment to cell cycle and in G2 for control of mitosis in fission yeast. *Nature.* 1981;292(5823):558–560.

72. Hindley J, Phear GA. Sequence of the cell division gene CDC2 from Schizosaccharomyces pombe; patterns of splicing and homology to protein kinases. *Gene.* 1984;31(1–3):129–134.

73. Nurse P. Genetic control of cell size at cell division in yeast. *Nature.* 1975;256(5518):547–551.

74. Beach D, Durkacz B, Nurse P. Functionally homologous cell cycle control genes in budding and fission yeast. *Nature.* 1982;300(5894):706–709.

75. Reed SI, Wittenberg C. Mitotic role for the Cdc28 protein kinase of Saccharomyces cerevisiae. *Proc Natl Acad Sci USA.* 1990;87(15):5697–5701.

76. Piggott JR, Rai R, Carter BL. A bifunctional gene product involved in two phases of the yeast cell cycle. *Nature.* 1982;298(5872):391–393.

77. Meyerson M, Enders GH, Wu CL, et al. A family of human cdc2-related protein kinases. *EMBO J.* 1992;11(8):2909–2917.

78. Harper JW, Adams PD. Cyclin-dependent kinases. *Chem Rev.* 2001;101(8):2511–2526.

79. Hartwell L, Weinert T, Kadyk L, Garvik B. Cell cycle checkpoints, genomic integrity, and cancer. *Cold Spring Harb Symp Quant Biol.* 1994;59:259–263.

80. Elledge SJ, Harper JW. Cdk inhibitors: on the threshold of checkpoints and development. *Curr Opin Cell Biol.* 1994;6(6):847–852.

81. Weinert T, Hartwell L. Control of G2 delay by the rad9 gene of Saccharomyces cerevisiae. *J Cell Sci.* 1989;12:145–148.

82. Hollstein M, Sidransky D, Vogelstein B, Harris CC. p53 mutations in human cancers. *Science (New York, NY).* 1991;253(5015):49–53.

83. Kuerbitz SJ, Plunkett BS, Walsh WV, Kastan MB. Wild-type p53 is a cell cycle checkpoint determinant following irradiation. *Proc Natl Acad Sci USA.* 1992;89(16):7491–7495.

84. Fidler IJ. The pathogenesis of cancer metastasis: the "seed and soil" hypothesis revisited. *Nat Rev.* 2003;3(6):453–458.

85. Chambers AF, Groom AC, MacDonald IC. Dissemination and growth of cancer cells in metastatic sites. *Nat Rev.* 2002;2(8):563–572.

86. Gupta GP, Nguyen DX, Chiang AC, et al. Mediators of vascular remodelling co-opted for sequential steps in lung metastasis. *Nature.* 2007;446(7137):765–770.

87. Pantel K, Brakenhoff RH. Dissecting the metastatic cascade. *Nat Rev.* 2004;4(6):448–456.

88. Christofori G. New signals from the invasive front. *Nature.* 2006;441(7092):444–450.

89. Guo W, Giancotti FG. Integrin signalling during tumour progression. *Nat Rev Mol Cell Biol.* 2004;5(10):816–826.

90. Hanahan D, Folkman J. Patterns and emerging mechanisms of the angiogenic switch during tumorigenesis. *Cell.* 1996;86(3):353–364.

91. Yang J, Mani SA, Donaher JL, et al. Twist, a master regulator of morphogenesis, plays an essential role in tumor metastasis. *Cell.* 2004;117(7):927–939.

92. Al-Mehdi AB, Tozawa K, Fisher AB, Shientag L, Lee A, Muschel RJ. Intravascular origin of metastasis from the proliferation of endothelium-attached tumor cells: a new model for metastasis. *Nat Med.* 2000;6(1):100–102.

93. Kim YJ, Borsig L, Varki NM, Varki A. P-selection deficiency attenuates tumor growth and metastasis. *Proc Natl Acad Sci USA.* 1998;95(16):9325–9330.

94. Khanna C, Wan X, Bose S, et al. The membrane-cytoskeleton linker ezrin is necessary for osteosarcoma metastasis. *Nat Med.* 2004;10(2):182–186.

95. Yu Y, Khan J, Khanna C, Helman L, Meltzer PS, Merlino G. Expression profiling identifies the cytoskeletal organizer ezrin and the developmental homeoprotein Six-1 as key metastatic regulators. *Nat Med.* 2004;10(2):175–181.

96. Criscuoli ML, Nguyen M, Eliceiri BP. Tumor metastasis but not tumor growth is dependent on Src-mediated vascular permeability. *Blood.* 2005;105(4):1508–1514.

97. Muller A, Homey B, Soto H, et al. Involvement of chemokine receptors in breast cancer metastasis. *Nature.* 2001;410(6824):50–56.

98. Gupta GP, Massague J. Cancer metastasis: building a framework. *Cell.* 2006;127(4):679–695.

99. Mundy GR. Metastasis to bone: causes, consequences and therapeutic opportunities. *Nat Rev.* 2002;2(8):584–593.

100. Boyle WJ, Simonet WS, Lacey DL. Osteoclast differentiation and activation. *Nature.* 2003;423(6937):337–342.

101. Kang Y, Siegel PM, Shu W, et al. A multigenic program mediating breast cancer metastasis to bone. *Cancer Cell.* 2003;3(6):537–549.
102. Logothetis CJ, Lin SH. Osteoblasts in prostate cancer metastasis to bone. *Nat Rev.* 2005;5(1):21–28.
103. Minn AJ, Gupta GP, Siegel PM, et al. Genes that mediate breast cancer metastasis to lung. *Nature.* 2005;436(7050):518–524.
104. Saha S, Bardelli A, Buckhaults P, et al. A phosphatase associated with metastasis of colorectal cancer. *Science (New York, NY).* 2001;294(5545):1343–1346.
105. Hurwitz HI, Fehrenbacher L, Hainsworth JD, et al. Bevacizumab in combination with fluorouracil and leucovorin: an active regimen for first-line metastatic colorectal cancer. *J Clin Oncol.* 2005;23(15):3502–3508.

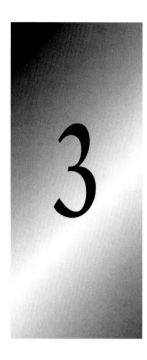

Principles of Chemotherapy

Vicky Makker
David Spriggs

Over the last two decades, there has been a steady improvement in the survival statistics for nearly all cancers due in large part to earlier detection and advances in surgery, radiation, and chemotherapy. In particular, chemotherapy has changed profoundly. While the entire discipline of medical oncology was founded on the management of serious toxicity, most of the newer agents that have been introduced into practice have had modified toxicity profiles with preserved efficacy (Table 3.1). Carboplatin has replaced cisplatin in many cancers, and the introduction of pegylated liposomal doxorubicin promises to do the same for anthracyclines. Nonetheless, the longer survival of patients with cancer has led to an increase in the chronic long-term toxicities associated with chemotherapy. The entire field is now increasingly focused on the problems of cancer survivors, and we are likely to see an expanding role for rehabilitation medicine in cancer centers and their programs.

In this chapter, we have focused primarily on the subacute and chronic toxicities associated with chemotherapy treatment. The acute toxicities, like myelosuppression and acute allergic reactions, are primarily the responsibility of the chemotherapist and unlikely to be treated by rehabilitation specialists. Rehabilitation practitioners, however, should be familiar with these acute toxicities. We have linked the characteristic organ toxicities to specific agents, both in the text and in tables, which should provide ready access to an extensive literature. Clearly, the huge numbers of drug entities in clinical development will continue to cause novel toxicities that are not anticipated in this chapter, which focuses on approved drugs.

CARDIAC TOXICITY

Cardiomyopathy

Anthracyclines include daunorubicin, doxorubicin, epirubicin, and idarubicin, and are utilized in the treatment of breast cancer, ovarian cancer, endometrial cancer, soft tissue sarcomas, Hodgkin and non-Hodgkin lymphoma, non-small cell lung cancer (NSCLC) and small cell lung cancer (SCLC), hepatomas, thyroid cancer, and gastric cancer. The incidence of anthracycline-induced cardiotoxicity is related to the cumulative dose administered. The risk is increased in patients with underlying heart disease, when anthracyclines are used concurrently with other cardiotoxic agents or radiation, and in patients undergoing hematopoietic cell transplantation. Cardiovascular complications can arise acutely (during administration), early (several days to months following administration), or years to decades following exposure (Table 3.2).

Anthracyclines intercalate into deoxyribonucleic acid (DNA) of replicating cells, resulting in inhibition of DNA synthesis and inhibition of transcription

KEY POINTS

- Over the last two decades, there has been a steady improvement in the survival statistics for nearly all cancers due in large part to earlier detection and advances in surgery, radiation, and chemotherapy.
- Longer survival of patients with cancer has led to an increase in the chronic long-term toxicities associated with chemotherapy.
- Anthracycline-induced cardiovascular complications can arise acutely (during administration), early (several days to months following administration), or years to decades following exposure.
- Bleomycin therapy can result in life-threatening interstitial pulmonary fibrosis in up to 10% of patients.
- Cisplatin is used to treat testicular, ovarian, bladder, esophageal, and head and neck cancers, as well as non-small cell lung cancer (NSCLC), small cell lung cancer (SCLC), non-Hodgkin lymphoma, and trophoblastic disease, and is commonly associated with peripheral neuropathy and ototoxicity.
- Lhermitte sign is a shocklike, nonpainful sensation of paresthesias radiating from the back to the feet during neck flexion, can develop in patients receiving cisplatin, and typically occurs after weeks or months of treatment.
- Taxane-induced motor and sensory neuropathies are cumulative and dose- and schedule-dependent.
- A peripheral neuropathy develops in approximately 75% of patients who receive prolonged thalidomide treatment.
- The dose-limiting toxicity of vincristine is an axonal neuropathy, which results from disruption of the microtubules within axons and interference with axonal transport.
- Chemotherapeutic agents can affect the glomerulus, tubules, interstitium, or the renal microvasculature, with clinical manifestations that range from an asymptomatic elevation of serum creatinine to acute renal failure requiring dialysis.
- Almost any chemotherapeutic agent can result in post-chemotherapy rheumatism, and this is a fairly common clinical phenomenon.

through inhibition of DNA-dependent ribonucleic acid (RNA) polymerase. These agents also inhibit topoisomerase II, which results in DNA fragmentation, and form cytotoxic free radicals, which result in single- and double-stranded DNA breaks with subsequent inhibition of DNA synthesis. Myocyte injury has been attributed to the production of toxic oxygen free radicals and an increase in oxidative stress, which cause lipid peroxidation of membranes. This, in turn, leads to vacuolation and myocyte replacement by fibrous tissue (1). Doxorubicin is also associated with a decrease of endogenous antioxidant enzymes, such as glutathione peroxidase, which are responsible for the scavenging of free radicals (2,3).

The strongest predictor of anthracycline-induced cardiotoxicity is cumulative dose administered, but age over 70, prior irradiation, concomitant administration of other chemotherapeutic agents (particularly paclitaxel and trastuzumab), concurrent chest irradiation, and underlying heart disease are also important factors (4–6). In addition, female gender has been demonstrated to be an independent risk factor (7).

Early reports in adults showed that with cumulative doxorubicin doses of 400, 550, and 700 mg/m^2 the percentage of patients who developed cardiotoxicity was 3%, 7%, and 18%, respectively (6). Subsequent series suggested that the incidence of doxorubicin-related cardiotoxicity was underestimated in these studies. A report that included 630 patients treated with doxorubicin alone in three controlled trials estimated that as many as 26% of patients receiving a cumulative doxorubicin dose of 550 mg/m^2 would develop doxorubicin-related heart failure (8). The use of a single threshold dose has been replaced by monitoring for early evidence of cardiotoxicity using better surveillance techniques. Therapy thus should be stopped at a lower cumulative dose if there is evidence of cardiotoxicity.

Age extremes predispose to cardiotoxicity at lower cumulative anthracycline doses (8). In older patients, it is not clear whether preexisting heart disease increases susceptibility to anthracycline-induced damage or whether there is less functional reserve to tolerate additional myocardial damage. Prior mediastinal irradiation may increase the susceptibility to anthracycline-induced cardiotoxicity by inducing endothelial cell damage and compromising coronary artery blood flow. The magnitude of increased risk may depend upon the anthracycline dose. The administration of nonanthracycline agents that also cause cardiotoxicity may result in synergistic toxicity when anthracyclines are given concurrently, and the most important agents in this regard are the taxanes (paclitaxel and docetaxel) and trastuzumab.

TABLE 3.1
Alphabetical List of Common Chemotherapy Agents

GENERIC NAME	TRADE NAME	CLASSIFICATION
Albumin-bound paclitaxel	Abraxane	Taxane
Aldesleukin	Proleukin, Interleukin-2, IL-2	Biological response modifier
Alemtuzumab	Campath, Hexalen, Hexamethylmelamine, HMM	Anti-CD 52 monoclonal antibody altretamine, alkylating agent
Amifostine	Ethyol	Organic thiophosphate analog
Anastrozole	Arimidex, Trisonex	Nonsteroidal aromatase inhibitor arsenic trioxide antineoplastic differentiating agent
Asparaginase	Elspar, L-Asparaginase	Antitumor antibiotic
Bacillus Calmette-Guerin (BCG)	Immucyst, Oncotice	Biological response modifier
Bevacizumab	Avastin	Anti-VEGF monoclonal antibody
Bicalutamide	Casodex	Nonsteroidal antihormone
Bleomycin	Blenoxane	Antitumor antibiotic
Bortezomib	Velcade	Reversible inhibitor of 26S proteosome, cytotoxic
Busulfan	Myleran, Busulfex	Alkylating agent
Capecitabine	Xeloda	Antimetabolite, cytotoxic
Carboplatin	Paraplatin, CBDCA	Platinum
Carmustine	BCNU, Bischloronitrosurea, BICNU	Alkylating agent
Cetuximab	Erbitux	EGF-R tyrosine kinase inhibitor
Chlorambucil	Leukeran	Alkylating agent
Cisplatin	Platinol, CDDP, CIS-Diamminedichloroplatinum	Platinum
Cladribine	Leustatin, 2-Chlorodeoxy-adenosine, 2-CDA	Antimetabolite
Clofarabine	Clolar	Antimetabolite
Cyclophosphamide	Cytoxan, CTX	Alkylating agent
Cytarabine	Cytosar U, Cytosine-arabinoside, ARA-C	Antimetabolite
Dacarbazine	DTIC-DOME Carboxamide, DIC, Imidazole, Carboxamide	Alkylating agent
Dactinomycin	Cosmegen, Actinomycin-D	Antitumor antibiotic
Dasatinib	Sprycel	Signal transduction inhibitor
Daunorubicin	Cerubidine, Daunomycin, Ruidomycin	Anthracycline
Daunorubicin Liposome	Daunoxomed	Anthracycline
Decitabine	Dacogen, 5-AZA-2-Deoxycytidine	Antimetabolite
Denileukin Diftitox	Ontak	Biologic response modifier
Dexrazoxane	Zinecard	Cardioprotectant
Docetaxel	Taxotere	Taxane
Doxorubicin	Adriamycin	Anthracycline
Doxorubicin Liposome	Doxil	Anthracycline *(Continued)*

TABLE 3.1 *Alphabetical List of Common Chemotherapy Agents, Continued*

GENERIC NAME	TRADE NAME	CLASSIFICATION
Epirubicin	Ellence, 4 Epidoxorubicin	Anthracycline
Erlotnib	Tarceva	ERF-R tyrosine kinase inhibitor
Estramustine	EMCYT, Estracyte	Alkylating agent
Etoposide	Vepesid, VP-16	Topoisomerase II inhibitor
Exemestane	AROMASIN	Aromatase inhibitor
Filgrastim	Neupogen, G-CSF 5-Fluro-2-deoxyuridine, FUDR	Recombinant human granulocyte colony-stimulating factor floxuridine, antimetabolite
Fludarabine	Fludara, 2-Furo-ARA-AMP	Antimetabolite
5-Flurouracil	Efudex, 5-FU	Antimetabolite
Flutamide	Eulexine	Nonsteroidal antiandrogen
Fulvestrant	Faslodex	Estrogen receptor antagonist
Gefitinib	Iressa	EGF-R tyrosine kinase inhibitor
Gemcitabine	Gemzar	Antimetabolite
Gemtuzumab Ozogamicin	Mylotarg	Anti-CD33 monoclonal antibody
Goserelin	Zoladex	Gonadotropin-releasing hormone analog
Hydroxyurea	Hydrea	Alkylating agent
Ibritumomab	Zevalin	Radiopharmaceutical monoclonal
Idarubicin	Idamycin, 4-Demethoxydaunorubicin	Anthracycline
Ifosfamide	IFEX, Isophosphamide	Alkylating agent
Imatinib	Gleevec	Bcr-Abl tyrosine kinase inhibitor
Interferon alfa	-Intron-A	Biologic response modifier
Irinotecan	Camptosar, CPT-II	Topoisomerase I inhibitor
Lenalidomide	Revlimid	Antiangiogenesis agent
Letrozole	Femara	Aromatase inhibitor
Leukovorin	Lederle Leukovorin	Folic acid metabolite
Leuprolide	Lupron	Gonadotropin-releasing hormone analog
Lomustine	CCNU, Bischloronitrosoure	Alkylating agent
Mechlorethamine	Mustargen, Nitrogen mustard	Alkylating agent
Megestrol	Megace	Synthetic progestin
Melphalan	Alkeran	Alkylating agent
Mercaptopurine	Purinethol, 6-MP	Antimetabolite
Mesna	Mesnex	Chemoprotective agent
Methotrexate	MTX, Amethopterin	Antimetabolite
Mitomycin-C	Mutamycin, mitomycin	Antitumor antibiotic
Mitotane	Lysodren	Adrenolytic agent
Mitoxantrone	Novantrone	Antitumor antibiotic
Nilutamide	Nilandron	Antiandrogen
Octreotide	Sandostatin	Somatostatin analog
Oxaliplatin	Eloxatin, dach-platinum, diaminocyclohexane platinum	Platinum

(Continued)

TABLE 3.1 *Alphabetical List of Common Chemotherapy Agents, Continued*

GENERIC NAME	TRADE NAME	CLASSIFICATION
Paclitaxel	Taxol	Antimicrotubule agent, taxane
Pamidronate	Aredia	Bisphosphonate
Panitumumab	Vectibix	Anti-EGFR monoclonal antibody
Pegylated filgrastim	Neulasta	Recombinant human granulocyte colony-stimulating factor
Pemetrexed	Alimta	Antifolate antimetabolite
Pentostatin NIPENT, Antimetabolite	2-deoxycoformycin, DCF	
Procarbazine	Matulane, N-methylhydrazine	Alkylating agent
Rituximab	Rituxan	Anti CD-20 monoclonal antibody
Sorafenib	Nexavar	Multitarget tyrosine kinase inhibitor
Streptozocin	Zanosar	Antitumor antibiotic
Sunitinib	Sutent	Multitarget tyrosine kinase inhibitor
Tamoxifen	Nolvadex	Antiestrogen
Temozolomide	Temodar	Alkylating agent
Thalidomide	Thalomid	Immunomodulator, antiangiogenesis factor
Thioguanine	6-thioguanine, 6-TG	Antimetabolite
Thiotepa	Thioplex	Alkylating agent
Topotecan	Hycamtin	Topoisomerase I inhibitor
Toremifene	Fareston	Antiestrogen
Tositumomab	Bexxar	Radiolabeled monoclonal antibody
Trastuzumab	Herceptin	Her2Neu monoclonal antibody
Tretinoin	Atra	Retinoid
Vinblastine	Velban	Vinca alkaloid
Vincristine	Oncovin	Vinca alkaloid
Vindesine	Eldisine	Vinca alkaloid
Vinorelbine	Navelbine	Vinca alkaloid

Three stages of anthracycline cardiotoxicity have been identified: acute, subacute, and late.

In acute toxicity, electrocardiographic abnormalities, ventricular dysfunction, an increase in plasma brain natriuretic peptide, and a pericarditis-myocarditis syndrome have been reported during or immediately after the administration of anthracyclines (9). These events are rare and seldom of clinical importance since they usually resolve within a week (10). The relationship between acute toxicity and the subsequent development of early and late cardiotoxicity is unclear.

In subacute toxicity, the appearance of heart failure can occur from days to months after the last anthracycline dose. The peak time for the appearance of clinical heart failure is three months after the last anthracycline dose, and mortality has been reported as high as 60% (5,6). More recently, survival in patients who develop heart failure has improved due to more aggressive medical management with medications such as angiotensin-converting enzyme (ACE) inhibitors and beta blockers.

In late toxicity, the onset of symptomatic heart failure can occur from 5 years to more than a decade after the last anthracycline dose. Serious arrhythmias, including ventricular tachycardia, ventricular fibrillation, and sudden cardiac death, have been identified in both symptomatic and asymptomatic patients with late cardiotoxicity. Late toxicity is primarily of concern where anthracyclines are used as part of a curative or adjuvant regimen. Late toxicity is most common in survivors of childhood malignancy, in whom late heart failure is due to a nonischemic dilated cardiomyopathy.

TABLE 3.2
Chemotherapy-Induced Cardiotoxicity

Toxicity type	Agent	References
Cardiomyopathy	Doxorubicin	(5,6,8,9)
	Epirubicin	(241)
	Trastuzumab	(13–16, 18, 19)
	Rituximab	(17)
	Bevacizumab	(7, 20)
	Cyclophosphamide	(11)
	Mitomycin	(242)
	Interferon-alfa	(25, 26)
	Sorafenib	(243)
	Sunitinib	(244)
	Imatinib	(245)
	Cisplatin	(246)
Rhythm disturbance	Paclitaxel	(27)
	Docetaxel	(247)
	Trastuzumab	(12)
	Ifosfamide	(11)
	Cisplatin	(246)
	Interferon-alfa	(22, 23)
	Methotrexate	(248)
	Cytarabine	(249)
	Interleukin-2	(34, 35)
	Arsenic Trioxide	(60)
	Alemtuzumab	(250)
	Rituximab	(17)
QT prolongation	Arsenic Trioxide	(48)
Vascular complications	Bleomycin	(251)
	Etoposide	(252)
	5-flurouracil	(39, 40)
	Capecitabine	(43)
	Vinca Alkaloids	(253, 254)
	Methotrexate	(248)
	Interleukin-2	(33)
	All-trans-retinoic acid	(255)
Hypertension	Bevacizumab	(44, 256)
	Sorafenib	(45)
	Sunitinib	(47)

In adults, other causes of heart failure must be excluded if delayed symptoms develop.

Approaches aimed at reducing the risk of anthracycline-induced cardiotoxicity have included the use of alternative administration schedules, the development of structural analogs (mitoxantrone, daunorubicin, idarubicin, and epirubicin), liposome encapsulation of the anthracycline molecule (liposomal doxorubicin), and the use of adjunctive cardioprotective agents (dexrazoxane).

The inability to develop safe ways to administer large doses of anthracyclines has made monitoring for the earliest evidence of cardiotoxicity necessary. Echocardiography and radionuclide angiography are the standard approaches for noninvasive monitoring. The prognosis in adults appears to be related to the severity of cardiac symptoms when cardiotoxicity is first diagnosed. Patients who present with clinical symptoms have a worse prognosis than those diagnosed with an asymptomatic decrease in left ventricular ejection fraction (LVEF).

Cyclophosphamide is a cell-cycle–nonspecific alkylating agent that is activated by the liver p450 cytochrome system and forms cross-links with DNA, resulting in inhibition of DNA synthesis. Cyclophosphamide is used for the treatment of breast cancer, non-Hodgkin lymphoma, chronic lymphocytic leukemia, ovarian cancer, bone and soft tissue sarcomas, and rhabdomyosarcoma, and has been associated with an acute cardiomyopathy. The incidence of cardiotoxicity may be particularly high in patients receiving cyclophosphamide as part of a high-dose chemotherapy program followed by autologous stem cell rescue. Other complications include hemorrhagic myopericarditis resulting in pericardial effusions, tamponade, and death, typically within the first week after treatment (11).

Trastuzumab is a recombinant humanized monoclonal antibody directed against the extracellular domain of the HER2/new human epidermal growth factor receptor, which down-regulates expression of HER2/new receptors and inhibits HER2/new intracellular signaling pathways. This receptor is overexpressed in 25%–30% of breast cancers, and in patients whose tumors overexpress HER2/neu, trastuzumab is effective, both as monotherapy and in combination with cytotoxic chemotherapy in the treatment of metastatic disease and in the adjuvant setting in combination with cytotoxic chemotherapy.

Trastuzumab-induced cardiomyopathy is most commonly manifested by an asymptomatic decrease in the LVEF and less often by clinical heart failure (11), though arrhythmias may also occur (12). The risk of any cardiac problem (asymptomatic decrease in LVEF or clinical heart failure) in patients receiving trastuzumab alone for metastatic breast cancer is between

2%–7% (13,14). The mechanism of trastuzumab-associated cardiac dysfunction is not fully understood, but data suggest that it is neither immune-mediated nor due to effects outside of the heart and that it does not result solely from exacerbation of anthracycline-induced cardiac dysfunction.

In a 2002 review of seven phase 2 and 3 trials of trastuzumab monotherapy involving 1,219 women, the incidence of cardiac dysfunction was between 3%–7%. The incidence of cardiomyopathy for patients receiving trastuzumab concurrently with chemotherapy was markedly higher in those receiving trastuzumab plus doxorubicin and cyclophosphamide (AC) than with AC alone (27% vs 8%, respectively). When trastuzumab was combined with paclitaxel, the increased risk of cardiomyopathy was substantially lower (13% vs 1% with paclitaxel alone). The incidence of moderate to severe heart failure (New York Heart Association [NYHA] class III to IV) was only 2%–4% with trastuzumab alone, 2% with paclitaxel plus trastuzumab (compared to 1% for paclitaxel alone), and 16% with AC plus trastuzumab (compared to 4% for AC alone) (14).

In randomized trials comparing chemotherapy plus trastuzumab with chemotherapy alone, a significant benefit for the addition of trastuzumab to adjuvant anthracycline-containing chemotherapy has been observed (15–18). In these trials, trastuzumab was administered sequentially after anthracyclines when anthracyclines were a component of the chemotherapy regimen due to concerns for increased cardiotoxicity. All trials included serial assessment of cardiac function at baseline, during, and after completion of treatment. Results suggest that approximately 5% of all patients treated with adjuvant trastuzumab, anthracycline, and taxane-containing therapy will develop some degree of cardiac dysfunction, 2% will develop symptomatic heart failure, and approximately 1% will develop NYHA class III or IV heart failure (19). These rates are substantially higher than those in control patients who did not receive trastuzumab.

In contrast to anthracycline-induced cardiotoxicity, trastuzumab-induced cardiotoxicity does not appear to be dose-related and usually responds to medical treatment for heart failure. Also, it may simply resolve with the discontinuation of trastuzumab (13,15). Continuation of trastuzumab therapy or resumption of treatment after resolution of cardiac abnormalities may be safe in some women with metastatic breast cancer who develop evidence of cardiac dysfunction (13,15). In the pivotal trial in women with metastatic breast cancer, 33 patients continued trastuzumab after developing cardiac dysfunction; of these, 21 (64%) had no further decrease in cardiac function (18).

Rituximab is a chimeric anti-CD 20 monoclonal antibody directed against the CD 20 antigen on malignant B lymphocytes. Rituximab is used to treat relapsed and/or refractory low-grade or follicular lymphoma and low-, intermediate- and high-grade non-Hodgkin lymphoma. Arrhythmias and angina have been reported during ≤1% of infusions, and acute infusion-related deaths occurring within 24th have a reported incidence of ≤0.1%. These deaths appear to be related to an infusion-related complex of hypoxia, pulmonary infiltrates, adult respiratory distress syndrome, myocardial infarction, ventricular fibrillation, and cardiogenic shock (17). Caution should be exercised when rituximab is used in patients with preexisting heart disease, as there is an increased risk of cardiotoxicity. Long-term cardiac toxicity has not been reported with rituximab administration.

Bevacizumab is a recombinant humanized monoclonal antibody directed against vascular endothelial growth factor (VEGF), blocking its activity. VEGF is a proangiogenic growth factor that is overexpressed in a myriad of solid-tumor malignancies. Bevacizumab is approved by the Food and Drug Administration (FDA) for the treatment of metastatic colorectal cancer and NSCLC, and is also used for the treatment of breast and ovarian cancers. Bevacizumab-induced cardiotoxicity includes angina, myocardial infarction, heart failure, hypertension, stroke, and arterial thromboembolic events. Grade 2 to 4 left ventricular dysfunction can occur in 2% of patients receiving treatment with single-agent bevacizumab. Concurrent use of anthracycline is associated with a 14% risk of heart failure, while prior anthracycline use is associated with an intermediate level of risk (7,20). Patients with an age >65 years and those with previous arterial thromboembolic events are at increased risk (7,20).

The interferons are a family of biologic response modifiers and are composed of interferon alpha (IFN β), interferon beta (IFN α), and interferon gamma (IFN γ). Cardiotoxicity of these agents appears to be a class effect, with IFN α being the most widely studied interferon in phase 1 and 2 trials. IFN α induces 2'5'-oligoadenylate synthetase and protein kinase, leading to decreased translation and inhibition of tumor cell protein synthesis, induction of differentiation, and modulation of oncogene expression. IFN α also causes indirect induction of host antitumor mechanisms mediated by cytotoxic T cells, helper T cells, natural killer (NK) cells, and macrophages. IFN α is used in the treatment of melanoma and renal cell carcinoma (RCC), and cardiotoxic effects of IFN α include myocardial ischemia and infarction, which are generally related to a prior history of coronary artery disease. These may be due to increased fever or associated flulike symptoms that increase myocardial oxygen requirements (21). Atrial and ventricular arrhythmias have reported in up to 20% of cases (22,23) and two cases of sudden death

have been reported (24). Prolonged administration of IFN α has been associated with cardiomyopathy, manifested by a depressed ejection fraction and heart failure, and is reversible upon cessation of IFN α infusion in some but not all cases (25,26).

Dysrhythmias

Paclitaxel is a cell-cycle–specific (active in M phase of the cell cycle) antimicrotubule agent that is used in the treatment of ovarian cancer, breast cancer, NSCLC, head and neck cancer, esophageal cancer, prostate cancer, bladder cancer, and AIDS-related Kaposi sarcoma. Paclitaxel has been associated with bradycardia and heart block, as reported in a phase 2 series of 140 women with ovarian cancer in whom transient asymptomatic bradycardia occurred in 29%. Serious cardiotoxicity (atrioventricular conduction block, ventricular tachycardia, cardiac ischemia) was reported in 5% (27). The risk of cardiotoxicity is higher when paclitaxel is combined with doxorubicin, and heart failure has developed in up to 20% of patients treated with this combination (28). The development of heart failure may occur at cumulative doxorubicin doses much lower than would be expected with doxorubicin alone (29,30).

Albumin-bound paclitaxel is a nano-particle (about 130 nm) form of paclitaxel, and is FDA-approved for treatment of advanced breast cancer, and has the same cardiac toxicity profile as non-albumin–bound paclitaxel. Asymptomatic electrocardiogram (ECG) changes, including nonspecific changes, sinus bradycardia, and sinus tachycardia, are most common (31).

Docetaxel is also an M-phase–specific antimicrotubule agent that is FDA-approved for the treatment of breast cancer and NSCLC, and is also indicated for the treatment of SCLC, head and neck cancer, gastric cancer, refractory ovarian cancer, and bladder cancer. Docetaxel has been associated with conduction abnormalities, cardiovascular collapse, and angina (37). Similar to paclitaxel, docetaxel appears to potentiate the cardiotoxicity of anthracyclines. This was illustrated in a trial of 50 women with stage III breast cancer who received neoadjuvant and adjuvant therapy with docetaxel and doxorubicin (32). In this study, congestive heart failure developed in 8%, with a mean decrease in ejection fraction of 20%, and total doxorubicin dose was <400 mg/m^2 in all patients.

Vascular Complications

Interleukin-2 (IL-2) is a biologic response modifier that has been used for the treatment of RCC, and is associated with capillary leak syndrome, manifested by increased vascular permeability and hypotension and a cardiovascular profile similar to septic shock. IL-2 has also been associated with direct myocardial toxicity, and in patients with underlying coronary artery disease, ischemia, myocardial infarction, arrhythmias, and death have been reported (33). Ventricular and supraventricular arrhythmias have been reported in 6%–21% of patients (34,35).

All-trans-retinoic acid (ATRA) is a derivative of vitamin A and differentiates leukemic promyelocytes into mature cells. ATRA is used to treat acute promyelocytic leukemia (APL), and approximately 10%–15% of patients develop the retinoic acid syndrome, which is marked by fever, weight gain, pulmonary infiltrates, pleural and pericardial effusions, myocardial ischemia/ infarction (20), hypotension, and renal failure. The majority of patients make a complete and rapid recovery if the syndrome is recognized early and ATRA is withdrawn.

5-fluorouracil (5-FU) is a fluorinated pyrimidine that impairs DNA synthesis by inhibiting thymidylate synthetase that is used to treat colorectal cancer, breast cancer, various gastrointestinal (GI) malignancies, and head and neck cancer, and is the second most common cause of chemotherapy-related cardiotoxicity, after anthracyclines (36). Chest pain, which can be nonspecific or anginal in nature, is the most common 5-FU–induced cardiotoxicity. Other cardiac manifestations can include arrhythmias (including atrial fibrillation, ventricular tachycardia, and ventricular fibrillation) and acute pulmonary edema due to ventricular dysfunction. Cardiogenic shock and sudden cardiac death have also been reported (20). The incidence of 5-FU–induced cardiotoxicity ranges from 1%–19% (36–38), although most series report a risk of ≤8% (20). Risk may be associated with the method of 5-FU administration, the presence of coronary artery disease, and the use of concurrent radiation or anthracyclines.

The underlying mechanism of toxicity is thought to be coronary artery vasospasm. However, other mechanisms, including myocarditis and a thrombogenic effect due to endothelial cytotoxicity, have also been postulated (39,40). Cardiac symptoms usually resolve with termination of 5-FU treatment and/or administration of nitrates or calcium channel blockers. Rechallenging patients who have had 5-FU–induced cardiotoxicity is controversial. If rechallenge is attempted, patients should be followed carefully during drug infusion, and in some instances changing from infusional to bolus 5-FU may allow treatment to be successfully resumed (41,42).

Capecitabine is a fluoropyrimidine that is metabolized in the liver and tissues to form 5-FU, which is the active moiety, and is FDA-approved to treat advanced breast and colorectal cancers. Capecitabine-induced cardiotoxicity profile is similar to that of infusional 5-FU. In clinical studies, reported cardiac complications have included angina, atrial fibrillation, myocarditis, myocardial infarction, and ventricular fibrillation (20,43).

Hypertension

Hypertension has emerged as one of the most common adverse effects of therapy with angiogenesis inhibitors such as bevacizumab, sorafenib, and sunitinib. Sorafenib is a signal transduction inhibitor that inhibits Raf kinase, VEGF receptor, and platelet-derived growth factor (PDGF) receptor, and is FDA-approved for the treatment of advanced RCC. Sunitinib is also a signal transduction inhibitor and inhibits VEGF receptor, PDGF receptor, stem cell receptor (KIT), Fms-like tyrosine kinse-3 (FLT-3), colony-stimulating factor receptor type 1 (CSF-IR), and glial cell line-derived neurotrophic factor receptor (RET), and is FDA-approved for the treatment of gastrointestinal stromal tumors (GIST) and advanced RCC.

Hypertension was observed in 22.4% of patients (11% with grade 3 hypertension) in a phase 3 trial of bevacizumab, irinotecan, fluorouracil, and leucovorin patients with colon cancer (51). In another study of renal cell carcinoma patients who were treated with high-dose bevacizumab, hypertension was reported in 36% (44).

A recent study evaluating the incidence of hypertension in patients with metastatic solid-tumor malignancies who were treated with sorafenib found that 75% of patients experienced an increase of ≥10 mmHg in systolic blood pressure and 60% of patients experienced an increase of ≥20 mmHg in systolic blood pressure (45). In a recent phase 3 trial of sorafenib in patients with advanced renal cell carcinoma, 17% of patients developed hypertension. Ten percent of patients experienced grade 2 hypertension, and 4% experienced grade 3 or 4 hypertension (46). A phase 1 trial of sunitinib revealed that at the maximum-tolerated dose, the most common side effects were grade 3 fatigue, grade 3 hypertension, and grade 2 bullous toxicity (47).

QT Prolongation

Arsenic trioxide induces differentiation of APL cells by degrading the chimeric PML/RAR-α protein, and is used to treat relapsed acute promyelocytic leukemia. Arsenic trioxide treatment can result in fluid retention, the "APL differentiation syndrome," which is similar to ATRA syndrome; QT prolongation (>500 msec) (48); complete atrioventricular block; and sudden death (49).

Management of Complications

Animal studies have suggested that the beta blocker carvedilol may protect against the cardiotoxicity of anthracyclines (50,51). Further support comes from a randomized trial of 50 patients undergoing anthracycline chemotherapy for a variety of malignancies. Patients were randomly assigned to carvedilol, 12.5 mg daily, or placebo. All patients underwent echocardiography prior to and six months after chemotherapy. Among the patients assigned to carvedilol, there was no change in the mean LVEF after chemotherapy (70% before and after therapy). In contrast, patients assigned to placebo had a statistically significant absolute reduction in LVEF of 17% (69% to 52%) (52).

ACE inhibitors have been shown to slow disease progression in patients with left ventricular systolic dysfunction due to a variety of causes. The potential protective effect of ACE inhibitors in patients with elevated serum cardiac troponin following chemotherapy was evaluated in a randomized trial (53). Of 473 patients treated with a variety of high-dose chemotherapy regimens, 114 patients with an elevated troponin T were randomly assigned to one year of treatment with the ACE inhibitor enalapril (2.5 mg daily, titrated to a maximum of 20 mg daily) or to no enalapril. After one year, an absolute reduction in LVEF of $\geq 10\%$ was found in 43% of the untreated patients, but in none of the patients treated with enalapril.

Hence, if patients undergoing treatment with cardiotoxic chemotherapeutic agents develop a decline in cardiac function, initiation of beta blockers and ACE inhibitors is encouraged. Additionally, management of overt congestive heart failure may require diuretics (eg, furosemide) and/or spironolactone.

Dexrazoxane is an FDA-approved, EDTA-like iron chelator, which may prevent anthracycline-induced cardiotoxicity by stripping iron from the doxorubicin-iron complex, thereby preventing free radical formation (54). In a meta-analysis of 1,013 adult and pediatric patients, dexrazoxane, initiated either with the start of anthracycline treatment or after a cumulative dose of 300 mg/m^2 had been attained, significantly reduced the incidence of congestive heart failure (relative risk = 0.28, 95% CI 0.18–0.42) (55). The cardioprotective effect of dexrazoxane is observed whether the drug is started initially or after 300 mg/m^2 of doxorubicin.

PULMONARY TOXICITY

Bleomycin is an antitumor antibiotic that contains a DNA-binding region and an iron-binding region at opposite ends of the molecule (Table 3.3). Cytotoxic effects result from the generation of an activated oxygen free-radical species, which causes single- and double-strand DNA breaks and eventual cell death. Bleomycin is used to treat cancers of the head and neck, cervix, and esophagus; germ cell tumors; and both Hodgkin and non-Hodgkin lymphoma. Bleomycin therapy can

---

TABLE 3.3
Chemotherapy-Induced Pulmonary Toxicity

TOXICITY TYPE	AGENT	REFERENCES
Acute toxicity	Gemcitabine	(114–116)
	Gefitinib	(110)
	Mitomycin C	(87,88)
	Cyclophosphamide	(107,108)
	Paclitaxel	(239,257)
	Docetaxel	(258,259)
Chronic toxicity	Bleomycin	(61)
	Methotrexate	(68,70,71)
	Chlorambucil	(81)
	Mitomycin C	(87,88)
	Carmustine, lomustine,	(96, 97)
	Cyclophosphamide	(107,109)

result in life-threatening interstitial pulmonary fibrosis in up to 10% of patients (56,57). Other, less common forms of pulmonary toxicity include hypersensitivity pneumonitis and nodular pulmonary densities.

Patient age; drug dose; renal function; severity of the underlying malignancy at presentation; and concomitant use of oxygen, radiation therapy, or other chemotherapeutic agents may influence the risk of developing bleomycin-induced pulmonary toxicity (57). Administration of higher doses of bleomycin increases the risk of lung injury, but damage can occur at doses less than 50 mg. Rapid intravenous infusion may also increase the risk of toxicity.

High concentrations of inspired oxygen increase the risk of developing bleomycin-induced pulmonary toxicity, whereas low oxygen concentrations substantially decrease the risk. Administration of high inspired fractions of oxygen may even result in pulmonary toxicity several years after bleomycin treatment (58). Thoracic irradiation increases the risk of bleomycin-induced pulmonary toxicity, whether it is administered prior to or simultaneously with bleomycin. It is not known whether a long interval between irradiation and administration of bleomycin eliminates the increased risk of pulmonary toxicity (59). Greater than 80% of bleomycin is eliminated by the kidneys, and renal insufficiency is a risk factor for bleomycin-induced toxicity (56,60).

Symptoms, physical signs, and pulmonary function abnormalities of bleomycin-induced pulmonary fibrosis are nonspecific and usually develop subacutely between one and six months after bleomycin treatment. Findings include nonproductive cough, dyspnea, pleuritic or substernal chest pain, fever, tachypnea, rales, lung restriction, and hypoxemia. Pneumothorax and/or pneumomediastinum are rare complications (61). Bleomycin-induced hypersensitivity pneumonitis may present with rapidly progressive symptoms. During bleomycin infusion, an acute chest pain syndrome arises in approximately 1% of patients, but does not predict the development of pulmonary fibrosis (62). Early radiographic findings can include bibasilar subpleural opacification with blunting of the costophrenic angles and fine nodular densities, and late findings can include progressive consolidation and honeycombing. Sputum analysis to rule out infection should be performed, and bronchoalveolar lavage (BAL) is encouraged in patients unable to expectorate sputum.

Bleomycin should be discontinued in patients with documented or suspected bleomycin-induced pulmonary toxicity. Reinitiation of treatment is contraindicated in patients with pulmonary fibrosis, but may be attempted in patients with hypersensitivity pneumonitis. Corticosteroid treatment of bleomycin-induced hypersensitivity pneumonitis usually results

in a rapid response. Case reports have also described substantial recovery when a significant inflammatory pneumonitis is present. Short-term improvement in symptoms may be followed by recurrence of symptoms when therapy is tapered. Also, pulmonary function abnormalities may revert over a period of four to five years, even in patients with an initially positive response to corticosteroids (63).

Methotrexate is a cell-cycle–specific antifolate analog, which is active in the S phase of the cell cycle, and competitively inhibits the enzyme dihydrofolate reductase and blocks the conversion of dihydrofolate to tetrahydrofolate. This results in depletion off folate and in impaired synthesis of thymidine, DNA, and RNA, and ultimately in reduced cellular proliferation. Methotrexate is used to treat breast cancer, head and neck cancer, gestational trophoblastic disease, meningeal leukemia and carcinomatous meningitis, bladder cancer, non-Hodgkin lymphoma, and osteogenic sarcoma.

Methotrexate-induced pulmonary toxicity may be classified as inflammatory, infectious, and possibly neoplastic. There is conflicting data regarding the influence of methotrexate on the development of malignancy (64).

Although the most common methotrexate-induced pulmonary toxicity is hypersensitivity pneumonitis, bronchiolitis obliterans with organizing pneumonia (BOOP), acute lung injury with noncardiogenic pulmonary edema, pulmonary fibrosis, and bronchitis have also been associated with methotrexate treatment (65,66). Both low- and high-dose methotrexate treatment and a variety of routes of administration can result in pulmonary toxicity. None of the proposed mechanisms of toxicity account for the observation that pulmonary toxicity may remit despite continued therapy and may not occur upon rechallenge (65,66). Hence, the mechanisms of methotrexate pulmonary toxicity are unresolved and may be multiple.

Methotrexate treatment may increase the risk for opportunistic infections by *Pneumocystis jiroveci*, cytomegalovirus, varicella-zoster virus, *Nocardia*, mycobacteria, or fungi (67). *Pneumocystis* is the most commonly reported pathogen, and has accounted for up to 40% of the infectious complications in some series (68,69).

Methotrexate-induced pulmonary toxicity may present in an acute, subacute, or chronic form. Subacute presentations are most common. The majority of patients who develop methotrexate pulmonary toxicity do so within the first year of therapy; cases have been reported as early as 12 days and as late as 18 years after the drug was initiated (68,70,71).

Acute methotrexate pneumonitis is generally nonspecific and progressive over several weeks, and is marked by fever, chills, malaise, cough, dyspnea, and chest pain (72,73). Rapid decompensation to respiratory failure may occur (65,66). Subacute pneumonitis is marked by dyspnea, nonproductive cough, fever, crackles, and cyanosis (74), and progression to pulmonary fibrosis is observed in approximately 10% of patients. Pleural effusions are uncommon, but can occur, with or without parenchymal involvement (75).

Pulmonary function testing reveals a restrictive pattern with a decrease in carbon monoxide diffusing capacity (DLCO), hypoxemia, and an increased alveolar-arterial (A-a) gradient (65,66). However, the majority of patients display no clinically significant deterioration of pulmonary function (76,77). BAL and lung biopsy are the primary modalities by which to establish diagnosis of methotrexate-induced lung disease, but are not necessary in all patients. BAL may be helpful in ruling out an infectious etiology of pneumonitis and in supporting the diagnosis of methotrexate pneumonitis.

Methotrexate-induced adverse reactions, including stomatitis and gastrointestinal and hematologic toxicity, can be alleviated or prevented by folic acid supplementation without altering the efficacy of methotrexate. Repletion of folate stores, however, does not reduce the risk for methotrexate-induced pulmonary or hepatic toxicity, suggesting that mechanisms other than folate depletion are involved in their pathogenesis (78,79).

Discontinuation of methotrexate is the initial step in management. Clinical improvement generally occurs within days of stopping the drug (75). Rechallenge with methotrexate is not recommended despite reports of successful rechallenge and even regression of pulmonary toxicity despite continued therapy (65,66). Exclusion of an infectious etiology and empiric antimicrobial therapy may be indicated while definitive procedures are performed. There have not been any prospective, randomized, placebo-controlled trials to support the use of corticosteroids in methotrexate-induced pulmonary toxicity, but anecdotal reports support this approach.

Chlorambucil is an alkylating cytotoxic agent used in the treatment of chronic lymphocytic leukemia, lymphomas, polycythemia vera, and amyloidosis. Chlorambucil-induced toxicity includes nausea, vomiting, hepatotoxicity, hallucinations, bone marrow suppression, and pulmonary toxicity. The incidence of chlorambucil-induced pulmonary toxicity is estimated at <1% (80).

The most common presentation of chlorambucil-induced pulmonary toxicity is chronic interstitial pneumonitis, and onset of symptoms varies from 5 months to 10 years (81). Patients present with insidious onset of nonproductive cough, dyspnea, weight loss, and fever, and physical examination often reveals bilateral inspiratory crackles.

The diagnosis of chlorambucil-induced pulmonary toxicity is one of exclusion, and specific markers or diagnostic clinical features are absent. Supporting signs include development of new pulmonary symptoms after beginning treatment, new chest radiograph abnormalities, a decrease in total lung capacity (TLC) or in DLCO, marked CD8+ lymphocytosis in BAL fluid, no evidence of infection, improvement in lung manifestations following withdrawal of the drug, and recurrence of interstitial pneumonia upon retreatment. Once chlorambucil-induced interstitial pneumonia is suspected, cessation of treatment should occur. Generally, patients improve within a few days of stopping treatment, but corticosteroid treatment is recommended in patients who do not improve rapidly after drug cessation and in those who develop acute respiratory failure (82,83).

Mitomycin C (MMC) is a cell-cycle–specific alkylating agent that cross-links DNA and results in inhibition of DNA synthesis and subsequent transcription by targeting DNA-dependent RNA polymerase. MMC is used to treat gastric, pancreatic, breast, cervical, bladder, head and neck, and NSCLCs. Adverse effects of MMC are dose-related, and include myelosuppression (most common) (84), nausea, vomiting, diarrhea, stomatitis, dementia, and alopecia (85,86). The frequency of pulmonary toxicity is between 3%–12%, and includes bronchospasm, acute pneumonitis, hemolytic uremiclike syndrome with acute lung injury, chronic pneumonitis manifested by the development of diffuse parenchymal, and pleural disease (87,88).

MMC-associated bronchospasm occurs at a frequency of 4%–6%, and most cases involve the concomitant use of vindesine and MMC (89,90). Bronchospasm typically develops within a few hours of treatment and resolves within 12–24 hours, either spontaneously or with bronchodilator administration (90). MMC-associated acute interstitial pneumonitis is characterized by sudden onset of dyspnea occurring on a day when a vinca alkaloid is administered. In a study of 387 patients with advanced NSCLC, there was a 6% incidence of acute dyspnea following treatment with mitomycin and vindesine or vinblastine (91). Significant improvement in dyspnea occurred over 24 hours, but approximately 60% experienced chronic respiratory impairment that only partially resolved with corticosteroid therapy.

MMC-induced thrombotic microangiopathy is similar to hemolytic uremic syndrome (HUS), but in 50% of cases is also associated with acute respiratory failure. This syndrome generally occurs during or shortly after treatment, and is characterized by microangiopathic hemolytic anemia, thrombocytopenia, renal insufficiency due to thrombotic occlusion of glomerular capillaries, and acute lung injury. The incidence of thrombotic microangiopathy is directly related to the total dose of drug administered, and prior blood transfusions or 5-FU treatment may increase the risk of developing this syndrome (102). In a review of 39 cases of MMC-associated thrombotic microangiopathy, 75% of patients developed the syndrome 6–12 months after starting chemotherapy. Approximately 50% of patients developed associated acute respiratory distress syndrome (ARDS) and had a significantly higher mortality rate, compared with patients who did not develop ARDS (95% vs 50%) (92).

MMC-associated interstitial fibrosis is marked dyspnea, nonproductive cough, tachypnea, and rales, and appears to be a dose-related condition that is unusual below a cumulative dose of 30 mg/m² (93). Chest radiograph may reveal bilateral diffuse reticular opacities with occasional fine nodularity, and pulmonary function testing reveals a restrictive pattern with a decrease in DLCO (94,95). Treatment with corticosteroids may result in rapid improvement of dyspnea and interstitial opacities, and abrupt cessation or early withdrawal of corticosteroids can result in a relapse of dyspnea and pulmonary opacities (94).

Pleural disease, characterized by exudative effusions, fibrinous exudates, and fibrosis over the pleural surfaces with occasional aggregates of lymphocytes and eosinophils, has been reported. Pleural effusion is often associated with underlying MMC-associated parenchymal lung disease (80,86).

The nitrosourea drugs include carmustine (BCNU), lomustine (CCNU), and semustine (methyl CCNU), and are a class of cell-cycle–nonspecific, DNA-alkylating agents. Nitrosourea drugs are used to treat Hodgkin and non-Hodgkin lymphoma, multiple myeloma, brain tumors, melanoma, and other solid tumors, including breast cancer. Carmustine is the most widely used nitrosourea, and can induce both acute and chronic pulmonary toxicity. Semustine has been associated with pulmonary fibrosis following treatment.

Although most patients develop pulmonary fibrosis within three years of carmustine treatment, some patients can present with fibrosis decades after exposure (96,97). The reported incidence of carmustine-induced pulmonary toxicity has ranged from 1% to 20%–30% (109). When carmustine is part of a preparative regimen for stem cell transplantation, the incidence of interstitial pneumonitis or idiopathic pneumonia has been reported to be 2%–23% (98,99). Lung fibrosis is most likely with very high doses, concurrent administration of other agents known to cause pulmonary toxicity, preexisting lung disease, localized chest wall radiotherapy, or atopy (98).

Patients with early-onset carmustine-induced lung fibrosis usually present with dry cough, breathlessness, and bilateral inspiratory crackles within weeks to months of treatment. Others may present with a fulminant disease similar to ARDS, and many others may have subclinical disease detected by pulmonary function testing (24,96,100). Radiographic imaging may reveal bilateral diffuse infiltrates or nodules, localized consolidation, localized or diffuse interstitial fibrotic changes, or ARDS. Apical pleural thickening, spontaneous pneumothoraces, and fibrotic stranding have also been described (101). Pulmonary function testing reveals decreased vital capacity (VC) and TLC, as well as reduced DLCO (96,102).

Corticosteroids have been beneficial in some studies if given early based upon symptoms or a fall in DLCO (24,100), but have been shown to be minimally effective in other reports (103,104). Patients with mild disease, and especially those who received low doses of carmustine or responded to steroid treatment, usually survive. However, these individuals may be at increased risk of late pulmonary fibrosis. Carmustine should be discontinued if lung fibrosis is suspected.

Patients with late-onset carmustine-induced lung fibrosis often have no symptoms for several years, although chest radiographs and lung function studies can reveal evidence of lung fibrosis (105). Severe fibrosis can result in breathlessness and sometimes cough at late stage of the disease. Radiographic changes can include upper-zone patchy linear opacities and volume loss due to apical pleural thickening. Pulmonary function testing reveals restricted lung volumes and reduced DLCO.

No treatment has proven to be efficacious in the management of late-onset carmustine-induced lung injury. Corticosteroids are not effective, and lung transplantation offers the best hope of long-term survival for severely debilitated patients. Prognosis is the worst for patients treated below the age of seven years, and patients who are treated beyond puberty appear to have the slowest rate of decline in pulmonary function (106).

Cyclophosphamide is cell-cycle–nonspecific alkylating agent that is used to treat breast and ovarian cancer, non-Hodgkin lymphoma, chronic lymphocytic leukemia, bone and soft tissue sarcomas, and rhabdomyosarcoma. The toxicity profile of cyclophosphamide includes leukopenia, hemorrhagic cystitis, infertility, the development of secondary malignancies, and pulmonary toxicity.

Cyclophosphamide-induced pulmonary toxicity is rare, but the risk may be increased by the concomitant administration of radiation, oxygen therapy, or other drugs with potential pulmonary toxicity. Two distinct patterns of pulmonary toxicity are associated with cyclophosphamide: an acute pneumonitis that occurs early in the course of treatment and a chronic, progressive, fibrotic process that may occur after prolonged therapy (107).

In acute pulmonary toxicity, patients present with cough, dyspnea, fatigue, and occasionally fever within one to six months after the onset of therapy. Radiographic imaging can show interstitial inflammation and/or a ground-glass appearance. Discontinuation of the drug and institution of corticosteroids usually result in complete resolution of symptoms (107,108).

Late-onset pulmonary toxicity typically develops in patients who have received treatment over several months to years with relatively low doses of cyclophosphamide (107,109), and is marked by progressive lung fibrosis. Symptoms arise insidiously and include slowly progressive dyspnea and nonproductive cough. Discontinuation of treatment and initiation of corticosteroids are minimally effective, and late-onset pneumonitis and fibrosis invariably lead to terminal respiratory failure. Radiographic imaging reveals bilateral reticular or nodular diffuse opacities with a fibrotic appearance. Bilateral pleural thickening of the mid- and upper lung zones is also a common feature (107). Pulmonary function testing typically displays a restrictive pattern with a reduced DLCO.

Gefitinib is an orally active selective epidermal growth factor receptor (EGFR) tyrosine kinase inhibitor, which is FDA-approved for the treatment of pancreatic cancer, NSCLC, breast cancer, and ovarian cancer, and is also used to treat bladder cancer and soft tissue sarcomas, and rarely results in dyspnea and interstitial lung disease (110,111). In a multi-institutional randomized phase 2 trial of gefitinib for previously treated patients with advanced NSCLC, 2 out of 106 patients experienced interstitial pneumonia and pneumonitis (112). In a recent retrospective analysis of 325 patients with NSCLC, 22 patients (6%) developed interstitial lung disease (ILD) after gefitinib treatment. The median toxicity grade of ILD was 3 (range 2–4), and 10 (3.1%) patients died. The median time to ILD after initiation of gefitinib treatment was 18 days (range 3–123), and half of the patients developing ILD manifested acute onset of dyspnea. Radiographic findings were characterized predominantly by diffuse groundglass opacities. Statistically significant factors affecting the occurrence of ILD by multivariate analysis were the presence of pulmonary fibrosis prior to gefitinib therapy and poor functional status. (113).

Limited evidence suggests that the combination of gemcitabine, an S phase cell cycle–specific antimetabolite, and taxanes may also lead to pulmonary toxicity. In one series, 4 of 12 patients with NSCLC who were treated with the combination of paclitaxel and gemcitabine developed pneumonitis (114), which was marked by increasing exertional dyspnea, a dry cough, malaise, and low-grade pyrexia that developed and progressed over a few days. None of the patients had received thoracic radiotherapy at any time during the course of their illness. Severe pulmonary toxicity has also been documented in patients receiving docetaxel in combination with gemcitabine for treatment of transitional cell bladder cancer (115,116).

Management of Complications

Management of chemotherapy-induced pulmonary toxicity involves prompt discontinuation of the offending chemotherapeutic agent and initiation of corticosteroids (as detailed previously). Oftentimes, there is a rapid improvement in pulmonary function with these measures, but depending on the agent, long-term pulmonary fibrosis and restricted pulmonary function can occur. In some instances, supplemental oxygen and referral to a pulmonary medicine specialist may be necessary. Pulmonary opportunistic infections should be managed with early judicious use of appropriate antibiotics.

NEUROTOXICITY

The platinum agents covalently bind to DNA and produce intrastrand (>90%) and interstrand (<5%) crosslinks, which result in inhibition of DNA synthesis and inhibition of transcription (Table 3.4). Cisplatin is used to treat testicular, ovarian, bladder, esophageal, and head and neck cancers, as well as NSCLC, SCLC, non-Hodgkin lymphoma, and trophoblastic disease, and is commonly associated with peripheral neuropathy and ototoxicity. Cisplatin induces an axonal neuropathy that predominantly affects large myelinated sensory fibers with damage occurring at dorsal root ganglion (primarily) and peripheral nerves (117–120). This leads to the subacute development of numbness, paresthesias, and occasionally pain, which begins in the toes and fingers and spreads proximally to affect the legs and arms, and also results in impairment of proprioception and loss of reflexes. Pinprick, temperature sensation, and power are usually spared. Nerve conduction studies reveal decreased amplitude of sensory action potentials and prolonged sensory latencies, consistent with a sensory axonopathy, and sural nerve biopsy reveals both demyelination and axonal loss. Cisplatin-induced neuropathy is usually generalized, but focal and autonomic neuropathies can rarely occur (121).

Patients with mild neuropathy can continue to receive full-dose cisplatin, but if the neuropathy interferes with neurologic function, the risk of potentially disabling neurotoxicity must be weighed against the

TABLE 3.4
Chemotherapy-Induced Neurotoxicity

TOXICITY TYPE	AGENT	REFERENCES
Central	Methotrexate	(130–133)
	Cytarabine	(155,156)
	5-flurouracil	(157)
	Ifosfamide	(162,163)
	Nitrosoureas	(167)
	Procarbazine	(168,169)
	Interferon alpha	(170,171)
	Interleukin-2	(177,178)
	Bevacizumab	(180, 181)
	Busulfan	(182)
	All-trans-retinoic acid	(184)
	Fludarabine	(186)
	Cladribine	(185)
	Pentostatin	(163, 185)
Vascular	Carboplatin	(120)
	Bevacizumab	(180,181)
Peripheral	Cisplatin	(180,181)
	Carboplatin	(180,181)
	Oxaliplatin	(126–128)
	Paclitaxel	(134–137)
	Docetaxel	(140,141)
	Thalidomide	(142)
	Vincristine (and, less frequently, other vinca alkaloids, such as vinorelbine, vinblastine, and vindesine)	(147–150)
	Cytarabine	(155,157)
	5-flurouracil	(159)
	Bortezomib	(146)
	Interferon alpha	(173,174)
	Interleukin-2	(179)
	Gemcitabine	(182)
	All-trans-retinoic acid	(186)

benefit of continued treatment. Alternatives include cisplatin dose reduction or replacement of cisplatin with a less neurotoxic agent, such as carboplatin. In 30% of patients, the neuropathy continues to deteriorate for up to several months even after cisplatin is discontinued (121), and in some cases, neuropathy may even begin after therapy is discontinued. Cessation of cisplatin use eventually results in improvement of neuropathy in most patients, although recovery is often incomplete.

Cisplatin-induced ototoxicity is characterized by a dose-dependent, high-frequency sensorineural hearing loss with tinnitus (122). Although symptomatic hearing loss affects only 15%–20% of patients receiving cisplatin, audiometric evidence of hearing impairment occurs in >75% of patients. Radiotherapy to the normal cochlea or cranial nerve VIII can result in sensorineural hearing loss, and concurrent administration of cisplatin results in synergistic ototoxicity, especially in the high-frequency speech range (123).

Lhermitte's sign is a shocklike, nonpainful sensation of paresthesias radiating from the back to the feet during neck flexion. It can develop in patients receiving cisplatin, and typically occurs after weeks or months of treatment. It has also been reported in patients receiving high cumulative doses of oxaliplatin (121).

Carboplatin is used to treat ovarian, endometrial, bladder, and head and neck cancers, as well as NSCLC, SCLC, germ cell tumors, and relapsed and refractory acute leukemia. Carboplatin is rarely associated with peripheral neuropathy and central nervous system (CNS) toxicity when given at conventional doses. However, a severe neuropathy can develop with higher-than-standard doses, as used in the setting of high-dose therapy with stem cell transplantation (124). Other neurotoxic manifestations include a microangiopathic hemolytic anemia resulting in progressive neurologic impairment and death (118), and retinal toxicity following intra-arterial administration to patients with brain tumors (125).

Oxaliplatin is a third-generation platinum complex that is FDA-approved for treatment of early-stage and advanced colorectal cancer and for the treatment of pancreatic and gastric cancers. The main dose-limiting toxicity of oxaliplatin is neuropathy. Oxaliplatin has been associated with two distinct syndromes: an acute neurosensory complex, which can appear during or shortly after the first few infusions; and a cumulative sensory neuropathy, with distal loss of sensation and dysesthesias. Ototoxicity is rarely associated with oxaliplatin. Infrequently, a neuromyotonialike hyperexcitability syndrome can occur, which can be marked by eyelid twitching, ptosis, visual field changes, teeth jittering, jaw stiffness, voice changes, dysarthria, hand shaking, and dysesthesias of the hands and feet. Acute transient neurotoxicity occurs in about 85%–95% of patients (126) and appears to be due to hyperexcitability of the peripheral nerves (127,128). Unusual pharyngolaryngeal dysesthesias, which can cause a feeling of difficulty in breathing or swallowing, have been described in 1%–2% of patients. Symptoms can be induced or aggravated by exposure to cold (126).

The dose-limiting cumulative sensory neuropathy develops in 10%–15 % of patients after a cumulative dose of 780–850 mg/m^2 (126). In about 75% of patients, the sensory neuropathy is reversible, with a median time to recovery of 13 weeks after treatment cessation (129).

Methotrexate (MTX)-induced neurotoxicity can be manifested as aseptic meningitis, transverse myelopathy, acute and subacute encephalopathy, and leukoencephalopathy. Aseptic meningitis is the most common neurotoxic effect of intrathecal (IT) MTX (130), and is characterized by headache, nuchal rigidity, back pain, nausea, vomiting, fever, and lethargy. Approximately 10% of patients are affected, but incidence rates as high as 50% have been reported. Symptoms usually begin 2–4 hours after drug injection, and may last for 12–72 hours (131). Cerebrospinal fluid (CSF) analysis usually demonstrates a pleocytosis with elevated protein content. Symptoms are usually self-limited, and treatment is usually not required. Some patients who develop aseptic meningitis can be subsequently retreated with MTX without further toxicity.

Transverse myelopathy is an uncommon complication of IT MTX manifested by isolated spinal cord dysfunction, which develops over hours to days in the absence of a compressive lesion. Transverse myelopathy is associated with IT MTX and is generally seen in patients receiving concurrent radiotherapy (RT) or frequent IT MTX injections. Affected patients typically develop back or leg pain followed by paraplegia, sensory loss, and sphincter dysfunction. The onset is usually between 30 minutes and 48 hours after treatment, but can occur up to two weeks later. The majority of cases show clinical improvement, but the extent of recovery is variable (132), and further administration of IT MTX is contraindicated.

Acute neurotoxicity is most frequently seen after high-dose MTX and is characterized by somnolence, confusion, and seizures within 24 hours of treatment. Symptoms usually resolve spontaneously without sequelae, and retreatment is often possible (131). Weekly or biweekly administration of high-dose MTX may produce a subacute "strokelike" syndrome, characterized by transient focal neurologic deficits, confusion, and occasionally seizures. Symptoms develop approximately six days after drug administration, last from 15 minutes to 72 hours, and then resolve spontaneously without sequelae. CSF analysis is usually normal, but the electroencephalogram (EEG) may show diffuse slowing and diffusion-weighted images may be abnormal. Subsequent administration of high-dose MTX may be accomplished without recurrent subacute encephalopathy (133).

The major delayed complication of MTX is leukoencephalopathy, which is dependent upon dose and route of administration (131). Although this syndrome may be produced by MTX alone, it is more common in the setting of concurrent or past RT. The mechanism is unknown, but it is possible that cranial irradiation either potentiates the toxic effects of MTX or disrupts the blood-brain barrier, allowing high concentrations of MTX to reach the brain.

The characteristic feature of leukoencephalopathy is a gradual impairment of cognitive function months to years following treatment with MTX. Clinical manifestations range from mild learning disability to severe progressive dementia accompanied by somnolence, seizures, ataxia, and hemiparesis. Many patients stabilize or improve following discontinuation of MTX, but the course is progressive in others and may be fatal. No effective treatment is available. The diagnosis is supported by cranial computed tomography (CT) and magnetic resonance imaging (MRI), which typically show cerebral atrophy and diffuse white-matter lesions. CT reveals characteristic hypodense nonenhancing lesions, while MRI reveals areas of high signal intensity on T2-weighted images.

Taxane-induced motor and sensory neuropathies are cumulative and dose- and schedule-dependent. Paclitaxel induces a neuropathy that involves sensory nerve fibers. The major manifestations include burning paresthesias of the hands and feet and loss of reflexes. Paclitaxel also causes a motor neuropathy, which predominantly affects proximal muscles (134). The incidence of grade 3 or 4 motor neuropathy is between 2%–10% (135). Other, less common manifestations include perioral numbness, autonomic neuropathies, severe myalgias and arthralgias, phantom limb pain, transient encephalopathies, and seizures (136,137).

Paclitaxel-induced neuropathies often do not progress even if treatment is continued, and there are reports of symptomatic improvement despite continued therapy. After completing treatment, approximately 50% of patients improve over a period of months (138). Additionally, the neurotoxicity of paclitaxel is synergistic with the concurrent platinum administration (139).

Docetaxel causes both sensory and motor neuropathies, although both of these occur less frequently than with paclitaxel. Any neuropathy occurs in less than 15% of patients, and grade 3 or 4 neuropathies occur in less than 5% (140). Lhermitte's sign has also been associated with docetaxel use (141).

Thalidomide is an antiangiogenic agent that is used in the treatment of multiple myeloma. A peripheral neuropathy develops in approximately 75% of patients who receive prolonged thalidomide treatment (142). This neuropathy is only partially reversible, and dose reduction or cessation of treatment is required in up to 60% of patients. Somnolence is also common, affecting 43%–55% of patients, and decreases in many patients after two or three weeks of continued therapy

(143). Other reported manifestations of neurotoxicity include tremor and dizziness (142) and, rarely, seizures (144). Lenalidomide, a thalidomide derivative, appears to be substantially less neurotoxic. In a phase 2 study in 70 patients with refractory or relapsed myeloma, significant peripheral neuropathy was seen in only two patients (145). Bortezomib is proteosome inhibitor that is used in the treatment of multiple myeloma, and has been associated with a sensory neuropathy. In a phase 2 study of 202 patients, 31% of patients developed a peripheral sensory neuropathy, in which 12% experienced grade 3 neuropathy (146).

Vincristine is a vinca-alkaloid used in the treatment of acute lymphoblastic leukemia, Hodgkin and non-Hodgkin lymphoma, multiple myeloma, rhabdomyosarcoma, neuroblastoma, Ewing sarcoma, chronic leukemias, thyroid cancer, brain malignancies, and trophoblastic neoplasms, whose dose-limiting toxicity is an axonal neuropathy, which results from disruption of the microtubules within axons and interference with axonal transport. The neuropathy involves both sensory and motor fibers, although small sensory fibers are especially affected (147). The earliest symptoms are usually paresthesias in the fingertips and feet, with or without muscle cramps. These symptoms often develop after several weeks of treatment, but can occur after the first dose. Also, symptoms may appear after the drug has been discontinued and progress for several months before improving (148).

Initially, in comparison to subjective complaints, objective sensory findings tend to be relatively minor, but loss of ankle jerks is common. Occasionally, there may be profound weakness, with bilateral foot drop, wrist drop, and loss of all sensory modalities. Neurophysiologic studies reveal a primarily axonal neuropathy (149). Patients with mild neuropathy can usually continue to receive full doses of vincristine, but progressive symptoms require dose reduction or discontinuation of drug. Discontinuation of treatment results in gradual improvement, which may take up to several months (150).

Vincristine can also cause autonomic neuropathies manifested by colicky abdominal pain and constipation, which can occur in almost 50% of patients, and rarely a paralytic ileus may result (150). Hence, patients receiving vincristine should take prophylactic stool softeners and/or laxatives. Less commonly, patients may develop impotence, postural hypotension, or an atonic bladder.

Vincristine may also cause focal neuropathies involving the cranial nerves (121). Most commonly, this affects the oculomotor nerve, but the recurrent laryngeal nerve, optic nerve, facial nerve, and auditory nerve may also be involved. Vincristine may also cause retinal damage and night blindness, and some patients may experience jaw and parotid pain during treatment.

Rarely, vincristine may cause syndrome of inappropriate antidiuretic hormone secretion (SIADH), resulting in hyponatremia, confusion, and seizures (151). Other rare CNS complications (unrelated to SIADH) include seizures, encephalopathy, transient cortical blindness, ataxia, athetosis, and parkinsonism (152).

Vindesine, vinblastine, and vinorelbine are associated with less neurotoxicity and have less affinity for neural tissue. Vinorelbine is associated with mild paresthesias in only about 20% of patients (153), and severe neuropathy is rare, occurring most often in patients with prior paclitaxel exposure (154).

Cytarabine is a pyrimidine analogue that is used to treat leukemias, lymphomas, and intrathecally for neoplastic meningitis. Conventional doses are associated with little neurotoxicity. However, high doses (3 g/m^2 every 12 hours) cause an acute cerebellar syndrome in 10%–25% of patients (155,156). Patients over the age of 40 who have abnormal liver or renal function, underlying neurologic dysfunction, or who receive a total dose of >30 g are particularly likely to develop cerebellar toxicity. The characteristic syndrome begins with somnolence and occasionally an encephalopathy that develops two to five days after beginning treatment. Immediately thereafter, cerebellar signs are noted on physical examination; symptoms range from mild ataxia to an inability to sit or walk unassisted. Rarely, seizures can occur.

High-dose cytarabine infrequently causes peripheral neuropathies resembling Guillain-Barré syndrome, brachial plexopathy, encephalopathy, lateral rectus palsy, or an extrapyramidal syndrome (155,157). Rarely, IT cytarabine can cause a transverse myelitis that is similar to that seen with IT MTX (157). IT cytarabine has also been associated with aseptic meningitis, encephalopathy, headaches, and seizures (121).

5-fluorouracil (5-FU) is rarely associated with an acute cerebellar syndrome (157) that is manifested by acute onset of ataxia, dysmetria, dysarthria, and nystagmus, and develops weeks to months after beginning treatment. 5-FU should be discontinued in any patient who develops cerebellar toxicity; over time, symptoms usually resolve completely. Other rarer neurologic side effects include encephalopathy, an optic neuropathy, eye movement abnormalities, focal dystonia, cerebrovascular disorders, a parkinsonian syndrome (152,158), peripheral neuropathy (159), or seizures (160). 5-FU derivatives doxifluridine, carmofur, and ftorafur have also been reported to rarely cause encephalopathies and cerebellar syndromes (152,161).

Ifosfamide is an analog of cyclophosphamide, and is used to treat recurrent germ cell tumors, soft tissue sarcomas, non-Hodgkin lymphoma, Hodgkin lymphoma, NSCLC and SCLC, bladder cancer, head and neck cancer, cervical cancer, and Ewing sarcoma. Ifosfamide had a systemic toxicity similar to cyclophosphamide, but unlike cyclophosphamide, about 10%–20% of patients treated with ifosfamide develop an encephalopathy. Patients at increased risk include those with a prior history of ifosfamide-related encephalopathy, renal dysfunction, low serum albumin, or prior cisplatin treatment (162,163). Other rare ifosfamide-associated neurologic toxicities include seizures, ataxia, weakness, cranial nerve dysfunction, neuropathies (147), or an extrapyramidal syndrome (164).

The nitrosoureas are lipid-soluble alkylating agents that rapidly cross the blood-brain barrier. High-dose intravenous (IV) carmustine, as used in the setting of hematopoietic cell transplantation, can cause an encephalomyelopathy and seizures, and these symptoms typically develop over a period of weeks to months following drug administration. Intra-arterial administration of carmustine produces ocular toxicity and neurotoxicity in 30%–48% of patients (165,166). Patients often complain of headache, eye, and facial pain. Confusion, seizures, retinopathy, and blindness also may occur. Concurrent radiotherapy increases the neurotoxicity of intracarotid carmustine (167).

Procarbazine is an alkylating agent that is used to treat Hodgkin lymphoma, non-Hodgkin lymphoma, cutaneous T-cell lymphoma, and brain tumors. At conventional doses, procarbazine can cause a mild reversible encephalopathy and neuropathy, and rarely psychosis and stupor (121,152). The incidence of encephalopathy may be higher in patients receiving higher doses of procarbazine, such as in the treatment of malignant gliomas (168). The combination of intravenous and intra-arterial procarbazine produces a severe encephalopathy (169). Procarbazine also potentiates the sedative effects of opiates, phenothiazines, and barbiturates. Concurrent use of alcohol or tyramine containing food with procarbazine can result in nausea, vomiting, CNS depression, hypertensive crisis, visual disturbances, and headache. Concurrent use of procarbazine with tricyclic antidepressants can result in CNS excitation, tremors, palpitations, hypertensive crisis, and/or angina.

IFN α is associated with dose-related neurotoxicity that is generally mild when low doses are used, as in the adjuvant treatment of malignant melanoma. In a study of 37 such patients treated with IFN α, the most frequent neurotoxicity observed in 22% of patients was tremor (170). At higher doses, IFN α can cause confusion, lethargy, hallucinations, and seizures (171). Although these effects are usually reversible, a permanent dementia or persistent vegetative state may result (172). Rarely, IFN α has been associated with oculomotor palsy, sensorimotor neuropathy (173), myasthenia gravis (188), brachial plexopathy, and polyradiculopathy (174).

IFN α-2a has been associated with depression and suicidal behavior/ideation (:15%), dizziness (21%), irritability (15%), insomnia (14%), vertigo (19%), and mental status changes (12%). Somnolence, lethargy, confusion, and mental impairment may also occur. Motor weakness may be seen at high doses, and usually reverses within a few days. Although IFN α-2b is associated with neurologic side effects similar to IFN α-2a, a particularly high incidence of neuropsychiatric toxicity has been noted in patients with CML treated with recombinant IFN α-2b. In one study of 91 patients, 25% experienced grade 3 or 4 neuropsychiatric toxicity that affected daily functioning. All patients recovered upon withdrawal of IFN α (175).

Intrathecal administration of IFN α has been evaluated for the treatment of meningeal and brain tumors and progressive multifocal leukoencephalopathy. An acute reaction (within hours of the first injection) consists of headache, nausea, vomiting, fever, and dizziness; these usually resolve over 12–24 hours. A severe dose-dependent encephalopathy develops in a significant number of patients within several days of the onset of treatment (176), and is worse in patients who have received cranial radiation (174).

Interferon beta and gamma have neurotoxicities that are similar to IFN α, although interferon beta appears to be better tolerated in general. Hypertonia and myasthenia have been reported with interferon beta (174).

IL-2 has been associated with neuropsychiatric complications in up to 30%–50% of patients, and these include cognitive changes, delusions, hallucinations, and depression (177). Transient focal neurologic deficits (178), acute leukoencephalopathy, carpal tunnel syndrome, and brachial neuritis (179) have been reported with IL-2.

Bevacizumab has been associated with a significant increase in the risk of serious arterial thromboembolic events (including transient ischemic attack, cerebrovascular accident, angina, and myocardial infarction). The incidence of such events is approximately 5%. Reversible posterior leukoencephalopathy syndrome (RPLS) occurs in ≤0.1% of patients (180,181), and symptoms can include headache, seizure, lethargy, confusion, blindness, and other visual and neurologic disturbances. The onset may occur from 16 hours to 1 year after initiation of therapy. Symptoms usually resolve with discontinuation of bevacizumab and control of any associated hypertension.

Other rare causes of neurotoxicity include the following chemotherapeutic agents. High-dose busulfan is a cell-cycle–nonspecific alkylating agent that is used in the treatment of chronic myelogenous leukemia (CML), and is also used in stem cell preparative regimens for refractory leukemia and lymphoma. Busulfan therapy, as used in the setting of hematopoietic stem cell transplantation, can cause seizures. Gemcitabine can cause mild paresthesias in up to 10% of patients. Occasionally, more severe peripheral and autonomic neuropathies can occur (182). An acute inflammatory myopathy has been reported following chemotherapy with gemcitabine and docetaxel, presenting as a symmetrical, painful, proximal muscle weakness (183). ATRA can rarely cause pseudotumor cerebri (184) and multiple mononeuropathies (164).

Fludarabine is a purine analog that is used to treat chronic lymphocytic leukemia (CLL) and indolent lymphomas, and can cause headache, somnolence, confusion, and paresthesias at low doses (185). A delayed progressive encephalopathy with seizures, cortical blindness, paralysis, and coma is more common at high doses, and rarely, a progressive multifocal leukoencephalopathy has been reported (186). Cladribine is also a purine analog, and is used to treat hairy cell leukemia, CLL, and Waldenström macroglobulinemia, and is associated with little neurotoxicity at conventional doses, but can produce a paraparesis or quadriplegia at high doses (185). Pentostatin, another purine analog, is used to treat hairy cell leukemia, cutaneous T-cell lymphomas, and CLL. At low doses, lethargy and fatigue are common, and at higher doses, severe encephalopathy, seizures, and coma can occur (146,185).

Management of Complications

Central toxicity induced by chemotherapeutic agents is managed with cessation of chemotherapy. Often this results in rapid improvement of toxicity. Peripheral symptoms such as numbness and pins-and-needles or burning paresthesias also often improve with drug cessation. In some patients, however, peripheral neuropathy often persists, and symptoms can be severe enough to affect quality of life. In these instances, agents such as gabapentin (Neurontin; Pfizer, Inc., New York, New York), pregabalin (Lyrica; Pfizer, Inc., New York, New York), amifostine (Ethyol; Medimmune, Gaithersburg, Maryland), acetyl L-carnitine, calcium and magnesium infusions, tricyclic antidepressants (amitriptyline), duloxetine (Cymbalta; Eli Lilly and Co.; Indianapolis, Indiana), venlafaxine (Effexor; Wyeth Pharmaceuticals, Philadelphia, Pennsylvania), and selective serotonin reuptake inhibitors (SSRIs) may be beneficial.

Gabapentin is an anticonvulsant, which is taken three times a day and can be quite effective for peripheral neuropathy, such as that induced by diabetes. However, in a recent phase 3 trial evaluating the efficacy of gabapentin in the management of chemotherapy-induced peripheral neuropathy (CIPN), 115 patients were randomly assigned to treatment with gabapentin or to the control arm. This study found that changes in symptom severity were statistically similar between the two groups and concluded that gabapentin was not effective in treating symptoms of CIPN (187).

Carbamazepine use has revealed conflicting results. In one study of oxaliplatin and capecitabine, 25 patients received detailed neurologic evaluation, including electromyography (EMG) and nerve conduction studies. Twelve of these patients were treated with carbamazepine during the second cycle of therapy, and all 12 patients had neurologic studies that included EMG and nerve conduction studies at baseline and after one cycle of therapy. Eleven patients were also evaluated after the second cycle of therapy. There was no evidence of nerve abnormalities at baseline in any patient. Abnormal EMG results were noted in 11 of 12 patients, and abnormal nerve conduction studies were reported in 8 of 12 patients after the first course of therapy (without carbamazepine). Carbamazepine was administered for five days before administration of oxaliplatin and continued for two days afterward. One of nine evaluated patients reported some reduction of cold-induced paresthesias. EMG and nerve conduction studies indicated no benefit from carbamazepine. Adverse effects associated with carbamazepine included ataxia, memory loss, dizziness, somnolence, fatigue, and unsteady gait (128).

In another trial of 40 patients treated with oxaliplatin, fluorouracil and leucovorin (FOLFOX), 10 patients received carbamazepine beginning one week before oxaliplatin administration. There were no cases of grade 2 or 3 neuropathy by World Health Organization (WHO) criteria after an average cumulative oxaliplatin dose of 722 mg/m². This was contrasted with a set of historical controls that received a cumulative dose of 510 mg/m² and experienced grade 2–4 neuropathy at a rate of 30% (188).

Pregabalin, a newer anticonvulsant, is titrated to three times a day dosing, with a maximum daily dose of 600 mg. Somnolence, dizziness, and ataxia can occur, but in general, pregabalin is well tolerated. In a report of a patient with stage IIB pancreatic cancer, pregabalin was successfully used to treat oxaliplatin-induced hyperexcitability syndrome with 72 hours of treatment (189). Randomized studies to further characterize the benefit of pregabalin are warranted.

Amifostine is an organic thiophosphate analog, and in a recent phase 2 trial of amifostine in the first-line treatment of advanced ovarian cancer with carboplatin/paclitaxel chemotherapy, a significant improvement in sensory neuropathy in accordance with National Cancer Institute Common Toxicity Criteria (NCI-CTC) was found ($P = 0.0046$), but amifostine failed to significantly improve the "global health status quality of life" score (190). Hypotension, nausea, and vomiting have been associated with intravenous amifostine, and these can largely be ameliorated with the use of the subcutaneous formulation (191).

Acetyl L-carnitine is an acetyl ester of L-carnitine, a naturally occurring compound that is synthesized from lysine and methionine amino acids. The effect of acetyl L-carnitine in paclitaxel- and cisplatin-induced peripheral neuropathy was evaluated in a study of 26 patients, and at least one WHO grade improvement in peripheral neuropathy was shown in 73% of patients (192).

The role of calcium and magnesium infusions was evaluated in patients with advanced colorectal cancer receiving FOLFOX. Fourteen patients were treated with infusions of calcium gluconate and magnesium sulfate before and after oxaliplatin treatment. Sensory neuropathy was noted in 57.1% of patients after four cycles of therapy. Hence, calcium and magnesium infusions may decrease acute oxaliplatin-induced neurotoxicity (193).

Tricyclic antidepressants, such as amitriptyline, may be effective in some patients, but their use has largely been replaced by SSRIs, venlafaxine (Effexor), and duloxetine (Cymbalta), due to significant side effects, including orthostatic hypotension, ECG changes, atrioventricular (AV) conduction delays, insomnia, sedation, ataxia, cognitive impairment, weight gain, and SIADH. In one report, venlafaxine at a 50-mg dose was effective in the management of oxaliplatin-induced peripheral neuropathy (194).

NEPHROTOXICITY

Chemotherapeutic agents can affect the glomerulus, tubules, interstitium, or the renal microvasculature, with clinical manifestations that range from an asymptomatic elevation of serum creatinine to acute renal failure requiring dialysis. The kidneys are one of the major elimination pathways for many antineoplastic drugs and their metabolites, further enhancing their potential for nephrotoxicity. Delayed drug excretion can result in increased systemic toxicity and is a major concern in patients with renal impairment. Many drugs, including azathioprine, bleomycin, carboplatin, cisplatin, cyclophosphamide, high-dose cytarabine, etoposide, hydroxyurea, ifosfamide, melphalan, methotrexate, mitomycin C, and topotecan, require dose adjustment when administered in the setting of renal insufficiency (Table 3.5).

Several factors can potentiate renal dysfunction and contribute to the nephrotoxic potential of antineoplastic drugs. These include intravascular volume depletion, either due to external losses or fluid

TABLE 3.5
Chemotherapy-Induced Nephrotoxicity

AGENT	TOXICITY	MANAGEMENT	REFERENCES
Cisplatin	Renal failure, renal tubular acidosis, hypomagnesemia	Vigorous saline hydration and diuresis	(195,196,198)
Carboplatin	Hypomagnesemia, renal salt wasting	Close laboratory monitoring and electrolyte replacement	(198,200)
Oxaliplatin	Renal tubular necrosis	Drug cessation and hydration	(202)
Cyclophosphamide	Hyponatremia and hemorrhagic cystitis	Hydration and mesna	(197,203)
Ifosfamide	Renal tubular acidosis, hemorrhagic cystitis, nephrogenic diabetes insipidus, Fanconi syndrome	Hydration and mesna	(209)
Nitrosoureas	Chronic interstitial nephritis and renal failure	Drug cessation	(204,205)
Mitomycin C	Hemolytic uremic syndrome	Drug cessation	(206,207)
Vinca alkaloids	SIADH	Drug cessation	(213)
Bevacizumab Sorafenib Sunitinib	Albuminuria and nephritic syndrome	Dose reduction or drug cessation	(217)
Interleukin-2	Capillary leak and resulting prerenal azotemia	Vigorous hydration and diuresis and urine alkalinization	(218)
Interferon-alpha	Minimal change nephropathy and massive proteinuria	Drug cessation	(219)
Methotrexate	Nonoliguric renal failure	Vigorous hydration and diuresis and urine alkalinization	(210,211)

sequestration (ascites or edema). The concomitant use of nonchemotherapeutic nephrotoxic drugs or radiographic ionic contrast media in patients with or without preexisting renal dysfunction can also potentiate renal dysfunction. Also, urinary tract obstruction secondary to underlying tumor and intrinsic idiopathic renal disease that is related to other comorbidities or to the cancer itself can also result in increased risk of renal dysfunction.

Cisplatin is a potent renal tubular toxin, and approximately 25%–42% of patients administered cisplatin will develop a mild and partially reversible decline in renal function after the first course of therapy (195). The incidence and severity of renal failure increases with subsequent courses, eventually becoming partially irreversible. Vigorous saline hydration with forced diuresis is the mainstay for preventing cisplatin-induced nephrotoxicity, along with the avoidance of concomitant use of other nephrotoxic drugs. Discon-

tinuation of therapy is generally indicated when a progressive rise in the plasma creatinine concentration is noted. In addition to the rise in the plasma creatinine concentration, potentially irreversible hypomagnesemia due to urinary magnesium wasting may occur in >50% of cases (196). Treatment generally consists of magnesium supplementation, and high doses may be required since raising the plasma magnesium concentration will increase the degree of magnesium wasting.

Cisplatin may also be associated with thrombotic microangiopathy with features of the hemolytic uremic syndrome or thrombotic thrombocytopenic purpura when combined with bleomycin (197). The onset of renal failure may be abrupt or insidious, and in the latter setting can develop months after treatment has been discontinued. The diagnosis of this form of nephrotoxicity is suggested by the concurrent presence of a microangiopathic hemolytic anemia and thrombocytopenia. Direct tubular injury leading to acute tubular necrosis is the primary mechanism. A less common renal side effect is renal salt wasting (198).

Carboplatin is significantly less nephrotoxic than cisplatin (199), and hypomagnesemia is the most common manifestation of nephrotoxicity, although it occurs less often than with cisplatin (200). Acute renal failure has been reported, particularly in patients previously treated with several courses of cisplatin (199). Direct tubular injury leading to acute tubular necrosis (ATN) is the primary mechanism. A less common renal side effect is renal salt wasting (198). Oxaliplatin has rarely been associated with ATN, (201), and limited data suggest that oxaliplatin does not cause exacerbation of preexisting mild renal impairment during treatment (202).

Cyclophosphamide is primarily associated with hemorrhagic cystitis, and the primary renal effect of cyclophosphamide is hyponatremia, which is due to an increased effect of antidiuretic hormone (ADH), impairing the kidney's ability to excrete water (203). Chemotherapy-induced nausea may also play a contributory role, since nausea is a potent stimulus for ADH release. Hyponatremia is usually seen in patients receiving high doses of intravenous cyclophosphamide (eg, 30–50 mg/kg or 6 g/m^2 in the setting of hematopoietic stem cell transplantation), and typically occurs acutely and resolves within approximately 24 hours after discontinuation of the drug. Hyponatremia poses a particular problem for patients undergoing high-dose intravenous cyclophosphamide treatment, who are often fluid-loaded to prevent hemorrhagic cystitis (197). The combination of increased ADH effect and enhanced water intake can lead to severe, occasionally fatal, hyponatremia within 24 hours.

The predominant urinary toxicity of ifosfamide is hemorrhagic cystitis. However, nephrotoxicity is more likely with ifosfamide than with cyclophosphamide. Ifosfamide-induced nephrotoxicity affects the proximal renal tubule, and is characterized by metabolic acidosis with a normal anion gap (hyperchloremic acidosis) due to type 1 (distal) or type 2 (proximal) renal tubular acidosis. Other toxicities include hypophosphatemia induced by decreased proximal phosphate reabsorption, renal glucosuria, aminoaciduria, and a marked increase in fl2-microglobulin excretion, all from generalized proximal dysfunction, polyuria due to nephrogenic diabetes insipidus, and hypokalemia resulting from increased urinary potassium losses. Preexisting renal disease is a risk factor for ifosfamide nephrotoxicity, and dose adjustments are recommended based upon renal function.

Prolonged therapy with the nitrosoureas can induce a slowly progressive, chronic interstitial nephritis that is generally irreversible (204). Although the exact mechanism of nephrotoxicity is not completely elucidated, these agents may produce nephrotoxicity by alkylation of tubular cell proteins. Their metabolites, which are thought to be responsible for nephrotoxicity, persist in the urine for up to 72 hours following administration (205).

MMC is associated with thrombotic thrombocytopenic purpura/hemolytic uremic syndrome (TTP-HUS) and resulting renal failure and microangiopathic hemolytic anemia (206). It most commonly occurs after at least six months of therapy, and the overall incidence is related to cumulative dose. Direct endothelial injury is the initiating event (207). Affected patients typically present with slowly progressive renal failure, hypertension, and relatively bland urine sediment, often occurring in the absence of clinically apparent tumor. MMC can be administered to patients with renal insufficiency, with close monitoring for signs and symptoms of TTP-HUS. Some guidelines suggest a 50% dose reduction for serum creatinine 1.6–2.4 mg/dL and avoidance of the drug for creatinine values >2.4 mg/dL (208). However, others note that urinary elimination accounts for only 20% of an administered dose and recommend dose reduction of 25% only for patients with creatinine clearance.

Low-dose methotrexate treatment (≤0.5–1.0 g/m^2) is usually not associated with renal toxicity unless underlying renal dysfunction is present. High-dose intravenous methotrexate (1–15 g/m^2) can precipitate in the tubules and induce tubular injury. Patients who are volume-depleted and those who excrete acidic urine are at particular risk. Maintenance of adequate urinary output and alkalinization will lessen the probability of methotrexate precipitation. Methotrexate can also produce a transient decrease in glomerular filtration rate (GFR), with complete recovery within six to eight hours of discontinuing the drug. The mechanism responsible for this functional renal impairment involves afferent arteriolar constriction or mesangial cell constriction that produces reduced glomerular capillary surface area and diminished glomerular capillary perfusion and pressure (210). In patients with renal insufficiency, methotrexate excretion is decreased and more significant bone marrow and gastrointestinal toxicity may result (211). Patients with ileal conduits and those with third-space fluid collections (eg, ascites, pleural effusion) may experience greater methotrexate toxicity, particularly if their creatinine clearance is low (212).

Vincristine, vinblastine, and vinorelbine are associated with SIADH (213). Topotecan is not associated with renal toxicity, but is predominantly cleared by the kidneys, and increased toxicity may result in patients with moderate renal insufficiency (214). Approximately 20%–40% of etoposide is excreted in the urine, and the dose should be reduced by 25% in patients with creatinine clearance 10–50 mL/min and by 50% for clearance Bevacizumab, sunitinib, and sorafenib produce albuminuria in 10%–25% of patients and occasionally result in nephrotic syndrome (217). This toxicity appears to be an effect common to all agents targeted at the VEGF pathway, but the factors associated with occurrence and severity of the proteinuria are unknown. If clinically significant, decreasing the dose or discontinuation of drug is recommended.

IL-2 can induce a relatively severe capillary leak syndrome, leading to edema, plasma volume depletion, and a reversible fall in glomerular filtration rate (218). Patients with normal renal function before treatment usually recover within the first week after discontinuing therapy. Patients with underlying renal dysfunction may take longer to recover from the renal failure. Therapy for renal failure secondary to IL-2 treatment is supportive. Interferon alfa and gamma have both been associated with renal insufficiency. Interferon alpha can cause massive proteinuria as a result of minimal-change nephropathy (219). Thrombotic microangiopathy is a rare complication, seen mostly in patients with chronic myelogenous leukemia treated with high doses of alpha interferon over a long time period (220). Interferon gamma has been associated with acute tubular necrosis when used for the treatment of acute lymphoblastic leukemia (221).

Management of Complications

Numerous chemotherapeutic agents can induce nephrotoxicity in a myriad of ways, and clinical manifestations can vary from asymptomatic elevation in creatinine to renal failure requiring dialysis. Hence, clinicians must follow renal function trends very carefully during chemotherapy treatment. It is also imperative to ensure that patients are not intravascularly depleted as a result of dehydration or third spacing of fluid (ie, ascites or peripheral edema). Concomitant use of nonchemotherapeutic nephrotoxic drugs (eg, nonsteroidal anti-inflammatory drugs [NSAIDs] and certain antibiotics), and contrast media should be minimized in the setting of even mild renal insufficiency. Also, extrinsic and intrinsic urinary obstruction and idiopathic renal disease (acute interstitial nephritis and glomerulonephritis) should be ruled out, and medical comorbidities (hypertension and diabetes) should be optimized. Referral to nephrology should be considered early should renal function not rapidly normalize with the previously described interventions.

AUTOIMMUNE TOXICITY

Autoimmune complications, including autoimmune hemolytic anemia (AIHA) and autoimmune thrombocytopenia, have been reported with the use of purine analogs (fludarabine, cladribine, pentostatin). One report described 24 patients with CLL who developed fludarabine-associated autoimmune hemolytic anemia (FA-AIHA) (241). Seventy-one percent of patients developed AIHA during the first three cycles of therapy, and one case occurred after six cycles. In six cases, AIHA was also associated with autoimmune thrombocytopenia (AITP). There are a myriad of case reports of AIHA in CLL or other lymphoproliferative disorders triggered by therapy with cladribine (242,243) or pentostatin (244). The two most important risk factors for developing AIHA are a positive direct antiglobulin test (Coomb test) and a prior history of AIHA. CLL patients are also at increased risk of acquiring AITP. The exact incidence of AITP is unknown, but is thought to be less frequent than AIHA (222).

IL-2 has been associated with a syndrome mimicking painless thyroiditis. In one study of 130 patients receiving IL-2–based immunotherapy, primary hypothyroidism occurred in 12% of patients before, 38% during, and 23% after immunotherapy. Hyperthyroidism occurred in 1%, 4%, and 7% of patients at those time intervals. Among patients initially euthyroid (n = 111), primary hypothyroidism developed in 32% during and 14% after immunotherapy, persisting a median of 54 days, and three patients required levothyroxine treatment. Hyperthyroidism developed in 2% of patients during immunotherapy and 6% after. Thyroid dysfunction was not a function of gender, diagnosis, type of treatment, or response to immunotherapy. Elevated titers of antithyroglobulin and antithyroid microsomal antibodies were detected after treatment in 9% and 7%, respectively (223).

In another study designed to evaluate the incidence and risk factors of this adverse autoimmune response, triiodothyronine, thyroxine, and thyrotropin levels were measured serially in 146 consecutive patients treated with IL-2 for refractory solid tumor (77 patients) or malignant hemopathy (69 patients). IL-2 was administered intravenously alone in 79 cases or in combination with autologous bone marrow transplantation in 26 cases, with interferon-gamma in 37 cases, with tumor necrosis factor-alpha in 13, and with cyclophosphamide in 5 cases. Some patients underwent more than one therapeutic treatment. Peripheral hypothyroidism was present upon entry in nine (6.2%) patients. Thyroid dysfunction appeared or worsened during IL-2 therapy in 24 (16.4%) patients. Sixteen (10.9%) patients exhibited peripheral hypothyroidism, out of which four exhibited biphasic thyroiditis. Another five (3.4%) patients developed transient hyperthyroidism. Thyroid dysfunction appeared early after one or two cycles, and all surviving patients recovered. Only gender and presence of antithyroid antibody were correlated significantly with IL-2–induced thyroid abnormalities. Antithyroid antibodies were detected in 60.9% of patients, and thyroid-stimulating antibodies were never detected (224).

Sunitinib-induced hypothyroidism has also been described. In one study of patients with metastatic renal cell carcinoma (RCC), 85% of patients had abnormalities in their thyroid function tests and 84% experienced symptoms related to hypothyroidism (225). In another study, 62% of patients had an abnormal level of thyroid-stimulating hormone (TSH) and 36% had hypothyroidism with sunitinib therapy for GISTs (226). However, in this study, 10% of patients were noted to have an elevated TSH before initiating sunitinib treatment and an additional 12% were being treated with L-thyroxine prior to enrollment. It has been theorized that increased thyroid function testing in patients treated with sunitinib may lead to increased detection of abnormalities in the absence of symptoms, a finding that may not necessarily have clinical consequences.

Management of Complications

AIHA treatment includes cessation of drugs and initiation of corticosteroids. In corticosteroid-resistant cases, immunosuppressive agents, such as cyclosporine A and azathioprine, may be utilized. Other agents, such as rituximab and intravenous immune globulin (IVIG), may also be efficacious (227,228). Splenectomy is considered for patients whose autoimmune disorder has proven refractory to the previously described treatments. Treatment of AITP is generally not indicated until platelet counts are <20,000 or bleeding occurs, and treatment is similar to that of AIHA (228, 229).

Thyroiditis treatment generally includes initiation of thyroid replacement therapy with L-thyroxine and frequent monitoring of thyroid function tests while on replacement therapy. It is also important to delineate whether symptoms of fatigue are due to sunitinib therapy (independent of thyroid dysfunction), underlying cancer itself, or due to clinical hypothyroidism, for, as stated, not all thyroid function derangements warrant treatment.

RHEUMATIC TOXICITY

Almost any chemotherapeutic agent can result in postchemotherapy rheumatism, and this is a fairly common clinical phenomenon. In one study of eight breast cancer patients receiving cyclophosphamide and 5-fluorouracil containing adjuvant combination chemotherapy, patients (ages 41–53) developed rheumatic symptoms (myalgias, arthralgias, joint stiffness, generalized musculoskeletal achiness, and periarticular tenderness) between one and four months after (one patient developed symptoms during treatment) chemotherapy treatment. Symptoms resolved between 2 and >16 months after completion of chemotherapy, and in all cases, recurrent cancer and rheumatic disorders (polymyositis, cancer-associated arthritis, systemic lupus erythematosus, polymyalgia rheumatica, and fibromyalgia) were ruled out as possible etiologies. In this study, NSAIDs were generally not beneficial, and one patient experienced prompt resolution of symptoms after initiation of low-dose oral corticosteroids (230).

Aromatase inhibitors (AIs) (anastrozole [Arimidex], letrozole [Femara], and exemestane [Aromasin]) are oral antiestrogen agents that are widely used as adjuvant endocrine treatment in postmenopausal women with early-stage breast cancer. AI-associated arthralgias are highly variable, and usually include bilateral symmetrical pain/soreness in the hands, knees, hips, lower back, shoulders, and/or feet, along with early-morning stiffness and difficulty sleeping. Typical onset is within two months of treatment initiation, and some patients develop more severe symptoms over time. Spontaneous symptom resolution is rare during treatment, but common after cessation of therapy (231). In the Arimidex and Tamoxifen Alone or in Combination (ATAC) trial, which had the longest median follow-up time, the incidence of musculoskeletal disorders was 30% with Arimidex and 23.7% with tamoxifen ($P < 0.001$). The incidence of arthralgia was 35.6% versus 29.4% ($P < 0.001$) with Arimidex versus tamoxifen, and the incidence of fractures was 11.0% versus 7.7% ($P < 0.001$) with Arimidex versus tamoxifen (232). The risk of important long-term skeletal problems, including osteoporosis, may increase with the use of aromatase inhibitors. The maintenance of bone density depends in part on estrogen, and aromatase inhibitors may enhance bone loss by lowering circulating estrogen levels. Short-term use of letrozole has been shown to be associated with an increase in bone-resorption markers in plasma and urine. However, it is possible that osteopenia might be prevented or modified with concurrent use of bisphosphonates (233).

Paclitaxel and docetaxel can also cause myalgias and arthralgias that are sometimes severe and can impair both physical function and quality of life. The incidence of these side effects is not known, although it has been reported to occur in up to 75% of patients (234–239). This still poorly understood process usually develops 24–48 hours following the completion of a paclitaxel infusion and may persist for 3–5 days. Occasionally, the symptoms of achiness and pain in the muscles and joints may last for a week or longer.

Management of Complications

There are no formal studies of treatment for chemotherapy-induced arthralgia syndrome. The most commonly prescribed treatment are NSAIDs, but chronic use of NSAIDs such as ibuprofen can contribute to adverse effects on the GI tract, heart, and kidneys. More potent NSAIDs, such as nabumetone, have also been prescribed in conjunction with a proton pump inhibitor in an effort to control GI side effects. Combinations of NSAIDs and other analgesics (both narcotic and non-narcotic) are also often used, but it is not clear to what extent these treatments improve chemotherapy-induced arthralgias. Cyclooxygenase 2 (COX-2) inhibitors had also been proposed as treatment of this syndrome, but have recently fallen out of favor due to their association with adverse cardiovascular events. Some data suggests that gabapentin may beneficial in the treatment of this syndrome (240). Gentle exercise may also be beneficial. The use of bisphosphonates to counter AI-induced bone loss is also recommended.

References

1. Singal PK, Deally CM, Weinberg LE. Subcellular effects of adriamycin in the heart: A concise review. *J Mol Cell Cardiol.* 1987;19(8):817–828.
2. Li T, Singal PK. Adriamycin-induced early changes in myocardial antioxidant enzymes and their modulation by probucol. *Circulation.* 2000;102(17):2105–2110.
3. Singal PK, et al. Adriamycin cardiomyopathy: pathophysiology and prevention. *FASEB J.* 1997;11(12):931–936.
4. Singal PK, Iliskovic N. Doxorubicin-induced cardiomyopathy. *N Engl J Med.* 1998;339(13):900–905.
5. Von Hoff DD, et al. Risk factors for doxorubicin-induced congestive heart failure. *Ann Intern Med.* 1979;91(5):710–717.
6. Von Hoff DD, et al. Daunomycin-induced cardiotoxicity in children and adults. A review of 110 cases. *Am J Med.* 1977;62(2):200–208.
7. Miller KD, et al. Randomized phase III trial of capecitabine compared with bevacizumab plus capecitabine in patients with previously treated metastatic breast cancer. *J Clin Oncol.* 2005;23(4):792–799.
8. Swain SM, Whaley FS, Ewer MS. Congestive heart failure in patients treated with doxorubicin: A retrospective analysis of three trials. *Cancer.* 2003;97(11):2869–2879.
9. Isner JM, et al. Clinical and morphologic cardiac findings after anthracycline chemotherapy. Analysis of 64 patients studied at necropsy. *Am J Cardiol.* 1983;51(7):1167–1174.
10. Lefrak EA, et al. A clinicopathologic analysis of adriamycin cardiotoxicity. *Cancer.* 1973;32(2):302–314.
11. Appelbaum F, et al. Acute lethal carditis caused by high-dose combination chemotherapy. A unique clinical and pathological entity. *Lancet.* 1976;1(7950):58–62.
12. Ferguson C, Clarke J, Herity NA. Ventricular tachycardia associated with trastuzumab. *N Engl J Med.,* 2006;354(6):648–649.
13. Keefe DL. Trastuzumab-associated cardiotoxicity. *Cancer.* 2002;95(7):1592–1600.
14. Seidman A, et al. Cardiac dysfunction in the trastuzumab clinical trials experience. *J Clin Oncol.* 2002;20(5):1215–1221.
15. Perez EA, Rodeheffer R. Clinical cardiac tolerability of trastuzumab. *J Clin Oncol.* 2004;22(2):322–329.
16. Esteva FJ, et al. Phase II study of weekly docetaxel and trastuzumab for patients with HER-2-overexpressing metastatic breast cancer. *J Clin Oncol.* 2002;20(7):1800–1808.
17. Millward PM, et al. Cardiogenic shock complicates successful treatment of refractory thrombotic thrombocytopenia purpura with rituximab. *Transfusion.* 2005;45(9):1481–1486.
18. Slamon DJ, et al. Use of chemotherapy plus a monoclonal antibody against HER2 for metastatic breast cancer that overexpresses HER2. *N Engl J Med.* 2001l;344(11):783–792.
19. Slamon D, Eiermann W, Robert N, et al. Phase III trial comparing AC-T with AC-TH and with TCH in the adjuvant treatment of HER2 positive early breast cancer: First planned interim efficacy analysis (abstract 1). In San Antonio Breast Cancer Symposium. 2005. San Antonio, TX.
20. Floyd JD, et al. Cardiotoxicity of cancer therapy. *J Clin Oncol.* 2005;23(30):7685–7896.
21. Sonnenblick M, Rosin A. Cardiotoxicity of interferon. A review of 44 cases. *Chest.* 1991;99(3):557–561.
22. Budd GT, et al. Phase-I trial of Ultrapure human leukocyte interferon in human malignancy. *Cancer Chemother Pharmacol.* 1984;12(1):39–42.
23. Martino S, et al. Reversible arrhythmias observed in patients treated with recombinant alpha 2 interferon. *J Cancer Res Clin Oncol.* 1987;113(4):376–378.
24. Chap L, et al. Pulmonary toxicity of high-dose chemotherapy for breast cancer: A non-invasive approach to diagnosis and treatment. *Bone Marrow Transplant.* 1997;20(12):1063–1067. Bone Marrow Transplant
25. Cohen MC, Huberman MS, Nesto RW. Recombinant alpha 2 interferon-related cardiomyopathy. *Am J Med.* 1988;85(4):549–551.
26. Sonnenblick M, Rosenmann D, Rosin A. Reversible cardiomyopathy induced by interferon. *BMJ.* 1990;300(6733):1174–1175.
27. Rowinsky EK, et al. Cardiac disturbances during the administration of Taxol. *J Clin Oncol.* 1991;9(9):1704–1712.
28. Gianni L, et al. Paclitaxel by 3-hour infusion in combination with bolus doxorubicin in women with untreated metastatic breast cancer: High antitumor efficacy and cardiac effects in a dose-finding and sequence-finding study. *J Clin Oncol.* 1995;13(11):2688–2699.
29. Biganzoli L, et al. Doxorubicin-paclitaxel: a safe regimen in terms of cardiac toxicity in metastatic breast carcinoma patients. Results from a European Organization for Research and Treatment of Cancer multicenter trial. *Cancer.* 2003;97(1):40–45.
30. Giordano SH, et al. A detailed evaluation of cardiac toxicity: A phase II study of doxorubicin and one- or three-hour-infusion paclitaxel in patients with metastatic breast cancer. *Clin Cancer Res.* 2002;8(11):3360–3368.
31. Abi 007. Drugs R D, 2004. 5(3): p. 155-9.
32. Malhotra V, et al. Neoadjuvant and adjuvant chemotherapy with doxorubicin and docetaxel in locally advanced breast cancer. *Clin Breast Cancer.* 2004;5(5):377–384.
33. Margolin KA, et al. Interleukin-2 and lymphokine-activated killer cell therapy of solid tumors: Analysis of toxicity and management guidelines. *J Clin Oncol.* 1989;7(4):486–498.
34. Crum E. Biological-response modifier—induced emergencies. *Semin Oncol.* 1989;16(6):579–587.
35. White RL, Jr. et al. Cardiopulmonary toxicity of treatment with high dose interleukin-2 in 199 consecutive patients with metastatic melanoma or renal cell carcinoma. *Cancer.* 1994;74(12):3212–3222.
36. Akhtar SS, Salim KP, Bano ZA. Symptomatic cardiotoxicity with high-dose 5-fluorouracil infusion: A prospective study. *Oncology.* 1993;50(6):441–444.
37. de Forni M, et al. Cardiotoxicity of high-dose continuous infusion fluorouracil: A prospective clinical study. *J Clin Oncol.* 1992;10(11):1795–1801.
38. Wacker A, et al. High incidence of angina pectoris in patients treated with 5-fluorouracil. A planned surveillance study with 102 patients. *Oncology.* 2003;65(2):108–112.

39. Kuropkat C, et al. Severe cardiotoxicity during 5-fluorouracil chemotherapy: A case and literature report. *Am J Clin Oncol.* 1999;22(5):466–470.
40. Sasson Z, et al. 5-Fluorouracil related toxic myocarditis: Case reports and pathological confirmation. *Can J Cardiol.* 1994;10(8):861–864.
41. Cianci G, et al. Prophylactic options in patients with 5-fluorouracil-associated cardiotoxicity. *Br J Cancer.* 2003;88(10):1507–1509.
42. Eskilsson J, Albertsson M. Failure of preventing 5-fluorouracil cardiotoxicity by prophylactic treatment with verapamil. *Acta Oncol.* 1990;29(8): 1001–1003.
43. Ng M, Cunningham D, Norman AR. The frequency and pattern of cardiotoxicity observed with capecitabine used in conjunction with oxaliplatin in patients treated for advanced colorectal cancer (CRC). *Eur J Cancer.* 2005;41(11): 1542–1546.
44. Hurwitz H, et al. Bevacizumab plus irinotecan, fluorouracil, and leucovorin for metastatic colorectal cancer. *N Engl J Med.* 2004;350(23):2335–2342.
45. Veronese ML, et al. Mechanisms of hypertension associated with BAY 43-9006. *J Clin Oncol.* 2006;24(9):1363–1369.
46. Escudier B, et al. Sorafenib in advanced clear-cell renal-cell carcinoma. *N Engl J Med.* 2007;356(2):125–134.
47. Faivre S, et al. Safety, pharmacokinetic, and antitumor activity of SU11248, a novel oral multitarget tyrosine kinase inhibitor, in patients with cancer. *J Clin Oncol.* 2006;24(1):25–35.
48. Chiang CE, et al. Prolongation of cardiac repolarization by arsenic trioxide. *Blood.* 2002;100(6):2249–2252.
49. Westervelt P, et al. Sudden death among patients with acute promyelocytic leukemia treated with arsenic trioxide. *Blood.* 2001;98(2):266–271.
50. Matsui H, et al. Protective effects of carvedilol against doxorubicin-induced cardiomyopathy in rats. *Life Sci.* 1999;65(12):1265–1274.
51. Santos DL, et al. Carvedilol protects against doxorubicin-induced mitochondrial cardiomyopathy. *Toxicol Appl Pharmacol.* 2002;185(3):218–227.
52. Kalay N, et al. Protective effects of carvedilol against anthracycline-induced cardiomyopathy. *J Am Coll Cardiol.* 2006;48(11):2258–2262.
53. Cardinale D, et al. Prevention of high-dose chemotherapy-induced cardiotoxicity in high-risk patients by angiotensin-converting enzyme inhibition. *Circulation.* 2006;114(23): 2474–2481.
54. Seifert CF, Nesser ME, Thompson DF. Dexrazoxane in the prevention of doxorubicin-induced cardiotoxicity. *Ann Pharmacother.* 1994;28(9):1063–1072.
55. van Dalen EC, et al. Cardioprotective interventions for cancer patients receiving anthracyclines. *Cochrane Database Syst Rev.* 2005;(1):CD003917.
56. O'Sullivan JM, et al. Predicting the risk of bleomycin lung toxicity in patients with germ-cell tumours. *Ann Oncol.* 2003;14(1):91–96.
57. Sleijfer S. Bleomycin-induced pneumonitis. *Chest.* 2001;120(2):617–624.
58. Blum RH, Carter SK, Agre K. A clinical review of bleomycin—a new antineoplastic agent. *Cancer.* 1973;31(4):903–914.
59. Berend N. Protective effect of hypoxia on bleomycin lung toxicity in the rat. *Am Rev Respir Dis.* 1984;130(2):307–308.
60. Kawai K, et al. Serum creatinine level during chemotherapy for testicular cancer as a possible predictor of bleomycin-induced pulmonary toxicity. *Jpn J Clin Oncol.* 1998;28(9): 546–550.
61. Sikdar T, MacVicar D, Husband JE. Pneumomediastinum complicating bleomycin related lung damage. *Br J Radiol.* 1998;71(851):1202–1204.
62. White DA, et al. Acute chest pain syndrome during bleomycin infusions. *Cancer.* 1987;59(9):1582–1585.
63. Maher J, Daly PA. Severe bleomycin lung toxicity: reversal with high dose corticosteroids. *Thorax.* 1993;48(1):92–94.
64. Conaghan PG, et al. Hazards of low dose methotrexate. *Aust N Z J Med.* 1995;25(6):670–673.
65. Cronstein BN, Molecular therapeutics. Methotrexate and its mechanism of action. *Arthritis Rheum.* 1996;39(12):1951–1960.
66. Lynch JP, 3rd, McCune WJ. Immunosuppressive and cytotoxic pharmacotherapy for pulmonary disorders. *Am J Respir Crit Care Med.* 1997;155(2):395–420.
67. Morice AH, Lai WK. Fatal varicella zoster infection in a severe steroid dependent asthmatic patient receiving methotrexate. *Thorax.* 1995;50(11):1221–1222.
68. Hilliquin P, et al. Occurrence of pulmonary complications during methotrexate therapy in rheumatoid arthritis. *Br J Rheumatol.* 1996;35(5):441–445.
69. Weinblatt ME. Methotrexate in rheumatoid arthritis: toxicity issues. *Br J Rheumatol.* 1996;35(5):403–405.
70. Golden MR, et al. The relationship of preexisting lung disease to the development of methotrexate pneumonitis in patients with rheumatoid arthritis. *J Rheumatol.* 1995;22(6):1043–1047.
71. Kremer JM, et al. Clinical, laboratory, radiographic, and histopathologic features of methotrexate-associated lung injury in patients with rheumatoid arthritis: A multicenter study with literature review. *Arthritis Rheum.* 1997;40(10):1829–1837.
72. Carroll GJ, et al. Incidence, prevalence and possible risk factors for pneumonitis in patients with rheumatoid arthritis receiving methotrexate. *J Rheumatol.* 1994;21(1):51–54.
73. Hassell A, Dawes P. Serious problems with methotrexate? *Br J Rheumatol.* 1994;33(11):1001–1002.
74. St Clair EW, Rice JR, Snyderman R. Pneumonitis complicating low-dose methotrexate therapy in rheumatoid arthritis. *Arch Intern Med.* 1985;145(11):2035–2038.
75. Searles G, McKendry RJ. Methotrexate pneumonitis in rheumatoid arthritis: Potential risk factors. Four case reports and a review of the literature. *J Rheumatol.* 1987;14(6):1164–1171.
76. Beyeler C, et al. Pulmonary function in rheumatoid arthritis treated with low-dose methotrexate: A longitudinal study. *Br J Rheumatol.* 1996;35(5):446–452.
77. Wall MA, et al. Lung function in adolescents receiving high-dose methotrexate. *Pediatrics.* 1979;63(5):741–746.
78. Dijkmans BA. Folate supplementation and methotrexate. *Br J Rheumatol.* 1995;34(12):1172–1174.
79. Morgan SL, et al. Supplementation with folic acid during methotrexate therapy for rheumatoid arthritis. A double-blind, placebo-controlled trial. *Ann Intern Med.* 1994;121(11):833–841.
80. Lane SD, et al. Fatal interstitial pneumonitis following high-dose intermittent chlorambucil therapy for chronic lymphocyte leukemia. *Cancer.* 1981;47(1):32–36.
81. Rosner V, et al. Contribution of bronchoalveolar lavage and transbronchial biopsy to diagnosis and prognosis of drug-induced pneumopathies. *Rev Pneumol Clin.* 1995;51(5): 269–274.
82. Crestani B, et al. Chlorambucil-associated pneumonitis. *Chest.* 1994;105(2):634–636.
83. Tomlinson J, et al. Interstitial pneumonitis following mitoxantrone, chlorambucil and prednisolone (MCP) chemotherapy. *Clin Oncol (R Coll Radiol).* 1999;11(3):184–186.
84. Verweij J, Pinedo HM. Mitomycin C: Mechanism of action, usefulness and limitations. *Anticancer Drugs.* 1990;1(1):5–13.
85. Folman RS. Experience with mitomycin in the treatment of non-small cell lung cancer. *Oncology.* 1993;50(Suppl 1):24–30.
86. Orwoll ES, Kiessling PJ, Patterson JR. Interstitial pneumonia from mitomycin. *Ann Intern Med.* 1978;89(3):352–355.
87. Castro M, et al. A prospective study of pulmonary function in patients receiving mitomycin. *Chest.* 1996;109(4):939–944.
88. Linette DC, McGee KH, McFarland JA. Mitomycin-induced pulmonary toxicity: Case report and review of the literature. *Ann Pharmacother.* 1992;26(4):481–484.
89. Kris MG, et al. Dyspnea following vinblastine or vindesine administration in patients receiving mitomycin plus vinca alkaloid combination therapy. *Cancer Treat Rep.* 1984;68(7–8):1029–1031.
90. Luedke D, et al. Mitomycin C and vindesine associated pulmonary toxicity with variable clinical expression. *Cancer.* 1985;55(3):542–545.

91. Rivera MP, et al. Syndrome of acute dyspnea related to combined mitomycin plus vinca alkaloid chemotherapy. *Am J Clin Oncol.* 1995;18(3):245–250.

92. McCarthy JT, Staats BA. Pulmonary hypertension, hemolytic anemia, and renal failure. A mitomycin-associated syndrome. *Chest.* 1986;89(4):608–611.

93. Verweij J, et al. Prospective study on the dose relationship of mitomycin C-induced interstitial pneumonitis. *Cancer.* 1987;60(4):756–761.

94. Chang AY, et al. Pulmonary toxicity induced by mitomycin C is highly responsive to glucocorticoids. *Cancer.* 1986;57(12):2285–2290.

95. Okuno SH, Frytak S. Mitomycin lung toxicity. Acute and chronic phases. *Am J Clin Oncol.* 1997;20(3):282–284.

96. Selker RG, et al. 1,3-Bis(2-chloroethyl)-1-nitrosourea (BCNU)-induced pulmonary fibrosis. *Neurosurgery.* 1980;7(6): 560–565.

97. Weiss RB, Poster DS, Penta JS. The nitrosoureas and pulmonary toxicity. *Cancer Treat Rev.* 1981;8(2):111–125.

98. Frankovich J, et al. High-dose therapy and autologous hematopoietic cell transplantation in children with primary refractory and relapsed Hodgkin's disease: Atopy predicts idiopathic diffuse lung injury syndromes. *Biol Blood Marrow Transplant.* 2001;7(1):49–57.

99. Wong R, et al. Idiopathic pneumonia syndrome after high-dose chemotherapy and autologous hematopoietic stem cell transplantation for high-risk breast cancer. *Bone Marrow Transplant.* 2003;31(12):1157–1163.

100. Cao TM, et al. Pulmonary toxicity syndrome in breast cancer patients undergoing BCNU-containing high-dose chemotherapy and autologous hematopoietic cell transplantation. *Biol Blood Marrow Transplant.* 2000;6(4):387–394.

101. Parish JM, Muhm JR, Leslie KO. Upper lobe pulmonary fibrosis associated with high-dose chemotherapy containing BCNU for bone marrow transplantation. *Mayo Clin Proc.* 2003;78(5):630–634.

102. Lind PA, et al. Predictors for pneumonitis during locoregional radiotherapy in high-risk patients with breast carcinoma treated with high-dose chemotherapy and stem-cell rescue. *Cancer.* 2002;94(11):2821–2829.

103. Rubio C, et al. Idiopathic pneumonia syndrome after high-dose chemotherapy for relapsed Hodgkin's disease. *Br J Cancer.* 1997;75(7):1044–1048.

104. Schmitz N, Diehl V. Carmustine and the lungs. *Lancet.* 1997;349(9067):1712–1713.

105. O'Driscoll BR, et al. Active lung fibrosis up to 17 years after chemotherapy with carmustine (BCNU) in childhood. *N Engl J Med.* 1990;323(6):378–382.

106. O'Driscoll BR, et al. Late carmustine lung fibrosis. Age at treatment may influence severity and survival. *Chest.* 1995;107(5):1355–1357.

107. Malik SW, et al. Lung toxicity associated with cyclophosphamide use. Two distinct patterns. *Am J Respir Crit Care Med.* 1996;154(6 Pt 1):1851–1856.

108. Segura A, et al. Pulmonary fibrosis induced by cyclophosphamide. *Ann Pharmacother.* 2001;35(7–8):894–897.

109. Hamada K, et al. Cyclophosphamide-induced late-onset lung disease. *Intern Med.* 2003;42(1):82–87.

110. Cohen EE, et al. Phase II trial of ZD1839 in recurrent or metastatic squamous cell carcinoma of the head and neck. *J Clin Oncol.* 2003;21(10):1980–1987.

111. Culy CR, Faulds D. Gefitinib. *Drugs.* 2002;62(15):2237–2248; discussion 2249–2250.

112. Fukuoka M, et al. Multi-institutional randomized phase II trial of gefitinib for previously treated patients with advanced non-small-cell lung cancer (The IDEAL 1 Trial) (corrected). *J Clin Oncol.* 2003;21(12):2237–2246.

113. Hotta K, et al. Interstitial lung disease in Japanese patients with non-small cell lung cancer receiving gefitinib: An analysis of risk factors and treatment outcomes in Okayama Lung Cancer Study Group. *Cancer J.* 2005;11(5):417–424.

114. Thomas AL, et al. Gemcitabine and paclitaxel associated pneumonitis in non-small cell lung cancer: Report of a phase I/II dose-escalating study. *Eur J Cancer.* 2000;36(18): 2329–2334.

115. Androulakis N, et al. Salvage treatment with paclitaxel and gemcitabine for patients with non-small-cell lung cancer after cisplatin- or docetaxel-based chemotherapy: a multicenter phase II study. *Ann Oncol.* 1998;9(10):1127–1130.

116. Dunsford ML, et al. Severe pulmonary toxicity in patients treated with a combination of docetaxel and gemcitabine for metastatic transitional cell carcinoma. *Ann Oncol.* 1999;10(8):943–947.

117. Mollman JE, et al. Cisplatin neuropathy. Risk factors, prognosis, and protection by WR-2721. *Cancer.* 1988;61(11):2192–2195.

118. Siegal T, Haim N. Cisplatin-induced peripheral neuropathy. Frequent off-therapy deterioration, demyelinating syndromes, and muscle cramps. *Cancer.* 1990;66(6):1117–1123.

119. van der Hoop RG, et al. Prevention of cisplatin neurotoxicity with an ACTH(4-9) analogue in patients with ovarian cancer. *N Engl J Med.* 1990;322(2):89–94.

120. von Schlippe M, Fowler CJ, Harland SJ. Cisplatin neurotoxicity in the treatment of metastatic germ cell tumour: Time course and prognosis. *Br J Cancer.* 2001;85(6):823–826.

121. Posner JB. *Side Effects of Chemotherapy; Neurologic Complications of Cancer.* Philadelphia: FA Davis; 1995.

122. Rademaker-Lakhai JM, et al. Relationship between cisplatin administration and the development of ototoxicity. *J Clin Oncol.* 2006;24(6):918–924.

123. Low WK, et al. Sensorineural hearing loss after radiotherapy and chemoradiotherapy: A single, blinded, randomized study. *J Clin Oncol.* 2006;24(12):1904–1909.

124. Heinzlef O, Lotz JP, Roullet E. Severe neuropathy after high dose carboplatin in three patients receiving multidrug chemotherapy. *J Neurol Neurosurg Psychiatry.* 1998;64(5): 667–669.

125. Stewart DJ, et al. Phase I study of intracarotid administration of carboplatin. *Neurosurgery.* 1992;30(4):512–516; discussion 516–517.

126. Gamelin E, et al. Clinical aspects and molecular basis of oxaliplatin neurotoxicity: Current management and development of preventive measures. *Semin Oncol.* 2002;29(5 Suppl 15):21–33.

127. Lehky TJ, et al. Oxaliplatin-induced neurotoxicity: acute hyperexcitability and chronic neuropathy. *Muscle Nerve.* 2004;29(3):387–392.

128. Wilson RH, et al. Acute oxaliplatin-induced peripheral nerve hyperexcitability. *J Clin Oncol.* 2002;20(7):1767–1774.

129. Cassidy J, Misset JL. Oxaliplatin-related side-effects: characteristics and management. *Semin Oncol.* 2002;29(5 Suppl 15):11–20.

130. Geiser CF, et al. Adverse effects of intrathecal methotrexate in children with acute leukemia in remission. *Blood.* 1975;45(2):189–195.

131. Phillips PC. Methotrexate toxicity. In: Rottenberg DA, ed. *Neurological Complications of Cancer Treatment.* Boston: Butterworth-Heinmann; 1991.

132. Gagliano RG, Costanzi JJ. Paraplegia following intrathecal methotrexate: Report of a case and review of the literature. *Cancer.* 1976;37(4):1663–1668.

133. Walker RW, et al. Transient cerebral dysfunction secondary to high-dose methotrexate. *J Clin Oncol.* 1986;4(12): 1845–1850.

134. Freilich RJ, et al. Motor neuropathy due to docetaxel and paclitaxel. *Neurology.* 1996;47(1):115–118.

135. Lee JJ, Swain SM. Peripheral neuropathy induced by microtubule-stabilizing agents. *J Clin Oncol.* 2006;24(10):1633–1642.

136. Akerley W, 3rd. Paclitaxel in advanced non-small cell lung cancer: An alternative high-dose weekly schedule. *Chest.* 2000;117(4 Suppl 1):152S–155S.

137. Perry JR, Warner E. Transient encephalopathy after paclitaxel (Taxol) infusion. *Neurology.* 1996;46(6):1596–1599.

138. Postma TJ, et al. Paclitaxel-induced neuropathy. *Ann Oncol.* 1995;6(5):489–494.

139. Piccart MJ, et al. Randomized intergroup trial of cisplatin-paclitaxel versus cisplatin-cyclophosphamide in women with advanced epithelial ovarian cancer: Three-year results. *J Natl Cancer Inst*. 2000;92(9):699–708.

140. Smith A, Rosenfeld S, Dropcho E, et al. High-dose thiotepa with hematopoietic reconstitution for recurrent aggressive oligodendroglioma (abstract). *Am Soc Clin Oncol*. 1997.

141. van den Bent MJ, et al. Lhermitte's sign following chemotherapy with docetaxel. *Neurology*. 1998;50(2):563–564.

142. Tosi P, et al. Neurological toxicity of long-term (>1 yr) thalidomide therapy in patients with multiple myeloma. *Eur J Haematol*. 2005;74(3):212–216.

143. Isoardo G, et al. Thalidomide neuropathy: clinical, electrophysiological and neuroradiological features. *Acta Neurol Scand*. 2004;109(3):188–193.

144. Clark TE, et al. Thalomid (Thalidomide) capsules: a review of the first 18 months of spontaneous postmarketing adverse event surveillance, including off-label prescribing. *Drug Saf*. 2001;24(2):87–117.

145. Richardson PG, et al. A randomized phase 2 study of lenalidomide therapy for patients with relapsed or relapsed and refractory multiple myeloma. *Blood*. 2006;108(10):3458–3464.

146. Richardson PG, et al. A phase 2 study of bortezomib in relapsed, refractory myeloma. *N Engl J Med*. 2003;348(26): 2609–2617.

147. Postma TJ, Heimans JJ. Chemotherapy-induced peripheral neuropathy. In: Vecht CJ, ed. *Handbook of Clinical Neurology*. Amsterdam: Elsevier Science; 1998:459.

148. Verstappen CC, et al. Dose-related vincristine-induced peripheral neuropathy with unexpected off-therapy worsening. *Neurology*. 2005;64(6):1076–1077.

149. McLeod JG, Penny R. Vincristine neuropathy: An electrophysiological and histological study. *J Neurol Neurosurg Psychiatry*. 1969;32(4):297–304.

150. Legha SS. Vincristine neurotoxicity. Pathophysiology and management. *Med Toxicol*. 1986;1(6):421–427.

151. Robertson GL, Bhoopalam N, Zelkowitz LJ. Vincristine neurotoxicity and abnormal secretion of antidiuretic hormone. *Arch Intern Med*. 1973;132(5):717–720.

152. Forsyth PA, Cascino TL. Neurologic complications of chemotherapy. In: Wiley RG, ed. *Neurologic Complications of Cancer*. New York: Marcel Dekker; 1995.

153. Paleologos N. Complications of chemotherapy. In: Biller J, ed. *Iatrogenic Neurology*. Boston: Butterworth-Heinemann; 1998:241.

154. Fazeny B, et al. Vinorelbine-induced neurotoxicity in patients with advanced breast cancer pretreated with paclitaxel—a phase II study. *Cancer Chemother Pharmacol*. 1996;39 (1–2):150–156.

155. Phillips PC, Reinhard CS. Antipyrimidene neurotoxicity: Cytosine arabinoside and 5-fluorouracil. In: Rottenberg DA, et al., eds. *Neurological Complications of Cancer Treatment*. Boston: Butterworth-Heinemann; 1991:97.

156. Smith GA, et al. High-dose cytarabine dose modification reduces the incidence of neurotoxicity in patients with renal insufficiency. *J Clin Oncol*. 1997;15(2):833–839.

157. Dunton SF, et al. Progressive ascending paralysis following administration of intrathecal and intravenous cytosine arabinoside. A Pediatric Oncology Group study. *Cancer*. 1986;57(6):1083–1088.

158. Brashear A, Siemers E. Focal dystonia after chemotherapy: A case series. *J Neurooncol*. 1997;34(2):163–167.

159. Stein ME, et al. A rare event of 5-fluorouracil-associated peripheral neuropathy: A report of two patients. *Am J Clin Oncol*. 1998;21(3):248–249.

160. Pirzada NA, Ali II, Dafer RM. Fluorouracil-induced neurotoxicity. *Ann Pharmacother*. 2000;34(1):35–38.

161. Ohara S, et al. Leukoencephalopathy induced by chemotherapy with tegafur, a 5-fluorouracil derivative. *Acta Neuropathol (Berl)*. 1998;96(5):527–531.

162. Meanwell CA, et al. Prediction of ifosfamide/mesna associated encephalopathy. *Eur J Cancer Clin Oncol*. 1986;22(7):815–819.

163. Pratt CB, et al. Ifosfamide neurotoxicity is related to previous cisplatin treatment for pediatric solid tumors. *J Clin Oncol*. 1990;8(8):1399–1401.

164. Yamaji S, et al. All-trans retinoic acid-induced multiple mononeuropathies. *Am J Hematol*. 1999;60(4):311.

165. Shapiro WR, Green SB. Reevaluating the efficacy of intra-arterial BCNU. *J Neurosurg*. 1987;66(2):313–315.

166. Shapiro WR, et al. A randomized comparison of intra-arterial versus intravenous BCNU, with or without intravenous 5-fluorouracil, for newly diagnosed patients with malignant glioma. *J Neurosurg*. 1992;76(5):772–781.

167. Rosenblum MK, et al. Fatal necrotizing encephalopathy complicating treatment of malignant gliomas with intra-arterial BCNU and irradiation: a pathological study. *J Neurooncol*. 1989;7(3):269–281.

168. Postma TJ, et al. Neurotoxicity of combination chemotherapy with procarbazine, CCNU and vincristine (PCV) for recurrent glioma. *J Neurooncol*. 1998;38(1):69–75.

169. Macdonald DR. Neurologic complications of chemotherapy. *Neurol Clin*. 1991;9(4):955–967.

170. Caraceni A, et al. Neurotoxicity of interferon-alpha in melanoma therapy: Results from a randomized controlled trial. *Cancer*. 1998;83(3):482–489.

171. Rohatiner AZ, et al. Central nervous system toxicity of interferon. *Br J Cancer*. 1983;47(3):419–422.

172. Meyers CA, Scheibel RS, Forman AD. Persistent neurotoxicity of systemically administered interferon-alpha. *Neurology*. 1991;41(5):672–676.

173. Rutkove SB. An unusual axonal polyneuropathy induced by low-dose interferon alfa-2a. *Arch Neurol*. 1997;54(7):907–908.

174. Delattre J, Vega F, Chen Q. Neurologic complications of immunotherapy. In: Wiley RG, ed. *Neurologic Complications of Cancer*. Marcel Dekker; 1995.

175. Hensley ML, et al. Risk factors for severe neuropsychiatric toxicity in patients receiving interferon alfa-2b and low-dose cytarabine for chronic myelogenous leukemia: Analysis of Cancer and Leukemia Group B 9013. *J Clin Oncol*. 2000;18(6):1301–1308.

176. Meyers CA, et al. Neurotoxicity of intraventricularly administered alpha-interferon for leptomeningeal disease. *Cancer*. 1991;68(1):88–92.

177. Denicoff KD, et al. The neuropsychiatric effects of treatment with interleukin-2 and lymphokine-activated killer cells. *Ann Intern Med*. 1987;107(3):293–300.

178. Bernard JT, et al. Transient focal neurologic deficits complicating interleukin-2 therapy. *Neurology*. 1990;40(1): 154–155.

179. Loh FL, et al. Brachial plexopathy associated with interleukin-2 therapy. *Neurology*. 1992;42(2):462–463.

180. Allen JA, Adlakha A, Bergethon PR. Reversible posterior leukoencephalopathy syndrome after bevacizumab/FOLFIRI regimen for metastatic colon cancer. *Arch Neurol*. 2006;63(10):1475–1478.

181. Ozcan C, Wong SJ, Hari P. Reversible posterior leukoencephalopathy syndrome and bevacizumab. *N Engl J Med*. 2006;354(9):980–982; discussion 980–982.

182. Dormann AJ, et al. Gemcitabine-associated autonomic neuropathy. *Lancet*. 1998;351(9103):644.

183. Ardavanis AS, Ioannidis GN, Rigatos GA. Acute myopathy in a patient with lung adenocarcinoma treated with gemcitabine and docetaxel. *Anticancer Res*. 2005;25(1B):523–525.

184. Selleri C, et al. All-trans-retinoic acid (ATRA) responsive skin relapses of acute promyelocytic leukaemia followed by ATRA-induced pseudotumour cerebri. *Br J Haematol*. 1996;92(4):937–940.

185. Cheson BD, et al. Neurotoxicity of purine analogs: a review. *J Clin Oncol*. 1994;12(10):2216–2228.

186. Gonzalez H, et al. Progressive multifocal leukoencephalitis (PML) in three patients treated with standard-dose fludarabine (FAMP). *Hematol Cell Ther*. 1999;41(4):183–186.

187. Rao RD, et al. Efficacy of gabapentin in the management of chemotherapy-induced peripheral neuropathy: A phase 3

randomized, double-blind, placebo-controlled, crossover trial (N00C3). *Cancer.* 2007;110(9):2110–2118.

188. Lersch C, et al. Prevention of oxaliplatin-induced peripheral sensory neuropathy by carbamazepine in patients with advanced colorectal cancer. *Clin Colorectal Cancer.* 2002;2(1):54–58.

189. Saif MW, Hashmi S. Successful amelioration of oxaliplatin-induced hyperexcitability syndrome with the antiepileptic pregabalin in a patient with pancreatic cancer. *Cancer Chemother Pharmacol.* 2007.

190. Hilpert F, et al. Neuroprotection with amifostine in the first-line treatment of advanced ovarian cancer with carboplatin/paclitaxel-based chemotherapy—a double-blind, placebo-controlled, randomized phase II study from the Arbeitsgemeinschaft Gynakologische Onkologoie (AGO) Ovarian Cancer Study Group. *Support Care Cancer.* 2005;13(10):797–805.

191. Penz M, et al. Subcutaneous administration of amifostine: A promising therapeutic option in patients with oxaliplatin-related peripheral sensitive neuropathy. *Ann Oncol.* 2001;12(3):421–422.

192. Maestri A, et al. A pilot study on the effect of acetyl-L-carnitine in paclitaxel- and cisplatin-induced peripheral neuropathy. *Tumori.* 2005;91(2):135–138.

193. Muto O, et al. Reduction of oxaliplatin-related neurotoxicity by calcium and magnesium infusions. *Gan To Kagaku Ryoho.* 2007;34(4):579–581.

194. Durand JP, Brezault C, Goldwasser F. Protection against oxaliplatin acute neurosensory toxicity by venlafaxine. *Anticancer Drugs.* 2003;14(6):423–425.

195. Ettinger LJ, et al. A phase II study of carboplatin in children with recurrent or progressive solid tumors. A report from the Children's Cancer Group. *Cancer.* 1994;73(4):1297–1301.

196. Ekhart C, et al. Flat dosing of carboplatin is justified in adult patients with normal renal function. *Clin Cancer Res.* 2006;12(21):6502–6508.

197. Bressler RB, Huston DP. Water intoxication following moderate-dose intravenous cyclophosphamide. *Arch Intern Med.* 1985;145(3):548–549.

198. Tscherning C, et al. Recurrent renal salt wasting in a child treated with carboplatin and etoposide. *Cancer.* 1994;73(6):1761–1763.

199. McDonald BR, et al. Acute renal failure associated with the use of intraperitoneal carboplatin: A report of two cases and review of the literature. *Am J Med.* 1991;90(3):386–391.

200. Vogelzang NJ. Nephrotoxicity from chemotherapy: prevention and management. *Oncology (Williston Park).* 1991;5(10):97–102, 105; discussion: 105, 109–111.

201. Levi F, et al. Oxaliplatin: Pharmacokinetics and chronopharmacological aspects. *Clin Pharmacokinet.* 2000;38(1):1–21.

202. Chollet P, et al. Single agent activity of oxaliplatin in heavily pretreated advanced epithelial ovarian cancer. *Ann Oncol.* 1996;7(10):1065–1070.

203. DeFronzo RA, et al. Proceedings: Cyclophosphamide and the kidney. *Cancer.* 1974;33(2):483–491.

204. Harmon WE, et al. Chronic renal failure in children treated with methyl CCNU. *N Engl J Med.* 1979;300(21):1200–1203.

205. Sponzo RW, DeVita VT, Oliverio VT. Physiologic disposition of 1-(2-chloroethyl)-3-cyclohexyl-1-nitrosourea (CCNU) and 1-(2-chloroethyl)-3-(4-methyl cyclohexyl)-1-nitrosourea (Me CCNU) in man. *Cancer.* 1973;31(5):1154–1156.

206. Price TM, et al. Renal failure and hemolytic anemia associated with mitomycin C. A case report. *Cancer,* 1985;55(1):51–56.

207. Groff JA, et al. Endotheliopathy: A continuum of hemolytic uremic syndrome due to mitomycin therapy. *Am J Kidney Dis.* 1997;29(2):280–284.

208. Chang AY, et al. Phase II evaluation of a combination of mitomycin C, vincristine, and cisplatin in advanced non-small cell lung cancer. *Cancer.* 1986;57(1):54–59.

209. Aronoff GM, et al. *Drug Prescribing in Renal Failure: Dosing Guidelines for Adults.* 4th ed. American College of Physicians; 2002.

210. Howell SB, Carmody J. Changes in glomerular filtration rate associated with high-dose methotrexate therapy in adults. *Cancer Treat Rep.* 1977;61(7):1389–1391.

211. Schilsky R. Renal and metabolic toxicities of cancer treatment. In: Perry M, Yarbro JW, eds. *Toxicity of Chemotherapy.* Grune & Stratton; 1984.

212. Bowyer GW, Davies TW. Methotrexate toxicity associated with an ileal conduit. *Br J Urol.* 1987;60(6):592.

213. Cutting HO. Inappropriate secretion of antidiuretic hormone secondary to vincristine therapy. *Am J Med.* 1971;51(2):269–271.

214. O'Reilly S, et al. Phase I and pharmacologic study of topotecan in patients with impaired renal function. *J Clin Oncol.* 1996;14(12):3062–3073.

215. Furuya Y, et al. Pharmacokinetics of paclitaxel and carboplatin in a hemodialysis patient with metastatic urothelial carcinoma—a case report. *Gan To Kagaku Ryoho.* 2003;30(7):1017–1020.

216. Menconi M, et al. Docetaxel pharmacokinetics with pre- and post-dialysis administration in a hemodyalized patient. *Chemotherapy.* 2006;52(3):147–150.

217. Sandler AB, Johnson DH, Herbst RS. Anti-vascular endothelial growth factor monoclonals in non-small cell lung cancer. *Clin Cancer Res.* 2004;10(12 Pt 2):4258s–4262s.

218. Belldegrun A, et al. Effects of interleukin-2 on renal function in patients receiving immunotherapy for advanced cancer. *Ann Intern Med.* 1987;106(6):817–822.

219. Selby P, et al. Nephrotic syndrome during treatment with interferon. *Br Med J (Clin Res Ed).* 1985;290(6476):1180.

220. Zuber J, et al. Alpha-interferon-associated thrombotic microangiopathy: A clinicopathologic study of 8 patients and review of the literature. *Medicine (Baltimore).* 2002;81(4):321–331.

221. Ault BH, et al. Acute renal failure during therapy with recombinant human gamma interferon. *N Engl J Med.* 1988;319(21):1397–1400.

222. Hamblin T. Disease and its management in chronic lymphocytic leukemia. In: Cheson B, ed. *Chronic Lymphoid Leukemias.* New York: Marcel Dekker; 2001.

223. Schwartzentruber DJ, et al. Thyroid dysfunction associated with immunotherapy for patients with cancer. *Cancer.* 1991;68(11):2384–2390.

224. Vialettes B, et al. Incidence rate and risk factors for thyroid dysfunction during recombinant interleukin-2 therapy in advanced malignancies. *Acta Endocrinol (Copenh).* 1993;129(1):31–38.

225. Rini BI, et al. Hypothyroidism in patients with metastatic renal cell carcinoma treated with sunitinib. *J Natl Cancer Inst.* 2007;99(1):81–83.

226. Desai J, et al. Hypothyroidism after sunitinib treatment for patients with gastrointestinal stromal tumors. *Ann Intern Med.* 2006;145(9):660–664.

227. Bussel JB, Cunningham-Rundles C, Abraham C. Intravenous treatment of autoimmune hemolytic anemia with very high dose gammaglobulin. *Vox Sang.* 1986;51(4):264–269.

228. Del Poeta G, et al. The addition of rituximab to fludarabine improves clinical outcome in untreated patients with ZAP-70-negative chronic lymphocytic leukemia. *Cancer.* 2005;104(12):2743–2752.

229. Hegde UP, et al. Rituximab treatment of refractory fludarabine-associated immune thrombocytopenia in chronic lymphocytic leukemia. *Blood.* 2002;100(6):2260–2262.

230. Loprinzi CL, Duffy J, Ingle JN. Postchemotherapy rheumatism. *J Clin Oncol.* 1993;11(4):768–770.

231. Donnellan PP, et al. Aromatase inhibitors and arthralgia. *J Clin Oncol.* 2001;19(10):2767.

232. Howell A, et al. Results of the ATAC (Arimidex, Tamoxifen, Alone or in Combination) trial after completion of 5 years' adjuvant treatment for breast cancer. *Lancet.* 2005;365(9453):60–62.

233. Smith IE, Dowsett M. Aromatase inhibitors in breast cancer. *N Engl J Med.* 2003;348(24):2431–2442.

234. Eisenhauer EA, et al. European-Canadian randomized trial of paclitaxel in relapsed ovarian cancer: High-dose versus low-dose and long versus short infusion. *J Clin Oncol.* 1994;12(12):2654–2666.

235. Garrison JA, et al. Myalgias and arthralgias associated with paclitaxel. *Oncology (Williston Park).* 2003;17(2):271–277; discussion 281–282, 286–288.

236. Gelmon K. The taxoids: paclitaxel and docetaxel. *Lancet.* 1994;344(8932):1267–1272.

237. McGuire WP, et al. Taxol: A Unique Antineoplastic Agent with Significant Activity in Advanced Ovarian Epithelial Neoplasms. *Ann Intern Med.* 1989;111(4):273–279.

238. Rowinsky EK, et al. Phase I and pharmacologic study of paclitaxel and cisplatin with granulocyte colony-stimulating factor: Neuromuscular toxicity is dose-limiting. *J Clin Oncol.* 1993;11(10):2010–2020.

239. Rowinsky EK, Donehower RC. Paclitaxel (Taxol). *N Engl J Med.* 1995;332(15):1004–1014.

240. Nguyen VH, Lawrence HJ. Use of gabapentin in the prevention of taxane-induced arthralgias and myalgias. *J Clin Oncol.* 2004;22(9):1767–1769.

241. Ryberg M, et al. Epirubicin cardiotoxicity: An analysis of 469 patients with metastatic breast cancer. *J Clin Oncol.* 1998;16(11):3502–3508.

242. Ravry MJ. Cardiotoxicity of mitomycin C in man and animals. *Cancer Treat Rep.* 1979;63(4):555.

243. Clinical Trial and prescribing information. (cited; Available from: www.fda.gov/cder/foi/label/2005/021923lbl.pdf.

244. Motzer RJ, et al. Activity of SU11248, a multitargeted inhibitor of vascular endothelial growth factor receptor and platelet-derived growth factor receptor, in patients with metastatic renal cell carcinoma. *J Clin Oncol.* 2006;24(1):16–24.

245. Kerkela R, et al. Cardiotoxicity of the cancer therapeutic agent imatinib mesylate. *Nat Med.* 2006;12(8):908–916.

246. Mortimer JE, et al. A phase II randomized study comparing sequential and combined intraarterial cisplatin and radiation therapy in primary brain tumors. A Southwest Oncology Group study. *Cancer.* 1992;69(5):1220–1223.

247. Fossella FV, et al. Phase II study of docetaxel for recurrent or metastatic non-small-cell lung cancer. *J Clin Oncol.* 1994;12(6):1238–1244.

248. Gasser AB, Tieche M, Brunner KW. Neurologic and cardiac toxicity following iv application of methotrexate. *Cancer Treat Rep.* 1982;66(7):1561–1562.

249. Hermans C, et al. Pericarditis induced by high-dose cytosine arabinoside chemotherapy. *Ann Hematol.* 1997;75 (1–2):55–57.

250. Lenihan DJ, et al. Cardiac toxicity of alemtuzumab in patients with mycosis fungoides/Sezary syndrome. *Blood.* 2004;104(3):655–658.

251. House KW, Simon SR, Pugh RP. Chemotherapy-induced myocardial infarction in a young man with Hodgkin's disease. *Clin Cardiol.* 1992;15(2):122–125.

252. Schwarzer S, et al. Non-Q-wave myocardial infarction associated with bleomycin and etoposide chemotherapy. *Eur Heart J.* 1991;12(6):748–750.

253. Harris AL, Wong C. Myocardial ischaemia, radiotherapy, and vinblastine. *Lancet.* 1981;1(8223):787.

254. Kantor AF, et al. Are vinca alkaloids associated with myocardial infarction? *Lancet.* 1981;1(8229):1111.

255. Warrell RP, Jr, et al. Acute promyelocytic leukemia. *N Engl J Med.* 1993;329(3):177–189.

256. Yang JC, et al. A randomized trial of bevacizumab, an anti-vascular endothelial growth factor antibody, for metastatic renal cancer. *N Engl J Med.* 2003;349(5):427–434.

257. Weiss RB, et al. Hypersensitivity reactions from Taxol. *J Clin Oncol.* 1990;8(7):1263–1268.

258. Read WL, Mortimer JE, Picus J. Severe interstitial pneumonitis associated with docetaxel administration. *Cancer.* 2002;94(3):847–853.

259. Wang GS, Yang KY, Perng RP. Life-threatening hypersensitivity pneumonitis induced by docetaxel (taxotere). *Br J Cancer.* 2001;85(9):1247–1250.

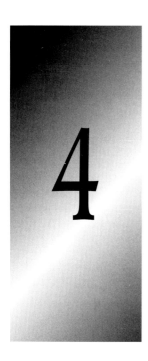

Principles of Immunotherapy

Guenther Koehne

The induction of a humoral and/or cellular immune response to antigens specifically expressed on malignant cells has been the ultimate goal in the approach to curing cancer or preventing its recurrence or development in patients at risk.

Historically, cancer therapy has included surgery, chemotherapy, and/or radiotherapy, either as a single-treatment approach or in combined treatment modalities. Complete surgical removal with negative margins remains a potentially curative approach for localized solid cancers. Also, a variety of solid tumors and hematologic malignancies can be cured by systemic cytotoxic chemotherapy. Adjuvant chemotherapy is the standard of care for breast cancer, colon cancer, and sarcomas, and chemotherapy is commonly given in combination with radiation therapy. High doses of chemotherapy for improved anticancer activity have been introduced, and require autologous stem cell support to shorten the interval of immune reconstitution afterward (1–4). This approach remains a treatment option for patients with relapsed indolent or diffuse large B-cell non-Hodgkin lymphoma (5–7) and relapsed Hodgkin disease, provided the tumor cells remain sensitive to chemotherapy at the time of relapse (8–10). This treatment of relapsed or refractory multiple myeloma has also resulted in an improved response rate and prolonged response duration (11–13).

After a high-dose myeloablative preparative regimen, allogeneic stem cell transplantations were traditionally performed for malignant hematologic malignancies in order to replace diseased bone marrow with stem cells from a healthy related or unrelated donor. Relapse rates following allogeneic stem cell transplantation were lower when acute or chronic graft-versus-host disease (GVHD) developed, and were greater when a syngeneic donor was used or T-cell depleted marrow transplantation was performed. This was evidence of an immunotherapeutic effect from allogeneic T lymphocytes that were transfused with the transplant or that developed after the engraftment occurred (14,15).

Significant progress in the development of cellular immunotherapeutic approaches occurred with patients who relapsed following allogeneic marrow transplant of chronic myelogenous leukemia using infusions of lymphocytes derived from the bone marrow donor (16–20) Consequently, improved laboratory-based methods permitted selective targeting of antigens that are expressed or overexpressed on malignant cell populations. Donor-derived antigen-specific T lymphocytes were generated for adoptive immunotherapeutic approaches in the treatment of minimal residual disease and relapse following an allogeneic marrow transplantation (21). Treatment of viral complications developing after an allograft, such as Epstein-Barr virus (EBV),-induced post-transplantation lymphoproliferative disorders (PTLDs), and cytomegalovirus (CMV) infections, refined the use and logistics of generating donor-derived, antigen-specific T lymphocytes for treatment of these diseases without inducing GVHD (22–24).

KEY POINTS

- Immunotherapies are rapidly evolving and will be increasingly integrated with standard therapies for the treatment of solid tumors and hematologic malignancies.
- The first proof of a graft-versus-leukemia effect resulted from the pioneering findings of Kolb, who demonstrated that patients who developed relapses of chronic myelogenous leukemia following an allogeneic marrow transplant were induced into durable molecular remissions by high doses of peripheral blood mononuclear cells derived from the original HLA-matched transplant.

- It is anticipated that natural killer cell–mediated immunotherapeutic approaches will be further developed and integrated into clinical trials to improve the outcome of hematological malignancies by allogeneic bone marrow transplantations.
- Monoclonal antibody-based therapies have emerged over the past decade for the treatment of hematological malignancies and solid tumors.
- The CD20 antigen is expressed on mature B cells and, therefore, on hematological malignancies derived from B lymphocytes, which can be targeted using rituximab as a single agent or in combination with chemotherapy.

Recently the immunotherapeutic effect of natural killer (NK) cells was advanced with the description of inhibitory and activating receptors (25,26). NK cells, mismatched for immunoglobulinlike receptors (KIRs) that are distinctly expressed on these cells, and HLA-class I molecules presented by recipient cells demonstrated NK-cell–mediated alloreactivity and enhanced NK-cell–mediated lysis of the recipient leukemic cell population. This resulted in improved overall survival in patients following haplotype mismatched and unrelated bone marrow transplantation (26–28). Results will soon be available from clinical trials integrating the NK-cell–mediated immune effect to improve marrow transplantation by use of KIR mismatched donors.

Monoclonal antibody-based therapy has increasingly played a role in the treatment of malignancies. The production of chimeric and humanized monoclonal antibodies has helped to overcome the generation of human antimouse antibodies, which resulted in rapid clearing and the need for multiple infusions of murine monoclonal antibodies. The anti-CD20 monoclonal antibody rituximab is administered as a single agent or in combination with systemic chemotherapy for the treatment of hematological malignancies (29,30). Radioimmunoconjugates of anti-CD20 monoclonal antibodies labeled with yttrium-90 or iodine-131 are being given for relapsed or refractory non-Hodgkin lymphomas (31–33). The CD33 antigen is expressed on myeloid cells and by the leukemic blasts of at least 90% of patients with acute myelogenous leukemia. Several trials targeting the antigen by humanized anti-CD33 monoclonal antibodies that are either unmodified or conjugated to radioisotopes, such as iodine-131 or yttrium-90, or the cell toxin calicheamicin, have been initiated to treat acute

myeloid leukemias or are integrated into a myeloablative conditioning regimen for allogeneic marrow transplants (34–37).

Advances in the identification of tumor-associated antigens and their conjugation to adjuvants have led to cancer vaccines with the potential to induce both cellular and/or humoral immune responses. Pioneering work by Levy et al. established the principle of generating specific immune responses against unique tumor-derived antigens after subcutaneous injections of custom-made vaccines. In these studies, the immunoglobulin idiotype, a unique amino acid sequence contained within the variable region of the immunoglobulin of B-cell non-Hodgkin lymphoma, was identified and complexed with adjuvant before injection to successfully induce anti-idiotype antibody responses (38–40). Advances in utilizing deoxyribonucleic acid (DNA) vaccines or cell based-vaccine strategies have led to clinical trials to assess the immune responses and potential clinical benefits in hematological malignancies and solid tumors (41–43). The enhancement of immune responses from administration of cancer vaccines is currently being addressed following immune manipulation with the blockade of cytotoxic T-lymphocyte–associated antigen (CTLA)-4, which is expressed on the cell surface of T lymphocytes with increased activation (44,45). Studies of the selective depletion of T regulatory cells, which have a capacity for inhibiting T-cell–mediated antitumor effects, are under way in order to improve cancer vaccine–induced immune responses (46).

This chapter describes current immunotherapeutic approaches for the treatment of malignancies. It does not claim to describe all experimental studies under investigation or to provide a complete overview of completed or currently ongoing clinical trials.

PRINCIPLES OF CELLULAR IMMUNE THERAPY

Adoptive Transfer of Donor Lymphocytes

First proof of a graft-versus-leukemia (GVL) effect resulted from the pioneering findings of Kolb et al. (16) and was later confirmed by several centers (17–20). Patients who developed relapses of chronic myelogenous leukemia (CML) following an allogeneic marrow transplant were induced into durable molecular remissions by high doses of peripheral blood mononuclear cells derived from the original HLA-matched transplant. These studies provided the first evidence that enhanced resistance to leukemia, accrued through a marrow allograft by comparisons of relapse rates following syngeneic vs HLA-matched allogeneic transplants, was indeed mediated by cells in the donor graft (14,47). The fact that more than 70% of patients with relapsed chronic myelogenous leukemia could be induced into remission by this approach altered the field of allogeneic bone marrow transplantation (17,48). While the specific effector cells that induced these remissions and the chronic myelogenous leukemia cells targeted by these cells remain only partially characterized, increasing evidence implicates alloreactive donor T cells as the principal mediators of adoptively transferred resistance to CML. More than 75% of the patients responding to these donor leukocyte infusions (DLIs) also developed GVHD. This was initially taken as evidence of the antileukemic effects of GVHD, which had also been proposed to explain the lower relapse rates among patients with acute or chronic GVHD following marrow allografts (15). Evidence of a separate GVL effect mediated by donor-derived, leukemia-specific T lymphocytes was provided by Falkenburg et al. (21). This study generated CD4+ T-cell clones on the basis of their capacity to lyse host leukemic cells and to inhibit the growth of (Philadelphia) Ph+CD34+ host CML precursors, and treated patients with CML relapse in the accelerated post-transplant phase who had failed to respond to donor leukocyte infusions. Three infusions providing a total of 3.2×10^9 total T cells from these T-cell lines induced molecular remission and reestablished complete donor chimerism (21).

Donor leukocyte infusions have also been attempted for AML relapses following allogeneic marrow transplants. Antileukemic effects of DLI have been less consistently observed and are often less durable than those in patients treated for CML. Results of donor leukocyte infusions at centers in the European Organization for Research and Treatment of Cancer (EORTC) (17) and other centers in the United States (14) were reported, with only 20%–29% of patients treated for AML relapses and 30% treated for recurrences of myelodysplastic syndrome (MDS) achieving complete remissions. While the majority of patients achieving remission also developed GVHD, a proportion of patients who developed clinically significant GVHD after DLI have not achieved AML remissions. Even patients with AML in relapse after initial treatment with chemotherapy to decrease tumor load, and who were subsequently treated with donor leukocyte infusions, achieved only marginally better response rates. In addition, most patients who achieved remissions following DLI relapsed within one to two years after treatment (49).

Apparent differences in sensitivity to DLI manifested by AML or acute lymphoblastic leukemia (ALL) and CML have been explained by quantitative differences in tumor load, the number of clonogenic AML or ALL blasts vs clonogenic Ph+ progenitors of chronic-phase CML present at clinical relapse, and differences in the expansion rate of these cells (49). Expansion of AML blasts appears to be rapid, and could outnumber the expansion rate of leukemia-reactive effector cells administered in the infusions of $1-5 \times 10^8$ donor T cells/kg. In addition, clinical responses are rarely observed before 8–12 weeks after infusion in CML post-DLI, and other features of AML may limit the capacity of these cells to induce a significant donor T-cell response. A characteristic feature of human AMLs and ALLs is their failure to express the costimulatory molecules B7.1 and B7.2, therefore likely limiting their capacity to elicit an immune response. Cardoso et al. (50) and others (51) showed that such B7.1 neg AML and ALL cells are incapable of inducing a proliferative or cytotoxic T-cell response in mixed leukocyte cultures with autologous HLA-matched or fully allogeneic T cells. The T cells emerging after sensitization with these B7.1 leukemic blasts appear to be anergized, are relatively refractory to restimulation, and are therefore incapable of mounting a significant antileukemic response.

Several groups have explored strategies to enhance the capacity of leukemic cells to present leukemia-associated antigens to autologous T cells and thereby to stimulate an antileukemic response. Choudhury et al. (52), confirmed by Smit et al. (53), described that Ph+CD34+ CML progenitor cells can be induced by granulocyte-microphage colony-stimulating factor (GM-CSF), tumor necrosis factor (TNF), and IL-4 to differentiate into dendritic cells capable of presenting antigens and eliciting an autologous leukemia-specific CD8+ T-cell–mediated cytotoxic response. Subsequent studies suggested that AML blasts and Ph+ B-ALL blasts may also be induced to form dendritic cells bearing appropriate costimulatory molecules for induction of a T-cell response (54,55). The direct modification of the antigen-presenting capacity of acute leukemic blasts has been evaluated by Dunussi-Joannnopoulos et al. (56) and Mutis et al. (57), describing that transient transfection of B7.1⁻ murine and human AML cells with a gene encoding human B7.1 permits the generation of T cells reactive against B7.1⁻ unmodified leukemic cells. In addition, culturing of human B7.1⁻ ALL cells on monolayers of murine 3T3 fibroblasts transduced to express CD40 ligand induced the expression of B7.1 on leukemic cells. Sensitization of either allogeneic or autologous T cells with the B7.1-expressing ALL cells elicits a specific proliferative and cytotoxic T-cell response (58). Based on information from these studies and refined laboratory methodologies of cell cultures and cell expansion, the generation of polyclonal antigen-specific T cells and T-cell clones for adoptive transfer rapidly evolved.

Immunotherapeutic Approaches with Donor-Derived, Antigen-Specific T Lymphocytes

Adoptive immunotherapeutic approaches with donor-derived, antigen-specific T lymphocytes were established by the treatment of Epstein-Barr virus (EBV) post-transplantation proliferative disorders (PTLD), and cytomegalovirus (CMV) infections complicating allogeneic marrow transplantation (59–61). EBV-associated lymphomas grow rapidly—a potentially lethal complication of marrow and organ allografts, and the majority of EBV-PTLD are of donor origin. The risk of developing an EBV lymphoma increases in recipients of HLA-disparate related or unrelated unmodified marrow grafts receiving prolonged immunosuppression or T-cell depleted marrow transplants. In 1994, it was reported that infusions of small numbers of peripheral blood mononuclear cells (PBMC) derived from a seropositive marrow donor could induce durable and complete regression of EBV lymphomas as a complication of related or unrelated T-cell–depleted marrow grafts, but infusions of donor-derived peripheral blood mononuclear cells, even in small numbers, also transferred alloreactive T cells sufficient to cause severe or even lethal GVHD, particularly if the donor and host differ at one or more HLA alleles (61–63). Rooney et al. reported the successful treatment of patients with EBV lymphoma in recipients of HLA-mismatched allografts using infusions of donor-derived, EBV-specific cytotoxic lymphocytes without inducing GVHD (23,64). In a follow-up study, 39 recipients of unrelated bone marrows were treated with the prophylactic administration of donor-derived, EBV-specific T cells. None of these patients developed a lymphoproliferative disorder, and only one patient experienced mild worsening of a preexisting GVHD (24).

In allogeneic bone marrow transplants, reactivation of latent CMV remains a major cause of morbidity and mortality (60). The contribution of virus-specific CD8⁺ cytotoxic T cells to control CMV infections has been suggested by the correlation between the reconstitution of CMV virus-specific CD8⁺ cytotoxic T cells and protection of the transplanted host from infection.

The generation, selection, and adoptive transfer of viral-antigen–specific T-cell clones for cytomegalovirus reactivation after allogeneic transplant, as shown by Riddell et al. (22,65) by extended culture in vitro, can markedly reduce or eliminate the risk of GVHD following adoptive T-cell transfer, even in HLA-disparate hosts. Other groups have tested donor-derived T cells sensitized with autologous monocyte-derived dendritic cells loaded with a commercially produced lysate of CMV infection. First, Peggs et al. (66) reported on 16 patients who had developed CMV viremia detected by quantitative polymerase chain reaction (PCR)-based analysis of blood for CMV DNA, who were then treated with donor T cells sensitized with autologous monocyte-derived dendritic cells generated by culturing PBMC with GM-CSF, IL-4, and thereafter TNF-α, which were loaded with a CMV lysate. No toxicities were observed following single infusions of 1×10^5 T cells/kg. Three patients were noted to have grade 1 skin GVHD, which cleared with topical steroid treatment. Of the 16 patients, all 16 cleared CMV viremia, 8 without concurrent treatment with ganciclovir. A second series reported by Einsele et al. (67) described a group of 8 patients with CMV viremia, detected by reverse transcription (RT)-PCR analysis, that persisted despite treatment with ganciclovir. These patients were treated with donor-derived T cells sensitized with CMV cell lysate and expanded with CMV antigen. Despite the resistance to antiviral therapy, five out of seven evaluable patients cleared the viral infection after transfusion of $10^7/m^2$ CMV-specific T cells and remained negative thereafter by RT-PCR analyses.

Clinical trials incorporating adoptive immunotherapeutic approaches are emerging for the treatment of minimal residual diseases and relapse following allogeneic grafts. Strategies for generating leukemia-reactive T cells for adoptive therapy have focused on the generation of T cells specific for peptides encoded by genes uniquely or differentially expressed on leukemic cells. The Wilms tumor gene (WT-1) is such a gene of interest, initially identified as a gene mutated in a Wilms tumor of the kidney in children. The WT-1 gene is a tumor-suppressor gene encoding a zinc finger transcription factor, which binds early growth-factor gene promoters, such as platelet-derived growth factor A chain, colony-stimulating factor-1, transforming growth factor-b1, and insulinlike growth factor II (68,69). The expression of the WT-1 gene is restricted to a limited number of normal tissues, including fetal kidney, ovary, testis, spleen, hematopoietic precursors, and the mesothelial cell lining of visceral organs (70,71). The WT-1 gene is overexpressed in 70%–80% of adult and pediatric AML as well as Ph⁺ ALL and CML in blast crisis, and recent studies indicate that peptides derived from WT-1 proteins are immunogenic (72–74). Initial studies have shown that specific WT-1 encoded peptides have a high affinity for HLA-A*2401 and HLA-A*0201. These peptides can stimulate WT-1-specific HLA-A*2401 or HLA-A*0201–restricted cytotoxic T-lymphocytes, with the capacity to kill WT-1–expressing leukemic cell lines in the context of the appropriate HLA-class I molecule in vitro (75,76). In one study, a WT-1 peptide-specific T-cell clone lysed WT-1, expressing HLA-A*0201 leukemic cell lines, but did not lyse normal HLA-A*0201+ CD34+ progenitor cells (77). In these studies, T-cell responses were generated against the WT-1-derived nonamers $_{126-134}$RMFP-NAPYL and $_{187-195}$SLGEQQYSV. The authors' group demonstrated that human lymphocytes sensitized to HLA-A*0201 and HLA-A*2402–binding WT-1 peptides, loaded on autologous cytokine-activated monocytes or EBV-transformed B cells, yielded HLA-restricted, WT-1 peptide-specific cytotoxic T cells that lysed primary WT-1+ leukemic cells in vitro and in vivo. These WT-1 peptide-specific T cells also homed to and induced regression of WT-1+ leukemic xenografts bearing the appropriate restricting HLA alleles (78).

Proteinase-3 is a myeloid tissue-restricted 26 kDa protease expressed in azurophilic granules in normal myeloid cells but overexpressed in leukemia cells (79,80). Molldrem et al. demonstrated that cytotoxic T-cell lines could be generated against an HLA-A*0201–restricted proteinase 3-derived nonamer, PR1. These PR1-specific T cells induced specific lysis of CML cells and inhibited CML progenitors (81,82). Using HLA-A*0201-PR1–restricted major histocompatibility complex (MHC) tetramers, these investigators illustrated the presence of circulating PR1-specific cytotoxic T lymphocytes in 11 out of 12 patients who responded to IFN-α2b therapy, whereas nonresponders as well as healthy HLA-A*0201+ individuals did not show any peptide-specific T cells (83). Subsequently, a correlation between the presence of PR1-specific T cells and clinical responses after IFN-α2b therapy and allogeneic bone marrow transplantation provided further evidence of the involvement of T-cell immunity in the remission of chronic myelogenous leukemia (82). As a consequence of these observations, early clinical trials to vaccinate patients with myeloid leukemia or myelodysplastic syndrome against PR-1 and/or WT-1 have been initiated. Most of these trials are ongoing, and only limited results have been published (84,85).

Minor histocompatibility antigens (mHA) are derived from normal cellular proteins and are the result of normal genetic variations of the human genome in single nucleotide polymorphisms (SNPs), leading to differences in amino acid sequences of proteins between donor and host cells (86). The mHA are presented by self major histocompatibility complexes

(MHC), and can trigger allogeneic T lymphocytes to recognize these peptides as foreign, despite a complete MHC match after allogeneic transplantation (87–89). The recognition of mHA by donor T lymphocytes can induce severe GVHD (87,90), which becomes relevant in the HLA-identical but sex-mismatched transplant from a female donor to a male recipient (91). Several mHAs (eg, SMCY, UTY) are encoded by genes of the Y chromosome, which can trigger a T-cell response from a female donor. Allogeneic transplants from a female donor to a male recipient have been associated with a higher rate of GVHD, but also with a reduced rate of leukemia relapse (91). Conversely, transplantation from a male into a female recipient was recently demonstrated to be associated with increased graft rejection (92). Several minor alloantigens, such as HA-1 and HA-2, are selectively expressed on hematopoietic cells (including leukemia cells) and their immunogenic peptides sequenced (93–97). These mHAs offer ideal targets for adoptive immunotherapeutic approaches, and clinical trials targeting the peptides by mHA-specific donor T lymphocytes have been initiated (98). The diallelic HA-1 minor alloantigens presented by HLA-A*0201 and selectively expressed on hematopoietic cells, including leukemia cells, have been described by den Haan et al. (90) Approximately 8%–13% of patients undergoing a marrow allograft would bear HLA-A*0201 and express an HA-1 disparity that could be recognized by a matched sibling donor (99,100). Disparities for HA-1 alleles have been correlated with GVHD by Goulmy et al. (93) and Tseng et al. (94) High frequencies of T cells binding HLA-A2 tetramers complexed with HA-1 peptides have been detected in HA-1-disparate, HLA-matched marrow graft recipients who develop GVHD (101). Results by Dickinson et al. and Marjit et al. (102,103) confirmed that mHA-specific cytotoxic T cells targeting antigens predominantly expressed on hematopoietic cells can induce complete remissions without inducing GVHD. Additional studies after allogeneic marrow transplantation demonstrated a high percentage of leukemia-reactive T cells targeting HA-1 or HA-2 expressed on the leukemic cell population following treatment with donor lymphocyte infusion (104). Genotyping of minor histocompatibility antigens may be included in the pretransplantation evaluation of the donor and recipient, and considered in the decision of donor selection to maximize the immunotherapeutic effect of allogeneic transplantations (97,105).

Immunotherapy with Natural Killer Cells

Natural killer (NK) cells are critical effector cells of the innate immune system. They have a capacity for direct lysis of virally infected cells and tumor cells in addition to mediating cellular cytotoxicity through their CD16 receptor that binds to the Fc portion of immunoglobulin G (106). NK cells are derived from CD34+ progenitor cells and are characterized by expression of CD56 and the absence of CD3. Early trials to stimulate antitumor effects of NK cells with differing concentrations of interleukin-2 (IL-2) have been disappointing (107–109), but the exploitation of NK cells for immunotherapeutic effect has gained interest with the description of inhibitory and activating receptors on CD56+CD3– effector cells (110–112). In contrast to the ability of alloreactive T lymphocytes to recognize antigens by presentation of minor or major histocompatibility complexes shared by normal tissue cells and tumor cells resulting in tumor cell killing and/or GVHD, the function of NK cells can be inhibited by the normal expression of matched MHC class I molecules binding to unique receptors, which are expressed on the NK cells. Killer cell immunoglobulinlike receptors (KIRs) are distinctly expressed on NK cells, and can be inhibitory or activating, although it appears that inhibitory KIRs have a greater affinity to MHC class I than the activating KIRs (25). NK-cell–mediated lysis is therefore inhibited when the inhibitory receptor expressed on the NK cell binds to the corresponding HLA-class I molecule. In contrast, mismatching of KIRs and HLA class I molecules would prevent the NK cell inhibition and could, therefore, be utilized for targeted NK-cell–mediated lysis (26). This principle has been explored by Ruggeri and Aversa et al., demonstrating a potent graft-versus-leukemia effect through uninhibited NK cell activity in recipients of HLA haplotype-mismatched transplants (27). When the donor NK cells could not encounter their inhibiting MHC allele, also not expressed in the leukemia cell population, the NK alloreactivity was primarily directed against the leukemia blasts, which led to a reduced leukemia relapse rate in the absence of GVHD (28,113). The NK alloreactivity was completely absent when the donors' KIR repertoire was found to match the corresponding HLA despite HLA haplotype-mismatched transplants. In these studies, patients undergoing haplotype-mismatched transplantations for acute myelogenous leukemia (AML) experienced a 79% five-year risk of relapse in the presence of KIR/HLA match, but only a 17% risk when the KIR repertoire was mismatched with the recipient's HLA allele (28,113). A study comparing KIR/HLA mismatches in 20 recipients of unrelated bone marrow transplants reported an improved 4½-year survival of 87% versus 39% for transplant recipients in which KIR repertoire and HLA matched (114). Analyses of the donors' KIR repertoire and the recipients' HLA also demonstrated a decreased relapse rate and improved overall survival in patients undergoing T-cell–depleted transplants from HLA-identical siblings for AML, in which donor KIRs were mismatched with the corresponding HLA allele

required for NK-cell inhibition (115). The decreased relapse rate could not be attributed to the effect of donor T lymphocytes in these T-cell–depleted transplantations. This outcome also confirms the feasibility of KIR/HLA mismatches despite HLA-matched sibling or matched unrelated transplantations because the KIR genotype, encoded on chromosome 19, is independently segregated from chromosome 6, which encodes the HLA genes (116). In all of these studies, however, the alloreactivity and NK-cell–mediated lysis was restricted to patients with AML, and no antileukemic effect of NK cells could be demonstrated against ALL. The differences in these outcomes are currently unexplained and may be multifactorial, such as varying susceptibility to NK-cell–mediated lysis or different expressions of activating receptors on NK cells. The lack of lymphocyte function antigen 1 (LFA-1) expression on ALL cells has been associated with reduced NK-cell–mediated lysis, indicating that additional factors may play a role in the activation of alloreactive NK cells (113). It is anticipated that NK-cell–mediated immunotherapeutic approaches will be further developed and integrated into clinical trials to improve the outcome of hematological malignancies by allogeneic bone marrow transplantations.

PRINCIPLES OF HUMORAL IMMUNE THERAPY

Monoclonal Antibody Therapy

Monoclonal antibody-based therapies have emerged over the past decade for the treatment of hematological malignancies and solid tumors. The limitations with murine monoclonal antibodies, such as the development of human antimouse monoclonal antibodies with rapid clearing from the body resulting in multiple administrations, could be overcome by chimeric and humanized antibodies. The anti-CD20 monoclonal antibody rituximab is a chimeric antibody with reduced immunogenicity and can be safely administered without the development of human antimouse antibodies. The CD20 antigen is expressed on mature B cells and, therefore, on hematological malignancies derived from B lymphocytes, which can be targeted using rituximab as a single agent or in combination with chemotherapy. Initial phase 2 studies administering the maximum tolerated rituximab dose of 375 mg/m² as a single agent to patients with indolent non-Hodgkin lymphoma (NHL) have demonstrated a 46%–48% response rate (29,30). Rituximab was subsequently evaluated for the treatment of relapsed and refractory diffuse large B-cell lymphoma (DLCBL) in combination with cyclophosphamide, doxorubicin, vincristine, and prednisone

(CHOP) chemotherapy (30,117), and is currently also administered for Epstein-Barr virus–associated lymphoproliferative disorder (EBV-PTLD) (118,119) and chronic GVHD (120,121). Only limited activity in the treatment of chronic lymphocytic leukemia (CLL) was demonstrated (122), which may be explained by the lower antigen density of CD20 expressed on CLL cells compared with the expression level on NHL or EBV-PTLD (123). In addition, circulating CLL cells may bind the monoclonal antibodies and, therefore, act as a sink, resulting in rapid clearance of the drug (124).

Campath-1 and the humanized monoclonal antibody Campath-1H (alemtuzumab) have specificity for CD52, a glycoprotein expressed on B and T lymphocytes that is highly expressed on CLL cells. Clinical trials with single-agent alemtuzumab have demonstrated activity in fludarabine-refractory patients with CLL (125–128). Campath-1H has been evaluated as front-line therapy for CLL as a single agent, with complete remissions of 19%–22% and overall remissions of 85%–87% (129,130). Treatment with alemtuzumab was associated with increased rates of opportunistic infections, particularly CMV reactivation.

CD33 is a 67-kD cell surface glycoprotein whose expression is largely restricted to cells of the monocytic/myeloid lineage (131,132). It is detected on promonocytes and monocytes in the monocytic lineage, on myeloblasts and promyelocytes, and on a proportion of metamyelocytes in the myeloid lineage. CD33 is expressed by the leukemic blasts of at least 90% of patients with acute myelogenous leukemia, but not by acute lymphocytic leukemia. Importantly, the expression is absent from mature granulocytes and primitive pluripotential stem cells, and may, therefore, be an interesting antigen for targeted immunotherapy (131–133). Unmodified antibodies used in the initial studies were limited in their activity against acute leukemia, largely because binding of the antibodies did not induce intracellular signaling and, therefore, did not induce cell death of the leukemic blasts (134). Furthermore, murine antibodies were not well recognized by human antigen-presenting cells, and induced only a weak, antibody-dependent cellular cytotoxicity (135). The humanized mouse IgG1, termed HuM195, was developed as a consequence and studied in a phase 1/2 trial (136). In this study, 60 patients with refractory or relapsed myeloid leukemia were treated with 12–36 mg/m^2 of HuM195 daily for four days, two weeks apart. Decreases in blast counts were observed, but only three complete remissions were obtained (137,138). The conclusion of that study was that unlabeled antibodies demonstrated clinical efficacy in patients with low tumor load and therefore might be most effective in patients with minimal residual disease. Since acute promyelocytic leukemia (APL) is strongly positive for CD33, in subsequent studies, HuM195 was given for consolidation or maintenance therapy in 31 patients with APL who were in complete remission and who had already been treated with all-trans-retinoic acid (ATRA) (139). In this trial, HuM195 was given twice a week for three weeks, followed by consolidation chemotherapy with idarubicin and cytarabine, followed by six months of maintenance therapy with HuM195 given twice a week every four weeks. Of the patients treated with ATRA and/or chemotherapy induction, 2 of 27 became PCR-negative. After treatment with HuM195, 12 of 24 evaluable patients (50%) were PCR-negative, and the probability of disease-free survival after a median follow-up of five years was 93%, compared with 73% obtained after treatment with ATRA and consolidation chemotherapy but without administration of HuM195 in the previous study (139,140).

In order to increase the antitumor effects of the native antibodies, drugs and bacterial toxins have been conjugated to the MoAbs. Sievers et al. studied a conjugate of the antitumor antibiotic, calicheamicin and the humanized anti-CD33 antibody, CMA-676, also known as gemtuzumab ozogamicin or Mylotarg (37). Binding of CD33 antigen causes internalization of the anti-CD33 and calicheamicin conjugate, and upon the release of the drug, causes DNA double-strand breaks and subsequently cell death via apoptosis (141). In an initial phase 1 trial, 40 patients with relapsed or refractory AML were treated with escalating doses of gemtuzumab. In 8 of the 40 patients (20%), leukemic blasts were eliminated and blood counts normalized in 8% of the patients (37). In a subsequent open-label multicenter phase 2 trial, 277 patients with CD33-positive AML in first relapse were treated with gemtuzumab at 9 mg/m^2 intravenously (IV) every two weeks for two doses. In this trial, 26% of patients achieved complete remission, characterized by no blasts in the peripheral blood and <5% in the bone marrow, neutrophils >1,500/mm^3, and independence from platelet infusion for one week. The median recurrence-free survival was 6.4 months for patients who achieved complete remission (142). Hyperbilirubinemia developed in 29% of patients, and hepatic veno-occlusive disease developed in 9% in this study who did not undergo subsequent stem cell transplantation.

The principal adverse effect from conjugated anti-CD33 monoclonal antibodies is myelosuppression. Grade 3–4 neutropenia (98%) and thrombocytopenia (99%) occurred in almost all patients in the postinfusion period. Other common adverse effects were fever, chills, gastrointestinal symptoms, dyspnea, epistaxis, and anorexia. Mucositis, sepsis (17%), and pneumonia (8%) were reported (142). Additional reports also describe evidence of hepatotoxicity induced by gemtuzumab ozogamicin (143,144). However, in some of these studies, the majority of the patients received gemtuzumab in combination with other investigational drugs (145).

Radioimmunotherapy

An alternative approach to enhance the antitumor activity of the anti-CD33 antibody was explored by conjugation with radioisotopes such as iodine-131 (^{131}I) or yttrium 90 (^{90}Y). In an initial phase 1 trial, 24 patients with relapsed or refractory myeloid leukemias were treated with escalating doses of ^{131}I-M195 (34). Twenty-two of the 24 patients had a reduction in leukemic burden, and gamma camera imaging demonstrated targeting to areas of leukemic involvement, such as vertebrae, pelvis, and long bones, as well as liver and spleen. Profound myelosuppression occurred at ^{131}I doses of 135 mCi/m^2 or greater, requiring bone marrow transplantation in eight patients. As in the initial trial with unconjugated murine M195 antibodies, 37% of the patients in this trial developed human anti-mouse antibodies. Subsequently, myeloablative doses of ^{131}I-M195 and ^{131}I-HuM195 (122–437 mCi) were studied in combination with busulfan (16 mg/kg) and cyclophosphamide (90 or 120 mg/kg) as a conditioning regimen for allogeneic bone marrow transplantation in 31 patients with relapsed or refractory AML, accelerated or blastic CML, or advanced MDS. These studies demonstrated that ^{131}I-M195 and ^{131}I-HuM195 have activity in myeloid leukemia, and can be used with standard chemotherapeutic agents without inducing additional toxicities (35).

Yttrium 90 offers several advantages over ^{131}I for myeloablation. ^{90}Y is a pure β-emitter with a half-life of 64 hours, compared with the 8 days half-life of ^{131}I, which is a β- and γ-emitter. Therefore, larger doses of ^{90}Y can be given safely in an outpatient setting. A phase 1 trial with ^{90}Y-HuM195 for patients with relapsed or refractory AML was performed. Nineteen patients were treated with escalating doses of ^{90}Y-HuM195 (0.1–0.3 mCi/kg) given as a single infusion. Myelosuppression lasted 9–62 days at a maximum tolerated dose of 0.275 mCi/kg, and 13 patients had reduction of bone marrow blasts. One patient achieved complete remission lasting five months (140). The inclusion of ^{90}Y-HuM195 in a reduced-intensity preparative regimen for allogeneic bone marrow transplantation in patients with CD33-expressing myeloid leukemia is currently under investigation (36).

CD45 is a pan-leukocyte antigen, and ^{131}I-labeled anti-CD45 has been investigated in a phase 1 trial in 44 patients with advanced leukemia or MDS (146). Thirty-four evaluable patients received escalating doses of ^{131}I-labeled anti-CD45 (76–612 mCi) followed by total body irradiation, cyclophosphamide, and allogeneic or autologous transplantation. Seven of 25 patients with AML or MDS remained alive and disease-free at 65-month follow-up, and 3 out of 9 patients with ALL remained in remission for 19, 54, and 66 months. A phase 1/2 trial was subsequently initiated combining ^{131}I-labeled anti-CD45 with busulfan and cyclophosphamide as a conditioning regimen in patients with AML in first remission (135).

The conjugation of radioisotope to anti-CD20 monoclonal antibodies has improved the activity induced by targeted radiation of CD20-expressing tumor cells. Anti-CD20 antibodies have been approved as radioimmunoconjugates, labeled with yttrium-90, Zevalin (ibritumomab) or iodine-131 Bexxar (tositumomab), for the treatment of relapsed or refractory low-grade or transformed NHL (33,147). The safety profile of these agents has been well characterized, with the principal side effect being reversible myelosuppression from the radiation. Durable responses have been obtained in patients who were proven resistant to chemotherapy (31,148–150). In addition, long-lasting responses were induced in patients refractory to previous treatments with the unlabeled anti-CD20 antibody (151,152). These results led to a phase 2 study to determine the effect of tositumomab in previously untreated patients with indolent lymphoma. Ninety patients with advanced-stage follicular lymphoma were treated with CHOP chemotherapy followed by I-131 tositumomab. An overall response rate of 90% with a complete remission of 67% was achieved, and treatment was well tolerated (32). In a five-year follow-up of this study, an overall survival of 87% and progression-free survival rate of 67% were recently reported, which compares favorably to CHOP chemotherapy alone (153). Chemotherapy in combination with radioimmunotherapy continues to be evaluated in ongoing clinical trials (154,155).

Monoclonal antibodies targeting epidermal growth factor receptor (EGFR) or blocking the binding of vascular endothelial growth factor (VEGF) to its receptor for the treatment of solid tumors are currently being evaluated in clinical trials.

PRINCIPLES OF CANCER VACCINES

The induction of a humoral and/or cellular immune response to antigens specifically expressed on malignant cells has been the ultimate goal in the approach to curing cancer or preventing its recurrence or development in patients at risk. For a cancer vaccine to be effective, the patient with a tumor or the healthy individual at risk has to mount a robust tumor-antigen–specific immune response after therapeutic or prophylactic vaccination. However, tumor cells are derived from host cells, and tumor antigens represent or are derived from normal self-antigens. The tumor antigen may not be expressed on the cell surface, therefore limiting the recognition of self-derived epitopes or the accessibility of the tumor-associated antigens to a potential immune response. Ideally, for a cancer vaccine to be effective, the targeted tumor-associated antigen would be exclusively expressed on the tumor cells, and the vaccination should overcome tolerance and permit induction of an immune response against the epitope. To modify the intensity of the immune response generated against a potential tumor-associated antigen, adjuvants are complexed with the antigen. A variety of adjuvants, such as lipopolysaccharide (LPS) derived from Gram-negative bacteria, aluminum salts-derived, emulsifier-derived, synthetic adjuvants or cytokines such as GM-CSF, have elicited an enhanced immune response (41–43,156,157). The adjuvants can have selective capacities for induction of specific immune responses, and therefore the appropriate choice of the adjuvant may be crucial in order to achieve the desired immune reaction. These immune reactions are believed to be the consequence of processing and presentation of tumor-associated antigens by antigen-presenting cells (APCs) through their major histocompatibility class I and/or class II molecules to CD8$^+$ or CD4$^+$ lymphocytes. The activated CD4$^+$ cells enhance the function of the CD8$^+$ cytotoxic T cells, support monoclonal antibody production, and promote survival of B lymphocytes. A humoral immune response and activation of CD8$^+$ cytotoxic lymphocytes can also be a directly induced immune response after tumor-associated antigen administration.

Anti-idiotype Antibody Vaccines

Anti-idiotype antibody vaccines and DNA vaccines derived from tumor-associated antigens complexed with adjuvants have demonstrated the capacity to induce specific immune responses, and a variety of clinical trials are under way. Immunoglobulin on the surface of B-cell lymphomas contains unique amino acid sequences within the variable region of its heavy and light chains (immunoglobulin idiotype) expressed in low-grade lymphomas, which can be specifically targeted by monoclonal antibodies recognizing the idiotype (anti-idiotype antibodies) (39). Pioneered by Levy et al. (38,40) the description of unique idiotypes on low-grade lymphoma prompted the development of vaccine strategies for patients with low-grade lymphomas who had minimal residual disease or complete remission following chemotherapy. In an initial clinical trial reported by Kwak et al. the immunoglobulin-idiotype protein derived from the tumor cells was conjugated to a protein carrier, mixed with an adjuvant, and the individually custom-made vaccines were injected in

nine patients (158). In seven of the nine, anti-idiotype–specific immune responses were observed. Two patients developed anti-idiotype–specific monoclonal antibody responses, four developed a cellular-mediated response, and one patient developed both a cellular-mediated and a humoral immune response against the idiotype. The two patients with minimal residual but measurable disease in this trial regressed completely, and the vaccine was well tolerated overall. These encouraging results led to a larger trial. Of 41 patients with low-grade lymphoma who received vaccination against the unique idiotype, 50% developed a humoral anti-idiotype antibody response (159). In a subsequent phase 2 clinical trial, previously untreated patients with follicular lymphoma were vaccinated with five monthly subcutaneous injections of the idiotype in combination with adjuvant Keyhole limpet hemocyanin (KLH). In this trial, GM-CSF was also injected subcutaneously near the vaccine site for five days to enhance the immune response. This study demonstrated the induction of tumor-specific CD8$^+$ and CD4$^+$ T-cell responses. In this trial, humoral immune responses were also observed in the majority of patients, and three patients developed a molecular remission with detectable antibody response, suggesting that an antibody response was not required to maintain molecular remissions. A sustained molecular remission was obtained in 8 of 11 treated patients who had detectable translocations in the blood by PCR after the completion of chemotherapy (160). A multicenter phase 3 clinical trial is under way for patients with follicular lymphoma in first complete remission, evaluating the clinical benefit of idiotype + KLH vaccine in combination with GM-CSF injections (161). In additional reports from these trials, Davis et al. described low levels of residual lymphomas as assessed by polymerase chain reactions for clonal rearrangement of immunoglobulin sequences in patients who had been in clinical remission for up to eight years. This suggests long-term control of the disease despite the persistence of residual malignancy (38). Weng et al. reported their observations in patients who developed an anti-idiotype antibody response with a longer progression-free survival after their last chemotherapy compared with those patients who did not have an antibody response. In contrast, the development of a cellular immune response did not lead to significant progression-free survival at five years after chemotherapy compared with patients without a cellular response (162). Further analyses of these studies demonstrated an association of clinical response to the vaccine and the IgG Fc receptor (FcγR) polymorphism. Anti-idiotype monoclonal antibodies binding to their respective lymphoma cell are usually recognized by effector cells (such as NK cells) via FcγR and mediate antibody-dependent cellular cytotoxicity (ADCC).

Favorable FcγR polymorphisms have higher affinities to the Fc fraction of the bound antibody, resulting in stronger activation of the effector cells and consequently more potent ADCC. Weng et al. clearly demonstrated a longer progression-free survival in patients with a FcγRIIIa 158 valine/valine genotype compared with the heterozygous valine/phenylalanine or homozygous phenylalanine/phenylalanine FcγRIIIa genotypes (162). The beneficial clinical outcome in patients receiving the vaccine who developed an anti-idiotype antibody production and those with a favorable FcγRIIIa 158 valine/valine genotype proved to be independent of partial or complete remission to induction chemotherapy (163).

Carcinoembryonic antigen (CEA) is a well-characterized, tumor-associated antigen expressed on neoplasms derived from gastrointestinal tract or other adenocarcinomas (164). Vaccination approaches to induce immune responses against this tumor-associated antigen have been initiated for patients with resected colon cancer. To overcome the limitations of anti-idiotype antibody responses against this self-antigen, a unique approach, described by Lindemann and Jerne as the network hypothesis (165,166), was explored by Foon et al. (167) The network hypothesis postulated that immunization with a tumor-associated antigen will induce monoclonal antibody production against this antigen, termed Ab1. Some of the anti-idiotype antibodies, Ab2, generated against the Ab1 antibodies, mimic the structure of the original carcinoembryonic antigen. Vaccinations with these anti-idiotypes, termed Ab2β, can induce immune responses, anti-anti-idiotype antibodies (Ab3), against the original antigen. This approach utilizes an anti-idiotype antibody vaccine to break immune tolerance and permit induction of immune response against the self-derived tumor-associated antigen. In a clinical phase 1 trial, Foon et al. vaccinated a total of 32 patients, 29 with resected Dukes B, C, and D and three with incompletely resected Dukes D disease, using the anti-idiotype antibody vaccine called CeaVac. They assessed the specific immune response against CEA. Four injections of 2 mg CeaVac were administered intracutaneously every other week and then monthly until disease progression. In addition, the impact of concurrent chemotherapy with 5-fluorouracil (5-FU) on the immune response was assessed in 14 patients. All 32 patients developed an antibody response, and 80% of the patients also developed a T-cell proliferative response against CEA, irrespective of concurrent 5-FU treatment, demonstrating the ability to overcome immune tolerance with this approach (167). Although some patients reportedly experienced prolonged progression-free survival, this study was not designed to draw clinical conclusions based on the results of individual patients, and a phase 3 study is required to capture beneficial outcome in these patients.

The principle of inducing anti-anti-idiotype antibodies is currently being tested against other tumor-associated antigens, such as anti-GD-2 (168,169), ACA125 (170), or anti-GD-3 (171).

DNA Vaccines

DNA vaccines consist of a plasmid DNA containing one or multiple genes. The DNA is typically administered intradermally or intramuscularly by needle injection or by use of a gene gun, which propels gold beads coated with plasmid DNA into the skin (172,173). The DNA is translated into the encoded proteins, then processed and presented by APCs, eliciting the vaccine-specific immune response. A variety of DNA vaccines are currently being tested in preclinical and early clinical trials, and only a limited selection of these trials have been included in this chapter to describe the principal approach of DNA immunization.

DNA vaccination against melanoma differentiation antigens has been intensively studied by Houghton et al. (174). The initial immunizations with the melanoma-derived tyrosine-kinase–related proteins TRP-2 and TYRP1 were complicated by development of autoimmunity, resulting in severe vitiligo (hypopigmentation) of the skin (175,176), whereas DNA immunizations against melanoma-derived antigen gp100 induced strong CD8+ T-cell responses with only minimal vitiligo (177). To overcome the poor immunogenicity of the self-antigen gp100, xenogeneic (mouse-derived) DNA vaccines were explored, demonstrating that antibody and T-cell responses induced by the xenogeneic DNA can cross-react with the original syngeneic DNA and induce effective immunity in a preclinical model (175–177). In addition, when plasmid DNAs of cytokines, proven to enhance immune responses, such as IL-2, IL-12, IL-15, IL-21, and GM-CSF, were co-injected with the gp100 plasmid DNA, increased CD8+ T-cell responses against gp100 and improved tumor-free survival were observed in a preclinical melanoma model (178). Clinical trials evaluating the clinical benefit in humans are currently ongoing. Powell and Rosenberg utilized a gp100-derived peptide, modified by substituting methionine for threonine at position 2 for increased HLA-A*0201 binding affinity, and thus elicited enhanced T-cell responses for multiple peptide vaccinations in five HLA-A*0201–positive patients with completely resected melanoma who remained at high risk for tumor recurrence after tumor resection. The initial three patients were vaccinated every three weeks for a total of 16 injections, and the final two patients were vaccinated weekly for 10 weeks followed by a 3-week break between treatment courses. After immunization, the patients developed high frequencies of gp100-specific CD8+ T lymphocytes, which were still functionally tumor-reactive and circulating in the blood at one year follow-up (179). The patients remained free of recurrence at one year after last immunization, and no autoimmune reactivity was observed in the study. Recently, these investigators studied nine patients with metastatic melanoma after vaccination with the modified gp100-derived peptide, followed by ex vivo expansion of the HLA-A*0201–restricted, gp100 peptide-specific T cells, and subsequent adoptive transfer of the expanded T-cell population in combination with high-dose interleukin-2 and the cancer vaccine after chemotherapy-induced lymphodepletion (180). Although the presence of circulating tumor-reactive $CD8^+$ T cells was demonstrated in the blood, no objective clinical response was described in these patients.

Prostate-specific membrane antigen (PSMA), initially thought to be a unique cancer antigen, is a self-antigen that is highly overexpressed on prostate cancer cells, but is also expressed on normal prostate cells, the brain, salivary glands, and biliary tree (181). PSMA is overexpressed on the neovasculature of other solid tumors, such as renal cancer, lung, bladder, pancreatic cancer, and melanoma, but is not found on normal vasculature (182). In a preclinical model, vaccination with xenogeneic PSMA DNA-induced monoclonal antibodies to both mouse and human PSMA provided the basis for evaluating PSMA DNA vaccination in clinical trials (183).

Cell-Based Vaccines

Cell-based vaccine strategies utilizing autologous or allogeneic tumor cells, genetically modified to secrete cytokines for enhanced antigen presentation and improved immune responses, were evaluated in the treatment of solid tumors. A phase 1 trial to assess the safety and feasibility of prostate cancer antigens was performed by Simons et al. (184) In this study, prostate tumor cells were surgically harvested from 11 patients with metastatic prostate cancer. Cells were cultured and complementary DNA (cDNA) encoding GM-CSF was retrovirally transduced into the tumor cells. Sufficient numbers of genetically modified cancer cells were obtained from 8 out of 11 patients. These GM-CSF–modified prostate cancer cells were lethally irradiated and injected intracutaneously up to six times every three weeks. The vaccine was well tolerated, although characterized by local inflammation of the vaccination sites. Biopsies of these infiltrates three days after the injection demonstrated the presence of autologous prostate cancer cells, dendritic cells, macrophages, eosinophils, and lymphocytes. A delayed-type hypersensitivity (DTH) reaction against challenge with irradiated, nontransduced, autologous tumor cells after completion of the vaccination series was newly induced in seven out of eight vaccinated patients. Biopsies of the DTH sites demonstrated infiltration with T lymphocytes as well as few B lymphocytes. In addition, monoclonal antibody responses against three prostate cancer-derived epitopes (not observed in the prevaccination sera from three of the eight vaccinated patients) was also documented (184). The broader application and a larger phase 2 clinical trial were limited by the impracticability of this approach, including the low yield of prostate cancer cells obtained after cell cultures and the necessity to manufacture the vaccine on an individual basis. A prostate cancer vaccine, termed GVAX, consisting of two allogeneic prostate cancer cell lines genetically modified to secrete GM-CSF, has been subsequently tested in a phase 2 clinical trial in hormone-refractory prostate cancer patients, and a phase 3 trial evaluating the vaccine alone or in combination with docetaxel in this patient cohort has been initiated (185).

The principle of using autologous tumor cells genetically modified to secrete GM-CSF was also explored in metastatic melanoma and metastatic non-small cell lung cancer (NSCLC). Vaccination with irradiated, autologous melanoma cells engineered to secrete GM-CSF, with a replication-defective adenoviral vector encoding human GM-CSF, was performed in 34 patients with metastatic melanoma. Vaccines were injected intradermally or subcutaneously at increasing doses from 1×10^6, 4×10^6, or 1×10^7, depending on overall yield at weekly intervals, until the vaccine supply was exhausted. Side effects were restricted to local skin reactions, and 25 patients could be assessed for DTH reaction. In this study, 17 of 25 patients developed a DTH reaction from autologous, nontransduced melanoma cells, and metastatic lesions that were resected after vaccination showed focal infiltration with T lymphocytes and plasma cells with tumor necrosis in 10 of 16 patients (186,187). A similar strategy was subsequently tested in a phase 1 trial of 35 patients with metastatic NSCLC. This produced DTH reaction to nontransduced autologous NSCLC cells in 18 of 22 assessable patients and improved clinical outcomes in some patients (188). To circumvent the requirement of genetic transduction of individual tumors, a phase 1=2 trial was conducted in which autologous NSCLC cells were admixed with an allogeneic bystander cell line (K562, a human erythroleukemia cell line) and genetically transduced to secrete GM-CSF at a cell ratio of 2:1 for intradermal vaccination. Forty-nine patients were vaccinated at two-week intervals for a total of 3–12 vaccinations, with doses ranging from $5–80 \times 10^6$ autologous NSCLC cells mixed with half the amount of GM-CSF–secreting K562 cells per vaccine (189). Although the GM-CSF secretion was found to be 25-fold higher compared with a previous trial vaccine derived from autologous NSCLC cells modified to secrete

GM-CSF (190), the frequency of vaccine site reactions, tumor response, and time to progression was inferior to the autologous cell vaccines of the previous trial.

PRINCIPLES OF T-CELL–MEDIATED IMMUNE RESPONSE MODIFICATION

In recent years, our knowledge of T-cell–induced lysis of tumor cells and persistence of antigen-specific T cells induced by vaccination has led to the integration of CTLA-4 blockade into clinical trials after vaccination. In addition, the immunoregulatory capacity of T-regulatory cells is currently under investigation. Studies are assessing the effects of selective depletion or infusion of this T-cell subset on enhanced T-cell–mediated tumor effect or amelioration of GVHD, respectively.

Cytotoxic T-Lymphocyte–Associated Antigen (CTLA)-4

T-cell responses are down-regulated by the stimulation of cytotoxic T-lymphocyte–associated antigen (CTLA-4) expressed on the cell surface of activated T lymphocytes. CTLA-4 protein is usually located in intracellular vesicles and increasingly expressed on the surface of T lymphocytes with increased activation of the cells. CTLA-4 expression serves as a counter-regulatory molecule to the activating receptor CD28 on T lymphocytes. The ligands CD80/B7.1 or CD86/B7.2, expressed on antigen-presenting cells, bind to CD28 on the T cells, either inducing their activation or binding to CTLA-4, which prevents overactivation and serves as a negative modulator of T-cell homeostasis (44,45). CTLA-4 activation induces antigen-specific cell death of activated T lymphocytes and prevents proliferation of autoimmune-reactive T cells (191,192). Blockade of CTLA-4 with nonagonistic antibodies to enhance DNA vaccine-mediated T-cell response has been tested in preclinical models (193–195), and the anti-CTLA-4 antibody ipilimumab has been found safe in early clinical trials with promising results, particularly in melanoma and renal cancer (196–198).

T-Regulatory Cells (Tregs)

T-cell tolerance is achieved through negative selection in the thymus of potentially autoreactive T lymphocytes (199). Despite this thymic selection, T cells can escape the process and are found in the peripheral blood of healthy individuals. T-regulatory cells (Tregs), characterized recently by their expression of CD4+CD25+FOXP3+, constitute a T-lymphocyte population that controls pathologic immune responses and is involved in the maintenance of lymphocyte homeostasis.

Several preclinical studies have demonstrated that Tregs prevent autoreactive T-cell responses (200,201), while other studies demonstrated that Tregs can inhibit antigen-specific T-cell responses and T-cell–mediated antitumor effects (46). Ex vivo expansion of these cells for the treatment of autoimmune diseases has been attempted, but these cells have poor in vitro proliferative potential (202,203), and the use of rapamycin, which induces preferential proliferation of Tregs, is currently under investigation (204). In contrast, the depletion of Tregs has been demonstrated to enhance T-cell–mediated antitumor effects in preclinical models (205). In a preclinical melanoma model, Sutmuller et al. combined CTLA-4 blockade with in vivo depletion of Tregs to obtain maximal tumor rejection by tyrosinase-specific T cells after vaccination with B-16-GM-CSF tumor-cell vaccine (206).

The immunoregulatory capacity of Tregs is currently also being investigated for control of GVHD following allogeneic bone marrow transplantation. Several groups have demonstrated that infusion of regulatory T cells can ameliorate GVHD without reducing the graft-versus-leukemia effect in preclinical models (207–209). Clinical trials investigating the potential of regulatory T cells in humans are anticipated.

CONCLUSIONS

Immunotherapies are rapidly evolving and will be increasingly integrated with standard therapies for the treatment of solid tumors and hematologic malignancies. However, the broader application of immunotherapies currently has limitations that need to be resolved. Biologic therapies, such as the production of cancer vaccines or the generation of antigen-specific T lymphocytes, have to be produced under strict manufacturing conditions, currently limiting these approaches to larger centers that provide an institutional environment for these therapeutic trials. Regulatory obstacles for these therapies have to be overcome. The generation of a cancer vaccine or of antigen-specific T lymphocytes includes the incorporation of novel agents needed for the production of the final product. These agents often require prior independent investigational new drug (IND) and Food and Drug Administration (FDA) approval. To facilitate the development of immunotherapies, the pharmaceutical industry must be involved in the production of materials and products that fulfill regulatory FDA criteria. An increased awareness of the implementation and integration of immunotherapies into clinical trials resulted in the first FDA/National Cancer Institute (NCI)–sponsored workshop in February 2007 entitled, "Bringing Therapeutic Cancer Vaccines and Immunotherapy to Licensure."

The workshop, attended by representatives from the FDA, investigators, and industry, discussed strategies to advance the approval process for these therapies.

An additional limitation of immunotherapies, once proven safe and effective, is associated with the time-consuming and labor-intensive process of production. Many cancer vaccines can be produced only on an individual basis, such as the anti-idiotype cancer vaccines, after the idiotype has been determined. The generation of antigen-specific T lymphocytes also has to be performed on an individual basis, targeting the antigen-derived peptide presented by the individuals' HLA type. For this reason, the individuals' HLA alleles and the peptide sequences derived from the antigen presented in these HLA alleles have to be determined prior to generating these peptide-specific T cells. Novel approaches for improving and overcoming some of these limitations are under investigation. Pulsing of antigen-presenting cells with overlapping pentadeca-peptides overspanning the entire amino acid sequence of known antigens for the generation of peptide-specific T cells circumvents prior knowledge of the HLA restriction of the peptide derived from the antigen. This strategy may be applied to generate specific T cells for all patients, independently of HLA type (210,211).

In addition, the identification and generation of more potent antigen-presenting cells has improved the cytotoxic potential of antigen-specific T cells and permits the generation of T lymphocytes targeting cancer-derived antigens with low immunogenicity (212,213). The development of artificial antigen-presenting cells consisting of nonimmunogenic mouse fibroblasts transduced to express selected HLA alleles and co-stimulatory molecules, which can be expanded without limit in vitro, may circumvent the necessity to repeatedly generate antigen-presenting cells for each individual, and may provide "off-the-shelf" access to these cells for the generation of antigen-specific T lymphocytes (214,215). Recent studies have demonstrated gene transfer of T-cell receptors, thereby redirecting the specificity of T cells to tumor antigens (216–219). This approach may produce antigen-specific T cells without the necessity of producing antigen-presenting cells.

Monoclonal antibodies are easily obtained and can be administered to all individuals who might benefit from this therapy. Current radioimmunotherapy trials that used β-emitting isotopes, such as ^{131}iodine and ^{90}yttrium, conjugated to anti-CD20, anti-CD33, or anti-CD45 monoclonal antibodies, demonstrated promising results and safe administration. The incorporation of α-emitters, such as ^{213}bismuth and ^{225}acinium, into trials for the treatment of minimal residual disease is currently under investigation and holds great promise because of the short range and high linear energy transfer (220,221).

It is anticipated that immunotherapies will continue to evolve, and as results of clinical trials become available, the benefits and limitations of these therapies will be better defined. Combination immunotherapies, such as the ex vivo expansion of antigen-specific T lymphocytes collected from patients after administration of a cancer vaccine and reinfusion of the expanded cell population and/or the administration of an immune response modifying agent, eg, anti-CTLA-4 antibody, could improve the outcome of these therapies once regulations limiting these approaches have been overcome.

References

1. Roberts MM, To LB, Gillis D, et al. Immune reconstitution following peripheral blood stem cell transplantation, autologous bone marrow transplantation and allogeneic bone marrow transplantation. *Bone Marrow Transplant.* 1993;12:469–475.
2. de Gast GC, Verdonck LF, Middeldorp JM, et al. Recovery of T cell subsets after autologous bone marrow transplantation is mainly due to proliferation of mature T cells in the graft. *Blood.* 1985;66:428–431.
3. Mackall CL, Fleisher TA, Brown MR, et al. Age, thymopoiesis, and CD4+ T-lymphocyte regeneration after intensive chemotherapy. *N Engl J Med.* 1995;332:143–149.
4. Koehne G, Zeller W, Stockschlaeder M, et al. Phenotype of lymphocyte subsets after autologous peripheral blood stem cell transplantation. *Bone Marrow Transplant.* 1997;19:149–156.
5. Pettengell R. Autologous stem cell transplantation in follicular non-Hodgkin's lymphoma. *Bone Marrow Transplant.* 2002;29(Suppl 1):S1–S4.
6. Kewalramani T, Zelenetz AD, Nimer SD, et al. Rituximab and ICE as second-line therapy before autologous stem cell transplantation for relapsed or primary refractory diffuse large B-cell lymphoma. *Blood.* 2004;103:3684–3688.
7. Hamlin PA, Zelenetz AD, Kewalramani T, et al. Age-adjusted International Prognostic Index predicts autologous stem cell transplantation outcome for patients with relapsed or primary refractory diffuse large B-cell lymphoma. *Blood.* 2003;102:1989–1996.
8. Diehl V, Josting A. Hodgkin's disease. *Cancer J.* 2000;6(Suppl 2):S150–S158.
9. Josting A. Autologous transplantation in relapsed and refractory Hodgkin's disease. *Eur J Haematol Suppl.* 2005;66:141–145.
10. Majhail NS, Weisdorf DJ, Defor TE, et al. Long-term results of autologous stem cell transplantation for primary refractory or relapsed Hodgkin's lymphoma. *Biol Blood Marrow Transplant.* 2006;12:1065–1072.
11. Barlogie B, Shaughnessy J, Tricot G, et al. Treatment of multiple myeloma. *Blood.* 2004;103:20–32.
12. Attal M, Harousseau JL, Facon T, et al. Single versus double autologous stem-cell transplantation for multiple myeloma. *N Engl J Med.* 2003;349:2495–2502.
13. Bruno B, Rotta M, Patriarca F, et al. A comparison of allografting with autografting for newly diagnosed myeloma. *N Engl J Med.* 2007;356:1110–1120.
14. Fefer A, Sullivan KM, Weiden P, et al. Graft versus leukemia effect in man: the relapse rate of acute leukemia is lower after allogeneic than after syngeneic marrow transplantation. *Prog Clin Biol Res.* 1987;244:401–408.
15. Weiden PL, Flournoy N, Thomas ED, et al. Antileukemic effect of graft-versus-host disease in human recipients of allogeneic-marrow grafts. *N Engl J Med.* 1979;300:1068–1073.

16. Kolb HJ, Mittermuller J, Clemm C, et al. Donor leukocyte transfusions for treatment of recurrent chronic myelogenous leukemia in marrow transplant patients. *Blood*. 1990;76:2462–2465.

17. Kolb HJ, Schattenberg A, Goldman JM, et al. Graft-versus-leukemia effect of donor lymphocyte transfusions in marrow grafted patients. *Blood*. 1995;86:2041–2050.

18. Mackinnon S, Papadopoulos EB, Carabasi MH, et al. Adoptive immunotherapy evaluating escalating doses of donor leukocytes for relapse of chronic myeloid leukemia after bone marrow transplantation: separation of graft-versus-leukemia responses from graft-versus-host disease. *Blood*. 1995;86:1261–1268.

19. Drobyski WR, Keever CA, Roth MS, et al. Salvage immunotherapy using donor leukocyte infusions as treatment for relapsed chronic myelogenous leukemia after allogeneic bone marrow transplantation: efficacy and toxicity of a defined T-cell dose. *Blood*. 1993;82:2310–2318.

20. Collins RH, Jr., Shpilberg O, Drobyski WR, et al. Donor leukocyte infusions in 140 patients with relapsed malignancy after allogeneic bone marrow transplantation. *J Clin Oncol*. 1997;15:433–444.

21. Falkenburg JH, Wafelman AR, Joosten P, et al. Complete remission of accelerated phase chronic myeloid leukemia by treatment with leukemia-reactive cytotoxic T lymphocytes. *Blood*. 1999;94:1201–1208.

22. Riddell SR, Watanabe KS, Goodrich JM, et al. Restoration of viral immunity in immunodeficient humans by the adoptive transfer of T cell clones. *Science*. 1992;257:238–241.

23. Heslop HE, Ng CY, Li C, et al. Long-term restoration of immunity against Epstein-Barr virus infection by adoptive transfer of gene-modified virus-specific T lymphocytes. *Nat Med*. 1996;2:551–555.

24. Rooney CM, Smith CA, Ng CY, et al. Infusion of cytotoxic T cells for the prevention and treatment of Epstein-Barr virus-induced lymphoma in allogeneic transplant recipients. *Blood*. 1998;92:1549–1555.

25. Vales-Gomez M, Reyburn HT, Mandelboim M, et al. Kinetics of interaction of HLA-C ligands with natural killer cell inhibitory receptors. *Immunity*. 1998;9:337–344.

26. Farag SS, Fehniger TA, Ruggeri L, et al. Natural killer cell receptors: new biology and insights into the graft-versus-leukemia effect. *Blood*. 2002;100:1935–1947.

27. Aversa F, Terenzi A, Tabilio A, et al. Full haplotype-mismatched hematopoietic stem-cell transplantation: a phase II study in patients with acute leukemia at high risk of relapse. *J Clin Oncol*. 2005;23:3447–3454.

28. Ruggeri L, Capanni M, Urbani E, et al. Effectiveness of donor natural killer cell alloreactivity in mismatched hematopoietic transplants. *Science*. 2002;295:2097–2100.

29. McLaughlin P, Grillo-Lopez AJ, Link BK, et al. Rituximab chimeric anti-CD20 monoclonal antibody therapy for relapsed indolent lymphoma: half of patients respond to a four-dose treatment program. *J Clin Oncol*. 1998;16:2825–2833.

30. Czuczman MS, Grillo-Lopez AJ, White CA, et al. Treatment of patients with low-grade B-cell lymphoma with the combination of chimeric anti-CD20 monoclonal antibody and CHOP chemotherapy. *J Clin Oncol*. 1999;17:268–276.

31. Witzig TE, Gordon LI, Cabanillas F, et al. Randomized controlled trial of yttrium-90-labeled ibritumomab tiuxetan radioimmunotherapy versus rituximab immunotherapy for patients with relapsed or refractory low-grade, follicular, or transformed B-cell non-Hodgkin's lymphoma. *J Clin Oncol*. 2002;20:2453–2463.

32. Press OW, Unger JM, Braziel RM, et al. A phase 2 trial of CHOP chemotherapy followed by tositumomab/iodine I 131 tositumomab for previously untreated follicular non-Hodgkin lymphoma: Southwest Oncology Group Protocol S9911. *Blood*. 2003;102:1606–1612.

33. Zelenetz AD. A clinical and scientific overview of tositumomab and iodine I 131 tositumomab. *Semin Oncol*. 2003;30:22–30.

34. Schwartz MA, Lovett DR, Redner A, et al. Dose-escalation trial of M195 labeled with iodine 131 for cytoreduction and marrow ablation in relapsed or refractory myeloid leukemias. *J Clin Oncol*. 1993;11:294–303.

35. Jurcic JG, Caron PC, Nikula TK, et al. Radiolabeled anti-CD33 monoclonal antibody M195 for myeloid leukemias. *Cancer Res*. 1995;55:5908s–5910s.

36. Jurcic JG, Scheinberg DA. Radionuclides as conditioning before stem cell transplantation. *Curr Opin Hematol*. 1999;6:371–376.

37. Sievers EL, Appelbaum FR, Spielberger RT, et al. Selective ablation of acute myeloid leukemia using antibody-targeted chemotherapy: a phase I study of an anti-CD33 calicheamicin immunoconjugate. *Blood*. 1999;93:3678–3684.

38. Davis TA, Maloney DG, Czerwinski DK, et al. Anti-idiotype antibodies can induce long-term complete remissions in non-Hodgkin's lymphoma without eradicating the malignant clone. *Blood*. 1998;92:1184–1190.

39. Levy R, Miller RA. Therapy of lymphoma directed at idiotypes. *J Natl Cancer Inst Monogr*. 1990;10:61–68.

40. Miller RA, Maloney DG, Warnke R, et al. Treatment of B-cell lymphoma with monoclonal anti-idiotype antibody. *N Engl J Med*. 1982;306:517–522.

41. Akbari O, Panjwani N, Garcia S, et al. DNA vaccination: transfection and activation of dendritic cells as key events for immunity. *J Exp Med*. 1999;189:169–178.

42. O'Hagan DT. Recent advances in vaccine adjuvants for systemic and mucosal administration. *J Pharm Pharmacol*. 1998;50:1–10.

43. Ulmer JB, DeWitt CM, Chastain M, et al. Enhancement of DNA vaccine potency using conventional aluminum adjuvants. *Vaccine*. 1999;18:18–28.

44. Tivol EA, Borriello F, Schweitzer AN, et al. Loss of CTLA-4 leads to massive lymphoproliferation and fatal multiorgan tissue destruction, revealing a critical negative regulatory role of CTLA-4. *Immunity*. 1995;3:541–547.

45. Waterhouse P, Marengere LE, Mittrucker HW, et al. CTLA-4, a negative regulator of T-lymphocyte activation. *Immunol Rev*. 1996;153:183–207.

46. Lanzavecchia A, Sallusto F. Regulation of T cell immunity by dendritic cells. *Cell*. 2001;106:263–266.

47. Gale RP, Champlin RE. How does bone-marrow transplantation cure leukaemia? *Lancet*. 1984;2:28–30.

48. Kolb HJ. Donor leukocyte transfusions for treatment of leukemic relapse after bone marrow transplantation. EBMT Immunology and Chronic Leukemia Working Parties. *Vox Sang*. 1998;74(Suppl 2):321–329.

49. Kolb HJ. Management of relapse after hematopoietic cell transplantation. In: Thomas ED BKG, Forman ST, eds. *Hematopoietic Cell Transplantation*. Blackwell Science Inc; 1999:929–936.

50. Cardoso AA, Schultze JL, Boussiotis VA, et al. Pre-B acute lymphoblastic leukemia cells may induce T-cell anergy to alloantigen. *Blood*. 1996;88:41–48.

51. Stripecke R, Cardoso AA, Pepper KA, et al. Lentiviral vectors for efficient delivery of CD80 and granulocyte-macrophage-colony-stimulating factor in human acute lymphoblastic leukemia and acute myeloid leukemia cells to induce antileukemic immune responses. *Blood*. 2000;96:1317–1326.

52. Choudhury A, Gajewski JL, Liang JC, et al. Use of leukemic dendritic cells for the generation of antileukemic cellular cytotoxicity against Philadelphia chromosome-positive chronic myelogenous leukemia. *Blood*. 1997;89:1133–1142.

53. Smit WM, Rijnbeek M, van Bergen CA, et al. Generation of dendritic cells expressing bcr-abl from CD34-positive chronic myeloid leukemia precursor cells. *Hum Immunol*. 1997;53:216–223.

54. Choudhury BA, Liang JC, Thomas EK, et al. Dendritic cells derived in vitro from acute myelogenous leukemia cells stimulate autologous, antileukemic T-cell responses. *Blood*. 1999;93:780–786.

55. Cignetti A, Bryant E, Allione B, et al. CD34(+) acute myeloid and lymphoid leukemic blasts can be induced to differentiate into dendritic cells. *Blood*. 1999;94:2048–2055.

56. Dunussi-Joannopoulos K, Weinstein HJ, Nickerson PW, et al. Irradiated B7-1 transduced primary acute myelogenous leukemia (AML) cells can be used as therapeutic vaccines in murine AML. *Blood.* 1996;87:2938–2946.

57. Mutis T, Schrama E, Melief CJ, et al. CD80-Transfected acute myeloid leukemia cells induce primary allogeneic T-cell responses directed at patient specific minor histocompatibility antigens and leukemia-associated antigens. *Blood.* 1998;92:1677–1684.

58. Cardoso AA, Seamon MJ, Afonso HM, et al. Ex vivo generation of human anti-pre-B leukemia-specific autologous cytolytic T cells. *Blood.* 1997;90:549–561.

59. Ljungman P, Aschan J, Lewensohn-Fuchs I, et al. Results of different strategies for reducing cytomegalovirus-associated mortality in allogeneic stem cell transplant recipients. *Transplantation.* 1998;66:1330–1334.

60. Boeckh M, Leisenring W, Riddell SR, et al. Late cytomegalovirus disease and mortality in recipients of allogeneic hematopoietic stem cell transplants: importance of viral load and T-cell immunity. *Blood.* 2003;101:407–414.

61. Papadopoulos EB, Ladanyi M, Emanuel D, et al. Infusions of donor leukocytes to treat Epstein-Barr virus-associated lymphoproliferative disorders after allogeneic bone marrow transplantation. *N Engl J Med.* 1994;330:1185–1191.

62. Bonini C, Ferrari G, Verzeletti S, et al. HSV-TK gene transfer into donor lymphocytes for control of allogeneic graft-versus-leukemia. *Science.* 1997;276:1719–1724.

63. Haque T, Wilkie GM, Taylor C, et al. Treatment of Epstein-Barr-virus-positive post-transplantation lymphoproliferative disease with partly HLA-matched allogeneic cytotoxic T cells. *Lancet.* 2002;360:436–442.

64. Rooney CM, Smith CA, Ng CY, et al. Use of gene-modified virus-specific T lymphocytes to control Epstein-Barr-virus-related lymphoproliferation. *Lancet.* 1995;345:9–13.

65. Walter EA, Greenberg PD, Gilbert MJ, et al. Reconstitution of cellular immunity against cytomegalovirus in recipients of allogeneic bone marrow by transfer of T-cell clones from the donor. *N Engl J Med.* 1995;333:1038–1044.

66. Peggs KS, Verfuerth S, Pizzey A, et al. Adoptive cellular therapy for early cytomegalovirus infection after allogeneic stem-cell transplantation with virus-specific T-cell lines. *Lancet.* 2003;362:1375–1377.

67. Einsele H, Roosnek E, Rufer N, et al. Infusion of cytomegalovirus (CMV)-specific T cells for the treatment of CMV infection not responding to antiviral chemotherapy. *Blood.* 2002;99:3916–3922.

68. Call KM, Glaser T, Ito CY, et al. Isolation and characterization of a zinc finger polypeptide gene at the human chromosome 11 Wilms' tumor locus. *Cell.* 1990;60:509–520.

69. Rauscher FJ, 3rd. The WT1 Wilms tumor gene product: a developmentally regulated transcription factor in the kidney that functions as a tumor suppressor. *Faseb J.* 1993;7:896–903.

70. Buckler AJ, Pelletier J, Haber DA, et al. Isolation, characterization, and expression of the murine Wilms' tumor gene (WT1) during kidney development. *Mol Cell Biol.* 1991;11:1707–1712.

71. Park S, Schalling M, Bernard A, et al. The Wilms tumour gene WT1 is expressed in murine mesoderm-derived tissues and mutated in a human mesothelioma. *Nat Genet.* 1993;4:415–420.

72. Gaiger A, Reese V, Disis ML, et al. Immunity to WT1 in the animal model and in patients with acute myeloid leukemia. *Blood.* 2000;96:1480–1489.

73. Miwa H, Beran M, Saunders GF. Expression of the Wilms' tumor gene (WT1) in human leukemias. *Leukemia.* 1992;6:405–409.

74. Tamaki H, Ogawa H, Inoue K, et al. Increased expression of the Wilms tumor gene (WT1) at relapse in acute leukemia. *Blood.* 1996;88:4396–4398.

75. Ohminami H, Yasukawa M, Fujita S. HLA class I-restricted lysis of leukemia cells by a CD8(+) cytotoxic T-lymphocyte clone specific for WT1 peptide. *Blood.* 2000;95:286–293.

76. Oka Y, Elisseeva OA, Tsuboi A, et al. Human cytotoxic T-lymphocyte responses specific for peptides of the wild-type Wilms' tumor gene (WT1) product. *Immunogenetics.* 2000;51:99–107.

77. Gao L, Bellantuono I, Elsasser A, et al. Selective elimination of leukemic CD34(+) progenitor cells by cytotoxic T lymphocytes specific for WT1. *Blood.* 2000;95:2198–2203.

78. Doubrovina ES, Doubrovin MM, Lee S, et al. In vitro stimulation with WT1 peptide-loaded Epstein-Barr virus-positive B cells elicits high frequencies of WT1 peptide-specific T cells with in vitro and in vivo tumoricidal activity. *Clin Cancer Res.* 2004;10:7207–7219.

79. Bories D, Raynal MC, Solomon DH, et al. Down-regulation of a serine protease, myeloblastin, causes growth arrest and differentiation of promyelocytic leukemia cells. *Cell.* 1989;59:959–968.

80. Dengler R, Munstermann U, al-Batran S, et al. Immunocytochemical and flow cytometric detection of proteinase 3 (myeloblastin) in normal and leukaemic myeloid cells. *Br J Haematol.* 1995;89:250–257.

81. Molldrem JJ, Clave E, Jiang YZ, et al. Cytotoxic T lymphocytes specific for a nonpolymorphic proteinase 3 peptide preferentially inhibit chronic myeloid leukemia colony-forming units. *Blood.* 1997;90:2529–2534.

82. Molldrem JJ, Lee PP, Wang C, et al. Evidence that specific T lymphocytes may participate in the elimination of chronic myelogenous leukemia. *Nat Med.* 2000;6:1018–1023.

83. Molldrem JJ, Lee PP, Wang C, et al. A PR1-human leukocyte antigen-A2 tetramer can be used to isolate low-frequency cytotoxic T lymphocytes from healthy donors that selectively lyse chronic myelogenous leukemia. *Cancer Res.* 1999;59:2675–2681.

84. Mailander V, Scheibenbogen C, Thiel E, et al. Complete remission in a patient with recurrent acute myeloid leukemia induced by vaccination with WT1 peptide in the absence of hematological or renal toxicity. *Leukemia.* 2004;18:165–166.

85. Oka Y, Tsuboi A, Taguchi T, et al. Induction of WT1 (Wilms' tumor gene)-specific cytotoxic T lymphocytes by WT1 peptide vaccine and the resultant cancer regression. *Proc Natl Acad Sci USA.* 2004;101:13885–13890.

86. Roopenian D, Choi EY, Brown A. The immunogenomics of minor histocompatibility antigens. *Immunol Rev.* 2002;190:86–94.

87. Korngold B, Sprent J. Lethal graft-versus-host disease after bone marrow transplantation across minor histocompatibility barriers in mice. Prevention by removing mature T cells from marrow. *J Exp Med.* 1978;148:1687–1698.

88. Wallny HJ, Rammensee HG. Identification of classical minor histocompatibility antigen as cell-derived peptide. *Nature.* 1990;343:275–278.

89. Goulmy E. Human minor histocompatibility antigens. *Curr Opin Immunol.* 1996;8:75–81.

90. den Haan JM, Sherman NE, Blokland E, et al. Identification of a graft versus host disease-associated human minor histocompatibility antigen. *Science.* 1995;268:1476–1480.

91. Randolph SS, Gooley TA, Warren EH, et al. Female donors contribute to a selective graft-versus-leukemia effect in male recipients of HLA-matched, related hematopoietic stem cell transplants. *Blood.* 2004;103:347–352.

92. Stern M, Passweg JR, Locasciulli A, et al. Influence of donor/recipient sex matching on outcome of allogeneic hematopoietic stem cell transplantation for aplastic anemia. *Transplantation.* 2006;82:218–226.

93. Goulmy E, Schipper R, Pool J, et al. Mismatches of minor histocompatibility antigens between HLA-identical donors and recipients and the development of graft-versus-host disease after bone marrow transplantation. *N Engl J Med.* 1996;334:281–285.

94. Tseng LH, Lin MT, Hansen JA, et al. Correlation between disparity for the minor histocompatibility antigen HA-1 and the development of acute graft-versus-host disease after allogeneic marrow transplantation. *Blood.* 1999;94:2911–2914.

95. Socie G, Loiseau P, Tamouza R, et al. Both genetic and clinical factors predict the development of graft-versus-host disease after allogeneic hematopoietic stem cell transplantation. *Transplantation*. 2001;72:699–706.

96. Lin MT, Gooley T, Hansen JA, et al. Absence of statistically significant correlation between disparity for the minor histocompatibility antigen-HA-1 and outcome after allogeneic hematopoietic cell transplantation. *Blood*. 2001;98:3172–3173.

97. Pietz BC, Warden MB, DuChateau BK, et al. Multiplex genotyping of human minor histocompatibility antigens. *Hum Immunol*. 2005;66:1174–1182.

98. Wu CJ, Ritz J. Induction of tumor immunity following allogeneic stem cell transplantation. *Adv Immunol*. 2006;90:133–173.

99. van Els CA, D'Amaro J, Pool J, et al. Immunogenetics of human minor histocompatibility antigens: their polymorphism and immunodominance. *Immunogenetics*. 1992;35:161–165.

100. Martin PJ. How much benefit can be expected from matching for minor antigens in allogeneic marrow transplantation? *Bone Marrow Transplant*. 1997;20:97–100.

101. Mutis T, Gillespie G, Schrama E, et al. Tetrameric HLA class I-minor histocompatibility antigen peptide complexes demonstrate minor histocompatibility antigen-specific cytotoxic T lymphocytes in patients with graft-versus-host disease. *Nat Med*. 1999;5:839–842.

102. Dickinson AM, Wang XN, Sviland L, et al. In situ dissection of the graft-versus-host activities of cytotoxic T cells specific for minor histocompatibility antigens. *Nat Med*. 2002;8:410–414.

103. Marijt WA, Heemskerk MH, Kloosterboer FM, et al. Hematopoiesis-restricted minor histocompatibility antigens HA-1- or HA-2-specific T cells can induce complete remissions of relapsed leukemia. *Proc Natl Acad Sci USA*. 2003;100:2742–2747.

104. Kloosterboer FM, van Luxemburg-Heijs SA, van Soest RA, et al. Direct cloning of leukemia-reactive T cells from patients treated with donor lymphocyte infusion shows a relative dominance of hematopoiesis-restricted minor histocompatibility antigen HA-1 and HA-2 specific T cells. *Leukemia*. 2004;18:798–808.

105. Allen RD. The new genetics of bone marrow transplantation. *Genes Immun*. 2000;1:316–320.

106. Trinchieri G. Biology of natural killer cells. *Adv Immunol*. 1989;47:187–376.

107. Foa R, Meloni G, Tosti S, et al. Treatment of residual disease in acute leukemia patients with recombinant interleukin 2 (IL2): clinical and biological findings. *Bone Marrow Transplant*. 1990;6(Suppl 1):98–102.

108. Meloni G, Vignetti M, Pogliani E, et al. Interleukin-2 therapy in relapsed acute myelogenous leukemia. *Cancer J Sci Am*. 1997;3(Suppl 1):S43–S47.

109. Fehniger TA, Cooper MA, Caligiuri MA. Interleukin-2 and interleukin-15: immunotherapy for cancer. *Cytokine Growth Factor Rev*. 2002;13:169–183.

110. Storkus WJ, Alexander J, Payne JA, et al. Reversal of natural killing susceptibility in target cells expressing transfected class I HLA genes. *Proc Natl Acad Sci USA*. 1989;86:2361–2364.

111. Shimizu Y, DeMars R. Demonstration by class I gene transfer that reduced susceptibility of human cells to natural killer cell-mediated lysis is inversely correlated with HLA class I antigen expression. *Eur J Immunol*. 1989;19:447–451.

112. Moretta A, Bottino C, Pende D, et al. Identification of four subsets of human CD3-CD16+ natural killer (NK) cells by the expression of clonally distributed functional surface molecules: correlation between subset assignment of NK clones and ability to mediate specific alloantigen recognition. *J Exp Med*. 1990;172:1589–1598.

113. Ruggeri L, Capanni M, Casucci M, et al. Role of natural killer cell alloreactivity in HLA-mismatched hematopoietic stem cell transplantation. *Blood*. 1999;94:333–339.

114. Giebel S, Locatelli F, Lamparelli T, et al. Survival advantage with KIR ligand incompatibility in hematopoietic stem cell transplantation from unrelated donors. *Blood*. 2003;102:814–819.

115. Hsu KC, Keever-Taylor CA, Wilton A, et al. Improved outcome in HLA-identical sibling hematopoietic stem-cell transplantation for acute myelogenous leukemia predicted by KIR and HLA genotypes. *Blood*. 2005;105:4878–4884.

116. Shilling HG, Young N, Guethlein LA, et al. Genetic control of human NK cell repertoire. *J Immunol*. 2002;169:239–247.

117. Coiffier B, Haioun C, Ketterer N, et al. Rituximab (anti-CD20 monoclonal antibody) for the treatment of patients with relapsing or refractory aggressive lymphoma: a multicenter phase II study. *Blood*. 1998;92:1927–1932.

118. Comoli P, Basso S, Zecca M, et al. Preemptive Therapy of EBV-Related Lymphoproliferative Disease after Pediatric Haploidentical Stem Cell Transplantation. *Am J Transplant*. 2007;7:1648–1655.

119. Savoldo B, Rooney CM, Quiros-Tejeira RE, et al. Cellular immunity to Epstein-Barr virus in liver transplant recipients treated with rituximab for post-transplant lymphoproliferative disease. *Am J Transplant*. 2005;5:566–572.

120. Cutler C, Miklos D, Kim HT, et al. Rituximab for steroid-refractory chronic graft-versus-host disease. *Blood*. 2006;108:756–762.

121. Ratanatharathorn V, Ayash L, Reynolds C, et al. Treatment of chronic graft-versus-host disease with anti-CD20 chimeric monoclonal antibody. *Biol Blood Marrow Transplant*. 2003;9:505–511.

122. Keating M, O'Brien S. High-dose rituximab therapy in chronic lymphocytic leukemia. *Semin Oncol*. 2000;27:86–90.

123. Huhn D, von Schilling C, Wilhelm M, et al. Rituximab therapy of patients with B-cell chronic lymphocytic leukemia. *Blood*. 2001;98:1326–1331.

124. Manshouri T, Do KA, Wang X, et al. Circulating CD20 is detectable in the plasma of patients with chronic lymphocytic leukemia and is of prognostic significance. *Blood*. 2003;101:2507–2513.

125. Keating MJ, Flinn I, Jain V, et al. Therapeutic role of alemtuzumab (Campath-1H) in patients who have failed fludarabine: results of a large international study. *Blood*. 2002;99:3554–3561.

126. Osterborg A, Dyer MJ, Bunjes D, et al. Phase II multicenter study of human CD52 antibody in previously treated chronic lymphocytic leukemia. European Study Group of CAMPATH-1H Treatment in Chronic Lymphocytic Leukemia. *J Clin Oncol*. 1997;15:1567–1574.

127. Rai KR, Freter CE, Mercier RJ, et al. Alemtuzumab in previously treated chronic lymphocytic leukemia patients who also had received fludarabine. *J Clin Oncol*. 2002;20:3891–3897.

128. Bowen AL, Zomas A, Emmett E, et al. Subcutaneous CAMPATH-1H in fludarabine-resistant/relapsed chronic lymphocytic and B-prolymphocytic leukaemia. *Br J Haematol*. 1997;96:617–619.

129. Lundin J, Kimby E, Bjorkholm M, et al. Phase II trial of subcutaneous anti-CD52 monoclonal antibody alemtuzumab (Campath-1H) as first-line treatment for patients with B-cell chronic lymphocytic leukemia (B-CLL). *Blood*. 2002;100:768–773.

130. Stilgenbauer S, Dohner H. Campath-1H-induced complete remission of chronic lymphocytic leukemia despite p53 gene mutation and resistance to chemotherapy. *N Engl J Med*. 2002;347:452–453.

131. Andrews RG, Torok-Storb B, Bernstein ID. Myeloid-associated differentiation antigens on stem cells and their progeny identified by monoclonal antibodies. *Blood*. 1983;62:124–132.

132. Griffin JD, Linch D, Sabbath K, et al. A monoclonal antibody reactive with normal and leukemic human myeloid progenitor cells. *Leuk Res*. 1984;8:521–534.

133. Matutes E, Rodriguez B, Polli N, et al. Characterization of myeloid leukemias with monoclonal antibodies 3C5 and MY9. *Hematol Oncol*. 1985;3:179–186.

134. Radich J, Sievers E. New developments in the treatment of acute myeloid leukemia. *Oncology (Williston Park)*. 2000;14:125–131.

135. Ruffner KL, Matthews DC. Current uses of monoclonal antibodies in the treatment of acute leukemia. *Semin Oncol.* 2000;27:531–539.

136. Scheinberg DA, Tanimoto M, McKenzie S, et al. Monoclonal antibody M195: a diagnostic marker for acute myelogenous leukemia. *Leukemia.* 1989;3:440–445.

137. Caron PC, Dumont L, Scheinberg DA. Supersaturating infusional humanized anti-CD33 monoclonal antibody HuM195 in myelogenous leukemia. *Clin Cancer Res.* 1998;4:1421–1428.

138. Feldman E, Kalaycio M, Weiner G, et al. Treatment of relapsed or refractory acute myeloid leukemia with humanized anti-CD33 monoclonal antibody HuM195. *Leukemia.* 2003;17:314–318.

139. Jurcic JG, DeBlasio T, Dumont L, et al. Molecular remission induction with retinoic acid and anti-CD33 monoclonal antibody HuM195 in acute promyelocytic leukemia. *Clin Cancer Res.* 2000;6:372–380.

140. Jurcic JG. Antibody therapy for residual disease in acute myelogenous leukemia. *Crit Rev Oncol Hematol.* 2001;38:37–45.

141. Zein N, Sinha AM, McGahren WJ, et al. Calicheamicin gamma 1I: an antitumor antibiotic that cleaves double-stranded DNA site specifically. *Science.* 1988;240:1198–1201.

142. Larson RA, Sievers EL, Stadtmauer EA, et al. Final report of the efficacy and safety of gemtuzumab ozogamicin (Mylotarg) in patients with CD33-positive acute myeloid leukemia in first recurrence. *Cancer.* 2005;104:1442–1452.

143. Bastie JN, Suzan F, Garcia I, et al. Veno-occlusive disease after an anti-CD33 therapy (gemtuzumab ozogamicin). *Br J Haematol.* 2002;116:924.

144. Rajvanshi P, Shulman HM, Sievers EL, et al. Hepatic sinusoidal obstruction after gemtuzumab ozogamicin (Mylotarg) therapy. *Blood.* 2002;99:2310–2314.

145. Giles FJ, Kantarjian HM, Kornblau SM, et al. Mylotarg (gemtuzumab ozogamicin) therapy is associated with hepatic venoocclusive disease in patients who have not received stem cell transplantation. *Cancer.* 2001;92:406–413.

146. Matthews DC, Appelbaum FR, Eary JF, et al. Phase I study of (131)I-anti-CD45 antibody plus cyclophosphamide and total body irradiation for advanced acute leukemia and myelodysplastic syndrome. *Blood.* 1999;94:1237–1247.

147. Witzig TE, Molina A, Gordon LI, et al. Long-term responses in patients with recurring or refractory B-cell non-Hodgkin lymphoma treated with yttrium 90 ibritumomab tiuxetan. *Cancer.* 2007;109:1804–1810.

148. Gordon LI, Molina A, Witzig T, et al. Durable responses after ibritumomab tiuxetan radioimmunotherapy for CD20+ B-cell lymphoma: long-term follow-up of a phase 1/2 study. *Blood.* 2004;103:4429–4431.

149. Kaminski MS, Zelenetz AD, Press OW, et al. Pivotal study of iodine I 131 tositumomab for chemotherapy-refractory low-grade or transformed low-grade B-cell non-Hodgkin's lymphomas. *J Clin Oncol.* 2001;19:3918–3928.

150. Fisher RI, Kaminski MS, Wahl RL, et al. Tositumomab and iodine-131 tositumomab produces durable complete remissions in a subset of heavily pretreated patients with low-grade and transformed non-Hodgkin's lymphomas. *J Clin Oncol.* 2005;23:7565–7573.

151. Horning SJ, Younes A, Jain V, et al. Efficacy and safety of tositumomab and iodine-131 tositumomab (Bexxar) in B-cell lymphoma, progressive after rituximab. *J Clin Oncol.* 2005;23:712–719.

152. Witzig TE, Flinn IW, Gordon LI, et al. Treatment with ibritumomab tiuxetan radioimmunotherapy in patients with rituximab-refractory follicular non-Hodgkin's lymphoma. *J Clin Oncol.* 2002;20:3262–3269.

153. Press OW, Unger JM, Braziel RM, et al. Phase II trial of CHOP chemotherapy followed by tositumomab/iodine I-131 tositumomab for previously untreated follicular non-Hodgkin's lymphoma: five-year follow-up of Southwest Oncology Group Protocol S9911. *J Clin Oncol.* 2006;24:4143–4149.

154. Gopal AK, Rajendran JG, Gooley TA, et al. High-dose [131I] tositumomab (anti-CD20) radioimmunotherapy and autolo-gous hematopoietic stem-cell transplantation for adults > or = 60 years old with relapsed or refractory B-cell lymphoma. *J Clin Oncol.* 2007;25:1396–1402.

155. Pantelias A, Pagel JM, Hedin N, et al. Comparative biodistributions of pretargeted radioimmunoconjugates targeting CD20, CD22, and DR molecules on human B-cell lymphomas. *Blood.* 2007;109:4980–4987.

156. Condon C, Watkins SC, Celluzzi CM, et al. DNA-based immunization by in vivo transfection of dendritic cells. *Nat Med.* 1996;2:1122–1128.

157. Randolph GJ, Inaba K, Robbiani DF, et al. Differentiation of phagocytic monocytes into lymph node dendritic cells in vivo. *Immunity.* 1999;11:753–761.

158. Kwak LW, Campbell MJ, Czerwinski DK, et al. Induction of immune responses in patients with B-cell lymphoma against the surface-immunoglobulin idiotype expressed by their tumors. *N Engl J Med.* 1992;327:1209–1215.

159. Hsu FJ, Caspar CB, Czerwinski D, et al. Tumor-specific idiotype vaccines in the treatment of patients with B-cell lymphoma—long-term results of a clinical trial. *Blood.* 1997;89:3129–3135.

160. Bendandi M, Gocke CD, Kobrin CB, et al. Complete molecular remissions induced by patient-specific vaccination plus granulocyte-monocyte colony-stimulating factor against lymphoma. *Nat Med.* 1999;5:1171–1177.

161. Neelapu SS, Gause BL, Nikcevich DA, et al. Phase III randomized trial of patient-specific vaccination for previously untreated patients with follicular lymphoma in first complete remission: protocol summary and interim report. *Clin Lymphoma.* 2005;6:61–64.

162. Weng WK, Czerwinski D, Timmerman J, et al. Clinical outcome of lymphoma patients after idiotype vaccination is correlated with humoral immune response and immunoglobulin G Fc receptor genotype. *J Clin Oncol.* 2004;22:4717–4724.

163. Weng WK, Czerwinski D, Levy R. Humoral immune response and immunoglobulin G Fc receptor genotype are associated with better clinical outcome following idiotype vaccination in follicular lymphoma patients regardless of their response to induction chemotherapy. *Blood.* 2007;109:951–953.

164. Gold P, Freedman SO. Demonstration of tumor-specific antigens in human colonic carcinomata by immunological tolerance and absorption techniques. *J Exp Med.* 1965;121:439–462.

165. Lindenmann J. Speculations on idiotypes and homobodies. *Ann Immunol (Paris).* 1973;124:171–184.

166. Jerne NK. Towards a network theory of the immune system. *Ann Immunol (Paris).* 1974;125C:373–389.

167. Foon KA, John WJ, Chakraborty M, et al. Clinical and immune responses in resected colon cancer patients treated with anti-idiotype monoclonal antibody vaccine that mimics the carcinoembryonic antigen. *J Clin Oncol.* 1999;17:2889–2895.

168. Cheung NK, Guo HF, Heller G, et al. Induction of Ab3 and Ab3' antibody was associated with long-term survival after anti-G(D2) antibody therapy of stage 4 neuroblastoma. *Clin Cancer Res.* 2000;6:2653–2660.

169. Foon KA, Lutzky J, Baral RN, et al. Clinical and immune responses in advanced melanoma patients immunized with an anti-idiotype antibody mimicking disialoganglioside GD2. *J Clin Oncol.* 2000;18:376–384.

170. Wagner U, Kohler S, Reinartz S, et al. Immunological consolidation of ovarian carcinoma recurrences with monoclonal anti-idiotype antibody ACA125: immune responses and survival in palliative treatment. See the biology behind: K. A. Foon and M. Bhattacharya-Chatterjee, Are solid tumor anti-idiotype vaccines ready for prime time? *Clin Cancer Res.* 2001;7:1112–1115, 1154–1162.

171. Yao TJ, Meyers M, Livingston PO, et al. Immunization of melanoma patients with BEC2-keyhole limpet hemocyanin plus BCG intradermally followed by intravenous booster immunizations with BEC2 to induce anti-GD3 ganglioside antibodies. *Clin Cancer Res.* 1999;5:77–81.

172. Johnston SA, Tang DC. Gene gun transfection of animal cells and genetic immunization. *Methods Cell Biol.* 1994;43 (Pt A):353–365.

173. Epstein JE, Gorak EJ, Charoenvit Y, et al. Safety, tolerability, and lack of antibody responses after administration of a PfCSP DNA malaria vaccine via needle or needle-free jet injection, and comparison of intramuscular and combination intramuscular/intradermal routes. *Hum Gene Ther.* 2002;13:1551–1560.

174. Houghton AN. Cancer antigens: immune recognition of self and altered self. *J Exp Med.* 1994;180:1–4.

175. Bowne WB, Srinivasan R, Wolchok JD, et al. Coupling and uncoupling of tumor immunity and autoimmunity. *J Exp Med.* 1999;190:1717–1722.

176. Weber LW, Bowne WB, Wolchok JD, et al. Tumor immunity and autoimmunity induced by immunization with homologous DNA. *J Clin Invest.* 1998;102:1258–1264.

177. Hawkins WG, Gold JS, Dyall R, et al. Immunization with DNA coding for gp100 results in CD4 T-cell independent antitumor immunity. *Surgery.* 2000;128:273–280.

178. Ferrone CR, Perales MA, Goldberg SM, et al. Adjuvanticity of plasmid DNA encoding cytokines fused to immunoglobulin Fc domains. *Clin Cancer Res.* 2006;12:5511–5519.

179. Powell DJ, Jr., Rosenberg SA. Phenotypic and functional maturation of tumor antigen-reactive CD8+ T lymphocytes in patients undergoing multiple course peptide vaccination. *J Immunother.* (1997) 2004;27:36–47.

180. Powell DJ, Jr., Dudley ME, Hogan KA, et al. Adoptive transfer of vaccine-induced peripheral blood mononuclear cells to patients with metastatic melanoma following lymphodepletion. *J Immunol.* 2006;177:6527–6539.

181. Silver DA, Pellicer I, Fair WR, et al. Prostate-specific membrane antigen expression in normal and malignant human tissues. *Clin Cancer Res.* 1997;3:81–85.

182. Chang SS, O'Keefe DS, Bacich DJ, et al. Prostate-specific membrane antigen is produced in tumor-associated neovasculature. *Clin Cancer Res.* 1999;5:2674–2681.

183. Gregor PD, Wolchok JD, Turaga V, et al. Induction of autoantibodies to syngeneic prostate-specific membrane antigen by xenogeneic vaccination. *Int J Cancer.* 2005;116:415–421.

184. Simons JW, Mikhak B, Chang JF, et al. Induction of immunity to prostate cancer antigens: results of a clinical trial of vaccination with irradiated autologous prostate tumor cells engineered to secrete granulocyte-macrophage colony-stimulating factor using ex vivo gene transfer. *Cancer Res.* 1999;59:5160–5168.

185. Simons JW, Sacks N. Granulocyte-macrophage colony-stimulating factor-transduced allogeneic cancer cellular immunotherapy: the GVAX vaccine for prostate cancer. *Urol Oncol.* 2006;24:419–424.

186. Soiffer R, Lynch T, Mihm M, et al. Vaccination with irradiated autologous melanoma cells engineered to secrete human granulocyte-macrophage colony-stimulating factor generates potent antitumor immunity in patients with metastatic melanoma. *Proc Natl Acad Sci USA.* 1998;95:13141–13146.

187. Soiffer R, Hodi FS, Haluska F, et al. Vaccination with irradiated, autologous melanoma cells engineered to secrete granulocyte-macrophage colony-stimulating factor by adenoviral-mediated gene transfer augments antitumor immunity in patients with metastatic melanoma. *J Clin Oncol.* 2003;21:3343–3350.

188. Salgia R, Lynch T, Skarin A, et al. Vaccination with irradiated autologous tumor cells engineered to secrete granulocyte-macrophage colony-stimulating factor augments antitumor immunity in some patients with metastatic non-small-cell lung carcinoma. *J Clin Oncol.* 2003;21:624–630.

189. Nemunaitis J, Jahan T, Ross H, et al. Phase 1/2 trial of autologous tumor mixed with an allogeneic GVAX vaccine in advanced-stage non-small-cell lung cancer. *Cancer Gene Ther.* 2006;13:555–562.

190. Nemunaitis J, Sterman D, Jablons D, et al. Granulocyte-macrophage colony-stimulating factor gene-modified autologous tumor vaccines in non-small-cell lung cancer. *J Natl Cancer Inst.* 2004;96:326–331.

191. Greenwald RJ, Oosterwegel MA, van der Woude D, et al. CTLA-4 regulates cell cycle progression during a primary immune response. *Eur J Immunol.* 2002;32:366–373.

192. Gribben JG, Freeman GJ, Boussiotis VA, et al. CTLA4 mediates antigen-specific apoptosis of human T cells. *Proc Natl Acad Sci USA.* 1995;92:811–815.

193. van Elsas A, Hurwitz AA, Allison JP. Combination immunotherapy of B16 melanoma using anti-cytotoxic T lymphocyte-associated antigen 4 (CTLA-4) and granulocyte/macrophage colony-stimulating factor (GM-CSF)-producing vaccines induces rejection of subcutaneous and metastatic tumors accompanied by autoimmune depigmentation. *J Exp Med.* 1999;190:355–366.

194. van Elsas A, Sutmuller RP, Hurwitz AA, et al. Elucidating the autoimmune and antitumor effector mechanisms of a treatment based on cytotoxic T lymphocyte antigen-4 blockade in combination with a B16 melanoma vaccine: comparison of prophylaxis and therapy. *J Exp Med.* 2001;194:481–489.

195. Gregor PD, Wolchok JD, Ferrone CR, et al. CTLA-4 blockade in combination with xenogeneic DNA vaccines enhances T-cell responses, tumor immunity and autoimmunity to self antigens in animal and cellular model systems. *Vaccine.* 2004;22:1700–1708.

196. Peggs KS, Quezada SA, Korman AJ, et al. Principles and use of anti-CTLA4 antibody in human cancer immunotherapy. *Curr Opin Immunol.* 2006;18:206–213.

197. Small EJ, Tchekmedyian NS, Rini BI, et al. A pilot trial of CTLA-4 blockade with human anti-CTLA-4 in patients with hormone-refractory prostate cancer. *Clin Cancer Res.* 2007;13:1810–1815.

198. Phan GQ, Yang JC, Sherry RM, et al. Cancer regression and autoimmunity induced by cytotoxic T lymphocyte-associated antigen 4 blockade in patients with metastatic melanoma. *Proc Natl Acad Sci USA.* 2003;100:8372–8377.

199. Van Parijs L, Abbas AK. Homeostasis and self-tolerance in the immune system: turning lymphocytes off. *Science.* 1998;280:243–248.

200. Curotto de Lafaille MA, Lafaille JJ. CD4(+) regulatory T cells in autoimmunity and allergy. *Curr Opin Immunol.* 2002;14:771–778.

201. Jonuleit H, Schmitt E. The regulatory T cell family: distinct subsets and their interrelations. *J Immunol.* 2003;171:6323–6327.

202. Earle KE, Tang Q, Zhou X, et al. In vitro expanded human CD4+CD25+ regulatory T cells suppress effector T cell proliferation. *Clin Immunol.* 2005;115:3–9.

203. Hoffmann P, Eder R, Kunz-Schughart LA, et al. Large-scale in vitro expansion of polyclonal human CD4(+)CD25high regulatory T cells. *Blood.* 2004;104:895–903.

204. Battaglia M, Stabilini A, Roncarolo MG. Rapamycin selectively expands CD4+CD25+FoxP3+ regulatory T cells. *Blood.* 2005;105:4743–4748.

205. Casares N, Arribillaga L, Sarobe P, et al. CD4+/CD25+ regulatory cells inhibit activation of tumor-primed CD4+ T cells with IFN-gamma-dependent antiangiogenic activity, as well as long-lasting tumor immunity elicited by peptide vaccination. *J Immunol.* 2003;171:5931–5939.

206. Sutmuller RP, van Duivenvoorde LM, van Elsas A, et al. Synergism of cytotoxic T lymphocyte-associated antigen 4 blockade and depletion of CD25(+) regulatory T cells in antitumor therapy reveals alternative pathways for suppression of autoreactive cytotoxic T lymphocyte responses. *J Exp Med.* 2001;194:823–832.

207. Jones SC, Murphy GF, Korngold R. Post-hematopoietic cell transplantation control of graft-versus-host disease by donor CD425 T cells to allow an effective graft-versus-leukemia response. *Biol Blood Marrow Transplant.* 2003;9:243–256.

208. Hanash AM, Levy RB. Donor CD4+CD25+ T cells promote engraftment and tolerance following MHC-mismatched hematopoietic cell transplantation. *Blood.* 2005;105:1828–1836.

209. Ermann J, Hoffmann P, Edinger M, et al. Only the CD62L+ subpopulation of CD4+CD25+ regulatory T cells protects from lethal acute GVHD. *Blood.* 2005;105:2220–2226.

210. Kern F, Faulhaber N, Frommel C, et al. Analysis of CD8 T cell reactivity to cytomegalovirus using protein-spanning

pools of overlapping pentadecapeptides. *Eur J Immunol.* 2000;30:1676–1682.

211. Trivedi D, Williams RY, O'Reilly RJ, et al. Generation of CMV-specific T lymphocytes using protein-spanning pools of pp65-derived overlapping pentadecapeptides for adoptive immunotherapy. *Blood.* 2005;105:2793–2801.

212. Ratzinger G, Baggers J, de Cos MA, et al. Mature human Langerhans cells derived from CD34+ hematopoietic progenitors stimulate greater cytolytic T lymphocyte activity in the absence of bioactive IL-12p70, by either single peptide presentation or cross-priming, than do dermal-interstitial or monocyte-derived dendritic cells. *J Immunol.* 2004;173:2780–2791.

213. Young JW, Merad M, Hart DN. Dendritic cells in transplantation and immune-based therapies. *Biol Blood Marrow Transplant.* 2007;13:23–32.

214. Latouche JB, Sadelain M. Induction of human cytotoxic T lymphocytes by artificial antigen-presenting cells. *Nat Biotechnol.* 2000;18:405–409.

215. Papanicolaou GA, Latouche JB, Tan C, et al. Rapid expansion of cytomegalovirus-specific cytotoxic T lymphocytes by arti-

ficial antigen-presenting cells expressing a single HLA allele. *Blood.* 2003;102:2498–2505.

216. Brentjens RJ, Latouche JB, Santos E, et al. Eradication of systemic B-cell tumors by genetically targeted human T lymphocytes co-stimulated by CD80 and interleukin-15. *Nat Med.* 2003;9:279–286.

217. Brentjens RJ. Novel Approaches to Immunotherapy for B-cell Malignancies. *Curr Oncol Rep.* 2004;6:339–347.

218. Rossig C, Brenner MK. Chimeric T-cell receptors for the targeting of cancer cells. *Acta Haematol.* 2003;110:154–159.

219. Savoldo B, Rooney CM, Di Stasi A, et al. Epstein Barr virus-specific cytotoxic T lymphocytes expressing the anti-CD30{zeta} artificial chimeric T-cell receptor for immunotherapy of Hodgkin's disease. *Blood.* 2007;110(7):2620–2630.

220. McDevitt MR, Ma D, Lai LT, et al. Tumor therapy with targeted atomic nanogenerators. *Science.* 2001;294:1537–1540.

221. Jurcic JG, Larson SM, Sgouros G, et al. Targeted alpha particle immunotherapy for myeloid leukemia. *Blood.* 2002;100:1233–1239.

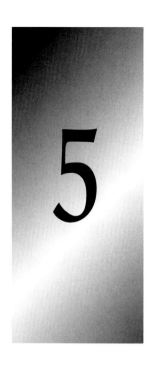

Principles of Radiotherapy

5

Yoshiya Yamada

The risk of radiation-induced secondary cancers is a difficult late effect of radiation therapy. Ever since the discovery of x-rays by Conrad Roentgen in 1895, radiation has been closely tied to medical applications, and it has been known to have significant biologic effects from the very beginning of the radiologic era. Antoine-Henri Becquerel, who discovered that uranium compounds emitted radiation in 1896, was the first to record the biological effect of radiation when he inadvertently left a vial of radium in his vest pocket, noting skin erythema two weeks later. This later turned into a skin ulcer, which took several weeks to heal. Pierre Curie repeated the experiment in 1901 by deliberately causing a radiation burn on his forearm. An Austrian surgeon, Leopold Freund, demonstrated in 1896 to the Vienna Medical Society that radiation could cause a hairy mole to disappear (1).

From these beginnings, radiation therapy has evolved into an important modality of treating benign and malignant illness. Radiotherapy has been shown to either contribute to the cure or be the primary curative therapy for cancers that affect every organ system in the body. Improvements in computer and imaging technology have expanded the role of radiotherapy, allowing for the effective noninvasive management of tumors without the morbidity commonly associated with surgical or chemotherapeutic strategies. Radiotherapy may offer curative options for patients who may not be able to tolerate radical surgery. Radiotherapy is not limited by the anatomic or functional constraints of surgical resection, and thus is able to treat cancer in a regional

paradigm, such as in the treatment of many lymphomas or spare significant morbidity and functional loss or deformity associated with radical resections. Because radiation effects are typically locoregional, patients can be spared the generalized toxicity associated with cytotoxic chemotherapy. Radiotherapy is not dependent upon the circulatory system to reach the target tissue. Hence, toxicity is limited to the tissues to which radiation is administered, but the benefits of radiation are also limited to the area to which radiation is given. Radiotherapy is also an integral part of combined modality therapy with systemic therapy and/or surgery. Nearly two-thirds of all cancer patients will receive radiation therapy at some point during their illness, and in 2004, nearly 1 million patients were treated with radiotherapy in the United States (2). As the incidence of cancer increases with an increasingly aging population, it is expected that even more patients will benefit from radiotherapy. Currently there are about 3,900 radiation oncologists in the United States.

RADIATION PHYSICS

Radiation therapy can be broadly defined as the use of ionizing radiation for the treatment of neoplasms. The most commonly utilized form of radiation is photon radiation, commonly known as x-rays (artificially produced) or gamma rays (emitted from naturally decaying isotopes). Photons are packets of energy that can interact with the atoms that make up the deoxyribonucleic

KEY POINTS

- Nearly two-thirds of all cancer patients will receive radiation therapy at some point during their illness, and in 2004, nearly 1 million patients were treated with radiotherapy in the United States.
- Improvements in computer and imaging technology have expanded the role of radiotherapy, allowing for the effective noninvasive management of tumors without the morbidity commonly associated with surgical or chemotherapeutic strategies.
- The most commonly utilized form of radiation is photon radiation, commonly known as x-rays (artificially produced) or gamma rays (emitted from naturally decaying isotopes).
- Radiation dose (Gray or Gy) is commonly defined as joules per kilogram (energy per unit mass) where 1 Gy equals 1 joule/kg.
- A technique called intensity modulated radiotherapy (IMRT) has allowed steep dose gradients around tumors, as high as 10% per millimeter.
- As opposed to treating tumors with the radiation source distant from the tumor, brachytherapy (placing radioactive sources inside of tumors) is another way to deliver very high-dose radiation and limit normal tissue doses.
- The effects of radiation therapy on tissues are dependent upon the inherent radiosensitivity of the tissue or organ in question, the dose of radiation given, and the volume of tissue irradiated.
- Radiation effects have been traditionally classified as early or late effects.
- Early effects are generally seen during the course of treatment or within six weeks of radiation therapy.
- Late effects are considered those that appear months to years after radiation, and are more likely in tissues with low proliferative potential, such as connective tissue (fibrosis) or neural tissue (neuropathy).
- Microvascular damage (endothelial thickening to the point that red blood cells are not able to pass through) has thought to play an important role in the late toxicity, causing hypoxic stress and cellular death.

acid (DNA) of a cell, causing disruption of chemical bonds and DNA strand breaks, which ultimately leads to irreparable damage (3). Cells not able to repair this damage may not be able to successfully complete mitosis, resulting in the death of both mother and daughter cells. Many cells will also undergo apoptotic death, when the cell detects DNA damage, without completing mitosis (4).

Radiation dose (Gray or Gy) is commonly defined as joules per kilogram (energy per unit mass) where 1 Gy equals 1 joule/kg (5). Since radiation is ionizing energy, radiotherapy does not induce heat or other manifestations of energy transfer that can be felt by patients. Thus, patients feel no pain during radiation administration. Because radiation effects are stochastic, they may cause similar effects on healthy normal cells. In order to reduce the side effects of radiotherapy, radiation oncologists attempt to concentrate the radiation in tumors and minimize the amount of radiation absorbed by surrounding normal tissues.

THE THERAPEUTIC RATIO

Tumor control probability and normal tissue complication probability is usually dose-dependent. Efforts to minimize radiation dose to normal tissue result in lower normal tissue complication probabilities, while increasing dose to the tumor should increase tumor control probabilities. Hence, a basic mantra of radiation oncology is to increase the gap between toxicity and tumor control probability curves (Fig. 5.1), commonly referred to as the therapeutic ratio.

One strategy to minimize radiation toxicity is to use the appropriate photon energy. Most radiation beams are created in machines that accelerate electrons to very high energies (typically 4–25 megaelectron volts or MV) called linear accelerators or linacs (3). Because of the very high energy of the resultant photons, they tended to penetrate deeper into the body as the energy increases. Thus, by choosing the appropriate beam energy, the radiation oncologist can limit radiation damage to superficial structures in the case of deep-seated tumors, or use lower-energy beams for superficial tumors to limit dose to deeper normal structures.

Another method of improving the therapeutic ratio is to shape radiation fields to match the three-dimensional shape of the target volume, thereby limiting the exposure of normal tissues to high doses of radiation (5). The shape of the radiation beam can also be manipulated by placing using thick lead or cerrobend blocks into the head of the linac to block out radiation except to the tumor. Modern linacs utilize a device known as the multileaf collimator (Fig. 5.2), which has multiple individually motorized leaves of thick tungsten 3–10 mm wide. These leaves can be pushed in or out of the radiation field to approximate the tumor outline and similarly block radiation

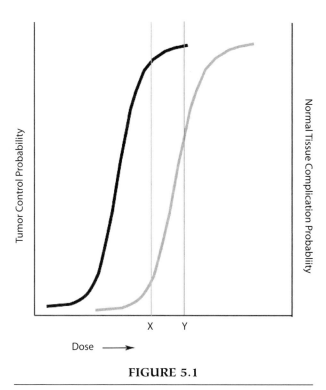

FIGURE 5.1

The therapeutic ratio. The aim of successful treatment is to increase the tumor control probability (black curve) while reducing the treatment complication (gray curve). Increase dose delivered to the tumor will typically increase the probability of cure, but will also increase the likelihood of toxicity. By reducing the amount of radiation given to normal tissues and/or the volume of normal tissue exposed to radiation, toxicity can be reduced (shifting the complication curve to the right of the tumor control curve). Because of the sigmoid nature of these curves, a moderate increase in dose (X to Y) can often result in a much higher probability of complications with only a modest gain in tumor control probability.

from areas where it is not necessary or desired. Most tumors are complex shapes, and will present different outlines when viewed from different angles. When multiple beams of shaped radiation fields intersect in the tumor, the result is a cloud of radiation where the high-dose volume is similar to the actual three-dimensional characteristics of the tumor. By conforming the high-dose region to just the tumor, higher doses of radiation can be delivered while the surrounding tissues can be relatively spared of high doses, and thus healthy tissue can be relatively spared the effects of higher doses, limiting the toxicity of treatment and improving the therapeutic ratio.

An important recent innovation has been the use of intensity modulation. By using fast computers, radiation doses can be changed or modulated within different regions of each radiation field. Hence, the radiation not only conforms to the three-dimensional

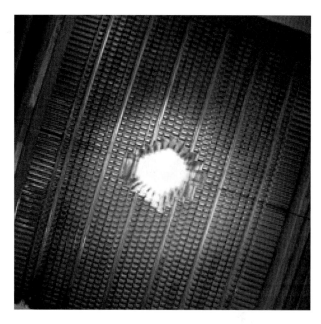

FIGURE 5.2

Multileaf collimator. The multileaf collimator is a device that is made up of many leaves of tungsten, each of which is individually motorized. This allows a computer to control the position of each leaf while the radiation beam is on. By adjusting the position of each leaf and the time spent at that position, the intensity of radiation at any particular part of the radiation field can be manipulated or modulated. When multiple beams of modulated radiation come from different directions and intersect in the target, the cumulative dose that results can be made to closely follow the three-dimensional characters of even complicated target volumes.

outline of the tumor, but can be modulated to reduce dose to areas of the field, which might approach a dose-sensitive normal structure that might be just in front or behind the field, or account for a change in the tumor outline, which may not be appreciable from different angles. This technique, called intensity modulated radiotherapy (IMRT), has allowed steep dose gradients around tumors as high as 10% per millimeter (5). Figure 5.3 illustrates how spinal cord doses are minimized relative to the tumor.

Uncertainty of where the radiation actually goes in relation to the intended target has always been a problem in radiation therapy. In traditional radiation therapy, patients undergo a procedure called simulation to radiographically identify the center of the target. During simulation, either two-dimensional (standard x-rays) or three-dimensional imaging (computed tomography [CT]/magnetic resonance imaging [MRI]/ positron emission tomography [PET] or a combination) is utilized to identify the target center in relation to the

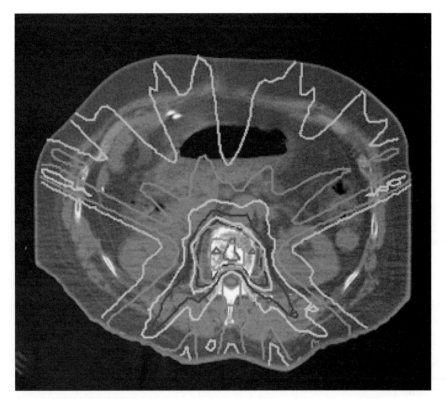

FIGURE 5.3

Radiation treatments are often represented by dose maps, called dose distributions, which depict different levels of dose intensity. The dose distribution shown is an example of a highly conformal radiation treatment plan that delivers 2400 cGy to the target while the spinal cord, which is an important dose-sensitive structure, receives less than 1400 cGy. Because the treatment was delivered using intensity-modulated techniques, the high-dose region of the treatment plan conformed very tightly to the tumor; hence, much less radiation was given to the spinal cord, even though it was only a few millimeters away. This was administered in a single treatment.

patient's anatomy. Small skin marks are made to allow the patient to be triangulated relative to the treatment machine to allow for daily administration of radiation. When patients are treated in this manner, a number of uncertainties must be accounted for. For example, respiration may cause substantial cranial-caudal displacement of a lung tumor during radiation administration. There are day-to-day variations in setting up the patient relative to the treatment machine. There may also be uncertainty regarding the true extent of disease. All of these must be taken into account when planning treatment. Allowances for potential positional errors during multiple radiation treatments (fractions) require that the radiation portals be enlarged beyond the dimensions of the target. Enlarging the margin of radiation around the tumor may result in unacceptably high doses of radiation to normal tissues. Reducing treatment-related uncertainties means less exposure of nearby normal tissues. Positional uncertainties can be reduced by the use of immobilization devices that are designed to minimize positioning errors and patient motion. Most recently, the advent of image-guided techniques, such as cone-beam CT of patients just about to undergo treatment, have greatly increased the accuracy of radiation to within a few millimeters of precision, allowing for even higher biologically effective doses to be delivered without a higher risk of toxicity (6).

Advances in imaging technology have also reduced the uncertainties associated with radiotherapy. When the tumor-bearing volume can be more precisely defined, tissue not needing treatment can be otherwise spared from radiation exposure. MRI and more recently PET imaging have been incorporated into the process of treatment planning to more accurately identify the volume at risk, as well as better visualization of normal tissues to be avoided.

Proton Beams

Charged particles, such as proton beam radiotherapy, are another type of ionizing radiation that is garnering more and more interest. Photons have no mass and therefore no kinetic energy. Charged particles do have mass and kinetic energy, and are subject to the physics of kinetic energy. One very useful aspect unique to charged particles is the Bragg peak effect (Fig. 5.4) in which accelerated particles such as protons deliver their inherent energy within a very narrow depth spectrum in tissue (3). Protons, in effect, have almost no "exit" dose, while photons are attenuated, as they interact with atoms within tissue but are likely to "exit" out of the back of the tumor. The kinetic energy of particle beams also results in higher amounts of energy deposition per linear distance, or linear energy transfer

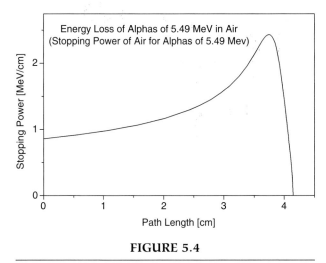

FIGURE 5.4

The Bragg peak effect. Because many charged particles have mass, they also have kinetic energy. Protons are accelerated to very high velocities. As they interact with other atoms, they tend to transfer their inherent energy to the atoms with which they interact. As they lose kinetic energy and slow down, they tend to give up more of their energy to the atoms they "bump into." Hence, towards the end of their trajectory, most of their energy is deposited over a very short distance. This phenomenon is call the Bragg peak effect. There is no "exit dose" after the peak effect. Photons (x-rays) have no mass, and hence have no kinetic energy, and do not demonstrate the Bragg peak effect.

(LET) (4). This depends upon the energy of the beam. For practical purposes, the conversion of proton beam doses to photon beam doses is expressed in Cobalt Gray equivalents by multiplying the proton beam doses by a factor of 1.1. However, other charged particles, such as carbon ions, have a much higher LET than photons and are more likely to inflict damage along the track the particle travels.

Brachytherapy

As opposed to treating tumors with the radiation source distant from the tumor, brachytherapy (placing radioactive sources inside of tumors) is another way to deliver very high-dose radiation and limit normal tissue doses. In brachytherapy, the dose falls off at an inverse to the square of the distance. Thus, the radiation dose quickly falls even a short distance from the implanted source. A commonly used isotope is iodine 125, which emits very weak gamma rays (29 KeV). The dose of radiation absorbed by the tissues immediately surrounding the source (within 1 cm) is very high; hence, if I 125 sources are placed strategically within a tumor, a very high dose can be given without exposing neighboring organs to much radiation (7).

Radiobiology

An understanding of radiobiology (how radiation affects different tissues) can also help improve the therapeutic ratio. The effects of radiation therapy on tissues is dependent upon the inherent radiosensitivity of the tissue or organ in question, the dose of radiation given, and the volume of tissue irradiated (1). The dose per fraction (treatment) is also an important determinant of toxicity. In general, a higher dose per fraction has a greater biologic impact, for both normal tissue as well as tumor. Thus, if larger doses of radiation are administered per fraction, the same probability of tumor control can be achieved with a lower total cumulative dose in comparison with a treatment schedule utilizing a small dose of radiation per fraction, which would require a higher total dose to achieve the same level of tumor control (8). A smaller dose per fraction may be desirable when it is important to spare radiosensitive organs that may be near the target volume or when a large volume of tissue needs to be treated. Since the total time required to deliver the prescribed radiation also has biologic effects, the dose rate, or how quickly radiation is given, is also important (9). This is especially significant in brachytherapy. The total dose prescribed may be reduced when using isotopes with a higher dose rate in comparison with an implant utilizing lower dose rate sources.

Time is thought to be critical because it may affect how well a cell can recover from radiation damage. A cell that has more time to repair damage is less sensitive to radiation effects. Thus, it is often noted that tissues that have a high rate of turnover, such as the bone marrow, are very sensitive to radiation. Time also allows the irradiated tissue to repopulate or replace cells lost to radiation. Because cells in different phases of the cell cycle have different sensitivities to radiation, giving time for cells to randomly distribute themselves to different phases of the cell cycle will ensure that at least some of the cells will be in more sensitive phases when the next fraction of radiation is delivered. Thus, fractionating radiation treatment allows time for reassortment and can make tissues more radiosensitive. Other factors, such as the oxygenation status of the tissue, may also be important. Hypoxic tissues are less sensitive to radiotherapy, and so allowing time to permit reoxygenation to increase the oxygen tension within the tumor is thought to increase the effects of radiation. Thus, most radiation schedules give radiation in multiple treatments or fractions to allow opportunity for normal tissues to repair radiation effects and repopulate. It also allows for reassortment of tumor cells into more radiosensitive phases of the cell cycle and reoxygenation of hypoxic tumors to increase the radiation effect (1).

There is great interest in the use of chemicals to increase the effect of radiation (radiosensitizers, such as many chemotherapeutic agents, which also target DNA) or protect normal tissues from the effects of radiation (radioprotectors such as amifostine) (10). The cell cycle appears to be regulated by a variety of protein kinases, which are under the control of complex signal transduction pathways. These may also be manipulated to increase the sensitivity of tumors to radiation (11).

Although dose is a significant contributor to the effects of radiation on normal tissue, another important factor to consider is the volume of irradiated tissue. In general, when a significant volume of an organ has been irradiated, the risk of radiation effects is higher. Whole-organ irradiation carries a much higher risk of organ failure compared to partial-organ irradiation. Hence, a higher dose or larger volume is more likely to result in radiation toxicity. For example, whole-brain radiation is typically much more morbid than stereotactic radiosurgery, which focuses a high dose of radiation to a very small volume (12).

Radiation effects have been traditionally classified as early or late (13). Early effects are generally seen during the course of treatment or within six weeks of radiation therapy. Early effects are usually manifest in tissues that are quite sensitive to radiation, such as the skin or oral mucosa, which are highly proliferative. Fortunately, most early or acute effects of radiation are temporary. Late effects are considered those that appear months to years after radiation, and are more likely in tissues with low proliferative potential, such as connective tissue (fibrosis) or neural tissue (neuropathy). Although the mechanisms involved are not completely well understood, the late effects of radiotherapy, such as fibrosis, are often irreversible. Often, microvascular damage (endothelial thickening to the point that red blood cells are not able to pass through) has thought to play an important role in late toxicity, causing hypoxic stress and cellular death. Endothelial thickening can take months to years to manifest. Loss of cells due to apoptosis after radiation-induced DNA damage also is likely to play a role. At high doses (>8 Gy) per fraction, there are likely greater effects on the endothelial lining mediated by the ceramide pathway, and could help explain the significantly higher risk of late radiation effects seen with higher doses per fraction (14).

Another difficult late effect of radiation therapy is the risk of radiation-induced secondary cancers. For example, radiation therapy represented the first curative treatment for Hodgkin disease, but requires regional radiation therapy of the lymph nodes. When breast tissue was included in these fields to treat mediastinal lymph nodes, the risk of subsequent breast cancer was found to be more than 10 times greater than in women who had never had such treatment (15 times greater in women who were irradiated between the ages of 20–30) (15). Overall, the risk of second cancers is approximately 2% higher over a patient's lifetime, but exposure to radiation at a younger age or to a large volume of normal tissue carries a higher risk (16).

PATIENT MANAGEMENT AND DECISION MAKING

A radiation oncologist must weigh many factors when approaching treatment of a patient. Radiation effects are dependent upon the inherent radiosensitivity and the volume of irradiated tissue, the dose of radiation delivered, and the dose fraction schedule employed for treatment, and must be considered when weighing the risks and benefits of such therapy. This requires a careful evaluation of the patient, paying particular attention to the potential toxicities of therapy weighed against the probabilities of benefit.

A common approach is to assess both patient factors and tumor factors associated with the case. Patient factors include the patient's ability to tolerate treatment, such as Karnofsky Performance Status (17), organ function, nutrition, or bone marrow reserve. Patient symptoms and signs are considered. The prognosis is also important to assess, and prior treatment must be considered. When evaluating tumor factors, histology, the extent of disease, location of the disease, and adjacent normal structures, as well as potentially involved areas of the body must also be factored in. A tissue diagnosis of a disease for which radiation can potentially be useful is critical.

An important decision point is to assess whether the intent of treatment is palliative or curative. In potentially curable disease, a higher level of toxicity is generally acceptable. However, with advances in systemic therapy, patients with incurable cancers may enjoy longer and longer survivals, and may warrant a more aggressive approach to controlling gross disease. Also, as patients live longer, quality of life is still an important issue. Aggressive treatment may add or detract to a patient's long-term quality of life, depending upon the situation. Hence, it is important for radiation oncologists to assess each patient thoroughly in order to recommend appropriate therapy.

SUMMARY

Cancer treatment is becoming increasingly complicated, and a multidisciplinary approach to treatment is appropriate in many cases. For example, radiation therapy can have adverse effects on wound healing (18), and if the patient is to undergo surgery after radiation,

radiation treatment should be planned in such a way as to minimize the effects on the surgical bed. Chemotherapy can also potentiate the effects of radiation on both normal tissue and tumor (19). Hence, evaluation of a patient from surgical and medical oncology perspectives, as well as radiation oncology, and input from other allied specialties, such as pathology, radiology, neurology, and physiatry, will often produce the most optimal approach.

References

1. Hall EJ, Giaccia, AJ. *Radiobiology for the Radiologist*, 6th ed. Philadelphia: Lippincott Williams & Wilkins; 2006.
2. American Society for Radiation Oncology. Fast Facts About Radiation Therapy; 2007. http://www.astro.org/pressroom/fastfacts/
3. Khan FM. *Physics of Radiation Therapy*, 3rd ed. Philadelphia: Lippincott Williams & Wilkins; 2003.
4. Tannock IH, Richard. *Basic Science of Oncology*. 3rd ed. New York: McGraw-Hill Professional; 1998.
5. Measures ICRU. Report 10b, Physical Aspects of Irradiation. Vol 10b: ICRU; 1964.
6. Yamada Y, Lovelock DM, Yenice KM, et al. Multifractionated image-guided and stereotactic intensity-modulated radiotherapy of paraspinal tumors: a preliminary report. *Int J Radiat Oncol Biol Phys*. 2005;62:53–61.
7. Nag S. *Principles and Practice of Brachytherapy*. Armonk: Futura Publishing Company; 1997.
8. Brenner DJ, Martinez AA, Edmundson GK, et al. Direct evidence that prostate tumors show high sensitivity to fractionation (low alpha/beta ratio), similar to late-responding normal tissue. *Int J Radiat Oncol Biol Phys*. 2002;52:6–13.
9. Fowler JF. The radiobiology of prostate cancer including new aspects of fractionated radiotherapy. *Acta Oncol*. 2005;44:265–276.
10. Brizel D, Overgaard J. Does amifostine have a role in chemoradiation treatment? *Lancet Oncol*. 2003;4:378–381.
11. Weinberg R. *The Biology of Cancer: Garland Science*. New York: Taylor and Francis Group; 2007.
12. Flickinger JC, Kondziolka D, Lunsford LD. Clinical applications of stereotactic radiosurgery. *Cancer Treat Res*. 1998;93:283–297.
13. Thames HD WH, Peters LJ, Fletcher GH. Changes in early and late radiation responses with altered dose fractionation: implications for dose-survival relationships. *Int J Radiat Biol Phys*. 1982;8:219–226.
14. Garcia-Barros M, Paris F, Cordon-Cardo C, et al. Tumor response to radiotherapy regulated by endothelial cell apoptosis. *Science*. 2003;300:1155–1159.
15. Hancock SL, Tucker MA, Hoppe RT. Breast cancer after treatment of Hodgkin's disease. *J Natl Cancer Inst*. 1993;85:25–31.
16. Hall EJ, Wuu CS. Radiation-induced second cancers: the impact of 3D-CRT and IMRT. *Int J Radiat Oncol Biol Phys*. 2003;56:83–88.
17. Karnofsky DA BJ. *The Clinical Evaluation of Chemotherapeutic Agents in Cancer*. New York: Columbia University Press; 1949.
18. Tibbs MK. Wound healing following radiation therapy: a review. *Radiother Oncol*. 1997;42:99–106.
19. Philips TL FK. Quantification of combined radiation therapy and chemotherapy effects on critical normal tissues. *Cancer*. 1976;37:1186–1200.

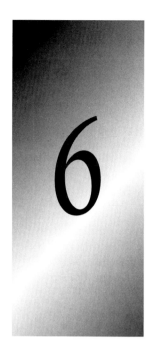

Principles of Neurosurgery in Cancer

6

Mark H. Bilsky

Metastatic spinal tumors are a major source of morbidity in cancer patients. The overriding goals for treatment are palliative in order to improve or maintain neurological status, provide spinal stability, and achieve local, durable tumor control. The principle treatments for spinal tumors are radiation and/or surgery. Recent advances in surgical and radiation techniques, such as image-guided intensity modulated radiation therapy (IGRT), have made treatment of spine metastases safer and more effective. Additionally, the development of newer chemotherapy, hormonal, and immunotherapy treatments has led to improved systemic control of many types of cancers. All interventions used to treat spinal tumors and their outcomes affect a patient's rehabilitation potential. Rehabilitative medicine plays a large role in achieving meaningful palliation and improved quality of life for patients with spinal tumors. A fundamental understanding of treatment decisions and outcomes will help in the assessment of cancer patients.

PRESENTATION

Spinal tumors typically present with pain (1). Three pain syndromes associated with spinal tumors are biologic, mechanical instability, and radiculopathy. All of these have important treatment implications. The vast majority of patients will present with a history of biologic pain, which is nocturnal or early morning pain that resolves over the course of the day. The pain

generator appears to be a reaction to inflammatory mediators secreted by the tumor. The diurnal variation in endogenous steroid secretion by the adrenal gland is decreased at night causing this flare-up of inflammatory pain. Biologic pain is responsive to exogenous steroids and very often responsive to radiation.

Differentiating biologic pain from mechanical pain is critically important to treating physicians. As opposed to biologic pain, mechanical pain, in broad terms, is movement-related pain and denotes significant lytic bone destruction. These patients often require surgery to stabilize the spine or possibly percutaneous cement augmentation with vertebroplasty or kyphoplasty. Physical therapy will typically not improve mechanical instability pain and may lead to an exacerbation of instability and neurologic progression.

The movement-related pain that denotes instability is dependent on the spinal level involved (1–3,8). Patients with atlantoaxial instability have flexion and extension pain, but also have a component of rotational pain. This is differentiated from the subaxial cervical spine, where flexion and extension pain are predominant with no rotational component. Our experience suggests that thoracic instability is worse in extension. While thoracic instability is relatively rare, it may be seen in patients with burst fractures with extension into a unilateral joint. These patients are very comfortable in kyphosis while leaning forward, but extension of the unstable kyphosis produces unremitting pain. Patients will often give a history of sitting in a reclining chair

KEY POINTS

- The overriding goals for treatment of spinal metastases are palliative in order to improve or maintain neurological status, provide spinal stability, and achieve local, durable tumor control.
- The three pain syndromes associated with spinal tumors are biologic, mechanical instability, and radiculopathy.
- Myelopathy indicates the presence of high-grade spinal cord compression that is treated with radiation for radiosensitive tumors (eg, multiple myeloma, lymphoma) or surgery for radioresistant tumors (non-small cell lung, renal cell, or thyroid carcinoma).
- The NOMS framework is designed to facilitate surgical and radiotherapeutic decision making into readily identifiable components: neurologic (N), oncologic (O), mechanical stability (M), and systemic disease and medical comorbidities (S).
- Spinal stabilization is dependent on instrumentation, with a very small expectation that patients will achieve arthrodesis. The instrumentation should be constructed with biomaterials that are magnetic resonance imaging (MRI)–compatible to facilitate imaging for recurrence.
- Typically, anterior resection and reconstruction are supplemented with posterior instrumentation in order to avoid subsidence of anterior grafts or to avoid losing anterior fixation in patients who have adjacent segment tumor progression.
- Currently, pedicle and lateral mass screw-rod systems are principally used to reconstruct cancer patients. These are placed a minimum of two levels superior and inferior to the level of the decompression.
- Distributing the load with multiple fixation points is more important in tumor reconstruction than saving motion segments, as is typically done for degenerative and trauma surgery.
- In the thoracic and lumbar spine, circumferential decompression and reconstruction is performed using a posterolateral transpedicular approach (PTA). This obviates the need to enter the chest or retroperitoneum, which is often poorly tolerated in the cancer population. This approach has relatively low morbidity and provides stabilization that allows patients to be mobilized early in the postoperative period. If patients are neurologically normal, the expectation is that they will sit in the chair postoperative day 1, walk day 2, stairs day 4, and home days 5 to 7. These patients are not placed in external orthoses.
- The ability to rehabilitate patients immediately after treatment takes on exaggerated significance in the cancer population, because nonambulatory patients are often excluded from further systemic therapy.
- Back or neck strengthening exercises are discouraged in patients who have undergone PTA due to the risk of creating hardware failure in patients with a low expectation of arthrodesis.

for several weeks because they cannot lie recumbent in bed. In the lumbar spine, the most common pattern of instability is mechanical radiculopathy (Fig. 6.1). These patients have searing radicular leg pain on axial load, such as sitting or standing. Radiographically, this is manifest as a burst or compression with extension into the neural foramen. This presentation is a mechanical problem as axial load narrows the neural foramen, resulting in compression of the nerve root. This pain does not typically respond to radiation therapy.

A large number of patients present with ongoing axial load pain resulting from a burst or compression fracture. These patients are not grossly unstable, but may benefit from percutaneous cement augmentation of the vertebral body with procedures such as vertebroplasty or kyphoplasty. The mechanism of pain relief is unclear, but a number of published series have shown significant pain relief in cancer patients (4). Technical limitations restrict the use of these procedures to the lumbar spine and thoracic spine below the T3 level and in the absence of epidural disease.

The third pain syndrome is radiculopathy, or nerve root pain. The recognition of radiculopathy pain is important, as it denotes that tumor extends into the neural foramen and very often is beginning to compress the spinal cord. Early recognition of radiculopathy that prompts MRI may avoid progression to high-grade spinal cord compression and myelopathy. Additionally, radiculopathy may mimic bone pain or brachial or lumbosacral plexopathy. For example, pain from an L2 radiculopathy and pathologic hip fracture both present with pain radiating to the groin. These can often be distinguished by using provocative tests, such as hip rotation, which elicits hip but not spine pain. However, metastatic disease often involves multiple bones, so spine and hip disease may occur concurrently. For this reason, the workup of pain radiating to the groin includes both hip films and an MRI of the spine. Diagnosis to differ-

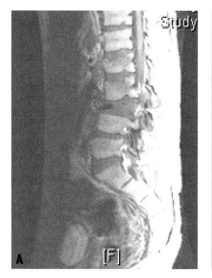 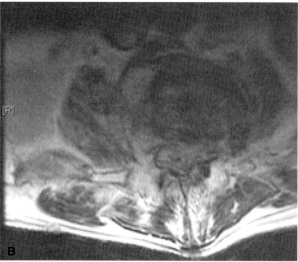

FIGURE 6.1

A. Sagittal T1: weighted image showing L3 burst fracture. B. Axial T2: weighted image showing high grade thecal sac compression.

entiate the pain generator may include electromyograms (EMGs) and nerve conduction studies.

The development of myelopathy should be treated with some degree of urgency prompting early MRI studies. Myelopathy indicates the presence of high-grade spinal cord compression that is treated with radiation for radiosensitive tumors (eg, multiple myeloma, lymphoma) or surgery for radioresistant tumors (non-small cell lung, renal cell, or thyroid carcinoma).

Early myelopathy is often manifest by involvement of the spinothalamic tracts with loss of pinprick, typically followed by loss of motor function. Dorsal column deficits are often a late finding with resultant loss of proprioception. Bowel and bladder loss are also lost late in the evolution of myelopathy except when tumor involves the conus medullaris at approximately T12-L1 or diffuse sacral replacement, where they may be a very early sign. Spinal cord compression that results in loss of bowel and bladder is most often associated with perineal numbness, which is absent with other causes, such as narcotics or prostate hypertrophy. Early recognition of myelopathy and therapeutic intervention improve the chance for meaningful recovery. This recovery often results in early return of motor function, although sensory modalities will often recover more slowly. Loss of proprioception is particularly difficult as recovery is often suboptimal and makes ambulation extremely difficult, despite normal motor function. Once a patient is paralyzed, meaningful recovery of ambulation and bowel and bladder function are rare (<5%).

DECISION FRAMEWORK: NOMS

The principle decisions in the treatment of spinal disease are radiation therapy or surgery. The NOMS framework is designed to facilitate decision making into readily identifiable components: neurologic (N), oncologic (O), mechanical stability (M), and systemic disease and medical comorbidities (S). The neurologic considerations include the severity of myelopathy, functional radiculopathy, and degree of epidural spinal cord compression. The oncologic consideration is based on tumor histology to establish the radiosensitivity of the tumor. Patients with radiosensitive tumors, such as multiple myeloma and lymphoma, can undergo radiation therapy as first-line therapy. Unfortunately, most tumors are resistant to conventional-dose radiation (eg, 30 Gy in 10 fractions). These tumors include most solid tumors, such as renal cell, lung, and colon carcinoma. For patients with tumor in the bone or dural impingement without spinal cord compression, stereotactic radiosurgery (SRS) can be used to effectively control tumors. Currently, SRS is being delivered at 24 Gy single fraction, with 95% local tumor control at a median follow-up of 16 months (9). This is significantly better than the 20% response rates seen using conventional external beam radiation in radioresistant tumors (5). Surgery in this population as initial therapy is based on data from the study published by Patchell et al. (6) comparing surgery and radiotherapy (RT) to RT alone in patients with solid, ie, radioresistant, tumors. Patients undergoing surgery and RT had significantly better outcomes with regard to maintenance and recovery of ambulation and survival. SRS is not a viable option in patients with high-grade spinal cord compression because the high dose is above spinal cord tolerance and would result in radiation-induced myelopathy. However, SRS is an effective postsurgical adjuvant for radioresistant tumors.

Mechanical instability is a second indication for operation. A number of principles have evolved for reconstruction of spinal tumors that may be somewhat different from those used for degenerative, trauma, or scoliosis surgery. Spinal stabilization is dependent on instrumentation, with a very small expectation that patients will achieve arthrodesis. The instrumentation should be constructed with biomaterials that are MRI-compatible to facilitate imaging for recurrence. Stainless steel is difficult to image using MRI and should be avoided in tumor patients. Anterior reconstruction is performed using a number of constructs, including polymethyl methacrylate (PMMA), titanium or polyetheretherketone (PEEK) carbon fiber cages, or allo- or autograft bone.

Typically, anterior resection and reconstruction are supplemented with posterior instrumentation in order to avoid subsidence of anterior grafts or to avoid losing anterior fixation in patients who have adjacent segment tumor progression. Currently, pedicle and lateral mass screw-rod systems are principally used to reconstruct cancer patients. These are placed a minimum of two levels superior and inferior to the level of the decompression. Distributing the load with multiple fixation points is more important in tumor reconstruction than saving motion segments, as is typically done for degenerative and trauma surgery. In the thoracic and lumbar spine, circumferential decompression and reconstruction is performed using a posterolateral transpedicular approach (PTA) (Fig. 6.2). This obviates the need to enter the chest or retroperitoneum, which is often poorly tolerated in the cancer population. This approach has relatively low morbidity and provides stabilization that allows patients to be mobilized very early in the postoperative period. If patients are neurologically normal, the expectation is that they will sit in the chair postoperative day 1, walk day 2, stairs day 4, and home days 5 to 7. These patients are not placed in external orthoses.

Finally, decision making is heavily dependent on what the patient can tolerate from a systemic cancer standpoint and the significance of medical comorbidities. Given the palliative nature of the surgery, with the overriding goal of improving quality of life, an assessment of the ability to tolerate radiation, surgery, or both is essential. Preoperative oncology assessment includes complete spinal axis imaging and extent of disease workup using either computed tomography (CT) of the chest, pelvis, and abdomen as well as bone scan or positron emission tomography (PET) scan. Medical workup may include Doppler ultrasound of the lower extremities and cardiology and pulmonary clearance. The ability to rehabilitate patients immediately after treatment takes on exaggerated significance in the cancer population because nonambulatory patients are often excluded from further systemic therapy.

REHABILITATIVE MEDICINE

The impact of rehabilitative medicine to optimize outcomes in spine oncology patients cannot be overstated. Early mobilization is essential for these patients. The majority of patients continue physical therapy following discharge to improve stamina and to improve gait if there are issues. We discourage back or neck strengthening exercises due to the risk of creating hardware failure in patients with a low expectation of arthrodesis. Early ambulation typically requires a walker, but the expectation at six weeks is that they will be independent. While physical therapists typically work with patients several days per week, physiatrists may only see patients on a weekly or biweekly basis unless ongoing pain or functional issues require closer attention. Careful assessment by the rehabilitation team is often instrumental in identifying changes in a patient's condition. A change in the patient's baseline pain may be a harbinger of recurrent disease or instrumentation failure. This pain prompts repeat plain radiographs and/or a repeat MRI of the spine.

Physiatrists have introduced therapeutic modalities that have significantly improved postradiation and surgical outcomes. Perhaps the most significant is the Botox injections for paraspinal muscle spasm (7). This agent has been remarkably useful in treating postradiation fibrosis, functional spasm, and postoperative muscle spasm, particularly in the cervical and thoracic spine to treat trapezius pain.

CONCLUSION

The treatment of spinal metastases is palliative and designed to improve a patient's quality of life. The NOMS decision framework helps delineate important decisions regarding treatment with radiation therapy and/or surgery. Currently, surgery is reserved for patients with high-grade spinal cord compression resulting from RT-resistant tumors and gross spinal

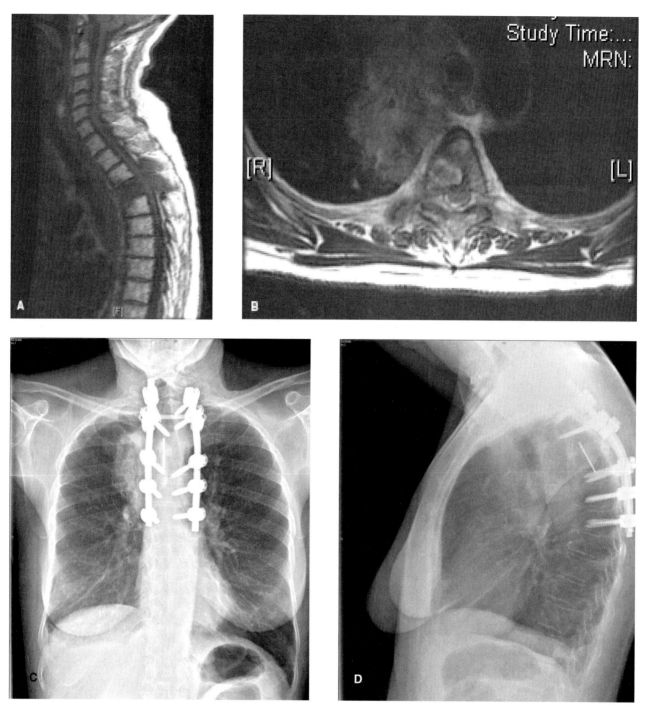

FIGURE 6.2

A. Sagittal T1-weighted image showing T4 burst fracture with circumferential bone disease. B. Axial T2-weighted image showing minimal epidural compression with circumferential bone disease and a large right-sided paraspinal mass. C. Post-operative AP radiograph. D. Post-operative lateral radiograph.

instability. Conventional external beam radiation is used for patients with radiosensitive tumors and radiosurgery for patients with RT-resistant tumors without spinal cord compression or as a postoperative adjuvant. Regardless of radiation or surgery, the goals of pain relief, restoration of neurologic function, and ambulation are essential to treatment in this patient population. Rehabilitative medicine plays an enormous role in meaningful palliation.

References

1. Bilsky M, Smith M. Surgical approach to epidural spinal cord compression. *Hematol Oncol Clin North Am.* 2006;20:1307–1317.
2. Bilsky MH, Boakye M, Collignon F, Kraus D, Boland P. Operative management of metastatic and malignant primary subaxial cervical tumors. *J Neurosurg Spine.* 2005;2:256–264.
3. Bilsky MH, Shannon FJ, Sheppard S, Prabhu V, Boland PJ. Diagnosis and management of a metastatic tumor in the atlantoaxial spine. *Spine.* 2002;27:1062–1069.
4. Hentschel SJ, Burton AW, Fourney DR, Rhines LD, Mendel E. Percutaneous vertebroplasty and kyphoplasty performed at a cancer center: refuting proposed contraindications. *J Neurosurg Spine.* 2005;2:436–440.
5. Maranzano E, Latini P. Effectiveness of radiation therapy without surgery in metastatic spinal cord compression: final results from a prospective trial. *Int J Radiat Oncol Biol Phys.* 1995;32:959–967.
6. Patchell RA, Tibbs PA, Walsh JW, et al. A randomized trial of surgery in the treatment of single metastases to the brain. *N Engl J Med.* 1990;322:494–500.
7. Stubblefield MD, Levine A, Custodio CM, Fitzpatrick T. The role of botulinum toxin type A in the radiation fibrosis syndrome: a preliminary report. *Arch Phys Med Rehabil.* 2008;89:417–421.
8. Wang JC, Boland P, Mitra N, et al. Single-stage posterolateral transpedicular approach for resection of epidural metastatic spine tumors involving the vertebral body with circumferential reconstruction: results in 140 patients. Invited submission from the Joint Section Meeting on Disorders of the Spine and Peripheral Nerves, March 2004. *J Neurosurg Spine.* 2004;1: 287–298.
9. Yamada Y, Bilsky MH, Lovelock DM, et al. High-dose, single-fraction image-guided intensity-modulated radiotherapy for metastatic spinal lesions. *Int J Radiat Oncol Biol Phys.* 2008;71(2):484–490.

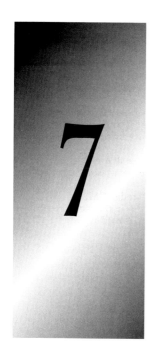

Principles of Orthopedic Surgery in Cancer

Carol D. Morris
Corey Rothrock

The musculoskeletal manifestations of cancer are far-reaching. Both benign and malignant tumors of bone can occur at any age and in any of the 206 bones in the human body. Soft tissue tumors follow a similar pattern, presenting in both pediatric and adult patients virtually anywhere in the body. The surgical management of bone and soft tissue tumors largely depends on the origin of the tumor. Both bone and soft tissue sarcomas are largely treated with curative intent in the form of limb salvage surgery or amputation. Secondary tumors of bone, or metastatic disease, are usually treated with palliative intent, which most often requires stabilization of the bone without removing the entire tumor. While tumors may metastasize to soft tissue, this pattern of spread is far less common. The role of the orthopedic oncologist is often twofold: (1) to eradicate cancer in muscle and bones and (2) rebuild the resulting defects in a functionally acceptable manner. This chapter will review the surgical principles of treating both primary and secondary musculoskeletal malignancies in the extremities.

GENERAL PRINCIPLES

Diagnosis and Staging

A thoughtful and methodical strategy for the diagnosis of bone and soft tissue tumors cannot be overemphasized. Because primary bone and soft tissue malignancies are relatively rare, they are diagnostically challenging, and a delay in diagnosis is not uncommon. An accurate diagnosis is based on a combination of clinical, imaging, and histological data.

Always start with a thorough history and physical exam. Most patients with malignant bone tumors present with pain. "Night pain," defined as pain that awakes one from sleep, is a classic complaint among patients with bone tumors and should always be investigated. Functional pain refers to pain with ambulation or certain activities, and can be indicative of an impending fracture. Most patients with functional pain should be placed on a restricted weight-bearing status. Pathologic fractures through primary bone sarcomas carry devastating consequences, often requiring immediate amputation of the affected limb to control tumor spread. In contrast, the majority of soft tissue sarcomas are painless unless nerve or bone involvement is present. Often, patients report a history of trauma that has brought attention to the affected area.

A patient's medical history can be contributory. In patients with a known diagnosis of cancer, bone pain must always be investigated to rule out metastatic disease. Certain clinical syndromes such as neurofibromatosis or Paget disease, are associated with sarcomas (1). Patients that have undergone radiation for other conditions are at risk of developing secondary sarcomas (2). Up to 10% of primary bone tumors will present pathologic fractures.

On physical examination, primary bone tumors are often associated with a painful mass. Other important aspects of the exam include altered gait, decreased range of motion of the adjacent joint, joint effusions, regional lymphadenopathy, overlying skin changes, and neurovascular status. When metastatic disease is suspected, the physical exam should also focus on the suspected primary site (thyroid, breast, etc.). For soft tissue tumors, the mass is evaluated for its size, mobility, and firmness in addition to more discreet findings, such as a Tinel sign, bruits, or transillumination. Large (>5 cm) and deep soft tissue masses should be considered malignant until proven otherwise (Fig. 7.1).

All bone tumors require an x-ray. In fact, despite advances in imaging modalities, the plane x-ray remains the most telling diagnostic study (Fig. 7.2). When a primary bone sarcoma is suspected, magnetic resonance imaging (MRI) of the entire bone, computed tomography (CT) scan of the chest, and whole-body bone scan are necessary for complete staging. For soft tissue tumors, MRI is the most revealing imaging modality, as it allows for excellent definition of the mass, including characteristic signal patterns and the relation of the mass to adjacent neurovascular structures (Fig. 7.3). In addition, soft tissue sarcomas (STS) are staged with CT of the chest, and more recently, positron emission tomography (PET) scans are being incorporated into staging protocols, though the role of PET scan has yet to be fully validated. For metastatic bone disease in which the primary cancer has already been identified,

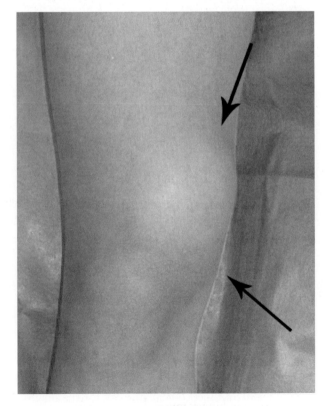

FIGURE 7.1

Clinical picture of a distal mesial thigh soft tissue mass.

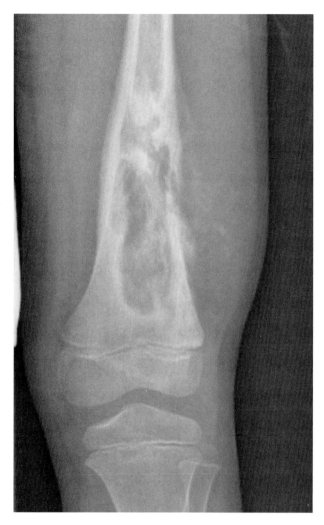

FIGURE 7.2

Classic x-ray appearance of an osteogenic sarcoma of the distal femur of a skeletally immature patient showing a permeative lesion with a wide zone of transition, cortical destruction with soft tissue extension, and periosteal elevation.

imaging is directed at the bone of interest to guide treatment. If the primary cancer is unknown, CT scan of the chest/abdomen/pelvis is performed to elucidate the primary cancer, as well as bone scan to identify other bony sites of disease.

Biopsy

The biopsy is an important part of the staging process. The purpose of the biopsy is to obtain tissue for pathologic analysis in order to make a diagnosis. Often referred to as the first step of a successful limb salvage operation, the biopsy must be done carefully so as not to adversely affect the outcome. It is preferentially performed by a surgeon with experience in musculoskel-

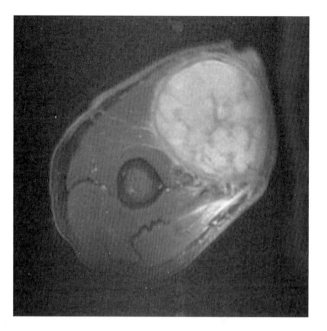

FIGURE 7.3

Typical MRI appearance of a high-grade soft tissue sarcoma in the upper extremity demonstrating a large heterogeneous mass.

etal oncology who will ultimately perform the definitive procedure. There are several types of biopsies: fine needle aspirates (FNA), core needle, open incisional, and open excisional (Fig. 7.4). The type of biopsy performed depends on a host of factors, including the size and location of the mass and the experience of the interpreting pathologist.

Needle biopsies are advantageous in that they can be performed in the office or by an interventional radiologist, are minimally invasive, and when done properly, are associated with minimal tissue contamination. Obviously, needle biopsy is associated with a small tissue sample, which can be problematic if special stains or studies are required to make an accurate diagnosis. In an open incisional biopsy, a generous tissue sample is obtained by surgically incising into the tumor. Open biopsies require considerable expertise, as several technical points must be considered: orientation along the limb salvage incision or directly adjacent to it, meticulous hemostasis, and avoidance of extra compartmental and neurovascular contamination. Any tissue exposed at the time of biopsy is theoretically contaminated and must be excised at the time of definitive surgery. A poorly performed open biopsy can have devastating consequences and is associated with more complex tumor resections, including unnecessary amputation (3,4). Open bone biopsies can create stress risers in the bone, which in turn, can result in pathologic fractures. Splinting and protected weight

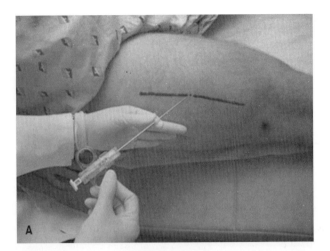
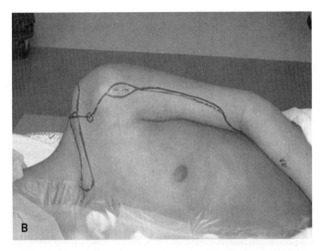

FIGURE 7.4

A: Needle biopsy of a thigh mass performed with a Tru-cut core needle. Note that the limb salvage incision is drawn out first. B: Open biopsy of the proximal humerus. The biopsy tract is incorporated into the definitive limb salvage incision.

bearing are often required following open bone biopsy to avoid such a complication. Excisional biopsy implies that the entire tumor is removed at the time of biopsy. Excisional biopsy is usually reserved for benign tumors, small malignant tumors (<3 cm), or situations in which incisional biopsy would cause considerable contamination. The decision to perform an excisional biopsy must be weighed carefully, as the potential associated complications when performed inadequately or unnecessarily are significant (Fig. 7.5).

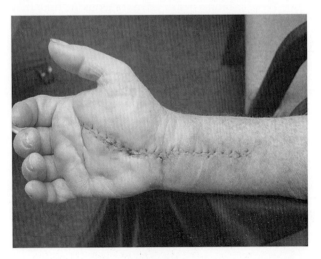

FIGURE 7.5

An open excisional biopsy was performed for a presumed benign tumor of the wrist, which turned out to be a sarcoma. The median nerve was isolated at the time of surgery. The area of contamination is quite large, making conversion to limb salvage difficult.

Oncologic Excisions

There are four types of oncologic excisions: intralesional, marginal, wide, and radical (5). The names of the excisions refer to the surgical margin by which the tumor is removed. In intralesional surgery, the surgeon enters the tumor, leaving microscopic and sometimes gross tumor behind. Intralesional excisions are usually reserved for benign bone tumors such as cyst. In selected instances, low-grade sarcomas, such as low-grade chondrosarcoma, can be treated with a combination of intralesional surgery and an effective adjuvant, such as liquid nitrogen (6). In marginal excisions, the tumor is excised through the "reactive" zone around the tumor or around the pseudocapsule of the tumor. This reactive zone is inflammatory in nature and theoretically contains tumor cells. Marginal excisions are typically performed for benign soft tissue masses such as lipoma. Most malignant tumors should be removed with wide or radical margins. A wide excision completely removes the tumor en bloc with a cuff of normal tissue around the tumor (Fig. 7.6A,B). The vast majority of bone and soft tissue sarcomas are removed by wide excision. Radical resections remove tumors en bloc by resecting the entire compartment: the entire bone or the entire muscle compartment from the origin to the insertion. Radical resections may be performed if "skip" lesions are present, but rarely need to be performed. Due to advances in superior imaging techniques as well as effective adjuvant treatments, such as chemotherapy and radiation, tumors can be excised with fairly narrow margins. Decreasing the amount of normal tissue that needs to be removed around the tumor improves functional outcomes without compromising oncologic results.

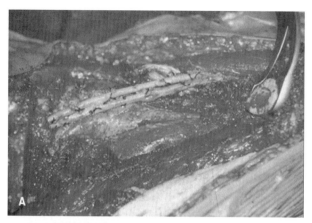

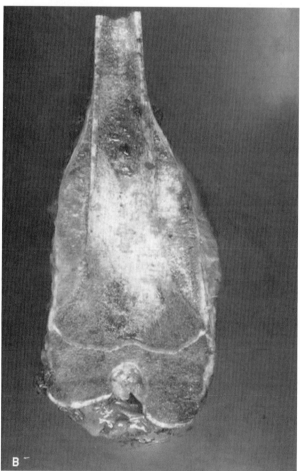

FIGURE 7.6

A: The resultant defect in the thigh following wide excision of a distal femur sarcoma. B: The gross pathology specimen of a distal femur sarcoma removed with wide margins.

SURGICAL MANAGEMENT OF PRIMARY BONE AND SOFT TISSUE SARCOMAS

Limb Salvage Surgery

Surgery is the cornerstone of treatment for bone and soft tissue sarcomas. Approximately 90% of all extremity sarcomas can be successfully removed without amputation. During the late 1970s and the 1980s, limb salvage surgery for sarcomas began to gain popularity. This was due to a variety of factors, including advances in imaging, effective adjuvant treatments, and advances in reconstruction. Several investigations have reported equivalent survival in patients undergoing limb salvage versus amputation (7,8). Limb salvage surgery requires that oncologic outcome is not compromised and the resultant limb has reasonable functional capacity. There are many variables to consider when deciding if an individual is an appropriate candidate for limb salvage surgery, such as vocational demands of the patient, response to neoadjuvant treatment, remaining skeletal growth in children, and cultural expectations.

Once a tumor has been removed, the resultant defect must be reconstructed. Soft tissue tumors may require soft tissue reconstructions, such as tendon transfers, nerve grafts, or flap coverage. In addition to soft tissue defects, bone tumors require reconstruction of the removed bone and often adjacent joint. Orthopedic oncologists typically utilize four reconstruction options in limb salvage surgery for bones: allografts, autografts, metallic prostheses, or allograft-prosthetic composites.

Allografts

Human bone allografts have been used for decades as a biologic solution for skeletal defects. They offer several advantages over synthetic implants, including attachments for host ligaments and muscle and the potential to serve as long-term solutions since the graft continues to incorporate with the host bone over time. Disadvantages of allografts include possible disease transmission, fractures, and nonunions at the host bone interface. Allografts can be used to reconstruct virtually any bone or joint. Clearly, certain anatomic sites have a more successful track record than others.

The American Association of Tissue Banks (AATB), in conjunction with the Food and Drug Administration (FDA), regulates the procurement, testing, and distribution of human allografts (9). Grafts are typically obtained though AATB-approved tissue banks. Once a decision has been made to use a structural allograft, the surgeon contacts a tissue bank to obtain a properly sized allograft that matches the dimensions of the patient's bone and possesses the desired soft tissue. Some medical centers have internal bone banks.

Osteoarticular allografts are large segments of bone with a cryopreserved articular surface (Fig. 7.7A). They can be used to reconstruct very large defects, with the adjacent joint most commonly around the knee and shoulder. Once the tumor is removed, the allograft is cut and sculpted to fit the defect. The allograft is then secured to the host bone using orthopedic hardware

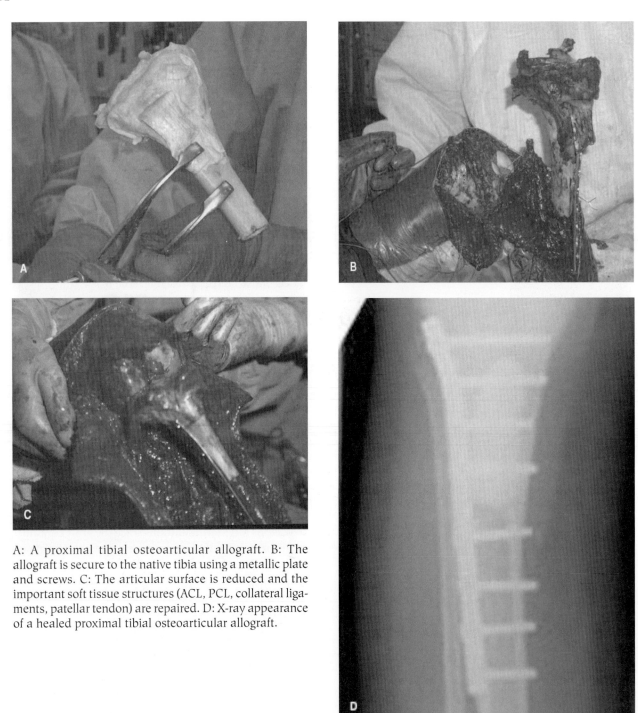

A: A proximal tibial osteoarticular allograft. B: The allograft is secure to the native tibia using a metallic plate and screws. C: The articular surface is reduced and the important soft tissue structures (ACL, PCL, collateral ligaments, patellar tendon) are repaired. D: X-ray appearance of a healed proximal tibial osteoarticular allograft.

FIGURE 7.7

(Fig. 7.7B). The surrounding ligaments and tendons are then attached to the allograft (Fig 7.7C). For example, in the knee, the anterior cruciate ligament (ACL), posterior cruciate ligament (PCL), collateral ligaments, and capsule would all be reapproximated giving rise to stable knee joint. With time, the allograft incorporates with the host bone creating a stable, durable limb (Fig. 7.7D). Allografts can also be used in an intercalary

fashion (Fig. 7.8) as well as for partial defects of long bones (Fig. 7.9).

The success of the allograft reconstruction is dependent on a variety of factors, but most importantly the ability to obtain union of the graft-host bone junction. Adequate internal fixation, external splints, and protected weight bearing all serve to enhance union rates, which are approximately 80% in most large series (10–12).

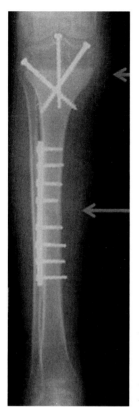

X-ray appearance of a healed intercalary allograft of the tibia. The arrows indicate the osteotomy sites proximally and distally. The patient's articular surface was preserved.

FIGURE 7.8

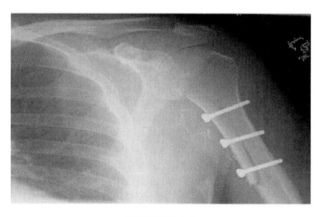

FIGURE 7.9

X-ray appearance of a hemicortical allograft used to reconstitute a partial defect on the medial proximal humerus.

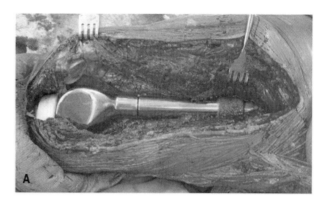

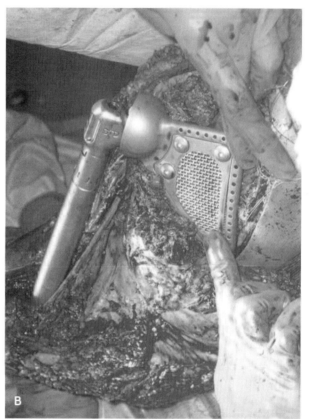

FIGURE 7.10

A: Intraoperative appearance of a distal femur replacement.
B: Intraoperative appearance of a total scapula and proximal humerus replacement.

Postoperatively, patients with allografts can mobilize fairly quickly. Almost all allograft reconstructions require an extended period of protected weight bearing until there is evidence of union at the allograft-host bone junction, as demonstrated on imaging. Progressive weight bearing is allowed relative to the amount of healing observed. When intra-articular soft tissue reconstructions are performed, as with osteoarticular allografts, the joint is typically immobilized for several weeks.

Metallic Prostheses

Megaprostheses are most commonly used to reconstruct large-segment bone defects. Historically, implants were fabricated on a custom basis for each patient. Currently, modular systems offering virtually limitless sizing options are widely available. Noncustom metallic implants are available for all commonly reconstructed anatomic sites: shoulder, elbow, hip, and knee (Fig. 7.10). Even smaller joints, such as the wrist and ankle, have "off-the-shelf" implant options.

Large megaprostheses are instantly durable, a quality that can be desirable in patients being treated for malignancies, since it can be difficult to maneuver assistive devices while undergoing chemotherapy or recovering from thoracotomy. In addition, modular systems give the operating surgeon great latitude during the reconstructive phase of the surgery. For example, if the proximal femur is found to be compromised by tumor or lack of bone quality following distal femoral resection, the entire femur can be replaced from hip to knee with minimal effort.

The major disadvantage of metallic prostheses is that they will all eventually fail when the patient is fortunate enough to be cured of disease. With increasing survival rates for most bone sarcomas, prosthetic revision has become increasingly common. Great research and development have gone into improving prosthetic designs. The weakest link in an endoprosthesis is where the metal stem attaches to bone. Currently, most stems are secured with cement or a press-fit technique that relies on bony in-growth of the stem. Both septic and aseptic loosening account for the vast majority of prosthetic failures (Fig. 7.11). Newer designs attempt to circumvent the problem of aseptic loosening.

Postoperatively, most patients with metallic prosthetic reconstructions can mobilize immediately. Exceptions might be reconstructions in which free flap or skin graft is required for wound closure. In general, cemented prostheses allow for immediate full weight bearing. Press-fit prostheses usually require a period of partial weight bearing, though this is highly dependent on surgeon preference and anatomic location. Joint mobilization is typically initiated when the surrounding soft tissue demonstrates adequate healing. Situations requiring soft tissue reconstruction will likely require longer periods of joint immobilization.

Allograft-Prosthetic Composites

Allograft-prosthetic composites (APCs) are the best of both worlds: the immediate structural integrity of a metallic prosthesis combined with the superior biologic soft tissue attachments of allografts. They have become an increasingly popular reconstruction method (13,14). Alloprosthetic composites are most commonly employed in the proximal tibia and proximal humerus. In the proximal tibia, the allograft provides for secure attachment of the patellar tendon, reconstituting an intact and sturdy extensor mechanism (15). In the proximal humerus, the rotator cuff tendons and capsule are attached to the remaining soft tissue on the allograft. This allows for a stable and hopefully functional joint. In addition, alloprosthetic composites have been used in the proximal femur to take advantage of the gluteus medius attachment to prevent a Trendelenburg gait.

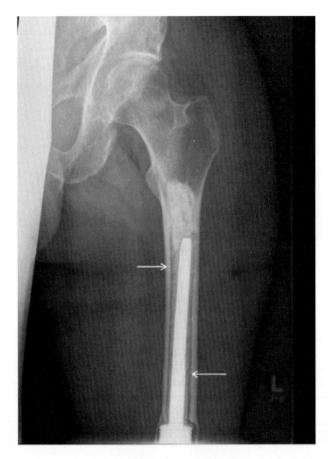

FIGURE 7.11

Aseptic loosening of a distal femoral prosthesis. The cement mantle is fractured and there is a lucency between the cement and the bone (arrows).

Regardless of the location, the surgical method is similar. The articular surface of the allograft is cut off and the stem of the implant placed in the allograft. The implant can be skewered through the bone (Fig. 7.12A) or simply into the allograft alone. The implant is typically cemented into the allograft, as bony in-growth is not expected. The skewered stem is then placed in the host bone by either press-fit or cemented techniques. Depending on the stability of the construct, the graft and host bone may or may not require additional fixation (Fig. 7.12B). The soft tissues, including tendon, ligaments, and capsule, are then reconstructed with heavy suture.

Alloprostheses offer many advantages. The soft tissue advantages are obvious, as the tendon and muscle attachments are functionally superior to those attached to metal. In addition, bone stock is reconstituted, allowing for greater revision options in the future. Also, the exact size matching of the allograft is not as crucial, since the articular surface is replaced with metal. The main disadvantage of APC reconstruc-

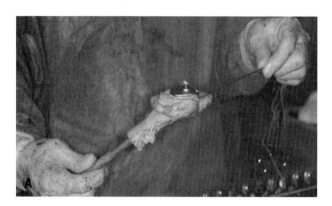

FIGURE 7.12

A: A proximal humerus alloprosthetic composite. A long-stemmed humerus component is skewered through the allograft. Sutures have been placed through soft tissue attachments on the allograft. B: X-ray appearance of a proximal humerus alloprosthetic composite. The construct was secured to the patient's bone with additional internal fixation, facilitating complete healing of the allograft and host bone junction.

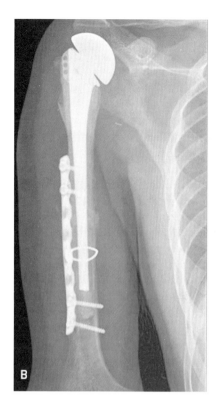

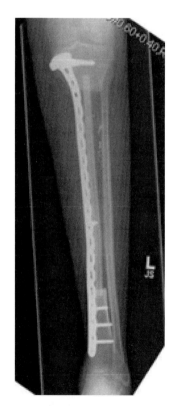

FIGURE 7.13

A vascularized fibular autograft used to reconstruct an intercalary segment of the contralateral tibia following wide excision of a chondrosarcoma.

tion is the lengthy operative time required compared to other techniques, which may theoretically lead to increased rates of infection (16).

Postoperatively, protected weight bearing is required to allow the allograft host bone junction to heal. In addition, the joint must be immobilized for an extended period to allow the soft tissue reconstruction to heal.

Autografts

Autografts are typically used to reconstruct intercalary defects. Tumors located in the diaphysis of the humerus and tibia are ideal for this reconstruction option. The most common autograft donor sites are the fibula and iliac crest. To enhance healing, often their corresponding vascular pedicle is transposed and reconnected by a microvascular anastomosis. Obviously, these types of procedures require a multidisciplinary team. The union rates of vascularized bone grafts are high, making them an attractive alternative (17). If the anastomosis is patent long-term, the graft tends to hypertrophy with time, assuming the diameter and strength of the replaced bone.

Autograft reconstructions usually require the longest period of protected weight bearing compared to other reconstruction options. Because the initial size mismatch between the autograft and the host bone (Fig. 7.13), extended periods (often greater than one year) of protected weight bearing and brace immobilization must be implemented to avoid fracture.

Special Considerations in Limb Salvage Surgery

CHILDREN. Skeletally immature patients are a particularly challenging group to reconstruct, as children require extremely durable constructs that allow for adjustments in longitudinal growth. The knee, the most common site for primary bone tumors, possesses the two most important growth plates to lower-extremity longitudinal growth. The distal femoral growth plate contributes approximately 1 cm a year, whereas the proximal tibia contributes approximately 0.6 cm a year. Obviously, obliterating these growth plates in a young child will lead to a considerable (and usually unacceptable) leg length discrepancy by skeletal maturity. In general, reconstruction strategies aim to (1) preserve growth plates when possible, (2) utilize extensible metallic prostheses, or (3) expand the remaining bone by a technique called bone transport. For example, a nine-year-old boy with a distal femoral osteogenic sarcoma has approximately 11 cm of growth remaining in the knee region, assuming he will grow until the age of 16. The complexity of the surgical management of this child is considerable. No doubt, above-knee amputation or rotationplasty will provide the most simple, most predictable, and least restrictive option. Limb salvage options might include using an extensible metallic prosthesis (Fig. 7.14) or an osteoarticular allograft. While these options seem attractive, they have considerable limitations, such as limited athletic activity to prolong the longevity of the implant, numerous future surgical procedures for lengthening and implant failure, and a lifetime risk of implant infection. Certainly, newer prosthetic designs with noninvasive expansion mechanisms attempt to address some of the current limitations.

PELVIS. Pelvic reconstruction following tumor excision probably represents the most complicated and technically difficult of orthopedic oncologic procedures. Patients often experience postoperative complications and require lengthy periods of immobilization. When the acetabulum can be spared, often, reconstruction can be avoided. When the acetabulum must be sacrificed, "hip replacement" is required. Reconstructions can be accomplished with metallic implants, allografts, and allograft-prosthetic composites (Figs. 7.15 and 7.16). Joint instability is a major problem following acetabular reconstruction. Usually, the majority, and in some cases all, of the surrounding muscles have

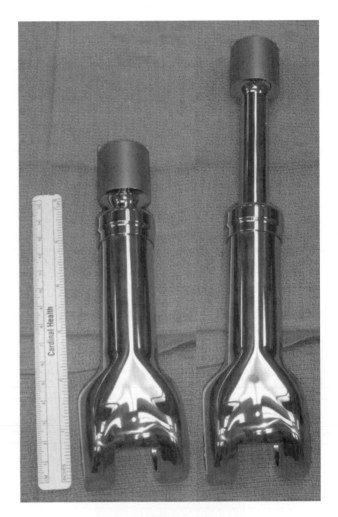

FIGURE 7.14

An expandable distal femoral prosthesis.

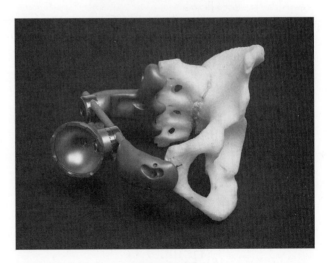

FIGURE 7.15

A custom metal pelvis prosthesis.

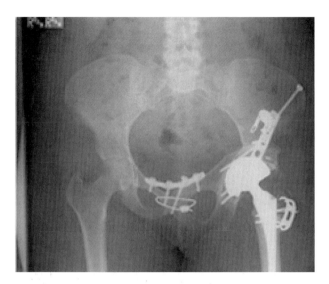

FIGURE 7.16

An x-ray of a pelvis allograft into which a bipolar hip prosthesis has been placed.

been transected or sacrificed, leading to both static and dynamic instability with minimal active control of the extremity. The disability is magnified if portions of the sciatic or femoral nerve are sacrificed or injured. In cases of severe instability, a hip orthosis may be required until adequate scarring of the surrounding soft tissue has been achieved. Patients status-post pelvic reconstruction require several months of rehabilitation to maximize their functional capacity.

Complications Following Limb Salvage Surgery

Unfortunately, complications following limb salvage surgery are plentiful. Approximately 10%–15% of all megaprostheses and/or allografts will become infected during a patient's lifetime. Infection is a particularly difficult problem to manage, requiring removal of the involved prosthesis, placement of an antibiotic-impregnated spacer, a lengthy period of intravenous antibiotics, followed by replacement of a new prosthesis. Cases in which the infection cannot be cleared or there is inadequate surrounding soft tissue, amputation may be required. Implant loosening or breakage is also common and almost guaranteed given enough time (Fig. 7.17). The more active the patient, the more quickly and more likely implant failure will occur. Prosthetic designs and biologic supplements are actively pursued areas of research aimed to prolong implant survival. Joint instability secondary to force mismatch from muscle or nerve resection can be problematic, leading to dislocation (Fig. 7.18). Solutions such as revision to a constrained implant or prolonged immobilization will usually solve this problem.

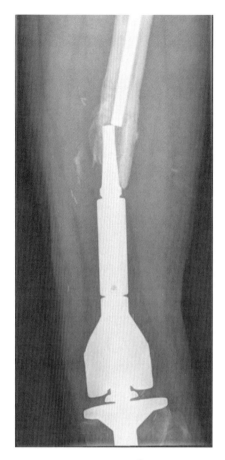

FIGURE 7.17

An x-ray of a broken cemented femoral stem.

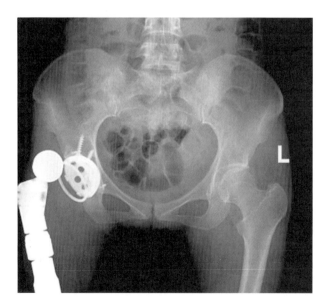

FIGURE 7.18

An unstable right hip following wide excision and reconstruction of the proximal femur and surrounding soft tissue.

Amputation

Only 10% of patients with primary bone and soft tissue sarcomas will require amputation for local tumor control. The main reason to perform amputation in the oncology setting is the inability to achieve negative tumor margins at the time of definitive surgery. This commonly occurs in cases of neglected tumors (Fig. 7.19) Other indications include recurrent disease, fracture, considerable remaining growth in a young child, superior function compared to limb salvage, and infected reconstructions. Tumors of the foot are often treated with below-knee amputation, not because of surgical margins, but rather because of superior function.

Levels of lower-extremity amputation and upper-extremity amputation are shown in Figures 7.20 and 7.21, respectively. The level of amputation in tumor surgery is entirely directed by the location of the tumor. In general, the higher the level of amputation, the greater the energy expenditure above baseline.

There are many advantages to amputation in cancer surgery. In certain tumors that are unaffected by adjuvants such as chemotherapy or radiation, amputation allows for the most complete removal of tumor. Local recurrence rates are lower with amputation. Usually, additional surgical procedures are not required following amputation compared to those needed for complications of limb salvage surgery. Finally, both upper- and lower-extremity prosthetic designs have enjoyed tremendous advancement in past decade with excellent function and cosmesis.

There are also disadvantages of amputation compared to limb salvage. Most amputees experience phantom sensation and some experience phantom pain. Phantom pain can be particularly debilitating and usually requires prolonged pharmacologic intervention.

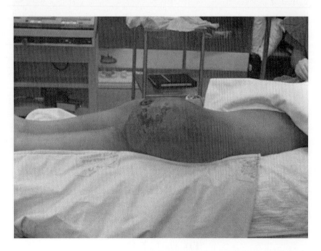

FIGURE 7.19

A very large osteogenic sarcoma of the distal femur with overlying skin compromise.

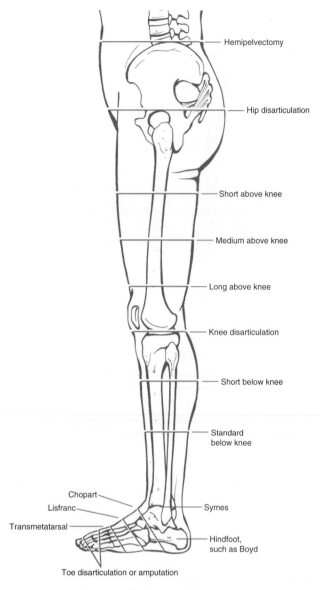

FIGURE 7.20

Amputation levels in the lower extremity.

Painful neuromas can occur at the stump of a transected nerve and can cause problems with weight bearing. Proprioception is compromised following amputation, leading to initial difficulties with gait training. Children with considerable remaining growth can get bony overgrowth at the terminal end of the bone, requiring surgical revision.

Lower-Extremity Amputations

Below-knee amputation (BKA) is typically performed for tumors of the foot, ankle, or distal tibia. The ideal length of residual tibia is 12–17 cm distal to the medial joint line (Fig. 7.22). BK amputees expend approximately

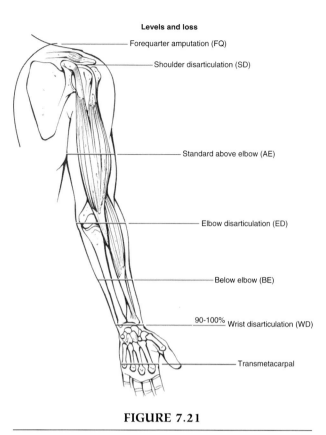

Levels and loss
- Forequarter amputation (FQ)
- Shoulder disarticulation (SD)
- Standard above elbow (AE)
- Elbow disarticulation (ED)
- Below elbow (BE)
- 90-100% Wrist disarticulation (WD)
- Transmetacarpal

FIGURE 7.21

Amputation levels in the upper extremity.

40% more kcal/min than nonamputees to maintain a normal gait and ambulate about 35% slower. Whereas a BKA performed for vascular compromise tends to use a large posterior flap, a BKA in cancer surgery utilizes a "fish-mouth" type incision for maximal tumor margins.

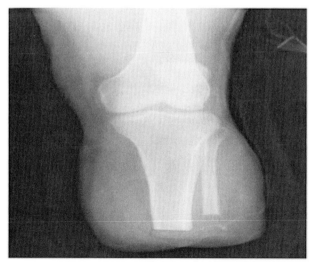

FIGURE 7.22

An x-ray of a below-knee amputation. The fibula is usually transected more proximally than the tibia.

Above-knee amputation (AKA) is performed for unresectable tumors of the proximal tibia, distal femur, and popliteal fossa. AKA amputees expend 89% more kcal/min than nonamputees and walk 43% slower. A "fish-mouth" incision is usually used, with an effort to make the anterior flap slightly larger than the posterior flap such that the distal incision is more posterior. Muscle balance is an important technical consideration. If amputation is performed proximal to the adductor tendon insertion, an adductor myodesis should be performed to balance the hip abductor proximally. Also, when the quadriceps myodesis is performed, the hip should be in full extension to avoid overtightening, leading to a hip flexion contracture.

In selected patients, both BKA and AKA are ideal for immediate prosthetic fitting following the definitive surgery. When the surgeon has closed the wound, a sterile dressing is applied. A prosthetist then applies an immediate postoperative prosthesis (IPOP) under the same anesthesia (Fig. 7.23). This temporary prosthesis is not meant to be used for weight bearing. The sensation and cosmetic appearance of an immediate artificial limb is thought to decrease the frequency and severity of phantom pain as well as assist in emotional acceptance. The IPOP typically comes off within a week after surgery once the swelling decreases. In patients with delayed healing secondary to radiation or chemo-

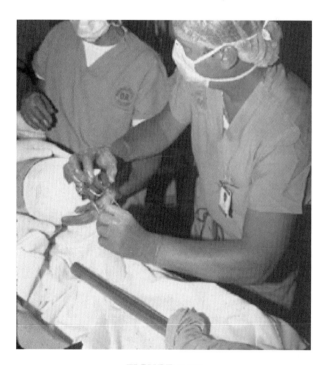

FIGURE 7.23

Following above-knee amputation, prosthetists place an immediate postoperative prosthesis (IPOP) while the patient is still under anesthesia.

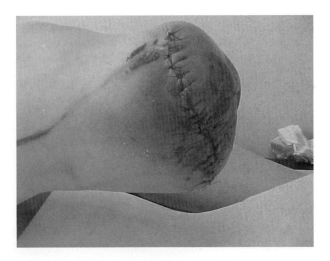

FIGURE 7.24

Wound breakdown following IPOP placement in a patient-post below-knee amputation. The patient had previously undergone radiation to the limb.

therapy, immediate prosthetic fitting can cause wound complications and is contraindicated (Fig. 24).

Hemipelvectomy is performed for tumors of the hip and pelvis. The resection can include the entire inominate bone (Fig. 7.25) or just portions of it. Hemipelvectomy is often preferred to limb salvage for pelvic tumors, as the associated complications are fewer. Wound complications following hemipelvectomy can be considerable, with rates greater than 50% in some

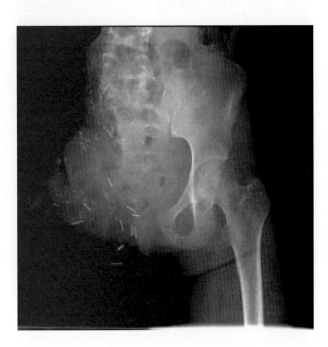

FIGURE 7.25

An x-ray following external hemipelvectomy.

series. Most patients who undergo hemipelvectomy do not ultimately use a prosthesis for ambulation.

Postoperatively, all patients that undergo amputation, regardless of level, are monitored for wound complications and phantom pain. These patients benefit greatly from early evaluation by rehabilitation or physiatry departments. Issues of standing balance and shaping of the residual limb are best addressed as early as possible. For hemipelvectomy patients in which the ischium has been removed, sitting balance needs to be addressed. The timing of prosthetic fitting and weight bearing is ultimately determined by the operating surgeon and is largely based on wound status.

Upper-Extremity Amputations

Upper-extremity amputations are far less common than lower-extremity amputations. Below-elbow amputations are quite functional. Successful prosthetic rehabilitation can be achieved in the majority of patients. Forearm strength and rotation are proportional to the maintained length. Even very short residual below-elbow limbs are preferable to through-elbow or above-elbow amputation. Maintenance of the biceps insertion is important. For above-elbow amputations, at least 5 cm of remaining humerus is required for prosthetic fitting. For proximal tumors, shoulder disarticulation is preferable to forequarter amputation when possible. The scapula provides cosmetic symmetry and is important for wearing clothes.

Rotationplasty

Rotationplasty is an innovative way to manage tumors around the knee that would otherwise require above-knee amputation. Originally described in the 1930s for limbs affected by tuberculosis, rotationplasty was performed for malignant tumors about the knee starting in the 1970s (18,19). The procedure involves removing the entire knee in continuity, with both the distal femur and proximal tibia en bloc, with all of the surrounding soft tissue except the popliteal artery and vein and the tibial and peroneal nerves. The distal portion of the extremity is then rotated 180 degrees, and the bones and soft tissues are reapproximated (Fig. 7.26). The resulting limb is functionally a below-knee amputation (Fig. 7.27A,B). Variations on the theme have been described around the hip and even in the upper extremity (20,21).

The most common indication for rotationplasty is a child with considerable remaining growth, as endoprosthetic reconstruction in skeletally immature patients will require multiple revisions for lengthening and failures. In addition, rotationplasty might be desirable for individuals with high physical demands.

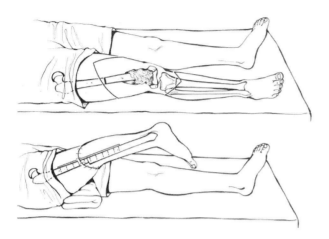

FIGURE 7.26

A schematic representation of a rotationplasty.

Other indications include compromised soft tissue around the knee, pathologic fractures, failed limb salvage procedures, and local recurrence. Compared to above-knee amputation, rotationplasty is void of phantom pain, demonstrates normal proprioception, and provides durable weight bearing without painful neuromas. The obvious disadvantage is the cosmetic appearance. While the procedure is still performed frequently in Europe, the advent of extensible endoprostheses has lead to decreased enthusiasm among parents who desire a more normal-appearing extremity for their child.

Postoperatively, patients are not permitted to bear weight through the extremity until the osteosynthesis site between the distal femur and proximal tibia has fully healed. Ankle range of motion and strengthening is initially restricted as well to allow tendon and muscle connections to heal.

SURGICAL MANAGEMENT OF SKELETAL METASTASES

The management of patients with skeletal metastases represents one of the most challenging aspects of orthopedic oncology. These patients are typically quite ill and in considerable pain. Bone pain from metastatic disease has a tremendous impact on the patient's quality of life. The role of the orthopedic oncologist is largely to maximize the patient's quality of life by treating impending and pathologic fractures for the purposes of pain control and to restore and maintain function and mobility. In certain instances of isolated bone metastases, cure, or at the very least lengthy disease-free intervals, may be achieved with surgical excision (22). A comprehensive overview of the multidisciplinary efforts required to care for patients with metastatic disease to bone is provided in Chapter 60.

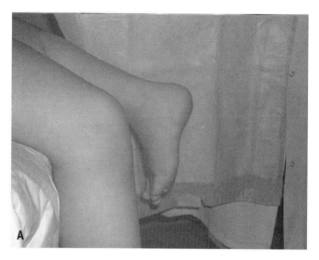

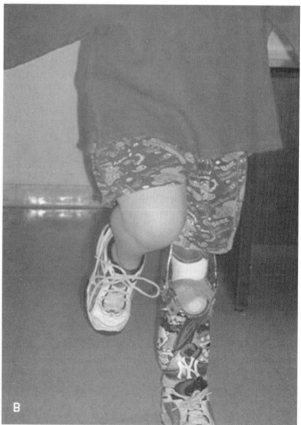

FIGURE 7.27

A: A clinical picture of a young boy post rotationplasty for a malignant tumor of the knee. Note that the heel is at the level of the contralateral knee. B: He has excellent physical coordination following prosthetic fitting of the rotated limb with a modified BKA prosthesis.

A pathologic fracture is a fracture that has occurred through diseased bone (Fig. 7.28). An impending fracture is one that is likely to occur with normal physiologic loading (turning in bed, ambulation, etc.) (Fig. 7.29). Today, numerous nonsurgical interventions

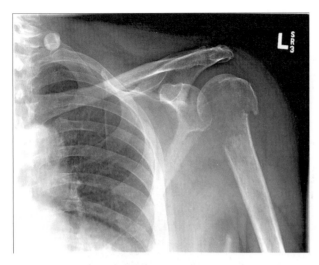

FIGURE 7.28

A pathologic proximal humerus fracture through metastatic renal cancer.

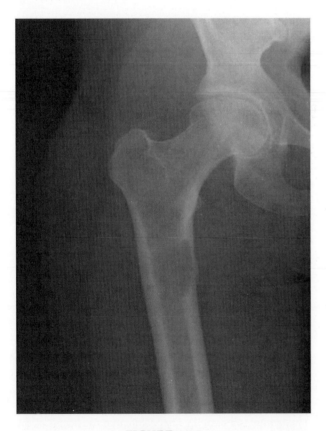

FIGURE 7.29

An impending pathological fracture of the femur through metastatic breast cancer.

are available to treat impending fractures or lesions at risk of evolving into impending fractures, including radiation, bisphosphonates, and a host of minimally invasive ablative techniques.

When is surgery indicated for pathologic bone lesions? Various investigations have attempted to quantify the risk of fracture depending on imaging and clinical characteristics (23–25). None of these scoring systems has the ability to accurately predict fracture risk. The decision to proceed with surgical fixation is largely dependent on a combination of imaging characteristics, pain, functional deficits, anatomic location of the lesion, and remaining life expectancy. As a rule, lower-extremity fractures should be surgically fixed if the patient's life expectancy is at least six weeks, whereas upper-extremity fractures are usually not fixed if the life expectancy is less than three months. Of course, many factors come into play when making such decisions.

When the decision is made to proceed with surgery, a few basic goals must be achieved:

1. The reconstruction must permit immediate weight bearing.
2. The reconstruction should last the patient's lifetime.
3. "One bone, one operation," meaning the entire bone and any other concerning lesions within the bone must be addressed at the time of surgery.

While these goals seem simple and intuitive, they can be difficult to achieve. New systemic biologic agents are changing the patterns of metastatic disease and the associated survival times. What was once thought to be an adequate fixation technique may not last long enough (Fig. 7.30). In general, the ends of long bones are treated with prosthetic replacements. This is especially true around the hip. Usually, oncologic prostheses are need as they possess varying stem lengths to splint the entire bone (Fig. 7.31). Diaphyseal lesions can be treated with standard intramedullary nails (Fig. 7.32). When possible, the metastasis should be excised. This potentially extends the longevity of the reconstruction, retarding local tumor progression. The remaining cavitary defect should be filled with cement, as it provides increased strength and prevents tumor reaccumulation. Even thermal and physical adjuvants, such as liquid nitrogen, can be used to supplement the surgery to halt local bone destruction (Fig. 7.33). An important aspect of the preoperative evaluation is considering other bones that may be at risk of fracture. For example, if a patient has a pathologic hip fracture, the upper extremities should be assessed for impending fracture, as the weight bearing will temporarily be transferred to the upper extremities during recovery.

Postoperative Care

Most patients will benefit from postoperative radiation to again prevent tumor progression and prevent loss of fixa-

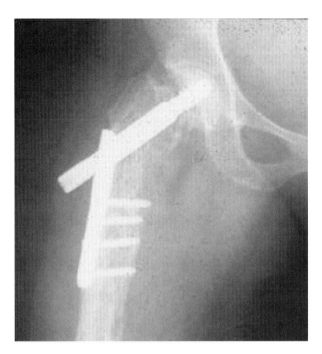

FIGURE 7.30

Failed internal fixation of a proximal femur fracture through metastatic thyroid cancer. The patient outlived the durability of the reconstruction. Revision to an endoprosthesis was performed.

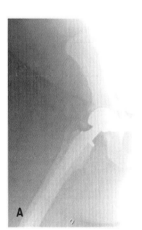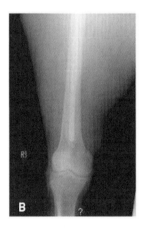

FIGURE 7.31

A long-stemmed cemented hemiarthroplasty of the hip. The shaft splints the entire bone prophylactically, addressing micrometastases in the remaining femur.

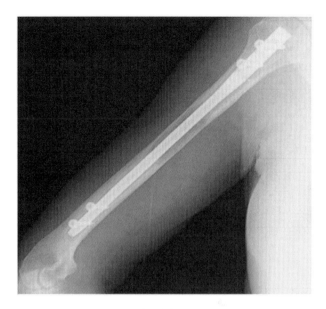

FIGURE 7.32

An intramedullary nail fixation of an impending humeral shaft fracture.

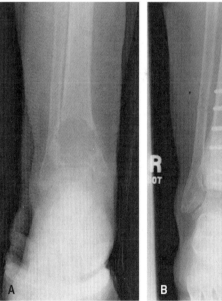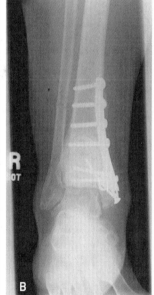

FIGURE 7.33

A pathological fracture (A) of the distal tibia through a plasma cell neoplasm. The lesion was treated with curettage, liquid nitrogen, cement, and internal fixation (B). The cement permitted immediate structural integrity, allowing full weight bearing.

tion (26). All patients should be mobilized immediately. Standard precautions should be observed for joint replacement to prevent dislocation, but otherwise there should be no weight-bearing restrictions. Postoperative complications are unfortunately common owing to the overall medical status of these patients. Infection and deep venous thrombosis are usually treated prophylactically. Aggressive pulmonary toilet is encouraged. Nutritional supplementation may be beneficial.

References

1. Mankin HJ, Hornicek FJ. Paget's sarcoma: a historical and outcome review. *Clin Orthop Relat Res.* 2005;438:97–102.
2. Brady MS, Gaynor JJ, Brennan MF. Radiation-associated sarcoma of bone and soft tissue. *Arch Surg.* 1992;127:1379–1385.
3. Mankin HJ, Lange TA, Spanier SS. The hazards of biopsy in patients with malignant primary bone and soft-tissue tumors. *J Bone Joint Surg Am.* 1982;64:1121–1127.
4. Mankin HJ, Mankin CJ, Simon MA. The hazards of the biopsy, revisited. Members of the Musculoskeletal Tumor Society. *J Bone Joint Surg Am.* 1996;78:656–663.
5. Enneking WF, Spanier SS, Goodman MA. A system for the surgical staging of musculoskeletal sarcoma. *Clin Orthop Relat Res.* 1980;153:106–120.
6. Marco RA, Gitelis S, Brebach GT, Healey JH. Cartilage tumors: evaluation and treatment. *J Am Acad Orthop Surg.* 2000;8:292–304.
7. Rougraff BT, Simon MA, Kneisl JS, Greenberg DB, Mankin HJ. Limb salvage compared with amputation for osteosarcoma of the distal end of the femur. A long-term oncological, functional, and quality-of-life study. *J Bone Joint Surg Am.* 1994;76:649–656.
8. Williard WC, Hajdu SI, Casper ES, Brennan MF. Comparison of amputation with limb-sparing operations for adult soft tissue sarcoma of the extremity. *Ann Surg.* 1992;215:269–275.
9. Accessed at http://www.aatb.org/.
10. Muscolo DL, Ayerza MA, Aponte-Tinao LA. Massive allograft use in orthopedic oncology. *Orthop Clin North Am.* 2006;37:65–74.
11. Hornicek FJ, Gebhardt MC, Tomford WW, et al. Factors affecting nonunion of the allograft-host junction. *Clin Orthop Relat Res.* 2001;382:87–98.
12. Mankin HJ, Gebhardt MC, Jennings LC, Springfield DS, Tomford WW. Long-term results of allograft replacement in the management of bone tumors. *Clin Orthop Relat Res.* 1996;324:86–97.
13. Gitelis S, Piasecki P. Allograft prosthetic composite arthroplasty for osteosarcoma and other aggressive bone tumors. *Clin Orthop Relat Res.* 1991;270:197–201.
14. Harris AI, Gitelis S, Sheinkop MB, Rosenberg AG, Piasecki P. Allograft prosthetic composite reconstruction for limb salvage and severe deficiency of bone at the knee or hip. *Semin Arthroplasty.* 1994;5:85–94.
15. Donati D, Colangeli M, Colangeli S, Di Bella C, Mercuri M. Allograft-prosthetic composite in the proximal tibia after bone tumor resection. *Clin Orthop Relat Res.* 2008;466:459–465.
16. Zehr RJ, Enneking WF, Scarborough MT. Allograft-prosthesis composite versus megaprosthesis in proximal femoral reconstruction. *Clin Orthop Relat Res.* 1996;322:207–223.
17. Pollock R, Stalley P, Lee K, Pennington D. Free vascularized fibula grafts in limb-salvage surgery. *J Reconstr Microsurg.* 2005;21:79–84.
18. Merkel KD, Gebhardt M, Springfield DS. Rotationplasty as a reconstructive operation after tumor resection. *Clin Orthop Relat Res.* 1991;270:231–236.
19. de Bari A, Krajbich JI, Langer F, Hamilton EL, Hubbard S. Modified Van Nes rotationplasty for osteosarcoma of the proximal tibia in children. *J Bone Joint Surg Br.* 1990;72:1065–1069.
20. Winkelmann WW. Hip rotationplasty for malignant tumors of the proximal part of the femur. *J Bone Joint Surg Am.* 1986;68:362–369.
21. Athanasian EA, Healey JH. Resection replantation of the arm for sarcoma: an alternative to amputation. *Clin Orthop Relat Res.* 2002:204–208.
22. Althausen P, Althausen A, Jennings LC, Mankin HJ. Prognostic factors and surgical treatment of osseous metastases secondary to renal cell carcinoma. *Cancer.* 1997;80:1103–1109.
23. Snell W, Beals RK. Femoral metastases and fractures from breast cancer. *Surg Gynecol Obstet.* 1964;119:22–24.
24. Harrington KD. New trends in the management of lower extremity metastases. *Clin Orthop Relat Res.* 1982;169:53–61.
25. Mirels H. Metastatic disease in long bones. A proposed scoring system for diagnosing impending pathologic fractures. *Clin Orthop Relat Res.* 1989;249:256–264.
26. Townsend PW, Smalley SR, Cozad SC, Rosenthal HG, Hassanein RE. Role of postoperative radiation therapy after stabilization of fractures caused by metastatic disease. *Int J Radiat Oncol Biol Phys.* 1995;31:43–49.

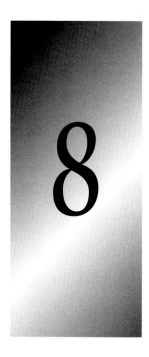

Principles of Breast Surgery in Cancer

8

Sarah A. McLaughlin
Tari A. King

While the earliest recorded descriptions of breast surgery date back to the ancient Egyptians, modern breast surgery practice is considered to have begun in the late 1890s with the work of Dr. William S. Halsted. In the 100 years since, the art of breast surgery has been a process in evolution, searching for a balance between what is the oncologically safest procedure and what is the least deforming one.

To date, the role of systemic chemotherapy and antiestrogen hormonal therapies has become increasingly important, but breast cancer remains largely a surgical disease. Surgery offers the best chance for a cure. This chapter covers the basic principles of breast surgery. Although some historical data is included, it focuses on the current concepts of screening, preoperative diagnosis by needle biopsy, surgical options for the breast, and sentinel lymph node (SLN) biopsy for axillary staging.

ANATOMY

The adult breast lies between the second and sixth ribs vertically and between the sternal edge medially and the midaxillary line laterally. The rounded breast has a lateral projection into the axilla, known as the axillary tail of Spence. The breast rests on the pectoralis major muscle and is separated from it by the retromammary space. This space represents a distinct plane between the investing fascia of the breast tissue and the pecto-

ralis major fascia, and is identified by a thin layer of loose areolar tissue through which small vessels and lymphatic channels pass. When a mastectomy is performed, the breast tissue is removed, incorporating the retromammary space and the pectoralis major fascia.

The glandular breast consists of segments of ducts (lobes) that are arranged radially and extend outward and posteriorly from the nipple-areolar complex. Each duct undergoes a complex system of branching, ultimately ending in the terminal ductal-lobular units (TDLU). The lobules are the milk-forming glands of the lactating breast; the ducts are the channels. It is in the TDLUs that most breast cancers arise (1).

The blood supply to the breast is primarily through superficial arteries branching from the internal thoracic (mammary) artery or the lateral mammary artery from the lateral thoracic artery. The venous drainage follows the arterial patterns, and these veins ultimately drain into either the internal thoracic or the axillary vein. The innervation of the breast is supplied via the anterior and lateral cutaneous branches of the second to sixth intercostal nerves.

The thoracic wall is comprised of 12 thoracic vertebrae, 12 ribs, costal cartilages, and sternum and associated muscles. Table 8.1 lists the muscles of the thoracic wall. The most common muscular variations seen in breast surgery include the finding of a rectus sternalis muscle or the finding of a Langer axillary arch. The rectus sternalis can be found in nearly 8% of patients and represents an extension of muscular

KEY POINTS

- The role of systemic chemotherapy and antiestrogen hormonal therapies has become increasingly important, but breast cancer remains largely a surgical disease.
- When a suspicious abnormality in the breast is palpated or identified by imaging, a biopsy should be obtained for tissue diagnosis.
- In 1894, William Halsted popularized the removal of the breast, pectoralis muscles, and axillary lymph nodes in levels 1, 2, and 3. This procedure was known as the radical mastectomy (RM) or Halsted mastectomy.
- In 1948, Patey and Dyson proposed leaving the pectoralis muscles and named the removal of only the breast and axillary contents the modified radical mastectomy (MRM).
- With more than 25 years of follow-up, it is well accepted that there is no survival difference between RM and MRM.
- Today, the treatment options for patients with early-stage (T1 or T2) breast cancer are total mastectomy (TM) or breast-conservation therapy (BCT).

- BCT involves excision of the tumor and a small portion of surrounding normal breast parenchyma to achieve negative surgical margins and whole-breast adjuvant radiation therapy.
- TM involves removal of the skin, nipple and areolar complex, and breast tissue, including the pectoralis major fascia.
- Sentinel lymph node mapping and biopsy has replaced axillary node dissection as the standard of care for staging the axilla in clinically node-negative patients.
- Intraoperative evaluation of the sentinel lymph node allows for immediate axillary lymph node dissection in cases with identifiable metastatic disease.
- Although sentinel lymph node (SLN) biopsy is considered less invasive than axillary lymph node dissection (ALND), lymphedema may still occur in roughly 3%–7% of patients undergoing an SLN biopsy as compared with 15%–20% of patients undergoing ALND.

and aponeurotic fibers from the rectus abdominus that run medial to the pectoralis major and parallel to the sternum. The sternalis is of anatomic interest only. Langer axillary arch is found in 3%–6% of patients and is a band of latissimus dorsi muscle fibers crossing the axilla superficially and inserting into the pectoralis major muscle medially. Langer arch can cause compression of the axillary artery or vein, or confusion during axillary dissection, but once identified, can be divided without risk.

The pectoralis minor muscle is enveloped in the clavipectoral fascia. It is by opening this fascia along the lateral border of this muscle that the axilla is entered. The axilla contains the axillary vessels and their branches, the brachial plexus, and lymph nodes. The borders of the axilla are listed in Table 8.2. The long thoracic, thoracodorsal, medial pectoral (located lateral to the pectoralis minor muscle), and intercostal brachial nerves are routinely identified during an axillary dissection. While the long thoracic nerve is always preserved

---

TABLE 8.1
Muscles of the Thoracic Wall and Axilla

MUSCLE	ACTION	NERVE
Pectoralis major	Flexion, adduction, medial rotation of arm	Medial and lateral pectoral
Pectoralis minor	Draws scapula down and forward	Medial pectoral
Subclavius	Draws shoulder down and forward	Long thoracic
Serratus anterior	Rotation of scapula; draws scapula forward	Long thoracic
Subscapularis	Medial rotation of arm	Upper and lower sub scapular
Teres major	Adduction, extension, medial rotation of arm	Lower subscapular
Latissimus dorsi	Adduction, extension, medial rotation of arm; draws shoulder down and backward	Thoracodorsal

TABLE 8.2 *Axillary Boundaries*	
BOUNDARIES	STRUCTURES
Anterior	Pectoralis major, pectoralis minor, clavipectoral fascia
Posterior	Subscapularis, teres major, latissimus dorsi
Medial	Serratus anterior, 1st–4th ribs, intercostal muscles
Lateral	Humerus, coracobrachialis, biceps muscles

(to avoid a "winged scapula"), the thoracodorsal and medial pectoral nerves are generally preserved, but can be sacrificed in cases of advanced disease when the nerves are encased in tumor. The intercostal brachial nerves run from medial to lateral through the axilla and supply sensation to the medial and posterior upper arm. Although these nerves can be saved, one or two are frequently sacrificed to allow better visualization and access to the subscapular nodes. As a result, patients may complain of varying degrees of regional patchy numbness in the medial and posterior upper arm, some of which may improve in time.

The lymph nodes in the axilla are divided into three levels. Level 1 is located lateral to the border of the pectoralis minor muscle and includes the external mammary, axillary, and scapular nodes. Level 2 is found deep in the pectoralis minor muscle and includes some central and subclavicular nodes. Level 3 is medial to the medial border of the pectoralis minor muscle and extends to Halsted ligament and the costoclavicular ligament of the first rib. This level includes the infraclavicular nodes and, rarely, a supraclavicular node. Interpectoral (Rotter) nodes are found between the pectoralis major and pectoralis minor muscles. While the exact number of axillary nodes is unknown and varies between patients, it is generally accepted that a complete axillary lymph node dissection (ALND) removes approximately 15–20 lymph nodes.

RISK ASSESSMENT, SCREENING, AND DIAGNOSIS

Breast cancer is the most common cancer in women and is second to lung cancer as the most common cause of cancer-related death in women. In 2006, the American Cancer Society (ACS) estimated that nearly 212,920 women would be diagnosed with the disease (2). According to National Cancer Institute (NCI) Surveillance Epidemiology and End Results (SEER) databases, one in eight women will develop breast cancer in her lifetime. Furthermore, breast-related symptoms, benign or malignant, are one of the most common reasons women seek medical care. For these reasons, an informed discussion regarding patient risk factors and appropriate screening tools should be undertaken with each patient.

It is important to distinguish women who may be at higher-than-normal risk for developing breast cancer. Many factors influence the development of breast cancer, most of which cannot be modified. These include older patient age, a family history of one or more first- or second-degree relatives with breast cancer, and a personal history of biopsy-proven atypical hyperplasia or lobular carcinoma in situ (LCIS). In addition, a history of mantle radiation can significantly increase a woman's risk of developing breast cancer over the next 10–15 years of her life. Modifiable risk factors include the use of postmenopausal hormone replacement therapy (HRT), which can increase one's risk of developing breast cancer by 30%, and possibly parity, with most data suggesting that a multiparous woman is at less risk of developing breast cancer than a nulliparous woman. The most commonly used risk assessment tool is the gail model, which can estimate a woman's overall risk of developing breast cancer over the next five years of her life and over her lifetime as a whole (3). However, this model is limited in patients with a strong family history.

The purpose of breast cancer screening is to facilitate early diagnosis and to decrease breast cancer mortality. The classic triad for routine breast cancer screening includes monthly breast self-exams, annual clinical breast exams, and annual mammography. Beginning at age 25, breast self-exams should be performed at approximately the same time each month or following the completion of menses, as this is the point when the breasts are the least tender. A breast self-exam is best performed while in the shower or while lying down with the ipsilateral arm above the head. An annual clinical breast exam can be performed by an internist, gynecologist, or surgeon. This exam should be a multipositional breast exam and include an evaluation of the axillary and supraclavicular lymph nodes.

The ACS and the NCI recommend annual mammography for all women 40 years and older. Women with a family history of a first-degree relative with breast cancer should begin annual mammography 10 years prior to the age of their relative's diagnosis of breast cancer or age 40, whichever comes first. Mammography is the ideal imaging modality to identify and evaluate both masses and calcifications. The sensitivity of mammography for breast cancer detection ranges between 70% and 85%, while its specificity exceeds 95% (4–6). A complete mammographic examination includes two views of each breast: a mediolateral oblique (MLO) view and a craniocaudal (CC) view. If an abnormality is seen, further images are obtained of the area in question using compression or magnification views.

Mammographic accuracy is limited in younger women and in women with dense breasts. Therefore, adjuncts to the routine screening mammogram include breast ultrasound and, in selected patients, magnetic resonance imaging (MRI) of the breast. Ultrasound can be used as a screening tool or for targeted assessment. Ultrasound cannot replace a screening mammogram because it cannot identify calcifications, which may be the earliest radiologic sign of carcinoma in situ, and because its interpretation is highly operator-dependent. If a mass is identified on mammogram or by palpation, ultrasound can help determine if it is solid or cystic and if its borders are regular or irregular. Malignant masses tend to be irregular, hypoechoic, and "taller than wide."

Data are accumulating to support MRI screening as an adjunct to screening mammography in certain high-risk populations. Currently, the only high-risk population that may derive a benefit from a screening MRI in addition to an annual mammogram is patients with a genetic predisposition to breast cancer, such as that conferred by a mutation in the BRCA 1 or 2 genes (7). The ACS has recently developed guidelines to standardize the recommendations for the use of MRI screening in addition to mammography (8) and plans to develop similar guidelines standardizing MRI techniques. While the sensitivity of MRI for detecting a breast cancer ranges from 86%–100%, the specificity is broad, ranging from 37%–97% (9), resulting in many false-positive biopsies. As a result, this limits its use as a screening modality.

When a suspicious abnormality in the breast is palpated or identified by imaging, a biopsy should be obtained for tissue diagnosis. Biopsy can be performed by direct palpation in a doctor's office, under image guidance, or in the operating room. A fine-needle aspiration (FNA) can be performed of a palpable mass by making several passes with a 22- or 25-gauge needle. The resulting specimen is then ejected onto a glass slide and smeared onto a second slide. The slides are placed into a 95% ethanol solution for fixation and transport to a cytopathologist. An FNA specimen will typically allow for determination between a benign or malignant mass. A core needle biopsy (CNB) employs a large-bore 14-gauge cutting needle that is passed through the mass or image abnormality and retrieves large cores of tissue. This process can be performed by palpation or with mammographic (stereotactic), ultrasound, or MRI

guidance. Vacuum assistance can be added as well to obtain larger volumes of tissue. After CNB, a titanium clip is commonly placed to mark the biopsy area. CNB is the preferred method of diagnosis, as it provides a tissue sample for definitive diagnosis and appropriate surgical planning prior to the operation. In addition to providing a diagnosis, tissue cores can be used to determine the estrogen (ER) or progesterone (PR) receptor, or *HER2/neu* status, of the cancer.

If a CNB cannot be completed, or if the results of the CNB are considered discordant from the image findings, an open surgical biopsy may be needed. Discordance suggests that radiologic images and pathologic diagnosis do not correlate, or that while the images suggest a malignant process, the biopsy pathology is benign. Surgical biopsy of nonpalpable lesions requires needle wire localization placed under stereotactic, sonographic, or MRI guidance. A specimen radiograph is then obtained in the operating room, documenting retrieval of the abnormality.

PATHOLOGY AND STAGING

It is generally believed that most breast cancers arise in the terminal duct-lobular units (TDLU). Breast cancers are then classified as being either in situ or invasive lesions. In situ cancers, specifically ductal carcinoma in situ (DCIS), develop from the epithelial cells lining the lactiferous ducts. Clusters of these cells are separated by orderly, distinct spaces, but all are confined within the basement membrane and surrounded by normal myoepithelial cells (Fig. 8.1). Because DCIS has not penetrated the basement membrane, it lacks the ability to metastasize. Invasive cancers also begin within the TDLU, but characteristically lack any uniform architecture. These tumors grow haphazardly without respect for the basement membrane boundaries, and thus infiltrate into the surrounding stroma (Fig. 8.1). Because invasive cancers extend outside of the TDLU, they have the potential to metastasize to regional lymph nodes or distant sites.

Lobular carcinoma in situ (LCIS) is an abnormal proliferative process arising from the epithelial cells lining the terminal lobules. LCIS cells have bland nuclei that expand and fill the acini of the lobules, but maintain the cross-sectional integrity of the lobular unit. Although LCIS retains the word "carcinoma" in its name, LCIS is not a cancer; instead, it is a multicentric marker of risk. The risk that a woman with LCIS will develop breast cancer is approximately 8- to 10-fold higher than the average woman, or about 25%–30% over her lifetime (Table 8.3). In women who develop cancer after a diagnosis of LCIS, more than 50% of the cancers will be of ductal origin. Classically, LCIS

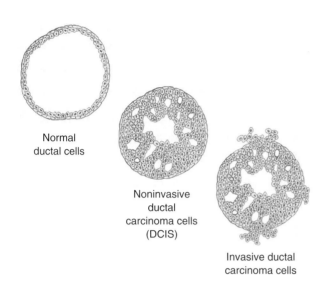

Normal
ductal cells

Noninvasive
ductal
carcinoma cells
(DCIS)

Invasive ductal
carcinoma cells

FIGURE 8.1

Pictorial illustration of normal breast duct, a duct filled with duct carcinoma in situ (*Note*: all cells are confined within the basement membrane of the duct), and invasive ductal carcinoma. Note that the cells have penetrated the basement membrane of the duct and are infiltrating into the surrounding stroma.

TABLE 8.3
Cancer Risk and Borderline Lesions

HISTOLOGY	RELATIVE RISK	ABSOLUTE RISK
Normal	1.0	10%
Hyperplasia, no atypia	~1.0	10%
ADH or ALH	~5.0	10%–20%
LCIS	~10.0	25%–30%

Abbreviations: ADH, atypical ductal hyperplasia; ALH, atypical lobular hyperplasia; LCIS, lobular carcinoma in situ.

Note: Relative risk is a *ratio of incidences* or (CA incidence with factor x)/(CA incidence without factor x). Absolute risk is a percentage or the proportion of a defined population who develop cancer.

lacks mammographic findings. Therefore, the finding of LCIS at biopsy is often incidental and, although controversial, a CNB diagnosis of LCIS should generally be surgically excised to rule out an associated malignant lesion. If LCIS is the only finding at excision, however, negative margins are not required because LCIS is a marker of risk and not a cancer.

Atypical ductal hyperplasia (ADH) and atypical lobular hyperplasia (ALH) represent borderline proliferative processes that histologically lie somewhere between the usual type of hyperplasia without atypia

and carcinoma in situ. In all likelihood, atypical hyperplasias are part of a spectrum of lesions that may have the potential to progress to carcinoma in situ. The challenge of distinguishing a severely atypical hyperplasia from an early DCIS is well known to pathologists. The risk that a woman with an atypical hyperplasia will develop breast cancer is about four to five times the average woman's risk (Table 8.3). However, if the woman has both atypical hyperplasia and a significant family history of breast cancer, her risk may be nine times higher than that of the average woman. If ADH or ALH is found at CNB, a surgical excision of that area is recommended to rule out an associated malignant lesion. The incidence of breast cancer at excisional biopsy is inversely related to the size of the core needle used for biopsy. For example, when ADH is diagnosed by 14-gauge CNB, cancer is found in the surgical specimen in 50% of patients; however, when ADH is diagnosed by 11-gauge CNB, cancer is found in the surgical specimen in 20% of patients (10). Furthermore, if ADH is diagnosed by a vacuum-assisted CNB, cancer is found in the surgical specimen in 10%–15% of patients. Of all patients who are upstaged from ADH to cancer after surgical excision, 75% will have DCIS and the remaining 25% will have invasive disease.

DCIS is the earliest form of breast cancer and accounted for 61,980 cases of breast cancer in 2006 (2). Over the last 20 years, there has been a dramatic rise in the incidence of DCIS, primarily due to the implementation of routine mammographic screening and the increasing capability of imaging to detect small lesions.

DCIS begins in the terminal ducts and is confined within them. As DCIS cells multiply, they are pushed centrally within the duct and away from their blood supply, causing cell death and calcification. These pleomorphic calcifications may be the first mammographic signs of DCIS. It is believed that most cases of DCIS will progress to invasive ductal cancer if they are left untreated.

Four subtypes of DCIS exist and are categorized according to their architectural structure: solid, micropapillary, cribriform, and comedo. In many published series, the comedo form predominates over the other three noncomedo forms. Comedo necrosis is characterized by its high nuclear grade, increased mitotic activity, and central necrosis.

Regardless of pathologic subtype, all forms of DCIS require surgical excision with negative margins for optimal treatment. While lumpectomy, with or without radiation therapy or mastectomy, may be appropriate, the ultimate treatment will depend on the amount of DCIS present, the patient's age and breast size, the ability to achieve negative margins, and the type of DCIS found. Lymph nodes are not routinely evaluated unless the DCIS presents as a mass (with a higher likelihood of microinvasion), or if a mastectomy is planned. In the TNM staging system, DCIS is categorized as a stage 0 breast cancer.

Invasive mammary cancer accounts for approximately 80% of all breast cancers. Invasive cancer is broadly divided into two categories based on their growth patterns: ductal or lobular. Ductal cancers tend to grow as a coherent mass and appear clinically as a palpable mass or mammographically as a mass, architectural distortion, or group of calcifications. Lobular cancers tend to permeate the breast in a single file, referred to as "Indian file" nature, making them harder to detect both clinically and mammographically. Invasive ductal cancer (IDC) is the most common type of breast cancer, accounting for 50%–70% of cases, followed by invasive lobular cancer (ILC) which represents 10%–15% of all invasive cancers. Less common variants of invasive ductal cancer include tubular, mucinous, papillary, medullary, and metaplastic carcinoma. While the first three are generally considered less aggressive due to their typically good prognostic features, like low nuclear grade and low mitotic index, medullary and metaplastic cancers tend to have poor prognostic features and are, therefore, considered more aggressive. Other, rarer tumors of the breast include squamous carcinoma, both benign and malignant phyllodes tumors, primary breast sarcoma or lymphoma, and metastases to the breast (most commonly from the contralateral breast, leukemia, lymphoma, lung, thyroid, cervix, ovary, and kidney).

The prognosis of invasive breast cancer is determined by the size of the tumor, histologic and nuclear grade, the presence of lymphovascular invasion, the number of nodal metastases, the hormone receptor status (ER or PR), and *HER2/neu* stains.

Inflammatory breast cancer (IBC) carries a poor prognosis and accounts for roughly 1%–6% of all invasive breast cancers. The incidence of IBC is highest among African Americans (10.1%), followed by Caucasians (6.2%), and then by other ethnic groups (5.1%) (11). IBC is a clinical diagnosis that implies the simultaneous development of inflammatory changes in the skin of the breast and the development of an aggressive tumor within the breast. The classic diagnosis as defined by Haagensen in 1971 includes diffuse erythema and edema of the skin, peau d'orange, tenderness, warmth, induration, and diffuse tumor within the breast (12). If IBC is suspected, a skin biopsy may confirm dermal lymphatic invasion by tumor emboli. However, a negative biopsy does not rule out the diagnosis of IBC. Patients with IBC generally present with a history of worsening erythema and skin changes, despite being treated with antibiotics for mastitis or cellulitis of the breast. IBC is regarded as stage IIIC

breast cancer. Optimal therapy includes neoadjuvant chemotherapy, followed by a modified radical mastectomy incorporating all involved skin, and postmastectomy chest-wall radiation. Overall five-year survival for IBC is approximately 40%.

Male breast cancer (MBC) accounts for less than 1% of all breast cancers and less than 0.5% of all cancers occurring in men. Male breasts lack lobules; therefore, nearly all male breast cancers are of ductal origin, and more than 80% are invasive. Most MBCs present as a palpable, retroareolar mass and are best treated with a mastectomy. Since routine screening is not performed for MBC, most MBCs present at a later stage than female breast cancer. However, MBC carries the same prognosis, stage for stage, as female breast cancer.

BREAST SURGERY

Historically, the first major advance in breast cancer surgery was described by William Halsted in 1894. Halsted theorized that breast cancer was a local-regional disease that spread in an orderly, centripetal fashion. In his manuscripts, he popularized the removal of the breast, pectoralis muscles, and axillary lymph nodes in levels 1, 2, and 3. This procedure was known as the radical mastectomy (RM) or Halsted mastectomy, and revolutionized the way 19th century surgeons approached breast cancer surgery. Following RM, Halsted documented a local recurrence rate of 6% at three years, which was significantly lower than the 70% shown by his 19th century colleagues (13); however, the operation was severely disfiguring. In 1948, Patey and Dyson proposed leaving the pectoralis muscles and named the removal of only the breast and axillary contents the "modified radical mastectomy" (MRM). With more than 25 years of follow-up, it is well accepted that there is no survival difference between RM and MRM (14).

In the 1970s, Bernard Fisher proposed an alternate theory, hypothesizing that breast cancer was, in fact, a systemic disease and that variations in local-regional therapy were unlikely to affect overall survival. He popularized breast conservation surgery (BCT), which was ultimately studied in a prospective, randomized fashion in thousands of women by The National Surgical Adjuvant Breast and Bowel Project (NSABP), NCI, and the Milan trialists groups. These groups compared MRM, lumpectomy alone, and lumpectomy plus radiation in a variety of study designs. Although local recurrences were higher in those patients having lumpectomy without radiation (approximately 4% per year vs 1% per year), there was no difference in overall or distant disease-free survival at 20 years follow-up between the groups (15).

Today, the treatment options for patients with early stage (T1 or T2) breast cancer are TM or breast-conservation surgery with adjuvant radiation therapy. Both options include an evaluation of the axillary lymph nodes. Approximately 80% of patients are eligible for BCT. Relative and absolute contraindications to BCT are listed in Table 8.4. BCT involves excision of the tumor and a small portion of surrounding normal breast parenchyma. Incisions are made along the lines of skin tension, and in general incision placement should be planned to facilitate subsequent excision if mastectomy is required. Unless the cancer is palpable, needle localization using mammographic (stereotactic), ultrasound (US), or MRI guidance is required to assist in surgical excision. Frequently, a specimen radiograph is performed to document retrieval of the cancer and the biopsy site marker. Surgical clips may be left to denote the extent of the excisional cavity to aid in radiation treatment planning. Successful BCT mandates achieving negative surgical margins, although the definition of a negative surgical margin continues to be a matter of debate. In all NSABP conservation trials, no tumor at the inked margin was considered negative. However, other studies report negative margins ranging from 1–3 mm. Regardless of definition, patients who are properly selected for BCT and have their cancer entirely removed have acceptable local recurrence rates, generally less than 10% at five years, when compared with patients who have undergone a mastectomy for similar sized early-stage breast cancer.

TM involves removal of the skin, nipple and areolar complex, and breast tissue, including the pectoralis major fascia. Many patients with early-stage breast cancer who have a TM (either by choice or out of necessity) are candidates for immediate breast reconstruction. When immediate reconstruction is chosen, a smaller ellipse or oval of skin is removed, incorporating the nipple and areolar complex. This procedure is called a skin-sparing mastectomy. By taking less skin, the breast retains its natural skin envelope and inframammary fold, which ultimately helps re-create a more natural and cosmetically acceptable reconstructed breast. Breast reconstruction can be performed with implant-based techniques or with tissue-transfer techniques, depending on the patient's body habitus and desired reconstructive outcomes.

All patients with an invasive cancer should undergo a pathologic evaluation of the axillary lymph nodes to allow for appropriate staging and treatment. Until the late 1990s, the standard of care was for each patient to undergo an axillary lymph node dissection (ALND) in addition to BCT or mastectomy. In 1997, Giuliano introduced the concept of the axillary sentinel lymph node (SLN) biopsy for patients with breast cancer and provided histopathologic validation of this hypothesis (16). This theory is based on the idea that the lymphatic drainage within the breast is uniform and constant, and that the breast drains in an orderly fashion to a "sentinel" node within the axilla. The SLN biopsy procedure entails the use of an intradermal injection of a radiolabeled isotope (technecium sulfur colloid) and a vital blue dye. Isotope can be injected intradermally or intraparenchymally with equal chances of success. Blue dye is injected intraparenchymally or into the sub-areolar plexus (Fig. 8.2). Any node that is found to be "hot" with the use of a gamma probe, or visualized as "blue," is considered a sentinel lymph node (17). In the Memorial Sloan-Kettering Cancer Center experience, the median number of SLNs removed per axilla is three. Intraoperative evaluation of the SLN, either by frozen section or by touch prep analysis, allows for immediate ALND in cases with identifiable metastatic

TABLE 8.4	
Absolute and Relative Contraindications to BCT	
ABSOLUTE	RELATIVE
Multicentric cancer	Poor cosmetic outcome
Inflammatory breast cancer	Tumor > 5 cm
Inability to receive radiation therapy[a]	

[a]May include history of previous irradiation to the breast, history of collagen vascular disease, or limited access to care.

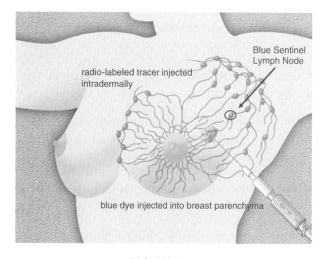

radio-labeled tracer injected intradermally

Blue Sentinel Lymph Node

blue dye injected into breast parenchyma

FIGURE 8.2

Pictorial illustration of the sentinel lymph node (SLN) mapping technique. Radiolabeled isotope is injected intradermally, and blue dye is injected intraparenchymally. The SLN is then identified in the axillary nodal basin as a hot and/or blue lymph node.

disease. If tumor is found, an immediate ALND can be performed. Subsequent routine pathologic analysis, with or without enhanced evaluation, including immunohistochemistry, is performed on all SLNs. If nodal metastases are identified, the standard of care at this time is delayed ALND.

The accuracy of SLN biopsy has been validated in multiple centers and with a variety of techniques—isotope or blue dye alone, intradermal or intraparenchymal injection, and injection of tracers over the tumor or into the subareolar plexus. Despite differing techniques, the accuracy of SLN biopsy has been demonstrated to be 97% and has been validated with "backup" ALND in 69 studies involving more than 8,000 women. Equally as important, the false-negative rate of SLN biopsy across these series has remained acceptable at 7% (18). The risk of axillary recurrence after negative SLN biopsy appears to be small and is reported at levels less than 1%; however, follow-up is limited at only two years (19). Longer follow-up is needed to compare the risk of local recurrence after SLN biopsy with the known risk of axillary recurrence after a full ALND, which is approximately 0%–2%, with follow-up ranging from 72 to 180 months (2,20,21).

Although SLN biopsy is considered less invasive than ALND, lymphedema may still occur in roughly 3%–7% of patients undergoing an SLN biopsy as compared with 15%–20% of patients undergoing ALND. There is also a small risk of isosulfan blue dye allergy, presenting most commonly as hives, in 1% of patients, but this has been reported to include anaphylaxis in less than 0.5% of patients. Additional morbidities of SLN biopsy include paresthesias in up to 7% of patients and decreased range of motion of the shoulder or arm in 3%–5% of patients. Longer follow-up of patients having SLN biopsy is ongoing, but the practice of SLN biopsy is considered the standard of care for staging the axilla in women with invasive breast cancer.

In patients with pure DCIS, an SLN biopsy is generally not indicated, as pure DCIS does not have metastatic potential. However, in less than 10% of cases, DCIS can present as a mass. In patients with DCIS presenting as a mass and diagnosed by CNB, SLN biopsy may be performed at the time of lumpectomy, as these cases have a much higher likelihood of harboring microinvasive disease, which carries the risk of nodal metastases in 5% of cases (22). Alternatively, patients can undergo excision of the DCIS alone for definitive diagnosis and return to the operating room (OR) for SLN biopsy should invasive disease be identified. In patients with DCIS who choose mastectomy or who have contraindications to BCT and must have a mastectomy, SLN biopsy should be strongly considered at the time of mastectomy because SLN mapping can-

not be performed after mastectomy. If a patient were diagnosed with a focus of invasive breast cancer, a traditional ALND would be the only option for axillary staging.

RADIATION THERAPY

Currently, radiation to the entire breast, known as whole-breast irradiation, is the standard of care following BCT. Radiation therapy is generally given after chemotherapy if this is also indicated. Radiation treatments can be administered to the breast with the patient lying supine or prone, depending on the original tumor location and the patient's body habitus. A total of 5000 Gy are given over six weeks. The first 25 treatments incorporate the entire breast, while the last 5 may or may not be given as a "boost" just to the tumor bed. At this time, a multicenter randomized trial (NSABP-39) is ongoing to determine the effectiveness of partial-breast radiation techniques compared with whole-breast irradiation.

Some patients require postmastectomy radiation treatments to the chest wall, with or without radiation to the regional lymph nodes. This is generally recommended in patients with locally advanced breast cancers, tumors larger than 5 cm, inflammatory breast cancer, and in patients with four or more positive lymph nodes. Radiation treatment to the axilla is rarely added, but may be used after complete axillary dissection in patients with more than 10 positive nodes. The combination of both ALND and radiation treatment to the axilla can greatly increase the risk of lymphedema, with reported rates of more than 50%.

References

1. Wellings SR, Jensen HM, Marcum RG. An atlas of subgross pathology of the human breast with special reference to possible precancerous lesions. *J Natl Cancer Inst.* 1975;55(2):231–273.
2. Louis-Sylvestre C, Clough K, Asselain B, et al. Axillary treatment in conservative management of operable breast cancer: dissection or radiotherapy? Results of a randomized study with 15 years of follow-up. *J Clin Oncol.* 2004;22(1):97–101.
3. Gail MH, Brinton LA, Byar DP, et al. Projecting individualized probabilities of developing breast cancer for white females who are being examined annually. *J Natl Cancer Inst.* 1989;81(24):1879–1886.
4. Poplack SP, Tosteson AN, Grove MR, Wells WA, Carney PA. Mammography in 53,803 women from the New Hampshire mammography network. *Radiology.* 2000;217(3):832–840.
5. Banks E, Reeves G, Beral V, et al. Influence of personal characteristics of individual women on sensitivity and specificity of mammography in the Million Women Study: cohort study. *BMJ.* 2004;329(7464):477.
6. Smith-Bindman R, Chu P, Miglioretti DL, et al. Physician predictors of mammographic accuracy. *J Natl Cancer Inst.* 2005;97(5):358–367.

7. Kuhl CK, Schrading S, Leutner CC, et al. Mammography, breast ultrasound, and magnetic resonance imaging for surveillance of women at high familial risk for breast cancer. *J Clin Oncol.* 2005;23(33):8469–8476.

8. Saslow D, Boetes C, Burke W, et al. American cancer society guidelines for breast screening with MRI as an adjunct to mammography. *CA Cancer J Clin.* 2007;57(2):75–89.

9. Morris EA, Schwartz LH, Dershaw DD, van Zee KJ, Abramson AF, Liberman L. MR imaging of the breast in patients with occult primary breast carcinoma. *Radiology.* 1997;205(2):437–440.

10. Liberman L, Cohen MA, Dershaw DD, Abramson AF, Hann LE, Rosen PP. Atypical ductal hyperplasia diagnosed at stereotaxic core biopsy of breast lesions: an indication for surgical biopsy. *AJR Am J Roentgenol.* 1995;164(5):1111–1113.

11. Levine PH, Steinhorn SC, Ries LG, Aron JL. Inflammatory breast cancer: the experience of the surveillance, epidemiology, and end results (SEER) program. *J Natl Cancer Inst.* 1985;74(2):291–297.

12. Haagensen C. *Diseases of the Breast,* 2nd ed. Philadelphia: Saunders; 1971.

13. Halstead W. The results of radical operations for the cure of carcinoma of the breast. *Ann Surg.* 1907(46):1–19.

14. Fisher B, Jeong JH, Anderson S, Bryant J, Fisher ER, Wolmark N. Twenty-five-year follow-up of a randomized trial comparing radical mastectomy, total mastectomy, and total mastectomy followed by irradiation. *N Engl J Med.* 2002;347(8):567–575.

15. Fisher B, Anderson S, Bryant J, et al. Twenty-year follow-up of a randomized trial comparing total mastectomy, lumpectomy, and lumpectomy plus irradiation for the treatment of invasive breast cancer. *N Engl J Med.* 2002;347(16):1233–1241.

16. Turner RR, Ollila DW, Krasne DL, Giuliano AE. Histopathologic validation of the sentinel lymph node hypothesis for breast carcinoma. *Ann Surg.* 1997;226(3):271–276; discussion 6–8.

17. Cody HS, 3rd, Borgen PI. State-of-the-art approaches to sentinel node biopsy for breast cancer: study design, patient selection, technique, and quality control at Memorial Sloan-Kettering Cancer Center. *Surg Oncol.* 1999;8(2):85–91.

18. Kim T, Giuliano AE, Lyman GH. Lymphatic mapping and sentinel lymph node biopsy in early-stage breast carcinoma: a metaanalysis. *Cancer.* 2006;106(1):4–16.

19. Naik AM, Fey J, Gemignani M, et al. The risk of axillary relapse after sentinel lymph node biopsy for breast cancer is comparable with that of axillary lymph node dissection: a follow-up study of 4008 procedures. *Ann Surg.* 2004;240(3):462–468; discussion 8–71.

20. Recht A, Pierce SM, Abner A, et al. Regional nodal failure after conservative surgery and radiotherapy for early-stage breast carcinoma. *J Clin Oncol.* 1991;9(6):988–996.

21. Veronesi U, Salvadori B, Luini A, et al. Conservative treatment of early breast cancer. Long-term results of 1232 cases treated with quadrantectomy, axillary dissection, and radiotherapy. *Ann Surg.* 1990;211(3):250–259.

22. Klauber-DeMore N, Tan LK, Liberman L, et al. Sentinel lymph node biopsy: is it indicated in patients with high-risk ductal carcinoma-in-situ and ductal carcinoma-in-situ with microinvasion? *Ann Surg Oncol.* 2000;7(9):636–642.

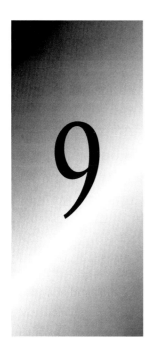

Principles of Breast Reconstruction in Cancer

Joseph J. Disa
Colleen M. McCarthy

Women who elect to undergo mastectomy for the treatment or prophylaxis of breast cancer may consider breast reconstruction in an attempt to improve their outward appearance, their sense of femininity, and ultimately, their self-esteem. For these women, the preservation of a normal breast form through breast reconstruction has been shown to have a positive effect on their psychological well-being.

RECONSTRUCTIVE OPTIONS

Contemporary techniques provide numerous options for postmastectomy reconstruction. These options include single-stage reconstruction with a standard or adjustable implant, tissue expansion followed by placement of a permanent implant, combined autologous tissue/implant reconstruction, or autogenous tissue reconstruction alone.

Procedure selection is based on a range of patient variables, including availability of local, regional, and distant donor tissues; size and shape of the desired breast(s); surgical risk; and most importantly, patient preference. Although autogenous tissue reconstruction is generally thought to produce the most natural-looking and feeling breast(s), the relative magnitude of these procedures is great. Many women will instead opt for a prosthetic reconstruction, choosing a less invasive operative procedure with a faster recovery time. Individualized selection of a reconstructive technique for each patient will be a predominant factor in achieving a reconstructive success.

TIMING OF RECONSTRUCTION

Immediate postmastectomy reconstruction is currently considered the standard of care in breast reconstruction. Numerous studies have demonstrated that reconstruction performed concurrently with mastectomy is an oncologically safe option for women with breast cancer (1). Immediate reconstruction is assumed to be advantageous when compared with delayed procedures based on improved cost-effectiveness and reduced inconvenience for the patient. Moreover, studies have shown that women who undergo immediate reconstruction have less psychological distress about the loss of a breast and have a better overall quality of life (2).

Technically, reconstruction is facilitated in the immediate setting because of the pliability of the native skin envelope and the delineation of the natural inframammary fold. The increasing use of postoperative radiotherapy for earlier staged breast cancers has, however, challenged this thinking. Adjuvant radiotherapy

KEY POINTS

- Women who elect to undergo mastectomy for the treatment or prophylaxis of breast cancer may consider breast reconstruction in an attempt to improve their outward appearance, their sense of femininity, and ultimately, their self-esteem.
- Breast reconstruction options include single-stage reconstruction with a standard or adjustable implant, tissue expansion followed by placement of a permanent implant, combined autologous tissue/implant reconstruction, or autogenous tissue reconstruction alone.
- Reconstruction performed concurrently with mastectomy is an oncologically safe option for women with breast cancer.
- Women who undergo immediate reconstruction have less psychological distress about the loss of a breast and have a better overall quality of life.
- Prosthetic reconstruction techniques include single-stage implant reconstruction with either a standard or adjustable permanent prosthesis, two-stage tissue expander/implant reconstruction, and combined implant/autogenous tissue reconstruction.

- To date, there is no definitive evidence linking breast implants to cancer, immunologic diseases, neurologic problems, or other systemic diseases.
- Reconstructive techniques using the lower abdominal donor site include the pedicled transverse rectus abdominis myocutaneous (TRAM) flap, the free TRAM flap, the free muscle-sparing TRAM, the deep inferior epigastric perforator (DIEP) flap, and the superficial inferior epigastric artery (SIEA) flap.
- There is some data to suggest that muscle- and fascia-sparing techniques, such as the use of DIEP flaps, result in measurably better postoperative truncal strength. Interestingly, however, muscle-sparing techniques do not appear to decrease the risk of abdominal bulging or hernia formation.
- Because surgical scars fade and tissue firmness subsides with time, the results of autologous breast reconstruction tend to improve as the patient ages rather than deteriorate, as with prosthetic reconstruction.

has been shown to increase the risk of postoperative complications (3,4). Based on the data, whether or not to perform immediate reconstruction for patients in whom radiation therapy is planned remains controversial. Similarly, for those who may be unwilling to decide about reconstruction while adjusting to their cancer diagnosis, delayed breast reconstruction may be an option.

IMPLANT-BASED RECONSTRUCTION

Techniques

Prosthetic reconstruction techniques include single-stage implant reconstruction with either a standard or an adjustable permanent prosthesis, two-stage tissue expander/implant reconstruction, and combined autogenous tissue/implant reconstruction.

Single-Stage Implant Reconstruction

Immediate single-stage breast reconstruction with a standard implant is best suited to the occasional patient with adequate skin at the mastectomy site and small, nonptotic breasts. Selection criteria for single-stage,

adjustable implant reconstruction is similar; yet, it is the preferred technique when the ability to adjust the volume of the device postoperatively is desired. In small-breasted women where the skin deficiency is minimal, the implant can be partially filled at the time of reconstruction and gradually inflated to the desired volume postoperatively.

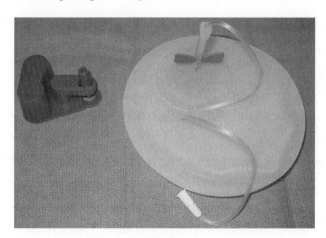

FIGURE 9.1

Textured surface, integrated valve, biodimensional-shaped tissue expander with a Magnasite fill port-locating device.

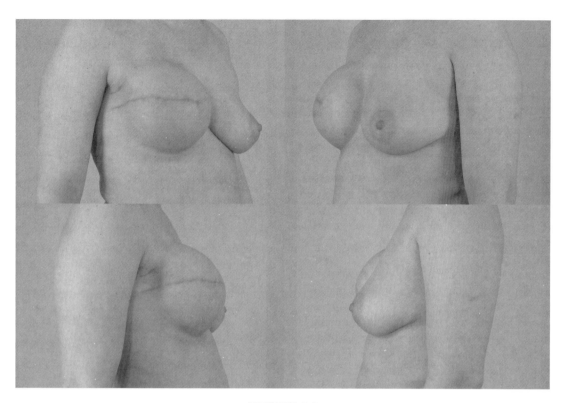

FIGURE 9.2

Unilateral right breast reconstruction with tissue expander. The expander is intentionally overfilled to maximize projection and inferior-pole skin.

Two-Stage Tissue Expander/Implant Reconstruction

While satisfactory results can be obtained with single-stage reconstruction, in the vast majority of patients, a far more reliable approach involves two-stage expander/implant reconstruction. Tissue expansion is used when there is insufficient tissue after mastectomy to create the desired size and shape of a breast in a single stage.

A tissue expander is placed under the skin and muscles of the chest wall at the primary procedure (Fig. 9.1). Postoperatively, tissue expansion is performed over a period of weeks or months, the soft tissues stretched until the desired breast volume is achieved (Fig. 9.2). Exchange of the temporary expander for a permanent implant occurs at a subsequent operation. A capsulotomy is often performed at this second stage. By releasing the surrounding scar capsule, breast projection and breast ptosis are increased. Similarly, precise positioning of the inframammary fold can be addressed (Fig. 9.3).

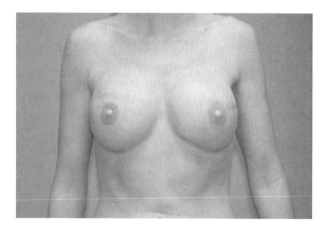

FIGURE 9.3

Bilateral breast reconstruction with silicone gel implants after nipple areola reconstruction.

Combined Autogenous Tissue/ Implant Reconstruction

Nearly every patient who undergoes a mastectomy is a candidate for some form of implant-based reconstruction. Implant reconstruction alone is contraindicated, however, in the presence of an inadequate skin envelope. A large skin excision at the time of mastectomy, due to previous biopsies or locally advanced disease, may preclude primary coverage of a prosthetic device. Similarly, previous chest wall irradiation and/or postmastectomy radiotherapy are considered by many a relative contraindication for implant-based breast reconstruction (5,6).

In patients with thin, contracted, or previously irradiated skin, the ipsilateral latissimus dorsi myocutaneous flap can provide additional skin, soft tissue, and muscle, obviating the need for or facilitating the process of tissue expansion. The skin island is designed under the bra line or along the lateral margin of the muscle, and the flap is tunneled anteriorly into the mastectomy defect. Although the latissimus dorsi myocutaneous flap is extremely reliable, the tissue bulk is usually inadequate. Thus, a permanent implant is often placed beneath the flap to provide adequate volume.

The latissimus dorsi flap is advantageous in that it can provide additional vascularized skin and muscle to the breast mound in a single operative procedure. Its disadvantages include the creation of new chest scars, a back donor scar, and the fact that the transfer of autogenous tissue does not, in this setting, eliminate the need for an implant.

Implant Selection

Currently, both saline and silicone gel implants are available for use in breast reconstruction. While the stigma surrounding the use of silicone-filled implants still exists, issues of silicone safety have been carefully investigated (7). To date, there is no definitive evidence linking breast implants to cancer, immunologic diseases, neurologic problems, or other systemic diseases. The use of silicone gel implants generally allows for a softer, more natural-appearing breast. Alternatively, the use of saline-filled implants allows for minor volume adjustments to be made at the time of implant placement. And while saline-filled implants may offer the greatest piece of mind for some patients in terms of safety, implant palpability and rippling is more likely.

Complications

Prosthetic breast reconstruction is a relatively simple technique that is generally well tolerated. Complications are generally centered on the breast, with minimal systemic health implications and minimal overall patient morbidity. Thus, implant reconstruction can often be performed on patients who might not be suitable candidates for the more complex surgical procedure required for breast reconstruction with autogenous tissue.

Perioperative complications, including hematoma, seroma, infection, skin flap necrosis, and implant exposure/extrusion, can occur. Late complications include implant deflation or rupture and capsular contracture. Capsular contracture occurs when the scar tissue or capsule that normally forms around the implant tightens and squeezes the implant. While capsular contracture occurs to some extent around all implants, in some, the degree of contracture will increase in severity over time (8). A pathologic capsular contracture or implant malfunction may require revisional surgery years following completion of reconstruction.

Advantages and Disadvantages

Implant reconstruction has the distinct advantage of combining a lesser operative procedure with the capability of achieving excellent results. The use of tissue expansion provides donor tissue with similar qualities of skin texture, color, and sensation compared to the contralateral breast. Donor-site morbidity is eliminated with use of a prosthetic device; by using the patient's mastectomy incision to place the prosthesis, no new scars are introduced.

Although implant techniques are technically easier than autologous reconstruction, with shorter hospitalization and a quicker recovery, they can provide additional reconstructive challenges. Patients who undergo tissue expander/implant breast reconstruction will experience varying degrees of discomfort and chest wall asymmetry during the expansion phase. In addition, patients must make more frequent office visits for percutaneous expansion. The breast mound achieved with implant reconstruction is generally more rounded, less ptotic, and will often require a contralateral matching procedure in order to achieve symmetry.

AUTOGENOUS TISSUE RECONSTRUCTION

Techniques

Numerous options exist for autogenous tissue reconstruction. Reconstructive techniques using the lower abdominal donor site include the pedicled transverse rectus abdominis myocutaneous (TRAM) flap, the free TRAM flap, the free muscle-sparing TRAM, the deep inferior epigastric perforator (DIEP) flap, and the superficial inferior epigastric artery (SIEA) flap. The TRAM or related flap is the most frequently used method for autogenous breast reconstruction. TRAM and TRAM-related flaps are designed so that the skin islands are oriented transversely across the lower abdomen and the resulting "abdominoplastylike scar" is camouflaged. Other autogenous tissue alternatives include the latissimus dorsi flap, gluteal flaps, the Rubens fat pad flap, and perforator flaps from the gluteal and lateral thigh donor sites.

Pedicled TRAM Flap Reconstruction

The blood supply of the pedicled TRAM flap is derived from the superior epigastric artery. The rectus muscle serves as the vascular carrier for a large ellipse of lower abdominal skin and fat. After harvest of the flap, a subcutaneous tunnel from the abdominal donor site to the mastectomy defect is created in order to accommodate the flap. The abdominal donor site is closed by reapproximating the anterior rectus sheath and by advancing the remaining superior skin edge of the donor site as a modified abdominoplasty. The ipsilateral, the contralateral, or bilateral rectus muscles may be used. The muscle-sparing TRAM flap, which is limited to the portion of muscle that encompasses the lateral and medial rows of perforating vessels, is a modification of the TRAM flap, which theoretically minimizes violation of the abdominal wall and the risk of donor-site morbidity. The muscle-sparing TRAM can be performed either as a pedicled flap or free tissue transfer.

Free TRAM Flap Reconstruction

The microvascular, or free, TRAM flap is based upon the more dominant inferior epigastric vascular pedicle, which permits transfer of larger volumes of tissue with

a minimal risk of fat necrosis. Similarly, because the blood supply to a free TRAM is more robust, the procedure can be used with a greater degree of safety in patients with risk factors such as tobacco use, diabetes, and obesity. Microvascular anastomoses are generally performed to the thoracodorsal or internal mammary vessels. Insetting of the free tissue transfer is facilitated because the flap is not tethered by a pedicle. In addition, the potential abdominal contour deformity arising from the bulk of the transposed pedicled flap is eliminated (Figs. 9.4 and 9.5).

DIEP Flap Reconstruction

The DIEP flap is a further refinement of the conventional muscle-sparing free TRAM flap. The overlying skin and subcutaneous tissues are perfused by transmuscular perforators originating from the deep inferior epigastric artery. When a perforating vessel is found, it is dissected away from the surrounding muscle and traced to its origin from the vascular pedicle. Because no muscle is harvested, donor-site morbidity is theoretically minimized (9,10). Harvest of the DIEP flap can be a tedious dissection, however, which can prolong surgical time. In addition, flap vascularity may be less than that of free TRAM flap because of the small size and number of the perforating vessels in some patients. A higher risk of venous insufficiency, partial flap loss, and fat necrosis compared with free TRAM flaps has been reported (11) (Fig. 9.6).

SIEA Flap Reconstruction

The SIEA flap can be used in breast reconstruction, with an aesthetic outcome similar to that of TRAM and DIEP flaps. The SIEA flap allows for transfer of a moderate volume of lower abdominal tissue based on

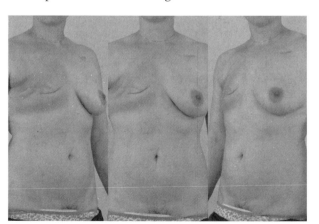 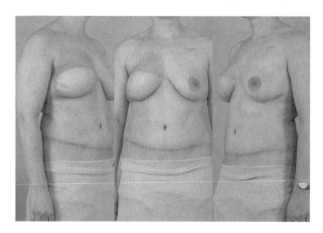

FIGURE 9.4

A: Right modified radical mastectomy and postoperative irradiation. Note radiation-induced skin changes on right chest wall. B: Delayed right breast reconstruction with a free TRAM flap. Photo taken prior to planned nipple areolar reconstruction.

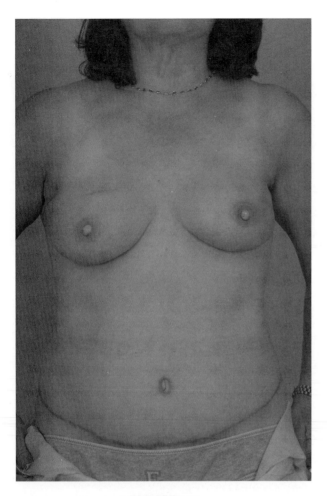

FIGURE 9.5

Bilateral free TRAM flap reconstruction was performed immediately following bilateral skin-sparing mastectomies. Bilateral nipple areolae reconstruction has been completed.

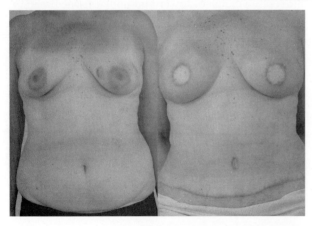

FIGURE 9.6

Bilateral free DIEP flap reconstruction following bilateral skin-sparing mastectomies, preoperative (left) and postoperative (right).

the superficial inferior epigastric artery. Based solely on the superficial system, the flap can be elevated off the anterior rectus sheath without excision or incision of the rectus abdominis muscle. Abdominal donor-site morbidity is theoretically eliminated. Because of the absence or inadequacy of the superficial epigastric vessels in up to 70% of patients, however, the use of the flap is limited (12).

Further Options in Autologous Tissue Reconstruction

A patient desiring a TRAM or related flap must have adequate tissues in the lower abdomen to be considered a candidate. Additionally, a patient's lifestyle must allow for the potential diminution of truncal strength. One of the primary reasons for use of an alternate flap includes inadequate abdominal fat in a patient with a slender body habitus. In addition, high-risk abdominal scars may predispose to flap necrosis and/or wound healing problems at the abdominal donor site. In a situation where a patient is an inappropriate TRAM flap candidate, yet still desires an autogenous reconstruction, alternate flap options include the Rubens fat pad flap, gluteal myocutaneous flaps, and perforator flaps from the gluteal and lateral thigh donor sites. These free flaps are much less commonly employed and have distinct disadvantages when compared with flaps from the abdominal donor site.

Complications

Autogenous reconstruction is more complex than implant-based reconstruction and requires a much lengthier, more invasive surgical procedure. Postmastectomy reconstruction with a TRAM or related flap generally requires a five-to-seven-day hospitalization and a four-to-six-week convalesce. Because of the magnitude of the procedure, complications do occur. Fortunately, major complications are uncommon.

Use of the free TRAM flap decreases the rate of complications compared to pedicled TRAM flaps. The incidence of both fat necrosis and partial flap loss is close to 5% in most series, as compared to 15%–20% in pedicled flaps (13,14). The rate of total flap loss is 1%–2% in most series and is comparable to those published for the pedicled TRAM flap (15). Smoking, chest wall irradiation, significant abdominal scarring, and obesity are associated with an increased complication rate (11).

There is some data to suggest that muscle- and fascia-sparing techniques, such as the use of DIEP flaps, result in measurably better postoperative truncal strength (9,10). Postoperative abdominal hernia, or more commonly, abdominal wall laxity remains a persistent issue for some patients choosing TRAM reconstruction. Interestingly, muscle-sparing techniques do not appear to decrease the risk of abdominal bulging or hernia formation (16).

Alterations in shape and size of the reconstructed breast are sometimes required, and donor site adjustments do exist. Common secondary adjustments include liposuction of the flap for improved contour, abdominal scar revision and hernia repair, and fat necrosis excision.

Advantages and Disadvantages

Breast reconstruction with autologous tissue can generally achieve more durable, natural-appearing results than reconstruction based on prosthetic implants alone. The breast mound reconstructed with autologous tissue is closer in consistency to the native breast. Because surgical scars fade and tissue firmness subsides with time, the results of autologous breast reconstruction tend to improve as the patient ages rather than deteriorate, as with prosthetic reconstruction. Complete restoration of the breast mound in a single stage is possible in most patients.

Permanent dependency on prosthesis can also lead to long-term complications, such as implant leak or deflation, often occurring many years after an otherwise successful reconstruction. Autogenous tissue reconstructions, therefore, may be especially appropriate for younger patients, who might be expected to live longer and be particularly susceptible to the longer-term problems of prosthetic reconstructions.

ADJUVANT THERAPY AND BREAST RECONSTRUCTION

Earlier breast cancers are being increasingly treated with adjuvant chemotherapy and radiotherapy in an attempt to increase survival. Chemotherapy does not increase the risk of postoperative complications. Previous reports have also demonstrated that patients who undergo immediate breast reconstruction are not predisposed to delays in administration of adjuvant chemotherapy compared with patients undergo mastectomy alone (17–19). The possible implications of adjuvant radiotherapy on the timing of breast reconstruction are, however, both profound and controversial.

Not only is tissue expansion difficult in the previously irradiated tissues, but the risks of infection, expander exposure, and subsequent extrusion are increased. Recent reports have demonstrated that patients who received postoperative radiotherapy had a significantly higher incidence of capsular contracture than controls. For these reasons, it is generally agreed

that autologous breast reconstruction is preferable in patients who have a history of previous chest wall irradiation and/or will require adjuvant postmastectomy radiotherapy.

Unfortunately, even though autologous tissue alone is preferred in this setting, autologous reconstructions may also be adversely affected by postmastectomy radiation. Contracture of the breast skin, development of palpable fat necrosis, and atrophy of the flap resulting in distortion of the reconstructed breast are described (20).

The increasing use of postmastectomy radiation and chemotherapy in patients with early-stage breast cancer necessitates increased communication between the medical oncologist, radiation oncologist, breast surgeon, and plastic surgeon during treatment planning. Paramount to a successful outcome is a frank discussion between the plastic surgeon and the patient about the potential risks of adjuvant radiotherapy on immediate reconstruction versus the additional surgery required for delayed reconstruction. There is no single "standard of care" in the setting of adjuvant radiotherapy, and each case must be individualized.

CONCLUSIONS

Breast reconstruction following mastectomy has been shown to have a positive impact on patients' physical and mental quality of life. Autologous tissue reconstruction has been advocated over implant-based reconstruction by some because of the potential for superior aesthetic results. In addition, the permanency of results and elimination of dependency on a permanent prosthesis are advantageous. Prosthetic reconstruction, however, has the capability of producing excellent results in the properly selected patient. Implant reconstruction is a less invasive surgical technique that is generally well tolerated.

The overriding goal of reconstructive breast surgery is to satisfy the patient with respect to her own self-image and expectations for the aesthetic result. Individualized selection of a reconstructive technique for each patient will be the predominant factor in achieving a reconstructive success.

References

1. Sandelin K, Billgren AM, Wickman M. Management, morbidity, and oncologic aspects in 100 consecutive patients with immediate breast reconstruction. *Ann Surg Oncol.* 1998;5:159–165.
2. Al Ghazal SK, Sully L, Fallowfield L, Blamey RW. The psychological impact of immediate rather than delayed breast reconstruction. *Eur J Surg Oncol.* 2000;26:17–19.

3. Spear SL, Onyewu C. Staged breast reconstruction with saline-filled implants in the irradiated breast: recent trends and therapeutic implications. *Plast Reconstr Surg.* 2000;105:930–942.

4. Cordeiro PG, Pusic AL, Disa JJ, McCormick B, VanZee K. Irradiation after immediate tissue expander/implant breast reconstruction: outcomes, complications, aesthetic results, and satisfaction among 156 patients. *Plast Reconstr Surg.* 2004;113:877–881.

5. Krueger EA, Wilkins EG, Strawderman M, et al. Complications and patient satisfaction following expander/implant breast reconstruction with and without radiotherapy. *Int J Radiat Oncol Biol Phys.* 2001;49:713–721.

6. Evans GR, Schusterman MA, Kroll SS, et al. Reconstruction and the radiated breast: is there a role for implants? *Plast Reconstr Surg.* 1995;96:1111–1115.

7. Hulka BS, Kerkvliet NL, Tugwell P. Experience of a scientific panel formed to advise the federal judiciary on silicone breast implants. *NEJM.* 2000;342:812–815.

8. Clough KB. Prospective evaluation of late cosmetic results following breast reconstruction: II. TRAM flap reconstruction. *Plast Reconstr Surg.* 2001;107:1710–1716.

9. Blondeel N, Vanderstraeten GG, Monstrey SJ, et al. The donor site morbidity of free DIEP flaps and free TRAM flaps for breast reconstruction. *Br J Plast Surg.* 1997;50:322–330.

10. Futter CM, Webster MH, Hagen S, Mitchell SL. A retrospective comparison of abdominal muscle strength following breast reconstruction with a free TRAM or DIEP flap. *Br J Plas Surg.* 2000;53:578–583.

11. Kroll SS. Fat necrosis in free transverse rectus abdominis myocutaneous and deep inferior epigastric perforator flaps. *Plast Reconstr Surg.* 2000;106:576–583.

12. Chevray PM. Breast reconstruction with superficial inferior epigastric artery flaps: a prospective comparison with TRAM and DIEP flaps. *Plast Reconstr Surg.* 2004;114:1077–1083.

13. Watterson PA, Bostwick J, III, Hester TR, Jr., Bried JT, Taylor GI. TRAM flap anatomy correlated with a 10-year clinical experience with 556 patients. *Plast Reconstr Surg.* 1995;95:1185–1194.

14. Kroll SS, Netscher DT. Complications of TRAM flap breast reconstruction in obese patients. *Plast Reconstr Surg.* 1989;84:886–892.

15. Serletti JM, Moran SL. Free versus the pedicled TRAM flap: a cost comparison and outcome analysis. *Plast Reconstr Surg.* 1997;100:1418–1424.

16. Nahabedian MY, Dooley W, Singh N, Manson PN. Contour abnormalities of the abdomen after breast reconstruction with abdominal flaps: the role of muscle preservation. *Plast Reconstr Surg.* 2002;109:91–101.

17. Nahabedian. Infectious complications following breast reconstruction with expanders and implants. *Plast Reconstr Surg.* 2003;112:467–476.

18. Vandeweyer E, Deraemaecker R, Nogaret JM, Hertens D. Immediate breast reconstruction with implants and adjuvant chemotherapy: a good option? *Acta Chir Belg.* 2003;103:98–101.

19. Wilson CR, Brown IM, Weiller-Mithoff E, George WD, Doughty JC. Immediate breast reconstruction does not lead to a delay in the delivery of adjuvant chemotherapy. *Eur J Surg Oncol.* 2004;30:624–627.

20. Tran NV, Evans GR, Kroll SS, et al. Postoperative adjuvant irradiation: effects on transverse rectus abdominis muscle flap breast reconstruction. *Plast Reconstr Surg.* 2000;106:313–317.

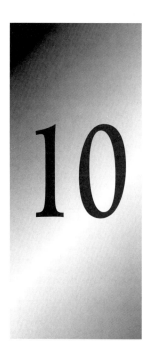

Principles of Spine Imaging in Cancer

10

Eric Lis
Christopher Mazzone

Cancer patients with symptoms referable to the spine present a unique imaging challenge. Metastatic disease can involve any portions of the spine. Most commonly, the epidural space is involved. Intradural disease, either leptomeningeal or intramedullary (spinal cord) metastasis, is less common. In addition, several complications of cancer therapy can affect the spine, sometimes mimicking metastatic disease. Problems that are often unique to cancer patients may be superimposed on more mundane and common processes that can involve any nonmalignant spine, particularly degenerative disease.

Metastatic disease to the spine is quite common, complicating the course of 5%–10% of cancer patients (1). As determined by autopsy, about 5% of patients that succumb to cancer exhibit spinal cord or cauda equina compression (2). The osseous spine is involved in about 30%–70% of patients with metastatic cancer (3). Overall, the spine is the most common site of bone metastasis, followed by the bony pelvis and femurs (4,5). The incidence of intradural metastasis (leptomeningeal and intramedullary) is much less than of epidural metastasis, accounting for fewer than 5% of metastatic disease to the spine (6).

The goal of this chapter is to impart an understanding of fundamental spine imaging anatomy to the clinician as well as to advance their knowledge of the most common lesions involving the spine in cancer patients. The choice of optimal imaging modalities for evaluation of such lesions will be discussed. Lesions that occur directly or indirectly from cancer treatment and may mimic metastatic disease will be reviewed. The diagnosis and treatment of spine metastasis and related processes in the cancer patient require a multidisciplinary approach and, with the proper use of imaging, will lead to earlier diagnosis, better management options, and ultimately improved neurological, functional, and potentially oncologic outcomes.

BASIC IMAGING ANATOMY AND TERMINOLOGY

The spine is best divided up into three anatomic spaces. The first and largest space is the epidural (extradural) space. The epidural space surrounds the thecal sac-dural sac and is everything outside of the thecal sac. Metastatic tumors that typically involve the epidural space usually arise within the osseous spine vertebrae. These are the typical vertebral-body metastases that expand into the epidural space and encroach upon the spinal canal and its contents. Less commonly, tumors such as leukemia and lymphoma can involve the epidural space without primary involvement of the osseous spine.

Intradural tumors can be broken down into two basic groups: intradural extramedullary and intramedullary lesions. Intradural extramedullary metastasis, more commonly referred to as leptomeningeal disease, is tumor that secondarily involves the leptomeninges and the subarachnoid (cerebrospinal fluid [CSF]) space. Occasionally, these lesions can be large enough to extrinsically deform or compress the spinal cord and are potentially confused with epidural disease. Least common is the intramedullary metastasis, which is a lesion arising within the substance of the spinal cord.

One of the best ways to understand the radiographic anatomy of the spine is with a postmyelogram computed tomography (CT) scan (Fig. 10.1A, C, and E). The thecal sac CSF space is opacified by contrast and is easily identified. The spinal cord is seen centrally, with the nerve route of the cauda equina also

easily identified. To review previously mentioned concepts, the epidural space would be everything outside of the opacified thecal sac. This space is predominately occupied by the vertebrae, but also includes epidural fat, ligaments, and vascular plexuses. Working inward, the next space is the intradural extramedullary space. This is everything between the spinal cord and the dura, and is, for practical purposes, the contrast-opacified CSF space. Typically, metastatic disease that involves the meninges of the spine would appear as

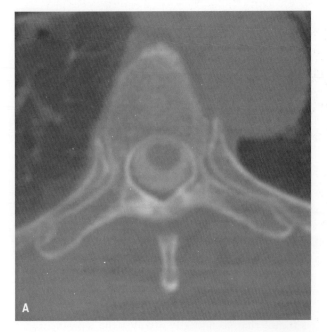 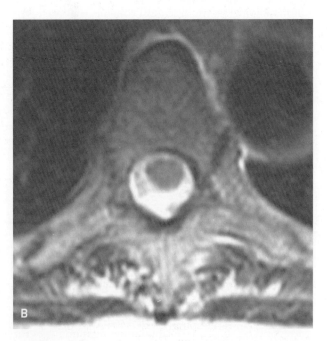

FIGURE 10.1 A–E

A: Axial postmyelogram CT through the mid-thoracic spine. B: Matching axial T2 weighted MRI.

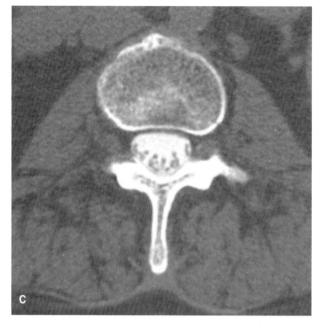

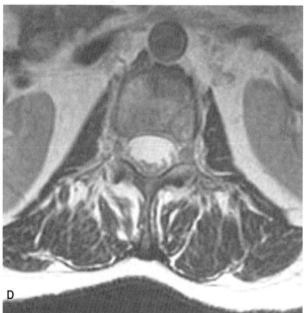

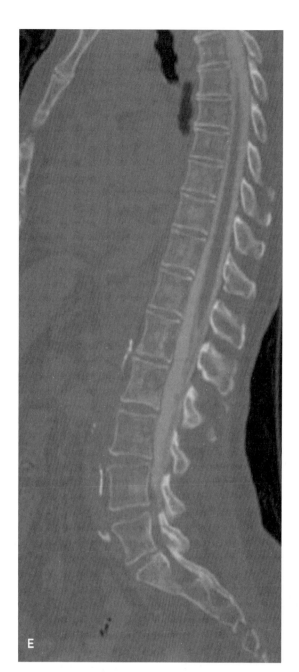

FIGURE 10.1 A–E (Continued)

Basic compartments of the spine. C: Postmyelogram axial CT through the cauda equina. D: Matching axial T2 weighted MRI. E: Postmyelogram CT reformatted in the sagittal plane. The postmyelogram images (A, C, E) show opacification of the subarachnoid space (intradural extramedullary), which is the space where leptomeningeal metastases are seen. The spinal cord (intramedullary) is outlined by the CSF. Similarly, the nerve roots of the cauda equina are well demonstrated (C, D). In simple terms, the epidural space is everything outside of the opacified thecal-CSF space, most of which is made up of bone vertebrae, fat, and ligaments.

filling defects or nodules along the surface of the cauda equina or spinal cord. The intradural intramedullary compartment is the spinal cord itself and is outlined by the opacified thecal sac. This basic understanding of spinal anatomy is easily applicable to magnetic resonance imaging (MRI).

DIAGNOSTIC SPINE IMAGING

The most common imaging modalities that are readily available to cancer patients with symptoms referable to the spine are plain films, CT, MRI, and CT-myelography. Adjunctive modalities, such as bone scans, positron emission tomography (PET) scans, and spinal angiography, are beyond the scope of this chapter.

Spine MRI

MRI is currently the most sensitive and specific imaging modality in evaluating spine tumors and, as such, is the modality of choice for imaging of the spine in cancer patients. Contraindications to MRI generally include the presence of any metallic material susceptible to magnetic fields. This includes a cardiac pacemaker, implanted cardiac defibrillator, cochlear implant, carotid artery vascular clamp, neurostimulator, insulin or infusion pump, implanted drug infusion device, bone growth/fusion stimulator, and certain aneurysm clips.

Adequate imaging of the entire spine can easily be performed with any of the commercially available MRI units. Thorough MR imaging of the spine usually requires both T1 and T2 weighted images obtained in the sagittal plane with selected axial images through regions of interest (7,8). Typically, the entire spine can be imaged in an hour or less by using a large field of view that essentially divides the spine into upper and lower halves, with slight overlap of the lower thoracic spine to ensure complete coverage (Fig. 10.2). Ideally, the part of the spine that is clinically symptomatic should be imaged first in case the patient is unable to complete the study. Axial images are prescribed as needed.

T1 weighted images provide anatomic definition, marrow detail, and a generally good overview of the spinal column. CSF is hypointense (dark), and fat is hyperintense (bright). Typically, most bone metastases are hypointense on T1 weighted sequences relative to the marrow, which is often slightly hyperintense secondary to its fat content in adults (Fig. 10.3). Fast spin echo (FSE) T2 weighted sequences have essentially replaced standard T2 weighted sequences secondary to a significant decrease in imaging time. CSF is hyperintense on T2 weighted images, with FSE T2 images providing excellent definition of both the spinal cord and CSF spaces. However, bone metastases are often less conspicuous on FSE T2 images, as fat is somewhat hyperintense. This can be compensated for by using the short tau inversion recovery (STIR) technique, which is essentially a fat-suppressed T2 image that makes many tumors appear hyperintense to adja-

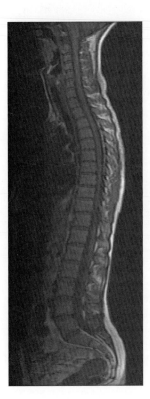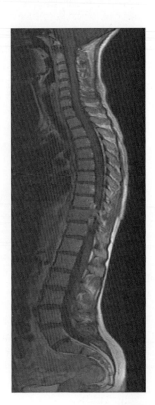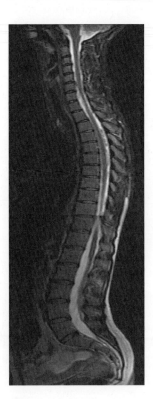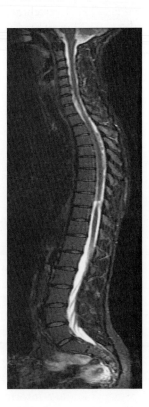

FIGURE 10.2

Normal MRI survey of the total spine in the sagittal plane. The images are merged from upper and lower spine studies and do not align perfectly. Left to right: Sagittal T1, matching postcontrast T1, FSE T2, and T2 STIR (D). Notice the hyperintense dorsal epidural fat, especially in the lumbar spine, as well as the hyperintense subcutaneous fat, both of which are suppressed on the T2 STIR images. Notice that the enhancement is limited to vascular structure, particularly the ventral epidural venous plexus.

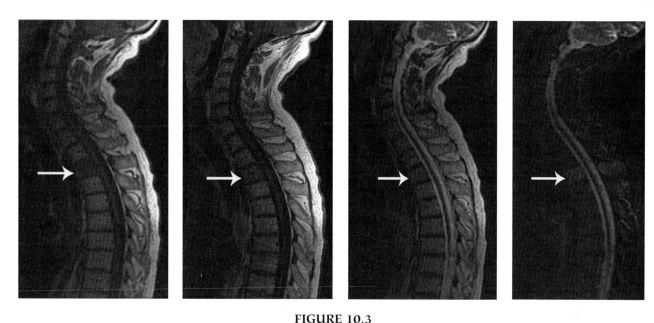

FIGURE 10.3

Typical MRI appearance of a T3 metastasis (arrow) in a patient with esophageal cancer. Left to right: Sagittal T1 with matching contrast-enhanced T1, T2, and T2 STIR images.

cent marrow and is also sensitive in identifying marrow edema. Most vertebral metastases are usually hypointense on T1 weighted images and hyperintense on T2 weighted images and also hyperintense, though generally more conspicuous, on T2 STIR images (Fig. 10.4). Sclerotic metastases are commonly hypointense on all pulse sequences (Fig. 10.5).

Other pulse sequences that are less common but are occasionally added to spine studies in certain situations include gradient echo (GRE) sequences, which are often useful in identifying blood products, or diffusion weighted images (DWI), which can play a role in spinal cord ischemia and the identification of bacterial abscesses. Some advanced MRI pulse sequences that are commonly utilized in brain imaging, such as DWI, perfusion imaging, and spectroscopy, are now being looked at on an investigational basis to evaluate neoplastic disease in the spine; however, they are generally limited by technical challenges. Ultra-fast sequences, such as half number of excitations (NEX) single-shot (SS) FSE T2 sequences, are useful when patient motion degrades standard images. This type of pulse sequence is able to image the lower or upper half of the spine in the sagittal or axial plane in less than 15 seconds. It comes at the cost of lesion conspicuity, but usually provides enough information to exclude any problem requiring immediate intervention (Fig. 10.6).

The use of gadolinium-based contrast agents are particularly useful in the identification of leptomeningeal disease or intramedullary spinal cord tumors, both of which typically enhance, as do most osseous

metastatic and epidural disease. Gadolinium may also be useful in the evaluation of the postoperative spine to differentiate scar from tumor and for the evaluation of infection abscess. Enhancement of the nerve roots of the cauda equina may sometimes be seen with the administration of gadolinium in patients with acute inflammatory demyelinating polyradiculoneuropathy (AIDP) and chronic idiopathic demyelinating polyradiculoneuropathy (CIDP).

Spine Plain Films

Plain films of the spine are readily available but generally a poor screening for metastatic disease. About 30%–50% bone destruction is needed before a lytic lesion can be identified on a radiograph. Vertebral compression fractures are easily identified, though the degree of canal compromise can be difficult to determine (Fig. 10.7). Plain films can be obtained while weight bearing, possibly identifying deformities or malalignments that would be otherwise undetected in supine non-weight bearing positions required for CT and MRI. In the postoperative patient, plain films are most useful in assessing the alignment of the spine and the structural integrity of the reconstruction hardware (Fig. 10.8).

Spine CT

Over the last decade, the introduction of multidetector helical CT scanners has greatly improved the use

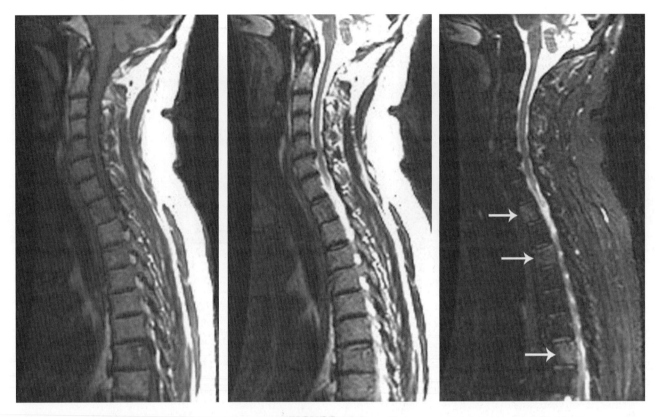

FIGURE 10.4

A patient with melanoma and multiple spine metastases. Left to right: Sagittal T1, FSE T2, and T2 STIR MRI showing multiple spine metastases. Notice that the metastases (arrows) are much more conspicuous on the T2 STIR image, especially when compared to the standard FSE T2 image.

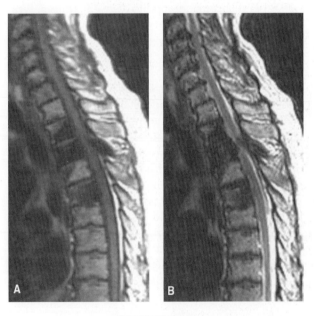

FIGURE 10.5

Sagittal T1 (A) and matching FSE T2 (B) MRI in a patient with metastatic prostate cancer and sclerotic metastasis that remain hypointense on both the T1 and T2 weighted sequences.

of CT as a spine imaging modality. Axial images can be quickly acquired through the entire spine in a matter of minutes and reconstructed in even thinner slice thicknesses for sagittal and coronal reformations. An unenhanced CT scan is not sensitive for the identification of epidural soft tissue tumor, especially when compared to MRI, but is extremely good at demonstrating lytic or sclerotic bony changes and cortical destruction (Fig. 10.9). Contrast will improve epidural soft tissue conspicuity, but is limited in identifying leptomeningeal and intramedullary tumor. Similarly, CT is not very good at identifying marrow infiltration without bony changes.

CT Myelography

Before MRI, myelography and then CT myelography was the diagnostic study of choice for the evaluation of the spine in regard to nerve root or spinal cord compression. The descriptive epidural, intradural, and intramedullary compartments were essentially brought to the forefront with myelography.

Myelography, when combined with a postmyelogram CT scan, is very sensitive in the detection of

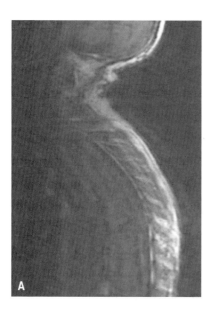
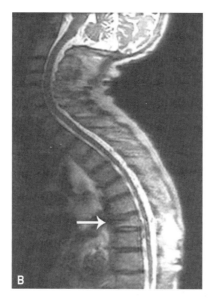
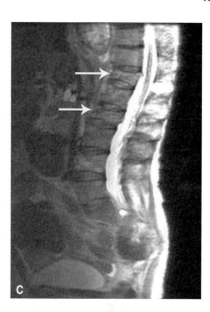

FIGURE 10.6

A patient with multiple myeloma with acute back pain. Sagittal T1 weighted MRI (A) is essentially nondiagnostic secondary to motion. Sagittal SS FSE T2 MRI of the upper and lower halves of the spine (B, C) demonstrates multiple partial collapse deformities (arrows) without cord compression.

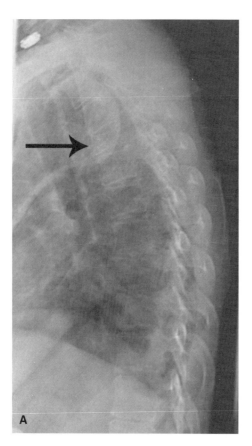
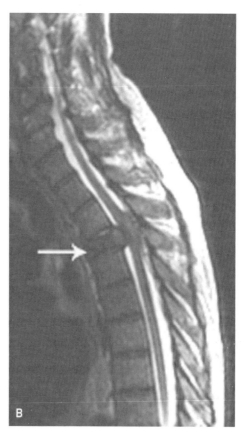

FIGURE 10.7

A: A lateral plain film of the thoracic spine in a patient with bladder cancer showing a T4 collapse deformity but essentially giving no information about the degree of canal compromise or the condition of the spinal cord. B: Sagittal T2 weighted MRI in the same patient showing spinal cord compression.

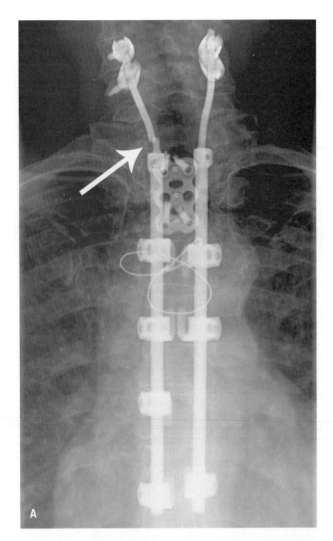
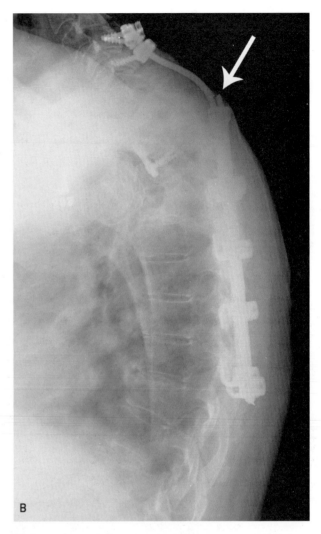

FIGURE 10.8

AP and lateral plain films (A,B) in a patient with multiple myeloma showing a broken posterior stabilization rod. Such a defect would not be detectable on MRI or CT.

epidural tumor and spinal cord compression. A myelogram consists of infusing a small amount of nonionic water-soluble contrast into the subarachnoid space via a lumbar puncture or, less commonly, a cervical C1-2 puncture (Fig. 10.10e). The intrathecal contrast is then advanced in a controlled fashion throughout the spinal column with fluoroscopic spot images obtained. Attention is given to regions of the spine where the flow of intrathecal contrast is either held up or "blocked," usually secondary to epidural tumor in cancer patients. A myelogram is usually followed by a CT scan of the spine, which adds much detail and anatomic definition. A small amount CSF is also obtained at the time of the procedure, which can sent for analysis. The presence of neoplastic cells on cytopathologic evaluation is indicative of leptomeningeal disease. Myelography is

generally safe, though it is an invasive procedure that can have side effects, including neurological decompensation in patients with high-grade blocks.

Although MRI has largely replaced CT myelography, it is still commonly performed on patients that have a contraindication to MRI or who have had prior spine reconstruction with instrumentation that results in artifact, making an MRI study nondiagnostic.

PUTTING THE IMAGING TOGETHER

Before proceeding to the specifics of the most common disease processes that involve the spine and cancer patients, it is worthwhile to discuss a patient with one typical spine lesion imaged with the previously

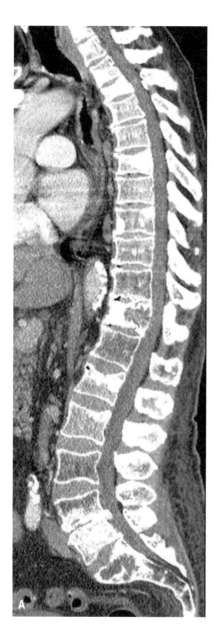 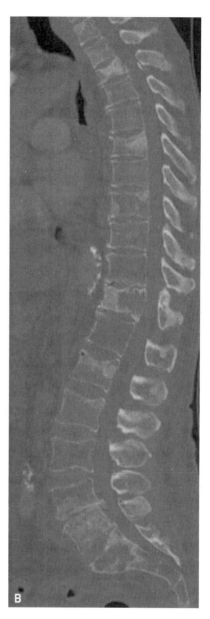

FIGURE 10.9

Reformatted contrast-enhanced CT scan in the sagittal plane in soft-tissue windows (A) and in bone windows (B) showing multiple lytic and sclerotic metastases, as well as several partial collapse deformities in this patient with an unknown primary.

discussed modalities. This will illustrate the clinical value and differences of each modality. The patient is a 61-year-old female with a history of breast cancer who presents to her oncologist with worsening back pain (Fig. 10.11).

EPIDURAL TUMOR

The epidural space is the most common compartment of the spine to be involved by metastatic disease, with the majority of epidural lesions arising from the verte-

brae. Back pain is the most common presenting symptom of metastatic epidural disease. Early and accurate diagnosis is of tremendous importance, as the treatments offered and the functional outcomes depend on the neurologic, oncologic, medical, and spinal stability status of the patient at the time of presentation.

At the Memorial Sloan-Kettering Cancer Center, spinal canal compromise is sometimes graded on MRI axial images using a standard scale: 0 to 3 (Fig. 10.12) (9). Grade 0 is vertebral body or posterior element disease with possibly early epidural involvement but

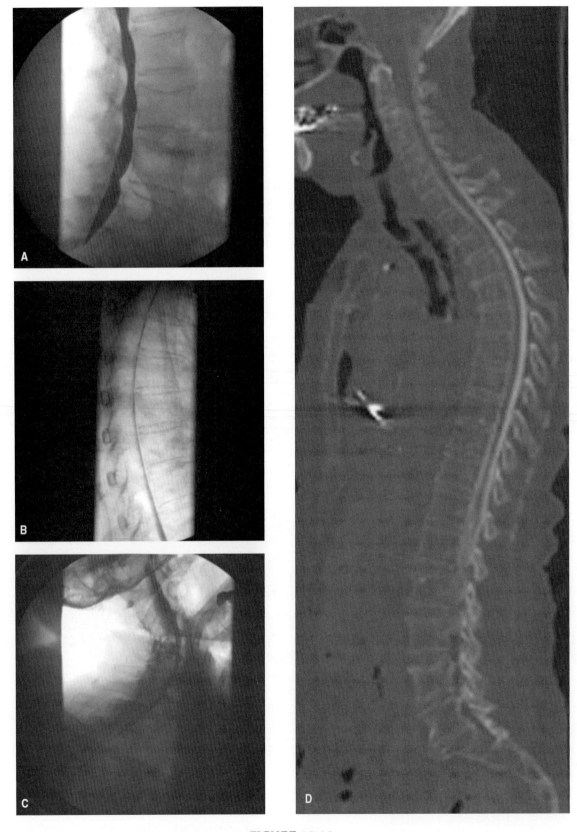

FIGURE 10.10

A–C: Lateral spot films obtained during a myelogram showing free passage of the intrathecal contrast throughout the spinal canal. D: A postmyelogram CT scan reformatted in the sagittal plane.

no mass upon the thecal sac. Essentially, there is no significant canal compromise. Grade 1 is when epidural disease results in partial effacement of the thecal sac but without spinal cord deformity or compression. Grade 1 disease usually is described as causing mild to moderate spinal canal compromise. Grade 2 epidural disease also partially obliterates the thecal sac, but without frank spinal cord compression. Grade 3 disease is complete obliteration of the thecal sac with spinal cord compression. Multiple examples of epidural disease are illustrated and discussed in Figures 10.13–10.19.

Leptomeningeal Metastases, Spinal Cord Metastasis, and Lesions Adjacent to the Spine.

When a patient presents with new or progressive spine symptoms but no epidural disease or non-neoplastic (ie, degenerative) causes are identified to explain their symptoms, a close inspection of the CSF spaces and spinal cord is indicated (Figs. 10.20–10.22). Also, it is usually worth evaluating areas adjacent to the spine (ie, paraspinally) when nothing centrally fits the patient's presentation.

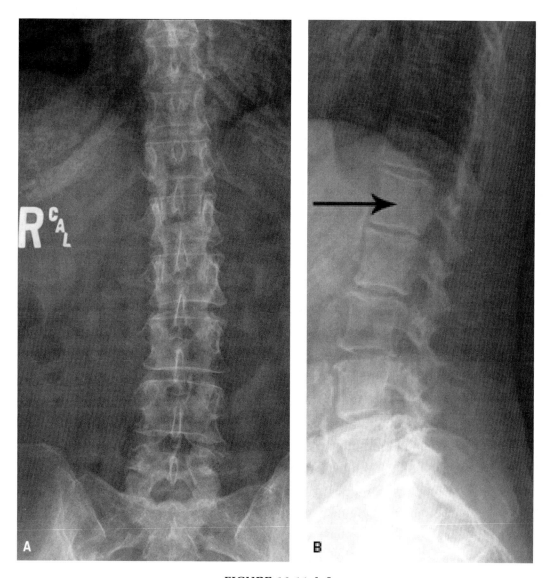

FIGURE 10.11 A–J

The patient is a 61-year-old female with a history of breast cancer with worsening back pain. AP and lateral plain films (A,B) of the lumbar spine show subtle lucency (arrow) along the posterior aspect of the L1 vertebral body.　　*(Continued)*

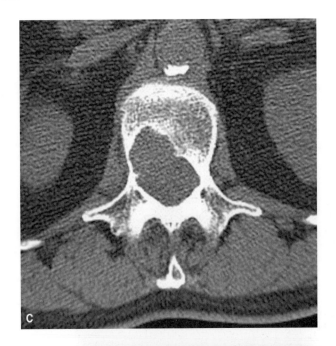

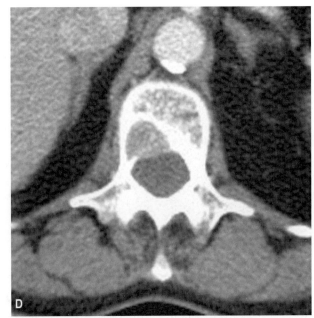

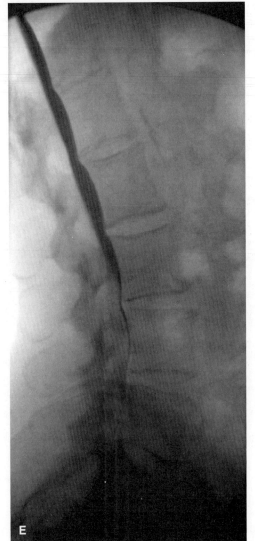

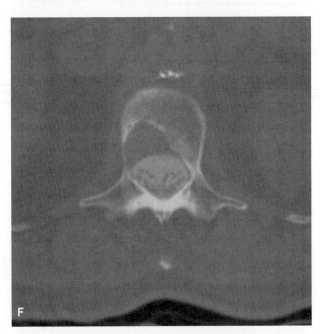

FIGURE 10.11 A–J (*Continued*)

A nonconstrast axial CT scan (C) through L1 shows a lytic metastasis with destruction of the posterior vertebral body cortex. Any significant epidural component cannot be determined by this image. A contrast-enhanced axial CT image (D) demonstrates enhancement of the metastasis with little epidural involvement and no significant canal compromise. A lateral plain film from a myelogram (E) shows free flow of the intrathecal contrast by L1 with an axial postmyelogram CT (F) through L1 showing the lesion that is without significant canal compromise. Notice the normal nerve roots of the cauda equina. The same lesion is seen in the sagittal plane on a noncontrast T1 and T2 STIR MRI (G, H) in the axial plane on T1 and T2 weighted images (I, J).

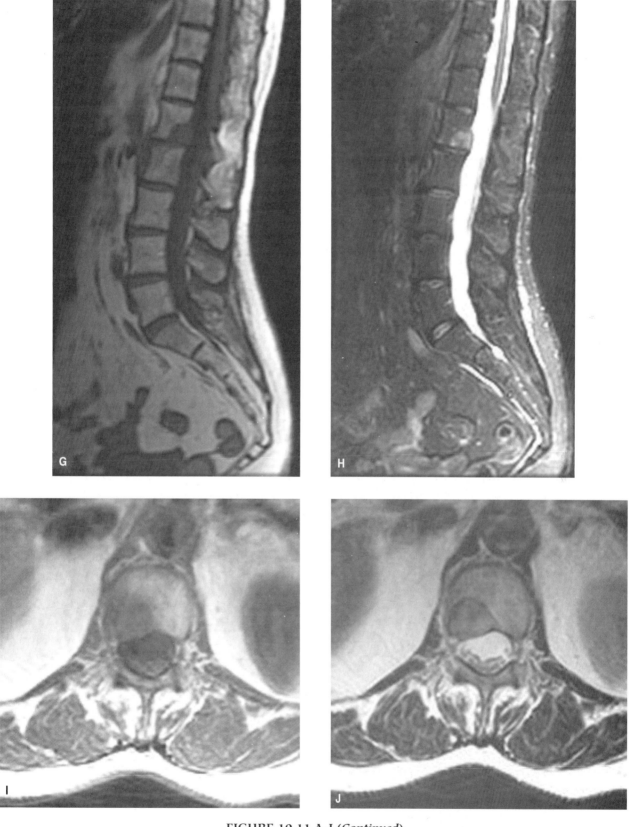

FIGURE 10.11 A–J (*Continued*)

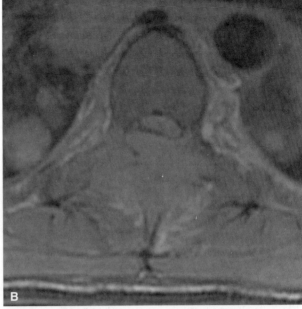

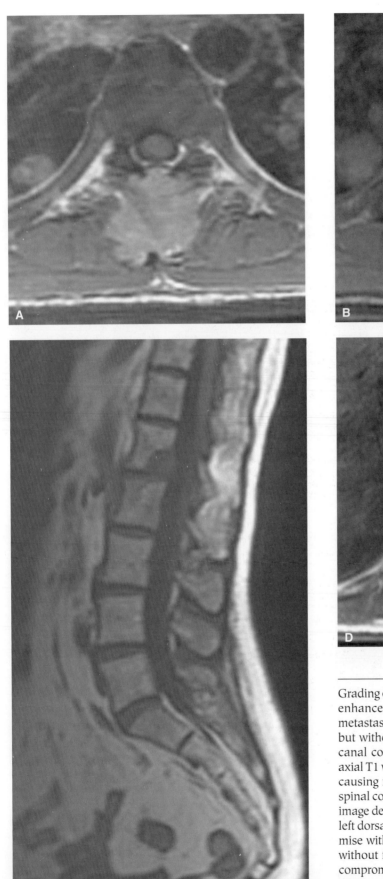

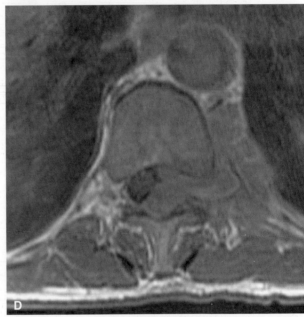

FIGURE 10.12

Grading epidural disease. A: Grade 0 as seen on a contrast-enhanced axial T1 weighted MRI showing an expansile metastasis extending just into the dorsal epidural space-fat but without any mass effect in the thecal sac. B: Grade 1 canal compromise as demonstrated by this postcontrast axial T1 weighted image showing left lateral epidural tumor causing mild to moderate canal compromise but without spinal cord compression. C: Postcontrast axial T1 weighted image depicts Grade 2 canal compromise by left lateral and left dorsal epidural tumor causing moderate canal compromise with spinal cord displacement and impingement but without frank spinal cord compression. D: Grade 3 canal compromise, as seen on this postcontrast axial T1 weighted image, where dorsal epidural tumor results in high-grade canal compromise and marked spinal cord compression.

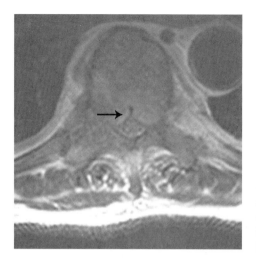

FIGURE 10.13

Axial T2 weighted MRI through the mid-thoracic spine showing biventral epidural tumor. Notice the posterior longitudinal ligament that contains the tumor and demonstrates an inverted V configuration secondary to its strong attachment to the mid-posterior vertebrae.

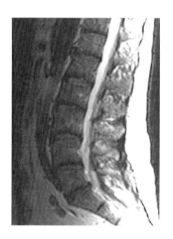 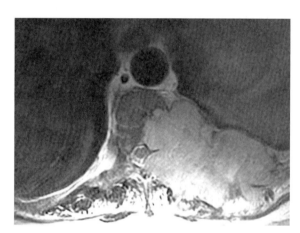 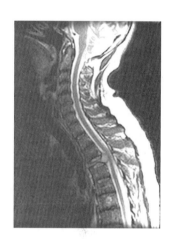

FIGURE 10.14

Tandem lesions. A patient with melanoma presented with worsening left-sided low back pain. Sagittal T2 weighted and axial T2 weighted (A, B) MRI show a left-side chest wall mass with vertebral and epidural involvement. A completion sagittal T2 MRI through the upper spine (C) shows a pathological collapse of T4 with cord compression that was relatively clinically silent but more critical. This is to emphasize the importance of imaging the entire spine in cancer patients.

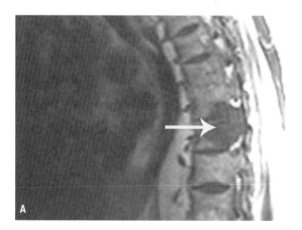 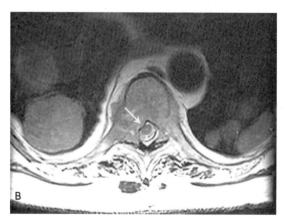

FIGURE 10.15

Metastatic leiomyosarcoma with right posterior chest wall pain that radiates anteriorly. A: Sagittal T1 weighted MRI demonstrates an expansile metastasis (arrow) encroaching upon the adjacent neural foramina. B: Axial T2 image showing epidural involvement with mild spinal canal compromise (arrow). Multiple pulmonary metastases are also visible.

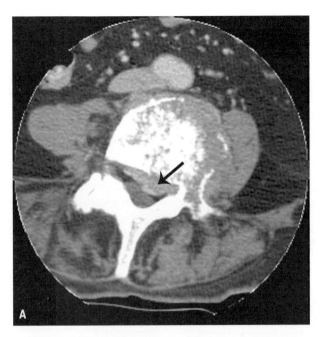

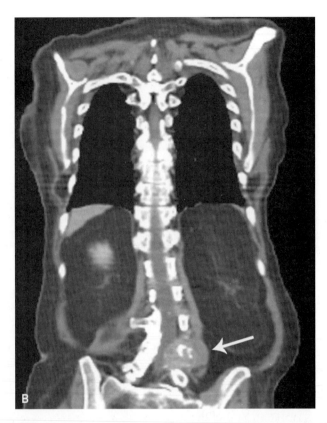

A patient with bladder cancer that has a worsening left L4 radiculopathy. A contrast-enhanced CT image through L4 (A) with coronal reformations (B) showing expansile metastatic disease involving L4, resulting in moderate canal compromise and involvement of the adjacent left-sided neural foramina.

FIGURE 10.16

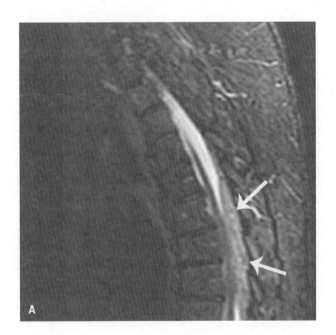

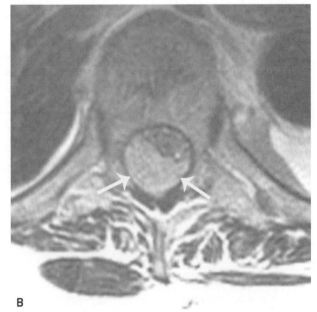

FIGURE 10.17

A patient presenting with back pain and weakness found to have lymphoma. A: Sagittal T2 STIR and B: axial T2 MRI demonstrate a thoracic dorsal epidural mass (arrows) causing high-grade spinal canal compromise and spinal cord compression. Notice that there is no obvious involvement of the vertebrae, a finding not uncommon with some of the hematologic malignancies, such as lymphoma.

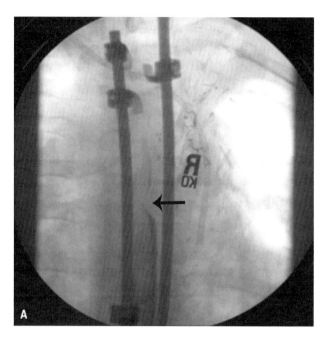

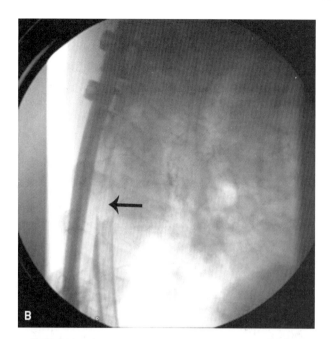

This patient has had multiple thoracic decompressive spine surgeries for recurrent sarcoma. Instrumentation degraded the MRI, so a myelogram was performed to evaluate for epidural disease. Spot images from a myelogram in the frontal and lateral projections (A, B) show epidural compression (arrows) of the thecal sac with a small amount of contrast sneaking past the region of spinal canal compromise. A postmyelogram CT scan (C) reformatted in the coronal plane showing a large paraspinal mass (arrows) with epidural extension into the spinal canal with spinal cord compression.

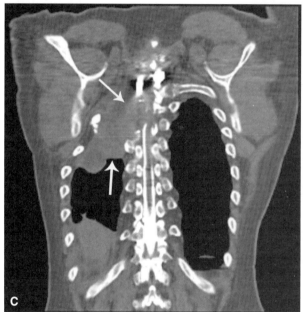

FIGURE 10.18

Lesions Mimicking Metastatic Disease

Cancer patients may present with spinal symptoms or imaging that is indeterminate for metastatic disease but which reflects direct or indirect sequelae of treatment. Spinal infections may occur in the immunocompro-mised patient, and secondary malignancies may occur because of prior radiation treatment. Nonmalignant osteoporotic type fractures of the spine are particularly common and may cause severe back pain (Figs. 10.23–10.31).

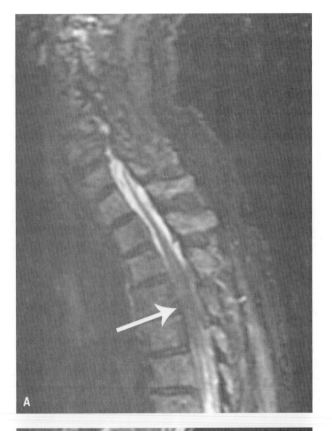

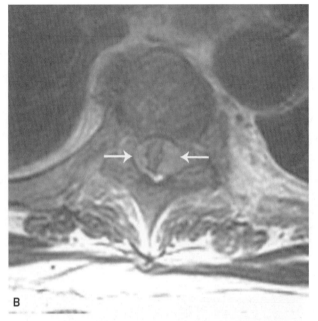

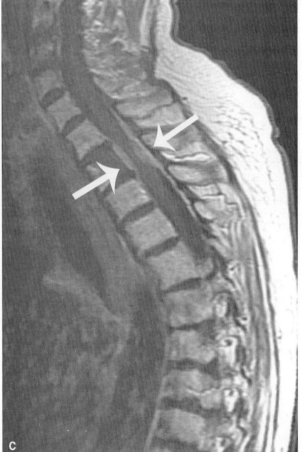

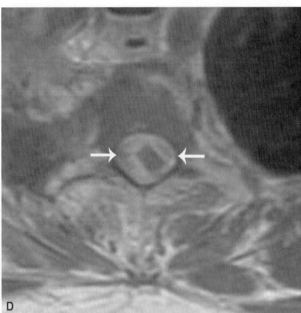

FIGURE 10.19

Sagittal T2 STIR MRI (A) revealing somewhat indistinct thoracic spinal cord. Axial T2 image (B) through this region showing bilateral lateral epidural tumor with cord compression (arrows). MRI from a different patient with lung cancer demonstrating circumferential epidural tumor with spinal cord compression (arrows) on postcontrast (C) sagittal and (D) axial T1 weighted images.

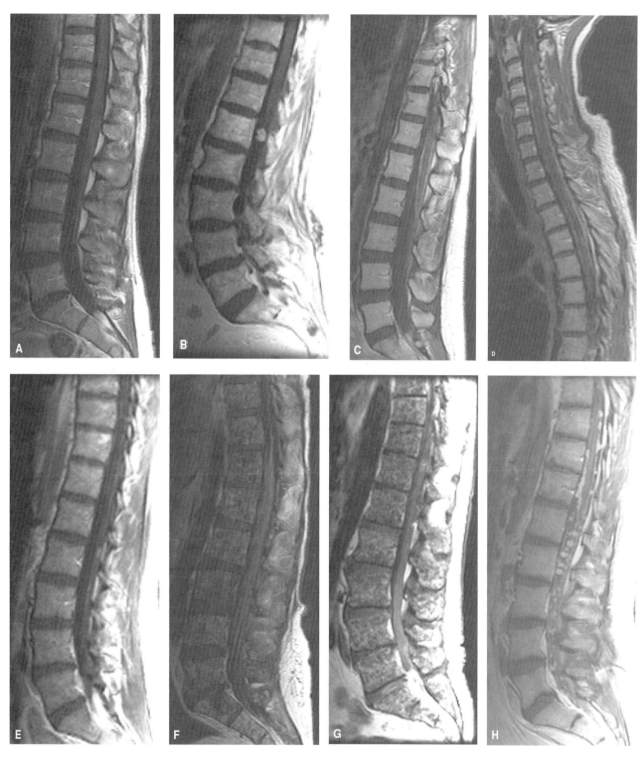

FIGURE 10.20

The variable appearance of leptomeningeal disease on MRI. This is a series of postcontrast sagittal T1 weighted MRIs of the spine in patients with documented leptomeningeal disease. A: Normal, no suspicious enhancement identified. B: Focal nodular enhancement. C, D: Plaquelike and nodular coating of the spinal cord. E: Scattered segmental plaques of enhancement. F: Confluent enhancing plaques of tumor extending along the cauda equina. G: Confluent-enhancing disease nearly filling the lumbar thecal sac. H: Extensive nodular leptomeningeal disease.

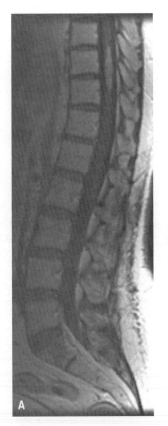
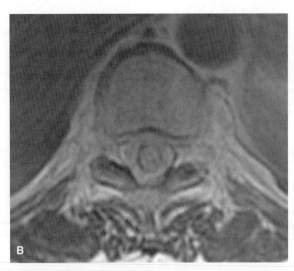
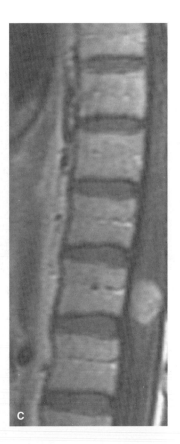

FIGURE 10.21

A patient with metastatic breast cancer and urinary incontinence. Contrast-enhanced sagittal T1 weighted MRI (A) showing a lower thoracic spinal cord metastasis. Axial T2 weighted image (B) showing the lesion within the spinal cord. A second patient with breast cancer and a metastasis to the conus as seen on a postcontrast sagittal T1 MRI (C).

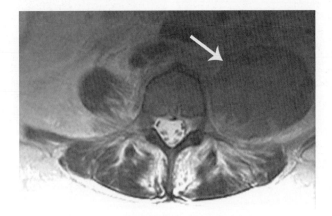

FIGURE 10.22

Lymphoma with left leg weakness. The MRI of the spine was essentially negative. A left psoas mass was identified and likely accounts for the symptoms.

CONCLUSION

MRI is generally the procedure of choice and the first imaging modality used to evaluate patients with symptoms referable to the spine. Exceptions include the presence of a contraindication to MRI, the suspicion of spinal stabilization hardware failure, or the presence of suspected tumor in an area where imaging is degraded, such as around hardware. Other imaging modalities can play a complementary role. It is important to remember that when the imaging is inconsistent with the clinical findings, a discussion and review of the imaging with the radiologist or neuroradiologist is indicated. Such collaboration can often lead to the elucidation of a subtle finding that will affect patient treatment and potential outcome.

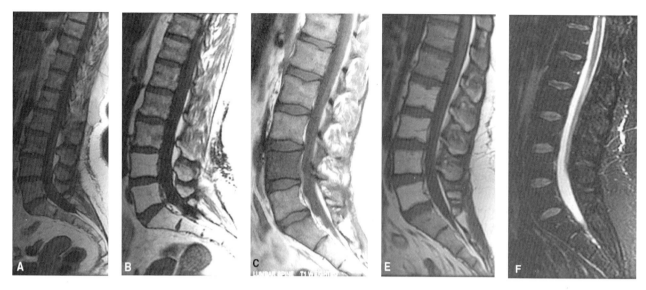

FIGURE 10.23

Radiation change. A: Sagittal T1 weighted MRI of the lumbosacral spine. B: The same patient three months after radiation to the pelvis showing the typical fatty change of the marrow, L4, L5, and the sacrum that now demonstrates homogenous hyperintensity on this T1 weighted image. The margins of the radiation port are usually well defined, as in this case. C: A second patient with L4 lymphoma as seen on this sagittal T1 weighted image. D: A postradiation sagittal T1 weighted image shows well demarcated radiation change-fatty change in the lumbar spine in addition to resolution of the L4 lesion and with homogenous suppression on the fat-suppressed T2 STIR image (E).

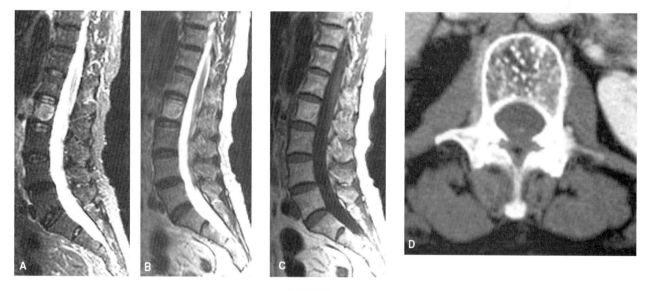

FIGURE 10.24

Hemangioma of bone. These benign lesions are common and should not be confused with metastatic disease. The patient has a history of lung cancer and focal bone scan activity in L2. Sagittal T2 STIR (A) and T2 weighted MRI (B) of the lumbar spine showing a focal hyperintense lesion in L2. A matching T1 weighted image (C) shows the lesion to be slightly hyperintense to isointense to adjacent marrow. An axial CT image through L2 (D) shows a coarsened trabecular pattern consistent with a hemangioma.

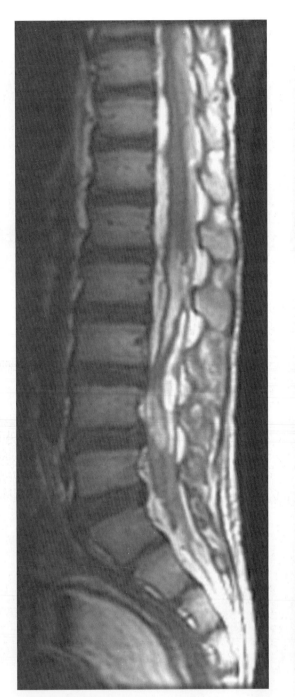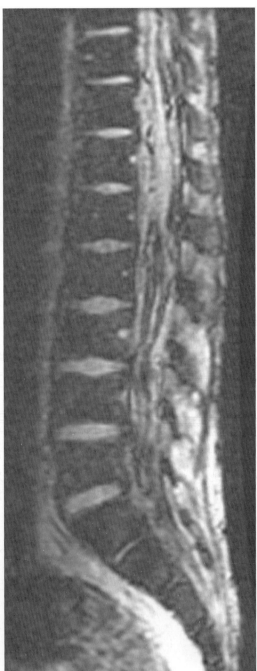

FIGURE 10.25

The patient has leukemia and developed lower-extremity weakness shortly after a lumbar puncture and intrathecal chemotherapy. Sagittal T1 weighted image (A) of the lumbar spine shows irregular hyperintensity in and about the thecal sac. A matching sagittal GRE image (B) shows regions of decreased signal supportive of hemorrhage.

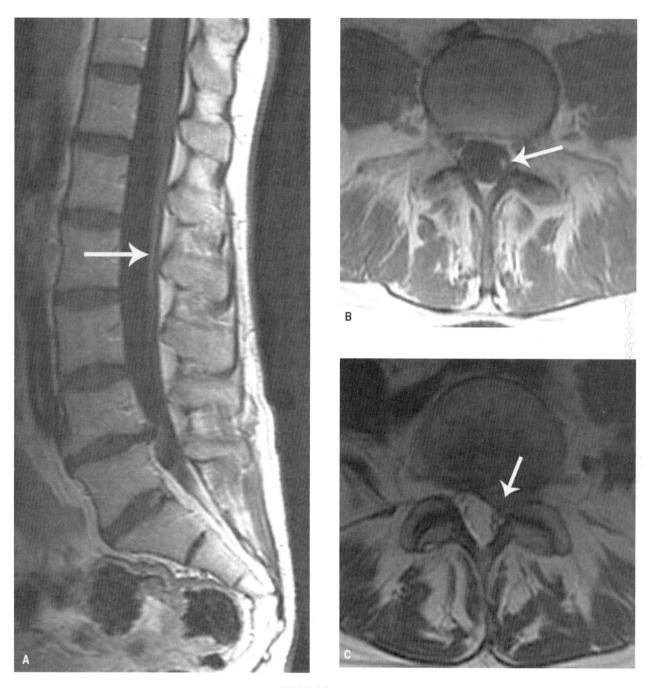

FIGURE 10.26

The patient has a history of lymphoma and developed an L5 radiculopathy. Postcontrast sagittal (A) and axial T1 weighted MRI (B) through the lumbar spine show segmental enhancement of the left L5 nerve root (arrows). This was determined to be reactive and secondary to impingement by a large left L4-5 disc herniation, as seen on an axial T2 weighted image (C, arrow), and not to represent leptomeningeal disease.

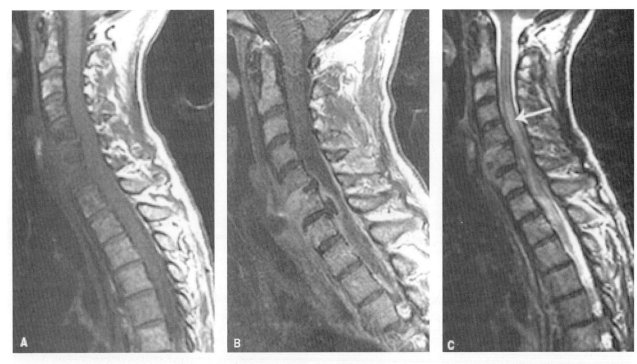

FIGURE 10.27

A patient with recurrent head and neck cancer that developed weakness and neck pain. Sagittal T1 weighted MRI (A) of the cervical spine followed by a contrast-enhanced sagittal T1 weighted image(B) and a matching sagittal T2 weighted image (C) showing discitis/osteomyelitis with C5-6 and C6-7 epidural abscesses. Note the spinal cord edema (arrow) on the T2 weighted images.

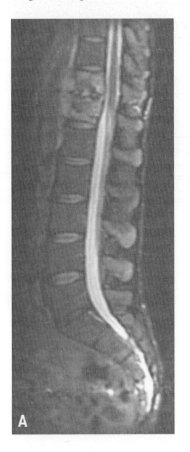

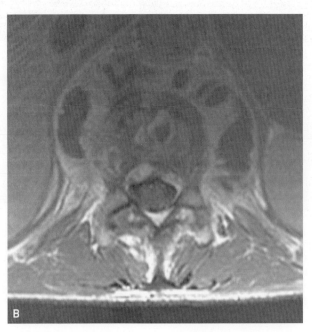

FIGURE 10.28

A patient with a remote history of lymphoma developed back pain and was thought to have a recurrence. Sagittal T2 STIR (A) demonstrates increased marrow signal in T11 and T12 with paraspinal soft tissue. Axial contrast-enhanced T1 weighted image (B) shows paraspinal disease with cystic change. CT-guided biopsy confirmed tuberculosis.

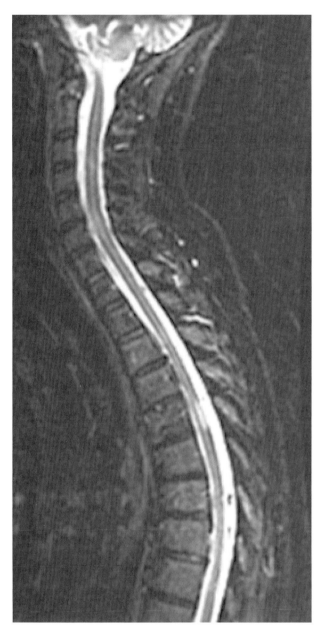

FIGURE 10.29

The patient is status-post bone marrow transplant for leukemia. Sagittal T2 STIR image of the spinal cord demonstrates nonspecific signal changes in the spinal cord. Subsequent biopsy revealed likely nonspecific demyelination.

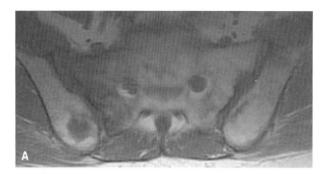

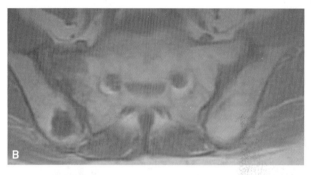

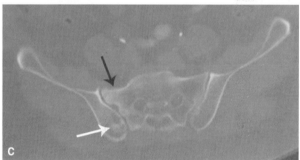

FIGURE 10.30

Osteoporotic fractures. Fractures of the spine, including the sacrum, commonly occur secondary to therapy-related or senile bone loss in cancer patients. A: A patient with a history of colon cancer presents with low back pain. An axial T1 weighted MRI demonstrates marrow changes in the right sacral ala. CT-guided biopsy was negative for tumor. Follow-up (B) axial T1 weighted MRI shows improvement with an axial CT image (C) showing patchy sclerosis (black arrow) most compatible with a healing stress fracture. Incidentally identified is a bone island in the right posterior iliac bone (white arrow).

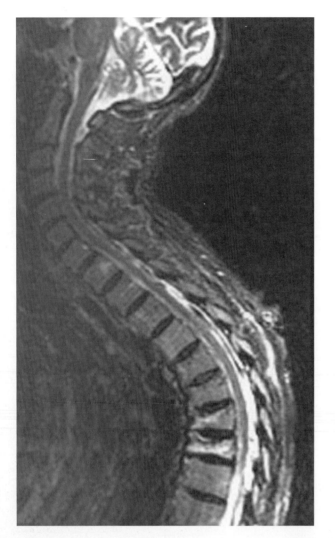 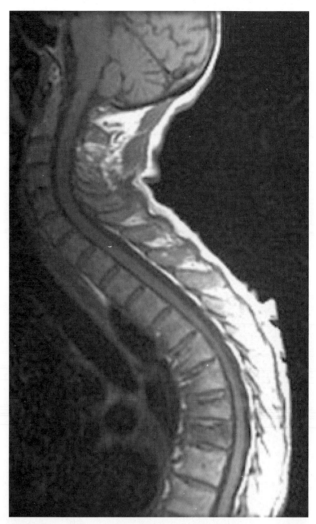

FIGURE 10.31

Typical-appearing osteoporotic fractures of the thoracic spine in a patient with a history of lung cancer. Sagittal T2 STIR (A) and sagittal T1 weighted MRI (B). Biopsy at the time of kyphoplasty was negative for tumor.

References

1. Bach F, Larsen BH, et al. Metastatic spinal cord compression: occurrence, symptoms, clinical presentations and prognosis in 398 patients with spinal cord compression. *Acta Neurochir.* 1990;170:37–43.
2. Barron KD, Hirano A, et al. Experiences with metastatic neoplasms involving the spinal cord. *Neurology.* 1959;8:91–106.
3. Fornasier V, Horne J. Metastases to the vertebral column. *Cancer.* 1975;36:590–594.
4. Galasko C. The anatomy and pathways of skeletal metastases. In: Weiss L, Gilbert H, eds. *Bone Metastasis.* Boston: GK Hall & Co; 1981:49–63.
5. Harrington K. Metastatic diseases of the spine. In: Harrington K, ed. *Orthopaedic Management of Metastatic Bone Disease.* St. Louis: CV Mosby; 1988:309–383.
6. Costigan D, Winkelman M. Intramedullary spinal cord metastasis. A clinicopathological study of 13 cases. *J Neurosurg.* 1985;62:227–233.
7. Algra PR, Bloem JL, et al. Detection of vertebral metastases: comparison between MR imaging and bone scintigraphy. *Radiographics.* 1991;11:219–232.
8. Riggieri PM. Pulse sequences in lumbar spine imaging. *Magn Reson Imaging Clin N Am.* 1999;7:425–437.
9. Bilsky M, Smith M. Surgical approach to epidural spinal cord compression. *Hematol Oncol Clin North Am.* 2006;20(6):1307–1317.

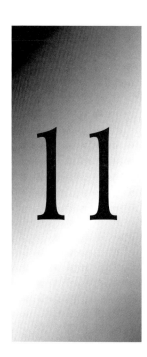

Principles of Plexus Imaging in Cancer

11

Jon Lewis
George Krol

Involvement of plexus in a patient with cancer may be due to a tumor arising directly from neural components, direct (contiguous) metastatic spread from adjacent organs, or compression by adjacent tumor masses (eg, enlarged nodes). Most common iatrogenically induced causes include sequelae or complications of surgical intervention or radiation therapy (RT). Clinical presentation in all these conditions is frequently similar, thus a common term "plexopathy" is used. Symptoms include pain, paresthesias, focal weakness, autonomic symptoms, sensory deficits, and muscle atrophy (1,2). Although history may suggest possible cause, physical examination is of limited value in evaluation of plexopathy. Conventional radiologic methods (plain radiographs) are usually negative, although may be helpful in advanced disease. Both computed tomography (CT) and magnetic resonance imaging (MRI) have been utilized all along, but in recent years, MRI has emerged as a leading method of imaging of plexus regions. Technical improvements (neurography) made it possible to visualize individual nerves directly (3–6). A reliable method of visualization of diseased nerve/plexus seems more difficult to find. As new techniques are introduced, improving resolution and depicting more detail and chemical composition of tissue, there arises a need for more thorough knowledge of utilization of imaging in normal and diseased state. This chapter will discuss the role of conventional and new modalities in the assessment of plexus disease, including indications, current techniques, advantages and pitfalls, and selection of methods of choice.

NORMAL ANATOMY OF PLEXUSES

Plexus is defined as a network of connections of nerve roots, giving rise to further interconnecting or terminal branches. As ventral (motor) and dorsal (sensory) roots leave the spinal cord, they soon unite within the spinal canal to form a spinal nerve. After exiting neural foramina, they form a network of interconnections (plexus), from ventral roots, trunks, and cords to individual nerves. Although there are many such stations in the body, the three main plexuses are cervical, brachial, and lumbosacral. Plexopathy may result when any of these segments of the plexus becomes involved. Since it may not be possible to visualize directly the abnormality within the nerve, one may have to rely on altered adjacent tissue to make a diagnosis. Thus, the knowledge of normal configuration, adjacent tissue characteristics, and spatial relationships of plexus components in reference to bony landmarks, vascular structures, and muscles is very important in detection of abnormality and interpretation of plexus disease.

Cervical and Brachial Plexus

The cervical plexus lies on the ventral surface of the medial scalene and levator scapulae muscles. It is formed by ventral rami of the cervical nerves C1 through C4. Each ramus at C2, C3, and C4 levels divides into two branches, superior and inferior. These, in turn, unite in the following way: superior branch of C2 with C1, inferior branch of C2 with superior branch of C3, inferior

KEY POINTS

- Involvement of plexus in a patient with cancer may be due to a tumor arising directly from neural components, direct (contiguous) metastatic spread from adjacent organs, or compression by adjacent tumor masses (eg, enlarged nodes).
- Magnetic resonance imaging (MRI), with and without contrast, has emerged as a leading method of imaging of plexus regions.
- Development of picture archiving and communication system (PACS) revolutionized the way the studies are viewed and interpreted by radiologists. Perhaps the best example is a cine mode option, which creates three-dimensional perception, allowing for better understanding of extent and configuration of lesions and their relation to adjacent normal structures, particularly vessels.
- The main advantages of MRI over computed tomography (CT) are ability of multiplanar scanning without change of patient's position, superior resolution, and tissue characterization.
- Primary plexus neoplasms, including schwannomas, perineuriomas, neurofibromas, and malignant peripheral nerve sheath tumors (MPNST), are usually present as well-defined, rounded, or oval masses orientated along the longitudinal axis of the nerve.
- Plexus may be compressed or infiltrated by an extrinsic neoplasm, arising from adjacent structures, with breast, neck, lung, and lymph node malignancies being most common offenders for brachial region and pelvic tumors for lumbosacral plexus.
- MRI in radiation-induced fibrosis (RIF) may reveal thickening and indistinct outline of plexus components, without identifiable focal mass.

---

branch of C3 with superior branch of C4, and inferior branch of C4 joins C5 to become part of the brachial plexus. Terminal cutaneous, muscular, and communicating branches supply skin and muscles in occipital area, upper neck, supraclavicular, upper pectoral region, and diaphragm.

The brachial plexus is formed by ventral rami of spinal nerves exiting through the neural foramina of the cervical spine at C5 to T1 levels (dorsal rami innervate posterior paravertebral muscles). Inconsistent contributions may arise from C4 and T2 segments. As the spinal nerves leave the foramina between vertebral artery anteriorly and facet joint posteriorly, they soon create the first station of connections between anterior and middle scalene muscles: C5 and C6 nerves unite to form superior trunk, C7 becomes middle trunk, and C8 and T1 form inferior trunk. Subclavian artery proceeds with the brachial plexus components within the triangle anteriorly to the trunks and subclavian vein courses in front of anterior scalene muscle. The trunks divide just laterally to the lateral margin of scalene muscles into three anterior and three posterior divisions. Pectoralis major and serratus anterior muscles constitute anterior and posterior boundaries, respectively. Anterior divisions of superior and middle trunks join to form lateral cord; anterior division of inferior trunk becomes medial cord, and posterior divisions of all three trunks unite to form posterior cord. The medial cord, which receives fibers from inferior C8 to T1 trunk, gives off the ulnar nerve. The lateral cord, containing contributions from superior and middle trunks (C5–C7) becomes the largest nerve of the upper extremity, the median nerve. The posterior cord contains fibers from all three trunks (C5–T1); its main pathway is the radial nerve. Other terminal branches include suprascapular, musculocutaneous, axillary, thoracodorsal, medial cutaneous, and long thoracic nerves (Figs. 11.1 and 11.2), (7,8).

Lumbosacral Plexus

The lumbosacral plexus is formed by ventral rami of the lumbar and sacral nerves, T12–S4. Lumbar part is formed by roots from T12—L4, and sacral component by L4–S4 roots. These divide into anterior and posterior divisions, which give rise to anterior and posterior branches, respectively. Anterior branches of the lumbar plexus include (in craniocaudal direction): iliohypogastric, ilioinguinal, genitofemoral, and obturator nerves; the same of sacral plexus are tibial component of sciatic nerve, posterior femoral cutaneous, and pudendal nerves. Posterior branches of lumbar plexus include lateral femoral cutaneous and femoral nerves, and those of sacral plexus are: peroneal component of sciatic nerve, superior and inferior gluteal, and piriformis nerves. The roots of lumbar plexus lie on the ventral surface of the posterior abdominal wall, proceeding in diagonal fashion anterolaterally, between fibers of psoas and iliacus muscles. The largest femoral nerve continues behind the inguinal ligament, supplying anterior and medial aspects of the thigh. The sacral plexus proceeds laterally along the posterior wall of the pelvis, where it lies between iliac vessels anterolaterally and piriform

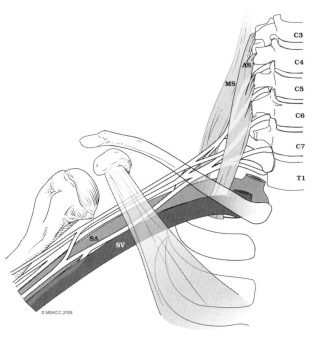

FIGURE 11.1

Brachial plexus proceeds laterally towards axillary fossa through the scalene triangle (bordered by anterior scalene [AS] and middle scalene [MS] muscles anteroposteriorly and first rib inferiorly), where it is located posteriorly to subclavian artery. Subclavian vein travels anteriorly to the anterior scalene muscle. SC—subclavian artery; SV—subclavian vein.

muscle posteromedially (Fig. 11.3). Terminal branches innervate pelvic organs, and the sciatic nerve, the largest nerve of the body, proceeds through the greater sciatic notch to supply regions of posterior thigh and below the knee (5).

RADIOGRAPHIC METHODS OF IMAGING

Evaluation of plexus with conventional radiography is difficult and yields little information (9). However, it may be used in preliminary evaluation of plexopathy, mainly to exclude major abnormality, such as bone destruction, fracture, lung infiltration, or ligamentous calcifications. Potential of computed tomography in detection of plexus disease has been realized by early investigators (10–15). Introduced in recent years, a new technique of multichannel scanning allows for uninterrupted data acquisition during continuous tube rotation and table advance (16). Further anatomical detail and tissue characteristics have been provided by MRI. Special sequences have been developed for selective imaging of nerve tissue (neurography). Sonography

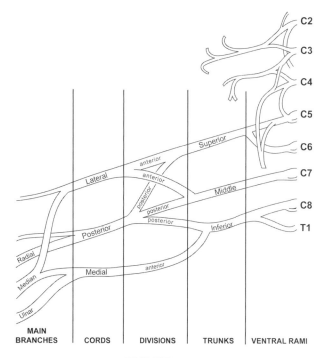

FIGURE 11.2

Schematic representation of cervical and brachial plexus network. Cervical plexus (C1–C4): Ventral rami C2, C3, and C4 divide, giving off superior and inferior branch at each level. Superior branch of C2 and C1 ramus unite to form ansa cervicalis. Adjacent inferior and superior branches of C2, C3, and C4 merge and give off lesser occipital, greater auricular, transverse cervical, supraclavicular, and phrenic nerves (unmarked). Brachial plexus (C5–T1): Superior, middle, and inferior trunks are formed by ventral rami of C5/C6, C7, and C8/T1, respectively. Each trunk divides into anterior and posterior divisions. Anterior divisions of superior and middle trunks form lateral cord; anterior division of inferior trunk becomes medial cord, and posterior divisions of all three trunks unite to form posterior cord. Major nerves of the arm—median, ulnar, and radial—receive contributions predominantly from lateral, medial, and posterior cords, respectively.

and positron emission tomography (PET) scanning also have been reported to provide valuable contributions (17–19). Development of picture archiving and communication system (PACS) revolutionized the way the studies are viewed and interpreted by radiologists. Perhaps the best example is a cine mode option, which enables three-dimensional perception, allowing for better understanding of extent and configuration of lesions and their relation to adjacent normal structures, particularly vessels. However, despite valuable contributions from these imaging methods, the assessment of plexus regions frequently presents a challenging problem for a clinician as well as a radiologist.

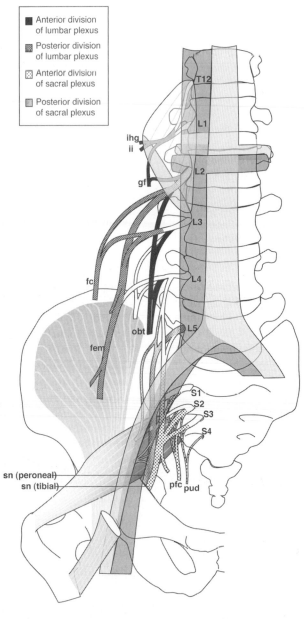

■ Anterior division
of lumbar plexus

▨ Posterior division
of lumbar plexus

▧ Anterior division
of sacral plexus

▨ Posterior division
of sacral plexus

FIGURE 11.3

Simplified coronal diagram of lumbosacral plexus depicted on a background of psoas, iliacus, and piriformis muscles. Anatomy of the lumbosacral plexus is much less intricate and more variable than that of brachial plexus. Anterior and posterior divisions unite and/or divide to form terminal branches (the trunks and cords are not distinguished). Anterior divisions of lumbar plexus unite to form iliohypogastric (ihg), ilioinguinal (ii), genitofemoral (gf), and obturator (obt) branches, whereas posterior divisions give rise to femoral cutaneous (fc) and femoral (fem) nerves. Of sacral plexus, anterior divisions divide to give rise to tibial component of sciatic nerve (sn), posterior femoral cutaneous (pfc), and pudendal nerves (pud), while posterior divisions give off peroneal component of sciatic nerve (sn), part of femoral cutaneous, gluteal, and piriformis nerves.

Technique

Because of its small size, the cervical plexus is rarely evaluated radiographically as a separate entity. Rather, it is included as a part of head, cervical spine, or neck examinations. Cervical plexus extends from C1 down to C4, thus scanning from skull base down to C5, utilizing small field of view (FOV) (25 cm), is sufficient. The anatomical brachial plexus extends approximately from C5 down to T2 vertebral levels. Adequate coverage of the plexus is provided by scanning the region from C4 to T3. However, we extend lower range with larger FOV down to T6 to include peripheral components within axillary fossas. Contiguous 4–5-mm spaced axial sections are obtained perpendicular to the table top. Coned-down view of the area in question may be added to the study. The elements of normal plexus are small and are depicted as nodular or linear areas of soft tissue density. They are difficult to identify and may not be outlined at all (20), particularly on inferior quality examination. Contrast injection is recommended (9), not only for identification of normal vascular structures and differentiation from lymph nodes, but also for more complete information on the enhancement pattern of the lesion. For this purpose, an intravenous injection in dynamic mode is preferred, using initial bolus of 50 cc, followed by contiguous infusion at the rate of 1 cc/second to a total of 100 cc of nonionic contrast (Omnipaque 300 or equivalent). The infusion should be administered on the site opposite to suspected pathology, since high concentration of intravenous contrast may produce streaking artifacts, obscuring detail (20).

Adequate coverage of the lumbosacral plexus includes axial sections from T12 down to the tip of the coccyx to visualize greater sciatic notches (GSN). Axial images with 4–5-mm slice thickness and FOV large enough to include both sacroiliac joints are usually sufficient. Intravenous contrast administration (100 cc of Omnipaque 300 or equivalent in dynamic mode or bolus injection) is recommended unless contraindicated. An intraoral contrast (Gastrografin, given two hours in advance) may be beneficial in assessment of plexus pathology, mainly to delineate distal urinary tract and colon, respectively.

MR Technique

The main advantages of MRI over CT are ability of multiplanar scanning without change of patient's position, superior resolution, and tissue characterization (21,22). Adequate anatomical coverage of the plexus must be assured. Thus, for brachial plexus, axial sections from levels of C3 down to T6 coronal sections, including glenohumeral joints and sagittal sections to cover both axillary fossas, should be obtained. For lumbosacral plexus, the coverage in axial plane needs to extend from T12 to coccyx. Sections of 5-mm thickness/0.25 gap are obtained in axial, sagittal, and coronal planes. We prefer scanning in direct axial, sagittal, and coronal planes (23), although oblique scanning planes have been advocated for brachial (24) and sacral plexus (25) to optimize visualization of plexus components and sciatic nerve. T1, fast spin echo T2, and short tau inversion recovery (STIR) (fat suppression) should be obtained. Use of phased-array coils is recommended for greater resolution of detail (26,27). Intravenous contrast (Magnevist or equivalent) is utilized routinely in a dose of 0.1 mmol/kg of body weight.

Visualization of Normal Plexus Components on CT and MRI

Conventional (noncontrast) CT offers rather poor definition of structures within the subarachnoid sac (spinal cord, roots of cauda equina). Nerve roots exiting laterally through foramina are more consistently seen, particularly in lumbar spine and sacrum, because of larger size and more abundant epidural fat. They are depicted as punctate or linear structures of muscle density, contrasting against the adjacent darker fat within the foramen or vicinity (Fig. 11.4). Trunks and cords of the brachial plexus are usually blended with muscle fibers and major vessels more distally. With

abundant fat tissue, individual nerve components may be visible as discrete, linear areas of soft tissue density, proceeding posteriorly along the subclavian artery (Fig. 11.5). Those of the lumbar plexus enter paraspinal musculature (psoas) and are difficult to identify with certainty. Femoral and obturator nerves may be visible, contrasted against the intrapelvic/intra-abdominal fat. The largest sciatic nerve (Fig. 11.6) is more consistently identified in the lateral aspect of GSN posteriorly to the ischial spine.

MRI depicts the plexus components with much greater accuracy (19,22,28), still improved when phased-array coils are used (27,29). Conventional T1 weighted sequences are routinely utilized for anatomic detail. Although individual nerves down to 2 mm in

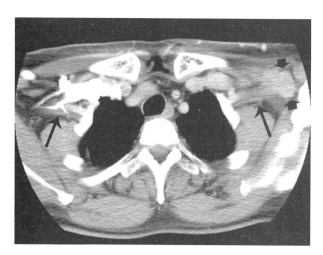

FIGURE 11.5

Axial CT image through thoracic inlet. Fibers of brachial plexus proceed posteriorly to vascular bundle (arrows). A lobulated mass (arrowheads) is visible more laterally on the left, representing recurrent metastatic breast cancer.

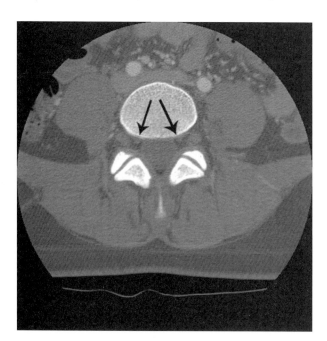

FIGURE 11.4

Axial CT section through inferior plate of L4. Nerve roots are clearly seen bilaterally (arrows) contrasting against a low-density background of fat tissue.

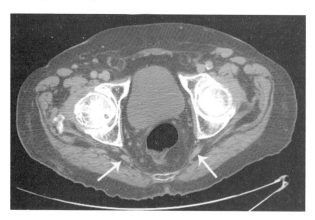

FIGURE 11.6

Axial CT section through the greater sciatic notch (GSN). Sciatic nerves (arrows) are visualized in the lateral aspect of GSN posteriorly to the ischial spine.

diameter can be seen (27), much of the success depends upon relaxation properties of adjacent tissues. Thus, even a smaller branch surrounded by fat or fluid (cerebrospinal fluid [CSF]) can be seen clearly, while a larger neural trunk encompassed by infiltrative process will blend with the abnormal tissue and may not be recognized at all. T2 weighted sequences (fast spin echo [FSE]) provide best detail of normal nerve when contrast interphase of fluid (CSF) or abnormal tissue (eg, edema) is present.

Thus, spinal nerves within the canal are demonstrated in good detail on T1 and T2 sequences because they contrast against fat (epidural) and fluid (CSF), respectively. Special sequences have been designed to create "myelographic effect," depicting the cord and roots within the thecal sac throughout the spine (30). Fat suppression sequences (STIR being most commonly used) null fat signal, thus rendering background fat tissue darker and nerve more clearly visible (31,32). The option can be applied to both T1 and T2 weighted sequences, and is most valuable in conjunction with contrast enhancement.

The normal neural components of plexus can be identified with various success on a good-quality MRI. Nerve roots within the foramina and immediate vicinity are routinely seen. As they descend with the muscle fibers, trunks and cords of the brachial plexus can be identified on axial images, proceeding between anterior and middle scalene group laterally to exit through the scalene triangle. Extended segments of the plexus may be demonstrated on one well-placed axial and/or coronal T1 weighted anatomic image (Fig. 11.7). Sagittal sections through and laterally to the scalene triangle outline the individual divisions as punctate areas of soft tissue intensity within the fat background, with subclavian artery and vein anteriorly (Fig. 11.8). Similarly, the lumbar and sacral roots within the subarachnoid space and neural foramina are seen in detail, while interconnecting network within the psoas complex is more difficult to identify. On axial sections, femoral nerve may be visualized as a single trunk proceeding anterolaterally along the ventral aspect of posterior abdominal wall. The greater sciatic nerve within the notch is more consistently seen, either as a single oval structure or as a cluster of several smaller individual nerves (Fig. 11.9), (6,22).

Abnormal Nerve

When involved by a disease, nerve tissue may exhibit swelling, focal or diffuse infiltration, edema, cyst formation, or necrosis. In the early stage, when there is no enlargement of peripheral nerve(s), these changes may not be appreciated on imaging modalities, but become more apparent as the process progresses. On

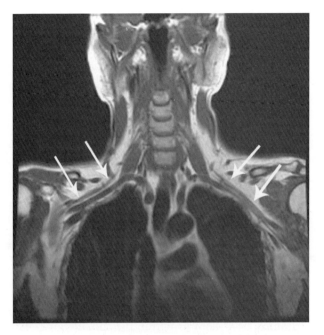

FIGURE 11.7

MRI of the brachial plexus. Long segments of plexus fibers (arrows) are demonstrated on coronal T1 weighted image.

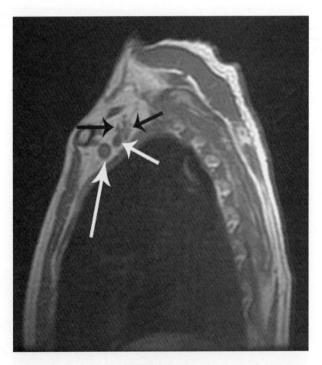

FIGURE 11.8

Sagittal T1 weighted image through the axillary fossa on the same patient as in Figure 11.7. Brachial plexus components (black arrows) depicted as nodular, somewhat irregular, soft tissue densities posteriorly to the artery (short white arrow) and vein (long white arrow), which are the rounded lower-intensity structures anteriorly.

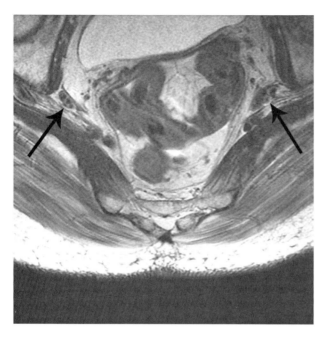

FIGURE 11.9

Sciatic nerves (arrows) depicted on axial T1 weighted MR image through the pelvic region as a conglomerate of individual fibers.

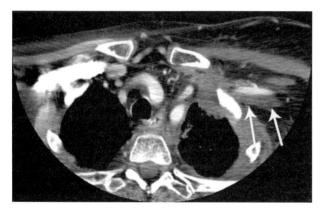

FIGURE 11.10

Recurrent breast cancer. Axial CT image demonstrates general thickening of the neurovascular bundle (arrows).

CT, abnormal nerve or plexus may appear locally or diffusely enlarged, or become indistinguishable from adjacent structures because of infiltrative process or fibrosis. In brachial plexus, this may be manifested as general thickening of neurovascular bundle (Fig. 11.10). Greater tissue discrimination allows MRI to assess the character and extent of disease more precisely. T1 weighted images may show segmental or diffuse enlargement, and increased T2 intensity may be seen within the nerve in case of involvement by infiltrative process or edema. The extent of the abnormal T2

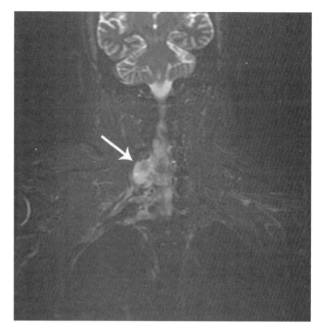

FIGURE 11.11

Coronal STIR MRI noncontrast sequence enhances visualization of the tumor tissue (arrow and bright areas on the right side).

signal may be demonstrated to the better advantage on fat suppression (STIR) sequences (Fig. 11.11). Contiguity (or disruption) of the nerve, increased diameter, change of course or contour (compression), altered intrinsic intensity, or enhancement within involved or compressed segment of the nerve may be observed. Neurography, utilizing combination of T1, T2, STIR, short inversion recovery (IR) sequences, and phased-array surface coils depict these changes with greater accuracy (4,33–35). In a study of 15 patients with neuropathic leg pain and negative or inconclusive conventional MRI conducted by Moore et al. (36), it proved definitely superior, revealing abnormality accounting for clinical findings in all cases.

An interesting phenomenon of increased T2 intensity within normal nerve(s), mimicking a diseased tissue, was reported by Chappell et al. (37) They observed raising intensity within the peripheral nerve as the orientation of longitudinal axis of the nerve approached 55 degrees to main magnetic field Bo. As the brachial plexus is usually scanned close to this "magic angle," T2 hyperintensity within the nerve or plexus should thus be interpreted with caution to avoid false-positive reading. Administration of contrast is essential in proper evaluation of extent of disease. Generally, enhancement of intraspinal or peripheral nerve after administration of conventional dose of gadolinium-based contrast is considered pathological.

Imaging Method of Choice

As x-rays yielded limited information on plexus involvement, early reports praised the ability of CT to demonstrate anatomic detail of normal and diseased plexus and its advantages over conventional radiography (10,14). As early as 1988, Benzel et al. considered CT a method of choice in evaluation of location and extent of nerve sheath tumors of sciatic nerve and sacral plexus, important in determination of resectability of these lesions. Hirakata et al. (15) found CT to be helpful in assessment of patients with Pancoast tumor. They reported obliteration of fat plane between scalene muscles on CT to be an indication of brachial plexus involvement. Addition of sagittal, coronal, and oblique reformatted images improved visualization of brachial plexus and helped to diagnose tumor recurrence (38). Soon after introduction of MRI, and as early as 1987, Castagno and Shuman (39) anticipated that new modality may have substantial clinical utility in evaluating patients with suspected brachial plexus tumor. The advantages of MRI over CT in assessment of plexus were reported in comparative studies by several investigators (40–42). In evaluation of 64 patients with brachial plexopathy of diverse cause by Bilbey et al. (43), the sensitivity of MRI was 63%, specificity 100%, and accuracy 77%. In subgroup of patients with trauma and neoplasm, these were even higher (81%, 100%, and 88%, respectively). Better anatomic definition provided by MRI was considered to improve patient care in the study by Collins et al. (44) In the study of patients with plexopathy following the treatment of breast cancer, Qayyum et al. (45) reported high reliability of MRI, with specificity of 95%, positive predictive value of 96%, and negative predictive value of 95%. MRI without and with contrast enhancement is also a method of choice in evaluating a patient with plexopathy at Memorial Sloan-Kettering Cancer Center.

PRIMARY PLEXUS NEOPLASMS

Primary tumors of peripheral nerve (plexus) are rare, constituting approximately 1% of all cancers. According to World Health Organization (WHO) classification proposed in 2000, four groups are distinguished: (1) schwannomas; (2) perineuriomas; (3) neurofibromas, and (4) malignant peripheral nerve sheath tumors (MPNST). Neurofibromas and schwannomas are most prevalent. On MRI, these tumors usually present as well-defined rounded or oval masses orientated along the longitudinal axis of the nerve (Fig. 11.12). Larger size or plexiform appearance favors neurofibroma, particularly in patients with neurofibromatosis (Fig. 11.13). Both are iso- or slightly hyperintense on T1 and hyperin-

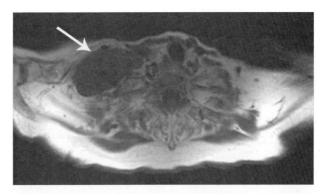

FIGURE 11.12

Brachial plexus schwannoma, depicted on axial T1 weighted MR image. Fusiform mass (arrows) is orientated along the longitudinal axis of the plexus.

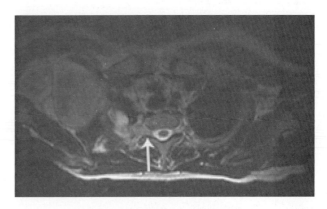

FIGURE 11.13

Patient with neurofibroma. Large mass is demonstrated in axillary fossa, involving brachial plexus and extending into the neural foramen (arrow).

tense on T2 weighted sequences, showing homogenous or inhomogeneous enhancement. Marked T2 hyperintensity may be seen in some patients (46–50). Capsule can be identified in approximately 70% of schwannomas and 30% of neurofibromas (45). A "target sign," consisting of central low-intensity area within the lesion on T2 weighted sequence, was found to be much more frequent in neurofibromas (51,52). On a CT, low density (in reference to the muscle) was a common feature of plexus tumors, and contrast enhancement varied from moderate to marked, as reported by Verstraete (53). MPNSTs are rare, arising either as spontaneous mutation or within preexisting neurofibroma, usually as a transformation to spindle cell sarcoma (54). It may be difficult to distinguish these tumors from their benign counterpart. Larger size, internal heterogeneity, poor definition of peripheral border, invasion of fat planes, and adjacent edema favor malignant variant

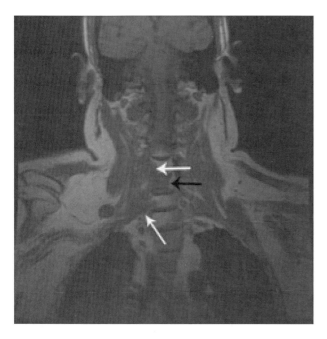

FIGURE 11.14

Malignant PNST, coronal T1 weighted MRI (the same patient as in Figure 11.11). The tumor (white arrows) is poorly defined and infiltrates adjacent cervical vertebrae (black arrow).

(Fig. 11.14) (55–58). Extremely rarely, other malignancies (eg, lymphoma) can arise from the nerve proper (59). There are no pathognomonic radiographic features that could be totally attributed to a particular group; thus, thorough knowledge of clinical information, such as age, gender, duration of symptoms, history of von Recklinghausen disease, etc., is helpful while interpreting the imaging studies.

EXTRINSIC PLEXUS TUMORS

Plexus may be compressed or infiltrated by an extrinsic neoplasm, arising from adjacent structures, with breast, neck, lung, and lymph node malignancies being most common offenders for brachial region and pelvic tumors for lumbosacral plexus (Fig. 11.15). Clinically, pain is a prominent feature of residual or recurrent tumor (1). Although local extent of the lesion may be depicted adequately by CT, infiltration of the plexus is difficult to diagnose, except for advanced disease with gross infiltration of the plexus region. In a study of 14 patients with Pancoast tumor (15), obliteration of fat planes between scalene muscles on CT was found to be suggestive of plexus involvement. The potential of MRI in evaluation of extent of thoracic malignancies and brachial plexus involvement was realized as early as 1989 (40). In the study of chest wall tumors by

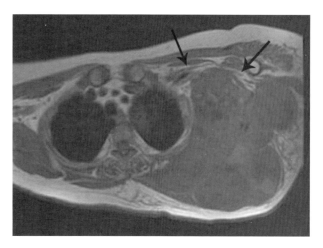

FIGURE 11.15

Axial CT section through thoracic inlet of patient with advanced osteogenic sarcoma of the scapula. Neurovascular elements (arrows) are compressed and displaced anteriorly.

Fortier (60), MRI clearly delineated the margins and revealed evidence of muscle, vascular, or bone invasion. T1 and T2 signal characteristics were nonspecific (apart for lipomas), not allowing for confident distinction of benign from malignant process. Qayyum (45) considered MRI to be a reliable and accurate tool in evaluation of brachial plexopathy due to tumor, reporting sensitivity, and positive predictive value of 96% and specificity and negative predictive value of 95%. Currently, MRI without and with contrast remains a method of choice for the assessment of local tumor extent and plexus involvement. PET scan is considered useful in evaluation of patients with plexopathy, mainly by excluding recurrent tumor (17,18).

RADIATION INJURY

Plexopathy is a recognized complication of radiation therapy, occurring most commonly in brachial plexus (Kori, 1981), following regional treatment of breast, lung, or neck cancers. Clinical presentation of radiation-induced fibrosis (RIF) is that of protracted course, with low-grade pain, as opposed to recurrent tumor, which is progressing more rapidly, with pain being a dominant symptom. Three forms are recognized: acute ischemic, transient, and delayed (radiation fibrosis), the latter being most common (61–63). Radiation-induced fibrosis occurs usually within the first few years after completion of treatment, although latent periods as long as 22 years have been reported (64,65). It is dose-dependent, more likely to occur above 6000 cGy and with larger fraction size. Younger patients and those

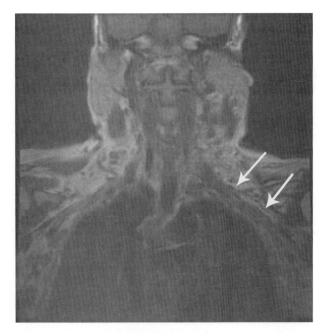

FIGURE 11.16

Patient with breast cancer and suspected postradiation left brachial plexopathy. MRI reveals matting and thickening of the left neurovascular bundle (arrows) without recognizable soft tissue mass, consistent with clinical diagnosis of RIF.

receiving cytotoxic therapy are more vulnerable (1,66). Changes are confined to the radiation port, with clearly demarcated margin from nonirradiated tissue. The main role of imaging is to distinguish this chronic iatrogenic process from a recurrent tumor, which generally carries unfavorable prognosis. CT may demonstrate poor definition of neurovascular bundle and increased density of regional fat without recognizable soft tissue mass (67), and MRI may reveal thickening and indistinct outline of plexus components, again without identifiable focal mass (Fig. 11.16). There is no uniform agreement as to signal intensity patterns and contrast enhancement of RIF. While some investigators reported low intensity of both on T1 and T2 weighted sequences (68), others described variable signal changes (69–71). Parascalene and interscalene T2 hyperintensity was reported by Bowen (72), and the degree of T2 hyperintensity was found to correspond with severity of fibrosis by Hoeller (71). Positive contrast enhancement was reported by most investigators, even in delayed cases (69).

SUMMARY

Clinical assessment of plexus involvement by primary neoplasm, metastases, or conditions related to treatment is limited, and imaging studies (CT, MRI) are routinely requested to further characterize the nature and extent of the process. With its many advantages

over CT, MRI, without and with contrast, is presently considered an imaging method of choice in evaluation of plexus disease. Utilizing high-resolution devices, we are now able to visualize individual nerves (MR neurography). However, there are still many limitations of MRI technique, such as inhomogenous fat suppression or vascular flow artifacts, making the interpretation difficult. Although abnormal signal or enhancement within the individual nerve can be depicted, the process cannot be further characterized (eg, benign or malignant). Recently introduced into clinical practice, higher field strength (3T) MRI may offer superior resolution and improved option for functional imaging. As the state of the art approach at present, it includes thorough clinical examination, followed by high-resolution phase-array MRI without and with contrast. Dynamic CT should be reserved for patients unable to have MRI and instances when additional information on bone detail or vascular anatomy is also needed. PET scan plays a complementary role to MRI in assessment of neoplastic involvement.

References

1. Kori SH, Foley KM, et al. Brachial plexus lesions in patients with cancer: 100 cases. *Neurology.* 1981;31(1):45–50.
2. Jaeckle KA. Neurological manifestations of neoplastic and radiation-induced plexopathies. *Semin Neurol.* 2004;24(4):385–393.
3. Filler AG, Howe FA, et al. Magnetic resonance neurography. *Lancet.* 1993;341(8846):659–661.
4. Filler AG, Kliot M, et al. Application of magnetic resonance neurography in the evaluation of patients with peripheral nerve pathology. *J Neurosurg.* 1996;85(2):299–309.
5. Aagaard BD, Maravilla KR, et al. MR neurography. MR imaging of peripheral nerves. *Magn Reson Imaging Clin N Am.* 1998;6(1):179–194.
6. Freund W, Brinkmann A, et al. MR neurography with multiplanar reconstruction of 3D MRI datasets: an anatomical study and clinical applications. *Neuroradiology.* 2007.
7. Clemente DC. The peripheral nervous system. In: *Gray's Anatomy, Thirtieth American Edition.* Philadelphia: Lea & Febiger Publishers; 1985:1149–1282.
8. Castillo M. Imaging the anatomy of the brachial plexus: review and self-assessment module. *AJR Am J Roentgenol.* 2005;185(6 Suppl):S196–S204.
9. Posniak HV, Olson MC, et al. MR imaging of the brachial plexus. *AJR Am J Roentgenol.* 1993;161(2):373–379.
10. Benzel EC, Morris DM, et al. Nerve sheath tumors of the sciatic nerve and sacral plexus. *J Surg Oncol.* 1988;39(1):8–16.
11. Cooke J, Cooke D, et al. The anatomy and pathology of the brachial plexus as demonstrated by computed tomography. *Clin Radiol.* 1988;39(6):595–601.
12. Dietemann JL, Sick H, et al. Anatomy and computed tomography of the normal lumbosacral plexus. *Neuroradiology.* 1987;29(1):58–68.
13. Gebarski KS, Glazer GM, et al. Brachial plexus: anatomic, radiologic, and pathologic correlation using computed tomography. *J Comput Assist Tomogr.* 1982;6(6):1058–1063.
14. Gebarski KS, Gebarski SS, et al. The lumbosacral plexus: anatomic-radiologic-pathologic correlation using CT. *Radiographics.* 1986;6(3):401–425.
15. Hirakata K, Nakata H, et al. Computed tomography of Pancoast tumor. *Rinsho Hoshasen.* 1989;34(1):79–84.

16. Rydberg J, Liang Y, et al. Fundamentals of multichannel CT. *Semin Musculoskelet Radiol*. 2004;8(2):137–146.

17. Graif M, Martinoli C, et al. Sonographic evaluation of brachial plexus pathology. *Eur Radiol*. 2004;14(2):193–200.

18. Hathaway PB, Mankoff DA, et al. Value of combined FDG PET and MR imaging in the evaluation of suspected recurrent local-regional breast cancer: preliminary experience. *Radiology*. 1999;210(3):807–814.

19. Ahmad A, Barrington S, et al. Use of positron emission tomography in evaluation of brachial plexopathy in breast cancer patients. *Br J Cancer*. 1999;79(3–4):478–482.

20. Krol G, Strong E. Computed tomography of head and neck malignancies. *Clin Plast Surg*. 1986;13(3):475–491.

21. Carriero A, Ciccotosto C, et al. Magnetic resonance imaging of the brachial plexus. Anatomy. *Radiol Med (Torino)*. 1991;81(1–2):73–77.

22. Gierada DS, Erickson SJ, et al. MR imaging of the sacral plexus: normal findings. *AJR Am J Roentgenol*. 1993;160(5):1059–1065.

23. Blake LC, Robertson WD, et al. Sacral plexus: optimal imaging planes for MR assessment. *Radiology*. 1996;199(3):767–772.

24. Panasci DJ, Holliday RA, et al. Advanced imaging techniques of the brachial plexus. *Hand Clin*. 1995;11(4):545–553.

25. Almanza MY, Poon-Chue A, et al. Dual oblique MR method for imaging the sciatic nerve. *J Comput Assist Tomogr*. 1999;23(1):138–140.

26. Kichari JR, Hussain SM, et al. MR imaging of the brachial plexus: current imaging sequences, normal findings, and findings in a spectrum of focal lesions with MR-pathologic correlation. *Curr Probl Diagn Radiol*. 2003;32(2):88–101.

27. Maravilla KR, Bowen BC. Imaging of the peripheral nervous system: evaluation of peripheral neuropathy and plexopathy. *AJNR Am J Neuroradiol*. 1998;19(6):1011–1023.

28. Blair DN, Rapoport S, et al. Normal brachial plexus: MR imaging. *Radiology*. 1987;165(3):763–767.

29. Bowen BC, Pattany PM, et al. The brachial plexus: normal anatomy, pathology, and MR imaging. *Neuroimaging Clin N Am*. 2004;14(1):59–85, vii–viii.

30. Gasparotti R, Ferraresi S, et al. Three-dimensional MR myelography of traumatic injuries of the brachial plexus. *AJNR Am J Neuroradiol*. 1997;18(9):1733–1742.

31. Tien RD, Hesselink JR, et al. Improved detection and delineation of head and neck lesions with fat suppression spin-echo MR imaging. *AJNR Am J Neuroradiol*. 1991;12(1):19–24.

32. Howe FA, Filler AG, et al. Magnetic resonance neurography. *Magn Reson Med*. 1992;28(2):328–338.

33. Dailey AT, Tsuruda JS, et al. Magnetic resonance neurography for cervical radiculopathy: a preliminary report. *Neurosurgery*. 1996;38(3):488–492, discussion 492.

34. Erdem CZ, Erdem LO, et al. High resolution MR neurography in patients with cervical radiculopathy. *Tani Girisim Radyol*. 2004;10(1):14–19.

35. Lewis AM, Layzer R, et al. Magnetic resonance neurography in extraspinal sciatica. *Arch Neurol*. 2006;63(10):1469–1472.

36. Moore KR, Tsuruda JS, et al. The value of MR neurography for evaluating extraspinal neuropathic leg pain: a pictorial essay. *AJNR Am J Neuroradiol*. 2001;22(4):786–794.

37. Chappell KE, Robson MD, et al. Magic angle effects in MR neurography. *AJNR Am J Neuroradiol*. 2004;25(3):431–440.

38. Fishman EK, Campbell JN, et al. Multiplanar CT evaluation of brachial plexopathy in breast cancer. *J Comput Assist Tomogr*. 1991;15(5):790–795.

39. Castagno AA, Shuman WP. MR imaging in clinically suspected brachial plexus tumor. *AJR Am J Roentgenol*. 1987;149(6):1219–1222.

40. Rapoport S, Blair DN, et al. Brachial plexus: correlation of MR imaging with CT and pathologic findings. *Radiology*. 1988;167(1):161–165.

41. Thyagarajan D, Cascino T, et al. Magnetic resonance imaging in brachial plexopathy of cancer. *Neurology*. 1995;45(3 Pt 1):421–427.

42. Taylor BV, Kimmel DW, et al. Magnetic resonance imaging in cancer-related lumbosacral plexopathy. *Mayo Clin Proc*. 1997;72(9):823–829.

43. Bilbey JH, Lamond RG, et al. MR imaging of disorders of the brachial plexus. *J Magn Reson Imaging*. 1994;4(1):13–18.

44. Collins JD, Shaver ML, et al. Compromising abnormalities of the brachial plexus as displayed by magnetic resonance imaging. *Clin Anat*. 1995;8(1):1–16.

45. Qayyum A, MacVicar AD, et al. Symptomatic brachial plexopathy following treatment for breast cancer: utility of MR imaging with surface-coil techniques. *Radiology*. 2000;214(3):837–842.

46. Baba Y, Ohkubo K, et al. MR imaging appearances of schwannoma: correlation with pathological findings. *Nippon Igaku Hoshasen Gakkai Zasshi*. 1997;57(8):499–504.

47. Cerofolini E, Landi A, et al. MR of benign peripheral nerve sheath tumors. *J Comput Assist Tomogr*. 1991;15(4):593–597.

48. Soderlund V, Goranson H, et al. MR imaging of benign peripheral nerve sheath tumors. *Acta Radiol*. 1994;35(3):282–286.

49. Saifuddin A. Imaging tumours of the brachial plexus. *Skeletal Radiol*. 2003;32(7):375–387.

50. Hayasaka K, Tanaka Y, et al. MR findings in primary retroperitoneal schwannoma. *Acta Radiol*. 1999;40(1):78–82.

51. Bhargava R, Parham DM, et al. MR imaging differentiation of benign and malignant peripheral nerve sheath tumors: use of the target sign. *Pediatr Radiol*. 1997;27(2):124–129.

52. Burk DL, Jr., Brunberg JA, et al. Spinal and paraspinal neurofibromatosis: surface coil MR imaging at 1.5 T1. *Radiology*. 1987;162(3):797–801.

53. Verstraete KL, Achten E, et al. Nerve sheath tumors: evaluation with CT and MR imaging. *J Belge Radiol*. 1992;75(4):311–320.

54. Antonescu C, Woodruff J. (2006). Primary tumors of cranial, spinal and peripheral nerves. In: McLendon RE, Rosenblum MK, Bigner DD, eds. *Russell and Rubinstein's Pathology of Tumors of the Nervous System*, 7th ed. Hodder Arnold Publisher; 2006:787–835.

55. Levine E, Huntrakoon M, et al. Malignant nerve-sheath neoplasms in neurofibromatosis: distinction from benign tumors by using imaging techniques. *AJR Am J Roentgenol*. 1987;149(5):1059–1064.

56. Fuchs B, Spinner RJ, et al. Malignant peripheral nerve sheath tumors: an update. *J Surg Orthop Adv*. 2005;14(4):168–174.

57. Geniets C, Vanhoenacker FM, et al. Imaging features of peripheral neurogenic tumors. *Jbr-Btr*. 2006;89(4):216–219.

58. Amoretti N, Grimaud A, et al. Peripheral neurogenic tumors: is the use of different types of imaging diagnostically useful? *Clin Imaging*. 2006;30(3):201–205.

59. Descamps MJ, Barrett L, et al. Primary sciatic nerve lymphoma: a case report and review of the literature. *J Neurol Neurosurg Psychiatry*. 2006;77(9):1087–1089.

60. Fortier M, Mayo JR, Swensen SJ, Munk PL, Vellet DA, Muller NL. MR imaging of chest wall lesions. *Radiographics*. 1994;14(3):597–606.

61. Gerard JM, Franck N, Moussa Z, Hildebrand J. Acute ischemic brachial plexus neuropathy following radiation therapy. *Neurology*. March 1989;39(3):450–451.

62. Salner AL, Botnick LE, et al. Reversible brachial plexopathy following primary radiation therapy for breast cancer. *Cancer Treat Rep*. 1981;65(9–10):797–802.

63. Maruyama Y, Mylrea MM, Logothetis J. Neuropathy following irradiation. An unusual late complication of radiotherapy. *Am J Roentgenol Ther Nucl Med*. September 1967;101(1):216–219.

64. Fathers E, Thrush D, et al. Radiation-induced brachial plexopathy in women treated for carcinoma of the breast. *Clin Rehabil*. 2002;16(2):160–165.

65. Nich C, Bonnin P, et al. An uncommon form of delayed radio-induced brachial plexopathy. *Chir Main*. 2005;24(1):48–51.

66. Olsen NK, Pfeiffer P, Johannsen L, Schroder H, Rose C. Radiation-induced brachial plexopathy: neurological follow-up in

161 recurrence free breast cancer patients. *Int J Radiat Biol Phys*. April 30, 1993;26(1):43–49.

67. Cascino TL, Kori S, et al. CT of the brachial plexus in patients with cancer. *Neurology*. 1983;33(12):1553–1557.

68. Wittenberg KH, Adkins MC. MR imaging of nontraumatic brachial plexopathies: frequency and spectrum of findings. *Radiographics*. 2000;20(4):1023–1032.

69. Wouter van Es H, Engelen AM, et al. Radiation-induced brachial plexopathy: MR imaging. *Skeletal Radiol*. 1997;26(5):284–288.

70. Dao TH, Rahmouni A, et al. Tumor recurrence versus fibrosis in the irradiated breast: differentiation with dynamic gadolinium-enhanced MR imaging. *Radiology*. 1993;187(3):751–755.

71. Hoeller U, Bonacker M, et al. Radiation-induced plexopathy and fibrosis. Is magnetic resonance imaging the adequate diagnostic tool? *Strahlenther Onkol*. 2004;180(10):650–654.

72. Bowen BC, Verma A, et al. Radiation-induced brachial plexopathy: MR and clinical findings. *AJNR Am J Neuroradiol*. 1996;17(10):1932–1936.

73. Garant M, Remy H, et al. Aggressive fibromatosis of the neck: MR findings. *AJNR Am J Neuroradiol*. 1997;18(8):1429–1431.

74. Gierada DS, Erickson SJ. MR imaging of the sacral plexus: abnormal findings. *AJR Am J Roentgenol*. 1993;160(5):1067–1071.

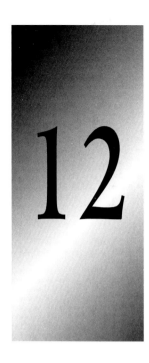

Cancer Statistics

Melissa M. Center
Ahmedin Jemal

Cancer is a complex constellation of hundreds of diseases (1) whose occurrence varies strikingly according to age, sex, race/ethnicity, socioeconomic status, geographic location, and time. Close examination of these variations has provided strong evidence that much of cancer is caused by environmental factors and is potentially avoidable (2). Monitoring time trends in cancer occurrence is also important to assess the effectiveness of cancer prevention and control efforts in the overall population and in subgroups that may be at higher risk. This chapter describes cancer occurrence patterns in the United States for all cancers combined and for seven select cancer sites, which together account for 58% of the total new cases in the United States (3).

DATA SOURCES

In the United States, the Surveillance, Epidemiology, and End Results (SEER) program has been collecting cancer incidence data in nine population-based cancer registries since 1975. These registries, which provide information on temporal trends, cover approximately 10% of the U.S. population. Subsequent expansions of the SEER program provide coverage of approximately 26% of the U.S. population (http://www.seer.cancer.gov) (4). The Centers for Disease Control and Prevention's National Program of Cancer Registries (NPCR) was established in 1994 to improve existing non-SEER

population-based cancer registries and to establish new statewide cancer registries (http://www.cdc.gov/cancer/npcr). Through the NPCR and SEER programs, cancer data are collected in almost all parts of the United States, although data quality varies across registries.

Mortality data have been collected for most of the United States since 1930, based on information from death certificates. The underlying cause of death is classified according to the most current International Statistical Classification of Diseases (ICD). Beginning with the 1999 mortality data, underlying causes of death are classified according to ICD-10 coding and selection rules, replacing ICD-9, which was used from 1979–1998 (5). The ICD-10 codes for malignant cancer are C00-C97 (6). Mortality data are available from the National Center for Health Statistics (http://www.cdc.gov/nchs/nvss.htm).

MEASUREMENTS OF CANCER OCCURRENCE

Incidence and Mortality

Incidence and mortality rates are two frequently used measures of cancer occurrence. These indices quantify the number of new cancer cases or deaths, respectively, in a specified population over a defined time period. They are commonly expressed as counts per

KEY POINTS

- Cancer is a complex constellation of hundreds of diseases whose occurrence varies strikingly according to age, sex, race/ethnicity, socioeconomic status, geographic location, and time.
- In the United States, the Surveillance, Epidemiology, and End Results (SEER) program has been collecting cancer incidence data in nine population-based cancer registries since 1975.
- Mortality data have been collected for most of the United States since 1930, based on information from death certificates.
- Incidence is the number of new cancer cases or deaths, respectively, in a specified population over a defined time period and is commonly expressed as counts per 100,000 people per year.
- Prevalence measures the proportion of people living with cancer at a certain point in time.
- The relative survival rate for a specific disease reflects the proportion of people alive at a specified period after diagnosis, usually five years, compared

to that of a population of equivalent age, sex, and race without the disease.
- The risk of developing cancer is affected by age, race, sex, socioeconomic status, geographic location, and calendar year.
- It is estimated that 1,444,920 new cancer cases and 559,650 new deaths due to cancer will occur in the United States in 2007.
- The probability of developing invasive cancer over a lifetime is about 45% for men and 38% for women.
- Survival rates for all cancers combined have increased significantly, from 50% during the period 1975–1977 to 66% during 1996–2003.
- The three most commonly diagnosed cancers in the United States in 2007 will be prostate, lung and bronchus, and colon and rectum in men and breast, lung and bronchus, and colon and rectum in females.
- Lung cancer accounts for the most cancer-related deaths in both men and women.

100,000 people per year and are age-standardized to allow comparisons across populations of varying age structure.

Prevalence

Prevalence measures the proportion of people living with cancer at a certain point in time. In principle, the number of prevalent cases includes newly diagnosed cases, those who are undergoing treatment, and people who are in remission. It is influenced by both the incidence rate of the cancers of interest and by survival or cure rates. In practice, estimates of the number of prevalent cases in the United States represent the total number of cancer cases diagnosed in a specified duration. Therefore, they cannot distinguish precisely between people who have been cured and those with active disease. There were 10.7 million people with a history of cancer (Table 12.1) in the United States in January 2004.

The Probability of Developing or Dying from Cancer

The probability that an individual will develop or die from cancer by a certain age is another measure used

to describe average risk in the general population. The probability, usually expressed as a percentage, can also be expressed as one person in X persons. These estimates are based on the average experience of the general population and may over- or underestimate individual risk because of family history or individual risk factors. The probability of developing cancer or dying of cancer are calculated using Probability of Developing Cancer Software (DevCan) developed by the National Cancer Institute (http://www.srab.cancer.gov/devcan/).

Estimated New Cancer Cases and Deaths

Each year, the American Cancer Society estimates the total number of new cancer cases and deaths that will occur in the nation and in each state in the current year. These estimates are of interest because actual mortality statistics do not become available for approximately three years. The American Cancer Society projections are more readily understood by the public than are projections of cancer rates, and are frequently cited by cancer control planners and researchers (7). The estimates are produced by modeling historic information on the observed number of cancer cases and deaths in past years and modeling trends over time (8,9).

Survival Rate

The relative survival rate for a specific disease reflects the proportion of people alive at a specified period after diagnosis, usually five years, compared to that of a population of equivalent age, sex, and race without the disease. It adjusts for normal life expectancy (events such as deaths from heart disease, accidents, and diseases of old age).

DEMOGRAPHIC AND GEOGRAPHIC FACTORS

As mentioned, the risk of developing cancer is affected by age, race, sex, socioeconomic status, geographic location, and calendar year.

Age

Age profoundly affects the risk of being diagnosed with cancer. For most cancers, the incidence rates increase with age because of cumulative exposures to carcinogenic agents such as tobacco, infectious organisms, chemicals, and internal factors, such as inherited mutations, hormones, and immune conditions. Figure 12.1 (left panel) depicts the age-related increase in the incidence rate from all cancer combined in men

and women. The incidence rate for age 0–4 years is twice that for ages 5–9 and 10–14 due to cancers such as acute lymphocytic leukemia, neuroblastoma, and retinoblastoma that have higher incidence rates among young children. The decrease in cancer incidence rates after age 84 may largely reflect underdiagnosis. The median age at diagnosis for most cancer sites is 60 or above. Cancers with median ages of diagnosis under 50 include cancers of the testis, bones and joints, thyroid, and cervix and Hodgkin disease.

Sex

Cancer affects both men and women, unless it is sex-specific. However, the incidence rates of most types of cancer are higher in men than in women (Table 12.2). The most extreme example is cancer of the larynx, for which the incidence rate is nearly five times as high in males as in females. The few exceptions in which cancers that affect both sexes are more common in women than men include breast, thyroid, and gallbladder (Table 12.2). Although overall cancer rates are lower in women than in men, the overall prevalence of cancer is higher in women. Of the 10.7 million prevalent cancer cases in 2004, 4.8 million were men, while 5.9 million were women (Table 12.1). This may reflect the high survival rates of women with early-stage breast cancers and the greater longevity of women than men.

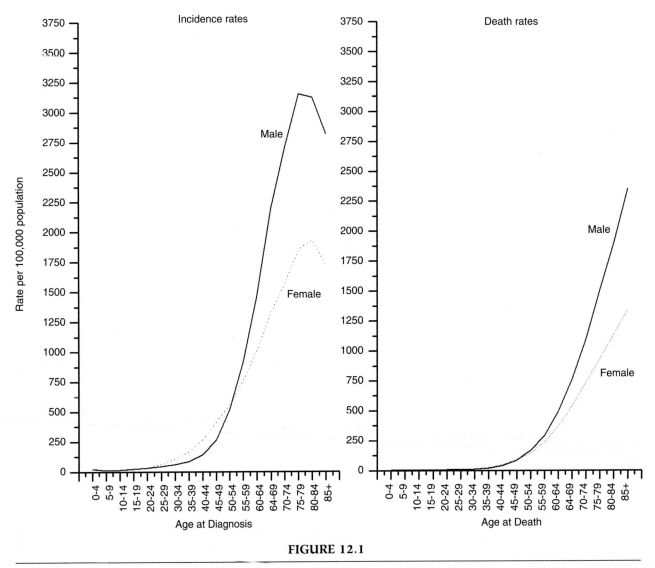

FIGURE 12.1

Age- and sex-specific incidence and death rates from all cancers combined, United States, 2004. Incidence rates from Surveillance, Epidemiology, and End Results (SEER) program statistics database for 1973–2004. Death rates from National Center for Health Statistics, Centers for Disease Control and Prevention.

Race

Cancer rates vary widely across racial and ethnic groups, and as Table 12.3 shows, blacks generally have higher cancer rates compared to whites. Cancer incidence and death rates are 16% and 27% higher, respectively, in black men than in white men. Similarly, cancer death rates are nearly 15% higher in black women than white women, despite lower incidence. While other racial ethnic groups, such as Asian American/Pacific Islanders, have lower incidence and mortality for all sites combined compared to whites and blacks, their rates of certain cancers (stomach, liver and intrahepatic bile duct, cervix) are generally higher. This is thought to reflect greater exposure to specific infectious agents (in the case of stomach and liver cancers), lower use

of screening (for cervical cancer), and higher consumption of preserved rather than fresh foods (for stomach cancer) (10).

Socioeconomic Status

Socioeconomic status (SES) is inversely correlated with death rates from cancer and many other causes because it is strongly associated with high-risk factors, such as smoking, drinking, lack of health insurance, access to care, and low screening rates (11–13). A study by Albano et al. found an inverse relationship between level of education and death rates from all cancers combined for African American and white men and for white women. Much of the variation in mortal-

TABLE 12.2
Average Annual Age-Standardized Cancer Incidence Rates[a] in Men Compared to Women, 2000–2004, United States

	MALE RATE	FEMALE RATE	RATE RATIO MALE VS. FEMALE
All sites	555.82	411.32	1.35
Oral cavity and pharynx	15.63	6.12	2.55
Esophagus	7.86	2.01	3.91
Stomach	11.43	5.58	2.05
Small intestine	2.17	1.49	1.46
Colon and rectum	60.76	44.57	1.36
Anus, anal canal, and anorectum	1.30	1.62	0.80
Liver and intrahepatic bile duct	9.51	3.39	2.81
Gallbladder	0.82	1.46	0.56
Pancreas	12.88	10.10	1.28
Larynx	6.64	1.37	4.85
Lung and bronchus	81.19	52.31	1.55
Bones and joints	1.04	0.78	1.33
Soft tissue, including heart	3.69	2.62	1.41
Melanoma of the skin	23.64	14.94	1.58
Breast	1.15	127.85	0.01
Urinary bladder	37.32	9.37	3.98
Kidney and renal pelvis	17.76	8.85	2.01
Eye and orbit	1.00	0.66	1.52
Brain and other nervous system	7.65	5.42	1.41
Thyroid	4.35	12.48	0.35
Hodgkin lymphoma	3.03	2.40	1.26
Non-Hodgkin lymphoma	23.21	16.25	1.43
Myeloma	6.96	4.54	1.53
Leukemia	15.99	9.51	1.68

[a]Rates are per 100,000 and age-adjusted to the 2000 U.S. standard population.

ity occurred between those with 12 or fewer years of education compared to those with additional schooling. The mortality rate ratio for all cancers combined in less educated persons compared to more educated persons was 1.43 for African American women, 1.76 for non-Hispanic white women, 2.24 for non-Hispanic white men, and 2.38 for African American men (14). In contrast, higher SES is positively associated with the incidence of some screening-related cancers. For example, the incidence of prostate cancer is higher in high and middle SES groups than in the poor, simply because of greater detection (12).

Geographic Location

Variability in cancer occurrence by place, together with surveillance data on cancer trends, has stimulated important hypotheses about the etiology and potential preventability of many cancers (2,15). High-risk areas for specific cancers may or may not be well characterized by official administrative boundaries, such as county, state, or national borders. For example, in the United States, the area with the highest death rates from cervical cancer spans much of Appalachia (16), where women historically lacked access to regular Pap testing or treatment. This observation motivated the

TABLE 12.3

Age-Standardized Incidence and Death Rates^a for Selected Cancer Sites by Race and Ethnicity, United States, 2000–2004

	WHITE	AFRICAN AMERICAN	ASIAN/PACIFIC ISLANDER	AMERICAN INDIAN/ ALASKA NATIVE	HISPANIC-LATINO[b]
Incidence					
All sites					
Males	556.7	663.7	359.9	236.3	421.7
Females	423.9	396.9	285.8	203.3	314.5
Breast (female)	132.5	118.3	89.0	51.0	89.4
Colon and rectum					
Males	60.4	72.6	49.7	29.1	47.6
Females	44.0	55.0	35.3	26.9	33.0
Esophagus					
Males	8.0	10.4	4.2	4.9	5.4
Females	1.9	3.2	1.2	1	1.2
Lung and bronchus					
Males	81.0	110.6	55.1	40.3	45.0
Females	54.6	53.7	27.7	27.6	25.3
Liver and bile duct					
Males	7.9	12.7	21.3	10.3	14.4
Females	2.9	3.8	7.9	4.4	5.7
Pancreas					
Males	12.8	16.2	10	7	11
Females	9.9	13.9	8.3	6.8	10
Prostate	161.4	255.5	96.5	52.5	140.6
MORTALITY					
All sites					
Males	234.7	321.8	141.7	187.9	162.2
Females	161.4	189.3	96.7	141.2	106.7
Breast (female)	25.0	33.8	12.6	16.1	16.1
Colon and rectum					
Males	22.9	32.7	15.0	20.6	17.0
Females	15.9	22.9	10.3	14.3	11.1
Esophagus					
Males	7.7	10.2	3.1	6.7	4.2
Females	1.7	3.0	0.8	1.5	1.0
Lung and bronchus					
Males	72.6	95.8	38.3	49.6	36.0
Females	42.1	39.8	18.5	32.7	16.1
Liver and bile duct					
Males	6.5	10.0	15.5	10.7	10.8
Females	2.8	3.9	6.7	6.7	5.0
Pancreas					
Males	12.0	15.5	7.9	7.6	9.1
Females	9.0	12.4	6.9	7.3	7.5
Prostate	25.6	62.3	11.3	21.5	21.2

^{a}Per 100,000, age-adjusted to 2000 U.S. standard population.
[b]Mortality rates for American Indian/Alaska Native are based on the CHSDA (Contract Health Service Delivery Area) counties.
[c]Hispanic-Latinos are not mutually exclusive from whites, blacks, Asian/Pacific Islanders, and American Indian/Alaska Natives.

Source: Reis LAG, Harkins D, Krapcho M, et al., eds. SEER Cancer Statistics Review, 1975–2004, National Cancer Institute, based on November 2006 SEER data submission, posted to the SEER Web site, 2007.

U.S. Congress to create the National Breast and Cervical Cancer Early Detection Program (NBCCEDP) to improve access to breast and cervical cancer screening and diagnostic services for low-income women (17).

Temporal Trends

Changes in cancer incidence over time may result from changes in the prevalence of risk factors and/or changes in detection practices due to the introduction or increased use of screening/diagnostic techniques. Furthermore, incidence trends can be affected by reporting delay and changes in disease classification. Trends in mortality rates may also be affected by most of the previously mentioned factors, with the exception of delay in reporting and artifacts of screening, in addition to improvements in cancer treatments over time.

CANCER OCCURENCE PATTERNS FOR ALL CANCERS COMBINED

All cancers combined include all malignant cases, except nonmelanoma skin cancers. It is estimated that 1,444,920 new cancer cases and 559,650 new deaths due to cancer will occur in the United States in 2007 (18). The probability of developing invasive cancer over a lifetime is about 45% for men and 38% for women (Table 12.4). Age-standardized incidence rates for all cancers combined are 26% higher in men than in women (Table 12.2) and 16% higher in black men than white men (Table 12.3). Survival rates for all cancers combined have increased significantly, from 50% during the period 1975–1977 to 66% during 1996–2003 (Table 12.5).

The interpretation of temporal trends for all cancers combined is complex because cancer is a constellation of more than 100 diseases, each of which is affected by several factors, including risk factors, screening, diagnosis, and treatment. However, the overall cancer trend is substantially influenced by trends of the major cancer sites. The increase in the incidence rate for all cancers combined among men from 1975–1988 (Fig. 12.2) reflects the rise in lung cancer from smoking and the diagnosis of prostate cancer from transurethral resection (19,20). In contrast, the sharp increase and subsequent decrease in the incidence of all cancers combined from 1988–1992 is driven by trends in prostate cancer incidence (Fig. 12.3, left panel) and reflect the introduction of prostate-specific antigen (PSA) testing, followed by the saturation and leveling off of PSA testing (21). The overall increase in incidence rates among women (Fig. 12.2), although slower during the most recent time period, predominantly reflects trends in lung and breast cancer incidence, which in turn, result from the increased consumption of cigarettes in women

born in the 1930s (19) and the increased utilization of mammography along with the increased prevalence of reproductive risk factors (22), respectively. Female breast cancer incidence rates are declining since 2000, likely due to reduction in use of mammography and hormone replacement therapy (23,24).

Among men, the long-term trend in overall cancer death rates (Fig. 12.2) is largely determined by trends in tobacco-related cancers, particularly lung cancer (19). Between 1930 and 1990, lung cancer death rates (per 100,000) rose from 4.3 to 90.4, representing a 21-fold increase (4). Thereafter, lung cancer death rates decreased to 70.3 per 100,000 in 2004 (4). These trends reflect historical smoking patterns. Cigarette consumption peaked during the mid-20th century and gradually decreased following the Surgeon General's report in 1964 (25). In addition to lung cancer, cigarette smoking has been linked to multiple other cancer types, including oral cavity, pharynx, larynx, esophagus, stomach, pancreas, urinary bladder, kidney, liver, cervix, and myeloid leukemia (26).

Improved treatments, increased screening, and changes in dietary habits may have also contributed to the reduction in death rates from all cancers combined since the early 1990s (27). Colorectal and prostate cancers are among the sites for which trends are shown in Figure 12.4 that may be affected by a combination of improved treatment and/or screening.

Among women, the overall cancer death rate decreased from the 1930s through early 1970s, increased until the early 1990s, and decreased thereafter (Fig. 12.2). The long-term decline before the 1970s reflects decreases in deaths from cancer of the stomach, cervix-uterus, and colon and rectum. The dramatic decrease in stomach cancer mortality, which has occurred in most industrialized countries, is thought to result from improvements in food preservation and reduced prevalence of *Helicobacter pylori* infection (28). Among women, the historic decreases in mortality from stomach and cervix-uterus cancers were offset by the increases in lung cancer mortality after 1960 (19). Decreases in the overall cancer death rates since the early 1990s reflect reduction in death rates from colorectal and breast cancers due to improved treatment and increased screening rates and plateauing of trends in lung cancer mortality rates (Fig. 12.4, right panel).

CANCER OCCURENCE PATTERNS FOR SELECT SITES

The three most commonly diagnosed cancers in the United States in 2007 will be prostate, lung and bronchus, and colon and rectum in men and breast, lung and

TABLE 12.4

Probability of (Percentage) Developing Invasive Cancers Over Specified Age Intervals, by Sex, United States[a]

	BIRTH TO 39 (%)	40 TO 59 (%)	60 TO 69 (%)	70 AND OLDER (%)	BIRTH TO DEATH (%)
All sites[b]					
Male	1.42 (1 in 70)	8.58 (1 in 12)	16.25 (1 in 6)	38.96 (1 in 3)	44.94 (1 in 2)
Female	2.04 (1 in 49)	8.97 (1 in 11)	10.36 (1 in 10)	26.31 (1 in 4)	37.52 (1 in 3)
Bladder[c]					
Male	0.02 (1 in 4477)	0.41 (1 in 244)	0.96 (1 in 104)	3.50 (1 in 29)	3.70 (1 in 27)
Female	0.01 (1 in 9462)	0.13 (1 in 790)	0.26 (1 in 384)	0.99 (1 in 101)	1.17 (1 in 85)
Breast					
Female	0.48 (1 in 210)	3.86 (1 in 26)	3.51 (1 in 28)	6.59 (1 in 15)	12.28 (1 in 8)
Colon and rectum					
Male	0.08 (1 in 1329)	0.92 (1 in 109)	1.60 (1 in 63)	4.78 (1 in 21)	5.65 (1 in 18)
Female	0.07 (1 in 1394)	0.72 (1 in 138)	1.12 (1 in 89)	4.30 (1 in 23)	5.23 (1 in 19)
Leukemia					
Male	0.16 (1 in 624)	0.21 (1 in 468)	0.35 (1 in 288)	1.18 (1 in 85)	1.50 (1 in 67)
Female	0.12 (1 in 837)	0.14 (1 in 705)	0.20 (1 in 496)	0.76 (1 in 131)	1.06 (1 in 95)
Lung and bronchus					
Male	0.03 (1 in 3357)	1.03 (1 in 97)	2.52 (1 in 40)	6.74 (1 in 15)	7.91 (1 in 13)
Female	0.03 (1 in 2964)	0.82 (1 in 121)	1.81 (1 in 55)	4.61 (1 in 22)	6.18 (1 in 16)
Melanoma of the skin					
Male	0.13 (1 in 784)	0.53 (1 in 190)	0.57 (1 in 175)	1.40 (1 in 72)	2.10 (1 in 48)
Female	0.21 (1 in 471)	0.42 (1 in 236)	0.29 (1 in 348)	0.64 (1 in 156)	1.40 (1 in 71)
Non-Hodgkin lymphoma					
Male	0.13 (1 in 760)	0.45 (1 in 222)	0.57 (1 in 174)	1.61 (1 in 62)	2.19 (1 in 46)
Female	0.08 (1 in 1212)	0.32 (1 in 312)	0.45 (1 in 221)	1.33 (1 in 75)	1.87 (1 in 53)
Prostate					
Male	0.01 (1 in 10553)	2.54 (1 in 39)	6.83 (1 in 15)	13.36 (1 in 7)	16.72 (1 in 6)
Uterine cervix	0.16 (1 in 638)	0.28 (1 in 359)	0.13 (1 in 750)	0.19 (1 in 523)	0.70 (1 in 142)
Uterine corpus	0.06 (1 in 1569)	0.71 (1 in 142)	0.79 (1 in 126)	1.23 (1 in 81)	2.45 (1 in 41)

TABLE 12.5
Changes in Five-Year Relative Survival Rates[a] (%), by Race and Year of Diagnosis in the United States from 1975–2003

Site	ALL RACES			WHITE			AFRICAN AMERICAN		
	1975–1977	1996–2003	Dif.	1975–1977	1996–2003	Dif.	1975–1977	1996–2003	Dif.
All cancers	50	66	16[b]	51	67	16[b]	40	57	17[b]
Brain	24	35	11[b]	23	34	11[b]	27	37	11[b]
Breast (female)	75	89	14[b]	76	90	14[b]	62	78	16[b]
Colon	51	65	14[b]	52	66	14[b]	46	55	9[b]
Esophagus	5	16	11[b]	6	18	12[b]	3	11	8[b]
Hodgkin disease	74	86	13[b]	74	87	13[b]	71	81	10[b]
Kidney	51	66	15[b]	51	66	15[b]	50	66	16[b]
Larynx	67	64	-3[b]	67	66	-1	59	50	-9
Leukemia	35	50	15[b]	36	51	15[b]	34	40	7
Liver and bile duct	4	11	7[b]	4	10	6[b]	2	8	6[b]
Lung and bronchus	13	16	3[b]	13	16	3[b]	12	13	1[b]
Melanoma of the skin	82	92	10[b]	82	92	10[b]	60	77	17
Multiple myeloma	26	34	8[b]	25	34	9[b]	31	32	1
Non-Hodgkin lymphoma	48	64	16[b]	48	65	17[b]	49	56	7
Oral cavity and pharynx	53	60	7[b]	55	62	7[b]	36	41	5
Ovary[c]	37	45	8[b]	37	45	8[b]	43	38	-5
Pancreas	2	5	3[b]	3	5	2[b]	2	5	3[b]
Prostate	69	99	30[b]	70	99	29[b]	61	95	34[b]
Rectum	49	66	17[b]	49	66	17[b]	45	58	13[b]
Stomach	16	24	8[b]	15	22	7[b]	16	24	8[b]
Testis	83	96	13[b]	83	96	13[b]	82	88	6
Thyroid	93	97	4[b]	93	97	4[b]	91	94	3
Urinary bladder	74	81	7[b]	75	81	7[b]	51	65	14[b]
Uterine cervix	70	73	3[b]	71	74	3[b]	65	66	1
Uterine corpus	88	84	-4[b]	89	86	-3[b]	61	61	0

[a]Survival rates are adjusted for normal life expectancy and are based in cases diagnosed from 1975–1977 to 1996–2003 and followed through 2004.
[b]The difference in rates between 1975–1977 and 1996–2003 is statistically significant ($p < 0.05$).
[c]Recent changes in classification of ovarian cancer, namely excluding borderline tumors, have affected 1996–2003 survival rates.

Note: "All sites" excludes basal and squamous cell skin cancers and in situ carcinomas except urinary bladder.

Source: Surveillance, Epidemiology, and End Results Program, 1973–2004, Division of Cancer Control and Population Sciences, National Cancer Institute, 2007.

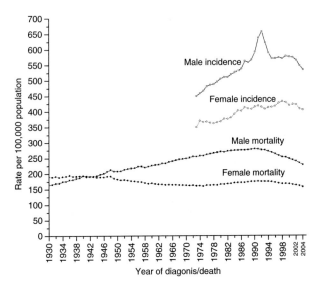

FIGURE 12.2

Trends in all cancers combined incidence and mortality rates, United States, 1930–2004. Incidence rates from Surveillance, Epidemiology, and End Results (SEER) program (http://www.seer.cancer.gov) SEER*Stat Database, 1973–2004. National Cancer Institute, 2007. Death rates from National Center for Health Statistics, Centers for Disease Control and Prevention, 2007.

bronchus, and colon and rectum in females (Fig. 12.5). These cancers account for more than 50% of the new cases in males and in females. Lung and bronchus cancer is the leading cause of cancer death in men and in women, followed by prostate cancer in men, breast cancer in women, and colorectal cancer in men and in women. For both sexes combined, colorectal cancer is the second leading cause of cancer death. The remainder of this section will focus on these four most common cancer sites, as well as three additional cancer sites (liver, esophagus, and pancreas) that are unique with respect to their risk factors, varying histologic types, and low survival rates. These cancers collectively account for 58% of the total new cases in the United States.

Lung and Bronchus Cancer

An estimated 213,380 new cases of lung and bronchus cancer are expected in 2007, accounting for about 15% of cancer diagnoses (18). Overall, men have higher rates of lung and bronchus cancer compared to women and blacks have the highest rates among racial/ethnic groups (Tables 12.2 and 12.3). Lung cancer accounts for the most cancer-related deaths in both men and women. An estimated 160,390 lung cancer deaths, accounting for about 29% of all cancer deaths, are expected to occur

in 2007 (18). The probability of developing invasive lung and bronchus cancer over a lifetime is 7.9% for men and 6.2% for women (Table 12.4).

The incidence rate of lung and bronchus cancer is declining significantly in men, from a high of 102.0 per 100,000 in 1984 to 72.6 per 100,000 in 2004 (4) (Fig. 12.3, left panel). In women, the rate is approaching a plateau after a long period of increase (Fig. 12.3, right panel). Lung cancer death rates have continued to decline significantly in men from 1991–2004 by about 1.9% per year (Fig. 12.4, left panel). Since 1987, more women have died each year from lung cancer than from breast cancer, although female lung cancer death rates are approaching a plateau after continuously increasing for several decades (27) (Fig. 12.4, right panel). These trends in lung cancer mortality reflect the patterns in smoking rates over the past 30 years. Cigarette smoking is by far the most important risk factor for lung cancer. Risk increases with quantity of cigarette consumption and years of smoking duration. Other risk factors include secondhand smoke, occupational or environmental exposures to radon and asbestos (particularly among smokers), certain metals (chromium, cadmium, arsenic), some organic chemicals, radiation, air pollution, and tuberculosis. Genetic susceptibility plays a contributing role in the development of lung cancer, especially in those who develop the disease at a younger age (18).

The five-year survival rate for all stages of lung cancer has slightly increased from 13% in 1975–1977 to 16% in 1996–2003 (Table 12.5), largely due to improvements in surgical techniques and combined therapies. The survival rate is 49% for cases detected when the disease is still localized; however, only 16% of lung cancers are diagnosed at this early stage (4).

Breast Cancer

Breast cancer is the most frequently diagnosed cancer in women, and an estimated 178,480 new cases of invasive breast cancer are expected to occur among women in the United States during 2007 (Fig. 12.5). Breast cancer occurs at higher rates among white women compared to other races/ethnicities, and incidence rates are substantially higher for women aged 50 and older (22). Breast cancer ranks second among cancer deaths in women, and an estimated 40,460 breast cancer deaths are expected among women in 2007 (18). Racial disparities in breast cancer death rates are observed, with black women having a 26% higher death rate than white women (Table 12.3). The higher death rate among black women, despite the lower incidence rate, is due to both later stage at diagnosis and poorer stage-specific survival (22).

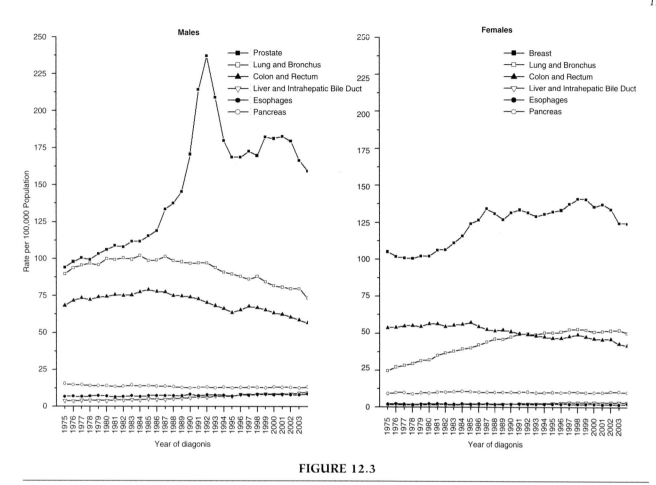

FIGURE 12.3

Annual age-adjusted cancer incidence rates among males and females for selected cancer sites, United States, 1975–2004. Rates are age-adjusted to the 2000 U.S. standard population and adjusted for delays in reporting. Incidence rates from Surveillance, Epidemiology, and End Results (SEER) program (http://www.seer.cancer.gov) SEER*Stat Database, 1973–2004. National Cancer Institute, 2007.

Breast cancer incidence rates increased rapidly among women from 1980–1987, a period when there was increasing uptake of mammography by a growing proportion of U.S. women, and then continued to increase at a slower rate through 1999. After continuously increasing for more than two decades, female breast cancer incidence rates decreased slightly and leveled off from 2001–2004 (Fig. 12.3, right panel). This may reflect the saturation of mammography utilization and reduction in the use of hormone replacement therapy (29). Death rates from breast cancer have steadily decreased in women since 1990 (Fig. 12.4, right panel), with larger decreases in women younger than 50 (a decrease of 3.3% per year) than in those 50 years and older (2.0% per year) (4). The substantial decreases in female breast cancer mortality are thought to reflect early detection (30) and improvements in treatment (31).

Aside from being female, age is the most important factor affecting breast cancer risk. Risk is also increased by inherited genetic mutations in the BRCA1 and BRCA2 genes, a personal or family history of breast cancer, high breast tissue density, biopsy-confirmed hyperplasia (especially atypical hyperplasia), and high-dose radiation to the chest as a result of medical procedures. Reproductive factors that increase risk include a long menstrual history, never having children or delayed childbearing (32), and recent use of oral contraceptives. Some potentially modifiable factors that increase risk include being overweight or obese after menopause, use of postmenopausal hormone therapy (especially combined estrogen and progestin therapy), physical inactivity, and consumption of one or more alcoholic beverages per day (22).

The five-year relative survival rate for all stages of breast cancer has increased from 75% in 1975–1977

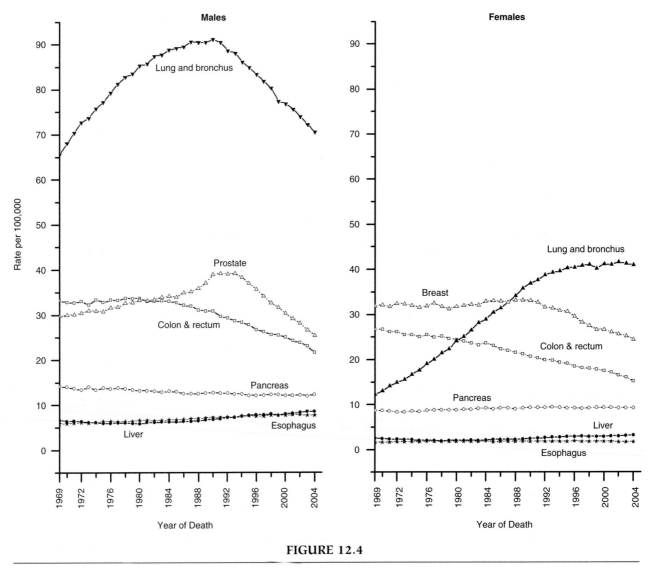

FIGURE 12.4

Trends in annual age-adjusted cancer death rates among males and females for selected cancer types, United States, 1969–2004. Death rates from National Center for Health Statistics, Centers for Disease Control and Prevention, 2007.

to 89% in 1996–2003 (Table 12.5). The five-year relative survival rate for localized breast cancer is 98%, while the rate for cancer that has spread regionally is 84% and that for distant spread is only 27% (4). Mammography can detect breast cancer at an early state, when treatment may be more effective. Numerous studies have shown that early detection saves lives and increases treatment options.

Prostate Cancer

An estimated 218,890 new cases of prostate cancer will occur in the United States during 2007 (Fig. 12.5) (18). Prostate cancer is the most frequently diagnosed cancer

in men. For reasons that remain unclear, incidence rates are significantly higher in black men than in white men (Table 12.3). More than 65% of all prostate cancer cases are diagnosed in men 65 years and older. With an estimated 27,050 deaths in 2007 (18), prostate cancer is a leading cause of cancer death in men.

Incidence rates of prostate cancer have changed substantially over the last 20 years: rapidly increasing from 1988–1992, declining sharply from 1992–1995, and increasing modestly since 1995 (Fig. 12.3, left panel). These trends, in large part, reflect increased prostate cancer screening with the PSA blood test (33). Moderate incidence increases in the last decade are most likely attributable to widespread PSA screening

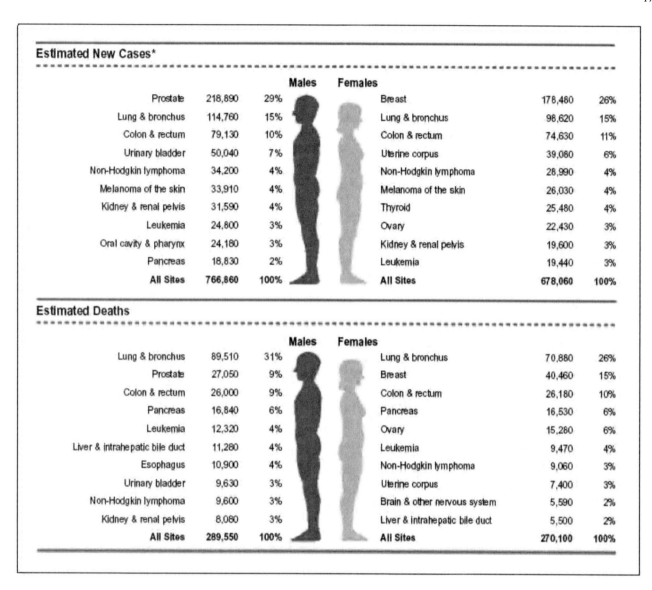

Estimated New Cases*

	Males				Females		
Prostate	218,890	29%		Breast	176,480	26%
Lung & bronchus	114,760	15%		Lung & bronchus	98,620	15%
Colon & rectum	79,130	10%		Colon & rectum	74,630	11%
Urinary bladder	50,040	7%		Uterine corpus	39,080	6%
Non-Hodgkin lymphoma	34,200	4%		Non-Hodgkin lymphoma	28,990	4%
Melanoma of the skin	33,910	4%		Melanoma of the skin	26,030	4%
Kidney & renal pelvis	31,590	4%		Thyroid	25,480	4%
Leukemia	24,800	3%		Ovary	22,430	3%
Oral cavity & pharynx	24,180	3%		Kidney & renal pelvis	19,600	3%
Pancreas	18,830	2%		Leukemia	19,440	3%
All Sites	**766,860**	**100%**		**All Sites**	**678,060**	**100%**

Estimated Deaths

	Males				Females		
Lung & bronchus	89,510	31%		Lung & bronchus	70,880	26%
Prostate	27,050	9%		Breast	40,460	15%
Colon & rectum	26,000	9%		Colon & rectum	26,180	10%
Pancreas	16,840	6%		Pancreas	16,530	6%
Leukemia	12,320	4%		Ovary	15,280	6%
Liver & intrahepatic bile duct	11,280	4%		Leukemia	9,470	4%
Esophagus	10,900	4%		Non-Hodgkin lymphoma	9,060	3%
Urinary bladder	9,630	3%		Uterine corpus	7,400	3%
Non-Hodgkin lymphoma	9,600	3%		Brain & other nervous system	5,590	2%
Kidney & renal pelvis	8,080	3%		Liver & intrahepatic bile duct	5,500	2%
All Sites	**289,550**	**100%**		**All Sites**	**270,100**	**100%**

FIGURE 12.5

Ten leading cancer types for the estimated new cancer cases and deaths, by sex, United States, 2007. Excludes basal and squamous cell skin cancer and in situ carcinomas except urinary bladder. Percentage may not total 100%. (Data from Cancer Facts and Figures, 2007. American Cancer Society.)

among men younger than 65. Prostate cancer incidence rates have leveled off in men 65 and older. Although death rates have been declining among white and African American men since the early 1990s, rates in African American men remain more than twice as high as those in white men (Table 12.3).

The only well-established risk factors for prostate cancer are age, ethnicity, and family history of the disease. Recent genetic studies suggest that strong familial predisposition may be responsible for 5%–10% of prostate cancers. International studies suggest that a diet high in saturated fat may also be

a risk factor (28,34). There is some evidence that the risk of dying from prostate cancer may increase with obesity (35).

More than 90% of all prostate cancers are discovered in the local and regional stages, and the five-year relative survival rate for patients whose tumors are diagnosed at these stages approaches 100% (4). The five-year survival rate for all stages combined has increased from 69% in 1975–1977 to 99% in 1996–2003 (Table 12.5). The dramatic improvements in prostate cancer survival are partly attributable to earlier diagnosis and improvements in treatment.

Colon and Rectum Cancer

An estimated 112,340 cases of colon and 41,420 cases of rectal cancer are expected to occur in 2007 (18). Colorectal cancer is the third most common cancer in both men and women, and it is estimated that in 2004, 1,076,335 persons were living with the disease, representing 10% of all prevalent cancer cases (Table 12.1). Males have a higher incidence of colorectal cancer compared to females (Table 12.2), and more than 90% of cases are diagnosed in individuals 50 and older. Black males and females have higher incidence rates of colorectal cancer compared to whites and all other racial/ethnic groups (Table 12.3). An estimated 52,180 deaths from colon and rectum cancer are expected to occur in 2007, accounting for about 10% of all cancer deaths (18).

Colorectal cancer incidence rates have been decreasing since 1985 for both sexes (Fig. 12.3). The more rapid decrease in the most recent time period (2.5% per year from 1998–2004 (4) partly reflects an increase in screening, which can detect and remove precancerous colorectal polyps (36,37), before they progress to cancer. Colorectal cancer mortality rates have continued to decline in both men and women over the past two decades (Fig. 12.4) because of detection and removal of precancerous polyps (36,37), earlier diagnosis, and improved treatment and supportive care. The risk of colorectal cancer increases with age and is also increased by certain inherited genetic mutations, a personal or family history of colorectal cancer and/or polyps, or a personal history of chronic inflammatory bowel disease. Several modifiable factors are associated with increased risk of colorectal cancer. Among these are obesity, physical inactivity, heavy alcohol consumption, a diet high in red or processed meat, and inadequate intake of fruits and vegetables (18). Beginning at age 50, men and women who are at average risk for developing colorectal cancer should begin screening.

When colorectal cancers are diagnosed at an early, localized stage, the five-year survival is 90%; however, only 39% of colorectal cancers are diagnosed at this stage, mostly due to low rates of screening. After the cancer has spread regionally to involve adjacent organs or lymph nodes, the five-year survival drops to 68%. For persons with distant metastases, five-year survival is 10% (4).

Liver Cancer

In 2007, it is estimated that there will be 19,160 new cases of liver cancer in the United States, accounting for approximately 1.3% of new cancer cases (18). The incidence of liver cancer is substantially greater among men than women. From 2000–2004, the incidence rate for liver cancer was 9.5 per 100,000 among males, while only 3.4 per 100,000 among females (Table 12.2). Incidence also varies by race and ethnicity, with Asian Americans, particularly those of Vietnamese and Korean ethnicities, experiencing the highest rates (10). Liver cancer incidence is highly correlated with age. The incidence peaks among individuals 75–79 years of age and is rare among those less than 50 years of age (Fig. 12.6). Approximately 16,780 deaths due to liver cancer are estimated to occur in 2007, representing 3% of all cancer deaths (18).

About 83% of liver cancers are hepatocellular carcinomas (HCC) affecting hepatocytes, the predominant type of cell in the liver. Worldwide, the major causes of liver cancer are chronic infection with hepatitis B virus (HBV) and hepatitis C virus (HCV). In developing countries, 37% of liver cancers are attributable to HBV, 25% to HCV, 10% to infection of the intrahepatic bile ducts by liver flukes, and 9% to other causes. In developed countries, 14% of liver cancers are attributable to HBV, 14% to HCV, and 71% to other causes, such as alcohol-related cirrhosis and possibly hepatitis

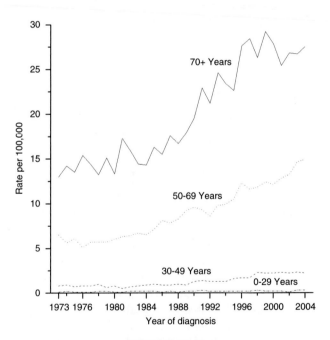

FIGURE 12.6

Age-specific liver cancer incidence, United States, 1973–2004. Incidence rates from Surveillance, Epidemiology, and End Results (SEER) program (http://www.seer.cancer.gov) SEER*Stat Database, 1973–2004. National Cancer Institute, 2007.

from obesity (38). Data for North America indicate that 6.2% of liver cancers are attributed to chronic infection with HBV, 23% are due to chronic infection with HCV, and a substantial portion of the remainder are due to alcohol-related cirrhosis (39). The majority of liver cancers occur in Eastern Asia and sub-Saharan Africa (40). The United States is considered a low rate area for liver cancer; however, the incidence in the United States has been steadily increasing, from 2.9 per 100,000 in 1984 to 6.1 per 100,000 in 2004 (41). Reasons for the increase in incidence are not entirely clear, but may be related to increased prevalence of HCV infection (42).

Survival rates for liver cancer are universally poor, and a five-year survival rate of only 11% was observed during the period 1996–2003 in the United States (Table 12.5). Because survival is so low, prevention mechanisms for the major causes of liver cancer are vitally important. A vaccine that protects against HBV has been available since 1982, and state laws mandating hepatitis B vaccination for middle school children have contributed to achieving high coverage rates among adolescents (43). Although progress in vaccination among adolescents has been made, hepatitis B infections among men over age 19 and women 40 and older have been rising since 1999. Increasing efforts to vaccinate high-risk individuals, including those with multiple sex partners, men who have sex with men, and injection drug users, are recommended to counteract this trend (44). There is no vaccine available for HCV. Universal precautions should be used among health care workers to prevent infection, and The Centers for Disease Control and Prevention (CDC) recommends that routine HCV testing be offered to individuals at high risk for infection.

Esophageal Cancer

It is estimated that 15,560 new cases and 13,940 new deaths due to esophageal cancer will occur in the United States in 2007 (18). Incidence rates for esophageal cancer rise with age and are very low among children and young adults. Males have higher rates of esophageal cancer compared to females, with the male to female ratio (3.91) nearly reaching four-fold (Table 12.2). Cancers of the esophagus typically have two distinct histologic types, squamous cell carcinoma and adenocarcinoma, that display remarkable racial and ethnic differences. Rates of esophageal adenocarcinoma are higher among whites than blacks, while the inverse is true for squamous cell carcinoma. Squamous cell carcinoma occurs in the upper third of the esophagus and is caused mainly by tobacco and alcohol consumption. Adenocarcinoma generally occurs in the lower third of

the esophagus and has risk factors that include obesity, gastroesophageal reflux disease (GERD), and Barrett esophagus, which is a premalignant condition involving chronic inflammation and dysplasia (45).

Trends in esophageal cancer have changed dramatically in recent years. The incidence of esophageal cancer has been rising in men and is stable in women (Fig. 12.3). Historically, squamous cell carcinoma has been the most common histologic type; however, its incidence has been decreasing since 1975, first among whites, followed by blacks. In contrast, adenocarcinoma, which used to be relatively rare throughout the world, has risen steeply among white males in the United States while remaining relatively stable among black males (Fig. 12.7) (46). Reasons for the sharp increase in esophageal adenocarcinoma among white men but not among black men are not fully understood; however, a higher prevalence of *Helicobacter pylori* infection in blacks, which may be protective against adenocarcinoma of the esophagus (47), has been suggested to be a factor (48). The increase in adenocarcinoma of the esophagus may also be related to the increase in obesity and GERD in the United States. As smoking is a primary cause of squamous cell carcinoma, the decrease in smoking rates in the United States most likely have contributed to the decrease in this type of esophageal cancer.

Survival from esophageal cancer is low, and survival rates do not differ by histologic type (45). In the United States, the five-year survival rate was 16% during the period 1996–2003. This was a significant improvement from the five-year survival rate of 5% from 1975–1977 (Table 12.5).

Pancreatic Cancer

An estimated 37,170 new cases and 33,370 new deaths due to pancreatic cancer are expected to occur in the United States in 2007 (18). Pancreatic cancer rates are slightly higher in men than in women, with a male-to-female ratio of 1.28 (Table 12.2). Age is an important predictor for pancreatic cancer, as both its incidence and mortality increase with age in a linear fashion. The median age of diagnosis is 72, and the majority of cases occur between ages 65 and 79 (49). In general, pancreatic cancer incidence rates are higher among blacks compared to whites in the United States (Table 12.3).

For both sexes combined, incidence rates increased slightly (by 0.5% per year) from 1993–2004 (4). The death rate from pancreatic cancer has continued to decline since the 1970s in men, while it has leveled off in women after increasing from 1975–1984. Tobacco smoking increases the risk of pancreatic cancer, and incidence rates are more than twice as high for cigarette

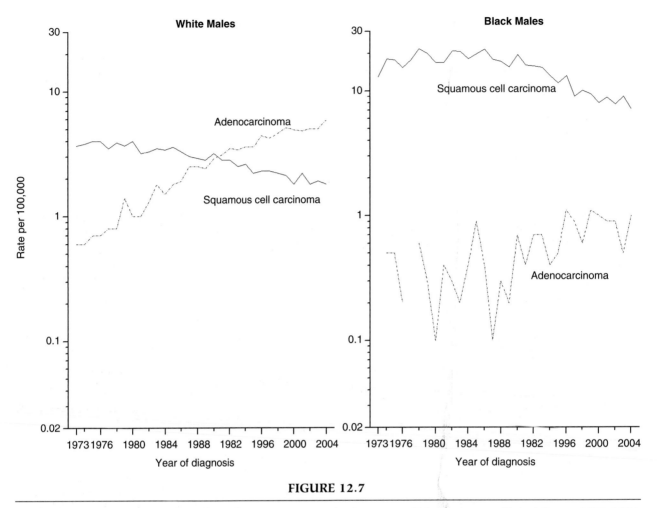

FIGURE 12.7

Age-adjusted incidence rates of esophageal cancer among males by race and histologic type, United States, 1973–2004. Incidence rates from Surveillance, Epidemiology, and End Results (SEER) program (http://www.seer.cancer.gov) SEER*Stat Database, 1973–2004. National Cancer Institute, 2007.

smokers than for nonsmokers. Risk also appears to increase with obesity, chronic pancreatitis, diabetes, and cirrhosis. Surgery, radiation therapy, and chemotherapy are treatment options that may extend survival and/or relieve symptoms in many patients, but seldom produce a cure.

Pancreatic cancer is highly lethal, and survival rates are among the lowest of any cancer. For all stages combined, the five-year survival rate is about 5% (Table 12.5). Even for those people diagnosed with local disease, the five-year survival rate is only 20% (4). Only about 7% of pancreatic cancers are diagnosed at the localized stage, whereas 52% are diagnosed at the distant stage (4). There is no screening test for early detection of pancreatic cancer, and early stages of the disease are usually asymptomatic. Difficulties in early detection, lack of effective treatments, and extremely low survival rates make cancer of the pancreas a serious medical and public health problem.

References

1. Extramural Committee to Assess Measures of Progress Against Cancer. Measurement of progress against cancer. *J Natl Cancer Inst.* 1990;82:825–835.
2. Doll R, Peto R. The causes of cancer: quantitative estimates of avoidable risks of cancer in the United States today. *J Natl Cancer Inst.* 1981;66:1191–1308.
3. Jemal A, Siegel R, Ward E, Murray T, Xu J, Thun MJ. Cancer statistics, 2007. *CA Cancer J Clin.* 2007;57:43–66.
4. Ries LAG, Melbert D, Krapcho M, et al., eds. *SEER Cancer Statistics Review, 1975-2004.* Bethesda, MD: National Cancer Institute, National Cancer Institute; 2007.
5. Anderson RN, Minino AM, Hoyert DL, Rosenberg HM. Comparability of cause of death between ICD-9 and ICD-10: preliminary estimates. *Natl Vital Stat Rep.* 2001;49:1–32.
6. World Health Organization. *International Statistical Classification of Diseases and Related Health Problems.* Geneva: WHO; 1992.
7. Thun MJ, Calle EE, Rodriguez C, Wingo PA. Epidemiological research at the American Cancer Society. *Cancer Epidemiol Biomarkers Prev.* 2000;9:861–868.

8. Tiwari RC, Ghosh K, Jemal A, et al. Derivation and validation of a new method of predicting U.S. and state-level cancer mortality counts for the current calendar year. *CA Cancer J Clin.* 2004;54:8–29.

9. Wingo PA, Landis S, Parker S. Using cancer registry and vital statistics to estimate the number of new cases cancer cases and deaths in the US for the upcoming year. *Journal of Registry Management.* 1998;25:43–51.

10. McCracken M, Olsen M, Chen MS, Jr., et al. Cancer incidence, mortality, and associated risk factors among asian americans of chinese, filipino, vietnamese, korean, and Japanese ethnicities. *CA Cancer J Clin.* 2007;57:190–205.

11. Ward E, Jemal A, Cokkinides V, et al. Cancer disparities by race/ethnicity and socioeconomic status. *CA Cancer J Clin.* 2004;54:78–93.

12. Singh GK, Miller BA, Hankey BF, Edwards BK, eds. *Area Socioeconomic Variations in U.S. Cancer Incidence, Mortality, and Survival, 1975–1999.* Bethesda, MD: National Cancer Institute, National Cancer Institute; 2003.

13. Howard G, Anderson RT, Russell G, Howard VJ, Burke GL. Race, socioeconomic status, and cause-specific mortality. *Ann Epidemiol.* 2000;10:214–223.

14. Albano J, Ward E, Jemal ARA, et al. Cancer mortality by education and Race in the United States *J Natl Cancer Inst.* 2007; 99:1364–1384.

15. Doll R. Epidemiological evidence of the effects of behaviour and the environment on the risk of human cancer. *Recent Results Cancer Res.* 1998;154:3–21.

16. Devesa SS, Grauman DJ, Blot WJ, Pennello GA, Hoover RN, Fraumeni JFJ. *Atlas of Cancer Mortality in the United States 1950–94.* Bethesda: National Institute of Health; 1999.

17. Centers for Disease Control and Prevention (2003), Available at: http://www.cdc.gov/cancer/nbccedp/about.htm.

18. American Cancer Society. *Cancer Facts & Figures 2007.* Atlanta, GA: American Cancer Society; 2007.

19. Thun MJ, Henley SJ, Calle EE. Tobacco use and cancer: an epidemiologic perspective for geneticists. *Oncogene.* 2002;21:7307–7325.

20. Potosky AL, Kessler L, Gridley G, Brown CC, Horm JW. Rise in prostatic cancer incidence associated with increased use of transurethral resection. *J Natl Cancer Inst.* 1990;82:1624–1628.

21. Potosky AL, Miller BA, Albertsen PC, Kramer BS. The role of increasing detection in the rising incidence of prostate cancer. *JAMA.* 1995;273:548–552.

22. Smigal C, Jemal A, Ward E, et al. Trends in breast cancer by race and ethnicity: update 2006. *CA Cancer J Clin.* 2006;56:168–183.

23. Jemal A, Ward E, Thun MJ. Recent trends in breast cancer incidence rates by age and tumor characteristics among U.S. women. *Breast Cancer Res.* 2007;9:R28.

24. Ravdin PM, Cronin KA, Howlader N, et al. The decrease in breast-cancer incidence in 2003 in the United States. *N Engl J Med.* 2007;356:1670–1674.

25. U.S. Public Health Service. *Smoking and Health. Report of the Advisory Committee to the Surgeon General of the Public Health Service.* Washington, DC: US Department of Health, Education, and Welfare, Public Health Service, Center for Disease Control; 1964.

26. US Department of Health and Human Services. *A Surgeon General's Report on the Health Consequences of Smoking.* Atlanta: US Department of Health and Human Services, Centers for Disease Control and Prevention, Office of Smoking and Health; 2004.

27. Howe HL, Wu X, Ries LA, et al. Annual report to the nation on the status of cancer, 1975–2003, featuring cancer among U.S. Hispanic/Latino populations. *Cancer.* 2006;107:1711–1142.

28. Parkin DM. The global health burden of infection-associated cancers in the year 2002. *Int J Cancer.* 2006;118: 3030–3044.

29. Jemal A, Clegg LX, Ward E, et al. Annual report to the nation on the status of cancer, 1975–2001, with a special feature regarding survival. *Cancer.* 2004;101:3–27.

30. Swan J, Breen N, Coates RJ, Rimer BK, Lee NC. Progress in cancer screening practices in the United States: results from the 2000 National Health Interview Survey. *Cancer.* 2003;97:1528–1540.

31. Mariotto A, Feuer EJ, Harlan LC, Wun LM, Johnson KA, Abrams J. Trends in use of adjuvant multi-agent chemotherapy and tamoxifen for breast cancer in the United States: 1975–1999. *J Natl Cancer Inst.* 2002;94:1626–1634.

32. Chu K, Tarone R, Kessler L, et al. Recent trends in U.S. breast cancer incidence, survival, and mortality rates. *J Natl Cancer Inst.* 1996;88:1571–1579.

33. Hankey BF, Feuer EJ, Clegg LX, et al. Cancer surveillance series: interpreting trends in prostate cancer—part I: evidence of the effects of screening in recent prostate cancer incidence, mortality, and survival rates. *J Natl Cancer Inst.* 1999;91:1017–1024.

34. Platz E, Giovannucci E. Prostate cancer. In: Schottenfeld D, Jr. Fraumeni JF, Jr. eds. *Cancer Epidemiology and Prevention Third Edition.* New York: Oxford University Press; 2006;1128–1150.

35. Gong Z, Agalliu I, Lin DW, Stanford JL, Kristal AR. Obesity is associated with increased risks of prostate cancer metastasis and death after initial cancer diagnosis in middle-aged men. *Cancer.* 2007;109:1192–1202.

36. Mandel JS, Bond JH, Church TR, et al. (1993) Reducing mortality from colorectal cancer by screening for fecal occult blood. Minnesota Colon Cancer Control Study. *N Engl J Med.* 1993;328:1365–1371.

37. Mandel JS, Church TR, Ederer F, Bond JH. Colorectal cancer mortality: effectiveness of biennial screening for fecal occult blood. *J Natl Cancer Inst.* 1999;91:434–437.

38. American Cancer Society. *Cancer Facts & Figures 2005.* Atlanta, GA: American Cancer Society; 2005.

39. Pisani P, Parkin DM, Munoz N, Ferlay J. Cancer and infection: estimates of the attributable fraction in 1990. *Cancer Epidemiol Biomarkers Prev.* 1997;6:387–400.

40. Parkin DM, Bray FI, Devesa SS. Cancer burden in the year 2000. The global picture. *Eur J Cancer.* 2001;37(Suppl 8):S4–S66.

41. Reis L, Melbert D, Krapcho M, et al. *SEER Cancer Statistics Review, 1975–2004.* Bethesda, MD: National Cancer Institute; 2007.

42. El-Serag HB, Davila JA, Petersen NJ, McGlynn KA. The continuing increase in the incidence of hepatocellular carcinoma in the United States: an update. *Ann Intern Med.* 2003;139:817–823.

43. Centers for Disease Cancer and Prevention (CDC). Hepatitis B vaccination—United States, 1982–2002. *MMWR Morb Mortal Wkly Rep.* 2002;51:549–552.

44. Centers for Disease Cancer and Prevention (CDC). Incidence of acute hepatitis B—United States, 1990–2002. *MMWR Morb Mortal Wkly Rep.* 2004;52:1252–1254.

45. Blot W, McLaughlin J, Fraumeni J, Jr. Esophageal cancer. In: Schottenfeld D, Fraumeni JF, Jr. eds. *Cancer Epidemiology and Prevention Third Edition.* New York: Oxford University Press; 2006; 647–706.

46. Ward EM, Thun MJ, Hannan LM, Jemal A. Interpreting cancer trends. *Ann N Y Acad Sci.* 2006;1076:29–53.

47. Ye W, Held M, Lagergren J, et al. Helicobacter pylori infection and gastric atrophy: risk of adenocarcinoma and squamous-cell carcinoma of the esophagus and adenocarcinoma of the gastric cardia. *J Natl Cancer Inst.* 2004;96:388–396.

48. Graham DY, Malaty HM, Evans DG, Evans DJ, Jr., Klein PD, Adam E. Epidemiology of Helicobacter pylori in an asymptomatic population in the United States. Effect of age, race, and socioeconomic status. *Gastroenterology.* 1991;100:1495–1501.

49. Anderson K, Mack T, Silverman D. Cancer of the pancreas. In: Schottenfeld D, Fraumeni JF, Jr. eds. *Cancer Epidemiology and Prevention Third Edition.* New York: Oxford University Press; 2006;721–762.

II

INTRODUCTION TO EVALUATION AND TREATMENT OF MALIGNANCY

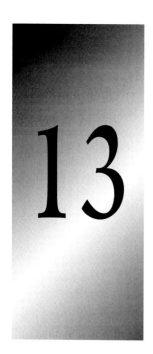

Evaluation and Treatment of Breast Cancer

Heather L. McArthur
Clifford A. Hudis

Breast cancer is the most common potentially life-threatening cancer among women in the United States, with more than 200,000 new cases and more than 40,000 breast cancer-related deaths anticipated in 2008 (1). The most well-defined risk factors for breast cancer include increasing age, prolonged endogenous or exogenous estrogen exposure, and family history. Significant estrogen exposure histories include nulliparity, early menarche, late menopause, obesity, oral contraceptive use, and hormone replacement therapy. Although as many as 20% of women with a new breast cancer diagnosis cite a positive family history, inherited genetic mutations that predispose to breast cancer are rare. For example, only 5%–10% of all breast cancers are attributable to inheritance of a breast cancer susceptibility gene (1,2). However, for those women who do inherit a gene mutation, the lifetime risk of developing breast cancer can be significant. For example, in a meta-analysis of 10 studies evaluating cancer risk among known BRCA1 and BRCA2 mutation carriers, the cumulative lifetime breast cancer risk was 57% in the BRCA1 cohort and 49% in the BRCA2 cohort (3). Other risk factors for developing breast cancer include a prior history of ductal carcinoma in situ (DCIS), lobular carcinoma in situ (LCIS), atypical ductal hyperplasia (ADH), a prior history of invasive breast cancer, and prior radiotherapy to the chest. Associations with environmental factors including smoking, alcohol consumption, and diet have also been established. Despite these risk factors and associations,

however, the etiology of most breast cancer diagnoses is unknown. The difficulty in identifying the majority of women who are at risk of developing breast cancer, combined with the significant burden of disease in the population, has resulted in the widespread adoption of breast cancer screening programs as a public health measure.

Annual mammography, in combination with annual clinical breast examination, is recommended for all women aged 40 years or older who are considered at average risk of developing breast cancer. Screening may be indicated earlier and more frequently for women at higher risk. When an abnormality is detected on screening, breast cancer diagnosis and management typically require a multidisciplinary approach that incorporates some combination of radiology, surgery, pathology, medical oncology, radiation oncology, and/or care by specialists in rehabilitation. This chapter provides an overview of the principles of breast cancer diagnosis and treatment.

DIAGNOSIS

Mammography

In the United States, the adoption of national screening programs accounts for a significant proportion of the improved breast cancer-specific mortality rates observed over the last three decades (4,5). The National Cancer Institute, American Cancer Society,

KEY POINTS

- Breast cancer is the most common potentially life-threatening cancer among women in the United States, with more than 200,000 new cases and more than 40,000 breast cancer-related deaths in 2008.
- The most well-defined risk factors for breast cancer include increasing age, prolonged endogenous or exogenous estrogen exposure, and family history.
- Annual mammography in combination with annual clinical breast examination are recommended for all women aged 40 or older who are considered at average risk of developing breast cancer.
- Patients with a suspicious abnormality on breast imaging and/or a clinically palpable mass should undergo a core needle biopsy to confirm the diagnosis and to facilitate appropriate surgical planning.
- For patients with evidence of breast cancer on core biopsy, definitive surgery is warranted.
- Malignant cells that are confined strictly to the breast ducts (ductal carcinoma in situ, DCIS) or lobules (lobular carcinoma in situ, LCIS), and therefore do not have metastatic potential, are designated as carcinoma in situ.
- A diagnosis of early-stage breast cancer denotes disease that is limited to the breast and/or axilla.
- Systemic chemotherapy is an integral component of the adjuvant treatment strategy for many women with early-stage breast cancer.
- Because of the significant risk of locoregional recurrence in the ipsilateral breast and/or axilla after breast conserving surgery, radiotherapy to the conserved breast is indicated. Radiotherapy to the axilla is also indicated when four or more lymph nodes are involved. The role of radiotherapy when one to three axillary lymph nodes are involved is uncertain.
- Metastatic breast cancer (MBC) is associated with a median survival of two to three years. Because MBC is generally incurable, the goals of therapy are to improve quality of life and ideally, improve survival.

American College of Radiology, American Medical Association, and American College of Obstetrics and Gynecology recommend breast cancer screening with routine mammography in conjunction with annual clinical breast examination for all women aged 40 years or older who are at average risk of developing breast cancer. Earlier screening, more frequent breast imaging, and/or adjunctive imaging may be indicated for women at increased risk. Furthermore, women with a strong family history or genetic predisposition may be considered for risk-reducing procedures. To facilitate individual risk estimations, the National Cancer Institute developed a computerized risk assessment tool that synthesizes information on age, race, age at menarche, age of first birth or nulliparity, number of first degree relatives with breast cancer, number of previous benign breast biopsies, and atypical hyperplasia in a previous biopsy into five–year and lifetime invasive breast cancer risk projections (www.cancer.gov/bcrisktool). Appropriate screening regimens may be planned accordingly.

It is important to note that although most breast cancer diagnoses are made as a result of abnormal screening mammograms (6), not all mammography findings represent cancer. If an abnormality is detected on a screening study, a variety of mammography techniques may be employed to better characterize suspicious lesions. These may include magnification views, spot compression views, and variations in angle views. Digital mammography, which has demonstrated superior diagnostic accuracy compared with traditional film techniques for young women, pre- or peri-menopausal women, and women with heterogenous breasts, is also increasingly utilized (Fig. 13.1) (7).

Mammography findings are summarized into diagnostic assessment categories using the American College of Radiology (ACR) Breast Imaging Reporting and Data System (BI-RADS) (www.acr.org). This system was developed in 1993 in order to standardize breast imaging terminology, communication, and reporting in clinical practice and in research. The BI-RADS system not only provides diagnostic and prognostic information, but also incorporates management recommendations (Table 13.1).

Ultrasound

Ultrasound imaging of the breast is sometimes employed as an adjunct to mammography. This imaging modality is frequently used to further characterize palpable or radiographically detectable masses (ie, by distinguishing between solid and cystic masses) and to guide interventional procedures. Ultrasound imaging is not routinely incorporated into the diagnostic paradigm, but has been demonstrated to improve diagnostic specificity by correctly downgrading the diagnosis, particularly among women with a palpable breast mass or an abnormal screening mammogram (8–10).

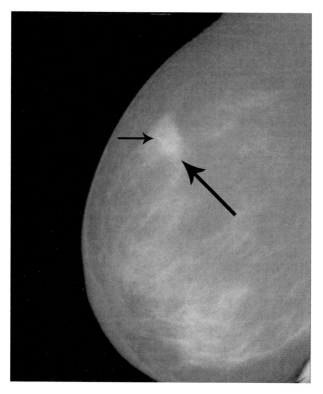

FIGURE 13.1

Digital mammogram obtained following an ultrasound guided biopsy and fine needle aspiration of a poorly differentiated invasive ductal carcinoma (large arrow). Note the clip placed at the biopsy site to facilitate surgical resection (small arrow).

Magnetic Resonance Imaging (MRI)

Almost all invasive breast cancers are visualized on gadolinium contrast-enhanced magnetic resonance imaging (MRI) (Fig. 13.2). Breast MRI has historically been associated with high sensitivity but variable specificity in detecting breast cancer among women are symptomatic, or those who are at high risk but are asymptomatic. In 2007, The American Cancer Society published guidelines for the use of breast cancer screening, suggesting MRI as an adjunct to mammography (11). Breast MRI was recommended for women with a greater than or equal to 20%–25% lifetime risk of developing breast cancer, including women with a known BRCA1 or BRCA2 mutation, a strong family history of breast or ovarian cancer, or a prior history of radiation therapy to the chest for the treatment of lymphoma. Outside of these indications, the role of MRI in breast cancer screening and management remains an ongoing area of investigation.

BREAST BIOPSY

Patients with a suspicious abnormality on breast imaging and/or a clinically palpable mass should undergo a core needle biopsy to confirm the diagnosis and to facilitate appropriate surgical planning. Fine needle aspiration (FNA) of suspicious breast lesions is typically less desirable than core biopsy because of the difficulty in distinguishing noninvasive (in situ) disease from invasive disease, the high incidence of false negative results, and the significant potential for yielding samples that are nondiagnostic. However, because identification of breast cancer that has spread to the axilla may have important clinical implications, FNA may be indicated for evaluation of suspicious axillary masses. Axillary involvement confirmed by FNA is typically managed

TABLE 13.1
Breast Imaging Reporting and Data System (BI-RADS) Mammographic Assessment Categories

ASSESSMENT CATEGORY	RECOMMENDATION	PROBABILITY OF MALIGNANCY
1. Negative	Routine follow-up	0%
2. Benign	Routine follow-up	0%
3. Probably benign	Short interval follow-up	<2%
4. Suspicious	Consider biopsy	2%–95%
5. Highly suggestive of malignancy	Appropriate management	≥95%
6. Incomplete	Further imaging evaluation	Not applicable

Source: Reprinted with permission of the American College of Radiology. No other representation of this material is authorized without expressed, written permission from the American College of Radiology.

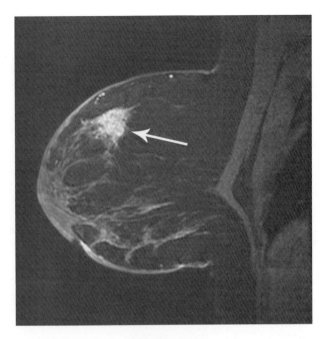

FIGURE 13.2

Breast MRI of the same poorly differentiated invasive ductal carcinoma illustrated on digital mammography in Figure 13.1.

with a complete axillary lymph node dissection, rather than sentinel lymph node biopsy alone, and may have implications for decisions regarding preoperative or neoadjuvant, chemotherapy.

Many centers have adopted stereotactic core needle biopsy techniques that utilize a specialized computer-guided imaging system or ultrasound guided core biopsy to investigate suspicious breast masses. Ultrasound guided biopsy is generally well tolerated and has the advantages of direct visualization of the target lesion and a relatively short study duration. Stereotactic methods are often reserved for patients with microcalcifications whose lesions are not well visualized on ultrasound, or for patients with deep masses close to the chest wall, where the biopsy needle can be inserted safely in parallel to the chest wall. Clips may also be inserted at the time of breast biopsy. Clips can provide radiographic correlation of the biopsied lesion, which may prove particularly important if the lesion is small and could be entirely removed by the biopsy procedure. Clips can also be useful in guiding further surgical interventions, or in following response to therapy for women with locally advanced disease undergoing neoadjuvant chemotherapy.

If breast cancer is identified on core biopsy, assays for hormone receptor status and HER2 status are typically performed on the biopsy specimen (see below). This practice may expedite decisions regarding post-

operative or adjuvant chemotherapy. However, given that breast cancers represent a heterogenous population of cells, and the potential for a false negative result is significant, these assays should be repeated on the excised surgical specimens if the assay results from the core biopsy specimens are reported as negative.

SURGERY

Breast: For patients with evidence of breast cancer on core biopsy, definitive surgery is warranted. Surgery may entail a lumpectomy (or breast conserving approach) or total mastectomy. Breast conserving surgery in combination with adjuvant radiotherapy to the breast is associated with an increased risk of local recurrence when compared to mastectomy, but there is no difference in overall survival (12).

Axilla: Historically, the standard approach to evaluation and management of the axilla was complete axillary dissection. However, surgical management of the axilla may now involve sentinel lymph node biopsy (SLNB), a technique that involves the injection of radioactive colloid or blue dye into the breast to identify the lymph nodes that first receive drainage from the tumor. If lymph node involvement is detected on SLNB, further surgery is typically warranted. The principles of breast surgery, perioperative imaging, and reconstruction are reviewed in detail elsewhere.

DUCTAL CARCINOMA *IN SITU* (DCIS)

Malignant cells that are confined strictly to the breast ducts (DCIS) or lobules (lobular carcinoma in situ, LCIS) are designated as carcinoma in situ (Fig. 13.3). Because there is no evidence of invasion into the surrounding stroma, these cells do not have the capacity for metastasis, a feature that distinguishes in situ from invasive disease. LCIS is not believed to be a direct precursor of invasive disease, but is considered a harbinger of increased risk (13–15). DCIS, however, is an established precursor of invasive disease, although the frequency of progression from untreated DCIS to invasive disease is uncertain. DCIS is treated with definitive local therapy comprised of mastectomy or breast conserving surgery with or without postoperative or adjuvant radiotherapy. If there is no evidence of invasive disease on the excised specimen, then evaluation of the axilla is generally not performed. Five years of additional treatment with tamoxifen, a selective estrogen receptor modulator, may be considered; however, the results of randomized trials have not been consistent (16,17). Furthermore, the potential benefits must be weighed against the risk for thromboembolic events

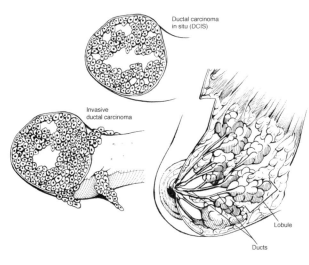

Ductal carcinoma in situ (DCIS)

Invasive ductal carcinoma

Lobule

Ducts

FIGURE 13.3

Ductal carcinoma in situ (DCIS) is an established precursor of invasive disease and is often treated with mastectomy or breast-conserving surgery with or without postoperative or adjuvant radiotherapy.

and the development of new uterine cancers associated with tamoxifen therapy.

STAGING FOR INVASIVE BREAST CANCER

The stage, or burden, of invasive disease at diagnosis is typically divided into either early-stage, locally advanced, or metastatic categories. However, a formal clinical and pathological staging system, developed by the American Joint Committee on Cancer (AJCC), is frequently used (18). In general, AJCC stages I and II are considered early; stage III, locally advanced; and stage IV, metastatic. These formal and informal staging categories endeavor to group together patients with a similar prognosis and may be used to guide further investigations. For example, women with small, node-negative, early-stage disease are at a low risk of distant spread. Consequently, the yield of further imaging studies is extremely low in this population. Women with large, bulky, node-positive disease, however, are at significant risk of distant spread and should therefore be considered for further evaluation at diagnosis to exclude established metastatic disease. The National Comprehensive Cancer Network currently recommends the following staging investigations for patients with early-stage (T1-2, N0-1) breast cancer: history and physical examination, complete blood count (CBC), liver function tests, chest imaging, and diagnostic mammogram (www.nccn.org/professionals/physician_gls).

Additional investigations with bone scan and abdominal imaging are recommended for patients with locally advanced or suspected metastatic disease. At present, the role of positron emission tomography imaging in the diagnosis and staging of women with breast cancer is uncertain. In addition, serum tumor marker assays, including CA 15-3 and CEA, lack sensitivity and specificity and are not recommended in the initial assessment of women with early-stage or locally advanced breast cancer.

The implication of accurate staging at diagnosis is that breast cancer that remains localized to the breast and/or axilla is potentially curable, whereas metastatic disease is not. Consequently, the therapeutic goals for localized versus metastatic disease are vastly different. In the treatment of early-stage disease, potentially toxic regimens associated with higher cure rates may be considered. Conversely, the goal of treatment for metastatic disease is to optimize quality of life and extend survival.

EARLY-STAGE DISEASE

Rationale for Adjuvant Chemotherapy

A diagnosis of early-stage breast cancer denotes disease that is limited to the breast and/or axilla. However, despite early detection, a significant proportion of these women will experience a distant relapse and later die of recurrence-related complications. These distant recurrences indicate that some women have undetectable micrometastatic disease at diagnosis. Consequently, locoregional therapy with surgery and/or radiotherapy is inadequate for cure in some women. Systemic chemotherapy, aimed at eradicating these subclinical micrometastases has thus become an integral component of the treatment strategy for some women with early-stage breast cancer. Adjuvant systemic therapy decisions are typically made by adopting a risk-benefit calculus, whereby an individual's risk of recurrence is weighed against the potential toxicity of the proposed regimen. Risk estimates are primarily derived from information on tumor size, nodal involvement, hormone receptor status, and HER2 status (see below). Other patient characteristics considered when designing an appropriate adjuvant strategy include age, comorbid conditions, patient preference, the acceptability of anticipated toxicity, and the desire for the expected benefits.

Risk Stratification

Historically, prognostic estimates for disease that remains clinically localized to the breast and/or axilla have been derived primarily from information on tumor size and lymph node status. However, prognostic profiling in the modern era is now frequently augmented by biologic data. Consequently, the risk stratification paradigm has become increasingly sophisticated for some women and treatment strategies are increasingly tailored to the biology of an individual's tumor.

Tumor Size and Nodal Status

Tumor size and the extent of nodal involvement are well-established prognostic factors for patients with early-stage breast cancer (19). Although nodal status has historically conferred the most compelling prognostic information, the advent of SLNB techniques has presented new challenges in risk stratification. When compared with traditional axillary dissection techniques, SLNB typically yields fewer lymph nodes for evaluation. Because of the important decision that hinges on proving that the sentinel nodes are negative, a more detailed evaluation of a fewer number of nodes is permitted. Isolated tumor cells or micrometastases that were undetectable by traditional staining techniques are now detected by immunohistochemistry (IHC), but the prognostic significance of such findings in conventionally negative lymph nodes has not yet been fully elucidated (20–24).

Hormone Receptor Status

Hormone receptor status is a well-established prognostic and predictive factor. The risk of recurrence for women with estrogen receptor (ER)-negative breast cancer peaks as high as 18.5% approximately one to two years after surgery and declines rapidly thereafter to 1.4% in years 8 through 12 (Fig. 13.4) (19).

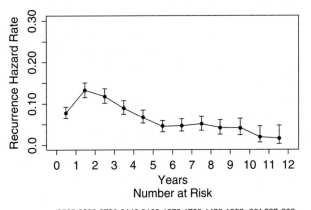

3585 3226 2786 2443 2168 1972 1739 1428 1089 801 527 328

FIGURE 13.4

Annual hazard of breast cancer recurrence by estrogen receptor (ER) status. Reprinted with permission from the American Society of Clinical Oncology.

Most women, however, have breast cancers that are ER-positive. For these women, the recurrence pattern is unique from that of their ER-negative counterparts, with a smaller and later recurrence risk peak of 11.0% in years two to three and a significant rate of persistent recurrence (approximately 5%) through to year 12. Thus, ER-status provides important information about the anticipated natural history of an individual's breast cancer.

ER status also provides important predictive information, not only to response to hormonal therapy, but also to systemic chemotherapy. In a retrospective subset analysis of three cooperative group adjuvant chemotherapy trials, investigators demonstrated that for women with node-positive breast cancer, the absolute benefit of chemotherapy was more pronounced for the ER-negative cohort compared to the ER-positive cohort (25). Similar findings have been reported in a large collaborative meta-analysis of more than 145,000 women who participated in 194 trials conducted by the Early Breast Cancer Trialists' Collaborative Group (EBCTCG) (26).

HER2 Status

The HER2 receptor is a member of the transmembrane human epidermal growth factor receptor (EGFR) family and is overexpressed in approximately 20%–25% of human breast cancers. Although HER2 overexpression has historically conferred a worse prognosis compared with non-overexpressing cohorts, the prognostic significance has become less relevant with the advent of HER2-targeted therapy (27,28). HER2 status remains an important predictive factor, however, for responses not only to trastuzumab (Herceptin), a recombinant monoclonal HER2-targeted antibody, but also to other chemotherapeutic agents. The most notable of these is an increased sensitivity to anthracycline-containing regimens among women with HER2-overexpressing breast cancer (29,30). Synergy and/or additive effects have also been demonstrated with the combination of trastuzumab and taxanes or vinorelbine (31,32). HER2-overexpressing breast cancers are also relatively resistant to treatment with tamoxifen, but not aromatase inhibitors (AIs) (33,34).

Risk Calculation Tools

Multiple tools have been developed to increase the accuracy of clinical risk-benefit estimations. The most notable web-based prognostic tool is Adjuvant! Online (www.adjuvantonline.com), which estimates 10-year relapse and mortality rates based on various patient/tumor characteristics and estimates the expected benefit of various adjuvant systemic treatment strategies.

Hormonal maneuvers are the therapeutic cornerstone for women with hormone receptor positive early-stage breast cancer. However, for women with small, node-negative, ER-positive, early-stage breast cancer for whom adjuvant hormone therapy is anticipated, it is often difficult to ascertain the potential additional benefit to be derived from adjuvant systemic chemotherapy. Several multigene assays have been developed to facilitate risk-benefit estimations for these women (35–38). For example, the Oncotype DX assay utilizes a 21-gene expression profile to categorize a woman's risk of recurrence as low, intermediate, or high, with average associated 10-year distant recurrence rates of 6.8%, 14.3%, and 30.5%, respectively (35). This assay enables some women who are truly at low risk to forgo overtreatment and exposure to the deleterious effects of chemotherapy, while women at a higher risk of recurrence may be considered for a more aggressive therapeutic strategy. However, the ideal management strategy for women at intermediate risk remains uncertain. The TailorRx trial was designed to address this question and is currently randomizing women at intermediate risk Oncotype DX to hormone therapy alone or in combination with chemotherapy. This test is performed on paraffin-embedded tumor specimens. The MammaPrint assay, which stratifies women into low risk or high risk categories based on a 70-gene assay developed in Europe, received United States Food and Drug Administration (FDA) approval in 2007 (36). This test is performed on fresh frozen material. Additional gene profile assays are in development.

Adjuvant Chemotherapy for Early-stage Disease

Systemic chemotherapy has been an integral component of the adjuvant treatment strategy for many women with early-stage breast cancer since investigators first reported benefits with single agent chemotherapy after radical mastectomy in the 1970s. Systemic chemotherapy regimens have since undergone a number of refinements in formulations, schedules, and dosage. Polychemotherapy, whereby a minimum of two agents are administered in combination, was an early modification and represents an approach that has since been supported by a number of studies, including the Early Breast Cancer Trialists' Collaborative Group meta-analysis (26). Modern polychemotherapy regimens often incorporate an anthracycline and/or a taxane (Table 13.2). However, because many modern regimens have not been directly compared in randomized control trials, the superiority of any singular regimen has not been clearly established, nor have the benefits of any specific regimens for specific subgroups been clearly delineated.

One significant innovation in systemic chemotherapy administration is the dose dense strategy, developed from the Norton-Simon model, whereby the interval between treatments is decreased in order to optimize tumor cell, thus improving the overall impact of therapy (39). Another innovation is in drug delivery. For example, the paclitaxel (Taxol) solvent, Cremophor, is associated with potentially life-threatening hypersensitivity reactions, and consequently requires specialized equipment and steroid premedication. Albumin-bound paclitaxel (nab-paclitaxel, Abraxane), is a Cremophor-free preparation that does not require steroid premedication or specialized intravenous tubing. When compared to the conventional formulation, nab-paclitaxel demonstrated improved response rates and time to progression in the metastatic setting (40); in 2008 the drug was evaluated in the adjuvant setting. The improved activity demonstrated in the metastatic setting is postulated to reflect the ability to administer higher doses of the active agent and potentially, the preferential delivery of albumin-bound paclitaxel to cancer cells.

Biologic/Targeted Therapy for Early-stage Disease

Breast cancer is not homogeneous, as indicated by the mix of hormone responsive and unresponsive tumor cells. Another distinction can be made, as discussed above, on the basis of HER2. Recognition of specific subtypes is important because it holds the promise of targeted therapies. In this regard, one of the most significant advances in breast cancer management has been the development of trastuzumab. This humanized HER2-targeted monoclonal antibody is the most extensively studied biologic therapy (after anti-estrogens) in the adjuvant setting to date. HER2 status is determined by IHC evaluation of the protein and/or fluorescence in situ hybridization (FISH) assay of the HER2 gene sequence. The addition of trastuzumab to various adjuvant chemotherapy backbones has been associated with significant survival benefits and is now a standard component of the adjuvant paradigm for this subgroup (27,28,32,41). In 2008, adjuvant studies of other promising biologic agents included bevacizumab (Avastin), an anti-VEGF antibody, and lapatinib (Tykerb), an orally active tyrosine kinase inhibitor that targets both the HER1 and HER2 receptors. It is hoped that the incorporation of generally well-tolerated targeted therapy into the adjuvant treatment strategy may permit some women to forgo some of the potentially toxic chemotherapeutic agents comprising conventional strategies.

TABLE 13.2
Selected Modern Adjuvant Chemotherapy Regimens

REGIMEN	AGENTS	DOSE	DAY OF ADMINISTRATION	FREQUENCY OF ADMINISTRATION	TOTAL NUMBER OF CYCLES
AC-T[53,54]	Doxorubicin	60 mg/m^2 IV	Day 1	Every 3 weeks or every 2 weeks with G-CSF support	4
	Cyclophosphamide	600 mg/m^2 IV	Day 1		
	Paclitaxel	175 mg/m2 IV	Day 1		4
CEF[55,56] (with cotrimoxazole prophylaxis)	Cyclophosphamide	75 mg/m^2/d PO	Days 1–14	Every 4 weeks	6
	Epirubicin	60 mg/m^2/d IV	Days 1 & 8		
	5-Fluorouracil	500 mg/m^2/d IV	Days 1 & 8		
CMF[57,58]	Cyclophosphamide	600 mg/m^2 IV	Day 1	Every 3 weeks	8
	Methotrexate	40 mg/m^2 IV	Day 1		
	5-Fluorouracil	600 mg/m^2 IV	Day 1		
FEC[59]	5-Fluorouracil	500 mg/m^2 IV	Day 1	Every 3 weeks	6
	Epirubicin	100 mg/m^2 IV	Day 1		
	Cyclophosphamide	500 mg/m^2 IV	Day 1		
FEC-D[60]	5-Fluorouracil	500 mg/m^2 IV	Day 1	Every 3 weeks	3
	Epirubicin	100 mg/m^2 IV	Day 1		
	Cyclophosphamide	500 mg/m^2 IV	Day 1		
	Docetaxel	100 mg/m^2 IV	Day 1	Every 3 weeks	3
TAC[61]	Docetaxel	75 mg/m^2 IV	Day 1	Every 3 weeks	6
	Adriamycin	50 mg/m^2 IV	Day 1		
	Cyclophosphamide	500 mg/m^2 IV	Day 1		

Abbreviations: AC-T, adriamycin/cyclophosphamide-paclitaxel; CEF, cyclophosphamide/epirubicin/5-fluorouracil; CMF, cyclophosphamide/methotrexate/5-fluorouracil; FEC, 5-fluorouracil/epirubicin/cyclophosphamide; FEC-D, 5-fluorouracil/epirubicin/cyclophosphamide-docetaxel; TAC, docetaxel/adriamycin/cyclophosphamide; G-CSF, granulocyte-colony stimulating factor; PO, by mouth; IV, intravenous.

Hormone Therapy for Early-stage Disease

Women with hormone-sensitive, early-stage breast cancer, as determined by estrogen and/or progesterone receptor status, are typically treated with adjuvant hormone therapy. The basic concept is that hormone-responsive cancers will not grow when estrogen-driven proliferation is inhibited. By "hormone therapy," we really mean anti-estrogen therapy, although the actual mechanisms of action for some hormone agents are too complex for such simple summation. Functionally, adjuvant hormone therapy for pre- or peri-menopausal women with hormone-sensitive tumors is comprised of tamoxifen or ovarian suppression. The efficacy of tamoxifen or an AI in combination with medical or surgical ovarian suppression is not well defined. The Sup-

pression of Ovarian Function Trial (SOFT) is currently randomizing pre-menopausal women with early-stage, hormone-sensitive breast cancer to tamoxifen, tamoxifen with ovarian suppression or an AI (exemestane, Aromasin) with ovarian suppression.

Prior to the early 2000s, tamoxifen was also considered the cornerstone of hormonal therapy for postmenopausal women with early-stage, hormone-sensitive disease. However, studies evaluating third-generation AIs in the adjuvant setting were reported as early as 2004. AIs inhibit the aromatase enzyme, which catalyzes the peripheral conversion of steroid precursors into active forms of estrogen. These drugs have been evaluated in a number of adjuvant strategies, including sequential strategies after two to three years of tamoxifen, upfront strategies, and extended strategies beyond five years of tamoxifen (42–47). Each of these demonstrated significant benefits; however, the superiority of any given strategy has not been determined. The most common AI-related toxicities include myalgias/arthralgias and decreased bone mineral density. However, AIs are not associated with the increased risk of thromboembolic events and new uterine cancers, which are associated with tamoxifen administration.

Adjuvant Radiotherapy

Because there is a significant risk of recurrence after breast conserving surgery, radiotherapy to the conserved breast is indicated in this setting to optimize local control (48). The addition of ipsilateral breast radiotherapy to breast conserving surgery is associated with a significantly lower rate of local recurrence (7% vs 26% at 15 years), and is thus an integral component of the breast conserving approach (12). Because of the increased risk of locoregional recurrence and the overall survival benefits demonstrated to date, radiotherapy post-mastectomy is indicated for women with large (5 cm or greater) tumors and/or four or more involved axillary lymph nodes (12,49). The benefits of radiotherapy for women with one to three involved lymph nodes is not well defined, and significant regional variability in practice patterns exist. By convention, radiotherapy is typically administered upon completion of adjuvant systemic therapy.

LOCALLY ADVANCED BREAST CANCER

Locally advanced breast cancer (LABC) is associated with a poorer prognosis than early-stage disease. The definition of LABC has not been consistent across clinical trials; however, the term generally denotes tumors that are large (greater than 5 cm), have extensive lymph node involvement, and/or involve the skin or chest wall. Inflammatory breast cancer (IBC) is a specific entity under the LABC umbrella, characterized by diffuse erythema, edema, and/or peau d'orange affecting the majority of the breast. IBC is primarily a clinical rather than pathological diagnosis, and portends a particularly poor prognosis.

LABC is represented by the stage III designation in the TNM classification system. LABC is typically treated with induction (neoadjuvant) chemotherapy followed by definitive locoregional therapy with surgery, radiotherapy or both. The practice of delivering neoadjuvant (preoperative) treatment (chemotherapy, hormone therapy, biologic therapy) affords a number of potential advantages. First, inoperable tumors can be rendered resectable. In addition, a neoadjuvant approach has the advantage of downstaging the cancer, thereby increasing the likelihood of a breast conserving approach as well as allowing procurement of pathologic specimens that may provide important correlative data regarding response to therapy. On the other hand, a number of potential benefits, including theoretically earlier eradication of micrometastases and the prevention of spontaneous somatic mutations postulated to lead to drug resistant cell populations, have not been observed. In research trials, response to neoadjuvant chemotherapy appeared to provide important prognostic information, which generally correlates with overall survival, but this form of treatment has not been generalized to standard practice (50).

Outside of a clinical trial, neoadjuvant chemotherapy is typically comprised of an anthracycline- and/or taxane-containing regimen followed by an assessment of response to therapy (46). Subsequent definitive locoregional therapy is indicated if a complete or near-complete clinical response is observed. However, in the absence of these findings, further neoadjuvant therapy with a non-cross-resistant chemotherapy regimen may be considered (ie, with a taxane if an anthracycline was previously administered, or vice versa). Although the optimal duration of trastuzumab administration in this setting is unknown, extrapolating from the survival benefits demonstrated with trastuzumab in the adjuvant setting, all women with HER2-overexpressing LABC should be considered for a 52-week course of trastuzumab therapy in the absence of any contraindication and regardless of whether treatment begins before or after surgery.

LOCOREGIONAL RECURRENCE

Despite adequate definitive therapy, a significant number of women with early-stage or LABC experience a locoregional recurrence, typically within the first 5 years after diagnosis (12). A recurrence in the ipsilateral preserved breast or chest wall is described as "local" whereas a recurrence in the ipsilateral axillary, supraclavicular, infraclavicular, and/or internal mammary nodes is described as "regional." If a locoregional recurrence is suspected, diagnostic re-evaluation with biopsy (including re-evaluation of hormone receptor and HER2 status) and repeat staging investigations to rule out distant recurrence should be considered. If recurrence occurs in the preserved breast after breast-conserving treatment, mastectomy is generally indicated. If recurrence occurs in the chest wall only, a wide local excision may be considered. Additional postexcision radiotherapy should also be considered, especially if postmastectomy radiotherapy was not previously administered. With regional recurrence after primary breast-conserving treatment or mastectomy, repeat axillary staging in the absence of clinically detectable nodal disease may be considered. ALND, if not previously performed, or resection (if ALND was previously performed) may be considered in the setting of clinically suspicious lymphadenopathy. The goal is to avoid under treating potentially curable second primary cancers that can arise in preserved duct epithelium. Very long-term disease control (and even cure) is reported for a subset of patients following local relapse only.

Systemic chemotherapy after definitive therapy for a locoregional recurrence is commonly recommended, although the benefits of this practice are not well defined. In a large, international, multicenter, phase III clinical trial led by International Breast Cancer Study Group and National Surgical Adjuvant Breast and Bowel Project investigators, women with a radically resected, locoregional breast cancer recurrence are currently being randomized to radiotherapy with or without chemotherapy. Until the results of this study are reported, systemic chemotherapy or in hormone-sensitive disease, hormone therapy, can be considered on an individual basis. As in the adjuvant setting, all women with HER2-overexpressing breast cancer should be considered for trastuzumab therapy.

METASTATIC BREAST CANCER

Metastatic breast cancer (MBC) represents approximately 5% of all new breast cancer diagnoses (1). In addition, the majority of women with early-stage or LABC who experience a relapse will relapse at a distant site. MBC is associated with a median survival of two to three years. Because MBC is generally incurable, the goals of therapy are to improve quality of life and ideally, improve survival. Consequently, the potential for treatment-related toxicity must be carefully weighed against the goals of therapy.

There is no consensus regarding the ideal treatment strategy for women with MBC; consequently, regional variations in practice patterns are observed. In general, however, reasonable MBC management strategies can be determined by considering a number of patient and tumor characteristics. The disease-free interval, prior adjuvant therapy prescription, number of metastatic sites, and potential for visceral crisis, as well as patient age, patient preference, comorbidities, performance status, hormone receptor status, and HER2 status, should all be considered when devising a treatment strategy. Bisphosphonate therapy should be considered in women with metastases to bone for the prevention of skeletal-related events (51). In general, endocrine therapies, which are generally well tolerated and associated

with favorable toxicity profiles, are recommended for women with hormone-responsive MBC who are not at risk for visceral crisis. Conversely, systemic chemotherapy is typically recommended for women with hormone-refractory disease, hormone-receptor negative disease, selected women with rapidly progressive disease, and/or women with significant cancer-related symptoms. All women with HER2-overexpressing MBC should be considered for trastuzumab therapy in the absence of any clear contraindication. In 2007, lapatinib, a small molecule tyrosine kinase inhibitor, was approved by the U.S. FDA for the treatment of anthracycline, taxane, and trastuzumab pretreated HER2-overexpressing MBC (40). For patients with HER2-normal disease, one trial suggested an advantage for the anti-angiogenic monoclonal antibody, bevacizumab, added to weekly paclitaxel as first-line therapy (52). The role of biologic therapy remains an active and promising area of investigation. Women should be considered for participation in clinical trials where appropriate.

CONCLUSIONS

Breast cancer is an important public health issue. The incidence and prevalence of breast cancer are significant. However, important strides in diagnosis and treatment have resulted in significant improvements in breast cancer-specific mortality rates (4,5). In the coming years, further improvements in screening and diagnostic technology are anticipated, with a particular focus on imaging modalities that exploit some of the biologic features of breast cancer. Similarly, clinical trials of promising biologic/targeted therapies as well as drug delivery and scheduling innovations continue in the adjuvant, neoadjuvant, and metastatic settings. It is hoped that these innovations in diagnosis and treatment will translate into ongoing improvements in breast cancer-specific outcomes.

References

1. American Cancer Society. *Cancer Facts & Figures*. http://www.cancer.org/docroot/STT/content/STT_1x_Cancer_Facts_and_Figures_2008.asp?from=fast
2. Claus EB, Schildkraut JM, Thompson WD, Risch NJ. The genetic attributable risk of breast and ovarian cancer. *Cancer.* 1996;77(11):2318–2324.
3. Chen S, Parmigiani G. Meta-analysis of BRCA1 and BRCA2 penetrance. *J Clin Oncol.* 2007;25(11):1329–1333.
4. Berry DA, Cronin KA, Plevritis SK, et al. Effect of screening and adjuvant therapy on mortality from breast cancer. *N Engl J Med.* 2005;353(17):1784–1792.
5. Elkin EB, Hurria A, Mitra N, Schrag D, Panageas KS. Adjuvant chemotherapy and survival in older women with hormone receptor-negative breast cancer: assessing outcome in a population-based, observational cohort. *J Clin Oncol.* 2006;24(18):2757–2764.

6. Smart CR, Hartmann WH, Beahrs OH, Garfinkel L. Insights into breast cancer screening of younger women. Evidence from the 14-year follow-up of the Breast Cancer Detection Demonstration Project. *Cancer*. 1993;72(4 Suppl):1449–1456.

7. Pisano ED, Gatsonis C, Hendrick E, et al. Diagnostic performance of digital versus film mammography for breast-cancer screening. *N Engl J Med*. 2005;353(17):1773–1783.

8. Soo MS, Rosen EL, Baker JA, Vo TT, Boyd BA. Negative predictive value of sonography with mammography in patients with palpable breast lesions. *AJR*. 2001;177(5):1167–1170.

9. Moy L, Slanetz PJ, Moore R, et al. Specificity of mammography and US in the evaluation of a palpable abnormality: retrospective review. *Radiology*. 2002;225(1):176–181.

10. Flobbe K, Bosch AM, Kessels AG, et al. The additional diagnostic value of ultrasonography in the diagnosis of breast cancer. *Arch Intern Med*. 2003;163(10):1194–1199.

11. Saslow D, Boetes C, Burke W, et al. American Cancer Society guidelines for breast screening with MRI as an adjunct to mammography. *CA Cancer J Clin*. 2007;57(2):75–89.

12. Early Breast Trialists' Collaborative Group. Effects of radiotherapy and of differences in the extent of surgery for early breast cancer on local recurrence and 15-year survival: an overview of the randomised trials. *Lancet*. 2005;366(9503):2087–2106.

13. Fisher ER, Land SR, Fisher B, Mamounas E, Gilarski L, Wolmark N. Pathologic findings from the National Surgical Adjuvant Breast and Bowel Project: twelve-year observations concerning lobular carcinoma in situ. *Cancer*. 2004;100(2):238–244.

14. Fisher B, Costantino JP, Wickerham DL, et al. Tamoxifen for the prevention of breast cancer: current status of the National Surgical Adjuvant Breast and Bowel Project P-1 study. *J Natl Cancer Inst*. 2005;97(22):1652–1662.

15. Chuba PJ, Hamre MR, Yap J, et al. Bilateral risk for subsequent breast cancer after lobular carcinoma-in-situ: analysis of surveillance, epidemiology, and end results data. *J Clin Oncol*. 2005;23(24):5534–5541.

16. Fisher B, Dignam J, Wolmark N, et al. Tamoxifen in treatment of intraductal breast cancer: National Surgical Adjuvant Breast and Bowel Project B-24 randomised controlled trial. *Lancet*. 1999;353(9169):1993–2000.

17. Houghton J, George WD, Cuzick J, Duggan C, Fentiman IS, Spittle M. Radiotherapy and tamoxifen in women with completely excised ductal carcinoma in situ of the breast in the UK, Australia, and New Zealand: randomised controlled trial. *Lancet*. 2003;362(9378):95–102.

18. American Joint Committee on Cancer (AJCC). *AJCC Cancer Staging Manual*, 6th ed. New York: Springer-Verlag; 2002.

19. Saphner T, Tormey DC, Gray R. Annual hazard rates of recurrence for breast cancer after primary therapy. *J Clin Oncol*. 1996;14(10):2738–2746.

20. Susnik B, Frkovic-Grazio S, Bracko M. Occult micrometastases in axillary lymph nodes predict subsequent distant metastases in stage I breast cancer: a case-control study with 15-year follow-up. *Ann Surg Oncol*. 2004;11(6):568–572.

21. Cummings MC, Walsh MD, Hohn BG, Bennett IC, Wright RG, McGuckin MA. Occult axillary lymph node metastases in breast cancer do matter: results of 10-year survival analysis. *Am J Surg Pathol*. 2002;26(10):1286–1295.

22. Millis RR, Springall R, Lee AH, Ryder K, Rytina ER, Fentiman IS. Occult axillary lymph node metastases are of no prognostic significance in breast cancer. *Br J Cancer*. 2002;86(3):396–401.

23. Elson CE, Kufe D, Johnston WW. Immunohistochemical detection and significance of axillary lymph node micrometastases in breast carcinoma. A study of 97 cases. *Anal Quant Cytol Histol*. 1993;15(3):171–178.

24. Herbert GS, Sohn VY, Brown TA. The impact of nodal isolated tumor cells on survival of breast cancer patients. *Am J Surg*. 2007;193(5):571–573; discussion 3–4.

25. Berry DA, Cirrincione C, Henderson IC, et al. Estrogen-receptor status and outcomes of modern chemotherapy for patients with node-positive breast cancer. *JAMA*. 2006;295(14):1658–1667.

26. Early Breast Cancer Trialists' Collaborative Group. Effects of chemotherapy and hormonal therapy for early breast cancer on recurrence and a 15-year survival: an overview of the randomised trials. *Lancet*. 2005;365:1687–1717.

27. Piccart-Gebhart MJ, Procter M, Leyland-Jones B, et al. Trastuzumab after Adjuvant Chemotherapy in HER2-Positive Breast Cancer. *N Engl J Med*. 2005;353(16):1659–1672.

28. Romond EH, Perez EA, Bryant J, et al. Trastuzumab plus adjuvant Chemotherapy for operable HER2-positive breast cancer. *N Engl J Med*. 2005;353(16):1673–1684.

29. Pritchard KI, Shepherd LE, O'Malley FP, et al. HER2 and responsiveness of breast cancer to adjuvant chemotherapy. *N Engl J Med*. 2006;354(20):2103–2111.

30. Paik S, Bryant J, Park C, et al. erbB-2 and response to doxorubicin in patients with axillary lymph node positive, hormone receptor-negative breast cancer. *J Natl Cancer Inst*. 1998;90(18):1361–1370.

31. Marty M, Cognetti F, Maraninchi D, et al. Randomized phase II trial of the efficacy and safety of trastuzumab combined with docetaxel in patients with human epidermal growth factor receptor 2-positive metastatic breast cancer administered as first-line treatment: the M77001 study group. *J Clin Oncol*. 2005;23(19):4265–4274.

32. Joensuu H, Kellokumpu-Lehtinen PL, Bono P, et al. Adjuvant docetaxel or vinorelbine with or without trastuzumab for breast cancer. *N Engl J Med*. 2006;354(8):809–820.

33. Schiff R, Chamness GC, Brown PH. Advances in breast cancer treatment and prevention: preclinical studies on aromatase inhibitors and new selective estrogen receptor modulators (SERMs). *Breast Cancer Res*. 2003;5(5):228–231.

34. Ellis MJ, Coop A, Singh B, et al. Letrozole is more effective neoadjuvant endocrine therapy than tamoxifen for ErbB-1- and/or ErbB-2-positive, estrogen receptor-positive primary breast cancer: evidence from a phase III randomized trial. *J Clin Oncol*. 2001;19(18):3808–3816.

35. Paik S, Shak S, Tang G, et al. A multigene assay to predict recurrence of tamoxifen-treated, node-negative breast cancer. *N Engl J Med*. 2004;351(27):2817–2826.

36. van de Vijver MJ, He YD, van't Veer LJ, et al. A gene-expression signature as a predictor of survival in breast cancer. *N Engl J Med*. 2002;347(25):1999–2009.

37. Buyse M, Loi S, van't Veer L, et al. Validation and clinical utility of a 70-gene prognostic signature for women with node-negative breast cancer. *J Natl Cancer Inst*. 2006;98(17):1183–1192.

38. Wang Y, Klijn JG, Zhang Y, et al. Gene-expression profiles to predict distant metastasis of lymph-node-negative primary breast cancer. *Lancet*. 2005;365(9460):671–679.

39. Norton L. A Gompertzian model of human breast cancer growth. *Cancer Res*. 1988;48:7067–7071.

40. Gradishar WJ, Tjulandin S, Davidson N, et al. Phase III trial of nanoparticle albumin-bound paclitaxel compared with polyethylated castor oil-based paclitaxel in women with breast cancer. *J Clin Oncol*. 2005;23(31):7794–7803.

41. Slamon D EW, Robert N, et al. Phase III randomized trial comparing doxorubicin and cyclophosphamide followed by docetaxel (ACT) with doxorubicin and cyclophosphamide followed by docetaxel and trastuzumab (ACTH) with docetaxel, carboplatin and trastuzumab (TCH) in HER2 positive early breast cancer patients: BCIRG 006 study. In: San Antonio Breast Cancer Symposium; San Antonio, TX; 2005.

42. Howell A, Cuzick J, Baum M, et al. Results of the ATAC (Arimidex, Tamoxifen, Alone or in Combination) trial after completion of 5 years' adjuvant treatment for breast cancer. *Lancet*. 2005;365(9453):60–62.

43. Coates AS, Keshaviah A, Thurlimann B, et al. Five years of letrozole compared with tamoxifen as initial adjuvant therapy for postmenopausal women with endocrine-responsive early breast cancer: update of study BIG 1-98. *J Clin Oncol*. 2007;25(5):486–492.

44. Coombes RC, Kilburn LS, Snowdon CF, et al. Survival and safety of exemestane versus tamoxifen after 2–3 years' tamoxifen treatment (Intergroup Exemestane Study): a randomised controlled trial. *Lancet*. 2007;369(9561):559–570.

45. Goss PE, Ingle JN, Martino S, Robert NJ, et al. Updated analysis of the NCIC CTG MA.17 randomized placebo (P) controlled

trial of letrozole (L) after five years of tamoxifen in postmenopausal women with early stage breast cancer. *Proc Am Soc Clin Oncol.* 2004;23:87.

46. Schwartz GF, Hortobagyi GN. Proceedings of the consensus conference on neoadjuvant chemotherapy in carcinoma of the breast, April 26-28, 2003, Philadelphia, Pennsylvania. *Cancer.* 2004;100(12):2512–2532.

47. Boccardo F, Rubagotti A, Puntoni M, et al. Switching to anastrozole versus continued tamoxifen treatment of early breast cancer: preliminary results of the Italian Tamoxifen Anastrozole Trial. *J Clin Oncol.* 2005;23(22):5138–5147.

48. Eifel P, Axelson JA, Costa J, et al. National Institutes of Health Consensus Development Conference Statement: adjuvant therapy for breast cancer, November 1–3, 2000. *J Natl Cancer Inst.* 2001;93(13):979–989.

49. Harris JR, Halpin-Murphy P, McNeese M, Mendenhall NP, Morrow M, Robert NJ. Consensus Statement on postmastectomy radiation therapy. *Int J Rad Oncol Biol Phys.* 1999;44(5):989–990.

50. Buzdar AU, Singletary SE, Booser DJ, Frye DK, Wasaff B, Hortobagyi GN. Combined modality treatment of stage III and inflammatory breast cancer. M.D. Anderson Cancer Center experience. *Surg Oncol Clin N Am.* 1995;4(4):715–734.

51. Hillner BE, Ingle JN, Chlebowski RT, et al. American Society of Clinical Oncology 2003 update on the role of bisphosphonates and bone health issues in women with breast cancer. *J Clin Oncol.* 2003;21(21):4042–4057.

52. Miller K, Wang M, Gralow J, et al. A randomized phase III trial of paclitaxel versus paclitaxel plus bevacizumab as first-line therapy for locally recurrent or metastatic breast cancer: a trial coordinated by the Eastern Cooperative Oncology Group (E2100). In: 28th Annual San Antonio Breast Cancer Symposium 2005; San Antonio, Texas: Breast Cancer Research and Treatment; 2005; S6.

53. Henderson IC, Berry DA, Demetri GD, et al. Improved outcomes from adding sequential Paclitaxel but not from escalating Doxorubicin dose in an adjuvant chemotherapy regimen for patients with node-positive primary breast cancer. *J Clin Oncol.* 2003;21(6):976–983.

54. Citron ML, Berry DA, Cirrincione C, et al. Randomized trial of dose-dense versus conventionally scheduled and sequential versus concurrent combination chemotherapy as postoperative adjuvant treatment of node-positive primary breast cancer: first report of Intergroup Trial C9741/Cancer and Leukemia Group B Trial 9741. *J Clin Oncol.* 2003;21(8):1431–1439.

55. Levine MN, Bramwell VH, Pritchard KI, et al. Randomized trial of intensive cyclophosphamide, epirubicin, and fluorouracil chemotherapy compared with cyclophosphamide, methotrexate, and fluorouracil in premenopausal women with node-positive breast cancer. National Cancer Institute of Canada Clinical Trials Group. *J Clin Oncol.* 1998;16(8):2651–2658.

56. Ejlertsen B, Mouridsen HT, Jensen MB, et al. Improved outcome from substituting methotrexate with epirubicin: results from a randomized comparison of CMF versus CEF in patients with primary breast cancer. *Eur J Cancer.* 2007;43(5):877–884.

57. Fisher B, Dignam J, Mamounas EP, et al. Sequential methotrexate and fluorouracil for the treatment of node-negative breast cancer patients with estrogen receptor-negative tumors: eight-year results from National Surgical Adjuvant Breast and Bowel Project (NSABP) B-13 and first report of findings from NSABP B-19 comparing methotrexate and fluorouracil with conventional cyclophosphamide, methotrexate, and fluorouracil. *J Clin Oncol.* 1996;14(7):1982–1992.

58. Fisher B, Anderson S, Tan-Chiu E, et al. Tamoxifen and chemotherapy for axillary node-negative, estrogen receptor-negative breast cancer: findings from National Surgical Adjuvant Breast and Bowel Project B-23. *J Clin Oncol.* 2001;19(4):931–942.

59. French Epirubicin Study G. Benefit of a high-dose epirubicin regimen in adjuvant chemotherapy for node-positive breast cancer patients with poor prognostic factors: 5-year follow-up results of french adjuvant study group 05 randomized trial. *J Clin Oncol.* 2001;19(3):602–611.

60. Roché H, Fumoleau P, Spielmann M, et al. Sequential adjuvant epirubicin-based and docetaxel chemotherapy for node-positive breast cancer patients: the FNCLCC PACS 01 Trial. *J Clin Oncol.* 2006;24(36):5664–5671.

61. Martin M, Pienkowski T, Mackey J, et al. Adjuvant docetaxel for node-positive breast cancer. *N Engl J Med.* 2005;352(22):2302–2313.

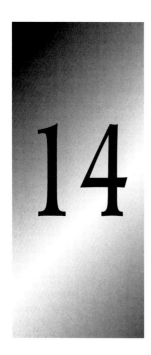

Evaluation and Treatment of Prostate and Genitourinary Cancer

Alexei Morozov
Susan F. Slovin

This chapter will begin with an overview of prostate cancer followed by a discussion of genitourinary cancers which include cancers of the urinary tract (bladder, urethra, and kidney) and the male genital tract (testis and penis). In the United States, it was estimated that over 186,000 new cases of prostate cancer would be diagnosed 2008, accounting for 29% of all new cancer diagnoses in men. For a man aged 70 or older, the estimated risk of developing prostate cancer is one in seven (1). Prostate cancer is the second largest cause of cancer mortality in men; in the United States, it was estimated that over 28,000 deaths from prostate cancer would occur in 2008. There has, however, been a steady decline in the prostate cancer death rate in the US since 1997 (1). Worldwide, there is wide variation in prostate cancer incidence rates among geographic and ethnic groups. The highest incidence of prostate cancer is seen in African-Americans and Caribbean men of African descent (2). Geographically, the highest rates are seen in North America and Western Europe, intermediate rates in Africa, and lowest rates in Asia. These trends were seen prior to the prostate-specific antigen (PSA) era as well (2,3). In addition to race and ethnicity, the presence of a first-degree relative with prostate cancer is a well-established risk factor for development of prostate cancer. Having an affected father confers a twofold risk of prostate cancer. The risk is further increased if multiple relatives are affected with prostate cancer, or if relatives with the disease were diagnosed before age 65 (4). Obesity was found to be positively associated with a risk of prostate cancer in a cohort analysis involving 900,000 patients. Patients with a BMI older than aged 35 were found to be 34% more likely to die from prostate cancer (5).

DIAGNOSIS

Following the introduction of PSA testing in the mid-1980s, the incidence of prostate cancer more than doubled, reaching its peak in 1992. Whereas in the pre-PSA era 50% of prostate cancers presented with metastatic disease, more than 90% of prostate cancers are now detected at the organ-confined stage. The American Cancer Society and the American Urological Association recommend screening PSA testing in men aged 50 or older with a life expectancy of at least 10 years, or starting at age 45 if any risk factors are present (6–8). Urinary symptoms such as hesitancy, nocturia, diminished urinary stream, as well as any change in erectile or ejaculatory function, perineal pain, or abnormal digital rectal exam (DRE) may prompt PSA testing in the appropriate clinical setting. Age-specific normal limits of PSA values have been described (9). The differential diagnosis for elevated PSA includes benign prostatic hypertrophy, prostatitis, and prostate cancer. A low free (unbound) PSA was approved by the U.S. Food and Drug Administration (FDA) as an indicator of likely malignancy in the setting of normal DRE and PSA between 4 and 10. A trial of antibiotics may help exclude the diagnosis of prostatitis. Poorly differentiated prostate carcinomas may produce minimal

KEY POINTS

- Prostate cancer is the second largest cause of cancer mortality in men, predicted to cause more than 28,000 deaths in the United States in 2008.
- The American Cancer Society and the American Urological Association recommend screening prostate-specific antigen (PSA) testing in men aged 50 or older with a life expectancy of at least 10 years, or starting at aged 45 if any risk factors are present.
- Many patients die with prostate cancer rather than from it.
- Androgen deprivation therapy (ADT), usually with a gonadotropin-releasing hormone (GnRH) analog, alone or in combination with an anti-androgen to block the castration testosterone flare, is highly effective at slowing tumor growth.
- After anti-androgen withdrawal, second-line anti-androgens, and adrenal suppression have been exhausted, the combination of the anti-microtubule inhibitor docetaxel along with prednisone is the standard of care.
- Pretreatment electromyography is being evaluated as a tool to assess for preexisting neuropathy, which may be exacerbated by docetaxel or similar agents such as the vinca alkaloids or estramustine.
- Bladder cancer is the fourth most common cancer in men and the eighth most common cause of cancer-related death in men.

- Germ cell tumor of the testis is the most common malignancy in young men.
- Long-term toxicity of chemotherapy in testicular cancer includes infertility, bleomycin-associated pulmonary toxicity, Raynaud's phenomenon, peripheral neuropathy, increased risk of cardiovascular disease, and secondary malignancy risk, which is highest in those treated with chemotherapy and radiation.
- Cancer of the kidney and renal pelvis is the seventh most common in men and ninth most common in women; in the United States, it was estimated that 33,000 new cases in men and 21,000 in women would occur in 2008.
- The tyrosine kinase inhibitors induce partial and complete remissions in patients with clear cell renal cell carcinoma, making them the standard of care for the metastatic setting.
- A unique feature of renal cell carcinoma is that approximately 20% of patients present with paraneoplastic symptoms, including anemia or erythrocytosis, weight loss, malaise, hypercalcemia, hepatic dysfunction in the absence of metastases, glomerulonephritis, neuromyopathy, and dermatitis.
- Carcinoma of the penis comprises less than 1% of all malignancies in men.

or no PSA, which can mask the diagnosis of prostate cancer. If clinical suspicion of malignancy is high, a transrectal ultrasound-guided biopsy of the prostate is performed. Metastatic disease may present with bone pain, spinal cord compression, or symptoms of visceral organ involvement.

The most common histologic type of prostate cancer is adenocarcinoma. The Gleason grading system is a measure of glandular differentiation determined at low magnification. The primary (most prevalent) and the secondary (second most prevalent) glandular patterns are graded from 1 (most histologically similar to normal prostate) to 5 (most undifferentiated and therefore most aggressive) (Fig. 14.1). The sum of the two values (the Gleason score), as well as the order of individual components (eg, 4 + 3 vs 3 + 4, the first number indicating the most predominant pattern), are powerful predictors of outcome (10). If suspicion for metastatic disease is high, a computed tomography (CT) scan of the abdomen and pelvis is performed to evaluate for soft tissue disease in the liver, lung, and lymph nodes. A CT scan is insufficient to evaluate the prostate itself. A bone scan complements the CT scan in evaluating for bone metastases. Proton emission tomography (PET) scan can detect actively metabolizing disease. It is FDA-

approved only for assessment of treatment response in patients receiving chemotherapy in the setting of a clinical trial. Magnetic resonance imaging (MRI) with an endorectal probe is useful to determine the extent of local disease (11). ProstaScint scan is an imaging modality using indium-111 oxine conjugated to a monoclonal antibody against prostate specific membrane antigen (PSMA). This imaging technique is FDA-approved for use in detecting occult recurrent disease. PSMA was originally thought to be a specific marker for prostate cancer. However, due to a high false positive rate, the use of this test remains controversial (12). The staging system for prostate cancer is presented in Table 14.1.

DEFINITIVE THERAPY

Prostate cancer is a heterogeneous disease. Many patients die with prostate cancer rather than from it (13). A clinical states model was proposed (14) to account for competing causes of death at any given state of cancer progression, and the likelihood of transitioning from one clinical state to the next (Fig. 14.2). For localized or regionally advanced prostate cancer, risk stratification is performed using clinical stage, Gleason

PROSTATIC ADENOCARCINOMA
(Histologic Grades)

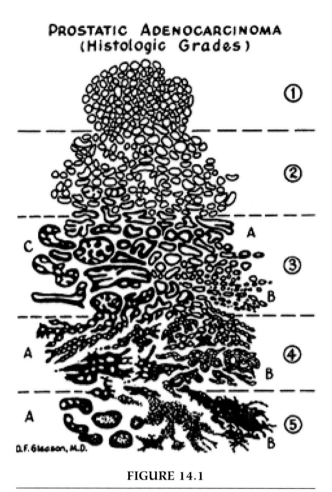

FIGURE 14.1

Gleason Grading System of Prostate Cancer. (From Ref. 42, with permission.)

score, and pretreatment PSA (Table 14.2). Advantages, disadvantages, and contraindications of the treatment approaches for localized or regional prostate cancer are outlined in Table 14.3. Neoadjuvant, concomitant, or adjuvant hormonal therapy may be considered for high-risk disease (15,16). The decision regarding optimal therapy for early-stage prostate cancer is made in consultation with a urologic surgeon, medical oncologist, and radiation oncologist (17). Assessment tools to estimate the rate of self-reported side effects following definitive therapy have been developed and validated extensively (18,19) (Table 14.3).

RISING PSA FOLLOWING DEFINITIVE THERAPY

Since the introduction of PSA, it became possible to identify a new subgroup of patients; that is, those who develop rising PSA levels following definitive therapy for prostate cancer without any radiographic evidence

TABLE 14.1
2002 AJCC TNM Staging of Prostate Cancer

PRIMARY TUMOR, CLINICAL (T)

TX Primary tumor cannot be assessed
T0 No primary tumor
T1 Clinically inapparent, not palpable or visible by imaging
  T1a Incidental histologic finding, ≤5% of resected tissue
  T1b Incidental histologic finding, >5% of resected tissue
  T1c Tumor identified by needle biopsy, for any reason (eg, elevated PSA)
T2 Palpable or visible tumor, confined within the prostate
  T2a ≤½ one lobe
  T2b One lobe
  T2c Both lobes
T3 Tumor extends through the capsule
  T3a ECE, unilateral or bilateral
  T3b Seminal vesicle involvement
T4 Tumor is fixed or invades adjacent structures
  T4a Invades bladder neck, external sphincter or rectum
  T4b Invades levator muscles or fixed to pelvic sidewalls

PRIMARY TUMOR, PATHOLOGIC (T)

pT2 Organ-confined
  pT2a Unilateral, involving half of one lobe or less
  pT2b Unilateral, involving more than half of one lobe but not both lobes
  pT2c Bilateral
pT3 Extraprostatic extension
  pT3a Extraprostatic extension
  pT3b Seminal vesicle involvement
pT4 Invasion of bladder or rectum
Regional lymph nodes (N)
NX Regional lymph nodes cannot be assessed
N0 No regional lymph node metastasis
N1 Metastasis in regional lymph node or nodes
Distant metastases (M)
MX Distant metastasis cannot be assessed
M0 No regional lymph node metastasis
M1 Distant metastasis
  M1a: Nonregional lymph nodes
  M1b: Bone(s)
  M1c: Other site(s)

Source: From Ref. 43, with permission.

TABLE 14.2
Risk Stratification for Clinically Localized and Regional Prostate Cancer[a]

	LOW RISK	INTERMEDIATE RISK	HIGH RISK	VERY HIGH RISK
Clinical stage	T1a-T2a	T2b-T2c	T3a-T3b	T3c-T4 or any T, N1-3
Gleason score	2–6	7	8–10	Any
PSA, ng/ml	<10	10–20	>20	Any

[a]One of three criteria is sufficient for a given risk category.
Source: From Ref. 17, with permission.

of local recurrence or detectable metastatic disease. This clinical state is referred to as biochemical relapse, or "rising PSA, non-castrate" (14) (Fig. 14.2). Following definitive therapy for early prostate cancer, PSA nadir is an important prognostic factor. After prostatectomy, the PSA should become undetectable within 30 days. Causes of persistent detectable PSA levels following prostatectomy include residual normal prostate glandular tissue versus systemic micrometastatic disease. Following definitive radiotherapy, PSA is expected to fall below 0.5 ng/ml (20). Nomograms have been published to predict the likelihood of biochemical relapse as a surrogate for metastatic disease. Nomograms developed by Memorial-Sloan Kettering Cancer Center are available at www.nomograms.org. In 2005, nomograms using more clinically relevant endpoints were developed to assess the risk of metastatic disease in the setting of biochemical relapse (21). The initial workup of a rising PSA following definitive therapy includes digital rectal examination and imaging tests to rule out local recurrence and distant metastases. In patients with local recurrence following prostatectomy with node-negative disease, salvage radiotherapy is indicated. Conversely, salvage prostatectomy may be considered for recurrence within the prostate following radiotherapy, but is recommended only in selected cases. The presence of metastases necessitates the initiation of hormonal therapy. In the absence of documented local recurrence or metastatic disease, the remaining options include hormonal therapy, expectant monitoring or investigational approaches. PSA doubling time (based on the log slope of the PSA) becomes a powerful prognostic factor. Patients with a PSA doubling time of less than 3 months are candidates for hormonal therapy (22).

METASTATIC DISEASE

Prostate cancer, as well as normal prostate tissue, is highly sensitive to testosterone through the action of androgen receptor. Androgen deprivation therapy

(ADT) usually with a gonadotropin-releasing hormone (GnRH) analog, alone or in combination with an anti-androgen to block the castration testosterone flare is therefore highly effective at slowing tumor growth. Several approaches to ADT have been developed (Table 14.4). ADT is highly effective at slowing progression of disease, but hormone-refractory disease usually develops within 18–24 months. After anti-androgen withdrawal (23), second-line anti-androgens, and adrenal suppression have been exhausted, cytotoxic chemotherapy may be necessary, although clinical trials are strongly advised in this setting. The combination of the anti-microtubule inhibitor, docetaxel, used along with prednisone, has been the standard of care (24,25). One of the main side effects of docetaxel is peripheral neuropathy (Table 14.5). Pretreatment electromyography (26) was evaluated in 2006 as a tool to assess for preexisting neuropathy, which may be exacerbated by docetaxel or similar agents, including the vinca alkaloids or estramustine. Mitoxantrone and prednisone (27,28) as well as estramustine are also approved by the FDA for hormone-refractory metastatic prostate cancer (see Table 14.5). Palliative measures include radiotherapy and ureteral stenting for urinary obstruction.

CARCINOMA OF THE BLADDER AND THE UPPER UROGENITAL TRACT

Epidemiology

It was projected that more than 68,000 (more than 51,000 in men and more than 18,000 in women) new cases of bladder cancer (including carcinoma in situ) would be reported in the United States in 2008. Projected death rates from bladder cancer numbered approximately 14,000 (almost 10,000 in men; more than 4,000 in women). Bladder cancer is the fourth most common cancer in men and the eighth most common cause of cancer-related death in men (1). There is a high degree of geographic and ethnic variation

TABLE 14.3
Main Treatment Options for Early Prostate Cancer

	ACTIVE OBSERVATION	RADICAL RETROPUBIC PROSTATECTOMY (RRP)	EXTERNAL BEAM RADIATION THERAPY (EBRT)	BRACHYTHERAPY
10-year PSA failure-free rate	Unknown	47%–78%	62%–83%	77%
Prevalence of side effects at 6 years follow-up[b]				
Urinary	N/A	8%	11%	16%
Bowel	N/A	3%	13%	10%
Sexual	N/A	39%	39%	55%
Other side effects	Anxiety side effects of surveillance re-biopsy	Perioperative complications (0%–5%)		Acute urinary retention (5%–34%) Rectal toxicity (2%–12%)
Advantages	Avoids or postpones treatment-related morbidity	■ Salvage radiation therapy remains an option ■ Improved prognosis based on pathologic features ■ Novel techniques (laparoscopic and robot-assisted) are being developed	■ Effective cancer control ■ Low risk of urinary incontinence ■ Available to patients with medical contra-indications to surgery	■ Equal cancer control rates for organ-confined tumors ■ Single treatment ■ Low risk of urinary incontinence (without prior TURP) ■ Available to patients with medical contra-indications to surgery
Disadvantages	■ Increased risk of metastases in intermediate-risk patients compared to prostatectomy ■ Anxiety-provoking	■ Significant risk of impotence ■ Risk of operative morbidity ■ Higher operator-dependence ■ Some risk of long-term incontinence	■ Significant risk of impotence ■ Lymph node involvement not determined ■ Salvage surgery is complicated by radiation changes ■ Prolonged treatment	■ Significant risk of impotence ■ Lymph node involvement not determined ■ Salvage surgery is complicated by radiation changes ■ Not appropriate for high-risk disease
Contraindications	■ High risk disease ■ Large prostate ■ Long life expectancy	■ Medical contra-indications to surgery ■ Neurogenic bladder	■ Previous pelvic XRT ■ Active inflammatory disease of rectum ■ Low bladder capacity ■ Chronic diarrhea	■ Previous pelvic XRT ■ Prior TURP ■ Large prostate ■ Significant voiding symptoms ■ Large tumor burden ■ Active inflammatory disease of rectum ■ Chronic diarrhea ■ Long life expectancy

[a]Retrospective study showed equivalent disease control rates with RRP and EBRT; randomized studies are in progress (44).
[b]Rates of adverse effects are unadjusted and therefore cannot be used to compare treatment modalities due to differences between groups(19)

Source: Modified from Ref. 17, with permission.

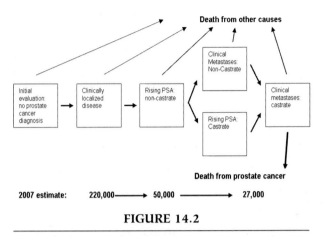

FIGURE 14.2

Clinical States Model of Prostate Cancer. (From Ref. 14 with permission.)

in the incidence rates, with the highest rates seen in non-Latino whites in the United States and Western Europe, and lowest rates in Asian-Americans (3). Cigarette smoking, occupational exposure to synthetic dyes, and prolonged use of an indwelling catheter are well-established risk factors for bladder cancer. Tumors of the upper urogenital tract, i.e. the renal pelvis and ureter, are about 17 times less common than bladder carcinoma, but have similar risk factors.

Diagnosis

Bladder cancer most commonly presents with total (present throughout the length of micturition), gross, painless hematuria. Alternatively, microhematuria may

TABLE 14.4
Forms of Androgen Deprivation Therapy

APPROACH (Ref)	AGENTS USED	INDICATIONS	MECHANISM OF ACTION	SIDE EFFECTS
Nonsteroidal anti-androgen monotherapy[45,46]	Bicalutamide	Biochemical relapse as an alternative to combined androgen blockade	Competes with testosterone for binding to androgen receptor	■ Hot flashes ■ Breast tenderness ■ Anemia ■ LFT abnormalities
Combined androgen blockade (CAB)[16]	GnRH agonist (goserelin acetate, leuprolide acetate) combined with anti-androgen (bicalutamide)	■ Metastatic disease ■ Neoadjuvant, concomitant or adjuvant therapy for early prostate cancer ■ Biochemical relapse	■ Supra-physiologic levels of GnRH agonist inhibit the anterior pituitary and thereby reduce circulating testosterone levels ■ Anti-androgen blocks the action of remaining testosterone and adrenal androgens ■ Anti-androgen protects from flair in testosterone upon initiation of GnRH agonist	■ Impotence, loss of libido ■ Osteoporosis ■ Accelerated atherosclerosis ■ Personality change ■ Weight gain ■ Hot flashes ■ Anemia ■ LFT abnormalities
Anti-androgen withdrawal[23]	Discontinuation of anti-androgen	Rising PSA on CAB	Prolonged exposure to anti-androgens leads to mutations in androgen receptor which cause anti-androgen to act as an agonist	N/A
Second-line anti-androgen therapy[47]	Flutamide, Nilutamide, Bicalutamide, Abiraterone	Rising PSA following anti-androgen withdrawal	Resistance mutations in androgen receptor are specific to particular anti-androgen	■ Hot flashes ■ Breast tenderness ■ Anemia ■ LFT abnormalities ■ Impaired dark adaptation (Nilutamide)
Adrenal suppression therapy	Ketoconazole	Rising PSA following second-line anti-androgen therapy	Suppresses production of adrenal androgens	■ Adrenal suppression—may require steroid supplementation ■ Nausea, vomiting ■ Need to avoid antacids

TABLE 14.5
Commonly Used Chemotherapy Regimens in Hormone-refractory Prostate Cancer

REGIMEN (REF.)	MEDIAN SURVIVAL (MONTHS)	SHORT-TERM SIDE EFFECTS	LONG-TERM SIDE EFFECTS
Mitoxanthrone and prednisone (24,27)	16.5	Nausea, vomiting (40%) Bone marrow suppression (22%) Fatigue (35%) Stomatitis (8%)	Cardiotoxicity (22%) Sensory neuropathy (7%) Change in taste (7%)
Docetaxel and estramustine (28)	17.5	Nausea, vomiting (20%) Bone marrow suppression (16%) Fatigue Stomatitis	Cardiovascular events (15%) Neurologic events (7%)
Docetaxel and prednisone every three weeks (27)	18.9	Nausea, vomiting (40%) Bone marrow suppression (32%) Fatigue (50%) Stomatitis (20%)	Alopecia (65%) Sensory neuropathy (30%) Change in taste (18%)
Weekly docetaxel (27)	17.4	Nausea, vomiting (40%) Bone marrow suppression (2%) Fatigue (50%) Stomatitis (17%)	Alopecia (50%) Sensory neuropathy (24%) Change in taste (24%)

be incidentally found on routine urinalysis. Although present in approximately 15% of the population, persistent microscopic hematuria on repeat evaluation should prompt further workup to exclude malignancy. In addition to urine cytology, new bladder tumor markers have been proposed for monitoring of patients with known bladder carcinoma (29). Cystoscopy or cystourethroscopy allow definitive diagnosis. For staging, transurethral resection of bladder tumor (TURBT) is required, along with CT scan of abdomen and pelvis, bone scan, and chest x-ray or CT of the chest. Staging of bladder cancer is reviewed in Table 14.6. The most common histological type of bladder cancer is transitional cell carcinoma.

Treatment

Low-risk superficial bladder cancer (Ta grade 1–2) is treated with TURBT with or without a single dose of intravesical mitomycin C (MMC). Other intravesical agents include interferon, gemcitabine, and cyclophosphamide (Cytoxan). High-risk superficial tumors are treated with a course of induction intravesical chemotherapy or immunotherapy with Bacillus Calmette-Guerin (BCG) vaccine. Intravesical therapy causes a local inflammatory reaction, resulting in a cytokine-mediated antitumor effect. Organ-confined disease (T2) is treated with radical cystectomy with possible neoadjuvant or adjuvant chemotherapy with methotrexate, vinblastine, doxorubicin, and cisplatin (MVAC) (30). Bladder-sparing approaches have been developed. For

non-organ-confined disease that is resectable, radical cystectomy is indicated (31). In unresectable disease, chemotherapy is administered and response is monitored with CT scan and cystoscopy. Postchemotherapy surgery may be feasible. For patients with advanced and metastatic disease, the choice of chemotherapy regimen depends on performance status and the presence of visceral metastases (32).

TESTIS CANCER

Epidemiology

Germ-cell tumor of the testis is the most common malignancy in young men. In 2008, approximately 8,000 cases were predicted in the United States, with only 380 deaths, illustrating relatively good prognosis and effective treatment of germ-cell tumors. Risk factors include undescended testis, which predisposes to bilateral testis cancer, albeit more likely in the undescended testis, as well as Klinefelter's syndrome.

Diagnosis

Testis cancer commonly presents with a painless or painful testicular mass. In addition to malignancy, differential diagnosis includes epididymitis, epididymo-orchitis, and testicular torsion as well as hernia, hydrocele, testicular torsion, varicocele, and spermatocele. Ultrasound is the next diagnostic step. Gynecomastia

TABLE 14.6
American Joint Committee on Cancer 2002 TNM Bladder Cancer Staging

Primary tumor (T)

Tx primary tumor cannot be assessed

T0 No evidence of primary tumor

Tis Carcinoma in situ

Ta Noninvasive papillary tumor

T1 Tumor invades the subepithelial connective tissue

T2 Tumor invades muscle

    pT2a Tumor invades superficial muscle (inner half)

    pT2b Tumor invades deep muscle (outer half)

T3 Tumor invades perivesical tissue

    pT3a Microscopically

    pT3b Macroscopically (extravesical mass)

T4 Tumor invades any of the following: prostate, uterus, vagina, pelvis or abdominal wall

    T4a Tumor invades prostate, uterus, vagina

    T4b Tumor invades pelvis or abdominal wall

Regional lymph nodes (N)

NX Regional lymph nodes cannot be assessed

N0 No regional lymph node metastasis

N1 Metastasis in a single lymph node, 2 cm or less in greatest dimension

N2 Metastasis in a single lymph node >2 cm but <5 cm in greatest dimension, or multiple lymph nodes, none >5 cm in greatest dimension

N3 Metastasis in a lymph node >5 cm in greatest dimension

Distant metastasis (M)

MX Distant metastasis cannot be assessed

M0 No distant metastasis

M1 Distant metastasis

Source: From Ref. 43, with permission.

TABLE 14.7
Testicular Cancer Staging System of the American Joint Committee of Cancer

Primary tumor (T)

pTX Primary tumor cannot be assessed (if no radical orchiectomy is performed, TX is used)

pT0 No evidence of primary tumor (histological scar in testis)

pTis Intratubular germ cell neoplasia (carcinoma-in-situ)

pT1 Tumor limited to the testis and epididymis and no vascular/lymphatic invasion

pT2 Tumor limited to the testis and epididymis with vascular/lymphatic invasion or tumor extending through the tunica albuginea with involvement of the tunica vaginalis

pT3 Tumor invades the spermatic cord with or without vascular/lymphatic invasion

pT4 Tumor invades the scrotum with or without vascular/lymphatic invasion

Regional lymph nodes (N): Clinical

Nx Regional lymph nodes cannot be assessed

N0 No regional lymph node metastasis

N1 Lymph node mass ≤2 cm in greatest dimension or multiple lymph node masses, none >2 cm in greatest dimension

N2 Lymph node mass >2 cm but not >5 cm in greatest dimension, or multiple lymph node masses, any one mass >2 cm but not >5 cm in greatest dimension

N3 Lymph node mass >5 cm in greatest dimension

Regional lymph nodes (N): Pathologic

pN0 No evidence of tumor in lymph nodes

pN1 Lymph node mass, ≤2 cm in greatest dimension and ≤5 nodes positive; none >2 cm in greatest dimension

pN2 Lymph node mass >2 cm but not >5 cm in greatest dimension, >5 nodes positive, none >5 cm, evidence of extranodal extension of tumor

pN3 Lymph node mass >5 cm in greatest dimension

Distant metastases (M)

M0 No evidence of distant metastases

M1 Nonregional nodal or pulmonary metastases

M2 Nonpulmonary visceral metastases

---

may be present due to secretion of beta-human chorionic gonadotropin (hCG) by the tumor. Metastatic disease may present with supraclavicular adenopathy, abdominal or back pain, bone pain, or CNS manifestations of brain metastases. Serum alpha fetoprotein (AFP), beta-hCG, and lactate dehydrogenase (LDH) are measured both to monitor treatment and to make the distinction between seminoma (which never causes AFP elevation) and non-seminomatous germ cell tumors (NSGCT). Staging according to The International Germ Cell Cancer Collaborative Group (33) is shown in Tables 14.7–14.10. Seminomatous and NSGCT demonstrate different clinical behavior and are treated differently.

Treatment

Radical orchiectomy through the inguinal approach is required for diagnosis and staging. Early-stage seminoma (stage cI and cIIA) is treated with adjuvant radiotherapy with near-100% cure rate. For early non-seminomatous tumors (stage cI and cIIA) retroperitoneal relapse is common. Treatment options include surveillance, retroperitoneal lymph node dis-

TABLE 14.8
Testicular Cancer Stage Grouping

STAGE	T	N	M	S
0	pTis	N0	M0	S0
Ia	T1	N0	M0	S0
Ib	≥T2	N0	M0	S0
Is	T any	N0	M0	S any
IIa	T any	N1	M0	S0, S1
IIb	T any	N2	M0	S0, S1
IIc	T any	N3	M0	S0, S1
IIIa	T any	N any	M1	S0, S1
IIIb	T any	N any	M0, M1	S2
IIIc	T any	N any	M0, M1	S3

Source: From Ref. 43, with permission.

TABLE 14.9
The International Germ Cell Cancer Collaborative Group Staging System

RISK	SEMINOMA	NON-SEMINOMA
Good risk	Nonpulmonary visceral metastases absent; any S stage; any primary tumor site	S stage 0 or 1; nonpulmonary visceral metastases absent; gonadal or retroperitoneal primary tumor
Intermediate risk (any criterion)	Nonpulmonary visceral metastases present; any S stage; any primary tumor site	S stage 2; nonpulmonary visceral metastases absent; gonadal or retroperitoneal primary tumor
Poor risk (any criterion)	–	Mediastinal primary tumor site; nonpulmonary visceral metastases present; S stage 3

TABLE 14.10
Definitions of Serologic (S) Staging for Germ Cell Tumors

STAGE	LDH	HCG	AFP
S1	<1.5 × upper limit of normal	<5000 IU/L	<1000 ng/ml
S2	1.5–10 × upper limit of normal	5000–50,000 IU/L	1000–10,000 ng/ml
S3	>10 × upper limit of normal	>50,000 IU/L	>10,000 ng/ml

Abbreviations: LDH, lactate dehydrogenase; HCG, human chorionic gonadotropin; AFP, alpha fetoprotein.
Source: From Ref. 43, with permission.

section (RPLND), and adjuvant chemotherapy (34). Features indicative of a high risk for retroperitoneal relapse, such as predominant embryonal carcinoma histology, the presence of lymphovascular invasion, or extension into the tunica or scrotum, necessitate a primary RPLND after normalization of markers. Patients with advanced disease are treated with chemotherapy, according to the risk-stratification scheme of The International Germ Cell Cancer Collaborative Group (1997) (Tables 14.8 and 14.9). Patients with good-risk disease are treated with three cycles of bleomycin, etoposide, and cisplatin (BEP) or four cycles of etoposide and cisplatin. High-risk patients are treated with four cycles of bleomycin, etoposide, and cisplatin. Long-term toxicity of chemotherapy includes infertility, bleomycin-associated pulmonary toxicity, Raynaud's phenomenon, peripheral neuropathy, increased risk of cardiovascular disease, and secondary malignancy risk, which is highest in those treated with chemotherapy and radiation (35).

RENAL CELL CARCINOMA

Epidemiology

Cancer of the kidney and renal pelvis is the seventh most common in men and ninth most common in women, with an estimated 33,000 new cases in men and 21,000 in women in predicted in the United States in 2008. Cigarette smoking, obesity, hypertension, and possibly, diuretic use have been linked to renal cell carcinoma. Two main genetic syndromes are associated with renal cell carcinoma. A germline mutation in the *VHL* gene predisposes to Von Hippel-Lindau (VHL) syndrome, which includes renal cell carcinoma of clear cell type. A germline mutation in the *MET* proto-oncogene is associated with hereditary renal cell carcinoma of papillary cell type.

Diagnosis

Over 50% of renal cell carcinoma cases are diagnosed incidentally on abdominal imaging. A unique feature of renal cell carcinoma is that approximately 20% of patients present with paraneoplastic symptoms including anemia or erythrocytosis, weight loss, malaise, hypercalcemia, hepatic dysfunction in the absence of metastases, glomerulonephritis, neuromyopathy, and dermatitis. The AJCC staging system for renal cell carcinoma is outlined in Tables 14.11 and 14.12.

Treatment

For localized renal cell carcinoma diagnosed by characteristic imaging appearance, biopsy is not indi-

---

TABLE 14.11
AJCC Staging of Renal Cell Carcinoma

Primary tumor (T)
TX Primary tumor cannot be assessed
T0 No evidence of primary tumor
T1 Tumor 7 cm or less in greatest dimension, limited to the kidney
T1a Tumor 4 cm or less in greatest dimension, limited to the kidney
T1b Tumor more than 4 cm but not more than 7 cm in greatest dimension, limited to the kidney
T2 Tumor more than 7 cm in greatest dimension, limited to the kidney
T3 Tumor extends into major veins or invades adrenal gland or perinephric tissues but not beyond Gerota's fascia
T3a Tumor directly invades the adrenal gland or perirenal and/or renal sinus fat but not beyond Gerota's fascia
T3b Tumor grossly extends into the renal vein or its segmental (muscle-containing) branches, or vena cava below the diaphragm
T3c Tumor grossly extends into vena cava above diaphragm or invades the wall of the vena cava
T4 Tumor invades beyond Gerota's fascia
Regional lymph nodes (N)
NX Regional lymph nodes cannot be assessed
N0 No regional lymph node metastases
N1 Metastases in a single regional lymph node
N2 Metastases in more than one regional lymph node
MX Distant metastasis cannot be assessed
M0 No distant metastasis
M1 Distant metastasis

---

cated. Radical nephrectomy is performed. Partial nephrectomy is performed for bilateral tumors or when radical nephrectomy would result in the need for dialysis. Renal cell carcinoma, thought to be an immunologically mediated disease, has shown spontaneous regressions over time including regression of metastatic lesions with removal of the primary renal mass. Low-volume metastatic disease can rarely be resected with curative intent. For the majority of patients with metastatic disease, systemic therapy remains the initial treatment of choice. Renal cell carcinoma is traditionally one of the most highly chemotherapy-resistant tumors. Metastatic renal cell carcinoma has a median survival of 9–15 months. Features associated with shortened survival include low Karnofsky performance status (1.5 times upper limit of normal), low hemoglobin (less than the lower limit of normal), high serum calcium, and

TABLE 14.12	
Stage Grouping for Renal Cell Carcinoma	
Stage I	T1 N0 M0
Stage II	T2 N0 M0
Stage III	T1 N1 M0
	T2 N1 M0
	T3 N0 M0
	T3 N1 M0
	T3a N0 M0
	T3a N1 M0
	T3b N0 M0
	T3b N1 M0
	T3c N0 M0
	T3c N1 M0
Stage IV	T4 N0 M0
	T4 N1 M0
	Any T N2 M0
	Any T Any N M1

Source: From Ref. 43, with permission.

absence of prior nephrectomy (36). Interferon and IL-2 are two traditional agents, with response rates of 10%–15%. In 2007, the standard of care for metastatic renal cell carcinoma changed with the introduction of sunitinib (Sutent) (37) as first-line therapy, demonstrating approximately 6-month prolongation of progression-free survival; and sorafenib (Nexavar) (38) showing three-month prolongation of progression-free survival in the second-line setting. Sunitinib and sorafenib are oral tyrosine kinase inhibitors designed to target the vascular endothelial growth factor VEGF pathway, which is activated in renal cell carcinoma due to loss of the VHL tumor suppressor gene (39).

PENILE CANCER

Carcinoma of the penis comprises less than 1% of all malignancies in men. Predisposing factors include the presence of foreskin and HPV exposure. The presenting lesion is usually painless. Squamous cell carcinoma is the most common histology. Penile conservation surgical techniques such as laser, Mohs surgery, and partial penectomy are used when feasible (40). Brachytherapy and external beam radiotherapy are alternatives to surgery for localized disease. Several chemotherapy agents are active for metastatic disease (41). This disease is most responsive to cisplatin. However, recurrent surgical resections are needed to debulk disease in regional lymph nodes.

References

1. American Cancer Society. *Cancer Facts and Figures*. Atlanta, GA: American Cancer Society; 2007.
2. Hsing AW, Tsao L, Devesa SS. International trends and patterns of prostate cancer incidence and mortality. *Int J Cancer*. 2000;85:60–67.
3. Parkin DM, Bray F, Ferlay J, Pisani P. Global cancer statistics, 2002. *CA Cancer J Clin*. 2005;55:74–108.
4. Giovannucci E, Platz EA. Epidemiology of prostate cancer. In: Vogelzang NJ, Scardino pT, Shipley WU, Debruyne FMJ, Linehan WM, eds. *Comprehensive Textbook of Genitourinary Oncology*. Philadelphia: Lippincott Williams and Wilkins; 2006:9.
5. Calle EE, Rodriguez C, Walker-Thurmond K, Thun MJ. Overweight, obesity, and mortality from cancer in a prospectively studied cohort of U.S. adults. *N Engl J Med*. 2003;348:1625–1638.
6. American Urological Association. Prostate-specific antigen (PSA) best practice policy. *Oncology*. 2000;14:267–272, 277–278, 280 passim.
7. Harris R, Lohr KN. Screening for prostate cancer: an update of the evidence for the U.S. Preventive Services Task Force. *Ann Intern Med*. 2002;137:917–929.
8. Smith RA, Cokkinides V, Eyre HJ. Cancer screening in the United States, 2007: a review of current guidelines, practices, and prospects. *CA Cancer J Clin*. 2007;57:90–104.
9. Oesterling JE. Age-specific reference ranges for serum PSA. *N Engl J Med*. 1996;335:345–346.
10. Gleason DF, Mellinger GT, Veterans Administration Cooperative Urological Research Group. Prediction of prognosis for prostatic adenocarcinoma by combined histological grading and clinical staging. 1974. *J Urol*. 2002;167:953–958; discussion 959.
11. Hricak H, Choyke PL, Eberhardt SC, Leibel SA, Scardino PT. Imaging prostate cancer: a multidisciplinary perspective. *Radiology*. 2007;243:28–53.
12. Thomas CT, Bradshaw PT, Pollock BH, et al. Indium-111-capromab pendetide radioimmunoscintigraphy and prognosis for durable biochemical response to salvage radiation therapy in men after failed prostatectomy. *J Clin Oncol*. 2003;21:1715–1721.
13. Sakr WA, Grignon DJ, Haas GP, Heilbrun LK, Pontes JE, Crissman JD. Age and racial distribution of prostatic intraepithelial neoplasia. *Eur Urol*. 1996;30:138–144.
14. Scher HI, Heller G. Clinical states in prostate cancer: toward a dynamic model of disease progression. *Urology*. 2000;55:323–327.
15. Messing EM, Manola J, Yao J, et al. Immediate versus deferred androgen deprivation treatment in patients with node-positive prostate cancer after radical prostatectomy and pelvic lymphadenectomy. *Lancet Oncol*. 2006;7:472–479.
16. Loblaw DA, Virgo KS, Nam R, et al. Initial hormonal management of androgen-sensitive metastatic, recurrent, or progressive prostate cancer: 2006 update of an American Society of Clinical Oncology Practice Guideline. *J Clin Oncol*. 2007;22(14):2927–2941.
17. Shipley WU, Scardino PT, Kaufman DS, Kattan MW. Treatment of early stage prostate cancer. In: Vogelzang NJ, Scardino pT, Shipley WU, Debruyne FMJ, Linehan WM, eds. *Comprehensive Textbook of Genitourinary Oncology*. Philadelphia: Lippincott Williams and Wilkins; 2006:153.
18. Talcott JA, Manola J, Clark JA, et al. Time course and predictors of symptoms after primary prostate cancer therapy. *J Clin Oncol*. 2003;21:3979–3986.
19. Miller DC, Sanda MG, Dunn RL, et al. Long-term outcomes among localized prostate cancer survivors: health-related quality-of-life changes after radical prostatectomy, external radiation, and brachytherapy. *J Clin Oncol*. 2005;23:2772–2780.
20. American Society for Therapeutic Radiology and Oncology. Consensus statement: guidelines for PSA following radiation

therapy. American Society for Therapeutic Radiology and Oncology Consensus Panel. *Int J Radiat Oncol Biol Phys.* 1997;37:1035–1041.

21. Slovin SF, Wilton AS, Heller G, Scher HI. Time to detectable metastatic disease in patients with rising prostate-specific antigen values following surgery or radiation therapy. *Clin Cancer Res.* 2005;11:8669–8673.

22. D'Amico AV. Management of rising PSA following surgery or radiation therapy. In: Vogelzang NJ, Scardino pT, Shipley WU, Debruyne FMJ, Linehan WM, eds. *Comprehensive Textbook of Genitourinary Oncology.* Philadelphia: Lippincott Williams and Wilkins; 2006:285.

23. Kelly WK, Scher HI. Prostate specific antigen decline after antiandrogen withdrawal: the flutamide withdrawal syndrome. *J Urol.* 1993;149:607–609.

24. Tannock IF, Osoba D, Stockler MR, et al. Chemotherapy with mitoxantrone plus prednisone or prednisone alone for symptomatic hormone-resistant prostate cancer: a Canadian randomized trial with palliative end points. *J Clin Oncol.* 1996;14:1756–1764.

25. Kantoff PW, Halabi S, Conaway M, et al. Hydrocortisone with or without mitoxantrone in men with hormone-refractory prostate cancer: results of the cancer and leukemia group B 9182 study. *J Clin Oncol.* 1999;17:2506–2513.

26. Stubblefield MD, Slovin S, MacGregor-Cortelli B, et al. An electrodiagnostic evaluation of the effect of pre-existing peripheral nervous system disorders in patients treated with the novel proteasome inhibitor bortezomib. *Clin Oncol (R Coll Radiol).* 2006;18:410–418.

27. Tannock IF, de Wit R, Berry WR, et al. Docetaxel plus prednisone or mitoxantrone plus prednisone for advanced prostate cancer. *N Engl J Med.* 2004;351:1502–1012.

28. Petrylak DP, Tangen CM, Hussain MH, et al. Docetaxel and estramustine compared with mitoxantrone and prednisone for advanced refractory prostate cancer. *N Engl J Med.* 2004;351:1513–1520.

29. Black PC, Brown GA, Dinney CP. Molecular markers of urothelial cancer and their use in the monitoring of superficial urothelial cancer. *J Clin Oncol.* 2006;24:5528–5535.

30. Grossman HB, Natale RB, Tangen CM, et al. Neoadjuvant chemotherapy plus cystectomy compared with cystectomy alone for locally advanced bladder cancer. *N Engl J Med.* 2003;349:859–866.

31. Herr HW, Donat SM. Role of radical cystectomy in patients with advanced bladder cancer. In: Vogelzang NJ, Scardino pT, Shipley WU, Debruyne FMJ, Linehan WM, eds. *Comprehensive Textbook of Genitourinary Oncology.* Philadelphia: Lippincott Williams and Wilkins; 2006:467.

32. Galsky M, Bajorin D. Chemotherapy for metastatic bladder, alone or in combination with other treatment. In: Vogelzang NJ, Scardino pT, Shipley WU, Debruyne FMJ, Linehan WM, eds. *Comprehensive Textbook of Genitourinary Oncology.* Philadelphia: Lippincott Williams and Wilkins; 2006:533.

33. International Germ Cell Cancer Collaborative Group. International Germ Cell Consensus Classification: a prognostic factor-based staging system for metastatic germ cell cancers. International Germ Cell Cancer Collaborative Group. *J Clin Oncol.* 1997;15:594–603.

34. Carver BS, Sheinfeld J. Germ cell tumors of the testis. *Ann Surg Oncol.* 2005;12:871–880.

35. Gilligan TD. Chronic toxicity from chemotherapy for disseminated testicular cancer. In: Vogelzang NJ, Scardino pT, Shipley WU, Debruyne FMJ, Linehan WM, eds. *Comprehensive Textbook of Genitourinary Oncology.* Philadelphia: Lippincott Williams and Wilkins; 2006:330.

36. Motzer RJ, Mazumdar M, Bacik J, Berg W, Amsterdam A, Ferrara J. Survival and prognostic stratification of 670 patients with advanced renal cell carcinoma. *J Clin Oncol.* 1999;17:2530–2540.

37. Motzer RJ, Hutson TE, Tomczak P, et al. Sunitinib versus interferon alfa in metastatic renal-cell carcinoma. *N Engl J Med.* 2007;356:115–124.

38. Escudier B, Eisen T, Stadler WM, et al. Sorafenib in advanced clear-cell renal-cell carcinoma. *N Engl J Med.* 2007;356:125–134.

39. Brugarolas J. Renal-cell carcinoma—molecular pathways and therapies. *N Engl J Med.* 2007;356:185–187.

40. Russo P, Horenblas S. Surgical management of penile cancer. In: Vogelzang NJ, Scardino pT, Shipley WU, Debruyne FMJ, Linehan WM, eds. *Comprehensive Textbook of Genitourinary Oncology.* Philadelphia: Lippincott Williams and Wilkins; 2006:809.

41. Pizzocaro G, Tan WW, Drieger R. Chemotherapy for penile cancer. In: Vogelzang NJ, Scardino pT, Shipley WU, Debruyne FMJ, Linehan WM, eds. *Comprehensive Textbook of Genitourinary Oncology.* Philadelphia: Lippincott Williams and Wilkins; 2006:827.

42. Tannenbaum MP. Histologic grading of prostate adenocarcinoma. In: Tannenbaum, M. (editor). *Urologic Pathology: The Prostate.* Philadelphia: Lea & Febiger; 1977:181.

43. Greene FL, American Joint Committee on Cancer. *AJCC Cancer Staging Atlas.* New York, NY: Springer; 2006.

44. Akakura K, Suzuki H, Ichikawa T, et al. A randomized trial comparing radical prostatectomy plus endocrine therapy versus external beam radiotherapy plus endocrine therapy for locally advanced prostate cancer: results at median follow-up of 102 months. *Jpn J Clin Oncol.* 2006;36:789–793.

45. Loblaw DA, Mendelson DS, Talcott JA, et al. American Society of Clinical Oncology recommendations for the initial hormonal management of androgen-sensitive metastatic, recurrent, or progressive prostate cancer. *J Clin Oncol.* 2004;22:2927–2941.

46. McLeod DG, Iversen P, See WA, et al. Bicalutamide 150 mg plus standard care vs standard care alone for early prostate cancer. *BJU Int.* 2006;97:247–254.

47. Beekman K, Tilley WD, Buchanan G, Scher HI. Beyond first-line hormones: options for treatment of castration-resistant disease. In: Vogelzang NJ, Scardino pT, Shipley WU, Debruyne FMJ, Linehan WM, eds. *Comprehensive Textbook of Genitourinary Oncology.* Philadelphia: Lippincott Williams and Wilkins; 2006:330.

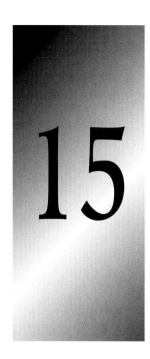

Evaluation and Treatment of Lung and Bronchus Cancer

15

Jorge E. Gomez

Approximately 213,380 cases of lung cancer were reported in 2007, accompanied by an estimated 160,390 deaths from the disease (1). The three other most common cancers, prostate, breast, and colon, were estimated at 511,740 cases, with 120,140 deaths. Lung cancer is the second most common cancer in men and women but is the leading cause of cancer mortality in both, surpassing prostate cancer in men and breast cancer in women. These statistics serve to emphasize the aggressive nature of lung cancer and the importance of efforts to both treat and prevent it. Although lung cancer incidence and death rates have been decreasing slightly in men, they have been increasing in women, likely related to increasing tobacco consumption.

EPIDEMIOLOGY

The majority of lung cancers are related to the consumption of tobacco products. Published studies have shown the association between smoking and the development of lung cancer. Smoking has also been strongly associated with an increased risk of death from lung cancer, which increases as the amount of tobacco consumption increases (2–4). However, approximately 15% of all lung cancers occur in nonsmokers. Asbestos and radon exposure has also been linked to the development of lung cancer (5,6), although their absolute contribution is difficult to calculate. Asbestos is a fibrous mineral used in many products including insulation, construc-

tion pipes, ceiling tiles, and other construction elements until the 1980s. Radon is a gas formed by the decay of radium that is naturally present in the environment, but can accumulate in homes. A meta-analysis published in 2004 showed a statistically significant increase in the risk of lung cancer with increased concentrations of radon (7). Although the major cause of lung cancer is likely environmental, some studies have suggested an inherited susceptibility to lung cancer. Specific genetic abnormalities have not been identified.

Lung cancer is a disease of the elderly and middle aged, with a median age at presentation of 70 (8). The incidence of lung cancer in women, which had traditionally been low, has been rapidly approaching the numbers seen in men. Approximately 46% of the estimated 213,380 lung cancers in 2007 occurred in women, along with 44% of the estimated deaths from this disease (1).

PATHOLOGY

Lung carcinoma is a pathologically heterogeneous tumor. The most important distinction is between small cell carcinoma and non-small cell carcinoma. Small cell carcinoma will be discussed later in this chapter. The World Health Organization (WHO) classification of lung tumors divides non-small cell lung cancer into different subtypes (Table 15.1) (9). The most common in order of incidence are adenocarcinoma, squamous

KEY POINTS

- Lung cancer is the second most common cancer in men and women, but is the leading cause of cancer mortality in both, surpassing prostate cancer in men and breast cancer in women.
- Smoking has been strongly associated with an increased risk of death from lung cancer, which increases as the amount of tobacco consumption increases.
- Lung carcinoma is a pathologically heterogeneous tumor. The most important distinction is between small cell carcinoma and non-small cell carcinoma.
- The most common non-small cell lung carcinomas, in order of incidence, are adenocarcinoma, squamous-cell carcinoma, and large-cell carcinoma.

- Lung cancer is usually diagnosed through a workup initiated because of one of the multiple symptoms caused by the disease.
- Treatment for early stage disease usually involves one or more modalities of treatment which include surgery, chemotherapy, and radiation therapy. Patients with advanced disease are treated with chemotherapy while other modalities are used for palliation of specific symptoms.
- Small cell lung cancer is almost exclusively a disease of smokers and a diagnosis of small cell lung cancer in a nonsmoker should raise significant doubts.
- As with non-small cell lung cancer, the treatment of small cell lung cancer depends on multiple modalities, mainly chemotherapy and radiation therapy. Surgery plays a minor role in this disease.

cell carcinoma, and large cell carcinoma. There are subtle clinical differences between these subtypes, but there is no clear evidence that tumor histology is an important prognostic variable in non-small cell lung cancer. Adenocarcinoma is the most common, making up approximately 30%–40% of lung cancers. It is more likely to be located in the periphery of the lung and to be associated with fibrous scarring. Squamous cell carcinoma tends to be centrally located, cavitates more commonly, and is more likely to be associated with hypercalcemia than most other lung cancers. Bronchoalveolar carcinoma is a subtype of adenocarcinoma characterized by slow growth and long periods of stable disease. (Fig. 15.1) Finding a mix of several of these histologies in a tumor sample is not uncommon.

SCREENING

Lung cancer is only curable in its early stages. Unfortunately, the majority of patients diagnosed with lung cancer have advanced disease that is incurable. Although there have been large strides in prevention of lung cancer by smoking cessation, smoking rates remain high in the United States and throughout the world. Therefore, early detection of lung cancer is important in subjects who are at high risk.

Three large, randomized controlled trials performed in the United States during the 1970s and 1980s were unable to prove a decrease in lung cancer mortality with chest x-ray and sputum cytology screening for lung cancer. These studies were, however, able to show a significant increase in the early detection of lung cancer lesions (10–12).

TABLE 15.1
1999 WHO Classification of Invasive Malignant Epithelial Lung Tumors

Squamous cell carcinoma
  Variants: papillary, clear cell, small cell, basaloid
Small cell carcinoma
  Variant: combined small cell carcinoma
Adenocarcinoma
  Acinar
  Papillary
Bronchioloalveolar carcinoma
  Nonmucinous (Clara cell/type II pneumocyte type)
  Mucinous (Goblet cell type)
  Mixed mucinous and nonmucinous (Clara cell/type II pneumocyte/goblet cell type) or indeterminate
  Solid adenocarcinoma with mucin formation
  Mixed
  Variants: well-differentiated fetal adenocarcinoma, mucinous ("colloid"), mucinous cystadenocarcinoma, signet ring, clear cell
Large cell carcinoma
  Variants: large cell neuroendocrine carcinoma, combined large cell neuroendocrine carcinoma, basaloid carcinoma, lymphoepithelioma-like carcinoma, clear cell carcinoma, large cell carcinoma with rhaboid phenotype
Adenosquamous carcinoma
Carcinomas with pleomorphic, sarcomatoid, or sarcomatous elements
  Carcinomas with spindle and/or giant cells
  Pleomorphic carcinoma
  Spindle cell carcinoma

Continued

TABLE 15.1
1999 WHO Classification of Invasive Malignant Epithelial Lung Tumors, Continued

Giant cell carcinoma
Carcinosarcoma
Blastoma (Pulmonary blastoma)
Carcinoid tumor
   Typical carcinoid
   Atypical carcinoid
Carcinomas of salivary gland type
   Mucoepidermoid carcinoma
   Adenoid cystic carcinoma
   Others
Unclassified carcinoma

Source: From Ref. 9.

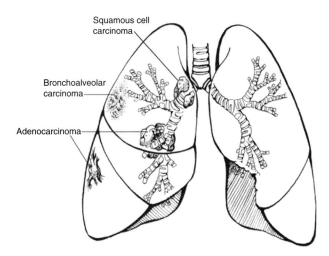

FIGURE 15.1

Illustration depicting several types of non-small cell lung carcinoma. Adenocarcinoma tends to be located in the periphery and associated with fibrous scarring; squamous-cell carcinoma is usually located centrally and may be associated with cavitation and with bronchoalveolar carcinoma, a subtype of adenocarcinoma that is often characterized by slow growth and potentially long periods of stable disease.

More recently, low-dose spiral CT has been shown to improve early detection of small lung cancer lesions over screening chest x-ray (13,14). Henschke at al. screened 1,000 subjects, aged 60 years or older and with at least 10 pack-years of cigarette smoking, with low-dose CT. Noncalcified pulmonary nodules were found in 233 subjects; of the 27 subjects found to have lung cancer, 26 had resectable lesions. The International Early Lung Cancer Action Program Investigators screened 31,567 asymptomatic persons at risk for lung cancer with low-dose CT. Of the 484 lung cancers that were diagnosed, 85% were clinical stage I. High risk for lung cancer was defined as having a history of cigarette smoking, occupational exposure (asbestos, beryllium, uranium, or radon), or exposure to secondhand smoke. It is clear that screening with CT for lung cancer in individuals at high risk can diagnose early stage, curable lung cancers. However, there is concern that this screening may also be associated with finding noncancerous lesions and may lead to additional testing, which can be both costly and invasive. Although no improvement in the overall survival from lung cancer has been found to date, it is important to continue efforts to improve early detection and treatment in the context of clinical trials.

PREVENTION

While the cause of most human cancers is not clearly understood, it is well recognized that exposure to tobacco smoke is the major cause of lung cancer. Although not all lung cancer is related to tobacco consumption, approximately 85% of lung cancer patients have had significant exposure. The risk of lung cancer decreases in subjects who have stopped smoking when compared to current smokers (15), although this risk never returns to the levels of an individual who has never smoked. Therefore, the most important preventive measure for non-small cell lung cancer is never consuming tobacco products. In a close second place is smoking cessation for individuals who already smoke. This modifiable behavioral factor should be where the greatest preventive efforts should be made by government and nongovernment health institutions.

Multiple large clinical trials have been performed with different agents in an attempt to prevent lung cancer. Approximately 70,000 people have participated in chemoprevention trials with beta carotene. Two of these large trials suggested an increased risk of lung cancer in patients receiving beta carotene (16,17). Multiple trials of retinoids in patients who have had non-small cell lung cancer have not shown improvement in recurrences or survival.

DIAGNOSIS

Lung cancer is usually diagnosed through a workup initiated because of one of the multiple symptoms caused by the disease. A significant number of patients, however, are diagnosed incidentally through chest x-rays performed in a routine health evaluation or as part of an evaluation for another health issue. Symptoms of lung cancer are related to the location of the disease.

Symptoms of local disease are as follows:

Dyspnea and cough can be related to lung collapse due to obstructing lesions or pericardial or pleural effusion.

Hemoptysis is related to bleeding from bronchial lesions.

Hoarseness can be caused by recurrent laryngeal nerve involvement causing vocal cord paralysis.

Pain can be caused by involvement of pleura or chest wall.

Symptoms of superior vena cava syndrome are caused by compression by tumor or lymph nodes.

Symptoms of metastatic disease include the following:

Brain metastases can produce headaches, nausea, vomiting, confusion, seizures, and focal neurologic symptoms.

Bone metastases can produce pain or fractures.

Paraneoplastic syndromes can be indicated as follows:

Hypercalcemia can cause confusion, nausea, and vomiting.

Pulmonary hypertrophic osteoarthropathy causes pain and bone deformity. Clotting abnormalities are not uncommon, and can cause deep venous thromboses and pulmonary emboli.

The standard workup for non-small cell lung cancer may include the following studies:

1. Bronchoscopy may help with the initial diagnosis of lung cancer by providing easy access to tissue and can assist in adequately staging patients with lung cancer.
2. Fine needle aspiration biopsy of lung lesions can easily diagnose most of lung cancers.
3. CT scan of the chest, including adrenal glands, with intravenous contrast can help determine stage and can serve as a baseline for the evaluation of response to treatment.
4. Radiographic imaging of the brain in patients with either early or locally advanced disease can help identify patients who have asymptomatic metastatic disease. In patients with advanced disease who have neurologic symptoms it can help assess the extent of disease and plan treatment.
5. PET scan is essential for staging of early disease and is useful for evaluating sites of metastatic disease.
6. Bone scan is useful for detecting metastatic disease in patients with bone symptoms or elevated alkaline phosphatase.
7. Pulmonary function tests can help assess the adequacy of postoperative pulmonary function in patients who are surgical candidates.
8. Mediastinoscopy—the direct evaluation of the mediastinum—is important to adequately confirm or exclude mediastinal lymph node involvement.

PARANEOPLASTIC SYNDROMES

Paraneoplastic syndromes are a combination of symptoms produced by substances formed by the tumor or produced by the body in response to the tumor. In non-small cell lung cancer the most common paraneoplastic syndromes are:

Hypercalcemia. Severe hypercalcemia in non-small cell lung cancer is usually due to the production of a parathyroid hormone related peptide (PTH rP). This protein binds to the same receptors as parathyroid hormone (PTH) and increases bone resorption of calcium and reabsorption of calcium in the kidney. This syndrome can be treated with intravenous hydration, diuretics, and bisphosphonates, and is usually an indicator of poor prognosis. Hypercalcemia can also be caused by metastatic disease to the bone.

Hypertrophic pulmonary osteoarthropathy. This syndrome is more common in adenocarcinoma and is characterized by abnormal proliferation of bone tissue at the distal extremities. This can take the form of mild arthralgias, or a more severe form that presents with swelling and pain of the bones of the extremities caused by proliferative periostitis.

Thrombotic phenomenon. Cancer has been associated multiple clotting abnormalities, including migratory superficial thrombophlebitis, deep venous thrombosis and pulmonary embolism, nonbacterial thrombotic endocarditis, and disseminated intravascular coagulation (18,19). The causes of these thrombotic events are multifactorial and are related both to the biology of the tumor and the prothrombotic properties of chemotherapeutic agents. Although there are no large randomized clinical trials to support this management, patients with active lung cancer who have a first episode venous or arterial thromboembolism should most likely be treated with anticoagulants for the remainder of their lives.

STAGING

As in most other cancers, stages are among the most important prognostic factors in non-small cell lung cancer. Stage depends on several important factors, such as primary tumor size and characteristics (T), the presence or absence of lymph nodes (N), and the presence or absence of metastatic disease (M). This system, known as TNM, was developed by The International Staging System for NSCLC and is the most commonly used in the United States (Tables 15.2 and 15.3). Clinical staging is performed by means of the standard radiologic imaging performed during the diagnosis. Pathologic confirmation of enlarged mediastinal lymph nodes by mediastinoscopy is critical in planning treatment in early-stage non-small cell lung cancer.

TABLE 15.2
Staging of Non-Small Cell Lung Cancer

Staging
As in most other cancers, stage is one of the most important prognostic factors in non-small cell lung cancer. The TNM staging system of The International Staging System for NSCLC is the most commonly used in the United States. Stage depends on several important factors such as primary tumor size and characteristics (T), the presence or absence of lymph nodes (N), and the presence or absence of metastatic disease (M)

Tumor (T)
TX Primary tumor cannot be assessed, or tumor proven by the presence of malignant cells in sputum or bronchial washings but not visualized by imaging or bronchoscopy
T0 No evidence of primary tumor
Tis Carcinoma *in situ*
T1 Tumor 3 cm or less in greatest dimension, surrounded by lung or visceral pleura, without bronchoscopic evidence of invasion more proximal than the lobar bronchus
T2 Tumor with any of the following features of size or extent: More than 3 cm in greatest dimension; Involves main bronchus, 2 cm or more distal to the carina; Invades the visceral pleura; associated with atelectasis or obstructive pneumonitis that extends to the hilar region but does not involve the entire lung
T3 Tumor of any size that directly invades any of the following: chest wall (including superior sulcus tumors), diaphragm, mediastinal pleura, parietal pericardium; or tumor in the main bronchus, 2 cm distal to the carina, but without involvement of the carina; or associated atelectasis or obstructive pneumonitis of the entire lung
T4 Tumor of any size that invades any of the following: mediastinum, heart, great vessels, trachea, esophagus, vertebral body, carina; or tumor with a malignant pleural or pericardial effusion, or with satellite tumor nodule(s) within the ipsilateral primary-tumor lobe of the lung

Lymph Nodes (N)
NX Regional lymph nodes cannot be assessed
N0 No regional lymph node metastasis
N2 Metastasis to ipsilateral mediastinal and/or subcarinal lymph node(s)
N3 Metastasis to contralateral mediastinal, contralateral hilar, ipsilateral or contralateral scalene, or supraclavicular lymph node(s)

Metastasis (M)
MX Presence of distant metastasis cannot be assessed
M0 No distant metastasis
M1 Distant metastasis present
 Stage Ia: a T1 lesion
 Stage Ib: a T2 lesion
 Stage IIa: a T1 lesion with N1 lymph nodes
 Stage IIb: a T2 or T3 lesion with N1 lymph nodes
 Stage IIIa: a T1-T3 lesion with N2 lymph nodes
 Stage IIIb: any T lesion with N3 lymph nodes, or a T4 lesion
 Stage IV: tumors with any metastatic disease

Source: Adapted from AJCC Cancer Staging Manual, 6th edition, New York, 2002.

TABLE 15.3
Stage Grouping for NSCLC

STAGE	T	N	M
Ia	T1	N0	M0
Ib	T2	N0	M0
IIa	T2	N1	M0
IIb	T2	N1	M0
	T3	N0	M0
IIIa	T3	N1	M0
	T1	N2	M0
	T2	N2	M0
	T3	N2	M0
IIIb	T4	N0	M0
	T4	N1	M0
	T4	N2	M0
	T1	N3	M0
	T2	N3	M0
	T3	N3	M0
	T4	N3	M0
IV	Any T	Any N	M1

Abbreviations: T, tumor; N, lymph nodes; M, metastasis.

Source: Adapted from: *AJCC Cancer Staging Manual*, 6th edition, New York, 2002.

TREATMENT

Non-small cell lung cancer is treated according to stage. Although the five-year overall survival for all patients diagnosed with non-small cell lung cancer is approximately 15%, the goal of treatment in early stages is to cure patients of their disease. Treatment for early stage disease usually involves one or more modalities of treatment, which include surgery, chemotherapy, and radiation therapy. Patients with advanced disease are treated with chemotherapy while other modalities are used for palliation of specific symptoms.

Stages I and II

Surgical resection is the best treatment for patients with stage I or II disease, with lobectomy producing a significantly decreased incidence of local recurrence over a limited resection (20). Although resection can be curative, many patients will recur within the first five years. Adjuvant chemotherapy has improved survival after surgery by 5%–12% in patients with stage II and III disease, and is a part of the standard treatment (21–24). Adjuvant chemotherapy is more controversial in stage I disease; one randomized trial showed improved disease-free survival but no improvement of overall survival (25). A meta-analysis of adjuvant chemotherapy including 4,584 patients showed a 5.3% improvement in survival at five years for patients receiving adjuvant chemotherapy versus those who did not (26). The most important large randomized clinical trials of adjuvant chemotherapy have been performed with regimens containing cisplatin and either etoposide or a vinca alkaloid, with the abovementioned meta-analysis suggesting superiority of the cisplatin/vinorelbine regimen.

Stage IIIA

The standard treatment of stage IIIa non-small cell lung cancer is controversial. Accepted modalities include preoperative or neoadjuvant chemotherapy followed by surgery; neoadjuvant chemotherapy and radiation followed by surgery; or definitive chemotherapy and radiation. The main controversy is based on the poor survival—between 13% and 23% at five years (27)—of patients with ipsilateral mediastinal lymph nodes positive for cancer that are treated with surgery alone. Trials comparing neoadjuvant chemotherapy followed by surgery to surgery alone have been small, but have suggested an improved survival for patients receiving chemotherapy (28–32). A phase III randomized trial of concurrent chemotherapy and radiotherapy versus concurrent chemotherapy and radiotherapy followed by surgical resection in stage IIIA non-small cell lung cancer performed by Albain and colleagues was reported at the 2005 American Society of Clinical Oncology meeting (33). Randomized patients numbered 429, and 396 patients were eligible. The authors found an improvement in progression-free survival but no improvement in overall survival. This increase in progression-free survival is present in spite of increased mortality in patients undergoing pneumonectomy. These two approaches, chemotherapy versus chemotherapy and radiation, before surgery, are currently being compared in randomized clinical trials.

Stage IIIB

Stage IIIB non-small cell lung cancer is treated with a combination of chemotherapy and radiation. Several studies in the late 1980s and early 1990s showed improved survival for sequential chemotherapy and radiation therapy over radiation therapy alone (34–38). Subsequent trials compared sequential chemotherapy and radiation to concurrent chemotherapy and radiation, showing an improvement in survival for the concurrent treatment arms (39,40). The five-year overall survival for patients who receive concurrent treatment is approximately 15%, with a median survival of 16–17 months. The chemotherapy used in the multimodality treatment of stage IIIb in these clinical trials was a combination of cisplatin and either etoposide or a vinca alkaloid. The advantage of this chemotherapy regimen over others is the ability to deliver full doses of chemotherapy during concurrent treatment. Since the major cause of death in these patients is systemic recurrence of their cancer, systemic treatment with effective chemotherapy is extremely important.

Stage IV

The mainstay of treatment in stage IV disease is chemotherapy. Multiple trials that have compared chemotherapy to best supportive care have shown an improvement in survival and quality of life in patients receiving chemotherapy. The overall survival difference is approximately 1.5 months (41). Standard chemotherapy regimens are composed of platinum-based doublets. A randomized trial of four platinum based doublets (cisplatin and gemcitabine, cisplatin and docetaxel, cisplatin and paclitaxel, or carboplatin and paclitaxel) showed no improvement in survival for any one regimen (42). The response rate to chemotherapy is approximately 17%–20% and the median survival for patients receiving chemotherapy is approximately nine months. Two recent trials have shown an improvement in survival by the addition of bevacizumab to either paclitaxel/carboplatin or gemcitabine/cisplatin (43,44). Second-line chemotherapies like docetaxel, erlotinib (Tarceva), and pemetrexed (Alimta) can also improve survival and/or quality of life. Erlotinib is an EGFR tyrosine kinase inhibitor that has recently been approved for the second line treatment of non-small cell lung cancer. There is strong evidence suggesting that patients who have specific mutations in EGFR have a significantly higher response rate to EGFR tyrosine kinase inhibitors (45).

Radiation therapy plays an important palliative role in stage IV disease by alleviating symptoms when treating brain metastases or leptomeningeal involvement, painful bone metastases, obstructive bronchial lesions, and superior vena cava syndrome.

Surgery can play a role in stage IV disease. There are multiple anecdotal reports of patients enjoying long-term survival after resection of single metastatic lesions in the brain, adrenals, lung, and other areas.

SPECIAL CLINICAL SCENARIOS

Superior Sulcus Tumors

In the 1920s and 1930s, Pancoast described lung tumors in the apex of the lungs. These tumors are important because of their significant potential for local extension and invasion of vertebral bodies, brachial plexus, the sympathetic chain, and ribs. The typically described presentation of Horner syndrome, shoulder pain, and upper extremity muscle atrophy is called Pancoast syndrome. Because of the difficult local control issues, the treatment of this tumor is usually a multimodality treatment that includes chemotherapy, radiation therapy, and both thoracic and spinal surgery, and usually begins with concurrent chemotherapy and radiation followed by surgical resection (46).

Malignant Pleural Effusions

The presence of a pleural effusion is a common finding a non-small cell lung cancer (Fig. 15.2). All effusions should be tested to test for the possibility of malignant effusion, which can cause significant morbidity in the form of dyspnea and rarely disappear spontaneously. The drainage of a malignant pleural effusion by thoracentesis may often alleviate symptoms of dyspnea, but this symptomatic improvement will frequently be short lived. In patients with lung cancer, a tube thoracostomy with pleurodesis may be the best procedure to prevent re-accumulation of fluid. Pleurodesis may be performed with different sclerosing agents including tetracycline, bleomycin, and talc. Thoracoscopy is a good alternative to thoracostomy, given the possibility of clearing adhesions that cause loculation.

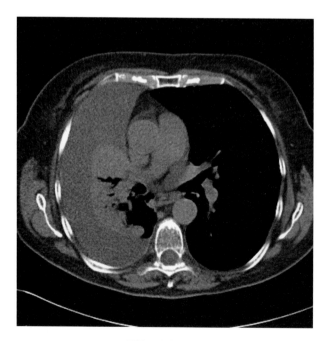

FIGURE 15.2

Computed tomography demonstrating pleural fluid surrounding a partially collapsed right lung.

Pericardial Effusion

The pericardial space is another area that can commonly accumulate fluid containing malignant cells (Fig. 15.3). Malignant cells can enter the pericardial space through the lymphatic drainage, through the arterial circulation, and by direct extension. Clinically, patients with pericardial effusion typically present with dyspnea, hypotension, tachycardia, and other signs of decreased cardiac output. The diagnosis is one that is suspected in patients with lung cancer and symptoms of shock. Most large pericardial effusions are readily visualized on CT scans of the chest; however, echocardiography is more specific and sensitive. Although pericardiocentesis can quickly relieve symptoms of shock and restore adequate circulation, fluid will quickly re-accumulate in patients with lung cancer. Open pericardiotomy can allow access to the pericardial sac for immediate drainage and placement of the drainage catheter. Sclerosis of the pericardial space can be performed with doxycycline, bleomycin, or thiotepa.

Superior Vena Cava Syndrome

Obstruction of the superior vena cava is a known complication of both small cell and non-small cell lung cancer (Fig. 15.4). In this disease, it is typically caused by compression or invasion of the superior vena cava by a right-sided tumor. The clinical presentation depends upon the length of evolution of the process. When there is an acute obstruction of the superior vena cava, patients present with facial, neck, and upper extremity swelling, dyspnea, orthopnea, and facial erythema. In a slow obstruction, symptoms of acute swelling are less apparent, and the symptoms of venous hypertension causing distention of collateral circulation are visible, in the form of dilated and prominent cutaneous veins. Superior vena cava syndrome can be adequately diagnosed in lung cancer through CT scan or MRI, although contrast venography is more accurate in identifying collateral circulation. In lung cancer, the treatment of severe vena cava syndrome is usually conservative, with radiation therapy being the best treatment for acute disease. Slowly progressive obstruction may sometimes respond to chemotherapy. In patients with complete obstruction who remain symptomatic after radiation therapy, stenting of the superior vena cava with a metallic stent can restore patency and adequately relieve obstructive symptoms (47).

SMALL CELL LUNG CANCER

Epidemiology

Small cell lung cancer is almost exclusively a disease of smokers, and a diagnosis of small cell lung cancer in a nonsmoker should raise significant doubts. This fact

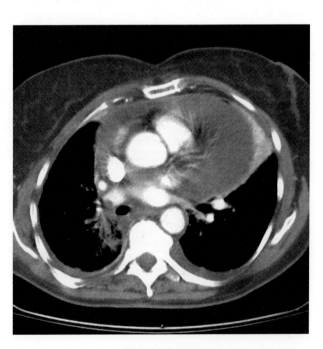

FIGURE 15.3

Computed tornography demonstrating fluid significantly dilating the pericardial sack.

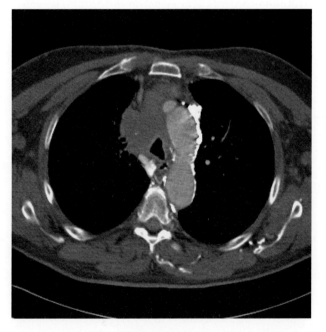

FIGURE 15.4

Computed tornography demonstrating tumor surrounding the superior vena cava. A pinpoint amount of contrast can be seen in the center of the collapsed vein.

may explain why the proportional incidence of small cell lung cancer in the United States has decreased over time. The Surveillance, Epidemiology, and End Results (SEER) database shows a decrease in the proportion of small cell lung cancer from 17% of all lung cancers in 1986 to 13% in 2002, parallel to a decrease in tobacco consumption in men. At the same time, the percentage of small cell lung cancer in women has increased from 28% in 1973 to 50% in 2002 (48).

Staging

The TNM staging system is generally not used for small cell lung cancer. Patients with small cell lung cancer are staged according to a classification developed by the Veterans Administration Lung Cancer Study Group in the 1970s. This classification divides patients into limited- or extensive-stage disease. Recent changes to this classification have improved its prognostic value.

Limited disease is defined as disease that is confined to one hemithorax with or without ipsilateral or contralateral mediastinal or supraclavicular lymph node metastases with or without ipsilateral pleural effusions independent of cytology. This has now been modified to exclude patients with a pleural or pericardial effusion, since these patients are unlikely to be cured with radiation therapy. Another modification that stresses the importance of radiation therapy in limited stage disease is that the tumor must be encompassed by a reasonable or tolerable radiation port.

Extensive disease is defined as any disease at sites beyond those defined in limited disease. The staging procedures and tests for small cell lung cancer are the same as those for non-small cell lung cancer. In patients with no radiographic signs of metastatic disease, but significant abnormalities in peripheral blood counts or elevation in alkaline phosphatase, a bone marrow biopsy may reveal metastases.

PROGNOSTIC FACTORS

Many groups have studied prognostic factors for small cell lung cancer. The most important prognostic factors found are performance status, stage of disease, age, and gender. The Southwest Oncology Group (SWOG) published a database of 2,580 patients with small cell lung cancer in 1990 showing that patients with good performance status, female sex, aged younger than 70 years, white race, and normal lactate dehydrogenase (LDH) were favorable independent predictors of outcome (49). In patients with limited disease, they found that high LDH, the presence of pleural effusion, and advanced age were important negative prognostic factors.

PARANEOPLASTIC SYNDROMES

Although paraneoplastic syndromes occur in non-small cell lung cancer, they are found more commonly in small cell lung cancer. Most of these syndromes are mediated by autoantibodies or by production of peptide hormones, allowing a classification into either endocrine or neurological syndromes. The most common endocrine syndrome is hyponatremia; it occurs in approximately 15% of patients, and has been linked to elevated levels of vasopressin (50) and atrial natriuretic factor in causing an SIADH like picture. Ectopic secretion of ACTH causing Cushing syndrome occurs in approximately 1%–3% of cases. Most neurological paraneoplastic syndromes are immune mediated. Multiple antibodies have been identified that are related to specific syndromes such as anti-Yo in cerebellar degeneration and anti-Hu in encephalomyelitis, sensory neuropathies, and autonomic dysfunction (51,52). The most common neurologic paraneoplastic syndrome is the Lambert–Eaton syndrome, believed to be related to antibodies against presynaptic voltage gated calcium channels, which occurs in approximately 3%–5% of small cell lung cancer patients, and causes a myasthenia syndrome.

TREATMENT

As with non-small cell lung cancer, the treatment of small cell lung cancer depends on multiple modalities, mainly chemotherapy and radiation therapy. Surgery plays a minor role in this disease.

Chemotherapy

Small cell lung cancer is an extremely chemotherapy-sensitive tumor. Response rates to standard agents are in the range of 60%–80%. The most accepted regimen in the United States is a common nation of etoposide (Eposin) and cisplatin, which has been the standard of care since the early 1990s (53). The median survival for patients with extensive disease in phase 3 trials is approximately 9–12 months. A trial by Noda showed superiority for a regimen containing irinotecan (Camptosar) and cisplatin, but subsequent trials have not shown the same results (54). Multiple high-dose chemotherapy strategies have not shown an advantage when compared to standard-dose treatments. Trials comparing etoposide and cisplatin with three drug combinations have either not shown a significant advantage, or have shown a small advantage at the cost of increased toxicity (53). The standard duration of treatment is approximately four cycles. The strategy of continuing treatment beyond four to six cycles has not been proven to be beneficial (55,56). In extensive disease, chemotherapy is given as a single modality. In limited disease it is given concurrently with radiation therapy.

Radiation Therapy

Radiation therapy as a single modality is not usually curative in small cell lung cancer. However, SCLC is highly sensitive to radiation therapy, and radiation therapy is an effective palliatives maneuver in many clinical situations, including:

Metastases causing pain
Obstructive bronchial lesions
Severe hemoptysis
Bone metastases at risk for fracture
Brain metastases

The most important use of radiation therapy in this disease is in combination with chemotherapy for limited stage disease. A meta-analysis published by Pignon et al. in 1992 showed a significant advantage in survival for patients receiving a combination of chemotherapy and radiation versus chemotherapy alone (57). Incorporating radiation therapy early in the course of chemotherapy confers a statistically significant survival advantage over incorporating radiation therapy in the latter cycles of chemotherapy (58–61). The median survival for patients with limited disease in phase III trials is 20–23 months with an overall five-year survival of approximately 20%.

Prophylactic Cranial Irradiation (PCI)

Isolated CNS metastases occur in approximately 15% of limited disease stage patients were treated with concurrent chemotherapy and radiation with curative intent. A meta-analysis published in 1999 showed a 5.4% increase in three-year survival in patients receiving PCI, as well as a 54% reduction in the risk of brain metastases (62). The PCI is delivered after completion of chemotherapy and radiation. A study presented at the American Society of Clinical Oncology meeting in 2007 showed an improvement in survival for patients with extensive disease receiving PCI after a documented response to chemotherapy compared to patients without PCI (63).

Surgery

Since small cell lung cancer is considered a systemic disease, with micrometastatic disease already present at the time of diagnosis, surgery as a single modality is not usually curative. A randomized trial studying the benefit of surgery in patients receiving both chemotherapy and radiation showed no increase in survival for patients who had a resection over patients who did not (64). Patients who are found to have small cell lung cancer at the time of surgery and have a complete resection, should receive adjuvant chemotherapy. Patients who do not have a complete resection should be treated with both chemotherapy and radiation.

References

1. Jemal A, Siegel R, Ward E, Murray T, Xu J, Thun MJ. Cancer statistics, 2007. *CA Cancer J Clin.* 2007;57(1):43–66.
2. Doll R, Peto R, Wheatley K, Gray R, Sutherland I. Mortality in relation to smoking: 40 years' observations on male British doctors. *BMJ (Clinical research ed).* 1994;309(6959):901–911.
3. Hammond EC. Smoking in relation to the death rates of one million men and women. *Natl Cancer Inst Monogr.* 1966;19:127–204.
4. McLaughlin JK, Hrubec Z, Blot WJ, Fraumeni JF, Jr. Smoking and cancer mortality among U.S. veterans: a 26-year follow-up. *Int J Cancer.* 1995;60(2):190–193.
5. Field RW, Steck DJ, Smith BJ, et al. Residential radon gas exposure and lung cancer: the Iowa Radon Lung Cancer Study. *Am J Epidemiol.* 2000;151(11):1091–1102.
6. van Loon AJ, Kant IJ, Swaen GM, Goldbohm RA, Kremer AM, van den Brandt PA. Occupational exposure to carcinogens and risk of lung cancer: results from The Netherlands cohort study. *Occup Environ Med.* 1997;54(11):817–824.
7. Darby S, Hill D, Auvinen A, et al. Radon in homes and risk of lung cancer: collaborative analysis of individual data from 13 European case-control studies. *BMJ (Clinical research ed).* 2005;330(7485):223.
8. Ries LAG MD, Krapcho M, Mariotto A, et al. SEER Cancer Statistics Review, 1975-2005, National Cancer Institute. Bethesda, MD, http://seer.cancer.gov/csr1975–2005/, based on November 2007 SEER data submission, posted to the SEER website, 2008.
9. The World Health Organization histological typing of lung tumors. *Am J Clin Pathol.* 1982;77:123–136.
10. Fontana RS, Sanderson DR, Taylor WF, et al. Early lung cancer detection: results of the initial (prevalence) radiologic and cytologic screening in the Mayo Clinic study. *Am Rev Respir Dis.* 1984;130(4):561–565.
11. Frost JK, Ball WC, Jr., Levin ML, et al. Early lung cancer detection: results of the initial (prevalence) radiologic and cytologic screening in the Johns Hopkins study. *Am Rev Respir Dis.* 1984;130(4):549–554.
12. Melamed MR.Lung cancer screening results in the National Cancer Institute New York study. *Cancer.* 2000;89(11 Suppl):2356–2362.
13. Henschke CI, McCauley DI, Yankelevitz DF, et al. Early Lung Cancer Action Project: overall design and findings from baseline screening. *Lancet.* 1999;354(9173):99–105.
14. Henschke CI, Yankelevitz DF, Libby DM, Pasmantier MW, Smith JP, Miettinen OS. Survival of patients with stage I lung cancer detected on CT screening. *N Engl J Med.* 2006;355(17):1763–1771.
15. Samet JM. Health benefits of smoking cessation. *Clin Chest Med.* 1991;12(4):669–679.
16. The effect of vitamin E and beta carotene on the incidence of lung cancer and other cancers in male smokers. The Alpha-Tocopherol, Beta Carotene Cancer Prevention Study Group. *N Engl J Med.* 1994;330(15):7.
17. Omenn GS, Goodman GE, Thornquist MD, et al. Effects of a combination of beta carotene and vitamin A on lung cancer and cardiovascular disease. *N Engl J Med.* 1996;334(18):1150–1155.

18. Blom JW, Vanderschoot JP, Oostindier MJ, Osanto S, van der Meer FJ, Rosendaal FR. Incidence of venous thrombosis in a large cohort of 66,329 cancer patients: results of a record linkage study. *J Thromb Haemost.* 2006;4(3):529–535.

19. Sack GH, Jr., Levin J, Bell WR. Trousseau's syndrome and other manifestations of chronic disseminated coagulopathy in patients with neoplasms: clinical, pathophysiologic, and therapeutic features. *Medicine.* 1977;56(1):1–37.

20. Ginsberg RJ, Rubinstein LV. Randomized trial of lobectomy versus limited resection for T1 N0 non-small cell lung cancer. Lung Cancer Study Group. *Ann Thorac Surg.* 1995;60(3):615–622; discussion 22–23.

21. Arriagada R, Bergman B, Dunant A, Le Chevalier T, Pignon JP, Vansteenkiste J. Cisplatin-based adjuvant chemotherapy in patients with completely resected non-small cell lung cancer. *N Engl J Med.* 2004;350(4):351–360.

22. Douillard J, Rosell R, Delena A, Legroumellec A, Torres F, Carpagnano F. ANITA: Phase III adjuvant vinorelbine (N) and cisplatin (P) versus observation (OBS) in completely resected (stage I-III) non-small cell lung cancer (NSCLC) patients (pts): Final results after 70-month median follow-up. On behalf of the Adjuvant Navelbine International Trialist Association. In: American Society of Clinical Oncology Annual Meeting; 2005; 2005.

23. Douillard JY, Rosell R, De Lena M, et al. Adjuvant vinorelbine plus cisplatin versus observation in patients with completely resected stage IB-IIIA non-small cell lung cancer (Adjuvant Navelbine International Trialist Association [ANITA]): a randomised controlled trial. *Lancet Oncol.* 2006;7(9):719–727.

24. Winton T, Livingston R, Johnson D, et al. Vinorelbine plus cisplatin vs. observation in resected non-small cell lung cancer. *N Engl J Med.* 2005;352(25):2589–2597.

25. Strauss Gea. Adjuvant chemotherapy in stage IB non-small cell lung cancer (NSCLC): Update of Cancer and Leukemia Group B (CALGB) protocol 9633. In: American Society of Clinical Oncology Annual Meeting; 2006.

26. Pignon JP. Lung Adjuvant Cisplatin Evaluation (LACE): a pooled analysis of five randomized clinical trials including 4,584 patients. In: American Society of Clinical Oncology Annual Meeting; 2006; Atlanta, GA; 2006.

27. Mountain CF. Revisions in the international system for staging lung cancer. *Chest.* 1997;111(6):1710–1717.

28. Depierre A, Milleron B, Moro D, Chevret D, Braun D, Quoix E. Phase III trial of neo-adjuvant chemotherapy (NCT) in resectable stage I (except T1N0), II, IIIa non-small cell lung cancer (NSCLC): the French experience. *Proc Am Soc Clin Oncol.* 1999;18:465a.

29. Depierre A, Milleron B, Moro-Sibilot D, et al. Preoperative chemotherapy followed by surgery compared with primary surgery in resectable stage I (except T1N0), II, and IIIa non-small cell lung cancer. *J Clin Oncol.* 2002;20(1):247–253.

30. Rosell R, Gomez-Codina J, Camps C, et al. A randomized trial comparing preoperative chemotherapy plus surgery with surgery alone in patients with non-small cell lung cancer. *N Engl J Med.* 1994;330(3):153–158.

31. Roth JA, Fossella F, Komaki R, et al. A randomized trial comparing perioperative chemotherapy and surgery with surgery alone in resectable stage IIIA non-small cell cancer. *J Natl Cancer Inst.* 1994;86:673–680.

32. Roth JA, Neely Atkinson E, Fossella F, et al. Long-term follow-up of patients enrolled in a randomized trial comparing perioperative chemotherapy and surgery with surgery alone in resectable stage IIIA non-small cell lung cancer. *Lung Cancer.* 1998;21:1–6.

33. Albain KS. Phase III study of concurrent chemotherapy and radiotherapy (CT/RT) vs CT/RT followed by surgical resection for stage IIIA(pN2) non-small cell lung cancer (NSCLC): outcomes update of North American Intergroup 0139 (RTOG 9309). . In: American Society of Clinical Oncology Annual Meeting; 2005; Orlando, FL; 2005.

34. Dillman R, Seagren S, Propert K, et al. A randomized trial of induction chemotherapy plus high-dose radiation versus radiation alone in stage III non-small cell lung cancer. *N Engl J Med.* 1990;323:940–945.

35. Dillman RO, Herndon J, Seagren SL, Eaton WL, Jr., Green MR.Improved survival in stage III non-small cell lung cancer: seven-year follow-up of cancer and leukemia group B (CALGB) 8433 trial [see comments]. *J Natl Cancer Inst.* 1996;88(17):1210–1215.

36. Le Chevalier T, Arriagada R, Quoix E, et al. Radiotherapy alone versus combined chemotherapy and radiotherapy in nonresectable non-small cell lung cancer: first analysis of a randomized trial in 353 patients. *J Natl Cancer Inst.* 1991;83:417–423.

37. Sause W, Kolesar P, Taylor SI, et al. Final results of phase III trial in regionally advanced unresectable non-small cell lung cancer: Radiation Therapy Oncology Group, Eastern Cooperative Oncology Group, and Southwest Oncology Group. *Chest.* 2000;117(2):358–364.

38. Sause WT, Scott C, Taylor S, et al. Radiation Therapy Oncology Group (RTOG) 88-08 and Eastern Cooperative Oncology Group (ECOG) 4588: preliminary results of a phase III trial in regionally advanced, unresectable non-small cell lung cancer. *J Natl Cancer Inst.* 1995;87(3):198–205.

39. Curran WJ, Scott C, Langer C, et al. Long term benefit is observed in a phase III comparison of sequential vs concurrent chemo-radiation for patients with unresected stage III nsclc: RTOG 9410. *Proc Am Soc Clin Oncol.* 2003;22:621.

40. Furuse K, Fukuoka M, Kawahara M, et al. Phase III study of concurrent versus sequential thoracic radiotherapy in combination with Mitomycin, Vindesine and Cisplatin in unresectbale stage III non-small cell lung cancer. *J Clin Oncol.* 1999;17:2692–2699.

41. Chemotherapy in non-small cell lung cancer: a meta-analysis using updated data on individual patients from 52 randomised clinical trials. Non-small Cell Lung Cancer Collaborative Group. *BMJ (Clinical research ed).* 1995;311(7010):899–909.

42. Schiller JH, Harrington D, Belani CP, et al. Comparison of four chemotherapy regimens for advanced non-small cell lung cancer. *N Engl J Med.* 2002;346(2):92–98.

43. Manegold C. Randomised, double-blind multicentre phase III study of bevacizumab in combination with cisplatin and gemcitabine in chemotherapy-na 239;ve patients with advanced or recurrent non-squamous non-small cell lung cancer. In: American Society of Clinical Oncology Annual Meeting; 2007; Chicago, IL; 2007.

44. Sandler A, Gray R, Perry MC, et al. Paclitaxel-carboplatin alone or with bevacizumab for non-small cell lung cancer. *N Engl J Med.* 2006;355(24):2542–2550.

45. Paz-Ares Lea. A prospective phase II trial of erlotinib in advanced non-small cell lung cancer (NSCLC) patients (p) with mutations in the tyrosine kinase (TK) domain of the epidermal growth factor receptor (EGFR). In: American Society of Clinical Oncology Annual Meeting 2006; Chicago, IL; 2006.

46. Rusch VW, Giroux DJ, Kraut MJ, et al. Induction chemoradiation and surgical resection for non-small cell lung carcinomas of the superior sulcus: Initial results of Southwest Oncology Group Trial 9416 (Intergroup Trial 0160). *J Thorac Cardiovasc Surg.* 2001;121:472–483.

47. Nagata T, Makutani S, Uchida H, et al. Follow-up results of 71 patients undergoing metallic stent placement for the treatment of a malignant obstruction of the superior vena cava. *Cardiovasc Intervent Radiol.* 2007;30(5):959–67.

48. Govindan R, Page N, Morgensztern D, et al. Changing epidemiology of small cell lung cancer in the United States over the last 30 years: analysis of the surveillance, epidemiologic, and end results database. *J Clin Oncol.* 2006;24(28):4539–4544.

49. Albain KS, Crowley JJ, LeBlanc M, Livingston RB. Determinants of improved outcome in small cell lung cancer: an analysis of the 2,580-patient Southwest Oncology Group data base. *J Clin Oncol.* 1990;8(9):1563–1574.

50. Johnson BE, Chute JP, Rushin J, et al. A prospective study of patients with lung cancer and hyponatremia of malignancy. *Am J Respir Crit Care Med.* 1997;156(5):1669–1678.

51. Graus F, Keime-Guibert F, Rene R, et al. Anti-Hu-associated paraneoplastic encephalomyelitis: analysis of 200 patients. *Brain.* 2001;124(Pt 6):1138–1148.

52. Peterson K, Rosenblum MK, Kotanides H, Posner JB. Paraneoplastic cerebellar degeneration. I. A clinical analysis of 55 anti-Yo antibody-positive patients. *Neurology*. 1992;42(10):1931–1937.

53. Roth BJ, Johnson DH, Einhorn LH, et al. Randomized study of cyclophosphamide, doxorubicin, and vincristine versus etoposide and cisplatin versus alternation of these two regimens in extensive small cell lung cancer: a phase III trial of the Southeastern Cancer Study Group. *J Clin Oncol*. 1992;10(2):282–291.

54. Hanna N, Bunn PA, Jr., Langer C, et al. Randomized phase III trial comparing irinotecan/cisplatin with etoposide/cisplatin in patients with previously untreated extensive-stage disease small cell lung cancer. *J Clin Oncol*. 2006;24(13):2038–2043.

55. Giaccone G, Dalesio O, McVie GJ, et al. Maintenance chemotherapy in small cell lung cancer: long-term results of a randomized trial. European Organization for Research and Treatment of Cancer Lung Cancer Cooperative Group. *J Clin Oncol*. 1993;11(7):1230–1240.

56. Spiro SG, Souhami RL, Geddes DM, et al. Duration of chemotherapy in small cell lung cancer: a Cancer Research Campaign trial. *Br J Cancer*. 1989;59(4):578–583.

57. Pignon JP, Arriagada R, Ihde DC, et al. A meta-analysis of thoracic radiotherapy for small cell lung cancer. *N Engl J Med*. 1992;327(23):1618–1624.

58. De Ruysscher D, Pijls-Johannesma M, Bentzen SM, et al. Time between the first day of chemotherapy and the last day of chest radiation is the most important predictor of survival in limited-disease small cell lung cancer. *J Clin Oncol*. 2006;24(7):1057–1063.

59. De Ruysscher D, Pijls-Johannesma M, Vansteenkiste J, Kester A, Rutten I, Lambin P. Systematic review and meta-analysis of randomised, controlled trials of the timing of chest radiotherapy in patients with limited-stage, small cell lung cancer. *Ann Oncol*. 2006;17(4):543–552.

60. Fried DB, Morris DE, Poole C, et al. Systematic review evaluating the timing of thoracic radiation therapy in combined modality therapy for limited-stage small cell lung cancer. *J Clin Oncol*. 2004;22(23):4837–4845.

61. Murray N, Coy P, Pater JL, et al. Importance of timing for thoracic irradiation in the combined modality treatment of limited-stage small cell lung cancer. The National Cancer Institute of Canada Clinical Trials Group. *J Clin Oncol*. 1993;11(2):336–344.

62. Auperin A, Arriagada R, Pignon JP, et al. Prophylactic cranial irradiation for patients with small cell lung cancer in complete remission. Prophylactic Cranial Irradiation Overview Collaborative Group. *N Engl J Med*. 1999;341(7):476–484.

63. Slotman Bea. A randomized trial of prophylactic cranial irradiation (PCI) versus no PCI in extensive disease small cell lung cancer after a response to chemotherapy (EORTC 08993-22993). In: American Society of Clinical Oncology Annual Meeting; 2007; Chicago, Il; 2007.

64. Lad T, Piantadosi S, Thomas P, Payne D, Ruckdeschel J, Giaccone G. A prospective randomized trial to determine the benefit of surgical resection of residual disease following response of small cell lung cancer to combination chemotherapy. *Chest*. 1994;106(6 Suppl):320S–323S.

Evaluation and Treatment of Colorectal Cancer

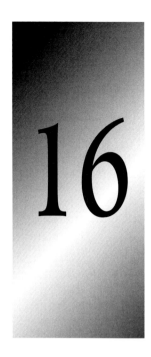

16

Leonard B. Saltz
Austin G. Duffy

Approximately 150,000 people are diagnosed with colorectal cancer (CRC) annually in the United States, making it the fourth most common cancer diagnosis, behind lung, breast, and prostate (1). A number of factors have resulted in an improved, and improving, outlook for patients diagnosed with this disease, although colorectal cancer still remains the number two cause of cancer death in this country.

The major modality for management of local-regional CRC is surgical resection. With the exception of the introduction and widespread adoption of total mesorectal excision (TME) for rectal cancer—which substantially improved local control of this disease (2)—the standard surgical techniques have changed little in recent years. Laparoscopic surgery has emerged as a treatment option, but this has not altered outcome or prognosis. Therefore, we must look at other areas to uncover the causes of this improved prognosis.

The wide adoption of the use of colonoscopic screening for polyps has undoubtedly had a reductive effect on the incidence of CRC and, with the earlier diagnosis of established cancers (3), has also led to improved survival times, both spurious (as a result of lead-time bias) and real (earlier diagnosis of more curable lesions and the earlier implementation of curative adjuvant therapies). Undoubtedly the most important factor has been the advent of a greater number of active systemic chemotherapy agents. This has led not only to prolonged survival for metastatic disease, but also to some increases in the numbers of patients that are actu-ally cured, through the incorporation of some of these agents into the adjuvant treatment following complete surgical resection.

The improvement in systemic therapy has altered the landscape in a number of ways. Patients with stage IV (metastatic) disease are surviving for longer periods (4), often with good functionality and quality of life, at least in the initial phases of treatment. However, long-term treatment of metastatic disease does appear to be resulting in a changing pattern of treatment failure. These patients are more likely to suffer events such as bone or brain metastases, or spinal cord compression, which have heretofore been unusual occurrences in CRC. In a sense, the natural history of the disease has been altered. In addition, more patients will have been exposed to the increased toxicities of the new therapies in the adjuvant setting. These patients have a high probability of cure; therefore, both the known and unknown long-term toxicities of therapy are of enormous significance for them. In addition, the wider use of more effective but potentially more toxic therapies means that more patients will be at risk for acute hospitalizations, with all the attendant morbidities and rehabilitation issues associated with this.

The aim of this chapter is to outline the therapeutic paradigm as it currently pertains to CRC, referencing briefly the major clinical trial milestones. In previous times, a patient with CRC receiving chemotherapy had, almost by definition, a very limited life expectancy. The role of rehabilitation medicine in such a patient was

KEY POINTS

- Approximately 150,000 people are diagnosed with colorectal cancer (CRC) annually in the United States, making it the fourth most common cancer diagnosis and the second leading cause of cancer death in the United States.
- The wide adoption of colonoscopic screening for polyps has had a reductive effect on the incidence of CRC and, with the earlier diagnosis of established cancers, improved survival times.
- The major modality for management of local-regional CRC is surgical resection, with the primary goal of removing the primary tumor and an adequate margin of healthy tissue along with the draining lymph nodes.
- A greater number of active systemic chemotherapy agents have led not only to prolonged survival for metastatic CRC, but also an increase in the numbers of patients that are cured.
- The postoperative management of CRC patients is dependent on two major factors—the performance status of the patient and the stage of the disease.

- The backbone of systemic therapy in this disease is 5-fluorouracil (5-FU) with two major cytotoxic additions being irinotecan and oxaliplatin.
- The addition of bevacizumab, a monoclonal antibody directed against vascular endothelial growth factor (VEGF)—an important mediator of tumor angiogenesis—to standard irinotecan-based chemotherapy improved the survival of patients by nearly five months.
- FOLFOX, the combination of oxaliplatin with the LV5FU2 (short-course infusion 5-FU with leucovorin incorporated into a 48-hour regimen given every other week) has been shown to be more effective than 5-FU therapy alone in patients with untreated metastatic colorectal cancer.
- The main toxicity of oxaliplatin, which is often dose-limiting, is neurotoxicity, which commonly manifests as a peripheral symmetrical cold sensitivity and paresthesias affecting the hands, feet, and throat.

likely to be very minimal given the competing priorities of symptom control in the context of a terminal illness. The black/white duality of that previous era has now been replaced by a gradation of grays as CRC is increasingly viewed as a chronic illness, in which the goals of rehabilitation medicine and oncology are likely to have increasing areas of overlap.

CLINICAL OVERVIEW

Approximately 80% of patients present with localized and, therefore, potentially curable disease (5). Prior to undergoing resection, patients should have staging computed tomography (CT) imaging of the chest and abdomen, and in the pelvis (in patients with rectal cancer, those with intrapelvic primaries, and all females) to rule out metastatic disease. A preoperative serum carcinoembryonic antigen (CEA) level should be drawn, as this has prognostic value and may help dictate postoperative treatment choices. For cancers outside of the rectum, initial surgery (ie, without preoperative, or neoadjuvant, therapy) is standard practice. The main principle of surgical oncology in colorectal, as in other cancers, is to remove the primary tumor with adequate margins of healthy tissue, in association with removal of the draining lymph nodes. The overwhelming majority of patients can be expected to have a surgical resection without a permanent colostomy; irreversible colostomy procedures such as abdominal

perineal resection (APR) are reserved only for a small subset of patients with distal rectal tumors on or very close to the anal verge.

The postoperative management of patients with CRC is dependent on two major factors—the performance status of the patient and the stage of the disease. Performance status, a numeric quantitation of the patient's overall state of well-being, is most commonly quantitated according to either the Eastern Cooperative Oncology Group (ECOG) or Karnofsky scoring systems. In the postoperative patient, performance status is a fluid variable that may be affected by surgical wound healing and by complications, but may improve with time.

CRC is staged according to the American Joint Commission on Cancer (AJCC) Tumor-Node-Metastasis (TNM) system (Table 16.1), which is primarily based on the pathological findings postresection but also takes into account the surgical and radiological findings (primarily for the metastatic [M] portion of the staging). Median expected survival times correlate with pathological stage. The broad paradigm of therapy is outlined in Table 16.2.

TREATMENT OF METASTATIC DISEASE

A meta-analysis of seven trials (866 patients) demonstrated convincingly that palliative chemotherapy was associated with an improvement in overall survival (6).

TABLE 16.1
TNM Staging for CRC

Primary Tumor (T)
Carcinoma in situ; intraepithelial (within glandular basement membrane) or invasion of lamina propria (intramucosal)
Tumor invades submucosa
Tumor invades muscularis propria
Tumor invades through the muscularis propria into the subserosa, or into nonperitonealized pericolic or perirectal tissues
Tumor directly invades other organs or structures, and/or perforates visceral peritoneum
Regional Lymph Node (N)
Regional nodes cannot be assessed
No regional nodal metastases
Metastasis in 1–3 regional lymph nodes
Metastasis in 4 or more regional lymph nodes
Distant Metastasis (M)
Distant metastasis cannot be assessed
No distant metastasis
Distant metastasis

TABLE 16.2
Therapies for Gastrointestinal Cancer According to Stage

Stage I: surgery only
Stage II: surgery ± adjuvant chemotherapy (controversial)
Stage III: surgery + adjuvant chemotherapy
Stage IV: chemotherapy only (occasionally surgery if resectable oligo-metastatic disease)

The chemotherapy used in these trials would today be considered suboptimal and the authors commented that the overall quality of evidence relating to treatment toxicity, symptom control, and quality of life measurement was poor by current standards. The field has moved on from this; however, this meta-analysis represents proof of principle that active systemic therapy is superior (compared to best supportive care) in terms of providing a survival benefit in this disease.

The backbone of systemic therapy in this disease is 5-FU, a fluoropyrimidine that acts by inhibiting thymidylate synthase, a critical enzyme in DNA synthesis. This drug was first patented in 1957. For much of the 1960s through the mid-1990s, investigational energies were focused largely on the various methods of administering and/or modulating 5-FU (7). These included bolus schedules on a daily or weekly basis or short course and prolonged infusional schedules that employed the use of semipermanent venous access devices. 5-FU was also combined with putative "biomodulating" compounds, such as leucovorin (Wellcovorin) or levamisole (Ergamisol), in an attempt to increase its efficacy. It is a fair summation to say that these different schedules had somewhat different toxicity profiles, but had approximate equivalence in terms of efficacy. Infusional schedules had, if anything, a slightly superior efficacy, with less hematologic toxicity. Leucovorin, a biomodulator that enhances 5-FU cytotoxicity by interacting with the enzyme thymidylate synthase, thereby prolonging inhibition of the enzyme by 5-FU, has remained a frequent component of 5-FU-based regimens. The combination of bolus and short-course infusional 5-FU with leucovorin has been incorporated into a 48-hour regimen given every other week (the de Gramont, or LV5FU2 regimen). This regimen has formed the backbone of several modern chemotherapy schedules for this disease, to which newer, active drugs have been added as they emerge from development. Oral formulations of fluoropyrimidines have also been developed, and these have been shown to have similar efficacy to parenteral leucovorin-modulated 5-FU regimens (8).

For several decades, the median survival times remained static at approximately one year. Towards the end of 1990s, as newer drugs were incorporated into practice, median survival times began to improve. The two major cytotoxic additions were irinotecan and oxaliplatin.

Irinotecan is an inhibitor of the enzyme topoisomerase 1. After early phase studies established its efficacy as a single agent in 5-FU-refractory disease, three major trials demonstrated the superiority of irinotecan combined with 5-FU compared to 5-FU alone in the first-line metastatic setting (9–11). The main toxicities of irinotecan are diarrhea and neutropenia.

Oxaliplatin is a platinum derivative that has synergistic activity with 5-FU. The combination of oxaliplatin with the LV5FU2 regimen (given the epithet FOLFOX) has been shown to be more effective than 5-FU therapy alone in patients with untreated metastatic colorectal cancer (12). The main toxicity of oxaliplatin, which is often dose-limiting, is neurotoxicity, which most commonly manifests as a peripheral symmetrical cold sensitivity and paresthesias affecting the hands, feet, and throat.

The emergence of irinotecan and oxaliplatin has added layers of complexity to treatment decisions that were simple when 5-FU was the only therapy available. A question that rapidly emerged was: which drug is the more active, and is the combination of both drugs together more efficacious than sequential therapy? Although FOLFOX out-performed irinotecan when the irinotecan was given with bolus 5-FU (13), when irinotecan is given with the LV5FU2 method (and given the epithet FOLFIRI), the regimens appear to be equivalent in terms of efficacy in the metastatic setting (14,15).

The study by Tournigrand et al. also answers the question about whether the order in which the treatments are given matters. This trial treated patients with either FOLFOX or FOLFIRI and then allowed them to cross over to the other therapy upon progression of their disease. There was no difference in survival between the two groups. The combination of irinotecan and oxaliplatin together (IROX) as first-line therapy has not been shown to be superior, and in the Intergroup study performed inferiorly to FOLFOX (13).

While the addition of these two effective chemotherapies to the armamentarium has prolonged median survival times modestly, the outcomes for patients with metastatic colorectal cancer remain poor, with cure being a vanishingly rare phenomenon. Clearly, additional and better therapies are still needed. For this reason, the so-called "targeted" therapies, an approach derived from an understanding of tumour biology, wherein drugs are rationally designed with a specific biological purpose in mind, have been investigated in colorectal cancer. This approach has yielded some modest improvements in treatment, although the benefits have been far more modest than had been hoped for.

The first pivotal study of a biologic, or targeted, therapy in CRC was presented in 2003, when the addition of bevacizumab, a monoclonal antibody directed against vascular endothelial growth factor (VEGF)—an important mediator of tumor angiogenesis—to standard irinotecan-based chemotherapy, improved the survival of patients by nearly five months (16). This study not only represented a change in standard first-line therapy of metastatic colorectal cancer, but also represented a proof of principle for anti-VEGF therapy. The efficacy of adding bevacizumab to oxaliplatin-based therapy, oral fluoropyrimidines, and also in the second-line setting has also been proven in large randomized trials (17,18). Of note, however, the addition of bevacizumab to oxaliplatin-based therapy in front-line therapy was not associated with a significant survival advantage in a recent large study (19).

Initially it was felt that these rationally-derived therapies would be less toxic than the older, cytotoxic chemotherapies. In a sense this is true, but as has been the case with trastuzumab in breast cancer, serious and important toxicities have surfaced. In addition, since these drugs have only modest activity on their own, the toxicity of all the older chemotherapy that must be used in conjunction with the targeted therapy remains. Bevacizumab is associated with a small risk of large or small bowel perforation and an increased frequency of arterial thrombotic events (myocardial infarction, cerebrovascular accident, transient ischemic attack, or angina). It also causes hypertension in 15%–18% of individuals, and can interfere with wound healing.

The second major target in colorectal cancer therapeutics has been the epidermal growth factor receptor (EGFR). Cetuximab is a monoclonal antibody directed against EGFR, and was shown to have modest activity as a single agent in irinotecan-refractory colorectal cancer (20). Intriguingly, cetuximab appears to overcome irinotecan-refractoriness, as shown in two trials that demonstrated superiority for the combination of irinotecan and cetuximab over cetuximab alone in patients who had already progressed on irinotecan (20,21). The role of cetuximab in the first-line therapy of colorectal cancer has not yet been established. A recent study demonstrated a very modest benefit (under one month) for the combination of cetuximab with FOLFIRI versus FOLFIRI alone (22). This disappointing result makes it difficult to recommend routine use of this therapy in the first-line setting. Unlike the case of trastuzumab in breast cancer, there is no correlation between immunohistochemical staining of EGFR and response to anti-EGFR therapy; therefore, EGFR staining should not be used for clinical decision making (and in the authors' opinion should not be done) (23). The most common toxicity of cetuximab is an acneiform rash, which in up to 20% of patients can be quite severe. Interestingly, those who get the more severe rash are more likely to benefit from therapy. Recently, panitumumab, a fully humanized monoclonal antibody, has been approves by the U.S. Food and Drug Administration for therapy in refractory colorectal cancer. In the registration trial, it demonstrated an 8% single-agent response rate and a very modest improvement in progression-free survival over best supportive care alone (24).

The emergence of these new therapies in a relatively contracted period of time has engendered much optimism for the patient diagnosed with advanced colorectal cancer. There is a greater complexity to managing this disease, however, with more potential toxicities, and that optimism must be tempered by the reality that the advances, hard fought for though they have been, are modest. The relative placing of each new agent within the therapeutic paradigm has not been fully elucidated. Until that process occurs, we at least have data which tell us that the fact of exposure to the maximum amount of available active therapies is an important factor associated with prolonged survival (25).

Adjuvant Therapy

A certain proportion of patients will have a recurrence of their colorectal cancer in the months and years following surgery. Excluding de novo second primary colon cancers (so-called metachronous primary cancers, which occur in 1.5%–3% of colorectal cancer patients in the first five years) it is reasonable to assume that for patients who relapse, the tumor had already metastasized prior to (or at the time of) resection, and had existed at a microscopic level. The biological hypothesis underlying the strategy of adjuvant therapy is that the eradication of these micrometastases is achievable and that cure can be effected in patients who were otherwise destined to relapse.

Since 1990, the use of systemic chemotherapy following potentially curative resection has been standard practice in patients with stage III (local regional lymph node metastases only) and some stage II (full-thickness tumors, clean lymph nodes) disease, based on major trials which demonstrated a survival benefit for adjuvant chemotherapy compared to no treatment or ineffective treatment (26–28). The basic component of this therapy is 5-FU. As outlined above in the metastatic setting, a great deal of investigational energy was expended on the question of how best to administer the treatment in terms of method and duration of administration, and what best to combine it with. A large Intergroup study was among those that showed no additional benefit for prolonging chemotherapy beyond six months (29). As yet, there is no way to predict who will benefit from the addition of chemotherapy following curative surgery. It must be remembered that in evaluating studies in common diseases such as colorectal cancer or breast cancer, small differences in therapeutic arms often translate into large absolute numbers when applied to the population at large.

The clear survival gains demonstrated in the adjuvant trials apply to those with nodal involvement, for whom the risk of recurrence is higher. The use of chemotherapy in patients at stage II is more controversial. Most of the adjuvant studies have shown a trend towards improved survival, but have had insufficient power to detect statistically significant differences. It is accepted practice to offer adjuvant therapy to those with stage II disease who have high-risk features (high CEA, perforation, presentation with obstruction, or microvascular invasion). Molecular markers are not routinely used to delineate which patients in stage II would benefit from chemotherapy. An ECOG study in 2008 aimed to prospectively stratify stage II patients into risk categories based on microsatellite instability and loss of heterozygosity of 18q, assigning high-risk patients to randomization with FOLFOX with or without bevacizumab and low-risk patients to observation alone.

An important development in adjuvant studies has been the demonstration that three-year disease-free survival is a surrogate for five-year overall survival (30). This has the practical effect of shortening the length of time taken for questions to be answered by clinical trials, and in adjuvant studies where the majority of patients will be cured and the number of events are less, this is crucial to the development of the field. This is of particular importance in the current era of multiple active agents whose role(s) in the adjuvant setting need to be explored.

The rational belief that therapies which are effective in the metastatic setting should prove beneficial in the adjuvant setting is a dominant philosophy in the design of adjuvant studies in medical oncology. Logically, a therapy which is effective in the advanced setting should be even more effective where the disease burden is less (microscopic, if present at all), thus increasing the proportion of people cured with adjuvant treatment. Thus, some studies have focused on moving some of the treatments that have emerged in recent years to an earlier stage in the therapeutic paradigm, although some results have been quite disappointing.

Oxaliplatin-based therapy has been proven to be more effective than 5-FU/LV alone (31). In the pivotal study, 2,246 patients with resected colorectal cancer were randomized to de Gramont 5-FU with or without oxaliplatin. There was an absolute difference in disease-free survival of 7% reported at three years, which has persisted on longer follow-up (32). The NSABP C-07 trial has confirmed the benefits of adding oxaliplatin to 5-FU in the adjuvant setting (33).

Surprisingly, given its equivalent efficacy in the metastatic setting, irinotecan-based regimens have been shown to be ineffective in the adjuvant setting (34–36). Trials incorporating bevacizumab and cetuximab into adjuvant therapy are currently underway. The irinotecan experience should serve as a cautionary note that just because some benefit from these agents has been seen in the metastatic setting does not mean that they will be effective in the adjuvant setting. We must wait for the trial results. It should be noted that the long terms effects of any of the agents used in the treatment of CRC are not known. Even 5-FU has only been consistently given to patients with curable disease for less than two decades. Whether late sequelae from exposure to these drugs will be seen remains unknown at this time.

CONCLUSIONS

The field of treating gastrointestinal cancer has changed enormously in a short period of time and this has engendered much optimism. The unexpected toxicities of many of these new agents must sound a note of caution however. Likewise, the negative adjuvant data with irinotecan speaks to the importance of conducting well-designed clinical trials to rigorously evaluate the plethora of potential therapies in all settings before reaching conclusions regarding safety or efficacy. We urgently need predictive testing to prevent patients from being exposed to therapies from which they will not benefit. Microarray technology offers the possibility of profiling tumors according to their inherent biology, rather than our current pathological staging which is more a function of when the patient happens to present. The design of our clinical trials will need to incorporate these technologies so that they are evaluated in a prospective manner.

References

1. Jemal A, Siegel R, Ward E, Murray T, Xu J, Thun MJ. Cancer statistics, 2007. *CA Cancer J Clin.* 2007;57(1):43–66.
2. Tzardi M. Role of total mesorectal excision and of circumferential resection margin in local recurrence and survival of patients with rectal carcinoma. *Dig Dis.* 2007;25(1):51–55.
3. Winawer SJ, Zauber AG, Ho MN, et al. Prevention of colorectal cancer by colonoscopic polypectomy. The National Polyp Study Workgroup. *N Engl J Med.* 1993;329(27):1977–1981.
4. Goldberg RM. Advances in the treatment of metastatic colorectal cancer. *Oncologist.* 2005;10(Suppl 3):40–48.
5. Jessup JM, McGinnis LS, Steele GD, Jr., Menck HR, Winchester DP. The National Cancer Data Base. Report on colon cancer. *Cancer.* 1996;78(4):918–926.
6. Simmonds PC. Palliative chemotherapy for advanced colorectal cancer: systematic review and meta-analysis. Colorectal Cancer Collaborative Group. *BMJ.* 2000;321(7260):531–535.
7. Saltz LB. Another study of how to give fluorouracil? *J Clin Oncol.* 2003;21(20):3711–3712.
8. Hoff PM, Ansari R, Batist G, et al. Comparison of oral capecitabine versus intravenous fluorouracil plus leucovorin as first-line treatment in 605 patients with metastatic colorectal cancer: results of a randomized phase III study. *J Clin Oncol.* 2001;19(8):2282–2292.
9. Douillard JY, Cunningham D, Roth AD, et al. Irinotecan combined with fluorouracil compared with fluorouracil alone as first-line treatment for metastatic colorectal cancer: a multicentre randomised trial. *Lancet.* 2000;355(9209):1041–1047.
10. Saltz LB, Cox JV, Blanke C, et al. Irinotecan plus fluorouracil and leucovorin for metastatic colorectal cancer. Irinotecan Study Group. *N Engl J Med.* 2000;343(13):905–914.
11. Kohne CH, van Cutsem E, Wils J, et al. Phase III study of weekly high-dose infusional fluorouracil plus folinic acid with or without irinotecan in patients with metastatic colorectal cancer: European Organisation for Research and Treatment of Cancer Gastrointestinal Group Study 40986. *J Clin Oncol.* 2005;23(22):4856–4865.
12. de Gramont A, Figer A, Seymour M, et al. Leucovorin and fluorouracil with or without oxaliplatin as first-line treatment in advanced colorectal cancer. *J Clin Oncol.* 2000;18(16):2938–2947.
13. Goldberg RM, Sargent DJ, Morton RF, et al. A randomized controlled trial of fluorouracil plus leucovorin, irinotecan, and oxaliplatin combinations in patients with previously untreated metastatic colorectal cancer. *J Clin Oncol.* 2004;22(1):23–30.
14. Tournigand C, Andre T, Achille E, et al. FOLFIRI followed by FOLFOX6 or the reverse sequence in advanced colorectal cancer: a randomized GERCOR study. *J Clin Oncol.* 2004;22(2):229–237.
15. Colucci G, Gebbia V, Paoletti G, et al. Phase III randomized trial of FOLFIRI versus FOLFOX4 in the treatment of advanced colorectal cancer: a multicenter study of the Gruppo Oncologico Dell'Italia Meridionale. *J Clin Oncol.* 2005;23(22):4866–4875.
16. Hurwitz H, Fehrenbacher L, Novotny W, et al. Bevacizumab plus irinotecan, fluorouracil, and leucovorin for metastatic colorectal cancer. *N Engl J Med.* 2004;350(23):2335–2342.
17. Saltz LBea. Bevacizumab (Bev) in combination with XELOX or FOLFOX4: Efficacy results from XELOX-1/NO16966, a randomized phase III trial in the first-line treatment of metastatic colorectal cancer (MCRC). In: GI Cancer Symposium; 2007; Orlando, Florida; 2007.
18. Giantonio BJ, Catalano PJ, Meropol NJ, et al. High-dose bevacizumab improves survival when combined with FOLFOX4 in previously treated advanced colorectal cancer: Results from the Eastern Cooperative Oncology Group (ECOG) study E3200. *ASCO Meeting Abstracts.* 2005;23(16 Suppl):2.
19. Saltz LB. Bevacizumab (Bev) in combination with XELOX or FOLFOX4: Updated efficacy results from XELOX-1/NO16966, a randomized phase III trial in first-line metastatic colorectal cancer. In: ASCO; 2007; Chicago, IL; 2007.
20. Saltz LB, Meropol NJ, Loehrer PJ, Sr., Needle MN, Kopit J, Mayer RJ. Phase II trial of cetuximab in patients with refractory colorectal cancer that expresses the epidermal growth factor receptor. *J Clin Oncol.* 2004;22(7):1201–1208.
21. Cunningham D, Humblet Y, Siena S, et al. Cetuximab monotherapy and cetuximab plus irinotecan in irinotecan-refractory metastatic colorectal cancer. *N Engl J Med.* 2004;351(4):337–345.
22. Van Cutsem E. Randomized phase III study of irinotecan and 5-FU/FA with or without cetuximab in the first-line treatment of patients with metastatic colorectal cancer (mCRC): The CRYSTAL trial. In: ASCO; 2007; Chicago, IL; 2007.
23. Chung KY, Shia J, Kemeny NE, et al. Cetuximab shows activity in colorectal cancer patients with tumors that do not express the epidermal growth factor receptor by immunohistochemistry. *J Clin Oncol.* 2005;23(9):1803–1810.
24. Van Cutsem E, Peeters M, Siena S, et al. Open-label phase III trial of panitumumab plus best supportive care compared with best supportive care alone in patients with chemotherapy-refractory metastatic colorectal cancer. *J Clin Oncol.* 2007;25(13):1658–1664.
25. Grothey A, Sargent D, Goldberg RM, Schmoll HJ. Survival of patients with advanced colorectal cancer improves with the availability of fluorouracil-leucovorin, irinotecan, and oxaliplatin in the course of treatment. *J Clin Oncol.* 2004;22(7):1209–1214.
26. Wolmark N, Rockette H, Fisher B, et al. The benefit of leucovorin-modulated fluorouracil as postoperative adjuvant therapy for primary colon cancer: results from National Surgical Adjuvant Breast and Bowel Project protocol C-03. *J Clin Oncol.* 1993;11(10):1879–1887.
27. Efficacy of adjuvant fluorouracil and folinic acid in colon cancer. International Multicentre Pooled Analysis of Colon Cancer Trials (IMPACT) investigators. *Lancet.* 1995;345(8955):939–944.
28. O'Connell MJ, Mailliard JA, Kahn MJ, et al. Controlled trial of fluorouracil and low-dose leucovorin given for six months as postoperative adjuvant therapy for colon cancer. *J Clin Oncol.* 1997;15(1):246–250.
29. Haller DG, Catalano PJ, Macdonald JS, et al. Phase III study of fluorouracil, leucovorin, and levamisole in high-risk stage II and III colon cancer: final report of Intergroup 0089. *J Clin Oncol.* 2005;23(34):8671–8678.
30. Sargent DJ, Wieand HS, Haller DG, et al. Disease-free survival versus overall survival as a primary end point for adjuvant colon cancer studies: individual patient data from 20,898 patients on 18 randomized trials. *J Clin Oncol.* 2005;23(34):8664–8670.
31. Andre T, Boni C, Mounedji-Boudiaf L, et al. Oxaliplatin, fluorouracil, and leucovorin as adjuvant treatment for colon cancer. *N Engl J Med.* 2004;350(23):2343–2351.
32. de Gramont Aea. Oxaliplatin/5FU/LV in adjuvant colon cancer: updated efficacy results of the MOSAIC trial, including survival, with a median follow-up of six years. In: ASCO; 2007.
33. Wolmark N, Wieand S, Kuebler JP, Colangelo L, Smith RE. A phase III trial comparing FULV to FULV + oxaliplatin in stage II or III carcinoma of the colon: results of NSABP Protocol C-07. *ASCO Meeting Abstracts.* 2005;23(16 suppl):LBA3500.
34. Saltz LB, Niedzwiecki D, Hollis D, et al. Irinotecan plus fluorouracil/leucovorin (IFL) versus fluorouracil/

leucovorin alone (FL) in stage III colon cancer (intergroup trial CALGB C89803). *ASCO Meeting Abstracts.* 2004;22 (14 suppl):3500.

35. van Cutsem E, Labianca R, Hossfeld D, et al. Randomized phase III trial comparing infused irinotecan/5-fluorouracil (5-FU)/folinic acid (IF) versus 5-FU/FA (F) in stage III colon cancer patients (pts). (PETACC 3). *ASCO Meeting Abstracts.* 2005;23(16 suppl):LBA8.

36. Ychou M, Raoul JL, Douillard JY, et al. A phase III randomized trial of LV5FU2+CPT-11 vs. LV5FU2 alone in adjuvant high risk colon cancer (FNCLCC Accord02/FFCD9802). *ASCO Meeting Abstracts.* 2005;23(16 suppl):3502.

Evaluation and Treatment of Melanoma

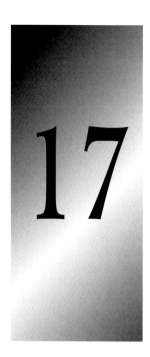

17

Jedd D. Wolchok
Yvonne Saenger

Prominent clinical features of the "black cancer" were first recorded by physicians in the early 19th century. At that time, Dr. William Norris of Stourbridge of England noted that melanoma could spread rapidly and widely throughout the body, that patients generally remain in good health until the final stages, and that the disease affects individuals with fair complexions and many nevi (1). Unfortunately, despite tremendous advances in cancer biology, Dr. Norris' description of the natural history of melanoma remains essentially accurate at the present time. It has, however, long been known that melanoma is an unpredictable syndrome and that rare patients live for years and even decades in symbiosis with the disease. The reasons for this remain unclear, although genetic profiling is now beginning to sort out different melanoma subtypes (2). Melanoma, in this sense, is a cancer which has frustrated and mystified generations of patients and clinicians.

Melanoma is treated with surgery, chemotherapy, radiotherapy, and immunotherapy, as well as experimental targeted therapies in development. Surgery remains the mainstay of clinical management for limited disease. The observation, first documented by Dr. Alexander Breslow, that tumor depth is a key determinant of prognosis, allows surgeons to tailor surgery based on the patient's risk. Once the cancer has metastasized, however, conventional chemotherapy and radiotherapy provide clinical benefit only to a minority of patients. Immunotherapy plays an important role in the clinical management of melanoma and remains a highly active

area of ongoing research. Finally, an understanding of the genetic aberrations in the signaling pathways driving melanomas is beginning to emerge, and this lays the groundwork for the development of effective targeted therapies.

RELEVANT ASPECTS OF MELANOCYTE BIOLOGY

Melanoma is presumed to develop from melanocytes, cells whose normal physiologic role is to produce pigment. Precursor cells originate in the neural crest and during embryologic development they migrate to their target tissues, most prominently the skin. It has been hypothesized that this migratory developmental program may be reactivated in metastatic malignant melanoma (3). Once located in the skin, the melanocyte "stem cell" resides in hair follicles, while more differentiated progeny home to the dermal epidermal junction, where they associate with keratinocytes. Melanocytes are not only found in the skin, however, but are also present in the conjunctiva, gastrointestinal and genital mucosa, leptomeninges, and even the capsules of lymph nodes. This explains why primary melanomas occasionally arise in the eye and areas other than the skin.

The primary function of melanocytes is to modulate the organism's exposure to potentially damaging solar radiation. Melanocytes accomplish this by pro-

KEY POINTS

- Prominent clinical features of the "black cancer" were first recorded by physicians in the early 19th century.
- Melanoma is treated with surgery, chemotherapy, radiotherapy, and immunotherapy, as well as experimental targeted therapies in development.
- Surgery remains the mainstay of clinical management for limited disease.
- Tumor depth is a key determinate of prognosis.
- Melanoma is presumed to develop from melanocytes found not only in the skin, but the conjunctiva, gastrointestinal and genital mucosa, leptomeninges, and even the capsules of lymph nodes.
- The incidence of melanoma among white populations has increased substantially over the past century.
- Children in particular should be protected from the sun, since there is some evidence that exposure early in life is more likely to lead to melanoma.

- The ABCD rule, which describes lesions that are *a*symmetric, have blurred *b*orders, are non-uniform in *c*olor, and have a *d*iameter greater than 5 mm. However, evolution (or enlargement) is the most sensitive indicator of a lesion in need of biopsy.
- In up to 20% of cases, the first melanoma symptom is from a metastatic lesion.
- One distinguishing feature of melanoma is the propensity to metastasize to the small bowel and manifest as gastrointestinal bleeding.
- Brain metastases are common and generally hemorrhagic, frequently causing seizures, which are occasionally the first manifestation of disease.
- Median survival for patients with metastatic disease is approximately 8.5–11 months, although there are occasional long-term survivors.
- There continues to be intense investigation of melanoma vaccines and other immunotherapies.

ducing melanin which adsorbs light in the UV spectrum. Melanin is only produced by melanocytes, and there is unique enzymatic machinery involved in melanin synthesis. Melanin is produced from tyrosine in membrane bound vesicles called melanosomes, and these granules are then packaged and transferred to keratinocytes via export of the entire melanosome. Intriguingly, it has been observed that melanosomes are positioned in response to UV radiation within the keratinocyte to form a parasol-like structure protecting the nucleus (4). Importantly, skin pigmentation is determined by the number and quality of the melanosomes—not by the number of melanocytes. Darker skinned individuals are therefore better shielded from UV radiation but do not have a higher total number of melanocytes.

The molecular basis for the susceptibility of pale individuals to melanoma is partially understood at this time (5). Tanning is essentially an increase in pigment production triggered by sun exposure. The exact mechanism whereby this occurs is unclear, although there is significant evidence that DNA damage directly induces tanning (6). Mutations in the MC1R melanocortin 1 receptor (MC1R) gene are associated with poor tanning and predispose some fair-skinned individuals to melanoma. Over 30 MC1R gene alleles have been identified in human populations (7). MC1R is a membrane bound G-protein coupled receptor that activates cyclic adenosine monophosphate (AMP) responsive element binding protein (CREB) transcription factors (8). These in turn up-regulate multiple gene products including

microphthalmia transcription factor (MITF), a master regulatory gene implicated in melanin production, melanocyte differentiation, and malignant transformation (9). Signaling via MC1R modulates pigmentation by increasing the relative levels of eumelanin (brown/black) versus pheomelanin (red/yellow). Pheomelanin both provides inferior UV adsorption and is a source of reactive oxidative byproducts which can cause DNA damage (10).

As a lineage, melanocytes appear in some aspects to be primed for tumorigenesis. They are constantly exposed to oxidative tyrosine metabolites, byproducts of melanin synthesis (11), and are remarkably resistant to apoptosis, perhaps due to high levels of expression of anti-apoptotic genes, including bcl-2 (12). Cultured melanocytes will grow and display some phenotypic features of melanomas before senescing (13). Melanocytes isolated from benign nevi, however, have been reported to form colonies in soft agar, an assay commonly used as a test for oncogenic transformation (14). Some of these features are suppressed by coculture with keratinocytes, highlighting the importance of tissue stroma in regulation of melanocyte growth and differentiation (15).

EPIDEMIOLOGY

The incidence of melanoma among white populations has increased very substantially over the past century.

This increase is now tapering off, although rates remain much higher than they were a generation ago. In the United States, the Surveillance, Epidemiology, and End Results program (SEER) estimated that in the period from 2000 to 2004, the incidence of melanoma would reach 18.5/100,000 persons per year, with white men having the highest incidence of 27.2/100,000/year. This puts the average lifetime risk at about 1.7% (16). Incidence varies widely around the globe, and the high incidence rates seen in Australia (40.5 per 100,000/year) suggest that the combination of fair skin and a sunny tropical climate predisposes to melanoma (17). Other regions with relatively high incidence are Northern Europe and Israel. Comparisons between populations with differing generational demographics are complicated because melanoma, despite being among the most common cancers in young people, is in fact, like most other cancers, a disease of older adults (median age of diagnosis is 59 in the United States).

In general, there appear to be two major factors underlying trends in melanoma incidence over the past century. The first is increasing sun exposure due to cultural factors among white populations, including the partial abandonment of pallor as a symbol of status and an increased willingness to display naked skin. The evidence that melanoma is related to sun exposure is epidemiologically robust, and includes the correlation between incidence among whites in North America and Australia with proximity to the equator, the increased rates among European migrants to sunny regions, particularly if they migrated at an earlier age, and evidence that, with heightened awareness of the risk of sun exposure, rates are now starting to decline among younger people (18). Studies also suggest that intermittent sun exposure may be worse, partially accounting for increased melanoma incidence in higher socioeconomic groups (19).

The second major factor underlying the increase in melanoma incidence over the past century is heightened awareness and screening. Cancer registries around the world have reported that the average thickness of melanoma at diagnosis has decreased over recent decades (18). Mortality rates, meanwhile, have gradually stabilized in the United States and elsewhere. These trends in the absence of major therapeutic advances, suggest that early detection artificially elevated incidence rates over the past 20–30 years, and is now having an impact on mortality since lesions, which would have been causing deaths, were removed.

If sunlight is the primary environmental factor contributing to melanoma genesis in whites, genetic factors also play an important role. Accordingly, a reported family history of melanoma confers the same increase in risk, which is approximately a twofold increase, as

a reported history of intense sun exposure (20). A diagnosis of xeroderma pigmentosum meanwhile increases risk by 1,000-fold in individuals younger than aged 20. There are undoubtedly certain families in whom the increased risk is much higher than others, although the molecular basis for this is largely unknown. Mutation in CDKN2A has been associated with melanoma and pancreatic cancer, but genetic testing is generally not recommended, because individuals from families with a high incidence of melanoma should receive dermatologic screening regardless of genotype. Phenotypic features correlating most closely with melanoma risk in the white population include skin type (difficulty tanning and propensity to burn), frequency of atypical nevi, frequency of common nevi, freckling, and light skin and/or hair (16). Nevi and freckling, however, reflect childhood sun exposure as well as genetic factors. Ethnic African populations rarely develop melanoma, and when they do it is usually on the palms and soles of the feet. Risk factors for melanoma in Africans are unknown. Asians, even pale individuals, have an exceedingly low rate of melanoma (17).

PREVENTION

Given the scope of epidemiologic evidence that sun exposure causes melanoma, basic precautions aimed at minimizing sunburn are advisable. Children in particular should be protected from the sun, because there is some evidence that exposure early in life is more likely to lead to melanoma. Individuals with fair complexions and/or many moles, poor tanners, individuals with red hair, and members of families at high risk should be especially cautious. Patients should also be cognizant of any atypical moles and bring any rapidly changing or unusual appearing lesions to medical attention. While there is no definitive study proving that hats and sunscreen prevent melanoma, epidemiologic trends including declining incidence in younger populations, and a stabilization of the death rate from melanoma in the United States in the absence of significant therapeutic advances, suggests that public health prevention measures have had a positive impact.

There is controversy regarding routine screening for melanoma, but it seems eminently reasonable for individuals at high risk. This would include at a minimum, people with a personal history of melanoma, a strong family history or known genetic predisposition, and numerous or atypical moles. While there is no large scale population based study that conclusively proves that screening benefits patients, the fact that depth is critical to prognosis and that screening leads to detection of thinner melanomas is a logical justification for screening.

CLINICAL PRESENTATION

The diagnosis of cutaneous malignant melanoma is difficult even for experienced dermatologists. Several general principles are useful to physicians confronted with a suspicious lesion. First, if the lesion is worrisome to the patient, it should probably be excised. Patients may be more sensitive to the fact that a lesion is an "ugly duckling," different from their other moles, and there are many substantiated reports of patients reporting itching or other more nonspecific symptoms associated with subsequently confirmed melanomas. Second, the lesion is suspicious if it has changed over weeks or months in terms of size, shape, or pigmentation. Third, any lesion that appears disordered or unusual and does not fit the profile of any known benign skin lesion should be biopsied, particularly if it is ulcerated, bleeding, or pruritic. Fourth, lesions are more concerning if the patient has a personal or family history of melanoma, atypical nevi, a history of intense sun exposure, or visibly sun damaged skin. Fifth, it is important to remember that not all melanomas are pigmented. If a lesion is of questionable concern and there are reasons to avoid biopsy, photography can be useful for monitoring. Finally, the ABCD rule can be applied, as melanomas are generally *a*symmetric, have blurred *b*orders, are black in *c*olor, and have a *d*iameter greater than 5 mm.

Melanoma can arise in rare atypical locations that escape monitoring by patients or physicians, and male patients are less likely to notice abnormal skin lesions than are female patients. Melanoma arising on the scalp, soles of the feet, palms of the hand, nail beds, oral cavity, genitals, and ocular conjunctiva often escapes attention. Nailbed melanomas sometimes have the appearance of hematomas and the patient may even give a history of trauma to the nail, while lesions on the palms and feet may be camouflaged by thickened skin. Ocular melanomas usually present as visual disturbances or are detected incidentally on ophthalmologic exam. Mucosal melanoma of the head and neck generally presents with epistaxis, obstruction, or odynophagia, or they may be noticed by the patient because of their color. Vaginal melanomas are sometimes found incidentally on pelvic exam, but often present with bleeding.

In up to 20% of cases, the first melanoma symptom is from a metastatic lesion (16). Most commonly, the patient notices a swollen lymph gland. In 5% of these cases, a primary lesion is never identified and has presumably regressed. Melanoma with distant spread, similar to other advanced cancers, presents with organ dysfunction. One distinguishing feature of melanoma is the propensity to metastasize to the small bowel and manifest as gastrointestinal bleeding. Brain metastases are common and generally hemorrhagic, frequently causing seizures, which are occasionally the first manifestation of disease. Finally, in patients diagnosed with a second skin melanoma, it is important to confirm the presence of an in situ component within the pathologic specimen in order to exclude an epidermotrophic metastasis.

HISTOPATHOLOGIC DIAGNOSIS

When evaluating a suspicious cutaneous lesion, an excisional biopsy is best, preferably 1–3 mm in diameter so as not to obscure drainage patterns for sentinel lymph node sampling. Shave biopsies should generally be avoided when melanoma is suspected because they do not provide a good estimate of tumor thickness, the key prognostic variable. There are unfortunately no definitive criteria for microscopic interpretation of melanocytic lesions; therefore, an experienced pathologist is essential, particularly for difficult or uncertain cases. Cytologic features and tissue architecture must be interpreted within the clinical context. Essential information to be obtained from biopsy include status of peripheral and deep margins, Breslow thickness, histologic ulceration, Clark level (measures the penetration through epidermal and dermal layers), the presence or absence of satellite lesions, and the presence or absence of an in situ component. These factors are all critical in estimating prognosis in the setting of localized disease. The presence of satellite lesion(s), in particular, confer a higher risk of recurrence. Other features of interest include location, regression, mitotic rate, tumor infiltrating lymphocytes, vertical growth phase, angiolymphatic invasion, neurotropism, and histologic subtype.

CLINICAL MANAGEMENT

The clinical management of melanoma is summarized in Table 17.1 and is a function of tumor burden. Localized disease less than 1 mm in depth is treated by wide local excision (WLE) only unless adverse prognostic factors are present in which case a sentinel lymph node biopsy (SLNB) may be offered to the patient. Intermediate thickness melanomas are treated with WLE and SLNB; however, SLNB is controversial in deep lesions or in the presence of satellite lesion(s). If disease is detected in a lymph node, completion lymph node dissection (CLND) is generally recommended. Regional and/or systemic metastases are also resected if feasible. Regional recurrences may be treated with isolated limb perfusion and/or intralesional therapies. Radiation is used for brain metastases and occasionally to achieve

TABLE 17.1
Clinical Management of Malignant Melanoma

EXTENT OF DISEASE	TREATMENT PLAN
In situ melanoma	Wide local excision (WLE) with 0.5-cm margins
Melanoma <1 mm in depth	WLE with 1-cm margins. Consider sentinel lymph node biopsy (SNLB) if adverse pathologic features present
Melanoma >4 mm in depth	WLE with 2 cm margins. SNLB. Optional adjuvant therapy if >2 mm and ulcerated
Melanoma >4 mm in depth and/or with satellite lesion	WLE with 2-cm margins. Optional SNLB. Optional adjuvant therapy
Melanoma metastatic to lymph nodes	WLE of primary lesion. completion lymph node dissection (CLND). Optional adjuvant therapy
Melanoma with regional metastasis	Surgical excision of all lesions with clear margins if feasible, with optional adjuvant therapy. If lesions cannot be excised, consider alternative local therapies or systemic therapy as below
Melanoma with systemic metastasis	Surgical excision of isolated metastasis or low burden of disease or for palliation. Excision and/or irradiation of any brain metastasis. Systemic chemotherapy and/or immunotherapy

local control. Systemic therapies for non-resectable disease include chemotherapy and immunotherapy. More detailed explanations are provided below.

Clinical Management of Localized Disease

It was readily apparent to those physicians who first described melanoma in the 18th and 19th centuries that these dangerous pigmented lesions should be surgically eliminated. While these pioneering clinicians advocated radical procedures such as amputation, the scale of the recommended surgical intervention has gradually declined over the past 200 years. Current recommendations are for wide local excision (WLE) with margins of 0.5 cm for in situ disease, 1 cm for lesions less than

1 mm in thickness, and 2 cm for lesions greater than 2 mm (21).

The primary concern for patients diagnosed with melanoma is the potential for disease recurrence. For patients with lesions less than 1 mm in thickness, prognosis is excellent, with a five-year survival rate of 93%. If the primary lesion is greater than 1 mm, the five-year survival rate decreases to 68%. The predictive power of tumor thickness was confirmed in a multivariate analysis of 13,581 patients performed by The American Joint Committee on Cancer (AJCC) (22). Ulceration suggests that the malignant cells are able to cross tissue barriers, and was the most accurate secondary predictive factor for all tumors except for very thin melanomas. In these lesions, the Clark level was more highly prognostic. Other factors affecting prognosis include age (better in those younger than aged 60), site (better for lesions located in the extremities), and gender (prognosis is better for females).

Lymph node status, however, when known, is superior to all prognostic indicators. This was shown in a Cox regression analysis of 1,201 patients in the AJCC melanoma database, and is the primary rationale for SLNB (22). The prognostic value of SLNB was recently prospectively validated in the third interim analysis of the Multicenter Selective Lymphadenectomy Trial (MSLT), in which 1,347 patients with intermediate depth melanoma were randomized to WLE with or without SLNB (23). In this study, melanoma specific mortality was 26.2% in patients with a positive SLNB, as compared to 9.7% in patients with a negative SLNB. While SLNB has not been proven to improve overall survival, the procedure is generally well tolerated and consideration of SLNB is recommended for patients with intermediate thickness and/or ulcerated primaries, and may also be considered for some patients with high-risk thin melanomas, particularly if the patient is young and high-risk features are present (Clark level IV or V, regression, high mitotic rate). SLNB for patients with thick melanomas and/or satellite lesions is controversial.

Routine surveillance is recommended for patients with a history of localized cutaneous melanoma. All patients with more than in situ disease should receive follow-up physical examinations, and patients with deep primaries and/or positive lymph nodes should be seen at least every six months for two to three years of follow-up. The risk of recurrence decreases over time, with most patients experiencing recurrence within two years. Recurrences in patients with thin melanomas are rare and occur later on average. Recommendations for imaging to screen for metastatic disease vary by institution and are not grounded in epidemiologic evidence. Dermatologic screening and sun exposure precautions are advised for all patients.

Clinical Management of Local Recurrence and Regional Metastases

The distinction between local recurrence and regional metastasis has historically been subjective; traditionally, lesions within 2 cm of the scar were categorized as local recurrence. According to the more current definition, a lesion must contain in situ disease or a radial growth phase in order to be classified as a true local scar recurrence (21). In any case, recurrence near the site of a previously excised melanoma is predictive of a poor prognosis, and in the Intergroup Melanoma Surgical Trial was associated with a five-year survival of 9% (24). The detection of local recurrence or regional metastasis should therefore be followed by full body imaging prior to resection. If the lesion is a true local recurrence rather than a metastasis, and there is no evidence of systemic spread, surgical margins should be wide.

For regional and nodal metastases, surgery is the mainstay of treatment. If disease is bulky and not amenable to resection, alternative local and systemic therapies may be considered. Local therapies in current use include isolated limb perfusion or infusion with melphalan, intralesional injection with immune modulating agents and/or chemotherapy, radiation, and laser ablation. Systemic therapy using biologic agents and/or chemotherapy may also be employed in this setting.

In patients who have melanoma which has spread to the lymph nodes, the burden of disease in the nodes is highly prognostic (22). A patient with a micrometastasis in one node, for example, has a far better outcome than one with clinically palpable disease in many nodes. Removal of all lymph nodes in the affected basin is the standard of care, although a prospective randomized trial is underway to determine the value of this procedure in patients with a positive SLNB and no clinical evidence of residual nodal disease (MSLT II) (25). Radiation is generally given if there is suspicion that residual tumor remains after surgery, and adjuvant therapy may be considered as described below.

The Question of Adjuvant Therapy

Once the melanoma lesion has been excised and the patient has been educated about the risks of sun exposure and advised to visit the dermatologist for screening along with his or her immediate family members, the question of possible adjuvant therapy emerges. Adjuvant therapy is generally considered for patients with positive lymph nodes, satellite lesions, primary lesions greater than 4 mm in thickness or ulcerated lesions that are greater than 2 mm in thickness, or previously resected metastatic lesions. There is no therapy conclusively proven to prevent disease recurrence; therefore, observation remains an acceptable choice for anyone with a history of melanoma and no evidence of disease.

High-dose interferon alpha is the only U.S. Food and Drug Administration (FDA)-approved adjuvant therapy for melanoma; however, there is considerable controversy surrounding its use because of limited efficacy and significant toxicity (26,27). There is no evidence that interferon improves overall survival, although there is some evidence that it does delay recurrence (28). Interferon may be more effective in patients who develop autoantibodies while on therapy, but these patients cannot be selected for prospectively (29). High-dose interferon is associated with many side effects, most prominently fatigue, flulike symptoms, depression, and liver toxicity. Low-dose interferon is less toxic, but it does not have established efficacy. There is no evidence that chemotherapy in the adjuvant setting is beneficial. A recent trial of biochemotherapy showed no advantage relative to high-dose interferon (30). Temozolomide (Temodar) is sometimes used in the adjuvant setting for patients at high risk of recurrence, but this is based on an extrapolation of data in patients with metastatic disease. Granulocyte-macrophage colony stimulating factor (GM-CSF), a stimulant of bone marrow production of immune cells, is sometimes offered based on a small study suggesting a possible benefit (31). Experimental vaccines may be given in the adjuvant setting, although none have been proven effective to date.

Clinical Management of Systemic Metastases

Median survival for patients with metastatic disease is approximately 8.5–11 months, although there are occasional long-term survivors. Survival correlates with site and number of metastases, remission duration, surgical resectability, response to systemic therapy, and serum lactic dehydrogenase (LDH) levels (32). Metastatic melanoma is highly aggressive, versatile, and grows in many organs, including lung, liver, bone, brain, gastrointestinal tract (small bowel in particular), spleen, kidney, heart, bone marrow, pancreas, peritoneum, adrenal glands, thyroid, breast, and placenta. Metastases are generally detected by clinical and radiologic criteria, as there are currently no reliable serum markers for metastatic disease.

Due to the diversity of sites of metastases, patients develop a variety of constellations of symptoms, many of which require palliative care. Prominent oncologic complications in melanoma include seizures and neurologic impairment due to hemorrhagic brain metastases and/or leptomeningeal disease, venous thrombosis and pulmonary embolism, GI bleeding and/or obstruction due to small bowel disease, liver necrosis and hemorrhage, rupture of a splenic metastasis, bony disease impinging on the spinal cord, marrow failure due to infiltration by melanoma, and urinary obstruction.

In many institutions, surgery remains the treatment of choice for patients who have resectable disease and a moderate rate of disease progression (tumor doubling time). There are multiple published studies documenting long-term survival, and even apparent cures, in selected patients after metastasectomy (33). The difficulty is that there are no large prospective randomized trials conclusively showing a benefit of surgery; however, it seems that patients who have limited metastases and more indolent disease do benefit from surgical intervention. Metastasectomy is particularly recommended for limited brain metastases, although stereotactic radiosurgery (SRS) is an excellent alternative. Partial or whole brain radiation may then be given as an adjuvant. Metastasectomy is also often used for a solitary lung metastasis where five-year survival rates of 20% have been reported (34).

Patients with widely disseminated disease are not candidates for surgical treatment and are treated with systemic medication, generally chemotherapy, immunotherapy, or a combination of both. Dacarbazine (DTIC) is the only FDA-approved cytotoxic agent for melanoma, and yields an estimated 7%–20% response rate (35). Temozolomide is an oral formulation of a similar drug, with a similar activity profile and an advantage of higher central nervous system penetrance (36). Response rates are higher with combination chemotherapy regimens such as the cisplatin, vinblastine, and DTIC regimen; the Dartmouth regimen, consisting of cisplatin, dacarbazine, carmustine (BiCNU), and tamoxifen; and the BHD regimen, consisting of BiCNU, hydroxyurea, and dacarbazine). However, none of these regimens have been shown to prolong overall survival. Biochemotherapy, a combination of chemotherapy and cytokine therapy with interleukin 2 (IL-2) and interferon, yielded highly promising results in phase II trials, but similar to chemotherapy did not yield reproducible improvements in overall survival. It is worth noting, however, that melanoma trials are smaller than breast cancer trials, for example, and therefore not powered to detect subtle differences in survival. Nonetheless, the choice of "aggressive" combination therapy versus single agent temozolomide or dacarbazine is often made based on the perceived need for rapid palliation.

Immunotherapy is an alternative to chemotherapy in metastatic melanoma, and yields similar therapeutic benefit. Interferon alpha, in the metastatic setting, produced a 16% response rate, with occasional durable responses (37), and improved response rates (although not overall survival) when given in combination with temozolomide (38). The most widely used immunotherapy in the metastatic setting is high dose IL-2, which in a trial conducted in the late 1980s yielded a 17% response rate with a small percentage of participants alive at five years, leading to speculation of possible cure (39). High-dose IL-2 is extremely toxic, and must be given in a monitored setting. Finally, the anti-angiogenic agent bevacizumab was recently shown to have some efficacy in metastatic melanoma (40).

EXPERIMENTAL IMMUNOTHERAPIES IN MELANOMA

A wide array of immune therapies is under development in both the adjuvant and metastatic setting. In the metastatic setting, the most promising for general application is checkpoint blockade with anti-CTLA-4 antibodies. CTLA-4 is a surface molecule expressed by activated T cells, and it functions as a "brake" on the immune system, signaling via an inhibitory tyrosine associated motif (ITIM) to down-regulate T-cell responses. By inhibiting CTLA-4, immune responses against melanoma can be generated. This strategy has been evaluated in several published phase I and phase II trials, with an overall response rate of 15% in pretreated patients (41). As was seen with IL-2, some of these responses appear to be quite durable. Anti-CTLA-4 therapy is associated in some patients with immune related adverse events, including rash, diarrhea, and more rarely, colitis, which can cause perforation (42). Therefore, extremely close monitoring of patients' bowel habits is essential. Responses to anti-CTLA-4 therapy appear to be different from responses to cytotoxic therapy; they may develop over weeks to months and sometimes "progression" is noted on scans prior to response. The development of inflammation in metastatic deposits complicates radiologic interpretation in these patients.

There continues to be intense investigation of melanoma vaccines. Vaccination against cancer is a difficult challenge because the immune systems of cancer patients are usually tolerant of the tumor and considers it self. Phase III trials of vaccines in melanoma patients have yielded disappointing results to date (43). Many strategies have been explored, including whole cell, protein, and, most recently, dendritic cell (DC)-based vaccines and DNA vaccines. DCs are the most potent antigen-presenting cell (APC) in the immune system, and multiple strategies are under investigation whereby they are generated ex vivo from the patient, coated with melanoma antigens, and reinfused. In DNA vaccination, cDNA encoding the antigen of interest is introduced into the skin, lymph node, or muscle, where it is taken up by APCs. DNA vaccination has advantages, both because CpG sequences in the DNA itself are inherently immunogenic, and because DNA is easy to manipulate to enhance the intrinsic immunogenicity of the encoded protein (44). One strategy to overcome self-tolerance is to vaccinate using xenogeneic (cross-species) antigen. It has been shown, for example, that vaccination against human melanoma antigens generate lymphocytes which are then cross reactive against mouse melanoma antigens (45).

Adoptive T-cell therapy using T cells isolated from tumor specimens, (tumor infiltrating T cells or TILs), has also been under intense investigation in recent years, and yielded a 51% response rate in a phase I study in selected pretreated patients (46). This study highlighted several factors which are important for the engraftment of transferred T cells. First, lymphodepletion with conditioning chemotherapy appears to be critical. This may be due to the phenomenon of homeostatic proliferation, whereby there is a compensatory proliferation of T cells when their numbers are low. Second, transfer of a combination of CD4+ and CD8+ T cells appears to be essential to the development of a robust CD8+ T-cell response, which was critical to efficacy. Third, the differentiation status of the CD8+ T cells is important for successful engraftment. Experimental approaches using transgenic T-cell receptors have also been used in this setting (47). Further studies in this area should yield better understanding of the antimelanoma T-cell response and to the development of newer and more widely applicable protocols for adoptive T-cell transfer in patients.

GENETIC LESIONS IN MELANOMA

It is evident from clinical and epidemiological data that melanoma is a genetically heterogeneous disease. Genetic profiling data has been used in the classification of melanomas into four different subtypes (2). These genetic profiles are characterized by distinct patterns of genetic aberration and correlate with melanomas arising in sun damaged skin, in normal skin, acral, and mucosal melanomas. Some of the defining mutations in these cancers are thought to be "driving mutations," in that they are required for the initiation of tumor growth. Moreover, the "oncogene addiction" hypothesis postulates that cancer cells become so dependent on the aberrant activation of particular signaling pathways that they cannot survive in their absence. The hope is that treatment with small molecule inhibitors targeted to particular signaling pathways can be tailored for individual patients based on melanoma genotype.

The RAS-RAF-MEK-ERK (MAP kinase) signaling pathway has received particular attention because it mediates diverse effects, including cell growth, and is frequently constitutively active in human tumors. In melanoma, mutations in B-Raf are reported in 66% of cases, while a further 15% have mutations in N-Ras (48). Mutations in these two signaling molecules are mutually exclusive, suggesting that two hits to this pathway would be redundant and confer no further selective advantage. Moreover, cell lines with a B-Raf mutation are sensitive to MEK inhibition, whereas cells with N-Ras are not, demonstrating that regulation of this pathway is highly complex (49). Phase I clinical trials of MEK and B-Raf inhibitors are underway. Amplification and mutations in the oncogenic tyrosine kinase, c-kit, have also been detected in a subset of melanomas and clinical trials with Imatinib, a c-kit inhibitor, are ongoing (50). Multiple other pathways including the Wnt pathway, the fibroblast growth factor pathway, and the PI3-AKT pathway, have been implicated in melanoma growth and metastasis (51). Further study of in vitro and in vivo models will deepen our understanding of the molecular biology of melanoma, leading to new biologic therapies for clinical application.

References

1. Norris W. *Eight Cases of Melanomsis with Pathological and Therapeutical Remarks on that Disease.* London: Longman, Brown, Green, Longman and Roberts; 1857.
2. Curtin JA, Fridlyand J, Kageshita T, et al. Distinct sets of genetic alterations in melanoma. *N Engl J Med.* 2005; 353(20):2135–2147.
3. Gupta PB, Kuperwasser C, Brunet JP, et al. The melanocyte differentiation program predisposes to metastasis after neoplastic transformation. *Nat Genet.* 2005;37(10):1047–1054.
4. Boissy RE. Melanosome transfer to and translocation in the keratinocyte. *Exp Dermatol.* 2003;12(Suppl 2):5–12.
5. Lin JY, Fisher DE. Melanocyte biology and skin pigmentation. *Nature.* 2007;445(7130):843–850.
6. Eller MS, Yaar M, Gilchrest BA. DNA damage and melanogenesis. *Nature.* 1994;372(6505):413–414.
7. Healy E, Jordan SA, Budd PS, Suffolk R, Rees JL, Jackson IJ. Functional variation of MC1R alleles from red-haired individuals. *Hum Mol Genet.* 2001;10(21):2397–2402.
8. Mountjoy KG, Robbins LS, Mortrud MT, Cone RD. The cloning of a family of genes that encode the melanocortin receptors. *Science.* 1992;257(5074):1248–1251.
9. Steingrimsson E, Copeland NG, Jenkins NA. Melanocytes and the microphthalmia transcription factor network. *Annu Rev Genet.* 2004;38:365–411.
10. Hill HZ, Hill GJ. UVA, pheomelanin and the carcinogenesis of melanoma. *Pigment Cell Res.* 2000;13(Suppl 8):140–144.
11. Prota. Recent advances in the chemistry of melanogenesis in mammals. *J Invest Dermatol.* 1980;75(1):122–127.
12. McGill GG, Horstmann M, Widlund HR, et al. Bcl2 regulation by the melanocyte master regulator Mitf modulates lineage survival and melanoma cell viability. *Cell.* 2002;109(6):707–718.
13. Shih IM, Elder DE, Hsu MY, Herlyn M. Regulation of Mel-CAM/MUC18 expression on melanocytes of different stages of tumor progression by normal keratinocytes. *Am J Pathol.* 1994;145(4):837–845.
14. Mancianti ML, Herlyn M, Weil D, et al. Growth and phenotypic characteristics of human nevus cells in culture. *J Invest Dermatol.* 1988;90(2):134–141.
15. Scott GA, Haake AR. Keratinocytes regulate melanocyte number in human fetal and neonatal skin equivalents. *J Invest Dermatol.* 1991;97(5):776–781.

16. http://seer.cancer.gov/statfacts/html/melan.html?statfacts_page=melan.html&x=14&y=20. (Accessed at January 31, 2009).

17. Ferlay J, Bray F, Pisani P, Parkin DM. *GLOBOCAN 2000: Cancer Incidence, Mortality and Prevalence Worldwide, version 1.0.* IARC CancerBase No 5. In. Lyon: IARC Press; 2001.

18. Berwick M, Weinstock, M. Epidemiology: current trends. In: Balch CM HA, Sober AJ, Soong S, eds. *Cutaneous Melanoma.* St. Lousi, Missouri: QMP; 2003;15–23.

19. Elwood JM, Jopson J. Melanoma and sun exposure: an overview of published studies. *Int J Cancer.* 1997;73(2):198–203.

20. Cho E, Rosner BA, Feskanich D, Colditz GA. Risk factors and individual probabilities of melanoma for whites. *J Clin Oncol.* 2005;23(12):2669–2675.

21. Coit et al. Houghton Aea. NCCN Clinical Practice Guidelines in Oncology-Melanoma. (Accessed at January 31, 2009).

22. Balch CM, Soong SJ, Gershenwald JE, et al. Prognostic factors analysis of 17,600 melanoma patients: validation of the American Joint Committee on Cancer melanoma staging system. *J Clin Oncol.* 2001;19(16):3622–3634.

23. Morton DL, Thompson JF, Cochran AJ, et al. Sentinel-node biopsy or nodal observation in melanoma. *N Engl J Med.* 2006;355(13):1307–1317.

24. Karakousis CP, Balch CM, Urist MM, Ross MM, Smith TJ, Bartolucci AA. Local recurrence in malignant melanoma: long-term results of the multiinstitutional randomized surgical trial. *Ann Surg Oncol.* 1996;3(5):446–452.

25. Multicenter Selective Lymphadenectomy Triall II. 2007. (Accessed 2007, at http://www.clinicaltrials.gov/ct/show/NCT00297895?order=1.) (Accessed at January 31, 2009).

26. Hurley KE, Chapman PB. Helping melanoma patients decide whether to choose adjuvant high-dose interferon-alpha2b. *Oncologist.* 2005;10(9):739–742.

27. Tarhini AA, Shipe-Spotloe J, DeMark M, Agarwala SS, Kirkwood JM. Response to "helping melanoma patients decide whether to choose adjuvant high-dose interferon-alpha2b." *Oncologist.* 2006;11(5):538–539; author reply 9–40.

28. Kirkwood JM, Manola J, Ibrahim J, Sondak V, Ernstoff MS, Rao U. A pooled analysis of eastern cooperative oncology group and intergroup trials of adjuvant high-dose interferon for melanoma. *Clin Cancer Res.* 2004;10(5):1670–1677.

29. Gogas H, Ioannovich J, Dafni U, et al. Prognostic significance of autoimmunity during treatment of melanoma with interferon. *N Engl J Med.* 2006;354(7):709–718.

30. Kim KBea. A Phase III Randomized Trial of Adjuvant Biochemotherapy (BC) versus Interferon-alpha-2b (IFN) in Patients (pts) with High Risk for Melanoma Recurrence. *J Clin Oncol.* 2006; *ASCO Annual Meeting Proceedings Part I.* 24(18S):8003.

31. Spitler LE, Grossbard ML, Ernstoff MS, et al. Adjuvant therapy of stage III and IV malignant melanoma using granulocyte-macrophage colony-stimulating factor. *J Clin Oncol.* 2000;18(8):1614–1621.

32. Balch CM, Soong SJ, Murad TM, Smith JW, Maddox WA, Durant JR. A multifactorial analysis of melanoma. IV. Prognostic factors in 200 melanoma patients with distant metastases (stage III). *J Clin Oncol.* 1983;1(2):126–134.

33. Wong JH, Skinner KA, Kim KA, Foshag LJ, Morton DL. The role of surgery in the treatment of nonregionally recurrent melanoma. *Surgery.* 1993;113(4):389–394.

34. Friedel G, Pastorino U, Buyse M, et al. Resection of lung metastases: long-term results and prognostic analysis based on 5206 cases—the International Registry of Lung Metastases. *Zentralblatt fur Chirurgie.* 1999;124(2):96–103.

35. Anderson CM, Buzaid AC, Legha SS. Systemic treatments for advanced cutaneous melanoma. *Oncology.* 1995;9(11):1149–1158; discussion 63–64, 67–68.

36. Bleehen NM, Newlands ES, Lee SM, et al. Cancer Research Campaign phase II trial of temozolomide in metastatic melanoma. *J Clin Oncol.* 1995;13(4):910–913.

37. Keilholz U, Goey SH, Punt CJ, et al. Interferon alfa-2a and interleukin-2 with or without cisplatin in metastatic melanoma: a randomized trial of the European Organization for Research and Treatment of Cancer Melanoma Cooperative Group. *J Clin Oncol.* 1997;15(7):2579–2588.

38. Kaufmann R, Spieth K, Leiter U, et al. Temozolomide in combination with interferon-alfa versus temozolomide alone in patients with advanced metastatic melanoma: a randomized, phase III, multicenter study from the Dermatologic Cooperative Oncology Group. *J Clin Oncol.* 2005;23(35):9001–9007.

39. Rosenberg SA, Yang JC, Topalian SL, et al. Treatment of 283 consecutive patients with metastatic melanoma or renal cell cancer using high-dose bolus interleukin 2. *JAMA.* 1994;271(12):907–913.

40. Varker KA, Biber JE, Kefauver C, et al. A randomized phase 2 trial of Bevacizumab with or without daily low-dose interferon alfa-2b in metastatic malignant melanoma. *Ann Surg Oncol.* 2007;14(8):2367–2376.

41. Dranoff G. CTLA-4 blockade: unveiling immune regulation. *J Clin Oncol.* 2005;23(4):662–664.

42. Maker AV, Phan GQ, Attia P, et al. Tumor regression and autoimmunity in patients treated with cytotoxic T lymphocyte-associated antigen 4 blockade and interleukin 2: a phase I/II study. *Ann Surg Oncol.* 2005;12(12):1005–1016.

43. Parmiani G, Castelli C, Santinami M, Rivoltini L. Melanoma immunology: past, present and future. *Curr Opin Oncol.* 2007;19(2):121–127.

44. Weber LW, Bowne WB, Wolchok JD, et al. Tumor immunity and autoimmunity induced by immunization with homologous DNA. *J Clin Invest.* 1998;102(6):1258–1264.

45. Turk MJ, Wolchok JD, Guevara-Patino JA, Goldberg SM, Houghton AN. Multiple pathways to tumor immunity and concomitant autoimmunity. *Immunol Rev.* 2002;188:122–135.

46. Rosenberg SA, Dudley ME. Cancer regression in patients with metastatic melanoma after the transfer of autologous antitumor lymphocytes. *Proc Natl Acad Sci USA.* 2004;101(Suppl 2):14639–14645.

47. Morgan RA, Dudley ME, Wunderlich JR, et al. Cancer regression in patients after transfer of genetically engineered lymphocytes. *Science.* 2006;314(5796):126–129.

48. Davies H, Bignell GR, Cox C, et al. Mutations of the BRAF gene in human cancer. *Nature.* 2002;417(6892):949–954.

49. Solit DB, Garraway LA, Pratilas CA, et al. BRAF mutation predicts sensitivity to MEK inhibition. *Nature.* 2006;439(7074):358–362.

50. Curtin JA, Busam K, Pinkel D, Bastian BC. Somatic activation of KIT in distinct subtypes of melanoma. *J Clin Oncol.* 2006;24(26):4340–4346.

51. Kalinsky K, Haluska FG. Novel inhibitors in the treatment of metastatic melanoma. *Expert Rev Anticancer Ther.* 2007;7(5):715–724.

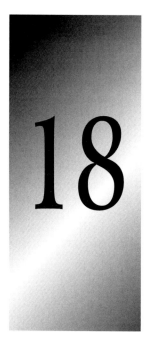

Evaluation and Treatment of Lymphoma

18

Enrica Marchi
Jasmine Zain
Owen A. O'Connor

The lymphomas represent one of the most heterogenous and diverse set of malignancies known to medicine. Underneath the umbrella of lymphoma exist some of the most rapidly growing cancers known to science, including diseases such as Burkitt lymphoma and lymphoblastic lymphoma/leukemia, as well as some of the slowest and most indolent cancers such as small lymphocytic lymphoma and follicular lymphoma. This remarkable diversity of diseases imposes significant challenges on pathologists and clinicians who seek to understand and elucidate what are sometimes subtle differences between the related subtypes of lymphoma. The understanding and diagnosis of lymphoma relies heavily on standard techniques of immunophenotyping, flow cytometry, cytogenetics, and the latest techniques in molecular biology, such as polymerase chain reaction (PCR) and fluorescent in situ hybridization (FISH). More recently, gene expression profiling of tumor samples has led to further understanding of these diseases. The improved understanding of the biological differences between the different forms of lymphoma has afforded us enormous opportunities to tailor specific treatments that are beginning to go well beyond simple CHOP-based chemotherapy.

All lymphomas are derived from lymphocytes, a form of white blood cell routinely generated by pluripotent hematopoietic stem cells, which reside in the intramedullary compartment of the bone marrow. There are three major lymphocyte populations that contribute to a functional immune system: B cells, T cells, and natural killer (NK) cells. These different types of lymphocytes mediate distinctly different immune effector functions. Surface proteins and receptors used in antigen recognition and mediating cellular immunity help differentiate these subsets of lymphocytes. For example, the B-cell receptor (BCR) and surface immunoglobulin (sIg) are found only on B cells, the T-cell receptor (TCR) is found on T cells, and clusters of differentiation (CD) are found on B cells, T cells, and NK cells. The variable expression of these and other proteins, form the basis for techniques in immunohistochemistry to differentiate the subpopulations of lymphocytes. While the details regarding the ontogeny of B cells and T cells is well beyond the scope of this chapter, the differentiation of these cells involves a multitude of steps in lymphoid organs, including the lymph node, spleen, thymus, and submucosal tissues (eg, Pyers patches in the gastrointestinal tract). During this complex process, lymphocytes "learn" to differentiate self from nonself, and in the process begin to form the major arms of our immune system: humoral immune responses, which are B-cell dependent, and cell mediated immunity, which is T-cell and NK-cell dependent. The type of lymphoma that develops typically depends on where in this ontogeny the cells become dysregulated. Figures 18.1 and 18.2 provide a schematic of B-cell and T-cell ontogeny, highlighting the different points in differentiation where different subtypes of lymphoma arise.

235

KEY POINTS

- All lymphomas are derived from lymphocytes, a form of white blood cell routinely generated by pluripotent hematopoietic stem cells.
- Non-Hodgkin lymphoma (NHL) comprises 5% of all malignancies and represents the fifth most common cancer in the United States. It is the most common hematologic malignancy in adults in the United States.
- Depending on the classification scheme used, there are considered to be more than 60 different subtypes of lymphoma.
- Immunosuppression, as a result of congenital or acquired medical conditions, a variety of autoimmune disorders, and certain infections is an acknowledged risk factor for the development of NHL.
- According to the WHO classification, NHLs are divided into: (1) B-cell neoplasms, which are further divided in *precursor* B-cell lymphoblastic leukemia/lymphoma and *mature* B-cell neoplasms; and (2) T-cell neoplasms, which are divided into the *immature* T-cell leukemia/lymphoma, and *mature* or postthymic T-cell and natural killer (NK)-cell neoplasms such as peripheral T-cell lymphoma not otherwise specified (PTCL NOS) (Tables 18.1 and 18.2).
- The most common clinical presentation of NHL is painless and slowly progressive peripheral lymphadenopathy.

- Perhaps the most critical element in the diagnosis and treatment of a patient with lymphoma is making the right histopathologic assessment.
- Chemotherapy remains the most important modality for managing most patients with lymphoma, and different regimens are employed depending upon the disease. Radiotherapy still plays a critical role in selected cases.
- Rituximab, the first monoclonal antibody approved by the U.S. Food and Drug Administration for the treatment of any cancer, targets the CD20 molecule presents on the surface of B cells. Randomized studies have demonstrated its activity in follicular lymphoma (FL), mantle cell lymphoma, and diffuse large B-cell lymphoma (DLBCL) in untreated or relapsing patients.
- Approximately two-thirds of patients with advanced Hodgkin disease (HD) can be cured with the current approaches to treatment.
- Because most HD patients can be cured with modern treatment modalities and will have a life expectancy equivalent to age-matched healthy individuals, it is important in the formulation of the treatment strategy to take into account not just the acute treatment-related toxicities, but also the long-term side effects of the chemotherapy and radiotherapy.

NON-HODGKIN LYMPHOMA

Introduction

Non-Hodgkin lymphoma (NHL) refers to all malignancies of the lymphoid system, with the exception of Hodgkin disease. The development of the lymphoid system is a highly regulated process, characterized by differential expression of innumerable cell-surface and intracytoplasmic proteins. Dysregulation of either the number or function of the cells can result in humoral deficiency, autoimmunity, or malignancy. Despite the variability in cell of origin and clinical presentation of these diseases, there are several clinical and pathologic features common to many lymphoproliferative diseases. Lymphadenopathy and splenomegaly, as well as changes in circulating lymphocytes and quantitative immunoglobulins, can be seen in malignant and benign lymphoproliferative diseases alike. However, all malignant diseases are characterized by an accumulation of proliferating lymphocytes, a process that can take years or hours, depending on the discrete subtype of lymphoma.

Although not all lymphomas originate in lymph nodes, most will invariably involve them at some point during the course of the disease. Historically, the cell of origin and the clinical behavior of the different subtypes of lymphoma have formed the basis for the widely differing nomenclatures used to classify these diseases. Over the past 100 years, many classification schemes have been proposed, leading to considerable confusion in communicating a specific diagnosis to patients and colleagues, a conundrum that has made interpreting the literature across eras of time virtually impossible. These classifications have evolved in parallel to our understanding of lymphoma biology. They reflect and encompass the immunological, cytogenetic, and clinical data that is available to describe these different subtypes. The most recent classification of NHLs, the revised American-European lymphoma (REAL) classification (1), was proposed in 1994 (Table 18.1), and has recently been updated by the World Health Organization (WHO) (2). This classification essentially divides these diseases into B-cell or T-cell/NK-cell neoplasms, which are yet further subdivided into precursor (ie, less differentiated) or mature (ie, more differentiated)

B- and T- Cell Development

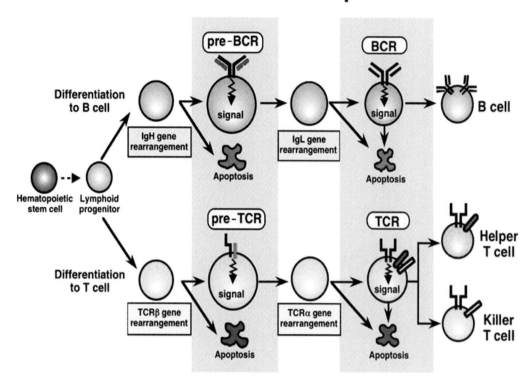

Schematic of B- and T-cell ontogeny.

FIGURE 18.1

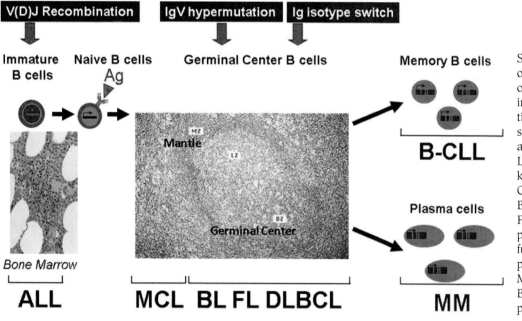

Schematic of B-cell ontogeny, with points of demarcation noting places in differentiation where various subtypes of B-cell arise.(ALL: Acute Lymphoblastic Leukemia; MCL: Mantle Cell Lymphoma; BL: Burkitt Lymphoma; FL: Follicular Lymphoma; DLBCL: Diffuse Large B-Cell Lymphoma; MM: Multiple Myeloma; B-CLL: B-Cell Chronic Lymphocytic Leukemia)

FIGURE 18.2

TABLE 18.1
Who Classification of Non Hodgkin Lymphomas

B-CELL NEOPLASMS

Precursor B-cell neoplasm
Precursor B-lymphoblastic leukemia/lymphoma (precursor B-cell acute lymphoblastic leukemia)
Mature (peripheral) B-cell neoplasms
B-cell chronic lymphocytic leukemia/small lymphocytic lymphoma
B-cell prolymphocytic leukemia
Lymphoplasmacytic lymphoma
Splenic marginal zone B-cell lymphoma (þ¹ villous lymphocytes)
Hairy cell leukemia
Plasma cell myeloma/plasmacytoma
Extranodal marginal zone B-cell lymphoma of MALT type
Nodal marginal zone B-cell lymphoma (þ¹ monocytoid B cells)
Follicular lymphoma
Mantle cell lymphoma
Diffuse large B-cell lymphoma
Burkitt lymphoma/ Burkitt cell leukemia

T- AND NK-CELL NEOPLASMS

Precursor T-cell neoplasm
Precursor T-lymphoblastic lymphoma/leukemia (precursor T-cell acute lymphoblastic leukemia)
Mature (peripheral) T-cell neoplasms
T-cell prolymphocytic leukemia
T-cell granular lymphocytic leukemia
Aggressive NK-cell leukemia
Adult T-cell lymphoma/leukemia (HTLV1þ)
Extranodal NK/T-cell lymphoma, nasal type
Enteropathy-type T-cell lymphoma
Hepatosplenic gd T-cell lymphoma
Subcutaneous panniculitis-like T-cell lymphoma
Mycosis fungoides/Sezary syndrome
Anaplastic large cell lymphoma, T/null cell, primary cutaneous type
Peripheral T-cell lymphoma, not otherwise characterized
Angioimmunoblastic T-cell lymphoma
Anaplastic large cell lymphoma, T/null cell, primary systemic type

forms of lymphoma. Depending on the classification scheme used, there are considered to be 30–35 different subtypes of lymphoma, comprising a diverse set of diseases with widely varying natural histories, each possessing its own subtleties in presentation, prognosis and management. Malignancies such as precursor B- or T-lymphoblastic leukemia/lymphoma evolve in the bone marrow, frequently giving rise to very high leukocyte counts (lymphocytosis) and generalized lymphadenopathy. Lymphoproliferative malignancies such as Burkitt lymphoma exhibit a penchant for involving the central nervous system. While potentially curable, these lymphomas are considered some of the most rapidly growing cancers known to science, and require aggressive chemotherapy that can continue for up to two years. In contrast, mature forms of B-cell and T-cell lymphoma, such as chronic lymphocytic leukemia (CLL) and mycosis fungoides, respectively, are more indolent diseases that often do not require treatment until they become symptomatic or threaten vital organ function.

Epidemiology and Etiology

NHL comprises 5% of all malignancies and represents the fifth most common cancer in the United States. It is the most common hematologic malignancy in adults in the United States. An estimated 66,000 cases of NHL were predicted for 2008, with an estimated 19,000 deaths, giving the disease a case fatality ratio of nearly 30%. Between 1950 and 1999, the incidence of NHL increased by about 3%–5% per year in the United States, accounting for a nearly 90% increase over those five decades. While the etiology for the increase in lymphoma is still poorly understood, HIV is thought to account for only a marginal component at best. Fortunately, this trend has changed over the recent past, with a nearly flat or decreasing incidence over the past five years. Despite the numerous claims, no specific etiology can explain these changes in incidence.

The overall incidence of lymphoma is higher in males (3). Irrespective of race, the incidence for males is approximately 23.5 per 100,000; in females, the incidence is approximately 16.3 per 100,000. The median age at the diagnosis across all forms of NHL is 67 years. Like many forms of cancer, there is a trend of increasing incidence as a function of age. Approximately 1.7% of cases of NHL are diagnosed under age 20; 4.1% of cases between ages 20 and 34; 7.4% of cases between ages 35 and 44; 14.0%–19% of cases between ages 45 and 64. The highest percentage, and approximately 23% of cases, are seen between ages 65 and 84. Interestingly, there is a significant decrease in NHL incidence for those older than age 85, where the incidence is only 8.5% of all cases. As noted earlier, the incidence of NHL has been rising over the past several decades (4), increasing from an age-adjusted rate of 11.1 per 100,000 in 1975 to 20.4 in 2004. Increases were seen in both nodal and extranodal subtypes of lymphoma. While increases were seen across both genders, the increase was greatest for female patients, with the male to female ratio changing from 1.26 in 1990–1992 to 1.13 in 2002–2004. Increases have been observed over time in the percentage of low-grade and T-cell/NK-cell subtypes compared with other aggressive histologic subtypes. Not surprisingly, incidence also varies significantly by race, with whites exhibiting a much higher risk of lymphoma compared to African-Americans and Asian Americans. In whites, the incidence rate is 24.3 and 17.1 per 100,000 males and females, respectively; while in African Americans, the incidence is 18.4 (males) and 12.1 (females) per 100,000; and 19.2 and 14.6 per 100,000 Hispanic males and females respectively. These differences in incidence across different ethnic groups are not uniform across all histologies. For example, the indolent lymphomas are far less common in African Americans, while diseases such as peripheral T-cell lymphoma, mycosis fungoides, and Sezary Syndrome are more common in African American populations.

The prognosis for patients with NHL improved significantly between 1990–1992 and 2002–2004 for both overall survival and age-specific survival. Overall, 5- and 10-year survival improved from 50.4% and 39.4%, respectively, in 1990–1992, to 66.8% (+16.4 percentage points) and 56.3% (+16.9 percentage points), respectively, in 2002–2004 ($P < .001$ for both). The greatest gains were seen in patients aged 15–44 years, for whom five-year relative survival increased by over 25%. NHL mortality rates peaked in 1997 at 8.9, after which they slowly decreased, reaching a rate of 7.0 in 2004.

While the etiologic factors contributing to lymphoma are generally not well defined, a number of risk factors have been described. Immunosuppression as a result of congenital or acquired medical conditions is an acknowledged risk factor. Immunosuppression associated with solid organ transplant is a well-known risk factor for lymphomas, in particular post-transplantation lymphoproliferative disorders (PTLD) (5,6). The overall incidence of PTLD is approximately 2%–8%, being highest in patients undergoing lung, gastrointestinal tract, and heart transplants, and lowest in patients receiving renal and liver transplants. For most of these patients, the disease develops approximately one or two years following the solid organ transplant, and it is frequently positive for Epstein-Barr virus (EBV), which is believed to result from impaired host immune surveillance of latently infected B cells. PTLD manifesting later is frequently EBV-negative, and carries a worse prognosis. Each transplant subtype has distinct features including organ source, duration and extent of immunosuppression, patient selection, risk of allograft involvement with PTLD, and variable merits for reduction of immunosuppression following a new diagnosis of PTLD. Consequently, each different type of transplant is unique with regard to the features of the associated PTLD (7).

Multiple autoimmune disorders (8,9), including Sjögren's disease (10), lupus, and rheumatoid arthritis, have also been linked with NHL. Most rheumatologists and oncologists consider autoimmune disorders and lymphoproliferative malignancies to exist on either end of a spectrum of lymphocyte dysregulation. That is, patients with autoimmune disorders are at higher risk for developing lymphoma, and patients with lymphoma are at higher risk for developing concomitant autoimmune disorders. Because many autoimmune disorders are treated with immunosuppressive therapy, it is often difficult to determine whether the underlying autoimmune disorder, or its immunosuppressive treatment, is responsible for the lymphoma.

Another increasingly important risk factor for lymphoma is infection, especially viral and bacterial infections. Patients who are HIV positive have a 59- to 104-fold higher risk of developing lymphoma compared to those who are HIV negative, with aggressive forms of NHL such as Burkitt and diffuse large B-cell lymphoma being the most likely (11–13). Variations in the geographic distribution of lymphoma have led to an improved understanding of many viral risk factors. Some lymphoma subtypes demonstrate marked geographic variation and association with very specific viruses. EBV is known to be a causal agent of a nasal subtype of NK-cell lymphoma in South America and Asia as well as endemic Burkitt lymphoma in Africa. These diseases, both very aggressive, require distinctly different treatments. Another retrovirus, human T-cell lymphotropic virus-1 (HTVL-1), is known to cause adult T-cell leukemia/lymphoma (HTLV-1 ATLL) in Caribbean, Asian, and African populations. Hepatitis C has been associated with B-cell lymphoma in northern Italy and Japan. In addition to viruses, other infectious agents have clear links to the development of NHL. For example, *Helicobacter pylori* is likely the etiologic agent leading to gastric mucosa-associated lymphoid tissue (MALT) lymphomas (14). MALT lymphomas were first described by Isaacson and Wright in 1983 in a small series of patients with low-grade B-cell gastrointestinal lymphomas. In *H. pylori*-related MALT lymphomas of the stomach, a course of antibiotics can not only eradicate the infection, but can induce cure of the lymphoma in approximately 75% of cases. The 25% that are unresponsive to antibiotics either carry a chromosomal translocation t(11;18)(q21;q21) or demonstrate a clinically advanced stage of the disease (15–17). Some studies suggest that eradication rates achieved by the first-line treatment with a proton pump inhibitor (PPI), clarithromycin, and amoxicillin have decreased to 70%–85%, in part due to increasing clarithromycin resistance in new strains of *H. pylori*. Eradication rates may also be lower with 7- versus 14-day regimens. Bismuth-containing quadruple regimens for 7–14 days are another first-line treatment option. Sequential therapy for 10 days has shown promise in Europe, but requires validation in North America. The most commonly used salvage regimen in patients with persistent *H. pylori* infection is bismuth quadruple therapy, though more recent data from Europe suggests that a PPI, levofloxacin, and amoxicillin for 10 days is more effective and better tolerated than bismuth quadruple therapy for persistent *H. pylori* infection (18).

Although MALT lymphomas occur most frequently in the stomach, they have also been described in various nongastrointestinal sites, such as the salivary gland, conjunctiva, thyroid, orbit, lung, breast, kidney, skin, liver, uterus, and prostate; some of these locations have also been linked to a specific infectious etiology. For example, *Borrelia burgdorferi*, transmitted by a tick, has been associated with some forms of extranodal marginal zone lymphoma of the skin (frequently referred to as skin-associated lymphoid tissue or SALT) (19), which has been successfully treated with doxycycline. Interestingly, however, nodal forms of these lymphomas do not appear to be associated with any infectious agents and may represent a genetically distinct subcategory of the marginal zone lymphomas.

Besides infectious etiologies, a number of different environmental factors have been associated with lymphoma, including exposure to pesticides and herbicides in farmers, and an array of occupational chemical exposures for those working in specific industries, such as chemists, dry cleaners, printing workers, wood workers, beauticians, and cosmetologists. While some of these associations are stronger than others, most links between lymphoma and a discrete environmental factor remain uncertain at best.

Classification

The histopathologic classification of lymphoma has evolved over the years as our understanding of the disease has improved. Despite this progress, lymphoma classification has been a source of confusion for clinicians and pathologists alike. In the last decade or so, much new information has become available regarding the morphological features, immunophenotype, and cytogenetic differences between many forms of lymphoma. This refined understanding has resulted in recognition of new entities and refinement of previously recognized disease categories. Prior to 1994, the National Cancer Institute (NCI) Working Formulation (20) and the Kiel (21,22) classification were used in the United States and in Europe, respectively. However, these classification schemes inadequately differentiated important subtypes of lymphoma, and were associated with a generally poor concordance among different hematopathologists. In 1994, the REAL classification was proposed as a mutually acceptable system, based on morphologic, immunophenotyping, and cytogenetic characteristics. The classification of NHLs has become a list of well-defined disease entities, each with its own distinctive clinical and biological features. Refinements of the REAL classification were recently incorporated into the WHO classification, in which morphologic, genetic, immunophenotypic, and clinical features are all used in defining discrete disease entities. According to the WHO classification, NHLs are divided into: (1) B-cell neoplasms, which are further divided in *precursor* B-cell lymphoblastic leukemia/lymphoma and *mature* B-cell neoplasms; and (2) T-cell neoplasms, which are divided into the *immature* T-cell leukemia/lymphoma, and *mature* or post-thymic T-cell and NK-cell neoplasms such as peripheral T-cell lymphoma not-otherwise-specified (PTCL NOS) (Tables 18.1 and 18.2).

Signs and Symptoms

Two-thirds of patients with any form of lymphoma present with lymphadenopathy; however, extranodal disease is common and can involve any organ. The presentation can be varied, depending on the subtype and location of the disease. In the case of indolent lymphomas (ie, chronic lymphocytic leukemia/lymphoma [CLL], follicular lymphoma, or marginal zone lymphoma), the most common clinical presentation is painless and slowly progressive peripheral lymphadenopathy. Primary extranodal presentation and symptoms including fever (ie, temperature higher than 38°C for three consecutive days, weight loss exceeding 10% of body weight in six months, and drenching night sweats, a grouping of symptoms known as B symptoms). B symptoms frequently arise as a consequence of cytokines released by the malignant disease; these symptoms might bring the disease to the physician's attention. However, B symptoms are uncommon at presentation, although both extranodal presentation and B symptoms can become common in patients with advanced stages of the disease. In the case of aggressive lymphoma, the clinical presentation can be more varied. Symptoms can be related to the rapid growth of the disease in a particular part of the body, causing compromise of some vital organ function (dyspnea in patients with primary mediastinal lymphoma; hydronephrosis or lower extremity edema in patients with diffuse large B-cell or Burkitt lymphoma in the pelvis). Alternatively, symptoms may be associated with an acutely enlarging lymph node associated with pain, or with a cosmetic finding. While superior vena cava syndrome is unusual in patients with lymphoma, even those with large bulky mediastinal disease, the development of pleural and pericardial effusions can be common in those with thoracic disease. These presentations are due to the presence of bulky lymphoma, or to its involvement of the parietal or visceral pleura. The very rapidly growing Burkitt

TABLE 18.2
Immunophenotypic Features and Molecular Characteristics of Non Hodgkin Lymphomas

SUBTYPE	FREQUENCY	IMMUNOPHENOTYPE	MOLECULAR LESIONS
DLBCL	31	CD20+	Bcl2, Bcl6,cMYC
FL	22	CD20+,CD10+,CD5-	Bcl2
SLL/CLL	6	CD20 weak, CD5+, CD23+	+12,del(13q)
MCL	6	CD20+,CD5+,CD23-	Cyclin D1
PTCL	6	CD20-,CD3+	Variable
MZL (MALT)	5	CD20+,CD5-,CD23-	Bcl10,+3,+18
PML	2	CD20+	Variable
ALCL	2	CD20-,CD3+,CD30+,CD15-,EMA+	ALK
LL (T/B)	2	T cell CD3+,B cell CD19+	Variable,TCL-3
Burkitt-like	2	CD20+,CD10-,CD5-	cMYC,Bcl2
MZL (Nodal)	1	CD20+,CD10-,CD23-,CD5-	+3,+18
SLL,PL	1	CD20+,cIg=,CD5-,CD23-	Pax-5
BL	1	CD20+,CD10+,CD5-	c-MYC
TOTAL	88		

DLBCL: Diffuse Large B-Cell Lymphoma; FL: Follicular Lymphoma; SLL: Small Lymphocytic Lymphoma; CLL: Chronic Lymphocytic Leukemia; MCL: Mantle Cell Lymphoma; PTCL: Peripheral T-Cell Lymphoma; MZL: Marginal Zone Lymphoma; PML: Primary Mediastinal Lymphoma; ALCL: Anaplastic Large Cell Lymphoma; LL: Lymphocytic Leukemia; PL: Prolymphocytic Leukemia; BL: Burkitt Lymphoma.

lymphoma (doubling time in a range of 36–48 hours) commonly presents as massive intra-abdominal disease, leading patients to experience a host of symptoms, ranging from bowel obstruction to hydronephrosis to lower extremity edema. Bone marrow involvement is more frequent in the indolent lymphomas, but can be seen in up to 25% of cases in diffuse large B-cell lymphoma (DLBCL). Patients presenting with intramedullary involvement of the bone marrow will often develop cytopenias, which are frequently detected incidentally on routine complete blood counts (CBC). The presence of B symptoms is considered an ominous sign, although it is not part of the International Prognostic Index (IPI), as discussed below.

Diagnosis and Staging

Perhaps the most critical element in the diagnosis and treatment of a patient with lymphoma is making the right histopathologic assessment. This requires consultation with an expert hematopathologist familiar with the latest techniques in immunophenotyping and cytogenetics. For this reason, it is imperative that every diagnosis of lymphoma be based on an adequate specimen, which should ideally include an excisional biopsy of an involved lymph node or an incisional biopsy of a large mass. Under no circumstances should a fine needle aspiration (FNA) be used to document a first-time diagnosis of lymphoma. In select cases, a bone marrow biopsy can be sufficient for a diagnosis in a patient with

CLL or acute lymphoblastic leukemia (ALL). Evaluation of lymph node architecture plays a crucial role in aiding the hematopathologist in differentiating normal from malignant cells.

NHL often involves discontiguous lymph node sites and extranodal areas. For this reason, total body computed tomography (CT) imaging of the neck, chest, abdomen, and pelvis are required to fully appreciate the extent of disease. CT imaging provides clear interpretation of anatomy and is best used to measure changes in size of abnormal lymph nodes or extranodal masses. However, given the "normal" presence of lymphatic tissue throughout the body, CT imaging can be unsatisfactory for delineating an enlarged fibrotic node that has resolved its lymphomatous infiltration from one with active NHL and cannot differentiate viable from dead disease. The (18)F-fluoro-deoxyglucose positron emission tomography (FDG-PET) has emerged as an important imaging tool in many forms of lymphoma based on the increased accumulation of FDG in the sites of active lymphoma (23). The increased sensitivity of PET imaging is capable of providing additional detail regarding extent of disease, and is especially useful in differentiating viable disease from fibrotic tissue. Unfortunately, it cannot distinguish lymphoma from sites of active inflammation, which also represents a collection of highly metabolically active, nonmalignant cells. Most recently, PET imaging has begun to play a major role in the prognostication of patients with diffuse large B-cell lymphoma and Hodgkin disease receiving active therapy. The PET scan in these cases serves as a means to evaluate true in vivo chemosensitivity. Patients who are able to convert their PET scan from positive to negative at the interim restaging analysis have been demonstrated to have superior outcomes compared to those patients who fail to convert their PET scan (25). This type of information is now being used to tailor and individualize therapy for patients based upon their functional imaging studies (26).

Almost all patients with NHL require a bone marrow biopsy at diagnosis. While there are some exceptions to this rule, a bone marrow biopsy will determine the presence of disease in the marrow before starting treatment, and can be important in determining whether a patient is responding or progressing through a particular treatment. Certainly, a patient with lymphoma presenting with cytopenia deserves a bone marrow biopsy to ascertain the cause of the bone marrow suppression. Evaluation of the gastrointestinal tract and examination of Waldeyer's ring might be warranted in patients MALT and mantle cell lymphoma, two diseases that frequently involve these particular sites. Although its use in this setting is controversial, lumbar puncture should be performed in patients with Burkitt lymphoma, patients with testicular or Waldeyer's Ring involvement, and certainly in any patient presenting with a focal neurological exam.

Compared to the solid tumor malignancies, the staging of lymphoma is relatively straightforward, and employs the Ann Arbor classification shown in Table 18.3. Staging is based on the involvement of broad lymph node regions. For example, stage I is comprised of involvement of a single lymph node region, whereas stage II disease involves more than one lymph node region on the same side of the diaphragm. Stage III disease is defined as disease both above and below the diaphragm, and stage IV disease is characterized by involvement of one or more extralymphatic organs, with or without associated lymph node involvement. The letter 'E' is added to the stage to denote involvement of an extranodal sites, the letter 'S' when there is the splenic involvement, and the letter 'X' when there is bulky disease (eg, <10 cm in greatest transverse diameter). Frequently, the letters A or B will denote the absence or presence of constitutional or B symptoms.

Prognostic Factors

Unlike most solid tumors, stage alone does not define the complete risk of a particular patient, an observation that should be intuitive when dealing with a malignancy born in the bone marrow and disseminated via hematogenous and lymphatic spread. Clearly, patients with similar diagnoses can have varied clinical presentations and outcomes. Reliable prognostic markers play

TABLE 18.3
Ann Arbor Staging Classification for Non Hodgkin Lymphomas

STAGE	AREA OF INVOLVEMENT
I	One lymph node region
IE	One extralymphatic organ or site
II	Two or more lymph node regions on the same side of the diaphragm
IIE	One extralymphatic organ or site (localized) in addition to criteria for stage II
III	Lymph node regions on both sides of the diaphragm
IIIE	One extralymphatic organ or site (localized) in addition to criteria for stage III
IIIS	Spleen in addition to criteria for stage III
IIISE	Spleen and one extralymphatic organ or site (localized) in addiction to criteria for stage III
IV	One or more extralymphatic organs with or without associated lymph node involvement (diffuse or disseminated); involved organs should be designed by subscript letters

a valuable role in aiding the clinician in discriminating these various subgroups of patients, sometimes by leading to different treatment recommendations based on the prognostic score. Historically, a large number of clinical and molecular prognostic factors have been reported in the literature (27–33). However, the recent introduction of monoclonal antibody-based therapies such as rituximab (Rituxan) have revolutionized the outcome of patients and reduced the reliability of the older prognostic scores, which were largely developed in the pre-rituximab era. As such, many of these prognostic models have had to be revalidated given the change in the standard treatment (34). Perhaps the most universally applied prognostic model is the IPI (35). This score was developed based upon 2,031 patients in 16 different institutions and cooperative groups in United States, Europe, and Canada, and has become the primary means by which clinicians predict outcome of patients with aggressive NHL. Based on the number of negative prognostic features present at the time of the diagnosis (aged 60 or older; Ann Arbor Stage III or IV; serum LDH level above normal; two or more extranodal sites; and performance status greater than or equal to ECOG 2), four prognostic groups were identified. The four risk groups (low, low-intermediate, high-intermediate, and high risk) had distinctly different rates of complete response, relapse-free survival, and overall survival. For example, the low-risk group exhibited a complete-response rate of 87% and a 5-year overall survival of 73%, whereas the high-risk group had a complete-response rate of only 44% and a 5-year overall survival of only 26%. Since the publication of the IPI, other groups have formulated their own more disease specific prognostic models. For example, in follicular lymphoma (FL), the Follicular Lymphoma International Prognostic Index (FLIPI) (36) stratifies patients similar to the IPI. In this case, a disease-specific prognostic index makes intuitive sense given the widely different behavior of these two diseases. Application of the IPI to patients with the FL does not differentiate the different prognostic categories well (ie, there is an over-representation of patients with low to low-intermediate risk). Again, based on a retrospective review of a large collection of patients with FL, a multivariate analysis led to the development of the following five independent risk factors: hemoglobin level lower that 12 g/dl, serum LDH higher than the upper normal value, Ann Arbor Stage III-IV, number of nodal sites higher than four, and aged older than 60 years. The FLIPI index defines three risk groups: low (0–1 risk factor), intermediate (2 risk factors), and high (≥3 risk factors). Similar to the IPI in aggressive lymphoma, the risk category effectively stratified patients; those patients in the low-risk group exhibited a five year overall survival of 90.6%; the intermediate-risk group exhibited a five year overall survival of 77.6%, and the high-risk group had a 5-year overall survival of only 52.5%.

This approach is gradually being applied to many individual subtypes of lymphoma, including the peripheral T-cell lymphomas. The concept is that the varying biological the 3 basis for different lymphomas will be reflected differentially across the diverse subtypes of the disease. For example, a prognostic index in peripheral T-cell lymphoma unspecified (PTCLU) called the Prognostic Index for PTCLU (PIT) (37) is based on four clinical variables: age (older than 60 years), PS (≥2), LDH level (more than 1× normal) and bone marrow involvement. The PIT differs from IPI because the variables related to the extension of the disease (stage and number of extranodal sites involved) do not seem to adversely affect prognosis. The PIT identified four groups of patients: group 1, with no adverse factors; group 2, with one factor; group 3, with two factors; and group 4, with three or four factors, and was successful in identifying groups with different clinical outcome. For the patients in the group 1, the 5-year survival rate was 62.3%; for patients in group 2, 52.9%; for patients in group 3, 32.9%; and for patients in group 4, 18.6%. The PIT does not include tumor-specific factors, and a new score was developed that integrates both clinical and tumor-specific characteristics (eg, Ki-67 marking ≥80%) (38). These prognostic scores are useful for designing risk-adapted therapy that is personalized to an individual's particular disease. Based on the fact

that aggressive lymphomas are considered curable and indolent lymphomas generally are not, the therapeutic approach for each kind of lymphoma, let alone specific patients, can differ dramatically. As such, for patients with generally curable disease, the tolerance for toxicity is higher given the return for possible cure, whereas for patients with an incurable disease, the tolerance for toxicity is typically much lower given the goals of treatment are oriented towards chronic management.

PRINCIPLES OF THERAPY

Chemotherapy remains the most important modality for managing most patients with lymphoma, and different regimens are employed depending upon the disease. While a detailed discussion of these different regimens is well beyond the scope of this chapter, suffice it to say that the selection of any given therapy is based upon an assessment of host morbidities and toxicity, with the goal of selecting the optimal treatment associated with the most favorable side effect profile (Table 18.4). Despite the implementation of various newer strategies, radiotherapy still plays a critical role in selected cases. However, modern treatment strategies, including monoclonal antibodies targeting lymphoma-associated antigens, radioimmunotherapy, therapeutic vaccination, high-dose chemotherapy combined with autologous stem-cell transplantation (ASCT), and allogenic hematopoietic stem cell transplantation, have the potential to profoundly impact clinical outcomes in lymphoma therapy. Rituximab, for example, the first monoclonal antibody approved by the U.S. Food and Drug Administration (FDA) for the treatment of any cancer, targets the CD20 molecule presents on the surface of B cells. Randomized studies have demonstrated its activity in follicular lymphoma (FL), mantle cell lymphoma, and DLBCL (39), in untreated or relapsing patients. Noncomparative studies have shown activity in all other subtypes of B-cell lymphoma. Because of its high activity and low toxicity ratio, rituximab has transformed the outcome of patients with B-cell lymphoma. A combination regimen consisting of chemotherapy, rituximab, cyclophosphamide, doxorubicin, vincristine, and prednisone (R-CHOP), has been found to have the highest efficacy ever described with any chemotherapy in DLBCL and FL. The role of rituximab in the treatment of B-cell lymphomas has rapidly emerged from the relapsed setting to the front line for virtually every B-cell subtypes of NHL. Presently, the role of maintenance rituximab in indolent lymphomas after first-line therapy is being defined as is the integration of radioimmunotherapy into the first-line therapeutic regimens.

Radioimmunotherapy (RIT) combines radiation delivered by radioisotopes with the targeting effect of

TABLE 18.4
Chemotherapeutic Regimens for Non Hodgkin Lymphoma

REGIMEN	DOSE	ROUTE	FREQUENCY
CVP ± Rituximab			Every 21 days
Cyclophosphamide	750–1,000 mg/m²	IV	Day 1
Vincristine	1.4 mg/m	IV	Day 1
Prednisone	100 mg or 100 mg/m²	PO	Day 1–5
Rituximab	375 mg/m²	IV	Day 1
CHOP ± Rituximab			Every 21 or 14 days (with G-CSF)
Cyclophosphamide	750 mg/m²	IV	Day 1
Doxorubicin	50 mg/m²	IV	Day 1
Oncovin (Vincristine)	1.4 mg/mL (max 2 mg)	IV	Day 1
Prednisone	40 mg/m² or 100 mg/d	PO	Day1–5
Rituximab	or 100mg/m²/d	IV	Day 1
	375 mg/m²		
CHOEP ± Rituximab			Every 21 days
Cyclophosphamide	750 mg/m²	IV	Day 1
Doxorubicin	50 mg/m²	IV	Day 1
Etoposide	100 mg/m²	IV	Day 1–3
Oncovin (Vincristine)	1.4 mg/mL (max 2 mg)	IV	Day 1
Prednisone	100 mg/m²	PO	Day1–5
Rituximab	375 mg/m²	IV	Day 1
FND			Every 21–28 days (depending on hematologic recovery)
Fludarabine	25 mg/m²	IV	Day 1–3
Novantrone	10 mg/m²	IV	Day 1
Dexamethasone	20 mg	PO/ IV	Day1–5

monoclonal antibodies (40). Two radioimmunoconjugates are currently approved for relapsed/resistant low-grade or transformed lymphoma: iodine-131 tositumomab and yttrium-90 ibritumomab tiuxetan. These agents are also effective in aggressive lymphoma, a transformed lymphoma arising from a preexisting low grade lymphoma. Their major toxicity is myelosuppression, although patients can also experience significant periods of thrombocytopenia following treatment with either of these agents. High-dose chemotherapy and ASCT has an established therapeutic role in the treatment of chemo-sensitive relapsed aggressive lymphoma, but has limited to no merit in chemorefractory disease. Recurrent disease is the major cause of treatment failure in all patient subsets not cured with the primary therapy. Methods for better eradication of underlying lymphoma are needed to improve outcome. Few effective treatment options exist for chemotherapy-

refractory indolent or transformed NHL. Nonmyeloablative allogeneic stem cell transplantation can produce durable disease-free survival in patients with relapsed or refractory indolent NHL, even in those patients who have relapsed following an ASCT. Generally, outcomes were good in patients with untransformed disease and related donors, whereas patients with transformed disease did poorly. Long-term survivors report good overall functional status. Allogeneic SCT has usually been employed in patients with relapsed or refractory disease, with the aim of providing both a tumor-free graft and the postulated graft-versus-lymphoma (GVL) effect. In support of the latter, the first retrospective studies comparing progression-free survival curves of patients undergoing autologous or allogeneic SCT showed a statistically significant difference in favor of allografted patients. Most retrospective studies on this issue showed that patients treated with allogeneic

SCT were usually affected by more advanced or refractory disease, thus suggesting the existence of immune-mediated antitumor activity (41–43). The additional evidence of clinical and molecular responses following the withdrawal of immunosuppressive therapy or donor lymphocyte infusions further supported the idea of an underlying GVL effect (44,45). However, the main obstacle to a wide application of myeloablative allogeneic SCT as a salvage strategy was the high incidence of transplant-related mortality (TRM) that offset the benefit of the GVL effect in terms of overall survival (46,47). Reduced intensity or nonmyeloablative allogeneic transplant have been developed to decrease the up-front mortality associated with an allogeneic transplant while maintaining the graft versus leukemia effect. While this approach allows the application of this modality to patients who are older than age 60, graft versus host disease remains a major challenge, with an incidence of 60%–70%.

IMPLICATION FOR REHABILITATION MEDICINE

There remains a host of concerns regarding the long-term management of patients who either have been cured of, or are being chronically managed for, their lymphoma that are significant for the practicing physiatrist. First of all, lymphoma patients are often elderly, entering a treatment program with an already compromised functional or performance status. In addition, many drugs used for the treatment of NHL exhibit toxicities that more often than not can have deleterious effects on a host of different organ systems. Many agents exhibit neurotoxicity, which may affect sensory, motor, or proprioceptive nerve fibers in a manner that contributes to a compromise in performance status. Many of these drugs render virtually all patients areflexive, the collective effects of which can lead to increase falls or tripping. Some patients with lymphoproliferative malignancies may experience involvement of the spinal cord or CNS, leading to pain, or compromised motor function, with lower or upper extremity weakness. These patients will obviously require more focused attention to address the collection of issues associated with spinal cord compression syndromes (48). An often overlooked side-effect of both the disease and its treatment involves the tendency for enhanced bone loss, leading to osteopenia and osteoporosis. Virtually every patient with lymphoma will require steroids, some for long-term management, which will further accelerate osteoporosis. Treatment-related bone loss is well recognized in prostate cancer, due to overt hypogonadism, and in breast cancer, but few studies have evaluated the effect of chemotherapy alone on bone mineral density (BMD) compared to the same population cross matched by age. The association of chemotherapy and an increased risk of fracture and osteoporosis in elderly patients with NHL is well described (49). At the very least, assuming no contraindications to therapy, these patients should all be on calcium, vitamin D, and a bisphosphonate.

Bone marrow toxicity is the most common side effect of chemotherapy. It might present as anemia, leucopenia, or thrombocytopenia. Many elderly patients already have some compromise in their normal hematopoietic function, and following treatment may be left with some compromise in their blood counts. In addition, most patients who receive chemotherapy may incur compromise in their normal immune function that can last for 9–12 months, and may be at risk for various infections. Collectively, these patients may present with symptoms attributable to one cell lineage or another, including asthenia, tachycardia, and fatigue and dyspnea in anemic patients; fever, tachycardia, pain, dyspnea, and cellulitis in patients with leucopenia; and ecchymosis or epistaxis in patients with thrombocytopenia. The use of cytokines such as granulocyte-colony stimulating factor (GCSF) may be indicated for those patients with neutropenia, although recently, the use of erythropoietic stimulating factors has not been recommended for patients who are not actively receiving chemotherapy due to the increased risk of mortality (50,51).

HODGKIN LYMPHOMA

Introduction

In 1832, Sir Thomas Hodgkin presented the clinical history and the postmortem findings of the massive enlargement of the lymph nodes and spleens of seven patients in the first description of the disease (52). As late as 1865, Sir Samuel Wilks linked Thomas Hodgkin's name to the disease that he described as "Cases of the Enlargement of the Lymphatic Glands and Spleen (or Hodgkin's Disease)." In 1878, Greenfield was the first to publish a drawing of the pathognomonic "giant cells" that would later become known as the Reed-Sternberg cells, named after Carl Sternberg and Dorothy Reed (1902), who contributed the first definitive microscopic descriptions of Hodgkin disease. Despite the very strong evidence for the malignant nature of HD over the past century, it was not until 1998 that Reed-Sternberg cells were shown to be clonally expanding, pre-apoptotic, germinal center-derived B lymphocytes that resemble true malignant lymphoid cells (53).

Epidemiology and Etiology

Hodgkin disease (HD) is an uncommon lymphoid malignancy that represents about 1% of all de novo neoplasms occurring every year worldwide, with an annual incidence of two or three cases per 100,000 persons in Europe and the United States. Between 2001 and 2005, the age-adjusted incidence rate was 2.8 per 100,000 men and women per year, while the age-adjusted death rate was 0.4 per 100,000 men and women per year. These rates are based on cases diagnosed from 17 SEER geographic areas (54). In industrialized countries, the onset of HD has a bimodal distribution, with a first peak occurring in the third decade of life and a second peak occurring after age 50 years. The age-specific incidence differs markedly in various countries; moreover, the incidence of HD by age also differs by histologic subtypes. In the group of young adults, the most common subtype is nodular sclerosis HD, which occurs at a higher frequency than the others subtypes as discussed below. More men than women (1.4:1) develop the disease. Compared to whites, HD is less common in African Americans.

The cause of HD remains unknown, and there are no clearly defined risk factors for the disease. However, familial factors and viruses seem to play a role in its development. For example, same-sex siblings of patients with HD have a 10 times higher risk for the disease, whereas the monozygotic twin sibling of patients with HD have a 99 times higher risk than a dizygotic twin sibling of developing HD. Familial aggregation may implicate genetic factors, but other epidemiologic findings suggest an abnormal reaction to a possible infectious agent, and both aspects have been implicated in the pathogenesis of HD. EBV has been implicated in the development of HD; however, the link of the relationship between symptomatic primary infection and HD remain unclear. The association of infectious mononucleosis and HD is strongest in young adults, but virus in tumor cells is least frequently detected in tumors in young adults. Finally, there are no conclusive studies regarding the possible increased incidence of HD in patients who are HIV positive (55), although several series have been reported that suggest a higher risk in these patients.

Signs and Symptoms

HD commonly presents as asymptomatic lymphadenopathy. However, about 30% of patients exhibit systemic symptoms, including night sweats, fever, weight loss, and pruritus at the beginning of the disease. More than 80% of patients with HD present with lymphadenopathy above the diaphragm, often involving the anterior mediastinum; in contrast, less than 20%–30% of patients present with a lymphadenopathy limited to regions below the diaphragm. The most commonly involved peripheral lymph nodes are located in the cervical, supracervical, and axillary regions. In contrast to NHL, lymphadenopathy tends to be contiguous in patients with HD.

Diagnosis and Staging

The initial diagnosis of HD can be made only by incisional or excisional biopsy of an enlarged lymph node. Because of the importance of the architecture, fine needle aspiration should never be used to make the diagnosis. The diagnosis is based on the identification of the characteristic multinucleate giant cells within an inflammatory milieu. As mentioned above, these multinucleate giant cells, termed Reed-Sternberg (RS) cells, are diagnostic. These RS cells are the malignant component of HD and are its diagnostic hallmark. Unique to HD, these malignant RS cells comprise approximately 1% or less of the cellular mass of the tumor mass. The remainder of the tumor consists of a variable number of mononuclear elements, including normal B cells and T cells. In 1994, based on many morphologic, phenotypic, genotypic, and clinical findings, HD was described in the REAL classification system and subdivided into two main types: lymphocyte-predominant HD and classical HD. The latter further included the following subtypes: (1) nodular sclerosis classical HD; (2) mixed cellularity classic HD; (3) lymphocyte depletion classic lymphoma; and (4) the lymphocyte-rich classical HD. This approach has been approved by the recently developed WHO scheme, which has promoted lymphocyte-rich classic HD from a provisional entity to an accepted entity (Table 18.5).

The assignment of stage is critical for the selection of the proper treatment in HD. The stage is based on the following characteristics: (1) number of involved sites; (2) presence of lymphadenopathy both above and below the diaphragm; (3) presence of bulky disease (?10 cm); (4) presence of contiguous extranodal involvement or disseminated disease; and (5) presence of B-symptoms. The classical staging system is the Cotswald staging classification, which describes four stages as follows: stage I describes the involvement of a single lymph node region or lymphoid structure (eg,

TABLE 18.5 *Classification of Hodgkin Disease*	
Lymphocyte-predominant Hodgkin lymphoma	Classic Hodgkin lymphoma
	1. Nodular sclerosis
	2. Mixed cellularity
	3. Lymphocyte depletion
	4. Lymphocite-rich

spleen, thymus, Waldeyer's ring); stage II describes the involvement of two or more lymph node regions on the same side of the diaphragm, where the number of anatomic sites should be indicated by a subscript; stage III refers to the involvement of lymph node or structures on both sides of the diaphragm, and can be divided into III_1 with or without involvement of splenic, hilar, celiac, or portal nodes; and stage III_2 denotes involvement of para-aortic, iliac, or mesenteric nodes. Finally, stage IV is defined as involvement of extranodal site(s) beyond that designated E. In the absence of B symptoms, the stage is defined A; in presence of B symptoms, it is defined as B (Table 18.6).

Prognostic Factors

Approximately two-thirds of patients with advanced Hodgkin disease can be cured with the current approaches to treatment. Prediction of outcome is important to avoid over treating some patients and to identify others in whom standard treatment is likely to fail. The international database on Hodgkin disease was used to develop a parametric model for predicting survival. The model was based on data from 5,023 patients who represented different stages of the disease. In brief, seven prognostic factors were identified based on a multivariate analysis, and included: (1) a serum albumin level of less than 4 g per deciliter; (2) a hemoglobin level less that 10.5 g per deciliter; (3) leukocytosis (white-cell count of at least 15,000/mm³); (4) a lymphopenia (a lymphocyte count of less than 600/

mm³); (5) male gender; (6) aged 45 years or older; and (7) stage IV disease. The score predicted the 5-year rate of freedom from progression of disease as follows: zero factors, 84%; one risk factor, 77%; two risk factors, 67%; three risk factors, 60%; four risk factors, 51%; and five or more risk factors, 42%. The international prognostic score, called the IPSS or Hasenclever (56), can be useful in establishing enrollment criteria in clinical trial, to describe study population, and to support decisions about treatment in individual patients.

Treatment

HD is typically considered a chemotherapy and radiation sensitive disease. However, up until the beginning of the 21st century, patients with advanced stages of HD were considered incurable. With the advent of more effective drugs, De Vita and colleagues at the NCI pioneered new treatment regimens with remarkable success, achieving a 50% cure rate for patients with advanced-stage disease with the drug combination MOPP (Mechlorethamine, Oncovin, Procarbazine, Prednisone). Despite the promising results with MOPP therapy, many investigators continued to identify other novel regimens and used different chemotherapy programs to improve the efficacy and reduce the toxicities (57–59). Over time, it was realized that the MOPP regimen was associated with significant acute toxicities and a high risk of sterility and acute leukemia secondary to the alkylating agents (namely the nitrogen mustard mechlorethamine). In 1975, Bonadonna and colleagues (60) introduced the doxorubicin,

TABLE 18.6
Cotswolds Staging Classification

STAGE	DESCRIPTION
Stage I	Involvement of a single lymph node region or lymphoid structure or involvement of a single extralymphatic region (IE)
Stage II	Involvement of two or more lymph node regions on the same side of the diaphragm; localized contiguous involvement of only one extra nodal organ or site and lymph node on the same side of the diaphragm
Stage III	Involvement of lymph node regions on both sides of the diaphragm (III), which may also be accompanied by involvement of the spleen (IIIS) or by localized contiguous involvement of only one extranodal organ site (IIIE) or both (IIISE)
Stage IV	Diffuse or disseminate involvement of one or more extra nodal organs or tissues, with or without associated lymph node involvement
Designation applicable to any disease stage:	
A	No symptoms
B	Fever, drenching night sweats, unexplained loss of > 10% of body weight within the preceding 6 months
X	Bulky disease (>10 cm)
E	Involvement of a single extranodal site that is contiguous or proximal o the known nodal site

bleomycin, vincristine, and dacarbazine (DTIC-Dome) (ABVD) regimen. Direct comparison of the MOPP and ABVD regimens revealed both to be highly active, though ABVD was associated with significantly less germ-cell and hematopoietic toxicity, and a lower risk of developing acute leukemia. Presently, the treatment is tailored to the stage of the disease. In North America, cooperative group trials have defined limited-stage disease in patients with clinical stage I-IIA and an absence of bulky disease (≥10 cm). Patients with stage IIB or those with stage I-II bulky disease are treated with the same protocols as those with stage III-IV disease, typically receiving full course of chemotherapy, and are collectively referred to as having advanced stage disease. In addition, patients with bulky disease are considered for radiation therapy to the site to bulky disease. Generally, a number of principles have emerged regarding the management of HD, including:

1. Surgical staging (eg, splenectomy) is no longer necessary.
2. Treatment with combined modality therapy is superior to treatment with radiation therapy as a single agent.
3. Inclusion of chemotherapy as a part of combined modality therapy allows for a reduction in the magnitude of radiation therapy.
4. Chemotherapy as a single modality in patients with limited-stage disease is effective.

In brief, the treatment of choice for early-stage classical HD consists of combination chemotherapy (ABVD) sometimes followed by involved-field radiotherapy (IFRT) for patients with bulky disease. On the other hand, for the treatment of stage III/IV disease or patients with high-risk disease based on Hasenclever score, combination chemotherapy regimens and dose-intense regimens such as BEACOPP (Bleomycin, Etoposide, Adriamycin, Cyclophosphamide Oncovin, Procarbazine, Prednisone) are increasingly recommended. Table 18.7 summarizes some of these chemotherapeutic regimens routinely used for the treatment of Hodgkin lymphoma, and Table 18.8 summarizes the toxicities associated with the combination chemotherapy and radiation therapy. Generally, the use of extended field radiotherapy is being abandoned by most groups, being replaced by the increasing use of involved field radiotherapy. The one-year relative survival rate is 93%, the five-year survival is 86%, and after 10 years the survival rate decreases slightly to 81%.

Late Complications of Therapy

Because most HD patients can be cured with modern treatment modalities and will have a life expectancy equivalent to age-matched healthy individuals, it is of importance to take into account not just the acute treatment-related toxicities, but also the long-term side

TABLE 18.7
Chemotherapeutic Regimens

REGIMEN	DOSAGE	SCHEDULE	FREQUENCY
MOPP			Every 28 days
Mechlorethamine	6 mg/m²	IV	Day 1
Oncovin	1.4 mg/m²	IV (max dose 2 mg)	Day 1
Procarbazine	100 mg/m²	PO	Day 1–7
Prednisone	40 mg/m²	PO	Day 1–14
ABVD			Every 28 days
Adriamycin	25 mg/m²	IV	Days 1,15
Bleomycin	10 mg/m²	IV	Days 1,15
Vinblastine	6 mg/m²	IV	Days 1,15
Dacarbazine	375 mg/m²	IV	Days 1,15
BEACOPP			Every 21 days
Bleomycin	10 mg/m²	IV	Day 8
Etoposide	100 mg/m²	IV	Days 1–3
Adriamycin	25 mg/m²	IV	Day 1
Cyclophosphamide	650 mg/m²	IV	Day 1
Oncovin	1.4 mg/mL	IV	Day 8
Procarbazine	100 mg/m²	PO	Days 1–7
Prednisone	40 mg/m²	PO	Days 1–14
G-CSF (Granulocyte-Colony Stimulating Factor) from day 8			

TABLE 18.8
Toxicities

ACUTE TOXICITIES	DELAYED TOXICITIES
Alopecia	Secondary malignancies (AML, ALL, NHL, melanoma, sarcoma, breast, gastric, lung, and thyroid cancer)
Nausea and vomiting	
Diarrhea	
Mucositis	
Paresthesias and neuropathies	Endocrine complications (infertility, hypothyroidism)
CNS confusion	
Anemia, leucopenia, thrombocytopenia	Pulmonary complication (pulmonary fibrosis)
Disulfiram like reaction following alcohol while taking procarbazine	Cardiac complications (cardiomyopathy, accelerated atherosclerotic heart disease, pericardial fibrosis)
Bleomycin-related lung toxicity	

effects of the chemotherapy and radiotherapy. The complications of the treatment could be mild, severe, or life-threatening, even for those cured of lymphoma. During the period from 1960s to the 1990s, the number of late-occurring sequelae of chemotherapy affected between 25% to 30% of patients after 10–20 years. This rate of complication balanced the initial success rates due to deaths that were consequences of treatment and not caused by the primary disease.

Modern combined-modality treatment strategies with reduced radiation fields, and declining intensities of induction chemotherapy have diminished the rate of late complications. Time will tell whether the still-aggressive drug combinations used in the early 21st century will be superior to the older treatment programs. Long-term complications of irradiation, including lung, heart, and thyroid dysfunction, in addition to secondary cancers of breast and lung, all remain important hurdles in our effort to not just cure the disease, but to decrease the morbidity and mortality of therapy. Some specific examples of these morbidities are discussed below.

Pneumonitis typically occurs 1–6 months after completion of mantle radiation therapy. The overall incidence of symptomatic pneumonitis is less than 5% after mantle irradiation. Patients with large mediastinal adenopathy or who received combined chemotherapy and radiation therapy have twofold or threefold greater risk (10%–15%) of developing this complication (61). After it resolves, there are usually no long-term sequelae. A mild nonproductive cough, low grade fever, and dyspnea characterize symptomatic radiation pneumonitis. Bleomycin-induced pneumonitis is typically an acute toxicity, though pulmonary fibrosis can be seen as a late complication.

Chemotherapy and radiotherapy have overlapping toxic effects on the heart. Modern treatment strategies

now avoid large radiation fields involving the heart, while efforts to limit excessive doses of cardiotoxic drugs such as anthracyclines have been incorporated into many new treatment programs. While these sequelae have become less common, they still affect 2%–5% of the patients. The risk of chronic cardiomyopathy increases as the cumulative dose of doxorubicin exceeds 400–450 mg/m^2. A careful cardiac evaluation using multi gated acquisition scans or echocardiograph patients treated with combined chemotherapy and radiotherapy is required, and probably should be performed as a workup for patients who developed unresolving dyspnea years after treatment.

The decline of the historical survival curves in HD in the second half of the 20th century was mainly attributed to the increasing number of secondary tumors. In the first three to five years after therapy, acute leukemias and lymphomas predominantly occur, whereas after 8–10 years, the number of solid tumors increases. The increasing incidence of secondary malignancies is potentiated by the administration of carcinogenic alkylating agents such as nitrogen mustard, procarbazine, and cyclophosphamide. Physicians should be aware that HD patients are at higher risk for developing secondary cancers, possibly because of some intrinsic genetic susceptibility to develop cancer compared to patients with other types of cancer. The incidence of solid tumors in treated HD patients increases with time and does not reach a plateau, even in the second decade after the treatment. The major risks appear to be lung and breast cancer (62–64). Other cancers include sarcomas, melanomas, connective tissue and bone marrow tumors, and skin cancers (65,66).

Gonadal dysfunction is another treatment-related disturbance that often occurs in young, sexually active HD patients. Loss of libido, sexual discomfort, impotence, and sterility are the major problems, and these symptoms afflict about 80% of the HD population (67,68). C-MOPP or C-MOPP-like chemotherapy induce azoospermia (69,70) in 50%–100% of male patients, and only 10%–20% will eventually recover after a long interval. A full course of C-MOPP chemotherapy causes approximately 50% of women (71) to have amenorrhea, with age-dependant premature ovarian failure. ABVD produces only limited and transient germ-cell toxicities in the men and rarely causes drug-induced amenorrhea.

CONCLUSIONS

Clearly, advances in the treatment of lymphoma have been significant, and may be among the most successful of any malignancy. As new drugs and new treatment paradigms emerge, our probability of curing or managing these patients will improve still further. The challenge moving forward is to make sure that we can nurture our elderly patients sufficiently enough that they are able to tolerate the noxious effects of our sometimes crude therapies. As the population ages, it is likely that the patients we treat will get older and older. These realities will most assuredly increase our reliance on those subspecialties of medicine that will be able to assist medical oncologists in formulating treatments that will allow for optimal outcomes.

*R*eferences

1. Harris NL, Jaffe ES, Stein H, et al. A revised European-American classification of lymphoid neoplasms: a proposal for the international lymphoma study group. *Blood*. September 1, 1994;84(5):1361–1392.
2. Jaffe ES, Harris NL, Stein H, Vardiman J. World Health Organization classification: tumours of hematopoetic and lymphoid tissues. In: Jaffe ES, Harris NL, Stein H, Vardiman JW, eds. Lyon: IARC Press; 2001.
3. Surveillance, Epidemiology, and End Results (SEER) Program. SEER*Stat Database: Mortality—All COD, Public-Use With State, Total US (1969–2004), National Cancer Institute, DCCPS, Surveillance Research Program, Cancer Statistics Branch, released April 2007. http://www.seer.cancer.gov. Underlying mortality data provided by NCHS (http://www.cdc.gov/nchs). Accessed May 1, 2007.
4. Pulte D, Gondos A, Brenner B. Ongoing improvement in outcomes for patients diagnosed as having Non-Hodgkin lymphoma from the 1990s to the early 21st century. *Arch Intern Med*. 2008;168(5):469–476.
5. Armitage JM, Kormos RL, Stuardt RS, et al. Posttransplant lymphoproliferative disease in thoracic organ transplant patients: ten years of cyclosporine-based immunosuppression. *J Heart Lung Transplant*. November–December 1991;10(6):877–886; discussion 886–887.
6. Leblonde V, Sutton L, Doren R, et al. Lymphoproliferative disorders after organ transplantation: a report of 24 cases observed in a single center. *J Clin Oncol*. April 1995;13(4):961–968.
7. Hourigan MJ, Doecke J, Molee PN, et al. A new prognosticator for post-transplant lymphoproliferative disorders after renal transplantation. *Br J Haematol*. April 13, 2008.

8. Ekstrom Smedby K, Vajdic CM, et al. Autoimmune disorders and risk of non-Hodgkin lymphoma subtypes: a pooled analysis within the InterLymph Consortium. *Blood*. April 15, 2008;111(8):4029–4038. Epub 2008 Feb 8.
9. Mellemkjaer L, Pfeiffer RM, et al. Autoimmune disease in individuals and close family members and susceptibility to non-Hodgkin's lymphoma. *Arthritis Rheum*. March 2008;58(3): 657–666.
10. Fain O, Aras N, et al. Sjögren's syndrome, lymphoma, cryoglobulinemia. *Rev Prat*. June 30, 2007;57(12):1287.
11. Beral V, Peterman T, et al. AIDS-associated non-Hodgkin lymphoma. *Lancet*. April 6, 1991;337(8745):805–809.
12. Rabkin CS, Biggar RJ, et al. Increasing incidence of cancers associated with the human immunodeficiency virus epidemic. *Int J Cancer*. March 12, 1991;47(5):692–696.
13. Ross R, Dworsky R, et al. Non-Hodgkin's lymphomas in never married men in Los Angeles. *Br J Cancer*. November 1985;52(5):785–787.
14. Wotherspoon AC. Gastric lymphoma of mucosa-associated lymphoid tissue and Helicobacter pylori. *Annu Rev Med*. 1998;49:289–299.
15. Parsonnet J, Isaacson PG. Bacterial infection and MALT lymphoma. *N Engl J Med*. January 15, 2004;350:213
16. Jaffe ES. Common threads of mucosa-associated lymphoid tissue lymphoma pathogenesis: from infection to translocation. *J Natl Cancer Inst*. April 21, 2004;96(8):571–573.
17. Ye H, Liu H, Attygalle A. Variable frequencies of t(11;18)(q21;q21) in MALT lymphomas of different sites: significant association with CagA strains of H pylori in gastric MALT lymphoma. *Blood*. August 1, 2003;102(3):1012–1018. Epub April 3, 2003.
18. University of Michigan Medical Center, Ann Arbor, Michigan 48109, USA American College of Gastroenterology Guideline on the Management of *Helicobacter pylori* Infection. *Am J Gastroenterol*. August 2007;102(8):1808–1825. Epub June 29, 2007.
19. Cerroni L, Zochling N, et al. Infection by Borrelia burgdorferi and cutaneous B-cell lymphoma. *J Cutan Pathol*. September 1997;24(8):457–461.
20. Krueger GR, Medina JR, Klein HO, et al. A new working formulation of non-Hodgkin's lymphomas. A retrospective study of the new NCI classification proposal in comparison to the Rappaport and Kiel classifications. *Cancer*. September 1, 1983;52(5):833–840.
21. Gerard-Marchant R, Hamlin I, Lennert K, et al. Classification of non Hodgkin lymphomas. *Lancet*. 1974;2:406–408.
22. Lukes RJ, Collins RD. Immunologic characterization of human malignant lymphomas. *Cancer*. October 1974;34(4 Suppl):1488–1503.
23. Cheson BD, Pfistner B, et al. Revised response criteria for malignant lymphoma. *J Clin Oncol*. February 10, 2007;25(5): 579–586.
24. Castellucci P, Zinzani PL, Pourdehnad M. 18F-FDG PET in malignant lymphoma: significance of positive findings. *Eur J Nucl Med Mol Imaging*. July 2005;32(7):749–756. Epub March 23, 2005.
25. Spaepen K, Stroobants S, Dupont P, et al. Early restaging positron emission tomography with (18)F-fluorodeoxyglucose predicts outcome in patients with aggressive non-Hodgkin's lymphoma. *Ann Oncol*. September 2002;13(9):1356–1363.
26. Gallamini A, Hutchings M, Rigacci S. Early interim 2-[18F] fluoro-2-deoxy-D-glucose positron emission tomography is prognostically superior to international prognostic score in advanced-stage Hodgkin's lymphoma: a report from a joint Italian-Danish study. *J Clin Oncol* August 20, 2007;25(24):3746–3752. Epub July 23, 2007.
27. Rosenberg SA. Validity of the Ann Arbor staging classification for the non-Hodgkin's lymphomas. *Cancer Treat Rep*. 1977;61:1023–1027.
28. Fisher RI, Hubbard SM, DeVita VT, et al. Factors predicting long-term survival in diffuse mixed, histiocytic, or undifferentiated lymphoma. *Blood*. 1981;58:45–51.

29. Shipp MA, Harrington DP, Klatt MM, et al. Identification of major prognostic subgroups of patients with large-cell lymphoma treated with m-BACOD or M-BACOD. *Ann Intern Med.* 1986;104:757–765.

30. Jagannath S, Velasquez WS, Tucker SL, et al. Tumor burden assessment and its implication for a prognostic model in advanced diffuse large-cell lymphoma. *J Clin Oncol.* 1986;4:859–865.

31. Coiffier B, Lepage E. Prognosis of aggressive lymphomas: a study of five prognostic models with patients included in the LNH-84 regimen. *Blood.* 1989;74:558–564.

32. Velasquez WS, Jagannath S, Tucker SL, et al. Risk classification as the basis for clinical staging of diffuse large-cell lymphoma derived from 10-year survival data. *Blood.* 1989;74:551–557.

33. Coiffier B, Gisselbrecht C, Vose JM, et al. Prognostic factors in aggressive malignant lymphomas: description and validation of a prognostic index that could identify patients requiring a more intensive therapy. *J Clin Oncol.* 1991;9:211–219.

34. Sehn L. Optimal use of prognostic factors in non-Hodgkin lymphoma. *Hematology Am Soc Hematol Educ Program.* 2006;295–302.

35. The International Non-Hodgkin's Lymphoma Prognostic Factors Project. A predictive model for aggressive non-Hodgkin's lymphoma. *N Engl J Med.* 1993;329:987–994.

36. Solal-Céligny P, Roy P, Colombat P. Follicular lymphoma international prognostic index. *Blood.* September 1, 2004;104(5):1258–1265.

37. Gallamini A, Stelitano C, Calvi R, et al. Peripheral T-cell lymphoma unspecified (PTCL-U): a new prognostic model from a retrospective multicentric clinical study. *Blood.* April 1, 2004;103(7):2474–2479. Epub November 26, 2003.

38. Went P, Agostinelli C, Gallamini A. Marker expression in peripheral T-cell lymphoma: a proposed clinical-pathologic prognostic score. *J Clin Oncol.* June 1, 2006;24(16):2472–2479. Epub April 24, 2006.

39. Coiffier B, Lepage E, Briere J, et al. CHOP chemotherapy plus rituximab compared with CHOP alone in elderly patients with diffuse large-B-cell lymphoma. *N Engl J Med.* January 24, 2002;346(4):235–242.

40. Press OW, Leonard JP, Coiffier B. Immunotherapy of non-Hodgkin's lymphomas; hematology. *Am Soc Hematol Educ Program.* 2001;221–240.

41. Chopra R, Goldstone AH, Pearce R, et al. Autologous versus allogeneic bone marrow transplantation for non-Hodgkin's lymphoma: a case-controlled analysis of the European Bone Marrow Transplant Group Registry data. *J Clin Oncol.* 1992;10:1690–1695.

42. Ratanatharathorn V, Uberti J, Karanes C, et al. Prospective comparative trial of autologous versus allogeneic bone marrow transplantation in patients with non-Hodgkin's lymphoma. *Blood.* 1994;84:1050–1055.

43. Verdonck LF, Dekker AW, Lokhorst HM, et al. Allogeneic versus autologous bone marrow transplantation for refractory and recurrent low-grade non-Hodgkin's lymphoma. *Blood.* 1997;90:4201–4205.

44. van Besien KW, de Lima M, Giralt S, et al. Management of lymphoma recurrence after allogeneic transplantation: the relevance of graft-versus-lymphoma effect. *Bone Marrow Transplant.* 1997;19:977–982.

45. Mandigers CM, Verdonck LF, Meijerink JP, et al. Graft-versus-lymphoma effect of donor lymphocyte infusion in indolent lymphomas relapsed after allogeneic stem cell transplantation. *Bone Marrow Transplant.* 2003;32:1159–1163.

46. Peniket AJ, Ruiz de Elvira MC, Taghipour G, et al. European Bone Marrow Transplantation (EBMT) Lymphoma Registry. An EBMT registry matched study of allogeneic stem cell transplants for lymphoma: allogeneic transplantation is associated with a lower relapse rate but a higher procedure-related mortality rate than autologous transplantation. *Bone Marrow Transplant.* 2003;31:667–678.

47. Farina L, Corradini P. Current role of allogeneic stem cell transplantation in follicular lymphoma. *Haematologica.* May 2007;92(5):580–582.

48. Chahal S, Lagera JE, Rider J, et al. Hematological neoplasms with first presentation as spinal cord compression syndromes: a 10-year retrospective series and review of the literature. *Clin Neuropathol.* November–December 2003;22(6):282–290.

49. Cabanillas ME, Lu H, Fans S, et al. Elderly patients with non-Hodgkin lymphoma who receive chemotherapy are at higher risk for osteoporosis and fractures. *Leuk Lymphoma.* August 2007;48(8):1514–1521.

50. Morrison VA. Non-Hodgkin's lymphoma in the elderly. Part 2: treatment of diffuse aggressive lymphomas. *Oncology.* September 2007;21(10):1191–1198; discussion 1198–1208, 1210.

51. Balducci L, Al-Halawani H, et al. Elderly cancer patients receiving chemotherapy benefit from first-cycle pegfilgrastim. *Oncologist.* December 2007;12(12):1416–1424.

52. Hodgkin T. On same morbid appearances of the absorbent glands and spleen. *Medico-Chirurgical Trans.* 1832;17:68–97.

53. Kuppers R, Rajewsky K. The origin of Hodgkin and Reed/Sternberg cells in Hodgkin's disease. *Annu Rev Immunol.* 1998;16:471–493.

54. Surveillance, Epidemiology, and End Results (SEER) Program. SEER*Stat Database: Mortality—All COD, Public-Use With State, Total US (1969–2004), National Cancer Institute, DCCPS, Surveillance Research Program, Cancer Statistics Branch, released April 2007. http://www.seer.cancer.gov. Underlying mortality data provided by NCHS (http://www.cdc.gov/nchs). Accessed May 1, 2007.

55. Engels EA, Biggar RJ, hall HI, et al. Cancer risk in people infected with human immunodeficiency virus in the United States. *Inter J Cancer.* July 1, 2008;123(1):187–194.

56. Hasenclever D, Diehl, et al. A prognostic score for advanced Hodgkin's disease. *N Engl J Med.* November 19, 1998;339:1506.

57. Nissen NI, Pajak TF, Glidewell O. A comparative study of a BCNU containing 4-drug program versus MOPP versus 3-drug combinations in advanced Hodgkin's disease: a cooperative study by the Cancer and Leukemia Group B. *Cancer.* January 1979;43(1):31–40.

58. Bakemeier RF, Anderson RJ, Costello W, et al. BCVPP chemotherapy for advanced Hodgkin's disease: evidence for greater duration of complete remission, greater survival, and less toxicity than with a MOPP regimen. Results of the Eastern Cooperative Oncology Group study. *Ann Intern Med.* October 1984;101(4):447–456.

59. Hancock BW. Randomised study of MOPP (mustine, Oncovin, procarbazine, prednisone) against LOPP (Leukeran substituted for mustine) in advanced Hodgkin's disease. British National Lymphoma Investigation. *Radiother Oncol.* November 1986;7(3):215–221.

60. Bonadonna G, Zucali R, Monfardini S, et al. Combination chemotherapy of Hodgkin's disease with adriamycin, bleomycin, vinblastine, and imidazole carboxamide versus MOPP. *Cancer.* July 1975;36(1):252–259.

61. Tardell N, Thompson L, Mauch P. Thoracic irradiation in Hodgkin's disease: disease control and long-term complications. *Int J Radiat Oncol Biol Phys.* February 1990;18(2):275–281.

62. Van leeuwen FE, Swerdlow AJ, et al. *Second Cancers after Treatment of Hodgkin's Disease.* Philadelphia: Lippincott Williams & Wilkins; 1999:607–632.

63. Tucker MA. Solid second cancers following Hodgkin's disease. *Hematol Oncol Clin North Am.* April 1993;7(2):389–400.

64. Valagussa P. Second neoplasms following treatment of Hodgkin's disease. *Curr Opin Oncol.* September 1993;5(5):805–811.

65. Van leeuwen FE, Somers R, et al. Increased risk of lung cancer, non-Hodgkin's lymphoma, and leukemia following Hodgkin's disease. *J Clinic Oncol.* August 1989;7(8):1046–1058.

66. Hancock LS, Hoppe RT. Long-term complications of treatment and causes of mortality after Hodgkin's disease. *Semin Radiat Oncol.* July 1996;6(3):225–242.

67. Bokemeyer C, Schmoll HJ, et al. Long-term gonadal toxicity after therapy for Hodgkin's and non-Hodgkin's lymphoma. *Ann Hematol.* March 1994;68(3):105–110.

68. Ortin TT, Shostak CA. Gonadal status and reproductive function following treatment for Hodgkin's disease in childhood: the Stanford experience. *Int J Radiat Oncol Biol Phys.* October 1990;19(4):873–880.

69. Tempest HG, Ko E. Sperm aneuploidy frequencies analysed before and after chemotherapy in testicular cancer and Hodgkin's lymphoma patients. *Hum Reprod.* February 2008;23(2): 251–258. Epub December 14, 2007.

70. Blumenfeld Z. Gender difference: fertility preservation in young women but not in men exposed to gonadotoxic chemotherapy. *Minerva Endocrinol.* March 2007;32(1):23–34.

71. Giuseppe L, Attilio G, et al. Ovarian function after cancer treatment in young women affected by Hodgkin disease (HD). *Hematology.* April 2007;12(2):141–147.

Evaluation and Treatment of Leukemia and Myelodysplasia

Heather J. Landau
Stephen D. Nimer

This chapter covers the common leukemias (AML, ALL, and CLL) and the myelodysplastic syndromes. We will describe the key features of these disorders and discuss how the various treatments affect the disease as well as the function of other organs, at times leading to acute or chronic organ dysfunction. With the advent of imatinib, dasatinib, and nilotinib, tyrosine kinase inhibitor therapy has dramatically changed the treatment of CML. Many excellent reviews have described the optimal approach to using these agents in CML, addressed how to best manage their side effects, and monitor the response to treatment (1,2). Therefore, CML will not be covered in this chapter.

ACUTE MYELOGENOUS LEUKEMIA (AML)

Unfortunately, the treatment of AML has not changed significantly in the past three to four decades (3,4), except for the treatment of acute promyelocytic leukemia (APL), a subtype of AML that is now eminently curable (5). The treatments for AML were initially designed based on the principles of nonoverlapping toxicities and, to some degree, different mechanisms of action. In the case of APL, the use of the vitamin A derivative all-trans retinoic acid (ATRA) has been a remarkable clinical advance. ATRA was also shown to represent targeted therapy, as the genetic abnormality underlying

APL involves translocation of the retinoic acid receptor alpha (RARa) gene (reviewed in Ref. 6).

Prognostic Features

The prognosis of AML depends on the age of the patient, the cytogenetic abnormalities detected, whether it occurs de novo or secondary to chemotherapy or environmental toxin exposure, and whether certain mutations or cell surface markers are found in the leukemia cell (7,8).

Specific cytogenetic abnormalities are associated with specific clinical syndromes, such as t(15;17) and with AML, M3 and t(8;21) with AML, M2. The core binding factor (CBF) leukemias are characterized by chromosomal translocations that involve either the CBFa gene (better known as the AML1 gene or the RUNX1 gene) or the CBFb gene. These genes encode proteins that form a complex at target gene promoters that can either turn on or turn off gene expression. The AML1 protein binds to DNA via its Runt domain, which is so named because of its homology to the drosophila gene Runt (9,10). It binds with a low affinity and is subject to ubiquitin-mediated proteasomal degradation, unless CBFb is also present. CBFb increases the affinity of AML1 for its DNA recognition sequence, and it protects AML1 from proteasomal degradation (11,12). The t(8;21) and the inv (16) or t(16;16), which is associated with AML, M4-Eo), generate the

KEY POINTS

- Acute leukemia manifests itself largely by its effects on normal hematopoiesis. Anemia, thrombocytopenia, and neutropenia, the result of marrow replacement by malignant cells, lead to increased fatigue, bruising or bleeding, and infection.
- Unfortunately, the treatment of acute myelogenous leukemia (AML) has not changed significantly in the past three to four decades, except for the treatment of acute promyelocytic leukemia (APL), a subtype of AML that is now eminently curable.
- The prognosis of AML depends on the age of the patient, the cytogenetic abnormalities detected, whether it occurs de novo or secondary to chemotherapy or environmental toxin exposure, and whether certain mutations or cell surface markers are found in the leukemia cell.
- Myelodysplastic disorders (MDS) are characterized by ineffective hematopoiesis, which most commonly manifests as a hypercellular bone marrow with peripheral blood cytopenias, but also by a variable tendency to progress to acute myelogenous leukemia.
- The clinical approach to patients with MDS should be based on (1) whether the patient has anemia only or also has significant neutropenia and/or thrombocytopenia; and (2) whether the patient has increased blasts and is therefore at risk for developing acute leukemia.
- Acute lymphoblastic leukemia (ALL) is the most common malignancy in children, but it is relatively uncommon in adults, with about 2,000 cases per year in the United States. Childhood ALL is cured with modern treatment regimens in approximately 80% of patients; however, only 20%–40% of adult patients are cured.
- Treatment of adult ALL is typically divided into four phases: induction, consolidation, maintenance, and central nervous system (CNS) prophylaxis.
- Treatment of ALL is complicated by toxicity, especially in older adults. Patients with diabetes, hypertension, or heart disease, which are common in the general population, are at increased risk for steroid-induced complications, vincristine-induced neuropathy, and anthracycline-associated cardiotoxicity.
- Chronic lymphocytic leukemia (CLL) is the most common leukemia in adults; approximately 10,000 new cases are diagnosed each year in the United States. The median age at diagnosis is approximately 70 years, with 80% of patients diagnosed at 60 years or older. Although the disease course is often indolent, each year approximately 4,600 patients die from complications of CLL, most commonly from infection.
- Conventional therapy for CLL is not curative and there is no evidence that patients with low or intermediate risk disease benefit from the early initiation of therapy. However, treatment is indicated for patients who have symptomatic progressive disease, bulky disease, or cytopenias.

leukemia-associated fusion proteins, AML1-ETO and CBFB-SMMHC, respectively. These AML subtypes tend to have a more favorable prognosis.

Treatment of AML

The treatment of AML in adults generally consists of combination therapy that includes an anthracycline (eg, Daunorubicin or Idarubicin) and cytosine arabinoside (Cytarabine). This treatment is often referred to as 7+3 because the cytosine arabinoside is given daily for seven days and the anthracycline given daily for three days. Once the diagnosis of AML is made, patients are quickly hospitalized, and treatment is initiated. Hydration and administration of allopurinol are started to prevent the infrequent occurrence of tumor lysis syndrome. The presence of an infection at the time of first presentation is a negative prognostic feature. It also complicates the initiation of treatment.

The most essential goal of therapy for AML is to achieve a complete remission (CR), which is defined by the disappearance of the leukemic blasts from the peripheral blood and the bone marrow (blasts must be less than 5%) and the return of the peripheral blood counts to normal levels (13). All of these features must last for at least one month to document a CR. In an attempt to induce a CR, induction chemotherapy may be given once or twice. Generally, the same chemotherapy drugs are repeated when leukemic cells persist after the first course of chemotherapy. As the rate of inducing a CR with a third course of induction chemotherapy is as low as 3%, a third course of similar chemotherapy is not recommended. Rather a distinct approach, using investigational agents (given the paucity of available drugs that have activity against AML blasts) is often considered for younger patients. For the elderly patients, who comprise the majority of patients with AML, a second course of induction chemotherapy is often not given because of concerns about toxicity. Additional myelosuppressive therapy can result in profound neutropenia and prolonged infection in these patients who are already quite compromised.

Once remission is achieved, further treatment is needed to prolong the remission duration and to offer the possibility of cure (which occurs in approximately 30%–40% of patients aged younger than 60 years). This treatment, called consolidation therapy, is intensive, although generally not as intensive as induction therapy. The optimal number of cycles of consolidation therapy is not known; however, patients who receive at least one cycle have a measurable cure rate (14). In general, patients are given two to four courses of consolidation therapy (15). In addition, both autologous and allogeneic transplantation can be offered to AML patients in first remission as a form of consolidation therapy, in an attempt to increase the cure rate. Several randomized trials (biologically randomized, based upon the availability of a suitable allogeneic donor, which historically meant an HLA-identical sibling) have been conducted and show better relapse-free survival but generally not better overall survival for patients who undergo autologous or allogeneic transplantation "upfront" (16–19). These studies suggest that patients aged younger than 60 years with poor prognosis AML seem to derive the greatest benefit from an allotransplant in first remission. Studies have shown that the CBF leukemia patients do best if given high dose cytosine arabinoside based consolidation therapy rather than a standard dose cytosine arabinoside based regimen (20).

What must be remembered when interpreting these studies is that the cure rates with the non-allotransplant approaches must include not only the cure rate from the initial therapy, but also the salvage rate when the allogeneic transplant is used to treat patients with relapsed disease (21).

Complications of AML Therapy

The side effects of induction chemotherapy include myelosuppression (which generally lasts weeks), GI toxicities due to breaking down of mucosal barriers, total alopecia, and the small possibility of long-term cardiac toxicity from the repeated administration of anthracycline-containing therapies. Patients with high risk AML often receive high dose cytabine as part of an induction regimen. Neurotoxicity (generally, cerebellar toxicity) occurs can, especially in the elderly or those with an elevated serum creatinine (ie, diminished renal function). Other than avoiding the use of the 3 gm/m² q12 hr dosing regimen for these types of patients, evaluating the patient's signature before each dose has been suggested as a way to avoid triggering severe cerebellar toxicity. Because cytosine arabinoside is excreted in tears, patients given high dose cytosine arabinoside require steroid eye drops before each dose of chemotherapy in order to avoid chemical conjunctivitis.

The toxicity of autologous transplantation is largely limited to the immediate post-transplant period, when patients have profound neutropenia. The transplant conditioning regimens for AML patients often include total body irradiation, which can cause severe mucositis, prolonged myelosuppression (nearly myeloablation), pulmonary toxicity (both acute and chronic), and premature cataract formation. High dose etoposide can cause profound hypotension during the prolonged drug infusion. Hemorrhagic cystitis and rarely, cardiopulmonary toxicity, can be seen with high dose cyclophosphamide.

The toxicity of allogeneic transplantation persists well beyond the initial 100 days post-transplant (22). In addition to complications from the profound immunosuppression that occurs post-transplant, both acute and chronic graft versus host disease (GVHD) result in liver, GI, and skin abnormalities that can also be severe. Chronic GVHD resembles an autoimmune disorder and can be very difficult to treat (23,24). Veno-occlusive disease of the liver (perhaps better described as sinusoidal obstruction syndrome, or SOS) is uncommon with autologous, but not allogeneic, transplantation (reviewed in 25).

Treatment of Acute Promyelocytic Leukemia (APL)

The most striking advances in the treatment of acute leukemia over the past decades have taken place in the treatment of APL, largely because of the use of all-trans retinoic acid (ATRA). APL has been more successfully treated than other subtypes of AML for years, but because patients with APL often present with disseminated intravascular coagulation (DIC), they can die from hemorrhage (or less commonly from thrombosis) before or during their induction chemotherapy, prior to achieving a complete remission (26). The remarkable ability of ATRA to both eliminate the leukemia cells, largely by triggering their differentiation into more mature myeloid cells, and to rapidly arrest the DIC process, has allowed more patients to survive induction chemotherapy and achieve a complete remission (27).

The diagnosis of APL may be obvious from the morphology of the cells involved and the presence of DIC, but the diagnosis is not always apparent during the initial workup of newly diagnosed AML. Detection of the PML-RARa fusion transcript in the leukemia cells not only confirms the diagnosis, but also confers an excellent prognosis because of the high response rate to ATRA plus chemotherapy (28). APL is classically accompanied by the t(15;17), which generates the PML-RARA fusion product, as well as a RARA-PML fusion protein. There are variant molecular forms of APL, including the t(5;17), which generates the PLZF-RARA fusion transcript and protein. Identifying this translocation is of great clinical importance because patients with the t(5;17) do not respond to ATRA based therapy. APL is a disease that is quite sensitive to anthracyclines; thus, many trials have focused on giving more anthracycline therapy (both for induction and consolidation) (29) rather than more cytosine arabinoside in an attempt to adequately treat the disease without causing repeated episodes of profound cytopenias. Nonetheless, cytosine arabinoside has clinical activity in APL (30).

Studies from the larger cooperative groups such as the Eastern Cooperative Oncology Group have shown that the inclusion of ATRA in the treatment of APL, either during the induction, consolidation, or maintenance phase of treatment, leads to a significant improvement in overall survival (31). Thus, the current standard approach to APL includes ATRA as part of an induction regimen, usually with chemotherapy using a regimen first reported by an Italian Leukemia Group, followed by consolidation therapy (two to four cycles of anthracycline containing treatment), followed by intermittent ATRA therapy given for 14 days every three months (32–34).

The relapse rate from this approach is perhaps 15%. For these patients, their disease can be very effectively treated with arsenic trioxide (ATO) (35). Relapsed APL patients are usually treated with an autologous transplant if their disease becomes undetectable by PCR, or with an allogeneic transplant, if PCR positivity persists despite various salvage treatments (36).

The most dramatic (and life threatening) side effect of ATRA therapy in APL is the retinoic acid (RA) syndrome (37). This side effect tends to occur in patients with higher baseline white blood cell (WBC) counts. Patients with APL tend to have low WBC counts, but in most patients treated with ATRA, the WBC count will begin to increase with the initiation of treatment. At times, the WBC count can reach very high levels, but even in patients who have only a modest rise in WBC count, the neutrophils and other earlier myeloid cells can infiltrate the lungs and cause a capillary leak syndrome that manifests itself with pulmonary infiltrates and hypoxia, and can progress to respiratory failure. This complication can be mitigated by the use of chemotherapy, and also by the use of corticosteroids, which are given at the first sign of pulmonary involvement (reviewed in Patatanian and Thompson) (38). This syndrome appears to be due to the differentiation and death of the APL cells, as it also occurs following treatment with ATO (39). Patients who develop leukocytosis from ATO (>10,000 cells/ml) are significantly more likely to develop the RA syndrome, but among patients with leukocytosis, there is no observed relation between the leukocyte peak and the probability of developing the syndrome. Given these findings, the syndrome has been renamed the "APL differentiation syndrome."

Side effects from ATO therapy include bradycardia and conduction disturbances, including prolonged QT interval. For this reason, it is particularly important to monitor electrolyte levels in patients receiving ATO, and to maintain serum potassium and magnesium levels at the high end of the normal range. Peripheral neuropathy, hyperglycemia, and skin rash are also seen in patients receiving ATO.

TREATMENT OF MYELODYSPLASTIC SYNDROMES

Over the past four years, three different drugs have been approved by the FDA for the treatment of patients with myelodysplastic syndromes (40–42). These disorders are characterized by ineffective hematopoiesis, which most commonly manifests as a hypercellular bone marrow with peripheral blood cytopenias, but also by a variable tendency to progress to acute myelogenous leukemia (43). Patients are classified by either the French-American-British (FAB) or the WHO classification systems, and prognosis is assigned using a score based on the key variables that predict survival. The most commonly used prognostic scoring system is the International Prognostic Scoring System (IPSS), which assigns a weighted score to each the following variables: cytogenetic abnormalities, percent bone marrow blasts, and the number of cytopenias (44). Other factors not taken into account in the IPSS but captured in the WHO classifications based prognostic scoring system (WPSS) are the transfusion requirements of the patients (those who require transfusion of either red blood cells or platelets have a poorer prognosis than transfusion-independent patients), and the influence of time on the course of the disease (45). In general, these classification systems separate myelodysplastic disorders (MDS) patients into relatively low-risk and high-risk groups. Because MDS is a disease of the elderly (with a median age of 70 or so), supportive care—meaning prompt administration of antibiotics and transfusions to provide symptomatic relief—has been the mainstay of therapy. However, the landscape of treatment options for MDS patients has changed, and so have the treatment algorithms.

The clinical approach to patients with MDS should be based on (1) whether the patient has anemia only or also has significant neutropenia and/or thrombocytopenia and (2) whether the patient has increased blasts and is therefore at risk for developing acute leukemia. If only anemia is present, patients may be given an erythropoietic stimulating agent (ESA) (46), immune modulatory therapy with lenalidomide, especially for 5q-patients (40) or ATG (47), or hypomethylating agents such as 5-azacytidine (42) or decitabine

(41). Patients who do not respond to these agents may be transfused on a regular basis. Patients at with low risk transfusion-dependent MDS are at risk for iron overload and should receive iron chelation therapy, using criteria such as those endorsed by the National Comprehensive Cancer Network or other organizations (48). Patients with significant thrombocytopenia or neutropenia can be treated with hypomethylating agents; however, for the younger patient with cytopenias and "refractory anemia" (by FAB classification), ATG can be used. At times, AML-like therapy may be the most appropriate form of therapy for some patients, despite its toxicity. Patients whose disease does not respond to these measures should be considered for an allogeneic transplant. MDS patients should be treated on clinical protocols whenever possible.

Patients with increased blasts are generally given hypomethylating agents, which seem to work best in patients with more advanced forms of MDS. These patients should not be given ATG, because they do not respond, and because it triggers prolonged immunosuppression. Allogeneic transplantation should be considered early for these patients.

ACUTE LYMPHOBLASTIC LEUKEMIA (ALL)

Although ALL is the most common malignancy in children, it is relatively uncommon in adults, with about 2,000 cases per year in the United States (49). Childhood ALL is cured with modern treatment regimens (50) in approximately 80% of patients; however, only 20%–40% of adult patients are cured (50,51). This large discrepancy in outcome reflects differences in the biology of the disease, with an increased incidence of unfavorable cytogenetic subgroups in adult patients (particularly Philadelphia chromosome-positive ALL patients) (52), along with an increased incidence of comorbidities that potentially limit the use of intensive therapy in adults.

Clinical Presentation and Diagnosis

Acute leukemia manifests itself largely by its effects on normal hematopoiesis. Anemia, thrombocytopenia, and neutropenia, the result of marrow replacement by malignant cells, lead to increased fatigue, bruising or bleeding, and infection. Although a marked elevation in WBC count is the classic hallmark of leukemia, pancytopenia is also common in adult patients with ALL. Mild hepatosplenomegaly and lymphadenopathy are seen in many cases.

Classification

While the FAB classification of ALL recognized three distinct subtypes (L1–L3) based on morphology and cytochemistry, most groups now characterize ALL based on immunophenotype and genetic features. Flow cytometric analysis defines three distinct subgroups that show considerable differences in presentation, clinical course, and prognosis.

Pre-B-cell ALL represents approximately 70% of patients and is manifested by immunoglobulin gene rearrangement and expression of an early B-cell markers such as CD19. Pro-B-cell disease is a more primitive B-cell leukemia that can be distinguished from the more common pre-B-cell ALL by the expression of CD10 (common ALL antigen or CALLA). Pre-B-cell and pro-B-cell ALL cells do not express surface immunoglobulin, the hallmark of the mature B cell. Pro-B-cell disease correlates with t(4;11). Overall, this subgroup has an intermediate prognosis when treated with standard chemotherapy regimens.

T-cell ALL is the second most common subtype, occurring in 20%–30% of patients. These lymphoblasts typically express T-cell antigens, including CD7, and variably express CD2, CD5, CD1a, and CD3. TdT is frequently expressed. CD4 and CD8 are sometimes expressed and are typically co-expressed, a pattern not found in mature T cells. The disease most often affects adolescents and young adults, and there is a significant male predominance. Patients typically present with mediastinal disease and there is a high frequency of central nervous system (CNS) involvement. With modern treatment regimens, patients with T-cell ALL have the most favorable prognosis of the ALL subtypes.

Mature B-cell disease is the least common ALL subtype representing less than 5% of adult ALL. The leukemic cells can be distinguished immunophenotypically from pre-B-cell lymphoblasts by surface immunoglobulin (Ig) expression. Karyotypically, these cells demonstrate t(8;14); rarely, the alternate translocations t(2;8) and t(8;22) can be seen. Adult patients typically present with extranodal disease, with the abdomen being the most frequent site of involvement. There is often early dissemination to the bone marrow and CNS infiltration occurs in up to 20% of adult patients (53). Patients who present with significant bone marrow involvement are said to have mature B-cell ALL, while those without bone marrow infiltration are said to have Burkitt lymphoma. Traditional ALL therapy is not appropriate for these patients; instead, a treatment regimen designed specifically for Burkitt lymphoma/leukemia should be used (54,55). Using regimens designed specifically for this rare disease, approximately 50% of adults with mature B-cell ALL can achieve long-term disease-free survival (55).

Prognostic Features

In general, older age is a continuous variable associated with a worse prognosis (56). The increased frequency of unfavorable cytogenetic subgroups such as Philadelphia chromosome-positive (Ph+) ALL, t(9;22) and t(4;11) in older patients with ALL contributes to their poor prognosis. Conversely, there is an increased incidence of favorable cytogenetic subgroups such as hyperdiploidy and t(12;21) in children compared to adults. A high WBC count at diagnosis is associated with a reduced likelihood of achieving a CR and decreased overall survival. Although a variety of WBC counts have been used to assign adults to a poor risk category, the most commonly used values are greater than 20,000/μl (57) or 30,000/μl (58).

The immunophenotype of the malignant cell is another prognostic factor (59). The rapidity of the response to therapy also has a significant impact on prognosis. Patients who require more than 4 or 5 weeks to achieve a CR during induction therapy have a lower likelihood of ultimately being cured (57, 58).

Treatment of ALL

Treatment of adult ALL is typically divided into four phases: induction, consolidation, maintenance, and CNS prophylaxis. With modern intensive therapy, complete responses are observed in 65%–90% of adults; however, most patients relapse, and only 20%–40% of adults with ALL are cured of their disease (60–68).

A combination of vincristine and prednisone has been the cornerstone of induction therapy for ALL, and achieves a complete response in approximately 50% of patients. The addition of an anthracycline increases the likelihood of achieving a complete response (83% compared to 47% without the anthracycline) (69). Further intensification with cyclophosphamide or L-asparaginase is widely accepted as improving remission induction rates. Therefore, most modern induction regimens contain four drugs (vincristine, glucocorticoid, anthracycline, and cyclophosphamide or asparaginase) or five drugs (vincristine, glucocorticoid, anthracycline, cyclophosphamide, and asparaginase). It has not yet been demonstrated that one multidrug regimen is superior to another. A novel approach to ALL induction combining cytosine arabinoside, an active agent most commonly used in the consolidation phase of ALL therapy, with a single very high-dose of mitoxantrone (80 mg/m²) has been compared to a standard four-drug induction regimen. Early results have been reported in abstract form and indicate an improved frequency of CR but similar overall survival at five years for the patients who received the cytosine arabinoside and high-dose mitoxantrone induction regimen (68).

Postinduction consolidation (sometimes called intensification) involves giving a combination of drugs, usually cytosine arabinoside combined with other active agents, such as anthracyclines, alkylators, epidophillotoxins, or antimetabolites. The clinical trials investigating intensive multidrug consolidation therapy have demonstrated superior outcomes with this strategy. In a phase III trial reported by Fiere et al., patients were randomized to receive cytosine arabinoside, doxorubicin, and asparaginase as consolidation therapy or to immediately receive maintenance therapy following remission induction. The three-year disease-free survival was markedly improved in the patients who received multiagent consolidation compared to no consolidation at 38% versus 0%, respectively (70).

Prolonged maintenance therapy is a feature unique to the treatment of ALL. In pediatric patients, the value of prolonged maintenance has clearly been established and attempts to shorten the duration of maintenance to 18 months or less has resulted in a higher rate of relapse (71,72). Extending maintenance beyond three years has not been shown to be beneficial, thus two years of maintenance therapy has become standard (73). In adults with ALL, the data to support maintenance therapy is less direct. Several phase II studies in which maintenance therapy was omitted reported poor long-term results suggesting that maintenance is important (74–76). A combination of methotrexate and mercaptopurine, typically administered orally, constitute the backbone of maintenance therapy. While these drugs alone are often sufficient for pediatric patients, most adult regimens incorporate other active agents such as vincristine, prednisone, anthracyclines, and cyclophosphamide (77).

Although CNS leukemia is uncommon in adults at diagnosis (5%–10%), patients who do not receive prophylactic therapy have a cumulative CNS risk of 35% during the course of their disease (77). Risk factors for developing CNS disease include a high WBC count or an elevated LDH at initial presentation, and either T-cell or mature B-cell immunophenotype (59,78). CNS directed prophylactic therapy (intrathecal chemotherapy with or without whole brain irradiation) has been demonstrated to reduce the cumulative incidence of CNS relapse to approximately 10% (79); it is now universally recommended.

Allogeneic transplants have been used in adults with ALL. This dose-intense treatment has the ability to eradicate leukemia in a small subset of patients with disease refractory to conventional chemotherapy, and is the only potentially curative option in the relapsed setting (87). However, the lack of availability of HLA-matched donors and the mortality (20%–40%) seen with its use has limited this approach in patients with ALL in first CR.

Two large studies comparing allogeneic transplant to standard chemotherapy for patients in first CR failed to demonstrate a survival benefit for the transplant group (80,81). However, in one study a subset analysis suggested a benefit in certain high-risk patients and this has been confirmed for patients with Ph+ ALL (80). Currently, patients with Ph+ disease or t(4;11) are recommended to undergo an allogeneic transplant for ALL in first CR. Recent data suggesting that matched unrelated-donor transplantation may yield similar results to matched related-donor transplantation in adults with ALL has expanded donor availability for these patients at high risk (83). Autologous transplantation has no established role in treating patients with ALL.

Treatment of Philadelphia Chromosome–Positive ALL

The outcome of patients with Ph+ ALL is extremely poor when treated with conventional chemotherapy and five-year overall survival is less than 10%. Thus, allogeneic transplantation is currently recommended as standard therapy. Imatinib, a potent bcr-abl tyrosine kinase inhibitor, induces responses in a substantial proportion of Ph+ ALL patients, although the responses are not durable (84). While studies investigating the combination of imatinib in addition to chemotherapy in Ph+ ALL patients are ongoing, initial reports suggest that this combination results in superior outcomes when compared to historical controls (82,85,86). A high proportion of patients (50%–75%) have been able to be transplanted in first CR, the best current option for long-term survival. Durable remissions have also been observed with imatinib and chemotherapy alone without allograft, although longer follow-up is required to determine the effect on survival. The role of allogeneic transplantation in Ph+ disease for patients with the era of effective BCR-ABL inhibitors may be redefined.

Treatment of Relapsed ALL

Treatment of relapsed adult ALL is a major challenge. Because most initial treatment protocols incorporate multiple active agents with different cytotoxic mechanisms, a selection for drug resistance occurs. The complete remission rate in the salvage setting is much lower than with initial therapy, approximately 30%–40%, and the median remission duration is only six months. Salvage strategies typically include reinduction with the initial regimen in patients with late relapse or high-dose cytosine arabinoside or methotrexate in those who relapse early. Clofarabine, another effective agent, is FDA approved for treating childhood ALL; while it

induces CRs in adults as well, its role in this setting is not yet clear. If a second CR is achieved, allogeneic transplantation has resulted in long-term, disease-free survival in a small subset of patients (87). Outcomes with high-dose therapy and autologous stem cell support have been poor. Experimental approaches include treating patients with monoclonal antibodies directed against leukemia-specific antigens, novel transplantation strategies, and investigational agents that target key abnormalities such as gamma secretase inhibitors in T-cell ALL that have activating Notch mutations.

Complications of ALL Therapy

Treatment of ALL is complicated by toxicity, especially in older adults. Patients with diabetes, hypertension or heart-disease, which are common in the general population, are at increased risk for steroid-induced complications, vincristine-induced neuropathy and anthracycline-associated cardiotoxicity.

Vincristine induces cytotoxicity by binding to tubulin, resulting in microtubule depolymerization, metaphase arrest, and ultimately, apoptosis of cells. Vincristine also binds to neuronal tubulin and interferes with axonal microtubule function, leading to neurotoxicity characterized by a peripheral, symmetric, mixed sensory-motor, and autonomic polyneuropathy. Patients initially develop symmetric sensory impairment and paresthesias of the distal extremities. With continued treatment, neuritic pain and loss of deep tendon reflexes may occur followed by foot drop, wrist drop, motor dysfunction, ataxia, and paralysis. Rarely, cranial nerves are affected, resulting in hoarseness, diplopia, and facial palsies. Autonomic neurotoxicity often manifests as constipation. High doses of vincristine (>2 mg/m^2) can lead to acute, severe neurologic dysfunction leading to paralytic ileus, urinary retention, and orthostatic hypotension (88).

Anthracyclines are associated with acute and chronic cardiac toxicity (89). The susceptibility of cardiac muscle to anthracyclines remains unclear, but it appears to be due, at least in part, to the interaction of these drugs with oxygen free radicals and intracellular iron. Acute effects include nonspecific ECG changes; however, rarely a pericarditis-myocarditis syndrome can occur. More commonly, dose-dependent cardiac myopathy occurs, which leads to congestive heart failure associated with high mortality. Monitoring for the onset of cardiomyopathy with serial measurement of the left ventricular ejection fraction allows for earlier detection of subclinical cardiac toxicity. The iron chelator, Dexrazoxane provides effective cardioprotection and its use is advocated when the cumulative doxorubicin dose exceeds 300 mg/m^2.

Conclusions

Despite more than three decades of experience with various potentially curative treatment strategies in adult ALL, no single regimen yields superior results. Although there is wide variation in reported outcomes, interpretation of the literature is complicated by the differences in patient mix and the duration of follow-up of patients enrolled in studies (50). Several studies observed an apparent survival advantage for adolescents treated on pediatric regimens rather than adult regimens (90,91). These findings have led some researchers to promote more aggressive treatment, even for older adults. Risk-adapted strategies are being investigated in children. The limited success of current regimens in adults suggests that novel agents and new treatment approaches will be required to improve the outcomes for these patients.

CHRONIC LYMPHOCYTIC LEUKEMIA (CLL)

Approximately 10,000 new cases of chronic lymphocytic leukemia (CLL) are diagnosed each year in the United States (92). The median age at diagnosis is approximately 70 years, with 80% of patients diagnosed at 60 years or older (93). Although the disease course is often indolent, each year approximately 4,600 patients die from complications of CLL, most commonly from infection. There are no clearly identifiable risk factors for developing CLL, and it is the only leukemia that has not been linked with previous exposure to radiation (104). Although family members do have a slight genetic predisposition to develop CLL and other lymphoproliferative disorders, no specific genetic predisposition has been elucidated (94).

Clinical Presentation

Approximately 50% of patients with CLL are asymptomatic at presentation, and these patients are usually identified based on finding an isolated peripheral lymphocytosis on blood work for obtained for an unrelated indication (95). Constitutional symptoms such as night sweats, weight loss, and fatigue are present in 15% of patients at diagnosis (96). The most common presenting complaint is lymphadenopathy that may wax and wane. Other physical findings include splenomegaly, and less frequently, hepatomegaly. Although the lymphocyte count in CLL can often exceed 100,000/μL, patients do not typically experience symptoms from leukostasis due to the small size of the malignant lymphocytes (97).

Diagnosis

The most updated diagnostic criteria from the International Workshop on Chronic Lymphocytic Leukemia (IWCLL) requires (1) an absolute lymphocyte count of 5,000 lymphocytes/μL or greater; (2) a blood smear showing small mature lymphocytes without visible nucleoli (often with smudge cells that are characteristic of CLL); and (3) a minimal panel of cell surface markers to distinguish CLL from other B cell malignancies including CD19, CD 20, CD 23, CD 5, Fmc7, and cell-surface Ig staining, which shows light chain restriction (105). A bone marrow evaluation, while not needed for the diagnosis, is useful to determine the extent of involvement and the etiology of cytopenias.

The natural history of CLL is highly variable, but survival has been shown to correlate with clinical staging (Table 19.1) (106–108), and patients with Rai intermediate-risk disease or Binet stage B, as a group, have a median life expectancy of five to eight years. Patients with Rai low-risk disease have a life expectancy comparable to age- and sex-matched controls with traditional therapy. Other prognosis features including chromosomal abnormalities, as determined by fluorescent in-situ hybridization (FISH) (109), mutational status of the IgV gene (110), surface expression of CD38 (111), and cytoplasmic expression of ZAP70 (112). These allow patients to be placed into various prognostic groups.

Management of CLL

Conventional therapy for CLL is not curative, and there is no evidence that patients with low- or intermediate-risk disease benefit from the early initiation of therapy. Therefore, the standard of care is to treat patients when the disease is symptomatic or progressive as defined by the National Cancer Institute Working Group 1996 criteria (113); the 2008 update of these criteria is now available online (99). Criteria for therapy include B symptoms (ie, fever, chills, night sweats), obstructive adenopathy, rapidly progressive enlargement of lymph nodes or hepatosplenomegaly, development of or worsening thrombocytopenia and anemia, and a rapid lymphocyte doubling time. A high lymphocyte count in the absence of a rapid doubling time or the above features is not an indication for treatment.

Patients with low- or intermediate-risk disease (approximately 75% of patients) at diagnosis should be educated about complications of CLL including the high risk for infection, the possibility of developing a Richter's transformation, and the risk of autoimmune phenomena, specifically autoimmune hemolytic anemia and immune thrombocytopenia. They should be fol-

TABLE 19.1
Modified Rai and Binet Staging Systems for Chronic Lymphocytic Leukemia with Approximate Median Survival Data by Stage

STAGE	CLINICAL FEATURES	MEDIAN SURVIVAL (YRS)
Modified Rai Staging System		
Low Risk	Lymphocytosis in blood and bone marrow	12.5
Intermediate Risk	Enlarged lymph nodes, spleen, or liver	7.2
High Risk	Anemia or thrombocytopenia	1.6
Binet Staging System		
A	Lymphocytosis + lymphadenopathy in <3 nodal groups	>10
B	Lymphadenopathy in >3 nodal groups	5
C	Anemia or thrombocytopenia	2

lowed by clinical evaluation and complete blood count every three to six months to determine the pace of the disease and to monitor for complications. In the setting of progressive cytopenias, a bone marrow evaluation is necessary in order to distinguish immune-mediated cytopenias from progressive CLL because immune-mediated cytopenias may require different therapy than cytopenias due to progressive CLL.

Treatment is indicated for patients who have symptomatic progressive disease, bulky disease, or cytopenias. Oral chlorambucil monotherapy, which is usually well tolerated, was the standard of care for many years but rarely led to complete responses (~5%), and ultimately, patients succumbed to progressive resistant disease (114). A large, randomized, multicenter trial demonstrated that treatment with the purine analog fludarabine was superior to chlorambucil based on a higher frequency of response and longer duration of remission (114). Thus, fludarabine has formed the basis of subsequent combination studies. Combining fludarabine with corticosteroids and chlorambucil led to significant toxicity, which precluded any real improvement in response frequency (115–117). However, the use of fludarabine with cyclophosphamide and/or rituximab has shown significant activity with acceptable toxicity (118–121). The combination of a purine analog, an alkylating agent, and rituximab—fludarabine, cyclophosphamide, and rituximab (FCR) or pentostatin, cyclophosphamide, and rituximab (PCR)—results in very high overall and complete response rates when used as initial therapy; response rates are between 90% and 96%, with complete responses seen in 50%–70% of patients (121–122). Based on the observation that patients who achieve complete responses are more likely to have improved progression-free and overall survival (123) combination regimens are often given as initial therapy, even though it is not yet known whether

patients who are treated with this approach upfront will ultimately live longer.

For patients with relapsed and/or refractory CLL, the choice of salvage therapy is based on response to prior therapies. Re-treatment with combination therapies using purine analogs, alkylating agents, and rituximab can be effective, but typically is associated with lower response rates and shorter response duration than is achieved with initial therapy. In patients with purine analog refractory disease, alemtuzumab used alone or in combination with rituximab, achieves responses, but these are rarely complete or durable (124). In October 2008, Bendamustine was approved by the FDA for the treatment of CLL. It has single agent activity and has been given with rituximab alone or with mitoxantrone.

Cyclophosphamide, vincristine, and prednisone (CVP), as well as cyclophosphamide, vincristine, adriamycin, and prednisone (CHOP)-based regimens (125–126) also have activity and are often used in patients with autoimmune complications of CLL or transformed disease, respectively. However, more effective salvage strategies are needed for patients with relapsed/refractory CLL.

Traditionally, stem cell transplantation has not played a significant role in treating CLL patients because the risk of transplant-related complications was considered too high for patients who had a relatively indolent disease and a favorable prognosis or were elderly and had other comorbidities. The role of transplantation is now being reevaluated to define its curative potential in CLL.

Complications of CLL

CLL can affect both humeral and cellular immunity and some patients will relate a history of frequent infections that precede the diagnosis of CLL. Hypogammaglobulinemia is associated with an increased susceptibility to severe infections (often with encapsulated organisms), and patients with documented low levels of Ig or recurrent infections are given intravenous Ig, which has been shown to decrease the incidence of serious bacterial infections. Defective cellular immunity often becomes evident as CLL progresses and patients receive cytotoxic therapy. Patients receiving treatment with purine analogs or alemtuzumab should receive herpes virus and pneumocystis pneumoniae prophylaxis (127). All patients should be advised to obtain early and aggressive antimicrobial therapy for symptomatic infection.

Immune dysregulation in patients with CLL is associated with an increased incidence of autoimmune phenomena, such as autoimmune hemolytic anemia (AIHA), immune thrombocytopenia (ITP), and pure red cell aplasia. These can occur at any time during the disease course, and their treatment is similar to the recommended therapy for de novo autoimmune disease. While treatment for the underlying CLL may also improve blood counts, treatment with purine analogs such as fludarabine has been associated with the development or worsening of AIHA or ITP and should be used with caution in these patients. The occurrence of these autoimmune conditions should be considered when monitoring the response to therapy with these agents. Other autoimmune disorders that have been reported in association with CLL include rheumatoid arthritis, Sjögren syndrome, systemic lupus erythematosus, ulcerative colitis, bullous pemphigoid, and Grave disease (128).

Patients with CLL have an increased risk of developing additional lymphoid malignancies as well as non-hematologic second malignancies. CLL transforms into a large cell lymphoma (Richter's transformation) in between 3% and 10% of patients. More rarely, CLL can transform into prolymphocytic leukemia (with >55% circulating prolymphocytes) and is associated with progression of cytopenias, splenomegaly, and refractoriness to therapy. Second malignancies such as Hodgkin lymphoma, lung, prostate, colon, and bladder cancers are increased in patients with CLL compared to the general population, and this risk is independent of initial treatment (129–130).

CLL is a common form of adult leukemia that causes considerable morbidity and mortality in some patients. Our understanding of CLL is evolving. Newer prognostic studies still do not influence the timing or type of treatment, and indications for therapy remain disease-related symptoms or significant cytopenias. Combination therapy with purine analogs, alkylating agents, and monoclonal antibodies have improved the likelihood of achieving complete remission and overall response rates, but no clear benefits in overall survival have been shown. Current research is focused on addressing these issues, and on establishing the role of stem cell transplantation in altering the natural history of this disease.

CONCLUSIONS

Signifiant advances have been made in our treatment of (APL), MDS, ALL, CML and CLL over the Past decade Hopefully in the decede to come we will better understand the basis of these designe and have better transplant and non-transplant oopptions to treat them.

References

1. Hughes T, Deininger M, Hochhaus A, Branford S, Radich J, Kaeda J, Baccarani M, Cortes J, Cross NC, Druker BJ, Gabert J, Grimwade D, Hehlmann R, Kamel-Reid S, Lipton JH, Longtine J, Martinelli G, Saglio G, Soverini S, Stock W, Goldman JM. Monitoring CML patients responding to treatment with tyrosine kinase inhibitors: review and recommendations for harmonizing current methodology for detecting BCR-ABL transcripts and kinase domain mutations and for expressing results. *Blood*. 2006;108:28-37.
2. Deininger MW. Optimizing therapy of chronic meyloid leukemia. *Exp Hematol*. 2007;35:144-154.
3. Gale RP, Cline MJ. High remission-induction rate in acute myeloid leukaemia. *Lancet*. 1977;1:497-499.
4. Rees JK, Sandler RM, Challener J, Hayhoe FG. Treatment of acute myeloid leukaemia with a triple ctyotoxic regime: DAT. *Br J Cancer*. 1977;36:770-776.
5. Wang ZY, Chen Z. Acute promyelocytic leukemia: from highly fatal to highly curable. *Blood*. 2008;111:2505-2515.
6. Scaglioni PP, Pandolfi PP. The theory of APL revisited. *Curr Top Microbiol Immunol*. 2007;313:85-100.
7. Estey E, Dohner H. Acute myeloid leukacmia. *Lancet*. 2006;368:1894-1907.
8. Lowenberg B. Prognostic factors in acute myeloid leukaemia. *Best Pract Res Clin Haematol*. 2001;14:65-75.
9. Peterson LF, Zhang DE. Thc 8;21 translocation in leukemogenesis. *Oncogene*. 2004;23:4255-4262.
10. Nimer SD, Moore MA. Effects of the leukemia-assocaited AML1-ETO protein on hematopoietic stem and progenitor cells. *Oncogene*. 2004;23:4249-4254.
11. Huang G, Shigasada K, Ito K, Wee HJ, Yokomizo T, Ito Y. Dimerization with PEBP2beta protects RUNX1/AML1 from ubiquitin-proteasome-mediated degradation. *Embo J*. 2001;20:723-733.
12. Wang Q, Stacy T, Miller JD, Lewis AF, Gu TL, Huang X, Bushweller JH, Bories JC, Alt FW, Ryan G, Liu PP, Wynshaw-Boris A, Binder M, Marin-Padilla M, Sharpe AH, Speck NA. The CBF-beta subunit is essential for CBFalpha2 (AML1) function in vivo. *Cell*. 1996;87;697-708.
13. Bruce D. Cheson, John M. Bennett, Kenneth J. Kopecky, Thomas Büchner, Cheryl L. Willman, Elihu H. Estey, Charles A. Schiffer, Hartmut Doehner, Martin S. Tallman, T. Andrew Lister, Francesco Lo-Coco, Roel Willemze, Andrea Biondi, Wolfgang Hiddemann, Richard A. Larson, Bob Löwenberg, Miguel A. Sanz, David R. Head, Ryuzo Ohno, Clara D. Bloomfield. Revised recommendations of the International Working Group for Diagnosis, Standardization of Response Criteria, Treatment Outcomes, and Reporting Standards for Therapeutic Trials in Acute Myeloid Leukemia. *J Clin Oncol*. 2003;21:4642-4649.

14. Rowe JM. Consolidation therapy: what should be the standard of care? *Best Pract Res Clin Haematol.* 2008;21:53-60.

15. Mayer RJ, Davis RB, Schiffer CA, Berg DT, Powell BL, Schulman P, Omura GA, Moore JO, McIntyre OR, Frei E. Intensive postremission chemotherapy in adults with acute myeloid leukemia. Cancer and Leukemia Group B. *N Engl J Med.* 1994;331:896-903.

16. Reiffers J, Stoppa AM, Attal M, Michallet M, Marit G, Blaise D, Huguet F, Corront B, Cony-Makhoul P. Gastaut JA, Laurent G, Molina L, Broustet A, Maraninchi D, Pris J, Hollard D, Faberes C. Allogeneic vs autologous stem cell transplantation vs chemotherapy in patients with acute myeloid leukemia in first remission: the BGMT 87 study. *Leukemia.* 1996;10:1874-1882.

17. Burnett AK, Goldstone AH, Stevens RM, Hann IM, Rees JK, Gray RG, Wheatly K. Randomised comparison of addition of autologous bone-marrow transplantation to intensive chemotherapy for acute meyloid leukaemia in first remission: results of MRC AML 10 trial. UK Medical Research Council Adult and Children's Leukaemia Working Parties. *Lancet.* 1998;351: 700-708.

18. Zittoun RA, Mandelli F, Willemze R, de Witte T, Labar B, Resegott L, Leoni F, Damasio E, Visani G, Papa G, Caronia F, Hayat M, Stryckmans P, Rotoli B, Leoni P, Peetermans M, Dardenne M, Vegna ML, Petti MC, Solbu G, Suciu S. Autologous or allogeneic bone marrow transplantation compared with intensive chemotherapy in acute myelogenous leukemia. European Organization for Research and Treatment of Cancer (EORTC) and the Gruppo Italiano Malattie Ematologiche Maligne dell'Adulto(GIMEMA) Leukemia Cooperative Groups. *N Engl J Med.* 1995;332:217-223.

19. Cassileth PA, Harrington DP, Appelbaum FR, Lazarus HM, Rowe JM, Paietta E, Willman C, Hurd DD, Bennett JM, Blume KG, Head DR, Wiernik PH. Chemotherapy compared with autologous or allogeneic bone marrow transplantation in the management of acute myeloid leukemia transplantation in the management of acute myeloid leukemia in first remission. *N Engl J Med.* 1998;339:1649-1656.

20. Bloomfield CD, Lawrence D, Byrd JC, Carroll A, Pettenati MJ, Tantravahi R, Patil SR, Davey FR, Berg DT, Schiffer CA, Arthur DC, Mayer RJ. Frequency of prolonged remission duration after high-dose cytarabine intensification in acute myeloid leukemia varies by cytogenetic subtype. *Cancer Res.* 1998;58:4173-4179.

21. Oliansky DM, Appelbaum F, Cassileth PA, Keating A, Kerr J, Nieto Y, Stewart S, Stone RM, Tallman MS, McCarthy PL Jr, Hahn T. The role of cytotoxic therapy with hematopoietic stem cell transplantation in the therapy of acute myelogenous leukemia in adults: an evidence-based review. *Biol Blood Marrow Transplant.* 2008;14:137-180.

22. Kansu E, Sullivan KM. Late effects of hematopoietic stem cell transplantation; bone marrow transplantation. *Best Pract Res Clin Haematol.* 2007;4:209-222.

23. Holler E. Risk assessment in haematopoietic stem cell transplantation: GvHD prevention and treatment. *Best Pract Res Clin Haematol.* 2007;20:281-294.

24. Pavletic SZ, Lee SJ, Socie G, Vogelsang G. Chronic graft-versus host disease: implications of the National Institutes of Health consensu development project on criteria for clinical trials. *Bone Marrow Transplant.* 2006;38:645-651.

25. McDonald GB. Review article: management of hepatic disease following haematopoeitic cell transplant. *Ailment Pharmacol Ther.* 2006;24:441-452.

26. Tallman MS, Abutalib SA, Altman JK. The double hazard of thrombophilia and bleeding in acute promyelocytic leukemia. *Semin Thromb Hemost.* 2007;33:330-338.

27. Sanz MA. Treatment of acute promyelocytic leukemia. *Hematology Am Soc Hematol Educ Program.* 2006;147-155.

28. Reiter A, Lengfelder E. Grimwade D. Pathogenesis, diagnosis and monitoring of residual disease in acute promyelocytic leukaemia. *Acta Haematol.* 2004;112:55-67.

29. Sanz MA, Vellenga E, Rayon C, Diaz-Mediavilla J, Rivas C, Amutio E, Arias J, Deben G, Novo A, Bergua J, de la Serna J, Bueno J, Negri S, Beltran de Heredia JM, Marin G. All-trans retinoic acid and anthracycline monochemotherapy for the treatment of elderly patients with acute promyelocytic leukemia. *Blood.* 2004; 104:3490-3493

30. Ades L, Chevret S, Raffoux E, de Botton S, Guerci A, Pigneux A, Stoppa AM, Lamy T, Rigal-Huguet F, Vekhoff A, Meyer-Monard S, Maloisel F, Deconinck E, Ferrant A, Thomas X, Fegueux N, Chomienne C, Dombret H, Degos L, Fenaux P. Is cytarabine useful in the treatment of acute promyelocytic leukemia? Results of a randomized trail from the European Acute Promyelocytic Leukemia Group. *J Clin Oncol.* 2006;24:5703-5710.

31. Tallman MS, Andersen JW, Schiffer CA, Appelbaum FR, Feusner JH, Ogden A, Shepherd L, Willman C, Bloomfield CD, Rowe JM, Wiernik PH. All-transretinoic acid in acute promyelocytic leukemia. *N Engl J Med.* 1997;337:1021-1028.

32. Sanz MA, Tallman MS, Lo-Coco F. Tricks of the trade for the appropriate management of newly diagnosed acute promyelocytic leukemia. *Blood.* 2005;105:3019-3025.

33. Fenaux P, Chastang C, Chevret S, Sanz M, Dombret H, Archimbaud E, Fey M, Rayon C, Huguet F, Sotto JJ, Gardin C, Makhoul PC, Travade P, Solary E, Fegueux N, Bordessoule D, Miguel JS, Link H, Desablens B, Stamatoullas A, Deconinck E, Maloisel F, Castaigne S, Preudhomme C, Degos L. A randomized comparison of all transretinoic acid (ATRA) followed by chemotherapy and ATRA plus chemotherapy and the role of maintenance therapy in newly diagnosed acute promyelocytic leukemia. the Eruopean APL Group. *Blood.* 1999;94: 1192-1200.

34. Mandelli F, Diverio D, Avvisati G, Luciano A, Barbui T, Bernasconi C, Broccia G, Cerri R, Falda M, Fioritoni G, Leoni F, Liso V, Petti MC, Rodeghiero F, Saglio G, Vegna ML, Visani G, Jehn U, Willemze R, Muus P, Pelicci PG, Biondi A, Lo Coco F. Molecular remission in PML/RAR alpha-positive acute promyelocytic leukemia by combined all-trans retinoic acid and idarubicin (AIDA) therapy. Gruppo Italiano-Malattie Ematologiche Maligne dell'Adulto and Associazione Italiana di Ematologia ed Oncologia Pediatrica Cooperative Groups. *Blood.* 1997;90:1014-1021.

35. Soignet SL, Maslak P, Wang ZG, Jhanwar S, Calleja E, Dardashti LJ, Corso D, DeBlasio A, Gabrilove J, Scheinberg DA, Pandolfi PP, Warrell RP Jr. Complete remission after treatment of acute promyelocytic leukemia arsenic trioxide. *N Engl J Med.* 1998; 339:1341-1348.

36. de Botton S, Fawaz A, Chevret S, Dombret H, Thomas X, Sanz, M, Guerci A, San Miguel J, de la Serna J, Stoppa AM, Reman O, Stamatoulas A, Fey M, Cahn JY, Sotto JJ, Bourhis JH, Parry A, Chomienne C, Degos L, Fenaux P. Autologous and allogeneic stem-cell transplantation as salvage treatment of acute promyelocytic leukemia initially treated with alltrans-retinoic acid: a retrospective analysis of the European acute promyelocytic leukemia group. *J Clin Oncol.* 2005;23:120-126.

37. Frankel SR, Eardley A, Lauwers G, Weiss M, Warrell RP, Jr. The "retinoic acid syndrome" in acute promyelocytic leukemia. *Ann Intern Med.* 1992;117:292-296.

38. Patatanian E, Thompson DF. Retinoic acid syndrome: a review. *J Clin Pharm Ther.* 2008;33:331-338.

39. Soignet SL, Frankel SR, Douer D, Tallman MS, Kantarjian H, Calleja E, Stone RM, Kalaycio M, Scheinberg DA, Steinherz P, Sievers EL, Coutre S, Dahlberg S, Ellison R, Warrell RP Jr. United States multicenter study of arsenic trioxide in relapsed acute promyelocytic leukemia. *J Clin Oncol.* 2001;19: 3852-3860.

40. List A, Dewald G, Bennett J, Giagounidis A, Raza A, Feldman E, Powell B, Greenberg P, Thomas D, Stone R, Reeder C, Wride K, Patin J, Schmidt M, Zeldis J, Knight R; Myelodysplastic Syndrome-003 Study Investigators. Lenalidomide in the myelodysplastic syndrome with chromosome 5q deletion. *N Engl J Med.* 2006;355:1456-1465.

41. Kantarjian H, Issa JP, Rosenfeld CS, Bennett JM, Albitar M, DiPersio J, Klimek V, Slack J, de Castro C, Ravandi F, Helmer R 3rd, Shen L, Nimer SD, Leavitt R, Raza A, Saba H. Decitabine improves patient outcomes in myelodysplastic

syndromes: results of a phase III randomized study. *Cancer.* 2006;106:1794-1803.

42. Silverman LR, Demakos EP, Peterson BL, Kornblith AB, Holland JC, Odchimar-Reissig R, Stone RM, Nelson D, Powell BL, DeCastro CM, Ellerton J, Larson RA, Schiffer CA, Holland JF. Randomized controlled trail of azacitidine in patients with the myelodysplastic syndrome: a study of the cancer and leukemia group B. *J Clin Oncol.* 2002;20:2429-2440.

43. Nimer SD. Myelodysplastic syndromes. *Blood.* 2008;111: 4841-4851.

44. Greenberg P, Cox C, LeBeau MM, Fenaux P, Moral P, Sanz G, Vallespi T, Hamblin T, Oscier D, Ohyashiki K, Toyama K, Aul C, Mufti G, Bennett J. International scoring system for evaluating prognosis in myelodysplastic syndromes. *Blood.* 1997;89:2079-2088.

45. Malcovati L, Germing U, Kuendgen A, Della Porta MG, Pascutto C, Invernizzi R, Giagounidis A, Hildebrandt B, Bernasconi P, Knipp S, Strupp C, Lazzarino M, Aul C, Cazzola M. Time dependent prognostic scoring system for predicting survival and leukemic evolution in myelodysplastic syndromes. *J Clin Oncol.* 2007;25:3503-3510.

46. Hellstrom-Lindberg E, Malcovati L. Supportive care and use of hematopoietic growth factors in myelodysplastic syndromes. *Semin Hematol.* 2008;45:14-22.

47. Sloand EM, Wu CO, Greenberg P, Young N, Barrett J. Factors affecting response and survival in patients with myelodysplasia treated with immunosuppressive therapy. *J Clin Oncol.* 2008;26:2505-2511.

48. Gattermann N. Guidelines on iron chelation therapy in patients with myelodysplastic syndromes and transfusional iron overload. *Leuk Res.* 2007;31(Suppl 3):S10-S15.

49. Jemal A, Murray T, Ward E, Samuels A, Tiwari RC, Ghafoor A, Feuer EJ, Thun MJ. Cancer statistics, 2005. *CA Cancer J Clin* 2005;55:10-30.

50. Lamanna N, Weiss M. Treatment options for newly diagnosed patients with adult acute lymphoblastic leukemia. *Curr Hematol Rep* 2004;3:40-6.

51. Hoelzer D, Gokbuget N, Digel W, Faak T, Kneba M, Reutzel R, Romejko-Jarosinska J, Zwolinski J, Walewski J. Acute lymphoblastic leukemia. *Hematology (Am Soc Hematol Educ Program)* 2002:162-92.

52. Pui CH, Relling MV, Downing JR. Acute lymphoblastic leukemia. *N Engl J Med* 2004;350:1535-48.

53. Soussain C, Patte C, Ostronoff M, Delmer A, Rigal-Huguet F, Cambier N, Leprise PY, Francois S, Cony-Makhoul P, Harousseau JL. Small noncleaved cell lymphoma and leukemia in adults. A retrospective study of 65 adults treated with the LMB pediatric protocols. *Blood* 1995;85:664-74.

54. Thomas DA, Cortes J, O'Brien S, Pierce S, Faderl S, Albitar M, Hagemeister FB, Cabanillas FF, Murphy S, Keating MJ, Kantarjian H. Hyper-CVAD program in Burkitt's-type adult acute lymphoblastic leukemia. *J Clin Oncol* 1999;17:2461-70.

55. Lee EJ, Petroni GR, Schiffer CA, Freter CE, Johnson JL, Barcos M, Frizzera G, Bloomfield CD, Peterson BA. Brief-duration high-intensity chemotherapy for patients with small noncleaved-cell lymphoma or FAB L3 acute lymphocytic leukemia: results of cancer and leukemia group B study 9251. *J Clin Oncol* 2001;19:4014-22.

56. Ohno R. Current progress in the treatment of adult acute leukemia in Japan. *Jpn J Clin Oncol* 1993;23:85-97.

57. Gaynor J, Chapman D, Little C, McKenzie S, Miller W, Andreeff M, Zalmen A, Berman E, Kempin S, Gee, T, Clarkson B. A cause-specific hazard rate analysis of prognostic factors among 199 adults with acute lymphoblastic leukemia: the Memorial Hospital experience since 1969. *J Clin Oncol* 1988;6:1014-30.

58. D Hoelzer, E Thiel, H Loffler, T Buchner, A Ganser, G Heil, P Koch, M Freund, H Diedrich and H Ruhl. Prognostic factors in a multicenter study for treatment of acute lymphoblastic leukemia in adults. *Blood* 1988;71:123-31.

59. C Boucheix, B David, C Sebban, E Racadot, MC Bene, A Bernard, L Campos, H Jouault, F, Sigaux and E Lepage. Immunophenotype of adult acute lymphoblastic leukemia, clinical

parameters, and outcome: an analysis of a prospective trial including 562 tested patients (LALA87). French Group on Therapy for Adult Acute Lymphoblastic Leukemia. *Blood* 1994;84:1603-12.

60. Schauer P, Arlin ZA, Mertelsmann R, Cirrincione C, Friedman A, Gee TS, Dowling M, Kempin S, Straus DJ, Koziner B, McKenzie S, Thaler HT, Dufour P, Little C, Dellaquila C, Ellis S, Clarkson B. Treatment of acute lymphoblastic leukemia in adults: results of the L-10 and L-10M protocols. *J Clin Oncol* 1983;1:462-70.

61. Hoelzer D, Thiel E, Loffler H, Bodenstein H, Plaumann L, Buchner T, Ubanitz D, Kock P, Heimpel H, Engelhardt R. Intensified therapy in acute lymphoblastic and acute undifferentiated leukemia in adults. *Blood* 1984;64:38-47.

62. **This article does not exist**

63. Linker C, Damon L, Ries C, Navarro W. Intensified and shortened cyclical chemotherapy for adult acute lymphoblastic leukemia. *J Clin Oncol* 2002;20:2464-71.

64. Larson RA, Dodge RK, Burns CP, Lee EJ, Stone RM, Schulman P, Duggan D, Davey FR, Sobol RE, Frankel SR. A five-drug remission induction regimen with intensive consolidation for adults with acute lymphoblastic leukemia: cancer and leukemia group B study 8811. *Blood* 1995;85:2025-37.

65. Thomas X, Danaila C, Le QH, Sebban C, Troncy J, Charrin C, Lheritier V, Michallet M, Magaud JP, Fiere D. Long-term follow-up of patients with newly diagnosed adult acute lymphoblastic leukemia: a single institution experience of 378 consecutive patients over a 21-year period. *Leukemia* 2001;15:1811-22.

66. Annino L, Vegna ML, Camera A, Specchia G, Visani G, Fioritoni G, Ferrara F, Peta A, Ciolli S, Deplano W, Fabbiano F, Sica S, Di Raimondo F, Cascavilla N, Tabilio A, Leoni P, Invernizzi R, Baccarani M, Rotoli B, Amadori S, Mandelli F; GIMEMA Group. Treatment of adult acute lymphoblastic leukemia (ALL): long-term follow-up of the GIMEMA ALL 0288 randomized study. *Blood* 2002;99:863-71.

67. Takeuchi J, Kyo T, Naito K, Sao H, Takahashi M, Miyawaki S, Kuriyama K, Ohtake S, Yagasaki F, Murakami H, Asou N, Ino T, Okamoto T, Usui N, Nishimura M, Shinagawa K, Fukushima T, Taguchi H, Morii T, Mizuta S, Akiyama H, Nakamura Y, Ohshima T, Ohno R. Induction therapy by frequent administration of doxorubicin with four other drugs, followed by intensive consolidation and maintenance therapy for adult acute lymphoblastic leukemia: the JALSG-ALL93 study. *Leukemia* 2002;16:1259-66.

68. Weiss M.A., Heffner L, Lamanna N, Kataycio M, Schiller G, Coutre S, Maslak P, Jurcic J, Panageas K, Scheinberg D.A.. A randomized trial of cytoarabine with high-dose mitoxantrone compared to a standard vincristine/prednisone-based regimen as induction therapy for adult patients with ALL. *Journal of Clinical Oncology.* 2005; 23:6516.

69. Gottlieb AJ, Weinberg V, Ellison RR, Henderson ES, Terebelo H, Rafia S, Cuttner J, Silver RT, Carey RW, Levy RN. Efficacy of daunorubicin in the therapy of adult acute lymphocytic leukemia: a prospective randomized trial by cancer and leukemia group B. *Blood* 1984;64:267-74.

70. Fiere D, Extra JM, David B, Witz F, Vernand JP, Gastaut JA, Dauriac C, Pris J, Marty M. Treatment of 218 adult acute lymphoblastic leukemias. *Semin Oncol* 1987;14:64-6.

71. Toyoda Y, Manabe A, Tsuchida M, Hanada R, Ikuta K, Okimoto Y, Ohara A, Ohkawa Y, Mori T, Ishimoto K, Sato T, Kaneko T, Maeda M, Koike K, Shitara T, Hoshi Y, Hosoya R, Tsunematsu Y, Bessho F, Nakazawa S, Saito T. Six months of maintenance chemotherapy after intensified treatment for acute lymphoblastic leukemia of childhood. *J Clin Oncol* 2000;18:1508-16.

72. Schrappe M, Reiter A, Zimmermann M, Harbott J, Ludwig WD, Henze G, Gadner H, Odenwald E, Riehm H. Long-term results of four consecutive trials in childhood ALL performed by the ALL-BFM study group from 1981 to 1995. Berlin-Frankfurt-Munster. *Leukemia* 2000;14:2205-22.

73. Duration and intensity of maintenance chemotherapy in acute lymphoblastic leukaemia: overview of 42 trials involving 12 000

randomised children. Childhood ALL Collaborative Group. Lancet 1996;347:1783-8.

74. Cassileth PA, Andersen JW, Bennett JM, Hoagland HC, Mazza JJ, O'Connell MC, Paietta E, Wiernik P. Adult acute lymphocytic leukemia: the Eastern Cooperative Oncology Group experience. Leukemia 1992;6 Suppl 2:178-81.

75. Cuttner J, Mick R, Budman DR, Mayer RJ, Lee EJ, Henderson ES, Weiss RB, Paciucci PA, Sobol R, Davey F, Bloomfield C, Schiffer C. Phase III trial of brief intensive treatment of adult acute lymphocytic leukemia comparing daunorubicin and mitoxantrone: a CALGB Study. Leukemia 1991;5:425-31.

76. Dekker AW, van't Veer MB, Sizoo W, Haak HL, van der Lelie J, Ossenkoppele G, Huijgens PC, Schouten HC, Sonneveld Wellemze R, Verdonck LF, van Putten WL, Lowenberg B. Intensive postremission chemotherapy without maintenance therapy in adults with acute lymphoblastic leukemia. Dutch Hemato-Oncology Research Group. J Clin Oncol 1997;15:476-82.

77. Scheinberg DA MP, Weiss M. Acute Leukemias. 7th ed. Philadelphia: Lipincott Williams and Wilkins; 2004.

78. Kantarjian HM, Walters RS, Smith TL, Keating MJ, Barlogie B, McCredie KB, Freireich EJ. Identification of risk groups for development of central nervous system leukemia in adults with acute lymphocytic leukemia. Blood 1988;72:1784-9.

79. Omura GA, Moffitt S, Vogler WR, Salter MM. Combination chemotherapy of adult acute lymphoblastic leukemia with randomized central nervous system prophylaxis. Blood 1980;55:199-204.

80. Sebban C, Lepage E, Vernant JP, Gluckman E, Attal M, Reiffers J, Sulton L, Racadat E, Michallet M, Maraninchi D, Dreyfus F, Fiere D. Sebban C, Lepage E, Vernant JP, et al. Allogeneic bone marrow transplantation in adult acute lymphoblastic leukemia in first complete remission: a comparative study. French Group of Therapy of Adult Acute Lymphoblastic Leukemia. J Clin Oncol 1994;12:2580-7.

81. Zhang MJ, Hoelzer D, Horowitz MM, Gale RP, Messerer D, Klein JP, Loffler H, Sobocinski KA, Thiel E, Weisdorf DJ. Long-term follow-up of adults with acute lymphoblastic leukemia in first remission treated with chemotherapy or bone marrow transplantation. The Acute Lymphoblastic Leukemia Working Committee. Ann Intern Med 1995;123:428-31.

82. Thomas X, Boiron JM, Huguet F, Dombret H, Bradstock K, Vey N, Kovacsovics T, Delannoy A, Fegueux N, Fenaux P, Stamatoullas A, Vernant JP, Tournilhac O, Buzyn A, Reman O, Charrin C, Boucheix C, Gabert J, Lhéritier V, Fiere D Outcome of treatment in adults with acute lymphoblastic leukemia: analysis of the LALA-94 trial. *J Clin Oncol.* 2004; 22: 4075-86.

83. Kiehl MG, Kraut L, Schwerdtfeger R, Hertenstein B, Remberger M, Kroeger N, Stelljes M, Bornhaeuser M, Martin H, Scheid C, Ganser A, Zander AR, Kienast J, Ehninger G, Hoelzer D. Diehl V, Fauser AA, Ringden O. Outcome of allogeneic hematopoietic stem-cell transplantation in adult patients with acute lymphoblastic leukemia: no difference in related compared with unrelated transplant in first complete remission. J Clin Oncol 2004;22:2816-25.

84. Ottmann OG, Druker BJ, Sawyers CL, Goldman JM, Reiffers J, Silver RT, Tura S, Fischer T, Deininger MW, Schiffer CA, Baccarani M, Gratwohl A, Hochhaus A, Hoelzer D, Fernandes-Reese S, Gathmann I, Capdeville R, O'Brian SG. A phase 2 study of imatinib in patients with relapsed or refractory Philadelphia chromosome-positive acute lymphoid leukemias. Blood 2002;100:1965-71.

85. Yanada M, Tekeuchi J, Sugiura I, Akiyama H, Usui N, Yagasaki F, Kobayashi T, Ueda Y, Takeuchi M, Miyawaki S, Maruta A, Emi N, Miyazaki Y, Ohtake S, Jinnai I, Matsuo K, Naoe T, Ohno R, Japan Adult Leukemia Study Group. High complete remission rate and promising outcome by combination of imatinib and chemotherapy for newly diagnosed BCR-ABL-positive acute lymphoblastic leukemia: a phase II study by the Japan Adult Leukemia Study Group. J Clin Oncol 2006; 24:460-6.

86. Lee KH, Lee JH, Choi SJ, Lee JH, Seol M, Lee YS, Kim WK, Lee JS, Seo EJ, Jang S, Park CJ, Chi HS. Clinical effect of imatinib added to intensive combination chemotherapy for newly diag-nosed Philadelphia chromosome-positive acute lymphoblastic leukemia. Leukemia 2005;19:1509-16.

87. Doney K, Fisher LD, Appelbaum FR, Buckner CD, Storb R, Singer J, Fefer A, Anasetti C, Beatty P, Bensinger W, Clift R, Hansen J, Hill R, Loughran TP Jr, Martin P, Petersen FB, Sanders J, Sullivan KM, Stewart P, Weiden P, Witherspoon R, Thomas ED. Treatment of adult acute lymphoblastic leukemia with allogeneic bone marrow transplantation. Multivariate analysis of factors affecting acute graft-versus-host disease, relapse, and relapse-free survival. Bone marrow transplantation 1991;7:453-9.

88. Haim N, Epelbaum R, Ben-Shahar M, Yarnitsky D, Simri W, Robinson E. Full dose vincristine (without 2-mg dose limit) in the treatment of lymphomas. Cancer 1994;73:2515-9.

89. Barry E, Alvarez JA, Scully RE, Miller TL, Lipshultz SE. Anthracycline-induced cardiotoxicity: course, pathophysiology, prevention and management. Expert Opin Pharmacother 2007;8:1039-58.

90. Boissel N, Auclerc MF, Lheritier V, Perel Y, Thomas X, Leblanc T, Rousselot P, Cayuela JM, Gabert J, Fegueux N, Piguet C, Huguet-Rigal F, Berthou C, Boiron JM, Pautas C, Michel G, Fiere D, Leverger G, Dombret H, Baruchel A. Should adolescents with acute lymphoblastic leukemia be treated as old children or young adults? Comparison of the French FRALLE-93 and LALA-94 trials. J Clin Oncol 2003;21:774-80.

91. de Bont JM, Holt B, Dekker AW, van der Does-van den Berg A, Sonneveld P, Pieters R. Significant difference in outcome for adolescents with acute lymphoblastic leukemia treated on pediatric vs adult protocols in the Netherlands. Leukemia 2004;18:2032-5.

92. Jemal A, Siegel R, Ward E, Murray T, Xu J, Smigal C, Thun MJ. Cancer statistics, 2006. CA Cancer J Clin 2006;56:106-30.

93. Jaffe ES HN, Stein H, Vardiman JW, editors. World Health Organization classification of tumours. Pathology and genetics of tumours of hematopoeitic and lymphoid tissues. Lyon (France): IARC Press; 2001.

94. Goldin LR, Pfeiffer RM, Li X, Hemminki K. Familial risk of lymphoproliferative tumors in families of patients with chronic lymphocytic leukemia: results from the Swedish Family-Cancer Database. Blood 2004;104:1850-4.

95. Molica S, Levato D. What is changing in the natural history of chronic lymphocytic leukemia? Haematologica 2001;86:8-12.

96. Pangalis GA, Vassilakopoulos TP, Dimopoulou MN, Siakantaris MP, Kontopidou FN, Angelopoulou MK. B-chronic lymphocytic leukemia: practical aspects. Hematol Oncol 2002;20:103-46.

97. Cukierman T, Gatt ME, Libster D, Goldschmidt N, Matzner Y. Chronic lymphocytic leukemia presenting with extreme hyper-leukocytosis and thrombosis of the common femoral vein. Leukemia & lymphoma 2002;43:1865-8.

98. Kantarjian HM, O'Brian S, Smith TL, Cortes J, Giles FJ, Beran M, Peirce S, Huh Y, Andreeff M, Koller C, Ha CS, Keating MJ, Murphy S, Freireich EJ. Results of treatment with hyper-CVAD, a dose-intensive regimen, in adult acute lymphocytic leukemia. *J Clin Oncol.* 2000; 18: 547-561.

99. Hallek M, Cheson BD, Catovsky D, Caligaris-Cappio F, Dighiero G, Dohner H, Hillmen P, Keating MJ, Montserrat E, Rai KR, Kipps TJ; International Workshop on Chronic Lymphocytic Leukemia. Guidelines for the diagnosis and treatment of chronic lymphocytic leukemia: a report from the International Workshop on Chronic Lymphocytic Leukemia updating the National Cancer Institute-Working Group 1996 guidelines. *Blood.* 2008; 111: 5446-5456.

100. Group CAC. Duration and intensity of maintenance chemotherapy in acute lymphoblastic leukaemia: Overview of 42 trials involving 12,000 randomized children. *Lancet.* 1996; 347: 1783-1788.

101. Scheinberg DA MP, Weiss M. *Acute Leukemias.* Philadelphia: Lipincott-Raven; 2005.

102. Sandherr M, Einsele H, Hebart H, Kahl C, Kern W, Kiehl M, Massenkeil G, Penack O, Schiel X, Schuettrumpf S, Ullmann AJ, Cornely OA; Infectious Diseases Working Party, German Society for Hematology and Oncology. Antiviral prophy-

laxis in patients with haematological malignancies and solid tumours: Guidelines of the Infectious Diseases Working Party (AGIHO) of the German Society for Hematology and Oncology (DGHO). *Ann Oncol.* 2006; 17: 1051-1059.

103. Hamblin TJ. Autoimmune complications of chronic lymphocytic leukemia. *Semin Oncol.* 2006; 33: 230-239.

104. Preston DL, Kusumi S, Tomonaga M, Izumi S, Ron E, Kuramoto A, Kamuda N, Dohy H, Matsui T, Nonaka H, Thompson DE, Soda M, Mabuchi K. Cancer incidence in atomic bomb survivors. Part III. Leukemia, lymphoma and multiple myeloma, 1950-1987. Radiat Res 1994;137:S68-97.

105. Diehl LF, Karnell LH, Menck HR. The American College of Surgeons Commission on Cancer and the American Cancer Society. The National Cancer Data Base report on age, gender, treatment, and outcomes of patients with chronic lymphocytic leukemia. Cancer 1999;86:2684-92.

106. Rai KR, Sawitsky A, Cronkite EP, Chanana AD, Levy RN, Pasternack BS. Clinical staging of chronic lymphocytic leukemia. Blood 1975;46:219-34.

107. Binet JL, Auquier A, Dighiero G, Chastang C, Piguet H, Goasguen J, Vaugier G, Potron G, Colona P, Oberling F, Thomas M, Tchernia G, Jacquillat C, Boivin P, Lesty C, Duault MT, Monconduit M, Belabbes S, Gremy F. A new prognostic classification of chronic lymphocytic leukemia derived from a multivariate survival analysis. Cancer 1981;48:198-206.

108. Rai: K. A critical analysis of staging in CLL, in Gale RP, Rai KR (eds): Chronic Lymphocytic Leukemia. Recent Progress and Future Direction. . New York, NY: Liss; 1987.

109. Dohner H, Stilgenbauer S, Benner A, Leupolt E, Krober A, Bullinger L, Dohner K, Bentz M, Lichter P. Genomic aberrations and survival in chronic lymphocytic leukemia. The New England journal of medicine 2000;343:1910-6.

110. Hamblin TJ, Davis Z, Gardiner A, Oscier DG, Stevenson FK. Unmutated Ig V(H) genes are associated with a more aggressive form of chronic lymphocytic leukemia. Blood 1999;94:1848-54.

111. Damle RN, Wasil T, Fais F, Ghiotto F, Valetto A, Allen SL, Buchbinder A, Budman D, Dittmar K, Kolitz J, Lichtman SM, Schulman P, Vinciguerra VP, Rai KR, Ferrarini M, Chiorazzi N. Ig V gene mutation status and CD38 expression as novel prognostic indicators in chronic lymphocytic leukemia. Blood 1999;94:1840-7.

112. Crespo M, Bosch F, Villamor N, Bellosillo B, Colomer D, Rozman M, Marcé S, López-Guillermo A, Campo E, Montserrat E.. ZAP-70 expression as a surrogate for immunoglobulin-variable-region mutations in chronic lymphocytic leukemia. The New England journal of medicine 2003;348:1764-75.

113. Cheson BD, Bennett JM, Grever M, Kay N, Keating MJ, O'Brian S, Rai KR. National Cancer Institute-sponsored Working Group guidelines for chronic lymphocytic leukemia: revised guidelines for diagnosis and treatment. Blood 1996;87:4990-7.

114. Rai KR, Peterson BL, Appelbaum FR, Kolitz J, Elias L, Shepherd L, Hines J, Threatte GA, Larson RA, Cheson BD, Schiffer CA . Fludarabine compared with chlorambucil as primary therapy for chronic lymphocytic leukemia. The New England journal of medicine 2000;343:1750-7.

115. O'Brien S, Kantarjian H, Beran M, Smith T, Koller C, Estey E, Robertson LE, Lerner S, Keating M. Results of fludarabine and prednisone therapy in 264 patients with chronic lymphocytic leukemia with multivariate analysis-derived prognostic model for response to treatment. Blood 1993;82:1695-700.

116. Elias L, Stock-Novack D, Head DR, Grever MR, Weick JK, Chapman RA, Godwin JE, Metz EN, Appelbaum FR. A phase I trial of combination fludarabine monophosphate and chlorambucil in chronic lymphocytic leukemia: a Southwest Oncology Group study. Leukemia 1993;7:361-5.

117. Weiss M, Spiess T, Berman E, Kempin S. Concomitant administration of chlorambucil limits dose intensity of fludarabine in previously treated patients with chronic lymphocytic leukemia. Leukemia 1994;8:1290-3.

118. Flinn IW, Byrd JC, Morrison C, Jamison J, Diehl LF, Murphy T, Piantadosi S, Seifter E, Ambinder RF, Vogelsang G, Grever MR. Fludarabine and cyclophosphamide with filgrastim support in patients with previously untreated indolent lymphoid malignancies. Blood 2000;96:71-5.

119. Byrd JC, Peterson BL, Morrison VA, Park K, Jacobson R, Hoke E, Vardiman JW, Rai K, Schiffer CA, Larson RA. Randomized phase 2 study of fludarabine with concurrent versus sequential treatment with rituximab in symptomatic, untreated patients with B-cell chronic lymphocytic leukemia: results from Cancer and Leukemia Group B 9712 (CALGB 9712). Blood 2003;101:6-14.

120. Wierda W, O'Brien S, Wen S, Faderl S, Garcia-Manero G, Thomas D, Do KA, Cortes Jk, Koller C, Beran M, Ferrajoli A, Giles F, Lerner S, Albitar M, Kantarjian H, Keating M. Chemoimmunotherapy with fludarabine, cyclophosphamide, and rituximab for relapsed and refractory chronic lymphocytic leukemia. J Clin Oncol 2005;23:4070-8.

121. Keating MJ, O'Brien S, Albitar M, Lerner S, Plunkett W, Giles F, Andreeff M, Cortes J, Faderl S, Thomas D, Koller C, Wierda W, Detry MA, Lynn A, Kantarjian H. Early results of a chemoimmunotherapy regimen of fludarabine, cyclophosphamide, and rituximab as initial therapy for chronic lymphocytic leukemia. J Clin Oncol 2005;23:4079-88.

122. Kay NE, Geyer SM, Call TG, Shanafelt TD, Zent CS, Jelinek DF, Tschumper R, Bone ND, Dewald GW, Lin TS, Heerema NA, Smith L, Grever MR, Byrd JC. Combination chemoimmunotherapy with pentostatin, cyclophosphamide, and rituximab shows significant clinical activity with low accompanying toxicity in previously untreated B chronic lymphocytic leukemia. Blood 2007;109:405-11.

123. Keating MJ, O'Brien S, Lerner S, Koller C, Beran M, Robertson LE, Freireich EJ, Estey E, Kantarjian H. Long-term follow-up of patients with chronic lymphocytic leukemia (CLL) receiving fludarabine regimens as initial therapy. Blood 1998;92:1165-71.

124. Faderl S, Thomas DA, O'Brien S, Garcia-Manero G, Kantarjian HM, Giles FJ, Koller C, Ferrajoli A, Verstovsek S, Pro B, Andreeff M, Beran M, Cortes J, Wierda W, Tran N, Keating MJ. Experience with alemtuzumab plus rituximab in patients with relapsed and refractory lymphoid malignancies. Blood 2003;101:3413-5.

125. Chemotherapeutic options in chronic lymphocytic leukemia: a meta-analysis of the randomized trials. CLL Trialists' Collaborative Group. J Natl Cancer Inst 1999;91:861-8.

126. Leporrier M, Chevret S, Cazin B, Boudjerra N, Feugier P, Desablens B, Rapp MJ, Jaubert J, Autrand C, Divine M, Dreyfus B, Maloum K, Travade P, Dighiero G, Binet JL, Chastang C; French Cooperative Group on Chronic Lymphocytic Leukemia. Randomized comparison of fludarabine, CAP, and ChOP in 938 previously untreated stage B and C chronic lymphocytic leukemia patients. Blood 2001;98:2319-25.

127. Sandherr M, Einsele H, Hebart H, Kahl C, Kern W, Kiehl M, Massenkeil G, Penack O, Schiel X, Schuettrumpf S, Ullmann AJ, Cornely OA; Infectious Diseases Working Party, German Soceity for Hematology and Oncology. Antiviral prophylaxis in patients with haematological malignancies and solid tumours: Guidelines of the Infectious Diseases Working Party (AGIHO) of the German Society for Hematology and Oncology (DGHO). Ann Oncol 2006;17:1051-9.

128. Hamblin TJ. Autoimmune complications of chronic lymphocytic leukemia. Seminars in oncology 2006;33:230-9.

129. Hisada M, Biggar RJ, Greene MH, Fraumeni JF, Jr., Travis LB. Solid tumors after chronic lymphocytic leukemia. Blood 2001;98:1979-81.

130. Kyasa MJ, Hazlett L, Parrish RS, Schichman SA, Zent CS. Veterans with chronic lymphocytic leukemia/small lymphocytic lymphoma (CLL/SLL) have a markedly increased rate of second malignancy, which is the most common cause of death. Leukemia & lymphoma 2004;45:507-13.

131. Doney K, Fisher LD, Appelbaum FR, et al. Treatment of adult acute

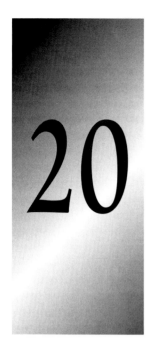

Evaluation and Treatment of Primary Central Nervous System Tumors

Sean A. Grimm
Lisa M. DeAngelis

Primary central nervous system (CNS) tumors encompass a heterogenous mix of histologies and sites of origin. Table 20.1 lists primary CNS tumors based on the World Health Organization (WHO) Classification. In this chapter, we will limit discussion to the presentation (Table 20.2), diagnosis, and treatment (Table 20.3) of the most common brain tumors: gliomas, meningiomas, and primary central nervous system lymphoma (PCNSL).

EPIDEMIOLOGY

Data concerning the incidence of primary CNS tumors are available from the American Cancer Society (ACS) and the Central Brain Tumor Registry of the United States (CBTRUS). Malignant tumors (excluding PCNSL) represented 1.4% of all CNS cancers diagnosed in 2007, but were projected to be the cause of death in 2.3% of all cancers (1). The incidence of brain tumors in 2006 was 20 cases per 100,000 adults (2). In adult men aged 20–39 years, CNS tumors were the second leading cause of death in 1998, 1999, 2001, and 2002, and the leading cause of death in 2000. The prevalence of CNS tumors in 2000 was: malignant 29.5 per 100,000; benign 97.5 per 100,000; and uncertain behavior 3.8 per 100,000 (3).

The most common types are gliomas (40% of all tumors and 78% of malignant tumors) and meningiomas (30% of all tumors) (2). Risk factors for the development of CNS tumors include ionizing radiation (4,5), familial syndromes (6), and immunosuppression (for PCNSL) (7).

CLINICAL PRESENTATION

CNS tumors can present with localized or generalized neurological dysfunction. Generalized symptoms and signs include headaches, seizures, and personality changes. Localized findings include focal weakness, sensory symptoms, gait ataxia, visual changes, or language dysfunction. Table 20.2 lists the relative frequency of each presenting symptom for the brain tumors discussed in this chapter. The neuro-anatomical location of the tumor determines the presenting symptoms and signs.

Contrary to popular perception, headache as the sole presenting symptom is rare. According to one prospective study of patients newly diagnosed with a brain tumor, isolated headache was the presenting symptom in only 8% (8). When associated with other symptoms or signs, headaches occurred at presentation in 37%–62% (9). Concurrent nausea, vomiting, an abnormal neurological examination, or significant change in a prior headache pattern, suggest a structural abnormality that warrants further investigation (10).

Seizures are the presenting symptom in 15%–30% of patients with a brain tumor (11). The location and histologic grade of a tumor correlate with seizure risk. Low-grade, slow growing tumors, and those located in

TABLE 20.1

World Health Organization Classification of Tumors of the Central Nervous System

Tumors of Neuroepithelial Tissue
Astrocytic tumors
    Astrocytoma
    Anaplastic astrocytoma
    Glioblastoma multiforme
    Pilocytic astrocytoma
    Subependymal giant-cell astrocytoma
Oligodendroglial tumors
    Oligodendroglioma
    Anaplastic oligodendroglioma
Mixed gliomas
    Oligoastrocytoma
    Anaplastic oligoastrocytoma
Ependymal tumors
    Ependymoma
    Anaplastic ependymoma
    Myxopapillary ependymoma
    Subependymoma
Choroid-plexus tumors
    Choroid-plexus papilloma
    Choroid-plexus carcinoma
Neuronal and mixed neuronal-glial tumors
    Gangliocytoma
    Dysembryoplastic neurepithelial tumor
    Ganglioglioma
    Anaplastic ganglioglioma
    Central neurocytoma
Pineal parenchymal tumors
    Pineocytoma
    Pineoblastoma
Embryonal tumors
    Medulloblastoma
    Primitive neuroectodermal tumor
Meningeal tumors
    Meningioma
    Hemangiopericytoma
    Melanocytic tumor
    Hemangioblastoma
Primary central nervous system lymphoma
Germ cell tumors
    Germinoma
    Embryonal carcinoma
    Yolk-sac tumor (endodermal-sinus tumor)
    Choriocarcinoma
    Teratoma
    Mixed germ-cell tumors
Tumors of the sellar region
    Pituitary adenoma
    Pituitary carcinoma
    Craniopharyngioma
Metastatic tumors

TABLE 20.2

Symptoms and Signs at Presentation

SYMPTOM	HIGH-GRADE GLIOMA	LOW-GRADE GLIOMA	PCNSL	MENINGIOMA
Seizures	++	+++	+	+++
Focal neurological dysfunction (eg, hemiparesis, visual field cut, hemisensory loss, aphasia)	+++	+	++	+
Cognitive/ behavioral changes	++	-	+++	+

the gray matter, are associated with the highest risk. Seizures are usually of focal onset, although secondary generalization often occurs. The clinical manifestation of focal seizures varies widely and is sometimes bizarre, but examples include isolated limb movements, tonic posturing, sensory symptoms, unpleasant smell, alteration of consciousness, déjà vu, or a sensation of fear.

DIAGNOSIS

In a patient suspected of harboring a CNS tumor, magnetic resonance imaging (MRI) scan with intravenous (I.V.) contrast is the preferred and only diagnostic test necessary. Head computerized tomography (CT) scan and non-contrast MRI are not adequate for a full evaluation, but CT must suffice for those unable to undergo an MRI (eg, patients who have a pacemaker). A normal contrast enhanced brain MRI essentially excludes a diagnosis of brain tumor. Once a tumor is identified, surgical biopsy or resection is necessary for histologic diagnosis because imaging characteristics are not definitive. Occasionally, positron emission tomography (PET) imaging, MR perfusion, or MR spectroscopy (MRS) are used to guide surgical biopsy to the most potentially malignant region of the tumor.

GLIOMAS

The gliomas are a morphologically and biologically heterogeneous group of primary CNS tumors that arise from neuroepithelial tissue. They are divided into two main histologic subgroups, astrocytoma and oligo-dendroglioma, and some tumors have mixed features that include both histologies. Both types can be low or high grade. High-grade tumors arise from previously low-grade lesions (secondary) or de novo (primary). Even though the low-grade tumors can be slow growing, most neuro-oncologists do not consider them benign because of diffuse infiltration of normal brain and confinement within the bony calvarium, limiting space for growth. In time (months to years), virtually all low-grade tumors will develop biologic characteristics and histologic features of aggressive gliomas. Although an individual tumor can have areas of low-grade and high-grade pathology, treatment is dictated by the highest grade identified. The third subgroup of gliomas, ependymoma, is less common and will not be discussed in this chapter.

Even when astrocytomas and oligodendrogliomas appear as discrete masses on neuroimaging, surgical cure usually is not possible because of diffuse microscopic infiltration of normal brain tissue. The most common classification and grading system used by neuropathologists is the WHO scheme, which grades gliomas based on nuclear atypia, mitosis, microvascular proliferation, and necrosis (12). The high-grade tumors are anaplastic astrocytoma, anaplastic oligodendroglioma, anaplastic oligoastrocytoma, and glioblastoma multiforme (GBM).

Astrocytic Tumors

Astrocytes are star-shaped supporting cells of the brain and spinal cord. In addition to forming a key component of the blood-brain barrier via their foot processes, they are thought to play an active role in creating and maintaining the microenvironment for neurons. The process by which an astrocyte transforms into a neoplastic cell is unknown, although several genetic abnormalities have been identified. Histologically, tumors of astrocytic origin can be identified by staining for glial fibrillary acidic protein (GFAP), a cytoplasmic fibrillary protein characteristic of astrocytes.

Glioblastoma Multiforme (GBM)

GBM (WHO grade IV) is thought to arise from astrocytes or their precursors (because GFAP can be identified in the cell cytoplasm), although the tumor cells are usually undifferentiated and have a bizarre morphology. It is the most common malignant primary brain tumor, and has a very poor prognosis; despite best treatment, most patients will not survive one year. Cures are rare and overall survival rates at two and

three years are 26% and 5%, respectively, in highly selected patients receiving the best treatment (13,14). The annual incidence in the United States is approximately 13,000 cases, making it the second most common primary brain tumor, representing 20% of all intracranial tumors. It is a tumor of the elderly, with a median age at onset of 64 years (2), although children and young adults are also affected.

GBM is usually localized to the cerebral hemispheres and presents with symptoms of increased intracranial pressure and focal neurological dysfunction. Seizures occur, but with less frequency than in low-grade tumors. On MRI (Fig. 20.1), the tumor appears as a heterogeneous contrast enhancing mass, with associated edema and mass effect. There is often a central area of necrosis, surrounded by a rim of contrast enhancement. The lesion is hypointense on T1- and hyperintense on T2-weighted sequences. The tumor often grows along white matter tracts and can cross the corpus callosum leading to the classic "butterfly" appearance. Although the MRI appearance may be characteristic, tissue diagnosis is essential. The surgical goal is to remove as much tumor as possible, although sometimes only a stereotactic biopsy is feasible when the tumor involves critical brain structures.

Grossly, the tumor appears as a necrotic, yellowish mass that diffusely infiltrates the normal brain. Microscopic features include increased cellularity, pleomorphism, atypia, mitoses, pseudo-palisading necrosis, and microvascular proliferation. Necrosis and vascular hyperplasia are the characteristic features that distinguish GBM from anaplastic astrocytoma.

Prognostic variables include age, extent of resection, performance status, and treatment. Although not curative, neurosurgery is the initial treatment modality. The goals of surgical resection are to improve patient function by decreasing mass effect and edema and to decrease the tumor volume to optimize the effectiveness of radiotherapy and chemotherapy (Table 20.3).

Following surgery, the standard of care is focal radiotherapy to a total dose of 60 Gy in combination with temozolomide (Temodar) chemotherapy (75 mg/m^2 daily during radiation), followed by 6–18 cycles of adjuvant temozolomide (150–200 mg/m^2 on a 5/28 day schedule). This treatment regimen is based on a phase III cooperative trial published by Stupp et al. in 2005, which was the first to demonstrate improved overall survival for GBM treated with radiotherapy plus chemotherapy versus radiotherapy alone (14). Patients in this study were randomized to radiotherapy alone (total dose of 60 Gy given as 2 Gy fractions, five days per week over six weeks) or concomitant daily temozolomide (75 mg/m^2/day) with standard radiotherapy followed

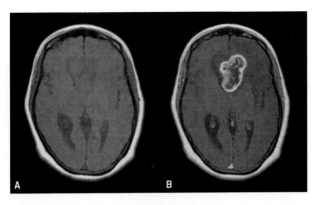

FIGURE 20.1

Glioblastoma multiforme. T1-weighted MRI pre- (A) and post- (B) contrast displaying a heterogeneous enhancing mass with associated edema and mass effect. Note the central area of necrosis, surrounded by a rim of contrast enhancement.

TABLE 20.3
Brain Tumor Initial Treatment

Low-Grade Glioma
　Maximal tumor resection and/or follow without treatment
　Focal radiotherapy
　Temozolomide for oligodendrogliomas
Anaplastic Astrocytoma, Anaplastic Oligoastrocytoma
　Maximal surgical resection
　Focal radiotherapy +/- concurrent temozolomide
　Adjuvant temozolomide chemotherapy
Glioblastoma Multiforme
　Maximal surgical resection
　Focal radiotherapy + concurrent temozolomide
　Adjuvant temozolomide
Primary Central Nervous System Lymphoma
　Methotrexate-based chemotherapy
　Whole brain radiotherapy
Meningioma
　Surgical resection
　Focal radiotherapy
　Stereotactic radiosurgery

---

extends survival about four to six months on average. Patients are not eligible for additional radiation treatment, and approved chemotherapeutic options are few. Active research is being conducted to discover and test promising agents. The current trend favors targeting specific cellular pathways thought to be important in tumor proliferation and survival. One example is the vascular endothelial growth factor (VEGF) pathway, which is important in tumor neovascularization. VEGF overproduction is commonly observed in gliomas, and the supporting vasculature is rich in VEGF receptors. A recent small phase II trial combined bevacizumab, an anti-VEGF antibody, with the cytotoxic agent irinotecan in patients with recurrent malignant gliomas. The authors of this study reported an impressive radiographic response in 63% of patients, a six-month progression-free survival probability of 38%, and six-month overall survival probability of 72% (15). Whether these results will be reproduced in larger trials remains to be seen.

Anaplastic Astrocytoma (AA) and Anaplastic Oligoastrocytoma

Anaplastic astrocytoma (WHO grade III astrocytoma) is a malignant tumor with a median survival of less than three years from diagnosis and estimated five-year survival of 28% despite best treatment (2). It is usually localized to the cerebral hemispheres and presents with seizures, symptoms of increased intracranial pressure and focal neurological dysfunction. The median age of onset is 41 years (16).

On MRI, the tumor presents as an ill-defined T1 hypointense and T2/FLAIR hyperintense mass. Heterogeneous contrast enhancement is usually present, although up to one-third of tumors may not enhance (17). PET imaging, MRS, and MRI with perfusion may assist in making a diagnosis but do not take the place of histology. Resection is advantageous therapeutically and diagnostically because a stereotactic biopsy may not be representative of the entire tumor.

Histologically, AAs are characterized by increased cellularity, nuclear atypia, marked mitotic activity, and microvascular proliferation. Although not curative, maximal resection is a positive prognostic factor. It reduces the mass effect responsible for neurological symptoms and the tumor burden for the subsequent chemotherapy and RT.

Standard treatment for AA consists of maximal surgical resection followed by focal radiotherapy. The standard radiotherapy approach is to treat the tumor bed and a surrounding margin to a total dose of 60 Gy in fractions. Higher doses and hyperfractionated/accelerated schedules have not shown benefit. The role of adjuvant chemotherapy in AAs is

by six cycles of adjuvant temozolomide (150–200 mg/m²/day on days 1–5 every 28 days). The important prognostic factors were equally balanced between the two groups. The group receiving chemoradiotherapy experienced significantly improved survival compared to the group receiving radiation therapy (RT) alone (median of 14.6 versus 12.1 months), with two-year survival rates of 26% and 10%, respectively.

At recurrence or progression, treatment options are limited. Re-resection can be helpful and probably controversial. Based on the large randomized trial in GBM, many neuro-oncologists treat AA patients with concurrent temozolomide chemotherapy and RT followed by adjuvant temozolomide chemotherapy. This practice has not been studied in randomized trials for AA. At recurrence, temozolomide has shown efficacy in AA that was treated initially with radiotherapy alone (18). Other options at recurrence include carmustine (BiCNU) or enrollment on an experimental protocol.

Astrocytoma

Diffuse fibrillary astrocytoma (WHO grade II) is the most common low-grade astrocytoma and should be distinguished from the more benign pilocytic astrocytoma (WHO grade I) and pleomorphic xanthoastrocytoma (WHO grade II). The discussion in this section is limited to fibrillary astrocytoma. Fibrillary astrocytomas can originate anywhere in the CNS, but show a preference for the white matter of the cerebral hemispheres. Mean age at diagnosis is 35–40 years, and only a small percentage of patients are younger than 19 years or older than 65 (19). Seizures occur in approximately 80% of patients, and are the most common presenting symptom (20–22). Other, less common presentations include focal neurological deficits and mental changes. Presentation with symptoms and signs of raised intracranial pressure (headache, vomiting, and papilledema) is rare.

On MRI (Fig. 20.2), low-grade astrocytomas are usually hyperintense on T2/FLAIR and hypointense on T1 sequences. Upon administration of I.V. contrast, there is usually no to little enhancement, and the presence of contrast enhancement is a poor prognostic factor (20,22). Because astrocytomas are highly infiltrative, tumor always extends beyond the abnormality observed on neuroimaging.

Fluorodeoxyglucose or methionine PET imaging, MRS, and MR perfusion assist in assessing tumor grade, but histopathology is necessary for diagnosis. Tissue can be obtained via craniotomy or stereotactic biopsy, although maximal resection is preferable if the lesion can be removed safely. Stereotactic biopsies may be confounded by sampling error and may miss regions of high-grade tumor intermixed with low-grade areas. In contrast, a resection provides more tissue for analysis, may treat focal neurological symptoms and seizures, and may prolong survival.

Grossly, the tumor is slightly discolored yellow or grey, with indistinct margins from normal brain. Under the microscope, there is increased cellularity compared to normal brain tissue with mild to moderate nuclear pleomorphism and no evidence of mitotic activity, vascular proliferative changes, or necrosis.

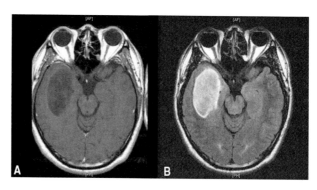

FIGURE 20.2

Astrocytoma. T1-weighted MRI post contrast (A) and FLAIR (B) sequence displaying a nonenhancing lesion in the right temporal lobe. Note that there is minimal mass effect or edema.

The type and timing of treatment for low-grade astrocytoma is controversial. The clinical course is difficult to predict, because tumor progression is highly variable among patients. Furthermore, studies are difficult to interpret because they are mostly retrospective in nature and include variable proportions of low-grade glioma subgroups.

RT is the most effective nonsurgical treatment, although the appropriate timing of its use has not been established. A large prospective study has shown that early radiotherapy prolongs progression-free survival but has no effect on overall survival, compared to reserving radiotherapy until disease progression. Clinically, it is difficult to predict whether early disease progression or the side effects of radiotherapy cause more disability to an individual patient. Consequently, some neuro-oncologists recommend treating early, while others advocate close monitoring, reserving treatment for disease progression.

Traditionally, chemotherapy has played a limited role in the treatment of low-grade astrocytoma because of the slow tumor growth rate. Since temozolomide has been shown efficacious in high-grade gliomas, enthusiasm for its use in low-grade gliomas has increased. To date, there are no good prospective trials to support its use, although it is the first choice for recurrent low-grade astrocytoma after radiotherapy.

Low-grade gliomas in patients aged 45 years or older tend to be biologically aggressive and often require immediate treatment consisting of maximum tumor resection followed by radiotherapy. Aggressive treatment may also be recommended for younger patients with medically intractable seizures, symptoms of increased intracranial pressure, or focal neurological deficits. Younger patients whose seizures are well controlled with anticonvulsant medications and who are neurologically normal may be followed closely and treatment held until there is clinical or radiographic progression. However, progression is often associated with transformation to a higher grade glioma.

The range of survival times for low-grade astrocytoma is large and unpredictable; some patients die early and others live for more than a decade. Most patients will die from their brain tumor once it progresses to a high-grade malignant glioma.

Oligodendroglioma

Oligodendroglioma makes up the other prominent category of glial cell tumors. Its cell of origin, the oligodendrocyte, is the glial cell that myelinates CNS axons. Oligodendroglioma is classified as low (WHO grade II) or high (anaplastic oligodendroglioma, WHO grade III) grade. They are less common than the astrocytic tumors, comprising only 3.7% of all primary brain tumors (2).

The oligodendrogliomas are usually supratentorial, arising in the frontal lobes. They also arise primarily in the white matter, but tend to infiltrate the cortex more than astrocytomas of similar grade. Diffuse infiltration of normal brain usually prohibits surgical cure.

On neuroimaging (Fig. 20.3), oligodendrogliomas cannot be distinguished from astrocytomas. Characteristically, the tumor is usually hypointense on T1- and hyperintense on T2-weighted sequences. The low-grade tumors typically do not enhance post-contrast, although the anaplastic tumors do. Contrast enhancement was a poor prognostic factor in several series. Oligodendrogliomas may be heavily calcified, which is often best appreciated on CT scan. MRS and PET imaging can help differentiate low-grade from high-grade lesions, although only histology is definitive.

On gross pathology, they appear similar to astrocytomas, although calcification is a more frequent find-

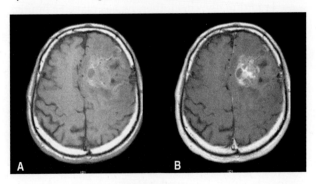

FIGURE 20.3

Anaplastic oligodendroglioma. T1-weighted MRI pre- (A) and post- (B) contrast displaying an enhancing lesion in the left frontal lobe. Note the hyperintense signal on the pre-contrast image consistent with hemorrhage or calcification, both of which are common findings in oligodendroglial tumors.

ing. Microscopically, the tumor cells have a classic "fried egg" appearance—uniform basophilic cells with cleared cytoplasm (perinuclear halos), distinct cell borders, and small bland hyperchromatic nuclei (23). Delicately branching vessels ("chicken wire" pattern) and microcalcifications are also common. Anaplastic oligodendrogliomas are characterized by high mitotic activity and microvascular proliferation.

Both low-grade and high-grade oligodendroglioma may show loss of heterozygosity for chromosomes (LOH) 1p and 19q. This genetic feature may predict a favorable response to chemotherapy or treatment in general. It is considered a positive prognostic factor and should be tested in all oligodendroglioma patients.

Low-Grade Oligodendroglioma

Low-grade oligodendroglioma presents most commonly as a focal seizure in a young adult (median age of onset is 41 years) (2). Because they grow more slowly than astrocytic tumors, there is often a prolonged period of symptoms (usually focal seizures) prior to diagnosis. Before modern neuroimaging, there are a few isolated case reports of patients experiencing seizures for decades, prior to a diagnosis of tumor. Presentation with focal neurological symptoms, such as hemiparesis or hemisensory symptoms occurs, although with lower frequency.

Young age, extent of resection, seizures as initial presenting symptom, high functional status, and presence of 1p and 19q LOH are all positive prognostic factors. In one study, patients diagnosed at younger than age 30 years had a 10-year survival of 75%, whereas those older than 50 years had a 10-year survival of 21%.

Treatment of low-grade oligodendrogliomas follows a paradigm similar to low-grade astrocytic tumors. If located in an accessible brain region, maximal resection is recommended. Asymptomatic patients or those with controlled focal seizures can be followed closely after surgery. Resection specimens should be sent for chromosomal analysis for prognostic considerations.

If the tumor is not resectable and the patient is asymptomatic (except for medically controlled seizures) a PET scan and MRS should be performed. If these confirm a low-grade tumor, the patient can be followed closely as above. If the patient is symptomatic, a biopsy or debulking should be performed followed by chemotherapy with temozolomide or radiotherapy. Oligodendroglioma, particularly associated with 1p and 19q LOH, often shows marked shrinkage of tumor and resolution of symptoms following chemotherapy. If chemotherapy fails, conformal radiotherapy to a total dose of 54 Gy is administered.

At recurrence, patients are treated with surgery if feasible, followed by RT (if not previously administered) and/or chemotherapy. Over time, low-grade oligodendrogliomas transform to anaplastic oligodendrogliomas, which is the cause of death in most patients.

Median overall survival is 16 years and not influenced by the sequence of chemotherapy or radiotherapy.

Anaplastic Oligodendroglioma

Anaplastic oligodendrogliomas present more commonly with focal neurological symptoms and signs than their low-grade counterparts. Seizures occur, but are often associated with hemiparesis, cognitive change, or hemisensory loss. The median age at diagnosis is 48 years (2) and median survival is three to five years (24,25).

Treatment of anaplastic oligodendroglioma is similar to AA. Like low-grade oligodendroglioma, 1p and 19q analysis may predict response to chemotherapy. Following maximal resection, patients are usually treated with conformal radiotherapy and adjuvant chemotherapy. The combination of procarbazine (Matulane), vincristine (Oncovin), and lomustine (CeeNU) in a regimen designated PCV is the only regimen that has been studied in prospective phase III trials of newly diagnosed patients (26,27). The addition of chemotherapy significantly prolongs progression-free survival but had no effect on overall survival. Because of the significant toxicity associated with PCV, most clinicians now use temozolomide, which is much better tolerated. The optimal number of chemotherapy cycles has not been established, but 6–18 cycles of adjuvant temozolomide are often used. Because oligodendroglioma can be exquisitely sensitive to chemotherapy, experimental protocols are underway to study treatment strategies using upfront chemotherapy and deferring radiotherapy. At recurrence, chemotherapeutic options include PCV, carboplatin, cisplatin, and carmustine. The 10-year survival rate is 29.6% (2).

MENINGIOMA

The term *meningioma* was coined by Harvey Cushing in 1922 to describe a tumor proximal to the meninges. Meningiomas are intracranial tumors that are thought to arise from the meningothelial arachnoid cap cells of the meninges. The overwhelming majority are benign, slow-growing tumors that compress the underlying brain but rarely invade it. They often invoke an osteoblastic response in surrounding bone, producing hyperostosis, which can be observed on head CT.

Meningiomas are the most common intracranial tumor, representing 30% (population-based studies) to 40% (autopsy studies) of all cases. They are diagnosed most often in late middle age; the median age is

64 years (2). Women (3:2 to 2:1) and African Americans predominate. Meningiomas are rare in children, accounting for less than 2% of pediatric brain tumors. Genetic predisposition (neurofibromatosis type 2) and prior exposure to ionizing radiation are the only definite predisposing risk factors. Sex hormones, history of breast cancer, and trauma have been proposed as risk factors, but evidence is incomplete.

Grossly, meningiomas are lobulated tumors with a rubbery consistency. When benign, they separate easily from brain tissue, although they can invade the sinuses and encase the cerebral arteries making surgical resection difficult. The tumor can penetrate the bone and present as a scalp mass. Growth patterns include a flat en plaque mass, infiltrating substantial portions of the meninges or, as a spherical mass lesion.

Microscopically, there is a wide range of benign pathologies (eg, meningothelial, fibrous, transitional, secretory, etc.), but most of the histologic subtypes do not have a clinical significance. In contrast, atypical (WHO grade 2), and anaplastic (WHO grade 3) meningiomas are aggressive tumors. Meningioma grading is based primarily on the mitotic count. High-grade meningiomas frequently invade the brain and can rarely metastasize (mostly to liver or bone).

Although there are a variety of presentations depending on tumor location, focal seizures and neurological deficits from brain or cranial nerve compression are most common. Other presenting symptoms and signs include anosmia, hemianopsia, cranial nerve dysfunction (II, III, IV, V, and VI), nuchal or suboccipital pain, tongue atrophy, monoparesis, behavioral change, urinary incontinence, and hearing loss.

MRI (Fig. 20.4) is the preferred neuroimaging test. Because meningiomas do not lie behind the blood-brain

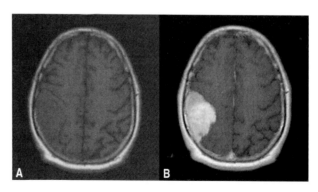

FIGURE 20.4

Meningioma. T1-weighted MRI pre- (A) and post- (B) contrast display an intensely enhancing mass in the right parietal region. Note that the lesion appears isointense prior to contrast administration, a differentiating feature from hemorrhage and metastasis, which are usually hyperintense and hypointense respectively.

barrier, they demonstrate intense, homogenous contrast enhancement, often with an enhancing dural tail. Meningiomas are usually hyperintense on T2 and isointense on T1-weighted imaging (a differentiating feature from metastases, hemorrhage, and schwannoma).

The differential diagnosis for a dural-based mass includes meningioma, lymphoma, metastases (commonly breast and prostate), myeloma, hematoma, inflammatory lesion (sarcoid, syphilis, or granulomatous infection), hemangiopericytoma, and hemangioblastoma.

If a patient is asymptomatic or has medically controlled seizures, meningiomas can be followed closely. If treatment is indicated, surgery is the mainstay and can be curative if the entire tumor is removed. In patients with unresectable tumors, conformal RT is the primary treatment modality. It is used following surgery in all instances of anaplastic meningioma, even if total resection was achieved. Radiosurgery is another option for recurrent benign, atypical, or anaplastic meningioma 3 cm or less in diameter.

There is no established chemotherapy for meningiomas. Isolated reports suggest that hydroxyurea, tamoxifen (Nolvadex), doxorubicin (Adriamycin), interferon-α, and mifepristone (RU486) may have efficacy in some patients.

Survival is widely variable and influenced by meningioma location and grade. In most patients, the tumor will not be the cause of their death.

PRIMARY CENTRAL NERVOUS SYSTEM LYMPHOMA (PCNSL)

PCNSL is a non-Hodgkin lymphoma that arises within and is restricted to the CNS (brain, spinal cord, meninges, and eye). It should be distinguished from metastatic systemic lymphoma because treatment differs. PCNSL occurs in two distinct patient populations—immunocompromised (HIV, transplant, etc.) and immunocompetent. The discussion in this chapter is limited to the immunocompetent group. During the period 1998–2002, PCNSL represented 3% of all primary brain tumors (2). The incidence rate increased more than 10-fold between 1973 and 1992 in presumably immunocompetent patients (28). Immunodeficiency is the only known risk factor; one study reported a 3,600-fold higher incidence rate in HIV patients than in the general population (29). Although prognosis is poor for most patients, survival has also improved in the last decade. The tumor is usually exquisitely sensitive to chemotherapy and radiation and approximately 20%–30% of patients may be cured with current strategies.

PCNSL is predominately a diffuse large B-cell (CD20+) tumor that is indistinguishable from high-grade, non-Hodgkin lymphoma occurring elsewhere in the body. Microscopically, there is a multifocal, angiocentric pattern of growth. As these areas of perivascular lymphocytes become confluent, a solid mass is formed. The diagnosis can be confused with an inflammatory process since a large number of reactive T-lymphocytes may coexist within the tumor, or a glioma, when a prominent astrocytic or microglial response accompanies the tumor.

The median age at diagnosis is 60 years (2). PCNSL appears multifocal on neuroimaging in 30% and predominately involves the frontal lobes, corpus callosum, and deep periventricular brain structures. As a consequence of this deep localization, cognitive impairment or behavioral changes are the most common presenting features; seizures are rare. Other symptoms include headache, hemiparesis, and hemisensory loss. Symptoms often progress over weeks to months before a diagnosis is made. Patients do not experience the classic "B" symptoms such as fever, night sweats, and weight loss associated with systemic lymphoma; therefore, the presence of these symptoms should prompt a careful investigation for systemic disease.

On MRI (Fig. 20.5), PCNSL is hypointense on T1 and hypo- to iso-intense on T2/FLAIR sequences, with

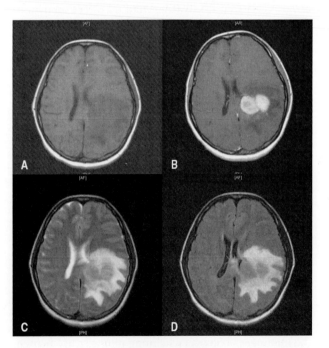

FIGURE 20.5

Primary central nervous system lymphoma. MRI, displaying T1 hypointense (A) a homogenously enhancing mass (B) in the deep left parietal lobe with associated edema and mass effect. The lesion is hypointense on T2 (C) and FLAIR (D) weighted sequences, a differentiating feature from glioma.

variable surrounding edema. There is usually homogenous enhancement with IV contrast. Ring enhancement is uncommon, except in immunocompromised patients. The appearance on T2 sequences and lack of central necrosis help to differentiate PCNSL from glioma.

Even with a "classic" MRI appearance, histology is essential for diagnosis. At presentation, corticosteroids should not be administered unless absolutely necessary (eg, impending brain herniation). With steroid treatment, PCNSL can transiently disappear (due to apoptosis), delaying diagnosis. In a patient suspected of harboring PCNSL, stereotactic needle biopsy is the best approach because, unlike other primary brain tumors, extensive resection does not improve survival.

Once a diagnosis of CNS lymphoma has been established, an extent-of-disease evaluation should be performed. At diagnosis, ocular and spinal fluid involvement are present in 20% and 25% of patients, respectively. Current staging recommendations include an enhanced cranial MRI, lumbar puncture for cytology, slit lamp examination (to look for ocular lymphoma), enhanced spine MRI (if spinal symptoms are present), HIV serology, body CT scan, and bone marrow biopsy to look for systemic lymphoma (30). Body PET may uncover a systemic site not appreciated by conventional imaging.

As previously mentioned, corticosteroids can decrease edema and induce apoptosis of lymphoid cells. There is a complete resolution of tumor in 15% and greater than 50% shrinkage in 25% of patients after dexamethasone administration and before use of definitive therapy. Eventually, the disease recurs despite continued steroids, usually within a few months. Without more definitive treatment, rapid tumor growth usually occurs, and median survival is three to four months.

PCNSL is exquisitely sensitive to radiotherapy and chemotherapy. In contrast to the gliomas, whole brain radiotherapy (WBRT) is more effective than focal radiotherapy because of the extensive infiltration of the disease throughout the brain. The optimal dose is 40–50 Gy, and there is no benefit of adding a boost to the tumor site (31,32). With WBRT alone, median survival is 12–18 months and the five-year survival rate is only 4%.

The standard systemic lymphoma chemotherapeutic regimens are ineffective for PCNSL. Four prospective trials failed to show any advantage of cyclophosphamide-doxorubicin-vincristine-prednisone (CHOP) or the modified regimen with dexamethasone instead of prednisone (CHOD) plus WBRT over WBRT alone (33–35). High-dose systemic methotrexate is the most effective and widely used drug. It is the only agent that has demonstrated significant advantage over WBRT alone. Protocols utilizing this agent have reported median survivals of 30–60 months (36). To achieve

sufficient drug concentrations in the CNS by overcoming the blood-brain barrier, IV methotrexate must be administered at a high-dose with a rapid infusion.

A median overall survival of 60 months was achieved in a prospective trial utilizing a regimen of five cycles of IV methotrexate 3.5 gm/m², vincristine, procarbazine (Matulane), and intrathecal methotrexate, followed by WBRT 45 Gy, and consolidation therapy with I.V. cytarabine (Cytosar) (37). With this treatment protocol, 87% of patients achieved a complete response. Unfortunately, the response is often short-lived with an approximately 50% relapse rate and a high incidence of treatment-related delayed neurotoxicity.

Neurotoxicity after PCNSL treatment is characterized by dementia, ataxia, and urinary incontinence occurring at a mean of seven months from diagnosis. Both methotrexate and radiotherapy can cause this syndrome, and the combination is synergistic. The risk is greatest in patients aged 60 years or older at diagnosis and when methotrexate is administered concurrently or following radiotherapy. In the trial mentioned above, patients 60 years or younger had a 100% incidence of neurotoxicity at 24 months, while those younger than 60 years had a 30% incidence at 96 months (37). On MRI (Fig. 20.6), treatment-related neurotoxicity is characterized by confluent periventricular T2/FLAIR hyperintensity and enlarged ventricles. There is no effective treatment for this complication, although some patients may benefit from ventriculoperitoneal

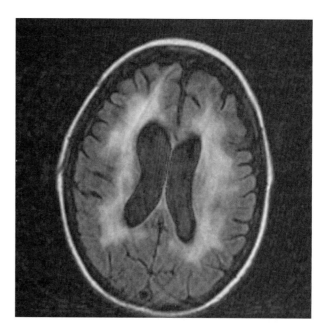

FIGURE 20.6

Leukoencephalopathy. MRI. FLAIR sequence displaying confluent periventricular white matter hyperintensity and large lateral ventricles.

shunt placement, even though intracranial pressure is not elevated; the situation is comparable to normal pressure hydrocephalus.

Recent work has focused on treatment strategies that reduce relapse risk and prevent neurotoxicity. In one PCNSL trial, withholding radiotherapy in patients aged 60 years and older did not worsen survival, eliminated treatment-related neurotoxicity but resulted in a higher relapse rate (41% vs 17%) (38). In 2008, studies investigated whether high-dose chemotherapy with autologous stem cell transplant can be a substitute for radiotherapy, and if lower dose WBRT can reduce the relapse rate without causing neurotoxicity. Rituximab (Rituxin), a monoclonal antibody to the CD-20 receptor of B-cells, is also being studied as an addition to methotrexate-based protocols.

More than 50% of patients who achieve a remission will eventually relapse. At recurrence, patients should undergo a repeat extent of disease evaluation. Chemotherapeutic options at relapse include a re-trial of high dose methotrexate, temozolomide, topotecan (Hycamtin), or the three drug regimen of procarbazine, vincristine, and lomustine. Some patients have an excellent response and prolonged survival to salvage therapy, but most will eventually die of tumor progression.

References

1. Jemal A, Siegel R, Ward E, Murray T, Xu J, Thun MJ. Cancer statistics, 2007. *CA Cancer J Clin.* 2007;57(1):43–66.
2. CBTUS. *Statistical Report: Primary Brain Tumors in the United States, 1998–2002.* Published by the Central Brain Tumor Registry of the United States; 2005.
3. Davis FG, Kupelian V, Freels S, McCarthy B, Surawicz T. Prevalence estimates for primary brain tumors in the United States by behavior and major histology groups. *Neurooncology.* 2001;3(3):152–158.
4. Amirjamshidi A, Abbassioun K. Radiation-induced tumors of the central nervous system occurring in childhood and adolescence. Four unusual lesions in three patients and a review of the literature. *Childs Nerv Syst.* 2000;16(7):390–397.
5. Ron E, Modan B, Boice JD, Jr., et al. Tumors of the brain and nervous system after radiotherapy in childhood. *N Engl J Med.* 1988;319(16):1033–1039.
6. Bondy M, Wiencke J, Wrensch M, Kyritsis AP. Genetics of primary brain tumors: a review. *J Neurooncology.* 1994;18(1):69–81.
7. Schabet M. Epidemiology of primary CNS lymphoma. *J Neurooncology.* 1999;43(3):199–201.
8. Vázquez-Barquero A, Ibáñez FJ, Herrera S, Izquierdo JM, Berciano J, Pascual J. Isolated headache as the presenting clinical manifestation of intracranial tumors: a prospective study. *Cephalalgia.* 1994;14(4):270–272.
9. Purdy RA, Kirby S. Headaches and brain tumors. *Neurol Clin.* 2004;22(1):39–53.
10. Forsyth PA, Posner JB. Headaches in patients with brain tumors: a study of 111 patients. *Neurology.* 1993;43(9):1678–1683.
11. Sperling MR, Ko J. Seizures and brain tumors. *Semin Oncol.* 2006;33(3):333–341.
12. Kleihues P, Cavenee WK. *International Agency for Research on Cancer. International Society of Neuropathology. Pathology and genetics of tumours of the nervous system.* Lyon: International Agency for Research on Cancer; 1998.
13. Scott JN, Rewcastle NB, Brasher PM, et al. Which glioblastoma multiforme patient will become a long-term survivor? A population-based study. *Ann Neurol.* 1999;46(2):183–188.
14. Stupp R, Mason WP, van den Bent MJ, et al. Radiotherapy plus concomitant and adjuvant temozolomide for glioblastoma. *N Engl J Med.* 2005;352(10):987–996.
15. Vredenburgh JJ, Desjardins A, Herndon JE, et al. Phase II trial of bevacizumab and irinotecan in recurrent malignant glioma. *Clin Cancer Res.* 2007;13(4):1253–1259.
16. See SJ, Gilbert MR.Anaplastic astrocytoma: diagnosis, prognosis, and management. *Semin Oncol.* 2004;31(5):618–634.
17. Henson JW, Gaviani P, Gonzalez RG. MRI in treatment of adult gliomas. *Lancet Oncol.* 2005;6(3):167–175.
18. Yung WK, Prados MD, Yaya-Tur R, et al. Multicenter phase II trial of temozolomide in patients with anaplastic astrocytoma or anaplastic oligoastrocytoma at first relapse. Temodal Brain Tumor Group. *J Clin Oncol.* 1999;17(9):2762–2771.
19. Wessels PH, Weber WEJ, Raven G, Ramaekers FCS, Hopman AHN, Twijnstra A. Supratentorial grade II astrocytoma: biological features and clinical course. *Lancet Neurol.* 2003;2(7):395–403.
20. Kreth FW, Faist M, Rossner R, Volk B, Ostertag CB. Supratentorial World Health Organization Grade 2 astrocytomas and oligoastrocytomas. A new pattern of prognostic factors. *Cancer.* 1997;79(2):370–379.
21. Leighton C, Fisher B, Bauman G, et al. Supratentorial low-grade glioma in adults: an analysis of prognostic factors and timing of radiation. *J Clin Oncol.* 1997;15(4):1294–1301.
22. Lote K, Egeland T, Hager B, et al. Survival, prognostic factors, and therapeutic efficacy in low-grade glioma: a retrospective study in 379 patients. *J Clin Oncol.* 1997;15(9):3129–3140.
23. Bruner JM. Neuropathology of malignant gliomas. *Semin Oncol.* 1994;21(2):126–138.
24. Cairncross G, Seiferheld W, Shaw E, et al. An intergroup randomized controlled trial (RCT) of chemotherapy plus radiation (RT) versus RT alone for pure and mixed anaplastic oligodendrogliomas: Initial report of RTOG 94-02. In: ASCO; 2004. *J Clin Oncol.* 2004;107S.
25. van den Bent MJ, Chinot O, Boogerd W, et al. Second-line chemotherapy with temozolomide in recurrent oligodendroglioma after PCV (procarbazine, lomustine and vincristine) chemotherapy: EORTC Brain Tumor Group phase II study 26972. *Ann Oncol.* 2003;14(4):599–602.
26. Cairncross G, Macdonald D, Ludwin S, et al. Chemotherapy for anaplastic oligodendroglioma. National Cancer Institute of Canada Clinical Trials Group. *J Clin Oncol.* 1994;12(10):2013–2021.
27. van den Bent MJ, Carpentier AF, Brandes AA, et al. Adjuvant procarbazine, lomustine, and vincristine improves progression-free survival but not overall survival in newly diagnosed anaplastic oligodendrogliomas and oligoastrocytomas: a randomized European Organisation for Research and Treatment of Cancer phase III trial. *J Clin Oncol.* 2006;24(18):2715–2722.
28. Corn BW, Marcus SM, Topham A, Hauck W, Curran WJ, Jr. Will primary central nervous system lymphoma be the most frequent brain tumor diagnosed in the year 2000? *Cancer.* 1997;79(12):2409–2413.
29. Coté TR, Manns AA, Hardy CR, Yellin FJ, Hartge P. Epidemiology of brain lymphoma among people with or without acquired immunodeficiency syndrome. AIDS/Cancer Study Group. *J Natl Cancer Inst.* 1996;88(10):675–679.
30. Abrey LE, Batchelor TT, Ferreri AJ, et al. Report of an international workshop to standardize baseline evaluation and response criteria for primary CNS lymphoma. *J Clin Oncol.* 2005;23(22):5034–5043.
31. DeAngelis LM, Yahalom J, Thaler HT, Kher U. Combined modality therapy for primary CNS lymphoma. *J Clin Oncol.* 1992;10(4):635–643.
32. Nelson DF, Martz KL, Bonner H, et al. Non-Hodgkin's lymphoma of the brain: can high dose, large volume radiation therapy improve survival? Report on a prospective trial by the

Radiation Therapy Oncology Group (RTOG): RTOG 8315. *Int J Radiat Oncol Biol Phys.* 1992;23(1):9–17.

33. Lachance DH, Brizel DM, Gockerman JP, et al. Cyclophosphamide, doxorubicin, vincristine, and prednisone for primary central nervous system lymphoma: short-duration response and multifocal intracerebral recurrence preceding radiotherapy. *Neurology.* 1994;44(9):1721–1727.

34. Schultz C, Scott C, Sherman W, et al. Preirradiation chemotherapy with cyclophosphamide, doxorubicin, vincristine, and dexamethasone for primary CNS lymphomas: initial report of radiation therapy oncology group protocol 88-06. *J Clin Oncol.* 1996;14(2):556–564.

35. Shibamoto Y, Tsutsui K, Dodo Y, Yamabe H, Shima N, Abe M. Improved survival rate in primary intracranial lymphoma treated by high-dose radiation and systemic vincristine-doxorubicin-cyclophosphamide-prednisolone chemotherapy. *Cancer.* 1990;65(9):1907–1912.

36. Shah GD, DeAngelis LM. Treatment of primary central nervous system lymphoma. *Hematol Oncol Clin North Am.* 2005;19(4):611–627, v.

37. Abrey LE, Yahalom J, DeAngelis LM. Treatment for primary CNS lymphoma: the next step. *J Clin Oncol.* 2000;18(17):3144–3150.

38. Gavrilovic IT, Hormigo A, Yahalom J, DeAngelis LM, Abrey LE. Long-term follow-up of high-dose methotrexate-based therapy with and without whole brain irradiation for newly diagnosed primary CNS lymphoma. *J Clin Oncol.* 2006; 24(28):4570–4574.

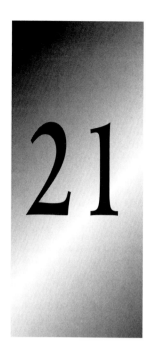

Evaluation and Treatment of Gynecologic Cancer

Meena J. Palayekar
Dennis S. Chi

Gynecologic cancers can originate from the uterus, ovaries, cervix, vulva, vagina, fallopian tubes, or peritoneum. Uterine cancers are the most common. They frequently arise from the endometrial lining of the uterus, and are usually diagnosed early, when the disease is confined to the uterus. Ovarian cancer is the second most frequent gynecologic malignancy. Its signs and symptoms are nonspecific; consequently, most ovarian cancers are not diagnosed until after the disease has spread to the upper abdomen or more distant sites. Invasive cervical cancer is one of the most common malignancies in developing countries, but has become increasingly more uncommon in the United States due to widespread screening using Papanicolaou (Pap) smears. Table 21.1 shows the stage at diagnosis and prognosis of the three most common gynecologic cancers. In this chapter, we will focus on these three gynecologic cancers, namely endometrial, ovarian, and cervical carcinomas. The interested reader is referred elsewhere for a more detailed description of these cancers and for information on the other less common gynecologic malignancies.

ENDOMETRIAL CANCER

Epidemiology

Endometrial cancer is the most common gynecologic malignancy in the United States, with an estimated 39,000 newly diagnosed cases expected in 2007 (1). It is most commonly diagnosed in affluent, obese, postmenopausal women of low parity. The incidence of endometrial cancer is higher in Western countries compared to developing countries. In the United States, white women have a twofold higher incidence of endometrial cancer compared to black women.

Etiology and Risk Factors

Endometrial adenocarcinoma is a cancer arising from the lining of the uterus. Two mechanisms are generally believed to be involved in the development of endometrial cancer. In approximately 75% cases, endometrial cancer develops in a background of endometrial hyperplasia due to exposure to unopposed estrogen, either endogenous or exogenous (type I). In these cases, the tumors tend to be well differentiated and associated with a favorable prognosis. Factors increasing exposure to estrogen, such as unopposed estrogen replacement therapy, obesity, anovulation, and estrogen-secreting tumors, increase the risk of type I endometrial cancer, whereas factors decreasing exposure to estrogens or causing an increase in progesterone levels, such as oral contraceptives and smoking, tend to be protective. Tamoxifen, used in the management of breast cancer, increases the risk of endometrial cancer two-to threefold due to its mild estrogenic effect on the female genital tract. Patients taking tamoxifen should be counseled about this risk, and any abnormal vagi-

KEY POINTS

- Gynecologic cancers can originate from the uterus, ovaries, cervix, vulva, vagina, fallopian tubes, or peritoneum.
- Endometrial cancer is the most common gynecologic malignancy in the United States, with an estimated 39,000 newly diagnosed cases expected in 2007.
- Tamoxifen, used in the management of breast cancer, increases the risk of endometrial cancer two- to threefold due to its mild estrogenic effect on the female genital tract.
- Patients with endometrial cancer commonly present with abnormal vaginal bleeding, usually, but not always, after menopause.
- Approximately 22,430 American women will be diagnosed with ovarian cancer in 2007, and an estimated 15,280 will die of the disease, making it the fifth most common cancer in women and the most common cause of gynecologic cancer mortality.
- Approximately 8%–13% of ovarian cancers are due to inherited mutations in the cancer susceptibility genes *BRCA1* and *BRCA2*.

- The majority of women with ovarian cancer present with advanced-stage disease, and these women are best treated in centers of excellence.
- State-of-the-art treatment for advanced ovarian cancer includes optimal primary tumor cytoreduction followed by systemic and intraperitoneal chemotherapy.
- Postoperative chemotherapy is known to significantly prolong survival in ovarian cancer, and the current data support the use of platinum and taxane-based regimens.
- Due to the widespread use of cervical cancer screening in the United States since the mid-1940s, the incidence of cervical cancer has steadily declined, with only 11,150 new cases expected in 2007.
- In June 2006, the Food and Drug Administration (FDA) approved Gardasil, the first quadrivalent vaccine to prevent cervical cancer and precancerous cervical lesions due to HPV-6, -11, -16, and -18.

nal bleeding should be investigated by an endometrial biopsy. In the other 25% of cases, endometrial adenocarcinoma appears relatively spontaneously without any clear transition from endometrial hyperplasia. These type II endometrial carcinomas generally arise in a background of atrophic endometrium, tend to be associated with a more undifferentiated cell type, and carry a worse prognosis.

Signs and Symptoms

Patients with endometrial cancer commonly present with abnormal vaginal bleeding, usually, but not always,

after menopause. Uncommonly, a hematometra may develop due to cervical stenosis, especially in elderly, estrogen-deficient patients, which may further progress to a pyometra, leading to a purulent vaginal discharge. Intermenstrual bleeding or prolonged heavy menstrual bleeding in premenopausal women should also arouse suspicion and should be further investigated with an endometrial biopsy.

Screening and Diagnosis

The American Cancer Society does not recommend routine screening for women with no risk factors or

---

TABLE 21.1
Stage at Diagnosis and Five-Year Survival Rate of Gynecologic Cancers, United States, 1995–2001[1]

SITE	STAGE AT DIAGNOSIS (%)			FIVE-YEAR SURVIVAL RATE (%)		
	Localized	Regional	Distant	Localized	Regional	Distant
Uterine corpus	72	16	8	96	66	25
Cervix	55	32	8	92	55	17
Ovary	19	7	68	94	69	29

Source: From Ref. 1.

for those at increased risk of endometrial cancer due to a history of exposure to unopposed estrogen (hormone replacement therapy, late menopause, tamoxifen therapy, nulliparity, infertility, obesity). However, these women should be educated about the symptoms of endometrial cancer, and any abnormal bleeding should be evaluated with an endometrial biopsy. Women with hereditary nonpolyposis colon cancer (HNPCC) syndrome have a 10-fold increased risk of endometrial cancer, with a cumulative risk for the disease of 43% by age 70. Therefore, it is recommended that these patients be offered annual screening with an endometrial biopsy starting at 35 years of age. On completion of childbearing, women with HNPCC who are undergoing surgery for colorectal cancer treatment or prevention should be offered the option of having a concurrent prophylactic hysterectomy. Prophylactic oophorectomy should also be considered, as these patients also have an increased risk of ovarian cancer.

Pathology

Adenocarcinoma

Endometrioid adenocarcinoma accounts for 75%–80% of endometrial carcinomas and is the most common type of endometrial cancer. It varies from well differentiated, with 95% glandular differentiation, to poorly differentiated, with less than 5% glandular differentiation. If the tumor has a malignant squamous component, it is called an adenosquamous carcinoma. Adenosquamous carcinomas are frequently associated with a poorly differentiated glandular component and therefore tend to have a worse prognosis.

Papillary Serous Carcinoma

Papillary serous carcinoma represents an aggressive form of endometrial cancer and accounts for 5%–10% of cases. It is usually found in older postmenopausal women. It has a tendency toward early myometrial invasion, extensive lymphatic space invasion, and early dissemination beyond the uterus.

Clear Cell Carcinoma

Clear cell carcinoma represents 1%–5% of endometrial carcinomas. Like serous carcinoma, it occurs in older postmenopausal women, presents at a higher stage, and has a poor prognosis due to its propensity for early intraperitoneal spread.

Secretory and Ciliary Adenocarcinoma

These are rare but well-differentiated types of endometrial carcinoma, with a good prognosis.

Mucinous Adenocarcinoma

Mucinous adenocarcinomas are tumors of low grade and stage, and are frequently seen in women treated with tamoxifen.

Sarcomas

Carcinosarcomas and other uterine sarcomas are uncommon tumors, accounting for less than 4% of all cancers of the uterine corpus.

Staging

In 1971, the International Federation of Gynecology and Obstetrics (FIGO) instituted clinical staging guidelines for endometrial cancer. Subsequently, seminal studies conducted by the Gynecologic Oncology Group (GOG) showed that information obtained at the time of surgery had significant impact on the accuracy of predicting prognosis and survival (2,3). Therefore, in 1988, FIGO introduced a surgical-pathologic staging system for endometrial cancer (Table 21.2). The surgical

---

TABLE 21.2
FIGO Surgical Staging for Endometrial Cancer

STAGE	GRADE	CHARACTERISTICS
IA	G1,2,3	Tumor limited to endometrium
IB	G1,2,3	Tumor invasion to less than half of the myometrium
IC	G1,2,3	Tumor invasion to more than half of the myometrium
IIA	G1,2,3	Endocervical glandular involvement only
IIB	G1,2,3	Cervical stromal invasion
IIIA	G1,2,3	Tumor invades serosa or adnexa or positive peritoneal cytology
IIIB	G1,2,3	Vaginal metastases
IIIC	G1,2,3	Metastases to pelvic or para-aortic lymph nodes
IVA	G1,2,3	Tumor invades the bladder and/or bowel mucosa
IVB		Distant metastases, including intra-abdominal and/or inguinal lymph nodes
		Histopathology: degree of differentiation
	G1	<5% of a nonsquamous or nonmorular solid growth pattern
	G2	6%–50% of a nonsquamous or nonmorular solid growth pattern
	G3	>50% of a nonsquamous or nonmorular solid growth pattern

Abbreviation: F160, International Federation of Gynecology and obstetrics.

staging procedure includes an abdominal exploration, peritoneal washings, biopsies of any suspicious lesions, total abdominal hysterectomy (TAH), bilateral salpingo-oophorectomy (BSO), and bilateral retroperitoneal pelvic and para-aortic lymph node dissection. In patients who are poor surgical candidates, the clinical staging system is still utilized.

Treatment

The cornerstone of treatment for endometrial cancer is a TAH-BSO, and this operation should be performed in all cases when feasible. Prospective surgical staging studies by the GOG have demonstrated that the incidence of lymph node metastasis is associated with the endometrial tumor grade and depth of invasion. With higher tumor grades and increasing depth of myometrial penetration, the likelihood of nodal metastasis increases (2,3). Given these findings, numerous authors have reported various preoperative and intraoperative strategies or algorithms that attempt to select patients for complete surgical staging based on tumor grade, depth of myometrial invasion, or intraoperative palpation of nodal areas. However, these strategies fail to detect at least 5%–10% of patients with high-risk factors who should have undergone comprehensive staging, and this inaccuracy could then lead to a second surgical procedure or the administration of unnecessary postoperative therapy (4). Therefore, we feel that comprehensive surgical staging should be considered for all patients with endometrial cancer when feasible. In patients with papillary serous and clear cell carcinoma, surgical staging also includes an omentectomy, as intra-abdominal disease is often found at this site.

Advances in minimally invasive surgical techniques have enabled surgeons to utilize laparoscopy to comprehensively stage patients with early-stage disease. A recently completed large, prospective, randomized trial conducted by the GOG (GOG LAP-2) confirmed prior studies that demonstrated that in well-trained hands, the laparoscopic approach, as compared to laparotomy, is associated with similar oncologic outcomes but decreases hospital stay and length of recovery time.

In patients who undergo surgical exploration for endometrial carcinoma and are found to have bulky retroperitoneal nodes or intra-abdominal metastasis, numerous studies have demonstrated a survival advantage to surgically debulking the metastasis to minimal residual disease prior to the initiation of postoperative therapy (5–7).

Stage I and II

Patients with stage IA/grade 1 or 2 tumors have an excellent prognosis, and no adjuvant therapy is necessary for this group. Patients with stage IA/grade 3 or stage IB disease of any grade are generally offered adjuvant vaginal vault radiation therapy to help prevent vaginal vault recurrence. For patients with stage IC, IIA, or IIB occult disease, postoperative therapy is tailored, usually involving whole-pelvic radiation therapy and/or vaginal brachytherapy, based on risk factors such as tumor grade, lymph-vascular space invasion, depth of myometrial penetration, and the patient's age (8). Patients with gross cervical involvement should undergo a radical hysterectomy instead of a simple hysterectomy, along with a BSO and pelvic and para-aortic lymphadenectomy. Postoperatively, adjuvant therapy is individualized.

Stage III and IV

The GOG recently reported the results of a randomized phase 3 trial of whole-abdominal radiation versus chemotherapy with doxorubicin and cisplatin in advanced endometrial carcinoma (9). Patients on the chemotherapy arm had significantly improved progression-free and overall survival rates. Distal recurrences were less for patients treated with chemotherapy. However, acute toxicity was greater with chemotherapy, and numerous prior studies have demonstrated excellent results with pelvic radiation therapy for isolated nodal and adnexal metastasis. In an attempt to improve efficacy and reduce toxicity, current studies are investigating combined radiation therapy and chemotherapy and other potentially less toxic chemotherapy regimens.

Recurrent Disease

Treatment for recurrent endometrial cancer needs to be tailored according to site of recurrence and prior therapy. Radiation therapy, surgery, endocrine therapy, or cytotoxic chemotherapy can be used alone or in combination. Patients who have not previously received radiation can be treated with radiation therapy. Surgical resection of isolated recurrences can be done. In patients with isolated, centrally located pelvic recurrence, pelvic exenteration can be considered (10,11).

OVARIAN CANCER

Epidemiology

Ovarian cancer is primarily a disease of postmenopausal women, with the majority of cases occurring in women between 50 and 75 years of age. Approximately 22,430 American women will be diagnosed with ovarian cancer in 2007, and an estimated 15,280 will die of the disease, making it the fifth most common cancer in women and the most common cause of gynecologic cancer mortality (1). Ovarian cancer is more common in Northern European and North American countries than in Asia, developing countries, or southern continents.

Etiology and Risk Factors

The etiology of ovarian cancer is unknown. Various risk factors have been reported, such as advancing age, infertility, endometriosis, use of assisted reproductive technologies, and application of perineal talc. Approximately 8%–13% of ovarian cancers are due to inherited mutations in the cancer susceptibility genes *BRCA1* and *BRCA2* (12,13). Women with mutations in *BRCA1* have a 35%–60% risk of developing ovarian cancer by the age of 70, whereas *BRCA2* mutation carriers have a 10%–27% risk of developing ovarian cancer by the age of 70. Approximately 1%–2% of ovarian cancers are associated with inherited defects in the mismatch repair genes *MLH1*, *MSH2*, and *MSH6*, associated with HNPCC syndrome. Carriers of this mutation have a 9%–12% risk of developing ovarian cancer by the age of 70. A family history of ovarian cancer is associated with a three- to fivefold increased risk of developing ovarian cancer compared with the general population (14). Multiple studies have shown multiparity and the use of oral contraceptives to be protective against ovarian cancer.

Signs and Symptoms

Ovarian cancer produces vague symptoms of abdominal pain, discomfort, and bloating. At a later stage, patients may present with weight loss, abdominal distension due to ascites, or a pleural effusion. Some patients may have menstrual irregularity or postmenopausal bleeding.

Screening and Diagnosis

Routine screening for ovarian cancer is not recommended. Women at an increased risk due to a family history of ovarian cancer but no proven genetic predisposition should be offered genetic counseling to help better clarify the risk of ovarian cancer. For this group, there is no clear evidence that currently available screening tests decrease mortality from ovarian cancer; therefore, routine screening is not recommended. Women with inherited mutations in *BRCA1* or the mismatch repair genes *MLH1*, *MSH2*, and *MSH6* should begin ovarian cancer screening between the ages of 30 and 35. For mutations in *BRCA2*, screening is initiated between the ages of 35 and 40.

Serum CA-125 and transvaginal ultrasound can be used for ovarian cancer screening, along with annual pelvic exams. Several studies have shown that a combination of transvaginal ultrasound and CA-125 results in a higher sensitivity for detection of ovarian cancer. A newer technology, proteomics, which involves evaluation of dozens to hundreds of low-molecular proteins simultaneously, is being developed. Newer serum markers, including osteopontin, YKL-40, prostasin, and lysophosphatidic acid (LPA), are being evaluated alone or in combination for ovarian cancer screening.

The diagnosis of ovarian cancer is generally made by histopathologic study following surgical evaluation. The stage of the disease can only be determined by surgery, as discussed next.

Pathology

Ovarian tumors are classified according to their tissue of origin. Eighty-five percent of ovarian cancers arise from the coelomic epithelium lining the ovary; 10% arise from germ cells; and approximately 5% are sex cord-stromal tumors, arising from ovarian mesenchymal tissue.

Epithelial Ovarian Tumors

Of the malignant epithelial ovarian tumors, 40%–50% are serous, 15%–25% are endometrioid, 6%–16% are mucinous, and 5%–11% are clear cell tumors. Less common types of epithelial cell tumors include transitional cell (Brenner), mixed epithelial, and undifferentiated carcinomas. Epithelial ovarian tumors can be benign, of low-malignant potential (borderline tumors), or frankly malignant. Borderline tumors have a much better prognosis than malignant epithelial cancers, but they are malignant and can result in death.

Germ Cell Tumors

Germ cell tumors are most commonly seen in the first two decades of life. The most common germ cell tumor is the mature cystic teratoma (dermoid), which is a benign tumor. Dysgerminoma is the most common malignant germ cell tumor, followed in incidence by the endodermal sinus tumor and the immature teratoma.

Sex Cord-Stromal Tumors

Sex cord-stromal tumors can either arise from the granulosa cells or the Sertoli-Leydig cells, and are named accordingly. More than 90% of malignant stromal tumors are granulosa cell tumors. These tumors can occur at any age, but are more common before menopause.

Staging and Prognosis

Ovarian cancer is surgically staged according to the FIGO staging system (Table 21.3). Surgical staging includes a complete abdominal and pelvic exploration with peritoneal washings, TAH-BSO, an infracolic omentectomy, and bilateral pelvic and para-aortic lymph node sampling. Peritoneal biopsies are taken from various peritoneal surfaces, and any suspicious lesions or adhesions are also sampled.

Laparoscopic surgical staging can be done in patients whose cancer is diagnosed during laparoscopy or in patients with apparently early cancer who are referred for evaluation after inadequate initial surgery (15). If laparoscopic staging is attempted but cannot be adequately performed, an open laparotomy must be performed for comprehensive staging.

Treatment

Surgery followed by postoperative chemotherapy is standard treatment for all patients with advanced-stage disease (stages III and IV) and for most patients with early-stage disease (stages I and II). Postoperative chemotherapy is known to significantly prolong survival, and the current data support the use of platinum- and taxane-based regimens.

Stage I and II

After a systematic and complete surgical staging is performed, the patient's appropriate stage, prognosis, and treatment can be established. In general, a patient with stage IA/grade 1 epithelial ovarian cancer (low risk) will not benefit from adjunctive chemotherapy. It is debatable as to whether stage IA/grade 2 cancer requires adjunctive chemotherapy. In other early-stage disease (high risk), some type of adjunctive treatment is usually required. Table 21.4 shows the classification of ovarian cancer patients within broad categories and their recommended treatment. In low-risk patients who wish to maintain fertility, a unilateral salpingo-oophorectomy with uterine preservation is acceptable.

Stage III and IV

In these patients with metastatic disease, the goal of surgery is to surgically remove or "debulk" all visible and palpable tumor. This level of "cytoreduction" is not always achievable, as there can be more than 1,000 tumor nodules encountered at the time of exploration. In cases in which all tumor cannot be completely removed, studies have shown that there still is a survival benefit if all disease is removed such that the largest tumor nodule remaining measures 1 cm or less in maximal dimension (16). Attaining this level of residual disease status is currently defined as "optimal cytoreduction," and these patients may be candidates for treatment with intraperitoneal chemotherapy in addition to systemic chemotherapy (17). However, if disease is identified outside of the peritoneal cavity (stage IV disease) or if cytoreduction is suboptimal, patients are treated with systemic chemotherapy without an intraperitoneal component.

TABLE 21.3
FIGO Surgical Staging for Ovarian Cancer

STAGE	CHARACTERISTICS
I	Growth limited to the ovaries
IA	Growth limited to one ovary; no ascites; no tumor on the external surfaces; capsule intact
IB	Growth limited to both ovaries; no ascites; no tumor on the external surfaces; capsule intact
IC	Tumor either stage IA or IB present on the surface of one or both ovaries; capsule ruptured; ascites containing malignant cells or positive peritoneal washings
II	Growth involving one or both ovaries with pelvic extension of disease
IIA	Extension of disease and/or metastases to the uterus and/or fallopian tubes
IIB	Extension of disease to other pelvic tissues
IIC	Tumor either stage IIA or IIB but present on the surface of one or both ovaries; capsule ruptured; ascites containing malignant cells or positive peritoneal washings
III	Tumor involving one or both ovaries with peritoneal implants outside the pelvis and/or positive retroperitoneal or inguinal nodes; superficial liver metastases equals stage III; tumor is limited to the true pelvis, but with histologically verified extension to small bowel or omentum
IIIA	Tumor grossly limited to the true pelvis with negative nodes but with histologically confirmed microscopic seeding of abdominal peritoneal surfaces
IIIB	Tumor of one or both ovaries; histologically confirmed implants on abdominal peritoneal surfaces, none >2 cm in diameter; nodes negative
IIIC	Abdominal implants >2 cm in diameter and/or positive retroperitoneal or inguinal nodes
IV	Growth involving one or both ovaries with distant metastases; if pleural effusion is present, there must be positive cytology to allot case to stage IV; parenchymal liver metastases equals stage IV

Chemotherapy

In the 1960s, single alkylating agents were the chemotherapy of choice for epithelial ovarian cancer. The most commonly used drugs were melphalan and chlorambucil. Overall response rates were 45%–55%, and complete clinical response was seen in 15%–20% of cases. Median survival was approximately 12 months. In the 1970s, multidrug regimens resulted in an improvement in overall response rates, complete clinical responses, and increased median survival of approximately 14 months. The introduction of cisplatin in the late 1970s resulted in combination chemotherapy regimens that achieved overall response rates of 70%–80%, with complete clinical response rates of approximately 50%. The median survival increased to approximately 24–28 months with cisplatin and cyclophosphamide. The replacement of cyclophosphamide with paclitaxel further increased the median survival to 36 months in patients with suboptimally cytoreduced advanced-stage disease.

The GOG then evaluated the combination of carboplatin and paclitaxel and found survival to be equivalent to the combination of cisplatin and paclitaxel (18). Toxicity (particularly neurotoxicity) was less in the carboplatin arm. Based on these studies, the standard primary chemotherapy regimen for advanced ovarian cancer then became carboplatin and paclitaxel.

The GOG recently published the results of a prospective randomized phase 3 trial that compared intravenous paclitaxel plus cisplatin to intravenous paclitaxel plus intraperitoneal cisplatin and paclitaxel in patients with optimally cytoreduced stage III ovarian cancer (17). The study arm receiving the intravenous/intraperitoneal regimen had a 16-month improvement from 50–66 months in median overall survival compared to the intravenous-only control arm. This trial, along with others that have demonstrated improved survival for the intravenous/intraperitoneal approach, led the National Cancer Institute (NCI) to issue an NCI Clinical Announcement in January 2006 that recommended that women with optimally debulked stage III ovarian cancer be counseled about the clinical benefit associated with combined intravenous and intraperitoneal administration of chemotherapy. Due to concerns regarding increased toxicity, however, studies are ongoing to determine the best drug dosing and the safest and efficacious combined intravenous/intraperitoneal regimen.

TABLE 21.4
Recommended Therapy for Epithelial Ovarian Cancer

CATEGORY OF OVARIAN CANCER	RECOMMENDED (STANDARD) THERAPY
Early Ovarian Cancer	
Low risk (stages IA and IB, grade 1[a])	TAH, BSO, full surgical staging
High risk (stages IA and IB, grades 2 and 3; stages IC, IIA, IIB, and IIC)	TAH, BSO[b] full surgical staging
	Adjunctive therapy with combination carboplatin/paclitaxel chemotherapy
Advanced Ovarian Cancer	
Stage III with optimal residual disease[c]	Maximal surgical cytoreduction
	Combination chemotherapy with systemic carboplatin/paclitaxel or systemic/intraperitoneal cisplatin and paclitaxel
Stage IV and/or suboptimal[d]	Maximal surgical cytoreduction
	Combination chemotherapy with carboplatin/paclitaxel

Abbreviations: BSO, bilateral salpingo-oophorectomy; TAH, total abdominal hysterectomy.
[a]Some investigators include grade 2 in the low-risk category.
[b]Unilateral salpingo-oophorectomy is permissible in patients who desire further childbearing.
[c]Optimal (≤1 cm residual tumaor).
[d]Suboptimal (stage III or IV, >1 cm residual tumor).

Recurrent Disease

Patients who develop recurrent disease are generally divided into one of two categories. Platinum-sensitive patients are defined as those who develop recurrent disease six months or more after completion of their primary platinum-based chemotherapy. Platinum-resistant patients relapse within six months of completion of their primary therapy. Patients with platinum-sensitive recurrent disease are usually retreated with platinum-based chemotherapy. These patients are frequently treated with combination chemotherapy with a taxane or gemcitabine added to the platinum compound. Some patients with platinum-sensitive recurrent disease may benefit from a second debulking surgery. The selection of patients for secondary cytoreduction should be based on the disease-free interval from completion of primary therapy, the number of recurrence sites, and the probability of achieving cytoreduction to minimal residual disease (19). Patients with platinum-resistant recurrence are generally not candidates for retreatment with platinum therapy or secondary cytoreduction. These patients are usually offered salvage chemotherapy with other agents or a clinical trial.

CERVICAL CANCER

Epidemiology

Due to the widespread use of cervical cancer screening in the United States since the mid-1940s, the incidence of cervical cancer has steadily declined, with only 11,150 new cases expected in 2007 (1). Cervical cancer still continues to be a significant health problem worldwide, especially in developing countries, where it is a leading cause of death among middle-aged women, primarily from the lower socioeconomic classes, with poor access to medical care and routine screening facilities. The peak age for developing cervical cancer is 47 years. Approximately 47% of women with invasive cervical cancer are aged <35 years at the time of diagnosis. Older women, aged >65 years represent only 10% of the patient population, but they are more likely to succumb to their disease due to more advanced stage at the time of diagnosis.

ETIOLOGY AND RISK FACTORS

Sexual Activity

Invasive cervical cancer can be viewed as a sexually transmitted disease. Early age-of-onset of sexual activity, especially before 16 years of age; onset of sexual activity within one year of menarche; multiple sexual partners; a history of genital warts; and multiparity increase the risk of invasive cervical carcinoma. This is because in early reproductive life, the cervical transformation zone is more susceptible to the oncogenic agent human papillomavirus (HPV). HPV-16 and HPV-18 are the types most commonly associated with cervical cancer. In June 2006, the FDA approved Gardasil, the first quadrivalent vaccine to prevent cervical cancer and precancerous cervical lesions due to HPV-6, -11, -16, and -18. This vaccine is given as three injections at zero, two, and six months, and is approved for use in females aged 9–26 years.

Cigarette Smoking

Cigarette smoking has been identified to be a significant risk factor for cervical cancer due to depression of the immune system, secondary to a systemic effect of cigarette smoke and its byproducts.

Oral Contraceptives

A higher incidence of cervical cancer, especially adenocarcinoma of the cervix, is observed in patients with prior oral contraceptive use.

Alterations in Immune System

Alterations of the immune system are associated with an increased incidence of cervical cancer, as exemplified by the fact that patients infected with human immunodeficiency virus (HIV) and those taking immunosuppressive medications are at an increased risk for developing both preinvasive and invasive cervical cancer.

Signs and Symptoms

The most common symptoms associated with cervical cancer are postcoital and intermenstrual bleeding. It can also present with postmenopausal bleeding, or may be asymptomatic until detected on routine cervical cancer screening. Less commonly, advanced cervical cancer presents with a foul-smelling vaginal discharge, pelvic pain and sciatica, or renal failure due to urinary tract obstruction.

Screening and Diagnosis

Papanicolaou (Pap) Smear

The cervical cytology, or Pap smear, is the paradigm for a cost-effective, easy-to-use, and reliable screening test for cervical cancer. The introduction of the Pap smear has resulted in a significant reduction in the incidence of invasive cervical carcinoma, as well as diagnosis at an earlier stage.

Current Screening Recommendations

The American College of Obstetricians and Gynecologists (ACOG) recommends that sexually active women aged 18 years or older be screened annually until three consecutive normal Pap smears, after which screening may be done less frequently, every two to three years. The American College of Surgeons (ACS) recommends that screening begin at least three years after the onset of vaginal intercourse, but no later than age 21, and should be performed every year with conventional cervical cytology smears, or every two years with liquid-based cytology until age 30. After age 30, HPV DNA testing may be added to cervical cytology for screening. Women older than 70 years with an intact cervix and three or more prior normal Pap smears within the past 10 years may elect to cease cervical cancer screening. Women with prior history of cervical cancer, in utero exposure to diethylstilbestrol (DES), and who are immunocompromised (including HIV positive) should continue cervical cancer screening for as long as they are in reasonably good health and do not have a life-limiting chronic condition. Women who have had a supracervical hysterectomy should continue cervical cancer screening as per the current guidelines.

Diagnosis

The diagnosis of invasive cervical cancer can be suggested by either an abnormal Pap smear or an abnormal physical finding. In the patient with an abnormal Pap smear but normal physical findings, colposcopy is indicated. Colposcopic findings of dense acetowhite epithelium, coarse punctuation and mosaic pattern, or atypical blood vessels are consistent with preinvasive or invasive cervical disease, and warrant biopsies for definitive diagnosis. If the biopsies demonstrate only precancerous changes, the patient should undergo an excisional biopsy of the cervix. The loop electrosurgical excision procedure (LEEP) is the most expedient method of performing an excisional biopsy. Patients with physical signs/symptoms of advanced invasive cervical cancer need a cervical biopsy for diagnosis and treatment planning.

Pathology

Squamous Cell Carcinoma

This accounts for 80% of all cervical carcinomas, and is the most common histology. Routine screening by Pap smears has resulted in a decline in the incidence of this histologic subtype.

Adenocarcinoma

This now accounts for about 20% of all cervical cancers. It has a similar prognosis to squamous cell carcinoma of the cervix when stratified by stage and size of tumor.

Aggressive Subtypes

Small cell or neuroendocrine tumors of the cervix are rare tumors that are very aggressive and have a poor prognosis, even when diagnosed at an early stage.

Rare Tumor Types

Lymphoma, sarcoma, and melanoma of the cervix are rare subtypes, which account for <1% of all cervical cancers.

Staging and Prognosis

Cervical cancer is staged clinically. After a histologic diagnosis of cervical carcinoma, an examination under anesthesia may determine whether the tumor is confined to the cervix or has extended to the adjacent vagina, parametrium, bladder, or rectum. Sometimes, the office examination gives enough information, and examination under anesthesia may not be necessary. According to the FIGO guidelines for clinical staging of cervical cancer (Table 21.5), diagnostic studies used for staging may include intravenous pyelography, cystoscopy, proctosigmoidoscopy, chest x-ray, and barium enema. Computed tomographic (CT) imaging and magnetic resonance imaging (MRI) are frequently used for pretreatment evaluation and treatment planning for

	TABLE 21.5 *FIGO Staging for Carcinoma of the Uterine Cervix*	
STAGE	**DESCRIPTION**
0	Carcinoma in situ, intraepithelial carcinoma
I	Carcinoma strictly confined to the cervix (extension to the corpus should be disregarded)
IA	Invasive cancer identified only microscopically; invasion is limited to stromal invasion with maximum depth of 5 mm and no wider than 7 mm
IA1	Measured stromal invasion no greater than 3 mm deep and no wider than 7 mm
IA2	Measured stromal invasion greater than 3 mm but less than 5 mm deep and no wider than 7 mm
IB	Clinical lesions confined to the cervix or preclinical lesions greater than stage IA
IB1	Clinical lesions no greater than 4 cm
IB2	Clinical lesions greater than 4 cm
II	Carcinoma extends beyond the cervix but not onto the pelvic side wall Carcinoma involves the vagina but not the lower third
IIA	No obvious parametrial involvement
IIB	Obvious parametrial involvement
III	Carcinoma has extended onto the pelvic side wall; there is no cancer-free space between the tumor and pelvic wall; tumor involves lower third of vagina
IIIA	No extension onto pelvic side wall, but lower third of vagina involved
IIIB	Extension to the pelvic side wall or hydronephrosis or nonfunctioning kidney
IV	Carcinoma has extended beyond the true pelvis or has clinically involved the mucosa of the bladder or rectum
IVA	Spread to adjacent organs
IVB	Spread to distant organs

patients with advanced disease (stage IIB and greater), but findings on CT/MRI are not used to assign a stage for cervical cancer. Similarly, although the benefits of laparoscopic extraperitoneal surgical staging have been reported, this approach has not yet been incorporated into the FIGO staging system.

Prognosis

Clinical stage is the most important determinant of prognosis. For patients with early disease (stage IB), the size of the lesion, percentage of cervical stromal invasion, histology, tumor grade, and lymph-vascular space involvement (LVSI) are important prognostic factors. For patients with advanced disease (stages II–IV), histology and size of the primary lesion are important prognostic factors.

Treatment

Stage IA1

These patients have microinvasive disease with <3 mm depth of tumor invasion, <7 mm of lateral invasion, and no LVSI. Patients desiring preservation of fertility can be treated with a cone biopsy alone, provided that the margins of the cone are negative. For patients not desirous of further childbearing, a simple hysterectomy is the standard therapy. Vaginal, abdominal, and laparoscopic hysterectomies are equally effective.

Stages IA2, IB1, and Nonbulky IIA Disease

The standard treatment for patients with small-sized cervical carcinomas (<4 cm) confined to the uterine cervix or with minimal vaginal involvement (stage IIA) is radical hysterectomy (removal of uterus, cervix, and parametrial tissue), pelvic lymphadenectomy, and aortic lymph node sampling. There is no difference in survival between patients undergoing radical hysterectomy and those undergoing radiation therapy for early cervical cancer. Radical hysterectomy, however, provides an improved quality of life.

Laparoscopic-assisted radical vaginal hysterectomy and total laparoscopic radical hysterectomy are less invasive alternatives to traditional radical hysterectomy, and results from centers that have the necessary surgical expertise are promising (20,21). In patients desirous of preserving fertility, laparoscopic pelvic lymphadenectomy followed by radical vaginal trachelectomy (removal of uterine cervix and bilateral parametria) and radical abdominal trachelectomy are options offered at a few select centers (22,23). Successful pregnancies after this procedure have been reported. The role of laparoscopic sentinel lymph node dissection in cervical cancer is an area of active investigation.

Adjuvant Therapy Following Radical Hysterectomy

Concurrent chemoradiation therapy (cisplatin + radiation) following radical hysterectomy has been shown to provide significant benefit in patients with positive nodes, margins, or parametria after radical hysterectomy for early-stage cervical cancer (24). Postoperative radiation therapy has been reported to be of benefit in patients with negative nodes but who are at risk for pelvic failure (primary tumor >4 cm, outer third cervical stromal invasion, LVSI, positive margins or parametria) (25).

Stages IB2 and Bulky IIA Disease

Patients with stage IB2 and bulky stage IIA cervical cancer are generally treated with either primary radical hysterectomy and bilateral pelvic lymphadenectomy, with adjuvant therapy based on risk factors, or primary concurrent radiotherapy and chemotherapy (26).

Stages IIB–IVA Disease

The standard therapy for patients with stage IIB–IVA cervical cancer is concurrent chemotherapy and radiation therapy. The chemotherapy is generally weekly cisplatin combined with external beam pelvic radiation.

Recurrent Disease

Pelvic exenteration is offered to patients whose disease recurs in the central pelvis after radiation therapy. Evidence of extrapelvic disease is a contraindication for pelvic exenteration. During surgery, careful exploration is carried out to confirm that there is no evidence of disease beyond the pelvis. In most cases, the operation involves removal of the bladder, uterus, cervix, vagina and rectum, with urinary and pelvic reconstruction. For patients undergoing successful pelvic exenteration, the five-year survival rates range from 25%–50%. For the rare patient who presents with a single isolated lung metastasis after treatment of invasive cervical carcinoma, pulmonary resection has been reported to be of benefit.

For patients with recurrent disease that is not confined to the pelvis or is thought to be unresectable, palliative chemotherapy is the only treatment that can be offered. A recent GOG study showed the combination of topotecan and cisplatin to have a significant survival advantage over single-agent cisplatin in this setting (27).

CONCLUSION

The three most common gynecologic cancers are carcinomas of the uterus, ovary, and cervix. Endometrial carcinoma is frequently diagnosed at an early stage when surgery alone or in conjunction with radiation therapy can be curative. Recent studies have demonstrated that chemotherapy may be more effective than radiation therapy for postoperative treatment of advanced-stage disease. The majority of women with ovarian carcinoma present with advanced-stage disease. These patients are best served by receiving their treatment in centers of excellence where comprehensive surgery and chemotherapy can be offered. The incidence of cervical carcinoma has decreased over the past 50 years and will most likely continue to decline due to the introduction of the HPV vaccine. Research is ongoing to develop innovative diagnostic, screening, surgical, and nonsurgical techniques for all of these malignancies. Significant advances have been made in our understanding of the molecular abnormalities associated with these diseases, and promising new drugs that target genetically defined abnormalities are being developed. Several such agents are undergoing phase 2 and 3 clinical trials, and offer new hope in the treatment of women with gynecologic cancers.

R*eferences*

1. Jemal A, Siegel R, Ward E, et al. Cancer statistics, 2007. *CA Cancer J Clin.* 2007;57:43–66.
2. Creasman WT, Morrow CP, Bundy BN, et al. Surgical pathologic spread patterns of endometrial cancer. A Gynecologic Oncology Group study. *Cancer.* 1987;60(8 suppl.):2035–2041.
3. Morrow CP, Bundy BN, Kurman RJ, et al. Relationship between surgical pathologic risk factors and outcome in clinical stage I and II carcinoma of the endometrium. A Gynecologic Oncology Group study. *Gynecol Oncol.* 1991;40:55–65.
4. Barakat RR, Lev G, Hummer AJ, et al. Twelve-year experience in the management of endometrial cancer: a change in surgical and post operative radiation approaches. *Gynecol Oncol.* 2007;105:150–156.
5. Chi DS, Welshinger M, Venkatraman ES, Barakat RR. The role of surgical cytoreduction in stage IV endometrial carcinoma. *Gynecol Oncol.* 1997;67:56–60.
6. Bristow RE, Zahurak ML, Alexander CJ, Zellars RC, Montz FJ. FIGO stage IIIC endometrial carcinoma: resection of macroscopic nodal disease and other determinants of survival. *Int J Gynecol Cancer.* 2003;13:664–672.
7. Lambrou NC, Gomez-Marino, Mirhashemi R, et al. Optimal surgical cytoreduction in patients with stage III and stage IV endometrial carcinoma: a study of morbidity and survival. *Gynecol Oncol.* 2004;93:653–658.
8. Keys HM, Roberts JA, Brunetto VL, et al. A phase III trial of surgery with or without adjunctive external pelvic radiation therapy in intermediate risk endometrial adenocarcinoma: a Gynecologic Oncology Group study. *Gynecol Oncol.* 2004;92:744–751.
9. Randall ME, Filiaci VL, Muss H, et al. Randomized phase III trial of whole-abdominal irradiation versus doxorubicin and cisplatin chemotherapy in advanced endometrial carcinoma: a Gynecologic Oncology Group study. *J Clin Oncol.* 2006;24:36–44.
10. Morris M, Alvarez RD, Kinney WK, Wilson TO. Treatment of recurrent adenocarcinoma of the endometrium with pelvic exenteration. *Gynecol Oncol.* 1996;60:288–291.
11. Barakat RR, Goldman NA, Patel DA, Venkatraman ES, Curtin JP. Pelvic exenteration for recurrent endometrial cancer. *Gynecol Oncol.* 1999;75:99–102.
12. Risch HA, McLaughlin JR, Cole DE, et al. Prevalence and penetrance of germline BRCA1 and BRCA2 mutations in a population series of 649 women with ovarian cancer. *Am J Hum Genet.* 2001;68:700–710.
13. Pal T, Permuth-Wey J, Betts JA, et al. BRCA1 and BRCA2 mutations account for a large proportion of ovarian carcinoma cases. *Cancer.* 2005;104:2807–2816.
14. Bergfeldt K, Rydh B, Granath F, et al. Risk of ovarian cancer in breast cancer patients with a family history of breast or ovarian cancer: a population based cohort study. *Lancet.* 2002;360:891–894.
15. Chi DS, Abu-Rustum NR, Sonoda Y, et al. The safety and efficacy of laparoscopic surgical staging of apparent stage I ovarian and fallopian tube cancers. *Am J Obstet Gynecol.* 2005;192:1614–1619.
16. Chi DS, Eisenhauer EL, Lang J, et al. What is the optimal goal of primary cytoreductive surgery for bulky stage IIIC epithelial ovarian carcinoma? *Gynecol Oncol.* 2006;103:559–564.
17. Armstrong DK, Bundy B, Wenzel L, et al. Intraperitoneal cisplatin and paclitaxel in ovarian cancer. *N Engl J Med.* 2006;354:34–43.
18. Ozols RF, Bundy BN, Greer BE, et al. Phase III trial of carboplatin and paclitaxel compared with cisplatin and paclitaxel in patients with optimally resected stage III ovarian cancer: a Gynecologic Oncology Group study. *J Clin Oncol.* 2003;21:3194–3200.
19. Chi DS, McCaughty K, Diaz JP, et al. Guidelines and selection criteria for secondary cytoreductive surgery in patients with recurrent platinum sensitive epithelial ovarian carcinoma. *Cancer.* 2006;106:1933–1939.
20. Spirtos NM, Eisenkop SM, Schlaerth J, Ballon SC. Laparoscopic radical hysterectomy (type III) in patients with stage I cervical cancer: surgical morbidity and intermediate follow-up. *Am J Obstet Gynecol.* 2002;187:340–348.
21. Abu-Rustum NR, Gemignani ML, Moore K, et al. Total laparoscopic radical hysterectomy with pelvic lymphadenectomy using the argon-beam coagulator: pilot data and comparison to laparotomy. *Gynecol Oncol.* 2004;93:275.
22. Plante M, Renaud MC, Roy M. Radical vaginal trachelectomy: a fertility-preserving option for young women with early stage cervical cancer. *Gynecol Oncol.* 2005;99:S143–S146.
23. Abu-Rustum NR, Sonoda Y, Black D, et al. Fertility sparing radical abdominal trachelectomy for cervical carcinoma: technique and review of literature. *Gynecol Oncol.* 2007;105:830–831.
24. Peters WA 3rd, Liu PY, Barrett RJ 2nd, et al. Concurrent chemotherapy and pelvic radiation therapy compared with pelvic radiation therapy alone as adjuvant therapy after radical surgery in high-risk early-stage cancer of the cervix. *J Clin Oncol.* 2000;18:1606–1613.
25. Sedlis A, Bundy BN, Rotman MZ, et al. A randomized trial of pelvic radiation therapy versus no further therapy in selected patients with stage IB carcinoma of the cervix after radical hysterectomy and pelvic lymphadenectomy: a Gynecologic Oncology Group study. *Gynecol Oncol.* 1999;73:177–183.
26. Keys HM, Bundy BN, Stehman FB, et al. Cisplatin, radiation and adjuvant hysterectomy compared with radiation and adjuvant hysterectomy for bulky stage IB cervical carcinoma. *N Engl J Med.* 1999;340:1154–1161.
27. Long HJ III, Bundy BN, Grendys EC Jr., et al. Randomized phase III trial of cisplatin with or without topotecan in carcinoma of the uterine cervix. A gynecologic Oncology Group study. *J Clin Oncol.* 2005;23:4626–4633.

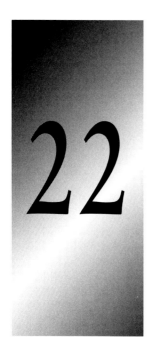

Evaluation and Treatment of Head and Neck Cancer

Laura Locati
Su Hsien Lim
Snehal Patel
David G. Pfister

Head and neck cancer (HNC) typically refers to malignant tumors arising from the mucosal lining of the upper aerodigestive tract, and encompasses primary sites within the oral cavity, larynx, and pharynx. Malignant tumors of the paranasal sinuses and nasal cavity are also sometimes included. Approximately 45,000 new cases of HNC (3% of all cancers) were diagnosed in the United States in 2007, with an associated 11,000 deaths (2% of all cancer deaths) (1). Worldwide, approximately 500,000 new cases of HNC are diagnosed annually, and the related mortality rate is over 50%. Squamous cell cancer or a variant is the histologic type in more than 90% of HNC. HNCs are associated with several challenges in their management, related to the direct involvement by these tumors of key anatomical areas involved with such vital functions as speech, breathing, chewing, and swallowing. Moreover, cosmesis can also be affected.

This chapter will provide a broad overview of the management of HNC with a focus on the anatomy, pathology, epidemiology, diagnostic evaluation, and treatment strategies. Salivary gland cancers will also be discussed, since these malignancies are unique to this body region. Thyroid cancers, also unique to this body region, are covered in another chapter of this text.

ANATOMIC SITES OF DISEASE

Knowledge of the related anatomy is critical to understanding the clinical presentation, patterns of spread, and management of HNCs.

The paranasal sinuses are air-filled spaces located within bones of the skull and face. The maxillary sinuses are the largest of the paranasal sinuses, and are located under the eyes. The frontal sinuses are located within the frontal bone above the eyes, while the ethmoid sinuses consist of several air cells within the ethmoid bones between the nose and the eyes. The sphenoid sinuses are positioned in the center of the skull base and lie superior to the nasopharynx and inferior-medial to the cavernous sinuses, which contain several important structures such as the internal carotid arteries and cranial nerves III (oculomotor nerve), IV (trochlear nerve), VI (abducens nerve), V_1 (ophthalmic nerve), and V_2 (maxillary nerve). Double vision is a typical symptom when a cavernous sinus is involved with tumor. The paranasal sinuses communicate with the nasal cavity.

The oral cavity is separated from the nasal cavity by the hard palate. It is bound anteriorly by the lips and posteriorly by the tonsillar pillars. The floor of the

KEY POINTS

- Head and neck cancer (HNC) typically refers to malignant tumors arising from the mucosal lining of the upper aerodigestive tract, and encompasses primary sites within the oral cavity, larynx, and pharynx.
- The vast majority of HNCs are of the squamous cell variety.
- Tobacco and alcohol use are the best established risk factors, and account for approximately 75% of all oral and pharyngeal cancers in the United States.
- Patients most commonly present with locoregional symptoms referable to the primary site or related spread to the neck and consistent with the anatomy of the region. A new ulcer that will not heal, pain, bleeding, dysphagia, odynophagia, changes in articulation, otalgia, hoarseness, nasal or ear congestion, epistaxis, diplopia, or a new lump in the neck are examples of common presenting symptoms.
- HNCs are associated with several challenges in their management, related to the direct involvement by these tumors of key anatomical areas with vital functions such as speech, breathing, chewing, and swallowing. Moreover, cosmesis can also be affected.
- Staging of HNC assesses the extent of disease, establishes prognosis, and guides management.

- Most commonly, the American Joint Committee on Cancer T (primary tumor) N (nodal disease) M (distant metastases) classification system (TNM system) is used for staging tumors of the head and neck.
- The aim of treatment for HNC is to maximize locoregional control and survival while minimizing functional and cosmetic alteration.
- Treatment plans are formulated optimally by a multidisciplinary team (ie, surgeon, radiation, and medical oncologist), particularly when more than one treatment option is available or when combined modality therapy is anticipated. Dental, speech, auditory, swallowing, and nutritional evaluations are commonly indicated before therapy.
- Surgery and radiation are both potentially curative treatments; chemotherapy by itself is generally considered a palliative modality.
- Comprehensive neck dissection involves removal of lymph node levels I–V; cranial nerve XI, the internal jugular vein, and the sternocleidomastoid muscle. A "modified" dissection spares some or all of these last three structures.
- Neck pain and shoulder dysfunction are potential sequelae to neck dissections, particularly comprehensive ones.

mouth is a U-shaped area bounded by the lower gum and the oral tongue. The mandible, the hard palate, the teeth, the anterior two-thirds of the tongue, and the retromolar trigone (located on the ascending portion of the mandible) are located in the oral cavity.

Posterior to the oral and nasal cavities is the pharynx. It is conventionally divided into three parts: nasopharynx, oropharynx, and hypopharynx. The nasopharynx lies behind the nasal cavity and extends from the skull base to the level of the junction of the hard and soft palates. Its lateral walls include the openings of the eustachian tubes within the fossae of Rosenmüller (pharyngeal recesses), which are located behind the torus tubari. Not surprisingly then, unilateral otitis media is a common presenting symptom for nasopharynx tumors. Inferiorly, the nasopharynx is continuous with the oropharynx and its inferior wall is formed, in part, by the superior surface of the soft palate.

The inferior surface of the soft palate and the uvula lie roughly at the level of C1, and they constitute the superior wall of oropharynx. The anterior wall consists of the base of the tongue, the vallecula, and glossoepiglottic folds, while the lateral wall is made up of the tonsil, tonsillar fossae, and tonsillar pillars. The surface of the base of the tongue appears irregular on exam due to scattered submucosal lymphoid follicles.

This lingual tonsillar tissue may harbor a clinically occult primary cancer. The musculature of the base of the tongue is continuous with that of the oral tongue. The posterior pharyngeal wall is continuous from the nasopharynx down to the hypopharynx. The plane of division between the posterior wall of the nasopharynx and the oropharynx is arbitrarily located at the Passavant ridge, a muscular ring that contracts to seal the nasopharynx from the oropharynx during swallowing. Lateral to the pharyngeal wall are the vessels, nerves, and muscles of the parapharyngeal space.

The oropharynx continues inferiorly into the hypopharynx and spans the area between C3 and C6, ending at the pharyngoesophageal junction. The hypopharynx comprises three subsites: the paired pyriform sinuses, the posterior pharyngeal wall, and the postcricoid area. The pyriform sinuses are grooves lateral to the larynx created by its intrusion into the anterior aspect of the pharynx. Each pyriform sinus has three walls—anterior, lateral, and medial—and communicates with the rest of the hypopharynx posteriorly. The medial wall of each pyriform sinus separates it from the larynx and is bordered superiorly by the aryepiglottic fold. The lateral walls of each pyriform sinus continue superiorly, with the lateral pharyngeal walls of the oropharynx behind the posterior tonsillar pillars. The transition from oropharynx to hypopharynx is located at the plane of the hyoid bone.

The larynx is divided into supraglottic, glottic, and subglottic regions. The supraglottic larynx consists of the epiglottis, false vocal cords, ventricles, aryepiglottic folds, and arytenoids. The glottis includes the true vocal cords and the anterior and posterior commissures. The subglottic larynx extends caudally from 5 mm below the free edge of the true vocal cords to the inferior border of the cricoid cartilage.

The lymphatic drainage of the mucosal surfaces of the head and neck is directed to the lymph nodes located within the fibroadipose tissues in the neck. These lymph nodes are grouped into levels I–VI (Fig. 22.1), corresponding to the submandibular and submental nodes (level I); upper, middle, and lower jugular nodes (levels II, III, and IV, respectively); posterior triangle nodes (level V); and the anterior or central compartment of the neck, located between the carotid arteries of the two sides (level VI). Lymph nodes at level VI receive lymphatics from the thyroid gland, subglottic larynx, cervical trachea, hypopharynx, and cervical esophagus.

With the exception of the glottic larynx and the paranasal sinuses, other sites within the head and neck

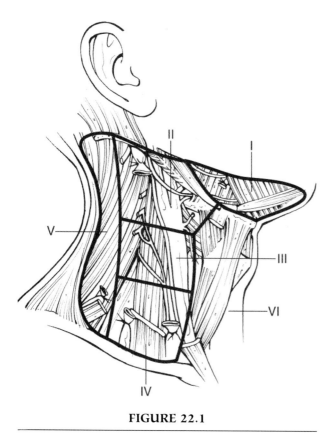

FIGURE 22.1

Superficial dissection of the right side of the neck, showing the carotid and subclavian arteries (Henry Gray, *Anatomy of the Human Body*, 20th ed, thoroughly revised and re-edited by Warren H. Lewis, Philadelphia: Lea & Febiger, 1918; New York: bartleby.com, 2000).

have a sufficient lymphatic network such that spread to the neck lymph nodes is common. The previous classification of cervical lymph nodes into levels is useful to predict the lymph node groups that are most likely to be involved with metastatic disease for different locations of primary tumors (2). For example, oral cavity cancers typically spread to lymph node levels I and II, while levels II, III, and IV are common sites for the dissemination of laryngeal carcinomas. The classification system is also fundamental in standardizing the terminology used to describe the different types of neck dissections (3). In the case of comprehensive neck dissections (removal of lymph node levels I–V; cranial nerve XI, the internal jugular vein, and the sternocleidomastoid muscle may be all removed or be selectively spared in a "modified" dissection), at least 10 or more nodes are included in the dissected specimen for pathological review. For selective neck dissection in which fewer than five lymph node levels are removed, at least six or more nodes must be removed (4). Neck pain and shoulder dysfunction are potential sequelae to neck dissections, particularly comprehensive ones.

The arterial supply of the head and neck is complex. The principal arteries are the two common carotid arteries and their branches. The common carotid arteries ascend in the neck and each divides into two branches: the external carotid, supplying the exterior of the head, face, and greater part of the neck; and the internal carotid, supplying to a great extent the contents of the cranial and orbital cavities.

With regard to the salivary glands, paired sublingual glands lie immediately underneath the mucosa of the anterior floor of the mouth, while the submandibular glands lie in the upper neck, resting on the external surface of the mylohyoid muscle between the mandible and the insertion of the mylohyoid. The submandibular duct (Wharton duct) exits in the anterior floor of the mouth near the midline. In the subcutaneous tissue of the face, overlying the mandibular ramus and anterior-inferior to the external ear, lie the parotid glands. They secrete saliva through Stenson ducts, opening into the buccal mucosa opposite the second upper molars. Collectively, the sublingual, submandibular, and sublingual glands are known as the major salivary glands. In addition, numerous minor salivary glands are distributed along the submucosa of the entire upper aerodigestive tract. Salivary gland malignancies may also spread to lymph nodes within the neck.

PATHOLOGY

Squamous Cell Cancer

As previously indicated, the vast majority of HNCs are of the squamous cell variety. Immunohistochemically, these tumors are positive for keratin. Carcinogenesis from normal epithelium starts with hyperplasia, with evolution to dysplasia, carcinoma in situ (restricted by the basement membrane and noninvasive) prior to invasive cancer. As such, squamous cell carcinomas may be preceded by various precancerous lesions. Erythroplakia (red, velvety plaque) and leukoplakia (a white plaque that does not rub off) are two widely appreciated premalignant entities. With erythroplakia, the incidence of dysplasia, carcinoma in situ, or invasive cancer is approximately 90%. Although overall, leukoplakia is less prognostically worrisome, a biopsy is recommended to evaluate the severity of dysplasia since the degree of atypia has a direct bearing on the prognosis and management (5).

The histologic grading of squamous cell carcinomas is based on the structure, degree of differentiation, nuclear polymorphism, and number of mitoses (6). Other parameters, such as mode and stage of invasion, presence of vascular invasion, and cellular response, are also assessed. Well-differentiated squamous cell carcinomas are easily recognizable. Epithelial pearls are commonly observed. Verrucous carcinoma, a variant of well-differentiated squamous cell carcinoma, is a low-grade tumor. The classic location of these lesions is the oral cavity (buccal mucosa and lower gingiva). Verrucous carcinomas are indolent neoplasms that may display malignant features such as basement membrane disruption without true signs of invasion. Regional lymph node metastases are rare, and the histology is not associated with distant metastases. Basaloid squamous cell carcinoma is an aggressive variant of squamous cell carcinoma. It is strongly associated with human papillomavirus (HPV) infection (7), and has a predilection for oral cavity, oropharynx, and larynx but can also occur in other sites outside the head and neck. Spindle cell carcinoma, adenoid squamous cell, adenosquamous, small cell, and lymphoepitheliomalike carcinoma are also derived from the surface epithelial tissue and are less frequently diagnosed variants of head and neck squamous cell carcinoma (HNSCC).

Nasopharynx Cancer (NPC)

Carcinomas account for about 85% of nasopharyngeal malignant tumors and are divided into three main histologic types according to the World Health Organization (WHO) classification: type I—keratinizing squamous cell carcinoma; type II—nonkeratinizing carcinoma; type III—undifferentiated, lymphoepithelioid carcinoma. Type I is identified in one-third to one-half of nasopharyngeal cancers, occurring in nonendemic areas of the world, such as North America, and has a more locoregional behavior not dissimilar to other squamous cell carcinomas of the head and neck. Types II and III predominate in endemic regions, such as southern

China, North Africa, and the far north hemisphere. These subtypes have a higher propensity for distant metastases. When a prominent lymphocytic infiltrate is present, the term lymphoepithelioma is applied, and the pathological distinction from lymphoma may be more difficult.

Nasal Cavity and Paranasal Sinus Cancer

Squamous cell carcinoma accounts for more than 50% of nasal cavity and paranasal sinus tumors, with the remainder consisting of minor salivary gland tumors, adenocarcinomas, and sinonasal neuroectodermal tumors (8–10). Squamous cell carcinoma comprises two basic histomorphologic subtypes: typical keratinizing and nonkeratinizing (cylindrical cell carcinoma, transitional-type carcinoma). Sinonasal neuroectodermal tumors include esthesioneuroblastomas, sinonasal neuroendocrine carcinomas (SNEC), and sinonasal undifferentiated carcinomas (SNUC) (11,12). This latter entity, possibly arising from the Schneiderian epithelium, has been recognized and clearly distinguished from esthesioneuroblastoma and undifferentiated nasopharyngeal carcinoma (13,14). Adenocarcinomas are relatively more common among ethmoidal sinus tumors and can be broadly classified into enteric and nonenteric subtypes based on their similarity to adenocarcinoma of the intestinal and seromucous glands, respectively.

Salivary Gland Cancer

Salivary gland cancers pose a particular challenge to the pathologist, primarily because of the complexity of the classification, which includes more than 20 different malignant histologies. The most commonly encountered are listed in Table 22.1. The situation is further compounded by the relative rarity of several entities and because there may be a broad spectrum of morphologic diversity within individual lesions.

TABLE 22.1
Histological Classification of Salivary Gland Carcinomas

MALIGNANT HISTOLOGY	INCIDENCE (%)
Mucoepidermoid	15.7
Adenoid cystic carcinoma	10.0
Adenocarcinoma	8.0
Malignant mixed tumor	5.7
Acinic cell carcinoma	3.0
Epidermoid carcinoma	1.9
Other	1.3

Adapted from Spiro RH. Salivary neoplasms: overview of a 35-year experience with 2,807 patients. *Head Neck Surg.* 1986;8:177–184.

Mucoepidermoid carcinoma (MEC) is the most common malignant salivary gland neoplasm, and is the predominant subtype observed in the parotid gland (15). MEC is a malignant epithelial tumor that is composed of various proportions of mucous, epidermoid (squamous), intermediate, columnar, and clear cells, and often demonstrates prominent cystic growth. MECs are histologically classified as low grade, intermediate grade, and high grade. High-grade MEC is an aggressive malignancy that both metastasizes and recurs locally. Although tumor grade may be useful, stage appears to be a better indicator of prognosis (16,17).

Adenoid cystic carcinoma (ACC) is a slow-growing but aggressive neoplasm with a remarkable capacity for recurrence (17). It is the most common malignant histology found in the minor salivary glands. Morphologically, three growth patterns have been described: cribriform, or classic pattern; tubular; and solid, or basaloid, pattern. Solid ACC is a high-grade lesion with reported recurrence rates of as much as 100%, compared with 50%–80% for the tubular and cribriform variants (18). Regardless of histologic grade, ACCs, with their unusually slow biologic growth, tend to have a protracted course characterized by neurotropic as well as distant spread, and ultimately a poor outcome. The 10-year survival is <50% for all grades (15,19,20). However, due to its indolent growth and poor response to chemotherapy, asymptomatic metastases, especially to the lungs, are frequently observed and not immediately treated. Clinical stage, particularly tumor size, is more critical than histologic grade in determining the outcome of ACC (21).

EPIDEMIOLOGY AND RISK FACTORS

Squamous cell HNC is more common among men than women. The incidence increases with age, and the age-adjusted incidence and mortality rates are higher among African Americans than members of other ethnic groups (22). Tobacco and alcohol use are the best established risk factors, accounting for approximately 75% of all oral and pharyngeal cancers in the United States (23), and may explain much of the variation in incidence rates among different ethnic groups and genders (24). The use of tobacco and alcohol is associated with so-called "field cancerization" of the upper aerodigestive tract, with an associated increased risk for synchronous lesions as well as second primary cancers.

More specifically, squamous cell HNC is six times more frequent in smokers than nonsmokers (25); continued tobacco use after successful treatment of the initial HNC is associated with a fourfold increased risk for a second primary cancer compared to those who stop smoking or never smoked (26). Smokeless tobacco and other chewed or ingested carcinogens, such as betel quid (Asia) and maté (South America), increase the risk of oral cancers (27,28). Alcohol appears to be a less potent carcinogen than tobacco (25); however, the combination of alcohol and tobacco is multiplicative not just additive (29). Of note, paranasal sinuses and the nasopharynx primary sites do not have a clear association with tobacco or alcohol usage.

There is a growing appreciation of the role of HPV infection as a risk factor for squamous cell HNC, particularly of the oropharynx in patients without a history of significant tobacco or alcohol use. The most commonly identified strains are HPV 16, -18, -31, -33, and -35, with HPV-16 being the most common. HPV genomic DNA has been detected in 26% of all squamous cell HNC and 50% of oropharyngeal cancer by polymerase chain reaction (PCR) methodology (7,30). HPV-positive HNC also seems to be a distinct entity in terms of epidemiologic, clinical, genomic, and histopathological characteristics when compared to the more common alcohol- and tobacco-related HNCs (7). HPV-positive HNSCC is more frequently seen in younger patients with high-risk sexual behavior, is characterized by poorly differentiated histology with basaloid histotype, and has a better overall prognosis compared to other HNCs related to more conventional risk factors (7).

Dietary factors may also contribute. The incidence of squamous cell HNC is highest among individuals with the lowest consumption of fruits and vegetables. Chronic nutritional deficiency as well as poor oral health may enhance the risk. Clinical findings consistent with poor oral hygiene (eg, mucosal irritation, dental caries, tartar) are associated with a two- to fourfold increase in the risk of oral cancer after adjustment for sex, age, diet, alcohol, and tobacco habits (31,32). The use of vitamin A and E supplementation may decrease the incidence of squamous cell HNC (33). Not surprisingly then, there has been keen interest in the use of certain vitamins and their analogues with chemopreventive intent.

With regard to other primary sites, certain occupational exposures, such as to nickel, wood, and leather dust, are associated with cancers of the sinonasal tract (25,34). Risk factors for salivary gland cancer are less well studied and established. However, prior exposure to ionizing radiation may increase the risk of salivary gland cancers, particularly MEC (35,36). An endemic form of nasopharyngeal cancer occurs in the Mediterranean basin and southern China, and appears linked to infection with the Epstein-Barr virus (EBV). EBV DNA levels seem to correlate with treatment response and may predict disease recurrence, suggesting that they may be an independent indicator of prognosis (37,38).

In nonendemic regions in which WHO type I is more common, the connection with EBV is more controversial (39). Diets high in smoked foods are also associated with an increased risk for nasopharynx cancer.

PRESENTATION AND DIAGNOSIS

Patients most commonly present with locoregional symptoms referable to the primary site and consistent with the anatomy of the region. A new ulcer that will not heal, pain, bleeding, dysphagia, odynophagia, changes in articulation, otalgia, hoarseness, nasal or ear congestion, epistaxis, diplopia, or a new lump in the neck are examples of common presenting symptoms. Whether a patient will present early or late is affected by the anatomy of the primary site. For example, glottic cancers tend to present early because patients will seek attention for new hoarseness; however, supraglottic cancers tend to present later because symptoms of dysphagia or throat discomfort may be more vague and discounted as not serious by the patient. With the exception of nasopharynx and hypopharynx primaries, distant metastases at presentation are uncommon. The lung, bone, or liver are the most common distant metastatic sites. Of note, an isolated lung nodule is commonly a new lung primary, given the risk of second or synchronous cancers, as opposed to a metastatic lesion from the primary HNC.

There are no compelling data that screening for HNC improves health outcomes, and as such, the United States Preventive Services Task Force (USPSTF) (40) has no specific recommendations regarding screening for these diseases in the general population. Similarly, there are no tests of serum or saliva that are routinely utilized. Nonetheless, direct inspection and palpation during routine dental examination is commonly recommended and frequently applied as a screen for oral cancer.

As mentioned in the pathology section, leukoplakia and erythroplakia are widely appreciated for their premalignant potential for the development of HNC. Their presence heralds the presence or development of invasive cancer and should be carefully evaluated.

For patients who are disease-free after treatment for their HNC, follow-up is needed due to a risk of relapse, particularly during the first three years, and also an increased rate of second primary cancers (3%–5% per year) among those patients who had an initial squamous cell primary. Per National Comprehensive Cancer Network guidelines (41), history and physical exams are performed every 1–3 months during the first year, every 2–4 months during the second year, every 4–6 months during the third to fifth years, and every 6–12 months thereafter. Thyroid function tests (if neck radiation was administered) are also recommended, as well as chest imaging as indicated. Once treatment is completed and the patient is felt to be disease-free, routine imaging of the primary site and neck are not routinely indicated in the absence of suspicious signs or symptoms.

Evaluation of a patient with suspected HNC is aimed at reaching a pathological diagnosis and ascertaining the stage of the disease. Tissue for pathological analysis can be obtained through biopsy performed on mucosal lesions during exam or endoscopy. Biopsies of tumors of the oral cavity and oropharynx can be obtained transorally under topical anesthetic; other tumors, such as those of the larynx and pharynx, that are not as easily accessible transorally require pharyngolaryngoscopy under general anesthesia. Fine-needle aspiration cytology (FNAC) is the least invasive and most expeditious method for investigating cervical lymph nodes (42). FNAC of smaller lymph nodes that are not definable on palpation can be performed using imaging guidance. Core biopsies of neck node/mass can be pursued when FNA yields equivocal or difficult to classify findings or lymphoma is suspected. Excisional biopsy of neck node may at times be necessary, but when squamous cell carcinoma is suspected and neck dissection is likely required, should be incorporated preferably into the definitive management plan.

STAGING OF HNC

Staging of HNC assesses the extent of disease, establishes prognosis, and guides management. Most commonly, the American Joint Committee on Cancer (AJCC, 2002) T (primary tumor) N (nodal disease) M (distant metastases) classification system (TNM system) is used for staging tumors of the head and neck. T staging is specific to different anatomical sites in the head and neck, while N staging is common to all head and neck sites (Table 22.2) except the nasopharynx. A final stage group (I–IV) is reached based on the aggregate TNM stage and is similar for all primary sites except NPC (Table 22.3). A detailed description of the TNM staging system for HNSCC is available elsewhere (43,44).

Clinical staging is assessed through physical exam, which often requires some type of endoscopic exam, and radiographic studies. Cross-sectional imaging with computed axial tomography (CAT) primary site and scan and/or magnetic resonance imaging (MRI) of the neck is routinely used to evaluate the locoregional extent of disease (T and N stages), except in case of T_1 laryngeal tumors confined to the vocal cords, where there is low likelihood that radiographic imaging improves the accuracy of clinical staging (45). The lungs are the most common

TABLE 22.2
Neck Staging for All Head and Neck Sites Except for Nasopharynx Cancer

N STAGE	DEFINITION
NX	Regional lymph node cannot be assessed
N0	No regional lymph node metastasis
N1	Metastasis in a single ipsilateral lymph node, 3 cm or less in greatest dimension
N2a	Metastasis in a single ipsilateral lymph node more than 3 cm but no more than 6 cm in greatest dimension
N2b	Metastasis in multiple ipsilateral lymph nodes, none more than 6 cm in greatest dimension
N2c	Metastasis in bilateral or contralateral lymph nodes, none more than 6 cm in greatest dimension
N3	Metastasis in a lymph node more than 6 cm in greatest dimension

TABLE 22.3
Stage Grouping

STAGE	T	N	M
0	Tis	N0	M0
I	T1	N0	M0
II	T2	N0	M0
III	T1-2/T3	N1/N0-1	M0
IVA	T1-3/T4a	N2/N0-2	M0
IVB	T4b	Nany	M0
	Tany	N3	
IVC	Tany	Nany	M1

Abbreviations: T, tumor; N, lymph node; M, metastasis.

site of distant metastasis from squamous cell HNCs, and a chest x-ray is used to evaluate for distant metastases to the lung, a second lung primary cancer, or other cardiopulmonary disease because medical comorbidity is common among many of these patients. Patients who are at a higher risk of distant spread, such as patients with N_2 disease below the level of the thyroid notch or N_3 disease, should be considered for a more detailed evaluation with CAT scan of the chest. No routine imaging of the liver or bones is performed unless indicated by abnormal biochemical markers or suspicious symptoms, such as pain.

Fluorodeoxyglucose-positron emission tomography (FDG-PET) is not routinely performed, but is helpful in selected circumstances: the detection of occult lymph node disease, the detection of subtle recurrences, and the identification of an unknown primary site (46). The intent is to obtain PET when the information obtained may change management.

Stage IV includes a wide spectrum of locoregionally advanced as well as distantly metastatic disease. Treatment decisions need to be carefully individualized for each patient by an experienced multidisciplinary team. A stage IVA tumor by virtue of treatable N_2 neck disease in the presence of a T1, T2, or even T3 lesion is still considered eligible for curative treatment, whereas a stage IVB patient with an advanced unresectable primary cancer (T4B) or far-advanced neck disease (N3) or both would have a lower probability of cure. Patients with stage IVC disease, because of distant metastases, have exceedingly poor prognosis, with a median survival of less than one year.

TREATMENT

The aim of treatment for HNC is to maximize locoregional control and survival while minimizing functional and cosmetic alteration. Treatment plans are formulated optimally by a multidisciplinary team (ie, surgeon, radiation, and medical oncologist), particularly when more than one treatment option is available or when combined modality therapy is anticipated. Dental, speech, auditory, swallowing, and nutritional evaluations are commonly indicated before therapy.

Surgery and radiation are both potentially curative treatments; chemotherapy by itself is generally considered a palliative modality. In patients who undergo primary surgical therapy, an oncologically adequate resection that obtains pathologically negative margins is the goal. Simply debulking a tumor, or compromising surgical margins in hopes of preserving function, potentially increases the risk of local failure. The following features are suggestive of disease that is likely not resectable for cure: (1) massive skull base invasion, (2) involvement of the prevertebral fascia, (3) direct infiltration of the cervical vertebrae or brachial plexus, (4) carotid artery encasement, (5) skin infiltration, and (6) rapid recurrence after prior extensive surgery.

With regard to radiation therapy, a curative dose of ≥70 Gy is delivered to the primary and gross adenopathy, with ≥50 Gy delivered to low-risk nodal stations. When adjuvant radiation is applied after surgery, the dose to areas of prior resected gross disease is closer to 60 Gy. Conventional fractionation involves delivery of 2 Gy once daily, five times a week. Radiation-related side effects include dry mouth, mucositis, hypothyroidism (when the thyroid is within the portal) (47), loss of taste, dysphagia, and Lhermitte syndrome (a self-limited, shocklike sensation induced by neck flexion, extending down the spine to the extremities). Certain drugs may be beneficial with regard to the treatment (ie, pilocarpine) or prevention (ie, amifostine) of xerostomia (48–50). Altered fractionation radiation is sometimes utilized, such as hyperfractionation (more than one fraction daily), which has been shown to increase efficacy but at the expense of added acute toxicity. Concurrent chemotherapy similarly improves efficacy. More recently, intensity-modulated radiotherapy (IMRT) has become widely available and allows a more conformal dose distribution. By decreasing toxicity to normal adjacent tissue, it allows for dose escalation and may improve locoregional control.

To organize the subsequent discussion, treatment options will be reviewed based on disease extent.

Stage I or II Disease

One-third of patients with HNC present with limited disease at diagnosis (ie, stages I or II, without lymph node involvement). Five-year overall survival in cases of limited disease ranges from 60%–90% (51), varying with primary site, stage, and histology. These patients are generally treated with single-modality surgery or radiotherapy if possible. The choice of treatment is often determined by the anatomical site of disease, available expertise, and the side effect profiles that can be expected with different treatment approaches.

Radiotherapy is preferred for less advanced laryngeal and oro-/hypopharyngeal cancers to preserve voice and swallowing. Similarly, radiation is the primary approach for small nasopharynx cancers, as these tumors are sensitive to radiation and the location makes surgical resection difficult. Surgery is generally favored in treatment of localized lesions of the oral cavity. This approach avoids the acute and late sequelae of radiotherapy treatment such as xerostomia, dental damage, and osteoradionecrosis of the jaw.

Surgery is also the preferred option for salivary gland cancers in general and for limited-stage disease of paranasal sinus and nasal cavity.

Most patients with limited squamous cell HNC are cured of their disease. As such, second primary cancers related to prior tobacco or alcohol exposure are a particular concern. Counseling patients regarding the role of tobacco or alcohol in the genesis of their disease and the importance of eliminating or at least decreasing these behaviors is important. There has been keen interest in chemoprevention to reduce the incidence of these second primaries. Vitamin A analogs have been the most widely investigated. An initial trial using isotretinoin compared to placebo was found to decrease the rate of second primaries (52). However, subsequent studies were not able to corroborate these results (53–55). Other agents are under investigation, but at present, the use of drugs with chemopreventive intent outside of a clinical trial after treatment is not recommended.

Stage III or IV, M0 Disease

Unfortunately, most patients with HNC present with locoregionally advanced disease at diagnosis and have an expected five-year overall survival of 30%–50% (51). Curative-intent treatment for patients with stage III or IVA-B disease requires a multimodality treatment strategy. As in patients with less advanced HNC, there is often more than one way to proceed with therapy, and the related side effects of different approaches are carefully considered.

In patients who undergo primary surgical treatment, in addition to surgical management of the primary site, surgical reconstruction is often necessary and neck dissection is frequently performed to address disease metastatic to neck lymph nodes. Although primary surgical management can be applied for resectable tumors at any primary site, it is arguably the preferred approach for advanced oral cavity and paranasal cancers, as good functional and cosmetic results after surgical removal can be obtained with flaps, grafts, and prostheses as indicated. Appropriate rehabilitation afterward remains nonetheless important. After surgical management of locoregionally advanced disease, adjuvant radiation is typically administered. The addition of concomitant chemotherapy (cisplatin) to postoperative radiotherapy has been demonstrated to improve locoregional disease control in patients with pathological features predicting high risk of failure, particularly: (1) microscopically involved resection margins and/or (2) extracapsular spread of tumor from neck nodes (56). The interval from surgery to completion of radiotherapy should be 10–11 weeks or less in the absence of any postoperative medical or surgical complications, since the cumulative time of combined therapy (from surgery to the completion of adjuvant radiotherapy) has been shown to affect locoregional control and survival in high-risk patients (57,58).

Primary chemoradiation, with surgery reserved for salvage, is preferred in settings where surgical treatment (eg, total laryngectomy) may lead to significant morbidity and available rehabilitative options (eg, esophageal speech, tracheoesophageal puncture [TEP]) may be viewed as not optimal by the patient. Under these circumstances, primary chemoradiation provides the benefit of possible organ and functional preservation without compromising survival. It is also pursued in patients with unresectable tumors. Radiation is the curative backbone of this treatment. In patients with advanced squamous cell head and neck cancer, concurrent chemotherapy with radiation appears to lead to superior disease control compared to the use of neoadjuvant (before radiation) or adjuvant (after radiation) chemotherapy (59,60). For example, concomitant chemoradiotherapy has resulted in better laryngectomy free-survival (organ preservation) compared to induction chemotherapy followed by radiotherapy or radiotherapy alone in a phase 3 trial in locally advanced laryngeal cancer (61). In patients with nasopharyngeal carcinoma, the addition of concomitant chemotherapy with cisplatin is also associated with therapeutic benefit, and for this site, adjuvant chemotherapy is also administered (62,63). Of note, newer triplet induction chemotherapy regimens appear superior to prior doublet ones (64–66), and the potential for integration of induction chemotherapy followed by concurrent chemoradiotherapy is being actively evaluated.

Cisplatin is the best established agent for concurrent use with radiation. Studies have found the most robust survival advantage using cisplatin, demonstrating an 11% absolute survival benefit at five years (59,60). Patients who are not optimal candidates for cisplatin therapy due to comorbidities such as preexisting renal insufficiency, neuropathy, or hearing loss can be considered for alternative concurrent options. One is cetuximab, a monoclonal antibody against the epidermal growth factor receptor (EGFR). In a recent phase 3 trial, concurrent administration of cetuximab resulted in a 10% improvement in overall survival at three years compared to radiotherapy alone without significantly increasing treatment-related local toxicities (67). However, cetuximab is not without its own side effects and can result in serious allergic reactions in a small minority of patients, and is also associated with an acneiform rash in the majority of patients.

It is important to appreciate that combined chemoradiotherapy is intense treatment and patients so treated often experience significant acute toxic effects. Mucositis, dysphagia, vomiting, dehydration, weight loss, anemia, and myelosuppression are commonly seen. The therapy is best done by an experienced multidisciplinary team with the availability of appropriate infrastructure to provide the necessary supportive care.

In patients who are treated with primary concurrent chemoradiation, persistent neck masses may require additional surgical management. Previously, studies found improved survival in patients with initial advanced nodal disease (N2–3) who underwent neck dissection following chemoradiation (68). However, more recently, the routine application of neck dissection under these circumstances independent of response has been questioned (69). Many centers will do such postchemoradiotherapy neck dissections more selectively based on observed response and radiographic imaging results.

Primary surgical management is preferred for advanced salivary gland cancers. Commonly applied indications for postoperative radiotherapy include: (1) microscopic (eg, R1 resection) or macroscopic (eg, R2 resection) residual disease after surgery; (2) multiple involved lymph nodes; (3) undifferentiated or high-grade tumors; (4) presence of perineural invasion; or (5) the presence of advance disease, for example, involvement of the deep lobe of the parotid (70). For unresectable salivary gland cancers, there are data to support the use of neutron therapy (71). Concomitant chemotherapy and radiation in this setting is less well studied.

Relapsed and/or Metastatic Disease

Most commonly, patients will have local or regional recurrent disease. If surgery or further radiotherapy (72) (possibly with concurrent chemotherapy) is feasible, these approaches offer the best chance for more durable disease control. Other patients with relapsed and/or metastatic disease are treated mainly with palliative chemotherapy and measures for best supportive care. The overall prognostic outlook for patients treated with the best available systemic therapies is worrisome. The expected major response rates to chemotherapy in this setting range between 10% and 40%, with median survivals consistently less than one year. Combination chemotherapy may improve the response rates, but at the expense of more toxicity and a disappointing impact on overall survival (73,74). Clinical trials evaluating new and promising agents are a particularly good option for many patients under these circumstances. There is keen interest in strategies that combine chemotherapy with newer targeted therapies. Preliminary results of a randomized trial comparing platinum-based chemotherapy with or without cetuximab in patients with recurrent or metastatic squamous cell HNC indicate a survival advantage with the addition of the cetuximab (75).

References

1. Jemal A, Siegel R, Ward E, et al. Cancer statistics, 2007. *CA Cancer J Clin.* 2007;57(1):143–166.
2. Shah JP. Patterns of cervical lymph node metastasis from squamous carcinomas of the upper aerodigestive tract. *Am J Surg.* October 1990;160(4):405–409.
3. Shah JP, Patel SG. *Head and Neck Surgery and Oncology*, 3rd ed. Edinburgh: Mosby; 2003.
4. Sobin LH, Wittekind C, eds. *TNM Classification of Malignant Tumors*, 6th ed. New York: Wiley-Liss; 2000.
5. Hellquist H, Lundgren J, Olofsson J. Hyperplasia, keratosis, dysplasia and carcinoma in situ of the vocal cords—a follow-up study. *Clin Otolaryngol Allied Sci.* 1982;7:11–27.
6. Schanmugaratnam K, Sobin LH. The World Health Organization histological classification of tumours of the upper respira-

tory tract and ear. A commentary on the second edition. *Cancer.* 1993;71:2689–2697.

7. Fakhry C, Gillison ML. Clinical implications of human papillomavirus in head and neck cancers. *J Clin Oncol.* June 10, 2006;24(17):2606–2611.

8. Katz TS, Mendenhall WM, Morris CG, et al. Malignant tumors of the nasal cavity and paranasal sinuses. *Head Neck.* September 2002;24(9):821–829.

9. Porceddu S, Martin J, Shanker G, et al. Paranasal sinus tumors: Peter MacCallum Cancer Institute experience. *Head Neck.* April 2004;26(4):322–330.

10. Dirix P, Nuyts S, Geussens Y, et al. Malignancies of the nasal cavity and paranasal sinuses: long-term outcome with conventional or three-dimensional conformal radiotherapy. *Int J Radiat Oncol Biol Phys.* November 15, 2007;69(4):1042–1050.

11. Silva EG, Butler JJ, Mac Kay B, et al. Neuroblastomas and neuroendocrine carcinomas of the nasal cavity: a proposed new classification. *Cancer.* 1982;50:2388–2405.

12. Haas I, Ganzer U. Does sophisticated diagnostic workup on neuroectodermal tumors have an impact on the treatment of esthesioneuroblastoma? *Onkologie.* 2003;26:261–267.

13. Frierson HF, Mills SE, Fechner RE, et al. Sinonasal undifferentiated carcinoma: an aggressive neoplasm derived from Schneiderian epithelium and distinct from olfactory neuroblastoma. *Am J Surg Pathol.* 1986;10:771–779.

14. Jeng J, Sung M, Fang C, et al. Sinonasal undifferentiated carcinoma and nasopharyngeal-type undifferentiated carcinoma: two clinically, biologically and histopathologically distinct entities. *Am J Surg Pathol.* 2002;26:371–376.

15. Speight PM, Barrett AW. Salivary gland tumours. *Oral Dis.* 2002;8(5):229–240.

16. Brandwein MS, Ivanov K, Wallace DI, et al. Mucoepidermoid carcinoma: a clinicopathologic study of 80 patients with special reference to histological grading. *Am J Surg Pathol.* 2001;25(7):835–845.

17. Ellis GL. Major and minor salivary glands. In: Rosai J, ed. *Ackerman's Surgical Pathology,* 8th ed. St. Louis: Mosby; 1996:815–856.

18. Tomich CE. Adenoid cystic carcinoma. In: Ellis GL, Auclair PL, Gnepp DR, eds. *Surgical Pathology of the Salivary Glands.* Philadelphia: Saunders; 1991:333–349.

19. Spiro RH. The controversial adenoid cystic carcinoma: clinical considerations. In: McGurk M, Renehan AG, eds. *Controversies in the Management of Salivary Gland Disease.* Oxford: Oxford University Press; 2001:207–211.

20. Friedrich RE, Bleckmann V. Adenoid cystic carcinoma of salivary and lacrimal gland origin: localization, classification, clinical pathological correlation, treatment results and long-term follow-up control in 84 patients. *Anticancer Res.* 2003;23(2A):931–940.

21. Spiro RH, Huvos AG. Stage means more than grade in adenoid cystic carcinoma. *Am J Surg.* 1992;164(6):623–628.

22. SEER registry. http://seer.cancer.gov, February 13, 2009.

23. Blot JW, McLaughlin JK, Winn DM, et al. Smoking and drinking in relation to oral and pharyngeal cancer. *Cancer Res.* June 1, 1988;46(11):3282–3287.

24. Day GL, Blot WJ, Austin DF, et al. Racial differences in risk of oral and pharyngeal cancer: alcohol, tobacco, and other determinants. *J Natl Cancer Inst.* March 17, 1993;85(6):465–473.

25. Decker J, Goldstein JC. Risk factors in head and neck cancer. *N Engl J Med.* 1982;306:1151–1155.

26. Day GL, Blot WL, Shore RE, et al. Second cancers following oral and pharyngeal cancers: role of tobacco and alcohol. *J Natl Cancer Inst.* January 19, 1994;82(2):131–137.

27. Ho PS, Ko YC, Yang YH, et al. The incidence of oropharyngeal cancer in Taiwan: an endemic betel quid chewing area. *J Oral Pathol Med.* 2002;31(4):213–219.

28. Goldenberg D, Golz A, Joachims HZ. The beverage maté: a risk factor for cancer of the head and neck. *Head Neck.* 2003;25(7):595–601.

29. Rothman K, Keller A. The effect of joint exposure to alcohol and tobacco on risk of cancer of the mouth and pharynx. *J Chronic Dis.* 1972;25:711–716.

30. Kreimer AR, Clifford GM, Boyle P, Franceschi S. Human papillomavirus types in head and neck squamous cell carcinomas worldwide: a systematic review. *Cancer Epidemiol Biomarkers Prev.* February 2005;14(2):467–475.

31. Talamini R, Vaccarella S, Barbone F, et al. Oral hygiene, dentition, sexual habits and risk of oral cancer. *Br J Cancer.* 2000;83:1238–1242.

32. Balaram P, Sridhar H, Rajkumar T, et al. Oral cancer in southern India: the influence of smoking, drinking, paan-chewing and oral hygiene. *Int J Cancer.* 2002;98:440–445.

33. Drigley G, McLaughlin JK, Block G, et al. Vitamin supplement use and reduced risk of oral and pharyngeal cancer. *Am J Epidemiol.* May 1992;135(10):1083–1092.

34. Barnes L. Intestinal-type adenocarcinoma of the nasal cavity and paranasal sinuses. *Am J Surg Pathol.* 1986;10: 192–202.

35. Ellis GL, Auclair PL. *Tumors of the Salivary Glands.* Washington, DC: Armed Forces Institute of Pathology; 1996. Atlas of Tumor Pathology

36. Guzzo M, Andreola S, Sirizzotti G, et al. Mucoepidermoid carcinoma of the salivary glands: clinicopathologic review of 108 patients treated at the National Cancer Institute of Milan. *Ann Surg Oncol.* 2002;9(7):688–695.

37. Lo YM, Chan LY, Chan AT, et al. Quantitative and temporal correlation between circulating cell-free Epstein-Barr virus DNA and tumor recurrence in nasopharyngeal carcinoma. *Cancer Res.* 1999;59:5452–5455.

38. Lin JC, Wang WY, Chen KY, et al. Quantification of plasma Epstein-Barr virus DNA in patients with advanced nasopharyngeal carcinoma. *N Engl J Med.* 2004;350:2461–2470.

39. Raab-Traub N. Epstein-Barr virus in the pathogenesis of NPC. *Semin Cancer Biol.* December 2002;12(6):431–441.

40. USPTF. http://www.ahrq.gov/clinic/uspstf/uspsoral.htm. (Accessed at February 13, 2009).

41. NCCN guidelines. http://www.nccn.org/professionals/ physician_gls/default.asp. (Accessed at February 13, 2009).

42. el Hag IA, Chiedozi LC, al Reyees FA, Kollur SM. Fine needle aspiration cytology of head and neck masses. Seven years' experience in a secondary care hospital. *Acta Cytol.* May–June 2003;47(3):387–392.

43. Greene FL, Page DL, Fleming ID, et al. *AJCC Cancer Staging Manual,* 6th ed. New York: Springer; 2002.

44. Patel SG, Shah JP. TNM staging of cancers of the head and neck: striving for uniformity among diversity. *CA Cancer J Clin.* 2005;55(4):242–258.

45. Kaanders JH, Hordijk GJ. Dutch Cooperative Head and Neck Oncology Group. Carcinoma of the larynx: the Dutch national guideline for diagnostics, treatment, supportive care and rehabilitation. *Radiother Oncol.* June 2002;63(3):299–307.

46. Regelink G, Brouwer J, de Bree R, et al. Detection of unknown primary tumours and distant metastases in patients with cervical metastases: value of FDG-PET versus conventional modalities. *Eur J Nucl Med Mol Imaging.* August 2002;29(8):1024–1030.

47. Turner SL, Tiver KW, Boyages SC. Thyroid dysfunction following radiotherapy for head and neck cancer. *Int J Radiat Oncol Biol Phys.* 1995;31(2):279–283.

48. Johnson JT, Ferretti GA, Nethery WJ, et al. Oral pilocarpine for post-irradiation xerostomia in patients with head and neck cancer. *N Engl J Med.* August 5, 1993;329(6):390–395.

49. Chambers MS, Posner M, Jones CU, et al. Cevimeline for the treatment of postirradiation xerostomia in patients with head-and-neck cancer. *Int J Radiat Oncol Biol Phys.* 2007;68(40):1102–1109.

50. Brizel DM, Wasserman TH, Henke M, et al. Phase III randomized trial of amifostine as a radioprotector in head and neck cancer. *J Clin Oncol.* October 1, 2000;18(19):3339–3345.

51. Vokes EE. Head and neck cancer. In: Kasper DL, Braunwald E, Hauser S, et al., eds. *Harrison's Principles of Internal Medicine,* 16th ed. New York: McGraw-Hill; 2005;503–506.

52. Hong WK, Lippman SM, Itri LM, et al. Prevention of second primary tumors with isotretinoin in squamous-cell carcinoma of the head and neck. *N Engl J Med.* September 20, 1990;323(12):795–801.

53. Bolla M, Lefur R, Ton Van J, et al. Prevention of second primary tumours with etretinate in squamous cell carcinoma of the oral cavity and oropharynx. Results of a multicentric double-blind randomized study. *Eur J Cancer*. 1994;30A(6):767–772.

54. Khuri FR, Lee JJ, Lippman SM, et al. Randomized phase III trial of low-dose isotretinoin for prevention of second primary tumors in stage I and II head and neck cancer patients. *J Natl Cancer Inst*. April 5, 2006;98(7):426–427.

55. Van Zanwijk N, Dalesio O, Patorino U, et al. EUROSCAN, a randomized trial of vitamin A and N-acetylcysteine in patients with head and neck cancer or lung cancer: for the European Organization for Research and Treatment of Cancer Head and Neck and Lung Cancer Cooperative Groups. *J Natl Cancer Inst*. 2000;92:977–986.

56. Bernier J, Cooper JS, Pajak TF, et al. Defining risk levels in locally advanced head and neck cancers: a comparative analysis of concurrent postoperative radiation plus chemotherapy trials of the EORTC (#22931) and RTOG (# 9501). *Head Neck*. October 2005;27(10):843–850.

57. Ang KK, Trotti A, Brown BW, et al. Randomized trial addressing risk features and time factors of surgery plus radiotherapy in advanced head-and-neck cancer. *Int J Radiat Oncol Biol Phys*. November 1, 2001;51(3):571–578.

58. Awwad HK, Lotayef M, Shouman T, et al. Accelerated hyperfractionation (AHF) compared to conventional fractionation (CF) in the postoperative radiotherapy of locally advanced head and neck cancer: influence of proliferation. *Br J Cancer*. February 12, 2002;86(4):517–523.

59. Pignon JP, Bourhis J, Domenge C, Designe L. Chemotherapy added to locoregional treatment for head and neck squamous-cell carcinoma: three meta-analyses of updated individual data. MACH-NC Collaborative Group. Meta-Analysis of Chemotherapy on Head and Neck Cancer. *Lancet*. March 18, 2000;355(9208):949–955.

60. Bouhris J, Amand C, Pignon JP. Update of MACH-NC (Meta-analysis of chemotherapy in Head & Neck cancer) database focused on concomitant chemoradiotherapy: 5505. *J Clin Oncol*, ASCO Annual Meeting Proceedings (Post-Meeting edition) 2004; 22 (145 (July 15 Supplement).

61. Forastiere AA, Goepfert H, Maor M, et al. Concurrent chemotherapy and radiotherapy for organ preservation in advanced laryngeal cancer. *N Engl J Med*. November 27, 2003;349(22):2091–2098.

62. Al-Sarraf M, LeBlanc M, Giri PG, et al. Chemoradiotherapy versus radiotherapy in patients with advanced nasopharyngeal cancer: phase III randomized Intergroup study 0099. *J Clin Oncol*. April 1998; 16(4):1310–1317.

63. Langendijk JA, Leemans CR, Buter J, et al. The additional value of chemotherapy to radiotherapy in locally advanced nasopharyngeal carcinoma: a meta-analysis of the published literature. *J Clin Oncol*. November 15, 2004;22(22):4604–4612.

64. Posner MR, Hershock DM, Blajman CR, et al. Cisplatin and fluorouracil alone or with docetaxel in head and neck cancer. *N Engl J Med*. 2007;357:1705–1715.

65. Vermorken JB, Remenar E, van Herpen C, et al. Cisplatin, fluorouracil, and docetaxel in unresectable head and neck cancer. *N Engl J Med*. 2007;357:1695–1704.

66. Hitt R, Lopez-Pousa A, Martinez-Trufero J, et al. Phase III study comparing cisplatin plus fluorouracil to paclitaxel, cisplatin, and fluorouracil induction chemotherapy followed by chemoradiotherapy in locally advanced head and neck cancer. *J Clin Oncol*. 2005;23:8636–8645.

67. Bonner JA, Harari PM, Giralt J, et al. Radiotherapy plus cetuximab for squamous-cell carcinoma of the head and neck. *N Engl J Med*. February 9, 2006;354(6):567–578.

68. Brizel DM, Prosnitz RG, Hunter S, et al. Necessity for adjuvant neck dissection in setting of concurrent chemoradiation for advanced head-and-neck cancer. *Int J Radiat Oncol Biol Phys*. April 1, 2004;58(5):1418–1423.

69. Goguen LA, Posner MR, Tishler RB, et al. Examining the need for neck dissection in the era of chemoradiation therapy for advanced head and neck cancer. *Arch Otolaryngol Head Neck Surg*. May 2006;132(5):526–531.

70. Licitra L, Locati LD, Bossi P, Cantu G. Head and neck tumors other than squamous cell carcinoma. *Curr Opin Oncol*. May 2004;16(3):236–241.

71. Laramore GE, Krall JM, Griffin BR, et al. Neutron versus photon irradiation for unresectable salivary gland tumors: final report of an RTOG-MRC randomized clinical trial. *Int J Radiol Oncol Bio Phys*. 1993;27:235–240.

72. De Crevoisier R, Bourhis J, Domenge C, et al. Full-dose reirradiation for unresectable head and neck carcinoma: experience of the Gustave-Roussy Institute in a series of 169 patients. *J Clin Oncol*. November 1998;16(11):3556–3562.

73. Jacobs C, Lyman G, Velez-Garcia E, et al. A phase III randomized study comparing cisplatin and fluorouracil as single-agents and in combination for advanced squamous cell carcinoma of the head and neck. *J Clin Oncol*. 1992;10:257–263.

74. Forastiere AA, Metch B, Schuller DE, et al. Randomized comparison of cisplatin plus fluorouracil and carboplatin plus fluorouracil versus methotrexate in advanced squamous-cell carcinoma of the head and neck: a Southwest Oncology Group study. *J Clin Oncol*. 1992;10:1245–1251.

75. Vermorken JB, Mesia R, Rivera F., et al. Platinum–based chemotherapy plus cetuximab in head and neck cancer. *NEJM*. 2008;359:1116–1127.

Evaluation and Treatment of Thyroid Cancer

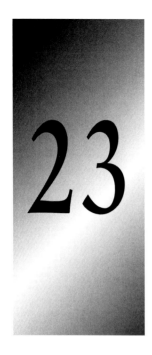

Robert Michael Tuttle
Rebecca Leboeuf

Accounting for more than 90% of all endocrine malignancies, thyroid cancer represents only about 1% of all human cancers. While there are five principal histological forms of thyroid cancer, more than 95% arise from thyroid follicular cells which, in the normal thyroid, concentrate iodine and synthesize thyroid hormone in response to TSH stimulation (1,2) (Table 23.1).

Although the incidence of very low disease-specific mortality for thyroid cancer has remained rather stable over the last 25 years, a dramatic rise in papillary thyroid cancer incidence has been seen over the last 20 years. In women, the incidence of thyroid cancer has risen from approximately 6 per 100,000 in the early 1970s to more than 12 per 100,000 by 2000–2003. A smaller, although statistically significant, rise has been seen in men over the same time frame (2.1 per 100,000 to 4.2 per 100,000) (3,4). Data from the same time period demonstrate no such rise in incidence in the other primary types of thyroid cancer.

It remains unclear whether this rise in thyroid cancer incidence is secondary to an unidentified environmental risk factor (5) or a product of more aggressive detection with more widespread use of neck ultrasound and other cross-sectional imaging over the last 20 years (3). While exposure to ionizing radiation is the best known risk factor for subsequent development of thyroid cancer after a 5–20 year latency period (6), it seems unlikely that most patients currently being diagnosed were exposed to significant radiation exposures during their lifetime.

	CELL OF ORIGIN	% OF ALL THYROID CANCERS	10-YR DISEASE-SPECIFIC SURVIVAL (%)
Papillary	Thyroid follicular cell	90	98
Follicular	Thyroid follicular cell	5	92
Anaplastic	Thyroid follicular cell	1	1–13
Medullary	C-cell (neuroendocrine)	3	80
Lymphoma	Lymphocytes	1	50–90

TABLE 23.1
Histology: disease specific survival

DIFFERENTIATED THYROID CANCER

Initial Presentation

Because the presentation, initial evaluation, and initial therapy of papillary and follicular thyroid cancer are quite similar, and because until the last 10–15 years these tumors were often lumped together by pathologists, they are often considered together as a group of malignancies knows as differentiated thyroid cancers.

In the past, differentiated thyroid cancer usually presented as a painless thyroid nodule detected either

KEY POINTS

- Thyroid cancer represents only about 1% of all human cancers, but 90% of all endocrine malignancies.
- There are five principal histological forms of thyroid cancer: papillary, follicular, anaplastic, medullary, and lymphoma.
- Most (95%) thyroid cancers arise from thyroid follicular cells.
- Because the presentation, initial evaluation, and initial therapy of papillary and follicular thyroid cancer are quite similar, they are often considered together as a group of malignancies knows as differentiated thyroid cancers.
- While the very low disease-specific mortality for thyroid cancer has remained rather stable over the last 25 years, a dramatic rise in papillary thyroid cancer incidence has been seen over the last 20 years.
- In the past, differentiated thyroid cancer usually presented as a painless thyroid nodule detected either by the patient, or a health care provider. With more widespread use of cross sectional radiologic imaging, thyroid cancer is now frequently detected as an asymptomatic incidental finding for unrelated medical conditions.
- Routine thyroid function tests (TSH, T4) are almost uniformly normal and are not used to confirm, nor can they rule out, the presence of thyroid cancer.
- Differentiated thyroid cancer usually responds very well to the standard initial therapy of thyroidectomy, lymph node dissection, and radioactive iodine (RAI) therapy. Tumor recurrence rates over a 20–30 year follow-up period remain as high as 15%–30%, particularly at both extremes of age.
- Clinically evident recurrences are not a trivial event, with as many as 8% of patients with local recurrence and 50% of patients with distant recurrence dying of the disease.
- The primary tool for detection of recurrent or persistent thyroid cancer is serum thyroglobulin (Tg).
- Since the vast majority of recurrent thyroid cancer occurs in cervical lymph nodes, and since they usually produce Tg very well, a combination of TSH stimulated Tg and careful neck ultrasonography has a very high sensitivity for detection of recurrent disease.
- RAI is often a very effective therapy for distant metastases.
- Unlike well-differentiated thyroid cancers, anaplastic thyroid cancer is a locally aggressive, poorly differentiated thyroid cancer that develops in older patients and has a disease specific mortality rate of more than 95% over 6–12 months after diagnosis.
- Primary thyroid lymphomas make up less than 2% of extranodal lymphomas, and are generally classified as either mucosa-associated lymphoid tissue (MALT) or diffuse large B-cell or mixed subtype lymphomas.
- Medullary thyroid cancer (MTC) is a neuroendocrine tumor arising from parafollicular C-cells within the thyroid gland.

by the patient or a health care provider. With more widespread use of cross-sectional radiologic imaging, thyroid cancer is now frequently detected as an asymptomatic incidental finding for unrelated medical conditions. With an average age at diagnosis of between 35 and 45, women are affected two to three times more commonly than men (7). Since more than 90% of all thyroid nodules are benign, fine-needle aspiration, often with ultrasound guidance, is used to establish a cytologic diagnosis and identify those malignant thyroid nodules that will require surgical resection (8). It is important to note that routine thyroid function tests (TSH, T4) are almost uniformly normal and are not used to rule in or cannot be used to rule out the presence of thyroid cancer.

At the time of diagnosis, differentiated thyroid cancer has metastasized to local cervical lymph nodes in at least 20%–50% of patients, but distant metastatic spread is seen in only about 2%–5% of all cases (4,9,10). Even though differentiated thyroid cancer usually responds very well to the standard initial therapy of thyroidectomy, lymph node dissection, and radioactive iodine (RAI) therapy, tumor recurrence rates over a 20–30 year follow-up period remain as high as 15%–30%, particularly at both extremes of age (9,10). Clinically evident recurrences are not a trivial event, with as many as 8% of patients with local recurrence and 50% of patients with distant recurrence dying of the disease (10).

Initial Therapy

The mainstay of thyroid cancer therapy is surgical resection of all gross evidence of disease with appropriate compartmental resection of involved cervical lymph node chains (11). Thyroid cancer patients who are at low risk of recurrence can be adequately treated with hemithyroidectomy while high risk patients usually require total thyroidectomy, resection of involved lymph node chains, and radioactive iodine ablation in the postoperative setting (8,12–15).

RAI is one of the oldest examples of targeted therapy. Because the thyroid follicular cells require iodine to synthesize thyroid hormone, they express a sodium iodine symporter in the cell membrane that very effectively transports iodine from the blood stream into the thyroid cell. Fortunately, at least 75% of malignant thyroid cells retain the function of this sodium iodine symporter and are therefore potential targets for RAI therapy. Since this transporter cannot differentiate stable iodine from RAI, we can effectively deliver a significant radiation dose to metastatic thyroid cancer cells while exposing the rest of the body to minimal radiation exposure. Low doses of RAI can be used for diagnostic whole-body scanning, whereas larger doses can be used for tumoricidal effects.

Maximal targeting of RAI to thyroid cells requires TSH stimulation (either thyroid hormone withdrawal or administration of recombinant human TSH) and depletion of stable iodine stores from the body, along with a low iodine diet for several days prior to treatment. It is necessary to avoid iodinated contrast (such as that used in CT scans) for several months before RAI treatment. If the whole body iodine stores are elevated, the relatively small amount of RAI is diluted out and will not effectively reach the metastatic thyroid cancer cells in sufficient quantity to result in cell death.

In the setting of initial therapy, external beam radiation therapy (EBRT) is seldom necessary in patients with differentiated thyroid cancer (16). EBRT is most often used for unresectable tumors that do not concentrate RAI, or older patients (older than aged 45 years) with evidence of gross extrathyroidal extension of the tumor into surrounding structures that are very likely to have microscopic or small volume macroscopic disease that is not amenable to RAI therapy. Similarly, traditional cytotoxic chemotherapy has a poor track record in differentiated thyroid cancer, and is seldom recommended in the initial management of all but the most aggressive thyroid cancers.

Since TSH is a growth factor to both normal and malignant thyroid cells, it is not surprising that retrospective studies demonstrate that TSH suppression with supraphysiologic doses of levothyroxine is associated with decreased recurrence rates. Therefore, following initial thyroid surgery and RAI treatment, TSH suppression has become a cornerstone of treatment for more than 40 years (17,18). In general, the TSH should be kept just below the reference range in most patients with differentiated thyroid cancer,

reserving high level suppression (undetectable TSH) for patients with advanced, progressive, or metastatic disease (8).

Detection of Recurrent Disease

Serum Tumor Marker

The primary tool for detection of recurrent or persistent thyroid cancer is serum thyroglobulin (Tg) (19,20). Tg is a protein synthesized and secreted by both normal and malignant thyroid cells into the peripheral circulation. The production of thyroglobulin by normal thyroid cells precludes the use of Tg as a diagnostic tool for thyroid cancer prior to FNA or surgery.

Since our initial therapies of total thyroidectomy and RAI ablation are designed to destroy all normal and malignant thyroid cells, patients cured of thyroid cancer should have nearly undetectable serum levels of Tg within 12–18 months of initial therapy. To improve the sensitivity for detection of low level thyroid cancer, serum Tg levels are often measured following TSH stimulation.

From a practical standpoint, it is critical that the Tg be measured serially in the same laboratory. Marked variations in serum Tg values are reported when the same blood samples are analyzed using different Tg assays (20). Additionally, the presence of anti-Tg antibodies in as many as 20% of thyroid cancer patients interferes with the sensitivity of Tg testing. Anti-Tg antibodies often result in falsely low Tg values through assay interference in patients that have persistent thyroid cancer.

Imaging Modalities

For many years, diagnostic RAI scanning was the primary follow up modality for patients with differentiated thyroid cancer. However, the last 15 years has seen a major paradigm shift away from routine RAI scanning and toward routine use of serum Tg and neck ultrasonography in the follow up of most of these patients (8,21). Because the vast majority of recurrent thyroid cancer is in cervical lymph nodes, which usually produce Tg very well, a combination of TSH-stimulated Tg and careful neck ultrasonography has a very high sensitivity for detection of recurrent disease.

Other imaging modalities such as CT, MRI, and 18 fluorodeoxyglucose positron emission tomography (FDG PET) scanning are generally reserved either for patients with aggressive thyroid cancers and very high risk, or patients in whom the serum Tg is elevated, but in whom the source of disease cannot be localized by physical examination or neck ultrasonography (22,23).

Treatment Options for Persistent/ Recurrent Disease

Locally Recurrent Disease

For structurally progressive, locally recurrent disease that is 1 cm or greater in size, surgical resection is generally considered the preferred treatment option. Recurrent disease less than 1 cm, or detected only on RAI scanning without associated structural disease, is often treated with additional RAI therapy (8,13). With the dramatic improvement in sensitivity for detecting persistent/recurrent disease using neck ultrasonography, and highly sensitive Tg assays, we are often finding small volume disease in cervical lymph nodes that progresses slowly, if at all. Often, these patients are carefully watched with serial ultrasounds with intervention reserved for only those documented disease progression.

In patients with a structurally significant local disease recurrence in which surgical resection would be associated with unacceptable morbidity or mortality, consideration is given to external beam irradiation. Unlike many other malignancies, surgical resection of locally recurrent disease for palliation and prevention of gross invasion into the aerodigestive tract is often considered even in the presence of untreatable distant metastases (8).

Distant Metastases

RAI is often a very effective therapy for distant metastases. Unfortunately, RAI is much less effective at destroying macroscopic pulmonary metastases, particularly when they arise in older patients with less-differentiated disease. While resection or EBRT to individual metastatic lesion in critical locations will not be curative, appropriate treatment can avert serious neurovascular symptoms or prevent seriously morbid complications. Patients with structurally progressive macroscopic metastatic disease that is not responsive to RAI should be referred for consideration of a clinical trial or other systemic therapy (24).

ANAPLASTIC THYROID CANCER

Unlike well-differentiated thyroid cancers, anaplastic thyroid cancer is a locally aggressive, poorly differentiated thyroid cancer that develops in older patients (mean age at diagnosis approximately 65 years) (25). In the vast majority of cases, the tumor is not resectable, does not concentrate RAI, and responds poorly to chemotherapy. Unfortunately, the disease specific mortality rate is more than 95% over 6–12 months after diagnosis. While unlikely to be curative, combina-

tion chemotherapy and external beam irradiation may result in a modest increase in progression-free survival from just a few days to at least a few months.

THYROID LYMPHOMA

Primary thyroid lymphomas make up less than 2% of extranodal lymphomas and are generally classified as either mucosa-associated lymphoid tissue (MALT) or diffuse large B-cell or mixed subtype lymphomas (26). They often present as a rapidly increasing thyroid mass in older patients with preexisting chronic lymphocytic thyroiditis.

While MALT lymphomas may follow a more indolent course and be amenable to single modality radiation therapy or total thyroidectomy diagnosed at an early stage, both the large B-cell and mixed subtype lymphomas are generally treated with multimodality therapy consisting of chemotherapy and hyperfractionated EBRT (25).

MEDULLARY THYROID CANCER

MTC is a neuroendocrine tumor arising from parafollicular C cells within the thyroid gland (27). Although these C cells cannot concentrate iodine nor produce thyroid hormones, they do synthesize calcitonin and CEA, which are commonly used as serum tumor markers in patients with MTC. In 75% of the cases, MTC presents as a sporadic (nonfamilial), unilateral thyroid mass, usually in the fourth to sixth decade of life, often with associated cervical lymphadenopathy (50% of patients), with no other associated endocrinopathies.

However, 25% of patients present with MTC as part of a well-defined clinical syndrome caused by germline mutation in the RET proto-oncogene. Although MTC is often the initial presentation in these clinical syndromes, patients may also present with hypertension associated with pheochromocytoma or with hypercalcemia associated with hyperparathyroidism. Therefore, screening for these diagnoses is essential in order to appropriately plan and sequence necessary surgical procedures. In addition, with the aid of commercially available genetic testing for carriers of the RET proto-oncogene, early detection of asymptomatic disease can be found in affected family members of patients with hereditary MTC.

After assessment for possible concurrent hyperparathyroidism and/or pheochromocytoma, the usual initial therapy for MTC is total thyroidectomy with compartmental dissection of potentially affected cervical lymph node chains. MTC is often a slow growing tumor with an indolent clinical course. The overall survival of patients with sporadic MTC ranges from 80%–85% at five years, 55%–65% at 10 years, and 45%–50% at 20 years.

CONCLUSIONS

Although generally considered a rare tumor, the incidence of thyroid cancer has dramatically increased over the last 20 years. The etiology of this rise in incidence remains elusive. While the 30-year disease-specific survival in thyroid cancer exceeds 90% in most patients, the risk of recurrent disease is as high as 30% over the same time period. Over the last 10–15 years, more widespread use of serum Tg and neck ultrasonography has resulted in earlier detection of locally recurrent disease, allowing more effective treatment of these recurrences. Unfortunately, treatment options for non-RAI avid, progressive, distant metastases are much less effective, resulting in a resurging interest in the development of novel systemic therapies.

*R*eferences

1. Gilliland FD, Hunt WC, Morris DM, et al. Prognostic factors for thyroid carcinoma. A population-based study of 15,698 cases from the Surveillance, Epidemiology and End Results (SEER) program 1973–1991. *Cancer.* 1997;79(3):564–573.
2. Hundahl SA, Cady B, Cunningham MP, et al. Initial results from a prospective cohort study of 5583 cases of thyroid carcinoma treated in the United States during 1996. U.S. and German Thyroid Cancer Study Group. An American College of Surgeons Commission on Cancer Patient Care Evaluation study. *Cancer.* 2000;89(1):202–217.
3. Davies L, Welch HG. Increasing incidence of thyroid cancer in the United States, 1973–2002. *JAMA.* 2006;295(18):2164–2167.
4. Ries LA, Harkins D, Krapcho M, et al. *SEER Cancer Statistics Review, 1975-2003, based on November 2005 SEER data submission.* 2006 [cited 2006 November 1]; Available from: http://seer.cancer.gov/csr/1975_2003/.
5. Nagataki S, Nystrom E. Epidemiology and primary prevention of thyroid cancer. *Thyroid.* 2002;12(10):889–896.
6. Schneider AB, Sarne DH. Long-term risks for thyroid cancer and other neoplasms after exposure to radiation. *Nat Clin Pract Endocrinol Metab.* 2005;1(2):82–91.
7. Sherman SI. Thyroid carcinoma. *Lancet.* 2003;361(9356):501–511.
8. Cooper DS, Doherty GM, Haugen BR, et al. Management guidelines for patients with thyroid nodules and differentiated thyroid cancer. *Thyroid.* 2006;16(2):109–142.
9. Hay ID, Thompson GB, Grant CS, et al. Papillary thyroid carcinoma managed at the Mayo Clinic during six decades (1940–1999): temporal trends in initial therapy and long-term outcome in 2444 consecutively treated patients. *World J Surg.* 2002;26(8):879–885.
10. Mazzaferri EL, Kloos RT. Clinical review 128: current approaches to primary therapy for papillary and follicular thyroid cancer. *J Clin Endocrinol Metab.* 2001;86(4):1447–1463.
11. Tuttle RM, Leboeuf R, Martorella AJ. Papillary thyroid cancer: monitoring and therapy. *Endocrinol Metab Clin North Am.* 2007;36(3):753–778, vii.
12. BTA. *British Thyroid Association and Royal College of Physicians: Guidelines for the Management of Thyroid Cancer in Adults.* 2002 [cited 2006 November 1]; Available from: british-thyroid-association.org.
13. Pacini F, Schlumberger M, Dralle H, et al. European consensus for the management of patients with differentiated thyroid carcinoma of the follicular epithelium. *Eur J Endocrinol.* 2006;154(6):787–803.
14. Sherman SI. *National Comprehensive Cancer Network, Clinical Practice Guidelines in Oncology, Thyroid Cancer V.2.2006.* 2006 [cited 2006 November 1]; Available from: http://www.nccn.org/professionals/physician_gls/PDF/thyroid.pdf.
15. ThyroidCarcinomaTaskForce. AACE/AAES medical/surgical guidelines for clinical practice: management of thyroid carcinoma. American Association of Clinical Endocrinologists. American College of Endocrinology. *Endocr Pract.* 2001;7(3):202–220.
16. Lee N, Tuttle RM. External beam radiation for differentiated thyroid cancer. *Endocrine Related Cancers,* 2006;13(4):971–977.
17. Biondi B, Filetti S, Schlumberger M. Thyroid-hormone therapy and thyroid cancer: a reassessment. *Nat Clin Pract Endocrinol Metab.* 2005;1(1):32–40.
18. McGriff NJ, Csako G, Gourgiotis L, et al. Effects of thyroid hormone suppression therapy on adverse clinical outcomes in thyroid cancer. *Ann Med.* 2002;34(7–8):554–564.
19. Spencer CA. Serum thyroglobulin measurements: clinical utility and technical limitations in the management of patients with differentiated thyroid carcinomas. *Endocr Pract.* 2000;6(6):481–484.
20. Spencer CA, Bergoglio LM, Kazarosyan M, et al. Clinical impact of thyroglobulin (Tg) and Tg autoantibody method differences on the management of patients with differentiated thyroid carcinomas. *J Clin Endocrinol Metab.* 2005;90(10):5566–5575.
21. Wong KT, Ahuja AT. Ultrasound of thyroid cancer. *Cancer Imaging.* 2005;5:157–166.
22. Larson SM, Robbins R. Positron emission tomography in thyroid cancer management. *Semin Roentgenol.* 2002;37(2):169–174.
23. Stokkel MP, Duchateau CS, Dragoiescu C. The value of FDG-PET in the follow-up of differentiated thyroid cancer: a review of the literature. *Q J Nucl Med Mol Imaging.* 2006;50(1):78–87.
24. Tuttle RM, Leboeuf R. Investigational therapies for metastatic thyroid carcinoma. *J Natl Compr Canc Netw.* 2007;5(6):641–646.
25. Green LD, Mack L, Pasieka JL. Anaplastic thyroid cancer and primary thyroid lymphoma: a review of these rare thyroid malignancies. *J Surg Oncol.* 2006;94(8):725–736.
26. Mack LA, Pasieka JL. An evidence-based approach to the treatment of thyroid lymphoma. *World J Surg.* 2007;31(5):978–986.
27. Ball DW. Medullary thyroid cancer: monitoring and therapy. *Endocrinol Metab Clin North Am.* 2007;36(3):823–837, viii.

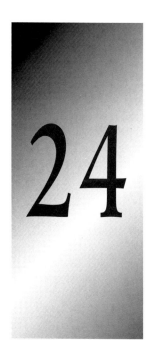

Evaluation and Treatment of Sarcoma

Robert G. Maki

Sarcomas constitute less than 1% of all cancers diagnosed annually, with ~12,000 people developing a sarcoma this year in the United States (census of 300 million people in 2006) (1). Approximately half of patients with newly diagnosed sarcoma will die of disease (2). The small number of cases seen and the diversity of histology (more than 50 histologies, the most common of which are shown in Table 24.1), anatomical site, and biologic behavior have made study of this family of tumors difficult. However, some features regarding treatment stand out, and those will be highlighted in this section. Loss of muscle or bone and its ability to heal will affect rehabilitation of the patient. The nature of the local therapy, whether radiation is involved, and whether periosteal stripping is employed can also make a difference in terms of risk to the limb of fracture, points that require discussion between treating physicians in a multidisciplinary setting.

ETIOLOGY

There is no clear cause for most sarcomas, the exception being those associated with radiation therapy (3,4). Radiation-associated sarcomas, often of the malignant fibrous histiocytoma (MFH) variety or "sarcoma not otherwise specified" are associated with diseases that are commonly treated with radiotherapy and in those in which a long survival period

---

TABLE 24.1
Common Soft-Tissue and Bone Sarcomas

Common Soft-Tissue Sarcomas
Gastrointestinal stromal tumor (GIST)
Liposarcoma
   Well-differentiated/dedifferentiated
   Myxoid/round cell
   Pleomorphic
Leiomyosarcoma
High-grade undifferentiated pleomorphic sarcoma (formerly termed MFH, malignant fibrous histiocytoma)
Synovial sarcoma
Fibrosarcoma
Malignant peripheral nerve sheath tumor (MPNST) also called malignant schwannoma
Common sarcomas of bone and cartilage
Osteogenic sarcoma (osteosarcoma)
   Osteoblastic
   Chondroblastic
   Fibroblastic
Ewing sarcoma
Chondrosarcoma
Malignant fibrous histiocytoma of bone
Leiomyosarcoma of bone
Chordoma

KEY POINTS

- Sarcomas constitute less than 1% of all cancers diagnosed annually, with ~12,000 people developing a sarcoma this year in the United States.
- Approximately half of patients with newly diagnosed sarcoma will die of disease.
- There are at least 50 soft-tissue sarcoma subclasses, many with distinctive features regarding anatomical distribution or responses to various chemotherapy agents.
- The small number of cases seen and the diversity of histology, anatomical site, and biologic behavior have made study of this family of tumors difficult.
- There is no clear cause for most sarcomas, the exception being those associated with radiation therapy.
- Radiation-associated sarcomas are associated with diseases that are commonly treated with radiother-

apy and in those in which a long survival period is expected, such as Hodgkin lymphoma and breast carcinoma.
- Surgery is the only curative modality for most sarcomas.
- Long-term sequelae resulting from larger radiotherapy doses and volumes are associated with increased fibrosis and edema, and possibly an increased rate of bone fractures.
- The orthopedic implications for primary bone sarcomas are often greater than those of soft-tissue sarcomas, due to extensive operations, such as those on the spine, internal or complete hemipelvectomies, and forequarter amputations.
- As with soft-tissue sarcomas, amputation is now uncommon for primary bone tumors, with allografts and increasingly sophisticated prostheses used for reconstruction.

is expected, such as Hodgkin lymphoma and breast carcinoma. Data regarding exposure to chemical compounds such as dioxins or herbicides, including Agent Orange, have not been conclusive (5). Other associations between patient exposures and subsequent sarcoma development include that of Kaposi sarcoma with human herpesvirus 8 (HHV-8, also termed Kaposi sarcoma herpesvirus, KSHV), whether in epidemic form associated with human immunodeficiency virus (HIV) infection or those endemic cases typically found in octogenarians of Mediterranean descent (6).

Familial syndromes associated with sarcomas give insight into the key genetic mediators. There is a high incidence of sarcomas, sometimes multiple asynchronous tumors, in patients with Li-Fraumeni syndrome (7). Li-Fraumeni syndrome is characterized by p53 genetic alterations and in second cancers in patients with retinoblastoma (Rb) who develop unilateral and oftentimes bilateral primary retinoblastomas. A genetic predisposition to soft-tissue sarcoma has also been associated with neurofibromatosis (8) (with germline NF1 alterations). What is perhaps surprising is that only ~5% of patients with neurofibromatosis (NF) develop malignant peripheral nerve sheath tumors (MPNSTs); primary tumors in the central nervous system, including acoustic neuromas and low-grade astrocytomas, are more typical of this syndrome. Familial adenomatous polyposis (FAP), a subset of which is termed Gardner syndrome, is associated with the development of intraabdominal deep fibromatoses, also termed desmoid tumors, tumors that are technically benign but that

can kill patients through involvement of local structures (9,10), as noted in a following section.

Finally, a familial gastrointestinal stromal tumor (GIST) syndrome has now been identified in fewer than 20 families worldwide to date (11,12). They often have multifocal and relatively indolent disease, though some can succumb to progression of one or many of the primary tumors. The syndrome, with a mutation in c-kit, is associated with pigment changes in the hands and feet as well as bowel dysmotility issues, in comparison to unaffected siblings, consistent with effect on the interstitial cells of Cajal, the pacemaker cells of the gut thought to be the origin of GISTs (13).

CYTOGENETIC ABNORMALITIES

While there have been associations between genetic syndromes and sarcomas, an entirely different group of sarcomas are interesting for the involvement of specific translocations, making sarcomas a solid tumor relative of hematalogic malignancies. The best examples include the Ewing sarcoma/primitive neuroectodermal tumor translocation t(11;22)(q24;q11.2-12) and the synovial sarcoma translocation t(X;18)(p11.2;q11.2) (Table 24.2). These genetic abnormalities can be used as a diagnostic tool. Multiple studies of genetic abnormalities have been published (14). For example, myxoid-round cell liposarcomas contain the translocation t(12;16)(q13;p11) FUS-DDIT3 (formerly called TLS-CHOP), which links these two morphologically distinct liposarcoma subtypes.

HISTOLOGY	CHROMOSOMAL ALTERATION	INVOLVED GENES	APPROXIMATE FREQUENCY (%)
Synovial sarcoma	t(X;18)(p11;q11)	SYT-SSX1, SYT-SSX2, SYT-SSX4	95
Myxoid—round cell liposarcoma	t(12;16)(q13;p11)	FUS(TLS)-DDIT3 (CHOP)	75
Ewing sarcoma	t(11;22)(q24;q12)	EWS-FLI1	85
Alveolar rhabdomyosarcoma	t(2;13)(q35;q14)	PAX3-FKHR	70
	t(1;13)(p36;q14)	PAX7-FKHR	20
Desmoplastic small round cell tumor	t(11;22)(p13;q12)	EWS-WT1	>90
Endometrial stromal sarcoma	t(X;17)(p15;q21)	JAZF1-JJAZ1	65

TABLE 24.2
Common Translocation-Associated Sarcomas

PATHOLOGIC CLASSIFICATION

There are at least 50 soft-tissue sarcoma subclasses, many with distinctive features regarding anatomical distribution or responses to various chemotherapy agents (15). Sarcoma histologic subtype is an important determinant of prognosis and an important predictor of distinctive patterns of behavior. For example, liposarcoma is characterized by five histologic subtypes (well differentiated, dedifferentiated, myxoid, round cell, and pleomorphic), each with its own biology, patterns of metastasis, and responsiveness to chemotherapy. The pattern of metastasis of most sarcomas is hematogenous. Some sarcomas, in particular extraskeletal myxoid chondrosarcoma and alveolar soft part sarcoma, spread in a characteristic fashion early in their course as innumerable small, round metastatic deposits that grow slowly over years. Patients with such diseases can live a surprisingly long time with a great burden of disease (Fig. 24.1). Lymph node metastases are uncommon, except for selected cell types most commonly associated with childhood sarcoma.

CLINICAL PRESENTATION

Soft-tissue sarcomas present as an enlarging mass, keeping in mind that benign tumors are at least 100 times more common than sarcomas. The mass is often large and painless, only coming to attention when more than 5 cm in maximum dimension (Fig. 24.2). A core-needle biopsy usually clinches the diagnosis, and when it does not, an incisional biopsy or planned resection of the entire mass en bloc is usually pursued next (16). Fine-needle aspiration is not often used for primary diagnosis in the United States; however, it is useful in defining recurrence of disease.

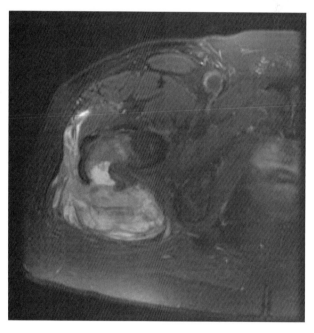

FIGURE 24.1

Axial T2 fat saturation Magnetic Resonance Imaging scan of a myxofibrosarcoma affecting the right hip. Deep tumors such as this can present late in their course.

IMAGING STUDIES

Magnetic resonance imaging (MRI) or computed tomography (CT) scans are the usual way to define the primary tumor and a means to examine for metastatic disease, seen in as many as 20% of patients at time of presentation. Imaging with multiple modalities, all focusing on the same entity, is not required. Positron emission tomography (PET) is occasionally employed

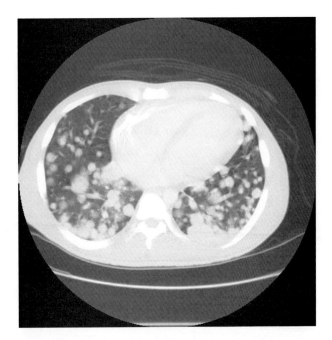

FIGURE 24.2

Chest Computed Tomograph scan from a young male patient with widespread lung metastases from alveolar soft part sarcoma. This is a characteristic pattern for this diagnosis.

to examine patients for evidence of distant disease at time of presentation prior to resection, but is not yet Food and Drug Administration (FDA)-approved for this indication (17). PET may also be helpful in following the development of GIST, but it is not yet clear if it is superior in detecting disease progression on imatinib or sunitinib than contrast-enhanced CT scans (18,19).

PATHOLOGICAL GRADE

After establishing the diagnosis of sarcoma, the most important piece of information the pathologist can provide is histologic grade. Grade comprises the overall assessment of cellularity, differentiation, pleomorphism, necrosis, and number of mitoses. Several grading scales and systems are used. Despite the presence of such criteria, the specific criteria that define a particular grade are not well defined. A four-grade system (Broders); a three-grade system, such as that of the French Federation of Cancer Centers Sarcoma Group; and a binary system (high- vs low-grade) are in use simultaneously at different institutions. Implications for the definition of grade, which heavily influences tumor staging, are clear. If "high grade" is defined differently at different centers, comparison of results between trials becomes difficult.

TABLE 24.3

AJCC Sixth Edition Staging System for Soft-Tissue Sarcoma

STAGE	GRADE	T SIZE	METASTASES
I	Low (1–2)	Any	M0
II	High (3–4)	T1a—b, T2a	M0
III	High (3–4)	T2b	M0
IV	Any	Any	N1 or M1

T1 ≤5 cm; T2 >5 cm; a, superficial to investing fascia; b, deep

Abbreviation: AJCC, American Joint Committee on Cancer.

STAGING

It is now clear that survival is defined by tumor grade, size, and location of tumor relative to a site's investing fascia (deep or superficial), and each factor helps define the risk of tumor spread to distant metastatic sites. New modalities, such as the presence of a specific genetic signature, may help stratify patient risk for recurrence in the future, but remain investigational.

Stage determines outcome in each commonly used staging system. In the United States, the American Joint Committee on Cancer (AJCC) version 6 staging system is most commonly used (20). This staging system is noted in Table 24.3. Risk is stratified first by grade of tumor, then by location (deep or superficial to the most superficial investing fascia of that site), size (cutoff of 5 cm), and presence or absence of metastatic disease. Lymph node metastasis carries a prognosis as poor or nearly as poor as that of bloodborne metastasis, and is included in stage IV disease.

SURGERY AS PRIMARY THERAPY

Surgery is the only curative modality for most sarcomas. In situations where surgery for en bloc resection is not feasible, such as the spine, some combination of local therapy employing definitive radiation is occasionally used. The idea of surgery is to perform an en bloc resection when feasible, which has now lowered the need for amputation for primary therapy of sarcomas to less than 10% (21). Importantly, local recurrence after a limb-sparing operation is nearly always feasible without affecting overall survival. For small primary lesions (under 5 cm), excision with wide margins is feasible and usually sufficient, with radiation reserved for local disease recurrence (after a repeat resection) (22,23).

Conversely, since high-grade, soft-tissue sarcomas more than 10 cm have a high risk of both local and distant recurrence, patients are good candidates for investigational approaches, such as neoadjuvant chemotherapy. Of note, all patients with primary soft-tissue sarcomas over 5 cm in size, high or low grade, should be considered for adjuvant radiation therapy, since it is proved to decrease the risk of local recurrence (24–27).

RADIATION THERAPY

Radiation therapy is used in the primary treatment of sarcomas to decrease the risk of local relapse, enhancing the effect of a definitive operation. Limb conservation using adjuvant external beam radiation therapy was shown to give local control similar to that of amputation in a randomized trial at the National Cancer Institute (NCI) (28). It is also worth noting that radiation should not be considered an acceptable option to make up for grossly positive tumor margins at time of primary resection.

External beam radiation therapy (EBRT) is the most commonly used form of radiation, since it is easy to perform relative to brachytherapy (temporary implants of radioactive seeds in the tumor bed) or more sophisticated planning techniques. Both EBRT and brachytherapy have been shown to decrease the risk of local recurrence for patients with high-grade sarcomas, but only EBRT provides improved local tumor control for low-grade sarcomas (25). Careful planning to ensure coverage of tumor margins and drain sites is paramount in maximizing the potential benefit of radiation therapy to a patient, while at the same time avoiding irradiation of such a large proportion of the cross-sectional area of the extremity that lymphedema becomes a more significant issue.

Few data are available to determine whether to give radiation before or after primary surgery. Radiation therapy before surgery employs a smaller radiation field and lower doses than postoperative radiation therapy, which often also employs a boost to the tumor bed. Radiation therapy before surgery is associated with a higher risk of wound complications than postoperative radiation therapy, nearly completely limited to lower extremity lesions (29–31). However, since higher doses and a larger volume of tissue is irradiated in the postoperative setting, the risk of chronic cicatricial and other wound changes was higher in the only randomized study of preoperative vs postoperative external beam irradiation for extremity sarcomas performed to date (29). There may also be a higher risk of bone fracture in patients receiving (higher dose, larger volume) postoperative irradiation therapy. This is of concern since this could affect the rehabilitation plan.

Special techniques for radiation therapy, including brachytherapy, intensity-modulated radiation therapy, combinations of chemotherapy and radiation, and investigational schedules of therapy, hold promise for the treatment of sarcoma but are beyond the scope of this chapter. One of the key complications of radiation therapy is the injury suffered by normal tissues that may reduce function in the long term.

ADJUVANT CHEMOTHERAPY

Despite good local control of disease, as many as half of patients with adequate local control of disease develop distant metastasis, usually to the lungs (extremity sarcomas) or liver (abdominal primary). It was the hope that adjuvant chemotherapy would decrease the frequency of distant metastases and thus increase overall survival. At least 15 randomized studies have examined adjuvant chemotherapy for soft-tissue sarcomas. Because anthracyclines are the most active agents in sarcoma therapy in the metastatic setting, they have been used in nearly all of the adjuvant trials, alone or in combination. Most of the studies are small and lack statistical power to detect small changes in overall survival.

Meta-analyses and more recent studies provide more data on the utility of chemotherapy combinations using the most active types of agents for most sarcomas, that is, anthracyclines and ifosfamide. The most rigorous meta-analysis regarding adjuvant doxorubicin-based chemotherapy is that published in 1997 (32). Median follow-up was 9.4 years. Analyses were stratified by trial, and hazard ratios were calculated for each trial and combined for each of the 14 trials, which allowed for an assessment of the risk of death or recurrence in comparison to control patients. Disease-free survival at 10 years was improved from 45% to 55% ($p = 0.0001$). Local disease-free survival at 10 years also favored chemotherapy, 81% versus 75% ($p < 0.02$). Although overall survival improved at 10 years from 50% to 54%, the difference was not statistically significant ($p = 0.12$). In an unplanned analysis, overall survival was shown to increase 7% in the subset of patients with extremity sarcomas receiving chemotherapy ($p = 0.029$).

Newer studies have examined ifosfamide combined with an anthracycline in the adjuvant or neoadjuvant setting. The largest of these studies (from Italy) showed a statistically significant overall survival advantage at five years, with borderline significance ($p = 0.07$) survival advantage overall (33,34). Two smaller studies, one of adjuvant and one of neoadjuvant chemotherapy, showed no survival advantage to the chemotherapy (35,36). Hence, based on these data, even if there is a benefit for the adjuvant use of chemotherapy, it appears a small one. The risks and benefits of adjuvant chemotherapy for any specific person should be discussed on a case-by-case basis.

COMPLICATIONS OF PRIMARY TREATMENT

Wound Complications

Assessment of the influence of preoperative chemotherapy on wound complications is difficult. The University of Texas M.D. Anderson Cancer Center compared morbidity of radical surgery for soft-tissue sarcoma in 104 patients receiving preoperative chemotherapy and 204 patients who had surgery first (37). The most common complications were wound infections and other wound complications, but the incidence of surgical complications was no different for patients who received chemotherapy or not.

One of the key features of the preoperative vs postoperative radiation study from Canada was inclusion of acute wound complication assessment in the study design from the outset and at defined time points for the initial four months after surgery (31). Using these criteria, postoperative radiotherapy also showed a significant risk of wound complications (17%). Furthermore, the wound complication rate after preoperative radiotherapy and primary direct wound closure was 16%, apparently lower than patients treated with a vascularized graft. Thus, in situations in which wound complications may be an issue, transpositional or free grafts should be considered before radiation therapy to attempt to decrease the local complication rate. It is notable that the risk of wound complication in the Canadian study appeared to be limited to lower extremity lesions.

Fracture

The question of weight bearing and the potential risk of fracture is common in the rehabilitation setting. A study of 145 patients with soft-tissue sarcoma undergoing limb-sparing surgery and postoperative radiation with or without chemotherapy demonstrated a 6% fracture rate (38). Patients treated with adjuvant beam radiation therapy (BRT) in a randomized trial from Memorial Sloan-Kettering Cancer Center (MSKCC) had a fracture rate of 4% versus 0% in the control arm, though this difference was not statistically significant (26).

One study highlighted the fracture risk associated with peritoneal stripping (39). Two hundred five patients with soft-tissue sarcoma of the thigh were examined for factors contributing to pathologic femur fracture after adjuvant radiation. One hundred fifteen patients were treated with BRT, 59 received EBRT, and 31 received a combination of EBRT and BRT. The five-year actuarial risk was 8.6%. On multivariate analysis of risk factors associated with fracture, only periosteal stripping was significant. Thus, while reha-bilitation is crucial to a patient's recovery after limb salvage surgery, particular attention should be paid to those patients who have periosteal stripping as part of their primary therapy.

QUALITY OF LIFE AND FUNCTIONAL OUTCOME

Quality of life (QOL) evaluations highlight the potential pitfalls of local therapy as it pertains to functional outcome. Obvious factors affecting QOL include those features associated with the primary tumor resection. Not surprisingly, there is a higher level of handicap in amputated patients compared to those treated with conservative surgery (40). Resection involving nerves was associated with poorer outcome on multivariate analysis ($p < 0.02$) in a separate study (41). Conventional chemotherapy has not had an impact on the functional outcome of patients with extremity sarcoma.

The best data regarding effects of radiation on functional outcome are again from the Canadian preoperative versus postoperative radiation therapy study, using well-examined instruments of outcome (29,31). Validated instruments, including the Musculoskeletal Tumor Society Rating Scale, Toronto Extremity Salvage Score, and the Short Form-36 Health Survey QOL instruments were used to evaluate patient outcomes and QOL. The preoperative group had inferior function, with lower bodily pain scores on all three rating instruments at six weeks. However, at later times up to one year after surgery, there were no differences in these scores. Thus, it appears that the timing of radiotherapy has little impact on the ultimate function of soft-tissue sarcoma patients. However, longer follow-up now indicates that late tissue sequelae resulting from larger radiotherapy doses and volumes are associated with increased fibrosis and edema, and possibly an increased rate of bone fractures. These late outcomes may ultimately override the influence of acute wound complications, although patients with acute wound complications can experience long-term functional impairment (29).

SURGERY FOR METASTATIC DISEASE

Median survival from the time metastases are recognized is 12–18 months, though the situation for patients with metastatic GIST has changed radically with the introduction of imatinib; for patients with non-GIST sarcomas, only 20%–25% of patients are expected to live more than two years, another factor in determining the appropriateness of patients for rehabilitation. Surgical resection can provide selected patients with prolonged periods of freedom from disease, and radiation therapy provides palliation for individual patients who have localized symptomatic metastases. Optimal treatment of patients with unresectable or metastatic soft-tissue sarcoma requires an appreciation for the natural history of the disease, close attention to the individual patient, and an understanding of the benefits and limitations of the therapeutic options. One such challenge, that of local-regionally recurrent angiosarcoma, can give surgeons fits (Fig. 24.3). The tumor, cleanly resected previously, recurred aggressively well clear of the negative margin, a frequent characteristic of angiosarcomas.

The MSKCC experience is emblematic of the situation for patients with lung-only metastatic disease. In their database of 716 patients with primary extremity sarcoma, pulmonary-only metastases occurred in 19%, or 135 patients. Of these 135 patients, 58% underwent thoracotomy, and 83% of those had a complete resection of their tumor. In the 65 patients who had a complete resection of their tumor, 69% had recurrence, with pulmonary metastases as their only site of disease. Median survival time from complete resection was 19 months, and three-year survival was 23% of those undergoing resection and 11% of those presenting with lung metastasis only. Patients who did not undergo thoracotomy all died within three years (42,43). Chemotherapy had no obvious impact on survival in either the patients who did or those who did not undergo resection. Thus, resection of limited metastatic disease, where feasible, remains a good standard of care for recurrent soft-tissue sarcoma. Not discussed here further are the equally important data that resection

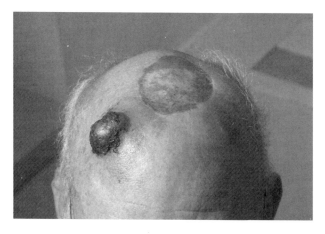

FIGURE 24.3

Regional recurrence of a scalp angiosarcoma following resection and skin graft of the primary site. Note the heaped-up nature of the tumor in this image, which is surrounded by tissue infiltrated with angiosarcoma.

of metastatic disease of osteogenic sarcomas can also be associated with cure.

SYSTEMIC THERAPY FOR METASTATIC DISEASE

Table 24.4 documents the expected response rate for selected systemic chemotherapy agents or combinations. Doxorubicin has been the workhorse of chemotherapy for advanced sarcoma. Liposomal forms of doxorubicin may have fewer side effects than doxorubicin itself. Response rates have been low, however, and in one randomized phase 2 study, the response rate to doxorubicin was as low as that of liposomal doxorubicin, perhaps owing to sarcoma subtypes enrolled on the study (44).

Ifosfamide has approximately the same efficacy as doxorubicin. During its development, ifosfamide administration was limited by hemorrhagic cystitis. The uroprotective agent mesna has markedly changed the ability to give both ifosfamide and cyclophosphamide, and ifosfamide doses as large as 14–18 g/m^2 or more have been given over one to two weeks (45). A third drug with modest activity in sarcoma is dacarbazine (DTIC) (46), whose activity was recognized more than 20 years ago. Temozolomide, an orally available version of dacarbazine, has demonstrated activity against leiomyosarcomas (47,48).

Combinations of doxorubicin and ifosfamide [and mesna, (AIM)] and of [mesna], doxorubicin, ifosfamide and dacarbazine (MAID) are used most frequently in patients in need of a response; the drugs appear to have additive benefit, but do not appear to synergize with one another. As for other single agents, excluding the remarkable story of the sensitivity of GIST to imatinib, the most significant investigational agent in soft-tissue sarcomas is presently ecteinascidin (ET-743), with an 8%–10% response rate in sarcomas (49,50), but striking activity against myxoid-round liposarcoma. mTOR inhibitors, such as temsirolimus, sirolimus, everolimus (RAD001), and deforolimus, have shown minor activity in sarcomas, as have sorafenib and other multi-targeted tyrosine kinase inhibitors; these new orally available agents remain investigational.

SARCOMAS OF BONE

Sarcomas of bone, mostly osteogenic sarcoma, Ewing sarcoma in children, and chondrosarcoma in adults, are only approximately one-fourth as common as soft-tissue sarcomas. Furthermore, primary bone tumors are, as a whole, much less common than metastatic carcinomas to bone, with their attendant complications.

TABLE 24.4

Selected Systemic Chemotherapeutic Agents
for Soft-Tissue Sarcoma and Approximate Response Rates

REGIMEN	DOSE	RESPONSE RATE (%)
Doxorubicin	60–75 mg/m^2	10–25
Ifosfamide	5–16 g/m^2	10–25
Dacarbazine	1000–1250 mg/m^2	10
AIM: (mesna) + Doxorubicin + Ifosfamide	varies	20–40
MAID: (mesna) + Doxorubicin + Ifosfamide + Dacarbazine	varies	20–40
Gemcitabine/Docetaxel	varies	15–20
Trabectedin (ET-743)	1.5 mg/m^2 over 24 h	10
Imatinib (for GIST only)	400–800 mg daily	50

Note: All drugs listed here except imatinib are given intravenously, typically on a 3-week repeating schedule. Imatinib is given daily by mouth.

However, like metastatic carcinoma to bone, the orthopedic implications for primary bone sarcomas are oftentimes greater than that of soft-tissue sarcomas, especially when factoring in extensive operations, such as those on the spine, internal or complete hemipelvectomies, and forequarter amputations. Functional loss with resection of a humeral osteogenic sarcoma oftentimes is greater than that of resection of a soft-tissue sarcoma affecting the shoulder girdle, and thus a few key points of management of these challenging tumors is warranted.

While not all bone tumors (eg, aneurysmal bone cyst, eosinophilic granuloma, and osteoid osteoma) require excision, surgery is the standard of care for more aggressive tumors, such as osteogenic sarcoma (osteosarcoma), chondrosarcoma, and Ewing sarcoma of bone. As a result, the reconstruction and its consequences have profound effects on the rehabilitation potential of patients. There are particularly important issues pertaining to children with osteogenic sarcoma. As with soft-tissue sarcomas, amputation is now uncommon for primary bone tumors, with allografts and increasingly sophisticated prostheses used for reconstruction, including those that can be extended at time of a followup surgery, or even via even newer devices that can extend themselves using strong external magnetic fields to drive an internal motor to extend the prosthesis (51).

Bone sarcomas are staged using a system similar to that for soft-tissue sarcomas (Table 24.5) (20). In comparison to soft-tissue sarcomas, the size cutoff for staging is 8 cm, not 5 cm, between small (A) and large (B) primary tumors. Stage IV is divided into two subsets: IVA (lung metastasis) and IVB (other metastatic disease), since patients with lung metastases can still be resected with curative intent.

TABLE 24.5

AJCC Sixth Edition Bone Sarcoma
Staging System

STAGE	GRADE	T SIZE	METS
IA	Low (1,2)	T1	M0
IB	Low (1,2)	T2	M0
IIA	High (3,4)	T1	M0
IIB	High (3,4)	T2	M0
III	Any	T3	M0
IVA	Any	Any	M1a
IVB	Any	Any	N1
	Any	Any	M1b

T1 ≤8 cm; T2 >8 cm; T3, discontiguous disease in one bone; M1a, lung; M1b other.

Abbreviation: AJCC, American Joint Committee on Cancer.

With the finding that tumor necrosis can serve as an indicator of responsiveness at the time of surgery, neoadjuvant chemotherapy is the standard of care for osteogenic sarcoma and for Ewing sarcoma of bone. Since chondrosarcomas are chemotherapy-insensitive, by and large, they are treated with surgery alone and occasionally with radiation as well. In the cases of osteogenic sarcoma and Ewing sarcoma, a period of chemotherapy is followed by definitive surgery, and then chemotherapy is continued to complete what is typically a 6-month (osteosarcoma) or nearly 12-month (Ewing sarcoma) course of therapy. Radiation is typically given during chemotherapy after the definitive surgery.

The standard of care for neoadjuvant chemotherapy for younger patients is doxorubicin, cisplatin, and methotrexate (52), although there is not particularly strong evidence that to support the contention that methotrexate is useful in the adjuvant setting (53). In older patients, cisplatin and doxorubicin form a reasonable combination for neoadjuvant/adjuvant therapy (54), although even this combination is difficult to administer to patients who develop osteosarcoma during the second peak of diagnosis of the disease in the eighth decade. Dose intensification of a standard doxorubicin-cisplatin backbone does not appear to improve survival (55). Ifosfamide is also active in osteosarcoma, though its use in a nonprotocol setting was called into question in the recent study from Meyers et al. in which ifosfamide and nonspecific immune-stimulate muramyl tripeptide were added to a standard doxorubicin-cisplatin-methotrexate backbone. Ifosfamide increased the cure rate in patients receiving chemotherapy, but only when given in conjunction with muramyl tripeptide (MTP), a bacterial cell wall component that is proinflammatory. In fact, survival in patients receiving ifosfamide was inferior to that of patients receiving the standard three-drug combination. Since MTP is not commercially available, the role of ifosfamide in the adjuvant setting is unclear, and remains investigational (52). Ifosfamide is active in metastatic disease and is often given in that setting. Other standard cytotoxic chemotherapy agents have little activity in osteogenic sarcoma, making this a ripe target for newer targeted therapeutics that may affect the ability of osteogenic sarcoma to metastasize.

Ewing sarcoma is most commonly treated with neoadjuvant chemotherapy, surgery, and postoperative radiation. It tends to spread locally without regard to tissue planes, so en bloc resection and adjuvant radiation must be carefully planned to involve a wide enough field. The standard of care for Ewing sarcoma is a five-drug regimen of vincristine, doxorubicin, cyclophosphamide (VAC), alternating with a combination of ifosfamide (with mesna) and etoposide (I/E) (56). The five-drug combination was shown superior to VAC in a large clinical trial and represents the best standard of care off-protocol. Topoisomerase I inhibitor combinations and cisplatin are somewhat active against Ewing sarcoma in the metastatic setting (57,58), and recent anecdotes of responses to insulinlike growth factor receptor inhibitors may form the basis for a new generation of studies combining targeted and standard cytotoxic agents in the near future.

Since both osteogenic sarcoma and Ewing sarcoma are common in younger patients, with peak age of incidence of both during adolescence, rehabilitation is a particularly important part of the multidisciplinary effort, especially in children without closure of their growth plates. Expandable prostheses and allograft reconstructions have helped minimize the residual dysfunction of the limb, but are still associated with episodes of nonunion, prosthesis failure, fracture, or wear and tear to the plastic parts of the prosthesis, requiring replacement (51). In some cases, poor local reconstruction options remain an inferior treatment to simple below-the-knee amputation, in which the rehabilitation potential ends up being greater with a good prosthesis, rather than a destabilizing operation, even if local control can be achieved.

DESMOID TUMORS (AGGRESSIVE FIBROMATOSES)

It is worth mentioning this soft-tissue neoplasm, as it can cause a great deal of morbidity, either from the primary tumor itself or from its treatment. Desmoid tumors are not quite sarcomas, belonging to a family of myofibroblastic tumors that are unusual in their bland histology and slow progression (15). Surgery remains the treatment of choice for these lesions, which cannot truly be called sarcomas due to their lack of metastatic potential. However, deaths have still been seen in patients with locally advanced disease, in particular in patients with desmoids associated with familial adenomatous polyposis (9). The complications of surgery can outweigh any perceived benefit from resection, however, and deaths in the series of patients treated at MSKCC have more frequently been iatrogenic rather than due to tumor per se. Whether this reflects the more aggressive nature of some desmoids versus others, these data indicate that one must proceed with great caution in the management of these lesions, which are occasionally seen to regress spontaneously. For truly resectable disease, surgery alone appears to be the optimal approach, especially in patients with negative microscopic margins. In advanced cases, a trial of nonsteroidal antiinflammatory drugs or hormonal therapy can be considered in most patients before moving to chemotherapy; those patients who are symptomatic and not a candidate for surgery should be given to radiation or chemotherapy.

CONCLUSION

A number of approaches will affect patient survival in the present and near future. Surgical approaches have benefitted from improvements in tumor imaging, which now make limb-sparing surgeries more routine. Improved techniques in tissue transfer make reconstruction of very large tissue defects feasible. Perhaps we will see in the next generation development of tissues in vitro to help with reconstruction of patients' wounds. Radiation therapy techniques have shown rapid increases in sophistication with the application of intensity-modulated external beam techniques to extremity tumors, minimizing toxicity while maintaining or improving local control (30). However, systemic therapy outside of GIST remains somewhat in a rut. Though there have been some particular success with synovial sarcoma and ifosfamide, angiosarcoma and paclitaxel, and trabectedin and myxoid-round cell liposarcoma, the truth is we still need better systemic agents to treat the bulk of sarcomas encountered in practice. Advances in the most important area of research, that is, basic and translational research, will hopefully have an impact on the treatment of a number of sarcoma subtypes in the near future.

References

1. Jemal A, Siegel R, Ward E, Murray T, Xu J, Thun MJ. Cancer statistics, 2007. *CA Cancer J Clin.* 2007;57(1):43–66.
2. Weitz J, Antonescu CR, Brennan MF. Localized extremity soft tissue sarcoma: improved knowledge with unchanged survival over time. *J Clin Oncol.* 2003;21(14):2719–2725.
3. Brady MS, Gaynor JJ, Brennan MF. Radiation-associated sarcoma of bone and soft tissue. *Arch Surg.* 1992;127(12):1379–1385.
4. Spiro IJ, Suit HD. Radiation-induced bone and soft tissue sarcomas: clinical aspects and molecular biology. *Cancer Treat Res.* 1997;91:143–155.
5. Fingerhut MA, Halperin WE, Marlow DA, et al. Cancer mortality in workers exposed to 2,3,7,8-tetrachlorodibenzo-p-dioxin. *N Engl J Med.* 1991;324(4):212–218.
6. Schwartz RA. Kaposi's sarcoma: an update. *J Surg Oncol.* 2004;87(3):146–151.
7. Li FP, Fraumeni JF, Jr. Soft-tissue sarcomas, breast cancer, and other neoplasms. A familial syndrome? *Ann Intern Med.* 1969;71(4):747–752.
8. D'Agostino AN, Soule EH, Miller RH. Sarcomas of the peripheral nerves and somatic soft tissues associated with multiple neurofibromatosis (Von Recklinghausen's disease). *Cancer.* 1963;16:1015–1027.
9. Lewis JJ, Boland PJ, Leung DH, Woodruff JM, Brennan MF. The enigma of desmoid tumors. *Ann Surg.* 1999;229(6):866–872; discussion 72–73.
10. Lotfi AM, Dozois RR, Gordon H, et al. Mesenteric fibromatosis complicating familial adenomatous polyposis: predisposing factors and results of treatment. *Int J Colorectal Dis.* 1989;4(1):30–36.
11. Maeyama H, Hidaka E, Ota H, et al. Familial gastrointestinal stromal tumor with hyperpigmentation: association with a germline mutation of the c-kit gene. *Gastroenterology.* 2001;120(1):210–215.
12. Robson ME, Glogowski E, Sommer G, et al. Pleomorphic characteristics of a germ-line KIT mutation in a large kindred with gastrointestinal stromal tumors, hyperpigmentation, and dysphagia. *Clin Cancer Res.* 2004;10(4):1250–1254.
13. Hirota S, Isozaki K, Moriyama Y, et al. Gain-of-function mutations of c-kit in human gastrointestinal stromal tumors. *Science.* 1998;279(5350):577–580.
14. Antonescu CR. The role of genetic testing in soft tissue sarcoma. *Histopathology.* 2006;48(1):13–21.
15. Fletcher CDM, Unni KK, Mertens F. *Pathology and Genetics of Tumours of Soft Tissue and Bone.* Lyon: IARC Press; 2002.
16. Heslin MJ, Lewis JJ, Woodruff JM, Brennan MF. Core needle biopsy for diagnosis of extremity soft tissue sarcoma. *Ann Surg Oncol.* 1997;4(5):425–431.
17. Schuetze SM. Imaging and response in soft tissue sarcomas. *Hematol Oncol Clin North Am.* 2005;19(3):471–487, vi.
18. Choi H, Charnsangavej C, de Castro Faria S, et al. CT evaluation of the response of gastrointestinal stromal tumors after imatinib mesylate treatment: a quantitative analysis correlated with FDG PET findings. *AJR.* 2004;183(6):1619–1628.
19. Van den Abbeele AD, Badawi RD. Use of positron emission tomography in oncology and its potential role to assess response to imatinib mesylate therapy in gastrointestinal stromal tumors (GISTs). *Eur J Cancer.* 2002;38(Suppl 5):S60–S65.
20. Greene FL, Page DL, Fleming ID, et al. *AJCC Cancer Staging Handbook*, 6th ed. New York: Springer; 2002.
21. Brennan MF. The management of soft tissue sarcomas. *Br J Surg.* 1984;71(12):964–967.
22. Lewis JJ, Leung D, Espat J, Woodruff JM, Brennan MF. Effect of reresection in extremity soft tissue sarcoma. *Ann Surg.* 2000;231(5):655–663.
23. Pisters PW, Leung DH, Woodruff J, Shi W, Brennan MF. Analysis of prognostic factors in 1,041 patients with localized soft tissue sarcomas of the extremities. *J Clin Oncol.* 1996;14(5):1679–1689.
24. Alekhteyar KM, Leung DH, Brennan MF, Harrison LB. The effect of combined external beam radiotherapy and brachytherapy on local control and wound complications in patients with high-grade soft tissue sarcomas of the extremity with positive microscopic margin. *Int J Rad Oncol Biol Phys.* 1996;36(2):321–324.
25. Alektiar KM, Leung D, Zelefsky MJ, Brennan MF. Adjuvant radiation for stage II-B soft tissue sarcoma of the extremity. *J Clin Oncol.* 2002;20(6):1643–1650.
26. Alektiar KM, Zelefsky MJ, Brennan MF. Morbidity of adjuvant brachytherapy in soft tissue sarcoma of the extremity and superficial trunk. *Int J Rad Oncol Biol Phys.* 2000;47(5):1273–1279.
27. Casper ES, Gaynor JJ, Harrison LB, Panicek DM, Hajdu SI, Brennan MF. Preoperative and postoperative adjuvant combination chemotherapy for adults with high grade soft tissue sarcoma. *Cancer.* 1994;73(6):1644–1651.
28. Rosenberg SA, Kent H, Costa J, et al. Prospective randomized evaluation of the role of limb-sparing surgery, radiation therapy, and adjuvant chemoimmunotherapy in the treatment of adult soft-tissue sarcomas. *Surgery.* 1978;84(1):62–69.
29. Davis AM, O'Sullivan B, Turcotte R, et al. Late radiation morbidity following randomization to preoperative versus postoperative radiotherapy in extremity soft tissue sarcoma. *Radiother Oncol.* 2005;75(1):48–53.
30. O'Sullivan B, Ward I, Catton C. Recent advances in radiotherapy for soft-tissue sarcoma. *Curr Oncol Rep.* 2003;5(4):274–281.
31. O'Sullivan B, Davis AM, Turcotte R, et al. Preoperative versus postoperative radiotherapy in soft-tissue sarcoma of the limbs: a randomised trial. *Lancet.* 2002;359(9325):2235–2241.
32. Sarcoma Meta-analysis Collaboration. Adjuvant chemotherapy for localised resectable soft-tissue sarcoma of adults: meta-analysis of individual data. *Lancet.* 1997;350(9092):1647–1654.
33. Frustaci S, De Paoli A, Bidoli E, et al. Ifosfamide in the adjuvant therapy of soft tissue sarcomas. *Oncology.* 2003;65(Suppl 2):80–84.
34. Frustaci S, Gherlinzoni F, De Paoli A, et al. Adjuvant chemotherapy for adult soft tissue sarcomas of the extremities and girdles: results of the Italian randomized cooperative trial. *J Clin Oncol.* 2001;19(5):1238–1247.
35. Brodowicz T, Schwameis E, Widder J, et al. Intensified adjuvant IFADIC chemotherapy for adult soft tissue sarcoma: a prospective randomized feasibility trial. *Sarcoma.* 2000;4:151–160.
36. Gortzak E, Azzarelli A, Buesa J, et al. A randomised phase II study on neo-adjuvant chemotherapy for "high-risk" adult soft-tissue sarcoma. *Eur J Cancer.* 2001;37(9):1096–1103.
37. Meric F, Milas M, Hunt KK, et al. Impact of neoadjuvant chemotherapy on postoperative morbidity in soft tissue sarcomas. *J Clin Oncol.* 2000;18(19):3378–3383.
38. Stinson SF, DeLaney TF, Greenberg J, et al. Acute and long-term effects on limb function of combined modality limb sparing therapy for extremity soft tissue sarcoma. *Int J Rad Oncol Biol Phys.* 1991;21(6):1493–1499.

39. Lin PP, Schupak KD, Boland PJ, Brennan MF, Healey JH. Pathologic femoral fracture after periosteal excision and radiation for the treatment of soft tissue sarcoma. *Cancer.* 1998;82(12):2356–2365.

40. Davis AM, Devlin M, Griffin AM, Wunder JS, Bell RS. Functional outcome in amputation versus limb sparing of patients with lower extremity sarcoma: a matched case-control study. *Arch Phys Med Rehabil.* 1999;80(6):615–618.

41. Bell RS, O'Sullivan B, Davis A, Langer F, Cummings B, Fornasier VL. Functional outcome in patients treated with surgery and irradiation for soft tissue tumours. *J Surg Oncol.* 1991;48(4):224–231.

42. Billingsley KG, Burt ME, Jara E, et al. Pulmonary metastases from soft tissue sarcoma: analysis of patterns of diseases and postmetastasis survival. *Ann Surg.* 1999;229(5):602–610; discussion 10–12.

43. Billingsley KG, Lewis JJ, Leung DH, Casper ES, Woodruff JM, Brennan MF. Multifactorial analysis of the survival of patients with distant metastasis arising from primary extremity sarcoma. *Cancer.* 1999;85(2):389–395.

44. Judson I, Radford JA, Harris M, et al. Randomised phase II trial of pegylated liposomal doxorubicin (DOXIL/CAELYX) versus doxorubicin in the treatment of advanced or metastatic soft tissue sarcoma: a study by the EORTC Soft Tissue and Bone Sarcoma Group. *Eur J Cancer.* 2001;37(7):870–877.

45. Patel SR, Vadhan-Raj S, Papadopolous N, et al. High-dose ifosfamide in bone and soft tissue sarcomas: results of phase II and pilot studies—dose-response and schedule dependence. *J Clin Oncol.* 1997;15(6):2378–2384.

46. Buesa JM, Mouridsen HT, van Oosterom AT, et al. High-dose DTIC in advanced soft-tissue sarcomas in the adult. A phase II study of the E.O.R.T.C. Soft Tissue and Bone Sarcoma Group. *Ann Oncol.* 1991;2(4):307–309.

47. Anderson S, Aghajanian C. Temozolomide in uterine leiomyosarcomas. *Gynecol Oncol.* 2005;98(1):99–103.

48. Garcia del Muro X, Lopez-Pousa A, Martin J, et al. A phase II trial of temozolomide as a 6-week, continuous, oral schedule in patients with advanced soft tissue sarcoma: a study by the Spanish Group for Research on Sarcomas. *Cancer.* 2005;104(8):1706–1712.

49. Garcia-Carbonero R, Supko JG, Maki RG, et al. Ecteinascidin-743 (ET-743) for chemotherapy-naive patients with advanced soft tissue sarcomas: multicenter phase II and pharmacokinetic study. *J Clin Oncol.* 2005;23(24):5484–5492.

50. Verweij J. Ecteinascidin-743 (ET-743): early test or effective treatment in soft tissue sarcomas? *J Clin Oncol.* 2005;23(24):5420–5423.

51. Cheng EY. Surgical management of sarcomas. *Hematol Oncol Clin North Am.* 2005;19(3):451–470, v.

52. Meyers PA, Schwartz CL, Krailo M, et al. Osteosarcoma: a randomized, prospective trial of the addition of ifosfamide and/or muramyl tripeptide to cisplatin, doxorubicin, and high-dose methotrexate. *J Clin Oncol.* 2005;23(9):2004–2011.

53. Bacci G, Gherlinzoni F, Picci P, et al. Adriamycin-methotrexate high dose versus adriamycin-methotrexate moderate dose as adjuvant chemotherapy for osteosarcoma of the extremities: a randomized study. *Eur J Cancer Clin Oncol.* 1986;22(11):1337–1345.

54. Souhami RL, Craft AW, Van der Eijken JW, et al. Randomised trial of two regimens of chemotherapy in operable osteosarcoma: a study of the European Osteosarcoma Intergroup. *Lancet.* 1997;350(9082):911–917.

55. Lewis IJ, Nooij MA, Whelan J, et al. Improvement in Histologic Response But Not Survival in Osteosarcoma Patients Treated With Intensified Chemotherapy: A Randomized Phase III Trial of the European Osteosarcoma Intergroup. In; 2007:112–128.

56. Grier HE, Krailo MD, Tarbell NJ, et al. Addition of ifosfamide and etoposide to standard chemotherapy for Ewing's sarcoma and primitive neuroectodermal tumor of bone. *N Engl J Med.* 2003;348(8):694–701.

57. Wagner LM, Crews KR, Iacono LC, et al. Phase I trial of temozolomide and protracted irinotecan in pediatric patients with refractory solid tumors. *Clin Cancer Res.* 2004;10(3):840–848.

58. Wagner LM, McAllister N, Goldsby RE, et al. Temozolomide and intravenous irinotecan for treatment of advanced Ewing sarcoma. *Pediatr Blood Cancer.* 2007;48(2):132–139.

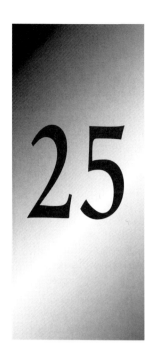

25

Evaluation and Treatment of Primary Bone Tumors

Gary C. O'Toole
Patrick J. Boland

Primary bone tumors are rare, with approximately 2,600 new malignant tumors of bone being diagnosed each year in the United States (1). The majority of these tumors arise in the lower limb, and the survival rate for children younger than 15 years with localized extremity disease is between 64% and 80%, as observed in specialized centers or multicentric groups (2,3).

There is a wide variety in histological subtype for primary bone tumors (Table 25.1). Osteogenic sarcoma is the most common of these tumors and represents the greatest paradigm of oncologic advancement in the 20th century. Historically, survival rates were 21% (4,5), and it was not until the 1970s, when chemotherapy was introduced into the treatment protocol, that survival rates improved (6). The advances in chemotherapy, coupled with improved radiological imaging techniques and surgical understanding of the disease behavior, have further helped improve survival rates. Despite this, the management of these patients from the initial biopsy through to the definitive resection is labor intensive and demanding, and should only be undertaken in a specialized center.

SURGICAL STAGING

The development of a staging system requires systematic accumulation and specialist interpretation of clinicopathologic data. Enneking (7) was the first to develop a universally accepted surgical staging system

TABLE 25.1 *Primary Bone Tumors*		
HISTOLOGIC TYPE	**BENIGN**	**MALIGNANT**
Hematopoietic		Myeloma
Chondrogenic	Osteochondroma	Primary chondrosarcoma
	Chondroma	Secondary chondrosarcoma
	Chondroblastoma	Dedifferentiated chondrosarcoma
	Chondromyxoid fibroma	Mesenchymal chondrosarcoma
Osteogenic	Osteoid osteoma	Osteosarcoma
	Benign osteoblastoma	Parosteal osteogenic sarcoma
Unknown origin	Giant cell tumor	Ewing's tumor
		Malignant giant cell tumor
		Adamantinoma
Fibrogenic	Fibroma	Fibrosarcoma
	Desmoplastic fibroma	
Notochordal		Chordoma
Vascular	Hemangioma	Hemangioendothelioma
		Hemangiopericytoma
Lipogenic	Lipoma	

KEY POINTS

- Primary bone tumors are rare, with approximately 2,600 new malignant tumors of bone being diagnosed each year in the United States.
- Osteogenic sarcoma is the most common primary bone tumor.
- Biopsy is often the most important procedure performed in the patient's management. Over 4% of cases required an amputation as a direct consequence of a poorly performed biopsy. Furthermore 8.5% of patients had their prognosis or outcome adversely affected as a result of a poorly planned biopsy.

- High dose methotrexate, adriamycin, cisplatin, and ifosfamide are the most commonly used as chemotherapeutic agents in osteogenic sarcoma and most other chemotherapy sensitive primary bone tumors.
- Radiation therapy has a limited role in the management of primary bone sarcomas.
- There are several reconstructive choices for the surgical management of malignant bone sarcomas including intercalary allografts, alloprosthetic composites, osteoarticular allografts, and endoprostheses. Other choices include rotationplasty and amputation.

for sarcomas of both bone and soft tissue lesions (Table 25.2). It was shown that the preoperative Enneking stage directly corresponds to five-year survival rates (8) (Fig. 25.1).

The Enneking staging system has been modified by the Musculoskeletal Tumor Society, and this newer system is accepted by most musculoskeletal oncologists (9) (Table 25.3).

The surgical staging system classifies bone and soft tissue tumors by a combination of grade (G0, G1, and G2), anatomic setting (T1 or T2), and the absence or presence of metastases (M0 or M1). The grade is determined by biopsy; the anatomic setting and metastases are determined by radiologic evaluation.

This staging system is used when planning definitive surgical resection. The primary aim of surgical intervention is to resect the tumor with wide negative margins, but benign bone tumors may be treated with intralesional therapy such as curettage, with or without cryotherapy as an adjunct. Wide negative margins remain the aim when intervening surgically in primary malignant bone sarcomas.

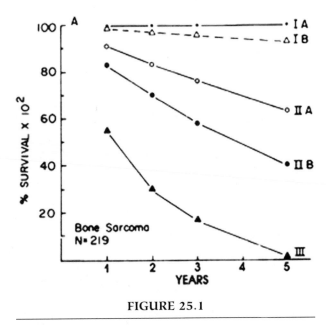

FIGURE 25.1

Preoperative Enneking stage, corresponds to five year survival rate.

TABLE 25.2 *Enneking Surgical Classification System*			
STAGE	GRADE	SITE	META-STASIS
IA	Low (G1)	Intracompartmental (T1)	M0
IB	Low (G1)	Extracompartmental (T2)	M0
IIA	High (G2)	Intracompartmental (T1)	M0
IIB	High (G2)	Extracompartmental (T2)	M0
III	Any G	Any T	M1

TABLE 25.3 *The AJCC Classification System*				
STAGE	GRADE	TUMOR	NODES	METASTASES
IA	Low	T1	N0	M0
IB	Low	T2	N0	M0
IIA	High	T1	N0	M0
IIB	High	T2	N0	M0
III	Any grade	T3	N0	M0
IVA	Any grade	Any T	N0	M1a
IVB	Any grade	Any T	N0/N1	M1b

Radiologic Evaluation

Conventional bone radiography remains the mainstay investigation in the evaluation of primary bone tumors (Fig. 25.2). However, primary bone tumors require further radiological investigations, such as magnetic resonance imaging (MRI) of the lesion. This MRI evaluates the proximity or involvement of the vascular structures of the limb and helps determine whether the lesion is suitable for limb salvage surgery (10). A bone scan and computed tomography (CT) scan of the thorax are helpful when looking for metastases (11,12) (Fig. 25.3).

The Biopsy

The biopsy of a primary bone tumor is not the easy operation many surgeons believe, but it is often the most important procedure performed in the patient's management. Members of the American Musculoskeletal Tumor Society (MSTS) assessed the hazards of biopsy in patients with malignant primary extremity bone and soft tissue tumors (13). For patients who had a biopsy prior to referral, there was an incidence of 18.2% major errors in diagnosis and a 17.3% incidence of skin, soft tissue, or wound problems. Over 4% of cases required an amputation as a direct consequence of a poorly performed biopsy. Furthermore, 8.5% of patients had their prognosis or outcome adversely affected as a result of a poorly planned biopsy. The authors recommended careful biopsy planning and execution, and advocated referral to a tumor center prior to biopsy when the surgeon was not prepared to proceed with definitive tumor treatment.

In 1996, the MSTS published a follow-up paper (14). Despite exhaustive educational efforts in the 10-year intervening period, the results were essentially the same. Furthermore, despite significant advances in radiological technology during this interval, the often innocuous clinical appearance of these tumors continued to deceive surgeons, and patients were often treated without any imaging studies. The findings prompted an editorial comment, "Has anyone been listening?" (15).

There are several simple rules for the surgical technique of carrying out a biopsy. For lesions of the periphery, where they allow for application of a tourniquet, only gravity exsanguination is permitted in order to avoid compression of the tumor. Fine-needle aspiration biopsy has been shown to be safe and an acceptable method for sampling pathological tissue (16).

When performing an open biopsy, biopsy tracts should be along the line with the definitive limb salvage surgical incision, so the biopsy tract can be later excised. Transverse incisions should be avoided because they compromise the definitive surgical procedure (Fig. 25.4). The incision should traverse the fewest possible

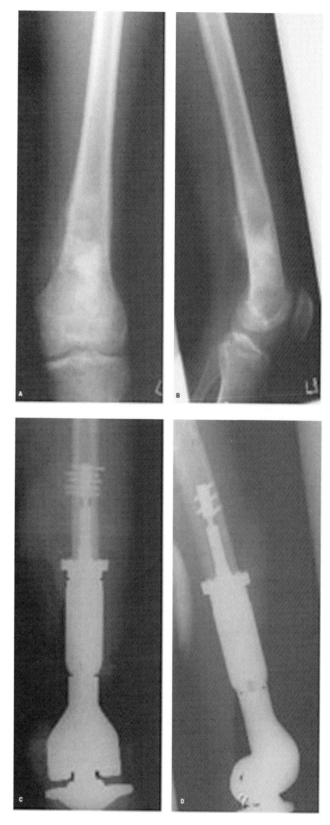

FIGURE 25.2

Conventional x-rays; preoperative anteroposterior (A); lateral (B); postresection anteroposterior (C); and lateral (D) of a malignant osteogenic sarcoma of the distal left femur.

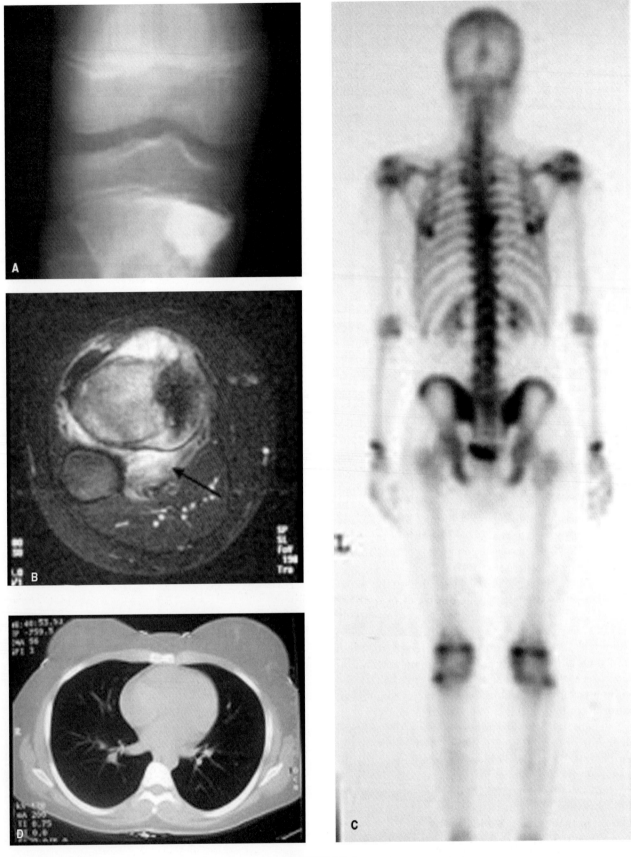

FIGURE 25.3

Preoperative radiologic studies for the investigation of a primary bone sarcoma of the proximal right tibia. In addition to plain radiographs (A), the patient underwent an MRI of the lesion (B), a whole body bone scan (C), and a CT scan of the chest (D).

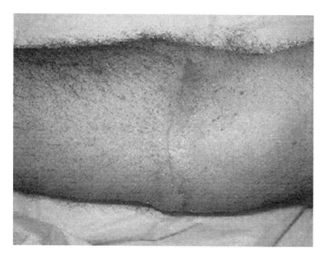

FIGURE 25.4

A biopsy of a lesion through a transverse incision, compromising future surgical intervention.

fascial compartments, and nerves and vessels should not be dissected or identified because this causes contamination and may necessitate amputation. Contamination of any joint should be avoided; where facilities allow, the biopsy should be sent for frozen section to ensure that it contains representative tissue. Biopsy material should be sent for culture and sensitivity to rule out infection. Meticulous hemostasis should be achieved prior to closing the skin to avoid a postoperative hematoma.

In addition to the above rules, bone biopsies necessitate that the defect created by the biopsy should be small and rounded in order to avoid a stress riser that could result in a postoperative fracture. Patients who undergo lower limb biopsies should be protected with crutches to avoid torsional stresses at the biopsy site.

TREATMENT PROTOCOL

Osteogenic sarcoma is the most common of the primary bone tumors and the tumor upon which the treatment protocol for primary bone tumors is based. Classically, once the tumor is confirmed by biopsy, the patient undergoes preoperative chemotherapy (17). No difference in survival has been demonstrated if preoperative chemotherapy is deferred in favor of surgery and only postoperative chemotherapy is given (18). High dose methotrexate (Trexall), doxorubicin (Adriamycin), cisplatin (Platinol), and ifosfamide (Mitoxana) are the most commonly used as chemotherapeutic agents.

Usually, after three cycles of preoperative chemotherapy the definitive surgery is undertaken, with chemotherapy being revisited again postoperatively. The resected specimen is then analyzed microscopically and can be compared to the biopsy specimen to evaluate the effect of the preoperative chemotherapy on the tumor. The percentage necrosis is graded according to the Huvos Classification (Table 25.3 and Fig. 25.5). A poor response to preoperative chemotherapy is predictive of a poor outcome, as is an elevated serum alkaline phosphatase at presentation, central (pelvic) location, older age, African American race, and radiation-induced bone sarcomas (19).

Such a protocol is acceptable for all chemotherapy-sensitive bone tumors and results similar to those demonstrated for osteogenic sarcomas have been demonstrated for Ewing sarcoma of bone (20). Chondrosarcomas are not chemosensitive, and there is no role for chemotherapy in primary malignant chondrosarcomas of bone (21); wide excision is the treatment of choice.

Radiation therapy has a limited role in the management of primary bone sarcomas. When surgery is not possible, radiotherapy has been used to help provide local control although results are not comparable to the gold standard chemotherapy and surgical combination (22,23).

Surgical Management

There are several reconstructive choices for the surgical management of malignant bone sarcomas. These choices include intercalary allografts (Fig. 25.6); alloprosthetic composites (Fig. 25.7); osteoarticular allografts (Fig. 25.8); and endoprostheses (Fig. 25.2). Other choices include rotationplasty (Fig. 25.9) and amputation. The choice depends on patient factors such as age, and tumor characteristics, such as size and position in bone and the presence or absence of a soft-tissue mass. The single most important factor is the ability to achieve negative margins at the time of surgery.

TABLE 25.4
The Huvos Classification System of Tumor Necrosis

Grade	Necrosis
I	Little or no effect
II	Areas of viable tumor, 60%–89% necrosis
III	Scattered foci, 90%–99% tumor necrosis
IV	No histological evidence of viable tumor—100%

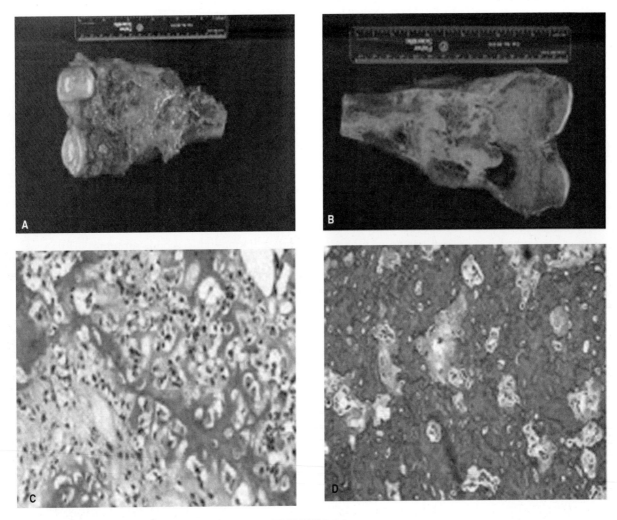

FIGURE 25.5

A typical resection specimen of a distal femoral osteogenic sarcoma. (A) and (B) show the gross resected specimen, (C) demonstrates the preoperative histological appearance, and (D) demonstrates a 40% necrosis rate as a result of the preoperative chemotherapy—a poor response to chemotherapy.

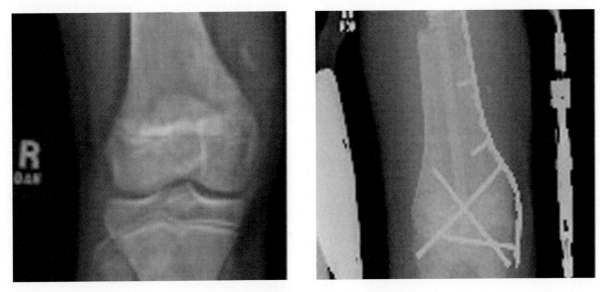

FIGURE 25.6

Physis sparing resection of osteogenic sarcoma of distal femur; preoperative picture (A) and postoperative picture (B). Reconstruction was achieved with intercalary bone graft, stabilized with a distal femur locking plate. The resection was achieved with negative margins and good knee function was achieved postoperatively.

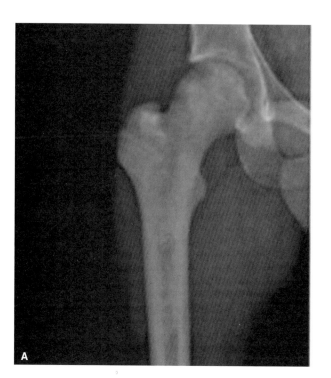
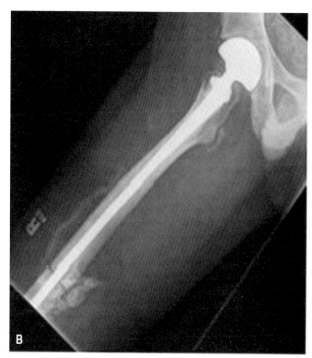

FIGURE 25.7

Osteogenic sarcoma proximal femur, resected with negative margins and reconstructed using an implant allograft (allo-prosthetic) composite.

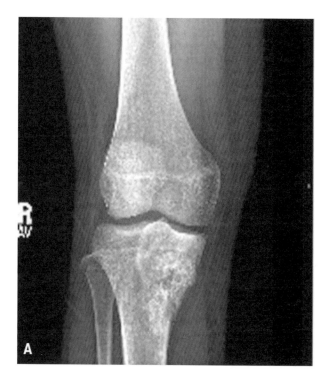
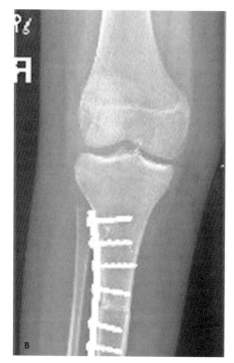

FIGURE 25.8

Primary osteogenic sarcoma of proximal tibia; negative resection margins were achieved and reconstruction was achieved using an osteoarticular allograft.

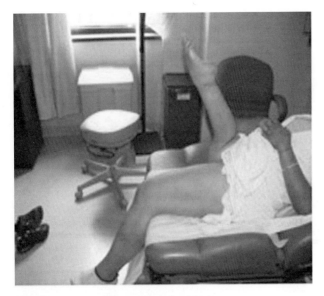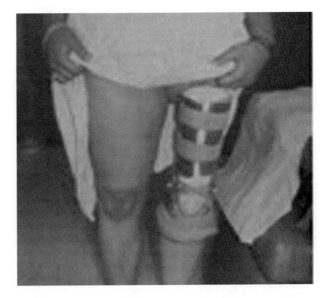

FIGURE 25.9

Postoperative rotationplasty patient.

*R*eferences

1. Cancer Facts and Figures. 2007. American Cancer Society (ACS). Atlanta Georgia 2007.
2. Bielack SS, Kempf-Bielack B, Delling G, et al. Prognostic factors in high-grade osteosarcoma of extremities or trunk: an analysis of 1,702 patients treated on neoadjuvant cooperative osteosarcoma study group protocols. *J Clin Oncol.* 2002;20(3):776–790.
3. Landis S, Murray T, Boldern S, Wingo P. Cancer statistics, 1999. *CA Cancer J Clin.* 1999;49:31.
4. Cade S. Osteogenic sarcoma: a study based on 33 patients. *J R Coll Surg Edinb.* 1955;1:79.
5. Friedman MA, Carter SK. The therapy of osteogenic sarcoma: current status and thoughts for the future. *J Surg Oncol.* 1972;4:482.
6. Rosen G, Murphy ML, Huvos AG, Gutierrez M, Marcove RC. Chemotherapy, en bloc resection, and prosthetic bone replacement in the treatment of osteogenic sarcoma. *Cancer.* January 1976;37(1):1–11.
7. Enneking W, Spanier S, Goodman M. Current concepts review. The surgical staging of musculoskeletal sarcoma. *J Bone Joint Surg.* 1980;62A:1027.
8. Enneking W, Spanier S, Malawer M. The effect of the anatomic setting on the results of surgical procedures for soft parts sarcoma of the thigh. *Cancer.* 1981;47:1005.
9. Enneking W. A system of staging musculoskeletal neoplasms. *Clin Orthop.* 1986;204:9.
10. Exner G, von Hochstetter A, Augustiny N, von Schulthess G. Magnetic resonance imaging in malignant bone tumors. *Int Orthop.* 1990;14:49.
11. Gosfield E, Alvai A, Kneeland B. Comparison of radionuclide bone scans and magnetic imaging in detecting spinal metastases. *J Nucl Med.* 1993;34:2191.
12. Simon M, Finn H. Diagnostic strategy for bone and soft tissue tumors. *J Bone Joint Surg.* 1993;75A:622.
13. Mankin HJ, Lange TA, Spanier SS. The hazards of biopsy in patients with malignant primary bone and soft tissue tumours. *J Bone Joint Surg Am.* 1982;64:1121.
14. Mankin HJ, Mankin CJ, Simon MA. The hazards of the biopsy, revisited. *J Bone Joint Surg Am.* May 1996;78(5):656–663.
15. Springfield DS, Rosenberg A. Biopsy: complicated and risky (an editorial). *J Bone Joint Surg (Am).* 1996;78(5):639–643.
16. Jelinek JS, Murphey MD, Welker JA, et al. Diagnosis of primary bone tumors with image-guided percutaneous biopsy: experience with 110 tumors. *Radiology.* 2002;223:731.
17. Goorin AM, Schwartzentruber DJ, Devidas M, et al. Presurgical chemotherapy compared with immediate surgery and adjuvant chemotherapy for nonmetastatic osteosarcoma: Pediatric Oncology Group Study POG-8651. *J Clin Oncol.* 2003;21:1574.
18. Link M, Goorin A, Miser A, et al. Adjuvant chemotherapy of high-grade osteosarcoma of the extremity. Updated results of the multi-institutional osteosarcoma study. *Clin Orthop.* 1991;270:8.
19. Myers PA, Heller G, Healey J, et al. Chemotherapy for non-metastatic osteogenic sarcoma: the memorial Sloan-Kettering experience. *J Clin Oncol.* 1992;10:5.
20. Wunder JS, Paulian G, Huvos AG, Heller G, Myers PA, Healey JH. The histological response to chemotherapy as a predictor of the oncological outcome of operative treatment of ewing sarcoma. *J Bone Joint Surg.* 1998;80(A):7, 1020.
21. Marco RAW, Gitelis S, Brebach GT, Healey JH. Cartilage tumors: evaluation and treatment. *J Am Acad Orthop Surg.* 2000;8:292.
22. DeLaney TF, Park L, Goldberg SI, et al. Radiotherapy for local control of osteosarcoma. *Int J Radiation Oncology Biol Phys.* 2005;61(2):492.
23. La TH, Meyers PA, Wexler LH, et al. Radiation therapy for Ewing's sarcoma: results from memorial Sloan-Kettering in the modern era. *Int J Radiation Oncology Biol Phys.* 2006;64(2):544.

III

MEDICAL COMPLICATIONS OF CANCER AND THEIR TREATMENT

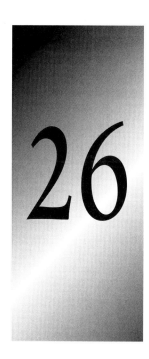

Pulmonary Complications of Cancer

Matthew N. Bartels
Megan L. Freedland

Pulmonary disease and pulmonary complications are major contributors to morbidity and mortality. This is also true with patients with cancer, whether they have primary lung cancer, secondary metastases, or complications with their treatment. The patient with cancer may have significant preexisting pulmonary disease that will need attention, or may develop pulmonary complications as a result of their primary oncologic disease. The discussion of primary lung cancer is not the focus of this chapter, but primary lung cancer is the leading cause of death in men and women in the United States (1). The issue of secondary metastases to the lungs and the accompanying complications cause significant morbidity and are commonly seen, since the lungs are one of the primary sites of metastatic disease. Other pulmonary issues are due to the effects of cancer treatment on the lungs, including lung resection, radiation therapy, chemotherapy, and complications such as pneumonia and pulmonary embolism. The rehabilitation focus is on preserving the function of the patient with cancer. Maintaining good pulmonary toilet practices, preserving overall conditioning, and focusing on strengthening and compensatory exercises will allow a patient to maintain their capacity in the face of their condition and its complications.

METASTATIC DISEASE

In patients who die of their tumors, lung metastases are common, reaching between 57% and 77% of breast cancer patients (2) and nearly half of patients with colorectal cancer (3). Similar levels of lung involvement are also seen in sarcoma and head and neck cancers. In fact, most patients who die of cancer die from metastatic disease rather than from continued growth of the primary tumor. The treatment of isolated lung nodules is often considered or pursued, but offers mixed results. Radiation treatment of lung nodules also has significant side effects due to the poor radiation tolerance of the lung (4), and surgical treatment is limited in that repeated surgery or multiple resections are often too strenuous to be tolerated by the patient.

Metastatic disease to the lung may be asymptomatic or can present dramatically with pleural effusions, bronchial obstruction, interstitial spread of the tumor, or even pneumothorax (5). Asymptomatic metastatic pulmonary disease is actually common, seen in 20%–54% of patients who die of extrathoracic malignancies (5). Tumors that are vascular are more likely to metastasize, and include real cell carcinoma, melanoma, choriocarcinoma, sarcomas, thyroid carcinoma, and testicular carcinoma. Commonly occurring tumors also frequently metastasize, including breast, hepatic, stomach, head, neck, prostate, and colorectal carcinomas (6–8). Most pulmonary metastases arise from hematogenous spread of the tumor through microemboli. Other methods of pulmonary metastases include lymphatic spread, direct invasion through the pleural space, and, in rare cases, via transbronchial aspiration (9–11).

KEY POINTS

- Beyond primary lung tumors, secondary metastases to the lungs and the accompanying complications cause significant morbidity and are commonly seen, since the lungs are one of the primary sites of metastatic disease.
- The treatment of isolated lung nodules is difficult because lung tissue has poor tolerance to radiation treatment and multiple surgical resections are often too strenuous to be tolerated by the patient.
- Restrictive lung disease may be seen as a result of the treatment of primary lung cancer and may be due to pleural effusions, kyphoscoliosis, neuromuscular disease complications, and phrenic nerve paralysis, and can lead to hypoventilation with symptoms of dyspnea.
- Bleomycin has been associated with acute-onset pulmonary edema and occurs in patients previously exposed to increased concentrations of inspired oxygen in concentrations as low 30%.
- Given that supplemental oxygen is a mainstay of pulmonary rehabilitation, patients with a history of Bleomycin exposure should avoid supplemental oxygen altogether, if possible, or use the lowest possible concentrations.
- Preexisting chronic obstructive pulmonary disease (COPD) is common in patients with lung cancer and can predispose to the development of radiation- and chemotherapy-associated pneumonitis.
- For patients who have had their tumor in remission for more than five years and appear to be disease-free, lung transplantation may be a reasonable treatment to offer in the setting of severe interstitial lung disease.

Most pulmonary metastases from a solid, nonpulmonary primary tumor are nodular, but about 7% occur in an interstitial form, presenting with lymphangitic carcinomatosis. Lymphangitic carcinomatosis can present unilaterally or bilaterally, and the symptoms include a dry persistent cough, dyspnea, and, in rare cases, hemoptysis. The clinical presentation can appear similar to a pneumonia, congestive heart failure, pulmonary embolism, sarcoidosis, or asthma (12). It is often difficult to detect the lymphangitic spread of a lung tumor, but it can often be seen with positron tomography and presents clinically with a limitation of the diffusion capacity of carbon monoxide (DL_{CO}) on pulmonary function test (PFT) studies, along with an intrinsic restrictive lung disease pattern (12). Other ways to diagnose the condition include high-resolution computed tomography (CT), and if all of these studies are not definitive, it may be necessary to consider a lung biopsy (13).

Nodular metastases are far easier to diagnose radiologically, and when present in isolation, can be treated with metastectomy, or resection of the nodule. This was not always an accepted treatment modality, but in recent years, with the advent of better chemotherapy regimens, resection of pulmonary nodules is performed for isolated lesions (14). The current feeling is that the lung is often the first filter for hematogenously spread tumors and that an isolated nodule resection might add to the benefit of the primary tumor treatment. Generally speaking, the criteria for surgical resection of lung metastases have been the following: (1) pulmonary disease completely resectable, (2) absence of nonresectable recurrent local disease or metastatic disease in other organs, (3) pulmonary function compatible with the proposed surgery, and (4) absence of other, more effective treatments (15). The role of rehabilitation is in the preparation of patients for possible resection. A pulmonary rehabilitation program can help to prepare the patient for surgery as well as allow a marginal patient to better tolerate the procedure and still have reasonable function after the surgery. In rare cases, even more radical approaches can be taken, including complete pneumonectomy for the metastases; but generally, the mortality and morbidity from this procedure makes it an unattractive option for most patients (16).

A final approach to isolated pulmonary metastatic disease is the use of transpulmonary chemoembolization, where chemotherapy is injected preferentially in vessels that feed metastases. This is a relatively new technique and takes advantage of the hematogenous nature of pulmonary metastases. This approach may be useful for patients who have surgically unresectable lesions or who could not tolerate lung surgery for other reasons. The procedure is well tolerated, and there is regression of disease, which may be associated with an increase in survival. This is not a curative approach, but is rather a palliative approach for lesions that cannot be otherwise addressed (17).

Extrapulmonary manifestations of metastatic malignant disease can be seen with pulmonary effusions. Malignant effusions are quite common. Approximately 175,000 cases are seen in the United States every year

(18), most commonly in lung and breast cancer (19). These malignant effusions often compromise pulmonary function through loss of functional lung volume, and can be a site for infection. The proper management of the effusion is important for the preservation of function for the patient, and should be coordinated to allow therapy to continue and to maximize quality of life. Simple aspiration of the effusion is only palliative, as the effusion will most likely recur, and is usually only advisable in patients with a short life expectancy and poor functional status (20,21). For patients who can tolerate pleurodesis, it is still an effective treatment. Although many different agents have been used for pleurodesis, sterile talc is still consistently shown to be one of the most effective agents (22,23). For patients who fail pleurodesis, indwelling catheters may be used, and there are long-term catheters that can allow a patient to return to home (24). An example of the most radical approach possible in patients who can tolerate the procedure is an extrapleural pneumonectomy. This is a radical surgery in which the parietal pleura, the pericardium, and diaphragm, and the lung on the affected side are removed. However, this treatment has a high operative mortality and morbidity. It is an approach that is only warranted if the patient can tolerate the procedure and there is a belief that it may be curative (Figs. 26.1 and 26.2) (25).

RESTRICTIVE LUNG CONDITIONS

Although it is not as commonly seen as metastatic disease, restrictive lung disease may be seen as a result of the treatment of the primary malignancy. In addition to the effects of malignant pleural effusions discussed previously, the extrapulmonary causes of pulmonary restriction include kyphoscoliosis, neuromuscular disease complications, and phrenic nerve paralysis. All of these conditions lead to a decreased ability to expand

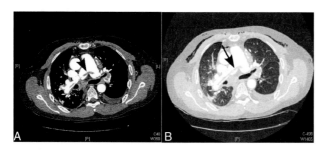

FIGURE 26.1

Saddle pulmonary embolus visible on the standard (A) and lung window (B) sections of a Computed Tomography. Embolism indicated with an arrow within the pulmonary artery.

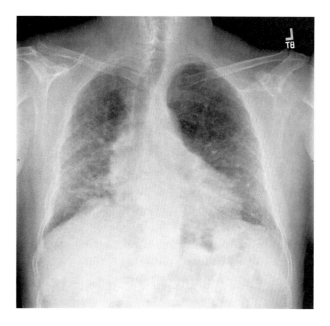

FIGURE 26.2

Chest x-ray of diffuse interstitial lung disease. Note the small lung volumes and the diffuse changes.

the chest wall and lead to hypoventilation with symptoms of dyspnea. In severe cases, they can even lead to respiratory failure.

Kyphoscoliosis can be seen in patients with cancer, and is usually caused by either metastatic lesions to the thoracic spine or by osteoporosis from treatment for the primary tumor. The presence of osteoporotic fractures is an indicator of poorer prognosis in postmenopausal women (26), and is also likely for patients with cancer, regardless of gender. The common causes of bone loss in cancer patients would be antiestrogen therapy after breast cancer and compromised nutritional status in older patients or in nutritional compromise from the primary cancer. Another group at particular risk of osteoporotic kyphosis is the group of survivors of acute leukemia. The treatment regimens for leukemia often include radiotherapy and systemic administration of corticosteroids for long periods of time (27). These can lead to abnormal bone growth or decreased activity of osteoclasts and a lowered bone mineral content. Methotrexate, a commonly used agent in hematogenous cancer therapy, also increases the risk of osteopenia (28,29). Additional risks inherent to the patient include a history of smoking (30), poor nutrition, female gender, and Caucasian race—the same as the general risk factors for osteoporosis in individuals without cancer (27). Treatment for the kyphosis and impaired ventilatory function is supportive. In cases of muscular failure, bilevel positive airway pressure support can be done as a form of noninvasive ventilation, and the use of supplemental oxygen may be helpful. The preferred medical treatment for the loss of bone mineral density is calcium, 1,25 dihydroxy-vitamin D supplementation, and bisphosphonates (31–33).Calcitonin and weight-bearing exercise should also be added to the patient's regimen, as they have an important role in the prevention of the progression of loss of bone mineral density (34). Low-dose parathyroid hormone and fluorides are also considered in select cases (39).

A long-term complication of radiation therapy in children and adolescents with cancer can be kyphosis with associated restrictive pulmonary disease. Kyphosis occurs in approximately 7% of children who have had radiation for Wilms tumor (35), and has a similar incidence in other childhood cancers where mantle irradiation is given. The incidence of scoliosis is even higher in children who have received irradiation, and can be as high as 61.2% in long-term follow-up, compared to 9.4% in matched children who had not received irradiation (36). The severity of scoliosis is also dependent upon the intensity and frequency of the dose of radiation (37). Patients with radiation doses of less than 2,400 centigray (cGy) had a lower incidence than those above that dose (34). Of interest, irradiation in solid tumors of childhood other than Wilms tumor resulted in even higher incidence of kyphoscoliosis, approaching 90% in some series (39). Although the rehabilitation professional will not change the course of the early irradiation in childhood tumors, it is good to be aware of the complications that might occur so that the appropriate management of resultant kyphoscoliosis can be anticipated and treatment started as required.

Neuromuscular disease is another unusual presentation of pulmonary disease in cancer. It is usually associated with Lambert-Eaton myasthenic syndrome (LEMS), and is associated with small cell lung cancer in about 60% of cases (39). The pulmonary manifestations of the condition include possible aspiration and pneumonia from dysphagia (40). Later in the course of the condition, frank respiratory failure may occur (41). Of interest, LEMS associated with malignancy tends to be more severe than LEMS that is idiopathic (42,43). The management from a rehabilitation perspective can include the diagnosis of the condition and then modification of exercise programs to accommodate for the needs of the patient. The features of LEMS are discussed in detail in Chapter XX. Blood tests to help clarify the diagnosis of LEMS include creatinine kinase, thyroid function studies, and calcium channel antibodies. The condition is especially prevalent in patients with lung tumors, so LEMS needs to be considered in any patient presenting with weakness, dysphagia, and respiratory muscle weakness who has a history of lung tumors. Medical treatment is limited to either 3,4-DAP

or IVIg, but with only limited evidence to support the efficacy in these treatments (44). Treatment results generally show improvement in muscle strength, but not a resolution of the syndrome.

Another important pulmonary complication of cancer is the development of phrenic nerve paralysis. This is a rare complication in extrathoracic tumors, but is seen relatively frequently in primary lung tumors that invade the mediastinum or in mediastinal tumors. It can also be seen as the result of surgery (45,46), either for the lung or in radical neck dissections (47). There are also isolated reports of phrenic nerve paralysis as a result of toxicity from chemotherapy, such as 5-fluorouracil or doxorubicin for breast cancer (48,49). The symptoms of phrenic nerve injury are dyspnea, which is far worse while lying supine and relieved somewhat when erect. Fortunately, the response to surgical treatment with plication of the affected diaphragm can be good, and the surgery can be done via video-assisted thoracoscopic surgery (VATS), minimizing the invasiveness of the procedure (50).

Interestingly, there may also occasionally be a role for causing a phrenic nerve paralysis in cancer patients in order to provide symptomatic relief. There are reports of the use of a phrenic nerve block to help to relieve the discomfort of intractable hiccups that may be the result of chemotherapy (51) or tumor metastases. Phrenic nerve paralysis can be done safely in a controlled setting, with preservation of pulmonary function (52). There also are reports of chronic shoulder pain in patients with cancer that can be relieved with palliative mediastinal radiotherapy when there is tumor invasion of the phrenic nerve (53). Obviously these are not common treatments, but in the palliation of symptoms, they may be considered.

The intrinsic lung conditions that can lead to restrictive lung disease include lymphangitic tumor spread and metastatic disease, leading to replacement of the lung parenchyma with tumor, as discussed previously. A common, and often severe, cause of pulmonary restriction in cancer patients that is not related to metastases or tumor is pulmonary fibrosis, which is often the result of radiation or chemotherapy for the treatment of the primary malignancy.

RADIATION PNEUMONITIS

Radiation-induced pulmonary injury can be both genetic and nongenetic. The nongenetic damage is usually most apparent in capillary endothelial and type I pneumocytes (54). The molecular pathways that are activated by the radiation injury include sphingomyelin hydrolysis, which, in turn, generates ceramide as a second messenger that leads to apoptotic deoxyribonucleic acid

(DNA) degradation. Nonlethal radiation also causes up-regulation of multiple stress response genes, which initiates a cellular repair process that involves cytokines, fibroblast growth factors, interleukin-1, and transforming growth factor-beta (TGF-beta). With time, the capillaries regenerate, but the lung does not regenerate type I pneumocytes, and these are replaced with type II pneumocytes (surfactant-producing cells) (55). Direct genetic damage from radiation causes apoptosis and loss of integrity of capillary and alveolar surfaces, leading to exudation of fluid into the alveoli. Clinically this presents as a loss of lung compliance (stiffer lungs), decreased gas exchange (decreased DL_{CO}), and in severe cases, pulmonary failure can result. The complex mechanisms of the combined genetic and nongenetic damage may also explain the time course of the presentation of radiation pneumonitis, which may be acute to chronic (56).

Radiation pneumonitis develops in 5%–15% of patients who receive high-dose external beam radiation for lung cancer (57), and in 10%–20% of individuals receiving external beam chest radiation for other tumors (58). However, there may actually be underreporting of pneumonitis, as many patients have nonspecific symptoms, such as cough or mild dyspnea, that may be attributed to a cardiovascular or respiratory disorder. As would be expected, the incidence of pneumonitis is dose-related and with higher doses, there is more severe involvement (59). Adjuvant, concomitant, or consolidation chemotherapy seems to also increase the incidence of pneumonitis, although it may be an additive effect since chemotherapy alone can often cause lung inflammation with selected agents (60). When the symptoms are mild, they are often self-limited and resolve in time with mild supportive treatment, such as inhaled corticosteroid therapy (61). However, severe pneumonitis may have a mortality rate as high as 50% (62), and can lead to long-term pulmonary disability, even if the patient survives, due to the resulting fibrosis and restrictive lung disease. Patients who experience severe radiation pneumonitis also have a significantly lower overall survival rate than similar patients with mild or absent radiation lung inflammation after radiation therapy (63).

In the diagnosis of radiation pneumonitis, pulmonary function studies usually do not have great sensitivity in detecting the condition, with the exception of DL_{CO}, which can decline dramatically. It is the clinical picture of cough and dyspnea which are essential in establishing the diagnosis. There are also several toxicity criteria for determining the level of pulmonary toxicity from radiation. The commonly used scales are listed in Table 26.1. In patients with radiation toxicity to the lung, the DL_{CO} is usually affected by more than 13% after radiotherapy for lung cancer, while

the Forced Expiratory Volume in one second (FEV1) was usually affected by less than 12% (61). Paradoxically, in patients with lung cancer, there may actually be an improvement in the flow volume loop of the PFT, even in the presence of radiation pneumonitis, since the radiation may have decreased the size of the tumor and reduced any obstruction that may have been present (64). However, the presence of radiation pneumonitis does have negative effects on function in milder cases, and a general estimation of the effect of radiation on total lung capacity and DL_{CO} can be made with the following calculations. For every 1% of lung volume receiving 20 or more grays (Gy) of radiation, the total lung capacity decreases by 0.8% and DL_{CO} decreases by 1.3% (65). Additionally, it should be remembered that DL_{CO} decreases can be seen whenever the total local radiation dose exceeds 13 Gy and occurs no matter how the radiation is fractionated (66). Given these findings, supplemental oxygen should be used when needed. For patients with a symptom of cough after undergoing radiation therapy that involves the lungs, inhaled steroids should be considered. Additionally, in view of how common radiation injury is, any new pulmonary symptoms in a patient who has had radiation therapy should be taken seriously lest they progress to severe and life-threatening levels.

Radiologic evaluation can help in making the diagnosis of radiation pneumonitis. Radiographs often will show ground glass opacification, diffuse haziness, or indistinct normal pulmonary markings over the irradiated area. Later in the course of the condition, there may be alveolar infiltrates or dense consolidation. Eventually, as the pneumonitis progresses to pulmonary fibrosis, fibrotic changes may appear, often in the pattern of the area of irradiation. Overall, chest CT is more sensitive than chest x-ray in the detection of the radiation pneumonitis (Figs. 26.3 and 26.4) (57).

There are several features in patient selection that can help to predict the possibility of the development of radiation pneumonitis. Patient characteristics that lead to a higher risk of pneumonitis include concurrent or antecedent chemotherapy, a history of smoking, tumor location (lower lobe), female gender, increased age, and low pulmonary functional status. Decrease in risk was seen in individuals who had surgery for their tumor (64). Chemotherapy with cisplatin and paclitaxel are the most likely to increase the incidence of radiation pneumonitis (64). Other agents that have been implicated in potentiating radiation pneumonitis include mitomycin C, gemcitabine, irinotecan, and docetaxel (64). Overall, however, the data is not as clear as would be desired, and there is still some controversy. However, it is relatively clear that chemotherapy concurrent with radiotherapy is more likely to cause pneumonitis than radiation given separately from chemotherapy.

TABLE 26.1
Assessment Scales for Pulmonary Toxicity

CRITERIA	1	2	3	4	5
CTCAE	Asymptomatic Radiologic findings only	Symptomatic Not interfering with ADL	Symptomatic Interfering with ADL Oxygen required	Life-threatening Ventilatory support needed	Death
RTOG	Asymptomatic Mild symptoms Has radiographic findings	Moderate symptoms Severe cough Fever	Severely symptomatic	Severe respiratory insufficiency Continuous oxygen needed Ventilatory support needed	Death
SWOG	Asymptomatic Symptoms not requiring steroids Has radiographic findings	Initiation or increase of steroid dose	Oxygen required	Ventilatory support needed	Death

Abbreviations: ADL, Activities of daily living; CTCAE, Common Terminology Criteria for Adverse Events; RTOG, Radiation Therapy Oncology Group; SWOG, Southwest Oncology Group.
Source: Modified from Ref. 58.

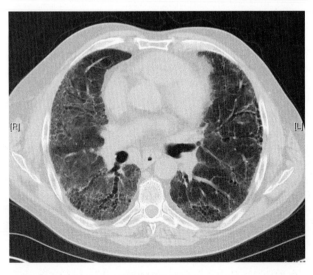

FIGURE 26.3

Representative slice of severe interstitial lung disease with traction bronchiectasis and honeycombing of the lung.

The time course of most cases of radiation pneumonitis is to present two to three months after the completion of the radiation treatment. When it presents at this point in time, the injury exists, with no way to reverse the damage. In an attempt to determine if there is injury much earlier, several biomarkers have been examined by trying to take advantage of the cytokine cascade discussed previously. The only biomarker found so far to have any value is significantly higher interleukin-1 alpha and interleukin-6 before, during, and after radiation treatment in patients who develop pneumonitis (67,68).

The prevention of radiation pneumonitis is a topic of great importance, as it can be such a serious complication. Many techniques can be used to decrease the intensity of the radiation dose to normal lung while still targeting the tumor. These include (1) continuous hyperfractionated accelerated radiotherapy (CHART; 54 Gy in 36 doses, 3 times a day, over 12 consecutive days) or CHARTWEL (60 Gy in 40 fractions of 1.5 Gy three times a day, excluding weekends) (69); (2) three-dimensional conformal radiotherapy, which is more accurate and has had lower episodes of grade 2 pneumonitis (70); (3) intensity-modulated radiotherapy (71); (4) boost radiotherapy (72); (5) single-dose stereotactic radiotherapy (73); (6) and proton radiotherapy (64). The selection of the appropriate type of radiotherapy for a patient is the decision of the radiation oncologist and oncologist for any given patient. The names of the different radiation-sparing treatment options are given here for information so that rehabilitation specialists can see if their patient has been on a radiation-sparing regimen.

An alternative to limiting radiation dose or alternate radiation therapy protocols is to administer cytoprotective medications to try to prevent radiation injury to normal tissues. Trials of prophylaxis with

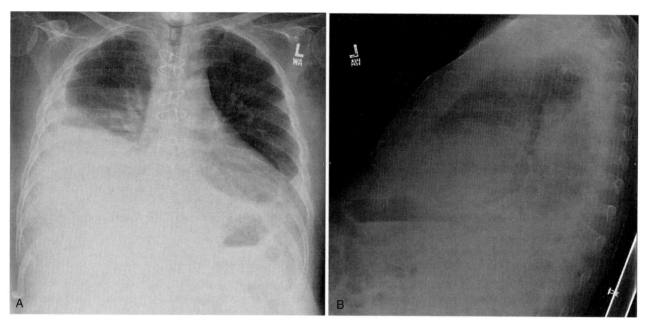

FIGURE 26.4

Postero-anterior (A) and lateral (B) chest x-rays of patient with bilateral effusions: right-sided, moderately to severely large; left-sided, mild to moderately large.

corticosteroids or azathioprine do not clearly reduce the incidence of radiation pneumonitis. However, in a few trials, no grade 3 pneumonitis has been reported. This may indicate that there is some benefit to considering these agents as a preventative treatment (75). Another agent is amifostine, which is an aminothiol with broad cryoprotection that may have benefit in the prevention of acute radiation injury. It offers cryoprotection for normal cells, while not protecting the tumor cells (76). Clinical trial results have also shown a possible role in the prevention of the decline in DL_{CO} that is seen with high-dose radiation therapy. Another agent that has been studied is the angiotensin-converting enzyme (ACE) inhibitor captopril, which has a thiol component that may be protective against radiation pneumonitis. However, even though several studies have been able to demonstrate benefit in a rat model, human studies have shown no benefit of ACE inhibitors to date (77). Finally, several other agents are also being investigated, including pentoxifylline in patients with lung or breast cancer (78) and melatonin (79). These are still clearly experimental at this point, and both animal and human studies are underway.

CHEMOTHERAPY PNEUMONITIS

Occurring with about the same incidence as radiation pneumonitis is chemotherapy-induced pulmonary

injury. The severity of the reaction can be anywhere from mild to life-threatening, and is generally divided into early (immediate to two months after therapy) and late onset (greater than two months after chemotherapy) (57). Table 26.2 summarizes the common injuries and time courses for injuries, grouped with their causative agents.

Early-onset chemotherapy-induced pneumonitis is usually a hypersensitivity type of reaction with an inflammatory interstitial pneumonitis. The appearance of the reaction can be immediate or up to a few months after the initiation of chemotherapy. The most common chemotherapeutic agents to cause this reaction are methotrexate, bleomycin, procarbazine, and carmustine (57). Acute pneumonitis is also seen occasionally with taxane-paclitaxel and mitoxantrone (80). The patients who experience pneumonitis with taxane-paclitaxel have lung injury in association with a general hypersensitivity reaction. This is seen in between 3% and 10% of patients on taxane-paclitaxel or mitoxantrone. If recognized early, chemotherapy pneumonitis usually resolves when the causative agent is stopped, and usually there is a full return of lung function. In severe cases, there may be the need to use oral corticosteroids to control symptoms (57).

Another form of acute pulmonary injury from chemotherapy is acute noncardiogenic pulmonary edema. This is usually caused by endothelial injury and the resultant alveolar edema. It is most often associated

---

TABLE 26.2
Most Common Chemotherapy-Induced Lung Injuries and Time Courses

Acute Chemotherapy Pneumonitis	Acute Chemotherapy Edema	Acute Pulmonary Fibrosis
Taxane-paclitaxel Mitoxantrone	Cytosine arabinoside (Ara-C) Bleomycin with supplemental oxygen Interleukin-2 All trans-retinoic acid	Carmustine (BCNU)
Early Chemotherapy Pneumonitis Methotrexate Bleomycin Procarbazine	**Early Chemotherapy Edema** Bleomycin with supplemental oxygen	**Early Pulmonary Fibrosis** Bleomycin Cyclophosphamide Isophosphamide
Late Chemotherapy Pneumonitis Bleomycin Busulfan Carmustine (BCNU) Mitomycin-C Methotrexate Cisplatin with radiation Tamoxifen and radiation	**Late Chemotherapy Edema** Bleomycin with supplemental oxygen	**Late Pulmonary Fibrosis** Bleomycin Mitomycin-C Busulfan Chlorambucil Melphalan Carmustine (BCNU)

---

with infusions of cytosine arabinoside (Ara-C), and is treated with supplemental oxygen and diuresis (81). In severe cases, the patient may require mechanical ventilation. Interleukin-2 can also cause pulmonary edema through a capillary leak syndrome, which is more pronounced in the lungs than in any other tissues. The capillary leak is seen more often in patients with a low FEV1, previous chemotherapy, and bolus injections of the medication. The infiltrates and edema usually resolve in three to five days, and treatment can include prostaglandins, cyclooxygenase-2, or interleukin-1 inhibitors in addition to supportive care (57). Another agent associated with a pulmonary edema syndrome is all-trans-retinoic acid, which is used to treat acute promyelocytic leukemia. The incidence of vascular leak is as high as 23%–28% with this medication, and is caused by the sudden differentiation of leukemic blast cells into mature granulocytes, which then adhere to the pulmonary endothelium (57).

Finally, bleomycin has been associated with acute-onset pulmonary edema in a clinical presentation that resembles acute respiratory distress syndrome. It occurs in patients previously treated with bleomycin who are exposed to increased concentrations of inspired oxygen. It may occur even months to years after the treatment with bleomycin and with oxygen concentrations as low as 30% (57). Clearly, this severe reaction is of concern

to rehabilitation specialists, as supplemental oxygen is a mainstay of pulmonary rehabilitation and providing supplemental oxygen, even at a low concentration, may precipitate a severe pulmonary reaction in these patients. The best practice to follow when designing a rehabilitation program for patients with a history of bleomycin exposure is to avoid supplemental oxygen altogether, if possible, or use the lowest possible oxygen concentration you can.

Other acute-onset conditions in patients receiving chemotherapy include bronchospasm, which is seen with vinblastine and methotrexate, and pleurisy with methotrexate (82). Eosinophilic pneumonitis has been reported in patients receiving minocycline (82), and there are case reports of eosinophilic pneumonitis after oxaliplatin in combination with fluorouracil for colorectal cancer (83).

Late-onset chemotherapy-induced lung disease presents more than two months after the completion of the chemotherapy, and is usually manifested by pulmonary fibrosis. The agents with the highest incidence of fibrosis include bleomycin, busulfan, carmustine (BCNU), and mitomycin-C (57). Other agents that have been implicated include methotrexate, cisplatin with radiation (84), and tamoxifen in combination with radiotherapy in postmenopausal women (85). The symptoms of the condition are generally progressive dyspnea and the need for supplemental oxygen. Patients will have decreased DL_{CO} on pulmonary function testing, along with the development of restrictive pulmonary physiology with low vital capacity and preserved forced expiratory volume in 1 second/vital capacity (FEV1/VC) ratio.

Bleomycin is the classic causative agent for pulmonary fibrosis. The pulmonary toxicity leading to pulmonary fibrosis has a varying incidence, but is present in about 10% of patients, with mortality from fibrosis in 1%–2% of patients (57,86). The incidence of fibrosis from bleomycin may actually even be higher in children than adults, with up to 70% of children demonstrating significant restrictive changes over time (82). The onset of the fibrosis generally starts several months after the completion of therapy and may be through a mechanism of lipid peroxidation, which leads to interstitial edema and the influx of inflammatory cells. Pulmonary fibrosis can be the end result of this inflammation, and there are reports of excess collagen deposition and presence of excess fibroblast mediators (87). The risk factors for bleomycin toxicity include advanced age, prior or concomitant radiotherapy, renal insufficiency, combination chemotherapy, and intravenous administration of the medication. Cumulative doses greater than 400–500 mg/m² are also associated with increased toxicity (87). Fortunately, 20% of patients with bleomycin toxicity will be asymptomatic, but the other 80% may be left with long-term injury.

Mitomycin-C toxicity occurs in 12%–39% of patients, and is associated with the development of interstitial pneumonitis and fibrosis that occurs 3–12 months after completion of therapy. As with bleomycin, oxygen exposure, radiation and concomitant chemotherapy with cisplatin, vinca alkaloids, cyclophosphamide, and doxorubicin will increase the risk of toxicity. About 5% of patients will develop symptoms, while about 28% will develop PFT abnormalities. Drug cessation and steroids are the mainstays of treatment (57). A related medication, actinomycin D, exacerbates radiation-induced lung injury and can be present in a delayed "radiation-recall" effect. The pattern of injury seen is in the radiation port, and can occur even if the agent is given a long time after the radiation has been given (57).

The alkylating chemotherapy agents are also often associated with interstitial lung damage. Cyclophosphamide is commonly used and has only an incidence of about 1% for lung injury. It occurs after a total dose of 150–250 mg has been reached, and in its early presentation can resemble bleomycin (88). The early-onset form of toxicity occurs between one and six months, and initially looks like an infectious pneumonia. The late-onset toxicity has similar clinical findings, with a slow onset. On radiographic studies, there is interstitial lung disease with pleural thickening. The mortality with the late-onset form of toxicity can reach 60%, and the incidence of lung injury has been found to be increased with combination therapy with carmustine (57). Ifosfamide is an analog of cyclophosphamide and causes a similar pattern of toxicity.

Busulfan is an agent that has a 4% incidence of fibrosis, and there are no clear associations with dose or any clear risk factors. The disease has a late onset, after 24 months, and has the appearance of classical bleomycin toxicity. Mortality rates are 80% once the condition is established, and no effective treatments exist. Chlorambucil and melphalan also cause fibrosis, with similarly high mortality rates, especially after doses in the range of 2.0–7.5 mg (57).

Antimetabolite drugs that cause interstitial fibrosis include methotrexate, azathioprine, fludarabine, and mercaptopurine. Methotrexate causes an interstitial fibrosis, and the syndrome is similar to a hypersensitivity pneumonitis. This can develop into a fibrotic syndrome over time, and treatment with corticosteroids seems to decrease the course of the disease and may be associated with improvements in survival. The overall mortality rate in methotrexate fibrosis is 10% (57). The other agents are less commonly associated with chronic fibrosis, and are used for immunomodulation therapy for collagen vascular disease or even transplant (57).

The nitrosourea group of medications is also implicated in the development of interstitial lung disease after chemotherapy. Carmustine is the most commonly implicated agent, although lomustine, semustine, fotemustine, and chlorozotocin have also been implicated. Carmustine has three distinct clinical syndromes of interstitial lung disease: (1) early-onset fibrosing alveolitis, seen in 30% of patients on high-dose treatment; (2) late-onset fibrosis, as seen in bleomycin; and (3) as a contributing agent in combination therapy, often for bone marrow transplant, with incidences that run as high as 40% in two years. The risk is highest in total doses above 1,500 mg/m², and risk increases with concomitant radiotherapy or preexisting COPD. Up to 60% of cases are steroid-responsive, but even then, there is a mortality rate of up to 60% overall (57).

In all of the various causes of chemotherapy-induced pulmonary fibrosis, the common clinical feature is insidious onset of dyspnea and a nonproductive cough. Chest radiographs usually show basilar interstitial markings, and PFT shows a restrictive pattern. The DL_{CO} is also reduced, out of proportion to the restriction. Chest CT and gallium scans have a higher sensitivity at detection than pulmonary function

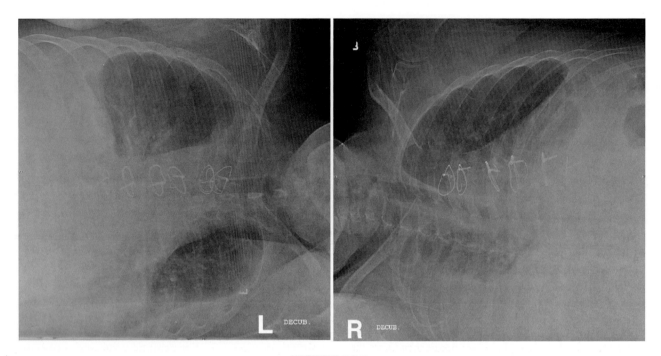

FIGURE 26.5

Left and right lateral decubitus films illustrating free-flowing effusions with no loculation.

studies. Thus, the diagnosis is often made on the basis of a combination of the history of exposure, the time course, the clinical presentation, the PFT, and the radiographic findings. In making the diagnosis, it is important to rule out infection, lymphangitic cancer spread, or other pulmonary diseases. In cases where the diagnosis is in doubt, biopsy may be needed to be sure of the diagnosis so that the appropriate treatment can be started.

OBSTRUCTIVE LUNG DISEASE IN CANCER PATIENTS

Other pulmonary issues to contemplate with patients with cancer are acute bronchospastic reactions to medications. This is relatively rare, but when it is present, it can be severe. The reaction is usually an acute episode during the administration of the medication. The most common chemotherapeutic cause of bronchospasm is seen with gemcitabine. It usually has onset within a few hours of administration and resolves after one to six hours. Supportive care is all that is required, and the medication usually can be continued (Figs. 26.5 and 26.6) (89,90).

Preexisting COPD is also fairly common in cancer patients, especially those with lung cancer. As discussed previously, the presence of COPD can be associated with a predisposition to the development of radiation- and chemotherapy-associated pneumonitis. Addition-

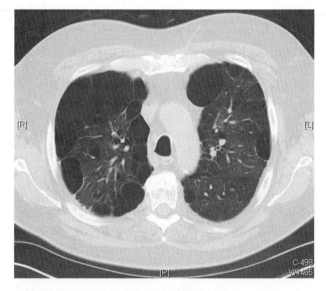

FIGURE 26.6

Computed Tomography scan with severe emphysema with large bullae, more on the right than the left.

ally, the limitations of COPD itself can present issues that complicate mobilization for patients with cancer. The techniques of pulmonary rehabilitation for COPD are well established, and are covered in numerous textbooks, so will not be reviewed again here (91–93).

Airway tumors can also present with obstructive lung disease symptoms, and are often diagnosed clinically. The obstruction can be from primary lesions or from metastases, and are confirmed with imaging, bronchoscopy, and biopsy. Treatment is symptomatic, and may involve focused radiotherapy and bronchial stenting. In primary or isolated lesions, there can be consideration of a lobectomy or pneumonectomy to try to achieve a cure, as long as the patient has sufficient pulmonary function to survive the procedure.

PULMONARY VASCULAR DISEASE

A major pulmonary complication of cancer is the occurrence of pulmonary embolism. Two types of pulmonary embolic disease can occur with tumors: thromboembolic emboli and tumor emboli. Thromboembolism is more likely in cancer patients due to the hypercoagulable state that many tumors create. Active cancer is the cause of approximately 20% of all venous thromboembolism that occurs in the community (94).The risk is highest in pancreatic cancer, lymphoma, malignant brain tumors, liver cancer, leukemia, colorectal, and other digestive system cancers (95). Increased risk of emboli formation also occurs in patients receiving cytotoxic chemotherapy. Tamoxifen, commonly used for breast cancer, is one of the most common noncytotoxic agents associated with thromboembolism (96). Another common risk factor for pulmonary thromboembolism is the presence of central venous catheters, which are common in patients who are undergoing chemotherapy or have infections associated with their cancer. These central lines account for 9% of community-based thromboembolism (95). Other risks that are often present in patients with cancer are a history of prior thromboembolism or major surgical procedures (Fig. 26.7) (97).

The appropriate prophylaxis and treatment of venous thromboembolism (VTE) are discussed in several authoritative references, and are covered with practice guidelines from the American College of Physicians (98). The key take-home points from the guidelines are as follows:

1. At-home treatment for VTE with low molecular weight heparin (LMWH) is as safe as in hospital treatment for appropriately selected patients with appropriate support services.
2. It is cost-effective to use LMWH versus unfractionated heparin for the treatment of VTE.
3. Compression stockings do have benefit in the prevention of post-thrombotic syndrome in patients with a history of deep venous thrombosis (DVT).
4. Vena caval filters are only modestly effective at reducing the recurrence of VTE and do not appear to reduce mortality.
5. Extended-duration treatment with oral vitamin K antagonists is most likely optimal for patients with unprovoked or recurrent VTE, as seen in cancer patients.
6. LMWH may be as efficacious as oral vitamin K antagonists for treatment of VTE in patients with cancer.

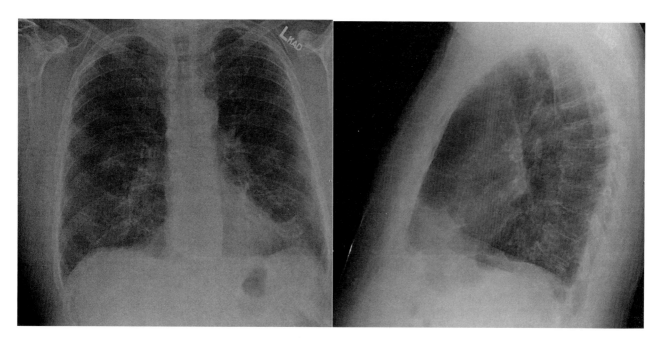

FIGURE 26.7

PA and lateral chest x-ray with emphysema; note the flattened diaphragms and the hyperinflation.

The treatment of the acute VTE event is supportive and includes the initiation of anticoagulation, ventilatory support, and supplemental oxygen. In severe cases, inotropic and circulatory support may be required. Up to 50% of cases of VTE involve massive pulmonary emboli, described as occluding more than 50% of the cross-sectional area of the pulmonary arterial tree (99). Since up to 70% of patients with VTE expire within the first hour after the onset of symptoms, rapid treatment and evaluation is important. Imaging studies are the mainstay of diagnosis, and include angiography, echocardiography, CT contrast angiography, and ventilation-perfusion scanning, among other studies. In extreme cases, thrombectomy can be done for acute embolism, but has had mixed reports on efficacy (100). Still, for a patient in extremis, thrombectomy can be a viable treatment option in select cases (101).

A rare, but possible, presentation of hypoxemia or progressive respiratory distress in a patient with a history of cancer is tumor pulmonary emboli. Most episodes of pulmonary tumor emboli are due to microemboli, and involve the small arteries, arterioles, and capillaries (102,103). Microembolization is usually asymptomatic, but on occasion it can be severe, with multiple emboli, and respiratory compromise can occur (104). The presentation can mimic VTE, and in some cases the diagnosis can only be made with a biopsy. The diagnosis of tumor pulmonary intravascular emboli may be made due to characteristic findings on chest CT scan. The images can demonstrate a multifocal dilatation and beading of the peripheral pulmonary arteries with possible associated distal infarcts (105). The source of the emboli is usually a vascularly invasive tumor, such as renal cell carcinoma, sarcoma, or an atrial myxoma. The incidence of tumor microemboli detected on autopsy has been reported to be between 2.4% and 26% in patients who have known malignancies (106). On the other end of the scale, a single massive tumor embolus to the lung is rare, but has also been reported to occur (107). Although it is a relatively rare cause of dyspnea after diagnosis with cancer, tumor emboli are worthwhile to consider, as lung metastases are common and most are hematogenous.

REHABILITATION TREATMENT OPTIONS

The role of rehabilitation in patients with pulmonary complications of cancer involves the usual areas of function and mobilization. Pain control is important with patients with lung-associated pain symptoms, since poor pain control in the chest can lead to impaired pulmonary toilet and impaired ventilation. In a patient with poor ventilatory reserve or hypoxemia, the standard pulmonary rehabilitation techniques of energy conservation and conditioning can help to restore func-

tion. A review of the basics of pulmonary rehabilitation techniques are reviewed in numerous standard rehabilitation textbooks and can be easily applied to the cancer patient with pulmonary complications (91–93).

Oxygen supplementation is an essential part of the care of individuals with pulmonary limitations and should be used as required in most patients. The only exception to liberal use of supplemental oxygen is in patients with a history of treatment with bleomycin, as acute pulmonary toxicity can be triggered with supplemental oxygen, even a long time after the administration of the agent (57). Otherwise, oxygen should be used as needed to allow for a saturation of >90% to be maintained. The patient with COPD should have low levels of supplemental oxygen at rest to prevent hypercarbia and oxygen as needed with exercise to prevent hypoxemia (108). In patients with severe interstitial disease, high-flow oxygen may be required, and as long as there is no history of bleomycin administration, it can be safely given (109).

For patients who have had their tumor in remission for more than five years and appear to be disease-free, lung transplantation may be a reasonable treatment to offer in the setting of severe interstitial lung disease. As many of the chemotherapy- and radiation-therapy-associated interstitial disease is progressive and has a high mortality over the short term, transplant can be considered. Most patients that eventually are assessed for transplantation are survivors of childhood tumors, Hodgkin disease, or other tumors that have a combination of high-dose chemotherapy and radiation therapy (110). Many patients have also had bone marrow transplantation, which makes their treatment unique and somewhat more complex, as graft versus host disease may have contributed to the pulmonary failure. A major concern in transplanting patients with a history of cancer is the possibility of recurrent tumor. The rate of recurrence of tumor in patients with lung transplant who have been more than five years after their treatment has been low with only a few sporadic cases of recurrence noted (111). This contrasts to the relatively high rate of recurrence of cancer in patients transplanted for primary unresectable bronchioloalveolar carcinoma of the lung (112). Although there are legitimate concerns about recurrence after a period of remission, with appropriate patient selection, the results of lung transplantation for lung disease after cancer treatment can approach the success of transplantation for other causes of lung disease.

ETHICAL CONSIDERATIONS

As with any terminal condition, decisions about end-of-life care need to be addressed in patients with metastatic or active primary cancer involving the lungs. In these patients, there is a good chance that their pulmonary disease may actually lead to a terminal event, and ventilatory support is a treatment that needs consideration before initiation. In order to avoid a situation of terminal life support that prolongs a patient's life unnecessarily, discussions about end-of-life issues and withdrawing ventilatory support should be discussed with terminally ill patients and their families prior to an acute event (113). At some point in the care of these patients, treatment goes from being curative to being palliative, and many patients need time to be able to settle their affairs and resolve financial and interpersonal issues (114). A realistic discussion of the actual prognosis and an understanding of the goals of the patient can allow for the design of a rehabilitation program that will allow the patient to achieve their goals and avoid unnecessary or burdensome end-of-life care. Management of pulmonary complications can also include management of pleural effusions, appropriate use of pain control, use of supplemental oxygen, noninvasive ventilatory support, bronchial stents, and use of targeted chemotherapy or radiotherapy.

In cases where end-of-life decisions need to be addressed when a patient is incapacitated, a strong prior relationship with the family helps to ease any discussions of end-of-life care. When the patient's choices and desires are not clear and when the family may have doubt about the right course of treatment, involvement of an ethics committee can be helpful. This is also a situation where advanced directives are especially helpful, as they can avoid unnecessary angst on the part of the patient's family and physicians (115).

In conclusion, the role of the rehabilitation specialist is to help to decrease disability in the patient with pulmonary complications of cancer. It is most important to help these patients achieve their goals, maximizing function, and improving the quality of life, while avoiding complications and minimizing discomfort. The specific rehabilitation approaches for pulmonary rehabilitation follow.

Considerations During Mobilization

When providing physical therapy for the oncology patient, several pulmonary factors should be taken into consideration. As outlined previously, these factors are directly related to the patient's treatment via chemotherapy, radiation, and surgery.

Chemotherapy

Several specific chemotherapeutic agents are responsible for pulmonary complications, including taxanes, busulfan, mytomycin-C, methotrexate, carmustine, bleomycin, and cyclophosphamide, and are described in detail in earlier sections. Depending on the agent, chemotherapy can cause either pneumonitis or fibrosis, both resulting in a restrictive pattern on pulmonary function testing.

The approach to treating chemotherapy-related pulmonary complications with chest physical therapy (CPT) is similar to that utilized with patients who have restrictive lung diseases. Because restrictive diseases are characterized by reduced lung volume with normal airflow and airway resistance, the focus of CPT sessions land largely on deep breathing exercises to assist in increasing or maintaining lung volumes. In addition, because the restrictive quality of lungs affected by chemotherapy is due to changes in the lung parenchyma, patients may present with reduced diffusion capacity, leading to lower resting oxygen saturation and desaturation with lower exercise workloads than typical. Although these patients may appear to require supplemental oxygen, it is important to recall that patients with a history of bleomycin treatment should not be exposed to increased concentrations of inspired oxygen, as this will increase the risk of acute-onset pulmonary edema. In addition to patients receiving chemotherapy, those receiving radiation therapy may be at risk for developing both pneumonitis and pulmonary fibrosis.

Radiation

Many patients receive radiation to the chest wall, including lung and breast cancer patients in addition to patients with hematologic malignancies undergoing total body irradiation. Radiation-induced lung injury continues to be the dose-limiting factor in chest irradiation (115,116). With radiation, as with chemotherapy, both pneumonitis and fibrosis are results of treatment and should be approached as outlined previously.

Surgery

Surgical interventions that directly affect the respiratory system (lung carcinoma resection) can have an impact on lung function and pulmonary health. In the case of pneumonectomies, postural drainage should be accomplished by positioning the patient on the side that has undergone surgery. This position allows the patient's sound lung to continue to expand and function fully in addition to preventing fluid, which typically collects in the postpneumonectomy space, from affecting the remaining healthy lung tissue. Positioning of a patient who has undergone a wedge resection would ideally be the opposite of those postpneumonectomy, lying on the unaffected side. This allows the affected lung to expand and secretions to drain through postural drainage. Both pneumonectomy and wedge resection patients should be instructed in the importance of upper extremity mobility and range of motion on the operative side to ensure continued mobility of the ribcage and thoracic wall.

Those who have undergone esophagectomy as a result of the surgical procedure must maintain a head-of-bed angle greater than 30? to assist in prevention of aspiration pneumonia. This positioning restriction prevents a patient from lying flat or being positioned in Trendelenburg, providing significant challenges regarding expansion and postural drainage for the lower lobes. Sessions with these patients must also include education regarding the importance of proper diaphragmatic breathing techniques to ensure continued expansion at the bases of the lungs.

Pulmonary function may also be compromised by surgeries that include large incisions in the thorax or abdominal areas. Pain from surgery may prevent these patients from engaging in deep breathing and pulmonary toileting activities, allowing secretions to accumulate. For these patients, the focus of CPT sessions is on coughing with splinting to reduce pain and encourage frequent and productive pulmonary toilet, in addition to deep breathing, postural drainage, percussion, and vibration to assist in the mobilization of secretions. Early participation in ambulation after surgery also plays a large role in postoperative pulmonary health (116). All patients who have undergone any thoracic or upper abdominal surgery should be encouraged to ambulate often and for significant distance. Thoracic surgery patients at the Memorial Sloan-Kettering Cancer Center (MSKCC) are encouraged to walk at least one mile per day within one to two days of surgery, depending on the intensity of the surgical procedure the patient endured and prior functional status. This focus on early mobilization has proven to decrease both incidence of pulmonary complications and length of hospital stay at MSKCC.

Oncology patients, who often become immunocompromised following their cancer therapies, are at risk for pneumonia and a variety of other pulmonary infections. Pneumonias must be treated with antibiotics and aggressive chest physical therapy consisting of postural drainage, percussion, and vibration targeting the site of pneumonia, in addition to deep breathing exercise and consistent participation in ambulation and out-of-bed mobility.

Cancer-Related CPT Precautions

Patients with increased pulmonary secretions will benefit from percussion and vibration. Care should be taken to avoid percussing directly over mediports or surgical incisions and drains; areas of bony metastases or active tumor also should be avoided. These patients can be effectively treated with a combination of gentle vibration, postural drainage, and deep breathing exercises.

References

1. ACS, Cancer Facts and Figures 2006. 2006.
2. Lee YT. Breast carcinoma: pattern of metastasis at autopsy. *J Surg Oncol.* 1983;23:175–180.
3. Kindler HL, Shulman KL. Metastatic colorectal cancer. *Curr Treat Options Oncol.* 2001;2:459–471.
4. Wang P, DeNunzio A, Okunieff P, O'Dell WG. Lung metastases detection in CT images using 3D template matching. *Med Phys.* 2007;34(3):915–922.
5. Dines DE, Cortese DA, Brennan MD, et al. Malignant pulmonary neoplasms predisposing to spontaneous pneumothorax. *May Clin Proc.* 1973;48:541–544.
6. Hirakata K, Nakata H, Nakagawa T. CT of pulmonary metastases with pathological correlation. *Semin Ultrasound CT MR.* 1995;16:379–394.
7. Libshitz HI, North LB. Pulmonary metastases. *Radiol Clin North Am.* 1982;20:437–451.
8. Seo JB, Im J, Goo JM, et al. Atypical pulmonary metastases: spectrum of radiologic findings. *Radiographics.* 2001;21:403–417.
9. Davis SD. CT evaluation for pulmonary metastases in patients with extrathoracic malignancy. *Radiology.* 1991;180:1–12.
10. Fraser R, Muller NL, Colman N, et al. *Diagnosis of Diseases of the Chest.* Philadelphia: WB Saunders; 1999:1381–1412.
11. Janower ML, Blennerhassett JB. Lymphangitic spread of metastatic cancer to the lung. A radiologic-pathologic classification. *Radiology.* 1971;101:267–273.
12. Acikgoz G, Kim SM, Houseni M, Cermik TF, Intenzo CM, Alavi A. Pulmonary lymphangitic carcinomatosis (PLC): spectrum of FDG-PET findings. *Clin Nucl Med.* 2006;31(11):673–678.
13. Avdalovic M. Thoracic manifestations of common nonpulmonary malignancies of women. *Clin Chest Med.* 2004;25:379–390.
14. Pastorino U, Buyse M, Friedel G, et al. Long term results of lung metastasectomy: prognostic analyses based on 5206 cases. *J Thorac Cardiovasc Surg.* 1997;113:37–49.
15. Abecasis N, Cortez F, Bettencourt A, Costa CS, Orvalho F, Mendes De Almeida JM. Surgical treatment of lung metastases: prognostic factors for long-term survival. *J Surg Oncol.* 1999;72:193–198.
16. Jungraithmayr W, Hasse J, Stoelben, E. Completion pneumonectomy for lung metastases. *Eur J Surg Oncol.* December 2004;30(10):1113–1117.
17. Vogl TJ, Wetter A, Lindemayr S, Zangos S. Treatment of unresectable lung metastases with transpulmonary chemoembolization: preliminary experience. *Radiology.* March 2005;234(3):917–922.
18. Marel M, Zrustova M, Stasny B, et al. The incidence of pleural effusion in a well-defined region: epidemiological study in central Bohemia. *Chest.* 1993;104:1486–1489.
19. Dibonito L, Falconieri G, Colautti I, et al. The positive pleural effusion. A retrospective study of cytopathological diagnosis with autopsy confirmation. *Acta Cytol.* 1992;36:329–332.
20. Atunes G, Neville E, Duffy J, et al. BTS guidelines for the management of malignant pleural effusions. *Thorax.* 2003;58:ii29.
21. American Thoracic Society. Management of malignant pleural effusions. *Am J Respir Crit Care Med.* 2000;162:1987–2001.
22. Maskell NA, Lee YCG, Gleeson FV, et al. Randomized trials describing lung inflammation after pleurodesis with talc of varying particle size. *Am J Respir Crit Care Med.* 2004;170:377–382.
23. Bennett R. Maskell N. Management of malignant pleural effusions. *Curr Opin Pulm Med.* 2005;11(4):296–300.
24. Ohm C, Park D, Vogen M, et al. Use of an indwelling pleural catheter compared with thoracoscopy talc pleurodesis in the management of malignant pleural effusions. *Am Surg.* 2003;69:198–202.
25. Sugarbaker DJ, Jaklitsch MT, Bueno R. Prevention, early detection, and management of complications after 328 consecutive

extrapleural pneumonectomies. *J Thorac Cardiovasc Surg.* 2004;128:138–146.

26. Kado DM, Browner WS, Palermo L, Nevitt MC, Genant HK, Cummings SR. Vertebral fractures and mortality in older women: a prospective study. Study of Osteoporotic Fractures Research Group. *Arch Intern Med.* 1999;159(11):1215–1220.

27. Haddy TB, Mosher RB, Reaman GH. Osteoporosis in survivors of acute lymphoblastic leukemia. *Oncologist.* 2001;6(3):278–285.

28. Schwartz AM, Leonidas JC. Methotrexate osteopathy. *Skeletal Radiol.* 1984;11:13–16.

29. Scheven BAA, van der Veen MJ, Damen CA, et al. Effects of methotrexate on human osteoblasts in vitro: modulation by 1,25-dihydroxyvitamin D3. *J Bone Miner Res.* 1995;10:874–880.

30. Krall EA, Dawson-Hughes B. Smoking increases bone loss and decreases intestinal calcium absorption. *J Bone Miner Res.* 1999;14:215–220.

31. Teegarden D, Lyle RM, Proulx WR, et al. Previous milk consumption is associated with greater bone density in young women. *Am J Clin Nutr.* 1999;69:1014–1017.

32. Fisher JE, Rogers MJ, Halasy JM, et al. Alendronate mechanism of action: geranylgeraniol, an intermediate in the mevalonate pathway, prevents inhibition of osteoclast formation, bone resorption, and kinase activation in vitro. *Proc Natl Acad Sci USA.* 1999;96:133–138.

33. Hochberg MC, Ross PD, Black D, et al. Larger increases in bone mineral density during alendronate therapy are associated with a lower risk of new vertebral fractures in women with post-menopausal osteoporosis. *Arthritis Rheum.* 1999;42:1246–1254.

34. Masi L, Bilezikian JP. Osteoporosis: new hope for the future. *Int J Fertil.* 1997;42:245–254.

35. Paulino AC, Wen BC, Brown CK, et al. Late effects in children treated with radiation therapy for Wilms' tumor. *Int J Radiat Oncol Biol Phys.* 2000;46(5):1239–1246.

36. Evans AE, Norkool P, Evans I, et al. Late effects of treatment for Wilms' tumor: a report from the National Wilms' Tumor Study Group. *Cancer.* 1991;67:331–336.

37. Riseborough EJ, Grabias SL, Burton RI, et al. Skeletal alterations following irradiation for Wilms' tumor. *J Bone Joint Surg.* 1976;58:526–536.

38. Makipernaa A, Heikkila JT, Merikanto J, Marttinen E, Siimes MA. Spinal deformity induced by radiotherapy for solid tumours in childhood: a long-term follow up study. *Eur J Pediatr.* March 1993;152(3):197–200.

39. Mareska M, Gutmann L. Lambert-Eaton myasthenic syndrome. *Semin Neurol.* June 2004;24(2):149–153.

40. O'Neill J, Murray N, Newsom-Davis J. The Lambert-Eaton myasthenic syndrome. *Brain.* 1988;111:577–596.

41. Wirtz P, Sotodeh M, Nijnuis M, et al. Difference in distribution of muscle weakness between myasthenia gravis and the Lambert Eaton myasthenic syndrome. *J Neurol Neurosurg Psychiatry.* 2002;73:766–768.

42. Wirtz PW, Wintzen AR, Verschuuren JJ. Lambert-Eaton myasthenic syndrome has a more progressive course in patients with lung cancer. *Muscle Nerve.* 2005;32(2):226–229.

43. Keesey J. Electrodiagnostic approach to defects of neuromuscular transmission. *Muscle Nerve.* 1989;12:613–626.

44. Maddison P, Newsom-Davis J. Treatment for Lambert-Eaton myasthenic syndrome. *Cochrane Database Syst Rev.* 2005;(2):CD003279 (online).

45. Willaert W, Kessler R, Deneffe G. Surgical options for complete resectable lung cancer invading the phrenic nerve. *Acta Chir Belg.* 2004;104(4):451–453.

46. Tanaka T, Kitamura H, Kunishima Y, et al. Modified and bilateral retroperitoneal lymph node dissection for testicular cancer: peri- and postoperative complications and therapeutic outcome. *Jpn J Clin Oncol.* June 2006;36(6):381–386.

47. de Jong AA, Manni JJ. Phrenic nerve paralysis following neck dissection. *Eur Arch Otorhinolaryngol.* 1991;248(3):132–134.

48. Munzone E, Nole F, Orlando L, et al. Unexpected right phrenic nerve injury during 5-fluorouracil continuous infusion plus cis-

platin and vinorelbine in breast cancer patients. *J Natl Cancer Inst.* 2000;92(9):755.

49. Twelves CJ, Chaudary MA, Reidy J, Richards MA, Rubens RD. Toxicity of intra-arterial doxorubicin in locally advanced breast cancer. *Cancer Chemother Pharmacol.* 1990;25(6):459–462.

50. Alkofer B, Le Roux Y, Coffin O, Samama G. Thoracoscopic plication of the diaphragm for postoperative phrenic paralysis: a report of two cases. *Surg Endosc.* May 2004;18(5):868–870.

51. Takiguchi Y, Watanabe R, Nagao K, Kuriama T. Hiccups as an adverse reaction to cancer chemotherapy. *J Natl Cancer Inst.* 2002;94:772.

52. Calvo E, Fernandez-La Torre F, Brugarolas A. Cervical phrenic nerve block for intractable hiccups in cancer patients. *J Natl Cancer Inst.* 2002;94(15):1175–1176.

53. Khaw PY, Ball DL. Relief of non-metastatic shoulder pain with mediastinal radiotherapy in patients with lung cancer. *Lung Cancer.* 2000;28(1):51–54.

54. Gross NJ. The pathogenesis of radiation induced-lung injury. *Lung.* 1981;159:115–125.

55. Kharbanda S, Ren R, Pandey P, et al. Activation of c-abl tyrosine kinase in the stress response to DNA-damaging stress agents. *Nature.* 1995;376:785–788.

56. Abid SH, Malhotra V, Perry MC. Radiation-induced and chemotherapy-induced pulmonary injury. *Curr Opin Oncol.* 2001;13(4):242–248.

57. Garipagaoglu M, Munley MT, Hollis D, et al. The effect of patient specific factors on radiation induced regional lung injury. *Int J Radiat Oncol Biol Phys.* 1999;45:3331–3338.

58. Roach M 3rd, Gandara DR, Yuo HS, et al. Radiation pneumonitis following combined modality therapy for lung cancer: analysis of prognostic factors. *J Clin Oncol.* 1995;13:2606–2612.

59. Huang EY, Wang CJ, Chen HC, et al. Multivariate analysis of pulmonary fibrosis after electron beam irradiation for post-mastectomy chest wall and regional lymphatics: evidence for non-dosimetric factors. *Radiother Oncol.* 2000;57:91–96.

60. Mehta V. Radiation pneumonitis and pulmonary fibrosis in non-small-cell lung cancer: pulmonary function, prediction, and prevention. *Int J Radiat Oncol Biol Phys.* 2005;63(1):5–24.

61. Magana E, Crowell RE. Radiation pneumonitis successfully treated with inhaled corticosteroids. *South Med J.* 2003;96:521–524.

62. Wang JY, Chen KY, Wang JT, et al. Outcome and prognostic factors for patients with non–small-cell lung cancer and severe radiation pneumonitis. *Int J Radiat Oncol Biol Phys.* 2002;54:735–741.

63. Inoue A, Kunitoh H, Sekine I, et al. Radiation pneumonitis in lung cancer patients: a retrospective study of risk factors and the long-term prognosis. *Int J Radiat Oncol Biol Phys.* 2001;49:649–655.

64. De Jaeger K, Seppenwoolde Y, Boersma LJ, et al. Pulmonary function following high-dose radiotherapy of non-small-cell lung cancer. *Int J Radiat Oncol Biol Phys.* 2003;55:1331–1340.

65. Gopal R, Starkschall G, Tucker SL, et al. Effects of radiotherapy and chemotherapy on lung function in patients with non–small-cell lung cancer. *Int J Radiat Oncol Biol Phys.* 2003;56:114–120.

66. Gopal R, Tucker SL, Komaki R, et al. The relationship between local dose and loss of function for irradiated lung. *Int J Radiat Oncol Biol Phys.* 2003;56:106–113.

67. Chen Y, Williams J, Ding I, et al. Radiation pneumonitis and early circulatory cytokine markers. *Semin Radiat Oncol.* 2002;12:26–33.

68. Chen Y, Rubin P, Williams J, et al. Circulating IL-6 as a predictor of radiation pneumonitis. *Int J Radiat Oncol Biol Phys.* 2001;49:641–648.

69. Bentzen SM, Saunders MI, Dische S. From CHART to CHARTWEL in non-small cell lung cancer: clinical radiobiological modeling of the expected change in outcome. *Clin Oncol (R Coll Radiol).* 2002;14:372–381.

70. Narayan S, Henning GT, Ten Haken RK, et al. Results following treatment to doses of 92.4 or 102.9 Gy on a phase I dose

escalation study for non–small cell lung cancer. *Lung Cancer.* 2004;44:79–88.

71. Dirkx ML, Heijmen BJ. Beam intensity modulation for penumbra enhancement and field length reduction in lung cancer treatments: a dosimetric study. *Radiother Oncol.* 2000;56:181–188.

72. Wu KL, Jiang GL, Liao Y, et al. Three-dimensional conformal radiation therapy for non–small-cell lung cancer: a phase I/II dose escalation clinical trial. *Int J Radiat Oncol Biol Phys.* 2003;57:1336–1344.

73. Lee SW, Choi EK, Park HJ, et al. Stereotactic body frame based fractionated radiosurgery on consecutive days for primary or metastatic tumors in the lung. *Lung Cancer.* 2003;40:309–315.

74. Bonnet RB, Bush D, Cheek GA, et al. Effects of proton and combined proton/photon beam radiation on pulmonary function in patients with resectable but medically inoperable non-small cell lung cancer. *Chest.* 2001;120:1803–1810.

75. Kwok E, Chan CK. Corticosteroids and azathioprine do not prevent radiation-induced lung injury. *Can Respir J.* 1998;5:211–214.

76. Komaki R, Lee JS, Milas L, et al. Effects of amifostine on acute toxicity from concurrent chemotherapy and radiotherapy for inoperable non–small-cell lung cancer: report of a randomized comparative trial. *Int J Radiat Oncol Biol Phys.* 2004;58:1369–1377.

77. Wang LW, Fu XL, Clough R, et al. Can angiotensin-converting enzyme inhibitors protect against symptomatic radiation pneumonitis? *Radiat Res.* 2000;153:405–410.

78. Ozturk B, Egehan I, Atavci S, et al. Pentoxifylline in prevention of radiation-induced lung toxicity in patients with breast and lung cancer: a double-blind randomized trial. *Int J Radiat Oncol Biol Phys.* 2004;58:213–219.

79. Vijayalaxmi, Reiter RJ, Tan DX, et al. Melatonin as a radioprotective agent: a review. *Int J Radiat Oncol Biol Phys.* 2004;59:639–653.

80. Tomlinson J, Tighe M, Johnson S, et al. Interstitial pneumonitis following mitoxantrone, chlorambucil and prednisolone (MCP) chemotherapy. *Clin Oncol (R Coll Radiol).* 1999;11:184–186.

81. Wesselius L. Pulmonary complications of cancer therapy. *Compr Ther.* 1999;25:272–277.

82. Camus P, Kudoh S, Ebina M. Interstitial lung disease associated with drug therapy. *Br J Cancer.* 2004;91(Suppl 2):S18–S23.

83. Gagnadoux F, Roiron C, Carrie E, Monnier-Cholley L, Lebeau B. Eosinophilic lung disease under chemotherapy with oxaliplatin for colorectal cancer. *Am J Clin Oncol.* 2002;25(4):388–390.

84. Kirkbride P, Hatton M, Lorigan P, Joyce P, Fisher P. Fatal pulmonary fibrosis associated with induction chemotherapy with carboplatin and vinorelbine followed by CHART radiotherapy for locally advanced non-small cell lung cancer. *Clin Oncol (R Coll Radiol).* 2002;14(5):361–366.

85. Koc M, Polat P, Suma S. Effects of tamoxifen on pulmonary fibrosis after cobalt-60 radiotherapy in breast cancer patients. *Radiother Oncol.* 2002;64(2):171–175.

86. Hay J, Shahzeidi S, Laurent G. Mechanisms of bleomycin-induced lung damage. *Arch Toxicol.* 1991;65(2):81–94.

87. Rossi SE, Erasmus JJ, McAdams HP, et al. Pulmonary drug toxicity: radiologic and pathologic manifestations. *Radiographics.* 2000;20:1245–1259.

88. Cooper Jr JA, White DA, Matthay RA. Drug-induced pulmonary disease. 1: cytotoxic drugs. *Am Rev Respir Dis.* 1986;133:321–340.

89. Danson S, Blackhall F, Hulse P, Ranson M. Interstitial lung disease in lung cancer: separating disease progression from treatment effects. *Drug Safety.* 2005;28(2):103–113.

90. Roychowdhury DF, Cassidy CA, Peterson P, et al. A report on serious pulmonary toxicity associated with gemcitabine-based therapy. *Invest New Drugs.* 2002;20:311–315.

91. Bartels MN. Pulmonary rehabilitation. In: Grant Cooper, ed. *Essential Physical Medicine and Rehabilitation.* Totowa, NJ: Humana Press; 2006:147–174.

92. Alba AS, Kim H, Whiteson JH, Bartels MN. Cardiopulmonary rehabilitation and cancer rehabilitation. 2. Pulmonary rehabilitation review. *Arch Phy Med Rehabil.* 2006;87 (3 Suppl):57–64.

93. Bartels MN. The role of pulmonary rehabilitation for patients undergoing lung volume reduction surgery. Minerva Pneumologica. Invited Review. Special issue distributed at the Congress of the Italian Society of Respiratory Medicine (Florence, October 4–7). *Minerva Pneumol.* 2006;45:177–196.

94. Heit JA, O'Fallon WM, Petterson TM, et al. Relative impact of risk factors for deep vein thrombosis and pulmonary embolism: a population-based study. *Arch Intern Med.* 2002;162:1245–1248.

95. Levitan N, Dowlati A, Remick SC, et al. Rates of initial and recurrent thromboembolic disease among patients with malignancy versus those without malignancy. *Medicine (Baltimore)* 1999;78:285–291.

96. Heit JA, Silverstein MD, Mohr DN, Petterson TM, O'Fallon WM, Melton LJ III. Risk factors for deep vein thrombosis and pulmonary embolism: a population-based case-control study. *Arch Intern Med.* 2000;160:809–815.

97. Heit JA. The epidemiology of venous thromboembolism in the community: implications for prevention and management. *J Thromb Thrombolysis.* 2006;21(1):23–29.

98. Segal JB, Streiff MB, Hoffman LV, Thornton K, Bass EB. Management of venous thromboembolism: a systematic review for a practice guideline. *Ann Intern Med.* 2007;146(3): 211–222.

99. Goldhaber SZ. Pulmonary embolism. *N Engl J Med.* 1998;339:93–104.

100. Aklog L, Williams CS, Byrne JG, Goldhaber SZ. Acute pulmonary embolectomy: a contemporary approach. *Circulation.* 2002;105:1416–1419.

101. Sadeghi A, Brevetti GR, Kim S, et al. Acute massive pulmonary embolism: role of the cardiac surgeon. *Texas Heart Inst J.* 2005;32(3):430–433.

102. Abbondanzo SL, Klappenbach RS, Tsou E. Tumor cell embolism to pulmonary alveolar capillaries: cause of sudden cor pulmonale. *Arch Pathol Lab Med.* 1986;110:1197–1198.

103. Kane RD, Hawkins HK, Miller JA, et al. Microscopic pulmonary tumor emboli associated with dyspnea. *Cancer.* 1975;36:1473–1482.

104. Jakel J, Ramaswamy A, Kohler U, Barth PJ. Massive pulmonary tumor microembolism from a hepatocellular carcinoma. *Pathol Res Pract.* 2006;202(5):395–399.

105. Shepard JA, Moore EH, Templeton PA, McLoud TC. Pulmonary intravascular tumor emboli: dilated and beaded peripheral pulmonary arteries at CT. *Radiology.* 1993;187(3):797–801.

106. Winterbauer RH, Elfenbein IB, Ball WC. Incidence and clinical significance of tumor embolization to the lungs. *Am J Med.* 1968;45:271–290.

107. Geschwind JF, Dagli MS, Vogel-Claussen J, Seifter E, Huncharek MS, Metastatic breast carcinoma presenting as a large pulmonary embolus: case report and review of the literature. *Am J Clin Oncol.* 2003;26(1):89–91.

108. Bartels MN. The role of pulmonary rehabilitation for patients undergoing lung volume reduction surgery. Minerva Pneumologica. Invited Review. Special issue distributed at the Congress of the Italian Society of Respiratory Medicine (Florence, October 4–7). *Minerva Pneumol.* 2006;45:177–196.

109. Bartels MN. Pulmonary rehabilitation. In: Grant Cooper, ed. *Essential Physical Medicine and Rehabilitation.* Totowa, NJ: Humana Press; 2006:147–174.

110. Pechet TV, de le Morena M, Mendeloff EN, Sweet SC, Shapiro SD, Huddleston CB. Lung transplantation in children following treatment for malignancy. *J Heart Lung Transplant.* 2003;22(2):154–160.

111. Kapoor S, Kurland G, Jakacki R. Recurrent medulloblastoma following pediatric double-lung transplant. *J Heart Lung Transplant.* 2000;19:1011–1013.

112. Garver RI, Zorn GL, Wu X, et al. Recurrence of bronchioloalveolar carcinoma in transplanted lungs. *N Engl J Med.* 1999;340:1071–1074.

113. Griffin JP, Nelson JE, Koch KA, et al. American College of Chest Physicians. End-of-life care in patients with lung cancer. *Chest.* January 2003;123(1 Suppl):312S–331S.

114. Steinhauser KE, Christakis NA, Clipp EC, et al. Factors considered important at the end of life by patients, family, physicians, and other care providers. *JAMA.* 2000;284:2476–2482.

115. Carruthers SA, Wallington MM. Total body irradiation and pneumonitis risk: a review of outcomes. *Br J Cancer.* 2004;90:2080.

116. Kim TH, Cho KH, Pyo RH, et al. Dose-volumetric parameters for predicting severe radiation pneumonitis after three-dimensional conformational radiation therapy for lung cancer. *Radiology.* 2005;235:308.

117. Reilly JJ Jr. Preoperative and postoperative care of standard and high risk surgical patients. *Hematol Oncol Clin North Am.* 1997;11:449.

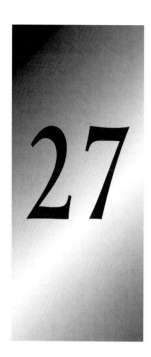

Cardiac Complications of Cancer

Matthew N. Bartels
Marsha Leight

Although the primary focus of this text is on the rehabilitation of patients with primary oncologic disease, the incidence of cardiac disease will still be high in this population and will account for a large percentage of the morbidity and mortality. This is especially true in many of the common oncologic diseases, as they often share in common advanced age, smoking, obesity, and other cardiac risk factors. The treatment of the primary oncologic disease can also cause cardiac comorbidity, and this must be kept in mind as a rehabilitation program is being created. The most common diseases will remain most common, and coronary artery disease is the most common coexisting condition that will be seen. The increased metabolic demands of surgery, chemotherapy, radiation therapy, and the underlying tumor will place an increased demand on cardiac function and can precipitate a myocardial infarction or angina. In patients with a decreased ejection fraction and CHF, these increased demands can precipitate frank heart failure, outside of any increase in myocardial injury from the treatments or the primary tumor (1–3).

With the contribution of preexisting or underlying cardiac disease kept in mind, this chapter will focus primarily on the *additional* cardiac morbidity from cancer and its treatments. The combination of advanced therapies allows more patients than ever to have extensive oncological treatments, and these are placing more individuals than ever at risk of cardiac complications. Awareness of toxicities has increased, and it is less common to see overt heart failure from

chemotherapy or radiation therapy. Still, there are many other comorbidities to explore and account for in the rehabilitation of patients with primary oncologic conditions.

CORONARY ARTERY DISEASE

Primary CAD is present in a large proportion of the population and is also present in individuals with cancer. Before most intensive surgical treatments, patients will have been screened for CAD. Any CAD, if known to be present, will have been treated in the usual fashion. It is a reasonable approach to aggressively treat with bypass surgery, coronary artery stenting, and medications, including cholesterol-lowering agents, beta blockers, and exercise. The stress of treatments (including surgery), fluid shifts with chemotherapy, and the emotional stress of the diagnosis can precipitate cardiac events. In the care of patients with cancer, all cardiac symptoms should be aggressively managed as long as the prognosis warrants intervention.

As a complication of cancer treatment, coronary artery disease may manifest in several ways. The patient with breast cancer is often taken off of hormones or started on agents that inhibit the effects of estrogen. Patients with endometrial or ovarian cancer are placed in premature menopause, thereby accelerating CAD. The precaution of managing risk factors is essential in these populations, including smoking cessation, weight

KEY POINTS

- The incidence of cardiac disease with cancer is high since the two conditions share many common risk factors, such as advanced age, smoking, and obesity.
- The increased metabolic demands of surgery, chemotherapy, radiation therapy, and the underlying tumor will place an increased demand on cardiac function, which can precipitate a myocardial infarction or angina.
- Before cancer surgery, it is reasonable to aggressively treat coronary artery disease (CAD) with bypass surgery, coronary artery stenting, and medications, including cholesterol-lowering agents, beta blockers, and exercise, as indicated.
- The mechanism of increase in CAD following radiation is thought to be via microcirculatory damage, which leads to accelerated atherosclerosis, among other cardiac issues.
- Clinicians should have an increased suspicion of CAD in any patient with a history of either radiation or chemotherapy who is undergoing a rehabilitation program where increased cardiac work will be anticipated.
- Cardiac transplant is usually not considered until the individual has been more than five years disease-free from their original tumor, as transplant immunosuppression would accelerate the development of metastatic disease.
- Cardiomyopathy in the setting of oncologic disease is usually associated with chemotherapy and is most often seen after treatment with doxorubicin or other anthracycline agents.
- Treatment of congestive heart failure (CHF) in chemotherapy-induced cardiomyopathy is the same as for other forms of cardiomyopathy: afterload reductions, volume reduction, low-dose beta blockers, and inotropic agents, as needed.
- Some of the medications and treatment regimens require high fluid loads and may tip a borderline patient into cardiac failure.
- The major issue with cardiac rehabilitation in the cancer patient is access. Practitioners must think to refer them for cardiac rehabilitation.

management, stress management, lipid lowering, and exercise (4,5).

Another major contributor to the development of coronary artery disease after cancer is the use of radiation therapy. In diseases where the heart may be in the field of irradiation, there is a great potential for cardiac injury and for accelerated CAD. The majority of experience regarding cardiac disease and radiation comes from breast cancer survivors. In the earlier days of radiation therapy, doses were often much higher, with less focused fields, and recent experience may be showing a decrease in the incidence of CAD due to radiation (6–8). Due to this, newer radiation techniques have decreased the cardiac exposure and likely also the incidence of CAD by using focused and oblique beams, with lower overall doses of radiation (9,10). The mechanism of the increase in CAD is thought to be via microcirculatory damage from the radiation, which leads to accelerated atherosclerosis, among other cardiac issues (11,12). There also can be the induction of clotting with subsequent fibrin deposition and then later development of endothelial proliferation. These changes are often seen in association with myocardial fibrosis and other changes that decrease cardiac efficiency (13). Despite improved radiation techniques, CAD is still a complication seen in a fair number of long-term breast

cancer survivors, and is most often seen in left-sided breast cancer survivors. There is an increase in CAD-associated mortality of 2% for left-sided breast cancer survivors, compared to a 1% increase for right-sided cancer survivors (14). Still, overall admissions for coronary artery disease are not statistically different for right-sided (9.7%) versus left-sided (9.9%) mastectomy with RT (adjusted hazard ratio of 1.05 [95% CI, 0.94–1.16]) in a survey of the Medicare database done over 1986–1993 (15). However, there is a higher rate of cardiac deaths in left-sided mastectomy patients, especially in long-term survivors (cumulative risk 6.4% [95% CI, 3.5%–11.5%] for left-sided, compared with 3.6% [95% CI, 1.8%–7.2%] for right-sided patients at 20 years) (10).

Another aspect of ischemic disease associated with cancer is the possibility of direct effects of chemotherapeutic agents. Although most agents are not clearly associated with coronary insufficiency or myocardial infarction, there have been reports of 5-fluorouracil causing acute cardiac events. The mechanism is not clear and it is a rare event, but the possibilities include acute coronary vasospasm (16,17). Cisplatinum has also had isolated reports of vascular events, including coronary artery spasm (18,19). There are also sporadic case and small series reports that indicate other agents may be associated with coronary artery disease in cancer patients, including paclitaxel in African American populations (20). The investigations into these possible interactions continue, but should be kept in consideration when a patient is still on active treatment with chemotherapy and receiving rehabilitation services.

The increased rate of cardiac death associated with coronary artery disease is also seen in patients with other diagnoses, including among younger patients in the pediatric and adolescent populations. There is an excess mortality from all causes in this younger age group, but nononcologic causes of death are led by cardiac disease, which is usually rare in teens and young adults. Among cardiac causes of disease, myocardial infarction is the greatest cause of death seen in the young cancer survivors (21–24). The other causes of cardiac mortality in this younger group of patients are cardiomyopathy from chemotherapy with anthracycline and/or bleomycin, and constrictive cardiac disease from mantle irradiation (21,25). Because myocardial infarction is the greatest cardiac cause of death in late (15-or-more-year survivors) pediatric and adolescent cancer patients, it is essential to attend to heart-healthy lifestyle modification (avoidance of smoking, low fat intake, reasonable exercise) since these interventions may help to decrease the possibility of later cardiac mortality.

Men with testicular cancer also have an excess rate of cardiac-related morbidity and mortality. There is an association of survival with testicular cancer and the development of hypertension, obesity, hypercholesterolemia, and vascular abnormalities such as Raynaud disease. This can be associated with an increase of myocardial infarction and coronary disease associated with the abnormal cardiac risk profile. One study showed an increase in odds ratio of 7.1 with 33% of individual patients having abnormal left ventricular function on echocardiogram (26). These findings and isolated reports in other types of cancer should increase the suspicion of CAD in any patient with a history of either radiation or chemotherapy who is undergoing a rehabilitation program where increased cardiac work will be anticipated.

CONSTRICTIVE CARDIAC DISEASE

Much more commonly recognized as a direct consequence of treatment with chemotherapy and radiation therapy is the possibility of constrictive cardiac disease. The etiologies of cardiac dysfunction come from a constrictive pericarditis, a pericardial effusion, or from myocardial injury with direct scarring. The causes of the injury to the myocardial tissue include direct

effects of radiation, the effects of chemotherapy, or from complications such as infection following immunosuppression or hematologic abnormalities that may lead to a pericardial effusion and complications. The full spectrum of disease that may cause a constrictive pericardial presentation is beyond the scope of this chapter, but a few of the more commonly seen conditions are discussed.

Although radiation-induced cardiac injury is less common now that the radiation protocols have been modified, it is still regularly seen. The most common situation for cardiac injury from radiation is after mantle irradiation for hematologic malignancies, especially Hodgkin's lymphoma, which now has a better survival and cardiac disease can manifest itself. Radiation injury to the heart is also often seen in breast cancer, especially after treatment of left-sided tumors. Constrictive cardiomyopathy was far less common than CAD or cardiomyopathy associated with combined chemotherapy and radiation. The pathophysiology of the constrictive cardiac injury is usually due to fibrosis of the pericardium or of the myocardium as a result of direct injury to the tissues, with the subsequent formation of scar tissue (6–11). Treatment for the constrictive pericarditis can include pericardial stripping and, for effusions, can include a window and correction of the underlying hematologic or infectious causes of the effusion. For constrictive cardiomyopathy, consideration may need to be given to heart transplantation. However, transplant is usually not considered until the individual has been more than five years disease-free from their original tumor, as transplant immunosuppression would accelerate the development of metastatic disease.

CARDIOMYOPATHY

Cardiomyopathy in the setting of oncologic disease is usually associated with chemotherapy and is most often seen after treatment with doxorubicin or other anthracycline agents. Most cases of toxicity are dose-related, with higher doses being associated with a higher likelihood of toxicity. Of interest, female patients, especially among pediatric and adolescent survivors, are more likely to develop cardiomyopathy (21–25). The mechanism of anthracycline-associated cardiotoxicity seems to be associated with the development of free radicals and associated mitochondrial enzymatic and nonenzymatic pathways (27,28). Free radicals damage the cell membranes, and cardiac cells are especially vulnerable due to their high levels of oxidation and poor antioxidant resistance. Finally, the anthracycline chemotherapeutic medications have a high affinity for cardiolipin, causing accumulation inside myocytes

(29). The most common histopathological features of anthracycline cardiomyopathies include loss of myofibrils and cytoplasmic vacuolization (30).

Cardiotoxicity due to anthracyclines presents in one of several ways. There is an acute toxicity that presents immediately after infusion and is present in less than 1% of patients. Stopping the infusion usually results in a return to normal cardiac function. However, a small number of patients have a permanent loss of cardiac function. The occurrence is related to the total lifetime dose of anthracycline agents (31). The next form of cardiomyopathy is seen as early-onset chronic progressive cardiomyopathy. This type of cardiac dysfunction appears in 1%–6% of treated individuals, and is associated with the total cumulative dose of the medication. Cumulative doses of greater than 550 mg/m^2 of doxorubicin, or 900 mg/m^2 of epirubicin are associated with up to a five times greater risk of cardiotoxicity (31). A combination of other agents, for example, trastuzumab, is associated with an increase in risk for individuals treated with anthracyclines (32). Late-onset toxicity starts more than a year after the completion of treatment with the agent, and is relatively common. Up to 65% of childhood survivors of cancer treated with anthracyclines have cardiac abnormalities (33). Unfortunately, no dose of anthracycline chemotherapy is guaranteed to be safe to prevent cardiac toxicity. This is especially true for late-onset toxicity, which can develop years later with even low doses. Once the cardiac toxicity starts, there is usually a progressive decline in cardiac function over time.

The best protection from anthracycline-induced cardiotoxicity is to try to help the natural defense of the body against oxidative damage. The use of antioxidants can help improve anthracycline tolerance. Table 27.1 outlines agents that are used to reduce anthracycline toxicity.

Other cardioprotective agents that are being explored in animal-based studies include Probucol, amifostine, carvedilol, vitamin A, vitamin C, selenium, and glutathione. The key to using a cardioprotective agent is that it does not interfere with the antitumor activity of the anthracycline medication. Active research continues in the evaluation of the effectiveness of these experimental agents, and new cardioprotective regimens will undoubtedly be developed.

Minimizing total dose is still the most important preventative measure, altering the dosing schedules, using agents that are anthracycline analogs, using dietary supplements, and adding cardioprotective agents to the regimen. It is felt that slower infusion may be safer and that the anthracycline analogs may have lower toxicity than doxorubicin. Some of the agents available include epirubicin, idarubicin, and mitoxantrone.

Once it is present, anthracycline-induced cardiomyopathy has a poor prognosis. Both asymptomatic and symptomatic cardiac dysfunction have poor outcomes. In asymptomatic individuals with incidentally discovered dilated cardiomyopathy, there is a 50%, seven-year mortality from cardiac disease (34). Patients with doxorubicin-induced heart failure have a one- and two-year mortality rate of 40% and 60%, respectively (35). Treatment of CHF in chemotherapy-induced cardiomyopathy is the same as for other forms: Afterload reduction with angiotensin-converting enzyme (ACE) inhibitors, volume reduction with diuretics, and the use of low-dose beta blocker and inotropic agents as needed. In long-term (>5 year) disease-free cancer survivors, cardiac transplantation may also be a possible therapeutic option for selected patients. In addition to these traditional medical treatments, lifestyle modification, weight control, and appropriate aerobic exercise, as found in a monitored cardiac rehabilitation program, are all beneficial (31).

Screening patients suspected of having cardiomyopathy or coronary artery disease from their cancer treatments should be done if a vigorous therapy program is anticipated. This is particularly true of individuals with high left chest radiation exposures, high anthracycline doses, or a combination of the two modalities. The screening can include an echocardiogram for

TABLE 27.1
Medical Treatments with Human Data to Decrease Anthracycline Toxicity

MEDICATION	ACTION	MECHANISM OF ACTION	RESEARCH-BASED DATA
Coenzyme Q-10	Dietary supplement	Antioxidant	Human
Carnitine	Dietary supplement	Antioxidant	Human
Vitamin E	Nutrient	Antioxidant	Human
N-acetylcysteine	Mucolytic agent	Increases antioxidant synthesis	Human
Dexrazoxane	Chelating agent	Prevents free radical formation	Human

Source: From Ref. 31.

possible cardiomyopathy to assess left and right ventricular function and rule out pericardial effusions, while Doppler echocardiography can help to assess valvular function. Radionuclide ventriculography can also be used to assess the left ventricular function. Exercise stress tests in patients who can perform them will help to assess for ischemia. In individuals unable to perform standard exercise tests, a pharmacological stress test with imaging can help to assess for cardiac disease. Cardiac catheterization can help to assess coronary disease and also be part of a heart failure assessment in patients with left ventricular failure. A baseline cardiogram is useful to assess for conduction abnormalities, and a lipid profile can help with secondary prevention and lipid management.

HYPERTENSIVE HEART DISEASE

It is also worth mentioning that noncardiac sequelae of oncologic disease and treatment can lead to cardiac issues in oncology patients. This is seen in the effects of hypertension on the heart, which is often due to the onset of renal disease. Additionally, some of the medications and treatment regimens require high fluid loads and may tip a borderline patient into cardiac failure. There is also the effect of the stress of dealing with an oncologic diagnosis, and that may contribute to hypertension. Whatever the cause, it is an aspect of the treatment of the patient that hypertension be addressed and treated as the patient enters a rehabilitation program. The specific details of treatment are not covered here, but the medications need to be customized to account for the toxicities of the treatments that the patient may be undergoing.

PERICARDIAL DISEASE

Pericardial disease leads to the development of constrictive heart disease physiology. It is most often seen in patients after radiation-induced injury. However, pericardial effusions can be due to primary or metastatic disease, infectious disease in immunocompromised patients, or due to postsurgical changes. The symptoms are shortness of breath, reduced cardiac output, and if untreated or recognized, cardiovascular collapse. Pericardial disease is divided into acute (<6 weeks), subacute (6 weeks to 6 months) or chronic disease (>6 months).

The most rapidly progressing form of pericardial disease is seen with pericardial effusions. The etiology is usually infectious, but may be due to an acute reaction to radiation treatment. The diagnosis is made most easily with echocardiography. Clinically, pericardial effu-

sion presents with pain in the chest, a friction rub on cardiac exam, and evidence of right-sided heart overload (distended neck veins, pulsus paradoxus) and may proceed to frank pericardial tamponade if not treated. Infection is the most common cause and must be ruled out. Treatment includes drainage and, if needed due to reaccumulating effusions, a pericardial window, pericardial stripping, or other surgical interventions.

Subacute pericarditis can be due to primary or metastatic neoplastic disease, infection, or any of the other common causes, such as uremia or anemia. This also requires treatment and will present similarly. Chronic pericarditis is usually associated with radiation-induced injury or previous surgery. This form of pericarditis usually requires a pericardial resection, as it is due to tissue limitations and not fluid accumulation.

PRIMARY AND METASTATIC CARDIAC TUMORS

Primary cardiac tumors are extremely rare and account for only 0.001%–0.28% of all tumors (36,37). Most of these are tumors of the valves and atria, and lead to heart valve pathology or to the need for a transplant for treatment in cases of local disease. Metastatic lesions are less rare, and have an incidence of 2.3%–18.3% in autopsy series (38). No tumors are known to have a predilection for metastasizing to the heart, but several are more common, including melanoma and local spread by primary mediastinal tumors. Most of the tumors seen in the heart are present through one of four mechanisms: (1) direct extension, (2) via the bloodstream, (3) via lymphatics, or (4) intravascularly via the pulmonary veins or vena cava. Most pericardial disease is via direct extension from the mediastinum or lungs, or more rarely, via retrograde lymphatic extension. Most myocardial or epicardial tumors are from lymphatic spread, and endocardial or valvular lesions come from intracavitary spread after lodging of the tumor from hematogenous spread (38). Pericardial metastases are most common, followed by epicardial and myocardial metastases. Primary cardiac tumors tend to be more frequent in younger patients, and metastatic lesions more common in males than females. The presenting symptoms of metastatic tumors to the heart vary, depending upon the location of the tumor. The most common presenting symptom of cardiac metastases is a pericardial effusion and often is the only presenting feature of this uncommon disorder. Intracavitary tumors may present with embolic events, particularly when there is an erosive surface to the lesion, or may present with valvular insufficiency or stenosis if the tumor is located near the valve. Endocardial tumors are rare, but when present are more common in the right heart and are usually due to endovascular growth, such as that seen in renal, liver, and uterine cancers. Most metastatic myocardial tumors are asymptomatic and are only recognized on autopsy.

ETHICAL ISSUES

The combination of cardiac and oncologic diagnoses in one patient can raise a host of ethical issues. The advancement of medical care has now allowed for the long-term survival of many individuals who will need treatment for two separate and potentially lethal disease processes. The patient must be informed and have an active role in the planning of their care to help to resolve these ethical issues. The following are a few cases with possible ethical issues.

Withdrawing Defibrillator Therapy in Patients with Cancer—Do not Resuscitate

The introduction of the automatic internal cardiac defibrillator (AICD) has provided patients with a life-prolonging device that can save patients from sudden cardiac death. It is not without consequences, however, and the shocks can be painful and the anxiety that the device can cause can be disabling for some patients. The group that often benefits from this treatment include individuals with left ventricular ejection fraction of <35%. Many patients will have AICD or have cardiac disease at the time of diagnosis with cancer or may, as a result of treatment of their cancer, have an AICD implanted. The patients treated with anthracycline medications or with radiation are the most likely oncology patients to benefit from AICD after development of subsequent cardiac disease. It is when there is a recurrence of cancer, or existing metastatic disease in a patient with arrhythmia, or in the end stages of cancer in the setting of preexisting cardiac disease that the ethical implications of the AICD and possible withdrawal of therapy become apparent.

It is not necessarily immoral, illegal, or unethical to withdraw a treatment once it has been established. In fact, withdrawal of a treatment is treated in the same manner as not initiating a treatment (39,40). In actual practice, it is common to withdraw life-sustaining interventions at the end of life, and AICD may be one of those treatments (41). In the case of advanced directives and with the consent of family members, the decision to withdraw care could be initiated and ultimately carried out. Discussions of these issues should be addressed while the patient is competent to make such decisions and advanced directives are particularly important. This is particularly true in instances where the wishes of the patient and family would preclude

cardiac resuscitation and defibrillation. In that setting, turning off the device would be most consistent with the care that the patient and family would desire (42). In a hospice setting, this issue may also arise, and the discontinuation of AICD should not stop mobilization of the patient and attempts to improve function. The main concern is the need to not provide a therapy that the patient does not wish to have provided. Each institution should review individual cases and establish policies to deal with end-of-life issues before they arise (43).

Potential Issues with Lvad—When to withhold Treatment

A similar situation may arise in the setting of the insertion of a left ventricular assist device (LVAD). Often, these devices are inserted in a patient in an emergency setting, with a plan for possible cardiac transplantation (44). Generally, outcomes are improved for these patients, but the potential exists for a patient with occult neoplasm to receive one of these devices. The subsequent evaluation may reveal a cancer that precludes transplantation, and the progress of the disease may be such that the patient is faced with an end-of-life dilemma. The patient may also chose to terminate the LVAD in this setting, under similar conditions that are present with AICD. The possibility of coexistent LVAD and terminal cancer is also increased as the LVAD has become an accepted treatment option for end-stage CHF as opposed to a bridge to transplant. Once again, the advanced directives and the frank discussions with patients and their families can ease the end-of-life transitions that may occur if the cancer progresses.

Offering Advanced Cardiac Surgery to Patients with Cancer—Ethical Issues and Considerations of Planning Interventions

When a patient has treatable cardiac disease in the setting of cancer, it is usually appropriate to treat this disease as long as the patient wishes to pursue that treatment. About 3.8% of cardiac surgical cases in one series had comorbid cancer at the time of surgery (45). This is especially true of cardiac disease that is a result of cancer treatment or occurs in apparently disease-free individuals. In the setting of advanced cancer, the treatment of the cardiac disease may place an undue burden on the patient and the option for palliative cardiac and cancer care may be most appropriate. This needs to be addressed on a case-by-case basis in consultation with the family and the patient. It is important to remember in the treatment of the original cancer that no future options are lost for the treatment of cardiac disease, as long-term cancer survivors still will face a high possibility of cardiac disease and cardiac mortality. An example may be the use of the internal mammary artery for breast reconstruction in a breast cancer survivor—removing the option of that vessel for treatment of CAD in the future or the effects of radiation on the outcomes of cardiac surgery (46,47).

A final consideration is that patients may benefit from simultaneous coronary surgery at the time of a primary tumor resection, and this should be considered for at-risk patients. An example is a patient with newly diagnosed lung cancer who may have coronary disease as well and would benefit from having a bypass at the time of the resection to allow for better tolerance of chemotherapy and other treatments that may follow. In some centers, this is becoming more common and is worthy of consideration in any patient undergoing a major thoracic procedure for cancer (48,49).

Cardiac Rehabilitation Treatment in the Setting of Oncologic Disease

The approaches to treatment of patients with cardiac disease in the cancer setting follow the same general principles used to rehabilitate the general patient with cardiac disease. These basic principles include emphasis on strengthening and conditioning while maintaining function and safety. The interested clinician is encouraged to review the many detailed references on the general principles of cardiac rehabilitation (3,50–53). A general outline of the essential principles applicable to the safe and effective cardiac rehabilitation in the oncology setting is presented here.

Over the past 35 years, the effectiveness of rehabilitation for patients with CAD has been established. A comprehensive program of cardiac rehabilitation now includes risk factor modification and patient education in addition to exercise and strengthening (54). Recent literature has demonstrated a variety of positive outcomes from these programs, including improved exercise tolerance, skeletal muscle strength, psychological status, and quality of life. Combined exercise and risk intervention programs can effectively reduce health care costs and hospitalization. Despite this volume of evidence, cardiac rehabilitation is often underutilized and should not be overlooked in a patient with cancer. A key element in all cardiac rehabilitation programs is smoking cessation, which is essential in cancer patients as well.

Cardiac rehabilitation for CAD patients reduces mortality by as much as 25%. The improvements in mortality rates are even better for CAD patients with multifactorial interventions than in patients exposed to exercise only (55). While reduction in morbidity with cardiac rehabilitation is not clearly proven, it is important to stress that exercise training does not result in an increase in morbidity. Exercise intervention has been shown to be safe, with low nonfatal cardiovascular event rates (3,50–53).

TABLE 27.2
Phases of a Cardiac Rehabilitation Program

PHASE	CHARACTERISTIC	CANCER-SPECIFIC EXAMPLE
Phase 1	(Acute Phase) Acute setting in the hospital; originally was a 14 d program of mobilization post-MI; now condensed to 2–3 d.	Patient has had a cardiac event after a tumor resection and is now post-CHF exacerbation or myocardial infarction.
Phase 1B	Often utilized for the elderly, this is a program of ongoing inpatient rehabilitation in either an acute or subacute rehabilitation setting. Most often used for patients with significant comorbidities.	Patient has had chemotherapy, amputation for tumor resection, or a prolonged intensive care unit stay, and has marked debility or a neurological event from their cancer.
Phase 2	(Training Phase) This is the traditional outpatient rehabilitation program.	Patients with radiation- or anthracycline-induced cardiomyopathy.
Phase 3	(Maintenance Phase) Often the poorest compliance part of the program, this is the part where the patient needs to keep up the exercise program and maintain the lifestyle modifications from the acute and training phases of the rehabilitation program. Enrollment in a maintenance program may help significantly with compliance.	Good cardiac health should be a part of the treatment of all patients with cancer. Good conditioning will help to fight recurrence of the disease.

Abbreviations: MI, myocardial infarction; CHF, congestive heart failure.

Emerging evidence indicates that intensive lifestyle modification may slow or reverse coronary artery disease in addition to the already proven benefits of exercise in lowering CAD. This effect has been difficult to isolate from the confounding contributions of dietary changes and lipid-lowering agents. Energy expenditures as low as ~1,800 kcal/week, or nearly four hours of moderate physical exercise, well below the threshold of most supervised exercise intervention programs, can be effective in reducing cardiac mortality (56,57).

Patients with cancer often have a greater degree of deconditioning, significantly lower exercise capacity, lower quality of life, and more depression than other patients with cardiac disease. Still, they can often show a marked increase in capacity, on par with their noncancer patient counterparts, and can have a marked improvement in quality of life with a decrease in depression indices. The major issues with cardiac rehabilitation in the cancer patient are those of access and participation. In addition, practitioners should remember to consider referral for cardiac rehabilitation when appropriate.

Tables 27.2 through 27.7 outline specifics for an effective cardiac rehabilitation program.

Cardiac rehabilitation can be an important and helpful part of a comprehensive care program of the patient with cancer. The crucial element to increase

---

TABLE 27.5
Goals of a Rehabilitation Program

1) Risk stratification
2) Improved emotional well-being
3) Lifestyle modification
   A) Reversible factors—Smoking cessation, diet, stress management, behavioral modifications
4) Psychological intervention
5) Energy conservation techniques
6) Improved conditioning
7) Improved muscle strength
8) Improved disease process understanding

TABLE 27.6
Elements of an Effective Rehabilitation Program

1) Strengthening exercises (free weight, Thera-Band, circuit training)
2) Stretching/calisthenic exercises
3) Endurance training (treadmill, bicycle, Air-Dyne, rowing machine, etc.)
4) Educational program
5) Lifestyle modification intervention (nutritional support, smoking cessation, etc.)
6) Medical supervision
7) Support group
8) Maintenance program availability

TABLE 27.3
Criteria for Cardiac Rehabilitation

ELIGIBLE CONDITIONS

Myocardial infarction
Post-coronary bypass surgery
Intracoronary revascularization
Intracoronary revascularization stable angina pectoris
Post-valve replacement
Chronic heart failure
All ages are eligible

TABLE 27.4
Medical Criteria

1) ECG-monitored exercise test
2) Strength measures (can be done by PT/physiologist)
3) Clinical review by referring physician
   a) Screen out unstable angina, uncompensated CHF
   b) Assess patient interest
4) Assess for depression or other psychological issues
5) Assess for other medical contraindications or limitations

TABLE 27.7
Memorial Sloan-Kettering Cancer Center Cardiovascular Precautions

Therapeutic interventions are suspended for:
DBP decrease of >10 mmHg from baseline
SBP decrease of >20 mmHg from baseline
DBP > 115 mmHg
SBP > 250 mmHg
Worsening
   Chest pain
   Fatigue
   Shortness of breath
   Onset of wheezing
   Leg cramps
   Claudication

---

the impact of cardiac rehabilitation in cancer patients is to increase physician referral and to increase patient participation through increased encouragement. One must remember that cardiac disease is still a significant issue in the treatment of the patient with a history of cancer.

References

1. Sawhney R, Sehl M, Naeim A. Physiologic aspects of aging: impact on cancer management and decision making, part I. *Cancer J.* 2005;11(6):449–460.

2. Gielen S, Adams V, Niebauer J, Schuler G, Hambrecht R. Aging and heart failure—similar syndromes of exercise intolerance? Implications for exercise-based interventions. *Heart Fail Monit.* 2005;4(4):130–136.

3. Bartels MN, Whiteson JH, Alba AS, Kim H. Cardiopulmonary rehabilitation and cancer rehabilitation. 1. Cardiac rehabilitation review. *Arch Phy Med Rehabil.* 2006;87(3 Suppl):46–56.

4. Kalantaridou SN, Naka KK, Bechlioulis A, Makrigiannakis A, Michalis L, Chrousos GP. Premature ovarian failure, endothelial dysfunction and estrogen-progestogen replacement. *Trend Endocrinol Metab.* 2006;17(3):101–109.

5. Muscari Lin E, Aikin JL, Good BC. Premature menopause after cancer treatment. *Cancer Pract.* 1999;7(3):114–121.

6. Giordano SH, Kuo YF, Freeman JL, et al. Risk of cardiac death after adjuvant radiotherapy for breast cancer. *J Natl Cancer Inst.* 2005;97:419–424.

7. Darby S, McGale P, Peto R. Mortality from cardiovascular disease after radiotherapy for breast cancer in 298,885 women registered in the SEER cancer registries. 27th Annual San Antonio Breast Cancer Symposium, San Antonio, TX, December 8–11, 2004 (abstr 32).

8. Cuzick J, Stewart H, Rutqvist L, et al. Cause-specific mortality in long-term survivors of breast cancer who participated in trials of radiotherapy. *J Clin Oncol.* 1994;12:447–453.

9. Korreman SS, Pedersen AN, Aarup LR, Nottrup TJ, Specht L, Nystrom H. Reduction of cardiac and pulmonary complication probabilities after breathing adapted radiotherapy for breast cancer. *Int J Radiat Oncol Biol Phys.* 2006;65(5):1375–1380.

10. Harris EE, Correa C, Hwang WT, et al. Late cardiac mortality and morbidity in early-stage breast cancer patients after breast-conservation treatment. *J Clin Oncol.* 2006;24(25):4100–4106.

11. Stewart JR, Fajardo LF, Gillette SM, et al. Radiation injury to the heart. *Int J Radiat Oncol Biol Phys.* 1995;31:1205–1211.

12. Early Breast Cancer Trialists' Collaborative Group: favourable and unfavourable effects on long-term survival of radiotherapy for early breast cancer: an overview of the randomised trials—Early Breast Cancer Trialists' Collaborative Group. *Lancet.* 2000;355:1757–1770.

13. Gyenes G, Rutqvist LE, Liedberg A, Fornander T. Long-term cardiac morbidity and mortality in a randomized trial of pre- and postoperative radiation therapy versus surgery alone in primary breast cancer. *Radiother Oncol.* 1998;48(2):185–190.

14. Paszat LF, Mackilliop WJ, Groome PA, Schultze K, Holowaty E. Mortality from myocardial infarction following post lumpectomy radiotherapy for breast cancer: a population based study in Ontario, Canada. *Int J Radiat Oncol Biol Phys.* 1999;43:755–761.

15. Patt DA, Goodwin JS, Kuo YF, et al. Cardiac morbidity of adjuvant radiotherapy for breast cancer. *J Clin Oncol.* 2005;23(30):7475–7482.

16. Tsibiribi P, Descotes J, Lombard-Bohas C, et al. Cardiotoxicity of 5-fluorouracil in 1350 patients with no prior history of heart disease. *Bull Cancer.* 2006;93(3):E27–E30.

17. Wacker A, Lersch C, Scherpinski U, Reindl L, Seyfarth M. High incidence of angina pectoris in patients treated with 5-fluorouracil. A planned surveillance study with 102 patients. *Oncology.* 2003;65(2):108–112.

18. Fukuda M, Oka M, Itoh N, et al. Vasospastic angina likely related to cisplatin-containing chemotherapy and thoracic irradiation for lung cancer. *Intern Med.* 1999;38(5):436–438.

19. Czaykowski PM, Moore MJ, Tannock IF. High risk of vascular events in patients with urothelial transitional cell carcinoma treated with cisplatin based chemotherapy. *J Urol.* 1998;160 (6 Pt 1):2021–2024.

20. Kamineni P, Prakasa K, Hasan SP, Akula R, Dawkins F. Cardiotoxicities of paclitaxel in African Americans. *J Natl Med Assoc.* 2003;95(10):977–981.

21. Green DM, Hyland A, Chung CS, Zevon MA, Hall BC. Cancer and cardiac mortality among 15-year survivors of cancer diagnosed during childhood or adolescence. *J Clin Oncol.* 1999;17(10):3207–3215.

22. Nicholson JS, Fears TR, Byrne J. Death during adulthood in survivors of childhood and adolescent cancer. *Cancer.* 1994;73:3094–3102.

23. Robertson CM, Hawkins MM, Kingston JE. Late deaths and nervous system after radiotherapy in childhood survival after childhood cancer: implications for cure. *BMJ.* 1994;309:162–166.

24. Hudson MM, Jones D, Boyett J, et al. Late mortality of long-term survivors of childhood cancer. *J Clin Oncol.* 1997;15:2205–2213.

25. Mertens AC, Yasui Y, Neglia JP, et al. Late mortality experience in five-year survivors of childhood and adolescent cancer: the Childhood Cancer Survivor Study. *J Clin Oncol.* 2001;19(13):3163–3172.

26. Meinardi MT, Gietema JA, van der Graaf WT, et al. Cardiovascular morbidity in long-term survivors of metastatic testicular cancer. *J Clin Oncol.* 2000;18(8):1725–1732.

27. Gianni L, Zweier J, Levy A, Meyers, CE. Characterization of the cycle of iron-mediated electron transfer from doxorubicin to molecular oxygen. *J Biol Chem.* 1985;259:6056–6058.

28. Olson R, Mushlin P. Doxorubicin cardiotoxicity: analysis of prevailing hypothesis. *FASEB J.* 1990;4:3076–3086.

29. Goormaghtigh E, Huart P, Praet M, Brasseur R, Ruysschaert JM. Structure of the doxorubicin-cardiolipin complex role in mitochondrial toxicity. *Biophys Chem.* 1990;35:247–257.

30. Arola OJ, Saraste A, Pulkki K. Kallajoki M, Parvinen M, Voipio-Pulkki LM. Acute doxorubicin cardiotoxicity involves cardiomyocyte apoptosis. *Cancer Res.* 2000;60:1789–1792.

31. Wouters KA, Kremer LC, Miller TL, Herman EH, Lipshultz SE. Protecting against anthracycline-induced myocardial damage: a review of the most promising strategies. *Br J Haematol.* 2005;131(5):561–578.

32. Slamon D, Pegram M. Rationale for trastuzumab (Herceptin) in adjuvant breast cancer trials. *Semin Oncol.* 2001;28:13–19.

33. Lipshultz SE, Lipsitz SR, Sallen SE, et al. Chronic progressive cardiac dysfunction years after doxorubicin therapy for childhood acute lymphoblastic leukemia. *J Clin Oncol.* 2005;23:2629–2636.

34. Redfield MM, Gersh BJ, Bailey KR, Rodeheffer RJ. Natural history of incidentally discovered asymptomatic idiopathic dilated cardiomyopathy. *Am J Cardiol.* 1994;74:737–739.

35. Haq MM, Legha SS, Choksi J, et al. Doxorubicin-induced congestive heart failure in adults. *Cancer.* 1985;56:1361–1365.

36. Virmani R. Tumours metastatic to the heart and pericardium. In: Burke A, Virmani R, eds. *Atlas of Tumour Pathology. Tumours of the Heart and Great Vessels.* 3rd Series Fascicle 16. Washington, DC: AFIP; 1995:195–209.

37. McAllister HA Jr. Tumors of the heart and pericardium. In: Silver MD, ed. *Cardiovascular Pathology.* Vol 2, 2nd ed. New York, NY: Churchill Livingstone; 1991:1297–1333.

38. Bussani R, De-Giorgio F, Abbate A, Silvestri F. Cardiac metastases. *J Clin Pathol.* 2007;60(1):27–34.

39. Fairman RP. Withdrawing life-sustaining treatment: lessons from Nancy Cruzan. *Arch Intern Med.* 1992;152:25–27.

40. American College of Physicians. Ethics Manual: fourth edition. *Ann Intern Med.* 1998;128:576–594.

41. Quill TE, Barold SS, Sussman BL. Discontinuing an implantable cardioverter defibrillator as a life-sustaining treatment. *AM J Cardiol.* 1994;75:205–207.

42. Mueller PS, Hook CC, Hayes DL. Ethical analysis of withdrawal of pacemaker or implantable cardioverter-defibrillator support at the end of life. *Mayo Clin Proc.* 2003;78(8):959–963.

43. Ballentine JM. Pacemaker and defibrillator deactivation in competent hospice patients: an ethical consideration. *Am J Hosp Palliat Care.* 2005;22(1):14–19.

44. Williams M, Casher J, Joshi N, et al. Insertion of a left ventricular assist device in patients without thorough transplant evaluations: a worthwhile risk? *J Thorac Cardiovasc Surg.* 2003;126(2):436–441.

45. Clough RA, Leavitt BJ, Morton JR, et al. The effect of comorbid illness on mortality outcomes in cardiac surgery. *Arch Surg.* 2002;137(4):428–432.

46. Nahabedian MY. The internal mammary artery and vein as recipient vessels for microvascular breast reconstruction: are we burning a future bridge? *Ann Plast Surg.* 2004;53(4):311–316.

47. Chang AS, Smedira NG, Chang CL, et al. Cardiac surgery after mediastinal radiation: extent of exposure influences outcome. *J Thorac Cardiovasc Surg.* 2007;133(2):404–413.

48. Danton MH, Anikin VA, McManus KG, McGuigan JA, Campalani G. Simultaneous cardiac surgery with pulmonary resection: presentation of series and review of literature. *Eur J Cardiothorac Surg.* 1998;13(6):667–672.

49. Gillinov AM, Greene PS, Stuart RS, Heitmiller RF. Cardiopulmonary bypass as an adjunct to pulmonary surgery. *Chest.* 1996;110(2):571–574.

50. Bartels MN. Cardiac rehabilitation. In: Grant Cooper, ed. *Essential Physical Medicine and Rehabilitation.* Totowa, NJ: Humana Press; 2006:119–146.

51. Humphry R, Bartels MN. Exercise, cardiovascular disease and chronic heart failure: a focused review. *Arch Phy Med Rehabil.* 2001;82(3 suppl 1):S76–S81.

52. Bartels MN. Cardiopulmonary assessment. In: Grabois M, ed. *Physical Medicine and Rehabilitation: The Complete Approach.* Chicago, IL: Blackwell Science, Inc.; 2000:chap 20; 351–372.

53. Bartels MN. Cardiac rehabilitation. In: Grabois M ed. *Physical Medicine and Rehabilitation: The Complete Approach.* Chicago, IL: Blackwell Science, Inc.; 2000:chap 79; 1435–1456.

54. Zwisler AD, Schou L, Soja AM, et al. DANREHAB group. A randomized clinical trial of hospital-based, comprehensive cardiac rehabilitation versus usual care for patients with congestive heart failure, ischemic heart disease, or high risk of ischemic heart disease (the DANREHAB trial)—design, intervention, and population. *Am Heart J.* November 2005;150(5):899e7–e16.

55. Lee S, Naimark B, Porter MM, Ready AE. Effects of a long-term, community-based cardiac rehabilitation program on middle-aged and elderly cardiac patients. *Am J Geriatr Cardiol.* 2004;13(6):293–298.

56. King ML., Williams MA, Fletcher GF, et al. American Association for Cardiovascular and Pulmonary Rehabilitation. American Heart Association. Medical director responsibilities for outpatient cardiac rehabilitation/secondary prevention programs. A statement for healthcare professionals from the American Association for Cardiovascular and Pulmonary Rehabilitation and the American Heart Association. *J Cardiopulm Rehabil.* 2005;25(6):315–320.

57. Leon AS, Franklin BA, Costa F, et al. American Heart Association. Council on Clinical Cardiology (Subcommittee on Exercise, Cardiac Rehabilitation, and Prevention). Council on Nutrition, Physical Activity, and Metabolism (Subcommittee on Physical Activity). American Association of Cardiovascular and Pulmonary Rehabilitation. Cardiac rehabilitation and secondary prevention of coronary heart disease: an American Heart Association scientific statement from the Council on Clinical Cardiology (Subcommittee on Exercise, Cardiac Rehabilitation, and Prevention) and the Council on Nutrition, Physical Activity, and Metabolism (Subcommittee on Physical Activity), in collaboration with the American Association of Cardiovascular and Pulmonary Rehabilitation. *Circulation.* 2005;111(3):369–376.

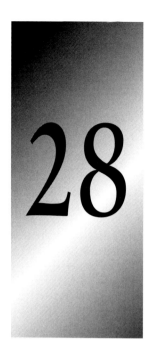

Gastrointestinal Complications of Cancer

James Han
Rebecca G. Smith
Kevin Fox
Argyrios Stampas

Gastrointestinal (GI) complications of cancer are significant and can be challenging to manage. Unfortunately, there is no safe harbor from cancer-related sequelae or side effects of treatments. Dysphagia, nausea, vomiting, diarrhea, constipation, fecal impaction, bowel obstruction, and infections are just a few of the adverse effects experienced by the cancer patient. Prolonged immobility causes additional complications that negatively impact morbidity, mortality, and quality of life. The following review will highlight the spectrum of potential gastrointestinal complications resulting from multimodal cancer treatments, including surgery, chemotherapy, and radiation. The current strategies for diagnosis and treatment will also be discussed.

CONSEQUENCES OF A MASS

Bowel Obstruction

Bowel obstruction of the upper and lower GI tract is a common cancer-related complication. Its incidence ranges from 5.5% to 42% in ovarian cancer and 10% to 28.4% in colorectal cancer. The overall incidence of intestinal obstruction from advanced cancer is 3% (1,2). Management of the obstruction depends upon the acuity, location, and severity of the obstruction. According to Khurana et al., complete versus partial obstruction is determined by the degree of distal collapse, proximal bowel dilatation, and transit of injected contrast material (3). The passage of contrast mate-

rial through the transition zone, described as the point between the dilated proximal portion and the collapsed distal portion, indicates a partial bowel obstruction (3). Furthermore, differentiating between small- and large-bowel obstructions is important in formulating their respective treatment strategies. In most cases, small-bowel obstructions are primarily due to adhesions from previous surgeries, hernias, and, less frequently, extrinsic compression from neoplasms. Large-bowel obstructions are due to carcinoma, volvulus, and diverticulitis (4,5). Colorectal, ovarian, and gastric tumors are the most common causes of small-bowel obstructions due to an intra-abdominal mass. More proximal gastroduodenal obstructions are commonly caused by gastric and pancreatic (6%–25%) carcinoma (6,7).

The suspicion of obstruction is initially based on a thorough history and physical examination. Complaints of nausea, vomiting (68%–100%), constipation, abdominal discomfort or pain (72%–76%), and distention (72%–76%) are common. The acute nature of these symptoms may help to differentiate a volvulus from an advanced cancer. Routine blood work, including a complete blood count and complete metabolic panel, is usually followed by supine and upright abdominal roentgenographs to evaluate further for constipation, as well as to confirm the cause and location of an obstruction. A barium enema and abdominal computer tomography may help further elucidate the cause of obstruction (3,5). It is important to note that the entire intestinal tract should be evaluated in all

KEY POINTS

- Small-bowel obstructions are primarily due to adhesions from previous surgeries, hernias, and extrinsic compression from neoplasms, whereas large-bowelobstructions are due to carcinoma, volvulus, and diverticulitis.
- Colorectal, ovarian, and gastric tumors are the most common causes of small-bowel obstructions due to an intra-abdominal mass and more proximal gastroduodenal obstructions are more likely than gastric and pancreatic (6%–25%) carcinoma.
- Ostomies require routine irrigation, and excessive odor and gas management is addressed by ensuring a good seal, odor-proof pouches, use of deodorizing agents, and via dietary modifications (avoiding legumes, asparagus, Brussels sprouts, onions, eggs, and garlic).
- Chemotherapy-induced nausea and vomiting is seen more often in women, children, and younger adults; those with a previous history of chemotherapy-induced nausea and vomiting (CINV); a history of motion sickness; emesis during pregnancy; and anxiety.
- How aggressively nausea and vomiting are prophylaxed depend on the emetogenicity risk of the che-

motherapeutic agent: (1) high (>90%) (2) moderate (30%–90%), low (10%–30%), and (4) minimal (<10%).
- Acute emesis may be prevented by administration of antiemetics prior to (but on the same day) as chemotherapy. For high- and moderate-risk agents, therapy should be continued for at least four days to help prevent delayed emesis.
- The management of uncomplicated diarrhea includes dietary management and initiation of loperamide; but if the diarrhea has progressed to National Cancer Institute (NCI) grades 3–4, it is recommended that the patient be admitted to an acute care hospital for octreotide, hydration, and further workup.
- Stomatitis is common in cancer patients undergoing chemotherapy or head and neck radiation therapy, and can progress to viral, fungal, or bacterial superinfections. Symptoms (mild discomfort to severe pain) can even limit food and fluid intake, and can be prevented by good oral hygiene with soft toothbrushes, removal of dental caries, mucosal barriers and coating agents, mucosal cell stimulants, and topical anesthetics for pain control.

patients suspected of having an obstruction because some (8.2%) will have both small- and large-bowel obstructions concurrently (7). While awaiting the final radiographic diagnosis, the patient should receive nothing by mouth and receive adequate intravenous supportive therapy to resuscitate their intravascular fluid volume and correct for any electrolyte disturbance that may have secondarily occurred from vomiting. If the patient continues to vomit or displays worsening distention, a nasogastric tube should be introduced for decompression.

Partial bowel obstructions may completely resolve with medical management (7). However, the patient's condition should be monitored with serial abdominal exams. Worsening symptoms or signs suggest progression of the bowel obstruction, and a tube decompression or percutaneous endoscopic gastrostomy (PEG) may need to be performed. These two options can provide symptomatic relief and serve as effective therapeutic alternatives after failed medical management. Endoscopic intervention with a stent bypass or surgical resection may be attempted if conservative methods fail and the patient's condition continues to decompensate. Even with the high mortality rates and the short mean survival time associated with surgery, it is the primary approach to malignant obstruction (6). Palliative surgery for the elderly (>70 years) in poor general health

with malignant ascites and a palpable mass should be considered with the understanding that the prognosis is poor. However, studies have shown that stent placement is an effective way to achieve safely immediate nonoperative decompression (6), as well as satisfactory palliative management of inoperable multiple partial obstructions and/or extensive tumors (4). Stent collapse has been documented, but remains an uncommon delayed complication that can be managed by restenting (8). Furthermore, patients with advanced disease can use opioids such as morphine for colicky pain control, antisecretory agents such as octreotide and hyoscine butylbromide for emesis and pain control, prokinetic agents such as metoclopramide for emesis control, antiinflammatory agents such as corticosteroids for edema reduction, total parenteral supplementation for nutritional support, and antispasmodic agents for symptomatic pharmacological palliation (4,7,9). These agents will be discussed in detail further in the chapter.

Management of Ostomies

Surgery plays an important role in the treatment of cancer. Postoperative complications, including infection, blood loss, embolism, and fistula formation may occur and require significant medical and/or surgical attention. The rehabilitation specialist caring for patients following GI surgery should be aware of these complications and be familiar with the specific issues involved in their management. Surgery involving the GI tract may necessitate a temporary or permanent fecal diversion, depending on the location and severity of surgery. The ostomy may be introduced at the distal ileum or differing levels of the colon. Each type of ostomy poses unique management issues. The different types have been extensively addressed in multiple surgical textbooks and will not be detailed here. We will discuss the management issues involved in ostomy care, the role of the rehabilitation team, the potential ostomy complications that both the rehabilitation team and the patient may encounter, and outline strategies to prevent and treat the complications if they arise.

Early patient education is important. Prior to the surgery, the patient should understand what the procedure entails, where the stoma will be placed, and how the fecal diversion will affect his or her daily function. They must also be informed whether the procedure is potentially temporary or permanent and whether "takedown," or reversal of temporary ostomies, is possible. Following the surgery, the physician and ostomy nurse can further ease the postoperative transition by encouraging the patient to participate actively in stoma management, skin care, and evacuation. Immediate and long-term quality-of-life studies have shown a strong correlation between having a good relationship with an enterostomal therapist and developing patient confidence with appliance changes (10,11). Continued emotional and psychosocial counseling by the appropriate specialists should be recommended to maintain patient morale and curb adjustment difficulties.

Following surgery, an appropriate pouch selection is made to minimize peristomal leakage. Significant attention to meticulous skin care will minimize maceration and breakdown. The patient should be taught how to properly apply adhesives, skin sealants, and barrier creams to the periostomy region. These basic hygiene techniques, in combination with a properly fitted and tape-bordered appliance, should minimize skin exposure and the likelihood of developing complications. Furthermore, the pouch seal is dependent on the patient's abdominal contour, with deep creases effectively reducing good contact (12).

A colostomy is placed to bypass the distal colon and rectum. It requires a good irrigation strategy along with adequate fluid and fiber intake to prevent constipation and food blockage. Routine irrigation requires instillation of lukewarm tap water through a cone tip irrigator, resulting in evacuation via a distention-activated peristalsis mechanism. Excessive odor and gas management can be addressed by ensuring a good seal with odor-proof pouches, by introduction of deodorizing agents such as bismuth or simethicone into the

appliance, and by dietary modifications. Foods known to increase gas production include legumes, asparagus, Brussels sprouts, and onions. Foods known to increase odor include eggs and garlic. Flatus vent caps have also been utilized as a mechanical deodorant (13–15).

The management of proximal intestinal ostomies, such as the ileostomy, placed to bypass the entire colon and rectum, as well as the cecostomy and ascending colostomy, present a different set of challenges. They produce high-output drainage rich in proteolytic enzymes and thereby increase the incidence of dehydration, electrolyte abnormalities, and skin breakdown. Thus, more attention must be made to ensure dry and nonirritated peristomal skin. If skin breakdown occurs, application of the pouch should follow a "crusting" procedure using pectin powder and alcohol-free plasticizing wipes to first allow the surface to dry, increasing its chance to heal (12). Fluid and electrolyte status should be regularly monitored by laboratory studies as well as by daily input and output volume recordings to minimize any gross imbalances. Fluctuations can be corrected by oral or intravenous supplementation as needed. Finally, certain medication preparations, which are enteric-coated or designed for slow release, will not have adequate time for absorption and may require regular monitoring of serum levels and/or changing the medication to a more dissolvable form, such as liquid.

Other potential complications include stomal herniations, stenosis, and prolapse (16). They may require further surgery if the conditions become incarcerated, severe, or persistent. Stomal retractions can usually be managed with special convex pouches that encourage stomal protrusion. Continued skin damage and breakdown with concomitant fungal or bacterial infections require the appropriate medication. A dermatology consultation may be necessary.

Fistulas

A fistula is an abnormal connection between two vessels or organs. The medical and surgical management of cancer may contribute to the formation of a fistula. Prolonged abscess, radiation therapy, and elective or palliative surgery are contributing factors. In such instances, the physiatrist may encounter a vomiting patient with significant weight loss or a deconditioned patient with complaints of generalized malaise, with or without observable cutaneous drainage on physical examination. Secondary symptoms of fistulas may include itching, malaise, and foul-smelling discharge.

The pathophysiology of a fistula is not completely understood, but a progression from an inflamed tissue segment to a fissure, exacerbated by increased intraluminal pressure due to distal stenosis is one explanation.

TABLE 28.1

Fistulas: Classification and Clinical Manifestations

Fistula Type	Risk Factor (Ref)	Clinical Manifestation (Ref)
Tracheoesophageal	Tracheostomy	Presents as coughing, choking, aspiration, or fever with abdominal distention from air collection
Gastrocolic or gastrojejunocolic	Stomach or intestinal malignancies and chronic NSAID use	Presents as epigastric pain, diarrhea, weight loss, feculent vomiting (33%), and GI bleeding (17,18)
Gastrocutaneous	Surgery	Recognized by the drainage of gastric fluid (19)
Enterocutaneous	Surgery, PEG tube (20)	Recognized by the drainage of intestinal/pancreatic fluid (21)
Enteroenteric or enterocolic	Surgery	Presents with epigastric pain, diarrhea, weight loss, and fecal halitosis, which is rare (2%) but pathognomonic (18,22)
Enterovaginal or Enterovesicular	Diverticulitis Abscess Hysterectomy	Presents with frequent vaginal or urinary tract infections or the passage of gas from the urethra during urination
Vesicovaginal	Irradiation Hysterectomy	Presents with continuous urinary incontinence
Anorectal	Abscess Irradiation	Presents with purulent discharge

Abbreviations: NSAID, nonsteroidal anti-inflammatory drug; PEG, percutaneous endoscopic gastrostomy.

Once a fistula forms, the abnormal connection serves as a conduit for the spread of infection and prevents healing. Fistulas can form throughout the entire alimentary tract and present with signs and symptoms unique to their location. They are classified as internal or external and complete or incomplete, indicating whether the fistula is completely or partially patent. Internal fistulas include tracheoesophageal, gastrocolic, enteroenteric, enterocolic, enterovaginal, enterovesical, and vesicovaginal fistulas. External fistulas include gastrocutaneous, enterocutaneous, colocutaneous, anorectal, and peristomal fistulas (Table 28.1) (17–22). Fistulas are diagnosed by barium enema (94% of gastrocolic and 77% of duodenocolic fistula), upper endoscopy, sigmoidoscopy, colonoscopy, intravenous pyelogram, or fistulogram (18).

Internal fistulas have been medically managed by aminosalicylates, corticosteroids, antibiotics (Flagyl), and immunosuppressants, particularly methotrexate, cyclosporine A, tacrolimus, and infliximab (18,22). Nutritional support via a feeding tube or intravenously may be necessary to counter malnutrition and deconditioning. Care must be taken to optimize skin integrity. If the fistula does not adequately resolve with these options, a site-dependent surgery, such as a fistulotomy or a partial bowel resection, may be required, necessitating a temporary ostomy. Surgical repairs of

fistulas have an inherent risk of forming a new fistula (20). Alternative options using sealants and plugging techniques have been studied and found to be a safe and effective strategy in certain populations (23).

Graft-versus-Host Disease

Graft-versus-Host Disease (GVHD) is a common and potentially life-threatening side effect that occurs when the donor T cells from the donor marrow or donor stem cells attack the host cells following allogeneic bone marrow transplantation (24). The gastrointestinal tract is frequently involved in acute GVHD and is classically characterized by a maculopapular skin rash, elevated liver enzymes, jaundice, crampy abdominal pain, and watery diarrhea (24,25).

VIPoma and Carcinoid Tumors

VIPomas are rare neuroendocrine tumors found mostly as an islet cell tumor within the pancreas that secretes vasoactive intestinal polypeptide (VIP). Also known as the watery diarrhea, hypokalemia (muscle cramps), and hypochlorhydria or achlorhydria (WDHA) syndrome, the metabolic derangement caused by the excessive secretion of VIP can be life-threatening if not managed appropriately (26). More frequent in females with a family history of multiple endocrine neoplasia (MEN) Type 1, patients may also present with flushing, nausea, vomiting, and dehydration lethargy.

Carcinoid syndrome is a rare manifestation due to the oversecretion of serotonin from a carcinoid tumor located most often in the GI tract. These tumors result from an idiopathic proliferation of enterochromaffin cells and are classified based on their embryonic origin. The appendix is the most common site of a GI carcinoid tumor, followed by intestinal and gastric carcinoids (27,28).

Both of these tumors can present significant GI complications that require early medical and/or surgical intervention. Their diagnoses should be included in the clinician's differential of possible causes when presented with diarrhea, nausea, vomiting, and flushing of the skin. Further in-depth discussion of the diagnosis and management of these tumors may be found in oncological textbooks and journal articles.

TREATMENT-INDUCED NAUSEA AND VOMITING

The treatment of cancer with chemotherapy agents and radiotherapy has dramatically improved the prognosis and survival of many patients diagnosed with cancer. However, these interventions may cause significant gastrointestinal side effects that can limit tolerability of treatment (29–31). These side effects include nausea, vomiting, diarrhea, and malabsorption. Those suffering from these adverse reactions may subsequently develop dehydration, electrolyte imbalances, mental status changes, and functional decline (30). The impact of these side effects on treatment and quality of life is significant. The initiation of 5-HT$_3$ antagonists, such as ondansetron, dolasetron, granisetron, tropisetron, and palonosetron has improved the statistics. However, nausea and vomiting continue to limit the tolerability of treatment and quality of life (30).

The clinician must also be aware of other causes of nausea and vomiting, including bacterial gastrointestinal infections, bowel obstruction, gastroparesis, brain metastases, vestibular dysfunction, irritable bowel disease, and the cancer itself. The onset and acuity of symptoms can help clarify the likely etiology, with routine blood tests, abdominal imaging studies, and/or endoscopy to confirm the ultimate diagnosis. Treatment is based on the underlying cause. Adequate measures to prevent complications of dehydration and electrolyte disturbance must be taken. With chronic and prolonged emesis, patients may need parenteral nutritional support and ongoing antiemetic therapy. The rehabilitation specialist may encounter patients who are experiencing gastrointestinal side effects of treatment with chemotherapy and/or radiation. These

adverse reactions may be limiting their patients' participation in therapy and ability to make functional gains. Knowledge of the proposed physiological mechanisms and their prevention and treatment strategies, as well as the special pharmacological considerations specific to the oncology patient population, is imperative to managing these side effects effectively and subsequently improving treatment outcomes and quality of life.

Chemotherapy-Induced Nausea and Vomiting

CINV can lead to significant morbidity affecting approximately 70%–80% of cancer patients receiving chemotherapy (30,32). The incidence, time of onset, severity, and duration of nausea and vomiting are influenced by a number of factors, including the specific chemotherapeutic agent used, dosage and schedule, concurrent medications, and individual variation of prevention/treatment strategies (30,32,33). Women, children, and younger adults are more likely to experience CINV, as are those with a previous history of CINV (32). Those with a history of motion sickness, emesis during pregnancy, and anxiety also have a higher incidence of CINV (34). Those that have a history of alcohol abuse are less likely to experience CINV (32,34).

Classification of Emetic Syndromes

Vomiting (emesis) is classified according to the time of onset and response to treatment, and includes anticipatory, acute, delayed, breakthrough, and refractory episodes Vomiting within 24 hours of chemotherapy is classified as acute. The delayed period occurs between 24 hours after chemotherapy and may continue for as long as seven days. Delayed episodes are more likely to occur if the acute period is not well tolerated or controlled. Anticipatory nausea and vomiting occurs prior to the administration of chemotherapy and is often related to a past experience of CINV. This is considered a learned response. Breakthrough emesis occurs despite administration of appropriate prophylaxis and rescue medication. Refractory emesis occurs when all pharmacological interventions have failed.

Pathophysiology

The pathophysiology of CINV is complex and not well understood. It involves both the central and peripheral nervous systems and includes a number of neurotransmitters. The central components within the brain known to have a role in the CINV mechanism include the vomiting center located in the medullary reticular formation and the chemoreceptor trigger zone (CTZ) in the area of the postrema of the fourth ventricle (32,34). The CTZ is comprised of many neurotransmitter receptors, most notably dopamine, serotonin, histamine, and substance P. Although knowledge of the precise mechanism is unclear, it is generally accepted that CINV is mediated through the CTZ. Stimulation of the CTZ by input from afferent fibers in the central cortex and/or peripherally from the GI tract, vestibular apparatus, and taste receptors may trigger the vomiting response (34).

The prevention and treatment strategies often utilize a combined pharmacological approach and target the receptors located in the CTZ and periphery. Although numerous neurotransmitters play a role in the vomiting response, serotonin and 5-hydroxytryptamine ($5\text{-}HT_3$) receptors are especially important in acute CINV. Substance P plays a predominant role in delayed CINV. Pharmacological prevention and treatment strategies utilize antagonists to these receptors (34).

Serotonin is released by enterochromaffin cells in the GI tract. It is suspected that chemotherapy increases the rate of turnover of these cells and high levels of serotonin are released into the bloodstream. Serotonin then stimulates the vomiting reflex via the vagus and greater splanchnic afferent nerves, both of which have $5\text{-}HT_3$ receptors (34). Commonly used $5\text{-}HT_3$ antagonists include metoclopramide, dolasetron, granisetron, ondansetron, palonosetron, and tropisetron (Fig. 28.1). Recent research supports the use of the $5\text{-}HT_3$ antagonists for prophylaxis of CINV. Further recommendations on the use of $5\text{-}HT_3$ antagonists will be discussed in a later section of this chapter.

Substance P exerts its emetic effects in the central nervous system by binding to the neurokinin-1 (NK1) receptors located in the brainstem (34,35). Hesketh

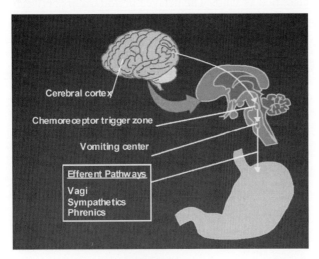

FIGURE 28.1

Anatomy of the vomiting reflex. Reprinted with permission from Ref. 32.

et al. demonstrated that serotonin-dependent mechanisms were responsible for the early acute emesis (first 8–12 hours post-cisplatin), and the substance P/NK1 mechanisms played a major role in late acute emesis (after 8–12 hours) and delayed emesis (36). Aprepitant, a novel NK1 antagonist, is currently recommended for the prevention of late acute and delayed CINV in selected cases when the emetogenicity of the chemotherapy agent is moderate to high (37,38).

Corticosteroids are also commonly used in the prophylaxis of CINV. A number of studies have demonstrated the efficacy of both dexamethasone and methylprednisolone as monotherapy and in combination with other agents to prevent CINV. Their mechanisms of action are not completely understood. There is evidence to suggest that corticosteroids may help reduce CINV by inhibiting the release of serotonin peripherally as well as acting centrally. However, the precise mechanism is unknown (39).

Additional agents that are frequently prescribed for the treatment of breakthrough and refractory CINV include dopamine receptor antagonists, anxiolytics, and cannabinoids. The widespread use of this broad spectrum of medications illustrates the complex nature of CINV and the various mechanisms that may be involved.

Prevention and Treatment Strategies

Current clinical practice guidelines seek to prevent CINV from occurring in an attempt to improve tolerance of treatment and quality of life. When CINV is present, prompt recognition and initiation of antiemetic therapy is paramount.

The most important factor influencing the occurrence of CINV is the emetogenicity of the chemotherapeutic agent or agents. The emetogenicity of chemotherapeutic agents is currently classified by a system based on the occurrence of acute emesis in a population of people who did not receive antiemetic prophylaxis. This system was developed by Hesketh et al. (40) and subsequently modified by Grunberg et al. (41) The current classification system divides the emetogenic potential of chemotherapeutic agents into four categories. They are (1) high emetic risk, 90% or more patients developed acute emesis; (2) moderate risk, 30%–90% of patients developed acute emesis; (3) low risk, 10%–30% of patients developed acute emesis; and (4) minimal risk, less than 10% of patients developed acute emesis (30,37). The emetogenic classification for commonly used intravenous and oral chemotherapy agents is summarized in Table 28.2. Acute emesis may be prevented by administration of antiemetics prior to but on the same day as the chemotherapy dose. For high- and moderate-risk agents,

TABLE 28.2
Emetogenic Potential of Single Intravenous (IV) and Oral (PO) Antineoplastic Agents

Degree of Emetogenicity (Incidence)	Agent
High (>90%)	IV: cisplatin, mechlorethamide, streptozocin, cyclophosamide ? 1500 mg/m², carmustine
	PO: hexamethylmelamine, procarbazine
Moderate (30%–90%)	IV: oxaliplatin, cytarabine > 1 g/m², carboplatin, ifosfamide, cyclophosphamide < 1,500 mg/m², doxorubicin, daunorubicin, epirubicin, idarubicin, irinotecan
	PO: cyclophosphamide, etoposide, temozolomide, vinorelbine, imatinib
Low (10%–30%)	IV: paclitaxel, docetaxel, mitoxantrone, topotecan, etopiside, pemetrexed, methotrexate, mitomycin, gemcitabine, cytarabine ≤ 100 mg/m², 5-fluorouracil, ortezomib, cetuximab, trastuzumab
	PO: capecitabine, fludarabine
Minimal (<10%)	IV: leomyine busulfan, bevacizumab, 2-chorodeoxyadenosine, fludarabine, vinbalstins, vinblastine, vincristies, vinorelnine
	PO: chlorambucil, hydroxyurea, L-phenylalanine mustard, 6-thioguanine, methotrexate, gefitinib

Source: From Ref. 41.

therapy should be continued for at least four days to help prevent delayed emesis. An outline of the principles of emesis control in cancer patients has been provided by the National Cancer Care Network and is further addressed in Chapter 70.

The current comprehensive and evidence-based guidelines for antiemetics are those established by the Multinational Association for Supportive Care in Oncology (MASCC) and are summarized in Tables 28.3 and 28.4. These guidelines were initially established during the MASCC Consensus Conference on Antiemetic Therapy at the Perugia International Cancer Conference VII in March 2004 and updated in April 2007. The following summarizes the guidelines for prophylaxis of CINV: (1) A three-drug regimen, including single doses of a 5-HT₃ antagonist, dexamethasone, and aprepitant, before chemotherapy is recommended to prevent acute CINV following chemotherapy of high emetic risk (HEC); (2) The combination of dexamethasone and aprepitant is suggested to prevent delayed CINV in patients receiving HEC rather than dexamethasone alone; (3) Prevention of acute CINV following chemotherapy of moderate emetic risk (MEC) depends on the chemotherapy agent. Women receiving anthracycline in combination with cyclophosphamide (AC) are at great risk of developing acute CINV and should receive a three-drug antiemetic regimen, including single doses of a 5-HT₃ antagonist, dexamethasone, and aprepitant, before chemotherapy. Patients receiving MEC, not including AC, as mentioned, should receive a 5-HT₃ receptor antagonist plus dexamethasone for prophylaxis of acute CINV. (4) The prevention of delayed CINV in patients receiving MEC depends upon the chemotherapy agent and the antiemetics used to prevent acute CINV. Dexamethasone or aprepitant is suggested to prevent delayed emesis in patients receiving a 5-HT₃ receptor antagonist, dexamethasone, and aprepitant to prevent acute CINV, while oral dexamethasone alone is the preferred treatment to prevent delayed CINV in patients who are receiving MEC without aprepitant as part of their prophylaxis for acute emesis. A 5-HT$_3$ receptor antagonist is an alternative if a corticosteroid cannot be used. (5) A single antiemetics agent is suggested to prevent acute CINV in patients receiving chemotherapy of low emetic risk (LEC). (6) Prophylactic antiemetic agents are not recommended for those patients who are receiving chemotherapy of minimal emetic risk and do not have a history of nausea or vomiting. (7) Patients receiving multiple-day treatment with cisplatin should receive a 5-HT$_3$ antagonist and dexamethasone for acute CINV and dexamethasone for delayed CINV. (8) Anticipatory CINV should be aggressively avoided by achieving the best possible control of acute and delayed emesis. Psychological interventions are recommended to treat anticipatory CINV. Benzodiazepines may also be given as needed (37).

Antiemetic Agents: Special Considerations

It is important to understand the mechanisms of action, potential side effects, and the drug-drug interactions of commonly used antiemetic agents to prevent and treat CINV. The older antiemetics include the phenothiazines (chlorpromazine), butyrophenones (haloperidol), and cannabinoids. They exhibit modest activity and have a number of side effects. They are not routinely used for CINV, but remain as options to consider for breakthrough or refractory nausea and vomiting. Phenothiazines are available in the oral and intravenous route. The intravenous route appears to be more active; however, it is occasionally associated with severe hypotension (34). Both phenothiazines and butyrophenones exert their antiemetics activity as dopamine (D2) antagonists. Unfortunately, they are also associated with acute dystonic reactions, including torticollis and trismus. Patients 30 years old and younger are at greater risk of experiencing these side effects (34). Torticollis and trismus are managed with intravenous diphenhydramine (Benadryl) or anticholinergics. Haloperidol is less sedating; however, it is associated with greater extrapyramidal reactions that may limit its use. The cannabinoids are predominantly centrally acting; however, they may also have an effect on gastrointestinal function by a peripheral mechanism (34,42). They include the semisynthetic agents, including dronabinol, nabilone, and levonantradol, as well as tetrahydrocannabinol (THC) and inhaled marijuana. They are often associated with autonomic side effects, including dizziness, dry mouth, and hypotension (34), as well as perceptual disturbance, confusion, and somnolence (42). Benzodiazepines may be used as an adjuvant medication to treat the anxiety associated with chemotherapy, but have little efficacy as a single agent in treating CINV (34). They may cause sedation.

The more active and better-tolerated agents include the 5-HT$_3$ antagonists, corticosteroids, and NK1 antagonists. Metoclopramide at high doses is thought to exert its effect as a 5-HT$_3$ antagonist. The newer selective 5-HT$_3$ antagonists include ondansetron, dolasetron, granisetron, tropisetron, and palonosetron. They provide good antiemetics control and have less severe side effects (34). The antiemetic efficacy and

---

TABLE 28.3
MASCC Recommendations for Prophylaxis of CINV

EMETOGENIC POTENTIAL	ACUTE CINV– ANTIEMETICS	DELAYED CINV-ANTIEMETICS
High	Serotonic antagonist + dexamethasone + aprepitant	Dexamethasone + aprepitant
Anthracycline (A)+ Cyclophosphamide (C)	Serotonin antagonist + examethazone + aprepitant	Dexamethasone or aprepitant
Moderate (Other than AC)	Serotonin antagonist + dexamethasone	Dexamethasone Serotonin antagonist is an alternative
Low	A single agent such as dexamethasone	No routine prophylaxis
Minimal	No routine prophylaxis	No routine prophylaxis

Abbreviations: CINV, chemotherapy-induced nausea and vomiting; MASCC, Multinational Association of Supportive Care in Oncology.
Source: From Ref. 37.

TABLE 28.4
MASCC Recommended Dosing for Prophylaxis of CINV

ANTIEMETIC	RISK	ACUTE EMESIS	DELAYED EMESIS
5-HT$_3$ antagonist			
	Ondansetron		IV 8 mg or 0.15 mg/kg PO 16 mg[a]
	Granisetron		IV 1 mg or 0.01 mg/kg PO 2 mg (or 1 mg[b])
	Dolasetron		IV 100 mg or 1.8 mg/kg PO 100 mg
	Tropisetron		IV 5 mg PO 5 mg
	Palonosetron		IV 0.25 mg
Dexamethasone	High	20 mg once (12 mg when used with aprepitant)[c]	8 mg twice a day for 3–4 d (8 mg once daily when used with aprepitant)
	Moderate	8 mg once (12 mg once daily when used with aprepitant)[c]	8 mg daily for 2–3 d
	Low		4–8 mg once
Aprepitant	125 mg orally, once		80 mg orally, once for 2 d

[a]Randomized studies have tested the 8-mg, twice-daily schedule.
[b]The 1-mg dose preferred by some MASCC panelists.
[c]The 12-mg dose of dexamethasone is the only one tested with aprepitant in large randomized trials.

Source: Adapted from: http://2006.confex.com/uicc/uicc/techprogram/P9944.HTM

adverse effects of these selective 5-HT$_3$ antagonists are comparable in controlled trials (29,35,37). Intravenous and oral formulations are equally safe and effective (35,37). Common side effects of the 5-HT$_3$ antagonists include mild headaches, usually self-limiting, as well as constipation and transient transaminase elevations (29,34,35).

Corticosteroids are effective antiemetics and are commonly used as single agents as well as in combination with other antiemetics, as described earlier. Their mechanism of action is not well understood. Caution should be taken in those with diabetes, as their serum glucose levels may be transiently elevated. Epigastric burning, sleep disturbances (38), and emotional liability may be reported.

The NK1 antagonist aprepitant is also a new, effective, and well-tolerated antiemetic. Aprepitant is a moderate inhibitor of CYP3A4. The metabolism of corticosteroids, which are 3A4 substrates, has been shown to be affected in normal volunteers when taken in combination with aprepitant (38). In current research studies, the treatment arm that combined aprepitant with corticosteroids was reduced, taking the known interaction into consideration and ensuring

comparable exposures (29). The recent 2006 update of guidelines for antiemetics in oncology formulated by the American Society of Clinical Oncology (ASCO) recommends the use of a lower dose of dexamethasone when administered as an antiemetic with aprepitant. This recommendation does not apply to the dose of prednisolone, dexamethasone, or any other steroid that is given as an anticancer therapy (35). Additionally, the serum levels of medications metabolized by cytochrome CYP2C9, such as phenytoin, tolbutamide, and warfarin, may be reduced, as well as the efficacy of oral contraceptives (29). Generally, aprepitant is well tolerated, and the most common adverse events reported in randomized trials were fatigue and asthenia. Other side effects reported include anorexia, nausea, constipation, diarrhea, and hiccups (42).

Radiation-Induced Nausea and Vomiting

Radiation-induced nausea and vomiting (RINV) is a serious concern for both oncologists and patients. An estimated one-third to three-fourths of patients receiving radiation therapy may experience RINV, with a potential greater incidence in females less than 50 years old with a previous history of RINV or CINV (37,43–45). The rehabilitation specialist may encounter cancer patients undergoing radiation therapy in a number of rehabilitation settings. An understanding of the strategies used to manage RINV is imperative to improve patient tolerance, ensure completion of radiation treatment, and successfully meet rehabilitation goals. Cancer patients are often admitted to the acute inpatient rehabilitation unit to continue both radiation therapy and physical rehabilitation. Understanding the management strategies for RINV is important for the rehabilitation specialist. This section will briefly discuss the current guidelines for emetogenic risk stratification as well as treatment and prevention recommendations for RINV. Similar to the discussion in the CINV section, the emetogenic risk of the therapeutic agent ultimately guides the physician's antiemetic treatment strategy. Furthermore, a risk-adjusted treatment for RINV has been proposed which takes into account not only emetogenic risk of the radiation, but also the added risk factors of the patient's age, sex, and history of chemoradiation-induced emesis (43).

The mechanism of RINV is still unclear, but is likely mediated by damage to the enterochromaffin cells within the GI tract, which sets off the serotonin pathway, similar to that described in CINV. Expectedly, the greater the body area being irradiated, along with greater treatment fractions, increases the risk and severity of RINV (44).

According to Feyer et al. (43), the international guidelines by ASCO, American Society of Health Systems Pharmacists (ASHP), MASCC, and National Comprehensive Cancer Network (NCCN) for antiemetic use in radiotherapy are conflicting and sufficient evidence in clear support of any one particular guideline is absent. The subsequent confusion over which guideline to use may contribute to the inadequate prophylaxis and treatment of RINV in the cancer patient population. According to a study done by the Italian Group for Anti-emetic Research in Radiotherapy (IGARR), only a small percentage of the studied patients received antiemetics (14%). Furthermore, more patients received rescue antiemetic doses instead of prophylactic doses (9% vs 5%), if they received any at all (43,44).

Recently in 2006, a panel of international oncology experts updated the guidelines previously published in an effort to decrease the confusion over emetogenic risk and antiemetic selection for both CINV and RINV. As efforts are continually made to reconcile previous organizational differences as well as to include new findings, the hope is to internationally standardize treatment and give every patient the most optimal care. The uses and mechanisms of 5-HT$_3$ receptor antagonists (5-HT3RA), as well as steroids, have been briefly described in the CINV section of this chapter

and will not be readdressed here. The Perugia Conference discussed the new derivatives of serotonin receptor antagonist and the comparison of one over the other in controlling emesis. At this time, the consensus is to continue using 5-HT3RA as the primary choice for both rescue and prophylaxis against RINV (37).

The latest international RINV treatment guidelines were updated at the Antiemetic Consensus Conference Perugia 2007. Further information is available at www.MASCC.org.

CANCER-TREATMENT-INDUCED DIARRHEA

Diarrhea is a common complication experienced by cancer patients. Diarrhea is defined as "frequent defecation, passage of loose or watery stools, fecal urgency, or a similar sense of incomplete evacuation" (46) and may occur as a side effect of chemotherapy or radiation, as well as be a sign of infection. The common causes of diarrhea among cancer patients are outlined in Table 28.5 (47). The common toxicity criteria used to determine grade or severity are outlined in Table 28.6 (48). Early recognition and treatment of diarrhea may prevent delays or interruption of cancer treatment and may potentially prevent life-threatening consequences,

---

TABLE 28.5
Common Causes of Diarrhea Among Cancer Patients

Drugs
  Laxatives
  Antibiotics
  Antacids
Chemotherapy
  5-fluorouracil
  Irinotecan (CPT-11)
  Docetaxel
Radiotherapy
  Pelvic Radiotherapy
Intestinal Obstruction
  Fecal impaction with overflow
Concurrent disease
  Inflammatory bowel disease
Malabsorption
  Pancreatic cancer
  Biliary obstruction
  Fistula
  Short bowel
Islet cell tumors
  Carcinoid
  VIPoma
  Gastrinoma

TABLE 28.6
National Cancer Institute's Common Toxicity Criteria for Grading Severity of Diarrhea

Toxicity	0	1	2	3	4
Patients without a colostomy	None	Increase of <4 stools/day over pretreatment	Increase of 4–6 stools/day of nocturnal stools	Increase of >7 stools/day	>10 stools/day
	None	None	Moderate cramping; not interfering with normal activity	Severe cramping and incontinence; interfering with daily activities	Grossly bloody diarrhea and need for parenteral support
Patients with a colostomy	None	Mild increase in loose, watery colostomy output compared with pretreatment	Moderate increase in loose, watery colostomy output compared with pretreatment, but not interfering with normal activity	Severe increase in loose, watery colostomy output compared with pretreatment; interfering with normal activity	Physiological consequences requiring intensive care; hemodynamic collapse

including dehydration, electrolyte imbalances, mental status changes, malnutrition, compromised immune function, perianal skin breakdown, and functional decline (47–51).

Vigilant monitoring of GI toxicities during chemotherapy was heightened following two independent prospective National Cancer Institute (NCI)–sponsored cooperative group trials investigating the combination regimen of irinotecan (CPT-11) plus bolus fluorouracil (FU)/leucovorin, known as IFL. The early death rates in the treatment arms that were receiving IFL were approximately two times higher than that of the controls and were determined by an independent panel to be caused by GI toxicity and cardiovascular events (48). The majority of the GI-associated deaths consisted of a GI syndrome with symptoms including severe nausea, vomiting, diarrhea, anorexia, and abdominal cramping. The subjects experienced severe dehydration, electrolyte imbalances, neutropenia, and fever. Abdominal cramping was determined to be a warning sign of imminent diarrhea (48). The independent panel recommended that diarrhea and other GI toxicities should be intensively monitored and treated, and furthermore, dose adjustments or discontinuation of chemotherapy should be made in future patients treated with IFL (48). Table 28.7 highlights the common chemotherapy agents with high rates of GI toxicities causing diarrhea.

The heightened awareness that potential GI toxicities causing diarrhea may occur during the course of chemotherapy and/or radiotherapy has led to a number of treatment strategies. Additional causes of diarrhea may include infections and obstructions of the GI tract. Evaluation and treatment strategies of infectious diarrhea will be discussed in a subsequent section. It is important for rehabilitation specialists to be aware of these potentially life-threatening complications and regularly monitor patients who are receiving chemotherapy or radiation therapy for diarrhea and other GI toxicities. Rehabilitation specialists must consider the spectrum of potential causes of diarrhea in the cancer patient and be vigilant to determine whether the etiology of the diarrhea is treatment-induced or of other origins. The following sections will highlight the pathophysiology of diarrhea, with specific reference to chemotherapy-induced and radiation-induced mechanisms, as well as the current management guidelines and special pharmacological considerations.

Pathophysiology

The pathophysiology of cancer-treatment-induced diarrhea (CTID) is not well understood, but thought to be multifactorial. Chemotherapy agents, such as CPT-11 and 5-FU, induce maturational arrest and cell death of the intestinal crypt cells responsible for the absorption of nutrients and other food substances. Damage to the crypt cells leads to the release of prostaglandins, cytokines, leukotrienes, and free radicals, with inflammation of the intestine. This leads to a loss of absorptive area and subsequent imbalance of absorption and secretion. The brush border enzymes responsible for the terminal digestion of proteins and carbohydrates are also damaged. It is felt that these processes increase the secretion of intestinal fluid and electrolytes and magnify this imbalance. Infection and antibiotic use may cause

TABLE 28.7
Incidence of Diarrhea Associated with Selected Chemotherapy Agents

AGENT	INCIDENCE OF DIARRHEA (%)	
	ALL[a] (GRADES 1 TO 4)	SEVERE[a] (GRADES 3 AND 4)
5-Fluorouracil		
Single-agent therapy		
IV bolus	43	9
Continuous infusion	26	5
Combination therapy		
IV bolus + low-dose		
leucovorin (20 mg/m^2)	48	10
IV bolus + high-dose		
leucovorin (200 mg/m^2)	56	23
Continuous infusion + low-dose leucovorin	34	9
INF-α-2a	41	
CPT-11		
100–125 mg/m2a	50–80	5–30
150 mg /m 2b	80	24
Topotecan	32	13
Capecitabine (5-FU prodrug)		30
Infusional 5-FU		12–21
Irinotecan/oxaliplatin		20
Oxaliplatin + infusional 5-FU/LV		11

Abbreviations: CPT-11, irinotecan; INF-α-2a, interferon alpha 2a; IV, intravenous; LV, leucovorin.
[a]National Cancer Institute Common Toxicity Criteria Grades

Source: Adapted from Kornblau and Viele (Refs. 49 and 50).

additional changes and damage of the gastrointestinal tract. The combination of these mechanisms results in an increased secretion of water and electrolytes in the diarrhea (50).

Assessment and Treatment Guidelines

The ASCO published updated recommendations in 2004 for the assessment and treatment of cancer-treatment-induced diarrhea. The ASCO guidelines for assessment (Fig. 28.2) emphasize the need for diligent monitoring of symptoms, including the myriad of symptoms, signs, duration, and severity, using the Common Toxicity Criteria (CTC), Version 2, for diarrhea (Table 28.7). The number of daily stools over baseline, presence of nocturnal diarrhea, and stool composition should also be assessed. The presence of added risk factors should be noted, including fever, abdominal pain/cramping, weakness, and orthostatic symptoms such as dizziness. The physical examination should include evaluation of

hydration status, serial abdominal exams, rectal exam, and regular assessment for perianal skin breakdown. Based on the significant mortality that occurred during the two NCI–sponsored cooperative group trials using the IFL regimen, it is also recommended that blood tests be performed on those receiving GI toxic chemotherapy no more than 48 hours before scheduled treatment to evaluate for neutropenia, as well as hydration and electrolyte status.

Once the assessment has been made, the diarrhea is classified as "uncomplicated" or "complicated" based on the constellation of symptoms and signs. This will determine the course of treatment. Patients with grade 1 or 2 diarrhea and no other complicating factors are classified as "uncomplicated" and managed conservatively. Patients with grade 1 or 2 diarrhea and one or more of the following risk factors are classified as "complicated" and should be managed more aggressively. The risk factors include moderate to severe cramping, ≥grade 2 nausea/vomiting, dehydration,

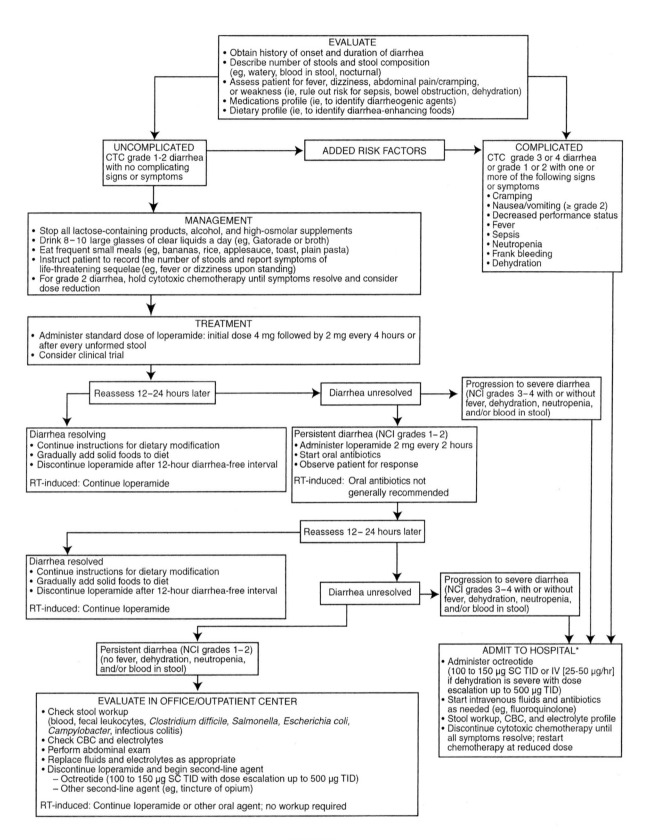

FIGURE 28.2

ASCO guidelines for treatment of cancer-treatment-induced diarrhea. Reprinted with permission from Ref. 6.

decreased performance status, fever, sepsis, neutropenia, or frank bleeding. Patients with grade 3 or 4 diarrhea are classified as "complicated" and require aggressive management (48). The ASCO guidelines emphasize the importance of recognizing warning signs of crampy abdominal pain that is often a harbinger of severe diarrhea and fever that may indicate an infection. Early detection and prompt initiation of treatment may prevent the potentially life-threatening consequences of CTID (48).

The management of uncomplicated grades 1 and 2 diarrhea includes dietary management and initiation of loperamide, with a standard initial dose of 4 mg followed by 2 mg every 4 hours or after every unformed stool. The patient should be reassessed in 12–24 hours, and further treatment depends on the persistence of diarrhea. If the diarrhea has progressed to NCI grades 3–4, with or without complicating factors, it is recommended that the patient be admitted to an acute care hospital for more intensive management, including the administration of the somatostatin analogue octreotide 100–150 μg subcutaneously three times a day or 25–50 μg/hour intravenously. Additional aggressive treatment includes hydration, possible initiation of antibiotics, stool workup, complete blood count, and electrolyte panel. Cytotoxic chemotherapy agents should be discontinued until all symptoms resolve for 24 hours. Subsequent doses of chemotherapy should be started at lower doses. The treatment with octreotide, as well as treatment of dehydration and other complicating factors should continue until the patient is free of diarrhea for 24 hours. Patients who initially demonstrate "complicated" grade 1 or 2, as well as either grade 3 or 4, should be admitted to an acute care hospital immediately to begin the aggressive protocol.

Patients who are undergoing pelvic or abdominal radiation are at risk of developing crampy abdominal pain and diarrhea due to acute enteritis. The incidence is reported to be as high as 50% (48) and even higher in those receiving concomitant chemotherapy. Symptoms commonly occur during the third week of fractionated radiation therapy (48). Those with radiation-induced diarrhea (RID) are evaluated and treated using the same ASCO protocol, with a few modifications. In those with uncomplicated grade 1 or 2 diarrhea, loperamide and, alternatively, diphenoxylate are the pharmacological agents of choice. The diarrhea with any associated symptoms and signs should be reassessed in 12–24 hours. If the diarrhea persists as an uncomplicated grade 1 or 2, loperamide administration should be intensified to 2 mg every two hours. In RID, oral antibiotics are not recommended unless an infection is definitively present. If the diarrhea is at any time a grade 3 or 4, or if it initially presents as a complicated grade 1 or 2, aggressive management should

be sought in an acute care hospital. Occasionally, outpatients experiencing uncomplicated RID of grade 3 or 4 are managed at home or at an intensive day hospital. There have been clinical trials evaluating the role of sucralfate, sulfasalazine, olsalazine, and octreotide in preventing RID. The results are inconclusive and are currently not recommended for the prevention of RID (48,52). The role of preparations with probiotic lactic-acid-producing bacteria administered prophylactically to patients receiving radiation has shown some promise in preventing and/or minimizing the severity of RID by restoring the gut flora that is potentially disturbed during radiation (52).

Pharmacological Considerations

As mentioned previously, octreotide (Sandostatin) is necessary for complicated or grade 3 or 4 diarrhea. It is approved by the U.S. Food and Drug Administration (FDA) for diarrhea secondary to carcinoid syndrome and vasoactive intestinal peptide-secreting tumors, but may be used "off-label" to control other cases of severe diarrhea, such as cancer-treatment-induced diarrhea. Octreotide is a synthetic analogue of somatostatin, a naturally occurring hormone produced in the brain and in the alimentary tract. It is an inhibitory hormone, suppressing the release of many gastrointestinal hormones responsible for diarrhea. Its actions resulted in a lower rate of gastric emptying and a reduction in smooth muscle contractions and blood flow within the intestine (53). It also acts by inhibiting growth-hormone-releasing hormone and thyroid-stimulating hormone, and its most common side effects are related to these actions. Hyperglycemia and hypoglycemia occur from a reported 1.5%–16%. Serious cardiovascular events, such as dysrhythmias, occur in about 10% of patients, and sinus bradycardia occurs in approximately 25%. A common potentially confounding side effect is the 22%–33% incidence of cholelithiasis that results from the overall reduced activity of the alimentary tract. Periodic electrocardiograms (ECGs), routine blood glucose levels, and thyroid function should be monitored throughout the course of octreotide. Octreotide is given in nonoral routes for those patients who have concurrent nausea and vomiting. It may be administered in the intravenous form as well as intramuscular and subcutaneous injections. A depot subcutaneous injection also exists. Octreotide should be renally dosed for those with poor kidney function.

Loperamide (Imodium, Imodium AD, Diamode, Imotil, Pepto) is a commonly used medication indicated to treat diarrhea of several etiologies. It is an opioid μ-receptor agonist that acts upon the myenteric plexus and does not affect the central nervous system. It acts by slowing peristalsis in the large colon and increasing transit time of fecal matter, allowing for greater water reabsorption and less frequent defecation. Diphenoxylate (Lomotil) is a similar antidiarrhea medication that functions as a μ and μ opioid receptor agonist in the gastrointestinal tract and does not readily cross the blood-brain barrier. Diphenoxylate has been shown to be habit-forming. Thus, Lomotil is prepared with a small dose of atropine. This strategy is employed to discourage the abuse of Lomotil by using the anticholinergic effects of atropine, nausea, and weakness if recommended dosages are exceeded. In adults, there are no serious adverse effects for loperamide, and the common side effects are somnolence, dizziness, fatigue, nausea, vomiting, hyperglycemia, and xerostomia (53). Diphenoxylate has a similar side-effect profile. In addition, it has three potentially serious adverse effects when combined with therapeutic doses of atropine, including toxic megacolon, pancreatitis, and anaphylaxis (53). Loperanide and diphenoxylate are both available in oral forms. Loperamide is reported to be two to three times more potent than diphenoxylate as an antidiarrheal agent on a per-milligram basis (54).

GASTROINTESTINAL INFECTIONS

The healthy individual with an intact immune system can ward off many of the infections that are introduced from the external environment. However, patients with cancer have a compromised immune system. Furthermore, treatments can be immunosuppressive and may leave the patients increasingly vulnerable to infections. A decreased appetite and progressive malnutrition following chemoradiation treatments can further weaken the immune system.

The hallmark sign of infection is fever. Temperatures greater than 100.5°F should prompt a thorough exam and blood workup for infection, with subsequent initiation of empiric broad-spectrum antibiotic therapy for those with concomitant neutropenia (55–58). According to the current guidelines, an absolute neutrophil count (ANC) of less than 1,000 cells/microL poses a moderate risk of infection. This risk becomes serious when the count drops below 500. At this point, the patient is unable to mount the necessary inflammatory response to fight many infectious agents (58). Additionally, one should be mindful of the noninfectious causes of fever specific to this patient population, such as tumor burden, drug reaction, and blood product hypersensitivity, and therefore manage the workup accordingly. Other classic signs and symptoms suspicious for infection include chills, shortness of breath, fatigue, cough, skin changes (especially around peripheral lines/drains/tubes), diarrhea, difficulty urinating,

and pain. The following section will briefly describe four common GI infections in the cancer patient.

Oral mucositis or stomatitis is an inflammation of the oral mucosal membrane commonly found in cancer patients undergoing chemotherapy or head and neck radiation therapy. If untreated, the inflammation can evolve into mucosal ulcerations, which can become superinfected by viral, fungal, or bacterial pathogens, leading to significant morbidity. The pathophysiology involves chemoradiation-therapy-induced cell damage and subsequent up-regulation of inflammatory cytokines that lead to ulceration of the mucosa. Symptoms range from mild discomfort to pain severe enough to limit food and fluid intake, which can understandably prevent continued cancer treatment. Therefore, a careful daily oral tissue examination in those at risk for developing stomatitis, as well as monitoring patient symptoms, can lead to early detection and treatment of ulcerative lesions (Table 28.8).

Prevention strategies include good oral hygiene with soft toothbrushes, removal of dental caries, mucosal barriers and coating agents, mucosal cell stimulants, and topical anesthetics for pain control (59). Benzydamine is currently recommended to prevent radiation-induced mucositis in those receiving moderate-dose radiation therapies. Sucralfate and antimicrobial lozenges are not recommended. Complete resolution of severe mucositis may require radiation treatment breaks (60). For standard-dose chemotherapy-induced mucositis prevention, patients receiving 5-fluorouracil (5-FU) should undergo 30 minutes of oral cryotherapy. Neither chlorhexidine nor acyclovir is recommended for routine prevention of mucositis (61,62).

Infectious esophagitis is common in immunocompromised cancer patients receiving steroids, antibiotics, and chemotherapy or radiation therapy. The etiology is usually viral and/or fungal in origin, with *Candida*, herpes simplex virus (HSV), and cytomegalovirus (CMV) occurring most frequently (63). Symptoms include neck

TABLE 28.8
World Health Organization Classification of Oral Mucositis

Grade	Signs and Symptoms
0	No symptoms
1	Sore mouth, no ulcers
2	Sore mouth with ulcers, but able to eat normally
3	Liquid diet only
4	Unable to eat or drink

Source: From Ref. 59.

and chest pain, usually aggravated by eating or swallowing. The patient may exhibit difficulty swallowing (dysphagia), painful swallowing (odynophagia), upper GI bleed, and/or oral ulcers. Currently, those predisposed to such infections receive prophylactic antifungal or antiviral medications, or both in cases of concomitant infection. In refractory cases, endoscopy with biopsy can reveal the exact causative organism and can help direct the appropriate treatment. Fluconazole, acyclovir, and ganciclovir are first-line treatments for *Candida*, HSV, and CMV esophagitis, respectively (63). Bacterial infections may coexist and can also be diagnosed through endoscopy and treated with the appropriate antibiotics.

Infectious pseudomembranous colitis due to *Clostridium difficile* (CD) is not uncommon in those receiving prophylactic or therapeutic antibiotics. The toxin has been reportedly found in as many as 25% of patients with antibiotic-associated diarrhea and 95% of patients with pseudomembranous colitis (64,65). The patient presents with frequent bouts of watery diarrhea with fever and leukocytosis, but in mild cases, the patient may remain afebrile. Antibiotic-associated CD colitis may produce symptoms 4–7 days after initiating or weeks after discontinuing the antibiotic. It can also be spread from person to person via fecal-oral transmission and is, therefore, preventable by wearing gloves and gowns when in direct contact with areas that may be contaminated (64). Attention to good hand hygiene by hospital staff and patient further decreases the rate of transmission. Diarrhea from CD colitis and chemotherapy-induced diarrhea may initially be difficult to distinguish. In both cases, CD toxins should be sent. If CD colitis is suspected, prophylactic oral metronidazole should be initiated after sending a stool culture for *C. difficile* toxins. The clinician must be aware that antidiarrheal or antiperistaltic agents, such as loperamide and Lomotil, indicated in chemotherapy-induced diarrhea, are contraindicated for symptomatic diarrhea control in CD colitis because

they can delay the clearance of CD toxins and lead to toxic megacolon (66,67). The original antibiotics that lead to the CD colitis should be discontinued and a new antibiotic should be initiated. Oral vancomycin is an effective alternative treatment of CD colitis in those who develop metronidazole-refractory CD colitis. Ensuring adequate intravenous or oral correction of potential fluid and electrolyte abnormalities from diarrhea is as important as antibiotic coverage. Institutions should have a policy on the management of CD infections. Many rehabilitation units require the patient to remain on contact and isolation precautions for at least 72 hours after being free of diarrhea and having negative repeat stool cultures. The patient should be allowed to continue therapy as long as the patient and the contaminants are contained. The patient should be thoroughly cleaned and outerwear decontaminated prior to active participation in therapy (65).

Finally, anorectal infections are serious complications of chemotherapy. A 2002 retrospective review of anorectal infections in 64 patients over a 12-year period at the NCI revealed that the overall incidence of perirectal abscess, perirectal or rectal cellulites, and anorectal infections was 34% in a variable cancer population (68). Whereas the morbidity and mortality of these infections were as high as 50% 30 years ago, improved early empiric interventions have dramatically improved prognosis and decreased mortality. Patients with anorectal infections may present with buttocks, pelvic, and/or rectal pain; fever; perianal erythema; and/or a draining abscess. The workup includes a wound culture to determine speciation and sensitivity. The patient should be started immediately on empiric antibiotics. Studies have used early broad-spectrum cephalosporins or a penicillin/aminoglycoside combination as first-line empiric therapy. Anaerobic coverage should be added if the infection does not respond to the initial antibiotics (68) (Table 28.9). Interestingly, *Pseudomonas* infections have been decreasing in multiple cancer centers nationwide.

TABLE 28.9
Antibiotic Choices for Anorectal Infections

Source	Initial Therapy	Severe/Refractory
Glenn et al. (1)	Broad-spectrum cephalosporin or combination of extended penicillin plus aminoglycoside	Anaerobic coverage
Pizzo et al. (2)	Ceftazidime, imipenem, or	Anaerobic coverage with
Freifeld et al. (3,4)	combination of oral cipro/augmentin or	metronidazole or clindamycin
Febrile neutropenic	aminoglycoside if drug sensitivity	

Source: Adapted from Ref. 68.

Infection control begins with prevention, and that responsibility falls on both the patient and the medical staff. Maintaining good personal hygiene and frequently washing hands are two important steps to mitigate infection risk (58), particularly in the immunocompromised cancer patient. When infection is suspected, starting early empiric antibiotic therapy is appropriate and can decrease associated morbidity. As the rehabilitation team controls infection, the patient gains more opportunity to work with the therapists to restore their maximal functional capacity.

CONCLUSION

Cancer rehabilitation includes vigilant monitoring for gastrointestinal complications of cancer. Gastrointestinal complications resulting from cancer treatment are variable in presentation and often multifactorial. Proper diagnosis of treatment-related symptoms and more serious sequelae is imperative. A thorough understanding of the complex nature of how cancer affects the gastrointestinal organ system allows the physician to provide a more complete and enhanced care. Consequently, the goal of preserving and perhaps improving one's quality of life while minimizing morbidity and mortality may be realized.

References

1. Baines M. ABC of palliative care: nausea, vomiting, and intestinal obstruction. *BMJ.* 1997;315:1148–1150.
2. Ripamonti C, DeConno F, et al. Management of bowel obstruction in advanced and terminal cancer patients. *Ann Oncol.* 1993;4(1):15–21.
3. Khurana B, Ledbetter S, et al. Bowel obstruction revealed by multidetector CT. *AJR.* 2002;178:1139–1144.
4. NCI. *Gastrointestinal Complications (PDQR), National Cancer Institute*, February 2003. National Cancer Institute February 26, 2005. http://www.nci.nih.gov.
5. Frager D, Medwid S, et al. CT of small-bowel obstruction: value in establishing the diagnosis and determining the degree and cause. *AJR.* 1994;162:37–41.
6. Dauphine C, Tan P, et al. Placement of self-expanding metal stents for acute malignant large-bowel obstruction: a collective review. *Ann Surg Oncol.* 2002;9(6):574–579.
7. Tang E, Davis J, et al. Bowel obstruction in cancer patients. *Arch Surg.* 1995;130(8):832–837.
8. Kim J, Song H, et al. Stent collapse as a delayed complication of placement of a covered gastroduodenal stent. *Am J Roentgenol.* 2007;188(6):1495–1499.
9. Ripamonti C, Fagnoni E, et al. Management of symptoms due to inoperable bowel obstruction. *Tumori.* 2005;91(3):233–236.
10. Marquis P, Marrel A, et al. Quality of life in patients with stomas: the montreux study. *Ostomy Wound Manage.* 2003;49(2):48–55.
11. Gooszen A, Geelkerken R, et al. Quality of life with a temporary stoma: Ileostomy versus colostomy. *Dis Colon Rectum.* 2000;43(5):650–655.
12. Doughty D. Principles of ostomy management in the oncology patient. *J Support Oncol.* 2005;3(1):59–69.
13. Colwell J. (2004). Principles of stoma management. Fecal and Urinary Diversions: Management Principles. Mo:Mosby: 240-262.
14. Colwell J, Goldberg M, et al. The state of the standard diversion. *J Wound Ostomy Continence Nurs.* 2001;28(1):6–17.
15. Floruta C. Dietary choices of people with ostomies. *J Wound Ostomy Continence Nurs.* 2001;28(1):8–31.
16. Park J, Del Pino A, et al. Stoma complications: The Cook County Hospital experience. *Dis Colon Rectum.* 1999;42(12):1575–1580.
17. Thyssen E, Weinstock L, et al. Medical treatment of benign gastrocolic fistula. *Ann Int Med.* 1993;118(6):433–435.
18. Pichney L. Gastrocolic and duodenocolic fistulas in Crohn's disease. *J Clin Gastroenterology.* 1992;15:205–211.
19. Pearlstein L, Jones C, et al. Gastrocutaneous fistula: etiology and treatment. *Ann Surg.* 1978;187(2):223–226.
20. Hitomi S, et al. Colocutaneous fistula after PEG. *Digestion.* 2007;75:103.
21. Chaudhry C. The challenge of enterocutaneous fistula. *Med J Armed Forces India.* 2004;60:235–238.
22. Present D. Crohn's fistula: current concepts in management. *Gastroenterology.* 2003;124:1629–1635.
23. Gage E, Jones G, et al. Treatment of enterocutaneous fistula in pancreas transplant recipients using percutaneous drainage and fibrin sealant: three case reports. *Transplantation.* 2006;82(9):1238–1240.
24. Gillis T, Donovan E. Rehabilitation following bone marrow transplantation. *Cancer.* 2001;92(4):998–1007.
25. Childs R. Allogenetic hematopoietic stem cell transplantation. In: *Cancer: Principles and Practice of Oncology.* Philadelphia, Lippincott, Williams and Wilkins; 2005:2423–2432.
26. O'Dorisio T, Mekhjian H, et al. Medical therapy of VIPomas. *Endocrinol Metabol Clin North Am.* 1989;18:545–556.
27. Modlin I, Lye K, et al. A 5-decade analysis of 13,715 carcinoid tumors. *Cancer.* 2003;97:934–959.
28. Kulke MH, Mayer RJ. Carcinoid tumors. *N Engl J Med.* 1999;340:858.
29. Aguilar A, Figueiras C, Cortes-Funes, et al. Clinical practice guidelines on antiemetics in oncology. *Expert Rev. Anticancer Ther.* 2005;5(6):963–972.
30. Ettinger D, Bierman P, et al. Antiemesis: clinical practice guidelines in oncology. *J Nat Comp Cancer Network.* 2007;5(1):12–33.
31. Lindley CM, Bernard S, et al. Incidence and duration of chemotherapy induced nausea and vomiting in the outpatient oncology clinic. *J Clin Oncol.* 1989;7(8):1142–1149.
32. Mitchell E. Gastrointestinal toxicity of chemotherapeutic agents. Elsevier Inc, *Semin Oncol.* 2006;33:106–120.
33. Antiemetic Subcommittee of the Multinational Association of Supportive Care in Cancer MASCC, Prevention of chemotherapy and radiotherapy-induced emesis: Results of the Perugia Consensus Conference. *Annal Oncol.* 2006;17:20–28.
34. Berger A, Rebecca A, et al. Chemotherapy-related nausea and vomiting. In: Berger AM, et al., eds., *Principles and Practice of Palliative Care and Supportive Oncology,* Third Edition. Philadelphia, PA: Lippincott, Williams, Wilkin; 2007:139–149.
35. Kris, M, Hesketh P, et al. Consensus proposals for the prevention of acute and delayed vomiting and nausea following high-emetic-risk chemotherapy. *Support Care Cancer.* 2005;13:85–96.
36. Hesketh PJ, et al. Differential involvement of neurotransmitters through the time course of cisplatin-induced emesis as revealed by therapy with specific receptor antagonists. *Eur J Cancer.* 2003;39:1074.
37. MASCC. Prevention of chemotherapy and radiotherapy induced emesis: results of the 2004 Perugia International Antiemetic Consensus Conference. *The Antiemetic Subcommittee of the Multinational Association of the Supportive Care in Cancer.* 2006;17:20–28.
38. Kris M, Hesketh P, et al. American Society of clinical oncology guidelines for antiemetics in oncology: update 2006. *J Clin Oncol.* 2006;24(18):2932–2947.

39. Grunberg S. Antiemetic activity of corticosteroids in patients receiving cancer chemotherapy: dosing, efficacy and tolerability analysis. *Ann Oncol.* 2007;18:233–240.

40. Hesketh, Paul J, et. al. Proposal for classifying the acute emetogenicity of cancer chemotherapy. *J Clin Oncol.* 1997;15:103–109.

41. Grunberg S, Osoba D, et al. Evaluation of new antiemetics agents and definition of antineoplastic agent emetogenicity—an update. *Support Care Cancer.* 2005;13:80–84.

42. Dalal S. *Principles and Practice of Palliative Care and Supportive Oncology.* Ed Burger, A, Third Edition, Philadelphia, PA: Lippincott, Williams & Wilkin; 2007.

43. Feyer P, Maranzano E, et al. Radiotherapy-induced nausea and vomiting (RINV): antiemetic guidelines. *Support Care Cancer.* 2005;13:122–128.

44. Urba S. Radiation induced nausea and vomiting. *J Natl Compr Canc Netw.* 2007;5(1):60–65.

45. Abdelsayed G. Management of radiation induced nausea and vomiting. *Exp Hematology.* 2007;35:34–36.

46. Hasler W, Owyang C. Approach to the patient with gastrointestinal disease. In: Kasper DL, Fauci AS, Longo DL, Braunwald E, Hauser, SL, Jameson JL, Isselbacher KJ, eds., *Harrison's Principles of Internal Medicine,* 16th ed. New York, NY: McGraw-Hill; 2005:271.

47. Solomon R, et al. Constipation and diarrhea in patients with cancer. *J Cancer.* 2006;12:355–364.

48. Benson A, Ajani J, et al. Recommended guidelines for the treatment of cancer treatment-induced diarrhea. *J Clin Oncol.* 2004;22:2918–2926.

49. Viele C. Overview of chemotherapy-induced diarrhea. *Sem Oncol Nurs.* 2003;19(4 Suppl 3):2–5.

50. Kornblau S, et al. Management of cancer treatment-related diarrhea: issues and therapeutic strategies. *J Pain Symp Man.* 2000;19:118–129.

51. Waldler S, et al. Recommended guidelines for the treatment of chemotherapy-induced diarrhea. *J Clin Oncol.* 1998;16:3169–3178.

52. Delia P, Sansotta G, et al. Use of probiotics for prevention of radiation-induced diarrhea. *World J Gastro.* 2007;13(6):912–915.

53. Micromedex (2007). USPDI Updates on-line. Available at: http://uspdi.micromedex.com

54. Pelemans W, Vantrappen F. A double blind crossover comparison of loperamide with diphenoxylate in the symptomatic treatment of chronic diarrhea. *Gastroenterology.* 1976;70(6):1030–1034.

55. Durnaa B, Dzierzanowska D. Infection in neutropenic cancer patients—etiology, microbiological diagnostics, treatment. *Wiad Lek.* 2006;59(708):506–511.

56. Bodey G, Rolston K. Management of fever in neutropenic patients. *J Infect Chemother.* 2001;7(1):1–9.

57. Kibbler C. Neutropenic infections: strategies for empirical therapy. *J Antimicrob Chemother.* 1995;36(B):107–117.

58. NCCN&ACS. Fever and neutropenia: treatment guidelines for patients with cancer. *National Comprehensive Cancer Network and American Cancer Society.* 2006:II.

59. Kowanko I, Long L, et al. Prevention and treatment of oral mucositis in cancer patients. *Best Practice.* 1998;2(3):1–6.

60. Johnson J. Prevention of radiation induced mucositis. *Curr Onc Rep.* 2001;3(1):56–58.

61. Rubenstein E, et al. Clinical practice guidelines for the prevention and treatment of cancer therapy induced oral and gastrointestinal mucositis. *Cancer.* 2004;100(9):2026–2046.

62. Keefe D, et al. Updated clinical practice guidelines for the prevention and treatment of mucositis. *Cancer.* 2007;109(5):820–831.

63. Mulhall B, Wong R. Infectious esophagitis. *Curr Treatment Options Gastroent.* 2003;6(1):55–70.

64. Sunenshine R, McDonald L. Clostridium difficile associated disease: new challenges from an established pathogen. *Cleveland Clinic J Med.* 2006;73(2):187–197.

65. Divison of Epidemiology and Immunization. Massachusetts Department of Public Health. Infection control guidelines for long term care facilities. http://www.mass.gov/dph/cdc/epii/sars/infosheets/infection_control.pdf (November 29) 2007;1–5.

66. McConnell E. Prevent the spread of clostridium difficile. *Nursing.* 2002;32(8):24–25.

67. PA-PSRS. Clostridium difficile: a sometimes fatal complication of antibiotic use. *Patient Safety Advisory.* 2005;2(2):1–8.

68. Lehrnbecher T, Marshall D, et al. A second look at anorectal infections in cancer patients in a large cancer institute: the success of early intervention with antibiotics and surgery. *Infections.* 2002;30(5):272–276.

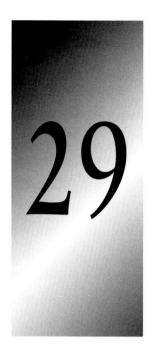

Renal Complications of Cancer

Michelle Stern
Ping Sun

Renal disease and electrolyte disorders are major causes of morbidity and mortality in the cancer setting. Renal dysfunction can cause fatigue, anemia, cognitive changes, muscle weakness, fluid overload, electrolyte abnormalities, fluctuating blood pressure, cardiac arrhythmias, and abnormal hormonal and metabolic states. Renal dysfunction may be unrelated to the patient's primary cancer or occur as a direct result of the malignancy or its treatments, including chemotherapy, bone marrow transplant, surgery, or radiation (1). Renal dysfunction and its complications can severely impact the cancer patient's function, mobility, quality of life, and ability to participate meaningfully in a rehabilitation program. Similarly, fluctuating volume status can complicate prosthetic fitting and the use of orthotics.

Renal failure can be classified by the anatomic location of pathology within the renal system (prerenal, intrinsic renal, and postrenal) or by chronicity (acute vs chronic). Prerenal failure is characterized by hypovolemia and may manifest clinically as resting and orthostatic hypotension, tachycardia, or syncope. Hypovolemia can result from depletion of extracellular fluid volume (vomiting, diarrhea, insensible fluid losses, and poor oral intake), third-space fluid accumulation (ascites, peripheral edema, lymphedema), hepatorenal syndrome (veno-occlusive disease, hepatic metastasis), and cardiovascular disease (heart failure, tamponade) (2,3). Medications that can contribute to a prerenal state

include angiotensin-converting enzyme (ACE) inhibitors, nonsteroidal anti-inflammatory drugs (NSAIDs), diuretics, and angiotensin receptor blockers (ARBs) (1,2). Intrinsic renal disease can occur at the level of the glomeruli, renal tubules, interstitial space, or vascular supply to the kidneys. A number of glomerular diseases are associated with malignancy, including membranous glomerulonephritis in lung and gastrointestinal cancers, minimal-change glomerulopathy in Hodgkin disease, and tubular-cast nephropathy with associated tubulointerstitial nephritis from the dysproteinemias associated with multiple myeloma and Waldenström macroglobulinemia (4). Postrenal dysfunction is caused by obstruction to urine flow, which can be due to tumor infiltration of the urethra, bladder, or ureters. Postrenal urinary obstruction is commonly seen as a result of progression of local tumors, such of those of the prostate, bladder, and ovaries. Retroperitoneal fibrosis and hematoma, as well as nephrolithiasis, can also cause obstruction (1).

Fluid and electrolyte disorders are exceedingly common in patients with cancer, particularly those with advanced disease or undergoing active treatment of their malignancy. Such abnormalities can result directly from the cancer or, more commonly, from its treatment. Regardless of etiology, fluid and electrolyte abnormalities can severely and adversely impact the patient's ability to participate in a rehabilitation program. The primary electrolyte abnormalities encoun-

KEY POINTS

- Renal dysfunction can cause fatigue, anemia, cognitive changes, muscle weakness, fluid overload, electrolyte abnormalities, fluctuating blood pressure, cardiac arrhythmias, and abnormal hormonal and metabolic states.
- Renal dysfunction and its complications can severely impact the cancer patient's function, mobility, quality of life, and ability to participate meaningfully in a rehabilitation program.
- Fluctuating volume status can complicate prosthetic fitting and the use of orthotics.
- Syndrome of inappropriate antidiuretic hormone secretion (SIADH) is most common in oat cell carcinoma of the lung or primary or secondary brain lesions.
- Multiple myeloma and bone marrow transplant are associated with renal dysfunction in 50% of patients.
- Current studies indicate that normalizing hemoglobin (Hb) improves exercise capacity.
- Dialysis may complicate physical therapy because of hypertension, cardiac arrhythmia, renal osteodystrophy, electrolyte disturbances, dialysis disequilibria syndrome, muscle cramps, restless leg syndrome, and fatigue.

tered in the cancer and cancer rehabilitation setting include hypercalcemia, hyperkalemia, hypokalemia, hyponatremia, and hypernatremia.

Hypercalcemia is common in the cancer setting. It can be seen as a result of noncancer conductions, such as primary hyperparathyroidism. Hypercalcemia also occurs as a direct result of extensive bony metastasis and osteolysis. Hypercalcemia from osteolysis was previously often seen in breast cancer, multiple myeloma, and lymphoma, but is now considerably less common due to widespread use of bisphosphonates. Hypercalcemia can also occur as a result of tumor secretion of parathyroid hormone-related peptide (PTH-RP). PTH-RP can be secreted by squamous cell carcinomas of the lung, head and neck, and esophageus as well as by carcinomas of the kidney, bladder, or ovaries. Symptoms of hypercalcemia include change in mental status (confusion, stupor, coma), easy fatigability, muscle weakness, gastrointestinal symptoms (anorexia, nausea, vomiting, constipation), and orthostasis due to volume depletion. Hypercalcemia can lead to heart block and cardiac arrest. Ambulation will help to minimize bone resorption that occurs with immobility (5).

Hyperkalemia is seen in patients with renal failure of any cause, adrenal insufficiency, acidosis, and tumor lysis syndrome. Hyperkalemia can cause muscle weakness, paresthesias, areflexia, ascending paralysis, and rapidly progressive and potentially dangerous cardiac arrhythmias, including bradycardia, asystole, prolongation of atrioventricular conduction block, complete heart block, and ventricular fibrillation. Hypokalemia in cancer patients is often caused by transcellular shifts (physiological stress, beta-agonist medications, alkalemia, excessive insulin, acute glucose loads), inadequate intake, extrarenal loss (vomiting, nasogastric drainage, fistulas, diarrhea), or renal loss (loop or thi-

azide diuretics, mineralocorticoid excess, amphotericin B, metabolic acidosis). Hypokalemia can cause malaise, fatigue, neuromuscular dysfunction (such as weakness, hyporeflexia, paresthesias, cramps, restless leg syndrome, paralysis, and respiratory failure), gastrointestinal (GI) disturbances (constipation, ileus, vomiting), rhabdomyolysis, and worsening hepatic encephalopathy. Cardiovascular abnormalities include orthostatic hypotension arrhythmias (especially on digitalis therapy), and electrocardiogram (ECG) changes (5,6).

Clinical manifestations of hyponatremia can range from malaise and headache to seizures, coma, and even death. Hyponatremia in cancer can be associated with conditions that decrease effective arterial volume or due to the syndrome of inappropriate antidiuretic hormone secretion (SIADH). SIADH causes fluid retention and inability to excrete diluted urine. It is most common in oat cell carcinoma of the lung and primary or secondary brain lesions. It is also seen in patients with severe dehydration, adrenal insufficiency due to metastatic disease, and can also be caused by the stress of pain (5). Symptoms from hypernatremia include lethargy, change in mental status, irritability, hyper-reflexia, and spasticity.

Hypernatremia in cancer patients can be due to significant water loss (such as from a febrile event or gastrointestinal losses) or by diabetes insipidus (DI). Central DI is characterized by decreased secretion of antidiuretic hormone (ADH) and causes polyuria and polydipsia. Primary brain tumors causing DI include craniopharyngioma or pineal tumors. Nephrogenic DI is characterized by a decrease in the ability to concentrate urine due to a resistance to ADH action in the kidney. Magnesium and phosphorus levels should also be monitored in cancer patients, as hypomagnesemia can decrease the kidneys' ability to retain other electrolytes, such as potassium and calcium, and hypophosphatemia can contribute to rhabdomyolysis (5,7).

Malignancies commonly associated with renal dysfunction include multiple myeloma, lymphoma, and leukemia. Multiple myeloma, for instance, is associated with renal disease in 50% of patients and can lead to complete renal failure and the need for dialysis. Myeloma patients with renal involvement have a worse prognosis for survival (1). Mechanisms of renal dysfunction include myeloma-cast nephropathy, amyloid depositions, and glomerular infiltration with light chains. For this group of patients, loop diuretics and nonsteroidal agents should be avoided. As previously noted, hypercalcemia is common in multiple myeloma from rapid bony destruction and reabsorption by tumor cells (2,8).

Tumor lysis syndrome is a potentially life-threatening condition that is most commonly associated with poorly differentiated lymphomas (Burkitt lymphoma), the leukemias (acute lymphoblastic leukemia, acute myeloid leukemia), and multiple myeloma (2). It usually arises from the initiation of cytotoxic chemotherapy, including cell death of malignant tissue, leading to rapid release of intracellular substances that overwhelm the renal excretion capacity. It is characterized by the rapid development of hyperkalemia, hyperuricemia, hyperphosphatemia, hypocalcemia, and lactic acidosis and can lead to renal failure. Prevention includes

aggressive hydration, prevention of urate production with the xanthine oxidase inhibitor allopurinol, or by the conversion of urate to allantoin with the recombinant urate oxidase rasburicase. If preventive therapy fails, urine flow should be maximized with hydration and diuretics. Dialysis may be required. The syndrome can lead to cardiac arrhythmia and seizures (2,9). Prognosis for renal recovery is good for most patients with treatment (2).

Hemolytic-uremic syndrome (HUS) and the related disorder thrombotic thrombocytopenic purpura (TTP) can occur in patients with malignancy. These disorders should be suspected in a patient with the triad of acute renal failure, thrombocytopenia, and a microangiopathic hemolytic anemia; fever and focal neurologic deficits also may be present. Mucin-secreting adenocarcinoma of the stomach, pancreas, or prostate and certain chemotherapy agents are known to cause HUS (10).

Many of the agents used in the assessment and treatment of cancer are commonly associated with renal dysfunction and even renal failure. These include bone marrow transplantation (BMT), several types of chemotherapy, and intravenous (IV) contrast agents used in diagnostic imaging.

BMT causes renal dysfunction in more than 50% of patients. Acute BMT nephropathy symptoms include severe hypertension, hemolytic anemia, thrombocy-

TABLE 29.1
Chemotherapy Agents and Renal Disease

Cisplatin	Mild and partially reversible decline in renal function that can increase in severity with subsequent courses Magnesium depletion leads to renal potassium wasting Thrombotic purpura/hemolytic uremic syndrome Carboplatin and oxaliplatin are less nephrotoxic
Ifosfamide	Causes proximal tubular defects (Fanconi syndrome) and chronic renal insufficiency. Monitor for hypokalemia, hyperchloremic metabolic acidosis hypophosphatemia Hemorrhagic cystitis
Cyclophosphamide	Hemorrhagic cystitis Also hyponatremia due to increased effect of ADH
Mitomycin C	Thrombotic purpura/hemolytic uremic syndrome
Methotrexate	Tubular injury
Cyclosporine A	Acute renal failure from renal vasoconstriction, chronic progressive renal dysfunction and hemolytic uremic syndrome. Also causes hyperkalemia and hyperuricemia
Streptozotocin	Proximal tubular toxicity
Vincristine, vinblastine and vinorelbine	SIADH
Bevacizumab, sunitinib, sorafenib	Albuminuria and nephrotic syndrome
Interleukin-2	Capillary leak syndrome

topenia, and elevated lactate dehydrogenase. Ten to 21 days after transplant, patients can develop hepatic veno-occlusive disease. Four weeks after transplant, patients are at risk for developing microangiopathic hemolytic anemia and thrombocytopenia due to total-body irradiation, calcineurin inhibitors (cyclosporine and tacrolimus), and chemotherapy agents. Patients also have a mild-to-moderate hypertension (1,11).

Chemotherapeutics represent a heterogeneous group of medications with widely varying clinical activity and thus effects on renal function. Disorders associated with some of the common agents are listed in Table 29.1. Interferon alpha is associated with minimal-change nephropathy or thrombotic microangiopathy. Interferon gamma has been associated with acute tubular necrosis, and rituximab is associated with acute renal failure. Other agents commonly used in the cancer setting that can cause significant renal dysfunction include the bisphosphonates, such as pamidronate or zoledronate (1,2,12). Radiocontrast is also a common cause of renal dysfunction and potentially failure in patients with cancer due to their frequent need for diagnostic imaging studies. Predisposing factors include age older than 60 years, diabetes mellitus, volume depletion, and concomitant nephrotoxic drug therapy (1). To reduce the risk of acute renal failure, hydration and *N*-acetylcysteine (Mucomyst; Apothecon, Princeton, New Jersey) (600 mg by mouth twice daily) on the day preceding and the day of the procedure are useful. Other nephrotoxic drugs should be withheld before the procedure (13).

REHABILITATION IMPLICATIONS

Renal dysfunction complicated by fatigue, anemia, cognitive changes, muscle weakness, fluid overload, electrolyte abnormalities, hypertension, hypotension, or cardiac arrhythmias can severely impact the therapist's treatment approach for a given patient. It is not uncommon for several of these impairments to coexist, further complicating rehabilitation efforts. Therapeutic interventions for the patient with renal dysfunction may involve endurance training, conditioning and aerobic exercises, stretching and flexibility exercises, gait training, and functional training in self-care and home management. Treatment frequency, duration, therapeutic activities, and exercise program should correspond to the patient's individual needs, as well as medical and physical condition. The anticipated therapy goals are to improve physical response to workloads, increase endurance and muscle strength, and improve functional performance related to self-care home management and sense of well-being.

There are several considerations for safe and effective physical and occupational therapy intervention. Anemia due to erythropoietin deficiency is common and can lead to decreased myocardial oxygenation and impaired exercise tolerance (14). Normalizing hemoglobin (Hb) may improve exercise capacity (15). Fluctuating blood pressure, arrhythmia, and heart failure are also commonly associated with renal dysfunction. Vital signs should be monitored and the patient observed for signs of dyspnea or chest pain. Activities should be discontinued if the heart rate becomes irregular or exceeds maximal heart rate parameters; systolic blood pressure exceeds 200 mmHg (millimeters of mercury) or falls below 90 mmHg; diastolic blood pressure (BP) exceeds 110 mmHg; oxygen saturation falls below 90%; or the patient shows signs of severe dyspnea, angina, or severe dizziness (16–18).

It can be exceptionally challenging working with patients undergoing dialysis. Complications of dialysis that may affect physical therapy treatments are hypertension, cardiac arrhythmia, renal osteodystrophy, electrolyte disturbances, dialysis disequilibria syndrome, dialysis-related amyloidosis (DRA), muscle cramps and restless leg syndrome, and the postdialysis fatigue syndrome (19,20). High-impact exercises and activities should be avoided in patients with severe renal osteodystrophy. A number of studies suggest that well-designed exercise training in patients on dialysis can be performed safely with proper supervision and patient education to improve muscle strength, mental, and physical function, and possible cardiac fitness (21–23).

The main treatment for nonmetastatic renal carcinoma is nephrectomy. Similar to other postabdominal surgery patients, postnephrectomy patients are at high risk of respiratory insufficiency. Atelectasis is a significant respiratory complication; initiation of chest physical therapy is beneficial (24,25). In addition, lower extremity active-range-of-motion (AROM) exercises and frequent ambulation showed a beneficial effect in reducing the risk of postoperative deep venous thrombosis (DVT) (26).

Therapy interventions to reduce orthostasis include early mobilization with abdominal strengthening and isotonic-isometric exercises for the lower extremities. Patients should try to keep their head at 15°–20° while supine. Patients should avoid sudden standing from the supine position, especially after eating. Antiembolic stockings (thromboembolism deterrent stockings, or TEDS), Ace wrapping of the lower extremity, or even abdominal binders can help to increase venous return and reduce orthostasis. The use of a tilt table may be required in some cases. Wheelchair adaptations can include elevating leg rests and a reclining back (27).

References

1. Kapoor M, Chan GZ. Malignancy and renal disease. *Crit Care Clin.* July 2001;17(3):571–598.
2. Lameire NH, Flombaum CD, Moreau D, Ronco C. Acute renal failure in cancer patients. *Ann Med.* 2005;37(1):13–25.
3. Weinamn EJ, Patak RV. Acute renal failure in cancer patients. *Oncology.* September 1992;6(9):47–52.
4. Alpers CE, Cortran RS. Neoplasia and glomerular injury. *Kidney Int.* 1986;30:465.
5. Kapoor M, Chan GZ. Fluid and electrolyte abnormalities. *Crit Care Clin.* July 2001;17(3):503–529.
6. Flombaum CD. Metabolic emergencies in the cancer patient. *Semin Oncol.* June 2000;27(3):322–334.
7. Thomas CR Jr, Dodhia N. Common emergencies in cancer medicine: metabolic syndromes. *J Natl Med Assoc.* September 1991;83(9):809–818.
8. Irish AB, Winearls CG, Littlewood T, et al. Presentation and survival of patients with severe renal failure and myeloma. *Q J Med.* 1997;90:773.
9. Coiffier B, Riouffol C. Management of tumor lysis syndrome in adults. *Expert Rev Anticancer Ther.* February 2007;7(2):233–239.
10. Elliot MA, Nichols WL. Thrombotic thrombocytopenic purpura and hemolytic uremic syndrome. *Mayo Clin Proc.* November 2001;76(11):1154–1162.
11. Otani M, Shimojo H, Shiozawa S, Shigematsu H. Renal involvement in bone marrow transplantation. *Nephrology.* October 2005;10(5):530–536.
12. Kintzel PE. Anticancer drug-induced kidney disorders. *Drug Saf.* 2001;24:19.
13. Tepel M, van der Giet M, Schwarzfeld C, Laufer U, Liermann D, Zidek W. Prevention of radiographic-contrast-agent-induced reductions in renal function by acetylcysteine. *N Engl J Med.* 2000;343:180.
14. Skinnner JS. *Exercise Testing and Exercise Prescription for Special Cases.* 3rd ed. Lippincott Williams & Wilkins; March 2005.
15. Muirhead N. A rational for an individualized haemoglobin target. *Nephrol Dial Transplant.* 2002;17(Suppl 6):2–7.
16. Gill TM, DiPietro L, Krumholz HM. Role of exercise stress testing and safety monitoring for older persons starting an exercise program. *JAMA.* 2000;284:342–349.
17. Fletcher BJ, Dunbar S, Coleman J, Jann B, Fletcher GF. Cardiac precautions for non-acute inpatient settings. *Am J Phys Med Rehabil.* June 1993;72(3):140–143.
18. Exercise & Physical Therapy Activity Guidelines Based on Best Available Evidence. American Physical Therapy Association. (Accessed April 10, 2007, at http://www.apta.org)
19. Pereira BJG, Sayegh MH, Blake PG. *Chronic Kidney Disease, Dialysis, & Transplantation.* 2nd ed. Elsevier Saunders. Lippincott Williams & Wilkins; November 2006.
20. Verrelli M, Mulloy L. Chronic Renal Failure. (Accessed April 13, 2007, at http://www.emedicine.com/med/topic374.htm)
21. Deligiannis A, Kouidi E, Tassoulas E, Gigis P, Tourkantionis A, Coast A. Cardiac effects of exercise rehabilitation in hemodialysis patients. *Int J Cardiol.* February 15, 2000;72(3):299–300.
22. Levendoglu F, Altintepe L, Okudan N, et al. A twelve-week exercise program improves the psychological status, quality of life and work capacity in hemodialysis patients. *J Nephrol.* November–December 2004;17(60):826–832.
23. Konstantinidou E, Koukouvou G, Kuouidi E, Deligianais A, Tourkantonis A. Exercise training in patients with end stage renal diseases on hemodialysis: comparison of three rehabilitation programs. *J Rehabil Med.* 2002;34:40–45.
24. Fagevik Olsen M, Hahn I, Nordgren S, Lonroth H, Lundholm K. Randomized controlled trial of prophylactic chest physiotherapy in major abdominal surgery. *Br J Surg.* November 1997;84(11):1535–1538.
25. Hall JC, Tarala RA, Tapper J, Hall JL. Prevention of respiratory complications after abdominal surgery: a randomized clinic trial. *BMJ.* January 20, 1996;312:148–152.
26. Agnelli G. Prevention of venous thromboembolism in surgical patients. *Circulation.* December 14, 2004;110(24 Suppl 1):IV4–12. Review.
27. Tan J. *Deconditioning in Practical Manual of Physical Medicine and Rehabilitation.* 2nd ed. Elsevier Mosby; 2006:459.

Endocrine Complications of Cancer

Juliana Khowong

The endocrine-related issues likely to be encountered by the physicians, therapists, and other health care providers who care for cancer patients are diverse and encompass complications arising from the endocrinopathy itself, from the cancer, and from cancer treatments.

DIABETES MELLITUS

Diabetes mellitus is a group of metabolic disorders of differing etiologies all of which cause altered glucose regulation. The two common categories are type 1 arising from insulin deficiency, primarily by autoimmune destruction of the beta cell, and type 2 characterized by a spectrum of disorders caused by insulin resistance and defects in insulin secretion. A third category also exists which includes hyperglycemia from drugs, pancreatic disease and genetic defects in insulin secretion and action. The diagnosis is made by measuring plasma glucose levels and using criteria established by the American Diabetes Association (1).

The goal of diabetic management is to keep serum glucose levels within normal range to prevent secondary complications from hyperglycemia, including cardiovascular disease, retinopathy, and nephropathy, which can be minimized or prevented with intensive glycemic control (2). This requires patient education, diet modification, exercise and pharmacological therapy with frequent monitoring of blood glucose levels.

Hypoglycemia

Hypoglycemia is usually due to iatrogenic factors when it occurs in the person with diabetes and it is often a consequence and limiting factor to tight glycemic control. It is primarily related to insulin treatment, and the Diabetes Control and Complications Trial showed a two- to six-fold increase in the risk of severe hypoglycemia in intensively treated type I diabetic patients compared with those undergoing conservative treatment (3). Hypoglycemia can be caused by inappropriate dosing of hypoglycemic medications; inadequate oral intake or fasting without adjusting medication dosage; and from drug interactions with nonsteroidal anti-inflammatory drugs (NSAIDS), sulfonamides, or monoamine oxidase inhibitors, which can increase the activity of certain oral hypoglycemic agents. Hypoglycemia has been defined as plasma glucose level <50 mg/dL in the presence of symptoms that can be grouped as autonomic (sweating, anxiety, tremors, tachycardia, palpitations, nausea) and those related to neuroglycopenia (seizures, fatigue, syncope, headache, behavioral and visual changes) and relief of symptoms after the ingestion of carbohydrates. The assessment of the hypoglycemic patient should include the patient's vital signs to help evaluate the urgency of the situation; review of recently administered hypoglycemic medications to determine the timing, severity, and chances of recurrence of the hypoglycemic episode following treatment; and physical examination. Laboratory data should include serum glucose levels, although treatment

KEY POINTS

- In the cancer population, increased insulin-like growth factor type II (IGF-II) precursor has been shown to occur in mesenchymal tumors, hepatocellular tumors, and other large tumors. Large tumors of the liver can also impair gluconeogenesis.
- Hyperglycemia often resolves within 48 hours of discontinuation or lowering of the corticosteroid.
- People with diabetes who are planning to undergo or who have had radiation therapy should be particularly vigilant in skin care overlying the irradiated area, as they are already susceptible to disrupted wound healing and chronic ulcers.
- Alterations in thyroid function can follow irradiation to the cervical area, resulting in primary hypothyroidism, or from irradiation to the cranial region, resulting in disturbance of the hypothalamic-pituitary axis, causing central hypothyroidism.
- Malignancy-related hypercalcemia is a common metabolic complication in the cancer population and has been reported to affect 20%–40% of cancer patients at some point in their illness. Hypercalcemia is by far the most common paraneoplastic endocrine syndrome and is seen with squamous cell cancers of the lung, head and neck and skin, esophageal, renal, bladder, and ovarian cancers.
- Syndrome of inappropriate antidiuretic hormone secretion (SIADH) is the second most common paraneoplastic endocrine disorder and results from excess production of vasopressin by certain tumor types, most often seen with small cell lung cancer, occurring in at least half of these patients.
- Severe hyponatremia or symptomatic patients presenting with seizure or mental status changes are treated with hypertonic saline infusion with carefully titrated sodium correction to prevent rapid fluid shifts and the development of osmotic demyelination or central pontine myelinolysis.

should not be postponed while waiting for results. Oral glucose can be given to patients that are awake, alert, and able to take fluids. Orange juice with sugar added and saltine crackers can be given for mild hypoglycemia. Intravenous (IV) glucose given as one ampoule of 50% dextrose can be given to those not able to tolerate fluids. If IV access is not available, glucagon 0.5–1 mg intramuscularly or subcutaneously may be given. This may induce vomiting; therefore, caution should be taken to protect the airway. Maintenance IV fluids with dextrose 5% in water (D5W) should be started and serial glucose levels followed.

In the cancer population, increased insulin-like growth factor type II (IGF-II) precursor has been shown to occur in mesenchymal tumors, hepatocellular tumors, and other large tumors. IGF-II precursor binds to insulin-like growth factor type I (IGF-I) receptors and acts similar to insulin to cause hypoglycemia. Secretion of a high molecular weight form of IGF-II (big IGF-II) has been implicated in causing non-islet cell tumor hypoglycemia. There is also evidence that IGF-II bioavailability is increased in these tumors, leading to increased insulin-like actions on target tissues and hypoglycemia. Laboratory investigation shows low serum glucose and suppressed insulin levels in the setting of clinical symptoms of hypoglycemia. IGF-II assays may not detect IGF-II precursors, but diagnosis can be confirmed with finding increased IGF-II messenger ribonucleic acid (mRNA) expression in the tumor and a high IGF II/IGF I ratio of >10:1 (4). Large tumors of the liver may also impair gluconeogenesis. Definitive treatment is with management of the underlying malignancy, and successful tumor excision has been correlated in some cases, with a significant decrease in big IGF-II levels and resolution of hypoglycemia (5). Frequent meals, intravenous glucose, glucagon, growth hormone, and glucocorticoids may help increase glucose production and levels in cases where tumor resection is not possible.

A large part of hypoglycemic management is patient education, and people with diabetes should be taught how to recognize the signs and symptoms of hypoglycemia and how to institute appropriate treatment and when to seek urgent medical attention.

Hyperglycemia

On the opposite end of the spectrum, uncontrolled hyperglycemia can also be an endocrine emergency. Diabetic ketoacidosis (DKA) and hyperglycemic hyperosmolar state (HHS) are two serious complications arising from uncontrolled hyperglycemia. DKA occurs when there is a lack of insulin in the presence of increased counter-regulatory hormones (glucagon, catecholamines, cortisol, and growth hormone), leading to gluconeogenesis, glycogenolysis, and lipolysis with ketone formation. Insulin deficiency results either from an interruption in insulin replacement or from an increased demand for insulin, which can occur during severe illness or infection. Symptoms of DKA develop rapidly over 24 hours and include nausea, vomiting, dyspnea, malaise, polyuria, polydipsia, and abdominal pain. Signs include dehydration, hypotension, tachycardia, and tachypnea with Kussmaul respirations and can progress to obtundation and coma if not quickly treated. Diagnostic evaluation includes glucose level, which is >250 mg/dL; serum electrolytes, which reveal a metabolic acidosis with an increased anion gap; and plasma ketones. Laboratory testing should also include complete blood count (CBC) and cultures to investigate for infectious etiology, as this is the most common precipitating cause of both DKA and HHS worldwide (6). Treatment is with aggressive IV fluid replacement and IV insulin administration titrated to serially drawn serum glucose levels. Potassium, phosphate, and magnesium are replaced as needed.

HHS is similar in presentation to DKA, but affects people with type II diabetes mostly and occurs subacutely over several days to weeks. A significant difference is the absence of severe ketoacidosis. In HHS, severe hyperglycemia causes an osmotic diuresis that is worsened in the setting of poor fluid intake. Causes include illness and infection, and patients clinically appear with mental status change, lethargy, or obtundation, and signs can indicate evidence of severe dehydration with poor skin turgor, hypotension, and tachycardia. Glucose levels are often >600 mg/dL, with serum hyperosmolarity and prerenal azotemia. Management is with aggressive rehydration, replacement of electrolytes as needed, and correction of hyperglycemia.

Hyperglycemia may also be precipitated by the use of steroids, which are often an integral part of palliative care in metastatic cancers. Glucocorticoids play an important role in oncologic treatment, particularly in the management of malignant primary and secondary brain tumors, neoplastic epidural spinal cord compression, adjuvant treatment in chemotherapy of selective central nervous system tumors, and perioperatively in brain surgery (7). Glucocorticoids can help reduce signs and symptoms resulting from increased intracranial pressure from cerebral tumors and the progression of neurological deficit, sensory loss, and pain resulting from epidural spinal cord compression (8). Glucocorticoids are the cornerstone of treatment of primary central nervous system (CNS) non-Hodgkin lymphoma, and studies have shown reduction in tumor size and even remission after glucocorticoid therapy.

The mechanism by which corticosteroid use causes hyperglycemia is not known, but may be from glucose metabolism inhibition or insulin resistance (9). Hyperglycemia often resolves within 48 hours of discontinuation or lowering of the corticosteroid. When hyperglycemia continues for more than one week after corticosteroid withdrawal, the diagnosis of diabetes is presumed. The management of steroid diabetes is similar to the patient with type II diabetes, and oral hypoglycemic agents and insulin can be used, depending on the severity of hyperglycemia. Chromium loss parallels stressful situations, such as from infection, exercise, and trauma, and a direct correlation between increased cortisol response to stress and chromium loss has been reported (10). Chromium supplementation has been shown to improve fasting and postprandial glucose, insulin, and hemoglobin A1c levels in people with type II diabetes (11) and was later found to have a similar beneficial effect on steroid diabetes, with reversal of steroid diabetes in some cases when administered at a dose of 200 micrograms three times a day (12). The mechanism of action is believed to be through potentiation of insulin action through an increase in insulin receptors and insulin binding to red blood cells (13).

Diabetes has wide-ranging effects on the peripheral nervous system and will be briefly discussed here and is discussed in further detail in Chapter 52. In addition to autonomic neuropathy, diabetes can damage the nerve root, plexus, large nerve fibers, and small nerve fibers. Clinical manifestations of diabetic peripheral neuropathy include distal symmetric large- and small-fiber neuropathies, mononeuropathy multiplex, diabetic amyotrophy, and mononeuropathies. The etiology of diabetic neuropathy is still under investigation, and some current theories suggest that it is due to microvascular insufficiency, oxidative stress, nitrosative stress, defective neurotrophism, and autoimmune-mediated nerve destruction in the setting of hyperglycemia (14). Diabetic polyneuropathy is the most common of the diabetic neuropathies, and the classic presentation is of a distal symmetric dysesthesia, first affecting the distal lower extremities and then the distal upper extremities as the nerves are affected in a length-dependent fashion. Weakness can also develop with progression of the neuropathy, again beginning distally as the longest nerves are affected first. Balance impairment may develop from low proprioception, and other sensory deficits may occur, including loss of vibration, touch, and temperature sensation. Diagnostic testing includes electromyogram, which can show a variety of abnormalities depending on which components of the peripheral nervous system are most affected. Polyradiculoneuropathies can present unilaterally or bilaterally, with involvement of multiple nerve roots, and can affect the intercostal nerves. Pain over the lower thoracic or abdominal wall is the usual presenting symptom and weakness is uncommon. Diabetic amyotrophy can be secondary to a lumbosacral radiculoplexopathy and presents with severe pain in the thigh and weakness of the muscles along the nerve distribution, most commonly the quadriceps. Mononeuropathies also present asymmetrically and can involve the cranial nerves, most often affecting the third cranial nerve, or can be due to entrapment of the median, ulnar, peroneal, and plantar nerve. Electrodiagnostic findings in polyradiculoneuropathies and mononeuropathies include evidence of denervation in the affected myotomes and nerve distribution. Autonomic neuropathy can involve multiple systems and can cause gastroparesis, neurogenic bladder, sexual dysfunction, and cardiac manifestations such as orthostatic hypotension.

Treatment strategies for diabetic neuropathy include improving glucose control, and the Diabetes Control and Complication Trial reported a 57%–69% risk reduction in the appearance of clinical and electrophysiologic evidence of neuropathy in the intensively treated diabetic group at five years (12). Symptomatic treatment includes nerve membrane stabilizers, such as gabapentin and pregabalin; tricyclic agents (amitriptyline, nortriptyline); and serotonin-norepinephrine reuptake inhibitors (duloxetine), all of which modulate the release of pain neurotransmitters in the central nervous system (15). Capsaicin is a topical analgesic that works by depleting the neurotransmitter substance P peripherally and may also be beneficial, particularly in individuals who cannot tolerate the side effects of the oral medications (15). Treatment of autonomic dysfunction in the diabetic patient is directed at symptomatic management. Recommendations for gastroparesis include small, frequent meals and an antiemetic. Timed voiding, a trial of bethanechol (a parasympathomimetic agent), and intermittent catheterization may improve toileting in neurogenic bladder. Phosphodiesterase type 5 inhibitors, including sildenafil (Viagra; Pfizer, New York, New York), tadalafil (Cialis; Eli Lilly, Indianapolis, Indiana), and vardenafil (Levitra; Bayer Pharmaceuticals, West Haven, Connecticut), are useful for erectile dysfunction. Compression stockings and pharmacological therapy with fludrocortisone, midodrine, and octreotide can reduce orthostatic hypotension.

Hyperglycemia has also been implicated in poor wound healing, and changes seen at the cellular level include increases in acute inflammatory cells; absence of cellular growth and migration of the epidermis over the wound, with narrowing of the vasculature within the wound edges; and reduced leukocyte response (16). Radiation therapy is also known to impair wound healing through its toxic effect on fibroblasts, and these changes may persist for long periods after irradiation. Skin that is irradiated prior to wounding in experimental studies shows similar decreased wound healing, whether the radiation is delivered 1 hour or up to 95 days prior to wounding (17). Diabetic patients who are planning to undergo or who have had radiation therapy should be particularly vigilant in skin care overlying the irradiated area, as they are already susceptible to disrupted wound healing and chronic ulcers.

THYROID DISORDERS

Endocrine complications may also arise from thyroid disorders, either from prior thyroid disease or, more commonly in this population, from cancer therapies. Acute thyroid complications from previously diagnosed disease do not often present themselves for urgent evaluation, but include uncontrolled hyperthyroid disease in thyrotoxicosis and thyroid storm and severe hypothyroid state that is seen with critical illness.

Hyperthyroidism

Thyroid storm and thyrotoxicosis present similarly and are characterized by fever, tachycardia, and delirium, with more acute and severe features in the former. Thyroid storm is usually preceded by a precipitating event, such as surgery or sepsis, in a patient with undiagnosed hyperthyroidism. Management involves reducing thyroid hormone synthesis and release, suppressing the effects of circulating thyroid hormone, and treating the underlying precipitant. Methimazole and propylthiouracil are used to block thyroid hormone production, and propylthiouracil additionally inhibits T4 to T3 conversion. Iodide and corticosteroids also block T4 to T3 conversion and can be given to inhibit release of stored thyroid hormone. Propranolol is used to reduce tachycardia and in patients with angina or myocardial infarction, but should be used cautiously in individuals with underlying congestive heart failure (CHF) or bronchospasm.

Hypothyroidism

Hypothyroidism can complicate severe illness by contributing to hypoventilation, hypotension, hypothermia, and bradycardia. Thyroid hormone levels may be low in critical illness and unrelated to thyroid disease in euthyroid sick syndrome, and plasma thyroid-stimulating hormone (TSH) levels with measurement of free T4 (FT4) by equilibrium dialysis should be obtained to establish true thyroid disease. These secondary complications are aggressively treated, and thyroid hormone replacement with thyroxine is given if hypothyroidism is diagnosed and only in extremely ill patients. Rapid thyroid replacement may cause exacerbation of heart disease, and vital signs and cardiac rhythm must be monitored. Hydrocortisone is recommended during the rapid replacement of thyroid hormone to prevent the precipitation of adrenal failure.

More commonly seen in the cancer population are thyroid disorders resulting from antineoplastic treatment from radiation and immune therapies.

Radiation Therapy

Head and neck irradiation is often a part of treatment for CNS malignancies, lymphoma, and head and neck cancers. Total body irradiation can also cause thyroid disorders, although less commonly, secondary to the low thyroid dose with total body irradiation. The mechanism by which radiation causes thyroid dysfunction is unknown. Histologic evaluation of thyroid tissue varies, depending upon the dose of radiation and the interval following exposure, and typically shows follicular changes ranging from decreased size to necrosis and vascular damage extending from vasculitis to sclerosis (18). Radiation injury to the blood supply to the thyroid can also cause ischemic changes. It has been proposed that early acute injury is from parenchymal cell damage and late injury is caused mainly by vascular damage (19).

Alterations in thyroid function can follow irradiation to the cervical area, resulting in primary hypothyroidism, or from irradiation to the cranial region, resulting in disturbance of the hypothalamic-pituitary axis, causing central hypothyroidism. The presentation is often subclinical with elevated TSH and normal serum FT4 levels in primary hypothyroidism. Clinical primary hypothyroidism causes increased TSH levels with reduced serum FT4, and patients may present with symptoms including fatigue, cold intolerance, decreased gastrointestinal motility, hair loss, weight gain, cognitive slowing, signs of periorbital and peripheral edema, pleural or pericardial effusions, delayed relaxation phase of deep tendon reflexes, and cool, dry skin on exam. Central hypothyroidism presents similarly, but laboratory values show low or inappropriately normal TSH and low serum FT4 levels. Other pituitary hormone deficiencies are often present. Although less common, hyperthyroidism can also develop postirradiation to the head and neck. Clinically, these patients may present with complaints of heat intolerance, weight loss, palpitations, and anxiety. Signs include brisk reflexes, tremor, stare and eyelid lag, sinus tachycardia, and atrial fibrillation. Thyroid cancers can also develop postirradiation, and these are usually well differentiated and less aggressive types that are rarely fatal (20).

Data from the Childhood Cancer Survivor Study obtained from survivors of Hodgkin disease who had undergone radiation treatment found that the incidence of underactive and overactive thyroid disease was significantly higher in the Hodgkin disease survivor group compared to sibling controls (21). The incidence of diagnosed thyroid nodule was also significantly increased. Of these cases, 7.5% were found to be cancerous. An additional nine cases of thyroid cancer were present in individuals who denied having a thyroid nodule. The calculated relative risk for developing thyroid cancer was again significantly higher.

Evaluation is recommended at least yearly and for a minimum of five years postirradiation. In patients who have received irradiation to the cervical region, primary hypothyroidism usually presents within the first five years after therapy, with peak incidence two to three years following treatment (22). During follow-up evaluations, patients should be questioned regarding changes in weight, thermal tolerance, skin and hair, and activity level. Baseline thyroid function tests measuring TSH and FT4 should be taken prior to initiating treatment and during annual exams. Physical examination should include palpation of the thyroid and fine-needle aspiration if nodules are present. Ultrasound is a sensitive but nonspecific diagnostic tool and often will show nodules that are nonpalpable by examination and which are ultimately found to be benign. Technetium scanning can help characterize nodules. Thyroid stimulation tests measuring the TSH response to thyroid-releasing hormone can also be performed and may be useful in suspected central hypothyroidism.

Treatment of hypothyroidism is with hormone replacement, and early repletion is recommended, including in subclinical thyroid disease, which often becomes overt hypothyroid disease. Recommendations for when to initiate thyroid hormone replacement vary. One study recommends starting therapy when TSH levels are >4.5 mIU/L (23). Thyroid replacement also avoids prolonged TSH thyroid stimulation, which may cause an increased risk of benign or malignant thyroid nodule development and also decreases complications from hypothyroidism, including atherosclerosis and hypercholesterolemia. The management of thyroid cancers includes surgery, radioiodine treatment, and suppression with thyroid hormone.

Immune Therapy

Immune therapies are frequent causes of thyroid disorders, and interleukin-2 (IL-2), which is used in the treatment of metastatic melanoma and renal cell carcinoma, has been associated with thyroiditis. Elevated levels of antithyroglobulin and antithyroid microsomal antibodies have been found, suggesting an autoimmune mechanism, and hypothyroidism is the most common thyroid complication (24). The length of IL-2 treatment has been positively correlated with the incidence of developing thyroid disease.

DISORDERS OF CALCIUM HOMEOSTASIS

Hypercalcemia

Malignancy is responsible for most causes of hypercalcemia in hospitalized patients, accounting for 65% of cases (25). Malignancy-related hypercalcemia is a common metabolic complication in the cancer population and has been reported to affect 20%–40% of cancer patients at some point in their illness (26). Two mechanisms have been identified in causing this calcium disturbance (27). Local osteolytic hypercalcemia results from stimulation of osteoclastic bone resorption by a variety of cytokines, including TGF-alpha, IL-1, IL-6, and tumor necrosis factor (TNF), all of which induce the formation and differentiation of osteoclasts. This occurs when there is extensive invasion of tumor into bone and is seen in breast cancer, myeloma, and lymphoma. Humoral hypercalcemia of malignancy occurs when tumors cells express humoral factors, including parathyroid hormone-related peptide (PTH-RP), osteolytic prostaglandins, cytokines, and osteoclast-activating factor, which cause increased bone resorption and decreased calcium excretion. It is by far the most common paraneoplastic endocrine syndrome and is seen with squamous cell cancers of the lung, head and neck and skin, esophageal, renal, bladder, and ovarian cancers. Parathyroid cancer is a rare malignancy, but can also cause markedly elevated serum calcium (>14 mg/dL) and parathyroid hormone levels (>5 times the normal value).

Hypercalcemia clinically presents when serum levels are >12 mg/dL, and symptoms are worse when the disturbance is acute. The range of presenting symptoms can be nonspecific, and anorexia, nausea, vomiting, constipation, polyuria, and weakness can be seen. In the cancer population, it is important to have a high level of suspicion, as these symptoms can be similar to side effects from concomitant cancer treatments. Patients can also present with neuropsychiatric signs ranging from confusion to stupor and coma. Renal failure and ectopic soft tissue calcification can develop when levels are >13 mg/dL. In general, renal calculi and osteitis fibrosa are not observed with malignancy-associated hypercalcemia because they are the result of long-standing hypercalcemia. However, in parathyroid carcinoma, nephrolithiasis and nephrocalcinosis are often seen secondary to the severity of the resulting calcium disorder (28). Osteopenia and fractures, pathologic or secondary to trauma, can also be presenting signs. Laboratory testing should include measurement of ionized calcium or calcium with a serum albumin and serum PTH. In hypercalcemia secondary to malignancy other than parathyroid carcinoma, PTH levels are suppressed.

The goal of hypercalcemia management is to lower calcium levels through increased calcium excretion via the kidneys and by promoting chelation and bone deposition. Pharmacological management is also directed at suppressing bone resorption and gastrointestinal absorption. Aggressive hydration is performed to restore the extra cellular fluid volume, followed by saline diuresis, which increases calcium excretion by inhibiting proximal tubule reabsorption. The bisphosphonates are used to inhibit osteoclastic bone resorption, and zoledronate is the drug of choice (29). Calcitonin can also be used to inhibit bone resorption and increase renal calcium excretion. It is administered via intramuscular or subcutaneous injections and has a rapid onset of action, decreasing serum calcium in 12–24 hours, but is less potent than the bisphosphonates, and serum calcium levels rapidly return to pretreatment levels within 48 hours. Gallium nitrate is a potent inhibitor of bone resorption and has been approved for use in correcting cancer-related hypercalcemia that is not responsive to hydration (30). Glucocorticoids are effective at lowering calcium levels through several mechanisms, including inhibiting bone resorption and intestinal calcium absorption, increasing urinary calcium excretion, and by cytolytic effects in lymphoma, myeloma, and leukemia (31). Multiple side effects can result from glucocorticoid therapy, as previously discussed, and limit their usefulness for long-term therapy. Dialysis is an effective method for treating hypercalcemia in resistant cases, particularly in patients with renal insufficiency or CHF.

Chronic management of hypercalcemia due to malignancy includes ensuring adequate hydration (recommended 3 L/day) with a high-salt diet of 8–10 g/day unless otherwise contraindicated. Dietary restriction of calcium has not been shown to be beneficial. Oral phosphates can also be used to decrease gastrointestinal calcium absorption and bone resorption, although results are usually modest. The definitive management is treatment of the underlying malignancy. In hypercalcemia related to parathyroid carcinoma, en bloc resection is the only treatment with a high rate of cure, and a relapse in hypercalcemia is often the initial signal of disease recurrence. Cinacalcet is a calcimimetic agent that binds to the calcium-sensing receptor on the surface of parathyroid cells and increases the receptor's sensitivity to extracellular calcium. PTH secretion is decreased, causing a reduction in serum calcium. Cinacalcet is administered orally and has been shown to improve calcium homeostasis in chronic hypercalcemia in patients with parathyroid carcinoma (32).

Hypocalcemia

Hypocalcemia can often be seen following thyroid surgery, and causative factors include surgical trauma, devascularization, and inadvertent excision of the parathyroid glands during surgery. The incidence rate varies widely, and in a review of the literature, Sippel et al. (33) found values ranging from 1.6%–50%. The incidence of permanent hypocalcemia secondary to hypoparathyroidism post-thyroid surgery was much smaller, occurring in 1.5%–4%. Incidental parathyroidectomy was reported to occur in 6.4% of thyroid resections, with risk factors including younger age, bilateral thyroid resection, and malignant pathology. Younger patients were more likely to undergo surgery for malignancy and require a more aggressive surgical approach.

The physical examination of patients with hypocalcemia can reveal increased nerve excitability with positive Trousseau sign (carpal spasm following blood pressure cuff inflation above the patient's systolic pressure for three minutes) and Chvostek sign (facial twitch after tapping the facial nerve anterior to the ear). Calcium gluconate is used in the acute management of symptomatic hypocalcemia. Chronic management requires calcium supplementation and vitamin D to increase gastrointestinal calcium absorption. Calcium carbonate 0.5–1.0 g by mouth three times a day should be taken with meals to increase absorption. Vitamin D is given at an initial dose of 50,000 IU by mouth every day, with usual maintenance dosages of 25,000–100,000 IU by mouth every day and requires weeks to achieve full effect. Calcitriol acts more rapidly and has a lower risk of toxicity, but is more expensive than vitamin D. The initial dosage is 0.25 micrograms my mouth, with a maintenance dose of 0.5–2.0 micrograms by mouth every day.

DISORDERS OF FLUID BALANCE AND SODIUM

Disorders of fluid balance and sodium occur in the syndrome of inappropriate antidiuretic hormone secretion (SIADH) and diabetes insipidus (DI).

Syndrome of Inappropriate Antidiuretic Hormone Secretion

SIADH is the second most common paraneoplastic endocrine disorder and results from excess production of vasopressin by certain tumor types, most often seen with small cell lung cancer, occurring in at least half of these patients (34). Carcinoids, other lung cancers, gastrointestinal, genitourinary, and ovarian tumors are other sources of ectopic vasopressin. Vasopressin is normally secreted by the posterior pituitary gland and promotes water retention in response to a drop in plasma volume or an increase in serum osmolality.

SIADH occurs when vasopressin is secreted in the absence of this stimuli, causing normovolemic hyponatremia. Patients present with symptoms from hyponatremia, including mental status changes, confusion, weakness, muscle cramps, and seizures. Symptoms are more severe when the onset is acute and when the sodium level is lower. Most patients are asymptomatic and are diagnosed on routine laboratory testing with hyponatremia; in these cases, it is usually chronic. Laboratory testing characteristic of SIADH reveals hypo-osmotic hyponatremia; inappropriately concentrated urine, with elevated urinary sodium usually >30 mEq/L; and normal renal, adrenal, and thyroid function. Other causes of vasopressin stimulation should be investigated, including hypotension, heart failure, hepatic cirrhosis, pulmonary disease, and neuropsychiatric disorders. Many chemotherapeutic agents, such as vincristine, vinblastine, cyclophosphamide, and cisplatin, have also been reported to cause SIADH.

In hyponatremia that has developed gradually, treatment consists of slow correction of sodium levels, initially by fluid restriction. Demeclocycline can be used to inhibit vasopressin action on the renal distal tubule. Side effects include photosensitivity and nephrogenic diabetes insipidus, and demeclocycline should be used with caution in patients with hepatic disease. The onset of action is relatively slow, over one to two weeks, and the medicine can be costly. Loop diuretics can be used to promote excretion of water and, when given with salt tablets, can increase free water excretion. Severe hyponatremia or symptomatic patients presenting with seizure or mental status changes are treated with hypertonic saline infusion with carefully titrated sodium correction to prevent rapid fluid shifts and the development of osmotic demyelination or central pontine myelinolysis. The definitive treatment of SIADH related to ectopic ADH secretion from tumor is to treat the underlying malignancy. Studies have shown that when small cell lung cancers respond to chemoradiotherapy, SIADH resolves in almost all cases and often before tumor regression is seen radiographically (35).

Neurogenic Diabetes Insipidus

Neurogenic DI occurs when there is inadequate production of ADH and can result from brain neoplasms. Patients present with polyuria, with urine volumes ranging from 2.5–6 L/day; polydipsia; and neurologic manifestations, such as seizures, headaches, and visual field defects. Signs of dehydration may also be present. Laboratory results show a low urine-specific gravity, low urine osmolarity, high serum osmolarity, and hypernatremia. The water deprivation test measures urine and plasma osmolarity after administration of vasopressin and is used to diagnose DI and distinguish between neurogenic DI and nephrogenic DI, which is due to renal tubule unresponsiveness to ADH. In neurogenic DI, urine osmolarity is less than plasma osmolarity and there is a >50% increase in urine osmolarity after vasopressin administration. In less severe partial neurogenic DI, urine osmolarity is greater than plasma osmolarity and there is a >10% increase in urine osmolarity after vasopressin. If neurogenic DI is confirmed, a magnetic resonance imaging (MRI) of the brain should be obtained.

Treatment of neurogenic DI includes desmopressin acetate (DDAVP), which can be administered intranasally, orally, subcutaneously, and intravenously. Vasopressin tannate in oil is another treatment option that can be used for long-term management because it is dosed intramuscularly every 24–72 hours. Milder cases of neurogenic DI can be managed with carbamazepine (increases vasopressin release), hydrochlorothiazide (decreases urine output in the absence of vasopressin), and chlorpropamide (enhances vasopressin action). Patients should be educated regarding the signs and symptoms of dehydration and should weigh themselves daily.

DISORDERS OF CORTISOL REGULATION

Adrenocorticotropic hormone (ACTH) is normally secreted by the anterior pituitary and is responsible for cortisol steroidogenesis and regulation. Ectopic ACTH secretion from nonpituitary tumors causes approximately 10% of cases of Cushing syndrome (36,136). The mechanism is due to increased expression of the proopiomelanocortin (POMC) gene, which is the precursor to ACTH and melanocyte-stimulating hormone (MSH) in addition to other peptides. Tumors in the lung account for nearly 50% of cases of paraneoplastic production of ACTH, with bronchial carcinoid tumors and small cell lung carcinoma (SCLC) as the predominant malignancies (37). The remainder is mostly caused by thymic carcinoid, islet cell tumors, other carcinoids, and pheochromocytomas. Corticotrophin-releasing hormone (CRH) can also be produced by SCLC, carcinoid tumors, medullary thyroid, and pancreatic tumors and can cause Cushing syndrome, but this occurs rarely.

Clinical features vary, depending on the underlying tumor. In patients with SCLC, the syndrome presents more acutely and prominent features include proximal myopathies, peripheral edema, hypokalemia, and glucose intolerance. Patients may also present with hyperpigmentation secondary to increased MSH activity from POMC overexpression. The typical cushingoid appearance with weight gain and central obesity is less often seen, likely because the duration of cortisol excess is relatively short and cancer patients tend towards weight loss and cachexia. Patients with carcinoid tumors present more typically with the classic symptoms of Cushing syndrome. Correlating with this, cortisol and ACTH levels are usually higher in patients with small cell carcinomas than in those with carcinoid tumors. Osteoporosis and fracture have also been reported in up to 50% of patients with ectopic ACTH secretion (36).

Laboratory evaluation consists of the high-dose dexamethasone suppression test and CRH test. Tumors causing ectopic ACTH secretion are characteristically unresponsive to glucocorticoid, and CRH feedback and cortisol levels are not suppressed. Bronchial and other carcinoids are exceptions and may exhibit feedback regulation and suppression of ACTH with glucocorticoid administration. Bilateral inferior petrosal sinus sampling is the most accurate method to differentiate excess ACTH secretion resulting from a pituitary adenoma from ectopic secretion, and has a sensitivity and specificity of 90%–100% (38). In pituitary adenomas, a gradient >3 (ACTH levels in the inferior petrosal sinus/peripheral vein) is present after CRH administration. Treatment consisting of medical therapy with agents to block steroid synthesis or action is recommended, and ketoconazole, metyrapone, and mitotane are commonly used. However, patients often require increasingly larger doses to maintain eucortisolism, with prolonged treatment and ultimately steroid blockade fails. Of the agents that inhibit steroidogenesis, ketoconazole is the drug of choice, and in a meta-analysis was shown to be effective in normalizing cortisol levels in 70% of cases (39,40). Liver toxicity was the main side effect and occurred in 15% of these cases. If the lesion is localized, surgical excision is the best treatment when possible, and in one series, Isidori et al. reported complete remission of hypercortisolemia in 83% of cases after resection of single primary lesions (41). Adrenalectomy can be considered if the underlying tumor is disseminated or not resectable and the prognosis is otherwise favorable, such as seen in carcinoid tumors.

References

1. Expert Committee on the Diagnosis and Classification of Diabetes Mellitus. Report of the expert committee on the diagnosis and classification of diabetes mellitus. *Diabetes Care.* 2003;26(Supp 1):5–20.
2. Diabetes Control and Complications Trial Research Group. The effect of intensive treatment of diabetes on the development and progression of long-term complications in insulin-dependent diabetes mellitus. *N Engl J Med.* September 30, 1993;329(14):977–986.
3. Diabetes Control and Complications Trial Research Group. Epidemiology of severe hypoglycemia in the diabetes control and complications trial. *Am J Med.* April 1991;90:450–459.

4. Lloyd RV, Erickson LA, Nascimento AG, Kloppel G. Neoplasms causing nonhyperinsulinemic hypoglycemia. *Endocr Pathol.* Winter 1999;10(4):291–297.

5. Fukuda I, Hizuka N, Ishikawa Y, et al. Clinical features of insulin-like growth factor-II producing non-islet-cell tumor hypoglycemia. *Growth Horm IGF Res.* 2006;16:211–216.

6. Kearney T, Dang C. Diabetic and endocrine emergencies. *Postgrad Med J.* 2007;83:79–86.

7. Koehler PJ. Use of corticosteroids in neuro-oncology. *Anticancer Drugs.* 1995;6:19–33.

8. Weissman DE. Glucocorticoid treatment for brain metastases and epidural spinal cord compression: a review. *J Clin Oncol.* March 1988;6(3):543–551.

9. Buchman AL. Side effects of corticosteroid therapy. *J Clin Gastroenterol.* October 2001;33(4):289–294.

10. Anderson BA, Bryden NA, Polansky MM, Thorp JW. Effects of carbohydrate loading and underwater exercise on circulating cortisol, insulin and urinary loss of chromium and zinc. Eur J Appl Physiol. 1991;63:146–150.

11. Anderson RA, Cheng N, Bryden NA, et al. Elevated intakes of supplemental chromium improve glucose and insulin variables in individuals with type 2 diabetes. *Diabetes.* November 1997;46(11):1786–1791.

12. Ravina A, Slezak L, Mirsky N, Bryden NA, Anderson RA. Reversal of corticosteroid-induced diabetes mellitus with supplemental chromium. *Diabet Med.* 1999;16:164–167.

13. Anderson RA, Polansky M, Bryden NA, Bhathena SJ, Canary JJ. Effects of supplemental chromium on patients with symptoms of reactive hypoglycemia. *Metab.* April 1987;36(4): 351–355.

14. Vinik A, Ullal J, Parson HK, Casellini CM. Diabetic neuropathies: clinical manifestations and current treatment options. *Nat Clin Prac Endocrinol Metab.* 2006;2(5):269–281.

15. Chong MS, Hester J. Diabetic painful neuropathy: current and future treatment options. *Drugs.* 2007;67(4):569–585.

16. Blakytny R, Jude E. The molecular biology of chronic wounds and delayed healing in diabetes. *Diabet Med.* 2006;23:594–608.

17. Bernstein EF, Sullivan FJ, Mitchell JB, Salomon GD, Glatstein E. Biology of chronic radiation effect on tissues and wound healing. *Clin Plast Surg.* July 1993;20(3):435–453.

18. Hancock SL, McDougall IR, Constine LS. Thyroid abnormalities after therapeutic external radiation. *Int J Radiat Oncol Biol Phys.* 1995;31(5):1165–1170.

19. Nishiyama K, Tanaka E, Tarui Y, Miyauchi K, Okagawa K. *Int J Radiat Oncol Biol Phys.* 1996;34(2):439–444.

20. Schneider AB, Recant W, Pinsky SM, Ryo UY, Bekerman C, Shore-Freedman E. Radiation-induced thyroid carcinoma: clinical course and results of therapy in 296 patients. Ann intern Med. 1986;105405:405–412.

21. Sklar C, Whitton J, Mertens A, et al. Abnormalities of the thyroid in survivors of Hodgkin's disease: data from the childhood cancer survivor study. *J Clin Endocrinol Metab.* 2000;85(9):3227–3232.

22. Jereczek-Fossa BA, Alterio D, Jassem J, Gibelli B, Tradati N, Orecchia R. Radiotherapy-induced thyroid disorders. *Cancer Treat Rev.* June 2004;30(4):369–384.

23. Garcia-Serra A, Amdur RJ, Morris CG, Mazzaferri E, Mendenhall WM. Thyroid function should be monitored following radiotherapy to the low neck. *Am J Clin Oncol.* 2005;28(3):255–258.

24. Weijl NI, Van Der Harst D, Brand A, et al. Hypothyroidism during immunotherapy with interleukin-2 is associated with antithyroid antibodies and response to treatment. *J Clin Oncol.* July 1993;11(7):1376–1383.

25. Kearney T, Dang C. Diabetic and endocrine emergencies. *Postgrad Med J.* 2007;(83):79–86.

26. Barri YM, Knochel JP. Hypercalcemia and electrolyte disturbances in malignancy. *Hematol Oncol Clin North Am.* August 1996;10(4):775–790.

27. DeLellis R, Xia L. Paraneoplastic endocrine syndromes: a review. *Endocr Pathol.* Winter 2003;14(4):303–317.

28. Rodgers SE, Perrier ND. Parathyroid carcinoma. *Curr Opin Oncol.* 2006;18:16–22.

29. Van Poznak C. Hypercalcemia of malignancy remains a clinically relevant problem. *Cancer J.* January/February 2006;12(1):21–23.

30. Cvitkovic F, Armand JP, Tubiana-Hulin M, Rossi JF, Warrell RP. Randomized, double-blind, phase II trial of gallium nitrate compared with pamidronate for acute control of cancer-related hypercalcemia. Cancer J, 2006;12:47–53.

31. Barri YM, Knochel JP. Hypercalcemia and electrolyte disturbances in malignancy. *Hematol Oncol Clin North Am.* August 1996;10(4):775–790.

32. Rodgers SE, Perrier ND. Parathyroid carcinoma. *Curr Opin Oncol.* 2006;18:16–22.

33. Sippel RS, Ozgul O, Hartig GK, Mack EA, Chen H. Risks and consequences of incidental parathyroidectomy during thyroid resection. *ANZ J Surg.* 2007;77:33–36.

34. Jameson JS, Johnson BE. Paraneoplastic syndromes: endocrinologic/hematologic. In: Braunwald E, Fauci AD, Kasper DL, Hauser SL, Longo DL, Jameson JL, eds. *Harrison's Principles of Internal Medicine*, 16th ed. New York: McGraw-Hill; 2005:Chapter 86.

35. List AF, Hainsworth JD, Davis BW, Hande KR, Greco A, Johnson DH. The syndrome of inappropriate secretion of antidiuretic hormone (SIADH) in small-cell lung cancer. *J Clin Oncol.* August 1986;4(8):1191–1198.

36. Ilias I, Torpy DJ, Pacak K, Mullen N, Wesley RA, Nieman LK. Cushing's syndrome due to ectopic corticotrophin secretion: twenty years' experience at the National Institutes of Health. *J Clin Endocrinol Metab.* 2005;90(8):4955–4962.

37. Isidori AM, Kaltsas GA, Pozza C, et al. The ectopic adrenocorticotropin syndrome: clinical features, diagnosis, management, and long-term follow-up. *J Clin Endocrinol Metab.* 2006;91(2):371–377.

38. Reimondo G, Paccotti P, Inetto M, et al. The corticotrophin-releasing hormone test is the most reliable noninvasive method to differentiate pituitary from ectopic ACTH secretion in Cushing's syndrome. *Clin Endocrinol.* 2003;58:718–724.

39. Nieman LK. Medical therapy of Cushing's disease. *Pituitary.* 2002;5:77–82.

40. Engelhardt D, Weber MM. Therapy of Cushing's syndrome with steroid biosynthesis inhibitors. *J Steroid Biochem Mol Biol.* 1994;49(4–6):261–267.

41.

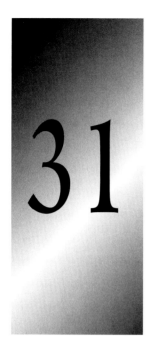

Hematologic Complications of Cancer

Argyrios Stampas
Rebecca G. Smith
Annelise Savodnik
Kevin Fox

The hematological complications of cancer and its treatment are profound, having potential involvement of all blood components. Anemia is frequently seen in oncology patients, regardless of treatment. Platelet count is also frequently affected due to both the primary cancer and the secondary iatrogenic intervention. White blood cells (WBCs) can exhibit overproduction as well as underproduction, each with its own specific risks and concerns. Chemotherapy remains the mainstay of cancer treatment, and because of its myelosuppressive properties, adverse events are known and should be expected. Because of this, the National Cancer Institute (NCI) has defined terminology for adverse events (Table 31.1) (1). Of more relevance to the rehabilitation physician are the consequences of these hematological abnormalities, from worsening quality of life (QOL) to

increasing morbidity and mortality. The rehabilitation team must be aware of these potential complications and their symptoms in order to heed the proper precautions and take the necessary measures to ensure patient safety.

The etiology, incidence, and treatment of each of the hematological complications will be discussed in the following sections based upon their effects on the three critical blood components: erythrocytes, leukocytes, and platelets.

ERYTHROCYTES

Anemia is a symptom of various diseases and can be defined most broadly, yet precisely, as a reduction in

TABLE 31.1
NCI Common Terminology Criteria for Adverse Events

	NEUTROPHILS/ GRANULOCYTES	HEMOGLOBIN	PLATELETS
Grade 1	<LLN–1,500 µL	<LLN–10.0 g/dL	<LLN–75,000/µL
Grade 2	<1,500–1,000 µL	<10.0–8.0 g/dL	<75,000–50,000/µL
Grade 3	<1,000–500 µL	<8.0–6.5 g/dL	<50,000–25,000/µL
Grade 4	<500 µL	<6.5 g/dL	<25,000/µL

Abbreviations: LLN, lower level of normal; NCI, National Cancer Institute.

KEY POINTS

- In oncology populations, anemia can be due to chronic disease, invasion of the bone marrow by the tumor, renal failure, and myelosuppressive therapy.
- Because of such variables as age, sex, lifestyle, and residential altitude, it is difficult to define anemia to a threshold for hemoglobin content.
- Neutropenia is defined as an absolute neutrophil count (ANC) of less than 2,000/μL and should be considered the most serious result of myelosuppression due to its mortality risk.

- Data supports that spontaneous hemorrhaging rarely occurs with platelet counts greater than 50,000/μl, and the risk increases considerably as the platelet count drops below 20,000/μl.
- Hyperviscosity syndrome may develop as a complication of erythrocytosis, leukocytosis, or thrombocytosis.
- Special consideration must be made and precautions observed when providing therapeutic interventions during an acute hospitalization, as well as during inpatient and outpatient rehabilitation programs.

the number of circulating red blood cells. In oncology populations, anemia can be due to chronic disease, invasion of the bone marrow by the tumor, renal failure, and myelosuppressive therapy. Because of such variables as age, sex, lifestyle, and residential altitude, it is difficult to define anemia to a threshold for hemoglobin content. This variability makes it particularly difficult to establish an association between the different cancers and anemia. Knight et al. made a valiant attempt at defining this association by reviewing the literature for the past 30 years, but a precise relationship was impossible (1). What can clearly be appreciated is that of the greater than 18 types of cancers that were reviewed in the literature, anemia is a significant symptom of cancer, correlating to a rate greater than 30% in most types of cancer (2).

Quantifying the rate of chemotherapy-induced anemia is equally as difficult. The incidence of grades 1 and 2 anemia for such common single agents as docetaxel, topotecan, and gemcitabine ranges from 55%–81% (3). Also, the adverse events that are usually reported are the NCI grades 3 and 4, largely under-representing many anemic patients with hemoglobin levels between 8–12 g/dL who still suffer symptoms.

The symptoms of anemia are well known and include dyspnea, fatigue, palpitations, tachycardia, and, when severe, may cause lethargy, confusion, angina, and life-threatening arrhythmias and myocardial infarctions. Much research has been devoted to the study of fatigue in cancer, of which anemia is a likely component. In one study of more than 400 oncology patients receiving chemotherapy or radiation, more than 78% reported fatigue during their treatment course and one-third suffered functional limita-

tions in their activities of daily living (4). Numerous studies have correlated anemia, hemoglobin levels, and QOL scores. This correlation is further supported by the improvement in QOL scores in patients who have responded to erythrocyte-stimulating growth factors. Finally, it has been implicated that anemia may be responsible for poor local control of tumors because tumor hypoxia is associated with resistance to chemotherapy and radiation. It has also been theorized that tumor hypoxia stimulates angiogenesis, which is a marker for increased tumor aggressiveness. For these reasons, improving anemia may not only have a significant impact on QOL, but also may improve morbidity and mortality (2).

To address the issue of improving anemia, the American Society of Clinical Oncology (ASCO) and the American Society of Hematology (ASH) published evidence-based clinical guidelines in 2002 on the use of erythropoietin. A summary of these recommendations can be found in Table 31.2 (5). These recommendations vary in strength of evidence, but are not level I or grade 1 recommendations. Therefore, it is up to the patient's oncologist to determine whether erythropoietin is appropriate in light of each individual's medical history and clinical situation. The three distinct erythrocyte growth factors available—erythropoietin alfa (Epogen, Procrit, Eprex), erythropoietin beta (Neo-Recormon, available in Europe), and darberythropoetin (Aranesp), are administered subcutaneously and require weekly monitoring of hemoglobin levels. Of note, erythropoietin alpha is administered three times per week, whereas erythropoietin beta is once weekly, and darberythropoietin can be given as infrequently as once every three weeks. The purpose of these growth factors is not to replace the need for blood transfusions

TABLE 31.2
Recommendations for the Use of Erythropoietin

1. The use of erythropoietin is recommended in chemotherapy-associated anemia and a hemoglobin concentration below 10 g/dL.[a]
2. For patients with declining hemoglobin levels ≥10 g/dL, the decision to use erythropoietin immediately should be based upon clinical circumstances.[a]
3. The recommended starting dose of erythropoietin is 150 μ/kg subcutaneously thrice weekly for a minimum of 4 wks. If the patient does not respond to this initial dosing, consider increasing to 300 μ/kg thrice weekly for an additional 4–8 wks. Less strong evidence exists for a weekly dosing regimen of 40,000 U/wk.
4. Continuing erythropoietin beyond 6–8 wks without a response (<1–2 g/dL rise in hemoglobin) is not beneficial and patients should be investigated for iron deficiency or tumor progression.
5. Erythropoietin should be titrated to maintain a hemoglobin level of or near 12 g/dL or restarted when the level falls to near 10 g/dL.
6. Baseline and periodic monitoring of iron studies, as well as repletion of iron when indicated, may be valuable in limiting the need for erythropoietin as well as determining the reason for erythropoietin failure.
7. There is an absence of published high-quality studies in the treatment of anemia with erythropoietin of myeloma, non-Hodgkin lymphoma, or chronic lymphocytic leukemia. Oncologists are advised to initiate chemotherapy first. If anemia persists after treatment, it is recommended that erythropoietin be initiated following the above guidelines.

[a]Blood transfusion is also a therapeutic option, depending on clinical circumstances.

Source: Adapted from American Society of Clinical Oncology and American Society of Hematology summaries

when necessary acutely, but to limit the need for this increasingly scarce resource.

Erythrocyte-stimulating growth factors are certainly not benign medications. Hemoglobin levels should be monitored weekly to ensure the appropriate response to erythropoietin. As the ASCO guidelines recommend, erythropoietin should be titrated to achieve a stable hemoglobin level of 12 g/dL. Ineffectiveness of erythropoietin will necessitate further workup, while the overproduction of hemoglobin requires holding or decreasing the usual dose of erythropoietin. It should be emphasized that any planned change to a patient's chemotherapy regimen should be thoroughly discussed with their oncologist.

The side effect profiles of all erythrocyte-stimulating growth factors are similar. Of the common adverse reactions listed on Lexi-Comp ONLINE, fever, nausea, and constipation can occur in up to 20% to more than 50% of patients (6). The rehabilitation team must also be aware that thrombotic events are increased in all cancer patients receiving erythrocyte growth factors, which may occur in nearly 25% of patients. This is compounded by the fact that oncology patients are often in a hypercoagulable state and in the setting of acute rehabilitation; they have experienced increased venous stasis from their hospital admission. The rehabilitation team should have a very low threshold for suspecting a deep venous thrombosis in these patients, including the less likely upper extremities.

LEUKOCYTES

Neutropenia is defined as an ANC of less than 2000/μL and should be considered the most serious result of myelosuppression due to its mortality risk. Neutropenia can also result spontaneously in hematologic malignancies as well as solid tumors that invade the bone marrow. The mortality risk in neutropenia is increased because of febrile neutropenia (FN), which is a medical emergency and usually a harbinger of sepsis. The established definition of FN is (1) a single oral temperature measurement of higher than 38.3°C (101°F) or a temperature of 38°C (100.4°F) or higher for longer than one hour and (2) neutropenia with an ANC of fewer than 500/L or fewer than 1,000/L with predicted rapid decline to fewer than 500/L. All patients treated with chemotherapy are at risk for neutropenic complications, and although it is difficult for physicians to predict which patients will have complications, numerous studies have identified risk factors to recognize patients at greater risk.

It has long been recognized that the degree and duration of neutropenia increases the risk of infection. For example, with grade 3 neutropenia, there is a 10% risk of serious infection within one week, a 30% risk in two weeks, and a 50% risk in four weeks (7). There have also been well-documented clinical factors that predispose patients to increased complications from prolonged neutropenia. Poor performance status is one of these clinical factors and will likely be present in all of the patients admitted to a rehabilitation service. Other predisposing clinical factors include patient age greater than 65 years; history of FN; extensive prior treatment, including large radiation ports, combined chemotherapy, and radiation; cytopenias due to bone marrow involvement by tumor; poor nutritional status; the presence of open wounds or active infections; more advanced cancer; chronic obstructive pulmonary disease; and any other serious comorbidity (7).

There have also been numerous studies associating types of cancers with their treatments and their risks for FN. The ASCO formulated a table that documents the rates of FN for commonly used chemotherapy regimens and further divided this by treatment diagnosis. Selected diagnoses and regimens have been included (Table 31.3) (8). The rehabilitation team should be aware of the potential for FN in their patients because this is an influential factor for receiving granulocyte colony-stimulating factors (G-CSF), as determined by their oncologist.

The nadir, or trough in the decline of the neutrophils, is generally expected seven days after chemotherapy. Oftentimes, the nadir neutrophil count and its timing are based upon its prior occurrence after chemotherapy cycle 1. In an attempt to reduce the rate of mortality secondary to FN, the ASCO released updated guidelines in 2006 for the prophylaxis against neutropenia, with the use of G-CSF partly based upon the documented rates of FN. Because the reduction of FN itself is a significant clinical outcome, the updated ASCO guidelines recommend primary prophylaxis (immediately after the first cycle of chemotherapy prior to neutropenia), with a G-CSF at a lower FN occurrence rate, from 40% to 20% (8). ASCO also recommends primary prophylaxis for those in whom a reduction in treatment intensity may compromise survival and those greater than 65 years of age receiving curative chemotherapy (cyclophosphamide, adriamycin, vincristine, and prednisone [CHOP] or more aggressive regimens) (8). Using these recommendations along with the clinical judgment of the oncologist, patients in a rehabilitation setting may have received or will need continued administration of G-CSF.

There are presently two forms of recombinant human G-CSF approved in the United States: filgrastim (Neupogen) and pegfilgrastim (Neulasta). Based upon the various indications (i.e., chemotherapy-induced neutropenia, bone marrow transplant, or severe chronic neutropenia), filgrastim is generally administered on a daily basis throughout the neutropenic period and discontinued when an indicated ANC has been achieved and remains stable. The duration of the treatment, as well as the goal ANC, should be delineated by the oncologist. Unlike filgrastim, pegfilgrastim is administered once after each chemotherapy cycle, at least 24 hours after cytotoxic therapy, with a mean time of maximum effect at day nine. Although the dosing between the two varies, they are otherwise similar in regards to efficacy, adverse reactions, and monitoring. The most frequent adverse reaction to G-CSFs is bone pain, occurring in 22%–33% of patients (6). With daily administration of filgrastim, WBCs should be monitored daily to prevent leukocytosis and to make dose adjustments if necessary.

FN is a medical emergency. If the patient is an inpatient, intravenous (IV) antibiotics should be initiated as soon as possible. Possible sources of infection should be located by a thorough physical exam and cultures sent prior to the initiation of antibiotics. The initial evaluation should include a complete blood count (CBC) with a differential; a complete metabolic panel, including liver function tests; urine culture; and two sets of blood cultures from two separate sites. As previously stated, this is a medical emergency and the prompt initiation of antibiotics should not be delayed in order to adequately culture the patient. Segal et al. have published an algorithm for the initial treatment of FN (Fig. 31.1) (10) based upon published clinical evidence (10). The rehabilitation physician should initiate this algorithm and decide whether vancomycin is indicated. Reasons to initiate vancomycin include (1) the patient is colonized by methicillin-resistant *Staphylococcus aureus* (MRSA) or other resistant Gram-positive organisms, (2) infected tunneled catheter, (3) blood cultures growing Gram-positive organisms, and/or (4) high risk for viridans group streptococcal infection (prior quinolone prophylaxis or active mucositis) (10). After promptly deciding upon and initiating antibiotics, it is appropriate to have the patient admitted to an inpatient medicine unit where further management and closer monitoring may be instituted. In the outpatient setting, the patient's oncologist should be contacted to determine the next step of the algorithm and the patient referred to the emergency room for further management.

In contrast to neutropenia, hyperleukocytosis may cause life-threatening complications because of leukostasis secondary to blood hyperviscosity. Hyperviscosity has also been documented in thrombocytosis as well as erythrocytosis, although less frequently. Leukostasis is the accumulation of leukemic blasts in the lumen of the vasculature. The sluggish capillary blood flow secondary to hyperleukocytosis has been attributed to both the increase in the number of WBCs and an abnormal expression of adhesion molecules. As expected, symptoms are found in an end-organ distribution with intraparenchymal brain hemorrhage and respiratory failure accounting for the majority of deaths (11).

TABLE 31.3
Incidence of Hematologic and Infectious Toxicities Associated with Selected Chemotherapy Regimens

CANCER HISTOLOGY	REGIMEN	NO. OF PATIENTS	FEBRILE NEUTROPENIA (%)	INFECTION (GRADE ≥3; %)	INFECTIOUS DEATH (%)
Kaposi sarcoma	VP-16	36	—	—	—
	(oral) paclitaxel	56	—	—	—
NHL	CHOP + G-CSF	25	0	-	
Bladder	GC	203	2	2.5	1
	MVAC	202	14	15.1	2.5
	CBDCA/Pac ± G-CSF	33	21	1	0
Breast	CA (60 mg/m²)	1,060	10	17	0
	CA → (all doses)	1,590	3	11	0
	CEF	351	8.5	—	0
	TAC	109	23.8	—	—
	A→T→C	484	3	3	0
	A→T→C + G-CSF	493	2	4	0
	AC→T	501	6	5	0
	AC→T + G-CSF	495	2	3	0
	A (75)	165	12.3	4.3	1
	Doc (100)	61	5.7	2.5	1
	AC	215	10	2	0.5
	AT	214	33	8	0
	TAC	54	34	2	0
Colorectal	5-FU/LV/L	449	—	—	<1
	5-FU/LV	116	—	—	1.7
	IFL	189	7.1	1.8	<1
	FL	226	14.6	0	1.4
	I	226	5.8	2.2	<1
Gastric	ECF (infusion)	289	-	6	<1
Head/neck	5-FU/CBDA	86	—	—	1.2
	Cis/Doc	36	6	11	0
	Cis/Doc/5-FU	43	19	2	0
Lung SCLC	Topo	107	28	4.7	
	CAV	104	26	4.8	1
Lung NSCLC	Cis/PAC (24 h)	288	16	10	2
	Cis/Gem	288	4	7	1
	Cis/Doc	289	11	9	
Lymphoma	MOPP	123	-	13	1
	ABVD	115	-	2	0
NHL	CHOP	216	-	5	1
	CHOP-R	33	18	6	0
Relapse NHL	VAPEC-B	39	44	5	2
	ESHAP	122	30	—	4.1
	DHAP	90	48	31	11
Multiple myeloma untreated	VAD ± Inf	169	—	—	1.2
MM recurrent/ refractory	VAD ± Inf	52	—	32.7	7.7

Abbreviations: 5-FU/CBDA, fluorouracil, carboplatin; 5-FU/LV/L, fluorouracil, leucovorin, levamisole; A, doxorubicin; ABVD, doxorubicin, bleomycin, vinblastine, decarbazine; CA, or AC, doxorubicin, cyclophosphamide; CAV, cyclophosphamide, doxorubicin, vincristine; CBDCA/Pac, carboplatin, paclitaxel; CEF, cyclophosphamide, epirubicin, fluorouracil; CHOP, cyclophosphamide, doxorubicin, vincristine, prednisone; CHOP-R, cyclophosph-amide, doxorubicin, vincristine, prednisone, rituximab; Cis/Doc, cisplatin, docetaxel; Cis/Gem, cisplatin, gemcitabine; Cis/Pac, cisplatin, paclitaxel; DHAP, dexamethasone, cisplatin, cytarabine; Doc, docetaxel; ECF, cyclophosphamide, epirubicin, fluorouracil; ESHAP, etoposide, methylprednisolone, Ara-C, cisplatin; GC, gemcitabine, cisplatin; G-CSF, granulocyte colony-stimulating factor; IFL, irinotecan, fluorouracil, leucovorin; inf, alpha interferon; MM, multiple myeloma; MOPP, mechlorethamine, vincristine, procarbazine; prednisone; MVAC, methotrexate, vinblastine, doxorubicin, cisplatin; NHL, non-Hodgkin lymphoma; NSCLC, non-squamous cell lung cancer; SCLC, squamous cell lung cancer; T, paclitaxel; TAC, docetaxel, doxorubicin, cisplatin; Topo, topocetan VAD, vincristine, doxorubicin, dexamethasone; VAPEC-B, vincristine, doxorubicin, prednisone, etoposide, cyclophosph-amide, bleomycin; VP-16, etoposide.

Source: Adapted from Ref. 8.

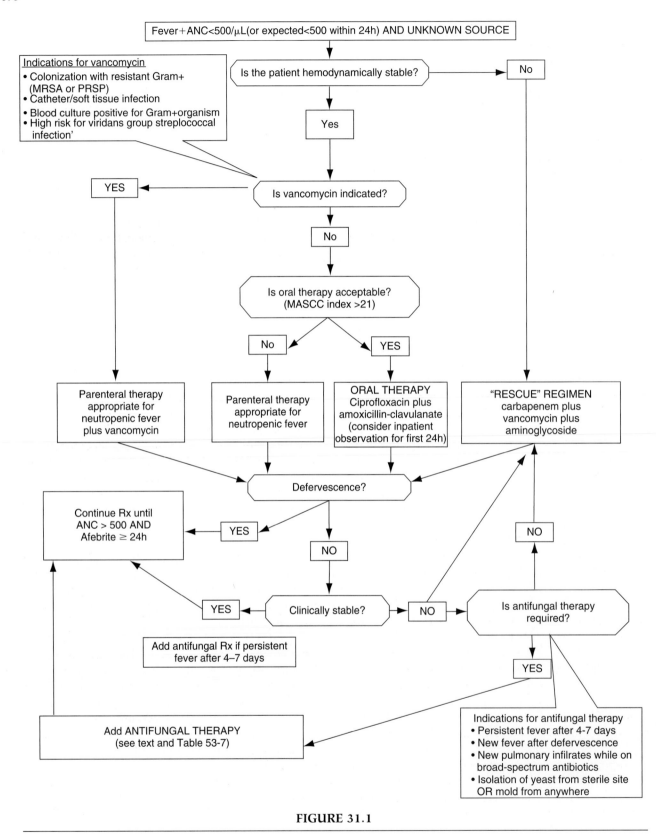

FIGURE 31.1

Algorithm for the treatment of febrile neutropenia.

Hyperleukocytosis is a well-documented phenomenon in acute leukemias, with greater symptomatology in myelogenic leukemias than in lymphoblastic leukemias. It is also far less symptomatic in chronic leukemias versus acute leukemias, despite the frequency of persistently elevated WBCs found in the former. The risk of mortality secondary to hyperleukocytosis ranges from 20%–40%. In acute myelogenous leukemia (AML), the frequency of hyperleukocytosis occurs in 5%–13% in adults and 12%–25% in pediatrics (11). In the French-American-British (FAB) classification system, myeloid leukemias with monocytic differentiation (M4, M5) have been associated with hyperleukocytosis. In acute lymphoblastic leukemia (ALL), the incidence of hyperleukocytosis ranges between 10%–30% and has a bimodal distribution, both in children less than one year of age and in patients in the second decade of life (11). Although hyperleukocytosis is more prevalent in ALL than in AML, leukostasis is rarely seen in ALL.

The diagnosis of leukostasis based on clinical exam alone can be indistinguishable from other disease presentations. The constellation of hyperleukocytosis and clinical exam findings are necessary to diagnose leukostasis and treat the patient urgently. Acute hyperleukocytosis has been defined as a WBC count and leukoblast count greater than 100,000/mm³. However, leukostasis has been documented to occur with far fewer WBCs. In both ALL and AML, a WBC count greater than 50,000/mm³ and 30,000/mm³, respectively, has been sufficient to cause leukostasis. Once leukostasis has occurred, fever is a nearly ubiquitous finding ($T > 39°C$ [102.2°F]), although infection is rarely the cause. The presenting symptoms are related to the respiratory system and the central nervous system. Respiratory distress and hypoxia may occur, with 50% of patients demonstrating pulmonary infiltrates on a chest radiograph. In the presence of a fever, this may be mistaken for an infection. Neurological symptoms may include confusion, lethargy, delirium, and coma. Complaints of headaches, dizziness, changes in visual acuity or field defects, tinnitus, or gait instability are frequent. On careful exam, papilledema and retinal hemorrhages may be seen, as well as cranial nerve defects and nuchal rigidity. Less common clinical findings, but of significance, include myocardial ischemia, priapism, limb ischemia, bowel infarction, and renal vein thrombosis (11).

Leukostasis can be further complicated with other concomitant hematologic abnormalities. Concurrent evidence of disseminated intravascular coagulation (DIC) has been seen in 40% of AML and 23% of ALL during leukostasis (11). Thrombocytopenia is generally found in leukostasis, yet underestimated in its documentation because automated cell analyzers often misread WBC fragments as platelets. Finally, spontaneous tumor lysis syndrome has occurred in both AML (10%) and ALL (18%) (11).

The mainstay of treatment of leukostasis is induction chemotherapy. However, because of the complication of tumor lysis syndrome, cytoreduction is also implemented concurrently. Both hydroxyurea and leukophoresis are often initiated with chemotherapy. Prompt leukoreduction can be most quickly achieved with leukopharesis, but there is much debate in the literature regarding guidelines for this intervention. The current standard of care, based upon a concise review of the literature by Porcu et al., is the emergent initiation of intravenous fluids, administration of allopurinol and hydroxyurea, as well as the correction of possible concurrent coagulopathy and thrombocytopenia (11). Induction chemotherapy should be sought as soon as possible.

PLATELETS

Platelet disorders in cancer patients may be seen as thrombocytosis, thrombocytopenia, and/or alterations of platelet function. As with the other blood components, platelet disorders may be caused by the cancer or its myelosuppressive treatment. Thrombocytopenia is broadly defined as a platelet count less than 150,000/μl and may present as poor hemostasis and an increased risk of bleeding. The greatest concern in thrombocytopenic patients is the risk for spontaneous bleeding, and the most worrisome of these are intracranial hemorrhages. Acute leukemias, hairy cell leukemia, myeloproliferative syndromes, and myelodysplasia are associated with thrombocytopenia and altered platelet function (12). Thrombocytopenia in malignancy is generally caused by decreased platelet production from myelosuppression due to chemotherapy or radiation or infiltration of the marrow by the malignancy. Other causes to be aware of include splenic sequestration, immune-mediated thrombocytopenia, or a consumptive process, as seen in DIC. It is important to recognize the multiple etiologies of thrombocytopenia that cancer patients may present with simultaneously.

The risk of bleeding in thrombocytopenic patients has been well documented in the literature since Gaydos et al. in 1962 (13). Since then, data supports that spontaneous hemorrhaging rarely occurs with platelet counts greater than 50,000/μl, and the risk increases considerably as the platelet count drops below 20,000/μl. It is now recognized that it is not only the absolute platelet count that increases bleeding risk, but also the nature of the underlying disease, the medications being used (which may alter platelet function), and also fever and coagulopathies that prohibit hemostasis. Thus, the function of the platelets is equally as important as the absolute number when assessing bleeding risk. However, there is no data in the literature to suggest that bleeding time can be used to assess bleeding risks.

Why not transfuse every thrombocytopenic patient with platelets prophylactically after chemotherapy and radiation to reduce the risk of bleeding? Unfortunately, this cannot be done, and the answer is multifactorial. First, prophylactic platelet transfusions have a brief duration of effect and multiple transfusions are often necessary if bleeding occurs. Second, the efficacy of transfusions is decreased as their frequency is increased. Finally, the risk to the patient is significant. Among transfusion products, bacterial contamination of platelets is the highest infective risk of all transfusion products, occurring in 1 in 2,000–3,000 transfusions of platelets (14). In the United States, transfusion mortality rates secondary to sepsis from bacteria-infected platelet products is second only to clerical error, with rates of 1–20,000 to 1–85,000 exposures (14). Thus, it is important to identify those patients who are at risk for bleeding and limit prophylactic transfusions to those patients only.

Efforts have been made to recognize those patients who are at risk for bleeding due to thrombocytopenia for the purpose of prophylactic platelet transfusions. Elting et al. developed a Bleeding Risk Index (BRI), published in 2002, that recognized certain factors predictive of bleeding in lymphomas and solid tumors after chemotherapy in a retrospective study (15). These factors were given a value, and based upon a patient's total score, the bleeding risk could be assessed on day 1

of chemotherapy (Table 31.4) (15). High-risk patients are transfused at 20,000/μl, moderate-risk patients at 10,000/μl, and low-risk patients at 5,000/μl. Although the BRI is helpful in identifying high-risk patients, several studies have demonstrated its limited clinical application (16). The ASCO developed guidelines for the transfusion of platelets in thrombocytopenic patients in 2001 (17). They reiterate that prophylactic transfusions of platelets in thrombocytopenia should rely on a threshold based upon "the patient's diagnosis, clinical condition, and treatment modality" (17). Essentially, clinical judgment dictates when a transfusion is necessary rather than platelet counts alone.

The clinical presentation of a bleeding patient may range from subtle skin and mucosal petechiae to more obvious ecchymosis, to frank epistaxis, hematuria, and hematochezia. Along with thrombocytopenia, there are a number of other reasons why a cancer patient may have spontaneous bleeding, including DIC, platelet dysfunction, decreased hepatic synthesis of coagulation factors, and autoimmune phenomena. The initial evaluation should include a CBC, liver function test, a coagulation panel, and a peripheral blood smear. After leukoreduced platelet transfusion is completed, a CBC should be drawn after 1 and 24 hours (17). If the platelets have not increased after one hour, alloimmunization or hypersplenism should be suspected. If the patient had an initial increase in platelets after 1 hour but the platelets return to their initial value after 24 hours, a consumptive process should be suspected secondary to continued bleeding, DIC, or platelet dysfunction resulting from paraprotein release from malignant cells (18). If bleeding persists or transfusion is ineffective in increasing the platelet count, it is appropriate to transfer the patient for further management and closer observation.

HYPERVISCOSITY SYNDROME

Hyperviscosity syndrome may develop as a complication of erythrocytosis, leukocytosis, or thrombocytosis. It may also occur when other blood components are increased, including circulating proteins. Approximately 20% of patients diagnosed with Waldenström macroglobulinemia (WM) have clinically evident hyperviscosity syndrome (19). WM is classified as a low-grade lymphoma and affects approximately 1,500 Americans each year, with a median age of about 65 years (20). WM is a neoplastic transformation of a lymphocyte, which continuously produces monoclonal immunoglobulin M (IgM). As the precursor to more specific antibodies in the lineage of the antibody response, IgM is a large molecule found in the intravascular space. At increased concentrations, IgM can increase plasma viscosity and

---

TABLE 31.4
Scoring the Bleeding Risk Index

Factor	Points[a]
Any prior bleeding episode	2
Receiving penicillin, cephalosporin, antihistamine, heparin, tricyclic, antidepressant, or phenothiazines	
Bone marrow metastasis	2
Baseline platelet count <75,000/mL	2
Genitourinary or gynecologic neoplasm	2
Baseline Zubrod score ≥ ⇑	2
Chemotherapy regimen, including any of the following: cisplatin, carboplatin, carmustine, lomustine, dacarbazine, mitomycin C	1

[a]Points are summed on day 1 of each chemotherapy cycle. Patients with 0 points are in the low-risk group, patients with 1–3 points are in the moderate-risk group, and patients with ≥ 4 points are in the high-risk group.

expand plasma volume, causing hyperviscosity syndrome. Clinically, hyperviscosity syndrome presents as a triad of bleeding, visual changes, and other neurologic deficits. Paradoxically, hyperviscosity syndrome causes thrombosis and patients are at risk for myocardial infarction and cerebrovascular accidents. Patients may also present with congestive heart failure. Tortuous, distended "sausage like" retinal veins are pathognomic for hyperviscosity syndrome. The treatment of hyperviscosity syndrome is prompt plasmapharesis to reduce the circulating concentration of IgM (21). This is a medical emergency, and immediate intervention will prevent life-threatening bleeding and irreversible neurologic deficits. Plasmapharesis is an interim treatment, and chemotherapy must be initiated concomitantly to suppress the underlying malignant process.

SPECIAL CONSIDERATIONS AND THERAPEUTIC PRECAUTIONS

Hematological complications of cancer and its treatment pose risks to a person's morbidity and mortality, as discussed earlier. Anemia may compromise cardio-

pulmonary stability and limit the patient's ability to tolerate activities. Neutropenia increases a patient's risk of developing infections. Thrombocytopenia increases the risk of spontaneous bleeding. Although research regarding these risks is limited, general recommendations (22) and guidelines (23) have been published to help guide activity and limit complications. Special consideration must be made and precautions observed when providing therapeutic interventions during an acute hospitalization, as well as during inpatient and outpatient rehabilitation programs. Table 31.5 (23) summarizes the precautions that are followed at many institutions, including Memorial Sloan-Kettering Cancer Center (MSKCC). Additionally, it is important to monitor vital signs and cardiopulmonary tolerance using scales such as the Borg or modified Borg Scale of Perceived Exertion to more accurately assess the patient's response to exercise and minimize complications.

A rehabilitation program should be individually tailored to accommodate hematological limitations. It is imperative for the therapist to monitor hemoglobin levels when working with these patients. Most medical institutions consider a hemoglobin of 8.0 g/dL a critical value. When hemoglobin levels are ≤8 g/dL,

---

TABLE 31.5
Exercise Precautions for Cancer Patients

MEDICAL PROBLEM	LABORATORY VALUES	RECOMMENDATIONS
Anemia Normal values: Hct 37–47%; Hb 12–16 g/dL	Hematocrit >35%; hemoglobin >10 g/dL	Ambulation, resistance exercise, and self-care as tolerated
	Hematocrit 25%–35%; hemoglobin 8–10 g/dL	Essential ADLs, assistance as needed for safety; light aerobics, light weights (1–2 lb)
	Hct < 25%, Hb < 8 g/dL	Light ROM exercise, isometrics; avoid aerobic or progressive resistance programs. Permission from primary oncology service is often obtained for additional limited activity if the pt has chronic anemia as seen in lymphoma and leukemia.
Thrombocytopenia Normal values: platelets 150,000–450,000/m³	150,000–450,00/m³	Unrestricted normal activity
	50,000–150,000/m³	Progressive resistance, swimming, bicycling
	30,000–50,000/m³	Moderate active exercise/ROM, light weights (1–2 lbs; no heavy resistance/isokinetics); ambulation, aquatic therapy, stationary bike
	20,000–30,000/m³	Self-care activity, light exercise (passive or active), functional mobility
	<20,000/m³	With permission from primary oncology service: ambulation and self-care with assistance as needed for endurance/balance safety; minimal or cautious exercise/activity; essential ADLs only

Abbreviations: ADLs, activities of daily living; Hct, Hematocrit; Hb, hemoglobin; pt, patient; ROM, range of motion.
Source: (Adapted from Ref. 23).

physical and occupational therapies are held. Exceptions to this general precaution are commonly made in patients with chronic anemia related to malignancies directly affecting the bone marrow, as seen in lymphoma and leukemia. In these populations, the primary oncology team should be involved in developing an individualized rehabilitation program.

Hospitalized patients with neutropenia are usually required to observe special precautions to minimize the risk and severity of infections. These may vary between institutions, but generally include isolation precautions and neutropenic precautions. During hospitalization, isolation precautions may require the patient wear a mask and gloves when leaving the hospital room for therapies or procedures. Reverse isolation precautions may require all visitors wear a mask and gloves when entering a patient's room. During certain times of the year, such as flu season, all visitors of patients with lymphoma and leukemia at many institutions, regardless of the patients' neutrophil counts, are required to follow reverse isolation precautions.

The neutropenic precautions followed at The Abramson Cancer Center of the University of Pennsylvania are initiated when the WBC count drops to 1,000/mm³ or below. Patients with neutropenia who are living at home are instructed to take their temperature four times daily and contact their physician if their oral temperature is above 100.5°F (38.1°C). Both hospitalized patients and those living at home with prolonged neutropenia are advised to eliminate uncooked foods from their diet secondary to the risk of its containing bacteria. These foods include raw vegetables; fresh, frozen, and dried fruits; raw meats and fish; natural cheeses; uncooked eggs; uncooked herbs, spices, and black pepper; and instant iced tea, coffee, or punch. Patients must avoid exposure to fresh flowers and plants that may have bacteria in the soil. Enemas, rectal suppositories, and rectal temperatures should not be administered. Unless an emergency, dental work should not be performed.

Although patients with neutropenia are generally able to leave their hospital rooms while following isolation precautions, there are medical circumstances when patients are confined to the hospital room unless given permission by the general oncology team to leave. This is especially true of those undergoing hospitalization for allogeneic bone marrow transplantations. This entails hospitalization for approximately one month, at which time the patients are predominantly confined to their rooms. This restricts the therapeutic options and requires a creative approach to maximize therapy in the limited space of the patient's room.

At most institutions, an uncomplicated patient confined to his or her room due to neutropenia or allogeneic bone marrow precautions will receive an initial physical therapy evaluation and instructions for a self-directed exercise program based on the patient's medical status and ability to tolerate exercise. A self-directed exercise program may include providing a sanitized stationary bicycle or an in-bed Pedo Cycle for the patient to maintain endurance (22). At MSKCC, the physical therapist evaluates the patient and provides level 1 and/or level 2 exercise programs. Additionally, the therapist instructs the patient on exercise guidelines and the use of the Pedo Cycle. Level 1 activities include gentle, active range-of-motion (AROM) exercises of both upper and lower extremities in a supine or supported seated position. Level 2 activities incorporate the use of a Thera-Band for resistive upper extremity exercises, as well as standing and lower extremity strengthening exercises. A team approach may be utilized to include nursing staff for regular daily monitoring of the patient's activity. The therapist will follow up regularly to monitor the patient's progress. If a patient experiences a decline in function, more frequent and formal therapy sessions will be initiated. Prior to discharge, a home exercise program is developed and reviewed with the patient.

Patients who have experienced significant medical complications during their hospitalizations may be debilitated and require an inpatient rehabilitation program prior to returning home. Communication between the primary oncology team, therapists, and consultants is imperative for minimizing functional decline and providing appropriate rehabilitation services.

When working with thrombocytopenic patients, the therapist must regularly monitor the platelet count and tailor the treatment plan accordingly. Most institutions consider a count of 20,000/μl a critical value. Generally, therapies are held for patients with counts of 20,000/μl or less. As with anemia, exceptions to the general precautions are made for patients with chronically low platelet counts. The therapist must be aware of the increased risk of spontaneous internal bleeding with a low platelet count and guard patients closely during all mobility to reduce the risk of falls. General guidelines for physical activity and thrombocytopenia are as follows: <20,000/μl, functional mobility/ADLs; 20,000–30,000/μl, light exercise, AROM, and functional mobility; 30,000–50,000/μl, moderate exercise, stationary bike; 50,000–150,000/μl, progressive resistive exercise, bicycling; >150,000/μl, unrestricted normal activity (23).

References

1. Daniel D, Crawford J. Myelotoxicity from chemotherapy. *Semin Oncol.* 2006;33:74–85.
2. Knight K, Wade S, Balducci L. Prevalence and outcomes of anemia in cancer: a systematic review of the literature. *Am J of Med.* 2004;116(7A):11S–26S.

3. Groopman JE, Itri LM. Chemotherapy-induced anemia in adults: incidence and treatment. *J Natl Cancer Inst.* 1999;91(19): 1616–1634.

4. Vogelzang NJ, Breitbart W, Cella D, et al. Patient, caregiver, and oncologist perception of cancer-related fatigue: results of a tripart assessment survey. *Semin Hematol.* 1997;34:4–12.

5. Rizzo JD, Lichtin AE, Woolf SH, et al. Use of epoetin in patients with cancer: evidence-based clinical practice guidelines of the American Society of Clinical Oncology and the American Society of Hematology. *J Clin Oncol.* 2002;20:4083–4107.

6. http://www.crlonline.com/crlsql/servlet/crlonline

7. Crawford J, Dale DC, Lyman GH. Chemotherapy-induced neutropenia: risks, consequences, and new directions for its management. *Cancer.* 2004;100:228–237.

8. Smith TJ, et al. Update of recommendations for the use of white blood cell growth factors: an evidence-based clinical practice guideline. *J Clin Oncol.* 2006;24:3187–3205.

9. Holmes FA, O'Shaughnessy JA, Vukelja S, et al. Blinded, randomized, multicenter study to evaluate single administration pegfilgrastim once per cycle versus daily filgrastim as an adjunct to chemotherapy in patients with high-risk stage II or stage III/IV breast cancer. *J Clin Oncol.* 2002;20(3):727–731.

10. Segal BH, Walsh TJ, Gea-B**anacloche JC,** Holland SM. Infections in the cancer patient. In: Devita VT, Hellman S, Rosenberg SA, eds. *Cancer: Principles and Practice of Oncology.* Philadelphia: Lippincott Williams and Wilkins; 2000:2488.

11. Porcu P, Cripe L, Ng E, et al. Hyperleukocytic leukemias and leukostasis: a review of pathophysiology, clinical presentation and management. *Leuk Lymphoma.* 2000;39(1–2):18.

12. Avvisati G, Tirindelli MC, Annibali O. Thrombocytopenia and hemorrhagic risk in cancer patients. *Crit Rev Oncol Hematol.* 2003;48S:S13–S16.

13. Gaydos LA, Freireich EJ, Mantel N. The quantitative relation between platelet count and hemorrhage in patients with acute leukemia. *N Engl J Med.* 1962;266:905–909.

14. Hillyer CD, Josephson CD, Blajchman MA, Vostal JG, Epstein JS,. Bacterial contamination of blood components: risks, strategies, and regulation: joint ASH and AABB educational session in transfusion medicine. *Hematology Am Soc Hematol Educ Program.* 2003;575–589.

15. Elting LS, et al. The bleeding risk index: a clinical prediction rule to guide the prophylactic use of platelet transfusions in patients with lymphoma or solid tumors. *Cancer.* 2002;94:3252.

16. Slichter, SJ. Relationship between platelet count and bleeding risk in thrombocytopenic patients. *Transfus Med Rev.* 2004;18(3):153–167.

17. Schiffer CA, et al. Platelet transfusion for patients with cancer: clinical practice guidelines of the American Society of Clinical Oncology. *J Clin Oncol.* 2001;19:1519–1538.

18. Green D. Management of bleeding complications of hematologic malignancies. *Semin Thromb Hemost.* 2007;33:427–434.

19. Hussein MA, Oken MM. Multiple myeloma, macroglobulinemia, and amyloidosis. In: Furie B, Atkins MB, Mayer RJ, Cassileth PA, eds. *Clinical Hematology and Oncology. Presentation, Diagnosis and Treatment.* Philadelphia: Churchill Livingstone; 2003:596–598.

20. In: Furie B, et al., eds. *Clinical Hematology and Oncology. Presentation, Diagnosis and Treatment.* Philadelphia: Churchill Livingstone; 2003:596–598.

21. Gertz MA, et al. Treatment recommendations in Waldenstrom's macroglobulinemia: consensus panel recommendations from the second international workshop on Waldenstrom's macroglobulinemia. *Semin Oncol.* 2003;30(2):121–126.

22. Gillis TA., Eileen SD. Rehabilitation following bone marrow transplantation. *Cancer Suppl.* 2001;92(4):998–1007.

23. Gerber L, Vargo M, Smith R. Rehabilitation of the cancer patient. In: Devita VT, Hellman S, Rosenberg SA, eds. *Cancer: Principles and Practice of Oncology.* Philadelphia: Lippincott Williams and Wilkins;7th Edition; 2005:2725–2726.

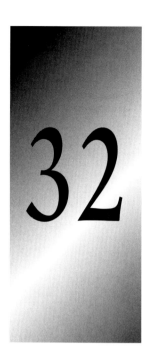

Infectious Complications of Cancer

Michelle Stern
Christine Laviano

Patients with cancer are susceptible to a variety of infections. Common infections include sepsis, cellulitis, pneumonia, urinary tract infections, and colitis. Infections can result in a decline in functional status, with subsequent debility, fatigue, and reduced oral intake. Common infections seen in the rehabilitation setting are presented in Table 32.1. Severe sepsis, defined as a systemic response to infection with acute organ dysfunction, causes about one in ten cancer deaths each year in the United States. Patients with underlying cancers have a 30% higher risk of death, compared with other severe sepsis patients (1,2).

<table>
<caption>

TABLE 32.1
Common Infections in the Rehabilitation Setting
</caption>
<tr><th>INFECTIONS</th><th>ASSOCIATION WITH TYPE OF CANCER</th><th>PRESENTING SIGNS</th><th>REHAB IMPLICATIONS</th></tr>
<tr><td>Bladder</td><td>Genitourinary/prostate Lower gastrointestinal Central nervous system lesions</td><td>Fever, burning on urination, cloudy and foul-smelling urine</td><td>Can lead to urosepsis with change in mental status and low blood pressure</td></tr>
<tr><td>Cellulitis</td><td>Breast cancer Head and neck cancers</td><td>Erythema Fever Edema of limb</td><td>Lymphedema Pain</td></tr>
<tr><td>Sepsis</td><td>Cancers and treatments causing neutropenia After bone marrow transplantation Patients who undergo splenectomy (Hodgkin disease)</td><td>Change in mental status Hypotension Fever</td><td>May be unable to participate due to weakness, fatigue, and low blood pressure</td></tr>
<tr><td>Pneumonia</td><td>Lung cancer Head and neck and brain tumors may be at risk for aspiration pneumonia</td><td>Coughing, sputum Decreased oxygen saturation Fever Abnormal chest sounds</td><td>Oxygen supplementation needed and close monitoring or saturation when mobilized</td></tr>
</table>

KEY POINTS

- An early sign of infection may be a change in the ability to tolerate therapy or a change in mental status.
- The cancer patient will have a broader differential diagnosis of an infection, including bacterial, fungal, viral, and parasitic etiologies.
- Pneumonia is common in patients with primary lung cancer or metastasis, due to partial obstruction of the airways causing atelectasis and post-obstructive pneumonia.
- Some of the techniques used during chest physical therapy include incentive spirometry, rhythmic

breathing and coughing, postural drainage, percussion, vibration, and aerobic exercise.
- Patients with *Clostridium difficile* require contact isolation, but should not prohibit therapy with contact precautions. Active diarrhea can interfere with therapy via electrolyte imbalances and dehydration.
- Compression garments, antiembolic stockings, and pneumatic pumps must be discontinued when a patient develops cellulitis, due to the increased risk of the infection spreading.

An early sign of infection may be a change in the ability to tolerate therapy or a change in mental status. Due to the heterogenous nature of cancer, certain factors place a patient at higher risk for infections. When evaluating a patient, it is important to note the type and stage of the cancer, risk of neutropenia, and alterations in humoral immunity and cell-mediated immunity. Critical information includes the timing and duration of cancer treatments such as chemotherapy, corticosteroids, radiation treatments, and stem cell/bone marrow transplant. Patients suffering from lymphoma, leukemia, or other blood cancers are more susceptible to severe sepsis than those suffering from cancer of a solid organ (3–5). Local factors also play a role in infection risk. Obstruction from metastases, operative procedures that disrupt normal anatomic barriers, and urinary and venous catheters can all lead to infections (6). The cancer patient will also have a broader differential diagnosis of the cause of an infection, which can include bacterial, fungal, viral, and parasitic etiologies (7).

Neutropenia (absolute neutrophil count [ANC]< 500/µL) is the most common cause of an infection in cancer patients. Patients at high risk for prolonged neutropenia include an initial treatment protocol in acute leukemia, patients undergoing bone marrow or stem cell transplantation, and after chemotherapy treatement (7). This is especially true in patients with testicular carcinoma, small cell carcinoma of the lung, and some lymphomas and sarcomas. Maximal neutropenia occurs 6–14 days after conventional doses of anthracyclines, antifolates, and antimetabolites. Alkylating agents differ widely in the timing of cytopenias. Nitrosoureas, dacarbazine, and procarbazine can display delayed marrow toxicity, first appearing six weeks after dosing. In patients undergoing bone marrow and/or hematopoietic stem cell transplantation, neutropenia typically lasts from one week before transplantation

(myeloablative or non-myeloablative regimens can be used) to three weeks after transplantation (7). The most common sites of infection include the lung, oropharynx, paranasal sinuses, blood, urinary tract, skin, and soft tissues, including the perirectal area (7-10).

Neutropenic patients may lack the usual signs of an infection due to their inability to mount a full inflammatory response, making diagnosis more difficult. Pneumonia may not present with x-ray changes or purulent sputum. Also, patients with a urinary tract infection may not have white blood cells in the urine, and patients with meningitis may lack typical meningeal signs. Peritonitis may present with abdominal pain, distention, and diminished-to-absent bowel sounds, but guarding and rebound may be absent (7,8). Neutropenia predisposes the cancer patient to many bacterial and fungal infections the most common are Gram-negative bacilli (*E. coli*, *Klebsiella*, and *Pseudomonas*), Gram-positive organisms (*Staphylococcus*, *Streptococcus viridans*, and *Enterococcus* species), and fungi (*Candida* and *Aspergillus*) (7,11,12). In addition to the customary supportive care for neutropenic patients, therapy with recombinant human granulocyte colony-stimulating factor (rG-CSF) (filgrastim) and pegfilgrastim (long-acting form of filgrastim) has been shown to be beneficial. Common reactions due to this medication that are often seen in rehab include fatigue, nausea, thrombocytopenia, bone pain, and myalgias. More serious complications that need to be monitored closely include allergic reactions, adult respiratory distress syndrome, and splenic rupture, especially in those that complain of upper-left abdominal pain or shoulder tip pain (13).

There is no established benefit for reverse isolation in most cases. Only patients with severe and prolonged neutropenia, such as remission induction therapy for acute leukemia or bone marrow transplantation, are treated in protected environments. Isolation should not limit the therapy program (7,14).

Cell-mediated immunity is regulated by T lymphocytes or mononuclear phagocytes. Patients with Hodgkin disease are likely to have impaired cell-mediated immunity, as are patients with chronic and acute lymphocytic leukemia (7). Defects in the mononuclear phagocytic system have been described in patients with monocytic leukemia. Immunosuppressive therapy with agents such as cyclosporine, tacrolimus, azathioprine, corticosteroids, and fludarabine can lead to impaired cellular immunity. Radiation therapy also results in depression of cell-mediated immunity, which can last for several months following treatment. These patients are especially susceptible to infection with intracellular organisms (7,15,16).

Humoral immunity is mediated by immunoglobulins with a binding specificity for microbial antigens and is produced by B lymphocytes. Multiple myeloma and Waldenström macroglobulinemia will cause lower levels of normal immunoglobulins. Hypogammaglobulinemia occurs in patients with chronic lymphocytic leukemia (7). Patients who have undergone splenectomy, such as those with Hodgkin disease, are also at greater risk for developing infections (17).

Pneumonia is common in patients with primary lung cancer or metastasis, due to partial obstruction of the airways with subsequent atelectasis and post-obstructive pneumonia. This may cause lung abscess formation with polymicrobial organisms (staphylococci, Gram-negative bacilli, anaerobes). If this occurs, treatment in addition to antibiotics is needed to ensure eradication of the infection, such as chemotherapy, radiation, stent placement, or endobronchial brachytherapy (18). Chest physical therapy may be beneficial to incorporate a variety of airway clearance techniques. Some of the techniques used during chest physical therapy include incentive spirometry, rhythmic breathing and coughing, postural drainage, and percussion and vibration. Aerobic exercise helps to improve pulmonary function and loosens mucus. When performing chest physical therapy, it is important to monitor for metastatic lesions to the ribs.

Pneumonia can also develop in patients at risk for aspiration, as in patients with head and neck cancers and those with brain lesions affecting swallowing. In these high-risk patients a flexible endoscopic evaluation of swallowing with sensory testing (FEEST) or modified barium swallow should be ordered to evaluate aspiration risk.

Mucositis is the inflammation of the mucosa that lines the digestive tract from the oral cavity to the anus and is a common complication in hematological malignancies on chemotherapy, radiation in head and neck cancers, and with hematopoietic stem cell transplantation. Mucositis significantly complicates cancer treatment by contributing to pain, dysphagia, weight loss, and increasing the risk of infection by facilitating microorganisms to enter the tissue and bloodstream (7). Antibiotics should be started promptly in these patients with signs of infections (19).

Infections of the urinary tract are common among patients with neurogenic bladder, catheter placement, or who have a compromise of ureteral excretion. Post-void residual and emptying of the bladder should be noted. Pyelonephritis should be differentiated from cystitis. Urine cultures taken with proper technique in patients without an indwelling catheter that reveal greater than 100,000 colonies should be treated in immunocompromised patients, regardless of symptoms (7). Patients may complain of urinary frequency, urgency, burning, or bladder incontinence.

Clostridium difficile colitis can occur in cancer patients due to chemotherapy or from the use of antibiotics (7). Patients with *Clostridium difficile* require contact isolation, which should not prohibit the patient from receiving therapy with contact precautions. While the patient is having active diarrhea, this can lead to electrolyte imbalance and dehydration, which may interfere with a therapy program and should be monitored closely.

Cellulitis occurs more often in patients with a history of lymph node dissection and can occur years after surgery. Intravenous catheters can also serve as a nidus for infection (7). Cellulitis presents as erythema, pain, swelling, and warmth and should be differentiated from venous thrombosis, which is also common in this patient population. Elevation of the limb while not in therapy can help reduce swelling.

Viral infections are most common following bone marrow transplant and in patients with leukemia and lymphoma. The herpes viruses are the most commonly involved, and treatment should begin immediately in patients with signs of infection who are at high risk. Typical lesions are most often found on the lips and oral mucosa, as well as in the genital and perianal region. When the skin lesions are visible, it is useful to differentiate from other causes of infections, but this is not always the case (7). Prophylaxis treatment can be considered to prevent reactivation in patients undergoing intensive chemotherapy or bone marrow transplant (20).

Antibiotic-resistant bacterial organisms are more common in persons with cancer, with the more common types being methicillin-resistant *Staphylococcus aureus* (MRSA) and vancomycin-resistant *Enterococcus faecalis* (VREF). These organisms have typically required isolation in a hospital setting, but studies are currently looking at the value of isolation on a rehabilitation floor (21–23).

There is still much debate in the current literature regarding the use of prophylactic antibiotics in these patients. It is not recommended routinely, but can be considered for high-risk patients (7).

PHYSICAL THERAPY IMPLICATIONS WITH INFECTIONS

Vital signs, including oxygen saturation, should be monitored closely during mobilization in patients with pneumonia. Adjustments in the intensity of the therapy program might be required if the patient is having difficulty maintaining an oxygen saturation at 90% or higher, or if they become short of breath. If the patient fails to maintain an oxygen saturation at that level after the intensity of the activity has been reduced, the session should be terminated for that day. Supplemental oxygen may be required to assist patients in maintaining oxygen saturation. If the patient requires the use of a non-rebreather mask, therapy is usually held until the mask is no longer required.

Decisions regarding the type and amount of supplemental oxygen required are determined after consultation with the rehab team.

Urinary tract infections and sepsis usually do not have far-reaching implications for a therapy program other than the ability for these infections to be accompanied by fever, low blood pressure, and an alteration in a patient's mental status. The intensity of the therapy program will be determined by the patient's ability to participate. Caution is warranted when exercising patients who have a fever. The patient's tolerance should be used as a guide. Patients with sepsis may have tachycardia or might have difficulty maintaining their blood pressure. Vital signs should be monitored closely in these patients and therapy held if the patient is not able to maintain their heart rate and blood pressure in response to activity. If this is the case, discussion with the medical team is important in order to establish appropriate blood pressure parameters for the patient during therapy. Oxygen saturation should also be monitored in patients with sepsis. Again, oxygen saturation levels should be maintained above 90%.

All compressive treatments, including compression garments, antiembolic stockings, and pneumatic pumps, must be discontinued when a patient develops cellulitis, due to the increased risk of the infection spreading (24). Once the infection has been treated with antibiotics, compressive treatments can be reinitiated.

References

1. Angus DC, Linde-Zwirble WT, Lidicker J, Clermont G, Carcillo J, Pinsky MR.Epidemiology of severe sepsis in the United States: analysis of incidence, outcome, and associated costs of care. *Crit Care Med.* 2001;29:1303–1310.

2. Williams MD, Braun LA, Cooper LM, et al. Hospitalized cancer patients with severe sepsis: analysis of incidence, mortality, and associated costs of care. *Crit Care.* 2004;8:R291–R298.

3. Casazza AR, Duvall CP, Carbone PP. Infection in lymphoma, histology, treatment and duration in relation to incidence and survival. *JAMA.* 1966;197:710–716.

4. Hersh EM, Bodey GP, Nies BA, Freireich EJ. Causes of death in acute leukemia. A ten-year study of 414 patients from 1954-1963. *JAMA.* 1965;198:105–109.

5. Bodey GP. Infections in cancer patients. A continuing association. *Am J Med.* 1986;81(Suppl 1A):11–26.

6. Maki DG. Infections associated with intravascular lines. In: Remington JS, Swartz MN, eds. *Current Clinical Topics in Infectious Diseases,* Vol. 3. New York: McGraw-Hill; 1980:309–363.

7. Rolston K, Bodey G. *Infections in Patients with Cancer.* Section 39 in Holland-Frei Cancer Medicine, 6th ed. Hamilton, Ontario: BC Decker; 2003.

8. Sickles EA, Greene WH, Wiernik PH. Clinical presentation of infection in granulocytopenic patients. *Arch Intern Med.* 1975;135:715–719.

9. Talcott JA, Siegel RD, Finberg R, Goldman L. Risk assessment in cancer patients with fever and neutropenia: a prospective, two center validation of a prediction rule. *J Clin Oncol.* 1992;10:316–322.

10. Rolston KV. Prediction of neutropenia. *Int J Antimicrob Agents.* 2000 October;16(2):113–115.

11. Koll BS, Brown AE. The changing epidemiology of infections at cancer hospitals. *Clin Infect Dis.* 1993;17(Suppl 2):S322–S328.

12. Bodey G, Bueltmann B, Duguid W, et al. Fungal infections in cancer patients: an international autopsy survey. *Eur J Clin Microbiol Infect Dis.* 1992;11:99–109.

13. Bhatt V, Saleem A. Drug-induced neutropenia—pathophysiology, clinical features, and management. *Ann Clin Lab Sci.* 2004;34(2):131–137.

14. Armstrong D. Symposium on infectious complications of neoplastic disease (Part II). Protected environments are discomforting and expensive and do not offer meaningful Protection. *Am J Med.* 1984 April;76(4):685–689.

15. Royer HD, Reinherz EL. T lymphocytes: ontogeny, function, and relevance to clinical disorders. *N Engl J Med.* 1987;317:1136–1142.

16. Hahn H, Kaufmann SHE. The role of cell-mediated immunity in bacterial infections. *Rev Infect Dis.* 1981;3:1221–1250.

17. Bohnsack JF, Brown EJ. The role of the spleen in resistance to infection. *Ann Rev Med.* 1986;37:49–59.

18. Rolston K. The spectrum of pulmonary infections in cancer patients. *Curr Opin Oncol.* July 2001; 13(4):218–223.

19. Silverman S Jr. Diagnosis and management of oral mucositis. *Support Oncol.* February 2007;5(2 Suppl 1):13–21.

20. Gold D, Corey L. Acyclovir prophylaxis for herpes simplex virus infection. *Antimicrob Agents Chemother.* 1987; 31:361–367.

21. Medeiros AA. Nosocomial outbreaks of multi-resistant bacteria: extended-spectrum beta-lactamases have arrived in North America. *Ann Intern Med.* 1993;119:428–430.

22. Murray BE. Vancomycin-resistant enterococci. *Am J Med.* 1997;102:284–293.

23. Mylotte JM, Kahler L, Graham R, Young L, Goodnough S. Prospective surveillance for antibiotic-resistant organisms in patients with spinal cord injury admitted to an acute rehabilitation unit. *Am J Infect Control.* August 2000;28(4):291–297.

24. Harris SR, Hugi MR, Olivotto IA, Levine M. Clinical practice guidelines for the care and treatment of breast cancer: 11. Lymphedema. *Canadian Medical Association Journal.* 2001;164(2):191–199.

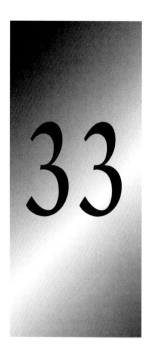

Thromboembolic Complications of Cancer

Julie Lin
Amanda Molnar

Thromboembolic events are well-recognized complications of malignancy. These events stem from any number of etiologies, including immobility, recent surgery, chemotherapy, and a hypercoagulability observed in cancer patients. Such hypercoagulable states are often characterized by thrombocytosis and increased plasma fibrinogen as well as markers of coagulation activation, including thrombin-antithrombin complex or prothrombin fragments 1 + 2 (1).

Events such as arterial and venous thromboembolism can result in significant morbidity and mortality. They can be a terminal event, occur following a diagnosis of malignancy, or, in some cases, can be a harbinger of occult cancer. It has been estimated that there is a 3- to 19-fold increase in prevalence of concomitant cancer in patients presenting with an idiopathic thromboembolic event (2). A large analysis of Medicare beneficiaries (3) found that patients who were hospitalized for DVT or pulmonary embolism (PE) had nearly 3.0 times the odds of being diagnored with colorectal carcinoina and more than 1.5 times the odds of being diagnosed with breast carcinoma respectively in the subsequent 24 months.

There is also some evidence that critical oncogenic events may initiate activation of the coagulation cascade, leading to a prothrombotic environment that not only manifests as venous thromboembolic disease, but also aids the progression of the malignancy (4). Although not currently recommended, this has led some to suggest that anticoagulation might play a role in cancer treatment.

There can be disastrous consequences of thromboembolic events, such as loss of limb with arterial thrombosis and even death. This chapter will focus on the effective prophylaxis and treatment of thromboembolic disease in the cancer setting to help minimize potential complications and maximize function.

TROUSSEAU SYNDROME

Trousseau syndrome is a term that was originally described by Trousseau in 1865 as the association of unexpected and/or unexplained migratory thrombophlebitis and malignancy. The definition now includes events with a wide range of presentations, including superficial thrombophlebitis, nonbacterial thrombotic endocarditis, arterial emboli, and disseminated intravascular coagulopathy (5). Trousseau syndrome is associated with many cancers, including pancreatic, gall bladder, gastric, colorectal, and pulmonary adenocarcinomas. Adenocarcinoma and metastatic cancer have been reported to be independently associated with PE risk (6). Additional at-risk categories in cancer include solid tumors, advanced age, infection, and leukopenia (7).

Recent research has suggested that malignant transformation, tumor angiogenesis, and metastasis can generate clotting intermediates, such as tissue factor (TF), factor Xa, and thrombin clotting; platelet function inhibitors; or fibrinolysis inhibitors, such as

KEY POINTS

- Thromboembolic events in cancer can be due to immobility, recent surgery, chemotherapy, or a hypercoagulable state.
- Low molecular weight heparin is favored over warfarin and unfractionated heparin for both the treatment and prophylaxis of thromboembolic events in the cancer.
- Cancer treatments such as thalidomide plus glucocorticoids and tamoxifen increase the risk of developing thromboembolic disease.
- Clinical presentation of deep venous thrombosis (DVT) includes pain, swelling, and erythema, but physical findings alone are unreliable to establish the diagnosis of DVT.
- Recent data demonstrates no significant differences in the new pulmonary events, fatal pulmonary embolism, or bleeding complications between those patients who were on bed rest versus those who were ambulatory after a new diagnosis of DVT.

plasminogen activator inhibitor type 1. In addition, it is felt that TF, Xa, and thrombin may induce important tumor cell-signaling cascades (8).

Medical treatment of Trousseau syndrome requires the use of anticoagulation treatment. Warfarin, unfractionated heparin, and most recently, low molecular weight heparin have all been used. Additional potential medications target various steps in the coagulation cascade, including direct thrombin inhibition and inhibition of factor Xa, factor IXa, the factor VIIa-tissue factor complex, and the factor Va-factor VIIIa complex. (9) Fondaparinaux, the first selective factor Xa inhibitor, represents one of these newer options. Its works by binding rapidly and strongly to antithrombin and catalyzes the inhibition of factor Xa, which results in inhibition of thrombin generation (10). Warfarin, for unknown reasons, is not as effective in preventing Trousseau syndrome (11).

Low molecular weight heparin (12) is favored over warfarin and unfractionated heparin for both the treatment and prophylaxis of thromboembolic events in the cancer patient. Advantages of low molecular weight heparin include the fact that it is more easily administered, does not require laboratory monitoring, has fewer adverse events, and is cost-effective than unfractionated heparin (13). As mentioned, there is also evidence to suggest that low molecular weight heparin exerts anticancer effects, including direct antitumor, antiangiogenic, and immune system modulatory actions (13).

TREATMENT-RELATED THROMBOEMBOLISM

Treatments such as cancer chemotherapy and various supportive therapies can increase the risk for throm-

boembolic events. Examples include thalidomide (14) or related compounds combined with glucocorticoids and/or cytotoxic chemotherapy in multiple myeloma patients (15). It has been estimated that thalidomide, dexamethasone, and both together significantly increase the risk of venous thromboembolic events among multiple myeloma patients by 2.6, 2.8, and 8 times, respectively (16). It is widely known that tamoxifen in breast cancer patients significantly increases risk for thromboembolic events. Some of the conventional risk factors for atherosclerosis may also increase risk for thromboembolic events. In a study by Decensi et al. (17), the authors demonstrated that the risk of thromboembolic events in patients taking tamoxifen was higher in women aged 55 or older, currently smoking, those with a family history of coronary heart disease, women with a body mass index ≥ 25 kg/m^2, those with elevated blood pressure, and total cholesterol ≥ 250 mg/dL, all compared with a placebo.

The third-generation aromatase inhibitors anastrozole, letrozole, and exemestane are associated with a significantly lower incidence of thromboembolic events compared to tamoxifen (18,19). Other treatments that increase risk for thromboembolic events include raloxifene (20) as well as cyclophosphamide, methotrexate, and fluorouracil (21).

ARTERIAL THROMBOSIS

Arterial thrombosis is a rare complication of cancer. Pathogenetic mechanisms of arterial thrombosis or embolism in malignancy include prolonged arterial spasm, precipitation of cryoglobulins or other abnormal proteins in small arteries, direct tumor invasion of arteries, embolization of intracardiac or intra-arterial metastases, and spontaneous arterial thrombosis due to hypercoagulability (22). There is a sparse literature, consisting primarily of case series, that describes the clinical course of such patients. Acute abdominal aortic thrombosis is typically caused by atherosclerosis, dissection, or aneurysm and is rare in the absence of these factors. Poiree et al. (23) reported two cases of acute aortic thrombosis in cancer patients whose only risk factor was cancer. Yeung and colleagues (24) reported a woman with repeated acute arterial thrombosis of the femoral arteries after intravenous carboplatin-based combination chemotherapy for metastatic ovarian carcinoma. Cases have been reported of the occurrence of limb ischemia in patients later diagnosed with acute lymphoblastic leukemia (25), acute promyelocytic leukemia (26), or acute myelogenous leukemia (27). Rigdon and associates (28) reported a case series of acute arterial thrombosis in three patients with breast, lung, and pancreatic cancer, all of whom ultimately required amputation. Another case series reported the presentations of seven patients with thromboembolism. Two clinical patterns were demonstrated, one with in situ thrombosis of small arteries and the other with occlusion of large arteries causing limb ischemia or fatal organ infarction (22).

Physical findings of limb ischemia include pain, pallor, pulselessness, paralysis, paresthesias, and cool skin. More advanced arterial occlusive disease is characterized by pain at rest or ischemic gangrene. Ischemic ulcers can develop, involving the tips of toes or heel of the foot. Appropriate treatment for advanced disease typically includes angiography and either angioplasty or surgery (29). Severe limb ischemia can result in tissue loss, including focal ischemic ulceration or nonhealing wounds (30). Gangrene and sepsis represent significant complications of chronic ischemia. The best patient outcomes are achieved when early diagnosis is determined and appropriate treatment administered. The differential diagnosis of limb ischemia includes lymphedema and cellulitis. Simple noninvasive tests, such as measurement of ankle-to-brachial indices or use of Doppler pressures, can help to determine the severity of limb ischemia. An ankle/arm systolic pressure index of <0.9 indicates severe disease. Subsequent diagnostic imaging studies, such as arteriography, magic resonance angiography, or ultrasound duplex scanning, provide detailed information needed to plan revascularization therapy. Contrast arteriography is used for definitive localization before intervention (31). Arteriography can be useful in mapping the extent and location of arterial pathology prior to revascularization (29). Treatment for limb ischemia includes heparinization and revascularization.

Balloon angioplasty and stenting work best for focal segments of narrowing or short occlusions of the iliac arteries and are less successful with longer and more distal lesions. Long segments of occlusion, especially those distal to the common femoral artery, are best treated with surgical bypass. Treatment for severe limb ischemia typically involves surgery. The best outcomes typically result from early amputation of nonviable limbs, heparinization, angiography, and immediate operative revascularization for threatened limbs (32).

DEEP VENOUS THROMBOSIS AND PULMONARY EMBOLISM

Venous thromboembolism (VTE) represents the most common thrombotic event in cancer patients. The incidence of concomitant cancer in patients with idiopathic venous thromboembolism ranges between 4%–24%, and the mean incidence of cancer within three years after that point is roughly 9% (33). Estimates of the prevalence of cancer among patients with venous thrombosis vary from 3%–18% (9,34). Concomitant VTE is considered a marker and potential mediator of increased risk of death among older cancer patients (35). In one study of VTE in nearly 9,500 glioma patients, it was associated with a 30% increase in the risk of death within two years (36). Conversely, Ziegler et al. (37) reported that unlike solid tumors, VTE before or at the time of diagnosis of acute leukemia is not associated with a worse prognosis. Additional risk factors for VTE in cancer include obesity; varicose veins; inflammatory bowel disease; fractures; surgery; use of oral corticosteroids, oral contraceptives, and opposed hormone therapy; and having indwelling central venous catheters (38,39).

Preventive measures for VTE consist of anticoagulation and compression stockings. Isolated studies and meta-analyses have consistently demonstrated the efficacy of pharmacologic prophylaxis, with higher doses of both low molecular weight and unfractionated heparin being more efficacious (40). In addition to pharmacological means, prophylaxis should include intermittent pneumatic compression and graduated compression, both of which have been shown to be effective in reducing VTE (41). Patients with new metastases or multiple episodes of neutropenia may be at increased risk for recurrent VTE. In these patients, vena cava filters may be appropriate (42).

Clinical presentation of deep venous thrombosis includes a painful swollen limb, positive Homan signs, and erythema. Unfortunately, physical findings alone are unreliable to establish the diagnosis. Confirmation should be made with compression ultrasonography or venography (42). Magnetic resonance venography is an option when ultrasound is inconclusive and, although not used often, contrast venography (44).

Radiologic diagnosis of PE includes ventilation-perfusion nuclear medicine scans, and chest computed tomography (CT). Chest x-ray and ventilation-perfusion scan can indicate the probability of pulmonary embolism. Patients with low-probability ventilation-perfusion (V/Q) scans have a 10–15% chance of having pulmonary embolus (45). In these patients, further diagnostic imaging, such as CT angiography, can be useful. Spiral CT angiography offers numerous advantages compared with other diagnostic tests (46). Specific calculations, such as the pulmonary arterial obstruction index, determined by embolus size and location on CT, may help to predict patient outcome (47). It has been shown that a D-dimer assay and CT pulmonary angiography together can be highly predictive for a negative CT pulmonary angiogram in suspected acute pulmonary embolus. In a study involving 101 patients undergoing both D-dimer assay and CT pulmonary angiography, a negative D-dimer could have prevented CT examinations from being performed in 36% of patients (48). Laboratory markers may aid in the diagnosis of VTE. Markers of thrombin generation and fibrinolysis have been utilized as first-line screening tests, with most elevated in acute thrombosis (49). Laboratory studies include D-dimer, factor V Leiden, prothrombin 20210A mutation, antiphospholipid antibodies, homocystinemia and antithrombin, protein C, or protein S (50). D-dimer has a high negative predictive value but poor specificity in the diagnosis of VTE. The rapid D-dimer enzyme-linked immunosorbent assays and the whole blood agglutination assay, SimpliRED D-dimer (Agen Biomedical, Brisbane, Australia) may be utilized as exclusionary tests for venous thrombosis (49). While the cost-effectiveness of D-dimers measurement in the diagnosis of *asymptomatic* DVT is unproven, D-dimers have been shown to be cost-effective in the diagnosis of *symptomatic* DVT (51). Laboratory markers may also be used to correlate response to anticoagulation and resolution of thromboembolism. In one case report of a patient with cholangiocarcinoma and pulmonary embolism, laboratory markers demonstrated elevated levels of fibrinogen, fibrinogen degradation product (FDP), D-dimer, and immunoglobulin M (IgM) anticardiolipin antibody (aCL Ab). After three weeks of low molecular weight heparin, the thromboembolism and follow-up laboratory studies demonstrated normalization of aCL Ab titer, FDP, and D-dimer levels (52).

Treatment for VTE includes anticoagulation with warfarin and eventually low molecular weight heparin and placement of vena cava filters in select cases. Inferior vena cava (IVC) filters may be useful in cancer patients at high risk for recurrent VTE who have contraindications to anticoagulation (11).

ADDITIONAL COMPLICATIONS

Additional thrombotic complications include cerebral sinus thrombosis and nonbacterial thrombotic endocarditis. Cerebral sinus thrombosis is a rare but devastating complication. In a review of the neurology database at Memorial Sloan-Kettering Cancer Center between 1994 and 1998, 20 patients were identified. Nine had hematologic malignancies and 11 had solid tumors. The most common symptom was headache. The most frequently involved cerebral sinus was the superior sagittal sinus. Multiple sinuses were affected in 8 of 19 patients. Five patients had a cerebral or subarachnoid hemorrhage and three had infarction. Disorders of coagulation were the most frequent etiology in patients with hematologic malignancies; compression or invasion of the cerebral sinus from dural/calvarial metastasis was the main cause in those with solid tumors. Ten of 20 patients improved clinically and 3 of 6 patients improved radiologically (53). Another study reported seven cases of sagittal sinus thrombosis over seven years in five patients with hematologic malignancies and two with solid tumors (54). Treatment for this condition includes anticoagulation therapy. Patients may improve, with resolution of hemiparesis reported in some cases (55).

Nonbacterial thrombotic or marantic endocarditis (NBTE) is another serious, potentially devastating, and underdiagnosed complication that can result in strokes (56). Two-dimensional echocardiography should be utilized to detect the presence of valvular thrombi. Findings are characterized by cardiac vegetations along valvular coaptation lines with preservation of leaflets (57). Treatment consists of systemic anticoagulation and control of the underlying malignancy whenever possible. Characteristic diagnostic findings are thrombocytopenia, elevated D-dimer levels, and a specific stroke pattern in magnetic resonance imaging (58). NBTE can be seen with many types of malignancies, including ovarian carcinoma. In one review of patients with nonbacterial thrombotic endocarditis, those with adenocarcinoma, especially pancreatic cancer, were at higher risk than patients with other malignant processes (59).

Extension of tumor mass into the inferior vena cava has been reported in patients with renal cell carcinoma, hepatocellular carcinoma, testicular tumors, or adrenal carcinoma (59). Ozben et al. (60) reported a case of pancreatic cancer associated with tumor extending from the inferior vena cava to the right atrium. Additional rare thromboembolic events in the cancer patient include disseminated intravascular coagulation, thrombotic thrombocytopenic purpura, or hemolytic uremic syndrome (61).

MOBILIZATION AND REHABILITATION OF CANCER PATIENTS AFTER DVT

Along with other measures discussed previously, prevention of VTE in a hospital setting is achieved, in great part, with early mobilization initiated by physical therapy and nursing. Encouraging ambulation, educating patients regarding extremity elevation and active movement, and providing compression garments to patients at risk for VTE are all appropriate interventions rehabilitation professionals can provide. Patients should also be educated on the signs and symptoms of acute vascular complications so they can notify medical staff immediately.

The more difficult decision is when and how to mobilize a patient with cancer following the diagnosis of DVT. Until recently, many patients newly diagnosed with DVT were placed on bed rest for several days. This clinical dogma was based on theory that it would take approximately three days for a new DVT to "mature" by forming fibrin cross links and thus be less prone to embolize. Recent data, however, demonstrated no significant differences in the new pulmonary events, fatal pulmonary embolism, or bleeding complications between those patients who were on bed rest versus those who were ambulatory (62). Though some contradicting evidence still exists, a majority of studies provide evidence that supports early mobilization and activity. Feldman (63) recently reviewed early mobilization after DVT and found the evidence supports mobilization "as soon as possible." In fact, early ambulation may assist the resolution of DVT-associated symptoms,

---

TABLE 33.1

MSKCC Guidelines for Physical, Occupational, and Lymphedema Therapy in Patients with Venous Thromboembolism

Lower-Extremity DVT

■ For patients with acute lower-extremity DVT, with or without PE, and no IVC filter, therapy (including physical, occupational, and lymphedema with bandaging and MLD) can be initiated once they are therapeutic on an anticoagulant. Resistive exercises should generally be deferred for 48–72 hours.

Definition of therapeutic anticoagulation by modality:

• LMWH preparations are preferred, as they are therapeutic immediately following the first injection. Monitoring is not required. Common preparations include enoxaparin (Lovenox), dalteparin (Fragmin), and tinzaparin (Innohep).

• Unfractionated heparin may take one to two days to become therapeutic and is more prone to bleeding complications than LMWH. The APTT should be monitored, and therapy can begin when it is between 50 and 70.

• Warfarin (Coumadin) may take several days to become therapeutic. The INR should be monitored, and therapy can begin when it is between 2 and 3.

■ For patients with acute lower-extremity DVT (with or without PE) and an IVC filter, therapy can be initiated immediately, regardless of their anticoagulation status.

■ For patients with acute lower-extremity DVT who cannot be anticoagulated and an IVC filter cannot be placed, therapy can be started immediately, but should be functional in nature (ambulation, balance, ADL training) and avoid resistive and repetitive exercises. Such patients are at very high risk for PE and death. Therapists are advised to discuss therapy interventions with the patient's primary attending or the rehabilitation medicine attending so that the relative risks and benefits of therapy can be better delineated.

Upper-Extremity DVT

■ Upper-extremity DVT carries the same risk for PE and death as lower-extremity DVT. IVC filters are not protective. For patients with acute upper-extremity DVT, with or without PE, therapy (including physical, occupational, and lymphedema with bandaging and MLD) can be initiated once they are therapeutic on an anticoagulant. Resistive exercises should generally be deferred for 48–72 hours. (See previous anticoagulation guidelines.)

■ For patients with acute upper-extremity DVT who cannot be anticoagulated, therapy should be functional in nature (ambulation, balance, ADL training) and avoid resistive and repetitive exercises. Such patients are at very high risk for PE and death. Therapists are advised to discuss therapy interventions with the patient's primary attending or the rehabilitation medicine attending so that the relative risks and benefits of therapy can be better delineated.

Abbreviations: ADL, activities of daily living; APTT, adjusted partial thromboplastin time; DVT, deep vein thrombosis; INR, international normalized ratio; IVC, interior vena cava; LMWH, low molecular weight heparin; MLD, manual lymphatic drainage; PE, pulmonary edema.

including pain and swelling (64,65). Unfortunately, most of the present data is based on lower-extremity DVT and there is little data concerning mobilization with upper-extremity DVT.

Before beginning any therapy session, the rehabilitation professional should review all recent lab values, special tests or procedures, and vital signs. It is also necessary to be vigilant for signs and symptoms of complications such as fever, dyspnea, chest pain, palpitations, and worsening fatigue, as they may be indicators of pulmonary embolism (66). There are general guidelines that the rehabilitation staff should consider when deciding upon the best rehabilitation strategy for patients who have newly diagnosed thromboembolism. The guidelines developed by Dr. Michael D. Stubblefield at the Memorial Sloan-Kettering Cancer Center to guide the safe and effective physical, occupational, and lymphedema therapy are presented in Table 33.1. It should be noted that these are only guidelines and that the clinical decision-making process used in a given patient may vary considerably and should be done on an individual basis, taking the patient's wishes, prognosis, current medical condition, etc. into consideration.

CONCLUSION

Patients presenting with arterial and venous thromboembolic events without demonstrable cause should be investigated for malignancy. Patients with malignancy should also be evaluated for evidence of hypercoagulability in an attempt to prevent VTE and arterial thromboembolic complications. Complications from thromboembolic events can significantly impact function and mobility, hindering quality of life, particularly following limb amputation and thromboembolic events. Appropriate rehabilitation, including early mobilization, can help to mitigate complications and maximize clinical outcomes. Rehabilitation professionals should be familiar with the potential complications of thromboembolic events in cancer patients and should be well versed in the management of their sequelae.

References

1. Zwicker JI, Furie BC, Furie B. Cancer-associated thrombosis. *Crit Rev Oncol Hematol.* 2007;62(2):126–136.
2. Otten HM, Prins MH. Venous thromboembolism and occult malignancy. *Thromb Res.* 2001;102(6):V187–V194.
3. Polite BN, Lamont EB. Are venous thromboembolic events associated with subsequent breast and colorectal carcinoma diagnoses in the elderly? A case-control study of Medicare beneficiaries. *Cancer.* 2006;106(4):923–930.
4. Lee AY. Thrombosis and cancer: The role of screening for occult cancer and recognizing the underlying biological mechanisms. *Hematology Am Soc Hematol Educ Program.* 2006;438–443.
5. Moody J, Scott B. Trousseau's syndrome. *Iowa Med* 1991;81(7):303–304.
6. Ogren M, Bergqvist D, Wahlander K, Eriksson H, Sternby NH. Trousseau's syndrome - what is the evidence? A population-based autopsy study. *Thromb Haemost.* 2006;95(3):541–545.
7. Lin J, Wakefield TW, Henke PK. Risk factors associated with venous thromboembolic events in patients with malignancy. *Blood Coagul Fibrinolysis.* 2006;17(4):265–270.
8. Rickles FR. Mechanisms of cancer-induced thrombosis in cancer. *Pathophysiol Haemost Thromb.* 2006;35(1–2):103–110.
9. Grudeva-Popova J. Cancer and venous thromboembolism. *J BUON.* 2005;10(4):483–489.
10. Mousa SA. Role of current and emerging antithrombotics in thrombosis and cancer. *Drugs Today (Barc).* 2006;42(5):331–350.
11. Streiff MB. Long-term therapy of venous thromboembolism in cancer patients. *J Natl Compr Canc Netw.* 2006;4(9):903–910.
12. Levine MN, Lee AY, Kakkar AK. From Trousseau to targeted therapy: New insights and innovations in thrombosis and cancer. *J Thromb Haemost.* 2003;1(7):1456–1463.
13. Burris HA, III. Low-molecular-weight heparins in the treatment of cancer-associated thrombosis: A new standard of care? *Semin Oncol.* 2006;33(2 Suppl 4):S3–S16.
14. Goz M, Eren MN, Cakir O. Arterial thrombosis and thalidomide. *J Thromb Thrombolysis.* 2008;25(2):224–226.
15. Zonder JA. Thrombotic complications of myeloma therapy. *Hematology Am Soc Hematol Educ Program.* 2006;348–355.
16. El Accaoui RN, Shamseddeen WA, Taher AT. Thalidomide and thrombosis. A meta-analysis. *Thromb Haemost.* 2007;97(6):1031–1036.
17. Decensi A, Maisonneuve P, Rotmensz N, et al. Effect of tamoxifen on venous thromboembolic events in a breast cancer prevention trial. *Circulation.* 2005;111(5):650–656.
18. Jonat W, Hilpert F, Kaufmann M. Aromatase inhibitors: A safety comparison. *Expert Opin Drug Saf.* 2007;6(2):165–174.
19. Mouridsen HT. Incidence and management of side effects associated with aromatase inhibitors in the adjuvant treatment of breast cancer in postmenopausal women. *Curr Med Res Opin.* 2006;22(8):1609–1621.
20. Deitcher SR, Gomes MP. The risk of venous thromboembolic disease associated with adjuvant hormone therapy for breast carcinoma: A systematic review. *Cancer.* 2004;101(3):439–449.
21. Pritchard KI, Paterson AH, Paul NA, Zee B, Fine S, Pater J. Increased thromboembolic complications with concurrent tamoxifen and chemotherapy in a randomized trial of adjuvant therapy for women with breast cancer. National Cancer Institute of Canada Clinical Trials Group Breast Cancer Site Group. *J Clin Oncol.* 1996;14(10):2731–2737.
22. Pathanjali Sharma PV, Babu SC, Shah PM, Seirafi R, Clauss RH. Arterial thrombosis and embolism in malignancy. *J Cardiovasc Surg (Torino).* 1985;26(5):479–483.
23. Poiree S, Monnier-Cholley L, Tubiana JM, Arrive L. Acute abdominal aortic thrombosis in cancer patients. *Abdom Imaging.* 2004;29(4):511–513.
24. Yeung KK, Coster E, Floris Vos AW, Van d, V, Linsen MA, Wisselink W. Repeated arterial thrombosis as a complication of carboplatin-based chemotherapy. *Vascular.* 2006;14(1):51–54.
25. Redmond EJ, Welch M, Durrans D, et al. Acute ischaemia of the lower limb: An unusual presenting feature of acute lymphoblastic leukaemia. *Eur J Vasc Surg.* 1993;7(6):750–752.
26. Kalk E, Goede A, Rose P. Acute arterial thrombosis in acute promyelocytic leukaemia. *Clin Lab Haematol.* 2003;25(4):267–270.
27. Chang VT, Aviv H, Howard LM, Padberg F. Acute myelogenous leukemia associated with extreme symptomatic thrombocytosis and chromosome 3q translocation: Case report and review of literature. *Am J Hematol.* 2003;72(1):20–26.

28. Rigdon EE. Trousseau's syndrome and acute arterial thrombosis. *Cardiovasc Surg.* 2000;8(3):214–218.

29. Halperin JL. Evaluation of patients with peripheral vascular disease. *Thromb Res.* 2002;106(6):V303–V311.

30. Dawson DL, Hagino RT. Critical limb ischemia. *Curr Treat Options Cardiovasc Med.* 2001;3(3):237–249.

31. Sontheimer DL. Peripheral vascular disease: Diagnosis and treatment. *Am Fam Physician.* 2006;73(11):1971–1976.

32. Yeager RA, Moneta GL, Taylor LM, Jr., Hamre DW, McConnell DB, Porter JM. Surgical management of severe acute lower extremity ischemia. *J Vasc Surg.* 1992;15(2):385–391.

33. Otten JM, Smorenburg SM, de Meij MA, van der Schoor CA, Brandjes DP, Buller HR. Screening for cancer in patients with idiopathic venous thromboembolism: The clinical practice. *Pathophysiol Haemost Thromb.* 2002;32(2):76–79.

34. Prandoni P, Piccioli A. Thrombosis as a harbinger of cancer. *Curr Opin Hematol.* 2006;13(5):362–365.

35. Gross CP, Galusha DH, Krumholz HM. The impact of venous thromboembolism on risk of death or hemorrhage in older cancer patients. *J Gen Intern Med.* 2007;22(3):321–326.

36. Semrad TJ, O'Donnell R, Wun T, et al. Epidemiology of venous thromboembolism in 9489 patients with malignant glioma. *J Neurosurg.* 2007;106(4):601–608.

37. Ziegler S, Sperr WR, Knobl P, et al. Symptomatic venous thromboembolism in acute leukemia. Incidence, risk factors, and impact on prognosis. *Thromb Res.* 2005;115(1–2):59–64.

38. Durica SS. Venous thromboembolism in the cancer patient. *Curr Opin Hematol.* 1997;4(5):306–311.

39. Huerta C, Johansson S, Wallander MA, Garcia Rodriguez LA. Risk factors and short-term mortality of venous thromboembolism diagnosed in the primary care setting in the United Kingdom. *Arch Intern Med.* 2007;167(9):935–943.

40. Leonardi MJ, McGory ML, Ko CY. A systematic review of deep venous thrombosis prophylaxis in cancer patients: Implications for improving quality. *Ann Surg Oncol.* 2007;14(2):929–936.

41. Patiar S, Kirwan CC, McDowell G, Bundred NJ, McCollum CN, Byrne GJ. Prevention of venous thromboembolism in surgical patients with breast cancer. *Br J Surg.* 2007;94(4):412–420.

42. Lin J, Proctor MC, Varma M, Greenfield LJ, Upchurch GR, Jr., Henke PK. Factors associated with recurrent venous thromboembolism in patients with malignant disease. *J Vasc Surg.* 2003;37(5):976–983.

43 Ho WK, Hankey GJ, Lee CH, Eikelboom JW. Venous thromboembolism: Diagnosis and management of deep venous thrombosis. *Med J Aust.* 2005;182(9):476–481.

44. Gomes MP, Deitcher SR. Diagnosis of venous thromboembolic disease in cancer patients. *Oncology (Williston Park).* 2003;17(1):126–135, 139.

45. Dunnick NR, Newman GE, Perlmutt LM, Braun SD. Pulmonary embolism. *Curr Probl Diagn Radiol.* 1988;17(6):197–237.

46. Remy-Jardin M, Mastora I, Remy J. Pulmonary embolus imaging with multislice CT. *Radiol Clin North Am.* 2003;41(3):507–519.

47. Wu AS, Pezzullo JA, Cronan JJ, Hou DD, Mayo-Smith WW. CT pulmonary angiography: Quantification of pulmonary embolus as a predictor of patient outcome—initial experience. *Radiology.* 2004;230(3):831–835.

48. Burkill GJ, Bell JR, Chinn RJ, et al. The use of a D-dimer assay in patients undergoing CT pulmonary angiography for suspected pulmonary embolus. *Clin Radiol.* 2002;57(1):41–46.

49. Lee AY, Ginsberg JS. Laboratory diagnosis of venous thromboembolism. *Baillieres Clin Haematol.* 1998;11(3):587–604.

50. Caprini JA, Glase CJ, Anderson CB, Hathaway K. Laboratory markers in the diagnosis of venous thromboembolism. *Circulation.* 2004;109(12 Suppl 1):I4–I8.

51. Crippa L, D'Angelo SV, Tomassini L, Rizzi B, D'Alessandro G, D'Angelo A. The utility and cost-effectiveness of D-dimer measurements in the diagnosis of deep vein thrombosis. *Haematologica.* 1997;82(4):446–451.

52. Jang JW, Yeo CD, Kim JD, et al. Trousseau's syndrome in association with cholangiocarcinoma: Positive tests for coagulation factors and anticardiolipin antibody. *J Korean Med Sci.* 2006;21(1):155–159.

53. Raizer JJ, DeAngelis LM. Cerebral sinus thrombosis diagnosed by MRI and MR venography in cancer patients. *Neurology.* 2000;54(6):1222–1226.

54. SigsbeeB, Deck MD, Posner JB. Nonmetastatic superior sagittal sinus thrombosis complicating systemic cancer. *Neurology.* 1979;29:139–146.

55. Akdal G, Donmez B, Cakmakci H, Yener GG. A case with cerebral thrombosis receiving tamoxifen treatment. *Eur J Neurol.* 2001;8(6):723–724.

56. el-Shami K, Griffiths E, Streiff M. Nonbacterial thrombotic endocarditis in cancer patients: Pathogenesis, diagnosis, and treatment. *Oncologist.* 2007;12(5):518–523.

57. Aryana A, Esterbrooks DJ, Morris PC. Nonbacterial thrombotic endocarditis with recurrent embolic events as manifestation of ovarian neoplasm. *J Gen Intern Med.* 2006;21(12):C12–C15.

58. Borowski A, Ghodsizad A, Gams E. Stroke as a first manifestation of ovarian cancer. *J Neurooncol.* 2005;71(3):267–269.

59. Gonzalez QA, Candela MJ, Vidal C, Roman J, Aramburo P. Non-bacterial thrombotic endocarditis in cancer patients. *Acta Cardiol.* 1991;46(1):1–9.

60. Ozben B, Papila N, Tanrikulu MA, Bayalan F, Fak AS, Oktay A. Inferior vena caval tumor thrombus extending into the right atrium in a patient with pancreatic cancer. *J Thromb Thrombolysis.* 2007;24(3):317–321.

61. Loreto MF, De MM, Corsi MP, Modesti M, Ginaldi L. Coagulation and cancer: implications for diagnosis and management. *Pathol Oncol Res.* 2000;6(4):301–312.

62. Trujillo-Santos J, Perea-Milla E, Jimenez-Puente A, et al. Bed rest or ambulation in the initial treatment of patients with acute deep vein thrombosis or pulmonary embolism: Findings from the RIETE registry. *Chest.* 2005;127(5):1631–1636.

63. Feldman LS, Brotman DJ. When can patients with acute deep vein thrombosis be allowed to get up and walk? *Clev Clin J Med.* 2006;73:893–896.

64. Aldrich D, Hunt DP. When can the patient with deep vein thrombosis begin to ambulate? *Phys Ther.* 2004;84:268–273.

65. Partsch H, Blatter W. Compression and walking versus bed rest in the treatment of proximal deep venous thrombosis with low molecular weight heparin. *J Vasc Surg.* 2000;32:861–869.

66. West MP, Paz JC. Vascular system and hematology. In: Paz JC, West MP, eds. *Acute Care Handbook for Physical Therapists,* 2nd ed. Boston, MA: Butterworth-Heinemann; 2002.

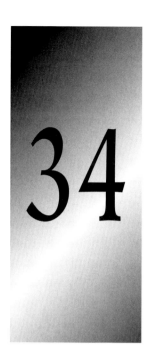

Paraneoplastic Complications of Cancer

Edward J. Dropcho

Neurologic paraneoplastic disorders are nonmetastatic syndromes that are not attributable to toxicity of cancer therapy, cerebrovascular disease, coagulopathy, infection, or toxic/metabolic causes. Paraneoplastic disorders are rare compared to metastases, neurotoxicities of chemotherapy and radiotherapy, and other neurologic complications of systemic cancer, but they have clinical importance for several reasons: (1) In most patients with paraneoplastic disorders, the neurologic symptoms are the presenting feature of an otherwise undiagnosed tumor. (2) Among patients with a known diagnosis of cancer, the paraneoplastic syndromes are an important part of the differential diagnosis of neurologic dysfunction. (3) Paraneoplastic disorders often cause severe and permanent neurologic morbidity. (4) Prompt recognition of a paraneoplastic disorder maximizes the likelihood of successful tumor treatment and a favorable neurologic outcome.

Almost any type of tumor can be associated with paraneoplastic disorders, but for most paraneoplastic neurologic syndromes there is an overrepresentation of one or more particular neoplasms. Myasthenia gravis associated with thymoma is the oldest known and most common neurologic paraneoplastic disorder; up to 20% of patients with myasthenia gravis have thymoma, and at least 10% of patients with thymoma have myasthenia gravis. Approximately 1%-3% of patients with small cell lung carcinoma develop Lambert-Eaton myasthenic

syndrome or another paraneoplastic syndrome. Other tumors over-represented among patients with paraneoplastic syndromes include breast carcinoma, ovarian carcinoma, Hodgkin lymphoma, and testicular germ cell tumors. Paraneoplastic opsoclonus-myoclonus occurs in 2%-3% of children with neuroblastoma.

Paraneoplastic disorders can affect any part(s) of the central or peripheral nervous systems. Many patients can be grouped into a recognizable clinical syndrome predominantly affecting one anatomic location or system (Table 34.1). Other patients may not neatly fit into this scheme because they have signs and symptoms of more than one syndrome. One view is that most if not all paraneoplastic disorders are subsets of a diffuse and multifocal paraneoplastic encephalomyeloneuritis, in which individual patients may show predominant involvement of particular parts of the nervous system.

Several syndromes should always raise the possibility of a paraneoplastic etiology, including limbic encephalopathy, subacute cerebellar degeneration, opsoclonus-myoclonus, severe sensory neuronopathy, Lambert-Eaton myasthenic syndrome, and dermatomyositis (1,2). It is important to keep in mind, however, that there is no neurologic syndrome that is absolutely pathognomonic for a paraneoplastic etiology; any of the disorders listed in Table 34.1 can occur in patients without a tumor.

KEY POINTS

- Neurologic paraneoplastic disorders are nonmetastatic syndromes that are not attributable to toxicity of cancer therapy, cerebrovascular disease, coagulopathy, infection, or toxic/metabolic causes.
- Most any type of tumor can be associated with paraneoplastic disorders, but the most common and best known are thymoma with myasthenia gravis and small cell lung carcinoma with Lambert-Eaton myasthenic syndrome.
- Neurologic paraneoplastic syndromes can affect every level of the nervous system, including the limbic system, cerebellum, brain stem, spinal cord, motor neuron, dorsal root ganglion, peripheral nerve, neuromuscular junction, and muscle.
- The clinical relevance of neurologic paraneoplastic disorders includes the following points: (1) In most patients with paraneoplastic disorders, the neurologic symptoms are the presenting feature of an otherwise undiagnosed tumor. (2) Among patients with a known diagnosis of cancer, the paraneoplastic syndromes are an important part of the differential diagnosis of neurologic dysfunction. (3) Paraneoplastic disorders often cause severe and permanent neurologic morbidity. (4) Prompt recognition of a paraneoplastic disorder maximizes the likelihood
- of successful tumor treatment and a favorable neurologic outcome.
- The central theory of autoimmunity for paraneoplastic disorders postulates that tumor cells express onconeural antigen(s) identical or antigenically related to molecules normally expressed by neurons, and that in rare instances an autoimmune response initially arising against the tumor subsequently attacks neurons expressing the same or related antigen.
- Most if not all paraneoplastic disorders are thought to be subsets of a diffuse and multifocal paraneoplastic encephalomyeloneuritis, in which individual patients may show predominant involvement of particular parts of the nervous system.
- Paraneoplastic limbic encephalitis generally has a subacute onset that evolves over days to weeks. Patients typically present either with an amnestic syndrome or psychiatric disorder; most patients eventually develop features of both.
- The most common clinical manifestation of subacute sensory neuronopathy reflects involvement of the dorsal root ganglia, presenting with asymmetric numbness and paresthesias, burning dysesthesias or lancinating pain with ambulatory disfunction due to pain, and profound loss of proprioception.

TABLE 34.1
Neurologic Paraneoplastic Disorders

CENTRAL NERVOUS SYSTEM	PERIPHERAL NERVOUS SYSTEM
Multifocal encephalomyelitis	Sensory neuronopathy
Cerebellar degeneration	Nerve vasculitis
Limbic encephalitis	Sensorimotor polyneuropathy
Opsoclonus-myoclonus	Motor neuropathy
Extrapyramidal syndrome	Neuromyotonia
Brainstem encephalitis	Autonomic insufficiency
Myelopathy	Lambert-Eaton syndrome
Motor neuron disease	Myasthenia gravis
Stiff person syndrome	Inflammatory myopathy
Optic neuritis	Necrotizing myopathy
Retinal degeneration	

AUTOIMMUNITY

Most neurologic paraneoplastic disorders are believed to be autoimmune diseases; however, with some exceptions, the exact immunopathogenetic mechanisms remain unclear. The central theory of autoimmunity for paraneoplastic disorders postulates that tumor cells express onconeural antigen(s) identical to or antigenically related to molecules normally expressed by neurons, and that in rare instances an autoimmune response initially arising against the tumor subsequently attacks neurons expressing the same or related antigen(s).

Since the mid-1980s there has been a steadily growing list of antineuronal antibodies identified in the sera of patients with paraneoplastic disorders (Table 34.2). The neuronal molecular targets of several of these autoantibodies have been cloned and characterized (3,4). Some paraneoplastic antibodies have selective neuronal reactivity and are found only in patients with a particular clinical syndrome, such as anti-Yo or anti-Tr antibodies in patients with cerebellar degeneration. Most paraneoplastic autoantibodies show a more widespread or pan-neuronal reactivity and are associated with a variety of clinical neurologic syndromes, or with multifocal encephalomyelitis. The most prevalent such antibodies are anti-Hu and anti-CV2. Patients with small cell lung carcinoma not infrequently have more than one type of autoantibody (5).

The proven or postulated immunopathogenetic mechanisms for paraneoplastic disorders fall into four main categories:

1. Autoantibodies against shared tumor-neuronal (onconeural) antigens are the direct cause of neurologic disease. For example, the Lambert-Eaton myasthenic syndrome is caused by antibodies that bind to and downregulate voltage-gated calcium channels at the presynaptic neuromuscular junction, leading to reduction in the quantal release of acetylcholine by a nerve impulse (6). Paraneoplastic neuromyotonia is probably caused by antibodies against voltage-gated potassium channels that cause prolonged motor neuron depolarization and spontaneous muscle activity (7). Antibodies against voltage-gated potassium channels (8) or N-methyl-D-aspartate (NMDA) receptors (9) may also cause neuronal injury or dysfunction in some patients with limbic encephalitis. Antibodies against voltage-gated calcium channels (10) or glutamate receptors (11) may directly mediate Purkinje cell injury in some patients with paraneoplastic cerebellar degeneration. Anti-amphiphysin antibodies may directly contribute to causing paraneoplastic stiff person syndrome (12).

2. A cellular immune reaction against onconeural antigens is the main cause of neuronal or nerve injury. This is probably true for most patients with paraneoplastic cerebellar degeneration (13), multifocal encephalomyelitis/sensory neuronopathy (14), and limbic encephalitis (15). It is postulated that onconeural antigens released by apoptotic tumor cells are presented to T lymphocytes in draining peripheral lymph nodes, initiating a Th1 helper response that eventually gains access to the CNS and attacks neurons expressing the antigens (16). If present, antineuronal antibodies in these patients (eg, anti-Hu or anti-Yo) are an epiphenomenon or "footprint" for autoimmunity but are probably not directly involved or are minor factors in causing neuronal injury.

3. Neoplastic plasma cells produce monoclonal paraproteins (immunoglobulins) that react with peripheral nerve antigens and cause neuropathy; for example, sensorimotor polyneuropathy is associated with anti-myelin-associated glycoprotein antibodies (17), and sensory ataxic neuropathy is associated with antidisialosyl ganglioside antibodies (18).

4. Some disorders arise from other (or poorly understood) immune mechanisms, such as paraneoplastic necrotizing myelopathy or vasculitic neuropathy. The pathogenesis of neuropathy in patients with osteosclerotic myeloma, also called polyneuropathy, organomegaly, endocrinopathy, monoclonal gammopathy, and skin changes (POEMS) syndrome, may be related to elevated serum levels of proinflammatory cytokines rather than to any direct effect of the paraprotein (19). The pathogenesis of myasthenia gravis associated with thymoma is complex and depends on intratumor production of autoreactive T lymphocytes (20).

CLINICAL SYNDROMES

Multifocal Encephalomyelitis

Small cell lung carcinoma is by far the tumor most commonly associated with paraneoplastic encephalomyelitis, with a scattering of patients with a variety of other neoplasms (21–23). Paraneoplastic encephalomyelitis is characterized clinically and pathologically by patchy, multifocal involvement of any or all areas of the cerebral hemispheres, limbic system, cerebellum, brainstem, spinal cord, dorsal root ganglia, and autonomic ganglia. Neuronal loss is accompanied by a variable degree of perivascular and leptomeningeal infiltration

TABLE 34.2
Paraneoplastic Disorders and Autoantibodies

CLINICAL SYNDROME	ASSOCIATED TUMOR(S)	AUTOANTIBODIES
Multifocal encephalomyelitis	SCLC	Anti-Hu (ANNA-1), anti-CV2 (CRMP-5), anti-amphiphysin, anti-Ri, ANNA-3
	Various carcinomas	Anti-Ma1, anti-Hu, anti-CV2
Limbic encephalitis	SCLC	Anti-Hu, anti-CV2, PCA-2, ANNA-3, anti-amphiphysin, anti-VGKC, anti-VGCC, anti-Zic4
	Testicular, breast	Anti-Ma2
	Thymoma	Anti–VGKC, anti-CV2
	Ovarian teratoma	Anti-NMDA receptor
Cerebellar degeneration	Breast, ovarian, others	Anti-Yo, anti-Ma1, anti-Ri
	SCLC, others	Anti-Hu, anti-CV2, PCA-2, ANNA-3, anti-amphiphysin, anti-VGCC, anti-Ri, anti-Zic4
	Hodgkin lymphoma	Anti-Tr, anti-mGluR1
Opsoclonus-myoclonus	Breast, ovarian	Anti-Ri, anti-Yo, anti-amphiphysin
	SCLC	Anti-Hu, anti-Ri, anti-CV2, anti-amphiphysin
	Neuroblastoma	Anti-Hu, others
	Testicular, others	Anti-Ma2
Extrapyramidal syndrome	SCLC, thymoma	Anti-CV2, anti-Hu
Brainstem encephalitis	SCLC, breast, others	Anti-Hu, anti-Ri
	Testicular	Anti-Ma2
Optic neuritis	SCLC	anti-CV2
Myelopathy	SCLC, thymoma	anti-CV2, anti-amphiphysin
Stiff person syndrome	Breast, SCLC, others	Anti-amphiphysin, anti-Ri, anti-GAD
Motor neuron disease	SCLC, others	Anti-Hu
Sensory neuronopathy	SCLC, others	Anti-Hu, anti-CV2, ANNA-3, anti-Ma1, anti-amphiphysin
Neuromyotonia	Thymoma, SCLC	Anti–VGKC
Sensorimotor polyneuropathy	SCLC, others	Anti-Hu, anti-CV2, ANNA-3
	Plasma cell dyscrasias	Anti-MAG, anti-disialosyl ganglioside
Autonomic insufficiency	SCLC	Anti-Hu, anti-ganglionic AchR
Lambert-Eaton syndrome	SCLC	Anti-VGCC

Abbreviations: SCLC, small cell lung cancer

of mononuclear cells, including T and B lymphocytes and plasma cells.

In most patients with paraneoplastic encephalomyelitis, the neurologic syndrome is the presenting feature of an otherwise occult tumor and precedes the discovery of the neoplasm by an average of several months. The most common clinical manifestation is subacute sensory neuronopathy reflecting involvement of the dorsal root ganglia. Other patients have a predominant clinical syndrome of focal cortical encephalitis, limbic encephalitis, extrapyramidal movement disorder, subacute cerebellar degeneration, brainstem encephalitis, or motor neuron disease. Regardless of individual patients' predominant clinical manifestations, nearly all display signs and symptoms of multifocal involvement of the CNS and dorsal root ganglia. Patients may additionally show involvement of the peripheral nervous system, including sensorimotor polyneuropathy, mononeuritis multiplex, autonomic system failure, or Lambert-Eaton syndrome.

Most patients with paraneoplastic encephalomyelitis have circulating antineuronal autoantibodies, the most common of which are anti-Hu antibodies reacting with a group of RNA-binding proteins (21,22,24,25), or anti-CV2 (CRMP-5) antibodies directed against a group of proteins expressed by neurons and oligodendrocytes (26). A minority of patients has one of several antibodies other than anti-Hu or anti-CV2 (Table 34.2), or has no detectable antineuronal autoantibodies.

The most common clinical course of paraneoplastic encephalomyelitis is deterioration over a period of weeks to months followed by stabilization at a level of severe neurologic disability, regardless of treatment. Subsequent stepwise or gradual neurologic deterioration is less common and tends to occur in patients with less than complete response of the associated small cell lung cancer to treatment (25). Fewer than 10% of patients show significant neurologic improvement despite successful tumor treatment and/or a variety of immunosuppressive therapies, including corticosteroids, cyclophosphamide, intravenous immunoglobulin (IVIg), or plasmapheresis (21,22,25,27).

Limbic Encephalitis

Approximately one-half of reported patients with paraneoplastic limbic encephalitis have small cell lung carcinoma (28–30). Other associated neoplasms include testicular germ cell tumors (15), thymoma (31,32), Hodgkin lymphoma (33), ovarian teratoma (9,34), and a variety of carcinomas.

The most consistent and severe neuropathologic abnormalities in autopsied cases of paraneoplastic limbic encephalitis are extensive neuronal loss, gliosis, and microglial nodules in the hippocampus and amygdala (15,29). Similar but less severe changes are often present in the parahippocampal gyrus, cingulate gyrus, insular cortex, orbital frontal cortex, basal ganglia, and diencephalon. Perivascular lymphocytic cuffing and leptomeningeal mononuclear cell infiltrates are patchy and variable. Most patients with paraneoplastic limbic encephalitis and small cell lung cancer, and many patients with other associated tumors, have multifocal encephalomyelitis.

Paraneoplastic limbic encephalitis generally has a subacute onset evolving over days to weeks. Patients typically present either with an amnestic syndrome or psychiatric disorder; most patients eventually develop features of both (28–30). The memory loss includes short-term anterograde amnesia and a variable period of retrograde amnesia. Denial of the deficit and confabulation are common. The affective disorder usually includes some combination of depression, anxiety, emotional lability, and personality change. Hallucinations and paranoid delusions may occur. Generalized or partial complex seizures occur in most patients, may be the initial neurologic feature, and can be medically intractable. Less common manifestations of limbic or diencephalic dysfunction include abnormal sleep-wake cycles, disturbed temperature regulation, labile blood pressure, inappropriate secretion of antidiuretic hormone, and elements of the Klüver-Bucy syndrome such as hyperphagia and hypersexuality. Some extralimbic clinical feaures have particular associations with certain tumors and antineuronal antibodies.

Most patients with paraneoplastic limbic encephalitis have circulating antineuronal autoantibodies, depending on the associated tumor (35) (Table 34.2). Among patients with limbic encephalitis and small cell lung carcinoma, approximately one-half have anti-Hu antibodies, some have other antibodies, and others have no identifiable antibodies (28,29). Anti-Hu-positive patients usually show additional signs and symptoms of multifocal encephalomyelitis. Several other antineuronal antibodies associated with paraneoplastic limbic encephalitis have a pan-neuronal or widespread reactivity (Table 34.2). None of these antibodies has a particular association with limbic encephalitis versus other neurologic syndromes.

A few antineuronal antibodies have a specific linkage to limbic encephalitis and are not commonly associated with other neurologic syndromes. Anti-Ma2 (anti-Ta) antibodies mainly occur in young men with testicular germ cell tumors (15). There are a few older women or men with breast carcinoma or non-small cell lung carcinoma (36,37). Some patients with anti-Ma2 antibodies have a clinically "pure" limbic encephalitis, whereas the majority present with a combined syndrome reflecting involvement of the limbic system, diencephalon (eg, sleep disorder or autonomic dysfunction), and brainstem (especially ocular motor disturbance).

Antibodies against voltage-gated potassium channels (VGKC) are found in some patients with limbic encephalitis, usually in association with thymoma or small cell lung cancer (38–40). To date, the majority of reported patients with limbic encephalitis and anti-VGKC antibodies actually do not have an identifiable neoplasm (41,42). Anti-VGKC antibodies are also found in patients with paraneoplastic or non-paraneoplastic neuromyotonia (see below), and in patients with the syndrome of Morvan fibrillary chorea, which features neuromyotonia, dysautonomia, insomnia, and encephalopathy (43).

Antibodies against NMDA receptors have recently been identified in young women with limbic encephalitis and a previously undiscovered ovarian teratoma (9,32,34). Anti-NMDA receptor antibodies stain the dendritic network and synaptic-enriched regions in the neuropil of the hippocampus. Some patients present with a typical limbic encephalopathy, although most have a more severe clinical course with some combination of acute psychosis, intractable seizures, depressed consciousness, movement disorder, autonomic instability, and central hypoventilation requiring extended mechanical ventilation. Most patients have evidence for multifocal limbic and extralimbic involvement on MRI or PET scans.

The neurologic course of paraneoplastic limbic encephalitis is variable. A few patients with clinically "pure" limbic encephalitis show spontaneous neurologic improvement prior to any treatment (23). Approximately 50% of patients with limbic encephalitis and small cell lung cancer improve after tumor treatment, with or without immunotherapy (21,28,29). Among patients with anti-Hu antibodies in whom limbic encephalitis is a component of multifocal encephalomyelitis, the limbic features may improve after tumor treatment, whereas the other neurologic features rarely do so. Among patients with limbic encephalitis, testicular germ cell tumors, and anti-Ma2 antibodies who receive tumor treatment and/or immunosuppressive therapy, approximately 25% have neurologic improvement and roughly the same percentage has neurologic stabilization (15). Successful tumor treatment is correlated with a better neurologic outcome. Most patients with limbic encephalitis and thymoma, including those with anti-VGKC or anti-CV2 antibodies, have significant neurologic improvement following successful tumor treatment and/or immunotherapy (32,38). Most patients with ovarian teratoma and anti-NMDA receptor antibodies have significant, and sometimes complete, neurologic recovery after resection of the teratoma and immunosuppressive therapy (9,32,34).

Cerebellar Degeneration

Most patients (90%) with paraneoplastic cerebellar degeneration have small cell lung carcinoma, Hodgkin lymphoma, or carcinoma of the breast, ovary, or female genital tract (44,45). The most striking and consistent neuropathologic finding is severe, diffuse loss of Purkinje cells throughout the cerebellar cortex. There may also be some neuronal loss in the granular cell layer and deep cerebellar nuclei. Some patients have perivascular cuffing and mononuclear cell infiltrates in the cerebellum and overlying leptomeninges.

The clinical onset of paraneoplastic cerebellar degeneration is typically fairly abrupt (45–47). Patients display signs and symptoms reflecting diffuse dysfunction of the cerebellum, including dysarthria and severe appendicular and gait ataxia. Abnormalities of oculomotor function are common and include nystagmus (particularly downbeat nystagmus), disruption of smooth pursuit movements, ocular dysmetria, and opsoclonus. Superimposed on the cerebellar deficits, many patients develop symptoms or signs of multifocal encephalomyelitis.

Virtually all paraneoplastic antineuronal antibodies react with antigens in the cerebellum and can be associated with clinical cerebellar dysfunction (Table 34.2). Anti-Yo, anti-Tr, and anti-mGlu1 glutamate receptor antibodies are associated with a pure cerebellar syndrome, whereas the other paraneoplastic antibodies occur in patients with a variety of clinical presentations, including cerebellar dysfunction or multifocal encephalomyelitis. Anti-Tr antibodies are present in some patients with cerebellar degeneration and Hodgkin lymphoma; these antibodies have not been found in association with other tumors or other clinical syndromes (48,49). Anti-Yo antibodies are almost entirely restricted to patients with cerebellar degeneration and carcinomas of the breast, ovary, or female genital tract, and to a few women and men with other adenocarcinomas (45,47,50).

The neurologic deficits in paraneoplastic cerebellar degeneration generally worsen over a period of several weeks to months and then stabilize at a level of severe disability. Significant neurologic improvement, either spontaneously or after successful treatment of the associated tumor, is distinctly unusual. Some patients with Hodgkin lymphoma, and exceptional patients with carcinoma, improve neurologically after successful tumor treatment (44–47,49,50).

Fewer than 10% of reported patients with paraneoplastic cerebellar degeneration show significant neurologic improvement after plasmapheresis, IVIg, corticosteroids, or cyclophosphamide (27,45,51). Exceptional patients do improve with immunotherapy (46,47,52). There are no apparent differences in the clinical presentation of the few responders versus the large majority of patients in whom immunotherapy is ineffective.

Opsoclonus-Myoclonus

The median age at onset of paraneoplastic opsoclonus-myoclonus in children is 18–24 months (53,54). In nearly all cases, the abrupt onset of the neurologic syndrome leads to discovery of an otherwise occult neuroblastoma. The cardinal feature of opsoclonus is continuous multidirectional rapid eye movements (saccadic oscillations) without an intersaccadic interval. In addition to opsoclonus, these children have some combination of moderate to severe multifocal myoclonus, limb and gait ataxia, and altered sensorium (53,54). There are no clinical, neuroimaging, or CSF findings that reliably differentiate paraneoplastic opsoclonus-myoclonus from postinfectious, or idiopathic, opsoclonus-myoclonus syndrome.

Opsoclonus as a paraneoplastic disorder is less common in adults than in children and most often occurs in association with small cell lung carcinoma or breast carcinoma (55,56). The neurologic symptoms and signs that accompany paraneoplastic opsoclonus in adults are heterogeneous and include multifocal limb myoclonus, pancerebellar dysfunction, and signs and symptoms of brainstem dysfunction, including vertigo, vomiting, dysphagia, and gaze palsy.

The pathologic substrate of paraneoplastic opsoclonus-myoclonus in adults or children remains unclear, as there are no distinctive or uniformly present lesions. Some of the very few published autopsied cases showed mild to severe loss of cerebellar Purkinje cells, and/or patchy neuronal loss and perivascular mononuclear cell infiltrates in the inferior olivary nuclei and other areas of the brainstem (55,57,58). A significant proportion of autopsied children and adults display no identifiable histopathologic abnormalities either in the cerebellum or brainstem (59,60).

Some children with paraneoplastic opsoclonus-myoclonus have serum autoantibodies that react with shared neuronal-neuroblastoma antigens, including anti-Hu antibodies in a few patients (61,62), or one of a number of antibodies with heterogeneous reactivities on immunocytochemical staining and immunoblots (62–64). The identity of the onconeural antigens remains to be shown. There is no universally observed antibody or antigen in published studies. Antineuronal antibody associations for adults with paraneoplastic opsoclonus are listed in Table 34.2. There are individual reports of adults with paraneoplastic opsoclonus and one of several unnamed atypical antibodies with different patterns of reactivity associated with small cell lung cancer or other neoplasms (65). A fairly high percentage of patients has no identifiable antineuronal antibodies.

The majority of children with paraneoplastic opsoclonus-myoclonus show neurologic improvement solely with tumor resection (61). Whether given before or after surgical resection, corticotropin produces rapid and dramatic neurologic improvement in at least two-thirds of children (66). Oral or intravenous corticosteroids are also used, but are probably less effective than corticotropin (66,67). Patients may also show improvement with IVIg (53), plasmapheresis (68) or rituximab (69), usually in combination with or following corticotropin and/or corticosteroids.

At least one-half of children with paraneoplastic opsoclonus-myoclonus have a protracted or fluctuating course. Exacerbations of neurologic symptoms may occur when corticotropin or corticosteroids are tapered or discontinued, or during febrile illnesses (66,70). At least two-thirds of children are left with some combination of residual motor deficits, speech delay, learning disability, impulsive or aggressive behavior, and sleep disturbance (61,71,72). An initial good neurologic response to tumor treatment and/or immunotherapy does not necessarily predict a better long-term neurologic outcome (53,61,73).

As a group, adults with paraneoplastic opsoclonus have a better neurologic outcome than patients with paraneoplastic cerebellar degeneration or encephalomyelitis. In some patients, the opsoclonus and other neurologic features spontaneously improve prior to any therapy (74). Patients may show significant neurologic improvement with successful treatment of the associated tumor (55,56). Some patients have significant neurologic improvement after corticosteroids, plasma exchange, IVIg, or protein A immunoadsorption therapy (74,75).

Extrapyramidal Syndromes

Chorea, athetosis, dystonia, or parkinsonism are rare manifestations of paraneoplastic encephalitis, occurring most often in association with small cell lung carcinoma (76–78) and also with lymphoma, thymoma, or other tumors. The extrapyramidal features may occur with or without other signs of multifocal encephalomyelitis. Some patients show neurologic improvement after tumor treatment or immunosuppression.

Brainstem Encephalitis

Paraneoplastic "brainstem encephalitis" manifests as a variety of gaze palsies or other ocular motor disturbances, possibly together with dysarthria, dysphagia, facial weakness, vertigo, central respiratory failure, or other signs and symptoms referable to the brainstem. This most commonly occurs in the setting of multifocal encephalomyelitis associated with small cell lung carcinoma (79), or in patients with testicular germ cell tumor, who generally have additional limbic and/or hypothalamic involvement (15). Other tumors have also been reported (80).

Optic Neuritis

Optic neuritis is a rare complication of breast carcinoma, small cell lung carcinoma, or other tumors. Nothing is clinically distinctive about the optic neuritis in these patients, who have decreased visual acuity, afferent pupillary defects, cecocentral scotomas, and disc edema (81,82). Some patients have serum anti-CV2 or other antineuronal antibodies (83). Paraneoplastic optic neuritis needs to be distinguished from paraneoplastic retinal degeneration occurring in association with melanoma or carcinoma (84,85).

Myelopathy

Patients with paraneoplastic encephalomyelitis associated with small cell lung cancer, breast carcinoma, thymoma, or other tumors may present with a predominant myelopathy syndrome. Some of these patients have myelopathy with rigidity, myeloradiculopathy, or myelopathy plus optic neuritis (Devic disease) (83,86–88). Associated antibodies include anti-CV2 (26) and anti-amphiphysin (87).

Paraneoplastic necrotizing myelopathy is a rare syndrome that is probably distinct from the multifocal patchy involvement of the spinal cord in cases of encephaloymelitis (89). This syndrome may occur in association with a variety of carcinomas and lymphoid tumors, without a clear preponderance of any specific tumor type. Patients present with subacute bilateral symptoms involving motor, sensory, and sphincter function with little or no pain. There are anecdotal reports of neurologic improvement after intrathecal corticosteroids (90,91), but most patients suffer rapid deterioration of function and a progressively ascending level of flaccid paralysis and numbness, often leading to death from respiratory failure or medical complications.

Stiff-Person Syndrome

A syndrome of muscle rigidity and spasms, which clinically resembles stiff person syndrome, is associated with a variety of neoplasms, including small cell lung carcinoma, thymoma, Hodgkin lymphoma, and carcinoma of the breast or colon. Rigidity is probably caused by

multifocal encephalomyelitis affecting the spinal cord and/or brainstem (92,93). Patients develop progressive aching and rigidity of the axial and proximal limb musculature, usually asymmetric at onset. There are superimposed painful and sometimes violent spasms, either occurring spontaneously or triggered by voluntary movement, passive movement, or sensory stimuli. Patients may eventually develop fixed flexion of the limbs or even opisthotonos and respiratory difficulty. Some patients have antibodies against glutamic acid decarboxylase (94,95) or against the synaptic vesicle-associated protein amphiphysin (87,93,96). High doses of diazepam, clonazepam, or baclofen may provide partial relief. Some patients improve after tumor treatment and/or immunosuppressive treatment (95,96).

Motor Neuron Disease

Paraneoplastic motor neuron dysfunction occurs in a variety of different settings. Lower motor neuron signs and symptoms are among the presenting or predominant manifestations in up to 25% of patients with multifocal encephalomyelitis associated with anti-Hu or other antibodies (21,22,97). Motor neuron involvement in these patients does not usually improve with treatment. A more problematic issue is how often, if ever, isolated motor neuron disease or, as it is sometimes called, amyotrophic lateral sclerosis (ALS), is a paraneoplastic syndrome (98). There is no convincing epidemiologic evidence that nonhematologic neoplasms occur in ALS patients any more frequently than would be expected in an age-matched control population. Despite the absence of a clear epidemiologic link between motor neuron disease and neoplasia, however, the relationship in small subsets of patients is probably more than coincidental. There are several well-described patients with a lower motor neuron syndrome or combined upper and lower motor neuron syndrome who had significant neurologic improvement after resection of lung or renal carcinomas (99,100).

There is an association between ALS, or progressive spinal muscular atrophy, and lymphoproliferative disease including Hodgkin lymphoma, non-Hodgkin lymphoma, and chronic lymphocytic leukemia (101). The frequency of lymphoproliferative disease in patients with motor neuron disorders has been estimated as high as 2%-5%. In roughly one-half of reported patients, the neurologic symptoms preceded diagnosis of the lymphoproliferative disease. Some patients have no systemic signs or symptoms, and the lymphoma is discovered only by bone marrow biopsy. Most patients with an ALS-like syndrome have progressive weakness leading to a fatal outcome despite treatment of the associated lymphoproliferative disease.

Subacute Sensory Neuronopathy

The most common clinical manifestation of paraneo-plastic encephalomyelitis is subacute sensory neuronopathy reflecting involvement of the dorsal root ganglia (21–23,102). More than 90% of reported patients have small cell lung carcinoma. Early symptoms are patchy or asymmetric numbness and paresthesias, often involving the face, the trunk, or the proximal limbs. The symptoms eventually spread to involve all limbs. Burning dysesthesias and severe aching or lancinating pain are common. Examination reveals severe sensory ataxia, predominant impairment of vibration sense and proprioception, frequent pseudoathetosis, and hypoactive or absent muscle stretch reflexes. Most patients cannot walk unassisted due to pain and profound loss of proprioception. Likewise, most patients have additional signs and symptoms that reflect a multi-focal encephalomyeloneuritis. Some patients develop concomitant Lambert-Eaton myasthenic syndrome, a component of motor neuropathy, or peripheral nerve microvasculitis presenting as mononeuritis multiplex (22,103).

The characteristic electrophysiologic profile of paraneoplastic sensory neuronopathy includes severely reduced amplitude or complete absence of sensory nerve potentials, with normal or only slightly reduced sensory nerve conduction velocities if a response is able to be elicited (102,104). Most patients do show at least minor abnormalities in motor nerve conduction studies, with or without symptoms of a mixed sensorimotor polyneuropathy (105,106).

The antibodies and tumors associated with para-neoplastic sensory neuronopathy are essentially the same as with paraneoplastic encephalomyelitis (Table 34.2). The most prevalent autoantibodies are anti-Hu antibodies, and the great majority of patients have small cell lung carcinoma. A minority of patients has no detectable antineuronal antibodies (107).

The clinical course of sensory neuronopathy in patients with small cell lung carcinoma is fairly stereotyped (22,23). By far the most common pattern is deterioration over a period of weeks to months, and then stabilization at a level of severe neurologic disability, regardless of treatment. Subsequent stepwise or gradual neurologic deterioration is less common. A few patients experience minimal CNS manifestations and a sensory neuronopathy that takes a relatively indolent course independent of any treatment (108,109). As with encephalomyelitis in general, patients with sensory neuronopathy rarely show significant neurologic improvement despite successful tumor treatment or a variety of immunosuppressive therapies (21–23,25,27,51,102). Patients with a relatively short

history of neurologic symptoms and who have successful treatment of the associated neoplasm may have a slightly better likelihood of neurologic stabilization or improvement (1,22,110).

Neuromyotonia

Patients with small cell lung carcinoma, thymoma, Hodgkin lymphoma, or plasmacytoma may develop peripheral nerve hyperexcitability which manifests as the cramp-fasciculation syndrome, or as a syndrome of diffuse muscle stiffness, cramps, and myokymia similar to neuromyotonia or continuous muscle fiber activity (Isaacs syndrome) (111–113). Needle EMG shows repetitive bursts of rapidly firing motor unit discharges (myokymic potentials) and/or very high frequency trains of discharges. Some patients have serum antibodies against voltage-gated potassium channels, which have also been identified in patients with non-paraneoplastic neuromyotonia (112,114). Successful tumor treatment may bring about significant neurologic improvement. Patients may also benefit from phenytoin, carbamazepine, plasmapheresis, and/or other immunosuppresive treatment.

Demyelinating Neuropathies and Carcinoma or Lymphoma

There are several reports of an acute, predominantly motor polyradiculoneuropathy occurring in the setting of a number of primary neoplasms, particularly lymphomas. The clinical features, electrophysiologic findings, CSF, and peripheral nerve pathology in these patients are indistinguishable from Guillain-Barre syndrome (115). There are several well-documented cases of patients with lymphoma or carcinoma who developed a sensorimotor polyneuropathy fulfilling the clinical and electrophysiologic diagnostic criteria for chronic demyelinating polyneuropathy (CIDP) (104,116,117). In some patients with acute or chronic demyelinating polyneuropathy, the tumor association may be fortuitous.

Demyelinating Neuropathy and Anti-MAG Antibodies

A significant proportion of patients presenting with an idiopathic polyneuropathy is discovered to have a monoclonal gammopathy. Most of these patients have monoclonal gammopathy of undetermined significance or nonmalignant monoclonal gammopathy. A minority has or will eventually develop multiple myeloma, plasmacytoma, Waldenstrom macroglobulinemia, non-Hodgkin lymphoma, chronic lymphocytic leukemia, or

Castleman syndrome (118). In 50%-60% of patients with IgM monoclonal gammopathy and neuropathy, the IgM paraprotein reacts with myelin associated glycoprotein (MAG) and several cross-reacting glycolipids (119,120).

Patients with anti-MAG antibodies generally develop a slowly progressive, predominantly sensory neuropathy which may be present for several years before the diagnosis is established. There is a male predominance with onset usually after age 60 years. Proprioception and vibratory sense are selectively affected. Intention tremor and ataxia are each present in up to one-half of patients at initial presentation. Muscle stretch reflexes are diminished or absent. Approximately 20% of patients have a predominantly motor neuropathy.

Electrophysiologic studies show slow nerve conduction velocities and low amplitude of compound muscle action potentials. Disproportionate prolongation of distal motor latencies may distinguish anti-MAG neuropathy from other acquired or hereditary demyelinating neuropathies (121). Biopsied nerves show segmental demyelination, characteristic widening of the myelin lamellae at the minor dense lines, and deposition of the anti-MAG IgM and complement on myelin sheaths (122).

Anti-MAG neuropathy is generally a chronic and slowly progressive condition, although patients often get at least partial and temporary benefit from treatment. Chemotherapy drugs such as chlorambucil, cyclophosphamide, or fludarabine reduce the serum paraprotein levels, but improvement or stabilization of the neuropathy does not always correlate with a reduction in paraprotein levels (123,124). Plasmapheresis may benefit some patients, whether alone or in combination with chemotherapy (125). IVIg usually produces modest short-term neurologic improvement (126). Recent studies show neurologic improvement after treatment with the monoclonal antibody rituximab which rapidly depletes circulating B-lymphocytes (127,128).

Demyelinating Neuropathy and Osteosclerotic Myeloma/POEMS Syndrome

Approximately one-half of individuals with osteosclerotic myeloma have a predominantly motor polyneuropathy (129). Examination shows weakness, disproportionate loss of vibration sense and proprioception, and diminished or absent muscle stretch reflexes. The neuropathy is usually slowly progressive but can be severely disabling. Electrophysiologic studies show primary demyelination (130).

Approximately 80% of patients with neuropathy and osteosclerotic myeloma have a paraprotein, usually of the IgG or IgA lambda type, which is often at a low

level and only detectable by immunofixation. Radiographic skeletal survey reveals the sclerotic myeloma (single in about one-half of patients) most often in the axial or proximal appendicular bones (129). In the great majority of patients, the osteosclerotic myeloma is only discovered through investigation of the neuropathy and is otherwise asymptomatic. Some patients with neuropathy and osteosclerotic myeloma have the multisystem POEMS syndrome (131,132).

Treatment of patients with osteosclerotic myeloma or POEMS syndrome includes some combination of surgical resection of the myeloma if possible, localized radiation, prednisone, or chemotherapy (usually including cyclophosphamide or melphalan) (131,132). Plasmapheresis or IVIg does not appear to be beneficial. When the myeloma responds to treatment patients usually have improvement of the neuropathy as well as all other multisystemic elements of the syndrome. There are anecdotal responses to tamoxifen, retinoic acid, or thalidomide. Selected patients may benefit from myeloablative chemotherapy with autologous stem cell transplantation (133).

Sensory Neuropathy and Anti-disialosyl Ganglioside Antibodies

This syndrome is rare relative to other neuropathies associated with plasma cell dyscrasias. Patients usually have an IgM nonmalignant monoclonal gammopathy. The paraprotein binds to GD1b and to several other gangliosides that bear disialosyl groups. Patients present with disporportinate loss of proprioception and vibratory sense and sensory gait ataxia (134,135). Weakness, if any, is mild. Some patients have ophthalmoparesis or other cranial nerve/bulbar involvement, including respiratory insufficiency. This syndrome resembles subacute sensory neuronopathy associated with small cell lung cancer. The clinical course may be steadily progressive, acute relapsing and remitting, or chronic worsening with acute relapses. Some of the small number of published patients responded to treatment with corticosteroids, cyclophosphamide, IVIg, or plasmapheresis.

Vasculitic Neuropathy

Peripheral nerve microvasculitis may occur in association with lymphomas or with carcinoma of the lung, prostate, uterus, kidney, or stomach (136,137). The clinical presentation and electrophysiologic findings are either those of mononeuritis multiplex, or of an asymmetric distal sensorimotor neuropathy. Patients with small cell lung cancer may additionally have encephalomyelitis or sensory neuronopathy (136). There are reports of neurologic improvement after tumor treatment and/or cyclophosphamide; corticosteroids alone do not seem to be beneficial.

Other Neuropathies

Rather than the more common sensory neuronopathy, a few patients with small cell lung cancer and anti-Hu antibodies have a mixed sensorimotor polyneuropathy with a mixed axonal-demyelinating electrophysiologic pattern (106). A few patients with anti-Hu antibodies have what appears to be a primary demyelinating polyneuropathy superimposed on sensory neuronopathy (138), or a mononeuritis multiplex with biopsy-proven nerve vasculitis (103). Patients with anti-CV2 antibodies (most of whom have small cell lung carcinoma) may develop a sensorimotor polyneuropathy with mixed axonal-demyelinating electrophysiologic features (139). Some of these patients have both anti-Hu and anti-CV2 antibodies.

Distal, slowly progressive axonal sensorimotor polyneuropathy occurs in patients with a wide variety of carcinomas and hematologic neoplasms (140). The majority of affected patients have suffered significant weight loss and are in an advanced or preterminal phase of their illness. The neuropathy itself is generally not a major source of disability. The exact etiology of the polyneuropathy in these patients is usually unclear and is probably multifactorial.

Autonomic Insufficiency

Paraneoplastic autonomic dysfunction most commonly occurs as a part of encephalomyelitis in patients with small cell lung carcinoma, or rarely in patients with other tumors. In some patients, the autonomic symptoms overshadow other manifestations of encephalomyelitis. These patients may develop severe and progressive gastrointestinal dysmotility, with gastroparesis, chronic intestinal pseudo-obstruction, and severe constipation/obstipation, presenting up to several months prior to discovery of the tumor (141,142). Patients may also have other features of sympathetic dysfunction (eg, orthostatic hypotension or anhidrosis) and/or parasympathetic dysfunction (eg, dry mouth, urinary retention, or impotence). Antineuronal antibodies include anti-Hu antibodies, which react with neurons in the sympathetic ganglia and myenteric plexus (142), and antibodies against neuronal ganglionic acetylcholine receptors (143). Improvement in autonomic function follows tumor resection or chemotherapy in some patients.

Lambert-Eaton Myasthenic Syndrome

Approximately one-half of patients with Lambert-Eaton syndrome have an associated neoplasm, which is small cell lung carcinoma in over 90% of well-documented cases (144–146). In most patients with paraneoplastic Lambert-Eaton syndrome, the neurologic symptoms precede discovery of the associated neoplasm; this interval may be as long as 5 years but is usually less than 12 months (6,144,147).

The clinical features of Lambert-Eaton syndrome are indistinguishable between paraneoplastic and nonparaneoplastic patients. Most patients have an insidious and gradual onset of weakness and fatigue. Early in the course there is often a discrepancy between patients' subjective weakness and easy fatigability and the relatively minor abnormalities seen on neurologic exam. Symmetric weakness predominantly affects proximal leg muscles, and to a lesser extent, shoulder girdle muscles. Muscle aches or distal paresthesias are not uncommon. Muscle stretch reflexes are characteristically diminished or absent. Approximately 75% of patients have symptoms of sympathetic or parasympathetic autonomic dysfunction, including dry mouth, impotence, blurred vision, constipation, difficulty with micturition, and reduced sweating (148). About one-third of patients have dysphagia, ptosis, or diplopia, which are generally mild and occur in the setting of significant limb weakness (149,150).

One feature that distinguishes paraneoplastic from nonparaneoplastic Lambert-Eaton syndrome is that some patients with a neoplasm have concomitant cerebellar degeneration, encephalomyelitis, sensorimotor polyneuropathy, or other overlapping syndromes. There is a particular association between Lambert-Eaton syndrome and cerebellar degeneration among patients with small cell lung cancer (151,152).

The characteristic electrophysiologic profile of Lambert-Eaton syndrome includes reduced amplitude of muscle action potentials, a significant increase in amplitude of compound muscle action potentials after several seconds of maximal voluntary contraction, a decremental response at low rates of repetitive nerve stimulation, and an incremental response at high rates of stimulation (145,153). Serum antibodies against P/Q-type voltage-gated calcium channels are found in over 90% of paraneoplastic or nonparaneoplastic Lambert-Eaton syndrome patients (154). The additional presence of antibodies against the SOX1 protein greatly raise suspicion for small cell lung carcinoma (155).

Most patients with paraneoplastic Lambert-Eaton syndrome improve neurologically with successful treatment of the associated tumor. Pyridostigmine is of benefit but is generally less effective for Lambert-Eaton syndrome than it is for myasthenia gravis. The potassium channel antagonist 3,4-diaminopyridine prolongs the action potential at motor nerve terminals and improves strength in nearly all patients with Lambert-Eaton syndrome (6,156). The combination of pyridostigmine and diaminopyridine often enhances the benefit and permits lower doses of both drugs. Diaminopyridine is an orphan drug in the United States but is available on a compassionate use basis.

For patients with paraneoplastic Lambert-Eaton syndrome who are receiving or will receive tumor treatment, it is usually reasonable to use pyridostigmine and/or diaminopyridine and to defer immunotherapy, since many of these patients will improve with successful tumor treatment. If this is not an option or patients still have severe weakness, prednisone and/or azathioprine are generally effective after a lag period of several weeks or longer (145). Cyclosporine may be used for patients who do not respond to or tolerate corticosteroids or azathioprine. Plasma exchange or IVIg produce improvement in most patients, usually lasting from two to three months (157).

Myasthenia Gravis

Median age at presentation for myasthenia gravis/thymoma patients is 40-50 years, which is older than for nonthymoma myasthenia patients. Patients with myasthenia/thymoma may have other systemic or neurologic autoimmune disorders, including neuromyotonia (see above) (158). The thymoma in myasthenia patients is almost never symptomatic of itself and is usually discovered radiographically shortly after the diagnosis of myasthenia. There is nothing distinctive about the clinical neurologic features of myasthenia among thymoma patients versus nonthymoma patients.

Nearly all patients with myasthenia/thymoma have anti-acetylcholine receptor antibodies. Autoantibodies against striated muscle are present in 80%-90% of patients with myasthenia/thymoma, and include antibodies against titin and the ryanodine receptor (159,160). These antibodies are also found with a much lower prevalence among myasthenia patients without thymoma.

Patients with myasthenia gravis and thymoma generally improve after thymoma resection. There are conflicting data as to whether myasthenia/thymoma patients have a worse or equivalent long-term neurologic outcome after thymectomy compared to nonthymoma patients (161,162). Myasthenia/thymoma patients usually require chronic immunosuppression therapy after thymectomy (158).

Myopathies

The weight of published evidence indicates a significantly higher than expected incidence of cancer among patients with dermatomyositis and, to a lesser degree, polymyositis (163–165). Except perhaps for ovarian carcinoma, there is no clear-cut over-representation of any particular tumor type compared with an age-matched control population. Elevated serum levels of the tumor markers CA19-9 and CA125 may be useful in identifying patients with an associated carcinoma (166). In most patients, the myositis and the associated neoplasm are diagnosed within a short time of each other. There is nothing distinctive about the neurologic symptoms, electromyogram (EMG) findings, muscle pathology, clinical course, or response to immunotherapy in patients with paraneoplastic myositis. In a few published reports, patients with polymyositis or dermatomyositis had significant neurologic improvement after treatment of the associated tumor without immunosuppressive therapy.

Severe necrotizing myopathy is a rare complication of lung carcinoma or other neoplasms (167). Patients develop severe, rapidly progressive weakness with marked elevation of serum creatine kinase. Muscle biopsy or autopsy show diffuse, extensive muscle fiber degeneration and necrosis with minimal or no inflammatory reaction. A few patients improved after tumor resection and corticosteroids, while others were severely disabled or died of bulbar and respiratory weakness.

PATIENT MANAGEMENT

The clincal management of patients with known or suspected paraneoplastic syndromes includes four components: (1) verification that the disorder is in fact paraneoplastic; (2) identification of the associated tumor; (3) treatment of the tumor; and (4) suppression of the autoimmune effectors causing neuronal injury.

Differential diagnosis of patients with a suspected paraneoplastic disorder varies according to whether there is a known cancer diagnosis. Among patients with neurologic dysfunction and a known cancer diagnosis, the level of suspicion for a paraneoplastic disorders depends on the neurologic syndrome, tumor histology, and presence of antineuronal antibodies. Tumor metastases and neurotoxicity of cancer treatments are far more common than paraneoplastic disorders and should always be considered, as should metabolic derangements and CNS infection. For patients without a previous cancer diagnosis, the level of suspicion for a paraneoplastic disorder depends on patient age, gender, risk factors (especially cigarette smoking), the neurologic syndrome, and the presence of antineuronal antibodies (2).

Neuroimaging and CSF evaluation are often abnormal in CNS paraneoplastic disorders but do not in themselves prove a paraneoplastic etiology. Brain MRI may (or may not) show focal lesions in the cerebral cortex, limbic system, basal ganglia, brainstem, or spinal cord in patients with corresponding clinical involvement. Brain MRI in patients with paraneoplastic cerebellar degeneration or opsoclonus-myoclonus is usually normal early in the course of the illness, and later shows nonspecific diffuse cerebellar atrophy. Brain MRI in at least two-thirds of patients with paraneoplastic limbic encephalitis shows areas of abnormal T2-weighted and/or FLAIR signal in the mesial temporal lobe and amygdala bilaterally, and less commonly in the hypothalamus and basal frontal cortex (15,30).

Most patients with CNS paraneoplastic syndromes have abnormal CSF, including some combination of mildly elevated protein, mild mononuclear pleocytosis, elevated IgG index, and/or oligoclonal bands. Normal CSF does not exclude a paraneoplastic diagnosis.

Nerve conduction studies and needle EMG are of great value in characterizing the clinical syndrome in patients with suspected paraneoplastic peripheral nervous system disorders, but cannot themselves differentiate a paraneoplastic versus non-paraneoplastic etiology.

The search for an associated tumor in adults should include CT or MR scans of the chest and abdomen, as well as mammography and pelvic imaging in women. In young men with limbic encephalitis testicular ultrasound may detect a small germ cell tumor, or may show only microcalcifications which orchiectomy reveals to be microscopic intratubular germ cell tumor (168). Total-body fluorodeoxyglucose (FGD)-PET scanning may demonstrate a neoplasm in patients with suspected paraneoplastic disorders (with or without autoantibodies) in whom other imaging studies are negative or equivocal (1,169,170). For patients with any of the syndromes, it is not uncommon for the tumor to be found only after repeated searches.

There are good but not perfect correlations among particular paraneoplastic syndromes, antineuronal antibody specificities, and associated tumor types (Table 34.2). The practical clinical value of antineuronal antibodies is that when present, they greatly increase the index of suspicion for a paraneoplastic condition, and the type of antibody can help guide the search for the associated tumor (2). Antineuronal antibody assays do, however, have important practical clinical limitations: (1) A given clinical syndrome may be associated with one of several autoantibodies. (2) Conversely, a given autoantibody may be associated with a variety of clinical presentations (5). (3) For most if not all neurologic syndromes, some patients have antineuronal autoantibodies and yet never develop a demonstrable tumor (1). The prime examples are Lambert-Eaton syndrome and limbic encephalitis. Presence of antibodies therefore does not absolutely indicate an underlying neoplasm. (4) Some autoantibodies are present at low titers in tumor patients without any accompanying clinical neurologic manifestations. (5) Patients with a suspected paraneo-

plastic syndrome may not have demonstrable antineuronal antibodies, or may have atypical or incompletely characterized antibodies not detected in commercially available assays. Some patients initially determined to be negative for the more common antibodies turn out eventually to have newly recognized antibodies as the list of paraneoplastic antibodies grows. A negative antibody assay, therefore, does not rule out the possibility of a paraneoplastic disorder and the presence of an underlying neoplasm.

Factors that interact in influencing the response of neurologic paraneoplastic disorders to immunotherapy include the neuroanatomic site (central vs peripheral), the cellular location of the onconeural target antigen(s) (neuronal cell surface vs intracellular), the mechanism(s) of neuronal injury (antibody-mediated vs cell-mediated), and treatment of the associated neoplasm. In general, syndromes affecting the peripheral nervous system are more likely to improve with tumor treatment and/or immunosuppressive treatment than are CNS syndromes. Syndromes caused by autoantibodies reacting with neuronal cell surface receptors or ion channels are more likely to respond to immunotherapy, probably because the antibodies do not usually cause axonal degeneration or neuronal cell death. For many if not most syndromes there is increasing evidence that successful tumor treatment is a major factor in determining neurologic outcome, and that immunotherapy is more likely to be effective when the tumor is also treated successfully (1,15,22,56).

Even for the "unfavorable" syndromes such as multifocal encephalomyelitis and cerebellar degeneration, there are a few patients who do show a meaningful neurologic response to immunotherapy. For these few responders, the only factors which sometimes correlate with neurologic improvement are successful tumor treatment, and the duration and severity of neurologic deficits prior to diagnosis and initiation of therapy. For patients who have already stabilized at a plateau of severe neurologic disability for more than several weeks, subsequent improvement with any intervention is not impossible but extremely unlikely. The decision whether to try immunosuppressive therapies must therefore be based on the particular syndrome and on the individual patient's circumstances.

There are several potential explanations for the disappointingly poor response to immunotherapy in many patients. As noted above, the continuing presence of even a small tumor burden seems to provide an antigenic drive for further neuronal injury. It is also likely that current immunotherapies do not adequately gain access to the central nervous system and do not effectively abrogate an ongoing autoimmune response that is sequestered in the central nervous system. Unfortunately, for many if not most central syndromes it is likely that patients have already suffered neuronal death or irreversible injury by the time the diagnosis of a paraneoplastic disorder is made.

There is theoretical concern that if paraneoplastic disorders arise from an immune response directed against the tumor, attempts to treat the neurologic disorder with immunosuppression may adversely affect the evolution of the tumor. At this time, there is no definite evidence that patients given immunosuppressive treatment have a worse tumor outcome (25,50).

References

1. Candler PM, Hart PE, Barnett M, Weil R, Rees JH. A follow up study of patients with paraneoplastic neurological disease in the United Kingdom. *J Neuro Neurosurg Psychiatr.* 2004;75:1411–1415.

2. Graus F, Delattre JY, Antoine JC, et al. Recommended diagnostic criteria for paraneoplastic neurological syndromes. *J Neuro Neurosurg Psychiatr.* 2004;75:1135–1140.

3. Musunuru K, Darnell RB. Paraneoplastic neurologic disease antigens: RNA-binding proteins and signaling proteins in neuronal degeneration. *Annu Rev Neurosci.* 2001;24:239–262.

4. Dropcho EJ. Remote neurologic manifestations of cancer. *Neurol Clin.* 2002;20(1):85–122.

5. Pittock SJ, Kryzer TJ, Lennon VA. Paraneoplastic antibodies coexist and predict cancer, not neurological syndrome. *Ann Neurol.* 2004;56:715–719.

6. Sanders DB. Lambert-Eaton myasthenic syndrome: diagnosis and treatment. *Ann NY Acad Sci.* 2003;998:500–508.

7. Tomimitsu H, Arimura K, Nagado T, et al. Mechanism of action of voltage-gated K+ channel antibodies in acquired neuromyotonia. *Ann Neurol.* 2004;56:440–444.

8. Kleopa KA, Elman LB, Lang B, Vincent A, Scherer SS. Neuromyotonia and limbic encephalitis sera target mature Shaker-type K+ channels: subunit specificity correlates with clinical manifestations. *Brain.* 2006;129:1570–1584.

9. Dalmau J, Tuzun E, Wu H, et al. Paraneoplastic anti-N-methyl-D-aspartate receptor encephalitis associated with ovarian teratoma. *Ann Neurol.* 2007;61:25–36.

10. Fukuda T, Motomura M, Nakao YK, et al. Reduction of P/Q-type calcium channels in the postmortem cerebellum of paraneoplastic cerebellar degeneration with Lambert-Eaton myasthenic syndrome. *Ann Neurol.* 2003;53:21–28.

11. Coesmans M, Sillevis Smitt PA, Linden DJ, et al. Mechanisms underlying cerebellar motor deficits due to mGluR1-autoantibodies. *Ann Neurol.* 2003;53:325–336.

12. Sommer C, Weishaupt A, Brinkhoff J, et al. Paraneoplastic stiff-person syndrome: passive transfer to rats by means of IgG antibodies to amphiphysin. *Lancet.* 2005;365:1406–1411.

13. Tanaka M, Tanaka K, Tsuji S, et al. Cytotoxic T cell activity against the peptide AYRARALEL from Yo protein of patients with the HLA A24 or B27 supertype and paraneoplastic cerebellar degeneration. *J Neurol Sci.* 2001;188:61–65.

14. Rousseau A, Benyahia B, Dalmau J, et al. T-cell response to Hu-D peptides in patients with anti-Hu syndrome. *J Neuro-Oncol.* 2005;71:231–236.

15. Dalmau J, Graus F, Villarejo A, et al. Clinical analysis of anti-Ma2-associated encephalitis. *Brain.* 2004;127:1831–1844.

16. Roberts WK, Darnell RB. Neuroimmunology of the paraneoplastic neurological degenerations. *Curr Opin Immunol.* 2004;16:616–622.

17. Monaco S, Ferrari S, Bonetti B, et al. Experimental induction of myelin changes by anti-MAG antibodies and terminal complement complex. *J Neuropathol Exp Neurol.* 1995;54:96–104.

18. Kusunoki S, Hitoshi S, Kaida K, Arita M, Kanazawa I. Monospecific anti-GD1b IgG is required to induce rabbit ataxic neuropathy. *Ann Neurol.* 1999;45:400–403.

19. Scarlato M, Previtali SC, Carpo M, et al. Polyneuropathy in POEMS syndrome: role of angiogenic factors in the pathogenesis. *Brain.* 2005;128:1911–1920.

20. Chuang WY, Strobel P, Gold R, et al. A CTLA4(high) genotype is associated with myasthenia gravis in thymoma patients. *Ann Neurol.* 2005;58:644–648.

21. Dalmau J, Graus F, Rosenblum MK, Posner JB. Anti-Hu-associated paraneoplastic encephalomyelitis/sensory neuronopathy: a clinical study of 71 patients. *Medicine.* 1992;71:59–72.

22. Graus F, Keime-Guibert F, Rene R, et al. Anti-Hu-associated paraneoplastic encephalomyelitis: analysis of 200 patients. *Brain.* 2001;124:1138–1148.

23. Sillevis Smitt P, Grefkens J, de Leeuw B, et al. Survival and outcome in 73 anti-Hu positive patients with paraneoplastic encephalomyelitis/sensory neuronopathy. *J Neurol.* 2002;249:745–753.

24. Lucchinetti CF, Kimmel DW, Lennon VA. Paraneoplastic and oncologic profiles of patients seropositive for type I antineuronal nuclear autoantibodies. *Neurology.* 1998;50:652–657.

25. Keime-Guibert F, Graus F, Broet P, et al. Clinical outcome of patients with anti-Hu-associated encephalomyelitis after treatment of the tumor. *Neurology.* 1999;53:1719–1723.

26. Yu Z, Kryzer TJ, Griesmann GE, et al. CRMP-5 neuronal antoantibody: marker of lung cancer and thymoma-related autoimmunity. *Ann Neurol.* 2001;49:146–154.

27. Keime-Guibert F, Graus F, Fleury A, et al. Treatment of paraneoplastic neurological syndromes with antineuronal antibodies (anti-Hu, anti-Yo) with a combination of immunoglobulins, cyclophosphamide, and methylprednisolone. *J Neurol Neurosurg Psychiatr.* 2000;68:479–482.

28. Alamowitch S, Graus F, Uchuya M, et al. Limbic encephalitis and small cell lung cancer: clinical and immunological features. *Brain.* 1997;120:923–928.

29. Gultekin SH, Rosenfeld MR, Voltz R, et al. Paraneoplastic limbic encephalitis: neurological symptoms, immunological findings and tumour association in 50 patients. *Brain.* 2000;123:1481–1494.

30. Lawn ND, Westmoreland BF, Kiely MJ, Lennon VA, Vernino S. Clinical, magnetic resonance imaging, and electroencephalographic findings in paraneoplastic limbic encephalitis. *Mayo Clin Proc.* 2003;78:1363–1368.

31. Fujii N, Furuta A, Yamaguchi H, Nakanishi K, Iwaki T. Limbic encephalitis associated with recurrent thymoma: a postmortem study. *Neurology.* 2001;57:344–347.

32. Ances BM, Vitaliani R, Taylor RA, et al. Treatment-responsive limbic encephalitis identified by neuropil antibodies: MRI and PET correlates. *Brain.* 2005;128:1764–1777.

33. Deodhare S, O'Connor P, Ghazarian D, Bilbao JM. Paraneoplastic limbic encephalitis in Hodgkin disease. *Can J Neurol Sci.* 1996;23:138–140.

34. Vitaliani R, Mason W, Ances B, et al. Paraneoplastic encephalitis, psychiatric symptoms, and hypoventilation in ovarian teratoma. *Ann Neurol.* 2005;58:594–604.

35. Bataller L, Kleopa KA, Wu GF, et al. Autoimmune limbic encephalitis in 39 patients: immunophenotypes and outcomes. *J Neurol Neurosurg Psychiatr.* 2007;78:381–385.

36. Blumenthal DT, Salzman KL, Digre KB, et al. Early pathologic findings and long-term improvement in anti-Ma2-associated encephalitis. *Neurology.* 2006;67:146–149.

37. Rojas-Marcos I, Graus F, Sanz G, Robledo A, Diaz-Espejo C. Hypersomnia as presenting symptom of anti-Ma2-associated encephalitis. *Neuro-Oncology.* 2007;9:75–77.

38. Buckley C, Oger J, Clover L, et al. Potassium channel antibodies in two patients with reversible limbic encephalitis. *Ann Neurol.* 2001;50:73–78.

39. Vernino S, Lennon VA. Autoantibody profiles and neurological correlations of thymoma. *Clin Cancer Res.* 2004;10:7270–7275.

40. Zuliani L, Saiz A, Tavolato B, et al. Paraneoplastic limbic encephalitis associated with potassium channel antibodies: value of anti-glial nuclear antibodies in identifying the tumour. *J Neurol Neurosurg Psychiatr.* 2007;78:204–205.

41. Thieben MJ, Lennon VA, Boeve BF, et al. Potentially reversible autoimmune limbic encephalitis with neuronal potassium channel antibody. *Neurology.* 2004;62:1177–1182.

42. Vincent A, Buckley C, Schott J, et al. Potassium channel antibody-associated encephalopathy: a potentially immunotherapy-responsive form of limbic encephalitis. *Brain.* 2004;127:701–712.

43. Liguori R, Vincent A, Clover L, et al. Morvan's syndrome: peripheral and central nervous system and cardiac involvement with antibodies to voltage-gated potassium channels. *Brain.* 2001;124:2417–2426.

44. Hammack JE, Kotanides H, Rosenblum MK, Posner JB. Paraneoplastic cerebellar degeneration: clinical and immunologic findings in 21 patients with Hodgkin's disease. *Neurology.* 1992;42:1938–1943.

45. Peterson K, Rosenblum MK, Kotanides H, Posner JB. Paraneoplastic cerebellar degeneration: a clinical analysis of 55 anti-Yo antibody-positive patients. *Neurology.* 1992;42:1931–1937.

46. Rojas-Marcos I, Rousseau A, Keime-Guibert F, et al. Spectrum of paraneoplastic neurologic disorders in women with breast and gynecologic cancer. *Medicine.* 2003;82:216–223.

47. Shams'ili S, Grefkens J, de Leeuw B, et al. Paraneoplastic cerebellar degeneration associated with antineuronal antibodies: analysis of 50 patients. *Brain.* 2003;126:1409–1418.

48. Bataller L, Wade DF, Graus F, Rosenfeld MR, Dalmau J. The MAZ protein is an autoantigen of Hodgkin's disease and paraneoplastic cerebellar dysfunction. *Ann Neurol.* 2003;53:123–127.

49. Bernal F, Shams'ili S, Rojas I, et al. Anti-Tr antibodies as markers of paraneoplastic cerebellar degeneration and Hodgkin's disease. *Neurology.* 2003;60:230–234.

50. Rojas I, Graus F, Keime-Guibert F, et al. Long-term clinical outcome of paraneoplastic cerebellar degeneration and anti-Yo antibodies. *Neurology.* 2000;55:713–715.

51. Uchuya M, Graus F, Vega F, Rene R, Delattre JY. Intravenous immunoglobulin treatment in paraneoplastic neurological syndromes with antineuronal antibodies. *J Neurol Neurosurg Psychiatr.* 1996;60:388–392.

52. Vernino S, O'Neill BP, Marks RS, O'Fallon JR, Kimmel DW. Immunomodulatory treatment trial for paraneoplastic neurological disorders. *Neuro-Oncology.* 2003;6:55–62.

53. Rudnick E, Khakoo Y, Antunes NL, et al. Opsoclonus-myoclonus-ataxia syndrome in neuroblastoma: clinical outcome and antineuronal antibodies: a report from the Children's Cancer Group. *Med Pediatr Oncol.* 2001;36:612–622.

54. Gambini C, Conte M, Bernini G, et al. Neuroblastic tumors associated with opsoclonus-myoclonus syndrome: histological, immunohistochemical and molecular features of 15 Italian cases. *Virchows Arch.* 2003;442:555–562.

55. Anderson NE, Budde-Steffen C, Rosenblum MK, et al. Opsoclonus, myoclonus, ataxia, and encephalopathy in adults with cancer: a distinct paraneoplastic syndrome. *Medicine.* 1988;67:100–109.

56. Bataller L, Graus F, Saiz A, Vilchez JJ. Clinical outcome in adult onset idiopathic or paraneoplastic opsoclonus-myoclonus. *Brain.* 2001;124:437–443.

57. Ziter FA, Bray PF, Cancilla PA. Neuropathologic findings in a patient with neuroblastoma and myoclonic encephalopathy. *Arch Neurol.* 1979;36:51.

58. Wong AM, Musallam S, Tomlinson RD, Shannon P, Sharpe JA. Opsoclonus in three dimensions: oculographic, neuropathologic and modelling correlates. *J Neurol Sci.* 2001;189:71–81.

59. Ridley A, Kennard C, Scholtz CL, et al. Omnipause neurons in two cases of opsoclonus associated with oat cell carcinoma of the lung. *Brain.* 1987;110:1699–1709.

60. Hersh B, Dalmau J, Dangond F, et al. Paraneoplastic opsoclonus-myoclonus associated with anti-Hu antibody. *Neurology.* 1994;44:1754–1755.

61. Hayward K, Jeremy RJ, Jenkins S, et al. Long-term neurobehavioral outcome in children with neuroblastoma and opsoclonus-myoclonus-ataxia syndrome: relationship to MRI findings and anti-neuronal antibodies. *J Pediatr.* 2001;139:552–559.

62. Korfei M, Fuhlhuber V, Schmidt T, et al. Functional characterisation of autoantibodies from patients with pediatric opsoclonus-myoclonus syndrome. *J Neuroimmunol.* 2005;170:150–157.

63. Antunes NL, Khakoo Y, Matthay KK, et al. Antineuronal antibodies in patients with neuroblastoma and paraneoplastic opsoclonus-myoclonus. *J Pediatr Hematol/Oncol.* 2000;22:315–320.

64. Blaes F, Fuhlhuber V, Korfei M, et al. Surface-binding autoantibodies to cerebellar neurons in opsoclonus syndrome. *Ann Neurol.* 2005;58:313–317.

65. Bataller L, Rosenfeld MR, Graus F, et al. Autoantigen diversity in the opsoclonus-myoclonus syndrome. *Ann Neurol.* 2003;53:347–353.

66. Hammer MS, Larsen MB, Stack CV. Outcome of children with opsoclonus-myoclonus regardless of etiology. *Pediatr Neurol.* 1995;13:21–24.

67. Rostasy K, Behnisch W, Kulozik A, et al. High-dose pulsatile dexamethasone therapy in children with opsolconus-myoclonus syndrome (abstract). *Ann Neurol.* 2005;58 (suppl 9):S109.

68. Yiu VW, Kovithavongs T, McGonigle LF, Ferreira P. Plasmapheresis as an effective treatment for opsoclonus-myoclonus syndrome. *Pediatr Neurol.* 2001;24:72–74.

69. Pranzatelli MR, Tate ED, Travelstead AL, et al. Rituximab (anti-CD20) adjunctive therapy for opsolconus-myoclonus syndrome. *J Pediatr Haematol Oncol.* 2006;28:585–593.

70. Mitchell WG, Brumm VL, Azen CG, et al. Longitudinal neurodevelopmental evaluation of children with opsoclonus-ataxia. *Pediatrics.* 2005;116:901–907.

71. Mitchell WG, Davalos Y, Brumm VL, et al. Opsoclonus-ataxia caused by childhood neuroblastoma: developmental and neurologic sequelae. *Pediatrics.* 2002;109:86–98.

72. Pranzatelli MR, Tate ED, Dukart WS, et al. Sleep disturbance and rage attacks in opsoclonus-myoclonus syndrome: response to trazodone. *J Pediatr.* 2005;147:372–378.

73. Russo C, Cohn SL, Petruzzi MJ, Alarcon PA. Long-term neurologic outcome in children with opsoclous-myoclonus associated with neuroblastoma: a report from the Pediatric Oncology Group. *Med Pediatr Oncol.* 1997;29:284–288.

74. Pittock SJ, Lucchinetti CF, Lennon VA. Anti-Neuronal nuclear autoantibody type 2: paraneoplastic accompaniments. *Ann Neurol.* 2003;53:580–587.

75. Batchelor TT, Platten M, Hochberg FH. Immunoadsorption therapy for paraneoplastic syndromes. *J Neuro-Oncol.* 1998;40:131–136.

76. Croteau D, Owainati A, Dalmau J, Rogers LR. Response to cancer therapy in a patient with a paraneoplastic choreiform disorder. *Neurology.* 2001;57:719–722.

77. Vernino S, Tuite P, Adler CH, et al. Paraneoplastic chorea associated with CRMP-5 neuronal antibody and lung carcinoma. *Ann Neurol.* 2002;51:625–630.

78. Kinirons P, Fulton A, Keoghan M, et al. Paraneoplastic limbic encephalitis and chorea associated with CRMP-5 neuronal antibody. *Neurology.* 2003;61:1623–1624.

79. Chong DJ, Strong MJ, Shkrum MJ, Kalapos P, Hammond RR. A 58 year-old woman with progressive vertigo, deafness and weakness. *Can J Neurol Sci.* 2005;32:103–108.

80. Rajabally YA, Naz S, Farrell D, Abbott RJ. Paraneoplastic brainstem encephalitis with tetraparesis in a patient with anti-Ri antibodies. *J Neurol.* 2004;251:1528–1529.

81. Thambisetty MR, Scherzer CR, Yu Z, Lennon VA, Newman NJ. Paraneoplastic optic neuropathy and cerebellar ataxia with small cell carcinoma of the lung. *J Neuro-Ophthalmol.* 2001;21:164–167.

82. Sheorajpanday R, Slabbynck H, van de Sompel W, et al. Small cell lung carcinoma presenting as CRMP-5 paraneoplastic optic neuropathy. *J Neuro-Ophthalmol.* 2006;26:168–172.

83. Cross SA, Salomao DR, Parisi JE, et al. Paraneoplastic autoimmune optic neuritis with retinitis defined by CRMP-5-IgG. *Ann Neurol.* 2003;54:38–50.

84. Keltner JL, Thirkill CE, Yip PT. Clinical and immunologic characteristics of melanoma-associated retinopathy syndrome: 11 new cases and a review of 51 previously published cases. *J Neuro-Ophthalmol.* 2001;21:173–187.

85. Ohguro H, Yokoi Y, Ohguri I, et al. Clinical and immunologic aspects of cancer-associated retinopathy. *Am J Ophthalmol.* 2004;137:1117–1119.

86. Antoine JC, Camdessanche JP, Absi L, Lassabliere F, Feasson L. Devic disease and thymoma with anti-central nervous system and antithymus antibodies. *Neurology.* 2004;62:978–980.

87. Pittock SJ, Lucchinetti CF, Parisi JE, et al. Amphiphysin autoimmunity: paraneoplastic accompaniments. *Ann Neurol.* 2005;58:96–107.

88. Ducray F, Weil R, Garcia PY, et al. Devic's syndrome-like phenotype associated with thymoma and anti-CV2 antibodies. *J Neurol Neurosurg Psychiatr.* 2007;78:325–327.

89. Ojeda VJ. Necrotizing myelopathy associated with malignancy: a clinicopathologic study of two cases and literature review. *Cancer.* 1984;53:1115–1123.

90. Dansey RD, Hammond-Tooke GD, Lai K, Bezwoda WR. Subacute myelopathy: an unusual paraneoplastic complication of Hodgkin's disease. *Med Pediatr Oncol.* 1988;16:284–286.

91. Hughes M, Ahern V, Kefford R, Boyages J. Paraneoplastic myelopathy at diagnosis in a patient with pathologic stage IA Hodgkin disease. *Cancer.* 1992;70:1598–1600.

92. Wessig C, Klein R, Schneider MF, et al. Neuropathology and binding studies in anti-amphiphysin-associated stiff-person syndrome. *Neurology.* 2003;61:195–198.

93. Petzold GC, Marcucci M, Butler MH, et al. Rhabdomyolysis and paraneoplastic stiff-man syndrome with amphiphysin autoimmunity. *Ann Neurol.* 2004;55:286–290.

94. Thomas S, Critchley P, Lawden M, et al. Stiff person syndrome with eye movement abnormality, myasthenia gravis, and thymoma. *J Neurol Neurosurg Psychiatr.* 2005;76:141–149.

95. Tanaka H, Matsumura A, Okumura M, et al. Stiff man syndrome with thymoma. *Ann Thorac Surg.* 2005;80:739–741.

96. Dropcho EJ. Antiamphiphysin antibodies with small cell lung carcinoma and paraneoplastic encephalomyelitis. *Ann Neurol.* 1996;39:659–667.

97. Verma A, Berger JR, Snodgrass S, Petito C. Motor neuron disease: a paraneoplastic process associated with anti-Hu antibody and small-cell lung carcinoma. *Ann Neurol.* 1996;40:112–116.

98. Rosenfeld MR, Posner JB. Paraneoplastic motor neuron disease. *Adv Neurol.* 1991;56:445–459.

99. Evans BK, Fagan C, Arnold T, Dropcho EJ, Oh SJ. Paraneoplastic motor neuron disease and renal cell carcinoma: improvement after nephrectomy. *Neurology.* 1990;40:960–962.

100. Forman D, Rae-Grant AD, Matchett SC, Cowen JS. A reversible cause of hypercapnic respiratory failure: lower motor neuronopathy associated with renal cell carcinoma. *Chest.* 1999;115:899–901.

101. Gordon PH, Rowland LP, Younger DS, et al. Lymphoproliferative disorders and motor neuron disease: an update. *Neurology.* 1997;48:1671–1678.

102. Chalk CH, Windebank AJ, Kimmel DW, McManis PG. The distinctive clinical features of paraneoplastic sensory neuronopathy. *Can J Neurol Sci.* 1992;19:346–351.

103. Eggers C, Hagel C, Pfeiffer G. Anti-Hu-associated paraneoplastic sensory neuropathy with peripheral nerve demyelination and microvasculitis. *J Neurol Sci.* 1998;155:178–181.

104. Antoine JC, Mosnier JF, Absi L, et al. Carcinoma associated paraneoplastic peripheral neuropathies in patients with and without anti-onconeural antibodies. *J Neurol Neurosurg Psychiatr.* 1999;67:7–14.

105. Camdessanche JP, Antoine JC, Honnorat J, et al. Paraneoplastic peripheral neuropathy associated with anti-Hu antibodies: a clinical and electrophysiological study of 20 patients. *Brain.* 2002;125:166–175.

106. Oh SJ, Gurtekin Y, Dropcho EJ, King P, Claussen GC. Anti-Hu antibody neuropathy: a clinical, electrophysiological, and pathological study. *Clin Neurophysiol.* 2005;116:28–34.

107. Molinuevo JL, Graus F, Serrano C, et al. Utility of anti-Hu antibodies in the diagnosis of paraneoplastic sensory neuropathy. *Ann Neurol.* 1998;44:976–980.

108. Graus F, Bonaventura I, Uchuya M, et al. Indolent anti-Hu-associated paraneoplastic sensory neuropathy. *Neurology.* 1994;44:2258–2261.

109. Byrne T, Mason WP, Posner JB, Dalmau J. Spontaneous neurological improvement in anti-Hu associated encephalomyelitis. *J Neurol Neurosurg Psychiatr.* 1997;62:276–278.

110. Oh SJ, Dropcho EJ, Claussen GC. Anti-Hu-associated paraneoplastic sensory neuronopathy responding to early aggressive immunotherapy: report of two cases and review of the literature. *Muscle Nerve.* 1997;20:1576–1582.

111. Lahrmann H, Albrecht G, Drlicek M, et al. Acquired neuromyotonia and peripheral neuropathy in a patient with Hodgkin's disease. *Muscle Nerve.* 2001;24:834–838.

112. Hart IK, Maddison P, Newsom-Davis J, Vincent A, Mills KR. Phenotypic variants of autoimmune peripheral nerve hyperexcitability. *Brain.* 2002;125:1887–1895.

113. Vernino S, Lennon VA. Ion channel and striational antibodies define a continuum of autoimmune neuromuscular hyperexcitability. *Muscle Nerve.* 2002;26:702–707.

114. Antozzi C, Frassoni C, Vincent A, et al. Sequential antibodies to potassium channels and glutamic acid decarboxylase in neuromyotonia. *Neurology.* 2005;64:1290–1293.

115. Vital C, Vital A, Julien J, et al. Peripheral neuropathies and lymphoma without monoclonal gammopathy: a new classification. *J Neurol.* 1990;237:177–185.

116. Vallat JM, De Mascarel HA, Bordessoule D, et al. Non-Hodgkin's malignant lymphomas and peripheral neuropathies-13 cases. *Brain.* 1995;118:1233–1245.

117. Antoine JC, Mosnier JF, Lapras J, et al. Chronic inflammatory demyelinating polyneuropathy associated with carcinoma. *J Neuro Neurosurg Psychiatr.* 1996;60:188–190.

118. Kyle RA, Therneau RM, Rajkumar SV, et al. A long-term study of prognosis in monoclonal gammopathy of undetermined significance. *New Engl J Med.* 2002;346:564–569.

119. Ponsford S, Willison H, Veitch J, Morris R, Thomas PK. Long-term clinical and neurophysiological follow-up of patients with peripheral neuropathy associated with benign monoclonal gammopathy. *Muscle Nerve.* 2000;23:164–174.

120. Eurelings M, Moons KG, Notermans NC, et al. Neuropathy and IgM M-proteins: prognostic value of antibodies to MAG, SGPG, and sulfatide. *Neurology.* 2001;56:228–233.

121. Lupu VD, Mora CA, Dambrosia J, et al. Terminal latency index in neuropathy with antibodies against myelin-associated glycoprotein. *Muscle Nerve.* 2007;35:196–202.

122. Lopate G, Kornberg AJ, Yue J, Choksi R, Pestronk A. Anti-MAG antibodies: variability in patterns of IgM binding to peripheral nerve. *J Neurol Sci.* 2001;188:67–72.

123. Nobile-Orazio E, Meucci N, Baldini L, Di Troia A, Scarlato G. Long-term prognosis of neuropathy associated with anti-MAG IgM M-proteins and its relationship to immune therapies. *Brain.* 2000;123:710–717.

124. Gorson KC, Ropper AH, Weinberg DH, Weinstein R. Treatment experience in patients with anti-myelin-associated glycoprotein neuropathy. *Muscle Nerve.* 2001;24:778–786.

125. Oksenhendler E, Chevret S, Leger JM, et al. Plasma exchange and chlorambucil in polyneuropathy associated with monoclonal IgM gammopathy. *J Neurol Neurosurg Psychiatr.* 1995;59:243–247.

126. Comi G, Roveri L, Swan A, et al. A randomised controlled trial of intravenous immunoglobulin in IgM paraprotein associated demyelinating neuropathy. *J Neurol.* 2002;249:1370–1377.

127. Pestronk A, Florence J, Miller T, et al. Treatment of IgM antibody associated polyneuropathies using rituximab. *J Neurol Neurosurg Psychiatr.* 2003;74:485–489.

128. Renaud S, Fuhr P, Gregor M, et al. High-dose rituximab and anti-MAG-associated polyneuropathy. *Neurology.* 2006;66:742–744.

129. Kelly JJ, Kyle RA, Miles JM, Dyck PJ. Osteosclerotic myeloma and peripheral neuropathy. *Neurology.* 1983;33:202–210.

130. Min JH, Hong YH, Lee KW. Electrophysiological features of patients with POEMS syndrome. *Clin Neurophysiol.* 2005;116:965–968.

131. Soubrier MJ, Dubost JJ, Sauvezie BJ. POEMS syndrome: a study of 25 cases and a review of the literature. *Am J Med.* 1994;97:543–553.

132. Dispenzieri A, Kyle RA, Lacy MQ, et al. POEMS syndrome: definitions and long-term outcome. *Blood.* 2003;101:2496–2506.

133. Dispenzieri A, Moreno A, Suarez GA, et al. Peripheral blood stem cell transplantation in 16 patients with POEMS syndrome. *Blood.* 2004;104:3400–3407.

134. Eurelings M, Ang CW, Notermans NC, et al. Antiganglioside antibodies in polyneuropathy associated with monoclonal gammopathy. *Neurology.* 2001;57:1909–1912.

135. Willison HJ, O'Leary CP, Veitch J, et al. The clinical and laboratory features of chronic sensory ataxic neuropathy with anti-disialosyl IgM antibodies. *Brain.* 2001;124:1968–1977.

136. Younger DS, Dalmau J, Inghirami G, Sherman WH, Hays AP. Anti-Hu-associated peripheral nerve and muscle microvasculitis. *Neurology.* 1994;44:181–183.

137. Oh SJ. Paraneoplastic vasculitis of the peripheral nervous system. *Neurol Clin.* 1997;15(4):849–863.

138. Antoine JC, Mosiner JF, Honnorat J, et al. Paraneoplastic demyelinating neuropathy, subacute sensory neuropathy, and anti-Hu antibodies: clinicopathological study of an autopsy case. *Muscle Nerve.* 1998;21:850–857.

139. Antoine JC, Honnorat J, Camdessanche JP, et al. Paraneoplastic anti-CV2 antibodies react with peripheral nerve and are associated with a mixed axonal and demyelinating peripheral neuropathy. *Ann Neurol.* 2001;49:214–221.

140. Gomm SA, Thatcher N, Barber PV, Cumming WJ. A clinicopathological study of the paraneoplastic neuromuscular syndromes associated with lung cancer. *Quart J Med.* 1990;75:577–595.

141. Condom E, Vidal A, Rota R, et al. Paraneoplastic intestinal pseudo-obstruction associated with high titres of Hu autoantibodies. *Virch Arch Pathol.* 1993;423:507–511.

142. Lee HR, Lennon VA, Camilleri M, Prather CM. Paraneoplastic gastrointestinal motor dysfunction: clinical and laboratory characteristics. *Am J Gastroenterol.* 2001;96:373–379.

143. Vernino S, Lennon VA. Neuronal ganglionic acetylcholine receptor autoimmunity. *Ann NY Acad Sci.* 2003;998:211–214.

144. O'Neill JH, Murray NM, Newsom-Davis J. The Lambert-Eaton myasthenic syndrome: a review of 50 cases. *Brain.* 1988;111:577–596.

145. Tim RW, Massey JM, Sanders DB. Lambert-Eaton myasthenic syndrome: electrodiagnostic findings and response to treatment. *Neurology.* 2000;54:2176–2178.

146. Wirtz PW, van Dijk JG, van Doorn PA, et al. The epidemiology of the Lambert-Eaton myasthenic syndrome in the Netherlands. *Neurology.* 2004;63:397–398.

147. Chalk CH, Murray NM, Newsom-Davis J, O'Neill JH, Spiro S. Response of the Lambert-Eaton myasthenic syndrome to treatment of associated small cell lung carcinoma. *Neurology.* 1990;40:1552–1556.

148. O'Suilleabhain P, Low PA, Lennon VA. Autonomic dysfuncton in the Lambert-Eaton myasthenic syndrome: serologic and clinical correlates. *Neurology* 1998;50:88–93.

149. Wirtz PW, Sotodeh M, Nijnuis M, et al. Difference in distribution of muscle weakness between myasthenia gravis and the Lambert-Eaton myasthenic syndrome. *J Neurol Neurosurg Psychiatr.* 2002;73:766–768.

150. Burns TM, Russell JA, LaChance DH, Jones HR. Oculobulobar involvement is typical with Lambert-Eaton myasthenic syndrome. *Ann Neurol.* 2003;53:270–273.

151. Mason WP, Graus F, Lang B, et al. Small-cell lung cancer, paraneoplastic cerebellar degeneration and the Lambert-Eaton myasthenic syndrome. *Brain.* 1997;120:1279–1300.

152. Graus F, Lang B, Pozo-Rosich P, et al. P/Q-type calcium-channel antibodies in paraneoplastic cerebellar degeneration with lung cancer. *Neurology.* 2002;59:764–766.

153. Oh SJ, Kurokawa K, Claussen GC, Ryan HF. Electrophysiological diagnostic criteria of Lambert-Eaton myasthenic syndrome. *Muscle Nerve.* 2005;32:515–520.

154. Motomura M, Lang B, Johnston I, et al. Incidence of serum anti-P/Q-type and anti-N-type calcium channel autoantibodies in the Lambert-Eaton myasthenic syndrome. *J Neurol Sci.* 1997;147:35–42.

155. Graus F, Vincent A, Pozo-Rosich P, et al. Anti-glial nuclear antibody: marker of lung cancer-related paraneoplastic neurological syndromes. *J Neuroimmunol.* 2005;165:166–171.

156. Sanders DB, Massey JM, Sanders LL, Edwards LJ. A randomized trial of 3,4-diaminopyridine in Lambert-Eaton myasthenic syndrome. *Neurology.* 2000; 54:603–607.

157. Rich MM, Teener JW, Bird SJ. Treatment of Lambert-Eaton syndrome with intravenous immunoglobulin. *Muscle Nerve.* 1997;20:614–615.

158. Lovelace RE, Younger DS. Myasthenia gravis with thymoma. *Neurology.* 1997;48(suppl 5):S76–S81.

159. Baggi F, Andreetta F, Antozzi C, et al. Anti-titin and antiryanodine receptor antibodies in myasthenia gravis patients with thymoma. *Ann NY Acad Sci.* 1998;841:538–541.

160. Buckley C, Newsom-Davis J, Willcox N, Vincent A. Do titin and cytokine antibodies in MG patients predict thymoma or thymoma recurrence? *Neurology.* 2001;57:1579–1582.

161. Durelli L, Maggi G, Casadio C, et al. Actuarial analysis of the occurrence of remissions following thymectomy for myasthenia gravis in 400 patients. *J Neurol Neurosurg Psychiatr.* 1991;54:406–411.

162. de Perrot M, Liu J, Bril V, et al. Prognostic significance of thymomas in patients with myasthenia gravis. *Ann Thor Surg.* 2002;74:1658–1662.

163. Buchbinder R, Forbes A, Hall S, Dennett X, Giles G. Incidence of malignant disease in biopsy-proven inflammatory myopathy: a population-based cohort study. *Ann Int Med.* 2001;134:1087–1095.

164. Hill CL, Zhang Y, Sigurgeirsson B, et al. Frequency of specific cancer types in dermatomyositis and polymyositis: a population-based study. *Lancet.* 2001;357:96–100.

165. Levine SM. Cancer and myositis: new insights into an old association. *Curr Op Rheumatol.* 2006;18:620–624.

166. Amoura Z, Duhaut P, Huong DL, et al. Tumor antigen markers for the detection of solid cancers in inflammatory myopathies. *Cancer Epidemiol Biomarkers Prev.* 2005;14:1279–1282.

167. Levin MI, Mozaffar T, Al-Lozi MT, Pestronk A. Paraneoplastic necrotizing myopathy: clinical and pathologic features. *Neurology.* 1998;50:764–767.

168. Mathew RM, Vandenberghe R, Garcia A, et al. Orchiectomy for suspected microscopic tumor in patients with anti-Ma2-associated encephalitis. *Neurology.* 2007;68:900–905.

169. Linke R, Schroeder M, Helmberger T, Voltz R. Antibody-positive paraneoplastic neurologic syndromes: value of CT and PET for tumor diagnosis. *Neurology.* 2004;63:282–286.

170. Younes-Mhenni S, Janier MF, Cinotti L, et al. FDG-PET improves tumour detection in patients with paraneoplastic neurological syndromes. *Brain.* 2004;127:2331–2338.w

IV

PAIN IN CANCER

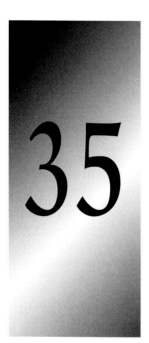

Approach to Evaluation of Pain Disorders in the Cancer Patient

35

Michael D. Stubblefield

The evaluation of pain in the cancer setting is one of the most important and challenging tasks faced by the rehabilitation physician and team. It is estimated that the prevalence of cancer pain is between 30% and 50% in patients undergoing chronic treatment and affects more than 70% in those with advanced disease (1). Quantity of life is of little value without a reasonable degree of quality of life. Pain may contribute significantly to decreased quality of life in cancer patients (2). While the physician usually bears primary responsibility for accurate diagnosis, each member of the rehabilitation team, including the nurses, therapists, social workers, and others, brings key insights into the potential cause of pain for a given patient. The experience, observations, and insights of team members are often instrumental in making the correct diagnosis. The challenge of adequately evaluating and treating pain in the cancer setting is often complicated by the multifactorial etiology and complex pathophysiological interrelationships among pain disorders.

The following chapters will discuss the pathophysiology of somatic, visceral, and neuropathic pain as well as the key components of effective pain management, including nonpharmacologic, pharmacologic, interventional, and complimentary modalities. This chapter is intended to provide a concise conceptual framework for the evaluation of pain. Failure to accurately and specifically determine the cause of pain will lead the clinician to pursue treatment strategies that may be ineffective, inappropriate, and potentially dangerous.

Pain in the cancer population is divided into that which is (1) caused by disease, (2) caused by treatment, and (3) unrelated to disease or treatment (3). All of these categories may coexist in a given patient. For instance, an older patient with prostate cancer is likely to have preexisting degenerative changes in his spine as well as a history of radiculopathy. If the prostate cancer metastasizes to the lumbar spine, and if treatments such as local radiation or neurotoxic chemotherapy are given, the patient's preexisting disorder may manifest as more significant back pain, radiculopathy, or neurological deficits (eg, foot drop) than a patient without significant preexisting degenerative spinal disease (4).

The World Health Organization (WHO) developed a three-step "ladder" to guide prescription of analgesics for relief of cancer pain (5). The ladder begins with nonopioids such as NSAIDS or acetaminophen, progresses as needed to mild opioids such as codeine, and ultimately, to strong opioids such as morphine. The pain ladder has been widely used and validated in the late-stage cancer pain setting with satisfactory pain control achieved in more than 70% of patents (6). While this WHO pain ladder has proven useful and effective in situations such as late-stage widely metastatic cancer, it does have limitations. Liberal use of escalating dose analgesics without regard to accurate diagnosis and the intention to discover and treat the primary cause of a given pain disorder is often not the way to produce the best outcome. A classic example of this is adhesive capsulitis (frozen shoulder), wherein

KEY POINTS

- The evaluation of pain in the cancer setting is one of the most important and challenging tasks faced by the rehabilitation physician and team.
- Pain in the cancer population is divided into that which is (1) caused by disease; (2) caused by treatment; and (3) unrelated to disease or treatment. All of these categories may coexist in a given patient.
- Liberal use of escalating dose analgesics without regard to accurate diagnosis and the intention to discover and treat the primary cause of a given pain disorder is often not the way to produce the best outcome.
- An accurate diagnosis of pain begins with a thorough history; the clinician should strive to fully understand all components of the patient's cancer diagnosis.

- Physical examination is often the most important diagnostic modality the clinician has in arriving at a correct diagnosis.
- The core of a good physical examination includes inspection, palpation, range of motion (ROM) assessment, neurological assessment, and special tests.
- Diagnostic testing is generally ordered by the rehabilitation physician to confirm that a neuromuscular or musculoskeletal disorder already suspected based on history and physical examination is present, determine its extent and etiology, and assist in predicting prognosis.
- A good diagnostician will endeavor to find anatomical congruence between the patient's history, physical examination, and any tests ordered.

treatment of pain in isolation—that is, use of opioids alone without therapeutic interventions to restore shoulder range of motion (ROM) and function—may be ineffective and can potentially worsen the primary disorder, leaving the patient less functional.

HISTORY

An accurate diagnosis of pain begins with a thorough history. The key historical elements of a comprehensive pain assessment are listed in Table 35.1. Like many aspects of medicine, eliciting an accurate history is both a skill and an art. The history should ultimately tell a comprehensive but concise, logically structured, and temporally accurate story of the patient's pertinent medical disorders and their treatments. Before details of the presenting pain complaint are discussed in detail, the clinician is advised to understand the background and context in which the pain exists for the patient. Events such as trauma, surgery, treatment of prior malignancies, and so forth, that predate the diagnosis and treatment of the patient's current cancer are often critically important. Similarly, a history of prior back pain, radiculopathy, fibromyalgia, depression, anxiety, and other disorders may be instrumental in understanding and treating current pain condition.

The clinician should strive to fully understand all components of the patient's cancer diagnosis, including when and how it was diagnosed, the type, stage, and grade of disease, and the patient's health status at diagnosis. Initial treatments including surgery, chemotherapy, immunotherapy, and radiotherapy as well

TABLE 35.1
Key Historical Elements of Pain Assessment

CHARACTERISTICS

Onset
Duration
Location(s)
Quality
Intensity
Associated symptoms
Exacerbating factors
Alleviating factors
Current management strategies
Previous management strategies
Medical history
Family history
Psychosocial history
Impact on function
Impact on quality of life
Expectations and goals

as how the patient tolerated or is tolerating treatment should be documented; if possible, the basic reasoning of the primary oncologist or surgeon in pursuing each course of treatment should likewise be documented. For patients who have already undergone primary treatment, the anticipated screening interval, screening modalities, and a general idea of prognosis for recurrence should be clarified. If there is metastatic or recurrent disease, the organs affected, treatment plan, and prognosis should be discussed with the primary provider.

Because cancer represents such a heterogeneous group of disorders with a vast number of rapidly evolving treatments, the rehabilitation physician is not expected to be familiar with all treatments for all cancers. That being said, it is incumbent upon the treating physician and other clinicians to understand the treatments that have been or will be provided to the patient they are treating. In many cases, unfamiliar disorders and treatments can be researched quickly, efficiently, and comprehensively on the internet, in textbooks, and in other references. It is potentially dangerous to provide treatment or render an opinion on a disorder that is unfamiliar to the practitioner.

A common pitfall in the elucidation of an accurate history is the failure to adequately guide the patient in presenting the history to you. Some patients are extremely sophisticated in understanding and relating their medical history. They may keep detailed notes with dates of symptom onset and severity as well as imaging, lab tests, medications, and other treatments. They may also be able to provide valuable insight into why certain treatments were chosen over others. Other patients may be unable to tell you the medicines they are currently taking, much less salient features of a complex medical history. Great care should be exercised in interpreting the history presented by the patient. A clinician who fails to critically evaluate the patient's preconceived notion of the origin of their pain can be easily misled and neglect to elicit additional information that might direct them to an alternative and potentially accurate diagnosis.

Past records should be reviewed to confirm the information presented by the patient. Patients may not always understand the thought processes of the clinicians who have treated them prior to their encounter with you. Additional and often extremely valuable information may come to light by discussing the case with the referring physician and other physicians involved. It is often the case that the documents and information most difficult to get prove to be the most important. For instance, the records detailing the dosage and fields of radiation given to a Hodgkin disease survivor may be buried in a 30-year-old file in the archives of a retired physician in another state. Despite the difficulties in retrieving such a file, it may bear heavily on the patient's current neuromuscular and musculoskeletal pain and functional disorders.

PHYSICAL EXAMINATION

There is an old adage in medicine: "when all else fails, examine the patient." In an era where increasingly sophisticated and powerful diagnostic tests have become an integral component of patient care, this medical pearl is easily forgotten. Physical examination is often the most important diagnostic modality the clinician has in arriving at a correct diagnosis. The clinician should become familiar with the common disorders likely to be encountered and the examination maneuvers that are important to their differentiation. The following chapters will help to clarify the disorders commonly seen in the cancer setting and help the examiner narrow the focus of their physical examination.

The core of a good physical examination includes inspection, palpation, ROM assessment, neurological assessment, and special tests intended to aid in diagnosis. These are often performed concomitantly but the clinician should strive to be consistent in their examination approach.

Inspection

Tremendous amounts of information can be gleaned by simple visual examination. In some cases, an obvious cause of new radicular symptoms such as a zoster eruption may be found. In other cases, subtle swelling, erythema, or muscular atrophy may point to the correct diagnosis. Failure to consistently incorporate a thorough inspection in the physical examination is a common factor in misdiagnosis.

Inspection will be more effective with practice and familiarity with commonly seen disorders. For instance, atrophy of muscles innervated by a specific myotome, plexus structure, or peripheral nerve is common in the cancer setting. A functional understanding of neuroanatomy is often key to localizing of lesion or lesions. For instance, atrophy of all the intrinsic muscles of the hand may point to a lower trunk plexopathy, whereas atrophy of the thenar eminence alone may be due to a median mononeuropathy and hand atrophy that spares the thenar eminence may be from an ulnar mononeuropathy. While all three disorders may be associated with hand pain and dysfunction, brachial plexopathy is commonly seen as a result of tumor or radiation fibrosis, while the other two are more likely to be benign. Effective treatment is likely to be different for each of the three diagnoses. Though any neuropathic pain disorders might benefit from a nerve stabilizing medication, tumor in the brachial plexus may also require surgery, chemotherapy, or radiation therapy. Carpel tunnel syndrome or an ulnar neuropathy might require splinting, physical therapy, anti-inflammatories, and potentially surgical release.

Palpation

Palpation is a natural extension of inspection and its importance cannot be overemphasized. The pathophysiological differences between nociceptive somatic and neuropathic pain will be discussed at length in following chapters. This distinction has major implications for both the diagnosis and treatment of pain. The basic rule for distinguishing the two clinically is:

1. If it hurts when you push on it, it is somatic pain.
2. If pushing where it hurts doesn't illicit pain, it is neuropathic pain.

For instance, a patient complaining of lateral hip pain may have trochanteric bursitis, which is easily diagnosed by eliciting tenderness on palpation of the bursa. Alternatively, they may have referred radicular pain, which would not reproduce pain by palpation of the area reported to be painful by the patient. While this simple rule is extremely useful in distinguishing neuropathic and somatic pain, it is not without caveat. The pain reproduced by palpation should be very similar in location, quality, and intensity to the pain the patient is complaining of. Also, neuropathic and somatic pain disorders commonly coexist and may have a causal relationship to one another. In the case of lateral hip pain, a patient may have both radiculopathy with pain radiating over the lateral hip and trochanteric bursitis precipitated by weakness and gait dysfunction from the radiculopathy. It is important to recognize when more than one pain disorder is present because their effective treatment is usually different, and both should be addressed simultaneously. The trochanteric bursitis may benefit from a potentially diagnostic and therapeutic bursal injection; anti-inflammatories, physical therapy for flexibility and strengthening, and modalities such as ultrasound may also be useful. Radiculopathy might require an epidural injection, nerve stabilizers, anti-inflammatories, physical therapy for flexibility, core stabilization, and modalities such as transcutaneous electrical nerve stimulation (TENS), or potentially surgery, and in the cancer setting, radiation therapy if the radiculopathy is from epidural disease.

Vigilance for cancer recurrence or new metastases is a major component of the cancer rehabilitation specialist's job. Patients with bony foci of metastatic disease usually complain of pain at and around the area of the metastases if there is significant cortical involvement, elevation of intraosseous pressure, or inflammation (7). Deep palpation of such areas often elicits tenderness and should raise the suspicion of metastatic disease, especially when the area is away from the usual locations of degenerative disorders such as the shoulder or knee.

Range of Motion Assessment

Assessment of ROM is also an important component of a good physical examination. In some conditions,

the location and extent of ROM abnormalities is diagnostic. For instance, adhesive capsulitis is a disorder or shoulder capsule tightness with subsequent restriction in ROM that is usually demonstrated on external rotation (8). While adhesive capsulitis is potentially painful and functionally disruptive in and of itself, it is often precipitated by other disorders such as cervical radiculopathy, rotator cuff tendonitis, axillary surgery, and local metastases, all of which should also be assessed and treated.

Neurologic Assessment

The importance of a comprehensive and insightful neurologic assessment to accurate evaluation and diagnosis of pain disorders cannot be overstated. A well done neurologic examination is often more sensitive and accurate than MRI and electrodiagnostic testing. The clinician should be able to reasonably differentiate classic presentations of radiculopathy, plexopathy, the various mononeuropathies as well as central neuropathic pain disorders based on the distribution of strength, sensation, and reflex abnormalities. Table 35.2 lists the common disorders of neurologic pain likely to be encountered in the cancer setting. The reader should keep in mind that there is tremendous variation from the "textbook" presentation among patients and that it is common for multiple disorders to coexist.

Special Tests

Special tests in physical examination are maneuvers designed to evaluate for and differentiate specific disorders. While dozens of named (often for the person who invented them) tests exist, only a few have been rigorously validated. Though none of them are 100% sensitive and specific, many of these tests are instrumental in determining the cause of pain and dysfunction. Table 35.3 lists several of the most common tests useful in the cancer setting. All readers are strongly encouraged to review Stanley Hoppenfeld's classic work on the physical examination of the spine and extremities for a more detailed review of key components of a comprehensive neuromuscular and musculoskeletal examination (9).

Diagnostic Testing

Diagnostic testing is generally ordered by the rehabilitation physician to confirm that a neuromuscular or musculoskeletal disorder already suspected based on history and physical examination is present, determine its extent and etiology, rule out other possibilities in the differential diagnosis, and assist in predicting prognosis. Electrodiagnostic testing is often extremely useful in

TABLE 35.2

Examination Findings in Painful Neurologic Disorders

LOCATION	PAIN/SENSORY ABNORMALITIES	WEAKNESS DISTRIBUTION	REFLEX ABNORMALITY
Central Nervous System			
Thalamus	Contralateral to lesion, varies from discrete, that is, arm only, to entire side of body	None (unless other structures involved)	None (unless other structures involved)
Spinal Cord			
Ascending spinothalamic tracts	Contralateral if small lesion or bilateral if larger lesion, varies from discrete, that is, arm only, to entire side of body	None (unless other structures involved)	None (unless other structures involved)
Root			
C-5	Posterior-lateral shoulder, lateral arm, lateral forearm	Rotator cuff, shoulder abduction > elbow flexion	Biceps tendon > brachioradialis tendon
C-6	Posterior-lateral shoulder, lateral arm, lateral forearm, thumb, index finger	Rotator cuff, shoulder abduction < elbow flexion	Biceps tendon < brachioradialis tendon
C-7	Posterior arm, posterior forearm, index/middle fingers	Elbow extension, wrist extension, finger extension	Triceps tendon
C-8	Posterior-medial arm, posterior-medial forearm, little/ring fingers	Long finger extensors, long finger flexors > hand intrinsics	Finger flexors
T-1	Anterior-medial arm, anterior-medial forearm (little/ring fingers generally spared)	Long finger extensors, long finger flexors < hand intrinsics	Finger flexors
T-2–T-12	Corresponding thoracic dermatome (ie, T4 nipples, T10 navel)	Corresponding thoracic myotome (rarely clinically evident)	None
L-1	Upper low back, lateral hip, groin	None	None
L-2	Upper/middle low back, lateral hip, groin, high anterior and medial thigh	Hip flexion > knee extension	Patellar tendon
L-3	Middle low back, lateral hip, middle anterior and medial thigh	Hip flexion < knee extension	Patellar tendon
L-4	Middle/low back, lateral hip, lateral thigh, knee, medial leg	Knee extension > ankle dorsiflexion	Patellar tendon
L-5	Low back, buttock, lateral hip, posterior/lateral thigh, lateral leg, dorsal foot, big toe	Hip abduction, knee flexion, ankle and toe dorsiflexion, foot inversion and eversion	Medial hamstring tendon

(Continued)

TABLE 35.2

Examination Findings in Painful Neurologic Disorders, Continued

LOCATION	PAIN/SENSORY ABNORMALITIES	WEAKNESS DISTRIBUTION	REFLEX ABNORMALITY
S-1	Low back, buttock, lateral hip, posterior thigh, posterior leg, lateral and plantar foot	Hip extension, knee flexion, plantar flexion, toe flexion	Achilles tendon, lateral hamstring tendon
S-2–S-5	Posterior leg (S2), saddle anesthesia	None	None
Cauda equina syndrome	Varies, all lumbar roots possible, saddle anesthesia common	Varies, all lumbar roots possible	Varies, all lumbar roots possible
Conus medullaris	Varies, all lumbar roots possible, loss of bladder function common	Varies, all lumbar roots possible	Varies, all lumbar roots possible
Plexus			
Anterior cervical	Anterior neck	None	None
Upper trunk brachial	Shoulder, lateral arm, lateral forearm, lateral hand	Rotator cuff, shoulder abduction, elbow flexion, radial wrist extension (rhomboid and serratus anterior spared)	Biceps tendon, brachioradialis tendon
Middle trunk brachial	Posterior arm and hand	Elbow extension (partial), wrist extension, finger extension (brachioradialis spared)	Triceps tendon
Posterior cord brachial	Posterior arm and hand	Shoulder abduction (past first 30 degrees), elbow extension, wrist extension, finger extension	Triceps tendon
Lower trunk brachial	Medial arm, medial forearm, little/ring fingers	Long finger extensors, long finger flexors, hand intrinsics	Finger flexors
Lumbar	Anterior thigh	Hip flexors, knee extensors, leg adductors	Patellar tendon
Lumbosacral trunk	Buttock, lateral leg, dorsum of foot	Hip extensors (variable), knee flexors (variable), dorsiflexion, ankle inversion, ankle inversion, toe flexion	Medial hamstring tendon
Sacral	Buttock, lateral hip, posterior thigh, posterior leg, lateral and plantar foot	Anal sphincter (variable), hip extensors, knee flexors, plantar flexors	Achilles tendon
Nerve			
Occipital	Posterior head	None	None
Trigeminal	Face	Masticatory muscles (rarely clinically evident)	None
Intercostobrachial	Axilla, medial arm	None	None

(Continued)

TABLE 35.2

Examination Findings in Painful Neurologic Disorders, Continued

LOCATION	PAIN/SENSORY ABNORMALITIES	WEAKNESS DISTRIBUTION	REFLEX ABNORMALITY
Axillary	Lateral arm	Shoulder abduction, external rotation	None
Musculocutaneous	Lateral forearm	Elbow flexion, supination	Biceps tendon
Radial	Distal posterior arm, posterior forearm, posterior-lateral hand	Elbow extension (spared if lesion below spiral groove), wrist extension, finger extension, supination	Triceps tendon (if above spiral groove), none (if below spiral groove)
Ulnar	Anterior-medial hand, posterior-medial hand	Finger flexion (4th–5th fifth digits), Finger abduction (spares thumb abduction)	Finger flexors
Median	Anterior-lateral hand	Forearm pronation, wrist flexion, finger flexion (2nd–3rd digits), thumb abduction (spares finger abduction)	None
Lateral femoral cutaneous	Anterior-lateral thigh (spares medial thigh)	None	None
Femoral	Anterior-medial thigh (spares lateral thigh), medial leg, medial foot	Hip flexion (if intrapelvic lesion, spared if at inguinal ligament), knee extension	Patellar tendon
Sciatic	Posterior buttock, posterior thigh, posterior-lateral leg, plantar foot	Hip extension < knee flexion, dorsiflexion, plantar flexion, foot eversion and inversion, toe flexion	Achilles tendon, hamstring tendons
Peroneal	Anterior-lateral leg, dorsum of foot	Dorsiflexion, foot eversion	None
Tibial	Plantar foot	Plantar flexion, foot inversion	None
Polyneuropathy	Generally distal symmetric in a "stocking and glove" distribution	Generally in distal muscle groups	Varies, generally distal tendon reflexes
Mononeuropathy Multiplex	Varies by nerves affected	Varies by nerves affected	Varies by nerves affected
Small fiber neuropathy	Generally distal symmetric in a "stocking and glove" distribution (affects pain/pinprick and temperature sensation but spares light touch, vibration and proprioception)	None	None

distinguishing between disorders of peripheral nervous system dysfunction, to determine if more than one disorder is present, to assess the severity of the disorder(s), and in some cases to predict prognosis. Electrodiagnostic testing can also assist in determining whether emergent neuropathic signs and symptoms in a given patient are a result of neurotoxic chemotherapy or other disorders such as radiculopathy. For instance, a

TABLE 35.3
Special Physical Examination Tests Useful in the Cancer Setting

LOCATION	TEST	PURPOSE	MANEUVER
Shoulder	Neer's Impingement Test	Rotator cuff tendonitis	The patient's arm is forcibly elevated and internally rotated through forward flexion while the scapula is depressed. Pain indicates rotator cuff tenonitis
	Hawkin's Impingement Test	Rotator cuff tendonitis	The patient's shoulder and elbow are flexed to 90° while the shoulder is internally rotated. Pain indicates rotator cuff tendonitis
	Supraspinatus Test (aka Empty Can Test)	Rotator cuff tendonitis	The shoulder is abducted to 90° with neutral rotation and then medially rotated and angled forward 30° so that the patient's thumbs point downward. Resistance to abduction if provided by the examiner. Pain and weakness indicate rotator cuff tendonitis
	Drop Arm Test	Supraspinatus muscle/tendon complex tear	Ask patient to fully abduct arm and then slowly lower it to the side. An abrupt drop of the arm to the side at about 90° indicates a tear of the supraspinatus muscle/tendon complex
Wrist	Finkelstein Test	De Quervain tenosynovitis	The thumb is tucked inside a closed fist and the hand deviated to the ulnar side. Pain over the wrist at the extensor pollicis brevis and abductor pollicis longus tendon indicates a positive test
Hip	FABER Test	Intrinsic pathology of the hip joint	The hip joint is flexed abducted and externally rotated with the patient supine. Pain radiating into the groin indicates intrinsics hip pathology

patient with multiple myeloma who suddenly develops worsening lower extremity pain while on thalidomide may have a radiculopathy from a spinal compression fracture as opposed to neuropathy from the chemotherapeutic agent. Such information may help in the decision to maintain a patient on a chemotherapy to which they are responding and potentially prolong their life and functional status.

Imaging is extremely important, particularly in the cancer setting, to determine or exclude the precise etiology of a pain disorder. The type of imaging ordered will depend on the area of interest and pathology anticipated. It is important to remember that imaging is not foolproof and in fact can easily mislead even the most experienced diagnostician. This is where the history and physical examination are most important. For instance, a patient complaining of leg pain could potentially have funicular pain from a thalamic or spinal cord lesion, radicular pain, lumbosacral plexopathy, asciatic neuropathy, small fiber neuropathy, or any of a number of musculoskeletal disorders. It is a well done clinical assessment that includes a comprehensive and accurate history and physical examination that will narrow the scope of likely disorders and make imaging more likely to be relevant.

CONCLUSION

The approach to evaluation is the key to an accurate assessment, correct diagnosis, and effective treatment of pain disorders. The approach should be logical, consistent, thorough, and encompass all the tools available to the clinician. A good diagnostician will endeavor to find anatomical congruence between the patient's history, physical examination, and any tests ordered. When these components do not initially meld, other diagnostic considerations should be actively pursued and excluded until the correct diagnosis is clarified. The diagnosis should be as specific as possible and the interrelationships between competing diagnoses, when present, should be clarified so that they can be more optimally impacted by treatment.

References

1. Goudas LC, Block R, Gialeli-Goudas M, Lau J, Carr DB. The epidemiology of cancer pain. *Cancer Invest*. 2005;23;182–190.
2. Manthy PW. Cancer pain and its impact on diagnosis, survival and quality of life. *Nat Rev Neurosci*. 2006;7:797–809.
3. Marcus NJ. Pain in cancer patients unrelated to the cancer or treatment. *Cancer Invest*. 2005;1:84–93.
4. Stubblefield MD, Slovin S, MacGregor-Cortelli B, et al. An electrodiagnostic evaluation of the impact of preexisting peripheral nervous system disorders in patients treated with the novel proteasome inhibitor bortezomib. *Clin Oncol*. 2006;18:410–418.
5. World Health Organization Pain Ladder (Accessed June 24 at http://www.who.int/cancer/palliative/painladder/en/index.html)
6. Zeck DFJ, Grond S, Lynch J, Hertel D, Lehmann KA. Validation of World Health Organization guidelines for cancer pain relief: a 10-year prospective study. *Pain*. 1995;63:65–76.
7. Chang VT, Janjan N, Jain S, Chau C. Update in cancer pain. *J Palliat Med*. 2006;9;1414–1434.
8. Stubblefield MD, Custodio CM. Upper-extremity pain disorders in breast cancer. *Arch Phys Med Rehabil*. 2006;87(3 Suppl):96–99.
9. Hoppenfeld S. *Physical Examination of the Spine & Extremities*. Norwalk: Appleton & Lange; 1976.

Somatic Pain in Cancer

Juan Miguel Jimenez-Andrade
Patrick W. Mantyh

Excluding skin cancer, more than 10 million people are diagnosed with cancer every year, and by 2020 it is estimated that 15 million new cases will be diagnosed each year (1). In 2005, cancer caused 7.6 million deaths worldwide (2). In the United States, cancer is a major health problem, being the second leading cause of death. Currently, 25% of U.S. deaths are cancer related (3).

Despite the increasing prevalence of cancer, improvements in the detection and treatment of most types of cancers have resulted in significantly increased survival rates (4). For many patients, pain is the first sign of cancer, and the majority of patients will experience moderate to severe pain during the course of their disease and into survivorship (5,6). Given the increasing life span of cancer patients, novel mechanism-based therapies need to be developed to reduce cancer-related pain if these cancer patients and survivors are to remain functional, integrated, and contributing members of society (7). Cancer-associated pain can be present at any time during the course of the disease, but the frequency and intensity of cancer pain tends to increase with advancing stages of cancer. Sixty-two to eighty-six percent of patients with advanced stage cancer experience significant amounts of cancer-induced pain (8).

Cancer pain may arise from different processes: by direct tumor infiltration/involvement, through diagnostic or therapeutic surgical procedures (eg, biopsies, resection), or as a side effect or toxicity related to therapies used to treat cancer (eg, chemotherapy, radiation therapy). Until recently, the management of cancer pain has been largely empirical, based on scientific studies of painful conditions other than cancer. In this chapter, we will focus on recent insights that have been provided by preclinical and clinical studies of cancer-induced pain. These studies have resulted in the beginning of a mechanism-based understanding of the factors that generate and maintain cancer-induced pain.

PRIMARY AFFERENT NEURONS AND CANCER-INDUCED PAIN

Primary afferent sensory neurons are the gateway by which sensory information from peripheral tissues is transmitted to the spinal cord and brain (Fig. 36.1). These sensory neurons innervate every organ of the body, with the exception of the brain. The cell bodies of sensory fibers that innervate the head and body are housed in the trigeminal and dorsal root ganglia (DRG), respectively, and can be divided into two major categories: large diameter myelinated A beta fibers and small diameter thinly myelinated A-delta and unmyelinated C fibers (Fig. 36.1).

Most small diameter sensory fibers (unmyelinated C fibers and finely myelinated A delta fibers) are sensory neurons known as nociceptors. Nociceptors express an extremely diverse repertoire of receptors and transduction molecules that can sense forms of noxious stimuli including thermal, mechanical, and chemical, albeit with varying degrees of sensitivity (9). These unmyelinated C fibers and finely myelinated A sensory neurons are involved in generating the chronic pain that accompanies many cancers (10). Following tissue injury induced by the tumor or tumor-associated cells, many nociceptors alter their pattern of neurotransmitter, receptor, growth factor expression, and response properties (Fig. 36.1). All these changes underlie, in part, the development of peripheral sensitization so that mild noxious sensory stimulation is perceived as highly noxious stimuli (hyperalgesia) and normally non-noxious sensory stimulation is now perceived as noxious stimuli (allodynia). Tumor or tumor-associated cell-induced sensitization of the C-fiber nociceptors leads to long-term changes in spinal excitability that may lead to secondary hyperalgesia, represented by the increased response of A fibers to mechanical stimulation outside of the site of direct injury. In contrast, large diameter myelinated A beta fibers originating in skin, joints, and muscles normally conduct non-noxious stimuli including fine touch, vibration, and proprioception. In a normal non-injured condition, these large sensory neurons do not conduct noxious stimuli.

This chapter will focus on involvement of sensory neurons in the generation and maintenance of bone tumor-induced pain. However, it should be stressed that following cancer-induced injury to sensory neurons, areas of the spinal cord and central nervous system involved in the processing of somatosensory information also undergo a variety of neurochemical and cellular changes known as central sensitization. These changes facilitate the transmission and conscious appreciation of both noxious and non-noxious sensory information.

TUMOR-INDUCED CANCER PAIN

Tumor-induced bone pain is the most common pain in patients with advanced cancer, and the most common symptom indicating that tumor cells have metastasized to sites beyond the primary tumor (11). Although bone is not a vital organ, most common tumors have a remarkable affinity to metastasize to bone. Tumor metastases to the skeleton are major contributors to the morbidity and mortality in metastatic cancer, as tumor growth in bone results in pain, bone remodeling, skeletal fractures, anemia, increased susceptibility to infection,

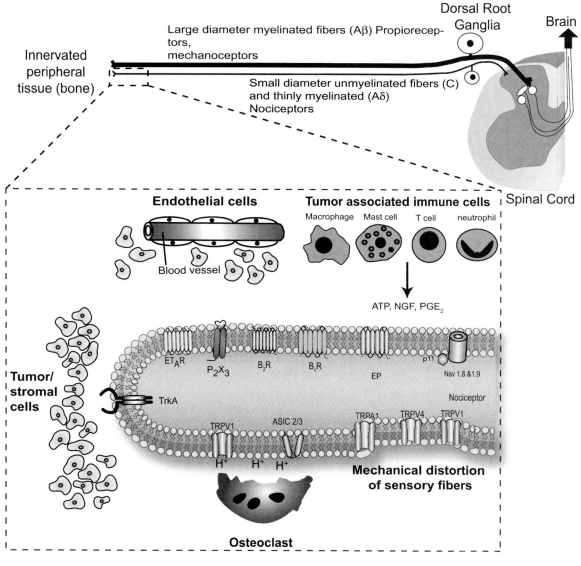

FIGURE 36.1

Primary afferent sensory nerve fibers involved in generating the cancer pain. Primary afferent neurons innervating the body have their cell bodies in the dorsal root ganglia (DRG) and transmit sensory information from the periphery to the spinal cord and brain. Myelinated A fibers (Aβ) containing large diameter cell bodies, which project centrally to the dorsal column nuclei and deep spinal cord, are involved in detecting non-noxious sensations including light touch, vibration, and proprioception. Unmyelinated C fibers and thinly myelinated A fibers contain small diameter cell bodies, which project centrally to the superficial spinal cord. These fibers are involved in detecting multiple noxious stimuli (chemical, thermal, and mechanical). Box: Nociceptors use several different types of receptors to detect and transmit signals about noxious stimuli that are produced by cancer cells (yellow), tumor associated immune cells (orange) or other aspects of the tumor microenvironment. Multiple factors may contribute to the pain associated with cancer. The transient receptor potential vanilloid receptor-1 (TRPV1) and acid sensing ion channels (ASICs) detect extracellular protons produced by tumor induced tissue damage or abnormal osteoclast mediated bone resorption. Several mechanosensitive ion channels may be involved in detecting high threshold mechanical stimuli that occurs when distal aspects of sensory nerve fiber are distended from mechanical pressure due to the growing tumor or as a result of destabilization or fracture of bone. Tumor cells and associated inflammatory (immune) cells produce a variety of chemical mediators, including prostaglandins (PGE$_2$), nerve growth factor (NGF), endothelins, bradykinin, and extracellular ATP. Several of these proinflammatory mediators have receptors on peripheral terminals and can directly activate or sensitize nociceptors. NGF and its cognate receptor, TrkA, may serve as a master regulator of bone cancer pain by modulating the sensitivity or increasing the expression of several receptors and ion channels contributing to increased excitability of nociceptors in the vicinity of the tumor.

and decreased mobility with resulting cardiovascular dysfunction, all of which compromise the patient's survival and quality of life (12). Once tumor cells have metastasized to the skeleton, the tumor-induced bone pain is usually described as dull in character, constant in presentation, and gradually increasing in intensity with time (11). As bone remodeling progresses, severe spontaneous pain frequently occurs (11), and given that the onset of this pain is both acute and unpredictable, this component of bone cancer pain can be particularly debilitating to the patient's functional status and quality of life (11). Breakthrough pain, which is an intermittent episode of extreme pain, can occur spontaneously but is more commonly induced by movement of the tumor-bearing bone(s) (6).

Currently, the treatment of pain from bone metastases involves the use of multiple complementary approaches including radiotherapy, chemotherapy, surgery, bisphosphonates, and analgesics (11). However, bone cancer pain is one of the most difficult of all persistent pains to fully control, as the metastases are generally not limited to a single site and the analgesics that are most commonly used to treat bone cancer pain, the nonsteroidal anti-inflammatory drugs (NSAIDS) (11) and opioids (11,13), are limited by significant adverse side effects. For example, nonselective NSAIDS can cause intestinal bleeding and have cardiovascular safety issues; selective cyclooxygenase (COX)-2 inhibitors may also increase the risk of cardiovascular events (14–17). Opioids are effective in attenuating bone cancer pain but are frequently accompanied by side effects such as constipation, sedation, nausea, vomiting, and respiratory depression (18). Individuals with primary bone tumors such as sarcomas, or those with breast or prostate tumors that metastasize primarily to bone and not other vital organs such as lung, liver, or brain, tend to live for a significant period of time (on average, 55 months for prostate cancer patients) beyond their initial diagnosis (19). Due to continuing increases in the length of survival for cancer patients, it is essential that new therapies be developed that can be administered over years to control bone pain without the side effects commonly encountered with the currently available analgesics.

In an effort to develop mechanism-based therapies to treat cancer pain, the first animal models of cancer pain have been developed. In these models, bone cancer pain is induced by injecting murine osteolytic sarcoma or osteoblastic prostate cells into the intramedullary space of the murine femur (Fig. 36.2). A critical component of cancer pain models is that the tumor cells are confined within the marrow space of the injected femur and do not invade adjacent soft tissues. Following tumor cells' proliferation, both ongoing and movement-evoked, pain-related behaviors develop and increase in severity with time. These pain behaviors correlate with the progressive tumor-induced bone destruction or bone formation that ensues and appears to mimic the condition in patients with primary or metastatic bone cancer. Cancer pain models will allow us to gain mechanistic insights into how cancer pain is generated, and how the sensory information it initiates is processed as it moves from sense organ to the cerebral cortex under a constantly changing molecular architecture. The insights gained from these models promise to fundamentally change the way cancer pain is controlled.

ACIDOSIS IN BONE CANCER PAIN

Recent reports in both murine and human bone cancer pain have suggested that osteoclasts play an essential role in cancer-induced bone loss and contribute to the etiology of bone cancer pain (20,21). Osteoclasts are terminally differentiated, multinucleated, monocyte lineage cells that resorb bone by maintaining an extracellular microenvironment of acidic pH (4.0–5.0) at the osteoclast-mineralized bone interface (22). Both osteolytic (bone destroying) and osteoblastic (bone forming) cancers are characterized by osteoclast proliferation and hypertrophy (23).

Bisphosphonates, a class of antiresorptive compounds that induce osteoclast apoptosis, have also been reported to reduce pain in patients with osteolytic (primarily bone destroying) and osteoblastic (primarily bone forming) skeletal metastases (24,25). Bisphosphonates are pyrophosphate analogues that display high affinity for calcium ions, causing them to rapidly target the mineralized matrix of bone (26). These drugs have been reported to act directly on osteoclasts, inducing their apoptosis by impairing either the synthesis of adenosine triphosphate or cholesterol, both which are necessary for cell survival (27). Studies in both clinical (24,25) and animal (28,29) models of bone cancer have reported antiresorptive effects of bisphosphonate therapy. The effect bisphosphonates have on tumor growth and long-term survival rate remains controversial.

In a recent study of the bisphosphonate alendronate in the murine 2472 sarcoma model (30), a reduction in the number of osteoclasts and osteoclast activity was noted, as evidenced by the reduction in tumor-induced bone resorption. Alendronate treatment also resulted in a reduction in the number of osteoclasts displaying the clear zone at the basal bone resorbing surface, which is characteristic of highly active osteoclasts. In this model, alendronate also attenuated ongoing and movement-evoked bone cancer pain as well as the neurochemical reorganization of the peripheral and central

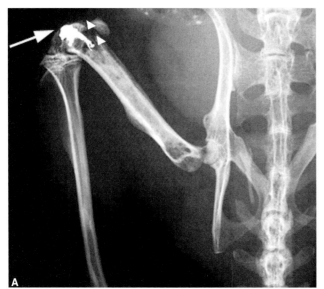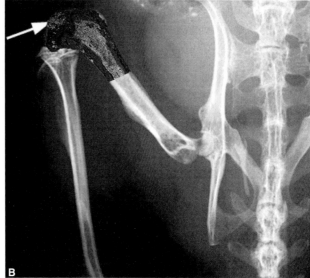

FIGURE 36.2

Development of murine bone cancer pain model. Low power anterior-posterior radiograph of mouse pelvis and hind limbs after a unilateral injection of sarcoma cells into the distal part of the femur and closure of the injection site with an amalgam plug (arrow) which prevents the tumor cells from growing outside the bone (A). As tumor progression continues, extensive bone destruction occurs, as characterized by multifocal radiolucencies and complete loss of trabecular bone regions as compared to contralateral hindlimb (arrowheads, A). Tumor burden may be visualized and quantified using sarcoma cancer cells genetically manipulated to express enhanced GFP, as shown in the overlapping confocal immunofluorescence picture. By day 14 post-injection, GFP-expressing tumor cells (dark gray) had completely filled the intramedullary space (B).

nervous system, while at the same time promoting both tumor growth and tumor necrosis. These results suggest that in bone cancer, alendronate can simultaneously modulate pain, bone destruction, tumor growth, and tumor necrosis, and that administration of alendronate along with a tumoricidal agent may synergistically improve the survival and quality of life of patients with bone cancer pain. Recent studies in humans with ibandronate, a novel nitrogen-containing bisphosphonate, have shown the agent to have remarkable effects in rapidly inducing long-lasting relief of bone cancer pain (31).

While bisphosphonates are currently being used to reduce tumor-induced bone destruction and bone cancer pain induced by both primarily osteolytic and osteoblastic tumors, the use of osteoprotegerin (OPG) or antibodies that have OPG-like activities holds significant promise for alleviating bone cancer pain. OPG is a secreted soluble receptor that is a member of the tumor necrosis factor receptor (TNFR) family (32). This decoy receptor prevents the activation and proliferation of osteoclasts by binding to and sequestering OPG ligand (OPGL; also known as receptor for activator of NFKB ligand [RANKL]) (32,33). While OPG has been shown to decrease pain behaviors in the murine sarcoma model of bone cancer (20), a monoclonal antibody (AMG-162) that also blocks the inter-

action of OPGL and RANKL is still being developed for use in treating skeletal pain. These results suggest that a substantial part of the actions of OPG results from inhibition of tumor-induced bone destruction via a reduction in osteoclast function.

The finding that sensory neurons (Fig. 36.1) can be directly excited by protons or acid originating from cells such as osteoclasts in bone has generated intense clinical interest in pain research. Studies have shown that subsets of sensory neurons express different acid-sensing ion channels (9). Two acid-sensing ion channels expressed by nociceptors are the transient receptor potential vanilloid-1 (TRPV1) (34) and the acid-sensing ion channel-3 (ASIC-3) (35). Both of these channels are sensitized and excited by a decrease in pH. Tumor stroma (36) and areas of tumor necrosis such as that observed in bone cancer typically exhibit lower extracellular pH than surrounding normal tissues. As inflammatory and immune cells invade the tumor stroma, they also release protons that generate a local acidosis.

It has been shown that TRPV1 is expressed by a subset of sensory neuron fibers that innervate the mouse femur, and that in an in vivo model of bone cancer pain, acute or chronic administration of a TRPV1 antagonist or disruption of the TRPV1 gene results in a significant attenuation of both ongoing and movement-evoked nocifensive behaviors (37). In addition, previous studies have also shown that in a sarcoma model of bone cancer pain, administration of a TRPV1 antagonist retains its efficacy at early, middle, and late stages of tumor growth (37). These results suggest that the TRPV1 channel plays a role in the integration of nociceptive signaling in a severe pain state, and that antagonists of TRPV1 may be effective in attenuating difficult-to-treat mixed chronic pain states, such as that encountered in patients with bone cancer pain.

In addition to acidosis, previous studies have suggested that a major source of bone pain is mechanical distortion of the periosteum (11,38). Thus, following fracture due to tumor-induced bone remodeling, the pain associated with the fracture is partially relieved if the bone and periosteum are repositioned and stabilized to their normal orientation (39).

TUMOR-DERIVED PRODUCTS AND BONE CANCER PAIN

The tumor stroma is made up of many different cell types apart from cancer cells, including immune cells such as macrophages, neutrophils, and T-lymphocytes. They secrete a variety of factors that have been shown to sensitize or directly excite primary afferent neurons, such as prostaglandins, tumor necrosis factor alpha (TNFα), endothelins, interleukins -1 and -6, epidermal growth factor, transforming growth factor beta, and platelet-derived growth factor (10). Receptors for many of these factors are expressed by primary afferent neurons.

Prostaglandins

Prostaglandins are lipid-derived eicosanoids that are synthesized from arachidonic acid by the COX isoenzymes COX-1 and COX-2. Cancer cells and tumor-associated macrophages have both been shown to express high levels of COX isoenzymes, leading to high levels of prostaglandins (40,41). Studies using the murine sarcoma model of bone cancer pain have shown that chronic inhibition of COX-2 activity with selective COX-2 inhibitors resulted in significant attenuation of bone cancer pain behaviors as well as many of the neurochemical changes suggestive of both peripheral and central sensitization (21). In addition, prostaglandins have been shown to be involved in tumor growth, survival, and angiogenesis (42–44). Therefore, COX-2 inhibitors are able to block cancer pain and retard tumor growth within bone (21). Chronic administration of a selective COX-2 inhibitor significantly reduced tumor burden in sarcoma-bearing bones and may, in turn, reduce factors released by tumor cells capable of exciting primary afferent fibers (45). Both acute and chronic administration of a selective COX-2 inhibitor significantly attenuated both ongoing and movement-evoked pain (21). Whereas acute administration of a COX-2 inhibitor presumably reduces prostaglandins capable of activating sensory or spinal cord neurons, chronic inhibition of COX-2 appears to simultaneously reduce osteoclastogenesis, bone resorption, and tumor burden. Together, suppression of prostaglandin synthesis and release at multiple sites by selective inhibition of COX-2 may synergistically improve the survival and quality of life of patients with bone cancer pain.

Endothelins

Endothelins (endothelin-1, -2, and -3) are a family of vasoactive peptides that are expressed at high levels by several types of tumors, including those that arise from the prostate (46). Clinical studies have shown a correlation between the severity of the pain and plasma levels of endothelins in prostate cancer patients (47). Endothelins may contribute to cancer pain by directly sensitizing or exciting nociceptors, as a subset of small unmyelinated primary afferent neurons express endothelin A receptors (48). Furthermore, direct application of endothelin to peripheral nerves induces activation of primary afferent fibers and an induction of pain-related behaviors (49). These findings suggest that endothelin antagonists may be useful in inhibiting bone cancer pain. In the sarcoma model of bone cancer pain, acute or chronic administration of an endothelin A receptor selective antagonist significantly attenuated ongoing and movement-evoked bone cancer pain. Chronic administration of this drug also reduced several neurochemical indices of peripheral and central sensitization without influencing tumor growth or bone destruction (50).

Kinins

Previous studies have shown that bradykinin and related kinins are released in response to tissue injury, and that they play a significant role in driving the acute and chronic inflammatory pain (51). The action of bradykinin is mediated by two receptors, termed B_1 and B_2. While the B_2 receptor is constitutively expressed at high levels by sensory neurons, the B_1 receptor is normally expressed at low but detectable levels by sensory neurons, and these B_1 receptors are significantly upregulated following peripheral inflammation and/or tissue injury (52). Tumor metastases to the skeleton induce significant bone remodeling with accompanying tissue injury, which presumably induces the release of bradykinin. Following the pharmacologic blockade of the B_1 receptor, both bone cancer-induced ongoing and movement-evoked nocifensive behaviors were reduced, and the therapeutic efficacy was retained even in advanced bone cancer (53).

Nerve Growth Factor

One important concept that has emerged over the past decade is that in addition to nerve growth factor (NGF) being able to directly activate sensory neurons, NGF also modulates expression and function of a wide variety of molecules and proteins expressed by sensory neurons that express the TrkA or p75 receptor. Some of these molecules and proteins include: neurotransmitters (substance P and calcitonin gene-related peptide), receptors (bradykinin R), channels (P2X3, TRPV1, ASIC-3, and sodium channels), transcription factors such as activating transcription factor-3, (ATF-3), and structural molecules (neurofilaments and the sodium channel anchoring molecule p11) (54). Additionally, NGF has been shown to modulate the trafficking and insertion of sodium channels such as Nav 1.8 and TRPV1 in the sensory neurons, as well as modulating the expression profile of supporting cells in the DRG and peripheral nerve, such as nonmyelinating Schwann cells and macrophages (55).

In light of the potential role that NGF may play in driving bone cancer pain, anti-NGF therapy was examined in a primarily osteolytic sarcoma and osteoblastic prostate model of bone cancer pain. In both models of bone cancer pain, it was demonstrated that administration of anti-NGF therapy was not only highly efficacious in reducing both early- and late-stage bone cancer pain-related behaviors, but that this reduction was greater than that achieved with acute administration of either 10 or 30 mg/kg of morphine sulfate (56,57). Given that the bone is primarily innervated by calcitonin gene related peptide (CGRP)/TrkA expressing sensory fibers (10), NGF sequestering therapies may be uniquely efficacious in attenuating the pain and improving the quality of life and function of patients with significant skeletal pain.

NEUROPATHIC COMPONENT OF BONE CANCER PAIN

To examine the interface of tumor cells and sensory nerve fibers as tumor cells invade the bone, osteosarcoma cells were injected and confined to the intramedullary space of the mouse femur. Using this model, it was noted that tumor cells were found to grow within the bone, come into contact, injure, and then destroy the distal processes of sensory fibers that innervate the bone marrow and mineralized bone (58). Thus, while sensory fibers were observed at and within the leading edge of the tumor in the deep stromal regions of the tumor, sensory nerve fibers displayed a discontinuous and fragmented appearance, suggesting that following initial activation by the osteolytic tumor cells, the distal processes of the sensory fibers were ultimately injured by the invading tumor cells. Tumor-induced injury to sensory fibers that normally innervated the tumor-bearing femur resulted in the expression of ATF-3 (which is upregulated following peripheral nerve injury) in the nucleus of sensory neurons that innervate the femur.

Tumor-induced injury of sensory nerve fibers by the invading sarcoma cells was also accompanied by an increase in ongoing and movement-evoked pain behaviors, upregulation of galanin by sensory neurons that innervate the tumor-bearing femur, upregulation of glial fibrillary acidic protein and hypertrophy of satellite cells surrounding sensory neuron cell bodies within the ipsilateral DRG, and macrophage infiltration of the DRG ipsilateral to the tumor-bearing femur (58). Similar neurochemical changes have been described following peripheral nerve injury and in other noncancerous neuropathic pain states (59,60). While chronic treatment with gabapentin in this model of bone cancer pain did not influence tumor growth, tumor-induced bone destruction, or the tumor-induced neurochemical reorganization that occurs in sensory neurons or the spinal cord, it did attenuate both ongoing and movement-evoked bone cancer-related pain behaviors (58). These results suggest that even when the tumor is confined within the bone, a component of bone cancer pain appears to be neuropathic in origin as tumor cells clearly induce injury or remodeling of the primary afferent nerve fibers that normally innervate the tumor-bearing bone.

CONCLUSIONS AND FUTURE PERSPECTIVES

Advances in cancer detection and therapies have dramatically increased the survival rates of patients with most cancers. With this increased survival there is an ever developing need to focus on cancer-associated pain and the impact it has on the cancer patient from initial diagnosis through therapy to survivorship. Pain can have a significant impact on the quality of life of both the cancer patient and cancer survivor. Animal models are now available that merge pain research and cancer research, and by working closely with clinicians who treat cancer patients, there is significant potential for synergistic translation research to occur at the interface of these two previously separate disciplines. By focusing and incorporating both preclinical and clinical pain research into mainstream cancer research and therapies, we have the opportunity to target and affect not only the tumor, but also the overall health, quality of life, and survival of the cancer patient.

References

1. Stewart B, Kleihues P, eds. *World Cancer Report*. Lyon, France: IARC Press; 2003.

2. WHO. Cancer control. http://www.who.int/cancer/en/. Accessed October 5, 2006.

3. Jemal A, Siegel R, Ward E, Murray T, Xu J, Thun MJ. Cancer statistics, 2007. *CA Cancer J Clin*. 2007;57:43–66.

4. Edwards B, Brown M, Wingo AH, et al. Annual report to the nation on the status of cancer, 1975–2002, featuring population-based trends in cancer treatment. *J Natl Cancer Inst*. 2005;97:1407–1427.

5. Portenoy RK, Payne D, Jacobsen P. Breakthrough pain: characteristics and impact in patients with cancer pain. *Pain*. 1999;81:129–134.

6. Mercadante S, Arcuri E. Breakthrough pain in cancer patients: pathophysiology and treatment. *Cancer Treat Rev*. 1998;24:425–432.

7. Aalto Y, Forsgren S, Kjorell U, Bergh J, Franzen L, Henriksson R. Enhanced expression of neuropeptides in human breast cancer cell lines following irradiation. *Peptides*. 1998;19:231–239.

8. van den Beuken-van Everdingen M, de Rijke J, Kessels A, Schouten H, van Kleef M, Patijn J. Prevalence of pain in patients with cancer: a systematic review of the past 40 years. *Ann Oncol*. 2007;18:1437–1449.

9. Julius D, Basbaum AI. Molecular mechanisms of nociception. *Nature*. 2001;413:203–210.

10. Mantyh PW. Cancer pain and its impact on diagnosis, survival and quality of life. *Nat Rev Neurosci*. 2006;7:797–809.

11. Mercadante S. Malignant bone pain: pathophysiology and treatment. *Pain* 1997;69:1–18.

12. Coleman RE. Metastatic bone disease: clinical features, pathophysiology and treatment strategies. *Cancer Treat Rev*. 2001;27:165–176.

13. Portenoy RK, Lesage P. Management of cancer pain. *Lancet*. 1999;353:1695–1700.

14. Chan AT, Manson JE, Albert CM, et al. Nonsteroidal antiinflammatory drugs, acetaminophen, and the risk of cardiovascular events. *Circulation*. 2006;113:1578–1587.

15. Graham DJ, Campen D, Hui R, et al. Risk of acute myocardial infarction and sudden cardiac death in patients treated with cyclo-oxygenase 2 selective and non-selective non-steroidal anti-inflammatory drugs: nested case-control study. *Lancet*. 2005;365:475–481.

16. Hippisley-Cox J, Coupland C. Risk of myocardial infarction in patients taking cyclo-oxygenase-2 inhibitors or conventional non-steroidal anti-inflammatory drugs: population based nested case-control analysis. *BMJ*. 2005;330:1366.

17. Mukherjee D, Nissen SE, Topol EJ. Risk of cardiovascular events associated with selective COX-2 inhibitors. *JAMA*. 2001;286:954–959.

18. Mercadante S. Problems of long-term spinal opioid treatment in advanced cancer patients. *Pain*. 1999;79:1–13.

19. Jemal A, Siegel R, Ward E, et al. Cancer statistics, 2006. *CA Cancer J Clin*. 2006;56:106–130.

20. Honore P, Luger NM, Sabino MA, et al. Osteoprotegerin blocks bone cancer-induced skeletal destruction, skeletal pain and pain-related neurochemical reorganization of the spinal cord. *Nat Med*. 2000;6:521–528.

21. Sabino MA, Ghilardi JR, Jongen JL, et al. Simultaneous reduction in cancer pain, bone destruction, and tumor growth by selective inhibition of cyclooxygenase-2. *Cancer Res*. 2002;62:7343–7349.

22. Delaisse JM, Vaes G, eds. *Mechanism of Mineral Solubilization and Matrix Degradation in Osteoclastic Bone Resorption*. Ann Arbor: CRC; 1992.

23. Clohisy DR, Perkins SL, Ramnaraine ML. Review of cellular mechanisms of tumor osteolysis. *Clin Orthop Rel Res*. 2000;373:104–114.

24. Fulfaro F, Casuccio A, Ticozzi C, Ripamonti C. The role of bisphosphonates in the treatment of painful metastatic bone disease: a review of phase III trials. *Pain*. 1998;78:157–169.

25. Major PP, Lipton A, Berenson J, Hortobagyi G. Oral bisphosphonates: a review of clinical use in patients with bone metastases. *Cancer* 2000;88:6–14.

26. Rogers MJ, Gordon S, Benford HL, et al. Cellular and molecular mechanisms of action of bisphosphonates. *Cancer* 2000;88:2961–2978.

27. Rodan G, Martin T. Therapeutic approaches to bone disease. *Science*. 2000;289:1508–1514.

28. Hiraga T, Tanaka S, Yamamoto M, Nakajima T, Ozawa H. Inhibitory effects of bisphosphonate YM175 on bone resorption induced by metastic bone tumor. *Bone*. 1996;18:1–7.

29. Sasaki A, Boyce B, Story B, et al. Bisphosphonate risedronate reduces metastic human breast cancer burden in bone in nude mice. *Cancer Res*. 1995;77:279–285.

30. Sevcik MA, Luger NM, Mach DB, et al. Bone cancer pain: the effects of the bisphosphonate alendronate on pain, skeletal remodeling, tumor growth and tumor necrosis. *Pain*. 2004;111:169–180.

31. Tripathy D, Body JJ, Bergstrom B. Review of ibandronate in the treatment of metastatic bone disease: experience from phase III trials. *Clin Ther*. 2004;26:1947–1959.

32. Simonet WS, Lacey DL, Dunstan CR, et al. Osteoprotegerin—a novel secreted protein involved in the regulation of bone density. *Cell*. 1997;89:309–319.

33. Yasuda H, Shima N, Nakagawa N, et al. Identity of osteoclastogenesis inhibitory factor (Ocif) and osteoprotegerin (Opg)—a mechanism by which Opg/Ocif inhibits osteoclastogenesis in vitro. *Endocrinology*. 1998;139:1329–1337.

34. Tominaga M, Caterina MJ, Malmberg AB, et al. The cloned capsaicin receptor integrates multiple pain-producing stimuli. *Neuron*. 1998;21:531–543.

35. Alvarez de la Rosa D, Zhang P, Shao D, White F, Canessa CM. Functional implications of the localization and activity of acid-sensitive channels in rat peripheral nervous system. *Proc Natl Acad Sci USA*. 2002;99:2326–2331.

36. Griffiths JR. Are cancer cells acidic? *Br J Cancer*. 1991;64:425–427.

37. Ghilardi JR, Rohrich H, Lindsay TH, et al. Selective blockade of the capsaicin receptor TRPV1 attenuates bone cancer pain. *J Neurosci*. 2005;25:3126–3131.

38. Mundy GR. *Bone Remodeling and Its Disorders*. 2nd ed. London: Taylor Francis; 1999.

39. Rubert Cynthia HR, Malawer Martin. Orthopedic Management of Skeletal Metastases. In: Body J-J, ed. *Tumor Bone Disease and Osteoporsis in Cancer Patients*. New York City: Marcel Dekker; 2000:305–356.

40. Kundu N, Yang QY, Dorsey R, Fulton AM. Increased cyclooxygenase-2 (cox-2) expression and activity in a murine model of metastatic breast cancer. *Int J Cancer*. 2001;93:681–686.

41. Molina MA, Sitja-Arnau M, Lemoine MG, Frazier ML, Sinicrope FA. Increased cyclooxygenase-2 expression in human pancreatic carcinomas and cell lines: growth inhibition by nonsteroidal anti-inflammatory drugs. *Cancer Res*. 1999;59:4356–4362.

42. Iniguez MA, Rodriguez A, Volpert OV, Fresno M, Redondo JM. Cyclooxygenase-2: a therapeutic target in angiogenesis. *Trends Mol Med*. 2003;9:73–78.

43. Williams CS, Tsujii M, Reese J, Dey SK, DuBois RN. Host cyclooxygenase-2 modulates carcinoma growth. *J Clin Invest*. 2000;105:1589–1594.

44. Masferrer JL, Leahy KM, Koki AT, et al. Antiangiogenic and antitumor activities of cyclooxygenase-2 inhibitors. *Cancer Res*. 2000;60:1306–1311.

45. Davar G. Endothelin-1 and metastatic cancer pain. *Pain Med*. 2001;2:24–27.

46. Nelson JB, Carducci MA. The role of endothelin-1 and endothelin receptor antagonists in prostate cancer. *BJU Int.* 2000;85:45–48.

47. Nelson JB, Hedican SP, George DJ, et al. Identification of endothelin-1 in the pathophysiology of metastatic adenocarcinoma of the prostate. *Nat Med.* 1995;1:944–949.

48. Pomonis JD, Rogers SD, Peters CM, Ghilardi JR, Mantyh PW. Expression and localization of endothelin receptors: implications for the involvement of peripheral glia in nociception. *J Neurosci.* 2001;21:999–1006.

49. Davar G, Hans G, Fareed MU, Sinnott C, Strichartz G. Behavioral signs of acute pain produced by application of endothelin-1 to rat sciatic nerve. *Neuroreport.* 1998;9:2279–2283.

50. Peters CM, Lindsay TH, Pomonis JD, et al. Endothelin and the tumorigenic component of bone cancer pain. *Neuroscience.* 2004;126:1043–1052.

51. Couture R, Harrisson M, Vianna RM, Cloutier F. Kinin receptors in pain and inflammation. *Eur J Pharmacol.* 2001;429: 161–176.

52. Fox A, Wotherspoon G, McNair K, et al. Regulation and function of spinal and peripheral neuronal B1 bradykinin receptors in inflammatory mechanical hyperalgesia. *Pain.* 2003;104:683–691.

53. Sevcik MA, Ghilardi JR, Halvorson KG, Lindsay TH, Kubota K, Mantyh PW. Analgesic efficacy of bradykinin B1 antag-

onists in a murine bone cancer pain model. *J Pain.* 2005;6: 771–775.

54. Pezet S, McMahon SB. Neurotrophins: mediators and modulators of pain. *Annu Rev Neurosci.* 2006;29:507–538.

55. Heumann R, Korsching S, Bandtlow C, Thoenen H. Changes of nerve growth factor synthesis in nonneuronal cells in response to sciatic nerve transection. *J Cell Biol.* 1987;104:1623–1631.

56. Halvorson KG, Kubota K, Sevcik MA, et al. A blocking antibody to nerve growth factor attenuates skeletal pain induced by prostate tumor cells growing in bone. *Cancer Res.* 2005;65:9426–9435.

57. Sevcik MA, Ghilardi JR, Peters CM, et al. Anti-NGF therapy profoundly reduces bone cancer pain and the accompanying increase in markers of peripheral and central sensitization. *Pain.* 2005;115:128–141.

58. Peters CM, Ghilardi JR, Keyser CP, et al. Tumor-induced injury of primary afferent sensory nerve fibers in bone cancer pain. *Exp Neurol.* 2005;193:85–100.

59. Woodham P, Anderson PN, Nadim W, Turmaine M. Satellite cells surrounding axotomised rat dorsal root ganglion cells increase expression of a GFAP-like protein. *Neurosci Lett.* 1989;98:8–12.

60. Hu P, McLachlan EM. Macrophage and lymphocyte invasion of dorsal root ganglia after peripheral nerve lesions in the rat. *Neuroscience.* 2002;112:23–38.

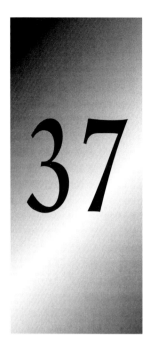

Visceral Pain in Cancer

Stacey Franz
Kristen E. Cardamone
Michael D. Stubblefield

Due to advances in clinical screening, diagnostics, and management, millions of people are now cancer survivors. These individuals not only live with cancer, but the majority also experience cancer-related pain. It is estimated that 65% to 90% of cancer patients experience pain (1–4), one of the most patient feared cancer-related complications (5,6).

Cancer pain can be classified into two broad categories: nociceptive pain and neuropathic pain. Nociceptive pain can be further subdivided into somatic and visceral pain (4,7). Various studies have documented the prevalence of visceral pain in the cancer population (8–11). It is estimated that 20% to 33% of cancer-related pain is visceral in origin (8,10), and certain cancer types appear to correlate with a higher affinity for visceral pain than others. In patients with lung cancer, for example, visceral pain may account for up to 42% of pain complaints (9). In patients with breast cancer, however, 15% of postmastectomy pain was found to be somatic or visceral in origin (11).

The literature suggests that health care providers commonly underestimate the severity of cancer-related pain (12). In order to provide optimal management, it is paramount that clinicians appropriately diagnose these pain syndromes through recognition of the respective pain generator. The purpose of this chapter is to elucidate the pathophysiology and clinical presentation of visceral pain as it relates to the cancer patient.

PATHOPHYSIOLOGY

Nociceptors, which transmit painful stimuli, are present in most of the bodily structures and viscera (13–15). The distribution of visceral nociceptors varies among the visceral structures. Generally hollow viscera (ie, esophagus, stomach, intestine, bladder, and uterus) contain nociceptors and are thus sensate to pain. The peritoneum, omentum, and parenchyma of the solid organs (ie, spleen, liver, kidney, and pancreas) have no nociceptors and are thus insensitive to pain. These insensate organs only signal awareness of pain if their capsules, which contain nociceptors, are distended and/or adjacent pain-sensitive structures are secondarily affected, such as with gross destruction by malignancy (16).

Visceral nociceptors are comprised of thinly myelinated A-delta fibers, which contribute to the perception of pricking pain when stimulated (17), or unmyelinated C fibers, by which stimulation results in burning or dull pain (18). At baseline, nociceptors are typically unresponsive, and can be described as "silent" nociceptors (19). However, with inflammation, nociceptors are sensitized and become active. Various other stimuli, including mechanical stimuli (compression, distension, and traction) and ischemia, have been associated with nociceptor sensitization.

Nociceptive information is relayed to the central nervous system via afferent fibers of both the sympa-

KEY POINTS

- More than half of all individuals with cancer experience cancer-related pain, and visceral pain may account for up to one-third of such pain.
- The distribution of nociceptors—sensory receptors which transmit the perception of pain—varies throughout the viscera, and some organs are insensate.
- Nociceptive information is relayed to the central nervous system via afferents of both the sympathetic and parasympathetic nervous system, primarily through the spinothalamic and spinoreticular tracts.
- Unlike somatosensitization, visceral systems do not operate via a "wind-up" mechanism; instead, central sensitization is achieved via increased release of neurotransmitters and various neural network feedback loops, which may account for enhanced motor and autonomic reflexes.

- True visceral pain is unrelenting and ranges in quality from vague, diffuse, deep pain to burning, aching, gnawing, cramping, or crushing pain. It may be accompanied by motor and autonomic reflexes and is not always linked to visceral injury, may not be evoked from all viscera, and may be referred to other locations.
- Referred visceral pain produces viscerosomatic reflexes through viscerosomatic convergence, a phenomenon that causes dermatomal hyperalgesia or myotomal somatic changes. Chapman's reflexes are the resulting tissue texture abnormalities, which reflect increased sympathetic activity in the corresponding spinal segmental region.
- Treatment of visceral pain is multi-factorial, including pharmacologic, manual, interventional, and complementary/alternative medicine techniques, as well as psychosocial support. Future treatment options may include receptor modulation.

thetic and parasympathetic nervous system. Central processing of visceral nociceptive information begins as the afferent fibers, or first-order neurons, of viscera enter the spinal cord at the level of the dorsal horn in lamina I and II, where they synapse on second-order neurons, most notably lamina V and X (13,20,21). Although visceral afferents comprise only 10% or less of all afferent input to the spinal cord (22–24), the amount of dorsal horn neurons that actually respond to visceral stimuli is considerable at an estimated to be 50% to 75% (25).

In the dorsal horn, the terminals of the visceral nociceptive afferent fibers express peptide neurotransmitters, such as substance P and calcitonin-gene-related peptide, which are integral in pain transmission. Similar to the somatic system, neurokinin and N-methyl-D-aspartic acid (NMDA) receptors are also involved in transmission of visceral pain. More recently, neurokinin (NK)1 and NK3 receptors have been shown to mediate visceral pain in cases of colonic distension (20).

Viscerosensory information is then conveyed through axons of second-order neurons that cross midline and ascend via the spinothalamic and spinoreticular tracts located in the anterolateral quadrant of the contralateral half of the spinal cord to higher levels of the neuraxis (26). These nociceptive projection neurons relay information to various regions of the brain, including the thalamus, brainstem, hypothalamus, amygdala, and sensory cortex. Contemporary

research suggests that the dorsal column pathway and spinohypothalamic pathway may also play a role in viscerosensory processing (27). Following central processing, the information is modulated via descending pathways that utilize neurotransmitters including opioids as well as serotonin and catecholamines produced in structures such as the periductal gray, locus ceruleus, nucleus raphe magnus, bulbar formation, and subceruleus (26).

Visceral pain systems do not mirror the somatic pain mechanism of "wind-up" to achieve central sensitization. Rather, visceral nociceptive systems generate central sensitization or hyperalgesia through increased release of neurotransmitters and various neural network feedback loops. Such feedback loops, which are abundant in the visceral system, may account for enhanced motor and autonomic reflexes. For example, these amplified reflexes may manifest as nausea and diaphoresis in the setting of pancreatic cancer.

CLINICAL IMPLICATIONS

Visceral pain can best be characterized as diffuse and poorly localized, accompanied by motor and autonomic reflexes, and referred to other locations (viscerosomatic convergence). Furthermore, it is not always linked to visceral injury or evoked from all viscera (not all viscera are innervated by nociceptors) (20,28).

True visceral pain quality is generally vague, deep, diffuse, burning, aching, gnawing, cramping, or crushing (29,30). The pain is usually unrelenting, forcing patients with visceral pain to appear unsettled as they continually change positions in an attempt to achieve a comfortable position. As a result of enhanced autonomic reflexes, patients with cancer who experience visceral pain may present with pallor, nausea, emesis, and hyperhidrosis, none of which are typical of somatic pain.

Referred Pain and Viscerosomatic Reflex Patterns

Referred visceral pain is described as the false localization of a noxious visceral stimulus to a somatic dermatome sharing the same spinal cord segment. The phenomenon known as viscerosomatic convergence is believed to be the neural basis for referred visceral pain (13,31–33). This mechanism can be explained by the absence of a specific sensory pathway in the brain for the viscera. Thus, an organ's nociceptive afferent information is transmitted to the appropriate dorsal horn relay neurons in spinal segments that also receive sensory information from skin and muscle (Fig. 37.1). This information is processed simultaneously, and the activity in the ascending spinal pathways may be misinterpreted as originating from the corresponding somatic structures (31–33). This in turn produces viscerosomatic reflexes, which may result in dermatomal hyperalgesia or myotomal somatic changes.

For example, a patient with pancreatic carcinoma may experience abdominal pain from the mass itself or referred pain into the midthoracic region. Specifically, visceral nociceptive information from the pancreas merges with the greater splanchnic nerves and synapses within the celiac ganglion, ultimately reaching its target spinal level at T5 to T9. Increased and prolonged input results in facilitation of the corresponding spinal segments, thereby leading to palpatory tissue changes and tenderness of the thoracic paraspinals (27,33).

Chapman's reflexes are predictable tissue texture abnormalities that appear to reflect viscerosomatic reflexes and indicate increased sympathetic activity in the corresponding spinal segmental region (33,34). These reflexes, which are used primarily for diagnostic purposes, are located anteriorly or posteriorly in the deep fascia or periosteum (Fig. 37.2). Palpation of the smooth, firm, discrete nodules generates a sharp, focal, nonradiating pain (33,34). To optimize management of visceral pain, it is essential that clinicians have a thorough knowledge of the visceral segmental innervation and referral patterns to facilitate localization of the pain etiology.

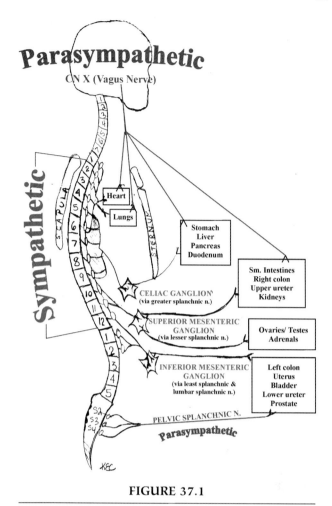

FIGURE 37.1

Autonomic innervation of the viscera.

TREATMENT OPTIONS

Subtherapeutic management of pain has been correlated with subsequent loss of function and decreased ability to participate in activities of daily living (3). Therefore, clinicians need to be familiar with options for pain control and symptom management. For those patients suffering from cancer-related visceral pain, treatment options include pharmacologic, manual, interventional, and complementary/alternative medicine techniques. Psychosocial support should also be an integral part of any treatment program.

Existing traditional approaches to visceral pain management will be discussed in subsequent chapters and include a combination approach to medications, including nonsteroidal anti-inflammatories (NSAIDs), opioids, and adjuvant medications. Interventional and surgical procedures may be employed for pain refrac-

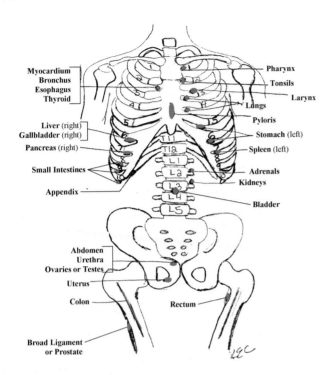

Anterior Chapman Reflex Points

(points are located bilaterally unless otherwise noted)

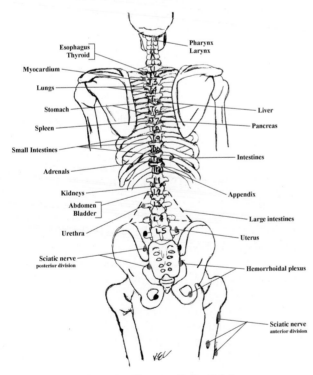

Posterior Chapman Reflex Points

(points are located bilaterally unless otherwise noted)

FIGURE 37.2

Anterior (top) and posterior (bottom) chapman reflex points. *Note:* Point are located bilaterally unless otherwise noted.

tory to more conservative approaches or limited by medication side effects. Such interventions include intrathecal anesthetic infusion, continuous epidural infusion, neurolytic blocks, or ablative neurosurgical procedures.

Although there is literature supporting the use of complementary/alternative medicine (CAM) in pain management of the general oncologic population (35–38), there is little, if any, evidence to support its use in patients who specifically suffer from visceral cancer pain. Despite the relative lack of evidence supporting its use for these patients, CAM should be considered when managing patients with visceral cancer pain. CAM options include acupuncture (36), chiropractic care (38), massage therapy (35,37), movement therapy, and relaxation techniques. Osteopathic manipulative treatment, performed by osteopathic physicians who are proficient in visceral osteopathic techniques, may also be helpful for those with visceral pain (33,39).

Future treatment options may include receptor modulation. Current research demonstrates that substance P has promising implications for visceral pain therapy, as substance P receptor knockout transgenic mice do not appear to develop hyperalgesia after visceral inflammation (28). Substance P is also the native ligand at the NK1 receptor; therefore, it is predicted that NK1 receptors will likely play a future role in management of visceral pain.

CONCLUSION

Both acute and chronic pain are common problems for individuals with cancer. It is not only the most feared symptom of advanced cancer, but may also be the rate-limiting factor in cancer management. Pain can have a serious impact on one's ability to function. It is imperative that clinicians are able to discuss, identify, and manage such cancer-related pain. The ultimate outcome of pain management in individuals with cancer is to relieve suffering and enable such individuals the best possible quality of life.

*A*dditional resources

Chang VC, Janjan N, Jain S, Chau C. Update in cancer pain syndromes. *J Palliat Med.* 2006;9(6):1414–1427.

Hobson AR, Aziz Q. Central nervous system processing of human visceral pain in health and disease. *News Physiol Sci.* 2003;18:109–114.

Ladabaum U, Minoshima S, Owyanh C. Pathobiology of visceral pain: molecular mechanisms and therapeutic implications. *Am J Physiol Gastrointest Liver Physiol.* 2000;79:G1–G6.

Purves D, Augustine G, Fitzpatrick D, Katz L, LaMantia A, McNamara J, eds. *Neuroscience.* Sunderland, MA: Sinauer Associates, Inc.; 1997.

References

1. Bonica JJ. Treatment of cancer pain: current status and future need. In: Fields ML, Dubner R, Cerrero F, Jones LE, eds. *Proceedings of the Fourth World Congress on Pain—Advances in Pain Research and Therapy.* New York: Raven Press; 1985:.

2. Daut RL, Cleeland CS. The prevalence and severity of pain in cancer. *Cancer.* 1982;50:1913–1918.

3. Foley KM. The treatment of cancer pain. *N Engl J Med.* 1985. 313:84–95.

4. Shaiova L. Difficult pain syndromes: bone pain, visceral pain and neuropathic pain. *Cancer J.* 2006;12:330–340.

5. Jacox A, Carr DB, Payne R. New clinical-practice guidelines for the management of pain in patients with cancer. *N Engl J Med.* 1994;330(9):651–655.

6. Greenhalgh T, Hurwitz B, eds. *Narrative Based Medicine. Dialogue and Discourse in Clinical Practice.* London: BMJ Publishing Group; 1998.

7. Portenoy RK. Cancer pain: pathophysiology and syndromes. *Lancet.* 1992;339:1026–1031.

8. Grond S, Zech D, Diefenbach C, Radbruch L, Lehmann KA. Assessment of cancer pain: a prospective evaluation in 2266 cancer patients referred to a pain service. *Pain.* 1996;64(1):107–114.

9. Mercadante S, Armata M, Salvaggio L. Pain characteristics of advanced lung cancer patients referred to a palliative care service. *Pain.* 1994;59(1):141–145.

10. Portenoy RK, Hagen NA. Breakthrough pain: definition, prevalence and characteristics. *Pain.* 1990;41(3):273–281.

11. Stevens PE, Dibble SL, Miaskowski C. Prevalence, characteristics, and impact of post-mastectomy pain syndrome: an investigation of women's experiences. *Pain.* 1995;61(1):61–68.

12. Cleeland CS, Gonin R, Hatfield AK, et al. Pain and its treatment in outpatients with metastatic cancer. *N Engl J Med.* 1994;330(9):592–596.

13. Cervero F. Sensory innervation of the viscera: peripheral basis of visceral pain. *Physiol Rev.* 1994;74(1):95–129.

14. Willis WD. Nociceptive pathways: anatomy and physiology of nociceptive ascending pathways. *Philos Trans R Soc Lond B Biol Sci.* 1985;308(1136):253–270.

15. Willis WD, Coggeshall RE. *Sensory Mechanisms of the Spinal Cord.* 2nd ed. New York: Plenum Press; 1991.

16. Regan JM, Peng P. Neurophysiology of cancer pain. *Cancer Control.* 2000;7(2):111–119.

17. Konietzny F, Perl ER, Trevino D, Light A, Hensel H. Sensory experiences in man evoked by intraneural electrical stimulation of intact cutaneous afferent fibers. *Exp Brain Res.* 1981;42:219–222.

18. Ochoa J, Torebjork E. Sensations evoked by intraneural microstimulation of C nociceptor fibers in human skin nerves. *J Physiol.* 1989;415:583–599.

19. Habler HJ, Janig W, Koltzenburg M. Activation of unmyelinated afferent fibers by mechanical stimuli and inflammation of the urinary bladder in the cat. *J Physiol.* 1990;425:545–562.

20. Al-Chaer ED, Traub RJ. Biological basis of visceral pain: recent developments. *Pain.* 2002;96:221–225.

21. Gebhart GF. Visceral pain mechanisms. In: Chapman CR, Foley K, eds. *Current and Emerging Concepts in Cancer Pain: Research and Practice.* New York: Raven Press; 1993:99–111.

22. Cervero F, Connel LA, Lawson SN. Somatic and visceral primary afferents in the lower thoracic dorsal root ganglia of the cat. *J Comp Neurol.* 1984;228:422–431.

23. Foreman RD, Weber RN. Responses from neurons of the primate spinothalamic tract to electrical stimulation of afferents from the cardiopulmonary region and somatic structures. *Brain Res.* 1980;186:464–468.

24. Jauanig W, Morrison JFB. Functional properties of spinal visceral afferents supplying abdominal and pelvic organs, with special emphasis on visceral nociception. In: Cervero F, Morrison JFB, eds. *Progress in Brain Research,* vol. 67. Amsterdam: Elsevier; 1986:87–114.

25. Cervero F, Tattersall JEH. Cutaneous receptive fields of somatic and viscerosomatic neurons in the thoracic spinal cord of the cat. *J Comp Neurol.* 1985;237:325–332.

26. Willis WD, Westlund KN. Neuroanatomy of the pain system and of the pathways that modulate pain. *J Clin Neurophysiol.* 1997;14:2–31.

27. Palecek J. The role of dorsal columns pathway in visceral pain. *Physiol Res.* 2004;53:S125–S130.

28. Cervero F, Laird JM. Visceral pain. *Lancet.* 1999;353:2145–2148.

29. Hardy JD, Wolff HG, Goodell H. Experimental evidence on the nature of cutaneous hyperalgesia. *J Clin Invest.* 1950;29:115–140.

30. Payne WW, Poulton EP. Visceral pain in the upper alimentary tract. *Q J Med.* 1923;17:53–80.

31. Fix J. Autonomic nervous system and pain. In: Fix J, ed. *Neuroanatomy,* 3rd ed. Philadelphia: Lippincott Williams & Wilkins; 2002.

32. Giamberardino MA. Referred muscle pain/hyperalgesia and central sensitization. *J Rehabil Med.* 2003;41(Suppl):85–88.

33. Kuchera ML, Kuchera WA. *Osteopathic Considerations and Systemic Dysfunction,* 2nd ed. Columbus, OH: Greyden Press; 1994.

34. Giamberardino MA, Vecchiet L. Pathophysiology of visceral pain. *Curr Pain Headache Rep.* 1997;1:23–33.

35. Cassileth BR, Vickers AJ. Massage therapy for symptom control: outcome study at a major cancer center. *J Pain Symptom Manag.* 2004;28(3):244–249.

36. Cohen AJ, Menter A, Hale L. Acupuncture: role in comprehensive cancer care—a primer for the oncologist and review of the literature. *Integr Cancer Ther.* 2005;4(2):131–143.

37. Corbin L. Safety and efficacy of massage therapy for patients with cancer. *Cancer Control.* July 2005;12(3):158–164.

38. Schneider J, Gilford S. The chiropractor's role in pain management for oncology patients. *J Manip Physiol Ther.* 2001;24(1):52–57.

39. DiGiovanna EL, Schiowitz S. *An Osteopathic Approach to Diagnosis and Treatment,* 2nd ed. Philadelphia: Lippincott Williams & Wilkins; 1997.

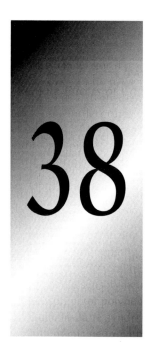

Neuropathic Pain in Cancer

38

Neel Mehta
Amit Mehta
Amitabh Gulati

DEFINITION OF NEUROPATHIC PAIN

Neuropathic pain is defined by the International Association for the Study of Pain as "pain initiated or caused by a primary lesion or dysfunction of the nervous system" (1). Nerve related pain, which is a direct consequence of a lesion or disease of the nervous system that signals pain, affects upwards of 3% of the population and can tremendously impact quality of life (2). Broadly, neuropathic pain can be classified as disorders of the peripheral nervous system or the central nervous system (brain and spinal cord) or as mixed (peripheral and central) neuropathic pain. However, attempts are being made to classify based on proposed underlying mechanisms to further improve specificity in diagnoses (3).

SYMPTOMS, PHYSICAL EXAMINATION, AND DIAGNOSIS

While the most common symptom of neuropathic pain is mechanical allodynia (painful responses to normally innocuous tactile stimuli), patients often experience hyperalgesia (increased responsiveness to noxious stimuli). Mechanical hyperalgesias can be divided into brush-evoked (dynamic), pressure-evoked (static), and punctuate, with sensory deficits occurring at varying degrees to sensory modalities such as light touch and

pain. Additionally, patients may have spontaneous pain, described as shooting, lancinating, or burning pain, with negative or positive motor phenomena. Negative motor phenomena include weakness, clumsiness, and fatigue, whereas positive motor phenomena include tremor, dyskinesias, ataxia, and dystonia.

Pain with and without apparent nerve injury can be diagnosed from the patient's description of symptoms and a comprehensive pain history. Furthermore, pain that improves from sympathetic nerve blocks may be sympathetically maintained pain. One may use the Leeds assessment of neuropathic symptoms and signs (LANSS), a scale based on the analysis of data obtained during bedside examination. The LANSS pain scale allows analysis of sensory description and sensory dysfunction, distinguishing nociceptive pain from neuropathic pain (4). It can be administered by a physician or given as a self-study questionnaire. Sensitivity and specificity of the scale were found to be 89.9% and 94.2%, respectively (5).

Examination should be comprehensive, consisting of thorough neurologic, musculoskeletal, and mental status assessments. Physical examination involves touch, pressure and palpation, pinprick, cold, heat, and vibration (6). Responses can be graded as normal, decreased, or increased to determine whether negative or positive sensory phenomena are involved (7). Mental status examination can aid in diagnosis when underlying disorders such as depression and anxiety are discovered.

KEY POINTS

- Neuropathic pain is defined by the International Association for the Study of Pain as "pain initiated or caused by a primary lesion or dysfunction of the nervous system."
- Broadly, neuropathic pain can be classified as disorders of the peripheral nervous system or the central nervous system (brain and spinal cord) or as mixed (peripheral and central) neuropathic pain.
- Recent evidence suggests that inflammation plays a central role in neuropathic pain.
- Peripheral sensitization in neuropathic pain occurs in primary afferent nociceptors.
- Two broad concepts of the pathophysiology of central pain have been theorized as central disinhibition and/or central sensitization.

- Medications commonly used in the treatment of neuropathic pain include tricyclic antidepressants, anticonvulsants, antiarrhythmics, opioid analgesics, N-methyl-D-aspartate (NMDA) antagonists, topical medications, and certain drugs that mimic the γ-aminobutyric acid (GABA) receptor.
- An expanding field, Neuromodulation therapy is being used to treat various neuropathic pain disorders, including Parthinson's disease, dystonia, obsessive-compulsive disorder, refractory pain, and complex regional pain syndrome (CBPS), which may be poorly managed with pharmacologic therapy.

There is a selection of diagnostic tools available for further investigation. For central pain syndromes, MRI and CT imaging may localize cerebral or spinal cord lesions. Nerve conduction studies may identify or confirm radiculopathy, plexopathy, or peripheral neuropathy. In addition, local anesthetic nerve blocks aid in diagnosis, especially for inconclusive conduction studies. Finally, skin biopsy of affected areas and histologic examination of nerve endings can help diagnosis. However, nerve biopsies, especially sural nerve biopsy, have fallen out of favor.

IMMUNE PATHOPHYSIOLOGY

It was previously thought that inflammatory and neuropathic syndromes were distinct and separate; however, recent evidence suggests inflammation plays a central role in neuropathic pain. Multiple inflammatory mediators released from damaged tissue acutely excite primary sensory neurons in the peripheral nervous system, producing ectopic discharge and leading to a sustained increase in their excitability.

Mast cells are a key component of allergic reactions and development of innate immunity (8). Upon nerve damage, mast cells near a peripheral nerve activate and degranulate, causing release of histamine, serotonin, cytokines, and proteases (9). Histamine sensitizes nociceptors (10) and when applied to the skin of patients with postherpetic neuralgia, can cause severe burning (11). Furthermore, neuronal histamine receptors are upregulated after a crush injury to the sciatic

nerve (12). Activated mast cells may recruit other key immune cell types, which in turn release pronociceptive mediators (13).

Neutrophils, absent in normal nerve tissue, are the first inflammatory cells to infiltrate damaged tissue and are the most important in the acute inflammatory stage (14). They cause phagocytosis and release proinflammatory factors, including cytokines and chemokines, which then activate and attract other inflammatory cell types, most notably macrophages (15). Recruited in response to peripheral nerve injury—such as inflammation and loss of axons, myelin, or both—neutrophils mainly phagocytose foreign material and microbes.

The macrophage population in the peripheral nerve consists of resident cells and hematogenously derived macrophages, only seen after tissue damage (16). In contrast to other tissue systems, resident macrophages do not need activation of precursor cells and respond rapidly to nerve injury (17), while recruited macrophages arrive later and aid in degeneration and subsequent regeneration of the nerve cell (18). Attenuation of macrophage recruitment into the damaged nerve has been shown to reduce neuropathic pain in models involving crush injury and nerve ligation (19–21).

Schwann cells surrounding degenerating axons during Wallerian degeneration begin to phagocytose myelin debris and synthesize other molecules such as nerve growth factor (NGF), tumor necrosis factor alpha (TNFα), interleukin-1 beta (IL-1β), interleukin-6 (IL-6), and adenosine triphosphate (22–26). In partial nerve injuries, which are often associated with neuropathic pain, axons that remain intact distal to the lesion (known as spared axons) are exposed to novel Schwann cell-derived factors. The distal ends of damaged axons are also exposed to some of these factors at the site of injury. There also has been circumstantial evidence that Schwann cells may contribute to some neuropathic pain states, such as that associated with human immunodeficiency virus (27).

Lymphocytes, specifically T cells (cellular immunity or natural killer cells), have been identified at nerve injury sites (28). T cells are delineated into helper T cells (CD4) and cytotoxic T cells (CD8) and are further divided into type 1 and 2, according to cytokine expression profile. Transfer of type 1 helper T cells in crush injury causes production of proinflammatory cytokines and increases in pain levels in rats, whereas transfer of type 2 helper T cells (producing anti-inflammatory cytokines) produces a reduction in pain sensitivity (29).

Cytokines may cause neuropathic pain in two primary ways: (1) proinflammation effects on primary afferent neurons directly, and (2) indirect actions via activation of signaling pathways of immune cells. These cytokines include, as mentioned above, TNFα, IL-6, leukemia inhibitory factor (LIF), and chemokine ligand 2 (CCL2).

TNFα causes a cascade of several further cytokines and growth factors. Studies have demonstrated a correlation between TNFα mRNA protein expression after injury and allodynia and hyperalgesia (30). Furthermore, initiation of the pain cascade has been shown after crush injuries, with increased sensitivity of injured and adjacent neurons, after expression of TNFα (31). Finally, increased levels of TNFα in the dorsal root ganglia may lead to neuropathic pain in some patients (32).

The subject of newer studies, IL-6 is a proinflammatory cytokine involved in development of neuropathic pain after both crushed nerve injury and peripheral nerve ligation (33). It has been proposed that IL-6 has direct excitatory effect on nociceptive neurons and causes adrenergic sprouting (34).

Studies have shown that LIF has de novo expression by Schwann cells at the site of injury after sciatic nerve transaction (35), and that nociceptive sensory fibers retrogradely transport and accumulate LIF in cell bodies (36). Finally, LIF has been shown to be involved in recruitment of macrophages and other immune cells to damaged nerves after crush injury (37).

In addition to recruiting immune cells to peripheral nerve damaged cells, CCL2 and its receptor may mediate neuropathic pain (38). It is expressed in Schwann cells, macrophages, and neurons, and is upregulated by the above mentioned chemokines (39). Furthermore, it has been proposed that there is more than one site where these receptors are activated, including nerve trunks, dorsal root ganglion, and the spinal dorsal horn (40).

NGF is known to regulate several functions of neurons, including survival and growth. Mutation in a high affinity receptor for NGF, tyrosine kinase A (TrkA), leads to congenital insensitivity to pain by interrupting signaling (41). NGF also produces sensitization of nociceptors via altered gene expression and post-translational regulation of receptors and ion channels, specifically transient receptor potential vanilloid 1 (TRPV1) (42) tetrodotoxin-resistant Na channels (43). NGF can also increase proliferation of B and T cells as well as eosinophils (44). After nerve injury, sensory neurons become disconnected from their targets, preventing retrograde transport of NGF and causing accumulation and non-neuronal cell expression of NGF mRNA (45).

CELL SIGNALING AND RECEPTOR PATHOPHYSIOLOGY

As a way of innate protection, noxious stimuli are immediately detected to prevent hazardous situations, enhancing survival. Multicellular organisms have evolved the nociceptor as a tool to aid in differentiation between innocuous and noxious stimuli. Much of this system is dependent on neurons and their channel-receptor relationship.

Sodium voltage-gated channels are a key component of neurons. Specifically, it has been shown that nine different genes (Nav 1.1 through 1.9) encode distinct channels and that their selective expression provides for different forms of the sodium channel. Pathology of these channels mainly occurs from mutation of the underlying genes that can produce abnormal channel proteins—leading to either failed or abnormal function. However, more frequently, pathology of channels occurs from traumatic events such as peripheral nerve injuries.

Peripheral sensitization in neuropathic pain occurs in primary afferent nociceptors. Pain sensations normally elicited by activity in normally silent unmyelinated (C) fibers or thinly myelinated (Aδ) primary afferent neurons become abnormally sensitive after a nerve lesion. Furthermore, they can develop spontaneous activity as a result of pathologic changes at the molecular and cellular level. These changes include increased expression of mRNA for voltage gated sodium channels in primary afferent neurons and ectopic impulse generation, which can lower action-potential thresholds and cause hyperactivity (46).

Following peripheral nerve damage, sodium channels can accumulate at the location of the nerve lesion and at the dorsal root ganglion. Membrane potential oscillations occur and cause ectopic firing due to alteration between voltage-dependent sodium channels (tetrodotoxin sensitive) and leaking voltage-independent potassium channels (47). Of note, the dorsal root ganglion lacks a blood-brain barrier and therefore may be easier to target with systemic therapy (48). Indirect evidence for ectopic afferent activity has been shown in neuropathic pain patients in whom lidocaine patches, a known sodium channel blocker, produce pain relief (49).

Peripheral nerve damage not only causes abnormal sodium channel function, but also upregulation of receptor proteins, some of which are not present in normal conditions. These changes occur at membranes of primary afferent neurons. An example includes vanilloid receptors (TRPV1), which are located on nociceptive afferent fibers known to detect heat greater than 43°C (50). Recent studies also provide evidence for an upregulation of TRPV1 in medium and large injured DRG cells (51) but novel expression of TRPV1 on uninjured C fibers and A fibers (52). Paclitaxel chemotherapy has been shown to cause mechanical hyperalgesia due to increased TRPV4 receptor, normally used to detect hypo-osmolarity and temperatures greater than 30°C (53). Furthermore, in cold and menthol-sensitive TRP channel (TRPM8) activated in the 8°C to 28°C range (54), upregulation occurs in the small diameter DRG neurons (55) after peripheral nerve injury sensitization, causing cold hyperalgesia (56).

In patients with complex regional pain syndrome (CRPS), it has been postulated that nerve injury triggers the expression of functional α1-adrenoceptors and α2-adrenoceptors on cutaneous afferent fibers. As a result, these neurons develop adrenergic sensitivity and have been shown to respond to sympathetic nerve block (57). Furthermore, noradrenergic sensitivity of human nociceptors occurs after partial or complete nerve lesion. In patients with postherpetic neuralgia, CRPS, and post-traumatic neuralgias, application of norepinephrine in physiological doses into a symptomatic skin area evokes or increases spontaneous pain and dynamic mechanical hyperalgesia (58,59).

During central sensitization, peripheral nerve hyperactivity causes secondary changes in the spinal cord dorsal horn, specifically increased general excitability. These spinal cord neurons can cause excitation of both nociceptive and non-nociceptive systems, leading to widespread neuronal excitation to many segments. These changes mainly occur in sensitized C fibers releasing glutamate, acting on postsynaptic N-methyl-D-aspartate (NMDA) receptors and the neuropeptide substance P. These changes may cause innocuous tactile stimuli to activate spinal cold pain-sensing neurons via Aδ and Aβ low-threshold mechanoreceptors (60). Central neuronal voltage-gated N-calcium channels located at the presynaptic sites on terminals of primary afferent nociceptors have an important role in central sensitization through the facilitation of glutamate and substance P release. These channels are overexpressed after peripheral nerve lesion. Furthermore, increased central sensitization has been shown in dorsal horn neurons, inhibited by γ-aminobutyric acid (GABA)-releasing interneurons decreasing in number after peripheral nerve injury (61).

NEUROPATHIC PAIN DISORDERS

While considering neuropathic pain disorders, it is often helpful to examine various diseases through their respective etiologies. Common etiologies include:

- Injury
- Compression
- Inflammation
- Ischemia
- Infection
- Demyelination
- Axonopathy
- Toxic/metabolic
- Neoplasm

This list can be arranged to aid in classification of the various disorders and to better categorize patients (Table 38.1).

- Peripheral focal and multifocal nerve lesions (traumatic, ischemic, or inflammatory)
- Peripheral generalized polyneuropathies (toxic, metabolic, hereditary, or inflammatory)
- Central nervous system (CNS) lesions (eg, stroke, multiple sclerosis, spinal cord injury)
- Complex neuropathic disorders (CRPS) (62).

Diabetic Neuropathy

Neuropathy is the leading cause of morbidity and mortality in patients with diabetes. It has a world prevalence of 20% and is often associated with 50% of nontraumatic amputations performed each year. The Diabetes Control and Complications Trial reported that, with tight glucose control, the annual incidence of diabetic neuropathy can be reduced from 2% to 0.56% (63).

TABLE 38.1

Common Classification and Causes of Neuropathic Pain in the Central and Peripheral Nervous System

FOCAL OR MULTIFOCAL LESIONS OF THE PERIPHERAL NERVOUS SYSTEM

Entrapment syndromes
Phantom limb pain, stump pain
Post-traumatic neuralgia
Postherpetic neuralgia
Diabetic mononeuropathy
Ischemic neuropathy
Polyarteritis nodosa
Radiation related injury
Cancer-related neuropathic pain

GENERALIZED LESIONS OF THE PERIPHERAL NERVOUS SYSTEM (POLYNEUROPATHIES)

Diabetes mellitus
Alcohol
Amyloid
Plasmocytoma
HIV neuropathy
Hypothyroidism
Hereditary sensory neuropathies
Fabry's disease
Bannwarth's syndrome (neuroborreliosis)
Vitamin B deficiency
Toxic neuropathies (arsenic, thallium, chloramphenicol, metronidazole, nitrofurantoin, isoniazid, vinca alkaloids, taxanes, gold)

LESIONS OF THE CNS

Spinal cord injury
Brain infarction (especially the thalamus and brainstem)
Spinal infarction
Syringomyelia
Multiple sclerosis

COMPLEX NEUROPATHIC DISORDERS

Complex regional pain syndromes type I and II (a.k.a.: reflex sympathetic dystrophy, causalgia)

Source: From Ref. 62.

Symptoms of diabetic neuropathy include numbness and tingling of extremities, dysesthesia, burning, and electric, stabbing pain. Mononeuropathies of thoracic or lumbar spinal nerves can lead to syndromes mimicking myocardial infarction, cholecystitis, or appen-

dicitis. Furthermore, diabetic have a higher incidence of entrapment neuropathies such as carpal tunnel syndrome.

These conditions are thought to result from diabetic microvascular injury, causing vasoconstriction and ischemia to nerves. Furthermore, glucose causes nonenzymatic bonding with proteins and glycosylation, leading to either abnormal or arrest of the protein function. Increased levels of glucose cause an increase in intracellular diacylglycerol, which activates protein kinase C and can lead to ischemia and decreased neuronal blood flow (63).

Postherpetic Neuropathy

Another common metabolic condition causing painful peripheral neuropathy results from reactivation of herpes zoster virus. Commonly known as shingles, the initial infection causes chickenpox. However, the virus can be latent in the nerve cell bodies and, less frequently, in the dorsal root, cranial nerve, or autonomic ganglion cells, without causing any symptoms (64). In an individual who is immunocompromised, perhaps years or decades after a chickenpox infection, the virus may break out of nerve cell bodies and travel down nerve axons to cause infection of the skin in the distribution of the nerve (65). The virus may spread from one or more ganglia along nerves of an affected segment and infect the corresponding dermatome, causing a painful rash (66). Although the rash usually heals within two to four weeks, some sufferers experience residual nerve pain for months or years, a condition known as postherpetic neuralgia (by definition, pain that continues for three months or more) (67).

Early symptoms of postherpetic neuropathy include nonspecific headache, fever, and malaise, and may result in an incorrect diagnosis (68). These symptoms are commonly followed by sensations of burning pain, itching, hyperesthesia, or paresthesia. The pain may be extreme in the affected dermatome, with sensations that are often described as stinging, tingling, aching, numbing, or throbbing, and can be interspersed with quick stabs of agonizing pain. In most cases, after one to two days (but sometimes as long as three weeks) the initial phase is followed by the appearance of the characteristic skin rash (69). A common location of pain and rash is on the torso, but the rash can also appear on the face, eyes, or other parts of the body. The rash initially appears similar to hives, but is not widespread but rather dermatomal in pattern, resulting in a stripe or belt-like pattern that is limited to one side of the body and does not cross the midline (70). With time, the rash becomes vesicular, forming small blisters filled with a serous exudate, as the fever and general malaise continue. The painful vesicles eventually become cloudy or darkened as they fill with blood. The lesions usually crust over within seven to ten days, after which the crust falls off and the skin heals. After severe blistering, scarring and discolored skin may remain.

Radiation Neuropathy

Radiation neuropathy may result from radiation therapy during treatment of various cancers, including breast and lung cancer, lymphomas, and metastatic disease. Symptoms include paresthesia, hypesthesia, muscle atrophy, weakness, decreased muscle stretch reflexes, pain, and edema of extremities (71). It is often classified based on the LENT-SOMA scale, assessing various grades of radiation therapy effects:

- Grade 1—Mild sensory deficits, no pain
- Grade 2—Moderate sensory deficits, tolerable pain, mild arm weakness
- Grade 3—Continuous paresthesia with incomplete motor paresis
- Grade 4—Complete motor paresis, excruciating pain, muscle atrophy.

Radiation-induced brachial plexus injuries are found to be a progressive process. Patients with grade 1 or 2 lesions may progress to grade 3 or 4 during the observation period, or up to 20 years (72). Diagnosis is based on clinical examination, electromyography, CT and MR imaging, and ultrasound examination. However, radiation neuropathy can often be confused with tumor-induced plexopathy, especially in the brachial plexus. Common risk factors include high radiation doses, overlapping fields, increased dose in axilla due to a smaller separation at that point, and concurrent chemotherapy (73).

Radiation of the peripheral nerves can cause several types of changes, including electrical and enzyme alterations, abnormal microtubule assembly, diminished vascular permeability, and fibrosis of tissue surrounding the nerve (73). Morphological changes include necrosis and hyalinization of the media of small arteries, fibrous replacement of nerve fibers, and demyelination and thickening of epineurium and perineurium. Infiltrating inflammatory cells, fibroblasts, and large amounts of various extra-cellular matrix components are found in fibrotic degenerated connective tissue. The incidence of neuropathy increases with time after radiation, as part of a slow process. The median interval between radiotherapy and occurrence of brachial neuropathy has been reported to be one to four years, but some neuropathies have occurred many years after completion of radiation treatment (from 6 to 22 years) (74).

Chemotherapy-associated Neuropathy

Similar to cancer patients receiving radiation therapy, patients receiving chemotherapy can develop peripheral neuropathies. Common chemotherapy drugs such as vinca-alkaloids, taxanes (paclitaxel), podophyllotoxins (etoposide), thalidomide, bortezomib, and interferon can cause symptoms promptly—sometimes after the first dose (75). However, platinum compounds have been shown to delay onset of symptoms, sometimes without effects until several weeks after the last dose. The severity of symptoms is often cumulative, and patients with preexisting neuropathy (due to alcoholism, diabetes, or malnutrition) may be more at risk for an increased severity or longevity of neuropathy (76).

The diagnosis of a toxic neuropathy is primarily based on the case history, the clinical and electrophysiological findings, and knowledge of the pattern of neuropathy associated with specific agents. In most cases, toxic neuropathies are length-dependent, with sensory or sensorimotor neuropathies often associated with pain. Although the mechanism for chemotherapy-induced neuropathy is not currently understood, in studies of vincristine-induced peripheral neuropathy in the rat, the animals experienced hyperalgesia to touch, and conduction velocities in sensory fibers were slowed (77). In other studies involving vincristine, large-diameter sensory neurons became swollen and neurofilaments in the cell bodies and axons increased in number, suggesting impaired anterograde axonal transport (78). The platinum compounds are unique in producing a sensory ganglionopathy. As more effective multiple drug combinations are used, patients will be treated with several neurotoxic drugs, providing a need for synergistic neurotoxicity to be investigated.

Plexopathy

Neuropathy related to a network of nerves is often referred to as a plexopathy. Common plexopathies occur at the brachial and lumbosacral nerve plexus, leading to sensorimotor deficits and significant pain syndromes. While plexopathies can be related to many etiologies such as diabetes, radiation, trauma (often during birth), they are commonly associated with cancer, occurring in upwards of 15% of patients with a cancer diagnosis.

Lumbosacral plexopathy commonly results from intra-abdominal tumor extension, and less often from metastases, lymph nodes, or bony structures. Of the tumors, colorectal is most common, followed by sarcomas, breast, lymphoma, cervical tumors, and multiple myeloma (79). Unilateral plexopathy is most common; however, in 25% of cases, it can be bilateral, usually from breast cancer metastasis. Symptoms most commonly include pain in the low back, buttocks, hips, and thighs, 90% being unilateral. With time, autonomic symptoms may present, with a "hot and dry foot" syndrome occurring with sympathetic components of the plexus being involved—most commonly temperature sensation (80).

Physical examination findings include muscle weakness, sensory loss, reflex impairment, and leg edema. Often there are gait abnormalities, weakness while getting up, or unilateral sensory deficits. Clinical diagnosis is aided with imaging modalities; with MRI is most accurate with soft tissues, whereas CT is helpful in abdominal and pelvic bony regions. Positron emission tomography (PET) scan can find active malignancy but has undetermined sensitivity and specificity.

Brachial plexopathies occur in 10% of all peripheral nerve lesions. Often it can be confused with radiation-induced brachial plexus lesions, but a lack of history of radiation above 50 Gy or a short duration of treatment can aid in differentiation. Some other characteristic features of brachial plexopathy are onset of limb pain less than six months following radiation, rapid development, Horner syndrome, severe pain (in addition to radition induced pain), and presence of other metastases (81). The most common causes are metastatic lesions from breast or lung, but it can also spread from the cervical spine. Primary tumors are less common, but are most often neural sheath tumors (82). Diagnosis of these neuropathies is similar to that of those lumbosacral in origin.

Complex Regional Pain Syndrome (CRPS)

CRPS consists of two types: type I (formerly known as reflex sympathetic dystrophy), where an obvious nerve lesion from trauma is unknown, or type II, where the lesion is known. Although a definitive mechanism has not been identified, it is thought that peripheral and central somatosensory, autonomic, and motor system changes occur along with pathology in the sympathetic and afferent systems. Current theories include autonomic dysfunction, presence of IgG in affected extremities, abnormal positive feedback circuits among the various nerve systems, abnormal mitochondrial enzyme activity, abnormal release of auto-antibodies, and presence of human lymphocyte antigen-DQ1 (HLA-DQ1) (83,84).

Symptoms include extreme pain (most common, often disproportionate), swelling, and symptoms related to sympathetic (alteration in blood flow leading to warmth) and motor nerves. CRPS I and II have much in common, including presence of spontaneous or evoked pain, allodynia, hyperalgesia, disproportionate pain, and pain not limited to a single nerve distribution. The condition affects upper extremities more often than lower extremities (85). Most commonly, CRPS is caused from trauma, but it can also be caused by surgery, herpes zoster infection, cancer, stroke, inflammation, myocardial infarction, but not excluding idiopathic origin (86).

Diagnosis includes a comprehensive history and physical examination, specifically looking for nature of trauma, presence of allodynia, hyperalgesia, hypoesthesia, hypothermesthesia, changes in proprioception, and anesthesia dolorosa. Physical findings include changes in skin color and temperature, edema, and restricted range of movement. One may also find dystrophic skin, nails, hair, muscle, or bone. Diagnostic tests can be as simple as recording skin temperature, sweat tests for autonomic dysfunction, and a quantitative sensory test for objective sensory findings. A diagnostic sympathetic ganglion nerve block can be performed, but cannot rule out other disorders and has inconsistent results. Imaging studies are limited to bone scans looking for diffuse increased activity, with juxta-articular accentuation uptake on the delayed images (87).

Central Pain Syndrome

Central pain syndrome was initially described following thalamic stroke; however, the syndrome has now been expanded to events following other types of stroke, spinal cord injury, multiple sclerosis, brain injury, amputations, or trauma to the CNS. Prevalence varies greatly, with approximately 1% to 8% of patients who have had stroke developing central pain, while 10% to 30% of patients with spinal cord injury are affected during the course of their illness (88).

Features of central pain consist of hypersensitivity at the site of the injury, allodynia, thermal hyperalgesia, autonomic dysregulation, and motor phenomena associated with CRPS. Two broad concepts of the pathophysiology of central pain have been theorized as central disinhibition and/or central sensitization. Both of these lead to neuronal hyperactivity and hyperexcitability of spinal and supraspinal nociceptive neurons. Furthermore, it is thought that disturbance of thalamocortical transmission is the main underlying pathology (89).

The pain of central pain syndrome can begin within days of the causative insult, or it can be delayed for years (particularly in stroke patients). While the specific symptoms of central pain syndrome may vary over time, the presence of a particular set of symptoms is essentially continuous once they begin. The pain is usually moderate to severe in nature and can be very debilitating. Symptoms may be made worse by a number of conditions, such as temperature change (especially exposure to cold), touching the painful area, movement, and emotions or stress.

Despite the pain being difficult to describe, diagnosis is usually made clinically based on prior history of spinal cord or brain injury and consequent development of the chronic pain syndrome. CT and MRI imaging of brain, spinal cord, or affected areas may be helpful, as well as nerve imaging studies, but in many cases these tests will add little to clinical knowledge.

INTRODUCTION TO TREATMENT OPTIONS

The various etiologies and mechanisms in neuropathic pain involve an interwoven dynamic relationship between the central nervous system and peripheral nervous system (91). Although one specific cause of neuropathic pain has not been identified, the concepts of central sensitization, sympathetically mediated pain, ectopic impulses from peripheral nerves, deafferentation hyperactivity, inflammation, and the reorganization of specific nerve fibers and central connections have been researched as possible triggers for the neuropathic pain cascade (90–94). Treatment modalities consist of pharmacologic methods as well as interventional procedures involving neuromodulation. Many new interventional modalities are on the horizon that may offer hope and relief to the millions of people suffering from neuropathic pain (90–94).

PHARMACOLOGIC TREATMENTS

A multitude of medications have been looked at for the treatment of neuropathic pain. Commonly used medications include tricyclic antidepressants, anticonvulsants, antiarrhythmics, opioid analgesics, NMDA antagonists, topical medications, and certain drugs that mimic the GABA receptor (90). The interrelationship between ionic channels and ectopic discharges from skin sensorial fibers and nerve tissue has been studied at the molecular level, as have the increases and changes in sodium channels and calcium channels (91–94). Early studies show tricyclic antidepressants (TCAs) as appropriate treatment for neuropathic pain, as they inhibit the reuptake of monoaminergic transmitters (90–93). Specifically, amitriptyline may relieve pain from diabetic neuropathy and postherpetic neuralgia (95). In the past few years, serotonin selective reuptake inhibitors (SSRI) and selective serotonin/norepinephrine reuptake inhibitors (SSNRI) have become common in the treatment of neuropathic pain, as their side effect profile is improved compared to the TCAs. While recent literature suggests SSRIs may have some efficacy for neuropathic pain, they may be less effective than TCAs (96–98). Research with SSNRIs is ongoing to determine relative efficacy compared to TCAs.

Anticonvulsants such as carbamazepine and phenytoin are effective in a select group of patients with neuropathic pain. Carbamazepine may be effective in trigeminal neuralgia, alleviating the lancinating electrical symptoms; however, is less helpful in other types of neuropathic pain (95). Gabapentin and its cousin pregabalin (both thought to modulate calcium channels in the CNS) have shown effectiveness in treating diabetic neuropathy and postherpetic neuralgia in recent placebo controlled trials (99,100). Lidocaine, mexiletine, and tocainide antiarrhythmics have an effect on neuropathic pain by blocking voltage-dependant sodium channels. It has been seen in certain studies that lidocaine infusions have alleviated pain from postherpetic neuralgia and diabetic neuropathy (101,102). Studies in 1988 and 1992 showed that mexiletine was effective in pain for diabetic neuropathy, and patients who received an intravenous lidocaine infusion along with mexiletine had longer duration of pain relief (103,104). Although these medications have been seen to alleviate pain in certain neuropathic pain syndromes such as postherpetic neuralgia and diabetic neuropathy, caution must be taken in prescribing these medications due to their side effect profiles.

Several drugs that mimic the inhibitory transmitter GABA, such as baclofen and clonazepam, have been shown to alleviate some pain symptoms. Baclofen is an agonist of the GABA-B receptor, and has been seen to prevent the release of excitatory neurotransmitters in alleviating pain with trigeminal neuralgia and muscle spasticity (105). Clonazepam, by modulating the GABA receptor, has been shown to be effective in certain cases of neuropathic pain as well (106).

The use of opioids for neuropathic pain is still controversial among many professionals in the field. Acute infusions of fentanyl and morphine have helped with postherpetic neuralgia as well as a certain population of neuropathic pain patients respectively (107,108). In addition, certain studies have shown the efficacy of oral oxycodone as well as tramadol in certain neuropathic syndromes (109,110). Although certain patient populations may benefit from opioid management, one must always use opioids with caution given the side effect profile and potential problems with chemical dependency.

Certain NMDA receptor blocking agents, such as ketamine, dextromethorphan, memantine, and amantadine have recently been researched extensively. Studies of small cohorts have shown that ketamine and dextromethorphan have efficacy in postherpetic neuralgia and diabetic neuropathy, respectively (111,112). Amantadine has been shown to be helpful in certain surgical neuropathies in cancer patients (113).

Certain topical medications, such as capsaicin and local anesthetics, have shown preliminary promise in alleviating certain types of neuropathic pain disorders.

Capsaicin has been helpful with postherpetic neuralgia as well as postmastectomy pain (114,115). However, the burning sensation of capsaicin limits its efficacy and overall effectiveness. Local anesthetics have been used in recent years, but more evidence is needed to prove its effectiveness in alleviating neuropathic pain.

Medical management of neuropathic pain consists of treatments using a variety of medications. Although some of these modalities are more effective than others, each medication must be titrated and evaluated with side effects profile in mind. Fortunately, new studies improve our knowledge of neuropathophysiology, with the hope of more precisely targeting neuropathic pain.

INTERVENTIONAL TREATMENTS

Many patients with neuropathic pain do not achieve satisfactory pain relief with medications alone. Recent reviews from the European Federation of Neurological Societies (EFNS) show that only 30% to 40% of patients obtain adequate relief from pharmacotherapy (116,117). Neuromodulation therapy is an expanding field; it is used to treat these various neuropathic conditions refractory to pharmacologic interventions, such as Parkinson disease, dystonia, obsessive-compulsive disorder, refractory pain, and CRPS. Techniques include transcutaneous electrical nerve stimulation (TENS) and peripheral nerve, spinal cord, deep brain, epidural motor cortex, and repetitive transcranial magnetic stimulation (118).

Deep Brain Stimulation

Electrical stimulation was used for pain control as early as 46 C.E., when Scribonius Largus suggested applying the live electric ray to the head of a patient suffering a headache (119). Recently, Fritsch and Hitzig noted various convulsions in response to electrical head stimulation (120). Since the 1950s, temporary electrodes had been implanted in various brain regions for control of pain via stimulation. Deep brain stimulation for the treatment of pain refractory to medical management was developed prior to the gate control theory (121). Deep brain targets in current use include the sensory (ventral posterior) thalamus and periventricular gray (PVG) matter. The targets used are contralateral to the pain if unilateral, or bilateral if indicated. Following use of MRI and stereotactic computer tomography for accurate target localization, an electrode is stereotactically inserted into the subcortical cerebrum. An implantable pulse generator (IPG) is placed subcutaneously in the chest or abdomen, and connected to these electrodes in an appropriate fashion (118).

Although deep brain stimulators have been studied for many years, the exact mechanisms of how they alleviate pain are still unclear. Studies in animals have shown that stimulation in the thalamic region suppresses deafferentation pain, possibly through thalamo-corticofugal descending pathways (118). Current research suggests ventral PVG stimulation engages nonopioid analgesia commensurate with coping behavior, while dorsal PVG stimulation may trigger "fight or flight" analgesia (122). Deep brain stimulation (DBS) was reported in the 1970s, when it was implanted in the thalamus for chronic pain (123,124). Irving Cooper performed multiple studies involving electrodes in the cerebellum and thalamic nuclei in over 200 patients in 1977. Although many of his studies were faulted for placebo effect and lack of efficacy, he showed that DBS studies had the advantage of being able to perform double blinded, prospective randomized trials (125).

In 1991, Blond and Siegfried reported thalamic DBS for tremor (126). Another study demonstrated that thalamic stimulation is safer than thalamotomy (127). In 2002, Pollak et al. evaluated novel sites for DBS, including the subthalamic nucleus of Luys (STN) (128). The use of DBS has been approved for general and segmental dystonia in 2003, and DBS trials for primary dystonia (PD) have shown efficacy (129). Since 1996, over 40,000 people worldwide have undergone placement of DBS systems for PD, essential tremor, and dystonia (125).

Due to the lack of conclusive evidence, the U.S. Food and Drug Administration removed approval for DBS for pain in 1989 (130). Furthermore, two multi-center ,open-labeled trials, which were completed in 1993 and 1998, showed only a 20% response rate (131). DBS may help patients who have medically refractory Parkinson disease, with prospective control trials showing improvement in both motor function and quality of life, but the effects of DBS on nonmotor aspects of Parkinson disease are unclear (132,133). Finally, refractory depression may be a target for DBS (134).

Many studies have looked at the treatment of DBS placement to alleviate neuropathic pain syndromes. Recently, a group from Milan has explored DBS of posterior hypothalamus for cluster headaches on the basis of PET studies that showed overreactivity in this region (135). DBS may be used after traumatic brain injury, epilepsy, and post-stroke central pain (136). Efficacy of DBS placement was evaluated in 47 patients with intractable neuropathic pain, including post-stroke, phantom limb, postherpetic, brachial plexus injury, anaesthesia dolorosa, and nerve damage. Phantom limb pain, head pain, and anaesthesia dolorosa showed improved pain relief. DBS of the PVG alone had the highest degree of pain alleviation (59%), and post stroke pain responded in 70% of patients (137).

However, long-term benefit from DBS for neuropathic pain remains controversial (138). Several reviews and one meta-analysis confirm that DBS is more effective for nociceptive pain compared to neuropathic pain (63%–47%) (139). Higher success rates for DBS are seen in patients with peripheral lesions such as phantom limb pain, radiculopathies, plexopathies, and neuropathies, with a mean long-term success rate of 46% (118). A meta-analysis was done in 2005 looking at six studies from 1977 to 1997, with long-term pain alleviation occurring with DBS of the PVG and/or periaqueductal grey matter (PAG) (79%).

Motor Cortex Stimulation (MCS)

Past studies have shown that electrical stimulation can exert strong inhibitory influences on the nervous system. Neuronal targets include large afferent peripheral fibers, spinal dorsal columns, thalamic sensory nuclei, or PAG (140). In the past decade, MCS has become a prominent modality in the treatment of drug resistant neuropathic pain. This technique consists of implanting epidural electrodes over the motor strip through a frontoparietal craniotomy or under a burr hole under local anesthesia. Following this, one or two quadripolar electrodes are placed over the motor representation of the painful region in appropriate relation to the central sulcus. Similar to the DBS, the electrode is then connected to a subcutaneous IPG (118).

MCS appears to trigger rapid activation in the lateral thalamus, which can lead to a cascade of subsequent events in the medial thalamus, anterior cingulated orbitofrontal cortices, and PAG (141–143). Activity in these structures relative to actual cortical neurostimulation becomes maximal during the hours that follow MCS arrest. One current hypothesis is that the emotional appraisal of pain may be modulated by activation of orbitofrontal and perigenual regions, and top down activation of brainstem PAG may lead to descending inhibition towards the spinal cord and possible release of endogenous opioids (118,141–143).

MCS was first reported by Tsubokawa et al., who showed that eight out of twelve patients had favorable pain relief one year after placement of motor cortex stimulation for deafferentation pain secondary to central nervous system lesions (144). In 2007, Lazorthes et al. discussed MCS as the treatment of choice in post-stroke pain, thalamic pain, facial anesthesia dolorosa, or brachial plexus avulsion. They concluded that the efficacy of MCS depends on accurate placement of the electrodes in the motor cortex and the programming of the stimulation parameters (145). Although randomized controlled studies for MCS have not been reported, case studies with over 200 patients indicate that 50% to 60% of patients with medically refrac-

tory neuropathic pain may benefit from the procedure (141,145). MCS was initially proposed to treat cases of central neuropathic pain caused by thalamic and suprathalamic lesions after failed treatment with dorsal column stimulation, periaqueductal, or thalamic stimulation (144).

Since initial reports in the 1990s, MCS of the M1 region of the cortex has been used to treat refractory pain conditions and a variety of movement disorders. Tsubokawa and Katayama found that 59% of patients who underwent DBS or MCS for post-stroke involuntary movements had benefit, while 19% of patients who underwent MCS primarily for pain control showed improvement (146). A recent randomized, double-blind trial looked at eleven patients with unilateral neuropathic pain; eight patients reported long-term pain relief from MCS placement (142). A retrospective study in 2006 evaluated 17 patients with chronic neuropathic pain (trigeminal neuropathic pain and post-stroke pain) with placement of unilateral MCS, showing long-term pain relief (143). MCS may also be beneficial for facial neuropathic pain and central post stroke pain (CPSP) (147,148). Katayama et al. showed success rates for 48% of patients with CPSP, and Nuti et al. reported a 52% success rate in 31 patients with various neuropathic pain conditions, mostly CPSP in origin (149,150).

Peripheral Nerve Stimulation (PNS)

Since the gate control theory proposed by Melzack and Wall, many electrical methods for stimulation to alleviate pain have been researched (151). TENS produces activation of Ab fibers to invoke paresthesias at a painful region. To provide a more stable and efficient stimulation, percutaneous electrodes can be implanted to contact the nerve and connected subcutaneously to a stimulation unit.

PNS was described in 1966 and 1967, with eight patients achieving pain relief as long as the stimulator was on (152). In 1976, Sweet et al. reported an overall success rate of 25%, and in 1982, Nashold et al. reported a success rate of 43% with PNS (153,154). Resurgence of the PNS approach may be credited to Weiner and Reed, who described the percutaneous technique of electrode insertion into the vicinity of the occipital nerves to treat occipital neuralgia (155). Since then, PNS has been used for neuropathic pain related to herniorrhaphy, low back pain, sacroiliac dysfunction, postherpetic neuralgia, post-surgical pain, migraines, occipital pain, CRPS, fibromyalgia, coccygodynia, and chronic abdominal pain (156).

The exact mechanisms of action are still unclear. However, certain animal studies have hinted that direct excitation of central pain processing systems and increases in excitability, as well as stimulation of the dorsal rostral pons and anterior cingulated cortex, may lead to responses to PNS (156,157).

The research with TENS units and neuropathic pain includes nine controlled trials in which approximately 200 patients with neuropathic pain participated (118,150). TENS units provided more alleviation of pain compared to placebo. For PNS, six clinical trials, totaling 202 patients with various neuropathies or mixed pains, reported an average success rate of 55% to 65% in relieving pain symptoms (118,150). Mobbs et al. concluded that over 60% of patients with pain in a peripheral nerve distribution had a significant improvement in their lifestyle and pain control following implantation of PNS (158).

Spinal Cord Stimulation (SCS)

Spinal cord stimulation has become accepted therapeutic modality for the treatment of intractable pain syndromes. SCS is an adjustable, nondestructive neuromodulatory procedure that delivers therapeutic doses of electrical current to the spinal cord for the management of neuropathic pain (159). The concepts behind this mode of treatment go back to concept of gate-control theory by Melzack and Wall and the stimulation of large myelinated nerve fibers (160). In 1967, Shealy inserted the first dorsal column stimulator, and since that time great advances have been made in the field (160,161).

The sympatholysis effect of SCS is the most obvious of its therapeutic effects. This is responsible in its effectiveness in treating peripheral ischemia, cardiac ischemia, CRPS, failed back syndrome, phantom pain, post amputation stump pain, diabetic neuropathy, postherpetic neuralgia, and multiple sclerosis (162). SCS is applied through an electrical generator that delivers pulses by means of electrodes placed in the epidural space adjacent to a targeted spinal cord area (Fig. 38.1). The electrodes can be implanted by laminectomy or percutaneously, and can be unipolar, bipolar, or tripolar. The parameters involved (amplitude, pulse width, electrode selection) and number of leads may vary with intensity of the pain and nerve roots.

SCS for CRPS was investigated by Kumar et al., who reported that all 12 patients with permanently implanted leads experienced good to very good results for pain control (163). In another series, Kemler et al. looked at an additional 23 cases, with 78% of the patients reporting improvement (164). A series of 54 patients who were randomized either to SCS with physical therapy or physical therapy alone showed a 67% pain relief in the SCS group, with five-year follow up (165). Overall, prospective studies demonstrate success rates of up to 84% (159–161, 166). In addition, in eight

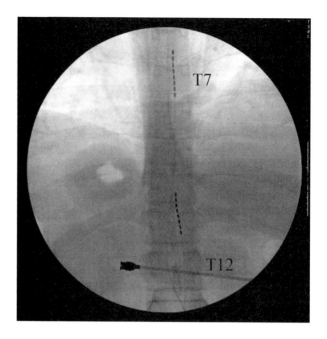

FIGURE 38.1

Spinal cord stimulator leads placed under fluoroscopic guidance. Needle is placed in the epidural space at T7 to cover abdominal pain and at T11 for testicular pain.

retrospective studies the overall success rate was 84% in 192 patients (162).

SCS has been evaluated most extensively for postlaminectomy pain syndromes. Systematic reviews of the literature show greater than 50% pain relief for 50% of patients (169). A prospective, multicenter study also reported a 55% success rate for stimulation after one-year follow up (170). Abdominal and visceral pain have also been looked at in the context of SCS. Khan et al. reported nine patients with refractory abdominal pain had significant improvement in pain scores as well as decreased narcotic use. Additionally, Nienke et al. conducted a prospective study for SCS in patients with angina pectoris, demonstrating improvement of quality of life and pain symptoms after three months of SCS placement (171).

Repetitive Transcranial Magnetic Stimulation (rTMS)

The use of rTMS in patients with chronic pain aims at noninvasive cortical stimulation to produce analgesic effects (172). The stimulation is performed by applying a coil of a magnetic stimulator on the scalp, above a targeted cortical region. Intensity of stimulation is measured and stimulation is performed just below motor threshold. One session should last 20 minutes and 1000 pulses, although frequency and pulses vary among patients. Stimulation is thought to activate fibers through the motor cortex and project to other processes in the neuropathic pain processing. Reviews of rTMS include 14 controlled studies looking at 280 patients with definite neuropathic pain. From these studies, there is moderate evidence that rTMS of the motor cortex using figure of eight coil and high frequency (5–20 Hz) induces significant pain relief in CPSP and other neuropathic pain conditions (118,150). However, because the results are modest and short-term, rTMS should not be used as the sole treatment. It has been observed that a positive response to high frequency rTMS is probably predictive of a positive outcome of subsequent MCS.

CONCLUSION

Although neuromodulation has been used for many years, new innovative ideas and studies are being published about this treatment modality. Peripheral, deep brain, motor, and spinal cord stimulation and rTMS for the alleviation of neuropathic pain give patients options that may be preferable to other treatment modalities. These scientific advances will be the building blocks for research in neuromodulation.

References

1. Merskey H, Bogduk N. *Classification of Chronic Pain*. Seattle: IASP Press; 1994.
2. Gilron I, Watson CP, Cahill CM, Moulin DE. Neuropathic pain: a practical guide for the clinician. *CMAJ*. 175(3):265–275.
3. Jensen TS, et al. The clinical picture of neuropathic pain. *Eur J Pharmacol*. 2001;429(1–3):1–11.
4. Bennet M. The LANSS Pain Scale: the Leeds assessment of neuropathic symptoms and signs. (St. Gemma's Hospice, Leeds, United Kingdom). *Pain*. 2004;92:147–157.
5. Yucel A. Results of the leeds assessment of neuropathic symptoms and signs pain scale in Turkey: a validation study. *J Pain*. 2003;5(8):427–432.
6. Bouhassira D, et al. Development and validation of the Neuropathic Pain Symptom Inventory. *Pain*. 2004;108:248–257.
7. Cruccu G, Anand P, Attal N. et al. EFNS guidelines on neuropathic pain assessment. *Eur J Neurol*. 2004;11:153–162.
8. Galli SJ, Nakae S, Tsai M. Mast cells in the development of adaptive immune responses. *Nat Immunol*. 2005;6:135–142.
9. Zuo Y, Perkins NM, Tracey DJ, Geczy CL. Inflammation and hyperalgesia induced by nerve injury in the rat: a key role of „m,ast cells. *Pain*, 2003;105:467–479.
10. Mizumura K, Koda H, Kumazawa T. Possible contribution of protein kinase C in the effects of histamine on the visceral nociceptor activities in vitro. *Neurosci Res*. 2000;37:183–190.
11. Baron R, Schwarz K, Kleinert A, Schattschneider J, Wasner G. Histamine-induced itch converts into pain in neuropathic hyperalgesia. *Neuroreport*. 2001;12:3475–3478.
12. Kashiba H, Fukui H, Morikawa Y, Senba E. Gene expression of histamine H1 receptor in guinea pig primary sensory neurons: a relationship between H1 receptor mRNA-expressing neurons and peptidergic neurons. *Brain Res Mol Brain Res*. 1999;66:24–34.
13. Thacker A, et al. Pathophysiology of peripheral neuropathic pain: immune cells and molecules. *Anasth Analg*. 2007;105(3):838–847.
14. Witko-Sarsat V, Rieu P, Scamps-Latscha B, Lesavre P, Halbwachs-Mecarelli L. Neutrophils: molecules, functions and pathophysiological aspects. *Lab Invest*. 2000;80:617–653.
15. Faurschou M, Borregaard N. Neutrophil granules and secretory vesicles in inflammation. *Microbes Infect*. 2003;5:1317–1327.
16. Griffin JW, George R, Ho T. Macro,-phage systems in peripheral nerves. A review. *J Neuropathol Exp Neurol*. 1993;52:553–560.
17. Perry VH, Brown MC, Gordon S. The macrophage response to central and peripheral nerve injury. A possible role for macrophages in regeneration. *J Exp Med*. 1987;165:1218–1223.
18. Taskinen HS, Roytta M. The dynamics of macrophage recruitment after nerve transection. *Acta Neuropathol (Berl)*. 1997;93:252–259.
19. Myers RR, Heckman HM, Rodriguez M. Reduced hyperalgesia in nerve-injured WLD mice: relationship to nerve fiber phagocytosis, axonal degeneration, and regeneration in normal mice. *Exp Neurol*. 1996;141:94–101.
20. Liu T, van Rooijen N, Tracey DJ. Depletion of macrophages reduces axonal degeneration and hyperalgesia following nerve injury. *Pain*. 2000;86:25–32.
21. Rutkowski MD, Pahl JL, Sweitzer S, van Rooijen N, DeLeo JA. Limited role of macrophages in generation of nerve injuryinduced mechanical allodynia. *Physiol Behav*. 2000;71:225–235.
22. Heumann R, Lindholm D, Bandtlow C, et al. Differential regulation of mRNA encoding nerve growth factor and its receptor in rat sciatic nerve during development, degeneration, and regeneration: role of macrophages. *Proc Natl Acad Sci USA*. 1987;84:8735–8739.
23. Wagner R, Myers RR. Schwann cells produce tumor necrosis factor alpha: expression in injured and non-injured nerves. *Neuroscience*. 1996;73:625–629.
24. Shamash S, Reichert F, Rotshenker S. The cytokine network of Wallerian degeneration: tumor necrosis factor-alpha, interleukin-1alpha, and interleukin-1beta. *J Neurosci*. 2002;22:3052–3060.
25. Bolin LM, Verity AN, Silver JE, Shooter EM, Abrams JS. Interleukin-6 production by Schwann cells and induction in sciatic nerve injury. *J Neurochem*. 1995;64:850–858.
26. Liu GJ, Werry EL, Bennett MR.Secretion of ATP from Schwann cells in response to uridine triphosphate. *Eur J Neurosci*. 2005;21:151–160.
27. Keswani SC, Polley M, Pardo CA, Griffin JW, McArthur JC, Hoke A. Schwann cell chemokine receptors mediate HIV-1 gp120 toxicity to sensory neurons. *Ann Neurol*. 2003;54:287–296.
28. Cui JG, Holmin S, Mathiesen T, Meyerson BA, Linderoth B. Possible role of inflammatory mediators in tactile hypersensitivity in rat models of mononeuropathy. *Pain*. 2000;88:239–248.
29. Moalem G, Xu K, Yu L. T lymphocytes play a role in neuropathic pain following peripheral nerve injury in rats. *Neuroscience*. 2004;129:767–777.
30. George A, Schmidt C, Weishaupt A, Toyka KV, Sommer C. Serial determination of tumor necrosis factor-alpha content in rat sciatic nerve after chronic constriction injury. *Exp Neuro*. 1999;160:124–132.
31. Schafers M, Svensson CI, Sommer C, Sorkin LS. Tumor necrosis factor-alpha induces mechanical allodynia after spinal nerve ligation by activation of p38 MAPK in primary sensory neurons. *J Neurosci*. 2003;23:2517–2521.
32. Lindenlaub T, Sommer C. Cytokines in sural nerve biopsies from inflammatory and non-inflammatory neuropathies. *Acta Neuropathol (Berl)*. 2003;105:593–602.
33. Banner LR, Patterson PH. Major changes in the expression of the mRNAs for cholinergic differentiation factor/leukemia inhibitory factor and its receptor after injury to adult peripheral nerves and ganglia. *Proc Natl Acad Sci USA*. 1994;91:7109–7113.

34. Thompson SW, Vernallis AB, Heath JK, Priestley JV. Leukaemia inhibitory factor is retrogradely transported by a distinct population of adult rat sensory neurons: co-localization with trkA and other neurochemical markers. *Eur J Neurosci.* 1997;9:1244–1251.

35. Sugiura S, Lahav R, Han J, et al. Leukaemia inhibitory factor is required for normal inflammatory responses to injury in the peripheral and central nervous systems in vivo and is chemotactic for macrophages in vitro. *Eur J Neurosci.* 2000;12: 457–466.

36. Boddeke EW. Involvement of chemokines in pain. *Eur J Pharmacol.* 2001;429:115–119.

37. Tofaris GK, Patterson PH, Jessen KR, Mirsky R. Denervated Schwann cells attract macrophages by secretion of leukemia inhibitory factor (LIF) and monocyte chemoattractant protein-1 in a process regulated by interleukin-6 and LIF. *J Neurosci.* 2002;22:6696–6703.

38. Abbadie C, Lindia JA, Cumiskey AM, et al. Impaired neuropathic pain responses in mice lacking the chemokine receptor CCR2. *Proc Natl Acad Sci USA.* 2003;100:7947–7952.

39. Indo Y, Tsuruta M, Hayashida Y, et al. Mutations in the TRKA/NGF receptor gene in patients with congenital insensitivity to pain with anhidrosis. *Nat Genet.* 1996;13:485–488.

40. Bonnington JK, McNaughton PA. Signalling pathways involved in the sensitisation of mouse nociceptive neurones by nerve growth factor. *J Physiol.* 2003;551:433–446.

41. Zhang YH, Vasko MR, Nicol GD. Ceramide, a putative second messenger for nerve growth factor, modulates the TTXresistant Na current and delayed rectifier K current in rat sensory neurons. *J Physiol.* 2002;544:385–402.

42. Otten U, Ehrhard P, Peck R. Nerve growth factor induces growth and differentiation of human B lymphocytes. *Proc Natl Acad Sci USA.* 1989;86:10059–10063.

43. Raivich G, Hellweg R, Kreutzberg GW. NGF receptormediated reduction in axonal NGF uptake and retrograde transport following sciatic nerve injury and during regeneration. *Neuron.* 1991;7:151–164.

44. Lai J, et al. The role of voltage-gated sodium channels in neuropathic pain. *Curr Opin Neurobiol.* 2003;13:291–297.

45. Amir R, et al. Oscillatory mechanism in primary sensory neurones. *Brain.* 2002;125:421–435.

46. Jacobs JM, et al. Vascular leakage in the dorsal root ganglia of the rat, studied with horseradish peroxidase. *J Neurol Sci.* 1976;29:95–107.

47. Meier T, et al. Efficacy of lidocaine patch 5% in the treatment of focal peripheral neuropathic pain syndromes: a randomized, double-blind, placebocontrolled study. *Pain.* 2003;106:151–158.

48. Catarina MJ, et al. Impaired nociception and pain sensation in mice lacking the capsaicin receptor. *Science.* 2000;288:306–313.

49. Hudson LJ, et al. VR1 protein expression increases in undamaged DRG neurons after partial nerve injury. *Eur J Neurosci.* 2001;13:2105–2114.

50. Hong S, Wiley JW. Early painful diabetic neuropathy is associated with differential changes in the expression and function of vanilloid receptor 1. *J Biol Chem.* 2005;280:618–627.

51. Alessandri-Haber N, et al. Transient receptor potential vanilloid 4 is essential in chemotherapyinduced neuropathic pain in the rat. *J Neurosci.* 2004;24:4444–4452.

52. Patapoutian A, et al. ThermoTRP channels and beyond: mechanisms of temperature sensation. *Nat Rev Neurosci.* 2003;4:529–539.

53. McKemy DD, et al. Identification of a cold receptor reveals a general role for TRP channels in thermosensation. *Nature.* 2002;416:52–58.

54. Wasner G, et al. Topical menthol—a human model for cold pain by activation and sensitisation of C nociceptors. *Brain.* 2004;127:1159–1171.

55. Price DD, et al. Analysis of peak magnitude and duration of analgesia produced by local anesthetics injected into sympathetic ganglia of complex regional pain syndrome patients. *Clin J Pain.* 1998;14:216–226.

56. Choi B, Rowbotham MC. Effect of adrenergic receptor activation on post-herpetic neuralgia pain and sensory disturbances. *Pain.* 1997;69:55–63.

57. Ali Z, et al. Intradermal injection of norepinephrine evokes pain in patients with sympathetically maintained pain. *Pain.* 2000;88:161–168.

58. Tal M, Bennett GJ. Extra-territorial pain in rats with a peripheral mononeuropathy: mechanohyperalgesia and mechano-allodynia in the territory of an uninjured nerve. *Pain.* 2004;57:375–382.

59. Moore KA, et al. Partial peripheral nerve injury promotes a selective loss of GABAergic inhibition in the superficial dorsal horn of the spinal cord. *J Neurosci.* 2002;22:6724–6731.

60. Baron R. Mechanisms of disease: neuropathic pain-a clinical perspective. *Nat Clin Pract.* February 2006;2(2):95–106.

61. Johnsoe R, et al. The effect of intensive diabetes therapy on the development and progression of neuropathy. The Diabetes Control and Complications Trial Research Group. *Ann Intern Med.* 1997;122(8):561–568.

62. Kennedy PG. Varicella-zoster virus latency in human ganglia. *Rev Med Virol.* 2002;12(5):327–334.

63. Gilden DH, Cohrs RJ, Mahalingam R. Clinical and molecular pathogenesis of varicella virus infection. *Viral Immunol.* 2003;16(3):243–258.

64. Peterslund NA. Herpesvirus infection: an overview of the clinical manifestations. *Scand J Infect Dis Suppl.* 1999;80:15–20.

65. Johnson RW, Dworkin RH. Clinical review: treatment of herpes zoster and postherpetic neuralgia. *BMJ.* 2003;326(7392):748.

66. Dworkin RH, Johnson RW, Breuer J, et al. Recommendations for the management of herpes zoster. *Clin Infect Dis.* 2007;44(Suppl 1):S1–S26.

67. Katz J, Cooper EM, Walther RR, Sweeney EW, Dworkin RH. Acute pain in herpes zoster and its impact on health-related quality of life. *Clin Infect Dis.* 2006;39(3):342–348.

68. Stankus SJ, Dlugopolski M, Packer D. Management of herpes 2000; zoster (shingles) and postherpetic neuralgia. *Am Fam Physician.* 61(8):2437–2444, 2447–2448.

69. Wadd NJ, Lucraft HH. Brachial plexus neuropathy following mantle radiotherapy. *Clin Oncol.* 1998;10:399–400.

70. Bajrovic A, Rades D, Fehlauer F, et al. Is there a life-long risk of brachial plexopathy after radiotherapy of supraclavicular lymph nodes in breast cancer patients? *Radiother Oncol.* 2004;71:297–301.

71. Pierce SM, Recht A, Lingos TI, et al. Long term radiation complications following conservative surgery (CS) and radiation therapy (RT) in patients with early stage breast cancer. *Int J Radial Oncol Biol Phys.* 1992;23:915–923.

72. Nich C, Bonnin P, Laredo JD, Sedel L. An uncommon form of delayed radio-induced brachial plexopathy. *Chir Main.* 2005;24:48–51.

73. Windebank A, Grisold W. Chemotherapy-induced neuropathy. *J Periph Nerv Syst.* 2006;13(1):27–46.

74. Chaudhry V, Chaudhry M, Crawford TO, Simmons-O'Brien E, Griffin JW. Toxic neuropathy in patients with pre-existing neuropathy. *Neurology.* January 28, 2003;60(2):337–340.

75. Tanner KD, Levine JD, Topp KS. Microtubule disorientation and axonal swelling in unmyelinated sensory axons during vincristine-induced pain neuropathy in rat. *J Comp Neurol.* 1998;395:481–492.

76. Topp KS, Tanner KD, Levine JD. Damage to the cytoskeleton of large diameter sensory neurons and myelinated axons in vincristine-induced painful peripheral neuropathy in the rat. *J Comp Neurol.* 2000;424:563–576.

77. Jaeckle KA. Neurological manifestations of neoplastic and radiation-induced plexopathies. *Semin Neurol.* December 2004;24(4):385–393.

78. Dalmau J, Graus F, Marco M. "Hot and dry foot" as initial manifestation of neoplastic lumbosacral plexopathy. *Neurology.* 1989;39:871–872.

79. Harper CM Jr, Thomas JE, Cascino TL, Litchy WJ. Distinction between neoplastic and radiation-induced brachial plexopathy, with emphasis on the role of EMG. *Neurology.* April 1989;39(4):502–506.

80. Kori SH, Foley KM, Posner JB. Brachial plexus lesions in patients with cancer: 100 cases. *Neurology.* January 1981;31(1):45–50.

81. Uceyler N, Eberle T, Rolke R, et al. Differential expression patterns of cytokines in complex regional pain syndrome. *Pain.* September 2007;132(1–8):195–205.

82. Blaes F, Tschernatsch M, Braeu ME, Matz O, Schmitz K, Nascimento D. Autoimmunity in complex-regional pain syndrome. *Ann N Y Acad Sci.* June 2007;1107:168–173.

83. Veldman PH, Reynen HM, Arntz IE, Goris RJ. Signs and symptoms of reflex sympathetic dystrophy: prospective study of 829 patients. *Lancet.* October 23, 1993;342(8878):1012–1016.

84. Maleki J, LeBel AA, Bennett GJ, et al. Patterns of spread in complex regional pain syndrome, type I (reflex sympathetic dystrophy). *Pain.* December 1, 2000;88(3):259–266.

85. Werner R, Davidoff G, Jackson MD, et al. Factors affecting the sensitivity and specificity of the three-phase technetium bone scan in the diagnosis of reflex sympathetic dystrophy syndrome in the upper extremity. *J Hand Surg [Am].* May 1989;14(3):520–523.

86. Schwartzman RJ, Maleki J. Postinjury neuropathic pain syndromes. *Med Clin North Am.* 1999;83:597–626.

87. Canavero S, Bonicalzi V. Central pain syndrome: Elucidation of genesis and treatment. *Expert Rev Neurother.* November 2007;7(11):1485–1497.

88. Melzack R, Wall P. *Handbook of Pain Management.* New York: Churchill Livingstone; 2003.

89. Janig W, Levine JD, Michaelis M. Interactions of Sympathetic and primary afferent neurons following nerve injury and tissue trauma. *Prog Brain Res.* 1996;113:161–184.

90. Wall PD, Gutnick M. Ongoing activity in peripheral nerves: the physiology and pharmacology of impulses originating from a neuroma. *Exp Neurol.* 1974;43:580–593.

91. Devor M, Rappaport ZH. Pain and pathophysiology of damaged nerves. In: Fields H1, ed., *Pain Syndromes in Neurology.* London: Butterworth; 1990:47–84.

92. Mollay B, Fishman S, Raja S, Liu S. *Essentials of Pain Medicine and Regional Anesthesia.* Second edition. Churchill living stone Inc. 2005.

93. McQuay H, Carroll D, Jadad A, Wiffen P, Moore A. Anticonvulsant drugs for management of pain: a systematic review. *Br Med J.* 1995;311:1047.

94. Max M, Lych S, et al. Effects of desipramine, amitriptyline and fluoxetine on pain in diabetic neuropathy. *N Engl J Med.* 1992;326:1250.

95. McQuay HJ, Tramer M, et al. A systematic review of antidepressants in neuropathic pain. *Pain.* 1996;68:217–227.

96. Sindrup S, Jensen T. Efficacy of pharmacological treatments of neuropathic pain: an update and effect related to mechanism of drug action. *Pain.* 1999;83:389–400.

97. Backonja M, Beydoun A, Edwards K, et al. Gabapentin for the symptomatic treatment of painful neuropathy in patients with diabetes mellitus: a randomized controlled trial. *J Am Med Assoc.* 1998;280:1831–1836.

98. Rowbotham M, Harden N, et al. Gabapentin for the treatment of postherpetic neuralgia: a randomized controlled trial. *J Am Med Assoc.* 1998;280:1837–1842.

99. Rowbotham MC, Reisner-Keller LA, Fields HL. Both intravenous lidocaine and morphine reduce the pain of postherpetic neuralgia. *Ann Neurol.* 1991;37:246–253.

100. Kastrup J, Petersen P, Dejgard A, Angelo HR, Hilsted J. Intravenous lidocaine infusion—a new treatment of chronic painful diabetic neuropathy? *Pain.* 1987;28:69–75.

101. Dejgard A, Petersen P, Kastrup P. Mexilitine for treatment of chronic painful diabetic neuropathy. *Lancet.* 1988;I:9.

102. Chabal C, Jacobson L, Mariano A, Chaney E, Britell CW. The use of oral mexiletine for the treatment of pain after peripheral nerve injury. *Anesthesiology.* 1992;76:513–517.

103. Fields H. Treatment of trigeminal neuralgia. *New Engl J Med.* 1996;334:1125.

104. Bartusch S, Sanders B, Dalessio J, Jernigan J. Clonazepam for the treatment of lancinating phantom limb pain. *Clin J Pain.* 1996;12:59–62.

105. Rowbotham MC, Reisner-Keller LA, Fields HL. Both intravenous lidocaine and morphine reduce the pain of postherpetic neuralgia. *Ann Neurol.* 1991;37:246–253.

106. Dellemijn P, Vanneste J. Randomized double blind active placebo controlled crossover trial of intravenous fentanyl in neuropathic pain. *Lancet.* 1997;349:753–758.

107. Watson C, Babul N. Efficacy of oxycodone in neuropathic pain: a randomized trial in postherpetic neuralgia. *Neurology.* 1998;50:1837–1841.

108. Harati Y, Gooch C, Swenson M, et al. Maintenance of the long term effectiveness of tramadol in treatment of the pain of diabetic neuropathy. *J Diabetes Complications.* 2000;14:65–70.

109. Eide P, Stubhaug A, Stenehjam A. Central dysesthesia pain after traumatic spinal cord injury is dependant on N-methyl-D-aspartate activation. *Neurosurgery.* 1995;37:1080–1087.

110. Nelson K, Park K, Robinovitz E. High-dose oral dextromethorphan versus placebo in painful diabetic neuropathy and postherpetic neuralgia. *Neurology.* 1997;48:1212.

111. Pud D, Eisenberg E, et al. The NMDA receptor antagonist amantadine reduces surgical neuropathic pain in cancer patients: a double blind, randomized placebo controlled trial. *Pain.* 1998;75:349–354.

112. Bernstein JE, Korman NJ, Bickers DR, Dahl MV, Millikan LE. Topical capsaicin treatment of chronic postherpetic neuralgia. *J Am Acad Dermatol.* 1998;21:265–270.

113. Watson C, Tyler K, Bickers D. A randomized vehicle-controlled trial of topical capsaicin in the treatment of postherpetic neuralgia. *Clinical Therapy.* 1993;15:510.

114. Finnerup NB, Otto M, McQuay HJ, et al. Algorithm for neuropathic pain treatment: an evidence based proposal. *Pain.* 2005;118:289–305.

115. Attal N, Cruccu G, Haanpaa M, et al. EFNS guidelines on pharmacological treatment of neuropathic pain. *Eur J Neurol.* 2006;13:1153–1169.

116. Cruccu G, Aziz TZ, Garcia-Larrea L, et al. EFNS guidelines on neurostimulation therapy for neuropathic pain. *Eur J Neurol.* 2007;14:952–970.

117. Rossi U. The history of electrical stimulation of eth nervous system for the control of pain. In: Simpson BA, ed. *Electrical Stimulation and the Relief of Pain,* 1st ed. Amsterdam: Elsevier B.V.; 2003:5–16.

118. Fritsch G, Hitzig E. The electrical excitability of the cerebrum. In: Wilkins RW, ed. *Neurosurgical Classics,* 1st ed. Thieme Medical Pubishers, Inc. American Association of Neurological Surgeons; 1992:15–27.

119. Heath RG, Mickle WA. Evaluation of seven years' experience with depth electrode studies in human patient. In: Ramey ER, ODoherty DS, eds. *Electrical Studies on the Unanesthetized Brain.* New York: Paul B. Hoeber; 1960:214–247.

120. Green AL, Wang S, Owen SL, et al. Stimulating the human midbrain to reveal the link between pain and blood pressure. *Pain.* 2006;124:349–359.

121. Hosobuchi Y, Adams JE, Rutkin B. Deep Barin stimulation for chronic pain. In: Burchiel KJ, ed. *Surgical Management of Pain,* 1st ed. New York: Thieme; 2002:565–576.

122. Mazars G, Merienne L, Cioloca C. Treatment of certain types of pain with implantable thalamic stimulators. *Neurochirurgie.* 1974;20:117–124.

123. Schwalb J, Hamani C. The history and future of deep brain stimulation. *Neurotherapeutics.* January 2008;5:3–13.

124. Blond S, Siegfried J. Thalamic stimulation for the treatment of tremor and other movement disorders. *Acta Neurochir Suppl (Wien).* 1991;52:109–111.

125. Schwalb JM, Lozano AM. Surgical management of tremor. *Neurosurg Q.* 2004;14:60–68.

126. Pollak P, Benabid AL, Gross C, et al. Effects of the stimulation of the subthalamic nucleus in Parkinsons disease. *Rev Neurol (Paris).* 1993;149:175–176.

127. Kupsch A, Benecke R, Muller J, et al. Pallidal deep-brain stimulation in primary generalized or segmental dystonia. *N Engl J Med.* 2006;355:1978–1990.

128. Gildenberg PL. History of movement disorder surgery. In: Lozano AM, ed. *Movement Disorder Surgery,* 1st ed. Basel: Karger; 2000:1–20.

129. Coffey RJ. Deep brain stimulation for chronic pain: results of two multicenter trials and a structured review. *Pain Med.* 2001;2:183–192.

130. Yu H, Neimat JS. The treatment of movement disorders by neural deep brain stimulation. *Neurotherapeutics.* 2008; 5:26–36.

131. Deuschl G, Schade-Brittinger C, Krack P, et al. A randomized trial of deep brain stimulation for Parkinsons disease. *N Engl J Med.* 2006;355:896–908.

132. Larson PS. Deep brain stimulation for psychiatric disorders. *Neurotherapeutics.* 2008;5:50–58.

133. Leone M, Franzini A, Felisati G, et al. Deep brain stimulation for treatment resistant depression. *Neuron.* 2005;45:651–660.

134. Schiff ND, Giacino JT, Kalmar K, et al. Behavioral improvements with thalamic stimulation after severe traumatic brain injury. *Nature.* 2007;448:600–603.

135. Owen S, Green A, Nandi D, et al. Deep Brain stimulation for neuropathic pain. *Acta Neurochirurgica.* 2007;97 (Pt 2):111–116.

136. Hamani C, Schwalb JM, Rezai AR, Dostrovsky JG, Davis KD, Lozano AM. Deep brain stimulation for chronic neuropathic pain: long term outcome and the incidence of insertional effect. *Pain.* 125(2006):188–196.

137. Bittar RG, Kar-Purkayastha I, Owen SL, et al. Deep brain stimulation for pain relief: a meta analysis. *J Clin Neurosci.* 2005;12:515–519.

138. Garcia-Larrea Luis, Peyron R,. Motor cortex stimulation for neuropathic pain: from phenomenology to mechanisms. *NeuroImage.* 37(2007):S71–S79.

139. Arle J, Shils J. Motor cortex stimulation for pain and movement disorders. *Neurotherapeutics.* January 2008;5:37–49.

140. Velasco F, Arguelles C, et al. Efficacy of motor cortex stimulation in the treatment of neuropathic pain:a randomized double blind trial. *J Neurosurg.* 2008;108:698–706.

141. Rasche D, Ruppolt M, et al. Motor cortex stimulation for long term relief of chronic neuropathic pain: a 10 year experience. *Pain.* 2006;121:43–52.

142. Tsubokawa T, Katayama Y, et al. Chronic motor cortex stimulation for the treatment of central pain. *Acta Neurochirurgica.* 1991;52:137–139.

143. Lazorthes Y, Sol JC, et al. Motor cortex stimulation for neuropathic pain. *Acta Neurochirurgica.* 2007;97(Pt 2): 37–44.

144. Katayama Y, Fukaya C, et al. Control of post stroke involuntary and voluntary movement disorders with deep brain or epidural cortical stimulation. *Stereotact Funct Neurosurg.* 1997;69:73–79.

145. Brown J, Pilitsis J, et al. Motor cortex stimulation for central and neuropathic pain. *Neurosurgery.* 2005;56:290–297.

146. Katayama Y, Yamamoto T, et al. Motor cortex stimulation for post stroke pain: comparison of spinal cord and thalamic stimulation. *Stereotact Funct Neurosurg.* 2001;77:183–186.

147. Nuti C, et al. Motor cortex stimulation for refractory neuropathic pain: four year outcome and predictors of efficacy. *Pain.* 2005;118:43–52.

148. Melzack R, Wall PD. Pain mechanisms: a new theory. *Science(NY).* 1965;150:971–979.

149. Wall PD, Sweet WH. Temporary abolition of pain in man. *Science.* 1967;155:108–109.

150. Sweet WH. Control of pain by direct stimulation of peripheral nerves. *Clin Neurosurg.* 1976;23:103–111.

151. Nashold BS Jr, Goldner JL, et al. Long term pain control by direct peripheral nerve stimulation. *J Bone Joint Surg Br.* 1985;67:470–472.

152. Weiner Rl, Reed KL. Peripheral neurostimulation for control of intractable occipital neuralgia. *Neuromodulation.* 1999;2:217–221.

153. Slavin K. Peripheral nerve stimulation for neuropathic pain. *Neurotherapeutics.* January 2008;5:100–106.

154. Bartsch T, et al. Stimulation of the greater occipital nerve induces increased central excitability of dural afferent input. *Brain.* 2002;125:1496–1509.

155. Mobbs RJ, Nair S, et al. Peripheral nerve stimulation for the treatment of chronic pain. *J Clin Neurosci.* 2007;14:216–221.

156. Falowski S, Celii A, et al. Spinal cord stimulation: an update. *Neurotherapeutics.* January 2008;5:86–99.

157. Shealy CN, Cady RK. Historical perspective of pain management. In: Weiner S, ed. *Pain Management: A Practical Guide for Clinicians.* 5th ed. Boca Raton FL: St. Lucie Press; 1998:7–15.

158. Shealy CN, Mortimer JT, et al. Electrical inhibition of pain by stimulation of the dorsal columns: preliminary clinical report. *Anesth Analg.* 1967;46:489–491.

159. Mailis-Gagnon A, Furlan AD, et al. Apinal cord stimulation for chronic pain (review). *Cochrane Database Syst Rev.* 2004;(3):CD003783.

160. Kumar K, Nath RK, et al Spinal Cord stimulation is effective in the management of reflex sympathetic dystrophy. *Neurosurgery.* 1997;40:503–508.

161. Kemler MA, Barensde GA, et al. Electrical spinal cord stimulation in reflex sympathetic dystrophy: retrospective analysis of 23 patients. *J Neurosurg.* 1999;90:79–83.

162. Kemler MA, Barendse GA, et al. Spinal cord stimulation in patients with chronic reflex sympathetic dystrophy. *N Engl J Med.* 2000;343:618–624.

163. Oakley JC, Weiner RL. Spinal cord stimulation for complex regional pain syndrome: a prospective study of 19 patients at two centers. *Neuromodulation.* 1999;2:47–50.

164. Turner JA, Loeser JD, Bell KG. Spinal Cord stimulation for chronic low back pain: a systematic literature synthesis. *Neurosurgery.* 1995;37:1088–1095.

165. Burchiel KJ, Anderson VC, et al. Propsective multicenter study of spinal cord stimulation for relief of chronic back and extremity pain. *Spine.* 1996;21:2786–2794.

166. Nienke C, Vulink C, et al. The effects of spinal cord stimulation on quality of life in patients with therapeutically refractory angina pectoris. *Neuromodulation.* 1999;2:33–40.

167. Lefaucheur JP. The use of repetitive transcranial magnetic stimulation in chronic neuropathic pain. *Neurophysiologie Clinique.* 2006;36:117–124.

39

Nonpharmacologic Pain Management in the Patient with Cancer

Julie K. Silver

Pain is often considered synonymous with cancer and its treatment. Essentially all survivors suffer from pain during their diagnosis, treatment and post-treatment phases. Previous chapters have defined the various types of pain encountered in the cancer setting. We can broadly categorize pain as malignant (related to tumor invasion or compression) and nonmalignant (related to treatment side effects or disorders unrelated to cancer).

This chapter addresses nonpharmacologic pain approaches in cancer survivors. It is important to note that effective pain management usually involves a multipronged approach that may include over the counter or prescription medications, injections, and potentially more invasive procedures such as radiation therapy and surgery. In fact, a combination of pharmacologic and nonpharmacologic treatment is the official standard of care, as presented in the World Health Organization guidelines (1). A multidisciplinary approach is also the classic rehabilitation model for pain management, and this may include physical and occupation therapy intervention as well as the input from various other rehabilitation specialists and mental health professionals.

One study evaluating the healthcare professionals' familiarity with nonpharmacologic strategies for managing cancer pain (2) found that of the 214 health care professionals surveyed (response rate was 67%; 141/214), respondents were least familiar with autogenic training, operant conditioning, and cognitive therapy. They most commonly recommended support groups (67%), imagery (54%), music or art therapy (49%), and meditation (43%) for managing cancer pain. Participants were the most interested in learning more about acupuncture, massage therapy, therapeutic touch, hypnosis, and biofeedback.

An important aspect of pain management in cancer survivors is recognizing what pain may or may not signal in terms of disease recurrence or progression. This is crucial for the clinician to understand and to work up appropriately. It is also vital for healthcare professionals to recognize and acknowledge that to cancer survivors, pain is an extremely threatening symptom. Even if the pain is not deemed to be a physical threat, it is often quite disabling emotionally because of the associated worry about disease recurrence and progression. Reassuring patients, while sometimes effective, may not be as psychologically effective as alleviating the pain symptoms through various measures. Understanding that cancer survivors, who might otherwise not complain or take much note of the pain they are having, may present with considerable anxiety surrounding this particular symptom.

To date, nonpharmacologic pain management has been only sparsely studied in the cancer setting. As with many other aspects of cancer research, nonpharmacologic pain management has been perhaps best studied in breast cancer survivors. While many of the studies cited in this chapter pertain to breast cancer, much of the information can be extrapolated to other types of cancer. The nonpharmacologic management of pain

in cancer patients can generally be divided into the
following categories:

- Physical medicine and modalities (eg, exercise,
ultrasound)
- Psychological interventions (eg, support groups,
mental health counseling)
- Complementary and alternative medicine (cognitive behavioral therapies such as hypnosis or
biofeedback, massage, acupuncture)

A separate chapter is devoted to complementary
and alternative medicine (CAM); thus, here the focus
will be the on the first two categories—physical medicine and modalities and psychological interventions.
Notably, some interventions may not clearly fit into
one of these categories, and the list of possible nonpharmacologic interventions is exceedingly long. Therefore,
this chapter will describe those therapies that are commonly prescribed and have some evidence to suggest
that they may be useful in reducing pain symptoms in
cancer survivors.

PHYSICAL MEDICINE AND MODALITIES

Therapeutic Exercise

Physical activity may play a role in preventing cancer
(3–7) and potentially reducing the incidence of cancer recurrence (8–10). Physical activity impacts physical function and may contribute to the improvement
of quality of life parameters such as fatigue (11,12)
and post-treatment body image (13). The relationship
between cancer, physical activity, and pain has not been
well documented or studied (14). Studies that have evaluated the benefits of exercise during and after cancer
treatment have generally concluded that when it is done
in a supervised setting and appropriate precautions are
taken (eg, monitoring of blood counts, cardiopulmo-

nary status, etc.), physical activity is safe and confers
positive effects on health and quality of life. The benefits of physical activity seem to span the continuum
of cancer care.

A study evaluating structured exercise in women
with early stage breast cancer (15), looked at 123
women with stages I and II breast cancer. These participants were placed into one of three groups: usual
care (control group), self-directed exercise, and supervised exercise. Quality of life, aerobic capacity, and
body weight measurements were taken at baseline and
at 26 weeks. Physical functioning in the control group
decreased over the course of the study, whereas in the
self-directed and supervised exercise groups physical
functioning increased. The researchers concluded that
exercise could blunt some of the negative side effects
of cancer treatment, such as reduced physical functioning. This is not a surprising result given the known
reduction in physical activity among cancer survivors
(16) and the positive effects of exercise on physical
functioning.

Exercise may be beneficial to patients near the end
of life, as evidenced by a study exploring the effects of
an exercise program on cancer patients with incurable
disease who had a short life expectancy (17). In one
study, 34 patients participated in a 50-minute group
program twice a week for six weeks. Physical performance was measured by three tests: a six-minute walk
test, timed repeated sit to stand, and functional reach.
Quality of life was assessed by the European Organization for Research and Treatment of Cancer Care
Quality of Life Questionnaire. Though there was no
control group, the researchers concluded that there was
a significant improvement in physical and emotional
functioning with the exercise intervention in palliative
care patients with a short life expectancy.

Many studies have shown that an exercise program focused on strength training, cardiovascular
conditioning, or both has positive physical and mental
health benefits (14,18–22). The effect of such programs

on pain has not been well evaluated. There are many unanswered questions when it comes to exercise and cancer. Not only are there deficits in our knowledge concerning the impact of exercise on pain, but it is not clear when it is safe for cancer survivors to exercise and how they should be screened. For example, the issues surrounding exercise and the development and worsening of lymphedema affect thousands of people. A few studies have looked at this issue, these studies were small, only preliminary in nature, and by no means definitive. Lane et al., for instance, examined the effect of a whole body exercise program and dragon boat training on changes in arm volume in breast cancer survivors (19). They studied 16 women for 20 weeks and concluded that there was a significant increase in upper extremity volume over time, but that this was symmetrical and likely due to gains in muscle hypertrophy rather than increasing lymphedema. The largest randomized trial to date on exercise and lymphedema was conducted by Ahmed et al. and included 45 women undergoing a strength training program. They concluded, "The results of this study support the hypotheses that a six-month intervention of resistance exercise did not increase the risk for or exacerbate symptoms of lymphedema" (23). One review suggests that exercise after breast cancer surgery should be delayed (24). Clearly more information on this subject is needed.

Safely prescribing exercise depends on factors including the patient's age, premorbid health status condition, current physical status, and comorbidities. Treatment complications or side effects such as cardiac morbidity (25) due to chemotherapy or radiation treatment, or pulmonary limitations secondary to surgical resection of a lung malignancy, are additional considerations (26). Therapeutic exercise that is supervised by a physical or occupational therapist is not the only way to have cancer survivors become more physically active. Studies investigating the use of dance (27) and yoga (28,29) have revealed positive mental and physical health benefits, although these activities do not specifically address pain relief.

Therapeutic exercise can certainly involve total body conditioning, but is often prescribed locally due to a particular problem a patient is experiencing. For instance, flexibility exercises may help improve range of motion and postoperative neck pain after thyroid surgery (30). There may be benefits to localized exercise in head and neck cancer patients who are experiencing shoulder dysfunction as well (31). This is also true for postoperative breast cancer patients (32).

It makes sense that physical activity would help reduce pain in cancer survivors, but there is not much literature to support this hypothesis. Instead, what we know currently is that exercise helps with both physi-

cal and emotional function. Of course in rehabilitation medicine, the saying "focus on function" applies to pain management as well, but there is clearly a void in the literature on this subject that will hopefully be explored further in the future.

Physical Modalities

Most physical modalities have not been well studied in cancer patients due to the concern of exacerbating an underlying malignancy. Those which are generally believed to be safe include cryotherapy (eg, the use of cold packs), biofeedback, iontophoresis and transcutaneous electrical nerve stimulation (TENS), and massage (33). Electrical stimulation, regardless of how it is delivered, is generally not done directly over a tumor site. The same is true for massage therapy and superficial heat. Deep heat (eg, ultrasound and phonophoresis) is usually contraindicated in cancer patients, though the evidence to support this is lacking and is generally based on a "standard of care" belief. Spinal traction is contraindicated in those patients with spinal metastases or with significant osteoporosis.

In a study conducted by Ahmed et al. evaluating percutaneous electrical nerve stimulation (PENS) in three terminal cancer patients with bony metastasis using acupuncture-like needle probes that were stimulated for 30 minutes at frequencies 4 to 100 Hz, the authors found that two of the three participants had good to excellent pain relief that lasted 24 to 72 hours after each treatment (34). Of course, this study is too small to conclude the effectiveness of PENS, but it does suggest that this might be an effective therapy in some instances.

In a randomized clinical trial conducted by Robb et al., 41 women who had chronic pain following breast cancer treatments were evaluated with TENS, transcutaneous spinal electroanalgesia (TSE), and a placebo (sham TSE) (35). None of the interventions were significantly better than the others, although all provided beneficial effects on pain and quality of life. This study suggested that there may be benefit resulting from the personal interaction involved in the treatment/placebo rather than a true effect of pain relief from electrical stimulation. However, again, this has not been studied to the extent that a definitive conclusion is reasonable.

Psychological Interventions

The vast majority of cancer patients experience psychological distress, and many go on to develop clinical depression or anxiety. Cancer pain can be intensified by psychological distress, as shown by a review of 19 studies conducted by Zaza and Baine (36). The fear of disease recurrence and progression is common, but the level of psychological distress varies among patients (37).

Keefe et al. pointed out three general categories of psychosocial interventions used to treat pain in cancer patients (38). These include education about cancer, hypnosis and imagery skills, and training in coping skills. Educational interventions include helping patients to comprehend pain assessment and overcome barriers to treatment for pain. Educational tools can include videos, tutorials, coaching, and didactic sessions, to name a few. The efficacy of education on pain management requires further study to determine whether it will be successful (38). The same is true for training in coping skills. Internet support groups may provide some benefit in terms of coping skills (39); however, they have not been studied sufficiently in the realm of how cancer pain is impacted.

CONCLUSIONS

In summary, in the management of pain in cancer, whether it is due to malignant cell growth or the side effects of treatment, the best approach is usually both multimodality and multidisciplinary. Pharmacologic management certainly has an important role, as do nonpharmacologic measures. While there is certainly some evidence to suggest that the nonpharmacologic interventions discussed in this chapter can be quite helpful to cancer survivors, there needs to be more investigation into these methods and others in the future.

*R*eferences

1. Jadad AR, Browman GP. The WHO analgesic ladder for cancer pain management: stepping up the quality of its evaluation. *JAMA.* 1995;274:1870–1873.
2. Zaza C, Sellick S, Willan A, Reyno L, Browman GP. Health care professionals' familiarity with nonpharmacological strategies for managing cancer pain. *Psycho-oncology.* 1999;8:99–111.
3. Dallal CM, Sullivan-Halley J, Ross RK, et al. Long-term recreational physical activity and risk of invasive and in situ breast cancer: the California teachers study. *Arch Intern Med.* 2007;167:408–415.
4. Larsson SC, Rutegard J, Bergkvist L, Wolk A. Physical activity, obesity, and risk of colon and rectal cancer in a cohort of Swedish men. *Eur J Cancer.* 2006;42:2590–2597.
5. Monninkhof EM, Elias SG, Vlems FA, et al. Physical activity and breast cancer: a systematic review. *Epidemiology.* 2007;18:137–157.
6. Lagerros YT, Hsieh S-F, Hsieh C-C. Physical activity in adolescence and young adulthood and breast cancer risk: a quantitative review. *Eur J Cancer Prev.* 2004;13:5–12.
7. Hannan LM, Leitzmann MF, Lacey JV, et al. Physical activity and risk of ovarian cancer: a prospective cohort study in the United States. *Cancer Epidemiol Biomarkers Prev.* 2004;13:765–770.
8. Meyerhardt JA, Heseltine D, Niedzwiecki D, et al. Impact of physical activity on cancer recurrence and survival in patients with stage III colon cancer: findings from CALGB 89803. *J Clin Oncol.* 2006;24:3535–3541.
9. Holmes MD, Chen WY, Feskanich D, Kroenke CH, Colditz GA. Physical activity and survival after breast cancer diagnosis. *JAMA.* 2005;293:2479–2486.
10. Enger SM, Bernstein L. Exercise activity, body size and premenopausal breast cancer survival. *Br J Cancer.* 2004;90:2138–2141.
11. Hewitt JA, Mokbel K, van Someren KA, Jewell AP, Garrod R. Exercise for breast cancer survival: the effect on cancer risk and cancer-related fatigue (CRF). *Int J Fertil.* 2005;50:231–239.
12. Mock V, Frangakis C, Davidson NE, et al. Exercise manages fatigue during breast cancer treatment: a randomized controlled trial. *Psychooncology.* 2005;14:464–477.
13. Pinto BM, Trunzo JJ. Body esteem and mood among sedentary and active breast cancer survivors. *Mayo Clin Proc.* 2004;79:181–186.
14. Stevinson C, Lawlor DA, Fox KR. Exercise interventions for cancer patients: systematic review of controlled trials. *Cancer Causes Control.* 2004;15:1035–1056.
15. Segal R, Evans W, Johnson D, et al. Structured exercise improves physical functioning in women with stages I and II breast cancer: results of a randomized controlled trial. *J Clin Oncol.* 2001;19:657–665.
16. Irwin ML, McTiernan A, Bernstein L, et al. Physical activity levels among breast cancer survivors. *Med Sci Sports Exerc.* 2004;36:1484–1491.
17. Oldervoll LM, Loge JH, Paltiel H, et al. The effect of a physical exercise program in palliative care: a phase II study. *J Pain Symptom Manag.* 2006;31:421–430.
18. Cheema BSB, Gaul CA. Full-body exercise training improves fitness and quality of life in survivors of breast cancer. *J Strength Cond Res.* 2006;20:14–21.
19. Lane K, Jespersen D, McKenzie DC. The effect of a whole body exercise programme and dragon boat training on arm volume and arm circumference in women treated for breast cancer. *Eur J Cancer Care.* 2005;14:353–358.
20. Daley AJ, Mutrie N, Crank H, Coleman R, Saxton J. Exercise therapy in women who have had breast cancer: design of the Sheffield women's exercise and well-being project. *Health Educ Res.* 2004;19:686–697.
21. Midtgaard J, Tveteras A, Rorth M, Stelter R, Adamsen L. The impact of supervised exercise intervention on short-term postprogram leisure time physical activity level in cancer patients undergoing chemotherapy: 1- and 3-month follow-up on the body & cancer project. *Palliat Support Care.* 2006;4:25–35.
22. Karvinen KH, Courneya KS, North S, Venner P. Associations between exercise and quality of life in bladder cancer survivors: a population-based study. *Cancer Epidemiol Biomarkers Prev.* 2007;16:984–990.
23. Ahmed RL, Thomas W, Yee D, Schmitz KH. Randomized controlled trial of weight training and lymphedema in breast cancer survivors. *J Clin Oncol.* 2006;24:2765–2772.
24. Shamley DR, Barker K, Simonite V, Beardshaw A. Delayed versus immediate exercises following surgery for breast cancer: a systematic review. *Breast Cancer Res Treat.* 2005;90:263–271.
25. Gaya AM, Ashford RFU. Cardiac complications of radiation therapy. *Clin Oncol.* 2005;17:153–159.
26. Win T, Groves AM, Ritchie AJ, Wells FC, Cafferty F, Laroche CM. The effect of lung resection on pulmonary function and exercise capacity in lung cancer patients. *Respir Care.* 2007;52:720–726.
27. Sandel SL, Judge JO, Landry N, Faria L, Ouellette R, Majczak M. Dance and movement program improves quality-of-life measures in breast cancer survivors. *Cancer Nurs.* 2005;28:301–309.
28. Culos-Reed SN, Carlson LE, Daroux LM, Hately-Aldous S. A pilot study of yoga for breast cancer survivors: physical and psychological benefits. *Psycho-oncology.* 2006;15:891–897.
29. Shannahoff-Khalsa DS. Kundalini yoga meditation techniques for psycho-oncology and as potential therapies for cancer. *Integr Cancer Ther.* 2005;4:87–100.

30. Takamura Y, Miyauchi A, Tomoda C, et al. Stretching exercises to reduce symptoms of postoperative neck discomfort after thyroid surgery: prospective randomized study. *World J Surg.* 2005;29:775–779.

31. McNeely ML, Parliament M, Courneya KS, et al. A pilot study of a randomized controlled trial to evaluate the effects of progressive resistance exercise on shoulder dysfunction caused by spinal accessory neurapraxia/neurectomy in head and neck cancer survivors. *Head Neck.* 2004;26:518–530.

32. Hase K, Kamisako M, Fujiwara T, Tsuji T, Liu M. The effect of zaltoprofen on physiotherapy for limited shoulder movement in breast cancer patients: a single-blinded before-after trial. *Arch Phys Med Rehabil.* 2006;87:1618–1622.

33. Watkins T, Maxeiner A. Musculoskeletal effects of ovarian cancer and treatment: a physical therapy perspective. *Rehabil Oncol.* 2003;21:12–17.

34. Ahmed HE, Craig WF, White PF, Huber P. Percutaneous electrical nerve stimulation (PENS): a complementary theory for the management of pain secondary to bony metastasis. *Clin J Pain.* 1998;14:320–323.

35. Robb KA, Newham DJ, Williams JE. Transcutaneous electrical nerve stimulaton vs. transcutaneous spinal electroanalgesia for chronic pain associated with breast cancer treatments. *J Pain Symptom Manage.* 2007;33:410–419.

36. Zaza C, Baine N. Cancer pain and psychosocial factors: a critical review of the literature. *J Pain Symptom Manage.* 2002;24:526–542.

37. Brietbart W, Payne D, Passik SD. Psychological and psychiatric interventions in pain control. In: Doyle D, Hanks NC, eds. *Oxford Textbook of Palliative Medicine,* 3rd ed. New York, NY: Oxford University Press; 2004:424–438.

38. Keefe FJ, Abernethy AP, Campbell LC. Psychological approaches to understanding and treating disease-related pain. *Ann Rev Psychol.* 2005;56:601–630.

39. Hoybye MT, Johansen C, Tjornhoj-Thomsen T. Online interaction. Effects of storytelling in an internet breast cancer support group. *Psycho-oncology.* 2005;14:211–220.

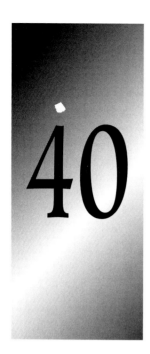

Pharmacologic Pain Management in the Patient with Cancer

Natalie Moryl

Pharmacologic cancer pain management requires the following skills: (1) making a pain diagnosis; (2) choosing and titrating an opioid; (3) choosing and titrating adjuvant analgesics; (4) addressing opioid side effects; (5) learning about opioid rotation; (6) accessing the institutional resources.

MAKING A PAIN DIAGNOSIS

Uncontrolled pain requires immediate intervention; rapid clinical assessment and establishing pain diagnosis should be done while providing immediate analgesia.

Pain diagnosis and differentiation of reversible from progressing or intractable causes of pain is essential in establishing the plan of treatment. Acute reversible pain related to a medical procedure, fracture, urinary retention, or other cause will require a different approach from the chronic progressing pain of pancreatic carcinoma or retroperitoneal carcinomatosis. Reversible causes of pain may require short-term, high-dose analgesics in oral, intravenous (IV), or epidural administration, under close monitoring, while progressive chronic pain requires comprehensive multidisciplinary approach and a combination of different analgesics and/or consecutive analgesic trials. Depending on the reversibility of the patient's pain, the patient and family may have different goals of care, leading to

the different acceptance of side effects such as sedation that may be desired by the patient in some instances and unacceptable in other situations. Usually unacceptable respiratory depression may not be a dose limiting side effect in a dying patient. Once an understanding of the patient's condition, prognosis, and priorities is clarified, the goals of care and treatment plan need to be communicated to the entire medical team.

CHOICE OF THE OPIOID AND TITRATION

The World Health Organization (WHO) Cancer Pain and Palliative Care Program endorses the use of opioids for moderate to severe pain. The effective use of analgesic medications should be a major part of every physician's armamentarium in managing cancer pain.

A few general principles have been endorsed by the National Comprehensive Cancer Network (NCCN) and American Pain Society (APS) and accepted by the medical community (1–4). Opioid dose, route, and titration schedule should be tailored to the patient's medical needs, treatment goals, and side effect profile. There is no minimum or maximum dose. The opioid dose needs to be titrated to maintain the patient's desired balance between pain relief and opioid-related side effects (Fig. 40.1).

Short-acting opioids are used for opioid titration and as needed (PRN) for breakthrough pain. In

KEY POINTS

- Uncontrolled pain requires immediate intervention; rapid clinical assessment and establishing pain diagnosis should be done while providing immediate analgesia.
- The effective use of analgesic medications should be a major part of every physician's armamentarium in managing cancer pain.
- When choosing a specific opioid for a patient with a history of opioid therapy, selection should be based on the patient's analgesic history, potential for the drug accumulation, side effects, and severity of pain.
- Methadone is an old opioid that has been increasingly used in cancer pain management over the last few years. It is a unique analgesic with effects thought to be due to N-methyl-D-aspartic acid

(NMDA) receptor antagonism, and has been found to provide effective analgesia for patients whose pain is uncontrolled with other opioids.
- The World Health Organization (WHO) Cancer Pain and Palliative Care Program advocates the three-step approach incorporating the use of nonopioid, opioid, and adjuvant analgesics alone, and in combination, titrated to the needs of the individual patient.
- Nausea, vomiting, sedation, and constipation are the most common opioid induced side effects.
- For patients unable to tolerate escalation of their current opioid dose because of dose-limiting side effects, an alternate opioid should be considered (opioid rotation).

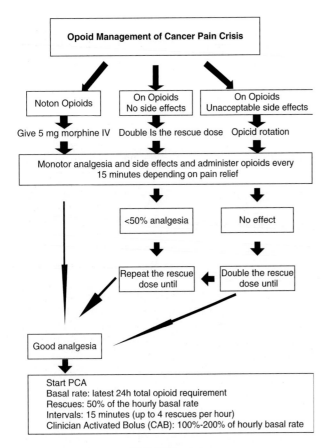

FIGURE 40.1

Opioid management of cancer pain crisis (rapid opioid titration needs to be done by the clinicians familiar with opioid side effects and their management).

chronic pain, long-acting opioids given in around-the-clock dosing are preferred to PRN opioids because it allows to achieve more consistent blood levels, reduce pain recurrence, improve compliance, and reduce the iatrogenic dependence.

When choosing a specific opioid for a patient with history of opioid therapy, selection should be based on the patient's analgesic history, potential for the drug accumulation, side effects, and severity of pain.

For a patient with moderate pain, who is not currently on opioids, a weak opioid agonist (codeine, hydrocodone, oxycodone, and tramadol) can be used alone or in combination with a nonsteroidal anti-inflammatory (NSAID) drug or acetaminophen (WHO analgesic ladder, step 2). In patients with severe pain, a strong opioid (morphine, hydromorphone, fentanyl, methadone, oxycodone, oxymorphone, or levorphanol), alone or in combination with adjuvant analgesics, is recommended by the WHO (step 3). It is critical that patients presenting with severe pain are treated with a strong opioid immediately.

Codeine is considered a weak opioid (about six times weaker than morphine) and has limited analgesic efficacy. It is used for the management of mild to moderate pain and has been included in step 2 of the analgesic ladder. In single-dose studies of cancer, dental, and postoperative pain, codeine 60 mg was found to be equianalgesic to acetylsalicylic acid (aspirin, ASA) 650 mg or acetaminophen 600 to 1,000 mg. Codeine is metabolized to morphine that is its main active metabolite. Approximately 15% of the population cannot convert codeine to morphine because of the lack of a specific enzyme and thus do not fully benefit from codeine. At the higher doses required to treat severe pain, codeine is poorly tolerated by patients because it produces significant nausea.

Oxycodone is included in both step 2 and step 3 of the analgesic ladder. Oxycodone is available in combination with acetaminophen (Percocet, Tylox) or alone in tablet form and liquid form. Bioavailability of oxycodone is about 50%. Oxycodone is about 10 times more potent than codeine; its potency compares with oral morphine, the ratio being about 3:2. Oxycodone is now available as 5, 15, and 30 mg immediate-release preparations, as well as extended-release OxyContin.

Morphine remains the drug of choice for the management of cancer pain because of its familiarity to physicians, wide availability, and variety of formulations (immediate release tablets, oral solutions, controlled-release tablets for 8, 12, or 24 hours, buccal tablets, rectal suppositories, and IV, subcutaneous, epidural, and intrathecal solutions). Morphine has approximately 35% oral bioavailability and a plasma half-life of two to three hours in a young patient with normal renal and liver function. Half-life of morphine and morphine-6-glucoronide (M6G), a morphine metabolite and mu-opioid agonist, may increase from 4 hours to few days in an elderly patient or a patient with significant renal or liver insufficiency, and may cause sedation that outlives its analgesic and sedating effects.

Hydromorphone is a strong opioid (1.5 mg of hydromorphone intravenously is equipotent to 10 mg of IV morphine), and is often used for the treatment of moderate to severe cancer pain. It may offer a better side effect profile in the setting of morphine toxicity. Hydromorphone-3-glucoronide (H3G), an active hydromorphone metabolite, can accumulate and cause myoclonus similar to morphine-3-glucoronide (M3G). Given its water solubility and availability in a high-potency formulation, hydromorphone is the drug of choice for chronic subcutaneous and intrathecal administration.

Fentanyl is an opioid with a short half-life and unique transdermal (TD) delivery system. If often becomes the opioid of choice for patients with renal or liver insufficiency, those who need to bypass gastrointestinal (GI) tract, or for patients who are noncompliant because of forgetfulness or other cognitive problems. It is available for IV use, in a TD patch, and in an oral transmucosal preparation. The TD fentanyl patch is contraindicated in opioid-naïve patients. After the patient is started on the fentanyl patch, there is a 6- to 12-hour delay in the onset of analgesia; therefore, patients need to have their pain controlled by the immediate release medication during this titration phase. TD fentanyl patch has to be changed every 72 hours. A small percentage of patients may experi-

ence end-of-dose failure, reporting escalation of pain on day three. Escalation of the dose or changing of the fentanyl patch every 48 hours should be considered if this occurs. Administration of a fentanyl patch may not eliminate or even significantly decrease the need for PRN short-acting opioids in some patients.

Oral transmucosal fentanyl citrate (OTFC) is a valuable option for the treatment of highly prevalent cancer-related breakthrough pain, a transient increase in pain over a well-controlled baseline pain. Two formulations of OTFC are currently approved for use in the United States. Fentanyl Actiq is available in a wide range of dosages (200–1600 μg) for the management of breakthrough pain in opioid-tolerant adults. Onset of relief may occur within 5 minutes. Fentora is another transmucosal fentanyl formulation, which is available as a buccal fentanyl tablet. Tablets contain 100, 200, 300, 400, 600, or 800 mcg of fentanyl. Fentora is designed to be placed and retained within the buccal cavity for a period sufficient to allow disintegration of the tablet and absorption of fentanyl across the oral mucosa.

When converting from Actiq to Fentora, the dosing conversion shown in Table 40.1 should be used.

Levorphanol is a second-line drug with the potential drug accumulation associated with its long half-life (12–16 hours). The d-isomer of levorphanol (dextrorphan) is thought to be devoid of opioid action but acts as an NMDA receptor antagonist that may offer additional value in pain management.

Methadone is an old opioid that has been increasingly used in cancer pain management over the last few years (5,6). It is a unique analgesic with effects thought to be due to NMDA receptor antagonism, and has been found to provide effective analgesia for patients whose pain is uncontrolled with other opioids. Additional advantages to the use of methadone in

TABLE 40.1
Actiq to Fentora Dosing Conversion

CURRENT ACTIQ (ORAL TRANSMUCOSAL FENTANYL CITRATE) DOSE(MCG)	INITIAL FENTORA DOSE (MCG)
200	100
400	100
600	200
800	200
1,200	400
1,600	400

TABLE 40.2 *Variability in Dose Ratios When Switching Oral Morphine, Oral Hydromorphone, and Transdermal Fentanyl to Methadone, Depending on the Prior Opioid Dose*	
MORPHINE DOSE	**MORPHINE→METHADONE RATIO(6)**
30–90 mg/24 h	4:1
91–300 mg/24 h	9:1
>300 mg/24 h	12:1
HYDROMORPHONE DOSE	**HYDROMORPHONE→METHADONE RATIO(8)**
<330 mg hydromorphone/24 h	0.95:1
>330 mg hydromorphone/24 h	1.6:1
FENTANYL DOSE	**FENTANYL→METHADONE RATIO(10)**
50 mcg/h–2,500 mcg/h	250 mcg/h: 1 mg/h(11)

Changing from oral morphine to oral methadone for a patient taking oral 80 mg morphine per day, the equivalent methadone dose based on this study (4:1 ratio) will be 20 mg oral methadone per 24 h. For a patient taking 800 mg oral morphine per day based on 12:1 conversion ratio, the equivalent methadone dose will be 67 mg per 24 h.

cancer pain include 48% to 96% bioavailability, lack of active metabolites, low cost, long half-life (allowing larger intervals between doses), and improved patient compliance (7).

When using methadone, the clinician must be aware of the highly variable and unpredictable half-life, which can vary between 17 and 24 hours, and has been reported to be up to 190 hours in some patients. Bioavailability of methadone varies twofold (46% to over 90%), further contributing to the complexity of titration. More importantly, when switching from another opioid to methadone, the equianalgesic dose ratios are variable, depending on the patient's previous experience with opioids (dose, length of exposure, and the degree of tolerance to the previous opioid (Table 40.2).

In rotating patients from morphine to methadone, Ripamonti and colleagues used a dose ratio of 4:1 for patients who received 30 to 90 mg of oral morphine daily, 9:1 for patients who received 90 to 300 mg daily, and 12:1 for patients who received 300 mg or more (8). Other studies suggest that as little as one-tenth the equianalgesic dose of methadone can provide effective analgesia in patients tolerant to other opioid analgesics (Fig. 40.2). Bruera and colleagues demonstrated that the hydromorphone/methadone ratio correlated with the total pre-switch opioid dose. In patients receiving more than 330 mg of hydromorphone prior to the switch, the dose ratio was 1.6:1, whereas in patients receiving less

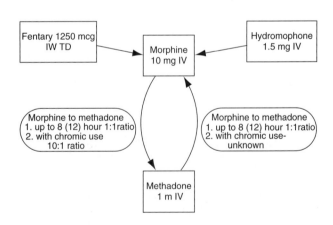

- For single doses: IV morphine to IV methadone ratio is 1:1
- For chronic use: IV morphine to IV methadone ratio is 10:1
- IV morphine to IV methadone ratio may be higher in morphoine to methadone rotation than is methadone to morphine rotation

FIGURE 40.2

With chronic use, methadone is expected to increase its potency, and morphine to methadone equianalgesic ratios change from 10 mg:10 mg to about 10 mg:1 mg; fentanyl 250 mcg:10 mg methadone changes to 250 mcg:1 mg and hydromorphone 1.5 mg:10 mg methadone to 1.5 mg:1 mg methadone.

than 330 mg of hydromorphone daily, the dose ratio was 0.95:1 (9). In two small studies analyzing dose ratio when rotating from fentanyl to methadone, 25 mcg/hour fentanyl was found to be equivalent to about 1 mg methadone IV/hour at the apparent methadone steady state (after completing the titration) (10,11). Thus, when changing from TD fentanyl to oral methadone, the dose ratio is reported to remain the same, independent of the fentanyl dose.

Opioid rotations from and to methadone may be challenging because of the unpredictable and variable half-life of methadone, its variable bioavailability, and the effect of the NMDA receptors. This may lead to drug accumulation a few days after analgesia is achieved on a stable dose. Sedation, confusion, and even death can occur when patients are started on an excessive dose of methadone that may be well tolerated for 1 or even 2 days. Methadone should therefore be used with caution, and a consultation with a pain or a palliative care team is strongly recommended when a rotation to (or from) methadone is considered.

Meperidine is an opioid with unique properties. It has recently been shown to block Na+ channels and has the molecular pharmacologic features of a local anesthetic. Repetitive dosing of meperidine in a patient with renal insufficiency can lead to accumulation of a toxic metabolite, normeperidine, resulting in central nervous system (CNS) hyperexcitability. This adverse effect is characterized by subtle mood changes followed by tremors, multifocal myoclonus, and occasionally seizures. Seizures have been reported even with therapeutic doses of meperidine in a patient with normal renal function.

OPIOID AGONISTS/ANTAGONISTS AND PARTIAL AGONISTS

Opioid agonist/antagonists have the main advantage of causing less respiratory depression and having less abuse potential. However, the clinical use of these agents in cancer pain management is limited by the ceiling analgesic effects. Pentazocine is a kappa-opioid agonist and a weak mu-opioid antagonist. When given to a patient tolerant to opioids, pentazocine may precipitate withdrawal symptoms. Nalbuphine and Butorphanol are similar to Pentazocine in agonist/antagonist opioid effects. Buprenorphine, partial mu-receptor agonist, is a semisynthetic opioid that is 25 to 50 times more potent than morphine. It is approved in the United States as substitute therapy for opioid addiction, but is widely used in Europe for pain.

CHOICE OF THE OPIOID IN PAIN CRISIS

As a general rule, when choosing an opioid during pain crisis or pain emergency management, it is helpful to have a long-term plan of analgesia in mind. If the patient has short bowel syndrome and significant malabsorption, oral long-acting opioids will not be an appropriate choice for long-term management. In a case like this, a TD fentanyl patch would be appropriate for long-term treatment, and IV fentanyl may be advantageous for the initial dose during pain crisis. Absence of long-acting hydromorphone makes it less attractive for acute pain management in a patient who requires long-acting opioids after discharge.

Temporary spinal analgesia may be a good short-term solution in a patient with pain crisis who can not tolerate therapeutic IV or oral opioid administration. Prior to considering a permanent infusion pump for the discharge, however, it is necessary to perform a detailed assessment of the caregiver's availability and willingness to be a responsible person for the infusion, as well as the insurance coverage that would have to cover both home care and the infusion company services. When spinal analgesia is not an option, IV and oral analgesia may need to be used both for pain emergency and opioid maintenance, regardless of the side effects. A discussion of the goals of care may be required in that case.

All of the clinically used opioids have similar mechanisms of analgesia. Thus, opioid choice depends mostly on the previous experience with the particular opioid, preferred route of administration (TD, oral, rectal, or spinal), and experienced or anticipated opioid-related side effects. Propensity to the opioid-related side effects depends on the liver and renal function of the patient, the age, baseline cognitive function, and comorbid conditions.

OPIOID TITRATION

Once an appropriate opioid has been selected, the dose should be rapidly titrated up until the patient experiences relief of pain or excessive side effects develop (Fig. 40.1). Since rapid opioid titration may be associated with development of side effects such as sedation, respiratory depression, and possibly, death, rapid opioid titration needs to be done by the clinicians familiar with opioid side effects and their management.

Based on the pharmacokinetics of morphine, fentanyl and hydromorphone, NCCN Cancer Pain Guidelines recommend that short-acting opioids need to be administered intravenously to the patient every 15 minutes, with dose adjustment as tolerated (Fig. 40.1).

TABLE 40.3
Adjuvant Analgesics in Pain Crisis Management

CATEGORY/DRUG	DOSAGE	INDICATION	COMMENTS
Acetaminophen	1,000 mg × 4 daily	Bone pain	No tolerance or physical dependence Additive analgesia when combined with an opioid Caution: Ceiling effect for analgesia Analgesia as in ibuprofen 600 mg × 4 daily
NSAIDS Ketorolac	15–30 IV q 4 h up to 3 d	Pain crisis equipotent with IV morphine time to analgesia—as morphine effective in bone, neuropathic, visceral and other pain	GI bleeding/renal failure Protrombotic effects
Topical analgesic Lidoderm patch	5% up to 3 every 24 h 12 h on, 12 h off	Neuropathic pain	
Tramadol	50–100 mg 6 h PRN	Neuropathic pain	NNT—3.4 Average effective dose—270 mg/d Increased risk of seizures
Antidepressants Amitriptyline/Nortriptyline (PO, liquid)	Start at 10–25 mg, effective 75–125 mg/d	Neuropathic burning pain	Analgesic effects usually takes 3–5 d, blood levels may need monitoring NNT—2.1–3.5
SSRIs			NNT similar to amitriptyline
Duloxetine	30–90 mg/d		51% (vs 31% placebo) reported 30% sustained pain reduction
Anticonvulsants Gabapentin (PO, liquid)	Start at 300 mg/d Effective—2,700–3,600 mg/d	Neuropathic pain	NNT—3.2–3.7 Analgesic effects usually takes days and titration
Pregabalin	Start at 50 mg/d Effective—300–600 mg/d		
Phenytoin (IV)	Start at 100 mg q6 h	Sharp, lancinating neuropathic pain	
Corticosteroids Dexamethasone	High dose regimen: 100 mg IV/po followed by 24 mg QID	Spinal/nerve compression	GI bleeding Hyperglycemia Psychosis

(Continued)

TABLE 40.3
Adjuvant Analgesics in Pain Crisis Management, Continued

CATEGORY/DRUG	DOSAGE	INDICATION	COMMENTS
	Low dose regimen: 10 mg IV/PO QID Anti-inflammatory: 2–4 mg/ every 6 h then taper	Neuropathic pain Bony metastasis	
Anxiolytics Lorazepam	0.5–1 mg PO/IV for an non-tolerant patient	Unremitting pain crisis that can not be controlled by other means.	Inform the patient/caregiver that sedation is common
Midazolam	1 mg IV slowly q2–3 min	Unremitting pain monitor for respiratory depression	Monitor for sedation and respiratory depression
Ketamine	0.02–0.05 mg/kg/h, titrate up by up to 100% every 4–6 h		Use an opioid-sparing agent when sedation/respiratory depression/intractable delirium limits opioid dose escalation

Abbreviation: NNT, number of patients needed to treat for at least 50% pain reduction.

CHOOSING AND TITRATING COANALGESICS

Use of Adjuvant Drugs as Coanalgesics

Table 40.3 shows adjuvant nalgesics used in pain crisis management. The World Health Organization (WHO), Cancer Pain and Palliative Care Program advocates the three-step approach advocating the use of nonopioid, opioid, and adjuvant analgesics alone, and in combination, titrated to the needs of the individual patient.

For mild pain alone (WHO step 1) or for moderate to severe pain (WHO steps 2, 3), NSAIDs and adjuvant medications are recommended. It is critical that patients presenting in severe pain should generally be treated with a strong opioid immediately.

Acetaminophen and NSAIDS

- Benefits
  - No tolerance or physical dependence
  - Additive analgesia when combined with an opioid
- Caution
  - Ceiling effect for analgesia

Acetaminophen 1000 mg four times per day is equivalent to ibuprofen 600 mg four times daily but inferior to naproxen 500 mg two times per day or ketoprofen 75 mg four times per day when evaluated in dental pain models (12–14).

Gastropathy

NSAIDS should be avoided in patients predisposed to gastropathy. Risk of gastrointestinal bleeding varies 20-fold, depending on the drug (lowest for ibuprofen, diclofenac, and indomethacin, followed by others). Misoprostol is the most effective protective regimen (9% vs 39% incidence of gastroduodenal ulceration). A combination of glucocorticoids with NSAIDS including cyclooxygenase (COX)-2 may significantly (up to four times) increase the risk of GI bleeding.

The nonacetylated salicylates (sodium salicylate, choline magnesium trisalicylate), are associated with a favorable toxicity profile since they do not interfere with platelet aggregation, are rarely associated with GI bleeding, and are well tolerated by asthmatic patients.

Cardiovascular Effects

In September 2006, the U.S. Food and Drug Administration (FDA) issued a warning that ibuprofen blocks ASA's cardioprotection: 400 mg ibuprofen may interact with low-dose ASA, thus decreasing the drug's therapeutic effects on platelets and its cardioprotective effects. To avoid the prothrombotic effect of ibuprofen, the FDA recommends taking ibuprofen only occasionally, or 8 hours before or 30 minutes after ASA. Other over-the-counter NSAIDS should be viewed as having the potential to interfere with antiplatelet effects of low-dose ASA as well. The COX-2 specific inhibitors do not bind to COX-1 and thus do not inhibit ASA's cardioprotective effect. All anti-inflammatories, including the nonspecific and COX-2 selective inhibitors, have a risk of cardiotoxicity with long-term use. While the mechanism of cardiotoxicity is unclear, it may be related to effects on renal perfusion and subsequent blood pressure elevations.

KETOROLAC Ketorolac is a potent NSAID that was shown to be equipotent to morphine in postoperative pain (1 mg ketorolac IV is equipotent to morphine IV 1 mg), with time to pain relief similar to morphine and a short-term side effect profile significantly better than the morphine group (15). Due to potential toxicity, however, this potent NSAID should be limited to three to five days in patients with normal renal functions and no GI contraindications.

LIDOCAINE PATCH A 5% lidocaine in the patch should be applied to painful areas of skin up to 12 hours within a 24-hour period (ie, 12 hours on, 12 hours off). the FDA approved its use for postherpetic neuralgia, but some analgesia has been reported in other neuropathic pain conditions and muscular skeletal pain. It can be applied only on intact skin up to a maximum of three patches at a time.

TRAMADOL Tramadol is a centrally active analgesic agent that inhibits reuptake of norepinephrine and serotonin and has mild effect on mu-opioid receptors. The number of patients needed to treat (NNT) to reach at least 50% analgesia for tramadol is 3.5. Tramadol has also been found to have significant therapeutic effect on paraesthesia, allodynia, and touch-evoked pain in neuropathic pain (16).

Extended release tramadol (Ultram ER), is now available. The average effective dose of extended release tramadol is 270 mg per day. Time to peak concentration for the immediate release tramadol is 1.5 hours, while for the extended release it is 12 hours. Tramadol may increase the risk of seizures even at the recommended dose, and may cause respiratory depression. When naloxone is administered to counteract respiratory depression, it may increase risk of seizures. Dizziness, nausea, and constipation are seen frequently (30% each).

Antidepressants: Amitriptyline

Amitriptyline is the mainstay of neuropathic pain treatment. For amitriptyline, NNT in diabetic neuropathy is 3.5, and 2.1 in postherpetic neuralgia. Average effective dose is 75 to 150 mg per day. Amitriptyline and nortriptyline levels may need to be monitored for toxic levels. Anticholinergic side effects need to be monitored, particularly in the elderly, especially in patients with benign prostate hypertrophy.

Selective Serotonin Reuptake Inhibitors (SSRIs)

In 186 randomized, controlled trials (RCT), amitriptyline was compared with other tricyclics/heterocyclics or with an SSRI. Efficacy of amitriptyline versus tricyclics/heterocyclics and SSRIs showed a 2.5% difference in the proportion of responders in favor of amitriptyline. Amitriptyline caused 11.6% to 13% more side effects than SSRIs (17).

Duloxetine is an atypical antidepressant that was approved in 2004 for major depression and neuropathic pain in diabetes. In a study of 1074 patients, 51% (vs 31% placebo), reported 30% sustained pain reduction. About 0.4% patients developed increases in alanine aminotransferase (ALT), aspartate aminotransferase (AST), creatinine phosphokinase (CPK), and alkaline phosphatase (ALP) (all within first 2 months), forcing them to stop duloxetine administration. Duloxetine is not recommended in patients with hepatic insufficiency, chronic insufficiency, and severe alcohol abuse. Serotonin syndrome has been described when duloxetine is used with SSRIs/SNRIs/triptans. Duloxetine has also been reported to increase suicide.

Anticonvulsant Medications

Gabapentin

Gabapentin was approved by the FDA for use as an adjunctive medication to control partial seizures in 1994, and in 2002, approval was added for treating postherpetic neuralgia and other painful neuropathies. It is also used in prevention of frequent migraine headaches and in the treatment of bipolar disorder. In patients with diabetic neuropathy, the NNT for gabapentin is 3.7, and in patients with postherpetic neuralgia the NNT is 3.2. Even a single 900 mg dose of gabapentin was shown to reduce acute pain and allodynia in patients with herpes zoster in a randomized, double-blind, placebo-controlled crossover study (900 mg);

493

pain severity decreased by 66% with gabapentin compared to 33% with placebo (18).

Pregabalin

Pregabalin, a newer anticonvulsant, was approved by the FDA for use in adjunctive treatment of patients with partial epilepsy and neuropathic pain associated with diabetic peripheral neuropathy, in 2004. It crosses the blood brain barrier and placenta, and is secreted in breast milk in animal studies. Its primary route of elimination is renal excretion (90%–98% unchanged), and the dose needs to be decreased in patients with renal insufficiency.

In a randomized, double-blind placebo-controlled trial study of 274 patients on pregabalin compared to 65 patients in placebo group, a significant reduction of pain score and improved pain-related sleep was demonstrated (19). The most common adverse effects include dizziness and drowsiness.

Ketamine is a potent analgesic that does not interfere with respiratory drive. Its analgesic action at low doses is thought to be due to noncompetitive blockade of the NMDA receptor complex. IV ketamine is an appropriate drug to use in moderate to severe pain when escalating doses of opioids are associated with severe toxicity, mainly sedation and respiratory depression. Multiple case series and prospective small studies using a double-blind placebo-controlled approach suggest that very low-dose ketamine may potentiate morphine analgesia and reduce pain (20–23). Cochrane's review reported its role as not yet established due to limited data (24). Future studies are necessary to develop evidence-based guidelines in cancer patients.

ADDRESSING OPIOID SIDE EFFECTS

Nausea, vomiting, sedation and constipation are the most common opioid-induced side effects.

Opioids that are associated with higher incidence of CNS toxicity include propoxifen, meperidine, and morphine due to their active metabolites, which accumulate, especially in patients with renal insufficiency. Morphine is glucoronized into mu-opioid active potent M6G and non-mu-active M3G, both of which can accumulate in patients with renal insufficiency. Neuroexcitatory side effects such as thost seen with M3G and H3G, and sedation seen with morphine and M6G, can be particularly poorly tolerated by the patients with marginal cortical function due to the previous brain injuries or atrophy.

Neurotoxicity may be seen more frequently in patients with history of brain injury, such as CVS, whole brain radiation, brain atrophy due to age, alcohol abuse, or head traumas.

Hydromorphone is glucoronized to H3G, which can cause anxiety, delirium, and other CNS side effects similar to M3G. Meperidine is metabolized to normeperidine, which is reported to cause seizures even at therapeutic dose in patients with normal renal function. Propoxifen has also been reported to cause seizures.

Although clinically significant respiratory depression in chronic opioid users is very uncommon, in patients with compromised pulmonary function, initiation of opioid therapy or rapid increase in the dose can impair compensation process and cause respiratory depression. Patients at risk include patients with COPD, patients after pneumonectomy or lobectomy, and patients with pulmonary fibrosis and other conditions compromising pulmonary function. Increased risk of respiratory depression can be seen in patients who compensate chronic hypercarbia by chronic hyperventilation and metabolic alkalosis. If rapid opioid titration precipitates CO2 narcosis, the respiratory depression will not respond to naloxone, and immediate intubation is indicated if congruent with the goals of care. In patients with increased risk of pulmonary compromise, the shortest acting opioids such as fentanyl or hydromorphone IV should be used until a stable safe and effective dose at the apparent steady state is established. Patients with compromised upper airways constitute another high-risk group for respiratory depression that is more likely to be seen in conjunction with sedation, such as with rapid opioid escalation in a patient with large laryngeal carcinoma who develops sedation and positions the neck to cause mechanical upper airway obstruction.

In terms of nausea and vomiting, there is no opioid that would predictably be better tolerated. Fortunately, tolerance to nausea usually develops quickly after the first few days, during which a routine antinausea medication such as metoclopramide or chlorpromazine may be required. In rare instances, consecutive opioid trials may be needed to determine a patient's sensitivity to different opioid in terms of nausea.

Constipation is the most common opioid-related side effect. The patient who experiences constipation should start laxatives at the same time as opioids, and the majority will require laxatives as long as opioids are used. In some instances, constipation may be debilitating to such an extent that the patients refuse opioids or require opioid rotation. In small studies and some case reports, TD fentanyl and methadone have been associated with less constipation than other strong opioids. Mixed agonists-antagonists may be advantageous in this setting if the patient is not at risk for withdrawal (chronic opioid use).

Sedation varies with the drug and dosage, and management includes reducing the individual dose but giving the drug more frequently or rotating to an opioid with a shorter plasma half-life. Discontinuing all other sedative drugs can be helpful. Psychostimulants, including caffeine, amphetamine, and methylphenidate have been demonstrated to counteract opioid-induced sedative effects. The use of pemoline, modafinil, and donepezil has also been reported anecdotally to improve sedative side effects. End-of-life sedation needs to be differentiated from unwanted opioid-related side effects.

Cardiac toxicity of methadone has been explored recently. There is a growing literature of the relationship between methadone and QTc prolongation. Published studies suggest that QTc prolongation is context dependent and occurs more frequently with high doses of methadone, concomitant administration of CYP3A4 inhibitors (which can inhibit the biotransformation of methadone) such as erythromycin, dicumarol, and others, hypokalemia, hepatic failure, and administration of other QTc prolonging agents such as chlorbutanol, the preservative in parenteral methadone preparations. Clearly the benefit of methadone in the individual patient needs to be weighed against the potential for increased cardiovascular risk. Each of the associated factors that could contribute to methadone toxicity need to be evaluated in patients with a history of significant QTc prolongation.

OPIOID ROTATION

For patients unable to tolerate escalation of their current opioid dosage because of dose-limiting side effects, an alternate opioid should be considered (opioid rotation). Studies in cancer patients demonstrate wide inter-individual variations in analgesic response and side effects. This variability is caused by environmental, psychological, and genetic factors that may regulate opioid pharmacokinetics (transporters and metabolizing enzymes) and pharmacodynamics (receptors and signal transduction elements). Also, the phenomena of incomplete cross tolerance, as evidenced by improved pain relief or a reduction in side effects following opioid rotation, is thought to be related in part to a range of interindividual pharmacogenetic factors, including genetic polymorphisms in the P-glycoprotein gene (*ABCB1*), the uridine 5'-diphosphate (UDP)-glucuronosyltransferase gene (*UGT2B7*), the mu-opioid receptor gene (*OPRM1*), and the catechol-O-methyl transferase gene (*COMT*), may be involved in the inter-patient variability in pain experience and analgesia.

In one prospective study, 80 of 100 patients referred to the Memorial Sloan-Kettering Cancer Center Pain Service required changes in either opioid or route of administration to obtain adequate analgesia with tolerable side effects. One opioid switch was required in 80% of patients, 44% of patients required two switches, and 20% of patients required three or more switches. When a new adverse effect appears in a previously stable patient, the clinician should suspect that another process may be contributing to the new adverse effects. Hypercalcemia, sepsis, worsening of renal function, and liver failure are among the most common comorbidities overlapping and worsening opioid-related side effects. Other sedatives, anticholinergics, and other centrally acting medications should be reviewed. In addition to clinicians' evaluation of the severity of the opioid-related side effects, patients' preferences and acceptability of the side effects may vary. In particular, a patient's preference regarding treatment-related side effects may change with changes in the trajectory of the disease. It is not uncommon for patients during active therapy to endure significant pain for the promise of a successful outcome. With advanced disease, however, when active antitumor therapy is no longer effective, it is common for patients and their families to request that if nothing else can be done, at least their pain should be adequately managed.

Besides inadequate analgesia and dose-limiting side effects, opioid rotations may be necessary for a number of other reasons, including:

- Improved efficacy
- Avoidance of toxicity
  - Cognitive failure, sedation;
  - Hallucinations, myoclonus;
  - Pruritus;
  - Urinary retention
- Change route of administration
  - Oral to parenteral opioids
  - Change to TD/transmucosal fentanyl
- Decrease costs

The main advantages of the opioid rotation are minimizing polypharmacy and improving analgesia. Among disadvantages are variable and unpredictable outcomes and potential need for consecutive opioid rotations and possibility of eventual need for a number of adjuvant analgesics.

Opioid Rotation and New Dosage Calculation

The concept of incomplete cross-tolerance relates to a decrease in effectiveness of a drug with its repeated administration and requires reduction in the dosage of the second opioid to which the patient may be less tolerant. In a patient tolerant to one opioid, the initial dosage of the second opioid needs to be reduced by 50% for incomplete cross tolerance.

If the patient reports good analgesia on the initial opioid prior to opioid rotation, the dose of the second opioid calculated on the basis of the equianalgesic opioid table needs to be decreased by half; for example OxyContin 30 mg orally three times per day (equivalent to TD fentanyl 50 mcg/hour), would be rotated to fentanyl 25 mcg/hour q 72 hours TD. The dose should then be titrated up to analgesia according to the NCCN or APS guidelines. If the patient has inadequate analgesia and the rotation is needed because of dose-limiting side effects, no dose reduction from the equianalgesic dose may be necessary and the new opioid may be started at the dose calculated based on the available single and chronic dose studies (Table 40.2). The dose then should be titrated up to effect according to the APS and NCCN guide lines (Fig. 40.1).

Opioid rotations from and to methadone may be particularly challenging. *Any rotation to (or from) methadone requires frequent monitoring of the patient for undertreatment, withdrawal symptoms, or oversedation.* A series of retrospective and prospective studies reviewed the rotation ratios when rotating from morphine, hydromorphone, and fentanyl to methadone (8–11). The ratio for calculating the dose conversion to methadone is different than the published single dose equianalgesic ratios which are 1:1 for parenteral morphine to methadone. With chronic use in the same patient, methadone's potency is expected to increase up to 10 times or higher with the same dose administered to the same patient (Fig. 40.2 and Table 40.2).

The dosage of the opioid to which the patient is switching depends on the length of exposure and the dosage of the previous opioid. In morphine, hydromorphone, and fentanyl to methadone dosage, ratios have been shown to be dependent on the previous opioid dose—the higher the previous opioid dose, the higher the ratio (Table 40.2), possibly due to incomplete cross tolerance.

Opioid rotations from methadone to other opioids could be more challenging in patients tolerant to methadone. In a series of 13 patients who were receiving methadone as a third- or fourth-line opioid, 12 of the 13, when rotated to an alternative opioid, had to be restarted on methadone because of pain escalation despite titration of the alternative opioid to the highest tolerated dosage. If rotation from high-dose methadone to an alternate opioid is necessary, a step-wise approach helps to prevent symptoms of withdrawal from methadone as well as side effects from rapid up titration of the alternate opioid. It allows the clinician to evaluate whether the new opioid is providing

adequate analgesia. A consultation with a pain or palliative care specialist for a safe and effective methadone titration schedule should be considered.

CONSULTATION

When the dosages or medications are not familiar to the clinician providing direct patient care, appropriate resources and experts should be sought (25–27). Each healthcare institution needs to create and adapt their own pain management guidelines and devote appropriate resources to address the needs of cancer pain patients. Institutional guidelines are important for resource allocation of staff time as well as for allotting designated beds to provide continuous monitoring of the opioid infusions. Availability of an expert clinician to provide direct supervision during cancer pain management is an essential part of the quality cancer care. NCCN developed guidelines for the treatment of cancer pain, and the Joint Commission on Hospital Accreditation has established pain treatment as an important priority in the delivery of high-quality inpatient care.

References

1. NCCN Clinical Practice Guidelines. Supportive Care Guidelines: cancer pain. http://www.nccn.org. Accessed December 6, 2006.
2. American Pain Society. *Principles of Analgesic Use in the Treatment of Acute Pain and Cancer Pain*, 5th ed. Glenview, IL: American Pain Society; 2007.
3. Moryl N, Carver A, Foley KM. Pain and palliation. In: Holland JF, Frei E, eds. *Cancer Medicine*, 6th Ed. Hamilton, Ontario: BC Decker Inc.; 2003:1113–1124.
4. National Consensus Project for quality palliative care: clinical practice guidelines for quality palliative care, executive summary. *J Palliat Med.* 2004;7(5):611–627.
5. Manfredi PL, Foley KM, Payne R, Houde R, Inturrisi CE. Parenteral methadone an essential medication for the treatment of pain. *J Pain Symptom Manage.* 2003;26(2):687–688.
6. Bruera E, Sweeney C. Methadone use for in cancer patients with pain: a review. *J Palliat Med.* 2002;5:127–138.
7. Davis MP, Walsh D. Methadone for relief of cancer pain a review of pharmacokinetics, pharmacodynamics, drug interactions and protocols of administration. *Support Care Cancer.* 2001;9:73–83.
8. Ripamonti C, Zecca E, Bruera E. An update on the clinical use of methadone for cancer pain. *Pain.* 1997;70(2–3):109–115.
9. Bruera E, Pereira J, Wantanabe S, Belzile M, Kuehn N, Hanson J. Opioid rotation in patients with cancer pain. A retrospective comparison of dose ratios between methadone, hydromorphone, and morphine. *Cancer.* 1996;78 (4):852–871.
10. Santiago-Palma J, Khojainova N, Kornick C, et al. Intravenous methadone in the management of chronic cancer pain: safe and effective starting doses when substituting methadone for fentanyl. *Cancer.* 2001;92:1919–1925.
11. Mercadante S, Villari P, Ferrera P, Casuccio A, Gambaro V. Opioid plasma concentrations during a switch from transdermal fentanyl to methadone. *J Palliat Med.* 2007;10(2):338–344.
12. Bjornsson GA, Haanaes HR, Skoglund LA. Naproxen 500 mg bid versus acetaminophen 1000 mg qid: effect on swelling and

other acute postoperative events after bilateral third molar surgery. *J Clin Pharmacol.* 2003;43(8):849–858.

13. Bjornsson GA, Haanaes HR, Skoglund LA. A randomized, double-blind crossover trial of paracetamol 1000 mg four times daily vs ibuprofen 600 mg: effect on swelling and other postoperative events after third molar surgery. *Br J Clin Pharmacol.* 2003;55(4):405–412.

14. Bjornsson GA, Haanaes HR, Skoglund LA. Ketoprofen 75 mg qid versus acetaminophen 1000 mg qid for 3 days on swelling, pain, and other postoperative events after third-molar surgery. *J Clin Pharmacol.* 2003;43(3):305–314.

15. Lai MW, Kauffman RE, Uy HG, Danjin M, Simpson PM. A randomized comparison of ketorolac tromethamine and morphine for postoperative analgesia in critically ill children. *Crit Care Med.* December 1999;27(12):2786–2791.

16. Duhmke RM, Cornblath DD, Hollingshead JR. Tramadol for neuropathic pain. *Cochrane Database Syst Rev.* 2004;2:CD003726.

17. Barbui C, Hotopf M. Amitriptyline v. the rest: still the leading antidepressant after 40 years of randomised controlled trials. *Br J Psychiatry.* February 2001;178:129–144.

18. Tenser RB, Dworkin RH. Herpes zoster and the prevention of postherpetic neuralgia: Beyond antiviral therapy. *Neurology.* 2005;65(3):349–350 (gabapentin).

19. Freynhagen R, Strojek K, et al. Efficacy of pregabalin in neuropathic pain evaluated in a 12-week, randomised, double-blind, multicentre, placebo-controlled trial. *Pain.* June 2005;115(3):254–263.

20. Visser E, Schug SA. The role of ketamine in pain management. *Biomed Pharmacother.* 2006;60(7):341–348.

21. Fine PG. Low dose ketamine in the management of opioid non-responsive terminal cancer pain. *J Pain Sympt Manage.* 2000;17:296–300.

22. Ben-Ari A, Lewis MC, Davidson E. Chronic administration of ketamine for analgesia. *J Pain Palliat Care Pharmacother.* 2007;21(1):7–14.

23. Mercandante S. Ketamine in cancer pain an update. *Palliat Med.* 1996;10(3):225–230.

24. Bell RF, Dahl JB, Moore RA, et al. Peri-operative ketamine for acute post-operative pain: a quantitative and qualitative systematic review (Cochrane review). *Acta Anaesthesiol Scand.* 2005;49(10):1405–1428.

25. Steinhauser KE, Christakis NA, Clipp EC, McNEilly M, McIntyre L, Tulsky JA. Factors considered important at the end-of-life by patients, family, physicians and other care providers. *JAMA.* 2000;284(19):2476–2482.

26. Coyle N. The hard work of living in the face of death. *J Pain Symptom Manage.* 2006;32(3):266–274.

27. Cohen MZ, Easley MK, Ellis C, et al. Cancer pain management and the JCAHO's pain standards an institutional challenge. *J Pain Symptom Manage.* 2003;25(6):519–527.

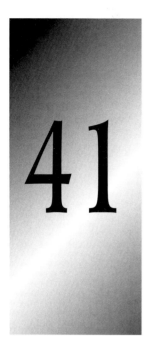

Interventional Pain Management in the Patient with Cancer

41

Laura Andima
Amitabh Gulati
Kenneth Cubert

Greater emphasis for adequate pain control and relief while still maintaining quality of life issues has led to the utilization of interventional pain procedures as an adjunct to pharmacologic therapy for cancer pain. Interventional procedures may lead to decreased consumption of pain medication, and thus, a better side effect profile, allowing for an improved rehabilitation process. Quality assurance studies have shown satisfaction with interventional pain procedures to be around 90%, supporting their use for the chronic pain patient (1). In an intriguing study, a population-based prospective cohort study conducted in England, patients who reported widespread pain had an increased incidence of cancer and an increased risk of death mainly from cancer over the subsequent eight years. Among those surveyed who developed cancer, those who originally reported widespread pain had a reduced survival versus those who originally reported no pain (2,3).

THERAPIES FOR MUSCULAR PAIN

While pain at the location of the tumor may be most prominent, patients with cancer may also have non-cancer related pain; for example, myofascial pain. Furthermore, inflammatory mediators released by tumors or resulting from cancer therapy may lead to various pain symptoms (4). Myofascial pain is pain or autonomic phenomena referred from active trigger points in muscles, fascia, and tendons. It is a common cause of regional pain syndromes such as headaches, neck pain, orofacial pain, and shoulder pain (5). Fortunately, myofascial pain syndromes (MPS) can be treated with varied interventional procedures.

The Trigger Point

One of the simplest methods to relieving myofascial pain is to treat a trigger point. Muscle may have areas of sustained contractions, taut bands that cause constant pain, which may radiate along the muscle when stimulated. Trigger points are located within these taut bands of skeletal muscle and are discrete, focal, hyperirritable spots. They are painful with compression and produce referred pain, referred tenderness, motor dysfunction, and autonomic dysfunction (6). Should pharmacologic or physical treatments (such as massage therapy) not release a taut band, needle injections may be utilized.

Using 22 to 30 gauge needles, combinations of local anesthetic, saline, and (rarely) steroids may be injected into taut bands. Various techniques have been described, with the goal of breaking the muscle spasm and providing durable (as long as 3–4 weeks) relief. The techniques of dry needling and injection of trigger points have become widely accepted. Both the use of dry needling and injection of lidocaine to treat trigger points were equally successful in reducing myofascial pain, which supports the consensus that the critical therapeutic factor is mechanical disruption by needling (7).

KEY POINTS

- Interventional pain procedures are an adjunct to pharmacologic therapy for cancer pain.
- One of the simplest methods to relieving myofascial pain is to treat a trigger point.
- Botulinum toxin injection is used as a treatment for spasticity, musculoskeletal pain, muscle spasms, migraines, neuropathic pain, and other disorders.
- Acupuncture treatments have been gaining acceptance in the medical profession as a modality to treat cancer pain and other related symptoms.
- Neurolysis can be performed with freezing, heating, or chemical techniques with either phenol or alcohol preparations.
- Due to technological improvements in image quality, ultrasonographic guidance for pain procedures has become increasingly common.

- As patients with cancer have oral or intravenous opiate regimens that are escalating and/or having significant side effects, physicians may choose to deliver medications neuroaxially.
- The role for epidural steroid injections in radicular pain is to facilitate earlier pain relief and an earlier return to full function.
- The main indications for use of spinal cord stimulators in the United States is lumbar radiculopathy, complex regional pain syndrome, and failed back syndrome.
- Kyphoplasty and vertebroplasty have been studied most extensively in stabilizing compression fractures from osteoporosis, but have also been used to treat fractures resulting from osteolytic metastasis, myeloma, vertebral osteonecrosis, and hemangioma.

Myofascial pain may result from scar formation from surgery. Nerve entrapment or neuromas at scar sites may elicit pain sensations along a nerve distribution. Injected healed scars along its entirety may relieve this type pain. These neuromas may present akin to trigger points, but they can be treated similarly with combinations of local anesthetics to interfere with pain signal transmission (8,9).

Botulinum Toxin

Botulinum toxin injection is used as a treatment for spasticity, musculoskeletal pain, muscle spasms, migraines, neuropathic pain, and other disorders (10). Botulinum toxin inhibits the release of acetylcholine from neurons at the motor end plate, causing paralysis of the innervated musculature. While this property of botulinum toxin has been used to treat spasticity for years, novel theories have immerged regarding the toxin's ability to block the release of pain mediators (eg, glutamate, substance P, calcitonin gene related peptide) at the site of peripheral inflammation, thereby inhibiting nociceptor sensitization and thus pain (11).

Potential targets for the use of botulinum toxin have been described for patients with radiation induced myokymia, proctitis, and spasticity (12). Botulinum toxin has been shown to reduce postoperative pain and narcotic use after muscular infiltration of the pectoralis major, serratus anterior, and rectus abdominis during mastectomy and tissue expander placement (13). Botulinum toxin A was used to reduce the pain of a series of patients who were suffering from neck muscle spasm and pain after radiotherapy for patients with head and neck cancer. An average of 22 units was injected with electromyogram (EMG) guidance into two sites of the sternocleidomastoid muscle (14). A recent study evaluated the efficacy of botulinum toxin A for radiation induced trismus, facial pain, and masseter spasms for patients with head and neck cancer. A total of 50 units were directly injected into both masseter muscles. At one-month follow up there was significant improvement of pain and cramping symptoms (15). A retrospective case series described the use of botulinum toxin A in radiation fibrosis syndrome. Furthermore, botulinum toxin A has been used to treat radiation induced cervical dystonia, trigeminal neuralgia, cervical plexus neuralgia, trismus, migraine, and thoracic pain, with 87% of patients reporting a benefit (16).

While no standard guidelines have been established, generally low doses of botulinum toxin (100–300 units, or about 3%–10% of the toxic intravenous dose) per treatment distributed among various muscles are delivered to muscle bellies. EMG or nerve stimulator guidance may be used to locate motor endplates or diseased muscle for placement of the botulinum toxin (Fig. 41.1). Relief may last from 6 to 12 weeks (17).

Acupuncture

Acupuncture treatments have been gaining acceptance in the medical profession as a modality to treat cancer pain and other related symptoms. Acupuncture involves stimulating specific discrete anatomic points by puncturing the skin generally with a needle. Indications for

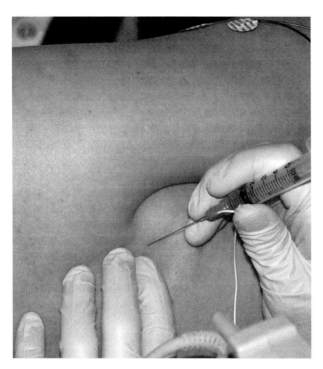

FIGURE 41.1

Botulinum toxin injection into muscles of the subscapularis using EMG guidance. EMG guidance allows for injection of medication at the motor end-plate zone.

its usage include, adjunct for pain control, nausea, xerostomia, vomiting post-chemotherapy, back pain, and vasomotor symptoms (19,20) While acupuncture treatment regimen and techniques are varied, short-term relief of pain appears promising in the current literature. Systemic reviews evaluating acupuncture role in relieving cancer pain have been equivocal; however, this is primarily due to a paucity of randomized controlled trials (21). Some trials have demonstrated the efficacy of reducing cancer related pain after two treatments of auricular acupuncture, with the second being given one month after the first (22). Acupuncture, as well as other modalities, is becoming an integral part to the multimodality treatment for pain control for patients with cancer (23).

THERAPIES FOR PERIPHERAL NERVE MEDIATED PAIN

Patients with cancer may not only experience myofascial pain, as discussed above, but may also suffer from pain with a neuropathic component. Pain may be generated by physical compression of nerves by tumors or inflammatory mediators related to tissue damage or host defenses. Neuropathic pain can result from abnor-

mal pain signal processing anywhere along the nervous system, either peripherally or centrally.

Local Blockade

Local anesthetics commonly used to anesthetize nerves include bupivacaine, ropivacaine, and lidocaine. Before proceeding to neurolysis, it is important to diagnose which peripheral nerve, if any, may be a generator of pain. The key to adequate diagnoses is the reliability of placement of local anesthetic near the nerve of interest. Commonly used methods for identifying nerves include paresthesia technique, nerve stimulation, and image guidance. A decrease in a patient's pain symptoms for a few hours after the procedure is an important endpoint before proceeding to neurolysis.

Nerves commonly subjected to neurolysis in cancer include the intercostal nerves (after thoracotomy), spinal median branch nerves (for malignant and non-malignant facet joint related pain), and cutaneous sensory nerves (such as the trigeminal and saphenous nerves). Neurolysis can be performed with freezing, heating, or chemical techniques with either phenol or ethanol preparations. Cryoanalgesia (freezing) involves the application of subzero temperatures to neurons. Current probes for neurolysis range in size from 1.4 to 3 mm and some have a built in nerve stimulator for localization of the nerve and a thermistor to identify tip temperature. Long-term pain relief from nerve freezing occurs because ice crystals create vascular damage to the vasa nervorum, which produces severe endoneural edema. This disrupts the nerve structure and induces wallerian degeneration, but leaves the myelin sheath and endoneurium intact. Cryoanalgesia has been reported in case series and case reports as being used for pain resulting from trigeminal neuralgia, to intercostal nerves for chest wall pain due to post-thoracotomy neuromas, persistent pain after rib fractures, and postherpetic neuralgia (Fig. 41.2). It has also been used to treat ilioinguinal, iliohypogastric, and various peripheral neuropathies including ulnar, medial, and sural nerves (24).

Radiofrequency ablation (RF) is a technique applying heat, via alternating electrical current at a frequency of 500,000 Hz, to nerves for neural cell death. Needle electrodes are directed onto target nerves exposing them to an electrode which is insulated along its length except for the 2 to 10 mm active tip. The current exiting the tip causes the formation of a static electric field and the generation of heat, typically 80°C to 90°C, to the surrounding tissues. Radiofrequency ablation has been used to treat sacroiliac joint pain, trigeminal neuralgia, thoracic zygapophyseal pain, sympathetically mediated pain, intercostal neuralgia, cervicogenic headache, occipital neuralgia, whiplash

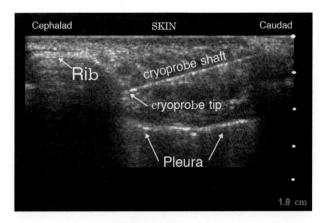

FIGURE 41.2

Cryoanalgesia of the intercostal nerve under ultrasound guidance. Shown is the inferior portion of the rib and the pleura. Notice the distance between the intercostal groove and pleura is less than 5 mm. Source: From Ref. 95.

injury and discogenic pain (25). A Cochrane review of radiofrequency denervation concluded reasonable evidence that radiofrequency denervation provided short-term relief chronic neck pain of zygapophyseal joint origin and chronic cervicobrachial pain. Furthermore, there is evidence on the short-term effect of RF on chronic low back pain of zygapophyseal joint origin (26).

Pulsed radiofrequency (PRF) is a modification of the RF technique. The tip of the electrode delivers a large current density in brief pulses to a nerve without thermal coagulation or histological lesion. Generally, two bursts of a 20 ms pulse is delivered per second, allowing for two silent phases of 480 ms for heat to dissipate. The resultant temperature is 42°C, which reduces the chance of permanent neural injury. Cahana and colleagues reviewed PRF prospective trials showing positive treatment outcomes for cervicogenic headache, cervicobrachialgia, sacroiliac lateral branches L4 to S3, and suprascapular nerve for chronic shoulder pain. Furthermore, successful use of PRF has been shown for lumbar and cervical zygapophyseal joint pain and at the dorsal root ganglion for cervical radiculopathy (27). Potential targets that have been evaluated include shoulder pain, sacroiliitis, sympathetically mediated pain, pelvic pain, postherpetic neuralgia, neuromas, and radicular pain (28,29).

Ultrasound Guided Procedures

Due to technological improvements in image quality, ultrasonographic guidance for pain procedures has become increasingly common. High frequency sound waves are generated within a transducer probe and sent

though tissue. Ultrasound waves are reflected off tissues and return to the transducer, where they are electronically transformed into an image. Tissue surfaces with high acoustic impedance (bone and bowel) reflect most sound waves and appear white, or hyperechoic. Tissues with high water content (muscles and fat), with limited reflection or low acoustic impedance, appear black, or hypoechoic (30).

As technology improves, ultrasound images with higher resolution and depth provide real time visualization of the needle, nerve, and surrounding vasculature. Ultrasonography may obviate the need for contrast dye or exposure to radiation. The use of ultrasound guidance can improve block success, reduce the likelihood of vascular puncture and intravascular injection, and avoid traumatic nerve injury. Multiple regional anesthetic techniques involve ultrasound guidance, including brachial plexus, femoral, and sciatic nerve blocks (Fig. 41.3) (30).

More recently, techniques have evolved using ultrasonography to guide interventional procedures for patients with chronic pain. The lateral femoral cutaneous nerve has been targeted by two reports, showing improvement of pain scores for meralgia paresthetica (31,32). Blockade of the pudendal nerve for perineal pain and use of ultrasonography for pelvic pain for pain relief have shown promising results (33,34). For the piriformis syndrome, ultrasound guided piriformis muscle injections have been described in a case series, all of whom experienced pain relief (35,36). Ultrasound guidance has also been described block the intercostal, ilioinguinal, and iliohypogastric nerves (37,38). Visualization of these nerves allows for more permanent

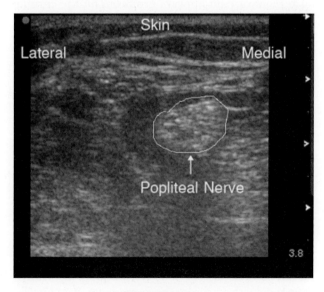

FIGURE 41.3

Ultrasound image of the popliteal nerve as a distinct mass that is hyperechoic relative to the surrounding tissue.

blocks using cryotherapy, chemical, or radiofrequency ablation (39).

The use of ultrasound is being expanded to guide joint injections (40). Hip injections have been performed via a longitudinal, anterior approach with no reported cases of inadvertent vascular or femoral nerve puncture (41). Ultrasound-guided hip injections have been confirmed with contrast and fluoroscopy (42). Another interesting case report describes the use of ultrasound-guided pulsed radiofrequency of the median nerve, which gave a patient with recurrent carpel tunnel syndrome pain relief lasting 12 weeks (43). The use of ultrasound guidance in interventional pain techniques continues to expand as research improves and machines become more portable and less expensive.

SYMPATHETIC BLOCKS

The sympathetic nervous system contributes to neuropathic, vascular, and visceral pain. Pain fibers innervating the perineal, pelvic, and abdominal regions travel with the sympathetic nervous system. First, diagnostic blocks with local anesthetic are performed to determine the extent of sympathetically mediated pain. Image-guided (fluoroscopy or CT guidance) permanent neurolytic procedures can be performed with ethanol or phenol. However, as pain fibers are damaged in this process, the region of interest is also sympathetically denervated (44).

The ganglion of impar is the fused terminus of the paired sympathetic chain at the level of the sacro-coccygeal junction (45). Blockade of the ganglion of impar has been reported for relief of chronic perineal pain, pain from vulvar, prostate, rectal and cervical cancer, and sacral postherpetic neuralgia (46–48). Most neurolysis is performed using phenol; however, use of cryoablation and radiofrequency ablation has been described (49,50).

The superior hypogastric plexus is located in the retroperitoneum below the aortic bifurcation on the anterior aspect of L5-S1junction and disc (51). The classic posterior approach for blockade of the superior hypogastric plexus was described by Plancarte et al in 1990. It is used mainly for chronic pelvic cancer pain (52). A more recent randomized study compared the classic posterior approach with a transdiscal approach, which was shown to be as effective with fewer side effects, such as urinary injury or intravascular puncture (53).

The celiac plexus is another common target for interventional pain techniques. The plexus is a group of nerve ganglia located beneath the diaphragm immediately adjacent to the aorta, below the take off of the celiac trunk at the level of T12-L1. The celiac plexus contains autonomic efferent nerves which innervate the abdominal viscera from the distal esophagus to the transverse colon. Afferent visceral nociceptive signals return to the spinal cord from the celiac plexus along the splanchnic nerves (54). The blockade of the celiac plexus has been used for cancer of the abdominal viscera to the splenic flexure and for chronic benign abdominal pain. Permanent blockade may cause transient hypotension and diarrhea and rarely pneumothorax, bleeding, bowel injury, paralysis, peripancreatic abscess formation, and nerve injury (55). Various block techniques are described utilizing fluoroscopy, computed tomography, percutaneous ultrasound, and endoscopic ultrasound. Wong et al. performed the largest randomized double-blinded study to date, studying 100 patients with unresectable pancreatic cancer and discovering that neurolytic celiac plexus blocks improved pain relief compared to optimized systemic analgesic therapy (56). Other studies have concluded neurolytic celiac plexus block for pancreatic cancer improves pain control and reduces narcotic usage and constipation (57).

Complex Regional Pain Syndrome

Sympathetically mediated pain, complex regional pain syndromes I and II, may present with symptoms of swelling, redness, and temperature changes at an extremity. Chronic changes include hair loss, muscle atrophy and disuse, and skin discolorations. Local anesthetic blocks and neuroablative techniques using local anesthetics targeting sympathetic fibers to the upper extremity (stellate ganglion at C7-T1) and lower extremity (lumbar sympathetics at L3-L5) can be used to treat these syndromes (44).

The stellate ganglion is star shaped and formed by the fusion of the inferior cervical and first thoracic sympathetic ganglia. It is located anterolateral to the C7 body at the neck of the first rib. A block can be performed with local anesthetic and/or steroid anatomically or with fluoroscopic guidance at the anterior tubercle of the C6 vertebra (Fig. 41.4). Neurolysis has been reported in the literature either thermally, with radiofrequency or pulsed radiofrequency, or chemically, with phenol (44,58–60). Stellate ganglion blockade has been used for complex regional pain syndrome of face and upper extremities, postherpetic neuralgia, facial causalgia, phantom tongue pain and causalgia, vasospastic disorders, and cluster headache (61–67).

The lumbar sympathetic chain is located at the anterolateral border of the lumbar vertebral bodies. There is anatomical variation of the size, number, and position on the vertebral bodies of the ganglia (68). While blockade of the lumbar sympathetic chain is most commonly indicated for complex regional pain

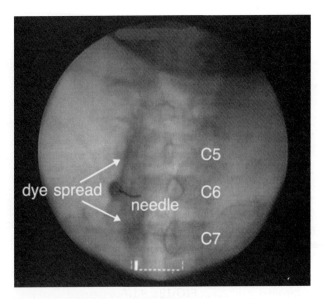

FIGURE 41.4

Stellate ganglion block under fluoroscopic guidance. The spinal needle is inserted at anterolateral aspect of C6 vertebra. Dye spread is confirmed to be lateral to vertebral midline and spread is toward the C7-T1 space under AP and lateral view (not shown).

syndromes I and II, it has also been performed for peripheral neuropathic pain and ischemia related pain. (69–72). Often this blockade is performed solely with local anesthetic at multiple visits. However, studies have sought efficacy for more permanent neurolysis. Phenol neurolysis has been shown to be both effective and superior to radiofrequency ablation for lumbar sympatholysis in reducing pain related to complex regional pain syndrome and ischemia (73,74).

SPINAL PROCEDURES

As patients with cancer have oral or intravenous opiate regimens that are escalating and/or having significant side effects, physicians may choose to deliver medications neuroaxially (75). Opiate side effects are often severe, which prevents adequate pain control and may lead to inadequate opioid prescription by physicians, resulting in underuse by patients (76,77). Both semipermanent epidural systems and permanent intrathecal pumps deliver local anesthetic, opiate, and adjunct medications directly to the spinal cord, thereby using fewer medications. Epidural systems have external components (which may lead to infection) that prevent long-term use beyond a few months. On the other hand, implantable intrathecal systems are placed within the body, thereby reducing the risk of infection and increasing longevity to the magnitude of years.

During patient selection, absolute contraindications include infection at the surgical or catheter site, patient refusal, and severe coagulopathy. Relative risks include increased intracranial pressure, sepsis, severe hypovolemia, and minor coagulopathies (78). Patient prognosis may guide which therapeutic strategy to pursue. If the patient's prognosis is greater than 3 to 6 months, many experts recommended an intrathecal implanted pump instead of an epidural system (79).

The intraspinal implantable drug delivery system consists of a small, battery powered, programmable pump which is placed subcutaneous layer, commonly in the anterior lower abdominal wall, with pump access through a port on the surface of the pump. It is connected to a small catheter, which is tunneled to the spinal canal. A prospective, multicenter randomized clinical trial concluded that implantable drug delivery systems improved clinical success in pain control, reduced pain, and significantly relieved common drug toxicities (80). A variety of analgesics that physicians use alone as first line agents or in combination in intrathecal pumps include morphine, hydromorphone, and ziconotide. Currently, clinicians use bupivacaine, clonidine, and fentanyl derivatives in combination with the above-listed medications (81).

Intrathecal granuloma formation at the tip of the catheter has been increasingly recognized as a serious adverse event for patients with an intrathecal pump. Granulomas are inflammatory masses that can compress the spinal cord, inducing neurologic injury and causing permanent damage to spinal cord. Symptoms have included paralysis, sensory loss, and impaired bowel and bladder function. Initial reports put the incidence of granulomas at 0.1%, but new data suggests the rate is at least 0.5%, and this new figure may still be underreported. An updated consensus panel recommended attentive follow up and monitoring neurological examinations. Physicians should maintain a low threshold for obtaining imaging studies and keep the drug dose and concentration as low as possible, because high doses and concentrations have been associated with granuloma formation (82). Other complications include wound or catheter site infections, bleeding, wound seroma, spinal headache, spinal catheter leak, rare epidural hematoma or abscess, meningitis, and transverse myelitis. Catheter and pump related complications include catheter occlusion, breakage, pump and battery failures, and pump filling/reprogramming errors (79).

Epidural Steroid Injections

Patients with cancer may suffer from inflammatory mediators released from disc herniations or compression of nerve roots from tumor or mechanical damage (eg, osteophytes). Acute disc herniation is associated with a marked inflammatory response in the epidural space adjacent to the spinal nerve. Glucocorticoid steroids injected into the epidural space may relieve this inflammatory response (Fig. 41.5) (83). Multiple studies evaluating epidural steroid injections for the treatment of acute radicular pain due to herniated nucleus pulposus show a more rapid resolution. The role for epidural steroid injections in radicular pain is facilitating earlier pain relief and an earlier return to full function. The transforaminal approach to epidural steroids has been advocated as a way to deliver a high concentration of steroid directly to the site of inflammation near the spinal nerve within the lateral epidural space (Fig. 41.6) (84). Epidural steroids can be a useful tool in treating radicular pain. However, in the cancer patient, procedures are contraindicated if placement of the steroids may introduce tumor cells into the epidural or spinal compartments.

Neuromodulation

Electrostimulation techniques disrupt the flow of pain signals to and within the spinal cord. Transcutaneous electrical nerve stimulation (TENS), spinal cord stimulators (SCS) at thoracic and lumbar regions, and deep brain stimulators at the thalamus or motor cortex interrupt conduction of pain signals to and from the central nervous system. Stimulation of large motor fibers inhibits the conduction of pain signals by small nerve fibers and has shown efficacy in various pain

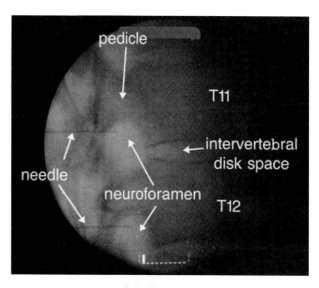

FIGURE 41.6

Transforaminal epidural steroid injection under fluoroscopic guidance, lateral view. The needles are in the superolateral aspect of the foramen to minimize needling of the thoracic nerve root during the procedure and injection.

syndromes. The main indications for use of spinal cord stimulators in the United States are lumbar radiculopathy, complex regional pain syndrome, and failed back syndrome (85,86). However, there is literature from Europe showing support for the use of spinal cords stimulators in patients with severe ischemic limb pain secondary to peripheral vascular disease and refractory angina pain (86).

Unfortunately, controversy exists related to performing magnetic resonance imaging (MRI) procedures for patients with spinal cord stimulation systems. There have been reports of injury including coma and permanent neurological impairment in patients with implanted neurological stimulators who underwent MRI procedures. The mechanism for these events is believed to involve heating of the electrodes at the end of the lead wires, resulting in injury to the surrounding tissue. Although these reports involved deep brain and vagus nerve stimulators, it is believed that this mechanism could occur in any type of implanted stimulator. This has led to reluctance to implant SCS in patients with cancer, who often require surveillance MRIs. There have been several studies indicating that MRIs that are performed at 1.5 Tesla in patients with deep brain stimulation systems are safe (87). Recently, a study of 31 patients with spinal cord stimulators who were scheduled to undergo MRI was conducted. Under an established protocol with the MRIs being performed at 1.5 Tesla, there were few complications, none of which were serious (88).

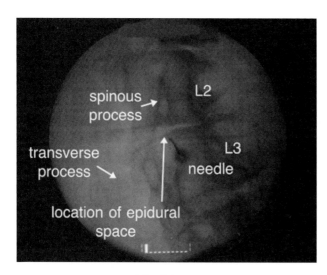

FIGURE 41.5

Epidural steroid injection under fluoroscopic guidance. Patient is shown to have severe scoliosis between L2 and L3. Using fluoroscopy, the entrance to the epidural space can be seen below the spinous process.

Vertebral Procedures

Another cause of back pain may result from tumor involvement of vertebrae. Tumors such as breast, multiple myeloma, and prostate cancer may infiltrate the vertebral body and result in spinal cord or nerve root compression and axial load pain, resulting in progressive and painful vertebral compression fractures at multiple levels (89). Both kyphoplasty and vertebroplasty procedures introduce cement to support vertebrae and increase interdiscal height, alleviating pain. These techniques have been studied most extensively in stabilizing compression fractures from osteoporosis, but have also been used to treat fractures resulting from osteolytic metastasis, myeloma, vertebral osteonecrosis, and hemangioma (90).

While vertebroplasty introduces cement to damaged vertebrae with a percutaneous technique, kyphoplasty precedes this process with balloon expansion of the vertebrae (91). Both techniques result in pain relief, in 87% of subjects with vertebroplasty and 92% of subjects with kyphoplasty (90). Kyphoplasty may better increase vertebral height and correct sagittal realignment, as well as have a lower risk of cement extravasation (92). In a study evaluating use of kyphoplasty for treatment of osteolytic vertebral compression fractures in multiple myeloma patients, there was a 34% average restoration of vertebral body height. The study also demonstrated a significant clinical improvement in pain and functioning (89).

Facet Arthropathy

Another source of pain may be the facet joints between two vertebrae. Both osteoarthritis and tumor damage may result in low back pain from movement such as bending or twisting. Treatments involve intra-articular injection of steroids into the joint or denervating the joint. Radiofrequency ablation of the medial branch nerves that innervate the joint may give pain relief for many months (26).

CONCLUSION

Most patients with cancer pain achieve good analgesia using traditional analgesics and adjuvant medications. The World Health Organization has developed guidelines to help physicians manage cancer pain and clinical trials have demonstrated that most patients (85%–90%) suffering from cancer-related pain syndromes can be well controlled using opioid and other analgesics by simple oral, transdermal, or parenteral routes of administration (93). Cancer physicians found that 10% of patients did not respond well to standard analgesic measures (94). The interventional techniques that have been discussed in this chapter are treatment options for this subset of cancer pain patients.

ACKNOWLEDGMENT

This chapter was funded by the Department of Anesthesiology and Critical Care at Memorial Sloan Kettering Cancer Center.

References

1. Zhou Y, Furgang FA, Zhang Y. Quality assurance for interventional pain management procedures. *Pain Physician.* April 2006;9(2):107–114.
2. McBeth J, Silman AJ, Macfarlane GJ. Association of widespread body pain with an increased risk of cancer and reduced cancer survival: a prospective, population-based study. *Arthritis Rheum.* June 2003;48(6):1686–1692.
3. Macfarlane GJ, McBeth J, Silman AJ. Widespread body pain and mortality: prospective population based study. *BMJ.* September 22, 2001;323(7314):662–665.
4. Lee BN, Dantzer R, Langley KE, et al. A cytokine-based neuroimmunologic mechanism of cancer-related symptoms. *Neuroimmunomodulation.* 2004;11(5):279–292.
5. Graff-Radford S. Myofascial pain:diagnosis and management. *Curr Pain Headache Rep.* December 2004;8(6):463–467.
6. Alvarez D, Rockwell P. Trigger points: diagnosis and management. *Am Fam Physician.* February 2002;65(4):653–650.
7. Houz CZ. Lidocaine injection versus dry needling to myofascial trigger point. The importance of the local twitch response. *Am J Phys Med Rehabil.* 1994;73:256–263.
8. Defalque RJ. Painful trigger points in surgical scars. *Anesth Analg.* June 1982;61(6):518–520.
9. Kotani N, Kushikata T, Suzuki A, Hashimoto H, Muraoka M, Matsuki A. Insertion of intradermal needles into painful points provides analgesia for intractable abdominal scar pain. *Reg Anesth Pain Med.* November–December 2001;26(6):532–538.
10. Royal MS. The use of botulinum toxins in the management of pain and headache. *Phys Med Rehabil Clin N Am.* 2003;14:805–820.
11. Aoki KR. Review of a proposed mechanism for the antinocipetive action of botulinum toxin type A. *Neurotoxicology.* 2005;26:785–793.
12. De Micheli C, Fornengo P, Bosio A, Epifani G, Pascale C. Severe radiation-induced proctitis treated with botulinum anatoxin type A. *J Clin Oncol.* July 2003;21(13):2627.
13. Layeeque R, Hochberg J, Siegel E, et al. Botulinum toxin infiltration for pain control after mastectomy and expander reconstruction. *Ann Surg.* October 2004;240(4):608–613; discussion 613–614.
14. Van Daele DJ, Finnegan EM, Rodnitzky RL, Zhen W, McCulloch TM, Hoffman HT. Head and neck muscle spasm after radiotherapy: management with botulinum toxin A injection. *Arch Otolaryngol Head Neck Surg.* August 2002;128(8):956–959.
15. Hartl D, Cohen M, Julieron M, Marandas P, Janot F, Bourhis J. Botulinum toxin for radiation-induced facial pain and trismus. *Arch Otolaryngol Head Neck Surg.* 2008;138:459–463.
16. Stubblefield M, Levine A, Custodio C, Fitzpatrick T. The role of botulinum Toxin type A in the Radiation Fibrosis Syndrome: a preliminary report. *Arch Phys Med Rehabil.* March 2008;89:417–421.
17. Lin EC-H, Seet RCS. Botulinum toxin:description of injection techniques and examination of controversies surrounding toxin diffusion. *Acta Neurol Scand.* 2008;117:73–84.

18. Lou JS, Pleninger P, Kurlan R. Botulinum toxin A is effective in treating trismus associated with postradiation myokymia and muscle spasm. *Mov Disord.* 1995;10(5):680–681.

19. Filshie J, Hester J. Guidelines for providing acupuncture treatment for cancer patients—a peer-reviewed sample policy document. *Acupunct Med.* December 2006;24(4):172–182.

20. Haake M, Muller H, Schade-Brittinger C, et al. German acupuncture trials for chronic lower back pain. *Arch Intern Med.* 2007;167(17):1892–1898.

21. Bardia A, Barton DL, Prokop LJ, Bauer BA, Moynihan TJ. Efficacy of complementary and alternative medicine therapies in relieving cancer pain: a systematic review. *J Clin Oncol.* December 1, 2006;24(34):5457–5464.

22. Almi D., Rubino C. Analgesic effect of auricular acupuncture for cancer pain: a randomized blinded controlled trial. *J Clin Oncol.* 2003;21:4120–4126.

23. Mansky PJ, Wallerstedt DB. Complementary medicine in palliative care and cancer symptom management. *Cancer J.* September–October 2006;12(5):425–431.

24. Trescot AM. Cryoanalgesia in interventional pain management. *Pain Physician.* July 2003;6(3):345–360.

25. Lord SM, Bogduk N. Radiofrequency procedures in chronic pain. *Best Pract Res Clin Anaesthesiol.* December 2002;16(4):597–617.

26. Niemisto L, Kalso E, Malmivaara A, Seitsalo S, Hurri H. Radiofrequency denervation for neck and back pain. *Cochrane Database Syst Rev.* 2003;(1).

27. Van Zundert J, Patijn J, Kessels A, Lame I, Van Suijlekom H, Van Kleef M. Pulsed radiofrequency adjacent to the cervical dorsal root ganglion in chronic cervical radicular pain: a double blind sham controlled randomized clinical trial. *Pain.* 2007;127:173–182.

28. Cahana A, Van Zundert J, Macrea L, Van Kleef M, Sluijter M. Pulsed radiofrequency: current clinical and biological literature available. *Pain Med.* 2006;7(5):411–423.

29. Wu H, Groner J. Pulsed radiofrequency treatment of articular branches of the obturator and femoral nerves for management of hip joint pain. *Pain Pract.* 2007;7(4):341–344.

30. Brull R, Perlas A, Chan V. Ultrasound-guided peripheral nerve blockade. *Curr Pain Headache Rep.* 2007;11:25–32.

31. Hurdle M, Weingarten T, Crisostomo R, Psimos C, Smith J. Ultrasound-guided blockade of the lateral femoral cutaneous nerve: technical description and review of 10 cases. *Arch Phys Med Rehabil.* October 2007;88:1362–1364.

32. Tumber P, Bhatia A, Chan V. Ultrasound-guided lateral femoral cutaneous nerve block for meralgia paresthetica. *Anesth Analg.* 2008;106(3):1021–1022.

33. Peng P, Tumber P. Ultrasound guided interventional procedures for patients with chronic pelvic pain—a description of techniques and review of literature. *Pain Physician.* March 2008;11(2):215–224.

34. Rofaell A, Peng P, Louis I, Chan V. Feasibility of real time ultrasound for pudendal nerve block in patients with chronic perineal pain. *Reg Anesth Pain Med.* March–April 2008;33(2):139–145.

35. Smith J, Hurdle MF, Locketz AJ, Wisniewski S. Ultrasound-guided piriformis injection: technique description and verification. *Arch Phys Med Rehabil.* December 2006;87:1664–1667.

36. Reus M, de Dios Berna, Vazquez V, Redondo MV, Alonso J. Piriformis syndrome: a simple technique for US-guided infiltration of the perisciatic nerve. Preliminary results. *Eur Radiol.* 2008;18:616–620.

37. Eichenberger U, Greher M, Kirchmair L, Curatolo M, Moriggi B. Ultrasound-guided blocks of the ilioinguinal and iliohypogastric nerve: accuracy of a selective new technique confirmed by anatomical dissection. *Br J Anaesth.* 2006;97(2):238–243.

38. Gofeld M, Christakis M. Sonographically guided ilioinguinal nerve block. *J Ultrasound Med.* 2006;25:1571–1575.

39. Byas-Smith MG, Gulati A. Ultrasound-guided intercostal nerve cryoablation. *Anesth Analg.* October 2006;103(4):1033–1035.

40. Qvistgaard W, Kristoffersen H, Terslev L, Danneskiold-Samsoe B, Torp-Pedersen S, Bliddal H. Guidance by ultrasound of intra-articular injections in the knee and hip joints. *Osteoarthritis Cartilage.* 2001;9:512–517.

41. Sofka C, Saboeiro G, Adler R. Ultrasound guided adult hip injections. *J Vasc Interv Radiol.* 2005;16(8):1121–1123.

42. Smith J, Hurdle MF. Office based ultrasound-guided intra-articular hip injection: technique for physiatric practice. *Arch Phys Med Rehabil.* February 2006;86:296–298.

43. Haider N, Mekasha D, Chiravuri S, Wasserman R. Pulsed radiofrequency of the median nerve under ultrasound guidance. *Pain Physician.* November 2007;10(6):765–770.

44. Day M. Sympathetic blocks: the evidence. *Pain Practice.* 2008;8(2):98–109.

45. Munir M, Zhang J, Ahmad M. A modified needle-inside-needle technique for the ganglion impar block. *Can J Anesth.* 2004;51(9):915–917.

46. Toshniwal G, Dureja G, Prashanth S.M. Transsacrococcygeal approach to ganglion impar block for management of chronic perineal pain: a prospective observational study. *Pain Physician.* 2007;10:661–666.

47. McAllister R, Carpentier B, Malkuch G. Sacral postherpetic neuralgia and successful treatment using a paramedical approach to the ganglion impar. *Anesthesiology.* 2004;101:1472–1474.

48. Ho K, Nagi P, Gray L, Huh B. An alternative approach to ganglion impar neurolysis under computed tomography guidance for recurrent vulva cancer. *Anesthesiology.* 2006;105:861–862.

49. Loev M, Varklet V, Wilsey B, Ferrante M. Cryoablation: a novel approach to neurolysis of the ganglion impar. *Anesthesiology.* 1998;88:1391–1393.

50. Reig E, Abejon D, del Pozo C, Insausti J, Contreras R. Thermocoagulation of the ganglion impar of Walther: description of a modified approach. Preliminary results in chronic, noncological pain. *Pain Pract.* 2005;5:103–110.

51. Bosscher H. Blockade of the superior hypogastric plexus block for visceral pelvic pain. *Pain Practice.* 2001;1(1):162–170.

52. Plancarte R, Amescua C, Patt R, Aldrete A. Superior hypogastric plexus block for pelvic cancer pain. *Anesthesiology.* 1990;73:236–239.

53. Gamal G, Helaly M, Labib Y. Superior hypogastric block: transdiscal versus classic posterior approach in pelvic cancer pain. *Clin J Pain.* 2006;22(6):544–547.

54. Noble M, Gress F. Techniques and results of neurolysis for chronic pancreatitis and pancreatic cancer pain. *Curr Gastroenterol Rep.* 2006;8:99–103.

55. Carroll I. Celiac plexus block for visceral pain. *Curr Pain Headache Rep.* 2006;10:20–25.

56. Wong G, Schroeder D, Carns P, et al. Effect of neurolytic celiac plexus block on pain relief, quality of life, and survival in patients with unresectable pancreatic cancer. *JAMA.* 2004;291(9):1092–1099.

57. Yan B, Myers R. Neurolytic celiac plexus block for pain control in unresectable pancreatic cancer. *Am J Gastroenterol.* 2007;102:430–438.

58. Racz G, Houlubec J. Stellate ganglion phenol neurolysis. In: Racz G, ed. *Techniques of Neurolysis.* Boston, MA: Kluwer Academic Publishers; 1989:133–144.

59. Forouzaner T, Van Kleef M, Weber W. Radiofrequency lesions of the stellate ganglion in chronic pain syndromes: retrospective analysis of clinical efficacy in 86 patients. *Clin J Pain.* 2000;16:164–168.

60. Kastler B, Michalakis D, Clair CH. Stellate ganglion radiofrequency neurolysis under CT guidance. Preliminary study. *JBR-BTR.* 2001;84:191–194.

61. Hanowell S, Kennedy S. Phantom tongue pain and causalgia: case presentation and treatment. *Anesth Analg.* 1979;58:436–438.

62. Jaeger B, Singer E, Kroening R. Reflex sympathetic dystrophy of the face: report of 2 cases and a review of the literature. *Arch Neurol.* 1986;43:693–695.

63. Ackerman W, Zhang J. Efficacy of stellate ganglion blockade for the management of type 1 complex regional pain syndrome. *South Med J.* 2006;99:1084–1088.

64. Milligan N, Nash T. Treatment of post-herpetic neuralgia. A review of 77 consecutive cases. *Pain.* 1985;23:381–386.

65. Khoury R, Kennedy S. Facial causalgia: report of case. *J Oral Surg.* 1980;38:782–783.

66. Albertyn J, Barry R, Odendall C. Cluster headache and the sympathetic nerve. *Headache.* 2004;44:183–185.

67. Arden R, Bahu S, Zuazu M, et al. Reflex sympathetic dystrophy of the face: current treatment recommendations. *Laryngoscope.* 1998;108:437–442.

68. Rauck R, de Leon-Casasola O. Interventional techniques. In: Raj P, ed, *Pain Medicine: A Comprehensive Review.* St. Louis: Mobsy; 2003:250–271.

69. Hugh–Davies D, Redman L. Chemical lumbar sympathectomy. *Anaesthesia.* 1976;31:1068–1075.

70. Plancarte R, Cavillo O. Complex regional pain syndrome type 2 (causalgia) after automated laser discectomy: a case report. *Spine.* 1997;22:459–461.

71. Alexander J. Chemical lumbar sympathectomy in patients with severe lower limb ischemia. *Ulster Med J.* 1994;63:137–143.

72. Furlan A, Lui P, Mailis A. Chemical sympathectomy for neuropathic pain: does it work? Case report and systematic literature review. *Clin J Pain.* 2001;17:327–326.

73. Haynsworth R, Noe, C. Percutaneous lumbar sympathectomy: a comparison of radiofrequency denervation versus phenol neurolysis. *Anesthesiology.* 1991;74:459–463.

74. Cross F, Cotton L. Chemical lumbar sympathectomy for ischemic rest pain. A randomized, prospective controlled clinical trial. *Am J Surg.* 1985;150:341–345.

75. O'Mahony S, Coyle N, Payne R. Current management of opioid related side effects. *Oncology.* 2001;15:61–82.

76. Meuser T, Pietruck C, Radbruch L, Stute P, Lehmann KL, Grond S. Symptoms during cancer pain treatment following WHO-guidelines: a longitudinal follow-up study of symptom prevalence, severity and etiology. *Pain.* 200l;93:247–257.

77. Miaskowski C, Dodd MJ, West C, et al. Lack of adherence with the analgesic regimen: a significant barrier to effective cancer pain management. *J Clin Oncol.* 2001;19:4275–4279.

78. Sloan P. Neuraxial pain relief for intractable cancer pain. *Curr Pain Headache Rep.* 2007;11:283–289.

79. Smith TJ, Coyne PJ. How to use implantable intrathecal drug delivery systems for refractory cancer pain. *J Support Oncol.* 2003;1:73–76.

80. Smith T, Staats P, Deer T, et al. Randomized clinical trial of an implantable drug delivery system compared with comprehensive medical management for refractory cancer pain: impact on pain, drug-related toxicity, and survival. *J Clin Oncol.* October 2002;20(19):4040–4049.

81. Deer T, Krames E, Hassenbusch S, et al. Polyanalgesic Consensus Conference 2007: recommendations for the management of pain by intrathecal (intraspinal) drug delivery: report of an interdisciplinary expert panel. *Neuromodulation.* 2007;10:(4):300–328.

82. Deer T, Krames E, Hassenbusch S, et al. Management of intrathecal catheter tip inflammatory masses: an updated 2007 consensus statement from an expert panel. *Neuromodulation.* 2008;11(2):77–91.

83. McLain R.F., Kapural L., Mekhail NA. Epidural steroid therapy for back and leg pain: mechanisms of action and efficacy. *Spine J.* 2005;5:191–201.

84. Young IA, Hyman GS, Packia Raj LN, Cole AJ. The use of lumbar epidural/transforaminal steroids for managing spinal disease. *J Am Acad Orthop Surg.* 2007;15(4):228–238.

85. North RB, et al. SCS versus repeated lumbosacral spine surgery for chronic pain. *Neurosurgery.* 2005;56:98–107.

86. Cameron T. Safety and efficacy of SCS for the treatment of chronic pain: a 20 year literature review. *J Neurosurg.* 2004;(56):254–267.

87. Rezal AR, Baker KB, Tkach J, et al. Is magnetic resonance imaging safe for patients with neurostimulation systems used for deep brain stimulation? *Neurosurgery.* 2005;57:1056–1062.

88. Andres J, Valia JC, Cerda-Olmedo G, et al. Magnetic resonance imaging in patients with spinal neurostimulation systems. *Anesthesiology.* 2007;106(4):779–786.

89. Dudeney S, Lieberman IH, Reinhardt MK, Hussein M. Kyphoplasty in the treatment of osteolytic vertebral compression fractures as a result of multiple myeloma. *J Clin Oncol.* May 2002;20(9):2382–2387.

90. Hulme P, Krebs J, Ferguson SJ, Berlemann U. Vertebroplasty and kyphoplasty: a systemic review of 69 clinical studies. *Spine.* 2006; 31(17):1983–2001.

91. Sabharwal T, Salter R, Adam A, Gangi A. Image–guided therapies in orthopedic oncology. *Orthop Clin North Am.* 2006;37:105–112.

92. Lieberman I, Reinhardt MK. Vertebroplasty and kyphoplasty for osteolytic vertebral collapse. *Clin Orthop Relat Res.* October 2003;415S:S176–S186.

93. Schug SA, Zech D, Dorr U. Cancer pain management according to WHO analgesic guidelines. *J Pain Symptom Manage.* 1990;5:27–32.

94. Sloan PA, Melzack R. Long term patterns of morphine dosage and pain intensity among cancer patients. *Hosp J.* 1999;14:35–47.

95. Byas-Smith M, Gulati A. Ultrasound-guided intercostal nerve cryoablation. *Anes Analg.* October 2006;103(4):1033–1035.

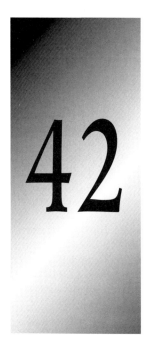

Complementary Therapies for Pain Management in the Patient with Cancer

Barrie Cassileth
Robin C. Hindery
Jyothirmai Gubili

Pain is an unfortunate reality for the majority of patients with cancer. It is estimated that up to 50% of patients undergoing active cancer treatment and up to 90% of patients in advanced stages of cancer suffer from pain on a daily basis (1). Cancer-related pain can take the form of chronic pain, resulting from a tumor or certain treatments, or acute pain, which most often follows surgery or other medical procedures.

Despite the prevalence of pain among patients with cancer, the issue is not always adequately recognized or properly approached. The National Cancer Institute attributes this to a variety of factors, including inadequate knowledge of pain management and poor assessment of pain by health care professionals; reluctance of patients to report pain; patient, family, and professional concerns about side effects and addiction resulting from use of analgesics; and poor adherence by patients to prescribed analgesic regimens (2).

The use of complementary and alternative medicine (CAM) therapies has become increasingly common among patients with cancer seeking to alleviate pain and other symptoms, such as nausea and fatigue. A systematic review of 26 surveys of patients with cancer from 13 countries found that 31% of patients used CAM therapies (3), most commonly dietary treatments, herbs, homeopathy, hypnotherapy, imagery or visualization, meditation, megavitamins, relaxation, and spiritual healing. Internationally, CAM use ranges from 7% to over 80% of patients with cancer across the numerous surveys conducted, depending on surveyor or patient definitions.

Unfortunately and as evidenced by the preceding list of therapies used, the term CAM embodies both viable, evidence-based therapies and unproved or disproved approaches. The latter category includes useless or potentially harmful interventions often touted as literal "alternatives" to mainstream care. Complementary therapies, conversely, are used adjunctively to control symptoms, not to cure or treat disease. It is likely that only a small percentage of patients seek alternative instead of mainstream treatment for malignant diseases.

The National Center for Complementary and Alternative Medicine (NCCAM) groups CAM therapies into four basic categories: mind-body medicine (such as meditation and hypnotherapy), biologically based practices (such as the use of dietary supplements and herbal products), manipulative and body-based practices (such as massage), and energy therapies (such as Reiki and therapeutic touch).

In addition, the NCCAM recognizes whole medical systems that overlap across these categories. Such systems include Ayurveda, the traditional system of India, and traditional Chinese medicine, which encompasses mind-body practices, manipulative techniques, herbal treatments, and acupuncture. Patients with cancer have looked to each of these categories and individual therapies to relieve pain. However, the number

KEY POINTS

- It is estimated that up to 50% of patients undergoing active cancer treatment and up to 90% of patients in advanced stages of cancer suffer from pain on a daily basis.
- Complementary and alternative medicine (CAM) therapies are grouped into four basic categories: mind-body medicine, biologically based practices, manipulative and body-based practices, and energy therapies.
- Fewer than 25% of CAM users received information on CAM therapy from their physician, and tend instead to rely on sources such as the Internet.
- When used properly, complementary therapies offer patients the opportunity to play a participatory role in their treatment, to control symptoms on their own, and to maintain or improve their quality of life after active cancer treatment.

- Studies performed to date support the utility of acupuncture as an effective treatment for cancer pain in some cases.
- The National Institutes of Health has judged hypnosis to be an effective intervention for alleviating pain from cancer and other chronic conditions.
- Hypnosis has been found to be especially effective among children.
- Caution should be exercised when considering the use of dietary supplements and herbal remedies to relieve pain. Many of these products have not yet been studied in patients with cancer and may interact negatively with chemotherapeutic agents or any prescription medication.
- The largely favorable risk-benefit ratio suggests that complementary therapies can play an important role in physical and emotional rehabilitation.

of high-quality randomized controlled trials (RCTs) evaluating CAM interventions for cancer pain remains small. Evidence supports the use of massage, acupuncture, hypnosis, and other mind-body therapies for the treatment of cancer pain, but further research and more rigorous trials are necessary.

Although patients previously often failed to discuss CAM therapies with their physicians, this is no longer the case. Both patients and physicians are more familiar with these modalities and today are more able and comfortable about discussing their use. Fewer than 25% of CAM users received information on CAM therapy from their physician (4), and tend instead to rely on sources such as the Internet.

Americans currently pay about $34 billion per year out of pocket for CAM therapies (5). The popularity of these therapies likely will continue to grow as health insurance programs increasingly cover them. Currently, coverage in the United States varies by state, and some require patients to obtain a prescription for CAM services or to utilize them under the supervision of a physician.

It is vital for physicians to understand the research behind CAM therapies in order to guide their patients through the range of options available for treating cancer pain. Misinformation and exaggerated claims of efficacy abound. The importance of informed decisions when integrating pharmacologic interventions and complementary medicine cannot be overstated. When used and understood properly, complementary therapies offer patients the opportunity to play a participatory role in their treatment, to control symptoms

on their own, and to maintain or improve their quality of life after active cancer treatment.

This chapter focuses on the current understanding of complementary therapies for the treatment of cancer pain, including acupuncture, massage therapy, hypnosis, music therapy, and dietary supplements and herbal remedies.

Acupuncture

Of all complementary therapies, acupuncture has been studied most extensively for pain control. It appears to be effective against cancer-related pain. Acupuncture is a technique of inserting and manipulating needles into various points on the body in order to restore health and well-being (Fig. 42.1). It is based on the ancient traditional Chinese medicine belief that the body's vital energy, or "qi," moves through interconnected vertical channels called "meridians." Illness was thought to occur when the individual's free flow of energy was blocked, and stimulating the qi with needles or pressure was believed to relieve the blockage and restore health.

No anatomic or histologic basis for the existence of meridians or qi has been uncovered. However, recent neuroscience research shows that acupuncture appears to induce analgesic effects and other clinical responses through modulation of the nervous system (6). Several animal and human studies demonstrate elevated serum and cerebrospinal fluid levels of endorphins and enkephalins following acupuncture treatment (7). In addition, a functional brain imaging study performed

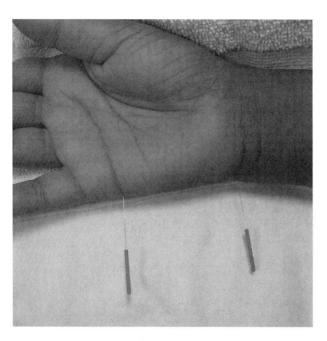

FIGURE 42.1

Acupuncture is safe and effective in controlling pain associated with cancer and cancer treatment.

on two groups of nine healthy subjects found that acupuncture stimulation of two different points—one on the leg and the other on the hand—activated the hypothalamus and nucleus accumbens and deactivated multiple limbic areas linked to pain association (8).

The World Health Organization supports the use of acupuncture as an effective intervention for problems such as adverse reactions to radiotherapy and chemotherapy, lower back pain, and postoperative pain (9), and a 1997 consensus conference at the National Institutes of Health found solid evidence for acupuncture as a treatment for nausea and osteoarthritic pain.

Many trials have evaluated acupuncture's effectiveness in treating chronic pain. One of the first was a study involving 183 patients with malignant pain (10), 82% of whom showed improvement over baseline pain after acupuncture treatment. More than half showed significant improvement, while the remaining 30% experienced shorter-term pain relief. This early study lacked controls and statistical analysis, but it helped lay the foundation for numerous future trials that investigated the efficacy of acupuncture for malignant cancer pain.

More recently, a randomized, blinded, controlled trial of 90 patients with cancer in Villejuif, France, examined the effects of auricular acupuncture on pain intensity (11). Auricular acupuncture uses the outer ear as a microsystem of the body. One group of patients in the trial received two courses of auricular acupuncture at points where an electrodermal signal had been detected.

Two other groups received treatment at placebo points. After two months, pain intensity had decreased 36% from baseline among patients receiving auricular acupuncture. In contrast, patients receiving placebo experienced only a 2% decrease. Most of the patients in the study suffered from neuropathic pain, which is often unresponsive to conventional medical treatment. The study relied on a single acupuncturist who was not blinded to the treatment, a factor that could limit the general applicability of its conclusions.

Another study, focusing specifically on women with breast cancer, suggests that acupuncture is an effective treatment to relieve pain after surgery (12). After undergoing ablation and axillary lymphadenectomy, 48 patients with breast cancer were treated with acupuncture, while a control group of 32 patients received no acupuncture after the same operation. On the fifth postoperative day, the women receiving acupuncture demonstrated significantly less pain in the area that was operated on compared to the control group ($P < 0.1$).

Studies performed to date support the utility of acupuncture as an effective treatment for cancer pain in some cases. This therapy merits further investigation, and appears worthy of pursuit as its risk-benefit ratio is favorable.

Massage Therapy

Massage therapy dates back thousands of years and is one of the complementary therapies used most by adults with cancer. There are multiple forms, including Swedish, sports, deep tissue, neuromuscular, and shiatsu massage.

In general, a therapeutic massage therapist uses his or her hands to rhythmically and methodically stretch and compress a patient's muscles and connective tissue. The end result includes increased circulation, stimulation of venous and lymphatic drainage, improved muscle tissue metabolism and elasticity, and greater relaxation through enhanced parasympathetic and reduced sympathetic nervous system activity (13).

A systematic review of research on massage therapy's impact on biochemistry found evidence of decreased levels of cortisol and increased levels of serotonin and dopamine associated with massage (14). The research reviewed included studies on depression, chronic fatigue, and breast cancer, among other conditions.

Patients with cancer have looked to massage not just for pain relief but also to reduce or relieve anxiety, emotional stress, muscular tension, and fatigue. A survey of 453 adult patients with cancer at The University of Texas M.D. Anderson Cancer Center in 2000 found that 26% had sought massage therapy (4). In 2004, a national survey of hospice programs found that 60% of 169 hospices offered complementary medicine services at their facilities, with massage being the most widely offered (15).

A systematic review of three years of data from 1290 patients at Memorial Sloan-Kettering Cancer Center examined patient-reported ratings of pain, fatigue, stress/anxiety, nausea, depression, and "other," both before and after they received massage therapy (16). After receiving massage, symptom scores among these patients were reduced by approximately 50%, even among patients reporting high baseline scores. In addition, the benefits persisted, with outpatients experiencing no return toward baseline scores over a 48 hour follow up period.

A crossover RCT of 87 patients with cancer assessed the subjects' levels of pain, nausea, and relaxation after two 10-minute foot massages (17) and one control period (18). Pain levels reported by patients decreased significantly during massage treatment.

Massage therapy may also reduce a patient's need for nonsteroidal anti-inflammatory drugs (NSAIDS). A randomized, prospective, two-period, crossover intervention study among 230 subjects tested the effects of therapeutic massage and healing touch in reducing symptoms and promoting relaxation (17). The study compared these therapies to presence of a therapist without massage or touch, and standardized care. After each of the four 45-minute sessions over a four week period, patients experienced reduced pain after receiving massage ($P < 0.001$) and healing touch ($P < 0.011$), compared to the control group. In addition, those in the massage group were able to reduce their use of NSAIDS over the course of the study.

Data from past studies indicate massage has an effect on physical symptoms, although in some cases its impact on pain was apparent in subgroups rather than the whole patient population. These studies, combined with the low likelihood of harmful side effects, support the use of massage as an adjunct to conventional care. However, the number of patients studied remains small, and further research would strengthen the evidence base.

Hypnosis

Mind-body therapies such as hypnosis are popular among patients with cancer not only because of their apparent effectiveness in relieving symptoms, but also because they are noninvasive techniques that can be tailored to each individual's needs and preferences. Patients can also be taught self-hypnosis to practice on their own.

Hypnosis is an altered state of consciousness, a state between wakefulness and sleep. It is most often achieved under the guidance of a trained hypnotherapist. The subject enters into a state where his attention is more focused and he is more open and responsive to suggestion. The goal is to help the subject gain more control over his behavior, thoughts or well-being. Hypnosis can be induced through a variety of methods, including progressive muscle relaxation or inviting the subject to fix his gaze while the therapist gives suggestions.

Hypnosis has been studied extensively and found useful for treating acute and chronic pain, nausea, anxiety, allergies, certain skin conditions, phobias, and posttraumatic stress disorder. In 1996 the National Institutes of Health judged hypnosis to be an effective intervention for alleviating pain from cancer and other chronic conditions.

Research suggests that hypnotic sensory analgesia is at least in part mediated by reduction in spinal cord antinociceptive mechanisms in response to hypnotic suggestion (19). In addition, studies show, hypnotic analgesia may be related to brain mechanisms that serve to prevent awareness of pain once nociception has reached higher centers via brain mechanisms. Finally, it may be related to a reduction in the affective dimension, perhaps as a result of the subject's reinterpretation of meanings associated with the painful sensation.

One RCT of 50 patients with cancer assigned some individuals to a month-long regimen of standard medical treatment and psychological support, and others to the same treatment regimen plus weekly hypnotherapy sessions (20). The researchers found a statistically significant reduction in physical distress scores for the hypnotherapy group compared with the standard care group ($P < 0.01$).

Hypnosis has been found to be especially effective among children. A 1988 RCT of 48 patients (children) with leukemia undergoing bone marrow aspirations tested the effectiveness of hypnosis and behavioral distraction (imaginative involvement) as compared to a control group that received standard care only (21). Results showed that for the younger patients (aged 3–6 years) hypnosis provided a significant reduction in pain, as compared to both the distraction and control groups. By contrast, among the older children (aged 7–10 years), both hypnosis and distraction showed significant reductions in observer-rated pain as compared to controls. Problems with this trial include the hospital nursing staff's possible contamination of the control group as staff members were inadequately blinded to group allocation.

In 1999, a three-armed RCT of 30 patients (children) with leukemia undergoing bone marrow aspiration evaluated the effect of hypnosis versus cognitive behavioral training and standard care controls (22). Pain and anxiety—both self-reported and observer-reported—were significantly less in the hypnosis and cognitive behavioral training groups than in the control group or than their own baseline recordings.

A later, four-armed RCT of 80 patients with leukemia undergoing lumbar punctures divided the children into four treatment groups: direct hypnosis, indirect hypnosis, therapist attention control, and standard treatment control (23). Those receiving hypnotherapy received both analgesic suggestions and ego strengthening, and treatment was varied according to the child's age, interests, and cognitive and social development. Patients in both hypnosis groups reported significantly less pain ($P < 0.01$). than the control groups. Self-hypnosis was found to be less effective.

Negative effects from hypnosis—including mild dizziness, nausea, or headache—are unusual and generally minimal.

Music Therapy

The use of music to ease pain, anxiety and depression is increasingly popular (Fig. 42.2). It is safe, low-cost, and easy to provide and obtain. In a study of 468 abdominal surgical patients in five U.S. hospitals, patients were assigned randomly to one of four groups: relaxation, music therapy, a combination of the two, and control (24). Music led to significant decreases in both pain intensity and related distress associated with pain.

However, a Cochrane systematic review of studies examining the effect of music on pain and opioid

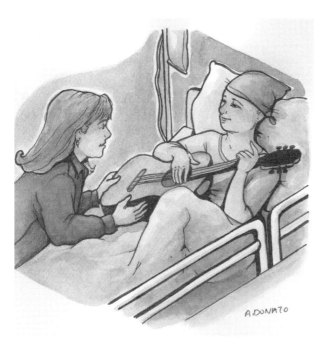

FIGURE 42.2

Music therapy reduces pain and other symptoms in cancer patients.

requirements found that many were of low quality and that there was unexplained heterogeneity within results (25). The clinical efficacy of music therapy for pain treatment requires further evaluation.

Opioid requirements were found to be reduced with music therapy, but not to a significant degree. NSAIDS with opioid-reducing effects have a far greater impact than the decrease seen with music therapy.

Dietary Supplements and Herbal Remedies

Patients with cancer should be cautious when considering the use of dietary supplements and herbal remedies to relieve pain. Many of these products have not yet been studied in patients with cancer and may interact negatively with chemotherapeutic agents or any prescription medication.

Dietary supplements such as S-adenosyl-L-methionine (SAMe), glucosamine, methylsulfonylmethane (MSM), chondroitin, and turmeric have been empirically tested as treatments for arthritic conditions and musculoskeletal pain such as chronic lower back pain and fibromyalgia. In addition, glucosamine and chondroitin sulfate have been shown to reduce osteoarthritis pain—a condition suffered by some patients with cancer. Glucosamine sulphate has positive effects on symptomatic and structural outcomes of knee osteoarthritis (26).

Supplementation with glutamine, a nonessential amino acid, was shown effective in reducing peripheral neuropathy induced by Paclitaxel in patients with cancer (27,28). There is also evidence that glutamine may decrease the toxicity associated with chemotherapy and radiation (29).

Herbal remedies that offer hope for pain relief include *Boswellia serrata* (known for its anti-inflammatory properties) and the Chinese herb *Corydalis yanhusuo* (known for its analgesic and sedating effects).

However, herbs and supplements whose effects mimic that of NSAIDS should not be used in place of those drugs until further studies confirm their safety and efficacy. Patients and their physicians should also take into consideration the possible effects of botanicals on other drugs when used simultaneously, as herb-drug interactions are common (30).

Symptom Management in Children

The use of complementary therapies for cancer pain is not limited to adult patients with cancer. A study of 75 children with cancer receiving conventional treatment at an urban academic medical center in the United States attempted to determine the prevalence of CAM use among them (31). Overall, 84% of the patients (or their parents) reported use of one or more complementary therapies, with the most common being mind/body therapies, nutritional and herbal agents, and changes in diet. Use of complementary therapies was not associated with specific demographic or clinical factors, or with participation in a clinical trial.

A systematic review of nine pain-related hypnosis studies conducted between 1982 and 1999 found reductions in pain among children with cancer (32). However, most of the trials did not use appropriate control groups, and results were inconsistent from study to study. Two more recent RCTs found therapist-guided hypnosis effective in reducing pain and anxiety among children with leukemia (22,23).

Only one controlled, child-focused acupuncture study exists. It focused on migraine pain, not cancer pain, but nonetheless demonstrated successful pain reduction among those receiving acupuncture treatment (33).

With massage, there is a similar absence of pediatric studies focused on cancer pain. Two small studies indicate that massage may be effective in reducing pain among children with juvenile rheumatoid arthritis (34) and children who are burn victims undergoing dressing changes (35). Child-focused trials of various complementary therapies lag behind those involving adults.

CONCLUSION

Complementary therapies serve as adjuncts to mainstream care, providing relief of physical and mental symptoms, addressing body, mind, and spirit and enhancing patients' quality of life. Increasing public interest in these therapies has created a multibillion dollar business in the United States and in other developed countries. Complementary therapies are diverse, minimally if at all invasive, comforting and amenable to patient self-choice. They enable patients to participate in their own care.

Although many have been practiced as part of traditional medicine systems for centuries, scientific research examining the safety and effectiveness of complementary modalities began less than two decades ago. The largely favorable risk-benefit ratio suggests that complementary therapies can play an important role in physical and emotional rehabilitation. These therapies should be tailored to the needs and preferences of each patient as part of patient-centered medical care.

References

1. Lesage P, Portenoy RK. Trends in cancer pain management. *Cancer Control.* 1999;6(2):136–145.
2. Pain (PDQ): Highlights of Pain Management. 2007. (Accessed at http://www.nci.nih.gov/cancertopics/pdq/supportivecare/pain/healthprofessional)
3. Ernst E, Cassileth BR. The prevalence of complementary/alternative medicine in cancer: a systematic review. *Cancer.* 1998;83(4):777–782.
4. Richardson MA, Sanders T, Palmer JL, Greisinger A, Singletary SE. Complementary/alternative medicine use in a comprehensive cancer center and the implications for oncology. *J Clin Oncol.* 2000;18(13):2505–2514.
5. Herman PM, Craig BM, Caspi O. Is complementary and alternative medicine (CAM) cost-effective? A systematic review. *BMC Complement Altern Med.* 2005;5:11.
6. Han JS. Acupuncture and endorphins. *Neurosci Lett.* 2004;361(1–3):258–261.
7. Grossman A, Clement-Jones V. Opiate receptors: enkephalins and endorphins. *Clin Endocrinol Metab.* 1983;12(1):31–56.
8. Wu MT, Hsieh JC, Xiong J, et al. Central nervous pathway for acupuncture stimulation: localization of processing with functional MR imaging of the brain—preliminary experience. *Radiology.* 1999;212(1):133–141.
9. Traditional medicine. 2003. (Accessed at http://www.who.int/mediacentre/factsheets/fs134/en/)
10. Filshie J, Redman D. Acupuncture and malignant pain problems. *Eur J Surg Oncol.* 1985;11(4):389–394.
11. Alimi D, Rubino C, Pichard-Leandri E, Fermand-Brule S, Dubreuil-Lemaire ML, Hill C. Analgesic effect of auricular acupuncture for cancer pain: a randomized, blinded, controlled trial. *J Clin Oncol.* 2003;21(22):4120–4126.
12. He JP, Friedrich M, Ertan AK, Muller K, Schmidt W. Pain-relief and movement improvement by acupuncture after ablation and axillary lymphadenectomy in patients with mammary cancer. *Clin Exp Obstet Gynecol.* 1999;26(2):81–84.
13. Field TM. Massage therapy effects. *Am Psychol.* 1998;53(12):1270–1281.
14. Field T, Hernandez-Reif M, Diego M, Schanberg S, Kuhn C. Cortisol decreases and serotonin and dopamine increase following massage therapy. *Int J Neurosci.* 2005;115(10):1397–1413.
15. Demmer C. A survey of complementary therapy services provided by hospices. *J Palliat Med.* 2004;7(4):510–516.
16. Cassileth BR, Vickers AJ. Massage therapy for symptom control: outcome study at a major cancer center. *J Pain Symptom Manage.* 2004;28(3):244–249.
17. Post-White J, Kinney ME, Savik K, Gau JB, Wilcox C, Lerner I. Therapeutic massage and healing touch improve symptoms in cancer. *Integr Cancer Ther.* 2003;2(4):332–344.
18. Grealish L, Lomasney A, Whiteman B. Foot massage. A nursing intervention to modify the distressing symptoms of pain and nausea in patients hospitalized with cancer. *Cancer Nurs.* 2000;23(3):237–243.
19. Kiernan BD, Dane JR, Phillips LH, Price DD. Hypnotic analgesia reduces R-III nociceptive reflex: further evidence concerning the multifactorial nature of hypnotic analgesia. *Pain.* 1995;60(1):39–47.
20. Liossi C, White P. Efficacy of clinical hypnosis in the enhancement of quality of life of terminally ill cancer patients. *Contemporary Hypnosis.* 2001;18:145–150.
21. Kuttner L, Bowman M, Teasdale M. Psychological treatment of distress, pain, and anxiety for young children with cancer. *J Dev Behav Pediatr.* 1988;9(6):374–381.
22. Liossi C, Hatira P. Clinical hypnosis versus cognitive behavioral training for pain management with pediatric cancer patients undergoing bone marrow aspirations. *Int J Clin Exp Hypn.* 1999;47(2):104–116.
23. Liossi C, Hatira P. Clinical hypnosis in the alleviation of procedure-related pain in pediatric oncology patients. *Int J Clin Exp Hypn.* 2003;51(1):4–28.
24. Good M, Stanton-Hicks M, Grass JA, et al. Relaxation and music to reduce postsurgical pain. *J Adv Nurs.* 2001;33(2):208–215.

25. Cepeda MS, Carr DB, Lau J, Alvarez H. Music for pain relief. *Cochrane Database Syst Rev.* 2006;2:CD004843.

26. Herrero-Beaumont G, Ivorra JA, Del Carmen Trabado M, et al. Glucosamine sulfate in the treatment of knee osteoarthritis symptoms: a randomized, double-blind, placebo-controlled study using acetaminophen as a side comparator. *Arthritis Rheum.* 2007;56(2):555–567.

27. Stubblefield MD, Vahdat LT, Balmaceda CM, Troxel AB, Hesdorffer CS, Gooch CL. Glutamine as a neuroprotective agent in high-dose paclitaxel-induced peripheral neuropathy: a clinical and electrophysiologic study. *Clin Oncol (R Coll Radiol).* 2005;17(4):271–276.

28. Vahdat L, Papadopoulos K, Lange D, et al. Reduction of paclitaxel-induced peripheral neuropathy with glutamine. *Clin Cancer Res.* 2001;7(5):1192–1197.

29. Savarese DM, Savy G, Vahdat L, Wischmeyer PE, Corey B. Prevention of chemotherapy and radiation toxicity with glutamine. *Cancer Treat Rev.* 2003;29(6):501–513.

30. AboutHerbs Web site (Accessed April 10, 2007, at http://www.mskcc.org/aboutherbs.)

31. Kelly KM, Jacobson JS, Kennedy DD, Braudt SM, Mallick M, Weiner MA. Use of unconventional therapies by children with cancer at an urban medical center. *J Pediatr Hematol Oncol.* 2000;22(5):412–416.

32. Wild MR, Espie CA. The efficacy of hypnosis in the reduction of procedural pain and distress in pediatric oncology: a systematic review. *J Dev Behav Pediatr.* 2004;25(3):207–213.

33. Pintov S, Lahat E, Alstein M, Vogel Z, Barg J. Acupuncture and the opioid system: implications in management of migraine. *Pediatr Neurol.* 1997;17(2):129–133.

34. Field T, Hernandez-Reif M, Seligman S, et al. Juvenile rheumatoid arthritis: benefits from massage therapy. *J Pediatr Psychol.* 1997;22(5):607–617.

35. Hernandez-Reif M, Field T, Largie S, et al. Childrens' distress during burn treatment is reduced by massage therapy. *J Burn Care Rehabil.* 2001;22(2):191–195; discussion 0.

V

NEUROLOGIC AND
NEUROMUSCULAR
COMPLICATIONS
OF CANCER

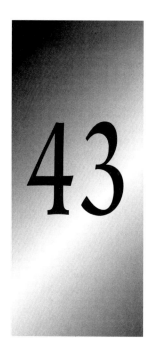

Rehabilitation of Patients with Brain Tumors

43

Michael W. O'Dell
C. David Lin
Eric Schwabe
Tara Post
Erin Embry

Within the field of cancer rehabilitation, interest in the functional management of persons with brain tumors has grown substantially over the past decade. This increased interest is likely the result of new chemotherapeutic treatments (1–4), less invasive resection techniques minimizing surgical morbidity (5–6), greater recognition of the importance of function by neuro-oncology professionals (7–11), and growing evidence of the efficacy of rehabilitation in this population (12–20). Several recent studies have demonstrated that inpatient rehabilitation outcomes in persons with brain tumors are comparable to those of case-matched subjects with stroke (14,18) and traumatic brain injury (TBI) (13,17,18).

The purpose of this chapter is to present an overview of disease management and impairments in persons with brain tumors and how they impact mobilization and performance. This chapter is organized into three sections: general information and models of brain tumor rehabilitation, management and treatment of disease and symptoms, and interdisciplinary rehabilitation issues.

EPIDEMIOLOGY, HISTOLOGY, AND DEMOGRAPHICS

About 9,000 cases of glioblastoma multiforme (GBM) and the same number of other primary brain tumors are diagnosed each year in the United States (Fig. 43.1) (1). The incidence of metastatic brain tumors appears to be increasing and is currently estimated at about 150,000 cases a year in the United States. The increase is probably related to earlier diagnosis, an increase in overall cancer survival that allows more time for metastases to occur, and disruption of the blood–brain barrier from chemotherapy (CT) used to treat the primary tumor (2,12) The most common primary tumors metastasizing to the brain are lung, renal cell, breast, and melanoma (2). From the rehabilitation perspective, brain tumor histology might be best viewed in three categories, as recently outlined by Giordana and Clara (10):

Group 1: *Nonprogressive* tumors frequently "cured" with surgical intervention, with or without residual impairments (cerebellar pilocytic astrocytomas in children, pituitary adenomas, schwannomas, and meningiomas).

Group 2: *More aggressive tumors*—but still with reasonable periods of disease-free survival (ie, low-grade astrocytomas, oligodendrogliomas, ependymomas, and cerebellar medulloblastomas).

Group 3: *Aggressive tumors*, which recur quickly and carry a poor prognosis (ie, GBM, anaplastic astrocytomas, and metastases to the brain).

It should be noted that the medical and surgical management may differ substantially within a given tumor group, that is, GBM and brain metastases.

517

KEY POINTS

- The incidence of metastatic brain tumors is increasing due to earlier diagnosis, an increase in overall cancer survival that allows more time for metastases to occur, and disruption of the blood–brain barrier from chemotherapy used to treat the primary tumor.
- Supportive rehabilitation occurs after a tumor has been controlled but there are permanent residual impairments, and is the model of care most familiar to rehabilitation professionals caring for other etiologies of acquired brain injury (ABI).
- Although overlapping impairment profiles suggest brain tumor survivors are like other ABIs, there are differences in natural history, medical management, and psychological response to the disease process.

- Functional gains by persons with brain tumors in inpatient rehabilitation are not statistically different from case-matched strokes or traumatic brain injury (TBI) subjects, they have shorter lengths of stay, 65%–85% return home, and 15%–30% require transfer back to acute care.
- Despite common practice to the contrary, there is no evidence that seizure prophylaxis is effective in patients with brain tumors.
- Prophylaxis of deep venous thrombosis is safe and effective in persons with brain tumors.
- Coping mechanisms in patients with malignant brain tumors may not differ substantially from those in other etiology of neurological disease.

Among the published inpatient brain tumor rehabilitation studies, about 20%–30% of admissions are GBM, 25%–30% are metastases (primary tumors mostly in lung and breast), and about 20% are meningiomas (13,15,16). Demographics differ from other acquired brain injuries (ABI), with brain tumor subjects being older and more likely female than TBI, but slightly younger than stroke patients. The only published outpatient rehabilitation study had 13 patients—8 male and 5 female, with an average age of 34 years, and 9 of whom had anaplastic glioma (20).

MODELS OF BRAIN TUMOR REHABILITATION

As discussed elsewhere (12,21–23), the process of general cancer rehabilitation can be grouped into one of four broad categories, often referred to as the Dietz Classification (24). *Preventative rehabilitation* emphasizes early intervention and education to help prevent or delay the symptoms of tumor progression or treatment (22,25). Interventions might include a home exercise program to minimize debility during radiation therapy (RT), splinting to maintain joint-range flexibility in a spastic extremity, safety awareness education to minimize injury from falls, prophylaxis for deep venous thrombosis (DVT) in inpatient rehabilitation, and substituting a sedating antiepileptic drug (AED) with a less sedating agent. *Restorative rehabilitation* focuses on patients who are expected to return to their premorbid functional status without substantial residual disability. This is exemplified in those patients who experience a resolution of motor, coordination, and

cognitive deficits three months following an uncomplicated frontoparietal meningioma resection. Goals in restorative rehabilitation ultimately emphasize community, educational, and vocational reintegration (22,26). *Supportive rehabilitation* occurs after a tumor has been controlled but there are permanent, residual impairments. This scenario is probably most familiar to rehabilitation professionals caring for other etiologies of ABI. The expectation here is to maximize functional independence in both the patient's home and community environments. For example, if the patient with a meningioma described previously experience permanent spastic hemiparesis and mild aphasia, then compensatory and communication strategies, bracing, use of the unaffected extremity, and adaptive equipment may be required. Cheville (21) has pointed out that primary and secondary cognitive deficits following craniotomy or RT can be addressed with cognitive rehabilitation in this supportive model. Finally, *palliative rehabilitation* occurs when intensive rehabilitation is no longer appropriate, as with the recurrence of a rapidly progressing tumor and functional decline (24). The goals here are comfort, caregiver education, minimizing burden of care, and appropriate equipment recommendations (see Chapter 70) (27). The rehabilitation focus will vary by tumor type (Table 43.1). This chapter will focus primarily on the preventative, restorative, and supportive phases of brain tumor rehabilitation.

Whatever the context, it is likely that rehabilitation services are underutilized given the association between functional status and quality of life in persons with brain tumors (28,29). Access to rehabilitation expertise may be a challenge due to lack of knowledge by patient,

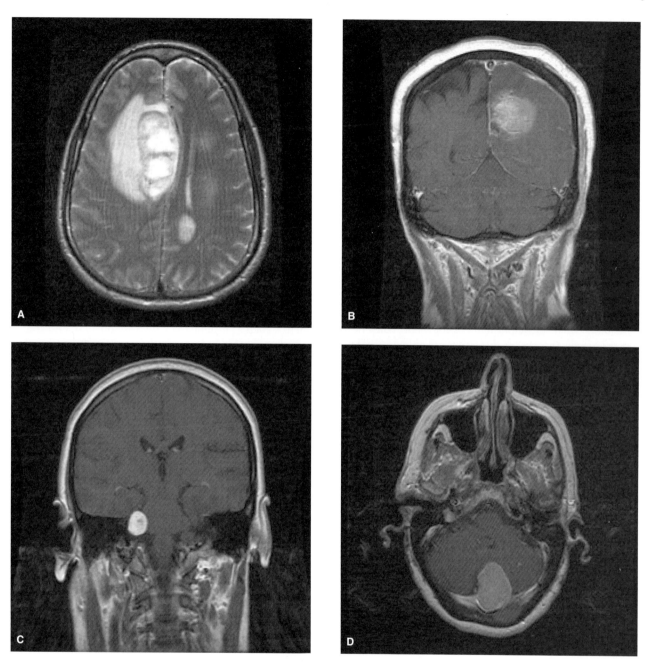

FIGURE 43.1

Magnetic resonance images of various brain tumor types. (A) glioblastoma multiforme, (B) colon cancer metastatic to the brain, (C) acoustic schwannoma, and (D) meningioma.

family, or neuro-oncologist. Ironically, rehabilitation professionals themselves may consciously or unconsciously limit access because they feel unprepared to provide care to this population (28,30,31).

The basic tenets of neurorehabilitation are heavily impairment-driven, with the goal to maximize function and minimize caregiver and societal burden for

all etiologies of ABI. Well-documented impairments in persons with brain tumors undergoing rehabilitation include weakness (hemiparesis and general debility), cognitive and visual-perceptive deficits, ataxia, cranial nerve dysfunction, bowel and bladder problems, aphasia, dysphagia, and dysarthria (15,16). These are typical impairments across the spectrum of ABI, includ-

TABLE 43.1
Tumor Groups versus Dietz Classification

Tumor Group	Survival Time	Preventative	Restorative	Supportive	Palliative	Neurorehab Model
1	Years to decades	XX	XX	XX		TBI[a]
2	Years	XX		XX	XX	Multiple sclerosis
3	Months to year(s)	XX		XX	XX	General cancer

[a]TBI: traumatic brain injury.

ing etiologies where rehabilitation is considered the standard of care.

Overlapping impairment profiles suggest that the rehabilitation team can approach brain tumor survivors much like other, more familiar etiologies of ABI. There are, however, important differences (Table 43.2). The natural history (ie, prognosis) of a given tumor greatly affects the rehabilitation management. Those survivors in tumor group 1 with nonprogressive tumors will be approached much like patients with TBI or stroke. They will have variable impairments, depending on the anatomy of the tumor, and their rehabilitation treatment will emphasize independence at home and in the community maintained over a substantial time period. Patients in tumor group 2 might be best characterized within a framework used for persons with relapsing-remitting multiple sclerosis (MS). After the initial tumor resection and treatment, there will likely be a core set of impairments and activity limitations, which decline over a variable time period. Depending on the histology and prognosis of the tumor, there will be recurrences associated with a drop in functional status somewhat analogous to an exacerbation of MS. The rehabilitation team will reevaluate at each recurrence and develop new goals based on the new set of impairments.

Although the model of care for progressive tumors in tumor group 3 is common in general cancer rehabilitation, it is somewhat unique in the rehabilitation of persons with ABI. These patients will require frequent reevaluation, as the importance of functional independence may decrease or disappear in the transition from supportive to palliative care (9). Goals are chosen that can be achieved over shorter time frames. Moreover, the need to *clearly* communicate *realistic* goals to patient and family is more important for brain tumor rehabilitation than other ABI etiologies. The team must recognize and address the psychological stress of patient, family, *and* of the rehabilitation team itself. Effective management of rapidly changing

medical comorbidities help mitigate symptoms directly or indirectly, limiting mobilization. Regardless of the tumor group being treated or the phase of rehabilitation care, there are common and challenging impairments, such as fatigue (32), depression (33), and cognitive demise (34), which are discussed in more detail in the following sections.

Brain tumor patients may require acute or subacute inpatient rehabilitation, outpatient rehabilitation, or home-based therapy (35). Most patients admitted to inpatient rehabilitation arrive after craniotomy, when they experience an acute decline in performance due to the tumor or side effects of treatment. In acute inpatient rehabilitation, fatigue and endurance deficits may be more limiting than neurological deficits, especially in preventing three hours per day of therapy participation. Most patients will clearly require daily medical and nursing care. The need for concomitant CT or RT during inpatient rehabilitation must be delineated, as both can compete and interfere with therapy treatment time. Every effort should be made to schedule RT and CT at the end of the day, after rehabilitation sessions. This may also have the added benefit of minimizing the impact of cancer-related fatigue often experienced by patients after these treatments.

If a patient cannot tolerate three hours of therapy but still has substantial medical and nursing needs, admission to a subacute rehabilitation facility may be required. However, the inability or unwillingness of some skilled nursing facilities to accommodate ongoing treatments, such as CT or RT; manage complicated medical needs; and provide skilled interventions related to cognitive, language, and visuoperceptive impairments may limit options. Those patients not requiring intensive multidisciplinary therapy or who need a "tune up" after treatment are candidates for outpatient or home-based therapy (35). Frank discussions with the treating neuro-oncologist or neurosurgeon are recommended before addressing hospice care with the patient and family.

TABLE 43.2

A Comparison of Brain Tumors to Other Acquired Brain Injuries

	BRAIN TUMOR	STROKE	TBI	MS
Onset	Insidious	Immediate	Immediate	Insidious
Age of onset[a]	Middle age to elderly	Elderly	Young	Young to middle age
Trajectory of functional evolution	Slowly to rapidly worsening	Stable to improving; possibility of second event	Stable to improving	Slowly worsening, with or without discreet exacerbations
Certainty of functional trajectory	High certainty of worsening with very aggressive and moderate with less aggressive tumors	Moderate certainty of improvement with risk for recurrence	High certainty of improvement	Intermediate to high certainty, but over a long time period
Neurologic presentation	UMN: focal and diffuse LMN: PN (chemo) or myopathy (steroids)	UMN: primarily focal LMN: unusual, occasional PN from DM	UMN: focal and diffuse LMN: traumatic nerve injuries	UMN: focal SC and brain and diffuse LMN: unusual
Surgical comorbidity	+	–[b]	+/–	–
Medical comorbidity	Fatigue, depression, seizures, cognitive impairment; complications of steroids, RT, chemo	HTN, cardiopulmonary and other age-related impairments, spasticity, language deficits	Seizures, cognitive and behavioral impairments, spasticity, traumatic fractures, visceral injury	Fatigue, cognitive and personality impairments, spasticity, complications of steroids
Dietz category addressed in rehabilitation	Preventative, restorative, supportive, or palliative depending on tumor type	Preventative, supportive (restorative in mild stroke)	Preventive, supportive (restorative in mild TBI)	Preventative, restorative, supportive, and palliative

Abbreviations: Chemo, chemotherapy; DM, diabetes mellitus; LMN, lower motor neuron; MS, multiple sclerosis; PN, peripheral neuropathy; RT, radiation therapy; SC, spinal cord;. TBI, traumatic brain injury; UMN, upper motor neuron.
[a]Estimate, highly variable in actuality.
[b]Except with some hemorrhagic stroke.

FUNCTIONAL OUTCOMES IN INPATIENT REHABILITATION

Table 43.3 provides a comparison of several published studies regarding inpatient rehabilitation outcomes in persons with brain tumors. Despite varying methodologies, several generalizations can be made. FIM (functional independence measure) admission scores cluster in the 60–70 range and FIM gains in the 20–25 point range. Functional gains are not statistically different for those studies that provide case-matched comparisons to stroke (14,18) and TBI (13,17,18). However, relatively small sample sizes might explain some of the lack of significance. Those same studies have consistently shown shorter lengths of stay among the tumor patients. Proposed explanations include better psychosocial support among tumor patients and a belief (stated or unstated) by the rehabilitation team that a rapid return home would positively impact quality of life. Sixty-five percent to eighty-five percent of patients

return home and 15%–30% required transfer back to acute care. Given that the transfer rates in general inpatient rehabilitation are about 10%, this underscores how important the medical management component is during inpatient rehabilitation (36). Despite being an area of great interest in the field, few conclusions can be drawn regarding factors that may predict outcomes at discharge. Marciniak and colleagues (15), with a larger small size (N =132) were able to conclude that outcomes were better among initial rather than recurrent tumors and among patients receiving RT compared with those not receiving such treatment. Little evidence supports the intuitive notion that gliomas (Group 3) might fare worse than meningiomas (Group 1) (13,15,18) or that metastatic (with prerequisite systemic disease) fare worse than primary disease (15,16). There is insufficient data to state whether the location of the tumor influences functional outcomes, although impairments will clearly differ on the basis of tumor location.

TABLE 43.3

Studies on Inpatient Rehabilitation: Outcomes in Brain Tumors

AUTHOR, Y (Y)	N	MEAN AGE (Y)	% F	HISTOLOGY (% GMB, MET, MEN, OTHER)	% RT	% CT	% T/H	FIM A/D/G/E	TA, LOS	COMMENTS
Feder, 1989 (1977–1986)	76	57.1	72	0/0/100/0	NS	NS	NS/85	NS	45ᵃ/106	Older Israeli data of historical interest addressing only post-operative meningioma, >70% "severe" neurological deficits, 28% had medical complications
Huang, 1998 (NS)	63	59.8	51	NS	NS	NS	NS/86	61/84.7/23.6/.84	19.6/25.3	Matched by age, gender & lesion side to 63 strokes, outcomes not statistically different, LOS shorter in tumors
O'Dell, 1998 (1994–1996)	40	53.1	40	20/12.5/20/47.5	17.5	12.5	7.5/82.5	71.5/96.9/25.4/1.5	11.1/17.8	Matched by admission FIM and age to 40 TBIs, outcomes not statistically different, LOS shorter in tumors, 25% recurrent tumors
Huang, 2000 (1992–1997)	78	57.2	56	NS	NS	NS	20/87	64.1/90.3/26.2/1.00	13.5/21.9	Matched by age and location with 78 TBIs, FIM gain greater in TBI, home discharge greater and LOS shorter in tumors, no difference in FIM efficacy
Marciniak, 2001 (1993–1996)	132	58	NS	26/33/16/25	15	3	24/65	60/82/23/.86ᵇ	NS/24.6	No functional difference between primary and metastatic tumors, 31% recurrent tumors and they did worse, radiation treatment did better, common impairments: hemiparesis 56%, cranial nerve 30%, dysphagia 26%
Mukand, 2001	51	59.7	35	31/26/26/17	??	??	15.7/68.6	67.2/87.1/19.9/NS	NS/19.7	Study cited incidence of RT and CT only prior to admission, common impairments: cognitive 80%, hemiparesis 78%, cranial nerve 29%, dysphagia 26%
Greenberg, 2006 (1993–2004)	168	58.5ᵇ	<50	23/0/67/0	0	0	NS/89	77/88/17.7/.81ᵇ	18/21.7ᵇ	Compared to 1660 strokes in database, no recurrent tumors, LOS shorter in tumors, FIM gains comparable among groups

Abbreviations: CT, chemotherapy; F, female; FIM, functional independence measure for admission (A), discharge (D), gain (G) and efficiency (E); GBM, glioblastoma multiforme; H, home discharge; LOS, rehab length of stay; MEN, meningiomas; MET, metastases; N, number of subjects; NS, not specified; RT, radiation therapy; T, transfer to acute care; TA, time from acute care admission to rehab transfer; Y, year published; (Y), years of data collection.

ᵃTime post-surgery.

ᵇData not reported but rather calculated from raw data provided in the study.

BRAIN TUMOR TREATMENT: REHABILITATION IMPLICATIONS

Details of specific medical and surgical treatment protocols for brain tumors are outlined in Chapters 5, 6, and 20. The following discussion is provided as an overview of common treatments and how they impact the rehabilitation process.

Surgery

Nearly all patients presenting for restorative and supportive rehabilitation will have already undergone surgery. For both primary and metastatic tumors, advances in surgical management have contributed to improved survival, provided tissue for pathology and treatment planning, and improved quality of life by decreasing symptoms associated with elevated intracranial pressure (37–39). Localization techniques, such as intraoperative and functional magnetic resonance imaging, magnetoencephalography, and diffusion tensor imaging, have allowed neurosurgeons to achieve more complete tumor resection and decreased surgical morbidity by sparing normal brain parenchyma. Brain mapping techniques have been particularly important to guide resection of tumors residing near the motor strip and language centers (38). The implication for the rehabilitation team may be fewer patients with focal neurological impairments and a greater proportion of more diffuse impairments. Beyond the tumor resection itself, adjuvant treatments can be surgically placed, including local CT delivered through sustained released polymers and placement of radioactive substances in the resected tumor bed. The techniques described previously have also contributed to the surgical management of brain metastasis, but patient selection for surgery is not necessarily as clear. The ideal candidates are probably patients with surgically accessible lesions, better functional status, younger age, and well-controlled primary tumor (39). Regardless of tumor types, almost all patients are placed on steroids to decrease cerebral edema.

Chemotherapy

Chemotherapy is not generally used for benign or metastatic brain tumors and has only recently become common in primary malignant tumors. This limitation stems from the need for CT to interrupt rapid cell division, whereas many brain tumors are slow-growing by nature and few agents can cross the blood–brain barrier to access the tumor. Published in 2005, Stupp and colleagues (4) presented class I evidence that treatment with temozolomide (Temodar) plus RT provides a survival benefit in the treatment of GBM compared to RT alone. Temozolomide is an oral alkylating agent used as monotherapy and has very few negative effects on quality of life (40). Common side effects include fatigue, headaches, alopecia, nausea, and vomiting (4). The benefit of adding temozolomide to RT was modest (12.1 vs 14.6 months mean survival and 10.4% vs 26.5% two-year survival), but some authors feel this early success will herald new advances in brain tumor CT over the next decade (3). Monitoring included complete blood counts for leucopenia (41). In addition to temozolomide, other oral agents include procarbazine and lomustine.

Nausea and vomiting is a side effect of CT that substantially affects rehabilitation. Antiemetic and antinausea medications (Compazine, ondansetron, granisetron, and metoclopramide) can be used prior to CT. Particularly for patients in tumor groups 1 and 2, some caution should be exercised with drugs such as metoclopramide that disturb dopaminergic activity and may impede the rate of neurologic recovery (42). Intravenous CT, such as cisplatin or bischloroethylnitrosourea (CBNU), will require intravascular access, usually through a mediport or peripheral intravenous line, which may require special certification by nursing staff or temporary transfer out of rehabilitation.

Thrombocytopenia from CT can cause bleeding from the nose, gums, urinary tract, or gastrointestinal tract. Platelet counts less than 20,000/mL of blood will generally result in bleeding and, at Weill Cornell Medical Center, rehabilitation therapy is held when counts are less than 10,000/mL. Patients with thrombocytopenia should avoid drugs that affect functioning of platelets, such as ibuprofen, aspirin, and naproxen. If counts are very low, platelet transfusions may be needed. In those patients with persistent thrombocytopenia, oprelvekin may prevent further falls in platelet counts (43). Neutropenia is also common after CT, and counts below 1,500/mL of blood may be associated with an increased the risk of infections. In order to speed up the recovery and activity of white blood cells, drugs such as colony-stimulating factors can be administered such as G-CSF and GM-CSF.

Radiation Therapy

Radiation therapy uses high-energy light beams (x-rays) or charged particles (proton beams) to damage critical biological molecules in tumor cells. The treatment is usually provided on an outpatient basis with each workday for a period of several weeks (44). RT is also commonly provided in inpatient rehabilitation units and has been cited as a factor influencing functional outcomes (15). Significant neurologic injury can be seen with therapeutic irradiation, with the symptoms depending on the location and dosage. RT is associated with local alopecia and skin erythema, fatigue, nausea and vomiting, loss of appetite, and alteration of taste. RT-induced fatigue may be persistent for several months. The most noticeable long-term side effect is a gradual decline of cognitive function and memory (45).

Acute RT reactions can be seen in both inpatient and outpatient rehabilitation, and are usually due to increased cerebral edema (which can be confirmed on brain imaging scans). Corticosteroids can help alleviate these symptoms, prompting some to advocate standing low-dose steroids while undergoing RT (46). Radiation necrosis is the most severe side effect, appearing from a few months to several years after RT is completed. Approximately 5% of patients irradiated for brain tumors develop clinically detectable radiation necrosis, which can be extremely difficult to differentiate from tumor recurrence (47).

MEDICAL MANAGEMENT OF BRAIN TUMORS

For nearly all inpatients, and a sizable number of outpatients, effective medical management is requisite to achieving optimal rehabilitation outcomes. Even in the best inpatient centers, general (48–50) and brain cancer (13,15,16) transfer rates back to the acute care services range up to 30%. The inpatient rehabilitation team must understand that medical complexity is intrinsic to this population and be willing to accept and manage complications that develop after admission. Likewise, the outpatient rehabilitation team should have a working knowledge of common medication and treatment side effects, as well as the clinical presentation consistent with tumor recurrence.

Steroids

Vasogenic edema surrounds brain tumors and contributes significantly to the morbidity experienced by patients. Edema results from the lack of tight endothelial junctions in the tumor blood vessels and increased permeability of tumor vessels. Peritumoral edema can lead to headaches, seizures, mass effect, and, if severe, fatal herniation. The mainstay of treatment is corticosteroids. Although the mechanism of action is not well understood, steroids may decrease edema by decreasing the permeability to tumor capillaries (51). Dexamethasone is generally used because of its low mineralocorticoid activity, lower infection risk, and less impairment of cognition than other steroids (52). The impact on wound healing is particularly important given that transfers from inpatient cancer rehabilitation

are often due to infection (53). Maintaining the lowest effective dose can help minimize insomnia, osteoporosis, hyperglycemia, essential tremors, and delayed wound healing, but requires constant vigilance to weigh risk versus benefit (54). Three complications of steroid treatment will be discussed more fully.

Dexamethasone is thought to increase the risk of gastrointestinal complications such as peptic ulceration and gastrointestinal bleeding, but the available data do not definitively support this association (55). Despite common practice to the contrary, H2 blockers and proton pump inhibitors should probably be restricted to the perioperative period, the elderly, those with a prior history of peptic ulcer disease, those receiving high doses of steroids or nonsteroidal anti-inflammatory drugs, or those on anticoagulants (56).

Steroid myopathy is a relatively common complication in brain tumor patients, with an estimated incidence of 2%–20% (57). The onset is usually subacute, occurring over several weeks and, therefore, is more likely to be seen in an outpatient rehabilitation setting. The patient will usually complain of gradual, painless proximal muscle weakness and wasting. Serum creatine phosphokinase levels are usually normal, and electromyography is usually unrevealing. Muscle biopsy may show atrophy of type II muscle fibers. Myopathy can be minimized by using the lowest possible dose of corticosteroids (57).

Immunosuppressed patients, including those with brain tumor treated with steroids, are at risk for *Pneumocystis carinii* pneumonia (PCP). The greatest risk is after about six weeks of treatment (46). The features of PCP are fever, shortness of breath, and dry cough, but sometimes can be subtle and nonspecific (58). Any unexplained drop in endurance associated with shortness of breath during mobilization should prompt a medical evaluation. Because of the increased risk of PCP, it may be prudent to consider prophylactic therapy against PCP with trimethoprim-sulfamethoxazole or dapsone.

Fatigue

Fatigue is a major detriment of quality of life in cancer (32) and, perhaps, even more prominent in patients with brain cancer. Cancer-related fatigue (CRF) has been defined by the National Comprehensive Cancer Network as a "persistent, subjective sense of tiredness related to cancer or cancer treatment that interferes with usual functioning." (59 This fatigue probably differs from that of generalized fatigue often seen in the patient with stroke or TBI. Even though fatigue is considered the most distressing symptom associated with cancer, it is consistently underreported to health care providers and overlooked as a treatable cause of cancer care (60). RT, AED, CT, anemia, depression, and chronic steroid use can all contribute. The initial workup should search for treatable causes, such as anemia and hypothyroidism (32).

Depending on severity, fatigue may be a much greater limiting factor in the rehabilitation process than focal sensorimotor, cognitive, or language deficits. CRF can interfere with a patient's basic and instrumental activities of daily living, communication, and functional mobility. In the acute care setting, sleep hygiene, rest, low-impact exercises, and pharmacological interventions are emphasized. Once in intensive rehabilitation, a flexible therapy schedule is necessary to accommodate fluctuating CRF. Behavioral techniques to enhance motivation can be helpful. Use of energy-conservation techniques during functional activities can minimize CRF while maintaining the greatest level of independence. Medication options are discussed in the next section.

Cognitive and Mood Impairment

Not surprisingly, cognitive and mood deficits are frequent and debilitating (61). Apart from tumor removal and resolution of the surrounding edema, treatment of primary cognitive deterioration is quite difficult. Cognitive function is an independent prognostic factor in patients with brain tumors and, especially in the outpatient rehabilitation setting, cognitive deterioration should be regarded as a potential indicator for tumor recurrence (62).

Minimizing and substituting sedating medications should be the first step in the management of cognitive deficits (42). If the patient experiences insomnia (ie, with steroid treatment) a soporific agent such as trazodone should be considered (32). Although the objective evidence is not outstanding, functional augmentation with various neurostimulant medication may be helpful in some cases. Methylphenidate was recently found to be associated with decreased "drowsiness scores" in a sample of general cancer rehabilitation inpatients (63). Meyers and colleagues (64) demonstrated significant improvements in cognitive function, mood, and fatigue in an open-label study of 30 brain tumor patients using methylphenidate (20–60 mg/day). Adverse effects were minimal and immediately resolved when treatment was discontinued. Rivera (65) reported a patient with intraventricular subependymoma where a postoperative Glasgow Coma Scale improved from 8 to 15 after receiving 400 mg/day of modafinil. Another recent case suggested that amantadine was useful to treat expressive aphasia in a patient after a partial resection of left-sided, parietal GBM (66). In a randomized clinical trial (RCT) of 83 children who were long-term survivors of cranial irradiation, methylphenidate therapy was associated with improvements in attention and social deficit (67). In another study, 24 adult patients with low-grade gliomas post-cranial radiation were treated with donepezil for 24 weeks showed improved cognitive function and mood compared to baseline (68). There is also some evidence that methylphenidate may be beneficial in reducing fatigue and improving depression and cognition (64). Modafinil and dextroamphetamine have also been used to treat CRF. In some cases, small increases in oral steroids can alleviate arousal deficits. A further discussion of cognition can be found in Chapter 79.

Depression and anxiety should be considered as a potential cause of secondary cognitive deficits and fatigue. This is especially important when deficits affect motivation, mobility, and self-care (69,70). One study found mood disorders to be common in the time period between surgery and starting RT (69). Research varies as to the most consistent predictors of depression in persons with brain tumors, but a frontal lesion (71) and lower functional performance (72) have been discussed. Selective serotonin reuptake inhibitors (SSRIs) (73) or methylphenidate (64) are reasonable drug treatments. One study found that SSRIs improved depression but not fatigue (73).

Seizure Prophylaxis and Treatment

Seizures occur more often than headache as the presenting symptom of a brain tumor (74). The risk of seizures is higher with primary brain tumors versus metastatic disease, supratentorial tumors and cortical tumors versus infratentorial tumors, and anterior tumors versus posterior lesions (56,74). In the more aggressive malignant gliomas, seizures contributed substantially to the neurologic morbidity in at least 25% of patients, and seizures at diagnosis were a strong predictor of subsequent recurrence (74,75).

Those patients with seizures should be treated with AEDs. Electroencephalogram may be useful, especially if the diagnosis of seizure is unclear. The most common complication of AEDs is a rash (Fig. 43.2). Other side effects include drowsiness, dizziness, high-level balance dysfunction, and impaired cognitive function. Phenytoin increases hepatic metabolism of dexamethasone, decreasing its anti-inflammatory effects. Conversely, dexamethasone may decrease phenytoin levels (76,77). As a rule, phenytoin and phenobarbital are less desirable due to their greater risk of cognitive side effects (78) and potential to decrease the rate of neurological recovery (79,80). We have found levetiracetam to have minimal cognitive effects in patients with brain tumor undergoing rehabilitation. Additionally, we know no of evidence regarding either a positive or negative impact on neurologic recovery.

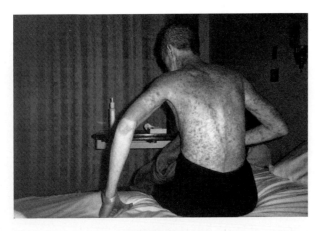

FIGURE 43.2

Diffuse, severe macular rash as a result of phenytoin allergy. The medication was used as prophylaxis in a woman following meningioma resection.

Patients with brain tumors are frequently given AED to prevent seizures. Glantz et al. (81) conducted an RCT in patients with newly diagnosed, mostly metastatic brain tumors prophylaxed with either valproic acid (VA) or placebo. Among 74 patients, there was no difference in the seizure rates (35% with VA vs 24% in placebo) or survival time. Forsyth and colleagues (82) studied prophylactic phenytoin in 100 newly diagnosed brain tumor patients (60% primary and 40% metastatic). Seizure and survival rates were not statistically different between groups in this randomized open trial. Cohen et al. (83) published a retrospective analysis of 195 patients with intracerebral metastasis. Patients receiving prophylactic phenytoin and no prophylaxis both had a 10% seizure frequency. DeSantis et al. (84) completed a prospective open-label study on 200 patients requiring elective craniotomy for supratentorial brain tumors and found that phenytoin given at dosages producing serum concentrations within the target range failed to prevent early postoperative seizures. Finally, Foy and associates (85) randomized 276 patients to treatment with carbamazepine or phenytoin for 6 or 24 months, or to no treatment. No significant differences in seizures were found among groups; however, drug-related side effects were common. In a position statement published by the American Academy of Neurology in 2000 (86), it was recommended that AEDs should be reserved for only those patients with brain tumors who actually experienced a seizure.

Deep Vein Thrombosis

In general, patients with cancer are predisposed to thromboembolism, and this holds true for persons with brain tumors. The incidence of symptomatic postoperative deep vein thrombosis (DVT) or pulmonary embolism in patients with high-grade gliomas ranges from 3%–60%, depending on the type of prophylaxis used (87). The risk of DVT is increased during the perioperative period for those with leg weakness, age greater than 60 years old, large tumor size, and during the use of CT (88). Using venous Doppler ultrasound as a screening tool for admissions to a mixed ABI rehabilitation unit, Yablon et al. (89) reported an incidence of 21.2%, well above the rates seen in stroke and TBI.

Ruff et al. (90) estimated the frequency of symptomatic bleeding into gliomas at 2%–4% without DVT prophylaxis. Metastases from melanoma, thyroid cancers, and renal cell cancers have a higher propensity for bleeding, while metastases from lung and breast cancer have less bleeding potential. Because of the high DVT risk, brain tumor patients undergoing surgery require adequate prophylaxis, but it is somewhat unclear which methods are superior. A meta-analysis of four RCT in (mainly) brain tumor patients found unfractionated heparin and low molecular weight heparin (LMWH) had a relative DVT risk reduction of 45% (91). In another large study of more than 2,000 patients undergoing intracranial neurosurgery, there was no association between LMWH and hemorrhage when begun within 24 hours after surgery (92). Schiff and colleagues (93) reported that only 3 out of 51 patients developed intracranial hemorrhage on Coumadin and, of those, two had supratherapeutic levels. Both an older study (94) and newer recommendations (95) would suggest very high complication and failure rates for IVC filters in brain tumors and that filters be reserved for only those patients with high risk for bleeding.

LMWH has become more important in the treatment of DVTs. The LMWHs have a longer half-life and are more predictable in dose response than unfractionated heparin. There is also a decreased frequency of heparin-induced thrombocytopenia, particularly important during CT, and osteopenia. LMWHs are also used for "coverage" while waiting for warfarin to reach therapeutic levels. In a large retrospective series of 203 cancer patients treated with LMWH for symptomatic DVTs (which included 45 with brain metastases), only one patient had an intracranial hemorrhage (96). Lee (97) studied cancer patients who had acute symptomatic proximal DVTs, pulmonary emboli, or both that were randomly assigned to receive an LMWH for five to seven days, then a warfarin derivative for six months (target international normalized ratio [INR] 2.5) or LMWH alone for six months. During the six-month period, 27 of 336 patients in the LMWH group developed recurrent DVTs as compared with 53 of 336 patients in the oral-anticoagulant group. No significant major bleeds occurred in either group, suggesting LMWH was more effective in reducing the risk of recurrent clots.

Wound Healing and Infection

Steroids and RT both delay healing and contribute to wound infections, particularly at the craniotomy site. CT also delays wound healing by decreasing proliferation of fibroblasts and contraction of wounds, causing neutropenia, and interfering with protein synthesis (98). The most frequent causative agent is staphylococcal organisms. Signs and symptoms of infection include redness and drainage from the wound, foul odor from the wound, fever, or elevated white blood cell count (99). Prophylactic antibiotics are prescribed for only a short time during and after the perioperative period (100). Cephalosporins and fluoroquinolones are reasonable choices to treat skin infections. Treatment may also include surgical irrigation and debridement.

Nutrition and Swallowing

For a variety of reasons, anorexia is common among brain tumors and usually worsens as the tumor grows and spreads. Postoperative pain and fatigue contribute to loss of appetite. Cachexia is a severe wasting syndrome that causes weakness and a loss of weight, fat, and muscle (101). Nutritionists advocate avoiding carbonated drinks and gas-producing foods such as beans and peas to avoid a feeling of fullness. High-protein and high-calorie foods such as eggs, cheese, milk, poultry, and fish have been shown to help wounds heal. Eating foods with fiber and adequate water intake should help with maintaining regular bowel movements (102).

Complaints of a change in the sense of taste, in particular a bitter taste, when undergoing CT are common. A sudden dislike of certain foods may occur. Painful mouth sores and dry mouth from CT, RT, and any number of medications will impair food intake. Proper hydration and eating moist foods may help (103).

There is a high risk for aspiration pneumonia in patients with brain tumors. This may occur as a direct result of motor, sensory, or cognitive changes from the tumor or complications from radiation, CT, or other treatment (104). Dysphagia can also contribute to dehydration and fatigue. In some cases when the swallow function is significantly impaired, a feeding tube may be necessary (105). A more comprehensive assessment of the patient's swallow function may be required through objective tests such as a modified barium swallow study or fiber-optic endoscopic evaluation of swallowing (106). Patients who experience dysphagia as a result of a brain tumor and participate in an intensive intervention program demonstrate similar improvements in swallow function compared to subjects with stroke (104).

Pain Management

Several different parts of the body may be sources of pain experienced by patients with neurologic deficits by brain tumors. Pain syndromes are discussed more thoroughly in Chapters 35–42. Thalamic pain and other central pain syndromes may be difficult to treat, but centrally acting neuropathic pain medications such as gabapentin, pregabalin, carbamazepine, and lamotrigine may be helpful (107). Pain with motion of the hemiparetic shoulder may be secondary to muscle imbalance or an inferior subluxation. Shoulder support is achieved with a lap tray or weight-bearing activities with activities of daily living (ADLs) and mobility. This will approximate the joint, decrease shoulder pain, and incorporate the affected extremity into the task. Physical and occupational therapy interventions, such as application of modalities, range of motion, and strengthening exercises, may improve shoulder function. Narcotic pain medications should be used at the lowest possible effective dose with vigilance for side effects of constipation and sedation (107).

INTERDISCIPLINARY REHABILITATION OF PERSONS WITH BRAIN TUMORS

Assessment

Whether in an inpatient or outpatient rehabilitation setting, review of the medical record or discussions with the referring or attending physicians will provide important information before assessment and treatment begins. Information helpful to the rehabilitation team includes initial presentation and premorbid functional status; the pathology, location, and prognosis of the tumor; surgical treatment and any complications, concomitant treatments (ie, CT, RT, steroids, AED, etc.); site and status of primary tumor (for brain metastases); medications; and response to rehabilitation in previous settings (ie, neurosurgical service, inpatient rehabilitation, outpatient, or home care). Location of the tumor will determine impairments such as side of hemiparesis, ataxia, cognitive and visual changes, aphasia, dysarthria, and dysphagia (15,16). For example, a GBM located in the frontal-parietal lobe may result in cognitive and motor dysfunction and have a poor prognosis for survival, whereas as an acoustic schwannoma may present with primarily equilibrium impairments and has a very good chance of survival. The relationship between tumor size and impairment is not straightforward, as slow-growing tumors can be quite extensive with relatively few symptoms (108).

A functional neurologic examination assesses strength, coordination, reflexes, muscle tone, and sensation. Particularly in the neurosurgical setting, it is best to avoid Valsalva maneuver as this increases intracranial pressure (22). Alertness, orientation, and mood are also assessed at this time. The clinician should consider how impairments in multiple areas (musculoskeletal, neurologic, mood, cognitive, visual, and vestibular) collectively affect limitations in activity and participation. For instance, a patient with metastatic lung cancer to the right parietal lobe may present with neglect and motor dysfunction further complicated by postcraniotomy pain and swelling, poor motivation due to depression, and chronic obstructive pulmonary disease limiting endurance.

Following the initial evaluation, impairment-specific tests may provide a more objective assessment to determine a functional baseline and develop a plan of care. Although we are not aware of brain tumor-specific assessment instruments, those used in other etiologies of ABI are probably adequate. In the patient with balance deficits (ie, cerebellar tumor or acoustic schwannoma), several tests may be useful to estimate fall risk, such as the Romberg Test (109), the Berg Balance Test (110,111), or the Dynamic Gait Index (112). The Mini-Mental State Examination or occupational therapy/speech language therapy (OT/SLP) cognitive screens may identify the need for more comprehensive neuropsychological assessments. Other functional assessments of cognition include the A-One (113), the Kohlman Evaluation of Living Skills (KELS) (114) focusing on safety awareness in the home, or the Ross Information Processing Assessment-2 (115) to assess linguistically based cognitive impairments. In addition, language and speech deficits can be further delineated with the Aphasia Diagnostic Battery (116) and the Apraxia Battery for Adults –2 (117). In the outpatient setting, frequent reevaluation is needed, as deficits in survivors of high-grade gliomas will progress quickly to impairments affecting independence in the home and community (118). It is interesting to note that given similar lesions, one study found subjects with brain tumors to have fewer impairments than those with stroke (119).

The team will then formulate a rehabilitation plan of care based on functional patient-driven goals. Before setting goals, it is appropriate to consider which Dietz category best describes the interventions and if they should be compensatory or remedial. It is essential that these goals be realistic, well defined, consider the prognosis, and involve the caregiver. Input from the referring or attending physicians may be required regarding anticipated future treatments and possible side effects. Oftentimes, the patient and family enter rehabilitation not fully aware of the diagnosis or prognosis. Indeed, inpatient rehabilitation will frequently begin before the pathological tissue analysis is complete and the treatment course is determined. The team *must* coordinate discussions of prognosis with the neurosurgical or neuro-oncology services to minimize conflicting or inaccurate information that adds to already high levels of patient and family stress. If the patient is unable or unwilling to articulate his or her own goals, the caregiver's goals should drive management.

Interventions

The same breadth of interventions used in other ABI can also be used in persons with brain tumors. Functional electrical stimulation, robotics, constraint-induced motor therapy, forced-use techniques, partial body weight-supported ambulation, advanced spasticity management, cognitive, and visual and vestibular (120) rehabilitation techniques will all be used in the appropriate clinical circumstance. This is especially true for patients in tumor groups 1 and 2, which hold a better prognosis for long-term survival. A few examples are offered. Similar to a TBI, a frontoparietal tumor may result in personality changes, social inappropriateness, and impaired judgment. Behavioral interventions and modification are used (121). Occipital lobe lesions with visual field deficits can be treated with prism glasses, corrective lenses, environmental adaptations, and compensatory strategies. Neuro-optometry consultation may be required. Dominant-side temporal lobe lesions may result in receptive language and memory impairments. Using a memory book and educating family and staff to utilize visual supports and nonverbal communication may be helpful. Persons with cerebellar tumors can have vestibular dysfunction, ataxia, dysmetria, and nystagmus and may benefit from incorporating vestibular adaptation and habituation activities as the primary focus. It has been suggested that vestibular deficits from cerebellopontine-angle tumors respond better than those related to posterior fossa tumors (122).

While traditional treatment approaches are widely used, there has been a recent interest to include a more holistic focus. The hospital experience leaves patients feeling hopelessness, frustrated, and out of control (20). Complementary and alternative medicine (CAM) therapies may be used in conjunction with traditional medical and rehabilitation approaches to reduce stress and anxiety and promote overall well-being. These methods are also beneficial in reducing pain, nausea, and other symptoms. In an effort to meet both the physical and emotional needs of the patient with a brain tumor, CAM therapies such as tai chi, yoga, and pet therapy groups have been instituted in the rehabilitation settings. Visual imagery, aromatherapy, medical acupuncture, music therapy, breathing techniques, and prayer and spirituality will be essential for certain patients.

Whatever the setting and strategy, the treating therapist(s) must remain flexible to accommodate fluctuations in patient status and schedule. On the inpatient unit, the team should schedule around radiation or CT if they cannot occur at the conclusion of the day. Therapy may need to be concentrated in the morning when a patient has the energy to tolerate and benefit from more intensive activity. Physician and nursing staff may need to strategically time analgesic medications before therapy. Sedating, but necessary, medicines should be given after therapy. Co-treatments are an effective way to efficiently address multidisciplinary goals in a single treatment session while maximizing patient participation. On days when a patient is psychologically overwhelmed, the time spent talking in therapy may be more important than the physical interventions provided.

Psychosocial Issues

The fluctuating status of a patient (arousal, pain, endurance, behavior, and motivation) can be disturbing to family and caregivers. Faced with clear deficits as mobilization is progressed, patients and families are forced to deal with the reality of functional and cognitive limitations (123). Coping mechanisms in patients with malignant brain tumors may not differ substantially from those in other etiology of neurologic disease (124). In addition, marital status appears to play a role in mood disturbances, with married patients more likely to report depression and single patients more likely to report anxiety (125). Although not well understood at this time, the rehabilitation team may be somehow affected by patients with cancer diagnoses being given consistently shorter lengths of stay compared to other ABI diagnoses across several studies (126). Social work will take the lead to assess a range of psychosocial issues, including mood and adjustment to disability, stage in the grieving process, social supports, and prior dynamics of the family unit (127). Other logistic issues related to discharge planning include insurance and benefits verification, social supports and supervision at home, and referrals to community-based resources. Psychology and psychiatry support is sometimes needed for patients to cope with an overwhelming diagnosis.

The increased burden of care for family requires a realistic assessment of the physical, psychological, and emotional abilities of the primary caregiver(s) (128,129). A family's perception of a patient's functional ability might differ greatly from the team's. An independent living experience (ILE) may be helpful to increase the patient's and caregiver's awareness of care needs after discharge home. Independent living is also

considered an important outcome measure after brain tumor treatment (130). It can also offer the patient a feeling of control sometimes absent in the hospital experience. An ILE consists of functional activities (ie, dressing, tracking therapy schedule, requesting medications, etc.) that empower the patient to be more independent in the hospital and mimics their everyday routine at home. It enables the team to assess the patient's cognitive and physical abilities to develop a realistic and manageable discharge plan. Community reintegration groups are another strategy to simulate the obstacles in a real-life situation after discharge. Other rehabilitation professionals, such as the recreational therapist, may also assess and modify leisure skills in preparation for discharge. Jones et al. (131) have suggested that interest in community-based exercise among subjects with brain tumor is far greater once treatments have ended. There is little guidance to the rehabilitation team when recommending the level of caregiver or home health aide assistance; however, the ILE and community groups can assist in making recommendations.

The provision of education and resources to the patient and family is the responsibility of the entire team. Family meetings with the team are an efficient method of communication. Educational resources include information on the tumor and treatment options and side effects. The family should be educated on the differing roles of the neuro-oncology, physiatry, and rehabilitation therapies (127). If appropriate and coordinated with the neuro-oncology service, community resources would include hospice and patient/caregiver support groups. Patients and caregivers may deal with harsh financial issues once home and may require assistance in planning. Financial resources must be considered when making recommendations for equipment, home care, and environmental modifications. Social workers can provide support and assistance in short- and long-term financial planning issues. They can also guide families toward appropriate referrals and help them access financial assistance programs and other community resources.

CONCLUSIONS

Rehabilitation in persons with brain tumors poses a great challenge within the spectrum of ABI. Recent developments in medical and surgical treatments have yielded a modest improvement in survival for GBM, and technology may play a great role over the next decade. The rehabilitation team will need to recognize and manage physical, cognitive, and behavioral impairments related to the tumor and its treatment. Aggressive management of the medical complications and comorbidities will be a key factor in the mobilization process. Given the complexity of the population, communication among physiatry, neuro-oncology, and the rehabilitation team is essential.

References

1. Robins HI, Chang S, Butowski N, Mehta M. Therapeutic advances for glioblastoma multiforme: current status and future prospects. *Curr Oncol Reports.* 2007;9:66–70.
2. Ranasinghe MG, Sheehan JM. Surgical management of brain metastases. *Neurosurg Focus.* 2007 22;E2.
3. Gilbert MR.Advances in the treatment of primary brain tumors: dawn of a new era? *J Neuro-Oncol.* 2006;8:45–49.
4. Stupp R, Mason WP, van der Bent MJ, et al. Radiotherapy plus concomitant and adjuvant temozolomide for glioblastoma. *N Eng J Med.* 2005;352:987–996.
5. Fox J, Kleinberg L. Evolving management of newly diagnosed brain metastases: expanding role of radiosurgery in lieu of whole brain radiation. *Future Oncology.* 2007;3:285–293.
6. Sarfaraz M. CyberKnife robotics arm stereotactic radiosurgery. *J Am Coll Radiol.* 2007;4:563–565.
7. Gilbert MR.Designing clinical trials for brain tumors: the next generation. *Curr Oncol Reports.* 2007;9:49–54.
8. Gababelli P. A rehabilitative approach to the patient with brain cancer. *Neurol Sci.* 2005;26:S51–S52.
9. Garrard P, Farnham C, Thompson AJ, Playford ED. Rehabilitation of the cancer patient: experience in a neurological unit. *Neurorehabil Neural Repair.* 2004;18:76–79.
10. Giordana MT, Clara E. Functional rehabilitation and brain tumor patients: a review. *Neurol Sci.* 2006;27:240–244.
11. Anonymous. Rehabilitation after brain cancer surgery. *Supp Oncol.* 2007;5:93.
12. Bell KR, O'Dell MW, Barr K, Yablon SA. Rehabilitation of the patient with brain tumor. *Arch Phys Med Rehabil.* 1998;79(Suppl 1):S37–S46.
13. O'Dell MW, Barr K, Spanier D, Warnick R. Functional outcomes in inpatient rehabilitation in persons with brain tumors. *Arch Phys Med Rehabil.* 1998;79:1530–1534.
14. Huang ME, Cifu DX, Keyer-Marcus L. Functional outcome after brain tumor and acute stroke: a comparative analysis. *Arch Phys Med Rehabil.* 1998;79:1386–1390.
15. Marciniak CM, Sliwa JA, Heinemann AW, Semik PE. Functional outcomes of persons with brain tumors after inpatient rehabilitation. *Arch Phys Med Rehabil.* 2001;82:457–463.
16. Mukand JA, Blackinton DD, Crincoli MG, Lee JJ, Santos BB. Incidence of neurological deficits and rehabilitation of patients with brain tumors. *Am J Phys Med Rehabil.* 2001;80:346–350.
17. Huang ME, Cifu DX, Keyer-Marcus L. Functional outcome in persons with brain tumor after inpatient rehabilitation: comparison with traumatic brain injury. *Am J Phys Med Rehabil.* 2000;79:327–335.
18. Greenberg E, Treger I, Ring H. Rehabilitation outcomes in patients with brain tumors and acute stroke. *Am J Phys Med Rehabil.* 2006;85:568–573.
19. Feder M, Ring H, Solzi P, Eldar R. Rehabilitation outcomes following craniotomy for intracranial meningiomas. *J Neuro Rehab.* 1989;3:15–17.
20. Sherer M, Meyers CA, Bergloff P. Efficacy of postacute brain injury rehabilitation for patients with primary malignant brain tumors. *Cancer.* 1997;80:250–257.
21. Cheville A. Cancer rehabilitation. *Sem Oncol.* 2005;32:219–224.
22. Hill C, Nixon SC, Ruehmeier JL, Wolf LM. Brain tumors. *Phys Ther.* 2002;82:496–502.
23. Broadwell DC. Rehabilitation needs of the patient with cancer. *Cancer.* 1987;60:563–568.
24. Dietz JH, Rehabilitation of the cancer patient: its role in the scheme of comprehensive care. *Med Clin N Am.* 1969;53:607–624.
25. Hinterbuchner C. Rehabilitation of physical disability in cancer. *NY State J Med.* 1978;78:1066–1069.
26. Kudsk EG, Hoffman GS. Rehabilitation of the cancer patient. *Prim Care.* 1987;14:381–390.
27. Dietz JH. Adaptive rehabilitation of the cancer patient. *Curr Probl Cancer.* 1980;5:1–56.
28. Davies E, Clarke CL. Malignant cerebral gliomas: rehabilitation and management. In: Greenberg RJ, Barnes MP, McMillan TM, Ward CD, eds. *Handbook of Neurological Rehabilitation.* 2nd ed. Hove and New York: Psychology Press/Taylor and Francis Group; 2006:595–609.
29. Brown PD, Ballman KV, Rummans TA, et al. Prospective study of quality of life in adults with newly diagnosed high-grade glioma. *J Neurooncol.* 2006;76:283–291.
30. Davies E, Hall S, Clarke C. Two year survival after malignant cerebral glioma: patient and relative reports of handicap, psychiatric symptoms and rehabilitation. *Disability Rehabil.* 2003;25:259–266.
31. Cruickshank GS, Wilkinson SC. Speech and language services for patients with malignant brain tumors: a regional survey of providers. *Health Bulletin.* 1998;56:659–666.
32. Franklin DJ, Packel L. Cancer-related fatigue. *Arch Phys Med Rehabil.* 2006;87(Suppl 1):S91–S93.
33. Pelletier G, Verhoef MJ, Khatri N, Hagen N. Quality of life in brain tumor patients: the relative contributions of depression, fatigue, emotional distress and existential issues. *J Neurooncol.* 2002;57:41–49.
34. Hahn CA, Dunn RH, Logue PE, King JH, Edwards CL, Halperin EC. Prospective study of neuropsychologic testing and quality-of-life assessment of adults with primary malignant brain tumors. *Int J Rad Oncology Biol Phys.* 2003;55:992–999.
35. Pace A, Parisi C, DiLelio M, et al. Home rehabilitation for brain tumor patients. *J Exp Clin Cancer Res.* 2007;26:297–300.
36. Unified Data System: 2007 Aggregate Data. University of Buffalo Foundation Activities, Inc.
37. Bussiere M, Hopman W, Day A, Pombo AP, Neves T, Espinosa F. Indicators of functional status for primary malignant brain tumors patients. *Can J Neurol Sci.* 2005;32:50–56.
38. Asthagiri AR, Pouratian N, Sherman J, Ahmed G, Shaffrey ME. Advances in brain tumor surgery. *Neurologic Clinics.* 2007;25:975–1003.
39. Kanner AA, Bokstien F, Blumenthal DT, Ram ZL. Surgical therapies and brain metastases. *Sem Oncol.* 2007;34:197–205.
40. Taphoorn MJ, Stupp R, Coens C, et al. Health-related quality of life in patients with glioblastoma: a randomized controlled trial. *Lancet Oncol.* 2005;12:937–944.
41. Jalali R, Basu A, Gupta T, et al. Encouraging experience of concomitant temozolomide with radiotherapy followed by adjuvant temozolomide in newly diagnosed glioblastoma multiforme: single institution experience. *Br J Neurosurg.* 2007;6:583–587.
42. Zafonte RD, Elovic E, Mysiw WJ, O'Dell MW, Watanabe T. Pharmacology in traumatic brain injury: fundamentals and treatment strategies. In: Rosenthal M, Griffith ER, Kreutzer JS, Pentland B, eds. *Rehabilitation of the Adult and Child with Traumatic Brain Injury.* 3rd ed. Philadelphia: FA Davis; 1999:536–555.
43. Adams VR, Brenner T. Oprelvekin (Neumega): first platelet growth factor for thrombocytopenia. *J Am Pharm Assoc (Wash).* 1999;39:706–707.
44. Stieber V, Mehta W, Minesh P. Advances in radiation therapy for brain tumors. *Neurologic Clinics.* 2007;25:1005–1033.
45. Laack NN, Brown PD, Ivnik RJ, et al. Cognitive function after radiotherapy for supratentorial low-grade glioma: A North Central Cancer Treatment Group prospective study. *Int J Radiat Oncol Biol Phys.* 2005, 63:1175.
46. Lassman AB, DeAngelis LA. Brain metastases. *Neurol Clin N Am.* 2003;21:1–23.
47. Ruben JD, Dally M, Bailey M. Cerebral radiation necrosis: incidence, outcomes, and risk factors with emphasis on radiation parameters and chemotherapy. *Int J Radiat Oncol Biol Phys.* 2006;65:499–508.

48. Cole RC, Scialla SJ, Bednarz L. Functional recovery in cancer rehabilitation. *Arch Phys Med Rehabil.* 2000;81:623–627.

49. O'Toole DM, Golden AM. Evaluating cancer patients for rehabilitation potential. *West J Med.* 1991;155:384–387.

50. Marciniak CM, Sliwa JA, Spill G, Heinemann AW, Semik PE. Functional outcome following rehabilitation of the cancer patient. *Arch Phys Med Rehabil.* 1996;77:54–57.

51. Kaal EC, Vecht CJ. The management of brain edema in brain tumors. *Curr Opin Oncol.* 2004;16:593–600.

52. Batchelor T, DeAngelis LM. Medical management of cerebral metastases. *Neurosurg Clin N Am.* 1996;7:435–446.

53. Alan E, Wilson RD, Vargo MM: In patient cancer rehabilitation: a retrospective comparison of trans for back and acute care between patients with heoplasm and other rehabilitation patients. *Arch Phys Med Rehabil.* 2008;89:1284–1289.

54. Hempen C, Weiss E, Hess CF. Dexamethasone treatment in patients with brain metastasis and primary brain tumors: do the benefits outweigh the side-effects? *Support Care Cancer.* 2002;10:322–328.

55. Nielsen GL, Sorensen HT, Mellemkhoer L, et al. Risk of hospitalization resulting from upper gastrointestinal bleeding among patients taking corticosteroids: a register-based cohort study. *Am J Med.* 2001;111:541–545.

56. Wen PY, Schiff D, Kesari S. Medical management of patients with brain tumors. *J Neurooncol.* 2006;80:313–332.

57. Dropcho EJ, Soong SJ. Steroid-induced weakness in patients with primary brain tumors. Neurology. 1991;41:1235–1239.

58. Pruitt AA. Treatment of medical complications in patients with brain tumors. *Curr Treat Options Neurol.* 2005; 7:323–336.

59. Mock V, Atikinson A, Barsevick A, et al. Cancer-related fatigue clinical practice guidelines to oncology. *J Natl Comp Cancer Network.* 2003;1:308–331.

60. Stone P, Richardson A, Ream E, et al. Cancer-related fatigue: inevitable, unimportant, and untreatable? Results of a multi-centre patient survey: cancer fatigue forum. *Ann Oncol.* 2000; 11:971.

61. Gleason JF, Case D, Rapp S, et al. Symptom clusters in patients with newly-diagnosed brain tumors. *J Supp Oncol.* 2007;5:427–433.

62. Taphoorn MJ, Klein M. Cognitive deficits in adult patients with brain tumors. *Lancet Neurol.* 2004;3:159–168.

63. Guo Y, Yopung B, Hainley S, Palmer JL, Bruera E. Evaluation and pharmacological management of symptoms in cancer patients undergoing acute rehabilitation in a comprehensive cancer center. *Arch Phys Med Rehabil.* 2007;88:891–895.

64. Meyers CA, Weitzner MA, Valentine AD, Levin VA. Methylphenidate therapy improves cognition, mood, and function of brain tumors patients. *J Clin Oncol.* 1998;16:2522–2527.

65. Rivera VM. Modafinil for the treatment of diminished responsiveness in a patients recovering from brain surgery. *Brain Injury.* 2005;19:725–727.

66. Barrett AM, Eslinger PJ. Amantadine for adynamic speech: possible benefit for aphasia? *Am J Phys Med Rehabil.* 2007;86:605–612.

67. Mulhern RK, Khan RB, Kaplan S, et al. Short-term efficacy of methylphenidate: a randomized, double-blind, placebo-controlled trial among survivors of childhood cancer. *J Clin Oncol.* 2004;22:4795–4803.

68. Shaw EG, Rosdhal R, D'Agostino RB Jr, et al. Phase II study of donepezil in irradiated brain tumor patients: effect on cognitive function, mood, and quality of life. *J Clin Oncol.* 2006;24:1415–1420.

69. Kilbride L, Smith G, Grant R. The frequency and cause of anxiety and depression amongst patients with malignant brain tumours between surgery and radiotherapy. *J Neurooncol.* 2007;84:297–304.

70. Litofsky NS, Farace E, Anderson F, et al. Depression in patients with high-grade glioma: results of the Glioma Outcomes Project. *Neurosurgery.* 2004;54:358–367.

71. Wellish DK, Kaleita TA, Freeman D, Cloughsey T, Goldman J. Predicting major depression in brain tumor patients. *Psychooncology.* 2002;11:230–238.

72. Mainio A, Hakko H, Niemela A, Koivukangas JJ, Rasanen P. Depression and functional outcome in patients with brain tumors: a population-based 1-year follow-up study. *J Neurosurg.* 2005;103:841–847.

73. Morrow GR, Hickok JT, Roscoe JA, et al. Differential effects of paroxetine on fatigue and depression: a randomized, double-blind trial from the University of Rochester Cancer Center Community Clinical Oncology Program. *J Clin Oncol.* 2003;21:4635–4641.

74. Van Breeman MSM, Wilms EB, Vecht CJ. Epilepsy in patients with brain tumors: epidemiology, mechanisms, and management. *Lancet Neurology.* 2007;6:421–430.

75. Moots PL, Maciunas R, Eisert DR.The course of seizure disorders in patient with malignant gliomas. *Arch Neurol.* 1995;52:717–724.

76. Gattis WA, May DB. Possible interaction involving phenytoin, dexamethasone, and antineoplastic agents: a case report and review. *Ann Parmacother.* 1996;5:520–526.

77. Rüeggs. Dexamethasone/phenytoin interactions: neurooncological concerns. *Swiss Med Rev.* 2002;132:425–426.

78. Dikman SS, Temkin NR, Miller B, Machamer J, Winn HR. Neurobehavioral effects of phenytoin prophylaxis of post-traumatic seizures. *JAMA.* 1991;265:1271–1277.

79. Brailowsky S, Knight RT, Efron R. Phenytoin increases the severity of cortical hemiplegia in rats. *Brain Res.* 1989;376:71–77.

80. Hernandez TD, Holling LC. Disruption of behavioral recovery by the anti-convulsant phenobarbital. *Brain Res.* 1994;635:300–306.

81. Glantz MJ, Cole BF, Friedberg MH. A randomized, blinded, placebo-controlled trial of divalproex sodium prophylaxis in adults with newly diagnosed brain tumors. *Neurology.* 1996;46:985–991.

82. Forsyth PA, Weaver S, Fulton D, et al. Prophylactic anticonvulsants in patients with brain tumour. *Can J Neuro Sci.* 2003;30:89–90.

83. Cohen N, Strauss G, Lew R. Should prophylactic anticonvulsants be administered to patients with newly-diagnosed cerebral metastases? A retrospective analysis. *J Clin Oncol.* 1998;10:1621–1624.

84. DeSantis A, Villani R, Sinisi M. Add-on phenytoin fails to prevent early seizures after surgery for supratentorial brain tumors: a randomized controlled study. *Epilepsia.* 2002;43:175–182.

85. Foy PM, Chadwick DW, Rajgopalan N. A randomized, blinded, placebo-controlled trial of divalproex sodium prophylaxis in adults with newly diagnosed brain tumors. *J Neurol Neurosurg Psychiatry.* 1992;55:753–757.

86. Glantz MJ, Cole BF, Forsyth PA. Practice parameters: anticonvulsant prophylaxis in patients with newly diagnosed brain tumors. Report of the quality standards subcommittee of the American Academy of Neurology. *Neurology.* 2000;54:1886–1893.

87. Marras LC, Geerts WH, Perry JR: The risk of venous thromboembolism is increased throughout the course of malignant glioma. Cancer. 2000;89:640–646.

88. Sawaya R, Zuccarello M, Elkalliny M, et al. Postoperative venous thromboembolism and brain tumors: Part I. Clinical profile. *J Neurooncol.* 1992;14:119–125.

89. Yablon SA, Rock WA, Nick TG, Sherer M, McGrath CM, Goodson KH. Deep venous thrombosis: prevalence and risk factors in rehabilitation admission with brain injury. *Neurology.* 2004;63:485–491.

90. Ruff RL, Posner JB. The incidence and treatment of peripheral venous thrombosis in patients with glioma. *Ann Neurol.* 1983;13:334.

91. Iorio A, Agnelli G. Low-molecular-weight and unfractionated heparin for prevention of venous thromboembolism: a meta-analysis. *Arch Intern Med.* 2000;160:2327–2332.

92. Gerlach R, Scheuer T, Beck J, et al. Risk of postoperative hemorrhage after intracranial surgery after early nadroparin administration: results of a prospective study. *Neurosurgery.* 2003;53:1028–1035.

93. Schiff D, DeAngelis LM. Therapy of venous thromboembolism in patients with brain metastases. Cancer. 1994;73:493–498.

94. Levin JM, Schiff D, Loeffler JS, et al. Complications of therapy for venous thromboembolic disease in patients with brain tumors. *Neurology.* 1993;43:1111–1114.

95. Walsh DC, Kakkar AK. Thromboembolism in brain tumors. *Curr Opin Pulm Med.* 2001;7:326–331.

96. Monreal M, Zacharski L, Jiminez JA, et al. Fixed-dose low molecular weight heparin for secondary prevention of venous thromboembolism in patients with disseminated cancer: a prospective cohort study. *J Thromb Haemost.* 2004;2:1311–1315.

97. Lee AY, Levine MN, Baker RI, et al. Low molecular weight heparin versus a coumarin for the prevention of recurrent venous thromboembolism in patients with cancer. *N Eng J Med.* 2003;349:146–153.

98. Drake DB, Oishi SN. Wound healing considerations in chemotherapy and radiation therapy. *Clin Plast Surg.* 1995;22:31–37.

99. Shinoura N, Yamada R, Okamoto K, et al. Early prediction of infection after craniotomy for brain tumors. *Br J Neurosurg.* 2004;18:598–603.

100. Korinek AM, Goldmard JL, Elcheick A, et al: Risk factors for neurosurgical site infections after craniotomy: a critical reappraisal of antibiotic prophylaxis on 4,578 patients. *Br J Neurosurg.* 2005;19:155–162.

101. Skipworth R, Stewart JE, Grant D. et al. Pathophysiology of cancer cachexia: much more than host-tumour interaction? *Clin Nutr.* 2007;26:667–676.

102. Marin Caro MM, Lvaiano A, Prichard C. Nutritional intervention and quality of life in adult oncology patients. *Clin Nutr.* 2007;26:289–301.

103. Smith GF, Toonen TR. Primary care of the patient with cancer. *Am Fam Physician.* 2007;75:1207–1214.

104. Wesling M, Brady S, Jensen M, et al. Dysphagia outcomes in patients with brain tumors undergoing inpatient rehabilitation. *Dysphagia.* 2003;18:203–210.

105. Newton HB, Newton C, Pearl D, Davidson T. Swallowing assessment in primary brain tumor patients with dysphagia. *Neurology.* 1994;44:1927–1932.

106. Doggett DL, Turkelson CM, Coates VR. Recent developments in diagnosis and intervention for aspiration and dysphagia in stroke and other neuromuscular disorders. *Curr Atheroscl Rep.* 2002;4:311–318.

107. Goldberg GR, Morrison RS. Pain management in hospitalized cancer patients: a systemic review. *J Clin Oncol.* 2007;25:1792–801.

108. Desmurget M, Bonnetblac F, Daffau H. Contrasting acute and slow-growing lesions: a new door to plasticity. *Brain.* 2007;130:898–914.

109. Garcin R. The Ataxias. In Vinken PJ, Bruyn GW, eds. *Handbook of Clinical Neurology.* New York: John-Wiley & Sons; 1969:311–313.

110. Berg K, Wood-Dauphinee S, Williams JI, Gayton D. Measuring balance in the elderly: preliminary development of an instrument. *Physiother Can.* 1989;41:304–311.

111. Berg KP, Maki BE, Williams JI, et al. Clinical and laboratory measures of postural balance in the elderly population. *Arch Phys Med Rehabil.* 1992;73:1073–1080.

112. Shumway-Cook A, Woolacott M. *Motor Control Theory and Application.* Baltimore, MD: Williams and Wilkins; 1995.

113. Arnadottir G. *The Brain and Behavior: Assessing cortical dysfunction through activities of daily living.* Philadelphia, PA: Mosby; 1990.

114. Thomson, LK. *Kohlman Evaluation of Living Skills.* 3rd ed. Washington, DC: AOTA Press; 1992.

115. Ross-Swain, D. *Ross Information Processing Assessment.* 2nd ed. Austin, TX: PRO-ED, Inc.; 1996.

116. Helm-Estabrooks, N. *Aphasia Diagnostic Profile.* Austin, TX: PRO-ED, Inc.; 1992.

117. Dabul, B. *Apraxia Battery for Adults.* 2nd ed. Austin, TX: PRO-ED, Inc.; 1986.

118. Archibald YM, Lunn D, Ruttan LA, et al. Cognitive functioning in long-term survivors of high-grade glioma. *Neurosurg.* 1994;80:247–253.

119. Anderson SW, Damasio H, Tranel D. Neuropsychological impairments associated with lesions caused by tumor or stroke. *Arch Neurol.* 1990;47:397–405.

120. Betker AL, Szturm T, Moussavi ZK, Cristabel N. Video game-based exercises for balance rehabilitation: a single subject design. *Arch Phys Med Rehabil.* 2006;87:1141–1149.

121. Meyers CA, Boake C. Neurobehavioral disorders in brain tumor patients: rehabilitation strategies. *Cancer Bull.* 1993;45:362–364.

122. Karakaya M, Kose N, Otman S, Ozgen T. Investigation and comparison of the effect of rehabilitation on balance and coordination problems in patients with posterior fossa and cerebellopontine angle tumors. *J Neurosurg Sci.* 2000;44:220–225.

123. Sherwood P, Given B, Schiffman, Murman D, Lovey M. Caregivers of persons with a brain tumor: a conceptual model. *Nursing Inquiry.* 2004;11:43–53.

124. Herrmann M, Curio N, Petz T, et al. Coping with illness after brain diseases—a comparison between patients with malignant brain tumors, stroke, Parkinson's disease and traumatic brain injury. *Dis Rehabil.* 2000;22:539–546.

125. Kaplan CP, Miner ME. Relationships: importance for persons with cerebral tumors. *Brain Injury.* 2000;14:251–259.

126. Kirshblum S, O'Dell MW, Ho C, Barr K. Rehabilitation of persons with central nervous system tumors. *Cancer.* 2001;92(Suppl):1029–1038.

127. Haut MW, Haut JS, Bloomfield SS. Family issues in rehabilitation of patients with malignant brain tumors. *NeuroRehabil.* 1991;1:39–47.

128. Steinbach JP, Herrlinger U, Wick W, et al. Surviving glioblastoma for more than 5 years: the patient's perspective. *Neurology.* 2006;66:239–242.

129. Pasacreta J, Barg F, Nuamah I, McCorkle R. Participant characteristics before and 4 months after attendance at a family caregiver cancer education program. *Cancer Nursing.* 2000;23:295–303.

130. Recht L, Glantz M, Chamberlain M, Hsieh CC. Quantitative measurement of quality outcome in malignant glioma patients using an independent living score (ILS). *J Neurooncol.* 2003;61:127–136.

131. Jones LW, Guill B, Keir ST, et al. Exercise interest and preferences among patients diagnosed with primary brain cancer. *Supp Care Cancer.* 2007;15:47–55.

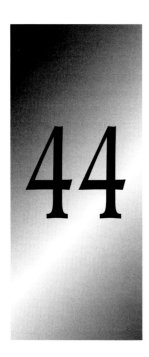

Rehabilitation of Patients with Spinal Cord Dysfunction in the Cancer Setting

44

William McKinley

Rehabilitation of individuals with spinal cord dysfunction in the cancer setting can be defined as a process that assists the person to obtain maximal physical, functional, social, and psychological abilities within the limits of the disease and its potential treatment. Spinal cord disease (SCD) can result from neoplastic spinal cord compression from epidural, intramedullary, or leptomeningeal tumor; as a consequence or radiation therapy; or from iatrogenic causes such as infection or hematoma (Fig. 44.1). The rehabilitation of SCD in the cancer setting involves negotiating several complex medical, functional, and psychosocial issues stemming from both the neoplastic effects and the neurological sequelae of the spinal cord involvement. These physical impairments and functional disabilities contribute to ongoing issues surrounding community reintegration and quality of life (QOL).

The incidence of rehabilitation patients admitted with spinal cord tumors is significant. In addition, their demographics, injury-related characteristics, and clinical presentation differentiate them from the more commonly seen traumatic spinal cord injury (SCI) individual. Early and comprehensive diagnosis and management are important, and several factors are related to survival along with neurologic and functional outcomes. Rehabilitation intervention utilizing an interdisciplinary team approach can improve an individual's mobility, activities of daily living (ADL), psychological adjustment, and community reintegration as well as reduce complications. Prevention and treatment of medical problems, such as pain, fatigue, spasticity, neurogenic bladder and bowel, pressure ulcers, infections, and thromboembolic disease, are important and will be discussed.

INCIDENCE AND DEMOGRAPHICS

Patients with cancer-related SCD represent a significant proportion of individuals with spinal cord injury/disease (SCI/D) admitted to rehabilitation settings. Though traumatic SCI (ie, motor vehicle accidents, falls, and acts of violence) accounts for the vast majority of SCI/D etiology, almost one-third of individuals admitted for inpatient rehabilitation have a diagnosis of nontraumatic SCD (such as spinal stenosis, tumors, infection, or ischemia) (1–6). Neoplastic cancer-related spinal cord compression injury has been reported to comprise up to 10%–14% of new-onset SCI (4,7,8) (Fig. 44.2). A better understanding of this population will assist in their medical management, rehabilitation, and long-term follow-up.

The demographic comparison between cancer-related SCD and traumatic SCI reveal several differences that may be of importance when considering functional outcome and discharge issues. Studies have revealed that these individuals are more likely to be significantly older, female, and unemployed when compared to those with traumatic SCI (Table 44.1) (4,7,9,10). Nontraumatic SCD comprised only 31%

KEY POINTS

- Cancer-related spinal cord disease can result from neoplastic spinal cord compression from epidural, intramedullary, or leptomeningeal tumor; as a consequence of radiation therapy; or from iatrogenic causes such as infection or hematoma.
- Spinal cord tumors are classified as being either primary (arising from central nervous [CNS] tissue such as neurons, supporting glial cells, and meninges) or metastatic (from sites distant to the spinal cord).
- Spinal metastases are seen in 15%–40% of all individuals with systemic cancer, cause epidural spinal cord compression in up to 5%, and comprise 10%–14% of new-onset spinal cord injuries.
- Breast, lung, prostate, and renal cancers, as well as lymphoma and multiple myeloma, commonly metastasize to the spine.
- Pain is the classic initial presentation of spinal cord neoplastic disease in about 90% of individuals.
- Once symptoms other than pain appear, its progression may become more rapid, resulting in permanent deficits.

- Magnetic resonance imaging (MRI) is the test of choice to evaluate for malignant spinal cord compression.
- The most significant factor for functional prognosis and survival appears to be pretreatment motor function, emphasizing the importance of early diagnosis and treatment.
- Spinal orthoses are rarely used in patients with spinal metastases, as pain from spinal instability or cord compression is generally treated emergently with surgical decompression and stabilization.
- Several studies have noted the importance of inpatient rehabilitation in the general spinal cord injury population and in patients with cancer.
- Medical complications in individuals with cancer-related spinal disease can be from the injury itself or treatment of the cancer, and can include neuropathic pain, pressure ulcers, infections, deep venous thrombosis, spasticity, fatigue, depression, and anxiety.

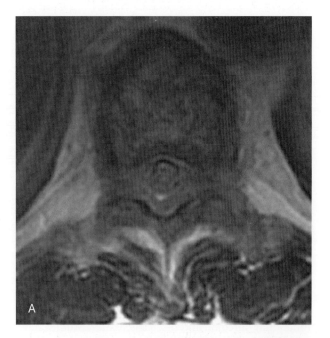 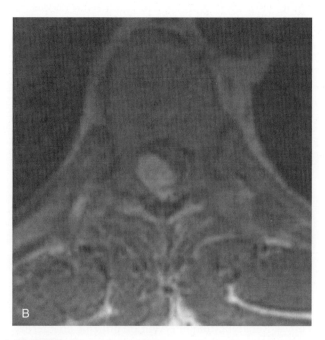

FIGURE 44.1 A and B

Magnetic resonance imaging (MRI) illustrating common causes of spinal cord disease (SCD) likely to be encountered in the cancer setting. A: Epidural tumor from metastatic prostate caner (axial T2). B: Intramedullary ependymoma (axial T1 with gadolinium enhancement).

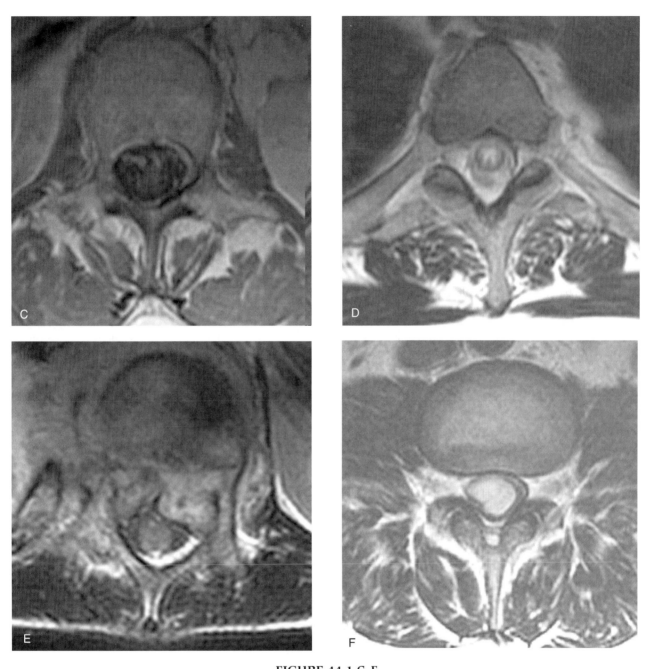

FIGURE 44.1 C–F

C: Leptomeningeal tumor from metastatic breast cancer (axial T1 with gadolinium enhancement). D: Radiation-induced myelopathy from treatment of an isolated vertebral metastasis in prostate cancer (axial T2). E: Tuberculosis of the spine in an immunocompromised patient (axial T2). F: Subdural hemorrhage in a patient with leukemia (axial T2).

of patients under 40 years old, but 87% of those over age 40, with neoplasm (53%) and spondylosis (25%) as the leading causes (11). Neoplastic spinal cord compression has a peak incidence between 50 and 70 years (7, 10,12–14).

Given the likelihood of cancer-related SCD to affect older individuals, consideration should be given to comorbid illnesses that may affect the patient's reha-

bilitation outcome. Older individuals may present with associated medical comorbidities, such as cardiovascular disease, arthritis, or depression, which could adversely affect their progress during rehabilitation and lead to decreased functional outcomes. Additionally, the use of medications, such as those utilized to control pain, depression, or anxiety following SCI/D, must be closely monitored to prevent sedative side effects, especially in

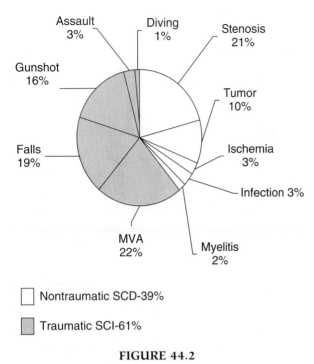

Assault 3%
Diving 1%
Stenosis 21%
Gunshot 16%
Tumor 10%
Falls 19%
Ischemia 3%
Infection 3%
MVA 22%
Myelitis 2%

☐ Nontraumatic SCD-39%

▨ Traumatic SCI-61%

FIGURE 44.2

Etiology of SCI rehabilitation admissions: non-traumatic SCD versus traumatic SCI.

elderly individuals who may have decreased tolerance. Memory retention may be diminished in older individuals and could result in diminished rehabilitation efficiency and long-term functional improvement.

PATHOPHYSIOLOGY OF NEOPLASTIC SCI

Spinal cord tumors are classified as being either primary (arising from CNS tissue such as neurons, supporting glial cells, and meninges) or metastatic (from sites distant to the spinal cord) (15–17). The vast majority (up to 85% of the cases) are metastatic lesions to the vertebrae or surrounding tissues causing spinal cord compression. Most primary spinal cord tumors do not disseminate widely through the body. Resultant neurologic compromise relates both to the degree of spinal cord involvement and neurological level of SCI.

Spinal metastasis is seen in 15%–40% of all individuals with systemic cancer and causes epidural spinal cord compression in up to 5%–10% (15–19). The pathogenesis is usually hematogenous spread of malignant cells to vertebral bone marrow through Batson epidural venous plexus via pelvic, abdominal, and thoracic veins (20). This type of spread is thought to be exacerbated by increased thoracic pressure, such as with

Valsalva or coughing, and is common in patients with prostate and other pelvic cancers. Subsequent spread into the epidural space may occur by means of tumor extension through the intervertebral foramina. The pathophysiology of SCD includes cord compression and ischemia with subsequent edema, demyelination, hemorrhage, and cystic (or cavitation) necrosis (21).

The primary cancer site for spinal metastasis is usually breast, lung, and prostate in greater than 50% (15,22). Other cancers include renal, lymphoma, and multiple myeloma, although nearly 10% have an unknown primary tumor site (14,23). In children, the common primary metastatic sites include lymphoma, sarcoma, and neuroblastomas(24). The thoracic region is the most common site for metastatic epidural SCD, accounting for about 70% of cases, with the lumbar spine involved in 20% (14). This distribution is largely determined by the volume of bone in a given region. Lung and breast cancers are more likely to metastasize to the thoracic spine, while gastrointestinal and pelvic malignancies more commonly affect the lumbosacral region likely due to dissemination through Batson plexus.

Neoplastic spinal cord compression is also often classified according to its anatomical proximity to the spinal cord and its surrounding meninges. Extramedullary (outside the cord) compression accounts for more than 90%, with the majority being epidural (primarily metastatic from the breast, lung, or prostate), and the remainder, intradural, often result from neurofibromas and meningiomas but can also be metastatic(25–27). Tumors that affect the paravertebral area may spread and compress the cord through expansion, particularly in an intervertebral foramen. Meningiomas arise from the meninges that surround the spinal cord and can cause spinal cord compression. About 85% of meningiomas are benign and can be cured with surgery, though about 15% are malignant or recur. Extramedullary metastases found in one segment of the spinal axis should prompt imaging of the entire spinal column to exclude tandem lesions. Leptomeningeal cancer refers to diffuse metastases to the tissues that surround the brain or spinal cord, and has been estimated to occur in up to 20% of patients diagnosed with cancer of the breast, lung, and melanoma (28). Without appropriate therapy, prognosis is poor.

Intramedullary (inside the cord) neoplastic compression accounts for less than 5% of spinal cord tumors and consists primarily of gliomas (29–31). Ependymomas represent a primarily benign tumor involving the ependymal cells, which line the spinal cord canal and CNS ventricles. Ependymomas may block the flow of cerebrospinal fluid (CSF), causing swelling and subsequent spinal cord compression. Astrocytomas (the most

TABLE 44.1
Demographics: Neoplastic SCD versus Traumatic Spinal Cord Injury

	NEOPLASTIC (N = 34)	TRAUMATIC (N = 159)	SIGNIFICANCE (000)
Age (years)	58.3	39.2	$P < 0.05$
Gender			
Male	50%	82%	$P < 0.05$
Female	50%	18%	
Ethnicity			
Caucasian	53%	41%	NS
Non-Caucasian	47%	59%	
Marital Status			
Married	59%	42%	NS
Not Married	41%	58%	
Work Status			
Employed	27%	60%	$P < 0.05$
Unemployed	73%	40%	

Abbreviations: NS, not significant; SCD, spinal cord disease.
Source: From Ref. 41, with permission.

common intramedullary spinal cord tumors in children) are often graded 1 through 4 by microscopic biopsy examination, related to their anaplastic characteristics (32). Grades 1 and 2 (slower growing) carry the best clinical prognosis for five-year survival (greater than 80%) and are seen most commonly. One-year survival rate for grades 3 and 4 (faster growing) astrocytomas are poor, with death often occurring within two years. Oligodendrogliomas, which originate from oligodendrocytes, typically spread along the CSF (though rarely outside the spinal cord) in a manner similar to that of astrocytomas.

Intramedullary spinal cord metastases are rare, but may be seen in patients with lung, breast, and gastrointestinal cancers as well as from malignant melanoma, lymphoma, renal, and adrenal tumors (16). A biopsy is often required for definitive diagnosis of the lesion as metastasis versus primary tumor and can help tailor therapeutic approach (33). Patients with intramedullary metastases commonly have undiscovered brain metastases. The entire central nervous system should be imaged if intramedullary metastases are found.

Additional primary spinal cord tumors consist of hemangioblastomas, dermoid tumors, and lipomas. Hemangioblastomas are benign tumors of the blood vessels, often in multiple locations, often associated with von Hippel-Lindau disease (34–36). They are usually asymptomatic and are commonly located in the thoracic region. Removal of the lesion is considered curative. Developmental tumors, such as dermoid,

epidermoid, and teratoma, occur in less than 5% and are slow-growing neoplasms, more commonly located within the thoracolumbar region. Lipomas are fatty depositions, not true neoplasms, which present in early life and may be associated with cutaneous abnormalities. Fibrous adhesions to the cord make surgical removal of developmental tumors and lipomas difficult.

CLINICAL PRESENTATION AND PHYSICAL EXAMINATION

An individual's clinical findings are very important in the early consideration for diagnosis of cancer-related SCD. Characteristic clinical presentations seen with symptomatic neoplastic spinal cord compression usually consist of pain, weakness, sensory loss, or bladder/bowel dysfunction (22,37–40). The differential diagnosis of neoplastic-related spinal cord compression includes such etiologies as mechanical low back pain, disc disorders, compression fractures, and myelopathy secondary to epidural hematoma, infection, spondylosis, syringomyelia, or transverse myelitis.

Pain is the classic initial presentation of spinal cord neoplastic disease in about 90% of individuals, often preceding additional symptoms associated with spinal cord compression (16). Spinal metastasis should be considered with an acute onset of localized back pain in a patient with cancer. Pain is initially localized to the cancer-involved area, is often insidious, and may follow a gradually progressive course over weeks to months. Thoracic pain is uncommon from degenerative causes and should raise suspicion of tumor or a compression fracture. This pain may worsen with a recumbent position in contrast to musculoskeletal back pain, which usually improves in this position. Pain may also worsen at night due to the circadian nadir of endogenous cortisol with a resultant increase in intratumoral pressure, decreased engorgement of Batson plexus, and decreased axial load on the tumor. Discogenic pain often worsens at night due to decreased axial load on the disk as well as cortisol nadir, and may be difficult to distinguish from tumor-related pain at initial presentation. Radicular pain, secondary to segmental nerve root irritation, may be present and can be exacerbated with movement or straining. Radicular pain is rarely seen without axial pain, but it can be the initial presentation of impending spinal cord compression.

The occurrence of leg weakness or paresthesias in the lower extremities and/or bowel or bladder dysfunction in patients with a history of cancer should evoke immediate concern for cord compression. Lower extremity weakness and bowel or bladder dysfunction (such as retention or incontinence) are usually late findings in malignant spinal cord compression. Bowel and bladder dysfunction can occur early with intramedullary tumors and from epidural compression when the conus medullaris, cauda equina, or sacrum is involved and may be accompanied by saddle anesthesia.

Physical examination is important in order to evaluate the spinal location of the tumor, along with the degree of cord impingement. Localized palpation tenderness over the posterior spinal region of cancerous involvement may be present. Hypoactive deep-tendon reflexes may be an indication of nerve root involvement (including at the cauda equina and conus medullaris), lower motor neuron injury, or spinal shock. Hyperreflexia, clonus, or a positive Babinski sign (upward movement of the toe in response to plantar stimulation) indicate upper motor neuron involvement, though these may be absent early in the course of compression. Diminished sensation with loss of pinprick, temperature, position, or vibratory sensation may occur early. Provocative physical exam maneuvers (such as straight leg raise or Lhermitte sign) may elicit findings indicative of neural/meningeal irritation. Valsalva maneuvers (induced by coughing or straining) may exacerbate radicular back pain from cord compression.

The clinical presentation of individuals with cancer-related SCD may reveal a pattern of insidious and less severe neurologic impairment as compared to those with traumatic SCI (10,41). They are much more likely to present with paraplegia (vs tetraplegia) and with motor incomplete (vs complete) lesions (Table 44.2). This can, most likely, be related to both etiology and the location of spinal involvement along with the insidious onset of nontraumatic SCD. Neoplastic spinal cord compression tends to involve the thoracic and lumbar regions more than the cervical region and thus, weakness tends to involve the lower extremities preferentially (13,42).

Almost one-half of patients with a tumor and subsequent spinal cord compression have some weakness in muscles below the level of neural involvement, with as many as 15% of patients having total paralysis at the time of diagnosis. Coexisting emergence of lower extremity weakness and sensory loss may cause ataxia or gait disturbance. Partial cord disorders, such as Brown-Séquard syndrome (unilateral motor and contralateral sensory deficits), arise from unilateral spinal cord compression. Lesions of the sacral spinal cord may lead to conus medullaris or cauda equina syndrome with a combination of upper and lower motor neuron signs. Ataxia from selective damage to the spinocerebellar tracts can cause severe gait dysfunction (43).

A comprehensive and detailed neurologic examination performed early and repeated often is important to document current findings and for predicting neurologic and functional outcomes. Key elements of the examination include motor and sensory testing, which allows for the designation of a neurologic level of injury and the completeness of injury (Fig. 44.3) (44). In addition, rectal examination is important to assess sacral motor and sensory function. The neurologic level of injury is defined as the most caudal (ie, lowest) level of the spinal cord that has normal motor and sensory function. Motor function is determined by manually testing key muscle groups. Sensory function is determined by examining key sensory points (within dermatomes) for both light touch and pin prick.

DIAGNOSIS AND EARLY MANAGEMENT

Spinal cord compression secondary to cancer is an emergency that requires early diagnosis and management to prevent permanent complications (45,46). Imaging techniques presently available for detection and monitoring of skeletal metastases include conventional radiography, bone scintigraphy (scan), computerized tomography (CT) scan, magnetic resonance imaging (MRI), and positron emission tomography (PET), as well as single-photon emission computed tomography (SPECT). Treatment of individuals with neoplastic spinal cord compression has been somewhat controversial, and the relative merits of interventions have been studied (47–51). Decisions regarding the level of therapeutic intervention involve factors

TABLE 44.2
Injury Characteristics: Neoplastic SCD versus Traumatic SCI

	NEOPLASTIC (N = 34)	TRAUMATIC (N = 159)	SIGNIFICANCE
Impairment			$P < 0.05$
Tetraplegia	12%	48%	
Paraplegia	88%	52%	
Level of Injury			$P < 0.05$
Cervical	12%	48%	
Thoracic	76%	38%	
Lumbosacral	12%	14%	
Complete/Incomplete			$P < 0.05$
Complete	12%	40%	
Incomplete	88%	60%	

Abbreviations: SCD, spinal cord disease; SCI, spinal cord injury.
Source: From Ref. 41, with permission.

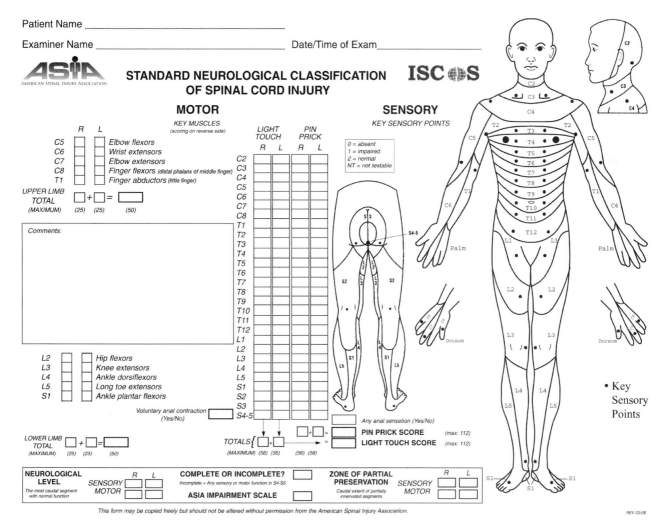

FIGURE 44.3

Standard neurological classification of spinal cord injury chart. Reprinted with permission from the American Spinal Injury Association, International Standards for Neurological Classification of Spinal Cord Injury, revised 2002.

relative to the patient's prognosis, as well as to the extent of disease in the spine. Intervention options typically include the use of steroids, radiation therapy, and surgery.

Plain radiographs provide limited information about the spinal cord compression, but may reveal bony destruction, though false negative findings comprise about 20% of cases. Roughly 50% of the bone must be destroyed to be visible on plain films. CT scan is superior to conventional radiographs and can more clearly demonstrate bone and soft tissue changes to assist in determining the extent of tumorous involvements. CT may also help in determining appropriate fields for radiation therapy of metastatic lesions. MRI provides soft tissue contrast superior to that of CT and may better define the lesion, vertebrae, epidural space, and spinal cord. It is the imaging study of choice for evaluating suspected metastatic spinal disease. Roughly one-third of people with spinal epidural metastases have multiple spinal metastases. MRI provides important information concerning location of secondary spinal tumors and integrity of adjacent vertebrae, all of which are essential for planning optimal treatment. Gadolinium-enhancement is needed for identification and evaluation of leptomeningeal disease, intramedullary disease, infection, sarcoid, acute inflammatory demyelinating polyradiculoneuropathy (AIDP), chronic inflammatory demyelinating polyradiculoneuropathy (CIDP), and in the postoperative spine to distinguish tumor from scar. CT myelography may be indicated in cases in which MRI is not readily available, is contraindicated, or in patients unable to tolerate MRI. It is also extremely useful for evaluating the patency of the spinal canal when epidural cord compression is suspected but hardware from previous surgery precludes adequate visualization due to artifact.

Bone scan is an excellent method for the early detection of skeletal metastases and can reveal metastatic lesions much earlier than conventional radiographs. Most tumors (excluding myeloma) exhibit increased activity on bone scans. Factors complicating the interpretation of bone scans include trauma, infection, and preexistent disease (such as osteoporosis or rheumatoid arthritis). Finding of a lesion on bone scan suggests the need for additional evaluation such as MRI, as soft tissue involvement is not seen well on bone scan. PET scan can assist with detection and confirmation of metastases in patients with cancer. Its role in the diagnostic therapeutic and prognostic value in metastatic bone disease is still in evolution, but it had proven useful in evaluating for recurrence in areas previously treated with surgery and/or radiation as it provides information on the metabolic activity of soft tissues. SPECT, with the use of injected metabolic radioactive tracers, may be useful in the diagnosis and management of metastatic disease, including skeletal metastasis.

Corticosteroids may alleviate pain acutely and preserve neurologic function in individuals with neoplastic spinal cord compression (52–54). Steroid administration is usually continued throughout radiation therapy at a tapering dose. Great care should be used when considering the administration of corticosteroids to patients with newly diagnosed tumors without a tissue diagnosis. Lymphomas (and potentially giant cell tumors, plasmacytomas, and eosinophilic granulomas) can undergo marked involution with steroids, delaying tissue diagnosis and thus the institution of optimal and potentially curative treatment. Steroids should be withheld in patients with newly identified spinal tumors and only minimal symptoms (ie, mild to moderate back pain and no neurologic deficits) until a definitive biopsy can be obtained.

Radiation therapy is the early treatment consideration in most cases of spinal cord compression, with a response rate reported at close to 80% (55,56). The primary aim of radiotherapy is relief of pain, restoration of function, and arrest of tumor growth. The extent of an epidural mass and neurologic involvement influence the response to radiation therapy. Patients presenting with complete SCI generally have residual neurologic impairment after radiation therapy greater than that of patients with partial SCI. Softening of bone can increase the risk of localized fracture, especially in the first few months until bone regains full strength. Spinal cord tolerance to radiation depends on the fraction size and cumulative dose. The radiation portal generally includes the area of spinal cord compression, plus a margin of two vertebral levels above and below the region involved by metastatic disease (28,57). Although a variety of schedules are used, the most common is 3,000 cGy, administered in 10 treatments (300 cGy per treatment) to the area of the spinal cord compression.

Radiation myelopathy may cause delayed necrosis of spinal or peripheral nerves (58–60). Its onset occurs anywhere from 6–48 months (most commonly 12–15 months) following radiation therapy to the vertebral or surrounding region, often with total radiation of 2,500–6,000 RADS. Damage to white matter (and sometimes the dorsal root ganglion) is associated with diffuse demyelination, swollen axons, and vascular necrosis. This has further demonstrated the importance of location and timing of radiation treatments and has led to recommendations for sites for radiation, along with daily, weekly, and total radiation quantities.

Surgical intervention in individuals with neoplastic SCD may be indicated in the following scenarios: to resect a tumor that is compressing the spinal cord and resulting in neurologic symptoms; for intractable pain; to ascertain a diagnosis from biopsy; to treat disease unrelieved with previously radiation therapy; or for stabilization of the spine (61,62). Some studies suggest that a combination of surgical decompression and radiotherapy may be more effective than radiotherapy alone (47,52,57,63). One should consider needle aspiration and cytologic evaluation biopsy to confirm metastatic disease in patients with a known primary tumor or to evaluate a lesion shown on conventional radiographs or bone scans.

NEUROLOGICAL AND FUNCTIONAL PROGNOSIS AND OUTCOMES

A review of the literature has identified several determinants of neurologic and functional prognosis in patients with SCD secondary to neoplasm, including early recognition of spinal cord compression, tumor type, neurologic status at the time of surgical intervention, completeness of the spinal cord insult, progression of neurologic symptoms, general medical status of the patient, bowel control at admission, and ambulatory ability (64–67).

The prognosis for recovery of neurologic deficits secondary to spinal cord compression is related to the duration and severity of the impairment at the start of treatment (68,69). Overall, less than 50% of patients regain lost functional capacity. The most significant factor for functional prognosis and survival appears to be pretreatment motor function, emphasizing the importance of early diagnosis and treatment. Normal bladder function is maintained in 30% of patients, but approximately 50% require catheterization before and after radiation therapy. Early consideration of radiation therapy and surgical decompression has been shown to be important to maintain neurologic integrity. Following radiation therapy, results reveal improvement of motor dysfunction in almost 50%, with stabilization of clinical status in an additional 30%. The potential for ambulation is 80% in patients who are ambulating at the initiation of radiation therapy, but 50% or less if they are unable or paraplegic at that time. Decompressive surgery plus postoperative radiotherapy is superior to radiotherapy alone for patients with spinal cord compression caused by metastatic cancer (47). Patients with spinal cord compression from radioresistent tumor should generally be offered surgery as initial therapy (48,70).

Disabling pain has been noted to occur in 64%–90% of patients with neoplastic SCD, and its successful management is important in the overall treatment of these individuals (4,12,42). Most studies on neoplastic SCD have focused on the treatment outcomes of decreased pain and ambulation following steroids, radiation, and surgery (12–14,42,43,65,71–73). Studies reveal pain improved in 78%–91%, while 18%–100% of patients studied remained nonambulatory following treatment.

More than 40% of patients who could ambulate before and after radiation therapy for spinal cord compression survived for one year, and 20% of this group survived for three years after treatment. In contrast, only 30% of patients who were nonambulatory at presentation and 7% of nonambulatory patients were alive at one year after treatment. Life expectancy has increased, both for cancer patients and following SCI/D, with both the level of injury and severity of neurologic lesion being important determinations. Persons sustaining traumatic paraplegia at age 20 years have an average subsequent life expectancy of 46 years, compared to 58 years for the general population (74). Mortality following SCI is highest in the first year after injury, after which rates decline. Despite encouraging results for many subsets, mortality remains high for older patients with new-onset SCI (75). Presently, the leading causes of death following SCI include pneumonia, heart disease, and sepsis. Pneumonia and pulmonary embolus are leading causes of death for younger patients and in the first year following injury.

REHABILITATION OUTCOMES

Recent studies have reviewed the rehabilitation outcome of neoplastic SCI with respect to functional changes in mobility, self-care skills, and bladder/bowel control (7,10,11,41,64,76–79). This may reflect, in part, a hesitancy to rehabilitate patients whose life expectancy may be shortened. Patients with metastatic spinal cord compression have a life expectancy that has been reported between 2 and 16 months following treatment. (13,42,78,79). Whereas, the one-year mortality in patients with neoplastic invasion of the spinal cord has been estimated to be over 80%, select patients may survive for extended periods, sometimes as long as four to nine years. Previous studies have noted the importance of inpatient rehabilitation in the general SCI population and in patients with cancer (80–84). Studies assessing metastatic disease of the spinal cord demonstrated functional improvement in the patient's ability to ambulate and to control bladder and bowel (14, 81,83). Marciniak and colleagues (81) compared admission to discharge functional abilities, and demonstrated significant functional gains in patients with SCI. Yoshioka et al. (83) found rehabilitation to be an effective component of care in the terminal cancer patient.

Functional improvements have been reported during the rehabilitation stay for individuals with neoplastic SCD in wheelchair mobility, ambulation, self-care, and transfer abilities (7). Patients demonstrated significant functional gains, and 84% returned home following rehabilitation. Follow-up surveys have indicated that the majority of patients maintained or improved upon their discharge level of function for mobility (either ambulation or wheelchair) and dressing at three months post-discharge.

Older age has been shown to effect rehabilitation outcome following SCI, with a higher prevalence of comorbidities and poorer outcomes (increased medical complications, rehospitalization, discharge to nursing homes, and need for attendant assistance) (85). Others have reported shorter hospital length of stay (LOS), lower hospital charges, decreased likelihood of divorce/separation, and decreased return to work for those of older age with new-onset SCI (86–89).

Patients with neoplastic SCD have been noted to have a shorter rehabilitation LOS compared to those with traumatic SCI. Factors that may have an influence in the shorter rehabilitation LOS in this group include differing patterns of neurologic recovery and a potential bias towards early discharge in patients with terminal cancer. Neoplasm affecting the spinal cord is primarily epidural in origin, causing compression due to a space-occupying lesion rather than actual spinal cord invasion. There is some potential for resolution of symptoms if the tumor is treated with surgical excision or radiation therapy, or if concomitant edema responds to treatment with steroids. The patient, family, or rehabilitation team may desire an earlier discharge given their potential limited life expectancy. This is especially pertinent given that spinal cord tumors often present secondary to metastasis and represent terminal illness. The shorter LOS allows patients to have more time at home with family and friends, thus enhancing QOL.

Further studies are necessary to more fully address functional outcome and QOL issues, to further access prognostic factors predictive of functional improvement during rehabilitation, to compare potential benefits of alternative therapeutic delivery systems such as outpatient and home health rehabilitation, and to address the maintenance of functional improvements.

REHABILITATION INTERVENTION AND GOALS

The objectives of rehabilitation of individuals with neoplastic spinal cord compression include maximizing an individual's medical, functional, and psychosocial outcomes and providing education to the patient and family. Rehabilitation approaches combine the management of both new-onset neurological impairments of SCI/D with general principles for cancer rehabilitation, with an emphasis on pain and psychological management. The rehabilitation process should begin as soon as possible after injury to maximize outcomes and reduce complications.

An interdisciplinary team approach is needed and involves a rehabilitation physician, nurse, therapists (physical, occupational, speech, recreational, and vocational), psychologist, nutritionist, and social worker. The health care team must develop rehabilitation goals within the limitations of the patient's illness, environment, and social support. Goals must be objective and attainable in a reasonable time. The SCI/D rehabilitation physician, often a specialist in physical medicine and rehabilitation, must be able to predict the potential functional outcomes of individuals with acute SCI/D. The primary oncologist's input on overall medical prognosis is also important in making this prediction in the cancer setting. This information assists in appropriately informing the patient and family, along with allowing formulating realistic functional team goals. Patient and family education stress an understanding of the unpredictable clinical course (with potential remissions and exacerbations) and the importance of compliance with the medical and rehabilitation program.

Intervention approaches during the rehabilitation of the cancer patient stress aspects of prevention, restoration, support, and palliation. Preventative interventions emphasize patient education, psychological counseling, physical conditioning, and maintaining general health status to lessen the effect of expected disabilities. Restorative interventions attempt to improve upon physical, psychological, social, and vocational functional abilities. If tumor progression leads to a functional decline, rehabilitation assumes a supportive role and its goals are adjusted to accommodate the patient's abilities and limitations. Education is important to teach patients to accommodate their disabilities, minimize potential complications, and provide emotional support associated with adjustment. With the onset of advanced disease, palliative interventions may be necessary to focus on minimizing complications (such as pain, contractures, and pressure sores) and providing comfort or psychological support for the patient and family.

Ongoing therapy can progress from the hospital and acute rehabilitation settings to outpatient and home health, depending on patient goals, functional progression, and tolerance. The majority of those with cancer-related SCD are discharged to private residences in the community. Community discharge can place a significant burden upon the patient's support system, but usually is preferable to a custodial care facility. Rehabilitation services must be considered on an outpatient or home-based basis to maintain gains and to prevent further deconditioning.

Mobility

Weakness, sensory deficits, fatigue, and pain may be impairments that limit mobility following both SCI and cancer, leading to a loss of functional independence. A major objective of rehabilitation is to enable the individual to maximize their mobility potential, including bed mobility, sitting tolerance, standing, transfers, and ambulation. Maintaining mobility is important for both QOL and preventing complications related to immobility. Therapy strategies must be employed to provide compensatory mobility techniques, increase strength, prevent disuse atrophy, and preserve joint (and soft tissue) range of motion. Patients are taught to modify their posture and body mechanics to capitalize on the strength of preserved muscle groups. Optimal therapy integrates motor and sensory reeducation techniques appropriate to each patient's unique ability. Provision of appropriate assistive devices (such as canes or walkers) is important during ambulation to compensate for weakness and reduced sensation and to enhance stability. Motorized or manual wheelchairs may be important for maintaining community mobility.

The severity and distribution of muscle weakness is related to the neurologic level of injury, with cervical spinal cord compression involving the upper and lower extremities and compression in the thoracic, lumbar, and sacral regions involving the lower extremities only. Patients with proximal lower extremity weakness may exhibit difficulty arising from a chair and can be assisted by strengthening or adaptive equipment such as elevated seats. Weakness of the hand's intrinsic muscles leads to difficulty with grasp, and adaptive devices, such as openers and large-handled utensils, are useful. Upper and lower extremity orthotics help stabilize joints in position for optimal function. High thoracic and cervical SCI may result in weakness of the respiratory muscles and diminished pulmonary function. Respiratory muscle strengthening exercises, chest physical therapy, and positioning techniques may assist enhancing respiration.

Fatigue is a component that requires patient education of strategies for energy conservation and work simplification techniques to maximize function. In addition, the therapist must evaluate the patient's upper extremity function and coexisting upper extremity metastases before weight bearing through the upper extremities can be allowed. Exercise recommendations for patients with bone metastases focus on increasing their muscle strength and endurance while maintain-

ing bone-protection strategies. High-impact activities should be avoided.

Activities of Daily Living

Therapeutic exercise is generally integrated with compensatory strategies and proper use of assistive devices to maximize ability for patients to perform ADL skills. Occupational therapists help patients to improve upper extremity function, allowing them to perform ADLs such as dressing, feeding, bathing, and grooming. Many modified utensils for performing ADLs are available. For those with proximal upper extremity weakness, adaptive devices, such as long-handled reachers and brushes, may be useful. Dressing, bathing, and grooming aids minimize the amount of effort and coordination required for these self-care activities. Patients can bathe and toilet with greater ease and safety if appropriate tub seats and commodes are provided. Hoyer lifts allow the transfer of patients with extensive motor impairments by a single caretaker. Home modifications will enhance patient safety and independence, and may be the key to their return to home. Ramps can be purchased, allowing wheelchair-dependent patients independent access to their homes. Education and orthotics can be helpful for enhancing function of sensation-deficient extremities. Reliance on visual rather than tactile feedback is stressed for hand positioning. If proprioceptive deficits are severe, orthoses can maintain affected joints in functional alignment for ambulation or grasp.

Psychological Adjustment and Life Satisfaction

Adjustment and coping are important issues that accompany both cancer and SCI/D rehabilitation. Group and individual psychological counseling, including an approach to pain management, should be considered. Counseling of both patients and family is important to address coping strategies, especially dealing with crisis and fear. Significant depression occasionally occurs and may require counseling and pharmacologic intervention. There is an increased risk of death from suicide, particularly early on.

QOL following SCI is often influenced by the ability of the patient to resume activity levels, including community reintegration (90). Key elements in any QOL intervention include maximizing the individual's physical and functional abilities and emotional and spiritual well-being, along with satisfaction with sexuality, occupational functioning, and financial concerns. Maintaining physical fitness and relaxation exercises can be beneficial. Many recent societal and legislative changes (such as the Americans with Disabilities Act) have allowed for increased accessibility, though additional work is needed to remove barriers impeding the return of persons with SCI to active roles within the community. Referrals for vocational rehabilitation should be considered when it becomes clear that certain functional deficits are stabilized.

FUNCTIONAL OUTCOMES BY NEUROLOGICAL LEVEL OF INJURY

The neurologic level and completeness of injury are important factors that assist in predicting neurologic recovery and therefore functional outcomes following SCI. The more incomplete the injury, the more favorable the potential for neurologic recovery and functional ability (85,86,91). Neurologic recovery usually plateaus in the first three to six months (though changes have been reported greater than one year after injury). Additional favorable prognostic factors are age younger than 50 years at time of injury, good initial hand or lower extremity motor score, education, and rapid early improvement. Ideal outcomes may not always be achieved for each individual and may vary, depending on factors such as the cancer progression, associated medical complications (pain, fatigue, depression, spasticity, contractures), patient motivation, and family/financial resources. Advances in surgical reconstruction and functional electrical stimulation (FES) may also enhance the patient's functional abilities following SCI. The intensity of therapies has been shown to affect outcome, and may be diminished in individuals with cancer-related issues (92).

Several functional outcome measures are reliable and valid for use in those with SCI (93). A common scale for the measurement of functional ability is the Functional Independence Measure (FIM), which uses a 7-point scale to measure 18 items in 6 categories: mobility, locomotion, self-care, continence of the bowel and/or bladder, communication, and social cognition. On the FIM scale, a score of 1 indicates total dependence on a caregiver and 7 indicates independence. Numbers between 1 and 7 represent different levels of assistance required from a caregiver or assistive device to perform a specific skill. Additional functional assessment scales are (1) the Quadriplegic Index of Function (QIF), which is designed to detect small but clinically relevant changes in individuals with tetraplegia in 9 categories of ADL; (2) the Modified Barthel Index (MBI), a 15-item assessment of self-care and mobility skills; (3) the Walking Index for SCI (WISCI), a 21-level scale that has demonstrated validity and responsiveness to changes in neurologic/walking function after SCI; (4) the Capabilities of Upper Extremity Instrument (CUE), a 32-item measure for assessing upper extremity function with tetraplegia; (5) the Spinal Cord Independence Measure (SCIM), which was designed as an alternative to the FIM to assess 16 categories of self-care, mobility, and respiratory and sphincter function; and (6) the Canadian Occupational Performance Measure (COPM), which is used to assess outcomes in the area of self-care, productivity, and leisure.

Orthotics in Cancer-Related SCD

Spinal orthotics are rarely necessary in the thoracic and lumbar spine, as patients with instability or spinal cord compression should be treated emergently with surgical decompression and stabilization, obviating the need for bracing. Bracing may rarely be of benefit in the management of movement-related spinal pain by controlling spinal position through external forces, thus providing some stability and restriction of spinal segment movement. When prescribed, spinal orthosis should immobilize one level above and below the painful or unstable vertebrae and apply pressure to at least three points to allow for partial weight transfer to the trunk when in upright positioning. The cruciform anterior spinal hyperextension (CASH) and Jewett hyperextension orthoses are easily obtainable, comfortable, and provide good flexion control. Custom thoracolumbosacral orthoses (TLSOs) provide much better spinal stability but are timely to produce, restrictive, uncomfortable, and rarely an appropriate option in the cancer setting. Orthoses are more commonly used in the cervical spine when treatment entails radiation and immobilization as opposed to surgery. Cervical collars may also be prescribed for use while driving following cervical stabilization to help protect from hardware failure should a collision occur. The Miami-J design comes in a variety of sizes, has reasonable adjustability, is comfortable, and is often the cervical orthosis of choice in the cancer setting.

Upper extremity orthotics can help patients with paresis involving the distal extremity to grasp and manipulate objects, and have been previously discussed. A universal cuff allows the patient to hold objects for feeding, grooming, and hygiene despite the absence of strength in the finger flexors or hand-intrinsic muscles. Orthotics can also be used to maintain the wrist in extension so that the thumb and digits will oppose each other for functional pinch. A balanced forearm orthotic supplements weak shoulder abductors and forward flexors in patients with preserved distal extremity strength. Lower extremity orthoses can enhance joint stability and muscle function for safe ambulation. An ankle-foot orthosis (AFO) may prevent foot-drop during the swing phase of gait. Knee orthoses compensate for weak quadriceps to prevent knee buckling.

MEDICAL ISSUES RELATED TO SPINAL CORD TUMORS

Medical complications in individuals with cancer-related SCD can present as either a consequence of the SCI itself or in relation to the underlying cancer. The neurologic sequelae of SCI/D results in weakness, neurogenic bladder/bowel, and sexual dysfunction. In addition, secondary SCI-related medical complications play an important role in the continuum of care for these individuals and can lead to increased rehospitalization rates and costs of care, along with decreased QOL (7,9). Secondary SCI/D complications may include neuropathic pain, pressure ulcers, infections (most commonly urinary tract infections and pneumonia), deep venous thrombosis, spasticity, and others. (4,8–10). Secondary issues related to the underlying cancer include pain, fatigue, depression, and anxiety. An important objective of the rehabilitation process is directed towards the prevention and management of these issues. Model systems programs for SCI have shown a decline in LOS and rehospitalization rate, citing advances in the prevention of secondary medical complications and improved treatment efficiency (94).

Pain

Pain is a significant issue in individuals with spinal cord tumors and may interfere with rehabilitation efforts, ongoing function, and QOL (95). It may result from tumor-related instability, spinal cord or nerve root compression, or as a consequence of its treatment. Accurate evaluation and diagnosis of etiology is important to the optimization of treatment (96). Cancer-related nociceptive pain may originate from soft tissue, bone, muscle, or nerve. Management may include surgical decompression, radiation therapy, physical therapy, and spinal orthotics. Analgesic medications are often necessary and consist of opioids, nonopioids (anti-inflammatory agents, acetaminophen, or tramadol), and adjuvant drugs (antidepressants, anticonvulsants, benzodiazepines, neuroleptics, calcitonin, and alpha blockers).

Neuropathic pain is often associated with SCI and is believed to result from changes in central (funicular) and peripheral (radicular) neuronal function, including increased spontaneous activity and reduced thresholds of response (97). It can be located at or below the level of injury and is often described as feeling hot/cold, tingling, or like an electric shock. It is sometimes exacerbated by external stimulus, perceived as painful with nonpainful stimuli (allodynia), or excessive in response to a painful stimulus (hyperalgesia). Management of neuropathic pain must include consideration of potential underlying conditions (such as infection), which if reduced, may decrease noxious stimuli. Patient education is important to help them understand the nature of this pain and potential management options. They should be encouraged to continue activity, which may also be beneficial as a management option. Pharmacologic management of neuropathic pain includes the use of anticonvulsants, antidepressants, and other analgesics. Patients should be informed that relief with these agents might not be immediate, as the initial dose may require titration.

Cancer Fatigue

Cancer-related fatigue (CRF) is common with patients receiving various treatments related to their disease process and consists of a persistent sense of tiredness that interferes with usual functional ability (98). Fatigue may cause a reduction in activity level, such as ability to perform mobility and other ADL skills. Fatigue in patients with cancer is a complex condition with a variety of contributing factors, such as the malignancy, cancer treatment, anemia, malnutrition, deconditioning, pain, anxiety, depression, and insomnia. Management of CRF includes an assessment of treatable factors that are known to commonly contribute to fatigue. The nutritional status of individuals with cancer should be maximized, but is often complicated by side effects of treatments (nausea/vomiting, diarrhea, poor appetite, diminished taste, or dysphagia). Effective management can include nutritional supplementation along with antiemetic or appetite-stimulant medications. Spreading out the frequency of rehabilitation therapies (such as PT and OT) to minimize fatigue may be necessary.

Musculoskeletal

Debilitation secondary to deconditioning can occur rapidly in individuals with limited activity levels due to conditions such as SCI/D and cancer. Studies have noted that even healthy individuals on complete bed rest reveal strength declines at a rate of 1%–2% per day, or about 10% per week (99). Additionally, muscle strength may decline as much as 20% in lower extremity muscles after five weeks of bed rest. Use of steroids can result in steroid myopathy characterized by proximal muscle weakness (100). Muscle or soft tissue contracture (shortening) may occur in individuals with decreased muscle strength, increased spasticity, or edema. Individuals with SCI also experience osteoporosis following an injury due to immobility. Long bone fractures are an additional secondary medical complication seen following SCI.

Urinary calcium excretion increases within two to three days of bed rest and continues over the first few months (101). A shift of calcium from bone to the circulatory system sometimes results in hypercalcemia. Underlying skeletal metastatic disease or paraneoplastic syndrome may also place patients at risk for hypercalcemia. Many tumors release humoral factors, mainly parathyroid hormone (PTH)-related protein (PTHrP), which stimulates bone resorption and/or tubular calcium reabsorption leading to hypercalcemia (102).

Spasticity is defined as a velocity-dependent increase in muscle tone (hyperreflexia) and occurs commonly following SCI, involving muscles below the level of injury (103). It can manifest itself as "tightness" of muscle movement, exaggerated muscle-stretch (deep tendon) reflexes, or involuntary contraction of muscle groups. Spasticity may have some beneficial effects, such as improving functional abilities or circulation and decreasing the risk of blood clots. More often, however, it can interfere with functional activities and may lead to difficulties with positioning, hygiene, and discomfort. A decision to intervene must incorporate both the positive and negative aspects of overall spasticity.

Initial treatment of spasticity includes elimination of exacerbating factors (such as bladder infections or pressure ulcers) and regular muscle stretching and positioning, with inclusion or oral antispasticity medications (such as baclofen, valium, tizanidine, dantrolene, or clonidine), should symptoms persist or worsen. For generalized spasticity, intrathecal delivery of baclofen via a subcutaneous pump and catheter system is available for individuals in whom medications are ineffective(104). Patients with the intrathecal baclofen pump have noted improvement of mobility, daily care skills, continence, and QOL. For more localized problematic spasticity, peripheral neurolysis with botulinum toxin or phenol injections are useful. Central ablative procedures, such as rhizotomy and myelotomy, are less often utilized.

Pulmonary

Respiratory complications represent a leading source of morbidity following SCI. In addition, prolonged bed rest and cancer-related conditions can lead to deconditioning with decreased pulmonary function. Pneumonia is the primary cause of death during the first year after SCI (105). Pulmonary complications are influenced by respiratory muscle paralysis, restrictive ventilation, ineffective cough, and atelectasis (106, 107). Individuals who are older or who have sustained a higher neurologic level of injury have been shown to be most vulnerable. Patients with cancer may be at increased risk for respiratory complications. Coughing or deep inspiration may be painful for the patients with rib metastases or for those who have undergone surgical procedures of the chest or abdomen. Primary lung tumors, metastatic disease, malignant pleural effusion, or complications

of chemotherapy or radiation therapy may further contribute to respiratory compromise. Preventative treatment and clinical management are important for maintaining optimal respiratory function, and include postural drainage, incentive spirometry, positive pressure breathing, consideration of airway bronchodilator medications, cough techniques, secretion management, and resistive strengthening exercises.

Genitourinary

Neurogenic bladder is a common sequela of SCI. Innervation for bladder control comes from the lowermost part of the spinal cord (sacral region), and individuals are often classified with either reflexic (spastic) or areflexic (flaccid) bladders. Management options include bladder catheterization techniques, fluid intake maintenance programs, medications, and sometimes surgery. Recently, bladder management with functional electrical stimulation has shown some success. The goal of a successful bladder program is to minimize infection rate, allow for continence and appropriate bladder emptying at acceptable bladder pressures, and increase QOL.

Neurogenic bladder management has undergone significant advances over the past 50 years, which has lessened the incidence of renal disease (once a leading cause of patient morbidity and mortality). Urinary tract infections are common, with symptoms that include fever, chills, and malaise; foul-smelling urine; or discomfort. Initiation of antibiotic treatment may be necessary, though recurrent infections are often problematic. A greater understanding of potential bladder complications, their prevention, and management, combined with the integral role of patient education are important factors for long-term success of a bladder management program (108). For individuals with limited life expectancy, conservative bladder management, with indwelling catheters, is often considered. Long-term periodic surveillance of the urinary tract and renal function remains important for early detection of potential complications. A regimen that evaluates the anatomy and function of the upper and lower tracts may include radiographs, renal ultrasound, renal nuclear scan, cystogram, and urodynamic examination.

Gastrointestinal

Neurogenic bowel is common following SCI and can result in decreased awareness and control of bowel emptying. There are often intermittent episodes of constipation or loose bowel movements, and a poorly controlled bowel program may lead to incontinence and increased social isolation. In addition, certain medications (such as narcotics, anticholinergics, and antibiotics) utilized in pain control or in relation to secondary

SCI-related conditions may lead to side effects that can adversely affect the program's success. The administration of chemotherapy or radiotherapy may also result in nausea, vomiting, and anorexia.

The objectives of a successful bowel program include achieving patient continence and regularity. Important factors for its success include medications (to improve consistency and colonic transport), diet (high in fiber), timing (after meals, to take advantage of gastrocolic reflexes), and positioning (to include gravity). Patient and family education is important to allow for an intermittent adjustment of the program. Neurologic assessment, with examination of the sacral (bulbocavernosus) reflexes, can suggest the presence of upper or lower motor neuron bowel dysfunction, and may assist in specific bowel management strategies. With upper motor neuron injury, defecation can be triggered with application of digital stimulation or application of a suppository. With lower motor neuron bowel dysfunction, evacuation may be assisted with the use of Valsalva maneuver or digital removal.

Cardiovascular

SCI can result in clinically significant compromise of cardiovascular control (109). Sympathetic nervous system neurons (which originate in the intermediolateral cell column of the thoracolumbar neurologic levels) control vasoconstriction and heart contractility. Impaired control of the autonomic nervous system in individuals with high thoracic and cervical SCI can result in problems such as hypotension, bradycardia, and autonomic dysreflexia. Education of patients, their families, and staff members is important for recognizing and managing cardiovascular complications.

Hypotension in connection with upright positioning is often observed, especially in SCI above the mid-thoracic level, and especially with more complete lesions. Decreased compensatory vasoconstriction (secondary to changes in sympathetic activity), in association with lower extremity venous pooling, can lead to reduced venous blood return, stroke volume, and blood pressure, producing lightheadedness and syncope. Hypotension usually improves within days to weeks after SCI as compensatory changes occur in the vascular beds, skeletal muscle, and rennin–angiotensin aldosterone system. Acceptable and tolerated systolic blood pressures for individuals with cervical SCI may be 80–100 mmHg. Early management begins with assessment of potential exacerbating factors, including prolonged recumbency, rapid changes in positioning, underlying infection, and dehydration. Medications that should be avoided include antihypertensives, diuretics, tricyclic antidepressants, anticholinergics, and narcotic analgesics. Treatment options include slow increases in upright positioning, application of an abdominal binder, and thigh-high antiembolism stockings to decrease venous pooling. Pharmacologic intervention (such as salt tablets, midodrine, or fludrocortisone) can also be considered.

Persons with an SCI at T6 or above are at risk for the development of autonomic dysreflexia, which may be associated with potentially dangerous blood pressure elevation. The pathophysiology appears to involve an unmodulated sympathetic response to a noxious stimulus below the level of the lesion. The classic presentation is that of profound headache, flushing, and diaphoresis in the presence of elevated blood pressure and bradycardia. Management includes placing the patient in a sitting position (which decreases intracranial pressure), checking for an inciting stimulus (such as distended bladder), and, if necessary, administering antihypertensive medications such as topical nitroglycerin or nifedipine. For recurrent bouts of dysreflexia, prophylaxis with alpha-blocking agents may be warranted.

Thromboembolic Disease

Individuals with cancer are at increased risk for deep venous thrombosis (DVT), due to hypercoaguable states. DVT is also a common complication following SCI, with studies reporting incidence ranging from 14%–90%, especially during the first six months after injury. DVT may result in pulmonary embolism (PE), which generally arises from thrombosis within the proximal leg veins (110). Risk factors for DVT following SCI include paralysis, venous stasis, and hypercoaguability.

Classic symptoms of DVT, such as calf tenderness, may be lacking after SCI, due to sensory loss. Symptoms of PE, such as shortness of breath, may be incorrectly attributed to concurrent problems, such as atelectasis or underlying pulmonary malignancy. Screening studies should be considered in those at highest risk. Prophylactic management consists of pneumatic compression devices, lower extremity compression hose, early mobilization, and subcutaneous injectable medications such as unfractionated heparin or LMWH, administered for two to three months following injury (111). In patients with multiple risk factors (eg, lower limb fracture, history of DVT, cancer, heart failure, obesity, age >70 years), placement of an inferior cava filter can be considered.

Skin

Pressure ulcers are frequently seen in individuals with SCI. Associated cancer-related factors (such as malnutrition and skin fragility) will also increase risk for skin breakdown and poor wound healing. Sustained pressure, especially over bony prominences, results in ischemic tissue injury. Because muscle and subcutaneous tissues are more sensitive to injury than the epidermis, the initial appearance of a pressure ulcer may not reflect the severity of the underlying injury. Several factors contribute to skin breakdown; these include pressure, time, shearing forces, friction, and moisture. Older individuals are at particular risk for pressure ulcers because of the aging-associated loss of subcutaneous tissue and decreased connective tissue elasticity. The most common locations for pressure ulcers following SCI include the sacrum, ischium, heels, trochanters, and malleolus. They may interfere with functional and social abilities of an individual secondary to positioning or bed rest required for its management. In addition, costs of care can be staggering in terms of lost workdays, increased skilled care, specialized supplies, and possible hospitalizations or surgery.

Prevention of pressure ulcers involves the identification of high-risk patients and intervention with positioning schedules, pressure-reducing support surfaces, reduction of skin moisture, adequate nutrition, and patient education. Treatment of an established ulcer involves limiting pressure to the area and aggressive wound care. Local care may include debridement of necrotic tissue, wound cleansing, management of exudate, and appropriate wound dressings. Proper nutrition is important, and includes adequate provision of calories, protein, and vitamins. Deep ulcers can be treated surgically with debridement and repair by myocutaneous flap, but is best deferred until nutritional status is adequate.

Sexuality

Sexual dysfunction involves both physiological and psychological issues, and is an important issue. Although individuals with cancer-related SCI are typically older, consideration of sexuality issues may still be warranted and desirable (112). Sexual drive may be intact, though may be diminished in the presence of fatigue, pain, or depression. SCI can result in erectile and ejaculatory dysfunction, often related to the completeness of injury. The individual's perceptions of sexuality issues may undergo changes, leading to patient (and family) anxiety, if not addressed appropriately. Interdisciplinary team members are taught to identify and address sexuality issues and to adequately outline the potential functional changes that may occur. Pharmacologic (oral and injectable medication) and technological (vacuum and implantable devices) options for restoring erectile capabilities can be utilized. If male fertility issues are of interest, technological innovations, such as vibratory or electrical stimulation, have enhanced the ability for successful ejaculation that, when combined with insemination techniques, can lead to successful pregnancy.

CONCLUSIONS

Patients with cancer-related SCD represent a significant proportion of individuals with SCI/D admitted to rehabilitation settings. These individuals tend to be older and have a greater incidence of incomplete and paraplegic injuries than their traumatic SCI counterparts. Following rehabilitation, studies have noted that patients achieve comparable rates of functional gains, have a shorter rehabilitation LOS, and can achieve similar discharge to community rates. Medical management for individuals with cancer-related SCD continues to be an integral part of the long-term follow-up and coordinated continuum of care. The rising costs of SCI care, along with the associated personal, vocational, and family impacts, make further understanding of these issues important. Priority should be given to studies aimed at reducing the incidences of further identifying risk factors and treatment strategies for rehabilitation and medical management.

*R*eferences

1. Adams R, Salam-Adams M. Chronic nontraumatic diseases of the spinal cord. *Neurol Clin.* 1991;9:605–623.
2. Dawson D, Potts F. Acute nontraumatic myelopathies. *Neurol Clin.* 1991;9:585–602.
3. Schmidt R, Markovchick V. Nontraumatic spinal cord compression. *J Emerg Med.* 1992;10:189–199.
4. McKinley W, Hardman J, Seel R. Nontraumatic spinal cord injury: incidence, epidemiology and functional outcome. *Arch Phys Med Rehabil.* 1998;79:1186–1187.
5. Guttman L. *Spinal Cord Injuries.* Comprehensive Management and Research. Oxford: Blackwell; 1973.
6. Buchan A, Fulford G, Jellinek E, Kerr W, Newsam J, Stark G. A preliminary survey of the incidence and etiology of spinal paralysis. *Parplegia.* 1972;10:23–28.
7. McKinley W, Conti-Wyneken A, Vokac C, Cifu D. Rehabilitative functional outcome of patients with neoplastic spinal cord compression. *Arch Phys Med Rehabil.* 1996;77:892–895.
8. Gibson C. *Final Report of the Rochester Regional Model Spinal Cord Injury System. 9-30-85 to 7-29-90.* Rochester, NY: Rochester Regional Model Spinal Cord Injury System; 1991.
9. McKinley W, Tellis A, Cifu D, Johnson M, Kubal W, Keyser-Marcus L. Rehabilitation outcome of individuals with nontraumatic myelopathy resulting from spinal stenosis. *J Spinal Cord Med.* 1998;21:131–136.
10. McKinley W, Tewksbury M. Neoplastic vs. traumatic spinal cord injury: an inpatient rehabilitation comparison. *Am J Phys Med Rehabil.* 2000;79:138–144.
11. Murray P. Functional outcome and survival in spinal cord injury secondary to neoplasia. *Cancer.* 1985;55:197–201.
12. Sundaresan N, Galicich J, Bains M, Martini N, Beattie J Jr. Vertebral body resection in the treatment of cancer involving the spine. *Cancer.* 1984;53:1393–1396.
13. Helweg-Larsen S. Clinical outcome in metastatic spinal cord compression. A prospective study of 153 patients. *Acta Neurol Scand.* 1996;94:269–275.
14. Gilbert R, Kim J, Posner J. Epidural spinal cord compression from metastatic tumor: diagnosis and treatment. *Ann Neurol.* 1978;3:40–51.
15. Plotkin SR, Wen PY. Neurologic complication of cancer therapy. *Neurol Clin.* 2003;21:279–318.
16. Posner J. Spinal metastases. In: Davis F, ed. *Neurological Complications of Cancer.* F.A. Davis Company, Philadelphia, PA; 1995:111–141.

17. Abrahm J. Management of pain and spinal cord compression. In: Patients with Advanced Cancer ACP-ASIM End of Life Care Consensus Panel. *Ann Intern Med.* 1999;131:37–46.

18. Byrne T. Spinal cord compression from epidural metastases. *N Eng J Med.* 1992;327:614–619.

19. Arguello F, Baggs R, Duerst R. Pathogenesis of vertebral metastasis and epidural spinal cord compression. *Cancer.* 1990;65:98–106.

20. Batson OV. The function of the vertebral veins and their role in the spread of metastases. *Ann Surg.* 1940;112–138.

21. Ushio Y, Posner R, Posner J. Experimental spinal cord compression by epidural neoplasms. *Neurology.* 1977;27:422–429.

22. Posner J. Back pain and epidural spinal cord compression. *Med Clin N. Am.* 1987;71(2):185–204.

23. American Cancer Society. Cancer statistics 2000. *Cancer Journal for Clinicians.* 2000;50:6–16.

24. Lewis D, Packer R, Raney B. Incidence, presentation, and outcome of spinal cord disease in children with systemic cancer. *Pediatrics.* 1986;78:438–442.

25. Alter M. Statistical aspects of spinal tumors. In: Vinken PJ, Bruyn GS, eds. *Handbook of Clinical Neurology, Vol 19.* Amsterdam: North Holland Publishing; 1975:1–22.

26. Levy W, Bay J, Dohn D. Spinal cord meningioma. *J Neurosurg.* 1982;57:804–812.

27. Stein B, McCormick P. Spinal intradural tumors. In: Wilkins RH, Rengachary SS, eds. *Neurosurgery.* New York, NY: McGraw-Hill;1996:1769–1789.

28. Balm M, Hammack J. Leptomeningeal carcinomatosis. Presenting features and prognostic factors. *Arch Neurol.* 1996;53(7):626–632.

29. Levin V, Leibel S, Gutin P. Neoplasms of the central nervous system. In: Vincent T. Devita V, Jr, Hellman S, eds. *Cancer: Principles & Practice of Oncology.* 6th ed. Philadelphia, PA: Lippincott Williams & Wilkins; 2001:2100–2160.

30. Epstein F, Farmer J, Freed D. Adult intramedullary astrocytomas of the spinal cord. *J Neurosurg.* 1992;77(3):355–359.

31. McCormick P, Torres R, Post K. Intramedullary ependymoma of the spinal cord. *J Neurosurg.* 1990;72(4):523–532.

32. Schwartz TH, McCormick PC. Intramedullary ependymomas: clinical presentation, surgical treatment strategies, and prognosis. *J Neurooncol.* 2000;47:211–218.

33. Bradley WG, Daroff RD, Fenichel GM, Jankovic J. *Neurology in Clinical Practice: The Neurological Disorders.* 4th Ed. Philadelphia, PA: Elsevier, Inc, 2004:1447–1450.

34. Merenda JT. Other primary benign tumors and tumor-like lesions of the spine. *Spine: State of the Arts Reviews.* 1988;2(2):275–286.

35. Lee M, Rezai AR, Abbott R. Intramedullary spinal cord lipomas. *J Neurosurg.* 1995 Mar;82(3):394–400.

36. Stein B, McCormick P. Intramedullary neoplasms and vascular malformations. *Clin Neurosurg.* 1992;39:361–387.

37. Gilbert R, Minhas T. Epidural spinal cord compression and neoplastic meningitis. In: Johnson RT, ed. *Current Therapy in Neurologic Disease.* Philadelphia, PA: Mosby. 1997:253–259.

38. Schiff D, O'Neill P, Suman J. Spinal epidural metastasis as the initial manifestation of malignancy: clinical features and diagnostic approach. *Neurology.* 1997 Aug;49(2):452–456.

39. Schiff D. Spinal cord compression. *Neurol Clin.* 2003 Feb;21(1):67–86.

40. Bach F, Larsen B, Rohde K. Metastatic spinal cord compression: occurrence, symptoms, clinical presentations, and prognosis in 398 patients with spinal cord compression. *Acta Neurochir.* 1990;107:37–43.

41. McKinley W, Huang M, Brunsvold K. Neoplastic vs Traumatic Spinal Cord Injury: An Outcome Comparison after Inpatient Rehabilitation. *Am J Phys Med Rehabil.* 2001;80:

42. Kim R, Spencer S, Meredith R, Weppelmann B, Lee J, Smith J. Extradural spinal cord compression: analysis of factors determining functional prognosis. *Radiology.* 1990;176:279–282.

43. Tatli YZ, Stubblefield MD, Custodio CM. Spinal ataxia from Ewing's sarcoma: a case report. *Arch Phys Med Rehabil.* 2004;85:E49.

44. American Spinal Injury Association/International Medical Society of Paraplegia. International standards for neurological and functional classification of spinal cord injury patients. Chicago, IL: American Spinal Injury Association; 2001.

45. Byrne T, Waxman S. *Spinal Cord Compression: Diagnosis and Principles of Treatment: Contemporary Neurology Series.* Philadelphia, PA: FA Davis; 1990.

46. Brotchi J, Lefranc F. Current management of spinal cord tumors. *Contemporary Neurosurgery.* 1999;21(26):1–8.

47. Patchell RA, Tibbs PA, Regine WF, et al. Direct decompressive surgical resection in the treatment of spinal cord compression caused by metastatic cancer: a randomized trial. *Lancet.* 2004;336:643–648.

48. Stubblefield MD, Bilsky MH. Barriers to rehabilitation of neurosurgical spine cancer patient. *J Surg Oncol.* 2007;10.1002:1–8.

49. Livingston K, Perrin R. The neurosurgical management of spinal metastases causing cord and cauda equina compression. *J Neurosurg.* 1978;49:839–843.

50. Siegal T, Siegal T. Current considerations in the management of neoplastic spinal cord compression. *Spine.* 1989;14:2:223–228.

51. Young R, Post E, King G. Treatment of spinal epidural metastases. Randomized prospective comparison of laminectamy and radiotherapy. *J Neurosurg.* 1980;53:741–748.

52. Black P. Spinal metastasis: current status and recommended guidelines for management. *Neurosurgery.* 1979;5(6);726–746.

53. Siegal T, Siegal T, Shapira Y, et al. Indomethacin and dexamethasone treatment in experimental spinal cord compression. Part 1. *Neurosurgery.* 1988;22:328–333.

54. Siegel T, Shohami E, Shapira Y, et al. indomethacin and dexamethasone treatment in experimental spinal cord compression. Part II. *Neurosurgery.* 1988;22:334–339.

55. Sgouros S, Malluci CL, Jackowski A. Spinal ependymomas—the value of postoperative radiotherapy for residual disease control. *Br J Neurosurg.* 1996;10(6):559–566.

56. Rades D, Veninga T, Staplers LJA, et al. Prognostic factors predicting functional outcomes, recurrence-free survival, and overall survival after radiotherapy for metastatic spinal cord compression in breast cancer patients. *Int J Radiation Oncology Biol Phys.* 2006;64:182–188.

57. Fuller B, Heiss J, Oldfield E. Spinal cord compression. In: Devita VT Jr, Hellman S, Rosenberg SA, eds. *Cancer Principles & Practice of Oncology.* 6th ed. Philadelphia, PA: Lippincott-Raven Publishing; 2001:2617–2633.

58. Rubin P, Constine LS, Williams JP. Late effects of cancer treatment: radiation and drug toxicity. In: Perez CA, Brady LW, eds. *Principles and Practice of Radiation Oncology.* 3rd ed. Philadelphia, PA: Lippincott-Raven Publishing; 1997:155–211.

59. Patchell RA, Posner JB. Neurologic complications of systemic cancer. *Neurol Clin.* 1985;3:729–750.

60. Burns BJ, Jones AN, Robertson JS. Pathology of radiation myelopathy. *J Neurol Neurosurg Psychiatry.* 1972;35:888.

61. Cristante L, Herrmann HD. Surgical management of intramedullary spinal cord tumors: functional outcome and sources of morbidity. *Neurosurgery.* 1994;35(1):69–74.

62. Hoshimaru M, Koyama T, Hashimoto N. Results of microsurgical treatment for intramedullary spinal cord ependymomas: analysis of 36 cases. *Neurosurgery.* 1999;44(2):264–269.

63. Jyothirmayi R, Madhavan J, Nair MK. Conservative surgery and radiotherapy in the treatment of spinal cord astrocytoma. *J Neurooncol.* 1997;33(3):205–211.

64. Hacking H, Van As H, Lankhorst GJ. Factors related to the outcome of inpatient rehabilitation in patients with neoplastic epidural spinal cord compression. *Paraplegia.* 1993;31:367–374.

65. Greenburg HS, Kim J, Posner J. Epidural spinal cord compression from metastatic tumor: results with a new treatment protocol. *Ann Neurol.* 1980;8:361–366.

66. Barcena A, Lobato R, Coirdobes F, et al. Spinal metastatic disease: analysis of factors determining functional prognosis and the choice of treatment. *Neurosurgery.* 1984;15:6:820–827.

67. Fundlay G. Adverse effects of the management of malignant spinal cord compression. *J Neurol Neurosurg Psychiatry*. 1984;47:761–768.

68. Cowap J, Hardy J, Ahern R. Outcome of malignant spinal cord compression at a cancer center: implications for palliative care services, *J Pain Symptom Manage*. 2000;19(4):257–264.

69. Guo Y, Young B, Palmer J, Mun Y, Bruera E. Prognostic factors for survival in metastatic spinal cord compression: a retrospective study in a rehabilitation setting, *Am J Phys Med Rehabil*. 2003;82(9):665–668.

70. Wang JC, Boland P, Mitra N, et al. Single-stage posterolateral transpedicular approach for resection of epidural metastatic spine tumors involving the vertebral body with circumferential reconstruction: results in 140 patients. *J Neurosurg (Spine 1)*. 2004;3:287–298.

71. Leviov M, Dale J, Stein M, et al. The management of metastatic spinal cord compression: a radiotherapeutic success ceiling. *Int J Radiat Oncol Biol Phys*. 1993;27:231–234.

72. Maranzano E, Latini P. Effectiveness of radiation therapy without surgery in metastatic spinal cord compression: final results from a prospective trail. *Int J Radiat Oncol Biol Phys*. 1995;32:959–967.

73. Sundaresan N, Sachdev VP, Holland J, et al. Surgical treatment of spinal cord compression from epidural metastasis. *J Clin Oncol*. 1995;9:2330–2335.

74. Spinal Cord Injury Information Network Spinal cord injury facts and figures at a glance. *J Spinal Cord Med*. 2007;30(1):79–80.

75. Kirshblum S, Groah SL, McKinley WO, Gittler MS, Stiens SA. Spinal cord injury medicine. 1. Etiology, classification, and acute medical management. *Arch Phys Med Rehabil*. 2002;83(3 Suppl 1):S50–S57, S90–S58.

76. Sandalcioglu IE, Gasser T, Asgari S, et al. Functional outcome after surgical treatment of intramedullary spinal cord tumors: experience with 78 patients. *Spinal Cord*. 2005;43:34–41.

77. Eriks IE, Angenot EL, Lankhorst GJ. Epidural metastatic spinal cord compression: functional outcome and survival after inpatient rehabilitation. *Spinal Cord*. 2004 Apr;42(4):235–239.

78. Parsch D, Mikut R, Abel R. Postacute management of patients with spinal cord injury due to metastatic tumor disease: survival and efficacy of rehabilitation. *Spinal Cord*. 2003 Apr;41(4):205–210.

79. Bach F, Larsen B, Rohde K, Borgesen S, Gjerris F, Boge-Rasmussen T. Metastatic spinal cord compression: occurrence, symptoms, clinical presentations and prognosis in 398 patients with spinal cord compression. *Acta Neurochir*. 1990;107:37–43.

80. DeLisa JA. Rehabilitation of the patient with cancer or human immunodeficiency virus. In: DeLilsa, ed. *Rehabilitation Medicine: Principles and Practice*. Philadelphia, PA: Lippincott; 1993:916–933.

81. Marciniak C, Sliwa J, Spill G, Heinemann A, Semik P. Functional outcome following rehabilitation of the cancer patient. *Arch Phys Med Rehabil*. 1996;77:54–57.

82. LaBan MM. Rehabilitation of patients with cancer. In: Kottke FJ, Lehman JF, eds. *Krusen's Handbook of Physical Medicine and Rehabilitation*. 4th ed. Philadelphia, PA: Saunders; 1990:1102–1112.

83. Yoshioka H. Rehabilitation for the terminal cancer patient. *Am Phys Med Rehabil*. 1994;73:199–206.

84. O'Toole DM, Golden AM. Evaluating cancer patients for rehabilitation potential. *West J Med*. 1991;155:384–387.

85. DeVivo MJ, Kartus PL, Rutt RD, Stover Sl, Fine PR. The influence of age at time of spinal cord injury on rehabilitation outcome. *Arch Neurol*. 1990;47:687–691.

86. Yarkony GM, Roth EJ, Heinemann AW, Lovell LL. Spinal cord injury rehabilitation outcome: the impact of age. *J Clin Epidemiol*. 1988;41:173–177.

87. Charles ED, Fine PR, Stover SL, Wood T, Lott AF, Kronenfeld J. The costs of spinal cord injury. *Paraplegia*. 1978. 15:302–310.

88. Meyer AR, Feltin M, Master RJ. Re-hospitalization and spinal cord injury: a cross –sectional survey of adults living independently. *Arch Phys Med Rehabil*. 1985;66:704–708.

89. Devivo MJ, Fine PR. Spinal cord injury: its short-term impact on martial status. *Arch Phys Med Rehabil*. 1985;66:501–504.

90. Richards JS, Bombardier CH, Tate D, Dijkers M, Gordon W, Shewchuk R, DeVivo MJ. Access to the environment and life satisfaction after spinal cord injury. *Arch Phys Med Rehabil*. 1999;80:1501–1506.

91. Ditunno JF Jr, Cohen Me, Formal C, et al. Functional outcomes. In: Stover SL, DeLisa JA, Whiteneck GG, eds. *Spinal Cord Injury: Clinical Outcomes from the Model Systems*. Gaithersburg: Aspen Publications; 1995:1170–1184.

92. Spivak G, Spettell CM, Ellis DW, Ross SE. Effects of intensity of treatment and length of stay on rehabilitation outcomes. *Brain Inj*. 1992;6:419–434.

93. Kirshblum S and Donovan W. Neurologic assessment and classification of traumatic spinal cord injury. In: Kirshblum S, Compagnolo D, Delisa J, eds. *Spinal Cord Medicine*. Philadelphia, PA: Lippincott Williams and Wilkins;2002:82–95.

94. DeVivo MJ. Discharge disposition from model spinal cord injury care system rehabilitation programs. *Arch Phys Med Rehabil*. 1999;80:785–790.

95. Cheville AL. Pain management in cancer rehabilitation. *Arch Phys Med Rehabil*. 2001;82:S84–S87.

96. Portenoy RK, Lessage P. Management of cancer pain. *Lancet*. 1999;353:1695–1700.

97. Falah M, Schiff D, Burns TM. Neuromuscular complications of cancer diagnosis and treatment. *J Support Oncol*. 2005;3:271–282.

98. Portenoy RK, Itri LM. Cancer-related fatigue: guidelines for evaluation and management. *The Oncologist*. 1999;4:1–10.

99. Muller EA. Influence of training and inactivity on muscle strength. *Arch Phys Med Rehabil*. 1970;51:449–462.

100. Batchelor TT, Yaylor LP, Thaler HT, et al. Steroid myopathy in cancer patients. *Neurology*. 1997;48:1234–1238.

101. Maynard FM. Immobilization hypercalcemia following spinal cord injury. *Arch Phys Med Rehabil*. 1986;67:41–44.

102. Esbrit P. Hypercalcemia of malignancy, new insights into an old syndrome. *Clin Lab*. 2001;47(1–2):67–71.

103. Lance†JW. The control of muscle tone, reflexes, and movement: Robert Wartenberg lecture. *Neurology*. 1980;30:1303?1313.

104. Penn RD. Intrathecal baclofen for spasticity of spinal origin: seven years of experience. *J Neurosurg*. 1992;77:236–240.

105. Jackson AB, Groomes TE. Incidence of respiratory complications following spinal cord injury. *Arch Phys Med Rehabil*. 1994;75(3):270–275.

106. Ledsome JR, Sharp JM. Pulmonary function in acute cervical cord injury. *Am Rev Respir Dis*. 1981:124:41–44.

107. McMichan JC, Michel L, Westbrook PR. Pulmonary dysfunction following traumatic quadriplegia. *JAMA*. 1980;243:528–531.

108. Groah SL, Stiens SA, Gittler MS, McKinley WO. Spinal cord injury medicine. 5. Preserving wellness and independence of the aging patient with spinal cord injury: a primary care approach for the rehabilitation medicine specialist. *Arch Phys Med Rehabil*. 2002 Mar;83:S82–S89, S90–S98.

109. Furlan JC, Fehlings MG, Shannon P, Norenberg MD, Krassioukov AV. Descending vasomotor pathways in humans: correlation between axonal preservation and cardiovascular dysfunction after spinal cord injury. *J Neurotrauma*. 2003;20(12):1351–1364.

110. Merli G, Herbison G, Ditunno J, et al. Deep vein thrombosis: prophylaxis in acute spinal cord injured subjects. *Arch Phys Med Rehabil*. 1988;69:661–664.

111. Green D, Rossi E, Yao J, et al. Deep vein thrombosis in spinal cord injury: effect of prophylaxis with calf compression, aspirin, and dipyridamole. *Paraplegia*. 1982;20:227–234.

112. Burt K. The effects of cancer on body image and sexuality. *Nurs Times*. 1995 Feb 15–22;91(7):36-37.

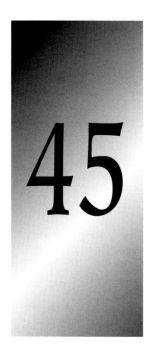

Radiculopathy in Cancer

Oksana Sayko
Tim Dillingham

Radiculopathy is a pathological process affecting the spinal nerve root. It is one of the most common causes of pain and dysfunction in the cancer setting. In the majority of cases, nerve root insult arises from direct compression. The most common etiology of compression in the general population is herniated nucleus pulposus, excess bony formation, and spurring from the uncovertebral joints (cervical region) or zygapophyseal joints, as well as hypermobility of the vertebral segment resulting in direct focal insult to the nerve roots exiting the spine (Figs 45.1 and 45.2). In elderly patients, the degenerative cascade of changes predisposes to lumbar spinal stenosis, which can compress many nerves in the cauda equina (Fig. 45.3). Degenerative causes of radiculopathy are as common in the cancer setting as in the general population and can predispose cancer patients to more significant signs and symptoms as these patients traverse the continuum of cancer care and are exposed to treatments such as radiation and neurotoxic chemotherapy. This chapter will focus on the cancer-specific etiologies of radiculopathy.

After intervertebral disc disease and spinal stenosis, tumors of the spine, adjacent soft tissues, and spinal cord, as well as infectious processes involving the spine, comprise other less common causes of compressive radiculopathy (1,2). In addition, noncompressive causes of radiculopathy resulting from vasculitic paraprotein-related phenomenon, radiation, and other causes can be seen in the cancer setting. They must be included in the differential diagnosis of the patient

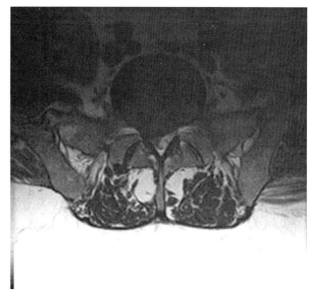

FIGURE 45.1

Axial T2 weighted MRI demonstrating a right paracentral herniated nucleus pulposus at L5–S1 with effacement of the ventral aspect of the thecal sac and mass effect on the right S1 nerve root.

with cancer presenting with radicular symptoms. Early diagnosis is crucial because the degree of pretreatment neurologic dysfunction is a strong predictor of treatment outcome (3–7).

KEY POINTS

- Radiculopathy is a pathological process affecting the spinal nerve root.
- Degenerative causes of radiculopathy are as common in the cancer setting as in the general population and can predispose cancer patients to more significant signs and symptoms as patients traverse the continuum of cancer care and are exposed to treatments such as radiation and neurotoxic chemotherapy.
- Spinal cord and nerve root damage may result from compression by tumor in the epidural space, by direct invasion of the spinal cord parenchyma, or by leptomeningeal involvement.
- Epidural compression, particularly from vertebral metastasis, is a relatively common neurologic complication of cancer occurring in 5%–10% of all patients with malignancies.
- 5. Epidural tumors damage the spinal cord and nerve roots by direct compression (with demyelination and axonal damage) and by secondary vascular compromise with resultant ischemia, edema, and infarction.
- Radiation treatment affects the peripheral nervous system, including the nerve root, by vascular endothelial damage and perivascular fibrosis within the radiation field with resultant nerve and muscle damage.
- The most common clinical presentation of radiculopathy includes pain and sensory impairment in the distribution of the affected nerve root.
- In case of epidural metastases, radicular pain is often preceded by local pain that is usually of subacute onset, aching in nature, and can become unbearable over time.
- Plain radiography has poor sensitivity in the identification of spinal tumors.
- Magnetic resonance imaging (MRI) is the most sensitive and specific diagnostic test to evaluate spinal lesions caused by cancer and is the test of choice to evaluate neurologic structures of the spine and vertebral column.
- MRI with gadolinium contrast enhancement is the preferred imaging technique when intramedullary tumors or leptomeningeal metastases are suspected and to evaluate the postoperative spine where scar is difficult to differentiate from tumor.
- Electromyography (EMG) and nerve conduction studies (NCS) are valuable diagnostic tools in evaluating patients with suspected nerve root compression from either benign or malignant processes, and can facilitate differentiating radiculopathies from plexopathies and peripheral nerve lesions, the clinical presentation of which can often be indistinguishable from radicular involvement.

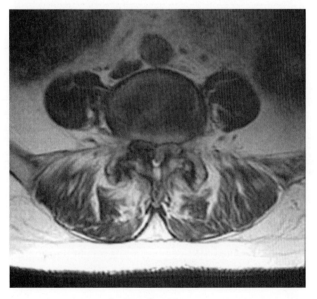

FIGURE 45.2

Axial T2 weighted MRI demonstrating advanced degenerative changes of the lumbar spine in a patient with grade 1 anterolisthesis of L4 on L5 and facet arthropathy, resulting in moderate to severe central canal compromise with compression and displacement of the thecal sac and mass effect on the right L5 nerve root.

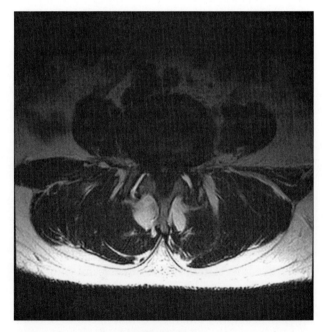

FIGURE 45.3

Axial T2 weighted MRI demonstrating severe central spinal stenosis from degenerative changes and hypertrophy of the ligamentum flavum with multiple nerve root compression.

COMPRESSIVE RADICULOPATHY

Epidural compression, particularly from vertebral metastasis, is a relatively common neurologic complication of cancer occurring in 5%–10% of all patients with malignancies (8,9). The thoracic spine is the most common location of epidural compression (59%–78%), followed by the lumbosacral (16%–33%), cervical (4%–15%), and sacral (5%–10%) spine (10–12). This distribution largely follows the volume of the spine. Multiple metastases are found in 10%–38% of patients (4,12). Intramedullary cord compression is relatively rare. All segments of spinal cord can be affected equally. Many patients with intramedullary spinal metastases also have parenchymal brain metastases (35%), and about 25% have concomitant leptomeningeal carcinomatosis (11).

Among the most common metastatic tumors that produce cord and nerve root compression are breast, prostate, and lung cancer. Other malignancies include lymphoma, renal cell carcinoma, myeloma, colorectal cancer, sarcoma, and thyroid cancer (Table 45.1).

Metastatic disease is the most frequent cause of spinal cord and associated nerve root compression as a result of cancer. It is the second most frequent cause of neurologic complications of cancer after brain metastases. With the improved treatments of many systemic cancers and the resultant increase in patient survival, spinal metastases and their sequelae are becoming increasingly common. Table 45.2 lists the common causes of spinal cord and nerve root involvement in patients with cancer. Spinal cord and nerve root damage may result from compression by tumor in the epidural space, by direct invasion of the spinal cord parenchyma, or by leptomeningeal involvement (Figs 45.4

and 45.5). Of these, metastatic epidural compression is the most common (6,13).

Epidural Metastases

Metastases can reach the epidural space in one of two ways. In the majority of cases, tumor metastasizes to the vertebral body and later forms space-occupying masses in epidural space that have the potential to compromise nerve roots to varying degrees (Fig. 45.4). Less commonly (characteristic of lymphomas and neuroblastomas), a paravertebral tumor grows into the spinal canal from the posterolateral direction through the intravertebral foramina, compressing the nerve roots first (6,14).

In most cases, metastases spread to the vertebral bodies by the hematogenous dissemination. Blood flow is high in red, marrow-rich vertebral bodies, accounting for the predilection of metastases for those areas. Furthermore, tumor cells produce adhesive molecules that bind them to stromal marrow cells and bone matrix (15). Spinal metastases tend to grow in the well-vascularized marrow space of the posterior vertebral body. They can produce spinal cord and related structure compression in two ways. The first is a result of continued tumor growth and subsequent obliteration of the marrow space with expansion into the epidural space and impingement on the anterior thecal sac and surrounding venous plexus. Alternatively, destruction of the cortical bone by tumor can result in vertebral body collapse, its anterior angulation, and subsequent posterior displacement of bony fragments into the epidural space, causing compression of the thecal sac and epidural venous plexus. Posterior compression of the spinal cord and related structures from the metastatic

TABLE 45.1
Frequency of Tumor Types Producing Cord Compression (De Vita, 2001)

AUTHOR	LUNG	BREAST	PROSTATE	MYELOMA	RENAL	LYMPHOMA	OTHER	SARCOMA	TOTAL
Katrini, 1998	19	15	11	10	3	7	33	3	101
Kovner, 1999	9	28	12	—	--	9	21	—	79
Solberg, 1999	11	9	30	5	6	—	25	—	86
Helweg-Larson, 1996	27	56	43	—	6	—	17	4	153
Maranzano, 1995	38	103	24	17	7	9	45	—	243
Gilbert, 1978	30	48	21	9	17	26	62	22	235
Stark, 1982	43	37	5	—	4	—	42	1	132
Total	177 (17.2%)	296 (29%)	146 (14.2%)	41 (4%)	43 (4.2%)	51 (5%)	245 (23.8%)	30 (2.9%)	1029 (100%)

Source: From Ref. 10.

TABLE 45.2

Common Causes of Spinal Cord/Nerve Roots Involvement in Cancer Patients

METASTATIC	NONMETASTATIC
I. Epidural lesions	I. Primary spinal tumors
1. From vertebral body	1. Extramedullary
2. Arising in epidural space	2. Intramedullary
3. From paravertebral structures	II. Infectious
II. Intradural lesions	III. Vascular disorders
1. Intramedullary metastases	1. Hemorrhage
2. Leptomeningeal metastases	2. Infarct
	IV. Side effects of cancer treatment
	1. Radiation therapy
	2. Chemotherapy

Source: Adapted from Ref. 18..

involvement of the neural arch also occurs but much less frequently (10).

Metastatic epidural tumors damage the spinal cord and nerve roots by direct compression (with demyelination and axonal damage) and by secondary vascular compromise with resultant ischemia, edema, and infarction (16,17). The edema of neurologic struc-

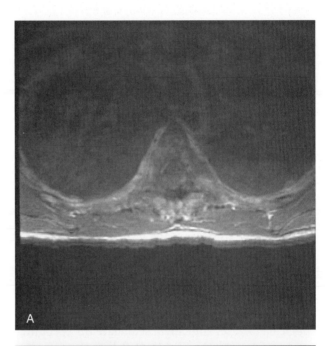

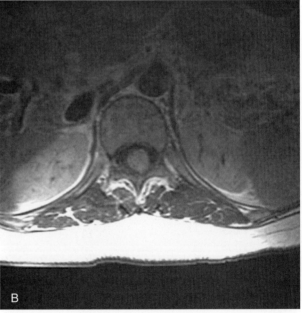

FIGURE 45.5 A and B

Axial T1 weighted gadolinium-enhanced MRI demonstrating (A) epidural tumor with spinal cord compression, (B) intramedullary metastasis.

FIGURE 45.4

Spinal metastases affecting spinal cord and nerve roots.

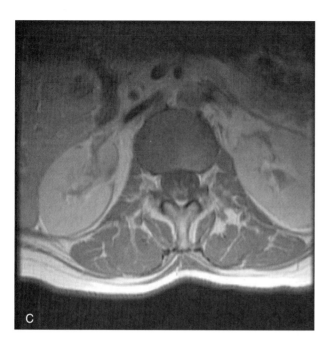

FIGURE 45.5 C

(C) leptomeningeal tumor (note the enhancement of the nerve roots within the cauda equina).

tures is thought to be a result of direct compression, venous congestion from compression of epidural venous plexus, or both. Compression of radicular arteries by tumor in the intervertebral foramen can lead to occlusion and result in infarction (18).

Intradural Metastases

Intradural metastatic disease (including leptomeningeal metastases and intradural metastases) is less common than epidural metastases, comprising less than 5% of all metastatic spinal cord tumors (6). Intradural metastases compromise spinal cord and nerve roots by compression or direct invasion. The mechanisms of metastatic invasion include tumor spread via subarachnoid space by hematogenous dissemination or from brain tumors via the cerebrospinal fluid (CSF) (19,20), by perineural growth along the nerve roots through the intervertebral foramina, or by invasion of the dura from the epidural mass.

Leptomeningeal metastases develop in about 8% of all patients with cancer (18). Any systemic cancer can spread to the leptomeninges. The most common tumors associated with leptomeningeal metastases are the hematologic malignancies (lymphoma, acute nonlymphocytic leukemia). Of the solid tumors, the most frequently seen are breast, lung, melanoma, and gastrointestinal cancers (21,22). U. Herrlinger et al. (23) in a study of 155 patients found leptomenin-

geal carcinomatosis in 61% of patients with primary brain tumors, 59% of patients with lymphoreticular tumors, 45% with primary lung malignancy, 38% with melanoma, and 27% with breast cancer. Leptomeningeal metastases are frequently accompanied by other metastatic central nervous system (CNS) tumors. They are usually a late manifestation of systemic cancer, although much less frequently may be a first finding in initial or recurrent disease. Patients can develop symptoms of leptomeningeal tumor spread many years after the initial diagnosis and treatment for primary tumor.

Malignant cells invade the meninges through different pathways, depending on histological type of the primary tumor. Hematogenous spread via the arterial circulation is more common in hematologic malignancies. Vertebral and paravertebral metastases, as well as head and neck cancers, may spread along peripheral or cranial nerves via endoneural/ perineural route or along the lymphatics or veins, then through the dural and arachnoid sleeves of nerve roots. Direct spread from CNS metastases is possible as well (18,22). Among primary neoplasms located in leptomeninges are primary lymphomas, melanomas, and rhabdomyosarcomas (18). Metastases located in the subarachnoid space can be multiple, but may also present as a single mass causing compression of neural structures.

Intramedullary metastases are much less common compared to leptomeningeal metastatic lesions. They spread either from subarachnoid space along nerve roots directly into the spinal cord or by hematogenous spread to the parenchyma of the cord. Small cell lung cancer, non-small cell lung cancer, breast cancer, melanoma, and lymphoma are the most common primary tumors, followed by gastrointestinal cancers and renal tumors (11,18). It is often difficult to differentiate intramedullary tumor spread from other intradural or epidural spinal cord compression based on clinical exam. Signs suggestive of intramedullary tumor include relatively more frequent sparing of sacral segment and early onset of autonomic dysfunction (loss of bladder control, impotence, etc). Clinically, pain may be less common compared to the compressive lesions. Rapid progression of symptoms may help distinguish intramedullary metastases from primary spinal cord tumors such as gliomas (11).

Primary Tumors of the Spine and Spinal Cord

Primary spine tumors are much less common than the metastatic tumors. Multiple myeloma, which arises from plasma cells within the bone marrow, is the tumor that most commonly affects the spine, comprising 45%. Multiple myeloma typically affects the vertebral body, sparing the posterior elements. Paraspinous and extradural extension may occur as well. Ewing sarcoma accounts for 10% of all primary bone tumors, with primary spine lesions in less than 5%. In osteogenic sarcoma, 2% of the lesions arise in the spine, mostly in lumbar segment. In 50%, they are secondary to previous irradiation or sarcomatous degeneration. Chondrosarcomas account for 10% of all malignant spine tumors, with most common sites of involvement in lumbosacral spine followed by thoracic region.

The frequency of primary spinal cord tumors is between 10%–19% of all primary CNS tumors. Although overall most spinal axis tumors are extradural, most primary spinal cord tumors are intradural. They have the potential to extend along nerve roots into extradural and extraspinal space and cause symptoms in radicular distribution.

Among primary tumors of the spinal cord, intradural extramedullary tumors comprise 60%–75%. Meningioma, a benign tumor that arises from the dura, is the most common in this group (50%), followed by neurofibromas (35%) and sarcomas (10%). Intramedullary primary spinal cord tumors comprise 20%–25% of all primary spinal neoplasms. The most common among them are astrocytomas (50%), ependymomas (30%), and hemangioblastomas (5%–10%) (24). Primary extradural spinal tumors are rare and include mostly benign tumors causing symptoms by compression of adjacent tissues.

Infection

The incidence of pyogenic infection of the spine is increasing secondary to increase in the number of patients at risk, as well as a result of advanced diagnostic methods able to identify it. The incidence of epidural abscess represents approximately 1.2 cases per 10,000 hospital admissions (25,26). Patients with known diagnosis of cancer, especially treated with chemotherapy and radiation, are among those at increased risk. Factors predisposing cancer patients to infection include impaired cellular immunity from T lymphocytes and mononuclear phagocytes dysfunction (lymphomas, cytotoxic drugs), neutropenia (leukemias, chemotherapy), impaired immunoglobulin synthesis (chronic lymphocytic leukemia [CLL], multiple myeloma [MM]). Invasive spinal procedures add to the risk of developing spinal abscess.

Purely radicular symptoms are rarely the initial presentation of spinal infection. Epidural abscess commonly presents with back pain (71%), local tenderness (17%), and limitation of movements in the related spinal segment. Fever develops in about two-thirds of the patients and is often associated with leukocytosis and elevated erythrocyte sedimentation rate (ESR) (26). Muscle weakness is present in about one-fourth of patients and sensory deficit in 13% (26). A high index of suspicion is required so that serious infection is not overlooked and treated in a timely manner. Infection in the lumbar spine accounts for the majority of cases and is more likely to be associated with radicular involvement (27).

It is believed that the most common mechanism of spinal infection is hematogenous spread from a distant source, followed in frequency by direct spread from local tissues or from trauma. The most common sites are lumbar > thoracic > cervical spine that seems to reflect the proportion of blood flow to different segments of the spine (24). Most of the time, infection begins near the anterior longitudinal ligament and subsequently extends to the vertebral body, causing its gradual destruction, also often involving the intervertebral disc. Local instability and deformity ensue. Isolated involvement of the posterior elements is rare and usually is the complication of surgery. Neurologic deficits are a result of direct extension of infection into the spinal canal or neuroforamen or compression of neural tissues as a result of spinal instability.

Many infective organisms can cause a spinal abscess. The most common organism in general is *Staphylococcus aureus*. In immunocompromised and postoperative patients Gram-negative rods are the most common pathogens identified. Less commonly, organisms of normal skin flora may be causative pathogens, especially in patients with previous spinal surgery. Mycobacterium tuberculosis and fungi are reported as causative organisms in some cases. Given overall high mortality (near 15%), early diagnosis and cause-directed treatment cannot be underemphasized. Surgical drainage of the abscess, together with antibiotic therapy, is a treatment of choice in the majority of cases.

Vascular Disorders

Epidural and subdural hematomas can potentially cause nerve root or spinal cord compression and be mistaken for compression caused by tumor. Spinal hemorrhage is almost always associated with platelet dysfunction and often follows lumbar puncture, but can also be spontaneous. In general, spontaneous bleeding occurs in patients with platelet count below 10,000/mm^3 or a rapidly dropping thrombocyte count. Symptoms of accumulating hematoma develop rapidly compared to epidural or subdural metastases. Patient experiences sudden onset of severe back pain, often accompanied by progressive sensory deficit and weakness that can lead to paraplegia. Symptoms can worsen within minutes to hours rather than days to weeks, as seen with tumor compression. MRI adds to clinical differential diagnosis. Imaging reveals an epidural mass usually extending over several spinal segments, tumor-free vertebral column, and difference in density between the hemorrhage and tumor.

The treatment is directed at prevention of hematoma by platelet transfusion in patients requiring lumbar puncture. Once bleeding occurs and patient develops weakness in lower extremities, needle aspiration or evacuation of hematoma can be considered after medical treatment fails. The decision must be made rapidly since neurologic deficits are likely to remain permanent even after the surgical treatment (18).

NONCOMPRESSIVE RADICULOPATHY

Radiation

Radiation treatment affects the peripheral nervous system by vascular endothelial damage and perivascular fibrosis within the radiation field, with resultant nerve and muscle damage. Damage to nerve structures thus occurs without extrinsic compression and is therefore noncompressive in nature. Radiation can also cause the development of nerve sheath tumors in the nerve roots, plexuses, or peripheral nerves. Radiation-induced tumors tend to occur decades after irradiation and include, among others, highly aggressive and infiltrating malignant peripheral nerve sheath tumors. Radiation treatment can also cause new tumors (sarcoma, meningioma) that may compress and potentially destroy neurologic structures.

Radicular upper extremity symptoms in a patient with history of local radiation treatment for cancer are often associated with nerve root damage as well as plexus involvement, either as a result of radiation plexopathy or a cancer recurrence. Patients with a history of mantle field radiation for Hodgkin disease and head and neck cancer commonly have both nerve root and plexus involvement (radiculoplexopathy). Radiation plexopathy may occur up to 30 years after the treatment with doses as low as 30 Gy. In brachial plexus, the upper trunk and, less commonly, the entire plexus can be affected. The relative resistance of the lower trunk to radiation is related to the protective effect of the clavicle and the pyramidal shape of the chest, as well as only a small part of the trunk being in the radiation field for some types of approaches (14). Patients typically present with progressive painless sensory deficit and weakness of arm and hand that can be associated with lymphedema in a significant percent of cases. The isolated lower trunk involvement is strongly suggestive

of metastatic plexopathy and is often associated with significant pain and Horner syndrome (14,28). The stellate ganglion—the peripheral ganglion of the cervical sympathetic chain—is located close to the C8 root. Lesions of the lower part of the brachial plexus located close to the vertebral column may thus invade sympathetic structures causing ipsilateral impaired sweating and vasomotor reaction on the face and neck (Horner syndrome) (21). This is the important clinical sign of neoplastic invasion of the lower plexus. MRI of the brachial plexus, with and without gadolinium, helps in differentiating tumor infiltration of the plexus from radiation plexopathy (29).

Electrodiagnostic testing can add to the diagnosis by better localizing the lesion and differentiating plexopathy from cervical radiculopathy or peripheral neuropathy. The initial electromyographic presentation may be solely low sensory nerve amplitude recorded in peripheral nerves originating from the involved part of the plexus; it may take months for spontaneous activity to appear (fibrillations, fasciculations, complex repetitive discharge). The presence of myokymic potentials on needle EMG favors radiation plexopathy over tumor-related plexus involvement, but does not exclude tumor.

Lumbosacral plexopathy is frequently associated with nerve root involvement (radiculoplexopathy) and often presents with painless unilateral or asymmetric bilateral lower extremity weakness. Distal muscles in the L5–S1 distribution are more frequently affected (30). The disease has the tendency to progress, causing severe disability. The absence of tumor on pelvic MRI and presence of electrodiagnostic signs of radiation plexopathy support the diagnosis.

Chemotherapy

Given that chemotherapeutic drugs are active against rapidly dividing cells, it is surprising that many of them have adverse effects on the peripheral nervous system. Potential toxic effect of antineoplastic medications should always be included in the differential diagnosis of a cancer patient with new neurologic symptoms (Table 45.3). In the majority of cases, there is no diagnostic test to separate iatrogenic causes from other etiologies.

The diagnosis of chemotherapy-related neurotoxicity is a clinical diagnosis based on temporal relationship between drug administration and clinical symptoms, knowledge of potential side effects of chemotherapeutic agents, and exclusion of other possible etiologies. The differentiation is even more important for the prognosis of functional recovery since the side effects of chemotherapy are often reversible and dose-dependent. Patients with symptomatic radicul-

TABLE 45.3
Chemotherapeutic Agents Associated With Neuropathies

DRUG	CLINICAL FEATURES	ELECTROPHYSIOLOGIC CHANGES
Vinca alkaloids (eg, vincristine)	Symmetric sensorimotor polyneuropathy; autonomic neuropathy; rarely cranial neuropathies	Axonal sensorimotor polyneuropathy; denervation in distal muscles
Cisplatin	Predominantly sensory neuropathy; sensory ataxia; Lhermitte sign	Low-amplitude or unobtainable SNAPs; motor NCS and EMG usually normal
Taxanes (eg, paclitaxel)	Symmetric predominantly sensory polyneuropathy; rare autonomic symptoms	Axonal sensorimotor polyneuropathy; denervation in distal muscles
Suramin: • Axonal neuropathy • Demyelinating neuropathy	Symmetric predominantly sensory polyneuropathy / Subacute sensorimotor neuropathy with diffuse proximal > distal weakness; areflexia; increased CSF protein	Axonal sensorimotor polyneuropathy; Acquired sensorimotor demyelinating neuropathy; EMG with decreased recruitment and denervation changes
Thalidomide	Symmetric sensorimotor polyneuropathy; autonomic neuropathy; sensory ataxia and spasticity in severe cases	Axonal sensorimotor polyneuropathy; denervation is distal muscles
Oxaliplatin	Predominantly sensory neuropathy; sensory ataxia; Lhermitte sign	Low-amplitude or unobtainable SNAPs; EMG with neuromyotonic discharges in acute cases

Abbreviations: CSF, cerebrospinal fluid; EMG, electromyography; NCS, nerve conduction studies; SNAP, synaptosomal associated protein.
Source: Form Ref. 30.

opathy as well as preexisting diabetic, alcoholic, or hereditary neuropathies are more likely to develop acute deterioration during or after treatment with neurotoxic chemotherapeutic agents (31–33).

Paraneoplastic Syndromes

Paraneoplastic syndromes are disorders of the central and peripheral nervous system that occur exclusively or in higher frequency in patients with cancer but are not caused by direct invasion of neurologic structures by primary or metastatic tumor. Small cell lung cancer is the tumor most often associated with paraneoplastic phenomena. Other tumors include breast, ovarian cancer, Hodgkin lymphoma, germ cell tumors, and thymoma (34). Incidence of most paraneoplastic diseases in patients with cancer is comparable to the general population. However, Eaton-Lambert myasthenic syndrome, subacute cerebellar degeneration, subacute sensory neuropathy, and dermatomyositis occur with significantly increased frequency in association with malignancy and require special attention in patients with known diagnosis of cancer. In the majority of cases, neurologic symptoms precede diagnosis of malignancy (18,34). In patients with known malignancy and suspected new paraneoplastic syndrome, metastatic disease and other systemic complications of cancer should be ruled out initially.

The pathogenesis of remote effects of malignancy is not known. The most accepted cause appears to be related to autoimmune mechanism mediated by T lymphocytes. The diagnosis is difficult when patients with clinical signs of paraneoplastic syndromes do not have diagnosis of cancer at presentation. The neurologic paraneoplastic syndromes can be separated by the location of anatomic structures predominantly involved (Table 45.4). Nerve root involvement is most commonly associated with subacute motor neuronopathy and Guillain-Barré syndrome.

Subacute motor neuronopathy is a process involving anterior horn cell degeneration as well as demyelination of nerve roots and spinal cord white matter. The condition is associated primarily with Hodgkin lymphoma, but can be seen in other lymphomas or thymoma. Clinical picture is characterized by the gradual onset of lower extremity weakness without significant sensory loss, pain, or upper motor neuron signs. Nerve conduction velocities recorded from the distal segments are usually normal; EMG is consistent with denervation in weak muscles. The syndrome usually develops after diagnosis of malignancy has been made and does not cause significant functional impairment. Clinically, weakness tends to improve spontaneously with the time. The cases examined at autopsy reveal patchy degeneration and loss of anterior horn cells; occasional inflammatory infiltrates; secondary thinning of ventral nerve roots; and widespread patchy

TABLE 45.4
Remote Effects of Cancer on the Nervous System

Brain
  Encephalomyelitis
  Cerebellar degeneration
  Opsoclonus-myoclonus syndrome
  Optic neuritis
  Retinal degeneration
Spinal cord
  Subacute necrotizing myelopathy
  Motor neuronopathy
Roots and peripheral nerves
  Subacute sensory neuronopathy
  Sensorimotor polyneuropathy
  Guillain-Barré syndrome
  Autonomic neuropathy
Neuromuscular junction
  Eaton-Lambert syndrome
  Myasthenia gravis (associated with thymoma)
Muscle
  Polymyositis
  Dermatomyositis
  Carcinoid myopathy
  Muscle weakness

Source: Form Ref. 16.

segmental demyelination of spinal roots, brachial, and lumbosacral plexuses (34).

Other Causes of Noncompressive Radiculopathy

Acute polyradiculoneuritis (Guillain-Barré syndrome) also occurs with higher incidence in patients with cancer, more frequently in association with Hodgkin disease and other lymphomas. Progressive ascending weakness develops with various preservation of sensation. Disease develops over a two- to four-week period and can involve respiratory muscles in 30% of patients. Electrophysiologic findings depend on the subtype of Guillain-Barré syndrome, which includes acute idiopathic demyelinating polyradiculoneuropathy (AIDP), acute motor axonal neuropathy (AMAN), and acute motor and sensory axonal neuropathy (AMSAN), as well as the Miller-Fisher variant. Electrophysiologic features of AIDP typically include slowing of nerve conduction in distal and proximal nerve segments or diffusely throughout the peripheral nerves. There is an early predilection for the proximal segments and nerve root involvement reflected in early F-wave abnormalities. Symptoms improve with steroid therapy or tumor resection, but many patients undergo spontane-

ous remission independent of the status of their underlying tumors (34).

Chronic inflammatory demyelinating polyradiculoneuropathy (CIDP) may be idiopathic or encountered in patients with lymphoproliferative disorders: lymphoma; monoclonal gammopathy of uncertain significance (MGUS); Castleman disease; and polyneuropathy, organomegaly, endocrinopathy, M-protein, skin changes (POEMS). It has been described also in association with solid tumors (small cell lung carcinoma, melanoma, gastrointestinal malignancies). The condition presents with chronic relapsing and remitting or progressive weakness and sensory loss in multiple limbs. Segmental demyelination and remyelination are the most prominent histologic findings, occasionally leading to onion-bulb formation and hypertrophic neuropathy. The process may involve spinal nerve roots, resulting in their gross enlargement and radicular symptoms overshadowing the primary distal nerve demyelination (35–37). Electrodiagnostic testing reveals prolonged distal motor latencies and F-wave latencies, slowed nerve conduction velocities, and conduction block with temporal dispersion. These changes can occur in a mononeuropathy multiplex distribution.

Rarely, systemic amyloidosis can present with localized deposition of kappa or lambda light chains (amyloidoma) in the respiratory tract, lungs, heart, skin, central, and peripheral nervous system even in the absence of any evidence of systemic disease (38–40). Other conditions that may potentially cause spinal nerve root infiltration and hypertrophy include neurofibromatosis and lymphoma. Secondary amyloidosis that occurs in various inflammatory conditions may result in serum amyloid protein A (acute phase reactant) deposition in peripheral nerves, heart, etc. When spinal roots are affected, clinical presentation is consistent with proximal and distal sensorimotor deficit localized in a root distribution with loss of muscle stretch reflexes. MRI examination demonstrating nerve roots with gadolinium enhancement would support the diagnosis (36,41). CSF examination is a crucial diagnostic tool, but often needs to be repeated a few times for tumor cells to be identified (41) in order to plan the treatment accordingly.

Sarcoidosis, a chronic granulomatous disease of unknown etiology, can affect any organ system, including the central and peripheral nervous system. In rare cases, the involvement is restricted to the nervous system only. Facial nerve palsy is the most frequent presentation. Spinal nerve roots may be affected as well, making the diagnostic process difficult since gadolinium-enhanced MRI findings and CSF examination are often nonspecific. A high index of suspicion is required for the diagnosis; root biopsy might be necessary in some cases (42,43).

Cancer patients with preexisting diabetes mellitus may be at increased risk for noncompressive radiculopathies due to vasculitic effects of diabetes on the nerve root. In addition, diabetic lumbosacral radiculoplexus neuropathy (diabetic amyotrophy) has to be considered in the differential diagnosis among other conditions. It can cause severe lowerextremity pain and weakness. Typically, symptoms develop in patients with type 2 diabetes mellitus early, when patients have relatively good glycemic control and no long-term complications of diabetic retinopathy, nephropathy, and peripheral neuropathy. Suggested pathophysiologic mechanism is immune-mediated microvasculitis of the nerves causing ischemic injury (44). Early in the disease, one segment is primarily involved. Other proximal and distal segments are eventually affected, as well as contralateral side. Electromyographic findings include decreased amplitude on sensory and compound motor action potentials, with only mild slowing of nerve conduction velocities and neuropathic changes on needle EMG. Paraspinal muscles are usually involved as well (44,45). Clinically, most of the patients improve, but recovery is often incomplete.

CLINICAL PRESENTATION

Comprehensive evaluation of patients presenting with lower back pain, neck pain, or radicular symptoms is important for establishing the diagnosis and starting the treatment early. The detailed history, physical exam, and imaging studies help to differentiate commonly seen degenerative joint arthropathy in the spine and intervertebral disc disease from rarer causes of spinal root involvement.

The most common clinical presentation of radiculopathy includes pain and sensory impairment in the distribution of the affected nerve root. It can be associated with weakness in corresponding myotome. Because of a wide overlap in dermatomal and myotomal distribution, it is unusual to see on the clinical exam severe sensory deficit and muscle paralysis rather than poorly defined sensory abnormalities and muscle weakness in the affected root distribution. Muscle stretch reflexes may be diminished or absent in the involved muscles.

CNS involvement by cancer and side effects of radiation and chemotherapy often include fatigue, headache, generalized weakness, and confusion. These clinical symptoms can coexist with radicular deficits and make clinical examination difficult unless findings are prominent.

In the case of epidural metastases, radicular pain is often preceded by local pain that is usually of subacute onset, aching in nature, and can become unbearable over time. It can be constant or have no clear association with activities and no relief with rest. Pain severity that is out of proportion to what usually is expected with mechanical lower back pain should cause concern about other causes. Local pain may be caused by tumor invasion of periosteum, paravertebral soft tissues, compression or invasion of dura, pathologic fracture of vertebrae, and by spinal cord compression itself. Worsening of pain at night or in supine position and relief with sitting or standing is suggestive of malignancy. Cancer pain may be related to the increased venous blood filling of spinal neural structures in supine position, as well as the nadir in endogenous cortisol that may increase the permeability of capillaries within the tumor and lead to increased intratumoral and intraosseous pressure. On the contrary, discogenic pain usually improves at least temporarily in supine position when the pressure on the discs decreases, but may also worsen at night as the circadian nadir of endogenous cortisol and decreased axial load allow the disk to swell.

While no clinical findings can reliably differentiate cancer pain from degenerative causes of pain, the location of the pain may be helpful. For instance, malignant epidural spinal cord involvement occurs most frequently in thoracic spine, while degenerative disease affects primarily cervical and lumbar segments. Osteoporotic compression fractures, however, are also more commonly seen in the thoracic spine. Only imaging can reliably differentiate malignant from degenerative causes of axial spinal pain and radiculopathy.

Leptomeningeal metastases can directly invade nerve roots, causing radicular symptoms that are often associated with bladder and bowel dysfunction (cauda equina is frequently involved) or signs of meningeal irritation (pain in the neck or back and nuchal rigidity). They tend to affect the CNS in multiple sites, causing neurologic symptoms simultaneously in separate anatomic areas: brain, cranial nerves, and spinal roots (18). Pain in radicular distribution is a presenting symptom in 12% of patients with leptomeningeal metastases, dermatomal sensory loss in 50%, and lower motor neuron weakness in 78% of patients at presentation (46,47).

DIAGNOSIS

Radiographic Imaging

Plain radiography has poor sensitivity in the identification of spinal tumors. Spinal metastases and primary malignant spine tumors have the tendency to invade the anterior elements, which have rich vascularity and bone marrow, while benign tumors occur more frequently in posterior elements. Plain films can identify osteolytic (lung, breast cancer, multiple myeloma) and osteoblastic lesions (prostate, breast cancer, lymphoma), but do not visualize soft tissue disease well. Approximately 30%–50% of vertebral body must be destroyed by the tumor before noticeable changes can be seen on radiographs (11,48). Spinal metastases and multiple myeloma more frequently involve multiple vertebrae, whereas primary tumors of the spine usually involve single vertebrae. Plain radiographs have some utility in differentiating the infectious process from cancerous—tumors tend to spare intervertebral discs and end plates, while infection tends to involve these structures.

Anteroposterior, lateral, and oblique views provide information about the anatomy of the spine and its integrity, and are the test of choice for evaluation of spinal instrumentation. Flexion and extension views help to diagnose dynamic spinal instability. Although the type of tumor and the location of metastases influence vertebral strength, fracture risk increases significantly when 40%–80% of vertebral body is involved. Number of vertebrae affected has a direct correlation with increased risk of fracture (49).

Magnetic Resonance Imaging

Magnetic resonance imaging (MRI) is the most sensitive and specific diagnostic test to evaluate spinal lesions caused by cancer and is the test of choice to evaluate neurologic structures of the spine and vertebral column (11,48,50,51). MRI with gadolinium contrast enhancement is the preferred imaging technique, especially when intramedullary tumors or leptomeningeal metastases are suspected and to evaluate the postoperative spine where scar is difficult to differentiate from tumor. Also, intradural tumors are often invisible on MRI without the contrast. Contrast enhancement in the basal cisterns, cauda equina, or ependyma on imaging in patients with clinical suspicion of leptomeningeal cancer involvement provides sufficient evidence for treatment even when result of lumbar puncture is nondiagnostic for malignant cells (18). Leptomeningeal tumor can also be suspected in the absence of contrast enhancement of the basal meninges in patients with radiologic signs of communicating hydrocephalus and strong clinical suspicion of cancer spread. Gadolinium enhancement also helps to distinguish extradural metastases from disc herniation, causing radicular compression (herniated discs do not enhance). The identification of nerve sheath tumors is significantly better with contrast use as well.

It should be noted that using higher doses of contrast material can lead to mild enhancement of normal-appearing spinal roots. In those cases, the level of clinical suspicion and results of other diagnostic tests should lead the physician in the diagnostic process.

Electrodiagnostic Studies

Electromyography (EMG) and nerve conduction studies (NCS) are valuable diagnostic tools in evaluating patients with suspected nerve root compression from either benign or malignant processes. The majority of compressive radiculopathies can be diagnosed by imaging studies. With advancing age, degenerative changes of the spine become increasingly common, and often can be incidental and unrelated to the patient's clinical symptoms. Electrodiagnostic examination helps to identify a functional involvement of neurologic structures and determine clinical relevance of anatomic findings. In true compressive root lesions, only EMG can help determine the severity of axonal loss and may provide some prognostic information regarding recovery of strength.

Noncompressive radicular involvement, especially if it is caused by leptomeningeal metastases, may be missed when MRI or myelography are normal. Since cancerous lesions initially occur on a microscopic level, there is no evidence of mass on imaging studies. CSF cytology, the gold standard test for leptomeningeal cancer involvement, is only 80%–90% sensitive even with repeated spinal fluid analysis (47,52). Similarly, other causes of noncompressive radiculopathy may be missed on imaging and CSF examination. Unless the physician's level of suspicion is high, nerve root involvement may be missed initially, at least until neurophysiologic testing demonstrates the presence of radiculopathy. It may potentially delay necessary treatment, influence morbidity, and affect the outcome. The electrodiagnostic study in these cases can delineate the type and extent of radicular involvement if motor axonal loss is occurring. In a study by J. Kaplan et al. (53), the diagnosis of leptomeningeal metastases was not suspected in 3 of 10 patients with a previous diagnosis of cancer. Myelography was performed in five patients and was normal in three of them, even when EMG studies demonstrated multilevel involvement. In no case did it add to the anatomic localization afforded by electrodiagnostic testing (Table 45.5).

In addition, electrodiagnostic testing can facilitate differentiating radiculopathies from plexopathies and peripheral nerve lesions, the clinical presentation of which can often be indistinguishable from radicular involvement (Table 45.6).

Motor nerve roots are formed by axons of primary motor neurons located in ventral gray matter of the spinal cord. They extend distally as a part of the spinal nerve to become the motor fibers in peripheral nerves. Sensory nerve roots are formed by centrally extending axons of neurons located in dorsal root ganglia (DRG) near the intervertebral foramina outside the spinal cord (Fig. 45.6). The sensory roots

TABLE 45.5
Comparison of Clinical, Electrophysiological, and Myelographic Findings

Tumor Type	Age	Late Responses		EMG Fibrillations		Nerve Conduction Studies		Clinical Abnormalities	Myelography
		Leg	Arm	Leg	Arm	Leg	Arm		
Breast									
1	54	AB	NL	L4-S2 innervated muscles	C6, 7	AB	NL	Back and leg pain; leg weakness, and numbness; vincristine five years earlier	NL
2	57	AB	AB	L4-S2	C6, 7	AB	NL	Arm pain and weakness; leg pain, weakness, and numbness	Intradural seeding
3	54	NL	NR	L5-S2	NR	NL	NR	Back pain; leg pain, weakness, and numbness	NL
Lung									
4	67	NR	NR	L2–4	NL	NR	NR	Arm weakness, numbness, and pain; back pain	NR
5	57	AB	NR	L4-S2	C5-T1	AB	NR	Distal leg weakness, pain	NR
Lymphoma									
6	47	AB	AB	NR	C5-T1	AB	NL	Back, leg and arm pain; arm and leg weakness; facial weakness; prior vincristine	
7	70	AB	NR	L2-S1	C6-T1	NL	NR	Leg weakness and numbness	NL
8	40	AB	NL	L4-S1	C6-T1	AB	NL	Back pain with leg pain, weakness, and numbness	Intradural seeding
Leukemia									
9	16	NL	NL	L2-S2	C7-T1	NL	NL	Leg weakness and sensory loss	NR
10	62	AB	NL	L2-S2	C5-T1	AB	NL	Leg and arm weakness and sensory loss	NR-MRI of spine with surface coils normal

Abbreviations: AB, abnormal; NL, normal; NR, not recorded.
Source: From Ref. 54.
Appendicular and paraspinal muscles sampled; denervation refers to the presence of fibrillations and/or positive sharp waves.

enter the spinal cord dorsally, and their axons either ascend in the posterior columns or synapse with sensory neurons located in the dorsal horn. The other axons originating from DRG extend peripherally as a part of mixed spinal nerves to form sensory fibers of peripheral nerves. Each spinal nerve divides into ventral and dorsal rami that contain sensory and motor fibers. The dorsal ramus innervates skin and paraspinal muscles at that segment. The ventral rami in cervical and lumbosacral regions form plexuses that provide sensory and motor innervation to the extremities (Fig. 45.7). In the thoracic region, ventral rami continue as intercostal nerves to provide sensory and motor innervation to the trunk. The anatomic differences in location of primary motor and sensory neurons result in a different pattern of motor and sensory nerve abnormalities on electrodiagnostic examination, depending on the location of the lesion—in the peripheral nerve or proximal to the DRG at the root level.

The American Association of Electrodiagnostic Medicine guidelines recommend that for optimal electrodiagnostic evaluation of patients with suspected radiculopathy, a needle EMG screen of a sufficient

TABLE 45.6

Typical Patterns of Electrodiagnostic Findings in Patients With Different Neurologic Manifestations of Malignancy

	SNAP	CMAP	EMG PARASPINAL MUSCLES	EMG LIMB MUSCLES
Radiculopathy	Normal	Normal	Fibrillations often seen	Fibrillations and/or neuropathic changes in the muscles innervated by involved spinal roots
Plexopathy	Reduced amplitudes or absent responses	Reduced amplitudes if large extent of plexus involved	Normal	Fibrillations and/or neuropathic changes in muscles innervated by involved part of the plexus
Peripheral neuropathy	Reduced amplitude or absent responses; slowed conduction velocities	Low amplitudes, temporal dispersion; slowed conduction velocities	Fibrillations can be seen in generalized polyneuropathy	Fibrillations and neuropathic changes in an axonal type polyneuropathy; normal in demyelinating neuropathy

Abbreviations: CMAP, ; EMG, electromyography; SNAP, synaptosomal associated protein.

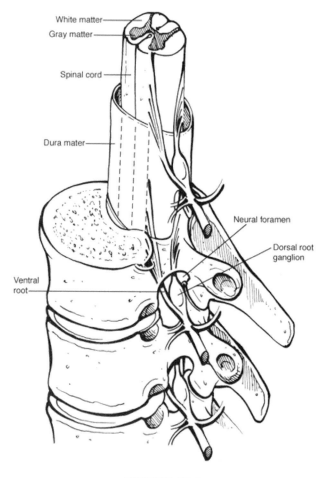

White matter
Gray matter
Spinal cord
Dura mater
Neural foramen
Dorsal root ganglion
Ventral root

FIGURE 45.6

Anatomy of spinal cord and nerve roots.

number of muscles and at least one motor and one sensory NCS should be performed in the affected limb (54). More extensive conduction studies are often needed in the cancer setting to exclude competing disorders, such as plexopathy and nonsymmetrical mononeuropathy multiplex-type neuropathies.

Nerve conduction studies are usually normal in patients with radiculopathies. They need to be performed in patients with suspected radicular lesions to exclude plexopathy or peripheral neuropathy. The synaptosomal associated protein (SNAP) is normal in lesions located proximally to DRG (nerve roots) even when there is a sensory loss on the clinical exam. On the contrary, lesions located distally to DRG (plexus, peripheral nerves) may present with decreased amplitude (axonal loss) or prolonged conduction velocity (demyelinating lesions) (see Table 45.6).

CMAP can be abnormal only if recorded from the muscles innervated by involved nerve root. Proximal axonal loss (root, plexus) may result in decreased CMAP amplitude and mild slowing of conduction velocity and distal latency. In the case of proximal demyelination (root, plexus), the axon itself remains intact, presenting with normal latency, conduction velocity, and CMAP amplitude if stimulated and recorded distally to the lesion. In this case, the abnormal F response would point to a demyelinating process at the corresponding root or plexus level.

Needle EMG is the most important and useful method of evaluating radiculopathies. It should include sampling of proximal, distal, and paraspinal muscles. Muscles innervated by the same nerve root but by dif-

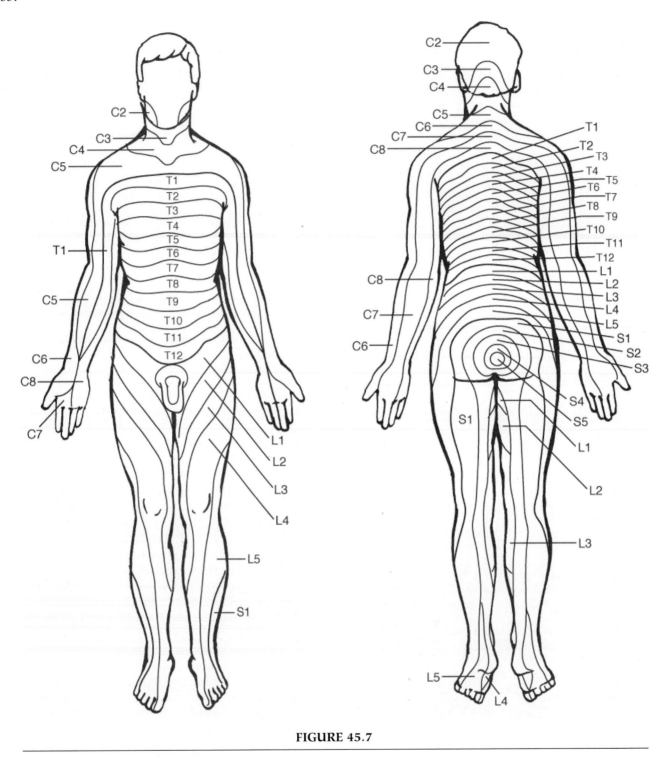

FIGURE 45.7

Cervical (C), thoracic (T), and lumbosacral (S) dermatomes.

ferent peripheral nerves need to be examined to rule out a mononeuropathy. Evaluation of proximal and distal muscles supplied by the same roots helps to distinguish radiculopathy from peripheral neuropathy. The importance of examining the paraspinal muscles cannot be underestimated. The presence of neuropathic changes in paraspinal muscles strongly indicates a lesion at that root level. On the other hand, EMG findings in paraspinal muscles can be abnormal in multiple conditions, so the full constellation of EMG findings must be taken into account to fully delineate a radiculopathy from plexopathy or polyneuropathy.

For evaluation of cervical and lumbosacral radiculopathy, the optimal number of muscles needs to be examined that represent all root level innervation and ideally include paraspinal muscles. Such an approach significantly increases the sensitivity of the examination and minimizes the patient's discomfort (55). An EMG study is considered diagnostic for a radiculopathy if EMG abnormalities are found in two or more muscles innervated by the same nerve root and different peripheral nerves, and muscles innervated by adjacent nerve roots are normal (56).

SUMMARY

Radiculopathy is an important cause of back pain in patients with a history of cancer. Most commonly, it is related to degenerative spine disease with incidence similar to the general population. Detailed history and physical exam is crucial to plan further workup. A high level of suspicion is necessary to promptly identify malignancy as a cause of radiculopathy in order to start treatment in a timely manner. Imaging is the diagnostic tool of choice to visualize the pathological process causing radicular symptoms, with electrodiagnostic testing being complementary to the imaging. Electrodiagnostics can localize the radicular lesion in cases when imaging is nondiagnostic and can identify a diffuse polyneuropathy. Timely establishment of a diagnosis of cancer as a cause of radiculopathy is critical since it determines further treatment and influences patients' quality of life.

REFERENCES

1. O'Connor MI, Currier BL. Metastatic disease of the spine. *Orthopedics.* 1992;15:611–620.
2. Radhakrishnan K, Litchy WJ, O'Fallon WM, Kurland LT. Epidemiology of cervical radiculopathy. A population-based study from Rochester, Minnesota, 1976 through 1990. *Brain.* 1994;117(Pt 2):325–335.
3. Falicov A, Fisher CG, Sparkes J, Boyd MC, Wing PC, Dvorak MF. Impact of surgical intervention on quality of life in patients with spinal metastases. *Spine.* 2006;31:2849–2856.
4. Gilbert RW, Kim JH, Posner JB. Epidural spinal cord compression from metastatic tumor: Diagnosis and treatment. *Ann Neurol.* 1978;3:40–51.
5. Katagiri H, Takahashi M, Wakai K, Sugiura H, Kataoka T, Nakanishi K. Prognostic factors and a scoring system for patients with skeletal metastasis. *J Bone Joint Surg Br.* 2005;87:698–703.
6. Schick U, Marquardt G, Lorenz R. Intradural and extradural spinal metastases. *Neurosurg Rev.* 2001;24:1–5; discussion 6–7.
7. Wang JC, Boland P, Mitra N, et al. Single-stage posterolateral transpedicular approach for resection of epidural metastatic spine tumors involving the vertebral body with circumferential reconstruction: results in 140 patients. Invited submission from the joint section meeting on disorders of the spine and peripheral nerves, March 2004. *J Neurosurg Spine.* 2004;1:287–298.
8. Bach F, Larsen BH, Rohde K, et al. Metastatic spinal cord compression. Occurrence, symptoms, clinical presentations and prognosis in 398 patients with spinal cord compression. *Acta Neurochir (Wien).* 1990;107:37–43.
9. Kim RY. Extradural spinal cord compression from metastatic tumor. *Ala Med.* 1990;60:10–15.
10. DeVita V, Hellman S, Rosenberg SA. *Cancer: Principles and Practice of Oncology.* 6th ed. Philadelphia, PA: Lippincott Williams & Wilkins; 2001.
11. Mut M, Schiff D, Shaffrey ME. Metastasis to nervous system: spinal epidural and intramedullary metastases. *J Neurooncol.* 2005;75:43–56.
12. Schiff D, O'Neill BP, Wang CH, O'Fallon JR. Neuroimaging and treatment implications of patients with multiple epidural spinal metastases. *Cancer.* 1998;83:1593–1601.
13. Clouston PD, DeAngelis LM, Posner JB. The spectrum of neurological disease in patients with systemic cancer. *Ann Neurol.* 1992;31:268–273.
14. Kori SH, Foley KM, Posner JB. Brachial plexus lesions in patients with cancer: 100 cases. *Neurology.* 1981;31:45–50.
15. Roodman GD. Mechanisms of bone metastasis. *N Engl J Med.* 2004;350:1655–1664.
16. Patchell RA, Posner JB. Neurologic complications of systemic cancer. *Neurol Clin.* 1985;3:729–750.
17. Schiff D. Spinal cord compression. *Neurol Clin.* 2003;21:67–86, viii.
18. Posner JB. *Neurologic Complications of Cancer.* Philadelphia, PA: F. A. Davis; 1995.
19. Mirimanoff RO, Choi NC. Intradural spinal metastases in patients with posterior fossa brain metastases from various primary cancers. *Oncology.* 1987;44:232–236.
20. Mirimanoff RO, Choi NC. The risk of intradural spinal metastases in patients with brain metastases from bronchogenic carcinomas. *Int J Radiat Oncol Biol Phys.* 1986;12:2131–2136.
21. Chad DA, Recht LD. Neuromuscular complications of systemic cancer. *Neurol Clin.* 1991;9:901–918.
22. Taillibert S, Laigle-Donadey F, Chodkiewicz C, Sanson M, Hoang-Xuan K, Delattre JY. Leptomeningeal metastases from solid malignancy: a review. *J Neurooncol.* 2005;75:85–99.
23. Herrlinger U, Forschler H, Kuker W, Meyermann R, Bamberg M, Dichgans J, Weller M. Leptomeningeal metastasis: survival and prognostic factors in 155 patients. *J Neurol Sci.* 2004 Aug 30;223(2):167–178.
24. Shelerud RA, Paynter KS. Rarer causes of radiculopathy: spinal tumors, infections, and other unusual causes. *Phys Med Rehabil Clin N Am.* 2002;13:645–696.
25. Johnston RA. Intraspine infection. In: Findlay G, Owen R, eds. *Surgery of the Spine.* St. Louis, MO: CV Mosby; 1997:621–627.
26. Reihsaus E, Waldbaur H, Seeling W. Spinal epidural abscess: a meta-analysis of 915 patients. *Neurosurg Rev.* 2000 Dec;23(4):175–204.
27. Shanahan MD, Ackroyd CE. Pyogenic infection of the sacro-iliac joint. A report of 11 cases. *J Bone Joint Surg Br.* 1985;67:605–608.
28. Jaeckle KA. Neurological manifestations of neoplastic and radiation-induced plexopathies. *Semin Neurol.* 2004;24:385–393.
29. Hoeller U, Bonacker M, Bajrovic A, Alberti W, Adam G. Radiation-induced plexopathy and fibrosis. Is magnetic resonance imaging the adequate diagnostic tool? *Strahlenther Onkol.* 2004;180:650–654.
30. Falah M, Schiff D, Burns TM. Neuromuscular complications of cancer diagnosis and treatment. *J Support Oncol.* 2005;3:271–282.
31. Hildebrandt G, Holler E, Woenkhaus M, et al. Acute deterioration of charcot-marie-tooth disease IA (CMT IA) following 2 mg of vincristine chemotherapy. *Ann Oncol.* 2000;11:743–747.
32. O'Connor OA, Wright J, Moskowitz C, et al. Phase II clinical experience with the novel proteasome inhibitor bortezomib in patients with indolent non-Hodgkin's lymphoma and mantle cell lymphoma. *J Clin Oncol.* 2005;23:676–684.

33. Stubblefield MD, Custodio CM. Upper-extremity pain disorders in breast cancer. *Arch Phys Med Rehabil.* 2006;87:S96–99; quiz S100–S101.

34. Dropcho EJ. Remote neurologic manifestations of cancer. *Neurol Clin.* 2002;20:85–122, vi.

35. Goldstein JM, Parks BJ, Mayer PL, Kim JH, Sze G, Miller RG. Nerve root hypertrophy as the cause of lumbar stenosis in chronic inflammatory demyelinating polyradiculoneuropathy. *Muscle Nerve.* 1996;19:892–896.

36. Pytel P, Rezania K, Soliven B, Frank J, Wollmann R. Chronic inflammatory demyelinating polyradiculoneuropathy (CIDP) with hypertrophic spinal radiculopathy mimicking neurofibromatosis. *Acta Neuropathol.* 2003;105:185–188.

37. Schady W, Goulding PJ, Lecky BR, King RH, Smith CM. Massive nerve root enlargement in chronic inflammatory demyelinating polyneuropathy. *J Neurol Neurosurg Psychiatry.* 1996;61:636–640.

38. Krishnan J, Chu WS, Elrod JP, Frizzera G. Tumoral presentation of amyloidosis (amyloidomas) in soft tissues. A report of 14 cases. *Am J Clin Pathol.* 1993;100:135–144.

39. Ladha SS, Dyck PJ, Spinner RJ, et al. Isolated amyloidosis presenting with lumbosacral radiculoplexopathy: description of two cases and pathogenic review. *J Peripher Nerv Syst.* 2006;11:346–352.

40. Laeng RH, Altermatt HJ, Scheithauer BW, Zimmermann DR. Amyloidomas of the nervous system: a monoclonal B-cell disorder with monotypic amyloid light chain lambda amyloid production. *Cancer.* 1998;82:362–374.

41. Viala K, Behin A, Maisonobe T, et al. Neuropathy in lymphoma: a relationship between the pattern of neuropathy, type of lymphoma and prognosis? *J Neurol Neurosurg Psychiatry.* 2007.

42. Burns TM, Dyck PJ, Aksamit AJ, Dyck PJ. The natural history and long-term outcome of 57 limb sarcoidosis neuropathy cases. *J Neurol Sci.* 2006;244:77–87.

43. Moore FG, Andermann F, Richardson J, Tampieri D, Giaccone R. The role of MRI and nerve root biopsy in the diagnosis of neurosarcoidosis. *Can J Neurol Sci.* 2001;28:349–353.

44. Dyck PJ, Windebank AJ. Diabetic and nondiabetic lumbosacral radiculoplexus neuropathies: New insights into pathophysiology and treatment. *Muscle Nerve.* 2002;25:477–491.

45. Dyck PJ, Norell JE, Dyck PJ. Non-diabetic lumbosacral radiculoplexus neuropathy: Natural history, outcome and comparison with the diabetic variety. *Brain.* 2001;124:1197–1207.

46. Olson ME, Chernik NL, Posner JB. Infiltration of leptomeninges by systemic cancer. A clinical and pathologic study. *Arch Neurol.* 1974;30:122–137.

47. Wasserstrom WR, Glass JP, Posner JB. Diagnosis and treatment of leptomeningeal metastases from solid tumors: Experience with 90 patients. *Cancer.* 1982;49:759–772.

48. Petren-Mallmin M. Clinical and experimental imaging of breast cancer metastases in the spine. *Acta Radiol Suppl.* 1994;391:1–23.

49. Shah AN, Pietrobon R, Richardson WJ, Myers BS. Patterns of tumor spread and risk of fracture and epidural impingement in metastatic vertebrae. *J Spinal Disord Tech.* 2003;16:83–89.

50. Burns AS, Dillingham TR. Importance of gadolinium enhancement when using MRI to evaluate spinal cord pathology. *Am J Phys Med Rehabil.* 2000;79:399–403.

51. Harrington KD. Orthopedic surgical management of skeletal complications of malignancy. *Cancer.* 1997;80:1614–1627.

52. Van Oostenbrugge RJ, Twijnstra A. Presenting features and value of diagnostic procedures in leptomeningeal metastases. *Neurology.* 1999;53:382–385.

53. American Association of Electrodiagnostic Medicine. Guidelines in electrodiagnostic medicine. *Muscle nerve.* 1999;Suppl 8:5–300.

54. Kaplan JG, Portenoy RK, Pack DR, DeSouza T. Polyradiculopathy in leptomeningeal metastasis: The role of EMG and late response studies. *J Neurooncol.* 1990;9:219–224.

55. Dillingham TR. Electrodiagnostic approach to patients with suspected radiculopathy. *Phys Med Rehabil Clin N Am.* 2002;13:567–588.

56. Wilbourn AJ, Aminoff MJ. AAEM minimonograph 32: the electrodiagnostic examination in patients with radiculopathies. American Association of Electrodiagnostic Medicine. *Muscle Nerve.* 1998;21:1612–1631.

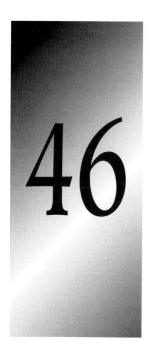

Plexopathy in Cancer

Mark A. Ferrante

The major peripheral nervous system (PNS) plexuses include the cervical, brachial, lumbar, and sacral plexuses; of these, the latter two typically are discussed as a single entity, the lumbosacral (LS) plexus. Through these structures pass nerve fibers that provide essentially all of the innervation to all four extremities, the shoulder girdle, and the pelvic girdle. Consequently, their involvement by neoplastic processes typically produces significant adverse effects on the quality of life of those affected individuals. With primary lesions, the tumor type, the plexus element involved, and the severity of that involvement dictate the impact of the lesion on the patient's quality of life. When the presenting symptoms are misdiagnosed as more benign orthopedic or neuromuscular conditions, diagnostic and therapeutic delays may contribute to a worsened outcome. Consequently, to enhance patient survival and quality of life, physicians caring for these patients require a complete understanding of plexus anatomy and the presentations associated with dysfunction of each plexus region. Integration of this information with a detailed clinical assessment dictates localization and the appropriate ancillary studies. The therapeutic options available are applied on an individual basis. Most patients with metastatic plexopathies are already known to harbor a malignancy and usually have already been treated. Consequently, most malignancies are quite advanced when the tumor involves

plexus fibers. Although many of these patients survive less than two years and typically die from systemic complications of cancer rather than neurologic ones, the role of the physician in pain relief, prevention of neuromuscular complications, and the maximization of any remaining neuromuscular function cannot be overemphasized.

CLASSIFICATION OF PERIPHERAL NERVOUS SYSTEM TUMORS

In 1969, Harkin and Reed pathologically detailed and classified the peripheral nerve tumors (PNTs) (1), and in 2000, the World Health Organization categorized them into four groups: (1) neurofibromas, (2) schwannomas, (3) perineuriomas, and (4) malignant neural sheath tumors (NSTs). NSTs were defined as any malignancy of peripheral nerve origin or with nerve sheath differentiation, excluding tumors of epineurial or vascular origin (2). Malignant NSTs are also referred to as neurogenic sarcomas. Neurofibromas are further divided into discrete and plexiform types and perineuriomas into intraneural and extraneural (ie, soft tissue perineuriomas). Plexiform neurofibromas are not neurofibromas of a PNS plexus, but are neurofibromas that involve multiple nerve fascicles. They are probable congenital lesions that may increase in size at any

KEY POINTS

- The World Health Organization categorizes peripheral nerve tumors into four groups: (1) neurofibromas, (2) schwannomas, (3) perineuriomas, and (4) malignant neural sheath tumors (NSTs).
- Peripheral nerve tumors can also be categorized based on their cell of origin and malignancy status into four categories: benign NSTs, benign non-NSTs, malignant NSTs, and malignant non-NSTs.
- Because of the segmental arrangement of the supraclavicular plexus, lesions involving the anterior primary ramus and trunk elements produce sensorimotor deficits of seemingly dermatomal and myotomal (ie, root) distributions, impeding localization.
- To lessen the demands of clinical localization and to foster communication among physicians prior to diagnostic testing, the supraclavicular plexus is divided into three parts: (1) the upper plexus (upper trunk; C5 and C6 roots), (2) the middle plexus (middle trunk; C7 root), and (3) the lower plexus (lower trunk; C8 and T1 roots).
- Schwannomas and neurofibromas are the most common benign NSTs, affecting males and females of any age or race.
- The incidence of metastatic plexopathies is unclear because plexus evaluations are not always performed when their outcome would not affect management or when patients are too ill or refuse them. The incidence also is underestimated when newly identified clinical features related to neoplastic plexus involvement are assumed to be due to an extraplexal structure or are simply dismissed as tumor progression. Consequently, the incidences reported must be underestimates.
- Although plexus fibers may be damaged in countless ways, their pathologic and pathophysiologic responses are much more limited. Wallerian degeneration follows focal axon disruption and renders the nerve fiber incapable of transmitting impulses, termed *conduction failure*. Conduction failure produces negative clinical features, such as weakness and sensory loss. With lesser degrees of insult, damage may be limited to the myelin coating. In this setting, either conduction block (termed *demyelinating conduction block*) or conduction slowing (termed *demyelinating conduction slowing*) occurs.
- The clinical manifestations associated with neoplastic plexopathies reflect the malignant status of the underlying etiology, the plexus region and nerve fiber types involved, and the severity of the lesion, as well as its rate of growth.
- Among patients with metastatic plexopathies, pain often overshadows any other clinical feature. Typically, it is severe and unrelenting, and it interferes with sleep. Neurologic deficits are frequent. Conversely, plexopathies following radiation therapy (x-ray therapy or XRT) usually are painless and frequently begin infraclavicularly, especially at the lateral cord.
- In contrast to other lung cancers, apical lung cancers are slow-growing, predominantly extrapulmonary (within the paravertebral gutter of the thoracic inlet), locally aggressive, radiosensitive lesions that infrequently metastasize.
- Neuralgic amyotrophy typically is heralded by severe shoulder pain that frequently interferes with sleep. It usually persists for 7–10 days and is followed by weakness and muscle atrophy, predominantly of proximal forequarter muscles. Often, a trigger precedes the onset of pain (eg, immunization, viral infection, unaccustomed or excessive activity).
- Although peripheral nerve fibers are relatively resistant to radiation damage, XRT may produce plexus fiber demyelination (with subsequent conversion to axon loss), impaired circulation, and fibrosis, a condition referred to as *radiation plexopathy*, which is a common component of the radiation fibrosis syndrome.
- Due to their resistance to XRT and chemotherapy and to their advanced stage at presentation, most metastatic plexopathies are incurable and treatment is palliative. Similarly, the pain associated with neoplastic plexopathies typically is severe, unrelenting, and difficult to treat. It represents one of the most formidable challenges to the physician, and it must be treated early and aggressively.
- In addition to pain, any functional loss resulting from the malignancy or its treatment may benefit from psychological counseling, physical and occupational therapy, and vocational rehabilitation. Assistive devices can maximize any remaining neurologic function, thereby enhancing quality of life. Limb edema may respond to compressive devices or elevation.
- The prognosis for patients with radiation plexopathy is poor because of inexorable progression, intraplexal expansion, and conversion from chronic demyelination to axon loss.

time (3). A more practical approach categorizes these tumors based on two features—their cell of origin and their malignancy status—thereby generating four categories: (1) benign NSTs, (2) benign non-NSTs, (3) malignant NSTs, and (4) malignant non-NSTs. The term malignant non-NSTs is applied to all malignant tumors of extraplexal origin that invade the plexus by either direct extension or metastasis (Table 46.1). An even simpler approach categorizes neoplastic plexopathies based on their (1) origin—within the plexus (primary) or external to it (secondary)—and (2) malignant status—benign or malignant. With this technique, four categories result: benign and malignant primary neoplastic plexopathies and benign and malignant secondary neoplastic plexopathies. In addition, the hereditary or sporadic nature of neurofibromas is considered because management varies between patients with and without neurofibromatosis type 1 (NF1). With NF1, conservative management with vigilant surveillance rather than frequent surgery, especially for cosmetic reasons, is recommended because the continued development of tumors is likely (4,5).

PERTINENT PLEXUS ANATOMY

The dorsal and ventral roots of each spinal cord segment traverse the intraspinal canal, enter the intervertebral foramen, and, just beyond the dorsal root ganglion (DRG), fuse to form a mixed spinal nerve (*mixed*, because it contains both sensory and motor nerve fibers). Almost immediately upon exiting the intervertebral foramen, the mixed spinal nerve terminates by dividing into two elements—a posteriorly directed one, the posterior primary ramus (PPR), and an anteriorly directed one, the anterior primary ramus (APR). The PPR provides sensorimotor innervation to the posterior one-third of the body, whereas the APR supplies the anterior two-thirds of the body and the extremities. Distal to the APR, the internal anatomy of the various plexuses differs and, thus, is individually addressed in the following section.

The Cervical Plexus

The cervical plexus is the smallest of the PNS plexuses (Fig. 46.1). It is located in the lateral aspect of the neck, adjacent to the lower four cervical vertebral bodies, and is composed of sensory and motor nerve fibers derived from the APR of the C1–C4 mixed spinal nerves. It lies deep to the sternocleidomastoid muscle and superficial to the scalenus medius and levator scapulae muscles. Its fibers form a series of anastomotic loops from which arise important nerve branches. Its sensory fibers form the lesser occipital (predominantly C2), greater auricular (C2 and C3), transverse cutaneous (C2 and C3), and supraclavicular nerves (C3 and C4). The latter emerge posterior to the sternocleidomastoid muscle and supply sensation to the back of the head (ie, that portion posterior to the interauricular line), the neck, and the cape region. Its motor fibers innervate the upper cervical paravertebral, scalenus medius, and infrahyoid

TABLE 46.1
Classification of Plexus Tumors

PRIMARY NEURAL SHEATH TUMORS (NSTs)		SECONDARY TUMORS (NON-NSTs)	
BENIGN	MALIGNANT	BENIGN	MALIGNANT
Neurofibroma	Fibrosarcoma	Brachial cleft cyst	Apical lung cancer
Schwannoma	Neurogenic sarcoma	Desmoid	Metastatic disease:
		Ganglion	Breast
		Hamartoma	Lung
		Hemangioma	Thyroid
		Lipoma	Testicular
		Lymphangioma	Bladder
		Myoblastoma	Gastrointestinal
		Osteochondroma	Lymphoma
			Melanoma
			Sarcoma
			Head and neck

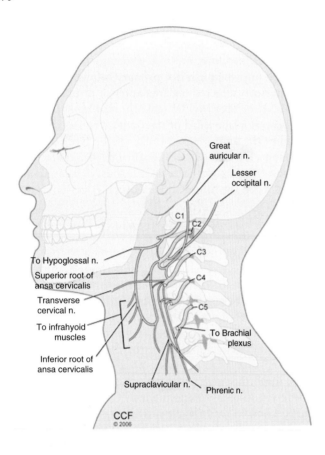

FIGURE 46.1

The cervical plexus.

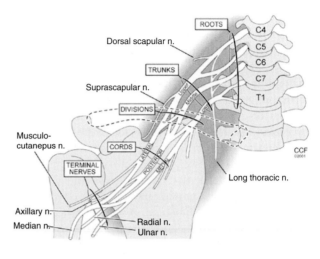

FIGURE 46.2

The brachial plexus.

muscles, as well as portions of the diaphragm, trapezius, and levator scapulae muscles. In addition, this plexus carries postganglionic sympathetic nerve fibers derived from the superior cervical ganglion (6,7).

The Brachial Plexus

The brachial plexus (BP) is the most complicated PNS structure (Fig. 46.2). Because it is the PNS plexus most often affected by malignancy, its anatomy is discussed in greater detail. This will permit the subsequent discussions of the clinical features associated with malignant invasion of its elements to be better appreciated. The BP contains several elements—five roots (C5–T1), three trunks (upper, middle, and lower), six divisions (three anterior and three posterior), three cords (lateral, medial, and posterior), and five terminal nerves (median, ulnar, radial, musculocutaneous, and axillary). Although anatomists consider the C5–T1 APR to be the most proximal elements (ie, the "roots") of the BP, clinicians specializing in BP lesions consider the roots to include, in addition to the APR, those PNS structures between the APR and the spinal cord (8).

Because of its clinical relevance, the more expansive definition of root is used in this chapter. The APR elements provide motor nerve fibers to the phrenic (C5), dorsal scapular (C5), and long thoracic (C5–C7 APR) nerves. Near the lateral edge of the anterior scalene muscle, the C5 and C6 APR fuse to form the upper trunk, the C7 APR continues as the middle trunk, and the C8 and T1 APR join to form the lower trunk. The trunk elements, which are named for their relationship to each other, are located in the anteroinferior aspect of the posterior cervical triangle. The suprascapular nerve, which exits from the proximal portion of the upper trunk, is the only nerve given off at this level. The trunks terminate by dividing into anterior and posterior divisions. The anterior divisions of the upper and middle trunks fuse to form the lateral cord, the anterior division of the lower trunk continues as the medial cord, and the three posterior divisions unite to form the posterior cord. The cords are the longest BP elements and are located in the proximal axilla. They are named for their relationship to the second portion of the axillary artery. The lateral cord gives off the lateral pectoral and musculocutaneous nerves before terminating as the lateral head of the median nerve; the posterior cord gives off the subscapular, thoracodorsal, and axillary nerves, and then continues as the radial nerve; and the medial cord gives off the medial pectoral, medial brachial cutaneous, medial antebrachial cutaneous, and ulnar nerves, before terminating as the medial head of the median nerve (7). Although the terminal nerves of the BP become the major nerves of the upper extremity, there is no anatomical landmark to identify this transition. Consequently, Wilbourn suggested that this demarcation be at the distal limit of the axilla (8).

A regional approach to plexus classification is particularly useful with neoplastic plexopathies because of the predilection of some malignancies to particular plexus regions. For example, most NSTs involve the proximal portions of the upper or middle plexuses, most apical lung tumors infiltrate the T1 APR or lower trunk, and cancer metastatic to the axillary lymph nodes usually infiltrates the medial cord or one of its neighboring nerves—the medial brachial, medial antebrachial, ulnar, and median nerves (9).

Lesion classification.

Because of its large size, it should not be surprising that different types of malignancy are associated with involvement of different BP regions. Thus, although BP lesions can be classified in a number of ways, classification by region is not only straightforward, but of clinical relevance. Because the divisions lie posterior to the clavicle (ie, they are retroclavicular), the BP is divided into supraclavicular and infraclavicular regions. Supraclavicular plexopathies are more common and, because of their frequent precipitation by severe traction, typically carry a worse prognosis, whereas infraclavicular lesions are less common, more frequently follow trauma, and tend to show better outcomes (10,11). Because of the segmental arrangement of the supraclavicular plexus, lesions involving the APR and trunk elements produce sensorimotor deficits of seemingly dermatomal and myotomal (ie, root) distributions, impeding localization. Localization by neurologic examination is further impeded by pain, mental status changes, and non-neural injuries (eg, fractures). Thus, to lessen the demands of clinical localization and to foster communication among physicians prior to diagnostic testing, the supraclavicular plexus is further divided into 3 parts: (1) the upper plexus (upper trunk; C5 and C6 roots), (2) the middle plexus (middle trunk; C7 root), and (3) the lower plexus (lower trunk; C8 and T1 roots). Upper plexopathies are more frequent and their prognosis is better than that associated with lower plexopathies because the former is more proximate to any denervated muscle fibers and the pathophysiology is more likely to have a demyelinating conduction block component (discussed below) (12). With this classification system, the infraclavicular plexus is not divided into regions, but, rather, is discussed in terms of its component cord and terminal nerve elements (Fig. 46.3).

The Lumbosacral Plexus

As previously stated, the LS plexus, which lies in the retroperitoneal space, actually consists of two smaller plexuses: the lumbar and sacral (Fig. 46.4). Although

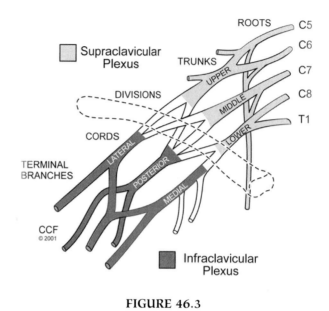

FIGURE 46.3

The supraclavicular and infraclavicular plexuses.

these structures have different origins and terminations, as well as unique anatomic relationships, typically they are discussed as a single structure. The lumbar plexus is formed from nerve fibers of the L1–L4 roots; the T12 root may also contribute. Some of the L4 APR nerve fibers merge with nerve fibers from the L5 APR and form the LS trunk. The LS trunk joins with the S1–S4 APR to form the sacral plexus. Unlike the APR of the BP, which intermingle to form trunk elements, those of the LS plexus divide into anterior and posterior divisions and fuse to form named nerves that innervate the lower torso, pelvic girdle, and lower extremity. These include the iliohypogastric (L1), ilioinguinal (L1), genitofemoral (L1–L2), obturator (anterior divisions of L2–L4), femoral (posterior divisions of L2–L4), lateral femoral cutaneous (posterior divisions of L2–L3), common peroneal (posterior divisions of L4–S2), tibial (anterior divisions of L4–S3), superior gluteal (posterior divisions of L4–S1), inferior gluteal (posterior divisions of L5–S2), pudendal (S2–S4), and posterior femoral cutaneous (posterior divisions of S1–S3) nerves, as well as motor branches to the quadratus lumborum, psoas major and minor, and iliacus muscles. The S4 APR contributes some fibers to the coccygeal plexus. Like the other PNS plexuses, the LS plexus conveys postganglionic sympathetic fibers. The lumbar plexus is situated within the posterior portion of the upper two-thirds of the psoas major muscle, anterior to the transverse processes of the lumbar vertebrae and within the psoas fascia. The iliohypogastric, ilioinguinal, and

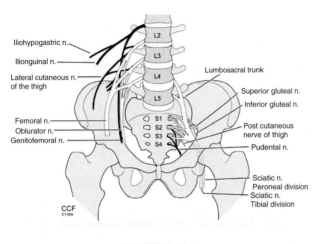

FIGURE 46.4

The lumbosacral plexus.

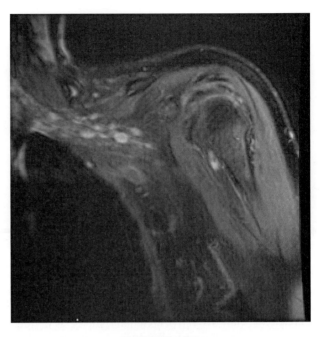

FIGURE 46.5

Coronal T2 fat saturation MRI in a patient with neurofibromatosis type I (NF1) and multiple neurofibromas along the course of the brachial plexus.

genitofemoral nerves descend along the anterior aspect of the iliopsoas muscle, posterior to the iliac fascia and the para-aortic and iliac lymph nodes. Thus, neoplastic involvement of these nodes places those nerves at risk (discussed in the following section). The sacral plexus lies within the bony pelvis on the anterior surface of the piriformis muscle, adjacent to the rectum, colon, and ipsilateral ureter. Thus, neoplastic involvement of these structures may affect the sacral plexus. The lumbar and sacral plexuses receive their blood supplies from lumbar arteries derived from the abdominal aorta and the internal iliac artery, respectively (7,13). Useful vascular landmarks for sacral plexus localization include the common iliac (anteromedial to the LS trunk), superior gluteal (passes between the LS trunk and the S1 APR or between the S1–S2 APR), and inferior gluteal (passes between the S1–S2 or the S2–S3 APR) vessels (14).

EPIDEMIOLOGY AND RISK FACTORS

Although cancer is the third leading cause of death, neoplastic plexopathies are uncommon. Moreover, neoplastic plexus involvement is not equally distributed. Among the major PNS plexus, malignancy most commonly involves the BP, least commonly the cervical plexus, and intermediately the LS plexus (15). Although most neoplastic plexopathies involve the BP, LS plexopathies are most likely to be neoplastic in origin, and neoplastic processes are a major cause of cervical plexopathies. In most series, benign lesions outnumber malignant ones and NSTs predominate over non-NSTs (16–18). Most primary BP tumors derive from the nerve sheath. Schwannomas and neurofibromas (Fig. 46.5) are the most common benign NSTs,

affecting males and females of any age or race (19). Schwannomas have a peak incidence in the fourth and fifth decades and are more frequent among women (11,17,18). However, when they involve the BP, their sex distribution is more uniform (17,18,20). Within the BP, schwannomas more commonly involve the upper plexus. Neurofibromas show a predilection for the PNS plexuses (21,22). Among non-NF1 patients, neurofibromas typically are sporadic, solitary lesions (much less frequently, they are localized to a single region of the body, termed segmental neurofibromatosis) that occur more frequently on the right side of the body, involve the supraclavicular plexus nearly twice as often as the infraclavicular plexus (usually the upper or middle plexus), show a female predominance, and have a low risk of malignant degeneration (11,16–18). Among NF1 patients, the incidence of neurofibromas is higher because defective neurofibromin predisposes to neurofibroma formation. Among NF1 patients, neurofibromas are larger and multiple, do not demonstrate gender or laterality bias, involve the BP more diffusely, have a much higher rate of malignant degeneration (15%), are more frequently plexiform (virtually pathognomonic for NF1), and tend to present at younger ages (11,16). In one series, the mean age at presentation for NF1 patients was nearly two decades earlier (25.1 years vs 41.7 years) (17). Up to 44% of NF1 patients develop plexiform neurofibromas, 5% of which undergo malignant transformation.

Malignant NSTs originate from Schwann cells or pluripotent neural crest cells and are quite rare, with an incidence of 1 per 100,000 in the general population (23). They do not show a gender bias or a laterality bias (21). About 50% of these tumors occur among NF1 patients, making NF1 the greatest risk factor for their development. Overall, NF1 patients have a cumulative lifetime risk of a malignant PNT of 4%–10% and suffer a life expectancy reduction of 10–15 years (23–27). Like neurofibromas, these tumors present in NF1 patients about one to two decades earlier than in non-NF1 patients (28). Irradiation, the second greatest risk factor, accounts for about 10% of cases (Fig. 46.6), and there may be a latency period ranging from 4 to 41 years (average, 15 years) (29,30). NF2 and schwannomatosis are other risk factors for primary neoplastic plexopathies (5).

The incidence of metastatic plexopathies is unclear because plexus evaluations are not always performed when their outcome would not affect management or when patients are too ill or refuse them. The incidence also is underestimated when newly identified clinical features related to neoplastic plexus involvement are assumed to be due to an extraplexal structure or are simply dismissed as tumor progression. Consequently, the incidences reported must be underestimates.

Regarding etiology, breast carcinoma is the most common metastatic lesion to involve peripheral nerve fibers, most commonly the BP via lymph node involvement (Fig. 46.7). Consequently, most neoplastic BP lesions affect middle-aged to elderly females. Apical lung cancer, through direct invasion, is the most common nonmetastatic malignancy to involve the BP, while squamous cell carcinoma of the cervix, via lymph node involvement, is the most common malignancy to involve the LS plexus (18,21).

PATHOGENESIS AND PATHOPHYSIOLOGY

Primary neoplastic plexopathies, of which NSTs (eg, schwannomas, neurofibromas) are most common, result from the uncontrolled growth of plexus fiber constituents, whereas secondary malignancies reflect plexus fiber invasion from an extraplexal source. Schwannomas arise from Schwann cells, especially at the myelination transition zone (ie, where Schwann cells and oligodendrocytes abut along the spinal nerve roots). They usually are benign, solitary paraneural lesions that grow slowly (1,19). As they grow, nerve fiber compression may occur. On rare occasions, they are multiple, undergo malignant transformation, or occur in NF1 patients (19). Solitary neurofibromas

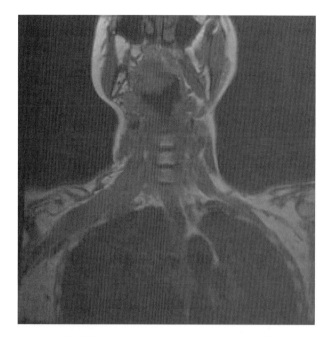

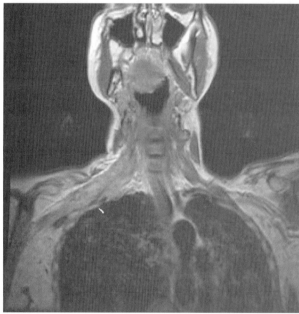

FIGURE 46.6

Coronal T1 (*top*) and T1 postgadolinium (*bottom*) MRI in a patient with a malignant peripheral nerve tumor (PNT) of the right brachial plexus resulting from remote treatment of Hodgkin disease with mantle field radiation therapy.

are intraneural rather than paraneural and frequently involve the entire cross-section of the nerve. They probably arise from perineural fibroblasts (17,18,21,31,). Neurofibromin, the protein product of the mutated gene in NF1 patients, has a role in tumor suppression. Its dysfunction permits overactivity of p21 *ras*, a promoter of cell growth and differentiation, to occur,

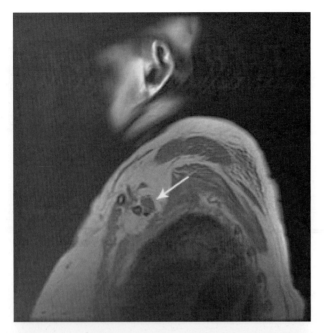

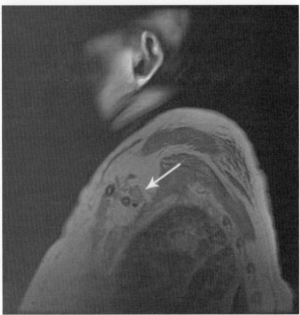

FIGURE 46.7

Sagittal T1 (*top*) and T1 postgadolinium (*bottom*) MRI of the brachial plexus in a patient with metastatic breast cancer and plexus involvement. Note the enhancing nodularity within the neurovascular bundle.

thereby increasing the incidence of tumors, mostly neurofibromas, in this group (32,33). Plexiform neurofibromas lack a capsule and, thus, are able to grow along tissue planes (ie, they are locally infiltrative). They can become quite large and in that setting, frequently damage the nerves from which they arise. Most malignant NSTs arise de novo or through the malignant transfor-

mation of a plexiform neurofibroma. Less commonly, these lesions arise from a solitary neurofibroma or ganglioneuroma. They rarely arise from a schwannoma (1). Most malignant NSTs lack p27 expression (an inhibitor of G1 phase to S phase) (34). Since nerve fibers do not contain obvious lymphatic ducts, dissemination of malignant NSTs occurs via direct extension or bloodborne metastasis (18,35).

Secondary neoplastic plexopathies follow plexus invasion from an extraplexal source, such as an adjacent primary (eg, apical lung cancer invading the lower plexus) or a metastatic lesion (eg, metastatic lung cancer invading the lower plexus). Neoplastic plexopathies also frequently follow invasion via adjacent lymph node metastases (eg, breast or cervical cancer). In addition, plexus fibers may be involved via hematogenous (eg, hematologic malignancies), cerebrospinal fluid (CSF; hematologic malignancies and solid tissue tumors, especially breast and lung cancer and melanoma), or lymphatic dissemination. Rarely, plexus fibers via a paraneoplastic phenomenon or by intraneural metastases or direct perineural spread (36). Neoplastic processes may also affect plexus fibers indirectly, such as by compressive forces (eg, an adjacent uterine leiomyoma or lymph node metastases), infection (eg, thoracic outlet infection related to immunosuppression), or ischemia (eg, leukemic infiltration) (37–42).

Although plexus fibers may be damaged in countless ways, their pathologic and pathophysiologic responses are much more limited. Wallerian degeneration follows focal axon disruption and renders the nerve fiber incapable of transmitting impulses, termed *conduction failure*. Conduction failure produces negative clinical features, such as weakness and sensory loss. With lesser degrees of insult, damage may be limited to the myelin coating. In this setting, either conduction block (termed *demyelinating conduction block*) or conduction slowing (termed *demyelinating conduction slowing*) occurs. Among neoplastic plexopathies, conduction failure related to axon disruption is, by far, the most common. Demyelination may predominate over axon loss in the setting of abrupt onset lesions, but isolated demyelination is unexpected.

CLINICAL FEATURES

The clinical manifestations associated with neoplastic plexopathies reflect the malignant status of the underlying etiology, the plexus region and nerve fiber types involved, and the severity of the lesion, as well as its rate of growth. The individual features associated with palpable masses reflect their underlying etiology. Due to their slow growth rate, benign NSTs usually present as painless, palpable masses overlying the course of a nerve, often with associated paresthesias that may be exacerbated or precipitated by motion or percussion (ie, Tinel sign). Their mobility may be limited longitudinally, but typically not laterally (16,43). Neurologic deficits are more frequent with neurofibromas than schwannomas (especially among NF1 patients), a reflection of their intraneural location as opposed to the paraneural location of schwannomas (1,18,43–45). NF1 patients may show café-au-lait spots, axillary or inguinal freckling, or Lisch nodules (iris hamartomas). Bony dysplasia, optic gliomas, and multiple or plexiform neurofibromas are other features of NF1. Plexiform neurofibromas may produce overlying soft tissue hypertrophy or skin hyperpigmentation. Unlike patients with benign NSTs, patients with malignant NSTs more typically present with painful, rapidly growing masses and progressive neurologic deficits. Rarely, metastatic involvement at presentation is noted (11).

Among patients with metastatic plexopathies, pain often overshadows any other clinical feature. Typically, it is severe and unrelenting and it interferes with sleep. Neurologic deficits are frequent (44). General examination may disclose lymphadenopathy. With the possible exceptions of head and neck cancer, neurotropic skin cancer, and lymphoma, most patients with metastatic plexopathies have already been treated for a known malignancy and have widely metastatic disease. In one series, however, approximately 35% (17 of 55) of patients with metastatic plexopathies presented without a history of underlying malignancy (46). The clinical features specific to each PNS plexus are discussed in the following sections.

The Cervical Plexus

When neoplastic plexopathies involve the cervical plexus, pain, often radiating to the neck, shoulder, or throat, is the primary symptom (47). It can occur in the distribution of any of the cervical plexus elements and may worsen with neck movement or swallowing. Sensory and motor disturbances are frequent, although the latter may go unrecognized when the affected muscles have multiple innervation (eg, trapezius, sternocleidomastoid), are difficult to assess (hyoid or deep cervical muscles), or are asymptomatic (eg, hemidiaphragmatic paralysis) (6,47–49). When these lesions extend into the intraspinal canal, epidural spinal cord compression may result in respiratory paralysis and sympathetic trunk involvement may produce Horner syndrome (ptosis, pupillary miosis, and facial anhidrosis).

The Brachial Plexus

As with other metastatic plexopathies, most of those involving the BP present with pain, usually involving the shoulder and axilla and radiating along the medial aspects of the arm, forearm, and hand (50). Malignant spread produces progressive neurologic deficits, the distribution of which reflects the plexus region affected. With upper plexus involvement, weakness occurs in muscles of the C5 and C6 myotomes (eg, serratus anterior, levator scapulae, rhomboids, spinati, deltoid, biceps, brachialis, brachioradialis, pronator teres, and flexor carpi radialis). If severe, the upper extremity may assume the "waiter's tip" position (ie, adduction and internal rotation of the shoulder, extension and pronation of the arm and forearm, and posterolateral rotation of the palm). Sensory disturbances occur along the lateral aspects of the arm, forearm, and hand, and the biceps and brachioradialis reflexes may be affected. With middle plexus involvement, weakness involves muscles of the C7 myotome (eg, triceps, anconeus, extensor carpi radialis, pronator teres, and flexor carpi radialis), sensory abnormalities involve the posterolateral aspect of the arm, the dorsal aspect of the forearm, and the lateral aspect of the hand, and the triceps muscle stretch reflex may be diminished. With lower plexus involvement, weakness involves muscles of the C8 and T1 myotomes; sensory disturbances occur along the medial aspects of the arm, forearm, and hand; and the finger flexor reflex may be diminished. Involvement of the T1 APR may produce ipsilateral Horner syndrome. (This also occurs with involvement of the paravertebral sympathetic trunk and indicates epidural tumor spread.) With lateral cord lesions, weakness occurs in the muscle domains of the musculocutaneous nerve (eg, biceps, brachialis) and the lateral head of the median nerve (eg, pronator teres, flexor carpi radialis), sensory disturbances lie in the distributions of the lateral antebrachial cutaneous nerve and the lateral head of the median nerve, and the biceps muscle stretch reflex may be involved. With posterior cord involvement, weakness occurs in the muscle domains of the subscapular, thoracodorsal, axillary, and radial nerves; sensory disturbances lie in the distributions of the upper and lower lateral brachial cutaneous, posterior brachial and antebrachial cutaneous, and superficial radial nerves; and the triceps muscle stretch reflex may be diminished. With medial cord lesions, weakness involves the muscle domains of the ulnar nerve, the medial head of the median nerve (eg, flexor pollicis longus, abductor pollicis brevis), and the C8-radial nerve fibers (eg, extensor indicis proprius, extensor pollicis brevis). Sensory disturbances in the medial brachial, medial antebrachial, and ulnar nerve distributions may be noted. The finger flexor reflex may be diminished. With terminal nerve involvement, the sensory and motor deficits are confined to the cutaneous and muscle domains of the affected nerve. The distribution of the sensory abnormalities associated with each BP element reflects the DRG from which its sensory nerve fibers originate (51). Upper extremity swelling from lymphedema is much more common following radiation therapy (XRT) than from metastatic plexus involvement (50).

The Lumbosacral Plexus

Although less than 1% of patients with cancer have spread to the LS plexus (47,52), the majority of LS plexopathies are likely malignant in etiology (15,53). About 15% of patients with LS plexus malignancies present without known malignancy (52). Pain, the most common and typically most disabling feature, often precedes other features by weeks to months (47,52,54,55). Its location varies with the plexus region involved. With lumbar plexopathies, it usually occurs in the lower torso, buttock, hip, anterolateral thigh, and medial leg regions, and it may be elicited or exacerbated by reversed straight leg testing. With sacral plexus involvement, it more commonly occurs in the posterolateral thigh, remainder of the leg, and foot; it may be elicited or exacerbated by straight leg testing (52,56). The *malignant psoas syndrome*, which is defined as intractable thigh pain and a positive psoas muscle stretch test, occurs when patients with advanced malignancy develop extensive para-aortic lymphadenopathy and secondary psoas muscle infiltration (57). Since hip extension exacerbates the pain, these patients often maintain their hip in flexion and cannot lie supine. The region of the LS plexus involved dictates the sensory and motor abnormalities observed. Lesions of the upper lumbar plexus produce sensory disturbances in the iliohypogastric, ilioinguinal, and genitofemoral nerve distributions. More inferior lesions are associated with deficits in femoral (anteromedial thigh and medial leg sensation, hip flexor and knee extensor strength, quadriceps reflex), obturator (superomedial thigh sensation, thigh adductor strength, adductor reflex), and lateral femoral cutaneous nerve distributions. A foot drop may occur when deep peroneal nerve fibers traversing the LS trunk or upper sacral plexus are involved. More inferior sacral plexus involvement may produce weakness (thigh extensors and abductors, leg flexors, all foot movements), sensory abnormalities (posterior aspect of thigh; leg, except medial aspect; foot), or ankle reflex changes. Hyperthermia and hypohidrosis of the foot, the *hot dry foot syndrome*, occurs when postganglionic sympathetic fibers traversing the LS plexus are disrupted. This syndrome also occurs with sympathetic ganglia involvement and may also lead to hyperhidrosis (58,59). With deep pelvic tumors (eg, cervical carcinomas, rectosigmoid tumors), sensory disturbances in the perineum and perianal area may precede lower extremity pain and weakness. Sciatic notch

tenderness, abnormalities of anal sphincter tone, palpable masses (lower abdominal, vaginal, rectal), bladder enlargement, urinary incontinence, lower extremity or penile edema (inferior vena cava or lymphatic system compression), hepatosplenomegaly, thrombophlebitis, ascites, and generalized lymphadenopathy are other features of pelvic malignancy (47,54–56,60). Vertebral body destruction, lower extremity edema, and ureteral obstruction are common features of retroperitoneal lymph node metastasis (61,62). About 25% of patients with features limited to just one side actually have bilateral involvement, especially in the setting of incontinence or impotence (52).

ASSOCIATED NEOPLASTIC DISORDERS

The particular neoplastic disorders associated with each PNS plexus primarily reflect the anatomical structures surrounding them.

The Cervical Plexus

Because of its relatively small size and the protection afforded it by overlying structures, closed injuries of this plexus frequently are due to malignancy. Most neoplastic cervical plexopathies represent local extension from squamous cell carcinoma of the head and neck, lymphoma, or from systemic cancers metastatic to neighboring lymph nodes or vertebrae, especially lung, breast, and lymphoreticular carcinoma (38,47). Both neoplastic meningitis and neoplastic involvement of cervical nerve roots in the epidural space can mimic cervical neoplastic plexopathy. Moreover, iatrogenic cervical plexopathies related to XRT for breast cancer can mimic tumor recurrence in the cervical plexus, as can cervical plexus damage related to radical neck dissection (47,63).

The Brachial Plexus

Primary neoplastic brachial plexopathies are rare, with NSTs outnumbering non-NSTs (17,21). Most NSTs are benign, whereas most non-NSTs are malignant (both metastatic and nonmetastatic disease). Schwannomas and neurofibromas are the most common benign NSTs, while desmoid tumors and lipomas are the most common benign non-NSTs. Solitary schwannomas occurring at the root level more commonly involve the sensory roots and, after growing through the neural foramen and expanding at both ends, take on a dumbbell shape (1). Secondary malignancies far outnumber primary ones. Breast and lung cancer, lymphoma, and melanoma account for the majority of metastatic brachial plexopathies (50). Apical lung cancer accounts for most of the nonmetastatic malignant BP lesions (64). Other common sources include thyroid, testicular, bladder, gastrointestinal, esophageal, pancreatic, sarcoma, rhabdomyosarcoma, and head and neck cancer (Table 46.1) (17,18,44). Unlike primary neoplasms of the BP, there is no particular plexus region predisposed to metastatic involvement (50). Head and neck, breast, and apical lung cancer are exceptions to this statement. Head and neck cancer tends to infiltrate the upper plexus because it advances from above the BP; breast cancer favors the infraclavicular plexus when it metastasizes to the lateral group of axillary lymph nodes; and, since it infiltrates from below, apical lung cancer favors the lower plexus. Intraneural metastases have been reported with carcinoid and hematologic malignancies (eg, leukemia, lymphoma, neurolymphomatosis, and angioendotheliomatosis) (65–71).

Pancoast syndrome.

In contrast to other lung cancers, apical lung cancers are slow-growing, predominantly extrapulmonary (within the paravertebral gutter of the thoracic inlet), locally aggressive, radiosensitive lesions that infrequently metastasize (Fig. 46.8) (72–74). About 3% of all lung cancers are of this type. Hare first described this tumor and its propensity to invade the spine, and Tobias first identified it as a lung primary (75,76). Henry Pancoast called attention to the full constellation of associated

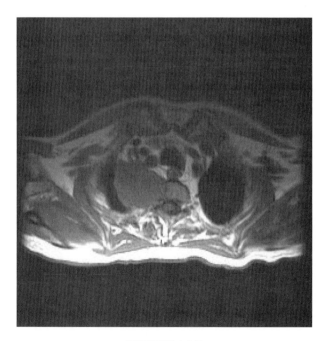

FIGURE 46.8

Axial T1 MRI demonstrating a Pancoast tumor in a patient with non-small cell lung carcinoma.

thoracic inlet abnormalities, hence the term *Pancoast syndrome* (77). The clinical features observed reflect the location of the tumor. Pleural involvement is associated with severe unrelenting shoulder pain that typically extends into the axilla and the medial aspect of the upper extremity (C8–T2), is worse at night, and interferes with sleep. Although it is initially aching or sharp, it quickly becomes dysesthetic (78). When it extends into the superior mediastinum or posterior primary rami, medial scapular pain develops (79). Since only the pleura lies between the lung tissue and the T1 APR and lower trunk elements of the BP, sensorimotor deficits have an initial T1 or lower trunk distribution. Horner syndrome follows T1 root or stellate ganglion involvement. When tumor involves the BP proximal to the C8 or T1 DRG, the clinical features can suggest a radiculopathy (64,80,81). However, the severity of the shoulder pain usually is out of proportion to typical radiculopathy pain. Supraclavicular fullness, venous distention, upper extremity edema, and bone destruction (upper thoracic ribs and, less often, the adjacent vertebral bodies) are other features of this syndrome (82,83). Although bronchogenic carcinoma is the most common cause of this disorder—a fact that accounts for the much higher incidence of this syndrome among middle-aged to elderly males with heavy smoking histories—it may occur with any disorder of the thoracic inlet (8,15,39,40,4282,84–88). Unlike most secondary neoplastic processes involving the BP, Pancoast syndrome often is the first manifestation of the malignancy. Consequently, its features must be recognized because earlier recognition leads to earlier treatment and greater survival (89).

The Lumbosacral Plexus

Neoplasms are responsible for the majority of LS plexus lesions (90). The LS plexus is involved by a variety of malignant carcinomas and lymphoreticular tumors, most commonly from the spread of local disease from the primary tumor or adjacent metastatic foci (52,56). Neoplastic involvement may be restricted to the lumbar (31%) or sacral (51%) plexus or involve both (18%) (52). Approximately 75% of secondary lesions follow direct invasion from primary malignancies (eg, abdominal, pelvic, or retroperitoneal tumors), the most common of which is colorectal carcinoma (91,92). Less commonly, metastatic spread (usually breast cancer) from adjacent lymph nodes or bone is responsible (52). Overall, lumbar plexus involvement more commonly follows direct extension from an intraabdominal source, whereas sacral plexus involvement usually is related to metastasis (52). Other common sources include gynecologic carcinoma, retroperitoneal sarcoma, lymphoma, melanoma, and myeloma, as well as lung, testicular, thyroid, renal, and bladder cancer (15,18,47,52,91). Malignant psoas syndrome frequently occurs with advanced genitourinary tract, prostate, and colorectal carcinomas, a reflection of their patterns of spread. The LS plexus may also be infiltrated by neoplastic processes involving the blood or CSF (eg, lung and breast cancer, lymphoma, melanoma). Finally, LS plexus involvement may also follow direct perineural spread (36). Benign neoplasms, mostly neurofibromas and schwannomas, infrequently involve the LS plexus (11,91,93,94) and usually are incidentally discovered when individuals with sensorimotor symptoms are referred for electrodiagnostic (EDX) testing that localizes the lesion and directs neuroimaging. Compressive forces related to benign tumors (omental dermoid cyst, uterine leiomyoma) may also disrupt LS plexus fibers (91).

DIFFERENTIAL DIAGNOSIS

The Cervical Plexus

When palpable neck masses are encountered that are associated with pain or paresthesias in a cervical plexus distribution, a primary neoplastic plexopathy must be considered. Other considerations include noncancerous cysts, nerve hamartomas, and traumatic neuromas. The presence of multiple neurofibromas is essentially pathognomonic of NF1, as are plexiform neurofibromas. Secondary neoplastic cervical plexopathies may be mimicked by neoplastic meningitis or by tumor spread to the epidural space with secondary nerve root involvement. When cervical plexopathies follow radical neck dissection for malignancy, the temporal relationship between the symptoms and the surgical procedure helps distinguish an iatrogenic process from tumor recurrence. Cervical plexopathies also may follow XRT for breast cancer (63).

The Brachial Plexus

Primary neoplastic plexopathies of the BP may be confused with secondary neoplastic and non-neoplastic plexopathies. With secondary malignancies (eg, metastatic spread or direct extension from an adjacent structure), the differential diagnosis is even more extensive. Among cancer patients with a history of XRT to the neck or shoulder region, the two most common causes of brachial plexopathy are metastatic plexopathy and radiation plexopathy (discussed next). As previously stated, metastatic plexopathies usually present with severe unrelenting pain that interferes with sleep and that more commonly involve the supra-

clavicular plexus. Conversely, plexopathies following XRT usually are painless and frequently begin infraclavicularly, especially at the lateral cord (95). As with cervical plexopathies, disorders related to the underlying cancer (eg, epidural metastases and neoplastic meningitis) can mimic neoplastic plexopathy, especially when multiple nerve roots are involved. With epidural spinal cord compression, spinal column tenderness and myelopathic signs usually are present, whereas patients with neoplastic meningitis usually have multifocal CNS involvement. Other plexopathies secondary to XRT include XRT-induced plexus tumors and XRT-induced subclavian artery occlusion with resultant plexus ischemia. Plexus involvement may also follow chemotherapy. In the postoperative setting, surgical trauma or trauma related to anesthetic administration must be considered. In the setting of severe shoulder pain, rotator cuff tears and neuralgic amyotrophy are possibilities. Neuralgic amyotrophy typically is heralded by severe shoulder pain that frequently interferes with sleep. It usually persists for 7–10 days and is followed by weakness and muscle atrophy, predominantly of proximal forequarter muscles. Often, a trigger precedes the onset of pain (eg, immunization, viral infection, unaccustomed or excessive activity) (8,30,50,96–99). Neoplastic brachial plexopathies may present with clinical features suggestive of a C8 or T1 radiculopathy or of an ulnar neuropathy. In this setting, EDX studies often identify atypical features that precipitate imaging studies and the recognition of the underlying process as neoplastic.

The Lumbosacral Plexus

LS plexopathies must be differentiated from lesions involving more proximal structures (ie, lower spinal cord, cauda equina, lumbosacral root) and more distal ones (eg, femoral and sciatic neuropathies). Careful strength assessment of the proximal lower extremity muscles is mandatory. (The tensor fascia lata and gluteal muscles are spared with sciatic neuropathies, and the iliopsoas muscle is spared with femoral neuropathies.) With known malignancy, metastatic plexopathy and other neoplastic complications (eg, epidural metastasis involving the cauda equina, neoplastic meningitis) are considered. Disc herniation is considered when severe unilateral, local, or radicular pain heralds the disorder, or when straight leg testing elicits or exacerbates the pain. Other entities associated with severe thigh pain include vasculitis and diabetic amyotrophy. Especially when the diabetic status of the patient is unknown, several of the features of diabetic amyotrophy may suggest malignancy, including progressive weight loss (often 10–30 pounds), older age, and persistent lower extremity pain interfering with sleep. In the setting of previous pelvic region irradiation (eg, for lymphoreticular, testicular, ovarian, cervical, or uterine malignancies), radiation fibrosis is another possibility. When chemotherapeutic agents are injected into the internal iliac artery to treat malignancies of the pelvic and lower extremity regions, LS plexus elements may be injured by an ischemic or, less likely, direct neurotoxic mechanism. Associated clinical features (eg, weakness, paresthesias, pain) can be immediate or delayed (up to 48 hours) and more frequently involve the sacral plexus (15,55,100). Intragluteal injections of analgesics also may damage the LS plexus. Pain usually is the first symptom, followed by sensorimotor disturbances in a sacral plexus distribution. The presumed etiology is ischemia from vasospasm or thrombosis of the blood supply to the affected sacral plexus elements (15,101). Patients with retroperitoneal hemorrhage (eg, leukemia, disseminated intravascular coagulation) frequently present with severe ipsilateral lower abdominal or groin pain radiating to the anterior thigh or medial aspect of the leg. Since hip movements aggravate their pain, the hip is held fixed, often with the thigh flexed and externally rotated. The distribution of the clinical deficits reflects the plexus elements involved. The most common presentation is of an isolated femoral neuropathy, usually with bleeding limited to the iliacus muscle or to the groove between the iliacus and psoas muscles (15). More extensive psoas muscle bleeding causes a lumbar plexopathy and, less commonly, an LS plexopathy (91,102,103). Patients with diabetic amyotrophy, similar to those with neoplastic LS plexus involvement, present with progressive weight loss and an inability to sleep due to persistent lower extremity pain. When the diabetic status of the patient is unknown, as is often the case, the diagnosis can be delayed. Other features of diabetic amyotrophy include anterior thigh pain, weakness, and atrophy in a lumbar or LS nerve root distribution and an absent or decreased patellar reflex. Like cancer, diabetic amyotrophy is more common among the elderly; it more commonly affects elderly males (sixth or seventh decade) with type 2 diabetes mellitus (104). Typically, the lower extremity pain exceeds the lower back pain. The disorder usually spreads to involve adjacent nerve roots located above, below, or contralateral to the initial site of involvement (*territorial extension*). The diagnosis may be more apparent when the thoracic nerve roots are involved (ie, diabetic thoracic radiculopathy). A disorder analogous to neuralgic amyotrophy but occurring in the lower extremity has been described and termed idiopathic LS plexopathy (105,106). Bradley and colleagues described what they believe to be a more severe variant of this disorder with persistent or recurrent pain and an elevated sedimenta-

tion rate (107). Similar to neoplastic LS plexopathies, patients with this variant typically present with severe, distally radiating buttock, groin, or thigh pain, with weakness and sensory loss following days to weeks later. Imaging studies and tests for diabetes are normal. Vasculitis only rarely involves the LS plexus (54). Some of its features, such as severe pain and concomitant weight loss, may suggest neoplastic involvement. Both can have a multifocal distribution. Infectious disorders (eg, Lyme disease) and the intravenous use of adulterated heroin may also cause painful LS plexopathies (108–110).

Radiation plexopathy.

Due to the clinical challenge of differentiating this entity from that of neoplastic plexopathy related to tumor recurrence, in those patients with a history of malignancy and XRT, this disorder warrants separate discussion. Although peripheral nerve fibers are relatively resistant to radiation damage, XRT may produce plexus fiber demyelination (with subsequent conversion to axon loss), impaired circulation, and fibrosis, a condition referred to as *radiation plexopathy*, which is a common component of the radiation fibrosis syndrome. (56,99,111–115). The first cases of this disorder were reported in 1964 (116). With the recognition that the incidence of this disorder increases with higher XRT doses and fraction sizes, shorter application times, use of the three-field technique, and concomitant chemotherapy, technical modifications were introduced to lessen these risk factors. The latter have resulted in a decline in the incidence of this complication over the past few decades (117,118). The plexus symptoms usually appear within 12–20 months of the last dose of XRT, but the range is wide (from a few weeks to more than 30 years) (8,38,99). With cervical anterior horn cell or plexus damage, patients may present with dropped head syndrome associated with neck and shoulder atrophy (119). Isolated paresthesias of one or more of the lateral three digits (ie, a lateral cord distribution) usually herald the disorder and reflect underlying demyelinating conduction block. This distribution of paresthesias may suggest a radiculopathy or carpal tunnel syndrome and, without EDX confirmation, result in unnecessary surgical interventions. Although pain at onset is infrequent, it ultimately develops in approximately two-thirds of patients, half of whom consider it a major issue (50). Sensory and motor deficits follow the paresthesias, sometimes with limb edema. Unlike most lesions manifesting demyelinating conduction block, those due to XRT tend to persist and convert to axon loss. Prior to this conversion, muscle atrophy is not present because the motor axons are in continuity with the muscle fibers they innervate. As the disorder extends throughout the plexus and axon loss supervenes, the upper extremity becomes flail, insensate, edematous, and often painful (8,15,56,115,120). Infrequently, XRT causes subclavian artery thrombosis, which in turn, produces plexus fiber ischemia and resultant permanent, painless weakness and sensory loss. Rarely, XRT causes transient paresthesias, usually of 6–12 months' duration (8). Lower motor neuron damage is a rare and untreatable complication of XRT to the cauda equina region. It presents with painless lower extremity wasting and fasciculations three to five years later (50,121). Even more rarely, XRT generates NSTs, mostly malignant ones, some 4–41 years afterward (30,91). In patients with a history of malignancy who received XRT to body regions encompassing plexus fibers, it can be challenging to distinguish radiation plexopathy from neoplastic plexopathy due to tumor recurrence. Features predictive of tumor recurrence include severe pain, rapid progression, and clinical or radiologic evidence of metastatic disease in other body regions. When recurrence occurs at the BP, lower plexus involvement and severe shoulder pain are common. Features suggesting radiation plexopathy include painless paresthesias, often in a lateral cord distribution; slow progression; and particular EDX findings, such as demyelinating conduction block, fasciculations, grouped repetitive discharges, and myokymic discharges) (46,50,95,121–123). Paraspinal muscle fibrillation potentials are more frequent with tumor recurrence (46). Not infrequently, the initial EDX examination is normal. With progression, low-amplitude median sensory responses are recorded from the symptomatic digits. Later, demyelinating conduction block appears between the supraclavicular fossa and axillary stimulation sites (eg, musculocutaneous motor nerve conduction study). Ultimately, axon loss supervenes (99,95,115). Neither Horner syndrome nor the time delay between radiation treatment and symptom onset helps to distinguish between these two possibilities (18). When radiation damage involves the LS plexus, bilateral, asymmetric, distal lower extremity weakness, often preceded by sensory disturbances, may occur. EDX abnormalities similar to those listed previously may also be noted. On MRI, the presence of nodular enhancement or a mass lesion strongly suggests recurrent tumor (22,98). Homogeneous enhancement or signal abnormality of the ipsilateral scalene muscles and other structures without nodularity suggests radiation plexopathy (Fig. 46.9) However, even surgical exploration with biopsy may be nondiagnostic (50,121). Importantly, the presence of radiation plexopathy never excludes tumor recurrence because the two conditions may exist simultaneously.

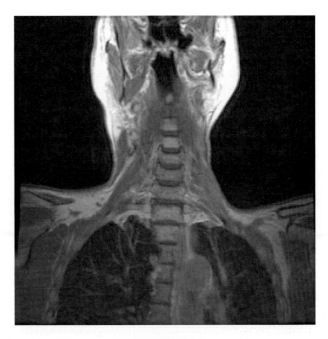

FIGURE 46.9

Coronal T1 postgadolinium MRI in a patient with head and neck cancer and a left brachial plexopathy from radiation therapy. Note the asymmetric enhancement of the left scalene muscles as compared with the right.

EVALUATION

General Evaluation

The accurate diagnosis of neoplastic plexopathies begins with the acquisition of pertinent historical data, including the growth rate of any masses and the presence of associated pain, neurologic deficits, or constitutional symptoms (eg, fever, weight loss). The patient is queried about a personal or family history of NF1 or cancer, as well as any cancer treatments rendered. On examination, the features of any masses, such as size, location, tenderness, Tinel sign, and mobility, is documented, as are any associated neurologic deficits and the presence of NF1 stigmata. In general, in addition to a comprehensive clinical evaluation, ancillary studies, especially radiographic and EDX examination, are required. The particular imaging studies employed reflect the site of the lesion, the presumed etiology, the urgency of the situation, and study availability. Bony changes related to neoplastic destruction (eg, intervertebral foraminal enlargement, vertebral erosion, spinal column stability) or to radiation exposure (ie, radiation osteitis) are recognizable by plain films and CT scans, and extraplexal metastases may be identified by radionuclide bone scanning. The limitations of CT scanning include poor soft tissue contrast, imaging restricted to the axial plane, beam hardening artifact, and the risks of ionizing radiation and iodinated contrast. Although thin-section CT myelography can image the axially oriented dorsal and ventral roots, the multiplanar imaging ability, lack of bony degradation, excellent soft tissue contrast, and noninvasivity of MRI make it the imaging modality of choice for defining the extent of the lesion, its relationship to its surrounding structures, and all related abnormalities (eg, lymphadenopathy) (124). Axial MRI best assesses the supraclavicular plexus, whereas coronal imaging is best for the infraclavicular plexus fat suppression typically is required. On MRI, NSTs appear as fusiform or spherical enlargements, and frequently the capsule and nerve or origin can be seen (125–127). NF1 is suggested by the presence of multiple neurofibromas or the multifocal nature of a plexiform tumor (16). Other roles of MRI include planning surgical and radiation therapy, monitoring treatment responses, and screening (eg, presymptomatic NF1 patients). Radiographic studies cannot be used to distinguish neurofibromas from schwannomas or benign lesions from malignant ones (19,128). Benign and malignant NSTs may both display heterogeneous signal and bone erosion, and irregular infiltrative borders may be observed with benign plexiform neurofibromas (129–131). Since MRI may not visualize the infiltration and tracking of malignant cells along the connective tissue sheaths of plexus elements, other imaging studies may be required. Other potentially useful radiographic studies include fluorodeoxyglucose positron emission tomography scanning to identify the malignant changes associated with plexiform neurofibromas, magnetic resonance neurography to differentiate intraneural and paraneural masses, and angiography to define tumor vascularity and any neighboring vessels (eg, for preoperative planning). Ultrasonography is less often helpful because it does not differentiate between various supraclavicular masses—most are hypoechoic—and it does not define the relationship of the tumor to the involved nerve (132,133). CSF examination for cytology is performed when neoplastic meningitis is suspected; it is most common with lung and breast cancer, melanoma, and lymphoma. (Prior to LP, a head computed tomography [CT] scan is obtained to exclude parenchymal metastases or hydrocephalus.) Although often considered an extension of the neurologic examination, EDX testing has several advantages over the latter, including the ability (1) to evaluate muscles not assessable clinically (eg, brachialis); (2) to identify subclinical muscle involvement; (3) to localize the lesion; (4) to determine its severity, chronicity, and rate of progression; (5) to differentiate tumor recurrence from radiation fibrosis syndrome; and (6) to exclude non-neurologic entities, such as orthopedic disorders (9). Since malignancies frequently infiltrate the BP from below, EDX assess

ment of the T1 nerve fibers is mandatory (ie, sensory study of the medial antebrachial cutaneous nerve and motor studies of the median nerve) (9,51,134). EDX studies frequently identify involvement beyond that determined radiographically, including contralaterally (eg, bilateral sacral plexus involvement). In this manner, EDX studies can further direct imaging studies. Serial EDX studies assess tumor progression and treatment response. Consequently, EDX studies provide important diagnostic and prognostic information critical to clinical decision making. Until sensorimotor deficits become persistent, however, EDX studies may be normal (16).

In general, the most accurate diagnostic information is derived from histologic study of tissue procured from tumor masses or enlarged lymph nodes. When benign plexus tumors are mistaken for non-neural lesions and biopsied or excised, severe and permanent neurologic deficits and pain may result. This mistake impedes subsequent excisions and may worsen the outcome and subsequent quality of life (16–18,44). Consequently, all plexus region masses that are associated with neurologic features (eg, Tinel sign, sensory or motor abnormalities) should be assumed to be neurogenic in origin, and consultation with a neurosurgeon experienced in the evaluation and treatment of such lesions should be obtained. When a malignant NST is suspected, definitive diagnosis is made by biopsy, usually at operation, and if confirmed, a metastatic evaluation—including chest films, bone scan, chest and abdominal CT scans, and magnetic resonance imaging [MRI] of the surrounding structures—is undertaken (21). When a malignant plexopathy is suspected and the MRI is normal, surgical exploration and studies to search for extraplexal involvement may be necessary; if the results are negative, reexploration should be performed three to six months later. Other aspects of the evaluation are more specific to the particular PNS plexus under study.

The Cervical Plexus

With cervical plexopathies, thorough examination of the head and neck (preferably by an otolaryngologist) is mandatory. Myelopathic features are sought to exclude epidural spinal cord compression (because of the proximity of this plexus to the spinal cord). Signs of cervical spine instability, bone erosion, lung masses, and hemidiaphragmatic paralysis are sought using plain films and CT scans of the neck and chest. Fluoroscopy may also identify hemidiaphragmatic involvement. The latter usually is secondary to a lesion of the phrenic nerve rather than the cervical plexus (15,16,132). Among the PNS plexuses, the cervical plexus is the least accessible to EDX assessment. One exception to this statement reflects those cervical plexus fibers contributing to the phrenic nerve, which are assessable by motor nerve conduction study of the phrenic nerve and needle electrode examination of the diaphragm. Unfortunately, these studies frequently are difficult to interpret and may yield inconclusive results (135). When tumor infiltration of the cervical plexus does not produce a recognizable mass (eg, squamous cell carcinoma), a repeat scan for evidence of enlargement or surgical exploration may be required (47).

The Brachial Plexus

With brachial plexopathies, the neck, supraclavicular fossa, shoulder, and axilla regions are palpated for masses. The features of Horner syndrome are sought because this syndrome is associated with epidural metastases and, thus, risk of spinal cord compression. In one series, Horner syndrome was observed in all 25 patients with epidural metastases (38). Plain films of the cervical spine, clavicle, scapula, shoulder, humerus, and chest help identify lung lesions (eg, superior sulcus masses) and bony changes related to malignancy and radiation. It is mandatory to visualize the lung apex. MRI determines the proximity of the lesion to the epidural space and spinal cord, and may directly (enhancement) or indirectly (eg, irregular borders, apical lung fat obliteration) identify the mass (98,128). Acquisition times are longer than with CT scanning, especially when multiple slices and planes are required (136). A newer MRI technique, *magnetic resonance myelography*, yields T2 weighted myelogramlike images of the proximal BP elements traversing the CSF following 3-D reconstruction (15,136,137,). The PNS plexus most suitable for EDX assessment is the BP. Typically, the specific elements involved, the severity, and the underlying pathophysiology are determined (51).

The Lumbosacral Plexus

With LS plexopathies, plain films of the spinal column and pelvis may reveal bony erosion or loss of clarity of the psoas shadow, thereby suggesting the presence of a retroperitoneal mass. Lower abdominal and pelvic CT scanning may identify solid tumors, including NSTs, metastases, calcifications, bony erosion, spinal column instability, bleeding, or radiation osteitis, and it is abnormal in up to 96% of those patients with metastatic disease (15,52,56). The increased sensitivity of modern scanners permits visualization of LS plexus elements, especially when oral, intravenous, and urographic contrast agents are administered. CT scanning does not indicate tumor etiology and does not recognize nonstructural lesions (eg, vasculitis). CT scanning may be used to guide percutaneous needles for tissue

procurement. CT myelography may identify neoplastic involvement of the cauda equina or epidural space (138). In one study, nearly half of patients with neoplastic plexopathies had epidural tumor extension (52). Despite advances in CT scanning, MRI remains more sensitive for identifying these lesions (92). Neoplastic plexus invasion, NSTs, and some metastatic lesions may not be visualized without gadolinium. Magnetic resonance myelography assesses structures proximal to the termination of the nerve root sleeve, such as the conus medullaris and cauda equina. Other useful radiographic techniques include bone scans (metastases), ultrasonography (lower abdominal and pelvic masses), and intravenous pyelography and barium enemas (distortion of bladder, ureter, or bowel). EDX testing is another useful study for the assessment of LS plexopathies (90). Because of the high innervation ratio of many lower extremity muscles, hundreds of fibrillation potentials are generated for each motor axon disrupted, making the needle electrode examination very sensitive toward even minimal motor axon loss. This technique also frequently identifies abnormalities outside the region of the imaged mass, including contralateral extension. Consequently, a normal EDX examination argues strongly against a lumbar plexopathy. Unfortunately, it may be impossible to distinguish lumbar plexopathies from lumbar radiculopathies due to the lack of reliable sensory nerve conduction studies at the lumbar level. (Sensory studies are abnormal with ganglionic and postganglionic disorders, such as plexopathies, but typically are normal with radiculopathies.) Some authors consider only the sural and superficial peroneal sensory studies to be reliable, at least in those individuals under the age of 60 years; neither of these assesses the lumbar plexus (90). Even when sensory response abnormalities are noted, fascicular involvement or reinnervation may render it impossible to differentiate a plexus lesion from a more distal neuropathy. EDX features of radiation fibrosis syndrome (ie, grouped repetitive discharges, myokymia, demyelinating conduction block) may be present (139,140). Again, their presence does not exclude concomitant malignancy. Tissue diagnosis of biopsy material procured from palpable masses or enlarged lymph nodes may be required. Serological testing may be helpful, including serum erythrocyte sedimentation rate, testing for diabetes, and specific antigen testing (eg, prostate-specific antigen [PSA], carcinoembryonic antigen [CEA], CA-125).

Pancoast Syndrome

With Pancoast syndrome, apical lordotic plain films may demonstrate an apical mass, the size of which reflects the stage of the disease. CT scanning and MRI of the neck, chest, and upper abdomen are useful to stage the tumor, which dictates the most appropriate surgical intervention (87,141). CT scanning assesses for bone destruction, and MRI defines the extent of the lesion and the presence of nodal involvement, epidural spread, and metastatic disease. Bone, liver, and brain imaging also assess for metastatic disease (87). Open biopsy, to delineate the tumor cell type prior to treatment, usually is unnecessary (87). When patients present with significant elbow pain or with symptoms restricted to a C8 or T1 distribution, EDX studies may be ordered. In this setting, however, the severity of the axon loss typically is too severe to be accounted for by cervical disc disease. Consequently, imaging is recommended and the tumor is identified.

MANAGEMENT

Introduction

The diversity of neoplastic plexopathies mandates individualized treatment plans for affected patients. Characteristics of the neoplasm, such as etiology, location, aggressivity, and sensitivity to radiation and chemotherapy, as well as the degree of involvement of adjacent structures and the general health and wishes of the patient, must be considered. Treatment goals include cure, restoration of function, symptom relief, palliation, and cosmetic improvement. Most nonmetastatic processes are treated surgically. Intralesional excisions (visible tumor remains) or marginal excisions (includes surrounding capsule or reactive zone) usually are applied to benign tumors, whereas malignant lesions typically require wide resection (includes a cuff of normal tissue) or radical resection (includes entire anatomical compartment). Chemotherapy and XRT serve adjunctive roles.

Benign Neural Sheath Tumors

Benign NSTs are treated conservatively when there is no neurologic dysfunction, pain, disfigurement, or suspicion of malignancy. Otherwise, surgical excision is employed, typically without additional neurologic insult (16,18). Schwannomas, which are well-encapsulated structures that do not arise from the fascicle, typically are excised without neurologic deficit and without recurrence. The management of neurofibromas varies somewhat between NF1 patients and those with sporadic tumors. With NF1, conservative management with vigilant surveillance rather than frequent surgery, especially for cosmetic reasons, is recommended because of the high likelihood that neurofibromas will continue to develop (4,5). Indications for excision of neurofibro-

mas among NF1 patients include rapid growth (ie, risk of malignant transformation), severe symptoms, and plexus fiber compression (16,18). Unlike the nonfunctioning parent fascicle, neighboring fascicles may still be functional. This determination is made using intraoperative EDX studies and permits the entire tumor and all of the nonfunctioning fascicles to be excised without added neurologic deficit (16,18). The chance of postoperative neurologic deficit is greater among NF1 patients than non-NF1 patients. Its frequency is about one-third for solitary neurofibromas and one-half for plexiform tumors (5). Due to the risk of malignant degeneration, whenever possible, all tumor fragments are removed (21). The poor delineation, increased vascularity, and infiltrative nature of plexiform neurofibromas reduce the likelihood of complete resection. These same features contribute to an increased incidence of postoperative neurologic deficits, even for palliative subtotal resections (16,21,142). When nerve function cannot be preserved, nerve grafting may be required. When patients with long-standing neurofibromas or known plexiform neurofibromas develop symptoms suggestive of sarcomatous transformation (eg, intractable pain, localized swelling, or new deficits), immediate MRI for evidence of malignant transformation (inhomogeneous gadolinium enhancement within the tumor) is required (32). Regionalized NF is a condition in which hundreds of smaller neurofibromas are situated both proximal and distal to the parent tumor and, occasionally, along other nerves in the same limb; it is treated palliatively (21). When benign non-NSTs grow extrinsic to their parent fascicles (eg, intraneural lipomas), epineurotomy and excision are usually performed without further neurologic deficit (143). The procedure is more challenging when the lesion is adherent to the epineurium (11,17,21,34).

Malignant Neural Sheath Tumors

Malignant NSTs are much more aggressive. Improved disease-free survival requires early and aggressive surgical intervention, the goal of which is complete resection with wide tumor margins (or the widest tumor margins possible with even larger tumors) or extremity amputation (141). Favorable prognosticators include tumor diameter below 5 cm, gross total tumor resection, and younger age (23). Resectability primarily reflects location and ranges from about 20% for tumors in a paraspinal location to about 95% for extremity tumors (23). More proximal tumors are also more likely to progress centripetally and infiltrate the spinal cord or brainstem. Neural sacrifice usually is unavoidable. Unfortunately, nerve grafting typically is precluded by the large area resected (graft length required is too long) and the adverse effects of postoperative radiotherapy on graft tissue (28). An international consensus statement suggested that adjuvant radiotherapy be used with low-grade tumors with marginal excisions and all medium- and high-grade tumors (144). This approach provides local control and delays recurrence, especially for those with incomplete resections, but does not increase long-term survival. Moreover, the XRT itself is a risk factor for the development of malignant NSTs, often with a latency period of 10 years or more (145,146). The roles of brachytherapy and intraoperative electron beam irradiation are unclear. Although these tumors may have a partial response to chemotherapy, a meta-analysis failed to show a survival difference despite improved progression-free survival and reduced 10-year relapse rates (147). It has no role in the initial treatment of patients without metastatic disease, but may be useful when complete resection is impossible, to avoid extremity amputation, as an alternative to radiotherapy, or with treatment failures (5,23,28). Moreover, extremity amputation may not prevent metastases or improve survival (22). Consequently, selected patients have more recently been offered limb-sparing approaches that include wide local resection, radiation, and chemotherapy, some of whom have shown good to excellent survival (21).

Metastatic Plexopathies

Due to their resistance to XRT and chemotherapy and to their advanced stage at presentation, most metastatic plexopathies are incurable and treatment is palliative. Although surgical resection for cure usually is impossible, subtotal resection for pain relief may be useful (21,47). With metastatic breast carcinoma, the malignancy may not invade the nerve beyond the epineurium, thereby permitting external neurolysis and removal of as much of the tumor as possible. With melanoma and lymphoma, tumor removal from epineurial attachments, followed by local irradiation, may be beneficial (21).

Pain

Unfortunately, the pain associated with neoplastic plexopathies typically is severe, unrelenting, and difficult to treat. It represents one of the most formidable challenges to the physician and it must be treated early and aggressively. Multiple medications, including nonsteroidal, steroidal (eg, dexamethasone), neuropathic (eg, anticonvulsants, tricyclics), and opioid analgesics, are usually required and should be used at dosages adequate to achieve control. Of these, opioid analgesics are the mainstay. Due to tolerance, the dosage usually must be increased over time. Other approaches include chemotherapy, XRT, transcutaneous electric nerve

stimulation, local anesthesia (eg, paravertebral nerve blocks), and implantable intrathecal pumps. The latter also reduce the required dosage. Surgical intervention may be required for severe and intractable pain (eg, dorsal root entry zone [DREZ] procedure, cordotomy, selective rhizotomy, celiac plexus block). Destructive procedures (eg, limb amputation) usually are ineffective (38,47,50). In addition to pain, any functional loss resulting from the malignancy or its treatment may benefit from psychological counseling, physical and occupational therapy, and vocational rehabilitation. Assistive devices can maximize any remaining neurologic function, thereby enhancing quality of life. Limb edema may respond to compressive devices or elevation.

Pancoast Syndrome

In the early part of the 20th century, when patients with Pancoast syndrome were considered inoperable and received only palliative radiotherapy, the average survival was about one year. Subsequently, resection with preoperative irradiation was shown to increase the five-year survival rate to 30%–40% (74,82,148–152). Those with less advanced disease had better outcomes. Preoperative irradiation improves surgical outcome in a number of ways: (1) it enhances resectability (the radiation necrosis produced functions as a pseudocapsule); (2) it diminishes tumor bulk; (3) it temporarily blocks the lymphatics, thereby blocking these vessels from absorbing cells during surgery; and (4) it reduces intraoperative seeding (by weakening any "spilled" cells) (87). Intraoperative brachytherapy has been reported to benefit those with more advanced disease (153). Advances in neurosurgery and imaging permit previously inoperable patients to receive curative resections, such as those with extensive BP or spinal column involvement (141,152). Consequently, the current goal is complete surgical resection for cure (141). En bloc resection includes removal of any involved lung, along with part of the chest wall (ie, adjacent portions of the first three ribs, upper thoracic vertebrae, intercostal nerves, lower trunk, stellate ganglion, dorsal sympathetic chain, and superior mediastinal and lower cervical nodes). Palliative surgery may be employed for patients with surgical contraindications or severe unresponsive pain (87,141). Aside from surgical resection, pain control usually is the primary focus. The radicular causalgic pain associated with this disorder may be unbearable. Unfortunately, combinations of nonsteroidal anti-inflammatory drugs, opioids, dexamethasone, tricyclic antidepressants, antiepileptics, ketamine, and transcutaneous electric nerve stimulation may not be effective. Although pain relief may follow radiotherapy and chemotherapy, it usually is short-lived. In one study, continuous administration of local anesthetics into the BP region was successful in six patients with unresponsive pain (154). Adequate pain relief may follow percutaneous cervical cordotomy, but the success rate of other, more invasive techniques, such as scalenotomy, spinothalamic tractotomy, myelotomy, cingulotomy, dorsal column stimulators, and subarachnoid instillation of phenol or alcohol, is unclear (154).

Radiation Plexopathy

There is no curative therapy for this entity and, thus, treatment is supportive. Physical therapy is employed to prevent contractures, capsulitis, muscle atrophy, and the formation of lymphedema. Pain is treated in a manner similar to that for neoplastic plexopathy. External neurolysis to remove as much scar tissue as possible may lessen unresponsive severe pain, but most patients treated in this manner note progression of their neurologic deficit (18). The long-term benefit of surgical procedures to restore plexus circulation and impede fibrosis, such as neurolysis with omental transfer, has not been demonstrated (8,155–158). The role of anticoagulation remains unclear (159).

PROGNOSIS

Neoplastic Plexopathies

The underlying malignancy is the primary determinant of outcome. Patients with benign plexus lesions typically do well, especially when the lesion is solitary. Following resection, new motor deficits and pain intensification are infrequent and recurrence occurs in less than 5%, with the exception of desmoid tumors, which tend to recur despite thorough excision (5,16,18,160,). As expected by their highly malignant nature, the recurrence rate and incidence of metastasis among patients with malignant NSTs is higher and their five-year survival is lower. Even with combined surgery and XRT, local recurrence occurs in 40%–65% and metastasis occurs in 40%–68% (161,162). The five-year survival rate is 42% for non-NF1 patients, but only 21% for NF1 patients (163). Since total removal causes loss of function and subtotal removal permits progression of tumor growth, the natural history of plexiform neurofibromas is functional loss of the involved nerve (16). The outcome for the majority of patients with metastatic plexopathies is uniformly poor. Typically, neurologic function worsens as the plexus lesion expands, pain severity increases and becomes more difficult to control, and metastatic disease disseminates to vital organs (15,47,52).

Pancoast Syndrome

Among patients with Pancoast syndrome, the degree of local invasion at presentation determines the resectability of the tumor and, thus, the likelihood of survival and cure (141). Favorable features include the absence of metastatic disease and lack of mediastinal or scalene node involvement (152). Pain resolution following preoperative radiation is also a good prognosticator (72). Extensive invasion of the BP, spinal column invasion, and cord compression portend a poor prognosis (152). The tumor cell type does not seem to influence survival (74). The hand intrinsic muscles are innervated via C8 and T1. When the T1 nerve root requires surgical resection, hand weakness results, but slowly improves via collateral sprouting. With lower trunk or combined C8 and T1 nerve root resections, the hand weakness is severe and permanent because neither mechanism of reinnervation is available (141). Future studies to determine whether prophylactic postoperative cranial irradiation lessens the incidence of brain metastases are needed.

Radiation Plexopathy

The prognosis for patients with radiation plexopathy is poor because of inexorable progression, intraplexal expansion, and conversion from chronic demyelination to axon loss (8,47,55,56,103). Since there is no effective treatment, most patients, especially those with upper extremity involvement, ultimately develop a functionally useless limb that is diffusely swollen, flail, anesthetic, and often painful (8,95). Even with incomplete lesions, the accompanying sensory ataxia usually renders the limb functionally useless (15).

Muscle Reinnervation

Reinnervation occurs by two mechanisms—collateral sprouting and proximodistal axonal regrowth. Collateral sprouting refers to the intramuscular branching of motor axons unaffected by the more proximally located lesion. Because collateral sprouting requires unaffected intramuscular axons, it does not occur in the setting of complete lesions. Proximodistal regrowth refers to axon regrowth from the proximal stump. For this mechanism to succeed, the lesion must lie within about 20 inches of the denervated muscle fibers, because regrowth occurs at a rate of about 1 inch per month and muscle fibers undergo irreversible degeneration after approximately 20 months in the denervated state. In addition, the degree of involvement of the supporting structures of the nerve—endoneurium, perineurium, and epineurium—affects the ability of advancing nerve fibers to traverse the lesion site. Their involvement, which leads to fibrosis, can impede reinnervation by axonal regrowth. Even when the disruption is limited to the endoneurial and perineurial regions, there may be too much internal scarring for axon advancement to occur. Consequently, the prognosis for motor nerve fiber recovery reflects the severity (ie, the completeness of the lesion), location (ie, the distance between the disrupted axons and the denervated muscle fibers), and the degree of connective tissue involvement. Consequently, the best outcomes are observed when both mechanisms of reinnervation are available—partial axon loss lesions (collateral sprouting can occur) proximate to their target organs (axonal regeneration can occur)—and connective tissue involvement is absent. The prognosis is intermediate for complete (or nearly complete) or distant lesions because only a single mechanism of reinnervation is available. The worst outcomes follow distant complete lesions because reinnervation cannot occur. Since sensory receptor degeneration does not follow denervation, there is no time or distance impediment to their reinnervation.

FUTURE PERSPECTIVES

Radiologic, oncologic, genetic, and surgical advancements continue to improve our diagnostic and therapeutic abilities. Over the past few decades, improvements in surgical technique, intraoperative EDX assessments, and the wide availability of MRI have significantly improved treatment outcomes. More recently, volumetric MRI was reported to be a sensitive measure of plexiform neurofibroma growth (164), and its utility has already been validated in a recent phase 1 trial of pirfenidone, an antifibrotic drug, in plexiform neurofibroma patients (165). Because younger patients demonstrate the fastest growth rates, clinical trials utilizing this technique must be stratified by age (164). In the near future, MR neurography may have an important role in the diagnosis of neoplastic plexopathies (166). In addition, as our understanding of the mechanism of action of tumor genes and the molecular principles underlying tumor growth increases, new targets for therapeutic intervention will undoubtedly lead to newer treatments that both prolong and improve the quality of life. For example, since dysfunctional neurofibromin produces p21 ras overactivity, clinical trials of anti-ras drugs (eg, farnesyl transferase inhibitors) have been initiated (5,32,144). In addition, a phase 1 clinical trial of interferon-alpha 2b for NF1 patients with plexiform neurofibromas is underway based on the premise that impeding angiogenesis will slow or halt tumor growth (5,167)

REFERENCES

1. Harkin JC, Reed RJ. Tumors of the peripheral nervous system. In: Atlas of Tumor Pathology, 2nd series, fascicle 3. Washington, DC: Armed Forces Institute of Pathology; 1969.
2. Kleihues P, Cavenee WK. World Health Organization Classification of Tumours: Pathology and Genetics of Tumours of the Nervous System. Lyon, France: AZRC Press; 2000.
3. Korf BR. Plexiform neurofibromas. Am J Med Genet. 1999;89:31–37.
4. Brooks DG. The neurofibromatoses: hereditary predisposition to multiple peripheral nerve tumors. Neurosurg Clin N Am. 2004;15:145–155.
5. Huang JH, Johnson VE, Zager EL. Tumors of the peripheral nerves and plexuses. Curr Treat Options Neurol. 2006;8:299–308.
6. Brazis PW, Masdeu JC, Biller J. Localization in Clinical Neurology. 2nd ed. Boston, MA: Little Brown; 1990.
7. Clemente CD. Gray's Anatomy. 30th ed. (American). Baltimore, MD: Williams & Wilkins, 1985.
8. Wilbourn AJ. Brachial plexus lesions. In: Dyck PJ, Thomas PK, eds. Peripheral Neuropathy. 4th ed. Philadelphia, PA: Elsevier Saunders; 2005:1339–1373.
9. Ferrante MA. Brachial plexopathies: classification, causes, and consequences (Invited Review). Muscle Nerve. 2004;30:547–568.
10. Birch R, Bonney G, Wynn Parry CB. Surgical Disorders of Peripheral Nerves. London: Churchill-Livingstone; 1998.
11. Kline DG, Hudson AR. Nerve Injuries. Philadelphia, PA: Saunders; 1995.
12. Ferrante MA, Wilbourn AJ. Electrodiagnostic approach to the patient with suspected brachial plexopathy. Neurol Clin N Am. 2002;20:423–450.
13. Hollingshead WH. Anatomy for Surgeons. The Back and Limbs. New York: Harper & Row; 1969:2.
14. Gierada DS, Erickson SJ. MR imaging of the sacral plexus: abnormal findings. AJR. 1993;160:1067–1071.
15. Wilbourn AJ, Ferrante MA. Plexopathies. In: Pourmand R, ed. Neuromuscular Diseases: Expert Clinicians' Views. Boston, MA: Butterworth Heinemann; 2001:493–527.
16. Donner TR, Voorhies RM, Kline DG. Neural sheath tumors of major nerves. J Neurosurg. 1994;81:362–373.
17. Ganju A, Roosen N, Kline DG, Tiel RL. Outcomes in a consecutive series of 111 surgically treated plexal tumors: a review of the experience at the Louisiana State University Health Sciences Center. J Neurosurg. 2001;95:51–60.
18. Lusk MD, Kline DG, Garcia CA. Tumors of the brachial plexus. Neurosurg. 1987;21:439–453.
19. Katz AD, McAlpin C. Face and neck neurogenic neoplasms. Am J Surg. 1993;166:421–423.
20. Pilavaki M, Chourmouzi D, Kiziridou A, Skordalaki A, Zarampoukas T, Drevelengas A. Imaging of peripheral nerve sheath tumors with pathologic correlation: pictorial review. Eur J Radiol. 2004;52:229–239.
21. Chang SD, Kim DH, Hudson AR, Kline DG. Peripheral nerve tumors. In: Katirji B, Kaminski HJ, Preston DC, Ruff RL, Shapiro BE, eds. Neuromuscular Disorders in Clinical Practice. Boston, MA: Butterworth Heinemann; 2002:828–837.
22. Park JK. Peripheral nerve tumors. In: Samuels MA, Feske SK, eds. Office Practice of Neurology, 2nd ed. Philadelphia, PA: Churchill-Livingstone; 2003:1118–1121.
23. Baehring JM, Betensky RA, Batchelor TT. Malignant peripheral nerve sheath tumor: the clinical spectrum and outcome of treatment. Neurology. 2003;61:696–698.
24. Collin C, Godbold J, Hajdu S, Brennan M. Localized extremity soft tissue sarcoma: an analysis of factors affecting survival. J Clin Oncol. 1987;5:601–612.
25. Ducatman BS, Scheithauer BW, Piepgras DG, Reiman HM, Ilstrup DM. Malignant peripheral nerve sheath tumors. A clinicopathologic study of 120 cases. Cancer. 1986;57:2006–2021.

26. Korf BR. Clinical features and pathobiology of neurofibromatosis 1. *J Child Neurol.* 2002;17:573–577.
27. Zoller M, Rembeck B, Akesson H, Angervall L. Life expectancy, mortality and prognostic factors in neurofibromatosis type 1. A twelve-year follow-up of an epidemiological study in Goteborg, Sweden. Acta Derm Venereol 1995;75:136–140.
28. Perrin RG, Guha A. Malignant peripheral nerve sheath tumors. Neurosurg Clin N Am. 2004;15:203–216.
29. Ducatman BS, Scheithauer BW. Postirradiation neurofibrosarcoma. *Cancer.* 1983;51:1028–1033.
30. Foley KM, Woodruff JM, Ellis FT, Posner JB. Radiation-induced malignant and atypical peripheral nerve sheath tumors. Ann Neurol. 1980;7:311–318.
31. Enzinger FM, Weiss SW. *Soft Tissue Tumors.* 2nd ed. St. Louis: CV Mosby; 1988.
32. Pacelli J, Whitaker CH. Brachial plexopathy due to malignant peripheral nerve sheath tumor in neurofibromatosis type 1: case report and subject review. *Muscle Nerve.* 2006;33:697–700.
33. Weiss B, Bollag G, Shannon K. Hyperactive ras as a therapeutic target in neurofibromatosis type 1. *Am J Med Genet.* 1999;89:31–37.
34. Woodruff JM. Pathology of tumors of the peripheral nerve sheath in type 1 neurofibromatosis. *Am J Med Genet.* 1999;89:23–30.
35. Russell DS, Rubenstein LJ. *Pathology of Tumors of the Nervous System.* Baltimore, MD: Williams & Wilkins; 1989.
36. Ladha SS, Spinner RJ, Suarez GA, Amrami KK, Dyck PJB. Neoplastic lumbosacral radiculoplexopathy in prostate cancer by direct perineural spread: An unusual entity. *Muscle Nerve.* 2006;34:659–665.
37. Felice KJ, Donaldson JO. Lumbosacral plexopathy due to benign uterine leiomyoma. *Neurology.* 1995;45:1943–1944.
38. Kori SH. Diagnosis and management of brachial plexus lesions in cancer patients. *Oncology.* 1995;9:756–765.
39. Shamji FM, Leduc JR, Bormanis J, Sachs HJ. Acute Pancoast's syndrome caused by fungal infection. *CJS.* 1988;31:441–443.
40. Simpson FG, Morgan M, Cooke NJ. Pancoast's syndrome associated with invasive aspergillosis. *Thorax.* 1986;41:156–157.
41. Van Echo DA, Sickles EA, Wiernik PH. Thoracic outlet syndrome, supraclavicular adenopathy, Hodgkin's disease. *Ann Int Med.* 1973;78:608–609.
42. Winston DJ, Jordan MC, Rhodes J. *Allescheria boydii* infections in the immunosuppressed host. *Am J Med.* 1977;63:830–835.
43. Dodge HW Jr, Craig, WM. Benign tumors of peripheral nerves and their masquerade. *Minn Med.* 1957;40:294–301.
44. Dart LH Jr, MacCarty CS, Love JG, Dockerty MB. Neoplasms of the brachial plexus. *Minn Med.* 1970;53:959–964.
45. Fisher RG, Tate HB. Isolated neurilemmomas of the brachial plexus. *J Neurosurg.* 1970;32:463–467.
46. Harper CM, Thomas JE, Cascino TL, Litchy WJ. Distinction between neoplastic and radiation-induced brachial plexopathy, with emphasis on the role of EMG. Neurology. 1989;39;502–506.
47. Jaeckle KA. Nerve plexus metastases. *Neurol Clin N Am.* 1991;9:857–866.
48. Haymaker W, Woodhall B. *Peripheral Nerve Injuries: Principles of Diagnosis.* Philadelphia, PA: Saunders; 1953.
49. Schaafsma SJ. Plexus Injuries. In: PJ Vinken, GW Bruyn, eds. *Handbook of Clinical Neurology, vol 7, Diseases of Nerves, Part 1.* Amsterdam: Elsevier; 1987:402–429.
50. Kori SH, Foley KM, Posner JB: Brachial plexus lesions in patients with cancer: 100 cases. *Neurology.* 1981;31:45–50.
51. Ferrante MA, Wilbourn AJ. The utility of various sensory nerve conduction responses in assessing brachial plexopathies. *Muscle Nerve.* 1995;18:879–889.
52. Jaeckle KA, Young DF, Foley KM. The natural history of lumbosacral plexopathy in cancer. *Neurology.* 1985;35:8–15.
53. Mumenthaler M, Schliack H. *Peripheral Nerve Lesions: Diagnosis and Therapy.* New York, Thieme; 1991.
54. Chad DA, Bradley WG. Lumbosacral plexopathy. *Semin Neurol.* 1987;7:97–107.
55. Pettigrew LC, Glass JP, Moar M, Zornoza J. Diagnosis and treatment of lumbosacral plexopathies in patients with cancer. *Arch Neurol.* 1984;41:1282–1285.
56. Thomas JE, Cascino TL, Earle JD. Differential diagnosis between radiation and tumor plexopathy of the pelvis. *Neurology.* 1985;35:1–7.
57. Stevens MJ, Gonet YM. Malignant psoas syndrome: recognition of an oncologic entity. *Australas Radiol.* 1990;34:150–154.
58. Dalmau J, Graus F, Marco M. "Hot and dry foot" as initial manifestation of neoplastic lumbosacral plexopathy. *Neurology.* 1989;39:871–872.
59. Gilchrist JM, Moore M. Lumbosacral plexopathy in cancer patients. *Neurology.* 1985;35:1392.
60. McKinney AS. Neurologic findings in retroperitoneal mass lesions. *South Med J.* 1973;66:862–864.
61. Saphner T, Gallion HH, Van Nagell JR, Kryscio R, Patchell RA. Neurologic complications of cervical cancer. *Cancer.* 1989;64:1147–1151.
62. Van Nagell JR, Sprague AD, Roddick JW. The effect of intravenous pyelography and cystoscopy on the staging of cervical cancer. *Gynecol Oncol.* 1975;3:87–91.
63. Westling P, Svensson H, Hele P. Cervical plexus lesions following post-operative radiation therapy of mammary carcinoma. *Acta Radiologica Therapy Physics Biology.* 1972;11:209–216.
64. Vargo MM, Flood KM. Pancoast tumor presenting as cervical radiculopathy. *Arch Phys Med Rehabil.* 1990;71:606–609.
65. Diaz-Arrastia R, Younger DS, Hair L, et al. Neurolymphomatosis: a clinicopathological syndrome reemerges. *Neurology.* 1992;42:1136–1141.
66. Glass J, Hochberg fibular head, Miller DC. Intravascular lymphomatosis: a systemic disease with neurologic manifestations. *Cancer.* 1993;71:3156–3164.
67. Grisold W, Jellinger K, Lutz D. Human neurolymphomatosis in a patient with chronic lymphatic leukemia. *Clin Neuropathol.* 1990;9:224–230.
68. Grisold W, Piza-Katzer H, Jahn R, Herczeg E. Intraneural nerve metastasis with multiple mononeuropathies. *JPNS.* 2000;5:163–167.
69. Levin KH, Lutz G. Angiotrophic large cell lymphoma with peripheral nerve and skeletal muscle involvement: early diagnosis and treatment. *Neurology.* 1996;47:1009–1011.
70. Liang R, Kay R, Maisey MN. Brachial plexus infiltration by non-Hodgkin's lymphoma. *Brit. J Radiol.* 1985;58:1125–1127.
71. van den Bent MJ, de Bruin HG, Bos GM, Brutel de la Rivere G, Sillevis Smitt PA. Negative sural nerve biopsy in neurolymphomatosis. *J Neurol.* 1999;246:1159–1163.
72. Kanner RM, Martini N, Foley KM. Incidence of pain and other clinical manifestations of superior pulmonary sulcus (Pancoast) tumors. In: Bonica JJ, Ventafridda V, Pagni CA, eds. *Advances in Pain Research and Therapy.* New York: Raven Press; 1982;4:27–39.
73. Komaki R, Roh J, Cox JD, et al. Superior sulcus tumors: results of irradiation in 36 patients. *Cancer.* 1981;48:1563–1568.
74. Ricci C, Rendina EA, Venuta F, Francioni F, De Giacomo T, Pescarmona EO, Ciriaco P. Superior pulmonary sulcus tumors: radical resection and palliative treatment. *Int Surg.* 1989;74:175–179.
75. Hare ES. Tumor involving certain nerves. London Med Gazette. 1838;23:16–18.
76. Tobias JW. Syndrome apico-costo-vertebral dolorosa por tumour, apexiamo: su valor diagnostico en el cancer primitivo pulmonar. *Rev Med Lat Am.* 1932;17:1522–1666.
77. Pancoast HK. Importance of careful roentgen-ray investigations of apical chest tumors. *JAMA.* 1924;83:1407–1411.
78. Yacoub M, Hupert C. Shoulder pain as an early symptom of Pancoast tumor. *J Med Soc N J.* 1980;77:583–586.
79. Hepper NGG, Herskovic T, Witten DM, Mulder DW, Woolner LB. Thoracic inlet tumors. *Ann Int Med.* 1966;64:979–989.
80. Hughes RK, Katz RI. Late recognition of bronchogenic carcinoma in the thoracic inlet. *JAMA.* 1965;192:964–966.

81. Rubin DI, Schomberg PJ, Shepherd RFJ, Panneton JM. Arteritis and brachial plexus neuropathy as delayed complications of radiation therapy. *Mayo Clin Proc.* 2001;76:849–852.

82. Attar S, Miller JE, Satterfield J, Ho CK, Slawson RG, Hankins J, McLaughlin JS. Pancoast's tumor: irradiation or surgery? *Ann Thor Surg.* 1979;28:578–586.

83. Pancoast HK. Superior pulmonary sulcus tumor. *JAMA.* 1932;99:1391–1396.

84. Omenn GS. Pancoast syndrome due to metastatic carcinoma from the uterine cervix. *Chest.* 1971;60:268–270.

85. Silverman MS, MacLeod JP. Pancoast's syndrome due to staphylococcal pneumonia. *Can Med Assoc J.* 1990;142:343–345.

86. Stathatos C, Kontaxis AN, Zafiracopoulos P. Pancoast's syndrome due to hydatid cysts of the thoracic outlet. *J Thorac Cardiovasc Surg.* 1969;58:764–768.

87. Urschel HC Jr. Superior pulmonary sulcus carcinoma. *Surg Clin.* 1988;68:497–509.

88. Wilson KS, Cunningham TA, Alexander S. Myeloma presenting with Pancoast's syndrome. *BMJ.* 1979;1:20.

89. Layzer RB. *Neuromuscular Manifestations of Systemic Disease.* Philadelphia, PA: FA Davis; 1985:434.

90. Ferrante MA, Wilbourn AJ. Plexopathies. In: Levin KH, Luders HO, eds. *Comprehensive Clinical Neurophysiology.* Philadelphia, PA: WB Saunders Company; 2000:201–214.

91. Donaghy, M. Lumbosacral plexus lesions. In: Dyck PJ, Thomas PK, eds. *Peripheral Neuropathy,* 4th ed. Philadelphia, PA: Elsevier Saunders; 2005:1375–1390.

92. Taylor BV, Kimmel DW, Krecke KN, Cascino TL. Magnetic resonance imaging in cancer-related lumbosacral plexopathy. *Mayo Clin Proc.* 1997;72:823–829.

93. Benzel EC, Morris DM, Fowler MR. Nerve sheath tumors of the sciatic nerve and sacral plexus. J Surg Oncol. 1988;39:8–16.

94. Hunter VP, Burke TW, Crooks LA. Retroperitoneal nerve sheath tumors: an unusual cause of pelvic mass. Obstet Gynecol. 1988;71:1050–1052.

95. Wilbourn AJ, Levin KH, Lederman RJ. Radiation-induced brachial plexopathy: electrodiagnostic changes over 13 years (Abstract). Muscle Nerve. 1994;17:1108.

96. Jackson L, Keats AS. Mechanisms of brachial plexus palsy following anesthesia. *Anesthesiology.* 1965;26:190–194.

97. Pezzimenti JF, Bruckner HW, DeConti RC. Paralytic brachial neuritis in Hodgkin's disease. *Cancer.* 1973;31:626–629.

98. Thyagarajan D, Cascino T, Harms G. Magnetic resonance imaging in brachial plexopathy of cancer. *Neurology.* 1995;45:421–427.

99. Wilbourn AJ. Brachial plexopathies. In, Katirji B, Kaminski HJ, Preston DC, Ruff RL, Shapiro BE, eds. *Neuromuscular Disorders in Clinical Practice.* Boston, MA: Butterworth Heinemann; 2002:884–906.

100. Castellanos AM, Glass JP, Yung WKA. Regional nerve injury after intra-arterial chemotherapy. *Neurology.* 1987;37:834–837.

101. Stoehr M, Dichgans J, Dorstelmann D. Ischaemic neuropathy of the lumbosacral plexus following intragluteal injection. *J Neurol Neurosurg Psychiatry.* 1980;43:489–494.

102. Emery S, Ochoa J. Lumbar plexus neuropathy resulting from retroperitoneal hemorrhage. *Muscle Nerve.* 1978;1:330–334.

103. Stewart JD. *Focal Peripheral Neuropathies.* 3rd ed. Philadelphia, PA: Lippincott Williams & Wilkins; 2000.

104. Bastron J, Thomas J. Diabetic polyradiculopathy. *Mayo Clin Proc.* 1981;56:725–732.

105. Evans BA, Stevens JC, Dyck PJ. Lumbosacral plexus neuropathy. *Neurology.* 1981;31:1327–1330.

106. Sander JE, Sharp FR. Lumbosacral plexus neuritis. *Neurology.* 1981;31:470–473.

107. Bradley WG, Chad D, Verghese JP, Liu HC, Good P, Gabbai AA, Adelman AS. Painful lumbosacral plexopathy with elevated erythrocyte sedimentation rate: a treatable inflammatory syndrome. Ann Neurol .1984;15:457–464.

108. Challenor YB, Richter RW, Bruun B, Pearson J. Nontraumatic plexitis and heroin addiction. *JAMA* .1973;225:958–961.

109. Garcia-Monco JC, Gomez-Beldarrain M, Estrade L. Painful lumbosacral plexitis with increased ESR and *Borrelia burgdorferi* infection. *Neurology.* 1993;43:1269.

110. Stamboulis E, Psimaras A, Malliara-Loulakaki S. Brachial and lumbar plexitis as a reaction to heroin. *Drug Alcohol Depend.* 1988;22:205–207.

111. Burns RJ. Delayed radiation-induced damage to the brachial plexus. *Clin Exp Neurol.* 1978;15:221–227.

112. Greenfield MM, Stark FM. Post-irradiation neuropathy. AJR. 1948;60:617–622.

113. Johannson S, Svensson H, Larson LG, Denekamp J. Brachial plexopathy after postoperative radiotherapy of breast cancer patients. Acta Oncol. 2000;39:373–382.

114. Stoll BA, Andrews JT. Radiation-induced peripheral neuropathy. *BMJ.* 1966;1:834–837.

115. Wilbourn AJ, Ferrante MA. Clinical electromyography. In: Joynt RJ, Griggs RC, eds. *Baker's Clinical Neurology on CD-ROM.* Philadelphia, PA: Lippincott; 2003.

116. Mumenthaler M. Armplexusparesen im anschluss an rontgenbestrahlung. *Schweiz Med Wochenschr.* 1964;94:1069–1075.

117. Olsen NK, Pfeiffer P, Johanssen L, Schroder H, Rose C. Radiation-induced brachial plexopathy: neurological follow-up in 161 recurrence-free breast cancer patients. *Int J Radiat Oncol Biol Phys.* 1993;26:43–49.

118. Pierce SM, Recht A, Lingos TI, et al. Long-term radiation complications following conservative surgery (CS) and radiation therapy (RT) in patients with early stage breast cancer. *Int J Radiat Oncol Biol Phys.* 1992;23:915–923.

119. Rowin J, Cheng G, Lewis SL, Meriggioli MN. Late appearance of dropped head syndrome after radiotherapy for Hodgkin's disease. *Muscle Nerve.* 2006;34:666–669.

120. Thomas JE, Colby MY. Radiation-induced or metastatic brachial plexopathy. *JAMA.* 1972;222:1392–1395.

121. Lederman RJ, Wilbourn AJ. Brachial plexopathy: recurrent cancer or radiation? *Neurology.* 1984;34:1331–1335.

122. Allen AA, Albers JW, Bastron JA, Daube JR. Myokymic discharges following radiotherapy for malignancy (Abstract). *Electroenceph Clin Neurophysiol.* 1977;43:148.

123. Esteban A, Traba A. Fasciculation-myokymic activity and prolonged nerve conduction block: a physiopathological relationship in radiation-induced brachial plexopathy. *Electroencephalogr Clin Neurophysiol.* 1993;89:382–391.

124. Rapoport S, Blair DN, McCarty SM, Desser TS, Hammers LW, Sostman HD. Brachial plexus: correlation of MR imaging with CT and pathologic findings. Radiology. 1988;167:161–165.

125. Cerofolini E, Landi A, DeSantis G, Maiorana A, Canossi G, Romagnoli R. MR of benign peripheral nerve sheath tumors. *J Comput Assist Tomogr.* 1991;15:593–597.

126. Friedman DP. Segmental neurofibromatosis (NF-5): a rare form of neurofibromatosis. *AJNR.* 1991;12:971–972.

127. Smith W, Amis JA. Neurilemmoma of the tibial nerve: a case report. *J Bone Joint Surg (Am).* 1992;74:443–444.

128. Mukherji SK, Castillo M, Wagle AG. The BP. *Sem US CT MRI.* 1996;17:519–538.

129. Kransdorf MJ, Jelinek JS, Moser RP, Utz JA, Brower AC, Hudson TM, Berrey BH. Soft tissue masses: diagnosis using MR imaging. *AJR.* 1989;153:541–547.

130. Levine E, Huntrakoon M, Wetzel LH. Malignant nerve sheath neoplasms in neurofibromatosis: distinction from benign tumors by using imaging techniques. *AJR.* 1987;149:1059–1064.

131. Petasnick JP, Turner DA, Charters JR, Gritelis S, Zacharias CE. Soft tissue masses of the locomotor system: comparison of MRI with CT. *Radiology.* 1986;160:125–133.

132. Gyhra A, Israel J, Santander C, Acuna D. Schwannoma of the brachial plexus with intrathoracic extension. *Thorax.* 1980;35:703–704.

133. Hughes DG, Wilson DJ. Ultrasound appearances of peripheral nerve tumors. *Br J Radiol.* 1986;59:1041–1043.

134. Seror P. Brachial plexus neoplastic lesions assessed by conduction study of medial antebrachial cutaneous nerve. *Muscle Nerve.* 2001;24:1068–1070.

135. Wilbourn AJ. Assessment of the brachial plexus and the phrenic nerve. In: Johnson EW, Pease WS, eds. *Practical*

Electromyography, 3rd ed. Baltimore: Williams & Wilkins; 1997:273–310.

136. Toshiyasu N, Yabe Y, Horiuchi Y, Takayama S. Magnetic resonance myelography in brachial plexus injury. *J Bone Joint Surg (Br)*. 1997;79B:764–769.

137. Krudy AG. MR myelography using heavily T2-weighted fast spin-echo pulse sequences with fat presaturation. *AJR*. 1992;159:1315–1320.

138. Gilbert RW, Kim JH, Posner JB. Epidural spinal cord compression from metastatic tumor: diagnosis and treatment. *Ann Neurol*. 1978;3:40–51.

139. Aho K, Sainio K. Late irradiation-induced lesions of the lumbosacral plexus. Neurology. 1983;33:953–955.

140. Albers JW, Allen AA Jr, Bastron JA, Daube JR. Limb myokymia. Muscle Nerve. 1981;4:494–504.

141. Bilsky MH, Vitaz TW, Boland PJ, Bains MS, Rajaraman V, Rusch VW. Surgical treatment of superior sulcus tumors with spinal and brachial plexus involvement. *J Neurosurg (Spine 3)*. 2002;97:301–309.

142. Tiel R, Kline D. Peripheral nerve tumors: surgical principles, approaches, and techniques. *Neurosurg Clin N Am*. 2004;15:167–175.

143. Louis DS. Peripheral nerve tumors in the upper extremity. *Hand Clin*. 1987;3:311–318.

144. Ferner RE, Gutmann DH. International consensus statement on malignant peripheral nerve sheath tumors in neurofibromatosis. *Cancer Res*. 2002;62:1573–1577.

145. Khanfir K, Alzieu L, Terrier P, LePechoux C, Bonvalot S, Vanel D, LeCesne A. Does adjuvant radiation therapy increase locoregional control after optimal resection of soft-tissue sarcoma of the extremities? Eur J Cancer. 2003;39:1872–1880.

146. Pollack A, Zagars GK, Goswitz MS, Pollock RA, Feig BW, Pisters PW. Preoperative vs. postoperative radiotherapy in the treatment of soft tissue sarcomas: a matter of presentation. Int J Radiat Oncol Biol Phys. 1998;42:563–572.

147. Tierney JF, Stewart LA, Parmar MKB, et al. Adjuvant chemotherapy for localised resectable soft tissue sarcoma of adults: meta-analysis of individual data. Sarcoma Meta-Analysis Collaboration. Lancet. 1997;350:1647–1654.

148. Binkley JS. Role of surgery and interstitial radon therapy in cancer of the superior sulcus of the lung. *Acta Un Int Cancer*. 1950;6:1200–1203.

149. Paulson DL. The importance of defining location and staging of superior pulmonary sulcus tumors (editorial). Ann Thor Surg. 1973;15:549–551.

150. Paulson DL. Carcinomas in the superior pulmonary sulcus. J Thorac Cardiovasc Surg. 1975;70:1095–1104.

151. Shaw RR, Paulson DL, Kee JL Jr. Treatment of the superior sulcus tumor by irradiation followed by resection. Ann Surg. 1961;154:29–40.

152. Sundaresan N, Hilaris BS, Martini N. The combined neurosurgical-thoracic management of superior sulcus tumors. *J Clin Oncol*. 1987;5:1739–1745.

153. Hilaris BS, Martini N. Multimodality therapy of superior sulcus tumors. In: *Advances in Pain Research and Therapy*. New York: Raven; 1982;4:113–122.

154. Vranken JH, Zuurmond WWA, de Lange JJ. Continuous brachial plexus block as treatment for the Pancoast syndrome. *Clin J Pain*. 2000;16:327–333.

155. Brunelli G, Brunelli F. Surgical treatment of actinic brachial plexus lesions: free microvascular transfer of the greater omentum. *J Reconstr Microsurg*. 1985;1:197–200.

156. Killer HE, Hess K. Natural history of radiation-induced brachial plexopathy compared with surgically treated patients. *J Neurology*. 1990;237:247–250.

157. LeQuang C. Postirradiation lesions of the brachial plexus: results of surgical treatment. *Hand Clin*. 1989;5:23–32.

158. Narakas AO. Operative treatment of radiation induced and metastatic brachial plexopathy in 45 cases, 15 having an omentoplasty. *Bull Hosp Jt Dis*. 1984;44:354–375.

159. Glantz MJ, Burger PC, Friedman AH, Radtke RA, Massey EW, Schold SC Jr. Treatment of radiation-induced nervous tissue injury with heparin and warfarin. *Neurology*. 1994;44:2020–2027.

160. Artico M, Cervoni L, Wierzbicki V, D'Andrea V, Nucci F. Benign neural sheath tumours of major nerves: characteristics in 119 surgical cases. Acta Neurochir. 1997;139:1108–1116.

161. Bilgic B, Ates lower extremity, Demiryont M, Ozger H, Dizdar Y. Malignant peripheral nerve sheath tumors associated with neurofibromatosis type 1. *Pathol Oncol Res*. 2003;9:201–205.

162. Weiss SW, Goldblum JR, Enzinger FM. *Enzinger and Weiss's Soft Tissue Tumors*. 4th ed. St. Louis: Mosby; 2001:1632.

163. Evans DG, Baser ME, McGaughran J, Sharif S, Howard E, Moran A. Malignant peripheral nerve sheath tumors in neurofibromatosis 1. *J Med Genet*. 2002;39:311–314.

164. Dombi E, Solomon J, Gillespie AJ, et al. NF1 plexiform neurofibroma growth rate by volumetric MRI: Relationship to age and body weight. *Neurology*. 2007;68:643–647.

165. Babovic-Vuksanovic D, Widemann BC, Dombi E, et al. Phase I trial of pirfenidone in children with neurofibromatosis type 1 and plexiform neurofibromas. *Pediatr Neurol*. 2007; 36:293–300.

166. Maravilla KR, Bowen BC. Imaging of the peripheral nervous system: evaluation of peripheral neuropathy and plexopathy. *AJNR*. 1998;19:1011–1023.

167. NIH Clinical Research Studies (protocol number: 05-C-0232). A phase 1 trial of peginterferon Alfa-2b (Peg-Intron) for plexiform neurofibromas. http://clinicalstudies.info.nih.gov/detail/ a_2005-c-0232.html.

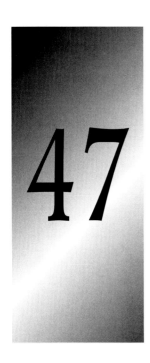

Peripheral Neuropathy in Cancer

47

Louis H. Weimer
Thomas H. Brannagan, III

Neuromuscular complications in patients with cancer are common and meaningfully affect function and quality of life. Recognition of specific processes is necessary for appropriate diagnosis and intervention. Complications can occur as a direct result of the underlying malignancy, complications of therapy, paraneoplastic effects, indirect effects of chronic illness, infection, or unrelated underlying medical conditions. Malignant processes can compress peripheral nervous structures or, less commonly, directly invade nerves. Many chemotherapeutic agents are toxic to peripheral nerve or muscle, usually in a dose-dependent manner. Radiation treatment can have effects on nerves, although they are usually delayed. Immune responses against the tumor may secondarily target neurologic structures, termed paraneoplastic syndromes—most commonly with small cell lung cancer and thymoma, discussed elsewhere in the book. These syndromes typically predate the cancer discovery and often prompt a timely diagnostic search for an underlying malignancy. Infections, increased in incidence in this population, can impede neurologic function and, on occasion, produce neuritis or radiculitis. Impairment of other organ systems may secondarily produce or predispose to neuropathy, such as renal or hepatic failure. Secondary effects of rapid weight loss, especially relative to vitamin deficiency, are potentially neurotoxic. Lastly, unrelated underlying medical conditions, such as diabetes or alcohol abuse, can enhance toxicity and independently produce neuropathy.

Because of the numerous possible neurologic complications, characterization of the pattern of symptoms and signs is critical for anatomical localization. Only then can a focused list of possibilities be compiled. Mononeuropathy affects a single named nerve, mostly commonly by nerve compression or entrapment. Polyneuropathy, often simply termed peripheral neuropathy, typically refers to a more generalized or systemic process. In most polyneuropathy cases, the longest nerves are most vulnerable to the inciting process and are primarily or predominantly affected—namely the nerves to the feet and lower legs. This process is often termed distal axonopathy and produces a clinical stocking-and-glove pattern of involvement. Other important features are the process acuity, symmetry, and affected modalities. Most commonly, small-diameter sensory nerve fibers are affected, producing symptoms of pain or temperature perception loss, dysesthesia, and temperature misperception. Clinical signs include cold, hairless, dry, and thinner skin. Impairment of large-diameter sensory fibers produces loss of vibration sense or proprioception, numbness, loss of fine touch, imbalance, and, when severe, sensory ataxia. Motor fibers are usually less affected and produce distal weakness and atrophy. Atypical patterns, such as predominant motor or large-diameter sensory impairment, rapid evolution, and asymmetry, are diagnostically useful and help narrow down possibilities. In addition to axonal loss or degeneration, relevant processes can directly

KEY POINTS

- Complications in cancer can occur as a direct result of the underlying malignancy, complications of therapy, paraneoplastic effects, indirect effects of chronic illness, infection, or unrelated underlying medical conditions.
- Careful clinical examination and in many cases electrodiagnostic studies are central to accurate diagnosis and characterization of neuropathy.
- Mononeuropathy affects a single named nerve, most commonly by nerve compression or entrapment.
- Polyneuropathy, often simply called peripheral neuropathy, typically refers to a more generalized or systemic process.
- Mononeuropathy (mononeuritis) multiplex is a distinct pattern of multiple evolving mononeuropathies and is produced by several processes.
- In most polyneuropathy cases, the longest nerves are most vulnerable to the inciting process and are primarily or predominantly affected—namely the nerves to the feet and lower legs. This process is often termed a distal axonopathy and produces a clinical stocking-and-glove pattern of involvement.

- In addition to axonal loss or degeneration, relevant processes can directly affect ganglionic neurons (ganglionopathy), especially certain toxins and paraneoplastic processes, which can occur in cancer patients. In this instance, the nerve length is a less critical factor for involvement.
- Some degree of induced neuropathy is tolerable in the treatment of life-threatening malignancies. However, the effect on quality of life for significant paresthesias, pain, and weakness should not be underestimated.
- Neurologic symptoms in cryoglobulinemia include peripheral neuropathy and rare cerebrovascular events.
- Neuropathy from multiple myeloma may be related to metabolic and toxic insults, chemotherapy, monoclonal protein, and/or amyloidosis.
- Amyloid is an insoluble extracellular aggregate of proteins that forms in nerve or other tissues when any of several proteins are produced in excess. Because the fibrils are arranged as insoluble beta-pleated sheets and accumulate with time, amyloid deposition destroys normal tissue architecture.

affect ganglionic neurons (ganglionopathy), especially certain toxins and paraneoplastic processes, which can occur in cancer patients. In this instance, the nerve length is a less critical factor for involvement. Less commonly, a primary demyelinating neuropathy is produced, which may produce weakness and potentially respond to treatment. Mononeuropathy (mononeuritis) multiplex is a distinct pattern of multiple evolving mononeuropathies and is produced by several processes discussed in this section. Careful clinical examination and, in many cases, electrodiagnostic studies are central to accurate diagnosis.

DIRECT COMPLICATIONS OF CANCER

Neurolymphomatosis

Primary tumor or metastatic mass lesions can compress peripheral nerve in focal sites, producing mononeuropathy, radiculopathy, or plexopathy, but not diffuse polyneuropathy, expect in rare circumstances. The term neurolymphomatosis is used to describe peripheral nervous system or spinal root disease resulting from infiltration by malignant lymphoma cells (1,2). The condition is quite rare and often not discovered prior to autopsy and usually predates lymphoma discovery.

The pattern of involvement can be one of peripheral neuropathy, mononeuropathy multiplex, or radicular involvement; some cases develop a cauda equina syndrome (3). A minority are more rapidly progressive, mimicking Guillain-Barré syndrome (4).

Nerve Tumors

Tumors, both benign and rarely malignant, can directly arise from nerve components or related tissues. These processes characteristically induce focal nerve or root involvement at a specific anatomical site that typically progressively worsens. Benign neoplasm examples include schwannomas and variants, neurofibromas, perineuriomas, and miscellaneous tumors of nearby tissues. The older terms neurilemoma and neurinomas are discouraged in the current World Health Organization classification (5). Rarely, malignant tumors arise from nerve sheath components and are termed malignant peripheral nerve sheath tumors; tumors arising from nearby fibroblasts, endothelial cells, and pericytes can produce similar findings, but are separately classified. Approximately half of these malignant nerve sheath tumors occur in patients with neurofibromatosis type-1 (NF-1). However, because only some tumors demonstrate Schwann cell components, the old term—malignant neurofibroma—is discouraged. Clinically, these tumors present as discrete firm mass lesions. More commonly, non-neoplastic neuromas arise after traumatic nerve injury. These structures are composed of reactive nerve sprouts attempting to regenerate the injured axon. These sites are frequently painful and can induce a Tinel sign when percussed.

COMPLICATIONS OF SECONDARY INFECTIONS

Patients with cancer are frequently immunosuppressed from chemotherapy or chronic illness and susceptible to secondary infection. Some conditions can produce neuropathy. Various patterns are possible, such as radiculitis from herpes zoster. Infectious diseases of the liver are also associated with peripheral neuropathy. Viral hepatitis (especially hepatitis C associated with cryoglobulinemia and hepatitis B-associated vasculitis are discussed more fully later). Other concerns, including HIV infection, cytomegalovirus infection, and infectious mononucleosis, may be associated with acute demyelinating neuropathy (Guillain-Barré syndrome), chronic demyelinating neuropathy, or mononeuropathy multiplex. However, possibly more relevant is that cancer patients frequently require antibiotic treatment. A number of agents are associated with toxic neuropathy; most, however, occur after extended use. The most relevant agents in this population are extended use of linezolid, metronidazole, and nitrofurantoin (6).

CHEMOTHERAPY-INDUCED NEUROPATHY

Predisposing Factors

Some degree of induced neuropathy is tolerable in the treatment of life-threatening malignancies. However, the effect on quality of life for significant paresthesias, pain, and weakness should not be underestimated (7). The incidence of chemotherapy-induced peripheral neuropathy (CIPN) is unknown, but is undoubtedly underestimated and can be a factor in successful rehabilitation. Most agents reviewed are neurotoxic in a dose-dependent manner, either of a single high dose or cumulative dose over an interval. Dose reduction can blunt or reduce toxicity, but potentially at the expense of treatment effectiveness (8,9). In addition, many malignancies can produce neuropathy directly or through an associated paraneoplastic process, complicating matters and, in some cases, predisposing to the neurotoxicity (10). Patients with cancer and peripheral neuropathy have increased vulnerability to other potential sources of neuropathy, including toxins, medications,

and focal nerve compression (10). The entities are too numerous to mention, but some important risk factors for toxic neuropathy susceptibility include impaired renal or hepatic function, increased age, genetic variations in drug metabolism, and underlying unrelated neuropathy. Some have rare genetic predispositions to certain agents, such as vincristine and Charcot-Marie-Tooth disease type 1 or neuroprotection, such as the slow Wallerian degeneration gene (Wld^s) that blunts Wallerian degeneration after toxic neuropathy or nerve injury (11,12). Patients also frequently have preexisting medical conditions that enhance vulnerability, such as diabetes, alcohol abuse, monoclonal gammopathy, renal disease, and numerous other problems. There is some controversy about neuropathy risk simply from the underlying cancer not related to paraneoplastic effects, infection, toxicity, or other measurable cause. However, peripheral neuropathy in general is prevalent in patients with cancer. Patients are also vulnerable to the effects of vitamin deficiency and occasionally vitamin excess. Pyridoxine (B6) can produce a significant large-fiber sensory neuropathy in excess dose (13). Renal failure may occur in cancer patients for various reasons, which can cause or contribute to peripheral neuropathy. Some degree of peripheral neuropathy is present in 70% of patients with chronic renal failure, but most are subclinical and are identified only by nerve conduction studies. Electrodiagnostic studies show a sensorimotor neuropathy with axonal features. Dialysis rarely reverses the neuropathy, but may stabilize symptoms; peritoneal dialysis is more effective than hemodialysis.

Numerous specific chemotherapeutic agents are associated with CIPN, but only the most clinically important or best-associated agents are discussed.

Vincristine

The vinca alkaloid vincristine is a widely used agent. A primary dose-limiting side effect is axonal neuropathy, which affects virtually all treated patients. Vincristine binds to tubulin, disrupts axonal microtubules, and interferes with axonal transport. Distal pain and paresthesias and loss of ankle jerks may be followed by weakness, sometimes severe, and generalized areflexia. Symptoms can occur after a single dose. Electrophysiologic studies demonstrate sensorimotor axonal neuropathy with reduced compound motor action potential (CMAP) amplitudes. Recovery after discontinuation of the drug may take up to two years. Coasting, which is worsening despite drug cessation, may occur. Vincristine must be specifically avoided in patients with known or suspected hereditary sensory motor neuropathy (Charcot-Marie-Tooth disease [CMT]) even if asymptomatic (14). Previously asymptomatic and unknown cases of hereditary sensory motor neuropathy type 1 (HSMN1) have been unmasked by vincristine treatment. Some have advocated CMT screening for patients with a suspicious phenotype or possible family history prior to chemotherapy onset (15). Autonomic neuropathy, which may cause constipation, postural hypotension, urinary retention, or impotence, is seen in some cases. Cranial neuropathies, sometimes affecting eye movements, can also occur.

Platins

Cisplatin, carboplatin, and oxaliplatin are important chemotherapeutic agents used to treat a variety of different cancers. There is a significant variation in susceptibility to cisplatin-induced neuropathy; patients with evident or subclinical neuropathy prior to starting chemotherapy are at particular risk, as are those with concurrent neuropathy risk factors, such as diabetes or alcoholism. Clinically, patients usually have minor tingling in the distal limbs with each treatment cycle that usually abates before the next dose. However, as the cumulative dose rises, subacute symptoms of numbness, paresthesias, and pain spread proximally and become more severe and potentially irreversible. Pin prick and temperature sensation may be spared, but proprioceptive loss is sometimes profound, causing severe incoordination and pseudoathetosis. Deep tendon reflexes are lost. Coasting may occur.

The chief site of neurotoxicity appears to be the dorsal root ganglion. Thus, both peripheral sensory nerve axons and ascending dorsal column pathways are affected. The primary drug effect is not precisely known, but the DNA binding leads to an arrest of cell division, prompting DNA repair (16). If the damage is sufficient, cell death is triggered either in a tumor cell or dorsal ganglia neuron (17). Animal models deficient in DNA repair show heightened neuropathy vulnerability. The blood–brain barrier blocks platinum, but high levels are measurable in the dorsal root ganglia and sural nerve axons (18). Nerve conduction studies typically show severely reduced sensory and normal motor nerve action potential amplitudes. This pattern may be problematic to distinguish from paraneoplastic sensory neuropathy associated with antinuclear neuronal antibodies (ANNA-1, anti-Hu), discussed elsewhere in this book, which should be assayed in the appropriate scenario. The propensity to trigger cell death supports the poor recovery in many cases, which is often limited or incomplete. The neurotoxic effects of taxoids may be additive. Ototoxicity is also common. Carboplatin toxicity appears to be similar to cisplatin.

Oxaliplatin

Structurally similar to cisplatin, oxaliplatin is a potent chemotherapeutic, platinum-containing complex, particularly important in the treatment of metastatic colorectal cancer. Oxaliplatin may cause a dose-limiting sensory neuropathy identical to that of cisplatin; however, a distinctive acute complex of reversible symptoms, starting with drug infusion and peaking within 24–48 hours, is commonly seen (19). The symptoms consist of acute cold-induced paresthesias and dysesthesias, throat and jaw muscle tightness, and limb cramps. On electrophysiological testing, hallmarks of peripheral nerve hyperexcitability are seen, including repetitive nerve discharges, multiple motor unit potentials, and neuromyotonic discharges (19). Other causes of acquired neuromyotonia, such as Isaacs syndrome, sometimes associated with thymoma, are due to antibodies against voltage-gated potassium channels. Oxaliplatin effects, however, are more likely due to sodium channel effects (19).

Suramin

Suramin remains an experimental, but well studied, chemotherapeutic agent used primarily for the treatment of refractory malignancies. Its usefulness against malignancies has been limited by side effects, including peripheral neurotoxicity in therapeutic cancer doses (20,21). Additionally, the extremely long half-life of suramin (40–50 days), a property that made it attractive as a prophylactic antiprotozoal agent, is particularly problematic if toxic symptoms occur. The peripheral neurotoxicity risk is estimated to be 15%–40% in patients with peak plasma levels exceeding 350 µg/mL (21). Generally, suramin may induce either a dose-dependent axonal neuropathy or a more acute demyelinating neuropathy with high cerebrospinal fluid (CSF) protein (20,22). Severity of symptoms varies; occasionally, progression to paralysis and respiratory failure is seen. Most commonly, patients slowly recover after drug discontinuation. The drug appears to induce nerve cell apoptosis thorough a ceramide-mediated pathway (23,24).

Bortezomib

Proteasomes are ubiquitous multienzyme complexes integral in pathways involved in cell survival, growth, migration, and drug resistance (25). Bortezomib (Velcade) is the first Food and Drug Administration (FDA)-approved member of a new class of anticancer drugs—proteasome inhibitors. Bortezomib received accelerated approval for the treatment of refractory progressive myeloma (25). Peripheral neuropathy is a common adverse event. Overall, 37% of 228 patients in a lymphoma trial receiving 1.3 mg/m^2 of the drug developed peripheral neuropathy; over one-third of these cases were severe (25). In a separate renal cell carcinoma trial, 47% developed neuropathy (26). The pattern is a length-dependent, often painful, mostly sensory axonal polyneuropathy with predominant small-fiber involvement. Development appears to be dose-related, and more than half of neuropathy cases seem to resolve after drug cessation. Monitoring for neuropathy signs and symptoms is necessary during bortezomib treatment. The neuropathy incidence is increased in patients with other causes of peripheral neuropathy or diabetes, and was surprisingly helped by a switch from thalidomide to lenalidomide in one study (27).

Thalidomide

Thalidomide was introduced in 1957 as a sedative-hypnotic drug. In addition to its infamous teratogenic effects, it caused a prevalent sensory neuropathy before the drug was withdrawn. Thalidomide has gradually reemerged over the past decade (FDA-approved in 1998) because of its useful anti-inflammatory and antiangiogenic properties in the treatment of a wide variety of dermatologic, rheumatologic, HIV-related, and neoplastic conditions. Because embryopathy can be avoided with contraception, neuropathy has become a primary dose-limiting side effect. The neuropathy is a length-dependent, heavily sensory axonal neuropathy affecting both small and large fibers, though minor motor and posterior column involvement is observed (28). Variable or incomplete recovery in many studies has been noted, suggesting a toxic effect on dorsal root ganglion neurons. A number of recent studies have examined neuropathy incidence in various disorders (29–31). In one prostate cancer study, virtually all individuals treated for more than six months developed either clinical or electrophysiological signs of neuropathy, though most stopped the drug because of lack of efficacy (32). Cavaletti et al. reported 65 patients, primarily with multiple myeloma (MM) and systemic lupus, studied before and during thalidomide treatment. The majority, including all 10 with mild existing neuropathy, developed neuropathy or had neuropathy progression (31). Risk and degree of neurotoxicity appears to correlate with cumulative dose (31,32), but the correlation was not found in some series (29). Similarly, a prospective study of patients with MM treated with thalidomide showed improvement in the myeloma but frequent sensory neuropathy (33). It has been proposed that a cumulative dose of 20 g is significant; studies examining patients below this threshold found no dose effect in contrast to studies above this level (31). The reported incidence of thal-

idomide-induced neuropathy varies from 25%–70%; this wide range is likely because of differing dosage levels and testing differences. Some individuals appear to tolerate high daily and cumulative doses without problem, implying genetic differences in drug metabolism. Because of lesser neuropathy improvement after cessation than many drugs, it is unclear whether dose reduction after neuropathy onset is a sufficient precaution or whether the drug should be stopped in all cases; treatment efficacy should be considered. Also, because of the high neuropathy incidence, careful monitoring for early neuropathy signs is advised. The mechanism of neurotoxicity is not known, but the drug inhibits (NF)-kB activation, which is important in sensory neuron survival.

A newer analog agent, lenalidomide, is more potent and possibly less neurotoxic.

Taxoids

The taxoids paclitaxel (Taxol) and the more potent docetaxel (Taxotere) are widely used agents against solid tumors, especially breast and ovarian cancers. Paclitaxel causes a dose-limiting, predominantly sensory peripheral neuropathy. Docetaxel-induced neuropathy is similar, but typically milder, though severe neuropathy after high doses is known (34). Symptoms are evident at low doses (<200 mg/m^2), but are usually not limiting. High doses are desirable for maximal efficacy, but increase the risk of neuropathy development. Unlike cisplatin neuropathy, which usually develops after a significant cumulative dose, patients given taxoids often develop symptoms within days of treatment. Risk of neurotoxicity increases with higher individual and cumulative doses, higher infusion rate, and coadministration of other neurotoxic agents, such as cisplatin (35). Sensory abnormalities and neuropathic pain beginning in the hands and feet are typical, and often persist after cessation of therapy. Autonomic and cranial nerve involvement may be seen. Motor involvement is typically minimal, except at high dose. Taxoids, in contrast to the microtubule disassemblers (colchicine, vincristine, podophyllin), promote assembly of large arrays of disordered microtubules in dorsal root ganglion cells, axons, and Schwann cells; electrophysiologic studies show predominantly axonal neuropathy signs. Inference with axonal transport is presumed to play a role in the neurotoxicity, but the precise mechanism and even the toxicity site—axon or sensory neuron—remains unknown. Both small and large fibers are affected. Abraxane (ABI-007; nab-paclitaxel), an albumin-bound, 130-nm particle form of paclitaxel that has a lower incidence of hypersensitivity, was FDA-approved in 2005. The formulation avoids the polyoxyethylated castor oil solvent Cremophor

EL required by the traditional paclitaxel infusion. The rates of neuropathy, however, appear to be similar or heightened compared to the parent drug, likely because of the higher dose enabled by the reduced systemic toxicity (36). Neuropathy remains a dose-limiting side effect in these newer preparations.

Promising preventative treatments include glutamine, acetyl-L-carnitine, and neurotrophins. Alpha-lipoic acid has diminished paclitaxel-induced neuropathy symptoms (37).

Misonidazole

This compound, used as a radiosensitizer to enhance radiation therapy efficacy, is chemically similar to metronidazole. A cumulative dose-related, painful, pansensory neuropathy is seen in more than one-third of patients, and is more common when the drug is given more frequently. Studies show a predominantly large-fiber axonal neuropathy, with secondary demyelination.

Epothilones

Epothilones are a newly emerging class of microtubule-stabilizing agents that are active against some multi-drug-resistant tumors (38). The agent ixabepilone was recently FDA-approved (October 2007), and toxic neuropathy appears to be a common side effect, mild in some, but more severe in up to 23% (39,40).

Other Agents

Selected other agents can cause neuropathy but predominantly only at high dose, usually in excess of typical therapeutic levels. Examples include etoposide and teniposide, which are semisynthetic analogs of podophyllotoxin, a well-established microtubular disassembly agent. Cytosine arabinoside in high dose is occasionally associated with demyelinating polyneuropathy. Gemcitabine is rarely associated with neuropathy, but is often combined with other agents such as platins. Ifosfamide, an alkylating agent and cyclophosphamide isomer, more commonly produces encephalopathy, but may produce other forms of neurotoxicity, possibly including neuropathy.

Various cancer treatments can trigger gouty attacks. Chronic use of colchicine is associated with myoneuropathy that can be quite severe.

Chemoprotectants

Because of the continued need for these important treatments, interest has focused on ways to eliminate or reduce neuropathy development by preventative means.

Cisplatin has been the primary target, but other agents have also been tried to a lesser degree, notably taxoids, vincristine, and pyridoxine. To date, amifostine is the only FDA-approved medication to blunt chemotherapeutic toxicity, primarily by reducing cisplatin renal toxicity and improving drug clearance. Other agents of note used experimentally or still undergoing study that show some promise include glutamate, radicicol, glutamine, glutathione, prosaptide, and others. The corticotropin (ACTH) analog Org 2766 showed early promise, but failed to affect cisplatin neuropathy in a large trial (41). Despite failures in other therapeutic areas, the only drug class that appears to markedly blunt or fully prevent neuropathy in experimental models is neurotrophins. Several studies of viral-mediated neurotrophin-3 and nerve growth factor (NGF) gene transfer have shown impressive preventative effects in rat models of cisplatin, pyridoxine, and acrylamide neuropathy (42). However, no human trials are ongoing at present.

NEUROPATHY ASSOCIATED WITH MONOCLONAL GAMMOPATHIES AND LYMPHOPROLIFERATIVE DISORDERS

Monoclonal Proteins (M-proteins)

Paraproteinemia

Monoclonal paraproteinemia (MP), also called monoclonal gammopathy, is present in many conditions, from benign to malignant, and occurs nonspecifically in chronic inflammatory and infectious diseases (43). Individual clones of antibody-producing cells (B cells) proliferate and produce excess antibody. These antibodies, called paraproteins or M-proteins, are monoclonal, and are identical in heavy and light chain types, idiotype, and antigen specificity (44).

Monoclonal paraproteinemia was first detected by electrophoresis (45), which became readily available in the 1950s when filter paper was introduced as a supporting medium. Cellulose acetate subsequently supplanted filter paper (46), and today serum is screened with agarose gel electrophoresis. Immunoelectrophoresis is performed when a lymphoproliferative disease is suspected, and immunofixation electrophoresis is used to determine immunoglobulin type (47). Bence-Jones protein, or free immunoglobulin light chain in urine, is demonstrated by immunoelectrophoresis or immunofixation of concentrated urine.

Monoclonal paraproteinemia occurs in 0.7%–1.2% of the normal adult population (48–51), is rare under age 50, but increases with each decade: 3.2% over the age of 50, 5.3% in the eighth decade, and 19% after age 95 (49,52). The M-proteins, named according to the heavy chain class, are IgG in 61%–73%, IgM in 8%–24%, and IgA in the remainder (49,52). The malignant IgG and IgA MP are usually associated with MM, whereas the IgM MP are associated with Waldenström macroglobulinemia (WM), or B-cell leukemia or lymphoma. Central nervous system (CNS) disease in the presence of MP is related to an underlying malignancy or amyloid; disease of the peripheral nervous system is more often associated with nonmalignant gammopathies (44).

Cryoglobulinemia

In 1947, Lerner et al. (53) used the term cryoglobulins to denote a group of serum proteins that precipitate when cooled and dissolve when heated, and further characterized the cryoproteins as gamma globulins. Cryoproteins have since been found in chronic infections, lupus, polyarteritis nodosa, viral hepatitis, rheumatoid arthritis, Sjögren syndrome, and hematologic malignancies, including MM, WM, chronic lymphocytic leukemia (CLL), and malignant lymphoma, and cryoglobulins may be found in low levels in normal people (54). Autoimmune diseases are the most frequently associated conditions (55). Mixed cryoglobulinemia can be inherited (56). If the cryoglobulins occur in the absence of an underlying disease, they are called essential.

There are three principal types of cryoglobulinemia: Type 1 is a monoclonal immunoglobulin. In type 2, or mixed, the cryoglobulins consist of both polyclonal (usually IgG) and monoclonal (usually IgM) immunoglobulins, with the latter having rheumatoid factor activity against the IgG. Type 3, also called mixed, includes polyclonal cryoglobulins, which are consistently heterogeneous; they are composed of one or more classes of polyclonal immunoglobulins, and are sometimes nonimmunoglobulin molecules, such as beta-1, C3, or lipoproteins (55). Cryoglobulins are type 1 in 25%, type 2 in 26%, and type 3 in 50% 3 (57). Type 3 cryoglobulins are associated mainly with infections and collagen vascular diseases, while Type 1, and to a lesser extent type 2, are associated with lymphoproliferative diseases (LPD), particularly MM and WM.

Type 1 cryoglobulins are typically present in large quantities and may even cause a hyperviscosity syndrome. The principal manifestations are circulatory. Patients present with purpura, Raynaud phenomenon, and hemorrhagic infarctions of the digits on exposure to cold. Immune complexes cause vasculitis, arthritis, and nephritis. Liver disease is a constant feature. The clinical features of types 2 and 3 cryoglobulinemia, whether essential or secondary, include purpura, arthralgias, hepatosplenomegaly, renal disease, and vasculitis of the skin. Peripheral neuropathy has been reported in 50%–70% of patients with mixed cryoglobulinemia (58,59).

The cryoglobulin concentration is measured directly by centrifugation (cryocrit) and radial immunodiffusion or indirectly by comparing the serum protein concentration before and after cryoprecipitation. Increasing the concentration of a purified cryoglobulin results in an increase of the temperature at which precipitation occurs (60), and IgM, which predominates in disease, generally undergoes cryoprecipitation at lower concentrations than IgG. Electrostatic (ionic) interactions are a major force in the cold-induced insolubility (61).

Treatment includes corticosteroids, plasma exchange, and immunosuppressive drugs (62). A vasculitic neuropathy associated with hepatitis C infection may improve with interferon alfa (63).

Neurologic symptoms in cryoglobulinemia include peripheral neuropathy and rare cerebrovascular events. The most common neurologic manifestation is a sensorimotor neuropathy, which occurs in 7%–15% of patients with cryoglobulinemia (63,64). Cryoglobulinemic neuropathy may be caused by immunologically mediated demyelination, microcirculatory occlusion, and vasculitis involving the vaso nervorum. Mononeuritis multiplex associated with human immunodeficiency (HIV) infection may improve with plasma exchange (65). Neurologic involvement is more frequent in those with type 3 cryoglobulinemia (57).

Plasma Cell Dyscrasia

Plasma cell dyscrasias include a spectrum of diseases characterized by the monoclonal proliferation of lymphoplasmacytic cells in the bone marrow. Typically, these cells produce an M-protein. The disorders include MM, plasmacytoma, WM, primary amyloidosis, and the rare condition of heavy-chain deposition disease. Other LPD, such as lymphoma and CLL, rarely produce M-protein (66). Monoclonal gammopathy of undetermined significance (MGUS) is a laboratory abnormality without evidence of malignancy, which sometimes evolves into one of the previously mentioned diseases (67).

Monoclonal Gammopathy of Undetermined Significance

Nonmalignant MGUS denotes the presence of MP in a patient who has no evidence of an underlying lymphoproliferative disorder. Three percent of the population older than 70 years and 1% of those older than 50 years have MP (48,49,68). In various series, MGUS accounted for 56%–99.5% of patients with

MP (48,49,52,68–70). The lower frequency reflects the experience in tertiary referral centers to which patients who are ill or with known malignancies are referred, and the higher frequency is from nonhospitalized population studies. The heavy-chain type is IgG in 69%, IgA in 11%, and IgM in 17%; and the type of light chain is kappa in 62% and lambda in 38% (52). Malignant transformation has been reported to occur in 15%–17% at 10 years and 11%–33% at 20 years (71–74). The risk of malignant transformation can be stratified based on the size of the M-protein, the type of immunoglobulin, and the free light chain ratio. Patients with three abnormal risk factors, a high serum level (>1.5 g/dL), a non-IgG monoclonal protein, and an abnormal free light chain (FLC) ratio have a risk of 58% of malignant transformation at 20 years (75). Malignant transformation results in MM in 56%–61% of patients, primary amyloidosis in 7%–14%, WM in 6%–12%, and other lymphoproliferative disorders in 8%–25% (66,75). No single factor predicts which patients with monoclonal gammopathy will develop a malignant plasma cell disorder, so periodic clinical evaluation and measurement of the M-protein should be considered.

Myeloma

Multiple Myeloma

Multiple myeloma (MM) is the most common plasma cell dyscrasia, affecting approximately 4.3 in 100,000 Americans each year. The median age at onset is 60 years, and black people are affected twice as often as whites (76).

Multiple myeloma is caused by neoplastic proliferation of a single line of plasma cells. Initial symptoms and signs are fatigue, weakness, lethargy, hypercalcemia, anemia, bone disease, renal failure, and immunodeficiency (77). Most patients with MM show evidence of bone marrow plasmacytosis (usually >15%) and bone disease (90%) (67)—either lytic bone lesions (60%) or generalized osteoporosis (30%) (78). Compression fractures of the spine are common and lead to localized pain, root compression, or spinal cord compression. Frank plasma cell leukemia occurs rarely.

More than 95% of patients have M-proteins in their serum or urine: 55% IgG, 25% IgA, 1% IgD, and 20% only kappa or lambda light chains (78). The concentration of the M component has prognostic significance, as it grossly reflects the tumor mass (79). Uninvolved normal immunoglobulin levels are usually suppressed, accounting for the increased susceptibility to infection (80).

The five-year relative survival rate is 45.7% for patients with plasmacytoma of bone marrow, 25.9%

for MM, and 13% for plasma cell leukemia (81). The overall median length of survival is three years (76,82).

Neuropathy may be related to metabolic and toxic insults, chemotherapy, MP, and amyloidosis (83).

Plasmacytoma

Plasmacytoma arises as part of the presentation of MM or as a solitary mass. Solitary plasmacytoma, which accounts for 5% of malignant plasma cell diseases (84), is a localized plasma cell tumor that occurs most often in the upper respiratory tract, but may also occur throughout the body (85). Magnetic resonance imaging (MRI) of the spine and pelvis is necessary to exclude occult bone or bone marrow disease elsewhere. Generalized myeloma develops in up to one-half of patients with solitary plasmacytoma of bone, usually within three years of the diagnosis, presumably as the result of occult disease not detected initially (86). Extramedullary plasmacytoma has a lower incidence of conversion to myeloma (87).

Eighty-two percent of patients with solitary plasmacytoma of bone have monoclonal paraproteinemia (88). Patients without paraproteinemia at presentation or whose paraprotein decreases after treatment progress to myeloma less often, and failure of the paraprotein to clear after local treatment suggests occult dissemination and predicts later development of overt myeloma (88). At least 36% of these cases progress to myeloma. Adjuvant chemotherapy does not appear to affect the incidence of conversion.

While 93% of cases respond to radiation therapy, 62% completely (86,89,90), combination therapy may be required to avoid radiation damage to the spinal cord in cases of spine tumor. In instances of local recurrence or dissemination with a progressive course, systemic chemotherapy is used (91). The prognosis is better than for MM, and the median survival is longer than 10 years (85).

Osteosclerotic Myeloma

Osteosclerotic myeloma is a plasma cell dyscrasia characterized by sclerotic bone lesions and progressive demyelinating polyneuropathy (92). It accounts for less than 3% of patients with myeloma, and produces a focal plasmacytoma in bone. The bone marrow aspirate contains fewer than 5% plasma cells, as opposed to >10% seen in typical myeloma (92). Raised protein levels in CSF, papilledema, and axonal and demyelinating neuropathy demonstrated by nerve conductions and nerve biopsy are common features (93). The M-protein is usually composed of IgA or IgG with lambda light chains (92).

Osteosclerotic myeloma may be associated with other systemic manifestations, and most patients develop one or more manifestations of the Crow-Fukase syndrome (94,95), also called the POEMS (polyneuropathy, organomegaly, endocrinopathy, M-protein, and skin changes) syndrome (96). Osteosclerosis is present in 3% of patients with MM versus 90% with POEMS syndrome. Skin changes are varied and include hypertrichosis, hyperpigmentation, diffuse skin thickening, hemangiomas, finger clubbing, and white nail beds (96,97). Endocrinopathy produces diabetes, hypothyroidism, and gynecomastia and impotence in men and amenorrhea in women. Organomegaly includes hepatosplenomegaly and generalized lymphadenopathy (98).

Diagnosis of osteosclerotic myeloma rests on the demonstration of monoclonal plasma cells in the biopsy of a sclerotic lesion (98,99). Occasional patients with POEMS syndrome may present without associated osteosclerotic myeloma. Elevated levels of interleukin-6 (100), and tumor necrosis factor-alfa (101) are detectable. The link between POEMS and osteosclerotic myeloma remains unexplained (96).

Clinical improvement of the neuropathy with reduced M-protein levels results from treatment of the plasmacytoma with surgical excision, radiation, and prednisolone (93,98). The neuropathy responds to treatment in nearly 50% of patients (96).

Waldenström Macroglobulinemia

Waldenström macroglobulinemia (WM) is a plasmacytoid lymphocytic lymphoma that accounts for 2% of hematologic cancers (102). The median age at diagnosis is 60 years (103). Symptoms and signs at onset include anemia, bleeding of mucous membranes, MP, and lymphocytosis. Lymphadenopathy, splenomegaly, and hepatomegaly develop eventually, and are detected in 40% by computed tomography (CT) or magnetic resonance imaging (MRI) of the abdomen (104). Plasmacytoid lymphocytic proliferation in bone marrow, lymph nodes, or spleen is evident on biopsy, and mast cells are also commonly found in the bone marrow. Bone marrow disease is present in more than 90% of patients (104).

Production of monoclonal IgM is characteristic, and circulating macroglobulin causes the hyperviscosity syndrome, cryoglobulinemia, amyloidosis, and hemolytic anemia. The hyperviscosity syndrome occurs in 15%–50% of patients (66,102). While type 1 cryoglobulins are detected in approximately 15% of patients with overt WM, less than 5% have symptoms (105,106). Five percent to 10 percent of patients with macroglobulinemia develop a chronic, predominantly demyelinating sensorimotor peripheral neuropathy (107).

Chronic Lymphocytic Leukemia

WM and CLL are at different ends of a spectrum of similar lymphoproliferative disorders, with marked leukemia uncommon in WM and MP uncommon in CLL. Chronic lymphocytic leukemia, the most common human leukemia in the United States (108), is known as an indolent disease that principally affects the elderly. The incidence ranges from rare before the fourth decade to 30.4 cases per 100,000 persons over the age of 80 years (109). The median age at diagnosis is 60 years (110). There is a male predominance, with a male-to-female ratio of 2:1.

The symptoms of CLL are varied. Frequently, the diagnosis is made by detecting lymphocytosis on a routine complete blood cell count. Symptomatic presentation includes fever, night sweats, weight loss, an increased susceptibility to viral or bacterial infections, and autoimmune hemolytic anemia. Likewise, physical findings range from no abnormalities to lymphadenopathy or organomegaly secondary to lymphocyte infiltration. As the disease progresses, neoplastic B lymphocytes accumulate and lymphadenopathy becomes widespread. In advanced cases, non-lymphoid organ infiltration also occurs. Anemia and thrombocytopenia, evidence of bone marrow failure, occur in the most advanced stages. Immunoglobulin abnormalities in CLL include panhypogammaglobulinemia (111) and monoclonal gammopathy, which occurs in 4%–31% of patients (112). Diagnosis is made by detecting an elevated absolute lymphocyte count greater than 30% replacement of the marrow cellularity by tumor cells or clonality of blood lymphocytes (109).

Ninety-five percent of patients with CLL exhibit a clonal expansion of B lymphocytes in the blood, bone marrow, lymph nodes, and spleen (113). Infiltrating CLL may cause peripheral neuropathy or cranial neuropathy (114).

NEUROPATHIES ASSOCIATED WITH MONOCLONAL GAMMOPATHIES OR LYMPHOPROLIFERATIVE SYNDROMES

Peripheral nervous system disease often results from the paraprotein itself, while disease of the CNS more often is caused by the direct effects of the underlying malignancy. Spinal cord, root, cauda equina, cranial nerve, and intracranial compression were known complications of lymphoproliferative disorders prior to modern methods of detecting MP (115). Leptomeningeal and nerve root infiltration may cause neuropathy, myelopathy, Guillain-Barré syndrome, and cranial neuropathy in lymphoma and CLL (1). Peripheral neuropathy, entrapment neuropathy, or nervous system compression may all be caused by amyloidosis. Autonomic dysfunction is particularly characteristic and leads to postural hypotension, impotence, and incontinence. Guillain-Barré syndrome (116) has long been recognized. Treatment carries its own set of complications. Neuropathy caused by vinca alkaloids is an example.

The difference between diseases of the perikaryon (motor neuron disease [MND]) and purely motor peripheral neuropathies is not always clear, however, and some of the patients with lower motor neuron syndromes may have motor neuropathy rather than motor neuron disease. The distinction is important, as motor neuropathy may improve with immunosuppression, whereas motor neuron disease does not.

The neuropathic syndromes associated with the monoclonal gammopathies are heterogeneous. Approximately 10% of patients with neuropathy of otherwise unknown etiology have a monoclonal gammopathy (117); 60% have IgM M-proteins, 30% have IgG M-proteins, and 20% IgA M-proteins (118–120) The IgM M-proteins frequently have autoreactive specificities against antigens in peripheral nerves and can be divided into several distinct clinical syndromes. The axonal neuropathies, which are associated with IgG or IgA lambda M-proteins or with osteosclerotic myeloma, form another distinct syndrome. In other cases, the monoclonal gammopathies are associated with amyloidotic or cryoglobulinemic neuropathy, or by infiltration of nerves by tumor cells. Other patients with monoclonal gammopathies have syndromes resembling chronic inflammatory demyelinating neuropathy (CIDP), whose relationship to the monoclonal gammopathy is unclear.

Neuropathy Associated with IgM Monoclonal Gammopathies

In patients with neuropathy and IgM M-proteins, the monoclonal gammopathy is usually nonmalignant, although it is sometimes associated with WM or CLL. The incidence of peripheral neuropathy in patients with IgM monoclonal gammopathies has been reported to be between 5% and 50% (121–124). In most cases, the IgM M-proteins have autoantibody activity and react with oligosaccharide determinants of glycolipids or glycoproteins (glycoconjugates) concentrated in peripheral nerve. Several distinct syndromes have been recognized and are described next. Occasional patients present with mononeuritis or mononeuritis multiplex resulting from cryoglobulinemia and vasculitis or from infiltration of nerve by tumor cells (122,125,126). In many cases, however, the M-proteins have no identifiable immunological or biological activity.

Demyelinating Neuropathy Associated with Anti-MAG Antibodies

In 50%–60% of patients with neuropathy and IgM monoclonal gammopathy, the M-proteins bind to myelin and to an oligosaccharide determinant that is shared by the myelin associated glycoprotein (MAG), the Po glycoprotein, the myelin protein PMP22, and the glycolipids sulfoglucuronyl paragloboside (SGPG) and sulfoglucuronyl lactosaminyl paragloboside (SGLPG) (127–129). The incidence of this type of neuropathy is estimated to be 1 to 5 per 10,000 adult population (129). Patients with anti-MAG antibodies have a slowly progressive distal symmetrical demyelinating neuropathy that affects the arms and legs. It typically is a sensory ataxic neuropathy, and tremor is frequent (130). Cranial nerves and autonomic functions are usually spared.

The CSF is acellular and protein concentration is usually increased. Visual evoked responses may reveal subclinical involvement of the optic nerves, particularly if the antibodies are present in the CSF (131).

Most patients have an IgM monoclonal antibody, though rare patients have not had monoclonal proteins. The monoclonal may be at a low level, and repeat testing and testing with protein immunoelectrophoresis or immunofluorescence is recommended. The majority of patients have a MGUS, but some patients have had WM, lymphoma, or CLL.

Nerve conduction studies show fairly uniform slowing with more pronounced distal involvement. No conduction block or temporal dispersion is seen, using strict criteria for conduction block (132–134). Investigators have demonstrated possible conduction blocks using less stringent definitions (121,135). Distal temporal dispersion can be demonstrated, as determined by a prolonged distal CMAP duration; however, this is rare compared with CIDP patients (136).

Pathological studies usually show demyelination with deposits of the monoclonal antibodies and complement on affected myelin sheaths (137). In some nerves, there is widening of the myelin lamellae at the minor dense line, an abnormality that is closely associated with the presence of anti-MAG antibodies (138–140).

Anti-MAG neuropathy is one of the best-characterized antibody-mediated autoimmune disorders, using the criteria proposed by Drachman (141). An autoantibody is present in patients with the disorder. The antigen is known and the antibody binds to the antigen. The neuropathy can be reproduced with injection of human antibodies into a chicken, with the characteristic pathological finding of the separation of the myelin lamellae at the minor dense line, similarly to that seen in the human disease (142).[Removal of the antibody with either plasmapheresis or chemotherapy improves the disease (129).

Anti-MAG antibodies are thought to be pathogenic. Deposits of IgM and complement are noted on myelin sheaths (137). The antibody may also interfere with the role of MAG in neurofilament spacing, which can disturb axonal transport and impair axonal survival (143).

For some patients, the anti-MAG neuropathy is not disabling or progressive and treatment is not necessary (144). The neuropathy associated with anti-MAG antibodies frequently improves, with therapy directed at lowering the autoantibody concentrations. Improvement has been associated with a 25%–50 % drop in the total IgM level (142,145). Plasmapheresis, chlorambucil, and cyclophosphamide have all been beneficial (142,144,146–148). Fludarabine is a chemotherapeutic agent that is also beneficial and may be better tolerated than cyclophosphamide (149,150). A placebo-controlled trial of intravenous immunoglobulin (IVIg) showed no benefit in the majority of patients, though some patients benefited (151). Another randomized controlled study did show reduced disability at four weeks as well as improvement in multiple other secondary outcome measures (152).

Rituximab, a monoclonal chimeric anti-CD20 antibody is used frequently now and is well tolerated (153–155). It has been shown to be efficacious in a randomized, double-blind, placebo-controlled clinical trial (156). Benefit can be seen for 6–12 months.

Motor Neuropathy and IgM Anti-GM1 Antibodies

Monoclonal IgM anti-GM1 antibodies were first reported in a patient with IgM monoclonal gammopathy and lower motor neuron disease syndrome (157) and in patients with motor neuropathy and multifocal conduction blocks. (158). Other patients with increased titers of monoclonal or polyclonal IgM anti-GM1 antibodies and motor neuropathy or motor neuron disease were later described (159–164)

Patients with multifocal motor neuropathy (MMN), with or without highly elevated anti-GM1 antibody titers, are typically characterized by progressive weakness with muscle wasting and fasciculations, and may resemble motor neuron disease. It can be generalized or involve one or several nerves. The motor axons or nerve fibers are primarily affected, which distinguishes it from motor neuron disease, in which the perikaryon or nerve cell body is primarily involved. MMN is often immunologically mediated, and can respond to immunosuppressive therapies, whereas motor neuron disease does not.

MMN can begin at any age, with onset reported between the ages of 15 years and 79 years. Men are more frequently affected than women. The arms are more frequently involved than the legs (165–167), and, unlike motor neuron disease, bulbar involvement or respiratory failure is rare (166,168). It is usually slowly progressive or progresses with stops and starts, and the course may be prolonged, often to more than 20 years (160,169,170). Deep tendon reflexes may be absent or reduced, but are sometimes hyperactive (160), although Babinski signs are absent. Some of the patients have mild distal paresthesias and sensory loss in the hands or feet.

Conduction studies frequently show one or more areas of conduction block in motor nerves; although in some patients, motor conductions are normal or diffusely slowed. Sensory conductions are typically normal, including over the regions of motor conduction block. CSF protein is usually normal but occasionally elevated. Monoclonal gammopathies are less common than polyclonal elevations of anti-GM1 antibodies; 4 of 14 of patients with highly elevated titers had IgM M-proteins (171). Serum IgM concentration may be elevated or normal. Estimates of the frequency of increased anti-GM1 antibody titers in patients with motor neuropathy and multifocal motor conduction block range from 18%–84%. The antibodies are sometimes in association with IgM monoclonal gammopathies, but usually as polyclonal antibodies (160).

In a review of patients with highly elevated anti-GM1 antibody titers, 5 of 14 patients had a single conduction block, 4 of 14 had multiple conduction blocks, and 1 had diffusely slowed motor conductions (172). In 4 of the 14 patients, however, conductions did not show signs of demyelination and the diagnosis would have been missed if not for the elevated anti-GM1 antibody titers. The disease is also different from CIDP, as it is purely or predominantly motor, nerve conduction velocities between regions of block are usually normal, the conduction blocks affect motor but not sensory fibers, CSF protein is not commonly elevated, and patients with typical CIDP and sensorimotor neuropathy do not have highly elevated titers of anti-GM1 antibodies.

Glycosphingolipids are composed of the long-chain aliphatic amine sphingosine (acylated ceramide), attached to one or more sugars. Gangliosides are complex glycosphingolipids containing sialic acid. Sialic acid is a generic term for N-acylneuraminic acid. Gangliosides are designated G for ganglioside, followed by M, D, T, or Q (for mono, di, tri, or quad), referring to the number of sialic acids. Arabic numbers and lower-case letters follow and refer to the sequence of migration by thin-layer chromatography (173,174).

In most patients, the anti-GM1 antibodies recognize the Gal(B1-3)GalNAc determinant, which is shared by asialo GM1 (AGM1) and the ganglioside

GD1b. The same determinant is also present on some glycoproteins and is recognized by the lectin peanut agglutinin (PNA). Some of the antibodies, however, are highly specific for GM1 or recognize internal determinants shared by GM2 (175–178).

Although GM1 and other Gal(B1-3)GalNAc– bearing glycoconjugates are highly concentrated and widely distributed in the central and peripheral nervous systems, they are mostly cryptic and unavailable to the antibodies. However, anti-GM1 antibodies bind to spinal cord gray matter and to GM1 on the surface of isolated bovine spinal motor neurons, but not to dorsal root ganglion neurons (172). In peripheral nerve, GM1 ganglioside and Gal(B1-3)GalNAc–bearing glycoproteins are expressed at the nodes of Ranvier (179–181). Two of the glycoproteins have been identified as the oligodendroglial-myelin glycoprotein (OMgp) in paranodal myelin, and a versicanlike glycoprotein in the nodal gap (182). The antibodies also bind to the presynaptic terminals at the motor endplate in skeletal muscle, where the antibodies might also exert an effect (183).

Pathological studies at postmortem in a patient who died with motor neuropathy and elevated titers of anti-GM1 antibodies revealed degeneration of the anterior roots, immunoglobulin deposits on myelin sheaths, and chromatolytic changes in spinal motor neurons (184). The predominant involvement of the anterior roots rather than the more distal nerve segments might explain the lack of correlation between the presence of conduction block and the distribution or severity of the weakness in many of the affected patients. The motor neurons may be secondarily involved to the anterior roots, as suggested by the presence of central chromatolysis.

It is not known whether the anti-GM1 antibodies cause or contribute to the disease or whether they are only an associated abnormality. The binding to motor but not sensory neurons correlates with the clinical syndrome, and GM1 is highly enriched in myelin sheaths of motor nerves and differs in its ceramides in comparison to sensory nerves (185,186). This might render the anterior roots more susceptible to the autoantibodies' effects. In one study, rabbits immunized with GM1 or Gal(1-3)GalNAc-BSA developed conduction abnormalities with immunoglobulin deposits at the nodes of Ranvier (187), and in another, serum from a patient with increased titers of anti-GM1 antibodies and IgM deposits at the nodes of Ranvier produced demyelination and conduction block when injected into rat sciatic nerve (188). The human anti-GM1 antibodies have also been shown to bind to and damage or kill mammalian spinal motor neurons in culture (189) and to block conduction at the motor endplate (190).

Though most patients with multifocal motor neuropathy do not have a malignant disease, several patients with non-Hodgkin lymphoma have been reported (162,191,192). Some of these patients have an IgM monoclonal protein reactive to GM1.

The treatment of choice for motor neuropathy is IVIg, which has been shown to be effective in placebo-controlled trials (193,194). A favorable response has been reported in 67%–100% of patients (195,196), and a reduction of the degree of conduction block or an increase in the CMAP may be seen (193).[

The therapeutic effect of IVIg is transient, and prolonged treatment is usually required. However, remissions following the use of IVIg (197), or occurring spontaneously (193), have also been reported. Prolonged benefit has been reported for years (117).

Motor neuropathy is also responsive to the chemotherapeutic agents chlorambucil (158,198,199), intravenous cyclophosphamide (149), or fludarabine (154), which lower autoantibody titers and serum IgM concentrations and reduce dependency on IVIg. Patients also have improved with the use of rituximab, a monoclonal antibody against the B cell marker CD20 (200,201). Oral cyclophosphamide, oral and intravenous corticosteroids, plasmapheresis, and immunoadsorption have generally been ineffective (198,202–205). In addition, corticosteroids and plasmapheresis have been associated with disease exacerbations (206).

Predominantly Sensory Neuropathy with Antibodies to GD1b and Disialosyl Ganglioside

Monoclonal IgM antibodies that react with GD1b and disialosyl gangliosides were first described in a patient with a predominantly sensory demyelinating neuropathy (206). The monoclonal IgM reacted best with GD3 and GT1b, but showed strong cross-reactivity with GD1b and GD2. Several other patients with predominantly sensory neuropathy and monoclonal IgM antibodies to one or more gangliosides of the same series have been reported since (200–206).

The syndrome has been designated CANOMAD for *c*hronic *a*taxic *n*europathy with *o*phthalmoplegia *m*-protein cold *a*gglutinins and *d*isialosyl antibodies. All the monoclonal antibodies reacted strongly with GD1b; in addition, some showed strong cross-reactivity with GT1b, GD3, GD1a, or GQ1b, or exhibited anti-Pr2 and cold agglutinin activity.(206,208,211) All had large-fiber sensory loss with areflexia, and most had gait ataxia and elevated CSF proteins. The neuropathy was of the demyelinating type, and IgM deposits were not detected in biopsied nerves using direct immunofluorescence. In one of the studies, the monoclonal IgM was found to bind to myelin in cross-sections of normal nerve (210). A mouse monoclonal anti-GD1b antibody was shown to bind to dorsal root ganglia neurons (212), possibly explaining the sensory neuropathy.

One of the patients developed an acute neuropathy as in the Guillain-Barré syndrome, but following initial improvement, the disease progressed in a stepwise fashion (207). Response to therapy was generally poor, although some improvement was reported with plasmapheresis, prednisone, IVIg, and rituximab (208,209). The antibodies are likely to be responsible for the disease, as immunization of rabbits with GD1b induced an experimental sensory ataxic neuropathy (213).

Sensory Neuropathy and Antisulfatide Antibodies

Monoclonal or polyclonal IgM antibodies to sulfatide have been reported in association with predominantly sensory neuropathy (214–217). In several of the patients, the clinical syndrome resembled that of ganglioneuritis or small-fiber sensory neuropathy, and electrophysiologic or nerve biopsy studies were normal and showed no abnormalities. Immunocytochemical studies using the anti-sulfatide antibodies from these patients revealed that the antibodies bound to the surface of rat dorsal root ganglia neurons (215,216). In several other patients, the antisulfatide antibodies cross-reacted with MAG and patients had a sensorimotor neuropathy, some with demyelination, widened myelin lamellae, and deposits of IgM on myelin sheaths (217–219). Antisulfatide antibodies may also sometimes cross-react with chondroitin sulfate C (206).

The role of the antisulfatide antibodies in the pathogenesis of the associated neuropathies is unknown and has not yet been examined in experimental systems. In immunofluorescence studies, several of the antisulfatide antibodies from the patients with demyelinating neuropathy bind to the surface of myelin in peripheral nerve, whereas the antibodies from the patients with ganglioneuritis bind to the surface of dorsal root ganglia neurons but not to unfixed peripheral myelin. It is likely that the antisulfatide antibodies differ in their fine specificities and cross-reactivities and that the antibodies could bind to sensory neurons, myelin, or both, depending on their fine specificities and the orientation of the sulfatide molecule on the surface of the target cells.

Neuropathy and Antichondroitin Sulfate Antibodies

Several patients with monoclonal or polyclonal IgM antichondroitin sulfate antibodies and predominantly sensory or sensorimotor axonal neuropathy have been described (216,220–225). In some, deposits of IgM in the endoneurium was demonstrated by immunofluorescence microscopy. Some of the chondroitin C antibodies cross-reacted with sulfatide (216).

Neuropathy and IgM Monoclonal Antibodies with Other Specificities or with No Identifiable Specificity

Neuropathy associated with monoclonal IgM antibodies to other glycolipids has also been reported. One patient had a monoclonal IgM that bound to sialosyl-lactosaminyl paragloboside (226,227). Two patients had IgM M-proteins specific for GM2, GM1b-GalNAc, and GD1a-GalNAc (228). One patient had a motor neuropathy with antibodies to GD1a (229). Another monoclonal IgM from a patient with CLL and neuropathy bound to myelin and cross-reacted with denatured DNA and with a conformational epitope of phosphatidic acid and gangliosides (223,230). Several patients with neuropathy and IgM antibodies to intermediate filaments have also been described (231).

In other patients with polyneuropathy and IgM monoclonal gammopathy, no demonstrable autoantibody activity can be detected. In these cases the antibody might be unrelated to the neuropathy or react with some as-yet-unidentified nerve component. In some of the cases, the monoclonal B cells may directly infiltrate the peripheral nerves (125). Many of these patients respond to immunosuppressive therapy, suggesting that the neuropathies in these patients may also be immune-mediated (107).

Neuropathy in Patients with IgM M-proteins and Cryoglobulinemia

IgM M-proteins may also function as cryoglobulins, which precipitate in the cold. In type 1 cryoglobulinemia, the cryoprecipitate contains the M-protein alone, whereas in type 2 cryoglobulinemia, the M-protein frequently has rheumatoid factor activity and is associated with polyclonal IgG or IgA. Type 3 cryoglobulinemia is associated with collagen vascular or chronic inflammatory disease and the cryoprecipitate is composed of polyclonal immunoglobulins (92). The neuropathy in cryoglobulinemia is thought to be due to vasculitis, and the skin is frequently, but not always, involved. The M-protein may have autoantibody activity in addition to its cryoprecipitability (232,233).

NEUROPATHIES ASSOCIATED WITH MYELOMA AND NONMALIGNANT IgG OR IgA MONOCLONAL GAMMOPATHIES

Neuropathy is estimated to occur in 1%–13% of all patients with myeloma (83,96,235). There is a particular association with osteosclerotic myeloma. Peripheral neuropathy is found in approximately 50% of patients with osteosclerotic myeloma and IgG or IgA monoclonal gammopathies. The significance of IgG or IgA monoclonal gammopathies is uncertain in the absence of myeloma, POEMS syndrome, amyloidosis, or cryoglobulinemia.

Neuropathy in Myeloma

Osteosclerosis is found in less than 3% of all myelomas, but approximately 50% of the patients have peripheral neuropathy, which is frequently the presenting complaint (235).

In other patients with MM, neuropathy may result from nerve compression by bony fractures or plasmacytomas, or from infiltrations of nerves by plasma cells, and present as cranial nerve palsies, mononeuritis, or mononeuritis multiplex (115,236). Patients with sensory neuritis or with CIDP have also been described (83,235). In later stages of MM, complicating factors such as renal failure or cachexia could contribute to or be responsible for the development of neuropathy.

Neuropathy in Nonmalignant IgG or IgA Monoclonal Gammopathies

In some cases of nonmalignant IgG or IgA monoclonal gammopathies, the neuropathy may be caused by some of the same mechanisms that are responsible for the neuropathy in myeloma because the nonmalignant monoclonal gammopathy may progress to overt myeloma (43), and nonmalignant gammopathies may be associated with the POEMS syndrome similarly to myeloma (96,98).

Nonmalignant monoclonal gammopathies are found more frequently in patients with neuropathy of otherwise unknown etiology; however, they are also present in approximately 1% of normal adults. The frequency increases with age or in chronic infections or inflammatory diseases, so the association with neuropathy could be coincidental in some. In a randomized, double-blind, sham-pheresis, controlled trial, plasmapheresis was beneficial for patients with neuropathy associated with IgA and IgG MGUS-associated neuropathy (237).

Other causes of neuropathy, particularly inflammatory conditions such as CIDP, should be considered. Patients present with a CIDP-like syndrome, and the association may be coincidental (66,238–240).

CIDP has been associated with IgG and IgA monoclonal gammopathies. These are usually monoclonal gammopathies of undetermined significance, but other disorders, such as CLL, may be present.

Peripheral Neuropathy Associated with Osteosclerotic Myeloma

Osteosclerotic myeloma is a plasma cell dyscrasia characterized by sclerotic bone lesions and a progressive demyelinating neuropathy. Focal sclerotic plasmacytoma accounts for less than 3% of patients with myeloma and produces a focal plasmacytoma in bone (92,241).

Unlike MM, patients rarely complain of bone pain. Fifty percent of patients with osteosclerotic myeloma have a peripheral neuropathy, which is often the presenting symptom. An IgG or IgA monoclonal protein with lambda light chains is usually present. The level of the monoclonal protein is often low and only detected on immunoelectrophoresis. It may be missed with serum protein electrophoresis (241).

Electrophysiologic and pathologic abnormalities are consistent with demyelination and axonal degeneration; patients are frequently misdiagnosed with CIDP.

Osteosclerotic myeloma may be associated with other systemic manifestations, and the term POEMS syndrome designates patients with a *p*olyneuropathy, *o*rganomegaly, *e*ndocrinopathy, *m*-protein, and *s*kin changes. Many patients do not have all of theses features, and edema, which is not in the eponym, is frequent (241). Hyperpigmentation of skin, excessive hair growth, hepatosplenomegaly, papilledema, elevated CSF protein content, hypogonadism, and hypothyroidism are seen in some patients. POEMS syndrome is sometimes associated with non-osteosclerotic myeloma or with nonmalignant monoclonal gammopathy. Vasoactive endothelial growth factor (VEGF) may play a role in the pathogenesis and can be measured in the serum and used as a diagnostic marker (242–244). The osteosclerotic lesion may be difficult to detect. Patients with a monoclonal gammopathy and a demyelinating neuropathy should have a skeletal survey, which is more sensitive than a bone scan, to detect osteosclerotic lesions (92).

Conventional immunomodulatory treatment for CIDP is rarely effective. Radiation, surgical removal of the plasmacytoma, or autologous peripheral blood stem cell transplant may result in improvement of the neuropathy (66,245).

AMYLOID NEUROPATHY

Amyloidosis refers to the accumulation of fibrillar proteins or protein-polysaccharide complexes (67). Amyloid is an insoluble extracellular aggregate of proteins that forms in nerve or other tissues when any of several proteins is produced in excess. Because the fibrils are arranged as insoluble beta-pleated sheets and accumulate with time, amyloid deposition destroys normal tissue architecture. The two principal forms of amyloid protein that cause neuropathy are immunoglobulin light chains in patients with primary amyloidosis and plasma cell dyscrasias, and transthyretin in hereditary amyloidosis.

The capital letter A is used to designate all amyloid proteins, and is followed by the letter abbreviation for the protein form. At least 13 different proteins have been identified. Classes include immunoglobulin-derived (AL) amyloidosis, secondary or reactive (AA) amyloidosis, heredofamilial amyloidoses, and senile systemic amyloidosis. Beta-2-microglobulin-derived amyloidosis has been recognized more recently in patients undergoing long-term hemodialysis with cuprophane membranes (67).

Secondary amyloidosis (AA), due to deposition of amyloid A, an acute-phase reactant, occurs in chronic infections and inflammatory diseases and does not cause peripheral neuropathy (246). The AA fibrils are derived from proteolytic cleavage of a low-molecular-weight protein precursor, serum amyloid A, which is synthesized by hepatocytes and circulates in association with plasma high-density lipoproteins. In the United States, rheumatoid arthritis is the most frequent cause (66). In the hereditary neuropathic amyloidoses, abnormal transthyretin (prealbumin) is deposited in nerves and causes autonomic and peripheral sensory neuropathies. Inheritance is autosomal dominant, except in familial Mediterranean fever (247).

Primary amyloidosis (AL) is caused by systemic deposition of amyloid and is part of the spectrum of plasma cell dyscrasias. The source of AL amyloid is always a single clone of the B lymphocyte. Primary amyloidosis is either idiopathic or secondary to MM or WM, and amyloidosis occurs in 15% of patients with MM (66). AL is the most common form of systemic amyloid deposition (246). After myeloma, primary systemic amyloidosis is the most common hematologic disease associated with MP. Nine percent of patients with an M-protein at a tertiary referral center had primary amyloidosis (247). Amyloid deposits in this form are fragments of antibody light chains, which may be produced by macrophage processing (248). Median age at onset is 65 years (246).

The syndrome is often a painful, small-fiber sensory neuropathy with progressive autonomic failure; symmetric loss of pain, temperature sensation, spared position, and vibratory senses; carpal tunnel syndrome; or some combination of these symptoms. Weakness and weight loss are the most common symptoms of primary amyloidosis (66). Patients usually present with symptoms of numbness or painful paresthesias distally in the hands or feet. The neuropathy progresses proximally in a symmetrical fashion, and the patients then develop motor weakness and autonomic symptoms of orthostatic hypotension, bowel and bladder dysfunction, and impotence. In many cases of systemic amyloidosis, patients present with symptoms of neuropathy, but they can also present with systemic diseases, such as cardiomyopathy, nephrotic syndrome, or gastrointestinal symptoms. Patients also develop macroglossia, purpura, cardiomyopathy, nephrotic syndrome, arthritis, carpal tunnel syndrome, peripheral neuropathy, and autonomic nerve infiltration with postural hypotension, gastrointestinal paresis, and impotence (247,249,250). Eighty-five percent of patients have MP (251), and 15%–20% have distal symmetric polyneuropathy (66). More than 95% have a demonstrable clonal excess of plasma cells in the bone marrow (252). Diagnosis should be suspected in patients with these symptoms and verified by Congo red stain of nerve biopsy or needle aspiration of subcutaneous fat. Rectal biopsy is positive in more than 70% (251). The proteins show apple-green birefringence under polarized light (66). The diagnosis of amyloid neuropathy can be established by histologic demonstration of amyloid in nerve, followed by immunocytochemical characterization of the deposits with the use of antibodies to immunoglobulin light chains or transthyretin. Mutation of the transthyretin gene is detected by DNA analysis. Other hereditary amyloidosis causes, such as apolipoprotein A1 and gelsolin, lead to less severe and less frequent neuropathy.

Electrophoresis of serum and urine with immunofixation can assist in the diagnosis of primary amyloid neuropathy. Patients with primary systemic amyloidosis and neuropathy frequently have an associated monoclonal gammopathy, and it is estimated that 25% of patients with monoclonal gammopathy and neuropathy have amyloidosis (247). In almost all cases, a monoclonal gammopathy can be discovered in the serum or blood of the affected patients. Amyloid neuropathy has been described in all types of monoclonal gammopathies, including in MM, WM, and nonmalignant monoclonal gammopathies, but is more common with IgG or IgA M-proteins. The disease is thought to be caused by the deposition of fragments of immunoglobulin light chains in peripheral nerve and other tissues. The mechanism of light chain deposition in amyloid formation is unknown.

Congestive heart failure (253) and increased serum beta-2-microglobulin (254) carry a poor prognosis, while the presence of peripheral neuropathy as the sole manifestation is associated with a better outcome (85,255). Overall, the median survival is 18 months; 6 months for those with overt congestive heart failure, to 50 months for those with peripheral neuropathy (256).

Liver transplantation has been reported to be beneficial for hereditary amyloidosis (257,258), and high-dose chemotherapy followed by hematopoietic stem cell transplantation has been reported to help some patients with primary amyloidosis (85). Patients that are ineligible for stem cell transplantation based on extensive organ involvement may be treated with melphalan, with or without dexamethasone.

REFERENCES

1. Diaz-Arrastia R, Younger DS, Hair L, et al. Neurolymphomatosis: a clinicopathologic syndrome re-emerges. *Neurology.* 1992;42(6):1136–1141.

2. Jellinger K, Grisold W. Unusual presentation of a primary spinal lymphoma. *J Neurol Neurosurg Psychiatry.* 2002;72:128–129.

3. Walk D, Handelsman A, Beckmann E, et al. Mononeuropathy multiplex due to infiltration of lymphoma in hematologic remission. *Muscle Nerve.* 1998;21(6):823–836.

4. Julien J, Vital C, Rivel J, et al. Primary meningeal B lymphoma presenting as a subacute ascending polyradiculoneuropathy. *J Neurol Neurosurg Psychiatry.* 1991;54(7):610–613.

5. Giannini C. Tumors and tumor-like conditions of peripheral nerve. In: Dyck PJ, Thomas PK eds. *Peripheral neuropathy*, 4th ed. Philadelphia, PA: Elsevier Saunders 2005;(Vol 1&2):2585–2606.

6. Pratt RW, Weimer LH. Medication and toxin-induced peripheral neuropathy. *Semin Neurol.* 2005;25(2):204–216.

7. Zauderer MG, Crew K, Weimer LH, Brafman L, Fuentes D, Sierra A, Hershman DL. Prospective evaluation of neurotoxicity in breast cancer patients treated with adjuvant paclitaxel. *Am Soc Clin Oncol.* 2008 [Abstract].

8. Windebank AJ. Chemotherapeutic neuropathy. *Curr Opin Neurol.* 1999;12:565–571.

9. Quasthoff S, Hartung HP. Chemotherapy-induced peripheral neuropathy. *J Neurol.* 2002;249:9–17.

10. Chaudhry V, Chaudhry M, Crawford TO, Simmons-O'Brien E, Griffin JW. Toxic neuropathy in patients with pre-existing neuropathy. *Neurology.* 2003;60:337–340.

11. Watanabe M, Tsukiyama T, Hatakeyama S. Protection of vincristine-induced neuropathy by WldS expression and the independence of the activity of Nmnat1. *Neurosci Lett.* 2007;411:228–232.

12. Wang MS, Fang G, Culver DG, Davis AA, Rich MM, Glass JD. The WldS protein protects against axonal degeneration: a model of gene therapy for peripheral neuropathy. *Ann Neurol.* 2001;50(6):773–779.

13. Weimer LH. Medication-induced peripheral neuropathy. *Curr Neurol Neurosci Rep.* 2003;3:86–92.

14. Weimer LH, Podwall D. Medication-induced exacerbation of neuropathy in Charcot Marie Tooth disease. *J Neurol Sci.* 2006;242:47–54.

15. Graf WD, Chance PF, Lensch MW, Eng LJ, Lipe HP, Bird TD. Severe vincristine neuropathy in Charcot-Marie-Tooth disease type 1A. *Cancer.* 1996;77:1356–1362.

16. Gill JS, Windebank AJ. Cisplatin-induced apoptosis in rat dorsal root ganglion neurons is associated with attempted entry into the cell cycle. *J Clin Invest.* 1998;101:2842–2850.

17. Ta LE, Espeset L, Podratz J, Windebank AJ. Neurotoxicity of oxaliplatin and cisplatin for dorsal root ganglion neurons correlates with platinum-DNA binding. *Neurotoxicology.* 2006;27(6):992–1002.

18. Krarup-Hansen A, Rietz B, Krarup C, et al. Histology and platinum content of sensory ganglia and sural nerves in patients treated with cisplatin and carboplatin: an autopsy study. *Neuropath Appl Neurobiol.* 1999;25:29–40.

19. Lehky TJ, Leonard GD, Wilson RH, et al. Oxaliplatin-induced neurotoxicity: acute hyperexcitability and chronic neuropathy. *Muscle Nerve.* 2004;29:387–392.

20. Chaudhry V, Eisenberger MA, Sinibaldi VJ, Sheikh K, Griffin JW, Cornblath DR. A prospective study of suramin-induced peripheral neuropathy. *Brain.* 1996;119:2039–2052.

21. Soliven B, Dhand UK, Kobayashi K, et al. Evaluation of neuropathy in patients on suramin treatment. *Muscle Nerve.* 1997;20:83–91.

22. Peltier AC, Russell JW. Recent advances in drug-induced neuropathies. *Curr Opin Neurol .*2002;15:633–638.

23. Russell JW, Gill JS, Sorenson EJ, Schultz DA, Windebank AJ. Suramin-induced neuropathy in an animal model. *J Neurol Sci.* 2001;192:71–80.

24. Gill JS, Windebank AJ. Ceramide initiates NFkappaB-mediated caspase activation in neuronal apoptosis. *Neurobiol Dis.* 2000;7:448–461.

25. Kane RC, Bross PF, Farrell AT, Pazdur R. Velcade: U.S. FDA approval for the treatment of multiple myeloma progressing on prior therapy. *Oncologist.* 2003;8:508–513.

26. Davis NB, Taber DA, Ansari RH, et al. Phase II trial of PS-341 in patients with renal cell cancer: a University of Chicago phase II consortium study. *J Clin Oncol.* 2004;22:115–119.

27. Badros A, Goloubeva O, Dalal JS, et al. Neurotoxicity of bortezomib therapy in multiple myeloma: a single-center experience and review of the literature. *Cancer.* 2007;110(5):1042–1049.

28. Giannini F, Volpi N, Rossi S, Passero S, Fimiani M, Cerase A. Thalidomide-induced neuropathy: a ganglionopathy? *Neurology.* 2003;60:877–878.

29. Briani C, Zara G, Rondinone R, et al. Thalidomide neurotoxicity: prospective study in patients with lupus erythematosus. *Neurology.* 2004;62:2288–2290.

30. Chaudhry V, Cornblath DR, Corse A, Freimer M, Simmons-O'Brien E, Vogelsang G. Thalidomide-induced neuropathy. *Neurology.* 2002;59:1872–1875

31. Cavaletti G, Beronio A, Reni L, et al. Thalidomide sensory neurotoxicity: a clinical and neurophysiologic study. *Neurology.* 2004;62:2291–2293.

32. Molloy FM, Floeter MK, Syed NA, et al. Thalidomide neuropathy in patients treated for metastatic prostate cancer. *Muscle Nerve.* 2001;24:1050–1057.

33. Plasmati R, Pastorelli F, Cavo M, et al. Neuropathy in multiple myeloma treated with thalidomide: a prospective study. *Neurology.* 2007;69(6):573–581.

34. Hilkens PH, Verweij J, Stoter G, Vecht CJ, van Putten WL, van den Bent MJ. Peripheral neurotoxicity induced by docetaxel. *Neurology.* 1996;46:104–108.

35. van Gerven JM, Moll JW, van den Bent MJ, et al. Paclitaxel (Taxol) induces cumulative mild neurotoxicity. *Eur J Cancer.* 1994;30A:1074–1077.

36. Robinson DM, Keating GM. Albumin-bound Paclitaxel: in metastatic breast cancer. *Drugs.* 2006;66(7):941–948.

37. Gedlicka C, Kornek GV, Schmid K, Scheithauer W. Amelioration of docetaxel/cisplatin induced polyneuropathy by alpha-lipoic acid. *Ann Oncol.* 2003;14:339–340.

38. Pronzato P. New therapeutic options for chemotherapy-resistant metastatic breast cancer: the epothilones. *Drugs.* 2008;68(2):139–146.

39. Denduluri N, Swain SM. Ixabepilone for the treatment of solid tumors: a review of clinical data. *Expert Opin Investig Drugs.* 2008;17(3):423–435.

40. Zhuang SH, Agrawal M, Edgerly M, et al. A Phase I clinical trial of ixabepilone (BMS-247550), an epothilone B analog, administered intravenously on a daily schedule for 3 days. *Cancer.* 2005;103(9):1932–1938.

41. Roberts JA, Jenison EL, Kim K, et al. A randomized, multi-center, double-blind, placebo controlled, dose-finding study of ORG 2766 in the prevention or delay of cisplatin-induced neuropathies in women with ovarian cancer. *Gynecol Oncol.* 1997;67:172–177.

42. Chattopadhyay M, Goss J, Wolfe D, et al. Protective effect of herpes simplex virus-mediated neurotrophin gene transfer in cisplatin neuropathy. *Brain.* 2004;127:929–939.

43. Kyle RA. Monoclonal gammopathy of undetermined significance—Natural-history in 241 cases. *Am J Med.* 1978;64:814–826.

44. Latov N. Pathogenesis and therapy of neuropathies associated with monoclonal gammopathies. *Ann Neurol.* 1995;37:S32–S42.

45. Longsworth LG, Shedlovsky T, MacInnes DA. Electrophoretic patterns of normal and pathological human blood serum and plasma. *J Exp Med.* 1939;70:399–413.

46. Kohn J. A Cellulose acetate supporting medium for zone electrophoresis. *Clin Chim Acta.* 1957;2:297–303.

47. Kyle RA, Rajkumar SV. Monoclonal gammopathy of undetermined significance. *Br J Haematol.* 2006;134:573–589.

48. Saleun JP, Vicariot M, Deroff P, Morin JF. Monoclonal gammopathies in the adult-population of Finistere, France. *J Clin Pathol.* 1982;35:63–68.

49. Axelsson U, Bachmann R, Hallen J. Frequency of pathological proteins (M-Components) in 6,995 sera from an adult population. *Acta Med Scand.* 1966;179:235–247.

50. Vladutiu AO. Prevalence of M-proteins in serum of hospitalized-patients—physicians response to finding M-proteins in serum-protein electrophoresis. *Ann Clin Lab Sci.* 1987;17:157–161.

51. Malacrida V, Defrancesco D, Banfi G, Porta FA, Riches PG. Laboratory investigation of monoclonal gammopathy during 10 years of screening in a General-Hospital. *J Clin Pathol.* 1987;40:793–797.

52. Kyle RA, Therneau TM, Rajkumar SV, et al. Prevalence of monoclonal gammopathy of undetermined significance. *N Engl J Med.* 2006;354:1362–1369.

53. Lerner AB, Barnum CP, Watson CJ. Studies of cryoglobulins .2. The spontaneous precipitation of protein from serum at 5-degrees-C in various disease states. *Am J Med Sci.* 1947;214:416–421.

54. Cream JJ. Cryoglobulins in vasculitis. *Clin Exp Immunol.* 1972;10:117–124.

55. Brouet JC, Danon F, Seligmann M. Immunochemical classification of human cryoglobulins. In: Chenas F, editor. *Cryoproteins.* Grenoble: Colloque; 1978:13–19.

56. Nightingale SD, Pelley RP, Delaney NL, et al. Inheritance of mixed cryoglobulinemia. *Am J Hum Genet.* 1981;33:735–744.

57. Brouet JC, Clauvel JP, Danon F, Klein M, Seligmann M. Biologic and clinical significance of cryoglobulins. A report of 86 cases. *Am J Med.* 1974;57:775–788.

58. Garcia-Bragado F, Fernandez JM, Navarro C, Villar M, Bonaventura I. Peripheral neuropathy in essential mixed cryoglobulinemia. *Arch Neurol.* 1988;45:1210–1214.

59. Ferri C, La Civita L, Cirafisi C, et al. Peripheral neuropathy in mixed cryoglobulinemia: clinical and electrophysiologic investigations. *J Rheumatol.* 1992;19:889–895.

60. Meltzer M, Franklin EC. Cryoglobulinemia—a study of twenty-nine patients. I. IgG and IgM cryoglobulins and factors affecting cryoprecipitability. *Am J Med.* 1966; 40:828–836.

61. Middaugh CR, Lawson EQ, Litman GW, Tisel WA, Mood DA, Rosenberg A. Thermodynamic basis for the abnormal solubility of monoclonal cryoimmunoglobulins. *J Biol Chem.* 1980;255:6532–6534.

62. Lippa CF, Chad DA, Smith TW, Kaplan MH, Hammer K. Neuropathy associated with cryoglobulinemia. *Muscle Nerve.* 1986;9:626–631.

63. Khella SL, Frost S, Hermann GA, et al. Hepatitis C infection, cryoglobulinemia, and vasculitic neuropathy. Treatment with interferon alfa: case report and literature review. *Neurology.* 1995;45:407–411.

64. Abramsky O, Slavin S. Neurologic manifestations in patients with mixed cryoglobulinemia. *Neurology.* 1974;24:245–249.

65. Stricker RB, Sanders KA, Owen WF, Kiprov DD, Miller RG. Mononeuritis multiplex associated with cryoglobulinemia in HIV infection. *Neurology.* 1992;42:2103–2105.

66. Gordon P.H., Brannagan TH, Latov N. Neurological manifestations of paraproteinemia and cryoglobulinemia. In: Aminoff MJ, Goetz CG, eds. *Handbook of Clinical Neurology.* Elsevier Science; Amsterdam. 1998:431–459.

67. Barlogie B, Alexanian R, Jagannath S. Plasma-cell dyscrasias. *JAMA.* 1992;268:2946–2951.

68. Fine JM, Lambin P, Leroux P. Frequency of monoclonal gammapathy ('M components') in 13,400 sera from blood donors. *Vox Sang.* 1972;23:336–343.

69. Radl J. Benign monoclonal gammopathy. In: Melchers F, Potter M, eds. *Mechanisms in B-Cell Neoplasia.* Berlin: Springer; 1985:p. 221–224.

70. Kahn SN, Riches PG, Kohn J. Paraproteinaemia in neurological disease: incidence, associations, and classification of monoclonal immunoglobulins. *J Clin Pathol.* 1980;33:617–621.

71. Fine JM, Lambin P, Muller JY. The evolution of asymptomatic monoclonal gammopathies. A follow-up of 20 cases over periods of 3–14 years. *Acta Med Scand.* 1979;205:339–341.

72. van de Poel MH, Coebergh JW, Hillen HF. Malignant transformation of monoclonal gammopathy of undetermined significance among out-patients of a community hospital in southeastern Netherlands. *Br J Haematol.* 1995;91:121–125.

73. Giraldo MP, Rubio-Felix D, Perella M, Gracia JA, Bergua JM, Giralt M. [Monoclonal gammopathies of undetermined significance. Clinical course and biological aspects of 397 cases]. *Sangre (Barc).* 1991;36:377–382.

74. Axelsson U. A 20-year follow-up study of 64 subjects with M-components. *Acta Med Scand.* 1986;219:519–522.

75. Rajkumar SV, Kyle RA, Therneau TM, et al. Serum free light chain ratio is an independent risk factor for progression in monoclonal gammopathy of undetermined significance. *Blood.* 2005;106:812–817.

76. Rajkumar SV, Kyle RA. Multiple myeloma: diagnosis and treatment. *Mayo Clin Proc.* 2005;80:1371–1382.

77. Osserman EF. Plasma-cell myeloma. II. Clinical aspects. *N Engl J Med.* 1959;261:952–960.

78. Bataille R, Chappard D, Klein B. Mechanisms of bone lesions in multiple myeloma. *Hematol Oncol Clin North Am.* 1992;6:285–295.

79. Durie BG, Salmon SE. A clinical staging system for multiple myeloma. Correlation of measured myeloma cell mass with presenting clinical features, response to treatment, and survival. *Cancer.* 1975;36:842–854.

80. Jacobson DR, Zolla-Pazner S. Immunosuppression and infection in multiple myeloma. *Semin Oncol.* 1986;13:282–290.

81. Hernandez JA, Land KJ, McKenna RW. Leukemias, myeloma, and other lymphoreticular neoplasms. *Cancer.* 1995;75:381–394.

82. Greipp PR. Prognosis in myeloma. *Mayo Clin Proc.* 1994;69:895–902.

83. Kelly JJ, Jr., Kyle RA, Miles JM, O'Brien PC, Dyck PJ. The spectrum of peripheral neuropathy in myeloma. *Neurology.* 1981;31:24–31.

84. Conklin R, Alexanian R. Clinical classification of plasma cell myeloma. *Arch Intern Med.* 1975;135:139–143.

85. Rajkumar SV, Dispenzieri A, Kyle RA. Monoclonal gammopathy of undetermined significance, Waldenström macroglobulinemia, AL amyloidosis, and related plasma cell disorders: diagnosis and treatment. *Mayo Clin Proc.* 2006;81:693–703.

86. Dimopoulos MA, Goldstein J, Fuller L, Delasalle K, Alexanian R. Curability of solitary bone plasmacytoma. *J Clin Oncol.* 1992;10:587–590.

87. Holland J, Trenkner DA, Wasserman TH, Fineberg B. Plasmacytoma. Treatment results and conversion to myeloma. *Cancer.* 1992;69:1513–1517.

88. Ellis PA, Colls BM. Solitary plasmacytoma of bone: clinical features, treatment and survival. *Hematol Oncol.* 1992;10:207–211.

89. Alexanian R. Localized and indolent myeloma. *Blood.* 1980;56:521–525.

90. Chak LY, Cox RS, Bostwick DG, Hoppe RT. Solitary plasmacytoma of bone: treatment, progression, and survival. *J Clin Oncol.* 1987;5:1811–1815.

91. Delauche-Cavallier MC, Laredo JD, Wybier M, et al. Solitary plasmacytoma of the spine. Long-term clinical course. *Cancer.* 1988;61:1707–1714.

92. Kelly JJ, Kyle RA, Miles JM, Dyck PJ. Osteosclerotic myeloma and peripheral neuropathy. *Neurology.* 1983;33:202–210.

93. Soubrier MJ, Dubost JJ, Sauvezie BJ. POEMS syndrome: a study of 25 cases and a review of the literature. French Study Group on POEMS Syndrome. *Am J Med.* 1994;97:543–553.

94. Shimpo S. [Solitary myeloma causing polyneuritis and endocrine disorders]. *Nippon Rinsho.* 1968;26:2444–2456.

95. Crow RS. Peripheral neuritis in myelomatosis. *Br Med J.* 1956;2:802–804.

96. Miralles GD, O'Fallon JR, Talley NJ. Plasma-cell dyscrasia with polyneuropathy. The spectrum of POEMS syndrome. *N Engl J Med.* 1992;327:1919–1923.

97. Waldenstrom JG, Adner A, Gydell K, Zettervall O. Osteosclerotic "plasmocytoma" with polyneuropathy, hypertrichosis and diabetes. *Acta Med Scand.* 1978;203:297–303.

98. Nakanishi T, Sobue I, Toyokura Y, et al. The Crow-Fukase syndrome: a study of 102 cases in Japan. *Neurology.* 1984;34:712–720.

99. Takatsuki K, Sanada I. Plasma cell dyscrasia with polyneuropathy and endocrine disorder: clinical and laboratory features of 109 reported cases. *Jpn J Clin Oncol.* 1983;13:543–555.

100. Mandler RN, Kerrigan DP, Smart J, Kuis W, Villiger P, Lotz M. Castlemans disease in POEMS syndrome with elevated interleukin-6. *Cancer.* 1992;69:2697–2703.

101. Gherardi RK, Belec L, Fromont G, et al. Elevated levels of interleukin-1 beta (IL-1 beta) and IL-6 in serum and increased production of IL-1 beta mRNA in lymph nodes of patients with polyneuropathy, organomegaly, endocrinopathy, M protein, and skin changes (POEMS) syndrome. *Blood.* 1994;83:2587–2593.

102. Dimopoulos MA, Alexanian R. Waldenstrom's macroglobulinemia. *Blood.* 1994;83:1452–1459.

103. Gertz MA, Kyle RA, Noel P. Primary systemic amyloidosis—a rare complication of immunoglobulin-M monoclonal gammopathies and Waldenstrom macroglobulinemia. *J Clin Oncol.* 1993;11:914–920.

104. Moulopoulos LA, Dimopoulos MA, Varma DG, et al. Waldenstrom macroglobulinemia: MR imaging of the spine and CT of the abdomen and pelvis. *Radiology.* 1993;188:669–673.

105. Facon T, Brouillard M, Duhamel A, et al. Prognostic factors in Waldenstrom macroglobulinemia: a report of 167 cases. *J Clin Oncol.* 1993;11:1553–1558.

106. MacKenzie MR, Fudenberg HH. Macroglobulinemia: an analysis for forty patients. *Blood.* 1972;39:874–889.

107. Kelly JJ, Adelman LS, Berkman E, Bhan I. Polyneuropathies associated with IgM monoclonal gammopathies. *Arch Neurol.* 1988;45:1355–1359.

108. Tefferi A, Phyliky RL. A clinical update on chronic lymphocytic leukemia. I. Diagnosis and prognosis. *Mayo Clin Proc.* 1992;67:349–353.

109. Faguet GB. Chronic lymphocytic leukemia: an updated review. *J Clin Oncol.* 1994;12:1974–1990.

110. Gale RP, Foon KA. Chronic lymphocytic leukemia. Recent advances in biology and treatment. *Ann Intern Med.* 1985;103:101–120.

111. Faguet GB, Marti GE, Agee JF, Bertin P. CD5 positive and negative B-CLL. Evidence supporting phenotypic heterogeneity in B-chronic lymphocytic leukemia (B-CLL). *Ann NY Acad Sci.* 1992;651:470–473.

112. Bernstein ZP, Fitzpatrick JE, O'Donnell A, Han T, Foon KA, Bhargava A. Clinical significance of monoclonal proteins in chronic lymphocytic leukemia. *Leukemia.* 1992;6:1243–1245.

113. Fialkow PJ, Najfeld V, Reddy AL, Singer J, Steinmann L. Chronic lymphocytic leukaemia: clonal origin in a committed B-lymphocyte progenitor. *Lancet.* 1978;2:444–446.

114. Cramer SC, Glaspy JA, Efird JT, Louis DN. Chronic lymphocytic leukemia and the central nervous system: a clinical and pathological study. *Neurology.* 1996;46:19–25.

115. Silverstein D, Doniger DE. Neurologic complications of myelomatosis. *Arch Neurol.* 1963;9:534–544.

116. Lisak RP, Mitchell M, Zweiman B, Orrechio E, Asbury AK. Guillain-Barre syndrome and Hodgkin's disease: three cases with immunological studies. *Ann Neurol.* 1977;1:72–78.

117. Latov N, Hays AP, Sherman WH. Peripheral neuropathy and anti-Mag antibodies. *Crit Rev Neurobiol.* 1988;3:301–332.

118. Suarez GA, Kelly JJ, Jr. Polyneuropathy associated with monoclonal gammopathy of undetermined significance: further evidence that IgM-MGUS neuropathies are different than IgG-MGUS. *Neurology.* 1993;43:1304–1308.

119. Gosselin S, Kyle RA, Dyck PJ. Neuropathy associated with monoclonal gammopathies of undetermined significance. *Ann Neurol.* 1991;30:54–61.

120. Yeung KB, Thomas PK, King RH, et al. The clinical spectrum of peripheral neuropathies associated with benign monoclonal IgM, IgG and IgA paraproteinaemia. Comparative clinical, immunological and nerve biopsy findings. *J Neurol.* 1991;238:383–391.

121. Nobileorazio E, Marmiroli P, Baldini L, et al. Peripheral neuropathy in macroglobulinemia—incidence and antigen-specificity of M-proteins. *Neurology.* 1987;37:1506–1514.

122. Logothetis J, Silverstein P, Coe J. Neurologic aspects of Waldenstrom's macroglobulinemia; report of a case. *Arch Neurol.* 1960;3:564–573.

123. Harbs H, Arfmann M, Frick E, et al. Reactivity of sera and isolated monoclonal IgM from patients with Waldenstrom's macroglobulinaemia with peripheral nerve myelin. *J Neurol.* 1985;232:43–48.

124. Kyle RA, Garton JP. The spectrum of IgM monoclonal gammopathy in 430 cases. *Mayo Clin Proc.* 1987;62:719–731.

125. Ince PG, Shaw PJ, Fawcett PR, Bates D. Demyelinating neuropathy due to primary IgM kappa B cell lymphoma of peripheral nerve. *Neurology.* 1987;37:1231–1235.

126. Arseth S, Ofstad E, Torvik A. Macroglobulinaemia Waldenstrom. A case with haemolytic syndrome and involvement of the nervous system. *Acta Med Scand.* 1961;169:691–699.

127. Nobileorazio E, Latov N, Hays AP, et al. Neuropathy and anti-Mag antibodies without detectable serum M-protein. *Neurology.* 1984;34:218–221.

128. Nobile-Orazio E, Francomano E, Daverio R, et al. Anti-myelin-associated glycoprotein IgM antibody titers in neuropathy associated with macroglobulinemia. *Ann Neurol.* 1989;26:543–550.

129. Latov N, Hays AP, Donofrio PD, et al. Monoclonal IgM with unique specificity to gangliosides Gm1 and Gd1B and to lacto-N-tetraose associated with human motor neuron disease. *Neurology.* 1988;38:763–768.

130. Pedersen SF, Pullman SL, Latov N, Brannagan TH. Physiological tremor analysis of patients with anti-myelin-associated glycoprotein associated neuropathy and tremor. *Muscle Nerve.* 1997;20:38–44.

131. Barbieri S, Nobile-Orazio E, Baldini L, Fayoumi Z, Manfredini E, Scarlato G. Visual evoked potentials in patients with neuropathy and macroglobulinemia. *Ann Neurol.* 1987;22:663–666.

132. Trojaborg W, Hays AP, Vandenberg L, Younger DS, Latov N. Motor conduction parameters in neuropathies associated with anti-Mag antibodies and other types of demyelinating and axonal neuropathies. *Muscle Nerve.* 1995;18:730–735.

133. Briani C, Brannagan TH, Trojaborg W, Latov N. Chronic inflammatory demyelinating polyneuropathy. *Neuromuscul Disord.* 1996;6:311–325.

134. Kaku DA, England JD, Sumner AJ. Distal accentuation of conduction slowing in polyneuropathy associated with antibodies to myelin-associated glycoprotein and sulfated glucuronyl paragloboside. *Brain.* 1994;117:941–947.

135. Kelly JJ. The Electrodiagnostic findings in polyneuropathies associated with IgM monoclonal gammopathies. *Muscle Nerve.* 1990;13:1113–1117.

136. Gondim FA, De Sousa EA, Latov N, Sander HW, Chin RL, Brannagan TH. Anti-MAG/SGPG associated neuropathy does not commonly cause distal nerve temporal dispersion. *J Neurol Neurosurg Psychiatry.* 2007;78:902–904.

137. Hays AP, Lee SSL, Latov N. Immune reactive C3D on the surface of myelin sheaths in neuropathy. *J Neuroimmunol.* 1988;18:231–244.

138. Takatsu M, Hays AP, Latov N, et al. Immunofluorescence study of patients with neuropathy and IgM M proteins. *Ann Neurol.* 1985;18:173–181.

139. Vital A, Vital C, Julien J, Baquey A, Steck AJ. Polyneuropathy associated with IgM monoclonal gammopathy. Immunological and pathological study in 31 patients. *Acta Neuropathol.* 1989;79:160–167.

140. Monaco S, Bonetti B, Ferrari S, et al. Complement-mediated demyelination in patients with IgM monoclonal gammopathy and polyneuropathy. *N Engl J Med.* 1990;322:649–652.

141. Drachman DB. How to recognize an antibody-mediated autoimmune disease: criteria. *Res Publ Assoc Res Nerv Ment Dis.* 1990;68:183–186.

142. Tatum AH. experimental paraprotein neuropathy, demyelination by passive transfer of human-IgM anti-myelin-associated glycoprotein. *Ann Neurol.* 1993;33:502–506.

143. Lunn MPT, Crawford TO, Hughes RAC, Griffin JW, Sheikh KA. Anti-myelin-associated glycoprotein antibodies alter neurofilament spacing. *Brain.* 2002;125:904–911.

144. Nobile-Orazio E, Meucci N, Baldini L, Di Troia A, Scarlato G. Long-term prognosis of neuropathy associated with anti-MAG IgM M-proteins and its relationship to immune therapies. *Brain.* 2000;123:710–717.

145. Gorson KC, Ropper AH, Weinberg DH, Weinstein R. Treatment experience in patients with anti-myelin-associated glycoprotein neuropathy. *Muscle Nerve.* 2001;24:778–786.

146. Leger JM, Oksenhendler E, Bussel A, et al. Treatment by chlorambucil with without plasma exchanges of polyneuropathy associated with monoclonal IgM—a prospective randomized control study in 44 patients. *Neurology.* 1993;43:A215–A216.

147. Meier C, Roberts K, Steck A, Hess C, Miloni E, Tschopp L. Polyneuropathy in Waldenstrom's macroglobulinaemia: reduction of endoneurial IgM-deposits after treatment with chlorambucil and plasmapheresis. *Acta Neuropathol.* 1984;64:297–307.

148. Haas DC, Tatum AH. Plasmapheresis alleviates neuropathy accompanying IgM anti-myelin-associated glycoprotein paraproteinemia. *Ann Neurol.* 1988;23:394–396.

149. Sherman WH, Latov N, Lange D, Hays R, Younger D. Fludarabine for IgM antibody-mediated neuropathies. *Ann Neurol.* 1994;36:326–327.

150. Wilson HC, Lunn MPT, Schey S, Hughes RAC. Successful treatment of IgM paraproteinaemic neuropathy with fludarabine. *J Neurol Neurosurg Psychiatry.* 1999;66:575–580.

151. Dalakas MC, Quarles RH, Farrer RG, et al. A controlled study of intravenous immunoglobulin in demyelinating neuropathy with IgM gammopathy. *Ann Neurol.* 1996;40:792–795.

152. Comi G, Roveri L, Swan A, et al. A randomised controlled trial of intravenous immunoglobulin in IgM paraprotein associated demyelinating neuropathy. *J Neurol.* 2002;249:1370–1377.

153. Renaud S, Gregor M, Fuhr P, et al. Rituximab in the treatment of polyneuropathy associated with anti-MAG antibodies. *Muscle Nerve.* 2003;27:611–615.

154. Levine TD, Pestronk A. IgM antibody-related polyneuropathies: B-cell depletion chemotherapy using rituximab. *Neurology.* 1999;52:1701–1704.

155. Pestronk A, Florence J, Miller T, Choksi R, Al Lozi MT, Levine TD. Treatment of IgM antibody associated polyneuropathies using rituximab. *J Neurol Neurosurg Psychiatry.* 2003;74:485–489.

156. Dalakas MC, Rakocevic G, Salajegheh MK, et al. A double-blind, placebo-controlled study of rituximab in patients with anti-MAG antibody-demyelinating polyneuropathy (A-MAG-DP). *Neurology.* 2007;68:A214.

157. Freddo L, Yu RK, Latov N, et al. Gangliosides Gm1 and Gd1B are antigens for IgM M-protein in a patient with motor-neuron disease. *Neurology.* 1986;36:454–458.

158. Pestronk A, Cornblath DR, Ilyas AA, et al. A treatable multifocal motor neuropathy with antibodies to Gm1 ganglioside. *Ann Neurol.* 1988;24:73–78.

159. Pestronk A, Chaudhry V, Feldman EL, et al. Lower motorneuron syndromes defined by patterns of weakness, nerve-conduction abnormalities, and high titers of antiglycolipid antibodies. *Ann Neurol.* 1990;27:316–326.

160. Kinsella LJ, Lange DJ, Trojaborg W, Sadiq SA, Younger DS, Latov N. Clinical and electrophysiologic correlates of elevated anti-Gm(1) antibody-titers. *Neurology.* 1994;44:1278–1282.

161. Lange DJ, Trojaborg W, Latov N, et al. Multifocal motor neuropathy with conduction block—is it a distinct clinical entity. *Neurology.* 1992;42:497–505.

162. Azulay JP, Blin O, Pouget J, et al. Intravenous immunoglobulin treatment in patients with motor-neuron syndromes associated with Anti-Gm1 antibodies—a double-blind, placebo-controlled study. *Neurology.* 1994;44:429–432.

163. Adams D, Kuntzer T, Burger D, et al. Predictive value of anti-GM1 ganglioside antibodies in neuromuscular diseases: a study of 180 sera. *J Neuroimmunol.* 1991;32:223–230.

164. Apostolski S, Latov N. Clinical syndromes associated with anti-GM1 antibodies. *Semin Neurol.* 1993;13:264–268.

165. Kaji R, Shibasaki H, Kimura J. Multifocal demyelinating motor neuropathy—cranial nerve involvement and immunoglobulin therapy. *Neurology.* 1992;42:506–509.

166. Magistris M, Roth G. Motor Neuropathy with Multifocal Persistent Conduction Blocks. *Muscle Nerve.* 1992;15:1056–1057.

167. Beydoun SR, Copeland D. Bilateral phrenic neuropathy as a presenting feature of multifocal motor neuropathy with conduction block. *Muscle Nerve.* 2000;23:556–559.

168. Parry GJ. Motor neuropathy with multifocal persistent conduction blocks (a reply). *Muscle Nerve.* 1992;15:1057.

169. Kaji R, Mezaki T, Hirota N, Kimura J, Shibasaki H. Multifocal motor neuropathy with exaggerated deep tendon reflex. *Neurology.* 1994;44:A180.

170. Evangelista T, Carvalho M, Conceicao I, Pinto A, Luis MDS. Motor neuropathies mimicking amyotrophic lateral sclerosis motor neuron disease. *J Neurol Sci.* 1996;139:95–98.

171. Brannagan TH, III. Immune-mediated chronic demyelinating polyneuropathies. In: Kalman B, Brannagan TH, III, eds. *Neuroimmunology in Clinical Practice.* Oxford: Blackwell; 2008:123–138.

172. Corbo M, Quattrini A, Latov N, Hays AP. Localization of Gm1 and Gal(Beta-1–3)Galnac antigenic determinants in peripheral-nerve. *Neurology.* 1993;43:809–814.

173. Willison HJ, Yuki N. Peripheral neuropathies and anti-glycolipid antibodies. *Brain.* 2002;125:2591–2625.

174. Svennerholm L. Designation and schematic structure of gangliosides and allied glycosphingolipids. *Prog Brain Res.* 1994;101:XI–XIV.

175. Ilyas AA, Willison HJ, Dalakas MC, Whitaker JN, Quarles RH. Identification and characterization of gangliosides reacting with IgM paraproteins in three patients with neuropathy associated with biclonal gammopathy. *J Neurochem.* 1988;51:851–858.

176. Sadiq SA, Thomas FP, Kilidireas K, et al. The spectrum of neurologic disease associated with anti-Gm1 antibodies. *Neurology.* 1990;40:1067–1072.

177. Baba H, Daune GC, Ilyas AA, et al. Anti-GM1 ganglioside antibodies with differing fine specificities in patients with multifocal motor neuropathy. *J Neuroimmunol.* 1989;25:143–150.

178. Kusunoki S, Shimizu T, Matsumura K, Maemura K, Mannen T. Motor dominant neuropathy and IgM paraproteinemia: the IgM M-protein binds to specific gangliosides. *J Neuroimmunol.* 1989;21:177–181.

179. Noguchi M, Mori K, Yamazaki S, Suda K, Sato N, Oshimi K. Multifocal motor neuropathy caused by a B-cell lymphoma producing a monoclonal IgM autoantibody against peripheral nerve myelin glycolipids GM1 and GD1b. *Br J Haematol.* 2003;123:600–605.

180. Stern BV, Baehring JM, Kleopa KA, Hochberg FH. Multifocal motor neuropathy with conduction block associated with metastatic lymphoma of the nervous system. *J Neurooncol.* 2006;78:81–84.

181. Garcia-Moreno JM, Castilla JM, Garcia-Escudero A, Izquierdo G. [Multifocal motor neuropathy with conduction blocks and prurigo nodularis. A paraneoplastic syndrome in a patient with non-Hodgkin B-cell lymphoma?]. *Neurologia.* 2004;19:220–224.

182. Apostolski S, Sadiq SA, Hays A, et al. Identification of Gal(beta 1–3)GalNAc bearing glycoproteins at the nodes of Ranvier in peripheral nerve. *J Neurosci Res.* 1994;38:134–141.

183. Thomas FP, Adapon PH, Goldberg GP, Latov N, Hays AP. Localization of neural epitopes that bind to IgM monoclonal autoantibodies (M-proteins) from two patients with motor neuron disease. *J Neuroimmunol.* 1989;21:31–39.

184. Adams D, Kuntzer T, Steck AJ, Lobrinus A, Janzer RC, Regli F. Motor conduction block and high titres of anti-GM1 ganglioside antibodies: pathological evidence of a motor neuropathy

in a patient with lower motor neuron syndrome. *J Neurol Neurosurg Psychiatry.* 1993;56:982–987.

185. Ogawa-Goto K, Funamoto N, Ohta Y, Abe T, Nagashima K. Myelin gangliosides of human peripheral nervous system: an enrichment of GM1 in the motor nerve myelin isolated from cauda equina. *J Neurochem.* 1992;59:1844–1849.

186. Ogawa-Goto K, Funamoto N, Abe T, Nagashima K. Different ceramide compositions of gangliosides between human motor and sensory nerves. *J Neurochem.* 1990;55:1486–1493.

187. Thomas FP, Trojaborg W, Nagy C, et al. Experimental auto-immune neuropathy with anti-GM1 antibodies and immunoglobulin deposits at the nodes of Ranvier. *Acta Neuropathol.* 1991;82:378–383.

188. Santoro M, Uncini A, Corbo M, et al. Experimental conduction block induced by serum from a patient with anti-GM1 antibodies. *Ann Neurol.* 1992;31:385–390.

189. Heiman-Patterson T, Krupa T, Thompson P, Nobile-Orazio E, Tahmoush AJ, Shy ME. Anti-GM1/GD1b M-proteins damage human spinal cord neurons co-cultured with muscle. *J Neurol Sci.* 1993;120:38–45.

190. Roberts M, Willison HJ, Vincent A, Newsom-Davis J. Multifocal motor neuropathy human sera block distal motor nerve conduction in mice. *Ann Neurol.* 1995;38:111–118.

191. Leger JM, Chassande B, Musset L, Meininger V, Bouche P, Baumann N. Intravenous immunoglobulin therapy in multifocal motor neuropathy: a double-blind, placebo-controlled study. *Brain.* 2001;124:145–153.

192. vandenBerg LH, Kerkhoff H, Oey PL, et al. Treatment of multifocal motor neuropathy with high-dose intravenous immunoglobulins—A double-blind, placebo-controlled study. *J Neurol Neurosurg Psychiatry.* 1995;59:248–252.

193. Azulay JP, Rihet P, Pouget J, et al. Long term follow up of multifocal motor neuropathy with conduction block under treatment. *J Neurol Neurosurg Psychiatry.* 1997;62:391–394.

194. Chaudhry V, Corse AM, Cornblath DR, et al. multifocal motor neuropathy—response to human immune globulin. *Ann Neurol.* 1993;33:237–242.

195. Chaudhry V, Corse AM, Cornblath DR, Kuncl RW, Freimer ML, Griffin JW. Multifocal motor neuropathy—electrodiagnostic features. *Muscle Nerve.* 1994;17:198–205.

196. Federico P, Zochodne DW, Hahn AF, Brown WF, Feasby TE. Multifocal motor neuropathy improved by IVIg—randomized, double-blind, placebo-controlled study. *Neurology.* 2000;55:1256–1262.

197. Chad DA, Hammer K, Sargent J. Slow resolution of multifocal weakness and fasciculation—a reversible motor-neuron syndrome. *Neurology.* 1986;36:1260–1263.

198. Feldman EL, Bromberg MB, Albers JW, Pestronk A. Immunosuppressive treatment in multifocal motor neuropathy. *Ann Neurol.* 1991;30:397–401.

199. Krarup C, Sethi RK. Idiopathic brachial-plexus lesion with conduction block of the ulnar nerve. *Electroencephalogr Clin Neurophysiol.* 1989;72:259–267.

200. Kaji R, Oka N, Tsuji T, et al. Pathological findings at the site of conduction block in multifocal motor neuropathy. *Ann Neurol.* 1993;33:152–158.

201. vandenBerg LH, Lokhorst H, Wokke JHJ. Pulsed high-dose dexamethasone is not effective in patients with multifocal motor neuropathy. *Neurology.* 1997;48:1135.

202. Donaghy M, Mills KR, Boniface SJ, et al. Pure motor demyelinating neuropathy—deterioration after steroid treatment and improvement with intravenous immunoglobulin. *J Neurol Neurosurg Psychiatry.* 1994;57:778–783.

203. Thomas PK, Claus D, Jaspert A, et al. Focal upper limb demyelinating neuropathy. *Brain.* 1996;119:765–774.

204. Carpo M, Cappellari A, Mora G, et al. Deterioration of multifocal motor neuropathy after plasma exchange. *Neurology.* 1998;50:1480–1482.

205. Finsterer J, Derfler K. Immunoadsorption in multifocal motor neuropathy. *J Immunother.* 1999;22:441–442.

206. Willison HJ, O'Leary CP, Veitch J, et al. The clinical and laboratory features of chronic sensory ataxic neuropathy with anti-disialosyl IgM antibodies. *Brain.* 2001;124:1968–1977.

207. Yuki N, Miyatani N, Sato S, et al. Acute relapsing sensory neuropathy associated with IgM antibody against B-series gangliosides containing a GalNAc beta 1–4(Gal3–2 alpha NeuAc8–2 alpha NeuAc)beta 1 configuration. *Neurology.* 1992;42:686–689.

208. Arai M, Yoshino H, Kusano Y, Yazaki Y, Ohnishi Y, Miyatake T. Ataxic polyneuropathy and anti-Pr2 IgM kappa M proteinemia. *J Neurol.* 1992;239:147–151.

209. Obi T, Kusunoki S, Takatsu M, Mizoguchi K, Nishimura Y. IgM M-protein in a patient with sensory-dominant neuropathy binds preferentially to polysialogangliosides. *Acta Neurol Scand.* 1992;86:215–218.

210. Younes-Chennoufi AB, Leger JM, Hauw JJ, et al. Ganglioside GD1b is the target antigen for a biclonal IgM in a case of sensory-motor axonal polyneuropathy: involvement of N-acetyl-neuraminic acid in the epitope. *Ann Neurol.* 1992;32:18–23.

211. Willison HJ, Paterson G, Veitch J, Inglis G, Barnett SC. Peripheral neuropathy associated with monoclonal IgM anti-Pr2 cold agglutinins. *J Neurol Neurosurg Psychiatry.* 1993;56:1178–1183.

212. Kusunoki S, Chiba A, Tai T, Kanazawa I. Localization of GM1 and GD1b antigens in the human peripheral nervous system. *Muscle Nerve.* 1993;16:752–756.

213. Kusunoki S, Shimizu J, Chiba A, Ugawa Y, Hitoshi S, Kanazawa I. Experimental sensory neuropathy induced by sensitization with ganglioside GD1b. *Ann Neurol.* 1996;39:424–431.

214. Pestronk A, Li F, Griffin J, et al. Polyneuropathy syndromes associated with serum antibodies to sulfatide and myelin-associated glycoprotein. *Neurology.* 1991;41:357–362.

215. Quattrini A, Corbo M, Dhaliwal SK, et al. Anti-sulfatide antibodies in neurological disease—binding to rat dorsal-root ganglia neurons. *J Neurol Sci.* 1992;112:152–159.

216. Nemni R, Fazio R, Quattrini A, Lorenzetti I, Mamoli D, Canal N. Antibodies to sulfatide and to chondroitin sulfate C in patients with chronic sensory neuropathy. *J Neuroimmunol.* 1993;43:79–85.

217. van den Berg LH, Lankamp CL, de Jager AE, et al. Anti-sulphatide antibodies in peripheral neuropathy. *J Neurol Neurosurg Psychiatry.* 1993;56:1164–1168.

218. Ilyas AA, Cook SD, Dalakas MC, Mithen FA. Anti-MAG IgM paraproteins from some patients with polyneuropathy associated with IgM paraproteinemia also react with sulfatide. *J Neuroimmunol.* 1992;37:85–92.

219. Nobile-Orazio E, Manfredini E, Carpo M, et al. Frequency and clinical correlates of anti-neural IgM antibodies in neuropathy associated with IgM monoclonal gammopathy. *Ann Neurol.* 1994;36:416–424.

220. Kabat EA, Liao J, Sherman WH, Osserman EF. Immunochemical characterization of the specificities of two human monoclonal IgMs reacting with chondroitin sulfates. *Carbohydr Res.* 1984;130:289–297.

221. Sherman WH, Latov N, Hays AP, et al. Monoclonal IgM kappa antibody precipitating with chondroitin sulfate C from patients with axonal polyneuropathy and epidermolysis. *Neurology.* 1983;33:192–201.

222. Freddo L, Hays AP, Sherman WH, Latov N. Axonal neuropathy in a patient with IgM M-protein reactive with nerve endoneurium. *Neurology.* 1985;35:1321–1325.

223. Freddo L, Sherman WH, Latov N. Glycosaminoglycan antigens in peripheral nerve. Studies with antibodies from a patient with neuropathy and monoclonal gammopathy. *J Neuroimmunol.* 1986;12:57–64.

224. Yee WC, Hahn AF, Hearn SA, Rupar AR. Neuropathy in IgM lambda paraproteinemia. Immunoreactivity to neural proteins and chondroitin sulfate. *Acta Neuropathol.* 1989;78:57–64.

225. Quattrini A, Nemni R, Fazio R, et al. Axonal neuropathy in a patient with monoclonal IgM kappa reactive with Schmidt-Lantermann incisures. *J Neuroimmunol.* 1991;33:73–79.

226. Baba H, Miyatani N, Sato S, Yuasa T, Miyatake T. Antibody to glycolipid in a patient with IgM paraproteinemia and polyradiculoneuropathy. *Acta Neurol Scand.* 1985;72:218–221.

227. Miyatani N, Baba H, Sato S, Nakamura K, Yuasa T, Miyatake T. Antibody to sialosyllactosaminylparagloboside in a

patient with IgM paraproteinemia and polyradiculoneuropathy. *J Neuroimmunol.* 1987;14:189–196.

228. Ilyas AA, Li SC, Chou DK, et al. Gangliosides GM2, IV4Gal-NAcGM1b, and IV4GalNAcGC1a as antigens for monoclonal immunoglobulin M in neuropathy associated with gammopathy. *J Biol Chem.* 1988;263:4369–4373.

229. Bollensen E, Schipper HI, Steck AJ. Motor neuropathy with activity of monoclonal IgM antibody to GD1a ganglioside. *J Neurol.* 1989;236:353–355.

230. Spatz LA, Wong KK, Williams M, et al. Cloning and sequence analysis of the VH and VL regions of an anti-myelin/DNA antibody from a patient with peripheral neuropathy and chronic lymphocytic leukemia. *J Immunol.* 1990;144:2821–2828.

231. Dellagi K, Brouet JC, Perreau J, Paulin D. Human monoclonal IgM with autoantibody activity against intermediate filaments. *Proc Natl Acad Sci U S A.* 1982;79:446–450.

232. Chad D, Pariser K, Bradley WG, Adelman LS, Pinn VW. The pathogenesis of cryoglobulinemic neuropathy. *Neurology.* 1982;32:725–729.

233. Thomas FP, Lovelace RE, Ding XS, et al. Vasculitic neuropathy in a patient with cryoglobulinemia and anti-MAG IGM monoclonal gammopathy. *Muscle Nerve.* 1992;15:891–898.

234. Driedger H, Pruzanski W. Plasma cell neoplasia with peripheral polyneuropathy. A study of five cases and a review of the literature. *Medicine (Baltimore).* 1980;59:301–310.

235. Kelly JJ, Kyle RA, Obrien PC, Dyck PJ. Prevalence of monoclonal protein in peripheral neuropathy. *Neurology.* 1981;31:1480–1483.

236. Hesselvik M. Neuropathological studies on myelomatosis. *Acta Neurol Scand.* 1969;45:95–108.

237. Dyck PJ, Low PA, Windebank AJ, et al. Plasma-exchange in polyneuropathy associated with monoclonal gammopathy of undetermined significance. *N Engl J Med.* 1991;325:1482–1486.

238. Noring L, Kjellin KG, Siden A. Neuropathies associated with disorders of plasmocytes. *Eur Neurol.* 1980;19:224–230.

239. Read DJ, Vanhegan RI, Matthews WB. Peripheral neuropathy and benign IgG paraproteinaemia. *J Neurol Neurosurg Psychiatry.* 1978;41:215–219.

240. Simmons Z, Albers JW, Bromberg MB, Feldman EL. Presentation and initial clinical course in patients with chronic inflammatory demyelinating polyradiculoneuropathy—comparison of patients without and with monoclonal gammopathy. *Neurology.* 1993;43:2202–2209.

241. Dispenzieri A, Kyle RA, Lacy MQ, et al. POEMS syndrome: definitions and long-term outcome. *Blood.* 2003;101:2496–2506.

242. Watanabe O, Maruyama I, Arimura K, et al. Overproduction of vascular endothelial growth factor—vascular permeability factor is causative in Crow-Fukase (POEMS) syndrome. *Muscle Nerve.* 1998;21:1390–1397.

243. Watanabe O, Arimura K, Kitajima I, Osame M, Maruyama I. Greatly raised vascular endothelial growth factor (VEGF) in POEMS syndrome. *Lancet.* 1996;347:702.

244. Dyck PJ, Engelstad J, Dispenzieri A. Vascular endothelial growth factor and POEMS. *Neurology.* 2006;66:10–12.

245. Kuwabara S, Misawa S, Kanai K, et al. Autologous peripheral blood stem cell transplantation for POEMS syndrome (Reprinted). *Neurology.* 2006;66:105–107.

246. Kyle RA, Gertz MA. Systemic amyloidosis. *Crit Rev Oncol Hematol.* 1990;10:49–87.

247. Kyle RA, Greipp PR. Amyloidosis (AL). Clinical and laboratory features in 229 cases. *Mayo Clin Proc.* 1983;58:665–683.

248. Durie BG, Persky B, Soehnlen BJ, Grogan TM, Salmon SE. Amyloid production in human myeloma stem-cell culture, with morphologic evidence of amyloid secretion by associated macrophages. *N Engl J Med.* 1982;307:1689–1692.

249. Trotter JL, Engel WK, Ignaczak FI. Amyloidosis with plasma cell dyscrasia. An overlooked caused of adult onset sensorimotor neuropathy. *Arch Neurol.* 1977;34:209–214.

250. Kelly JJ, Jr., Kyle RA, O'Brien PC, Dyck PJ. The natural history of peripheral neuropathy in primary systemic amyloidosis. *Ann Neurol.* 1979;6:1–7.

251. Gertz MA, Kyle RA. Amyloidosis—prognosis and treatment. *Semin Arthritis Rheum.* 1994;24:124–138.

252. Gertz MA, Greipp PR, Kyle RA. Classification of amyloidosis by the detection of clonal excess of plasma cells in the bone marrow. *J Lab Clin Med.* 1991;118:33–39.

253. Duston MA, Skinner M, Anderson J, Cohen AS. Peripheral neuropathy as an early marker of AL amyloidosis. *Arch Intern Med.* 1989;149:358–360.

254. Gertz MA, Kyle RA, Greipp PR, Katzmann JA, O'Fallon WM. Beta 2-microglobulin predicts survival in primary systemic amyloidosis. *Am J Med.* 1990;89:609–614.

255. Kyle RA, Greipp PR, O'Fallon WM. Primary systemic amyloidosis: multivariate analysis for prognostic factors in 168 cases. *Blood.* 1986;68:220–224.

256. Sharma P, Perri RE, Sirven JE, et al. Outcome of liver transplantation for familial amyloidotic polyneuropathy. *Liver Transplantation.* 2003;9:1273–1280.

257. Comenzo RL, Vosburgh E, Falk RH, et al. Dose-intensive melphalan with blood stem-cell support for the treatment of AL (amyloid light-chain) amyloidosis: Survival and responses in 25 patients. *Blood.* 1998;91:3662–3670.

258. Rajkumar SV, Gertz MA. Advances in the treatment of amyloidosis. *N Engl J Med.* 2007;356:2413–2415.

259. Richardson PG, Barlogie B, Berenson J, et al. A phase 2 study of bortezomib in relapsed, refractory myeloma. *N Engl J Med.* 2003;348:2609–2617.

260. Ilyas AA, Quarles RH, Dalakas MC, Fishman PH, Brady RO. Monoclonal IgM in a patient with paraproteinemic polyneuropathy binds to gangliosides containing disialosyl groups. *Ann Neurol.* 1985;18:655–659.

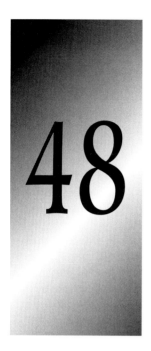

Neuromuscular Junction Disorders in Cancer

48

Mill Etienne
Clifton L. Gooch

Two common syndromes affecting the neuromuscular junction are of particular interest and can dramatically affect a patient's daily function: myasthenia gravis (MG) and Lambert-Eaton myasthenic syndrome (LEMS). MG affects 15%–30% of patients with thymoma or more, while LEMS affects 3% of patients with small cell lung cancer (SCLC). Conversely, 10% of patients with MG will have a thymoma, and 40% of patients presenting with LEMS will ultimately develop a cancer (1–5). Because of these strong associations and the significant functional disability these diseases can cause, it is critical that physicians participating in all aspects of cancer care have at least a basic understanding of these disorders.

MYASTHENIA GRAVIS

Pathophysiology

Myasthenia gravis is one of the best understood of all autoimmune diseases. It is caused by autoantibodies directed against epitopes on or around the acetylcholine receptor in the postsynaptic membrane of the neuromuscular junction. These antibodies can block the binding of acetylcholine (ACh) to its receptors or cause receptor malfunction through other mechanisms and may initiate immune-mediated degradation of the receptors, reducing receptor numbers and damaging the postsynaptic membrane (6–9). Decreased number and malfunction of the ACh receptors results in fewer miniature end plate potentials (MEPPs) and a lower end plate potential (EPP), reducing the likelihood of reaching the depolarization threshold necessary for muscle contraction.

Epidemiology

MG has a prevalence of 1 in 10,000 in the United States, occurring in all ethnic groups. Female incidence peaks in the third decade of life, with a mean age of onset of 28 years; while male incidence peaks in the sixth or seventh decade, with average age of onset of 42. The female-to-male ratio was originally described as 6:4 in a young cohort, but as this population has aged, the incidence has become equal between male and female. Recent advances in treatment and care of critically ill patients have resulted in a marked decrease in the mortality rate, from a natural history rate of 30% (before current treatments) to contemporary rates of 3%–4%. Risk factors for death from MG include age older than 40 years, rapidly progressive severe disease at onset, and malignant thymoma (10,11).

Myasthenia Gravis and Thymoma

Approximately 10%–15% of patients presenting with MG will have a thymoma, and 30%–65% of patients presenting with thymoma will have myasthenia (1–3,5).

KEY POINTS

- The two common syndromes that affect the neuromuscular junction are myasthenia gravis (MG) and Lambert-Eaton myasthenic syndrome (LEMS).
- MG affects 15%–30% of patients with thymoma or more, while LEMS affects 3% of patients with small cell lung cancer (SCLC). Conversely, 10% of patients with MG will have a thymoma and 40% of patients presenting with LEMS will ultimately develop a cancer.
- Myasthenia gravis is caused by autoantibodies directed against epitopes on or around the acetylcholine receptor in the postsynaptic membrane of the neuromuscular junction. These antibodies can block the binding of acetylcholine to its receptors or cause receptor malfunction through other mechanisms and may also initiate immune-mediated degradation of the receptors, reducing receptor numbers and damaging the postsynaptic membrane.
- The primary manifestations of MG are muscular weakness and fatigability, which variably affect the ocular, bulbar and respiratory, and extremity muscles.
- The antibody assays available for the diagnosis of MG include the acetylcholine receptor binding, modulating, and blocking antibodies.
- When all antibody assays are negative, the diagnosis of MG can be confirmed by electrophysiologic testing, the edrophonium test, or by clinical criteria.
- Patients with LEMS develop fluctuating proximal weakness due to a decrease in release of acetylcholine (ACh) from the presynaptic terminal at the neuromuscular junction.

- Antibodies directed at the P/Q type of voltage-gated calcium channel (VGCC) in the presynaptic neuronal membrane are seen in 85%–95% of patients with LEMS.
- The diagnosis of LEMS may be the presenting feature of cancer and proceed its diagnosis by two years or more; however, 40% of patients with LEMS will never develop a cancer.
- Patients with LEMS typically present with proximal limb weakness that begins in the legs and spreads to the arms. Associated symptoms, such as fatigue, myalgias, xerostomia (dry mouth), and orthostatic hypotension, are also common.
- Patients with LEMS may demonstrate mild improvement in strength after exercise (the "warm-up" phenomenon) that wanes with more continuous activity, though this may not be a significant clinical feature.
- Nerve conduction studies in LEMS show low motor amplitudes due to neuromuscular blockade, in contrast to MG, in which motor amplitudes are usually normal. In addition, motor nerve amplitude may dramatically fluctuate during repeated stimulation on routine nerve conduction studies in LEMS. Sensory nerve conductions, however, are normal, with no fluctuation in both disorders. Needle electromyogram (EMG) examination may reveal motor unit instability and subtle myopathic change in the proximal muscles, though less commonly in LEMS than in MG.
- Paraneoplastic LEMS typically responds to successful treatment of the underlying cancer, though symptoms may return with relapse of cancer.

The mean age of thymoma patients is 50 years, with a 1:1 male-to-female ratio. Ninety percent of these tumors are benign and easily treatable with resection, but 10% are malignant and will spread beyond the thymic capsule to local tissue, the lymphatic system, or the blood. Only 1%–5% metastasize distantly (12,13).

Patients with malignant thymoma should undergo a thorough surgical resection by an experienced thoracic surgeon, which may be followed postoperatively by radiotherapy, with or without chemotherapy, depending upon tumor grade and extent of invasion. Antistriated antibodies are strongly associated with concurrent myasthenia and thymoma and are elevated in 90% of these patients; thus, when this assay is posi-

tive, thymoma is more likely (14,15). With successful tumor therapy, antistriated antibody levels fall, and progressively increasing titers after initial treatment may be the first indicator of tumor recurrence.

Recurrence of benign tumors is rare, but malignant thymomas that have spread to the pleura or elsewhere have a 5–10-year average survival, despite surgery and radiotherapy (12). The majority of patients with MG and thymoma present with severe generalized extremity and bulbar weakness, whereas pure ocular disease is rare in this patient group (1). Some of these patients may have cardiac involvement (herzmyasthenia) with arrhythmia, bundle branch block, or cardiac failure with focal myocarditis (16). When thymoma is diagnosed late, myasthenics typically have more severe symptoms, more frequent exacerbations, and a higher mortality rate. In contrast, myasthenia associated with early-diagnosed thymoma has a slightly better prognosis than myasthenia gravis with thymic hyperplasia alone (17).

Thymomas are classified as lymphomas; according to their cells of origin, they are epithelial, carcinoid, or mesenchymal tumors. The epithelial thymic tumor is the classic "thymoma." It is often referred to as a lymphoepithelial tumor and graded according to lymphocytic infiltration, though the epithelial cell is the neoplastic element (1).

Clinical Features

The name myasthenia gravis is derived from the Greek, meaning "the great weakness." True to its name, the primary manifestations of myasthenia are muscular weakness and fatigability, which variably affect the ocular, bulbar and respiratory, and extremity muscles. This weakness typically worsens with exercise and improves with rest, often becoming more dramatic by the end of the day. Muscles that control eye and eyelid movement, facial expression, chewing, talking, swallowing, and respiration are especially susceptible.

Nearly all patients with myasthenia gravis will experience diplopia and/or ptosis. Fifty to 60 percent will present with diplopia and ptosis as early primary features, and an additional 30% will develop these symptoms as the disease progresses. Conversely 85%–90% of patients presenting with ocular symptoms will eventually develop more generalized weakness. Myasthenic patients may also develop weakness of the muscles of facial expression, resulting in a flat, depressed-appearing demeanor, diminished eyelid closure, masseter weakness, dysarthria, and hypernasality due to posterior pharyngeal and palatal weakness. They often develop difficulty with swallowing and may develop respiratory muscle weakness. Respiratory muscle weakness can lead to respiratory depression and failure, the most severe potential consequence of the disease.

A clinical classification scheme for myasthenia gravis has been established by the Medical Scientific Advisory Board of the Myasthenia Gravis Foundation of America to assist with standardization of severity rating for research and clinical care (Table 48.1) (18).

Neurologic Examination

Mental status testing and sensory examination are normal, and deep tendon reflexes are usually normal to mildly depressed. Common cranial nerve abnormalities include unilateral or bilateral ptosis. With more severe ptosis, patients may furrow their brows in an attempt to compensate for eyelid droop. If ptosis is not present at rest, it can often be elicited with sustained upgaze for 30–60 seconds. Patients may have diplopia due to extraocular muscle weakness, which may mimic many ophthalmologic or neuro-ophthalmologic syndromes, including internuclear ophthalmoplegia. Patients often will have a facial diplegia due to weakness of the muscles of facial expression. Weakness of palatal muscles may produce nasal speech and nasal regurgitation of fluids when drinking. Some patients may have weakness of the jaw with prolonged chewing, and the jaw may hang open after prolonged talking due to masseter fatigue.

TABLE 48.1

MGFA Clinical Severity Scale for Myasthenia

Class I	Any eye muscle weakness or ptosis without muscle weakness elsewhere
Class II	Mild weakness affecting other muscles, with or without ocular muscle weakness
IIa	Predominantly limb or axial muscle weakness
IIb	Predominantly bulbar and/or respiratory muscle weakness
Class III	Moderate weakness of other muscles, with or without ocular muscle weakness
IIIa	Predominantly limb or axial muscle weakness
IIIb	Predominantly bulbar and/or respiratory muscle weakness
Class IV	Severe weakness of other muscles, with or without ocular muscle weakness
IVa	Predominantly limb or axial muscle weakness
IVb	Predominantly bulbar and/or respiratory muscles (can also include feeding tube without intubation)
Class V	Neuromuscular respiratory failure requiring intubation to maintain airway

Source: From Ref. 18.
Abbreviation: MGFA, Myasthenia Gravis Foundation of America.

Muscle strength testing of the extremities typically reveals predominately proximal muscle weakness, usually more severe in the legs. Respiratory function must also be carefully evaluated by history and, often, by pulmonary function testing, as this may lead to potentially fatal respiratory failure without proper acute and chronic management. During hospital admission, pulse oximetry is not adequate to monitor respiratory status, as ventilatory weakness may produce serious carbon dioxide retention and narcosis before oxygen levels significantly decline. Consequently, the MG patient's vital capacity (VC) and/or negative inspiratory force (NIF) must be followed serially throughout admission during an exacerbation.

The Edrophonium (Tensilon) Test

The intravenous administration of edrophonium chloride (Tensilon), an acetylcholinesterase inhibitor, may transiently improve signs and symptoms in patients with myasthenia gravis by temporarily increasing the levels of acetylcholine at the neuromuscular junction. This test may be up to 90%–95% sensitive and 80%–95% specific in generalized myasthenia gravis and 80%–95% sensitive and 80%–90% specific for ocular myasthenia (19–23). However, these figures assume that the test is performed by an experienced examiner in a patient with an obviously weak muscle, which can be clearly tested both before and after edrophonium administration. Weakness caused by several other neuromuscular diseases (eg, amyotrophic lateral sclerosis) may also transiently improve with edrophonium. Though cholinergic overdose is rare in myasthenics in the age of immunotherapy, the edrophonium challenge test may also help distinguish weakness due to myasthenic crisis from that caused by cholinergic crisis due to pyridostigmine overdose, as patients with myasthenic crisis may improve with the drug, while those with cholinergic crisis will worsen.

In most patients, the edrophonium test can be performed easily, but appropriate preparations are critical. A crash cart and the ability to provide rapid intubation, mechanical ventilation, and defibrillation should be immediately available, as intravenous (IV) edrophonium can rarely cause sudden cardiac arrhythmia. A clearly weak muscle, which can be clearly assessed before and after edrophonium, must also be identified. Ptosis or a weak proximal muscle, such as the deltoid and biceps, are readily observable and easily tested. If indicated, pulmonary function can also be followed with forced vital capacity (FVC) or NIF before and after administration of edrophonium.

As edrophonium increases circulating acetylcholine levels, it may cause heart block, asystole, bradycardia, and syncope in rare instances, so the patient should be placed on a cardiac monitor for heart rate and rhythm assessment. Two 1-mL tuberculin syringes should be prepared, one containing 1 mL of normal saline to serve as placebo injection and the other containing 10 mg of edrophonium in 1 mL of solution (1 mg per 0.1 mL). This test can be done single blind (blinding the patient only) or double blind (blinding both the patient and examiner, with a third health care professional serving as an unblinded observer). An initial test dose (1 mg) of edrophonium is given to assess for side effects. Some patients may respond noticeably to this small dose. After one to two minutes, if there is no adverse reaction, another dose (4 mg) of edrophonium should produce noticeable improvement in muscle strength within one minute. If no improvement occurs, an additional dose of 5 mg can be administered (total dose should not exceed 10 mg). Patients who respond generally show dramatic improvement in muscle strength. In patients with less severe exacerbations, the degree of improvement with edrophonium may be subtle. Many authors recommend having several blinded observers assess the patient's response in these cases. When placebo is used, the placebo injection should be given first, using the same protocol as the edrophonium injection, which should be given last (if given as the first injection, residual edrophonium may influence muscle function during subsequent placebo injection).

Antibody Assays: Antiacetylcholine, Anti-MuSK, and Others

The antibody assays available for the diagnosis of MG include the acetylcholine receptor binding, modulating, and blocking antibodies (14,24–28). Although the binding antibody has high specificity for MG (up to 99%), it can be positive in patients with thymoma alone without myasthenic symptoms. Blocking antibodies are found in only 1% of myasthenic patients without binding antibodies. Both the blocking and modulating antibody assays are most useful when the acetylcholine receptor-binding antibody assay is negative. The modulating antibody assay may be more sensitive in patients with early, mild, or pure ocular disease. The sensitivity and specificity of each of these assays varies and improves with worsening disease severity. A positive ACh receptor antibody assay is up to 99% specific for myasthenia, with sensitivities ranging from 59% (blocking) to 90% (binding and modulating) in generalized disease, but only 30% (blocking) to 70% (binding and modulating) in pure ocular disease (24). Although there is not a strong correlation between absolute antibody titers and disease severity in the individual patient, mean antibody titers rise with increasing disease severity in large populations of myasthenics (28). However, decreasing titers below initial baseline in the individual patient are often seen following immunotherapy and correlate with symptomatic improvement (28). High antibody titers also may be seen in some patients with thymoma and early-onset MG.

In recent years, a new population of antibodies has been identified in patients with MG: the antibody against muscle-specific kinase (MuSK). One series found anti-MuSK antibodies in 47% of MG patients who did not have any ACh receptor antibodies (29,30) MuSK is a tyrosine kinase that has an important role in regulating and maintaining ACh receptors (AChRs) and their functional clusters at the neuromuscular junction. Its absence significantly disrupts the structure and function of the postsynaptic apparatus. The anti-MuSK antibody is a high-affinity antibody that binds to the extracellular domains of native MuSK, and is predominately of the IgG4 subclass. Passive transfer experiments show reductions in MEPP amplitude in murine models of myasthenia gravis in a fashion similar to that induced by antiacetylcholine receptor IgG (31).

Patients with anti-AChR antibodies almost never harbor anti-MuSK antibodies, and pure ocular myasthenics virtually never have anti-MuSK antibodies, regardless of whether they are positive for the anti-AChR antibody or not. Anti-MuSK antibodies do not appear in normal controls. Anti-MuSK–associated MG appears at an earlier age than other varieties and disproportionately affects the neck, shoulder, and respiratory muscles, with less limb weakness and rarer ocular symptoms. Some studies have shown that anti-MUSK disproportionately affects women (29–31). However, both anti-AChR and anti-MuSK antibody-positive myasthenics appear to respond equally well to acetylcholinesterase inhibitors and immunomodulatory therapy. Anti-MuSK myasthenia gravis patients are less likely to have thymic hyperplasia and rarely have thymoma (32). However, the efficacy of thymectomy in these patients is difficult to gauge because of the small numbers of patients reported thus far (29,30,33–36).

Another group of antibodies against striated muscle were the first reported autoantibodies in myasthenia gravis. These antibodies are reactive against thymic myoid cells as well as the contractile elements of skeletal muscle, and they are present in 27% of all patients with the disease, with high levels noted in up to 90% of patients with myasthenia gravis and concurrent thymoma (14,15). The myoid cells are muscle-like cells found mainly within the medulla of the thymus, and they contain nicotinic acetylcholine receptors, suggesting that the myoid cells may provide the primary antigens involved in the autoimmune response of MG. Progressive rises in antistriatal antibody titers can be the first indication of thymic tumor recurrence following resection. They may be also present in isolation

when AChR antibody assays are negative, making them a useful adjunctive test. Other antibodies found in a significant percentage of myasthenia gravis patients include antinuclear (20%–40%), thyroid (15%–40%), rheumatoid factor (10%–40%), gastric parietal cell (10%–20%), lymphocyte (40%–90%), and platelet (5%–50%) antibodies, as well as antismooth muscle, mitochondrial, red blood cell, and squamous epithelial antibodies, often without additional disease.

Despite these many assays, from 20%–40% of patients with the clinical diagnosis of MG may have not identifiable autoantibodies; this group has been dubbed "seronegative" myasthenia gravis. However, seronegativity by these assays does not by any means exclude an immunologic cause for MG in this patient group, as negative assays may result from unusually low levels of serum antibody or technical errors in performance of the assay. In some patients, high-affinity antibodies may aggressively adhere to their respective antigens in vivo, rendering standard assays negative because of extremely low serum levels of free antibody. Most importantly, as discoveries in recent years have shown, there are very likely other, as-yet-undiscovered pathogenic antibodies that cause MG (37). When all antibody assays are negative, the diagnosis can be confirmed by electrophysiologic testing, the edrophonium test, or by clinical criteria. Seronegative patients also respond to immunosuppression, though perhaps not as well as patients with detectable antibody (37).

Electrodiagnostic Testing: Repetitive Nerve Stimulation and Single-Fiber EMG

Two major electrodiagnostic tests are available to assess neuromuscular junction function: repetitive nerve stimulation (RNS) and single-fiber EMG (SFEMG). RNS involves repeated electrical stimulation of a selected peripheral nerve, with simultaneous recording of the electrical response produced by the muscle it innervates (Fig. 48.1). After baseline RNS, RNS is again delivered following 30–60 seconds of maximal voluntary contraction of the muscle, then again at set intervals every few minutes after this brief exercise. The size (amplitude or area) of the first waveform (compound motor action potential or CMAP) in a train is compared to one of the later waveforms to assess for decreases (decrement) or increases (increment) in CMAP size within each train.

In MG, the CMAP typically decreases in size (decrements) by 10%–15% or greater in the baseline train (Fig. 48.2). Conversely, the CMAP size remains stable in normal subjects during RNS and does not decline (38).

After exercise, the CMAP size may transiently improve in patients with MG by 10%–50% (postexercise facilitation) (38), and decrement may improve

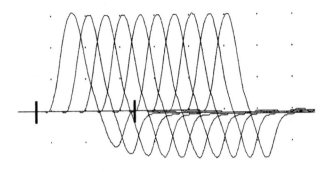

FIGURE 48.1

Repetitive nerve stimulation. This recording was made using slow (3 Hz) repetitive stimulation of the median nerve at the wrist while recording from the median-innervated thenar muscles in the hand of a healthy subject. Ten stimulations were given, generating a train of ten compound motor action potentials (CMAPs), which were recorded and are displayed in a row in the order of their stimulation (first generated waveform on the left, last on the right). Each individual CMAP in this train is normal, and no significant change in CMAP amplitude or area is observed during repetitive stimulation, a normal response. *Settings:* Sweep speed 5 milliseconds/division; sensitivity 5 millivolts/division.

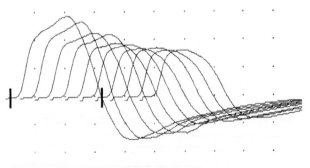

FIGURE 48.2

Decrement during repetitive nerve stimulation in myasthenia gravis. This recording was made using slow (3 Hz) repetitive stimulation of the median nerve at the wrist while recording from the median-innervated thenar muscles in the hand of a patient with active myasthenia gravis, using the same protocol as described for the tracing in Figure 48.1. Progressive decreases in CMAP size are seen, confirmed by loss in both measured amplitude and area of 40%–50%. These losses are due to transmission failure (block) at increasing numbers of neuromuscular junctions during repetitive nerve stimulation, consistent with significant neuromuscular junction dysfunction in the tested muscle (see text). *Settings:* Sweep speed 5 milliseconds/division; sensitivity 5 millivolts/division.

(decrement repair). This is followed within one to three minutes by transient worsening of CMAP decrement, dropping below baseline levels (postactivation exhaustion) (39). Within five minutes postexercise, the neuromuscular junction has re-equilibrated and all parameters typically return to baseline levels.

SFEMG (40) utilizes a needle engineered to record single muscle fiber discharges and indirectly provides precise quantitation of neuromuscular junction function known as "jitter." SFEMG provides a highly sensitive assay of neuromuscular junction function. In myasthenic patients, variability in neuromuscular junction (NMJ) transmission time (jitter) is considerably increased compared to controls. MG may also produce intermittent blocking of neuromuscular junction transmission, with failure of contraction in the muscle fiber; SFEMG can also quantitate this phenomenon and its frequency. Blocking should not occur in normal subjects.

The sensitivity and specificity of repetitive nerve stimulation and single-fiber electromyography differ considerably. Repetitive nerve stimulation in a hand or shoulder muscle has a sensitivity of approximately 75% in patients with generalized weakness due to myasthenia gravis, but is less than 50% in pure ocular disease. In contrast, single-fiber electromyography is the most sensitive single test in myasthenia gravis, with a sensitivity of 95% or greater in generalized, and 90% or greater in pure ocular myasthenia gravis, when weak muscles are tested (38,40). Because of its high sensitivity, single-fiber electromyography has its greatest diagnostic utility in cases of mild generalized, pure ocular, or seronegative myasthenia gravis. As jitter may be increased in a variety of other neuromuscular diseases, however, the specificity of this technique is limited, and other conditions must be appropriately excluded by routine electrodiagnostic testing prior to single-fiber electromyography studies.

Symptomatic Therapy: The Acetylcholinesterase Inhibitors

Mary Walker first documented the efficacy of acetylcholinesterase inhibitors as symptomatic treatment of MG in 1934 (41). Although physostigmine was used originally, the most commonly used acetylcholinesterase inhibitor for MG in the modern era is pyridostigmine. Acetylcholinesterase inhibitors block the breakdown of acetylcholine at the NMJ, thereby increasing acetylcholine concentration in the neuromuscular junction and facilitating acetylcholine receptor activation and subsequent muscle activation and contraction. These drugs take effect within 20–30 minutes of oral administration, usually reaching maximal efficacy within 45 minutes, and lasting for 2–3 hours or more. A typical starting dose is 30–60 mg every six hours, with gradual increases in frequency of administration until adequate symptomatic effect is achieved (eg, from every six hours to every four hours to every two to three hours while awake). An extended-release formulation of pyridostigmine is available in doses of 180 mg, and is most useful when administered before bedtime to prevent severe symptoms on awakening. The acetylcholinesterase inhibitors are primarily useful in contemporary management as adjunctive therapy in patients receiving primary immunomodulatory therapy. However, in mild, nonprogressive cases, such as pure ocular myasthenia, these drugs may be used as monotherapy The most common side effects of these drugs are autonomic, resulting from muscarinic receptor activation, and include gut hypermotility and diarrhea, diaphoresis, and excessive respiratory secretions. Bradycardia and other cardiac symptoms may occur in patients with preexisting heart disease, but significant arrhythmias are rare in normal patients in the absence of overdose. Though clinically insignificant, many patients also notice diffuse fasciculations while taking these agents, and may require reassurance that this symptom is not serious and does not suggest worsening neuromuscular disease.

Chronic Therapy: Oral Immunosuppressants

For the majority of MG patients, immunosuppressive therapy is the treatment of choice, as prevention of exacerbations is a cornerstone of management and should be the primary goal of managing physicians. Steroids remain the most effective chronic immunotherapy for MG and are often used as primary therapy (4). High-dose daily prednisone is the most common initial regimen in the United States, and is usually started at doses of 60–80 mg daily. Paradoxically, an exacerbation of MG symptoms occurs in up to 50% of patients shortly after initiation of high-dose oral steroids, usually starting within 5 days and typically lasting less than 4 days, though exacerbations may be delayed by up to 17 days (42). A more severe exacerbation may occur in 10% of patients starting on oral steroid therapy. Consequently, it is often useful to pretreat patients with a temporizing therapy (see next) before starting high-dose daily prednisone. Patients with more severe symptoms may require hospitalization during steroid initiation until a clear pattern of improved symptoms is established to appropriately monitor for worsening respiratory symptoms. Oral prednisone therapy usually begins to work within two weeks and becomes clearly effective within four weeks in most patients, providing dramatic relief in the majority.

Once significant improvement has begun, steroid taper is initiated at monthly intervals. Most patients can be tapered to reasonably low doses within 6–12 months. An alternative means of initiation of steroid therapy is to begin with low doses of steroids, with gradual increases on alternate days (eg, starting on 10–25 mg on alternate days, with gradual increase to 60–80 mg on alternate days). Patients with mild disease may be started at low daily doses, with gradual increments at monthly intervals until an adequate therapeutic response is obtained.

The side effects of steroids, especially at high doses, are numerous and include diabetes, weight gain, fluid retention, hypertension, anxiety and insomnia, psychosis, glaucoma and cataracts, myopathy, gastrointestinal hemorrhage and perforation, increased susceptibility to infections, and avascular joint necrosis, among others. Patients on high-dose daily prednisone should usually be placed on antiulcer prophylaxis and should be assessed for their risk of osteopenia/osteoporosis; most will require vitamin D and calcium supplementation, and may need other agents. An endocrinologist or bone metabolism specialist may be helpful for bone density monitoring and tailoring of an appropriate prophylactic regimen.

A variety of other immunosuppressive therapies are also effective for the treatment of MG. The most commonly used agents include azathioprine and, more recently, mycophenolate mofetil. These agents can be effective as primary therapy, but are most often used in refractory patients who cannot be tapered to acceptably low doses of steroids without experiencing an exacerbation ("steroid-sparing" agents). In these patients, secondary therapy with one of these agents is started while steroids are continued to allow taper of steroids to lower doses or to off. Third-line agents, which are effective but have significant toxicities, include cyclosporine A and cyclophosphamide.

Azathioprine is metabolized to 6-mercaptopurine, which inhibits DNA and RNA synthesis and interferes with T-cell function. This agent may take from 4–12 weeks to begin to work in MG and, therefore, is limited as a primary agent to patients who do not have severe or rapidly progressive symptoms. It is the most common steroid-sparing agent used in MG, and its role in this regard has been well studied (43,44). Its side effect profile is comparatively mild, and includes rare instances of myelosuppression and hepatotoxicity, both of which are typically reversible, as well as an acute flulike syndrome, with malaise, fever, and muscle aches. Patients must be monitored with regular blood counts and liver function tests. It also increases the risk of hematologic malignancy when used chronically. Cyclophosphamide is also effective, but has substantial toxicity, and MG symptoms typically recur when cyclophosphamide is tapered. Side effects include myelosuppression; hemorrhagic cystitis; malignancies of the blood, bladder, and skin; teratogenesis; alopecia; and nausea and vomiting, among others. It can be used as a steroid-sparing agent also, but there are better-tolerated alternatives (45). Cyclosporin inhibits calcineurin signaling and T-cell function. It is effective as both primary and steroid-sparing therapy, but also has substantial toxicity and is poorly tolerated by many patients, causing hypertension, renal dysfunction, and increasing generalized malaise. Consequently, it is not widely utilized today (4). Mycophenolate mofetil is metabolized to mycophenolic acid, which is a reversible inhibitor of inosine monophosphate dehydrogenase, an enzyme crucial for purine synthesis, playing a critical role in B- and T-cell proliferation (46,47). Mycophenolate's selectivity for B- and T-cell proliferation gives it a more favorable side effect profile when compared to most other agents, but side effects include possible myelosuppression, a 2% incidence of peptic ulcer disease, and an increased long-term risk of malignancy, especially melanoma and cancers of the blood. Blood counts must be performed at regular intervals, especially during the first weeks of therapy. Its precise efficacy in MG remains under active investigation, but it appears to work within 6–12 weeks in most patients, and is being increasingly employed as a steroid-sparing drug.

Temporizing Therapy: Plasma Exchange and IVIG

Patients who present with more severe symptoms, a rapidly progressive course, or respiratory compromise require immunotherapy, having a more rapid onset than the oral medications provide. More severe cases may also require hospitalization for respiratory monitoring and support. Two interventions provide rapid relief of symptoms in most MG patients: plasma exchange and IVIG. These approaches can also be helpful as pretreatment to prepare MG patients for surgery (reducing the risk of prolonged postoperative paralysis and/or respiratory weakness) and as pretreatment prior to the initiation of high-dose daily steroid therapy to reduce the risk of transient steroid exacerbation. These approaches, when used repeatedly, can also be considered for chronic therapy in patients who have failed or have major contraindications to the oral agents.

Plasma exchange removes many macromolecules, including acetylcholine receptor antibodies, from the blood. It has been shown to reduce perioperative morbidity when used as preparation for thymectomy and to successfully counter steroid-induced exacerbations (48). Typically, 2–4 liters of plasma are removed during each exchange. Three exchanges per week (usually on alternate days) are often given over a two-week period, for a total of six exchanges. Improvement is usually noted within days, usually peaking the week after exchange is completed. The duration of clear benefit is four to six weeks in most patients, though effects may persist longer in some (49–54). Plasma exchange is usually well tolerated, but complications can arise due to difficulties with vascular access, especially when a central line is required (infection, local thrombosis, and vascular perforation), removal of circulating clotting factors (bleeding), dehydration (hypotension and abnormal heart rate), and transient electrolyte disturbances, among others. Plasma exchange is personnel- and equipment-intensive and costly, but remains highly effective when a more rapid response is needed in the myasthenic patient.

High-dose intravenous immunoglobulin is a mixture of antibodies distilled from the sera of a number of human donors. It exerts its effects through a number of possible mechanisms, including the introduction of neutralizing anti-idiotypic antibodies directed against native pathogenic ones, modulation of B- and T-cell activity, and reduction of native pathogenic antibody production via negative feedback. Its time course of effect is similar to that of plasma exchange in most patients, with improvement starting within days, and it is equally efficacious. An initial course of IVIG is usually administered in daily infusions of 400 mg/kg of body weight per day for five days, for a total dose of 2 g/kg. Improvement appears in approximately 70% of patients within 5 days of initiation, with maximal effects at 8–9 days and a duration of 4–12 weeks (55). Side effects are typically mild and may include headache, chills, fever, and nausea, usually due to mild aseptic meningitis. Pretreatment with acetaminophen and diphenhydramine may prevent these minor reactions. Anaphylaxis and/or serum sickness is extremely rare with this agent, and the risk of an acute adverse event is likely less than such risk with most intravenous antibiotic preparations. Patients should be screened for IgA deficiency with quantitative immunoglobulin measurements. Though IgA deficiency is usually clinically silent in the general population, it may predispose patients treated with IVIG to serious allergic reactions. Acute renal failure is also a significant complication, usually occurring within days of infusion. All patients should be screened for renal insufficiency prior to infusion, although normal renal function before and during infusion does not guarantee that this complication can be avoided. Most of the early cases of acute renal failure following IVIG were in patients with known diabetes and involved IVIG preparations containing sucrose. Caution must be exercised in patients with either diabetes or renal insufficiency, and other treatment approaches (eg, plasma exchange) more carefully considered. Mild leucopenia and/or myelosuppression may occur during and for a few days after infusion, particularly in the elderly, but this is seldom of any consequence in patients without a preexisting hematologic disorder. IVIG infusion introduces a substantial fluid load and may be contraindicated in patients with congestive heart failure. The protein load during infusion also increases serum osmolarity, which, in concert with reports of thrombotic events during administration, has led to speculation that IVIG may increase cardiac and cerebrovascular risk during the infusion phase. The validity of this claim remains controversial, but IVIG should be used with caution in patients at high cardiovascular risk IVIG is also an expensive drug, but costs may be similar to plasma exchange, when equipment and personnel costs for each therapy are tabulated. If patients tolerate initial infusions well in a supervised setting (such as a hospital or infusion center) and inpatient monitoring of MG symptoms is not needed, subsequent infusions may be given at home, substantially reducing the cost of this intervention. Studies comparing IVIG to plasmapheresis have not shown a significant difference in efficacy for the treatment of myasthenic exacerbations or for preoperative therapy (56–58).

Hundreds of medications are known to worsen the symptoms of MG and can even precipitate a myasthenic crisis; these compounds should be avoided, if possible, or used with great caution if absolutely required. These agents include the aminoglycoside class of antimicrobial agents, as well as other antimicrobials (eg, ciprofloxacin, ampicillin), beta-adrenergic receptor blocking agents (eg, propranolol), verapamil, penicillamine, procainamide, lithium, magnesium, quinidine, chloroquine, anticholinergics (eg, trihexyphenidyl), and neuromuscular blocking agents (eg, vecuronium, curare), among many others. A reasonably comprehensive and useful reference list of these medicines may be found on the Web site for the Myasthenia Gravis Foundation of America (MGFA) at the following Web address: http://www.myasthenia.org/hp_edmaterials_reference.cfm#table1.

Surgical Therapy: Thymectomy

For almost a century, removal of the thymus gland has been considered a standard therapy for myasthenia gravis, though thymectomy is only now being studied in a controlled prospective clinical trial. Nevertheless, published clinical data over the last few decades suggest thymectomy is safe and effective for the treatment of myasthenia. Thymectomy yielded unexpected benefits following resection of a thymic tumor in patients with myasthenia gravis in the early part of the 21st century (59), inspiring many subsequent studies, which suggested it increased the chances of clinical remission in patients both with and without thymoma (60). As meta-analyses of studies of thymectomy in MG have been hindered by significant differences in both the variety of scoring used and in the definition of what constitutes a clinical response, the stricter criteria of complete remission rates (defined as the absence of any symptoms or signs in a patient on no other therapy) have been primarily employed for study-to-study comparisons. Natural history studies prior to effective medical immunotherapy or thymectomy reported spontaneous remission rates of 6%–20%. Several studies of thymectomy done prior to 1960 in myasthenics without thymoma reported modest remission rates of 11%–20%, with one study claiming 52%. With advances in critical care during the 1960s and 1970s, improved remission rates appeared in numerous studies, ranging from 27%–38% (61,62). Results reported during the 1980s in patients on adjunctive immunosuppressive therapy reported higher rates of remission, ranging from 54%–56% (63,64).

A variety of surgical approaches are employed for thymic resection, including the classic transsternal approach (splitting of the sternum with removal of the well-defined mediastinal lobes), the extended transsternal thymectomy (splitting of the sternum with wider exploration of the extrapleural and cervical regions), maximal transcervical and transsternal thymectomy (extensive exploration of the neck and mediastinum with direct visual inspection and removal of all suspected thymic tissue), and in recent years, less invasive techniques, including the transcervical approach (a more limited resection through a cervical incision instead of a sternotomy) and mediastinoscopic resections. Reported mean remission rates are 20%–30% for transcervical (65–69), 30%–40% for classic transsternal (17,68,70,71), and 50%–60% for both extended transsternal and maximal surgeries (64,72,73). The newer, less invasive methods have not been in widespread use long enough to assess their efficacy. The differences between remission rates for cervical and maximal thymectomy have a high level of statistical significance ($P = .0001$) (72), but because of the significant increase in complication rates with the maximal thymectomy, most centers favor the extended transsternal approach. When thymoma is present, myasthenic improvement following resection is less marked.

Numerous studies have also documented a decreased medication requirement and improved overall symptoms following thymectomy (71,74). Clinical improvement is typically delayed at least 6–12 months, and may not appear for several years (17,75–77). Traditional transsternal and extended thymectomies are safe when performed in experienced centers with appropriate preoperative and perioperative management, with complication rates approaching that of general anesthesia alone (6). Myasthenics undergoing thymectomy remained intubated only 1.4 days on average (78). However, if properly prepared, most MG patients in the modern era are not intubated longer following surgery than patients without MG.

The judicious selection of patients for thymectomy is critical, and chest computed tomography (CT) or magnetic resonance imaging (MRI) are a mandatory part of the MG workup. All patients with localized thymic tumors should undergo complete resection. Patients with widely metastatic disease, however, may not benefit from surgery, which should be performed only as a debulking maneuver to prolong survival. Thymectomy should be performed in most patients with new-onset myasthenia. However, patients with pure ocular myasthenia are not usually referred for surgery, as its benefits are unclear in this group. There is also a consensus that most benefit appears in patients ranging in age from early adulthood to 60 years. The thymus plays an integral role in the developing pediatric immune system, so thymectomy is not usually recommended for the rare cases of autoimmune myasthenia in children. Because the thymus progressively shrinks with age and because patients older than 60–65 years carry greater surgical risk, thymectomy is rarely performed in the elderly.

Appropriate preparation for any surgery, including thymectomy, is highly important in the myasthenic patient. Preoperative pulmonary function testing (including vital capacity measurements) should be done in addition to other routine preoperative tests. Ideally, the patient's disease should be stable enough to enable them to forego acetylcholinesterase inhibitor therapy for at least 24 hours prior to surgery. Acetylcholinesterase inhibitors should, in any case, be stopped no later than the morning of surgery. Muscle relaxants, especially depolarizing agents, should be avoided if possible, as they may induce prolonged paralysis. Postoperatively, a transient but dramatic increase in strength may be observed that may persist for several days. Patients on acetylcholinesterase inhibitor therapy may report up to a 25% reduction in dosage requirement during this period (60).

Thymoma will be found in 10%–15% of all myasthenic patients, and 40% of patients with thymoma will develop myasthenia (1). The mean age of thymoma patients is somewhat higher than that of patients with myasthenia alone, at 50 years. Approximately 90% of these tumors can be easily treated with resection. The remaining 10% are malignant and spread throughout the mediastinum, although distant metastasis occurs in only 1%–5% (12,13). Patients with malignant thymoma should undergo thorough surgical resection, with consideration of postoperative oncologic therapy

under the guidance of an oncologist. Despite treatment, patients with malignant thymomas that have spread to the pleura or elsewhere have a five- to ten-year average survival (14,61).

Antistriated antibodies are strongly associated with concurrent myasthenia and thymoma, and are elevated in 90% of these patients. As such, antibodies are seen in only in 27% of all patients with myasthenia; their presence raises suspicion for a possible tumor (14,15). With successful tumor therapy, antistriated antibody levels fall. Consequently, progressively increasing titers may serve as the first evidence of tumor recurrence.

The mechanisms through which thymectomy works remain controversial. Immunologically active tissue is so abundant elsewhere in the body that a gross reduction in immune system mass seems an unlikely explanation for the observed effects. Resection of the thymus does decrease the levels of the immunoactive thymic hormones, perhaps accounting for a more widely distributed immunosuppression (79). However, the presence of the quintessential elements for B- and T-lymphocyte autosensitization against the AChR within the thymus makes it a key location for the continued production of myasthenic antibodies, making its removal particularly efficacious in quelling that specific immune response (37).

LAMBERT–EATON MYASTHENIC SYNDROME (LEMS)

Pathophysiology and Epidemiology

The disorder now known as Lambert-Eaton myasthenic syndrome (LEMS) was first reported by Lambert and Eaton in 1957 (80). Eighty-five percent to 95 percent of patients with LEMS are seropositive for antibodies directed at the P/Q type of voltage-gated calcium channel (VGCC) in the presynaptic neuronal membrane (81,82). Anti-VGCC antibodies reduce numbers of VGCC in motor nerve terminals (83,84). By decreasing the influx of calcium triggered by each arriving action potential, anti-VGCC antibodies ultimately impair the calcium-dependent release of acetylcholine into the neuromuscular junction, causing clinical muscle weakness. Parasympathetic, sympathetic, and enteric neurons are all affected. In 1989, Lennon and colleagues developed an assay for anti-VGCC antibodies (85), and have found that these antibodies are present in the serum of 100% (32/32 patients) of paraneoplastic LEMS patients and 91% (30/33 patients) of non-paraneoplastic LEMS patients (82).

Nearly 60% of LEMS cases are paraneoplastic and are most commonly associated with small cell lung cancer (SCLC). A number of other cancers have been reported in association with LEMS, including non-SCLC; lymphosarcoma; malignant thymoma; and carcinomas of the breast, stomach, colon, prostate, bladder, kidney, and gallbladder. Only lymphoproliferative diseases such as lymphoma seem to occur in a significantly higher number of LEMS patients (4,86,87). The diagnosis of LEMS may be the presenting feature and may precede the development of a cancer. In these cases, the diagnosis of cancer is typically made within two years after the diagnosis. However, 40% of patients with LEMS will never develop a cancer, and the odds of a late malignancy appearing after two years are small, but not zero. LEMS is rare, making precise epidemiological estimates difficult to calculate, but its prevalence is probably between 1 in 500,000 and 1 in 1,000,000.

Clinical Features

Patients with LEMS typically present with proximal limb weakness that begins in the legs and spreads to the arms. Classically, patients have a mild improvement in strength after exercise (the "warm-up" phenomenon) that wanes with more continuous activity, though this may not be a significant clinical feature. Besides weakness, more vague symptoms, such as fatigue and myalgias, may be prominent, leading to psychiatric misdiagnoses. In addition, mild autonomic symptoms, such as xerostomia (dry mouth) and orthostatic hypotension, are common. In contrast to MG, respiratory muscles are usually not affected, although rare cases with severe respiratory failure have been reported. Oculobulbar weakness, producing symptoms such as diplopia and ptosis and less often dysarthria and dysphagia, is relatively common in LEMS patients, but these symptoms are typically described as transient and mild, and are rarely presenting complaints (4). However, in a small case series, Burns et al. (88) described the pattern of weakness of LEMS patients and found significant oculobulbar signs and symptoms in 78% of patients, in whom they were a presenting complaint in 30%. Interestingly, 6 of the 11 patients with diplopia in this series also had ataxia, an atypical symptom in LEMS; none of the patients without diplopia was found to have ataxia. The high number of patients with ataxia and diplopia suggest that several of the patients in this series may have had a combined paraneoplastic syndrome of both LEMS and subacute cerebellar degeneration (SCD).

Neurologic Examination

In LEMS, mental status and sensory examination are typically normal, although stocking and glove sensory loss may be seen if there is concurrent paraneoplastic sensory neuropathy (89). Deep tendon reflexes are typically reduced, but may transiently normalize following brief (15-second) exercise of the attached muscle (a phenomenon known as "reflex facilitation" or "reflex augmentation"). Strength testing usually demonstrates mild proximal weakness, most commonly affecting, and often isolated to, the hip flexor muscles. Though oculobulbar symptoms may be subtle, careful cranial nerve examination reveals ptosis and/or diplopia, usually mild, in 25% of patients. If a cancer patient has prolonged paralysis following the use of neuromuscular blocking agents following surgery, LEMS should be strongly considered and evaluated, with neurologic consultation and appropriate diagnostic testing. If symptoms of orthostasis or presyncope are reported, sitting and lying blood pressure and pulse should be measured.

Electrodiagnostic Testing: Routine Studies, Repetitive Stimulation, and SFEMG

Nerve conduction studies show low motor amplitudes due to neuromuscular blockade, in contrast to myasthenia gravis, in which motor amplitudes are usually normal. In addition, motor nerve amplitude may dramatically fluctuate during repeated stimulation on routine nerve conduction studies. Sensory nerve conductions, however, are normal, with no fluctuation. Needle EMG examination may reveal motor unit instability and subtle myopathic change in the proximal muscles, though less commonly than in MG.

In LEMS, RNS produces decrement similar to that seen in MG when low-frequency stimulation is used. However, brief exercise in LEMS patients classically produces dramatic increases in CMAP size (postexercise facilitation), typically exceeding 100%, much larger than those seen in MG. High-frequency RNS in the place of exercise usually also produces dramatic CMAP size facilitation in LEMS. CMAP facilitation exceeding 100% is relatively specific for LEMS, but is not 100% sensitive; therefore, a normal RNS study does not exclude the diagnosis.

The jitter and blocking measured by single-fiber EMG is increased markedly in LEMS, frequently out of proportion to the severity of weakness. In many endplates, jitter and blocking decrease as the firing rate increases. This pattern is not seen in all endplates or in all patients with LEMS. Because jitter and blocking may also decrease at higher firing rates in some endplates of patients with MG, this pattern does not confirm the diagnosis of LEMS. However, if this pattern is dramatic and seen in most muscles, it is highly suggestive of a LEMS diagnosis (90).

Symptomatic Therapies

Paraneoplastic LEMS typically responds to successful treatment of the underlying cancer, though symptoms may return with relapse of cancer. In SCLC, chemotherapy is the first choice, and this will have an additional immunosuppressive effect (4,91). The presence of LEMS in a patient with SCLC is associated with improved patient survival from the cancer. Reports of better prognosis in patients with other paraneoplastic syndromes have shown that patients with paraneoplastic syndromes have longer survival than those with histologically identical tumors without paraneoplastic syndromes, though not universally (92–94).

Cholinesterase inhibitors, guanidine hydrochloride, 3-aminopyridine (3AP), and most recently, 3,4-diaminopyridine (DAP) have been used as symptomatic therapy for LEMS. 3,4 DAP is only available in the United States on a compassionate-use basis from a single manufacturer (Jacobus Pharmaceutical Co., Inc., Princeton, New Jersey; fax: 609-799-1176) (4,95). A research protocol is usually required to use the drug in LEMS in the United States. 3AP is a potent inhibitor of ribonucleotide reductase, the rate-determining enzyme in the supply of deoxynucleotides for DNA synthesis. It has broad-spectrum antitumor activity and acts synergistically with antitumor drugs that target DNA. 3,4-diaminopyridine works by blocking potassium channel efflux in nerve terminals so that action potential duration is increased. Ca2+ channels can then be open for longer time and allow greater acetylcholine release, partially overcoming the VGCC blockade. Two randomized controlled trials have demonstrated the efficacy of 3,4 DAP in improving LEMS symptoms (96–99).

Immunomodulatory Therapies

Immunomodulatory therapy is not generally as effective in LEMS as in MG. Both plasma exchange and IVIG (100,101) seemed to provide some measurable improvement in strength in clinical trials, but do not generally provide significant functional improvement. Prednisone and azathioprine also appeared modestly effective in clinical trials, but most patients do not notice enough improvement in their symptoms to make these agents worthwhile (101). Other immunosuppressants, such as mycophenolate, cyclophosphamide, and tacrolimus, are sometimes used; however, data on the use of these agents is limited to case series reports (4,102) and efficacy appears limited.

Cancer Screening

If a patient is diagnosed with LEMS and has not been diagnosed with any malignancy, a thorough workup for primary cancer must be initiated. This evaluation may include a full-body PET scan, which may detect tumors that escape detection by standard imaging (103,104), and should include all routine cancer screens, as well as more intensive screens tailored to the patient's history and examination (eg, bronchoscopy in a smoker, colonoscopy in a younger patient with a family history of colon cancer, etc.). Even if a tumor is not found initially, oncologic surveillance should be continued every 6–12 months for two to five years.

References

1. Aarli JA. Myasthenia gravis and thymoma. In: Lisak RP, ed. *Handbook of Myasthenia Gravis and Myasthenic Syndromes.* New York: Marcel Dekker; 1994:207–249.
2. Evoli A, Minicuci GM, Vitaliani R, et al. Paraneoplastic diseases associated with thymoma. *J Neurol.* 2007;254:756–762.
3. Morgenthaler TI, Brown LR, Colby TV, Harper CM, Coles DT. Thymoma. *Mayo Clin Proc.* November 1993;68(11):1110–1123.
4. Skeie GO, Apostolski S, Evoli A, et al. Guidelines for the treatment of autoimmune neuromuscular transmission disorders. *Eur J Neurol.* 2006;13:691–699.
5. Souadjian JV, Enriquez P, Silverstein MN, Pépin JM. The spectrum of diseases associated with thymoma. Coincidence or syndrome? *Arch Intern Med.* 1974;134:374–379.
6. Drachman DB. Myasthenia gravis. *N Engl J Med.* 1994;330:1797–1810.
7. Fambrough D, Drachman DB, Satyamurti S. Neuromuscular junction in myasthenia gravis. Decreased acetylcholine receptors. *Science.* 1973;182:293.
8. Wolf SM, Rowland LP, Schotland DL, et al. Myasthenia as an autoimmune disease; clinical aspects. *Ann NY Acad Sci.* 1966;135:517.
9. Zacks SI, Bauer WX, Blumberg JM. The fine structure of the myasthenic neuromuscular junction. *J Neuropathol Exp Neurol.* 1962;21:335–347.
10. Phillips LH, Torner JC. Has the natural history of myasthenia gravis changed over the past 40 years? A meta-analysis of the epidemiological literature. *Neurology.* 1993;43:A386.
11. Treves TA, Rocca WA, Meneghini F. Epidemiology of myasthenia gravis, In: Anderson DW, Schoenberg DG, eds. *Neuroepidemiology: A Tribute to Bruce Schoenberg.* Boston: CRC Press; 1991:297.
12. Legolvan DP, Bell MR. Thymomas. *Cancer.* 1977;39:2142–2157.
13. Verley JM, Hollmann KH. Thymoma. A comparative study of clinical stages, histologic features, and survival in 200 cases. *Cancer.* 1985;55:1074–1086.
14. Limburg PC, The H, Hummel-Tappel E, Oosterhuis HJ. Anti-acetylcholine receptor antibodies in myasthenia gravis. Part I: their relation to the clinical state and the effect of therapy. *J Neurol Sci.* 1983;58:357.
15. Gilhus NE, Aarli JA, Christenson B, et al. Rabbit antisera to a citric extract of human skeletal muscle cross-reacts with thymomas from myasthenia gravis patients. *J Neuroimmunol.* 1984;7:55.
16. Rowland LP, Hoefer PF, Aranow H Jr, Merritt HH. Fatalities in myasthenia gravis. *Neurology.* 1956;6:307–326.
17. Oosterhuis HJ. Myasthenia gravis. A survey. *Clin Neurol Neurosurg.* 1981;83:105–135.
18. Task Force of the Medical Scientific Advisory Board of the Myasthenia Gravis Foundation of America 2000. Myasthenia Gravis: Recommendations for clinical research standards. *Neurology.* 2000;55:16–23.

19. Evoli A, Tonali P, Bartoccioni E, et al. Ocular myasthenia: diagnostic and therapeutic problems. *Acta Neurol Scand.* 1988;77:31.

20. Nicholson GA, McLeod JG, Griffiths LR. Comparison of diagnostic tests in myasthenia gravis. *Clin Exp Neurol.* 1983;19:45.

21. Osserman KE, Benkins G. Critical reappraisal of the use of edrophonium (Tensilon) chloride tests in myasthenia gravis and significance of clinical classification. *Ann NY Acad Sci.* 1966;135:212.

22. Phillips LH, Melnick PA. Diagnosis of myasthenia gravis in the 1990s. *Sem Neurol.* 1990;10:62–69.

23. Viets HR, Schwab RS. Problems in the diagnosis of myasthenia gravis, a 20-year report of the neostigmine test. *Trans Am Neurol Assoc.* 1955;80:36.

24. Howard FM, Lennon VA, Finley J, et al. Clinical correlations of antibodies than bind, block or modulate human acetylcholine receptors in myasthenia gravis. *Ann NY Acad Sci.* 1987;505: 526–538.

25. Lennon VA, Jones G, Howard FM, et al. Autoantibodies to acetylcholine receptors in myasthenia gravis. *N Engl J Med.* 1983;308:402–403.

26. Lennon VA, Howard FM. Serologic diagnosis of myasthenia gravis. In: Nakamura RM, O'Sullivan MB, eds. *Clinical Laboratory Molecular Analysis: New Strategies in Autoimmunity, Cancer and Virology.* New York: Brune and Stratton; 1985;29–44.

27. Lennon VA. Serological diagnosis of myasthenia gravis and the Lambert-Eaton myasthenic syndrome. In Lisak RP, ed. *Handbook of Myasthenia Gravis and Myasthenic Syndromes.* New York: Marcel Dekker Inc; 1994:249.

28. Limburg PC, Hummel E, The TH, Oosterhuis HJ. Relationship between changes in anti-acetylcholine receptor antibody concentration and disease severity in myasthenia gravis. *Ann NY Acad Sci.* 1981;377:859.

29. Evoli A, Tonali PA, Padua L, et al. Clinical correlates with anti-MuSK antibodies in generalized seronegative myasthenia gravis. *Brain.* 2003;126:2304–2311.

30. Evoli A, Tonali PA, Padua L, et al. Clinical correlates with anti-MuSK antibodies in generalized seronegative myasthenia gravis. *Brain.* 2003;126:2304–2311.

31. Padua L, Tonali P, Aprile I, Caliandro P, Bartoccioni E, Evoli A. Seronegative myasthenia gravis: comparison of neurophysiological picture in MuSK+ and MuSK- patients. *Eur J Neurol.* 2006;13:273–276.

32. Lauriola L, Ranelletti F, Maggiano N, et al. Thymus changes in anti-MuSK-positive and negative myasthenia gravis. *Neurology.* 2005;65:782–783.

33. Hoch W, McConville J, Helms S, Newsom-Davis J, Melms A, Vincent A. Auto-antibodies to the receptor tyrosine kinase MuSK in patients with myasthenia gravis without acetylcholine receptor antibodies. *Nat Med.* 2001;7:365–368.

34. Niks EH, Kuks JB, Verschuuren JJ. Epidemiology of myasthenia gravis with anti-muscle specific kinase antibodies in The Netherlands. *J Neurol Neurosurg Psychiatry.* 2007;78:417–418.

35. Sanders DB, El-Salem K, Massey JM, McConville J, Vincent A. Clinical aspects of MuSK antibody positive seronegative MG. *Neurology.* 2003;60:1978–1980.

36. Deymeer F, Gungor-Tuncer O, Yilmaz V, et al. Clinical comparison of anti-MuSK- vs anti-AChR-positive and seronegative myasthenia gravis. *Neurology.* 2007;68:609–611.

37. Vincent A, Hart ZL, Barrett-Jolley R, et al. Seronegative myasthenia gravis. Evidence for plasma factors interfering with acetylcholine receptor function. *Ann NY Acad Sci.* 1993;681: 529–538.

38. Howard JF, Sanders DB, Massey JM. The electrodiagnosis of myasthenia gravis and the Lambert-Eaton myasthenic syndrome. In: Sanders DB, ed. *Myasthenia Gravis and Myasthenic Syndromes. Neurologic Clinics of North America.* Vol. 12, No. 2. Philadelphia: WB Saunders Company; 1994: 305–329.

39. Sanders DB. Clinical neurophysiology of disorders of the neuromuscular junction. *J Clin Neurophysiol.* 1993;12:169.

40. Stalberg E, Eksted J, Broman A. Neuromuscular transmission in myasthenia gravis studied with single fibre electromyography. *J Neurol Neurosurg Psychiatry.* 1974;37:540–547.

41. Walker MB. Treatment of myasthenia gravis with physostigmine. *Lancet.* 1934;ii:1200–1201.

42. Pascuzzi RM, Coslett HB, Johns TR. Long-term corticosteroid treatment of myasthenia gravis. *Ann Neurol.* 1984;15:291.

43. Bromberg MB, Wald JJ, Forshew DA, Feldman EL, Albers JW. Randomized trial of azathioprine or prednisone for initial immunosuppressive treatment of myasthenia gravis. *J Neurol Sci.* 1997;150:59–62.

44. Palace J, Newsom-Davis J, Lecky B. A randomized double-blind trial of prednisolone alone or with azathioprine in myasthenia gravis. Myasthenia Gravis Study Group. *Neurology.* 1998;50:1778–1783.

45. Gladstone DE, Brannagan TH 3rd, Schwartzman RJ, Prestrud AA, Brodsky I. High dose cyclophosphamide for severe refractory myasthenia gravis. *J Neurol Neurosurg Psychiatry.* 2004;75:789–791.

46. García-Carrasco M, Escárcega RO, Fuentes-Alexandro S, Riebeling C, Cervera R. Therapeutic options in autoimmune myasthenia gravis. *Autoimmun Rev.* 2007;6:373–378.

47. Lim AK, Donnan G, Chambers B, Ierino FL. Mycophenolate mofetil substitution for cyclosporine-dependent myasthenia gravis and nephrotoxicity. *Intern Med J.* 2007;37:55–59.

48. Sanders DB, Howard JF Jr, Johns TR, et al. High dose daily prednisone in the treatment of myasthenia gravis. In: Dau PC, ed. *Plasmapheresis and the Immunobiology of Myasthenia Gravis.* Boston: Houghton Mifflin; 1979:225,289–306.

49. Dau PC, Lindstrom JM, Cassel CK, et al. Plasmapheresis and immunosuppressive drug therapy in myasthenia gravis. *N Engl J Med.* 1977;297:1134.

50. Hawkey CJ, Newsom-Davis J, Vincent A. Plasma exchange and immunosuppressive drug treatment in myasthenia gravis: no evidence of synergy. *J Neurol Neurosurg Psychiatry.* 1981;44:469.

51. Keesey J, Buffkin D, Kebo D, et al. Plasma exchange as therapy for myasthenia gravis. *Ann NY Acad Sci.* 1981;377:729.

52. Kornfeld P, Ambinder EP, Matta RJ, et al. Plasmapheresis in refractory generalized myasthenia gravis. *Arch Neurol.* 1981;38:478.

53. Newsom-Davis J, Wilson SG, Vincent A, Ward CD. Long-term effects of repeated plasma exchange in myasthenia gravis. *Lancet.* 1979;1:464–468.

54. Pinching AJ, Peters DK, Newsom-Davis J. Remission of myasthenia gravis following plasma exchange. *Lancet.* 1976;2:1373.

55. Arsura EL. Experience with intravenous immunoglobulins in myasthenia gravis. *Clin Immunol Immunopathol.* 1989;53:S170.

56. Gajdos P, Chevret S, Clair B, Tranchant C, Chastang C. for the Myasthenia gravis clinical study group. Clinical trial of plasma exchange and high-dose intravenous immunoglobulin in myasthenia gravis. *Ann Neurol.* 1997;41:789–796.

57. Gajdos P, Tranchant C, Clair B, et al. Treatment of myasthenia gravis exacerbation with intravenous immunoglobulin: a randomized double-blind clinical trial. *Arch Neurol.* 2005;62:1689–1693.

58. Pérez Nellar J, Domínguez AM, Llorens-Figueroa JA, et al. A comparative study of intravenous immunoglobulin and plasmapheresis preoperatively in myasthenia. *Rev Neurol.* 2001;33:413–416.

59. Blalock A, Mason MR, Morgan HJ, et al. Myasthenia gravis and tumors of the thymic region: report of a case in which the tumor was removed. *Ann Surg.* 1939;110:554–561.

60. Blalock A. Thymectomy in the treatment of myasthenia gravis: report of 20 cases. *J Thorac Surg.* 1944;13:316–339.

61. Perlo VP, Poskanzer DC, Schwab RS, Viets HR, Osserman KE, Genkins G. Myasthenia gravis: evaluation of treatment in 1,355 patients. *Neurology.* 1966;16:431–439.

62. Schwab RS. Thymectomy for myasthenia gravis. In: Viets HR, ed. *Myasthenia Gravis.* Illinois: Charles C. Thomas; 1961.

63. Olanow CW, Lane RJ, Roses AD. Thymectomy in late onset myasthenia gravis. *Arch Neurol.* 1982a;39:82–83.

64. Olanow CW, Wechsler AS, Roses AD. A prospective study of thymectomy and serum acetylcholine receptor antibodies in myasthenia gravis. *Ann Surg.* 1982b;196:113–121.

65. Donnelly RJ, Laquaglia MP, Fabri B, Hayward M, Florence AM. Cervical thymectomy in the treatment of myasthenia gravis. *Ann R Coll Surg Engl.* 1984;66:305–308.

66. Klingen G, Johansson L, Westerholm CJ, Sundstroom C. Transcervical thymectomy with the aid of mediastinoscopy for myasthenia gravis: eight years' experience. *Ann Thorac Surg.* 1977;23:342–347.

67. Masaoka A, Monden Y. Comparison of the results of transsternal simple, transcervical simple and extended thymectomy. *Ann NY Acad Sci.* 1981;377:755–764.

68. Matell G, Lebram G, Osterman PO, Pirskanen R. Follow up comparison of suprasternal vs. transsternal method for thymectomy in myasthenia gravis. *Ann NY Acad Sci.* 1981;377:844–855.

69. Paletto AE, Maggi G. Thymectomy in the treatment of myasthenia gravis: results in 320 patients. *Int Surg.* 1982;67:13–16.

70. Emery KB, Strugalska MH. Evaluation of results of thymectomy in myasthenia gravis. *J Neurol.* 1976;211:155–168.

71. Mulder D, Graves M, Herrman C. Thymectomy for myasthenia gravis: recent observations and comparisons with past experience. *Ann Thorac Surg.* 1989;48:551–555.

72. Jaretzki A, Penn AS, Younger DS. "Maximal" thymectomy for myasthenia gravis: results. *J Thorac Cardiovasc Surg.* 1988;95:747–757.

73. Rubin JW, Ellison RG, Moore HV, Pai GP. Factors affecting response to thymectomy for myasthenia gravis. *J Thorac Cardiovasc Surg.* 1981;82:720–728.

74. Frist WH, Shanti T, Doehring CB, et al. Thymectomy for the myasthenia gravis patient: factors influencing outcome. *Ann Thorac Surg.* 1994;57:334–338.

75. Kimura J, van Allen MW. Post-thymectomy myasthenia gravis. *Neurology.* 1967;17:413.

76. Lindberg C, Andersen O, Larsson S, Oden A. Remission rate after thymectomy in myasthenia gravis when the bias of immunosuppressive therapy is eliminated. *Acta Neurol Scand.* 1992;86:323–328.

77. Monden Y, Uyama T, Nakahara K, et al. Clinical characteristics and prognosis of myasthenia gravis with other autoimmune disease. *Ann Thorac Surg.* 1986;41:189.

78. Mier-Jedrzejowicz AK, Brophy C, Green M. Respiratory muscle function in myasthenia gravis. *Am Rev Respir Dis.* 1988;138:867–873.

79. Twomey JJ, Lewis VM, Patten BM. Myasthenia gravis, thymectomy and serum thymic hormone activity. *Am J Med.* 1979;66:639.

80. Eaton LM, Lambert EH. Electromyography and electrical stimulation of nerves in diseases of the motor unit: observations on a myasthenic syndrome associated with malignant tumours. *JAMA.* 1957;163:1117–1124.

81. Graus F, Lang B, Pozo-Rosich P, et al. P/Q type calcium-channel antibodies in paraneoplastic cerebellar degeneration with lung cancer. *Neurology.* 2002;59:784–766.

82. Lennon VA, Kryzer TJ, Griestmann GE, et al. Calcium channel antibodies in Lambert-Eaton myasthenic syndrome and other paraneoplastic syndromes. *N Engl J Med.* 1995;332:1467–1474.

83. Fukunaga H, Engel AG, Osame M, et al. Paucity and disorganization of presynaptic membrane active zones in the Lambert–Eaton myasthenic syndrome. *Muscle Nerve.* 1982;5:686–697.

84. Nagel A, Engel AG, Lang B, et al. Lambert-Eaton myasthenic syndrome IgG depletes presynaptic membrane active zone particles by antigenic modulation. *Ann Neurol.* 1988;24:552–558.

85. Lennon VA, Lambert EH. Autoantibodies bind solubilized calcium channel-omega-conotoxin complexes from small cell lung carcinoma: a diagnostic aid for Lambert-Eaton myasthenic syndrome. *Mayo Clin Proc.* 1989;64:1498–1504.

86. Argov Z, Shapira Y, Averbuch-Heller L, Wirguin I. Lambert-Eaton myasthenic syndrome (LEMS) in association with lymphoproliferative disorders. *Muscle Nerve.* 1995;18:715–719.

87. O'Neill JH, Murray NMF, Newsom-Davis J. The Lambert-Eaton myasthenic syndrome: a review of 50 cases. *Brain.* 1998;111:577–596.

88. Burns TM, Russell JA, LaChance DH, Jones HR. Oculobulbar involvement is typical with Lambert-Eaton myasthenic syndrome. *Ann Neurol.* 2003;53:270–273.

89. Tomiyasu K, Ito H, Kanazawa N, Saito T, Kowa H. Anti-Hu antibody in a patient with Lambert-Eaton myasthenic syndrome and early detection of small cell lung cancer. *Internal Medicine.* 1995;34:1082–1085.

90. AAEM Quality Assurance Committee. Literature review of the usefulness of repetitive nerve stimulation and single fiber EMG in the electrodiagnostic evaluation of patients with suspected myasthenia gravis or Lambert-Eaton myasthenic syndrome. American Association of Electrodiagnostic. *Muscle Nerve.* 2001;24:1239–1247.

91. Maddison P, Newsom-Davis J, Mills KR, Souhami RL. Favourable prognosis in Lambert-Eaton myasthenic syndrome and small-cell lung carcinoma. *Lancet.* 1999;353:117–118.

92. Altman AJ, Baehner RL. Favorable prognosis for survival in children with coincident opso-myoclonus and neuroblastoma. *Cancer.* 1976;37:846–852.

93. Hiyama E, Yokoyama T, Ichikawa T, et al. Poor outcome in patients with advanced stage neuroblastoma and coincident opsomyoclonus syndrome. *Cancer.* 1994;74:1821–1826.

94. Rojas I, Graus F, Keime-Guibert F, et al. Long-term clinical outcome of paraneoplastic cerebellar degeneration and anti-Yo antibodies. *Neurology.* 2000;55:713–715.

95. Verschuuren JJ, Wirtz PW, Titulaer MJ, Willems LN, van Gerven J. Available treatment options for the management of Lambert-Eaton myasthenic syndrome. *Expert Opin Pharmacother.* 2006;7:1323–1336.

96. Sanders DB, Howard JF Jr, Massey JM. 3,4-Diaminopyridine in Lambert-Eaton myasthenic syndrome and myasthenia gravis. *Ann N Y Acad Sci.* 1993;681:588–590.

97. Sanders DB. 3,4-Diaminopyridine (DAP) in the treatment of Lambert-Eaton myasthenic syndrome (LEMS). *Ann N Y Acad Sci.* May 13, 1998;841:811–816.

98. Sanders DB, Massey JM, Sanders LL, Edwards LJ. A randomized trial of 3,4-diaminopyridine in Lambert-Eaton myasthenic syndrome. *Neurology.* 2000;54:603–607.

99. Sanders DB. Lambert-Eaton myasthenic syndrome: Diagnosis and Treatment. Ann NY Acad sic 2003;998:500–508.

100. Bain PG, Motomura M, Newsom-Davis J, et al. Effects of intravenous immunoglobulin on muscle weakness and calcium-channel autoantibodies in the Lambert-Eaton myasthenic syndrome. *Neurology.* 1996;47:678–683.

101. Newsom-Davis J. Therapy in myasthenia gravis and Lambert-Eaton myasthenic syndrome. *Sem Neurol.* 2003;23:191–198.

102. Maddison P, Lang B, Mills K, et al. Long term outcome in Lambert-Eaton myasthenic syndrome without lung cancer. *J Neurol Neurosurg Psychiatry.* 2001;70:212–217.

103. Antoine JC, Cinotti L, Tilikete C, et al. 18F]Fluorodeoxyglucose positron emission tomography in the diagnosis of cancer in patients with paraneoplastic neurological syndrome and anti-Hu antibodies. *Ann Neurol.* 2000;48:105–108.

104. Rees JH, Hain SF, Johnson MR, et al. The role of [18F]fluoro-2-deoxyglucose-PET scanning in the diagnosis of paraneoplastic neurological disorders. *Brain.* 2001;124:2223–2231.

Myopathy in Cancer

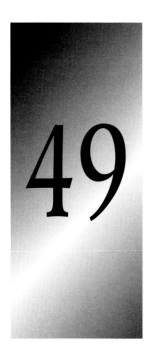

49

Edward J. Cupler
Eric Graf
Sakir Humayun Gultekin

Muscle weakness in cancer patients, especially those receiving aggressive life-saving therapies, is difficult to dissect (1). While muscle is rarely a primary organ affected by neoplasms in adults, direct invasion of muscle from a tumor or metastasis to muscle is more likely to occur. Either case can be the cause of specific myopathies. A generalized myopathy can also occur and usually is due to a paraneoplastic process, unintended side effects of therapy, or cachexia.

TUMOR INVASION AND METASTASES

Skeletal muscle metastases are rare, although single and multiple muscle metastases have been reported from many tumor types (2–7). Symptoms of muscle metastasis may include focal swelling, pain, or difficulty with muscle function. Case reports and small case series are published (8); however, incidence and prevalence rates of muscle metastasis are unknown. Primary tumor sites include lung, breast, melanoma, thyroid, liver, and others. Muscle magnetic resonance imaging (MRI) is the diagnostic tool of choice for muscle metastasis (Fig. 49.1) (4,8). Therapy for solitary muscle metastasis depends on the tumor type and may include excision, chemotherapy, or radiation therapy.

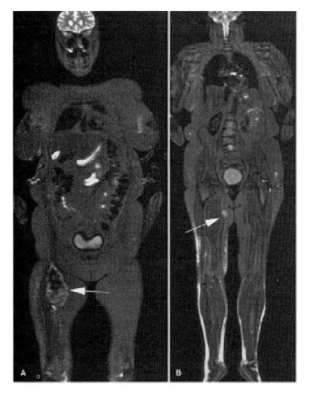

FIGURE 49.1

Coronal whole body STIRR showing evidence of a metastatic tumor in the right Sartorius muscle.

KEY POINTS

- A generalized myopathy can occur due to a para-neoplastic process, unintended side effects of cancer therapy, or cachexia.
- Skeletal muscle metastases are rare, although single and multiple muscle metastases have been reported from many tumor types.
- Amyloid myopathy is a rare complication of multiple myeloma.
- Chronic glucocorticoid use may cause a proximal myopathy in up to 60% of cancer patients.

- Electromyogram (EMG) in steroid myopathy may be normal or show short-duration motor units that are nonspecific.
- A number of chemotherapeutic agents have been associated with muscle weakness or myopathy to varying degrees, including alkylating agents, cisplatin (mitochondrial myopathy), antimetabolites (eg, fluorouracil), anthracyclines, topoisomerase inhibitors, and nitrosoureas.

PARANEOPLASTIC

Necrotizing Myopathy

An acute necrotizing myopathy has been described in patients with cancer (43). The onset is characterized by rapidly progressive proximal muscle weakness that occurs over months. Necrotizing myopathy has been associated with breast, small cell carcinoma of the lung, gastrointestinal (GI) malignancies (stomach, colon, pancreatic, and gallbladder), genitourinary (GU) cancer (kidney, bladder, ovarian, and prostate) melanoma, multiple myeloma, and head and neck cancer. The serum creatine kinase (CK) levels are usually markedly elevated, up to 100 times the upper limit of normal. Electromyography (EMG) usually reveals fibrillation potentials, occasionally positive sharp waves, and short-duration, small-amplitude, polyphasic motor units. Muscle histology reveals muscle necrosis, myophagocytosis, and the absence of lymphocytic inflammatory cells (Fig. 49.2). Immunohistochemical staining shows membrane attack complex present upon the sarcolemma. In addition to treating the underlying malignancy, there is a role for oral corticosteroids at dosages similar to those of idiopathic inflammatory myopathies: prednisone 60 mg daily or 1 mg/kg/day. Intravenous immunoglobulin (IVIG) has also been reported beneficial at dosages of 2 g/kg given over three to five days each month (9).

Inflammatory Myopathy: Polymyositis, Dermatomyositis, and Inclusion Body Myositis

Polymyositis (PM), dermatomyositis (DM), and inclusion body myositis (IBM) are primary inflammatory

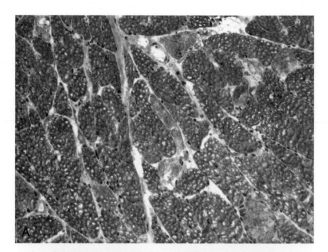
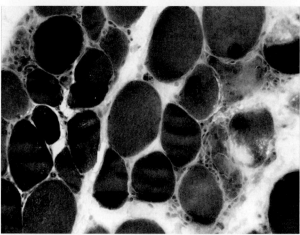

FIGURE 49.2

Paraneoplastic necrotizing myopathy. Scattered necrotic myofibers are present, but there is no accompanying inflammatory infiltrate. (*See color insert following page 736*)

disorders of muscle. Each of these disorders has a distinct clinical phenotype and unique myopathological features (10,11). Case reports of inflammatory myopathy in association with cancer appear in early 20th century literature (12,13). Subsequently, retrospective studies and case series have confirmed the association (14). A controversy exists in the literature as to whether there are increased incidences of neoplasm occurring in both PM and DM or if an increase is confined to DM (15,16). This confusion, in part, is due diagnostic criteria for PM and DM. Bohan and Peter criteria, published in 1975, do not require a muscle biopsy to establish a diagnosis of possible or probable PM or DM (17,18). Without muscle pathology, the incidence of PM may be overestimated (19). In 2001, Hill et al. reviewed hospital-based data from Scandinavia (20). Using Bohan and Peter criteria, 618 cases of DM and 918 cases of PM were identified. The risk of cancer was found to be 30% in DM and 15% in PM; the relative risk of cancer was 3.0 in DM and 1.4 in PM. In 60% of cases, PM or DM was diagnosed prior to malignancy. Patients with IBM have not been found to have an increased risk of cancer (21).

Polymyositis

PM is an immune-mediated myopathy in which patients develop progressive proximal muscle weakness. Symptoms of symmetrical weakness involving the shoulder and pelvic girdle muscles develop insidiously. Muscle pain may be present. Serum CK, aldolase, and aspartate aminotransferase (AST) are usually elevated, but may on occasion be normal. EMG reveals an abundance of small-amplitude, short-duration, polyphasic motor units with early recruitment, fibrillation potentials, positive sharp waves, and possibly complex repetitive discharges. Muscle biopsy shows CD8+ T cells surrounding and invading normal-appearing muscle fibers that abnormally express major histocompatibility complex (MHC) class 1 markers on the sarcolemma (Fig. 49.3).

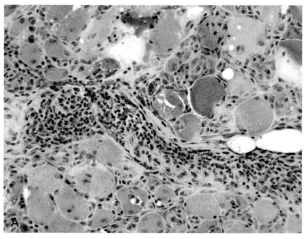
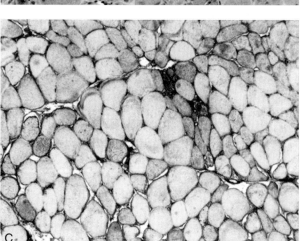
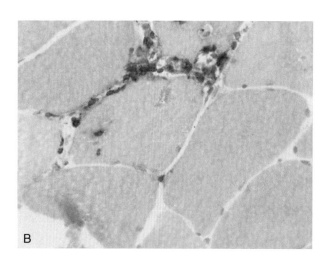

Polymositis. Marked chronic inflammation, necrosis, and regeneration of muscle fibers (A). Autoaggresive inflammation in polymyositis. T cells attacking an intact muscle fiber (B). Diffuse de novo membraneous MHC-1 expression in muscle fibers (C). (*See color insert following page 736*)

FIGURE 49.3

In addition, there are areas of myophagocytosis, necrosis, internalized nuclei, and atrophy of both fiber types. Treatments for PM include high-dosage corticosteroid therapy, prednisone 60 mg/day or 1.0 mg/kg/day; other immunosuppressant medications (eg, azathioprine 2–3 mg /kg/day); and IVIG 2.0 g/kg divided over three to five days monthly.

Dermatomyositis

Patients with dermatomyositis present with proximal muscle weakness, myalgias, and skin lesions that may occur simultaneously or in tandem (19). The typical heliotrope rash is usually over the eyelids. Rash can also occur on the face, neck, elbows, and knees. Gottran papules, a red, scaly rash over the knuckles, may also be present. Dilated capillary loops in the nail beds and cuticle damage may also be present. Subcutaneous calcifications occur in more severe cases. Additionally, there may be signs and symptoms of systemic vasculitis. The serum CK is usually elevated and may be up to 100 times the upper limit of normal. However, the serum CK may also be normal. EMG shows evidence of a myopathy that is usually irritative in nature and includes increased insertional activity and small-amplitude, short-duration, polyphasic motor units. Fibrillations and positive sharp waves may be present.

Dermatomyositis is an immune-mediated disorder with complement and membrane attack complex deposited on the capillary endothelium and the sarcolemmal membrane. This leads to reduction of capillary density, myonecrosis, muscle ischemia, and perifascicular atrophy (Fig. 49.4). MHC class 1 molecules are up-regulated on the sarcolemma. More recently, gene expression profiles in muscle from DM patients reveal up-regulation of interferon (IFN) alpha/beta inducible genes (22). Dendritic cells are present and produce IFN alpha/beta. These findings suggest an immune-mediated rather than an ischemic process in DM. Therapy for DM includes high-dosage corticosteroid therapy, prednisone 60 mg/day or 1.0 mg/kg/day; other immunosuppressant medications such as,

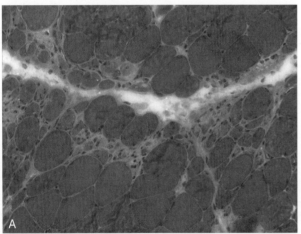

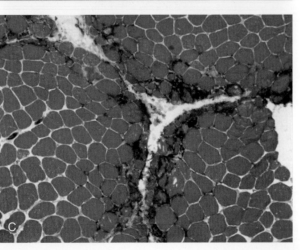

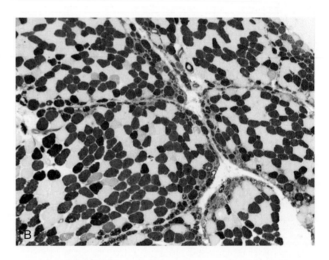

Dermsromyositis (A) Selective atrophy and necrosis of the perifascieular myofibers H&E Stain x400 (B) Distinct perifascieular distribution of atrophic myofibers. ATPase (9.4 x200). (C) Perifaseicular myofibers show regenerative changes, and the connective tissue is also labeled (bluck). Alkaline Phosphatase Stain x200. (*See color insert following page 736*)

FIGURE 49.4

azathioprine 2–3 mg /kg/day; and IVIG 2.0 g/kg divided over three to five days monthly (23,24).

Inclusion Body Myositis

Inclusion body myositis (IBM) is the most common acquired myopathy occurring over the age of 50 years. Patients present with symptoms of hand weakness, quadriceps weakness, and dysphagia. IBM does not have an increased association of malignancy in contrast to PM and DM. The serum CK may be modestly elevated, but can be normal. The EMG may demonstrate fibrillation potentials and positive sharp waves. Motor units can be mixed with both large-amplitude, long-duration and small-amplitude, short-duration polyphasic motor unit potentials demonstrated. The muscle biopsy shows CD8+ lymphocytes surrounding and invading MHC class 1 expression muscle fibers. In addition, there are red-rimmed vacuoles, amyloid deposits, ragged red fibers, and angulated fibers. Electron microscopy reveals filaments that may be associated with vacuoles or within the nucleus. There are no effective pharmacotherapies for IBM.

Other Myopathies

Amyloid Myopathy

Amyloid myopathy is a rare complication of multiple myeloma (25,26). The diagnosis is often overlooked unless the myopathy is the presenting symptom of the disorder (25,27,28). Patients present with mild proximal weakness and diffusely enlarged muscles. The serum CK is usually within normal limits. The EMG may show small-amplitude, short-duration, polyphasic motor units. In amyloid myopathy, muscle biopsies reveal nonspecific myopathic changes, such as atrophy, myofiber necrosis, and regeneration (29). Amyloid deposits can be identified with light microscopy with Congo Red stain or by fluorescence microscopy using Thioflavin S (Fig. 49.5). The abnormal deposits typically involve the endomysium surrounding individual myofibers or appear as mural deposits in blood vessels of the perimysium. Electron microscopy can also be used to identify amyloid deposits in the form of fibrillary deposits. Amyloid myopathy generally is a gradually progressive disorder. Therapy is directed at the underlying multiple myeloma.

Antidecorin Antibody Myopathy

A myopathy has been described in Waldenström macroglobulinemia that is slowly progressive in nature (30). In this myopathy, monoclonal IgM antibodies are

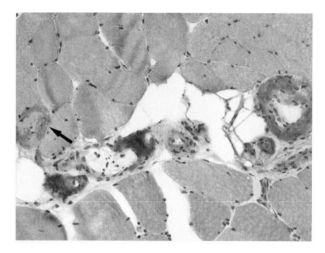

FIGURE 49.5

Amyloid myopathy. Amyloid deposits (arrow) surrounding a muscle fiber, and as intramural/perivascular deposits in the perimysial fibroadipose tissue. (*See color insert following page 736*)

directed against decorin. The role of this antibody in the pathogenesis of the myopathy is not clear.

Granulomatous Myositis in Thymoma

Thymomas are the most common anterior mediastinal tumors and are epithelial cell tumors. About half of patients with thymoma will have autoimmune myasthenia gravis. Rarely, granulomatous myositis and myocarditis will occur in conjunction with thymoma (31).

THERAPY-INDUCED MYOPATHY

Steroid Myopathy

Chronic glucocorticoid use may cause a proximal myopathy in up to 60% of cancer patients (32). Women seem to be more susceptible to developing steroid myopathy than men. The onset of steroid myopathy is insidious. Initial symptoms include difficulty climbing stairs or raising the arms up for extended time periods. Muscle weakness tends to be symmetrical (33). The cumulative dosage and duration of steroid use seems to be related to the development of the myopathy. The serum CK is usually normal. The EMG may be normal or show short-duration motor units that are nonspecific. Spontaneous activity is lacking. The muscle biopsy shows a pattern of type 2 atrophy that is not specific in nature. In time, there may be increased lipid content in type-1 fibers (Fig. 49.6). Therapy is directed to minimize or eliminate glucocorticoid exposure, if possible.

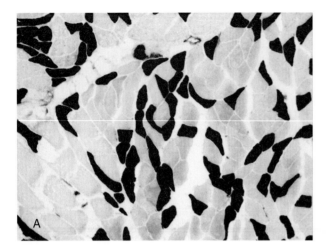 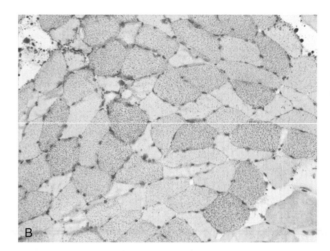

FIGURE 49.6

Steroid myopathy. Selective atrophy of type 1 fibers (A). Type 1 myofibers have increased lipid content (B). (*See color insert following page 736*)

Other Medications

A number of other chemotherapeutic agents have been associated with muscle weakness or myopathy to varying degrees (34,35). These include alkylating agents, cisplatin (mitochondrial myopathy), antimetabolites (eg, fluorouracil), anthracyclines, topoisomerase inhibitors, and nitrosoureas.

MUSCLE WEAKNESS IN CACHEXIA

Muscle weakness is common in patients with cachexia associated with cancer (36,37). These patients present with decreased proximal muscle strength and diffusely decreased muscle bulk. Muscle protein loss results from both increased muscle catabolism and impaired muscle anabolism (37,38). Three process have been identified that increase muscle catabolism; up-regulation of the ubiquitin-proteasome proteolytic system (39), dysregulation of the dystrophin glycoprotein complex (40), and tumor expression of proteolysis-inducing factor (41,42). Impaired muscle anabolism results from an imbalance in the amino acid pool, reduced myosin expression, and up-regulation of myostatin. The serum CK is usually normal or decreased. EMG may be normal or may show short-duration motor units. Spontaneous activity is lacking. Muscle pathology reveals type 2 fiber atrophy, a nonspecific finding. There is no specific therapy to improve this type of myopathy.

CONCLUSIONS

The muscle disorders occurring in the setting of cancer are rare. Defined paraneoplastic myopathies occur in the setting of cancer. These tend to be necrotizing myo-pathy, dermatomyositis, and polymyositis. Weakness also occurs as part of cachexia or as side effects of therapy. Treatments always include therapy directed at the underlying neoplasm and, in some cases, immunotherapy similar to that used in idiopathic cases. Supportive therapies, including nutritional, physical therapy, and occupational therapy, improve quality of life.

References

1. Sliwa JA. Acute weakness syndromes in the critically ill patient. *Arch Phys Med Rehabil.* 2000;81(3 Suppl 1):S45–S52.
2. Viswanathan N, Khanna A. Skeletal muscle metastasis from malignant melanoma. *Br J Plas Surg.* 2005;58(6):855–858.
3. Nabi G, Gupta NP, Gandhi D. Skeletal muscle metastasis from transitional cell carcinoma of the urinary bladder: clinicoradiological features. *Clin Radiol.* 2003;58(11):883–885.
4. O'Brien JM, et al. Skeletal muscle metastasis from uterine leiomyosarcoma. *Skeletal Radiol.* 2004;33(11):655–659.
5. Wu G, et al. PET detection of solitary distant skeletal muscle metastasis of esophageal adenocarcinoma. *Clin Nucl Med.* 2005;30(5):335–337.
6. Heyer CM, et al. Metastasis to skeletal muscle from esophageal adenocarcinoma. *Scand J Gastroenterol.* 2005;40(8):1000–1004.
7. Wu M-H, Wu Y-M, Lee P-H. The psoas muscle as an unusual site for metastasis of hepatocellular carcinoma: report of a case. *Surg Today.* 2006;36(3):280–282.
8. Tuoheti Y, et al. Skeletal muscle metastases of carcinoma: a clinicopathological study of 12 cases. *Jap J Clin Oncol.* 2004;34(4):210–214.
9. Sampson, J.B., et al., Paraneoplastic myopathy: response to intravenous immunoglobulin. *Neuromuscul Disord.* 2007;17(5):404–408.
10. Greenberg SA, Amato AA. Uncertainties in the pathogenesis of adult dermatomyositis. *Curr Opin Neurol.* 2004;17(3):359–364.
11. Greenberg SA, et al. Molecular profiles of inflammatory myopathies. [see comment]. *Neurology.* 2002;59(8):1170–1182.
12. Kankeleit. Uber primaire nichteitrige polymyositis. *Dtsch Arch Klin Med.* 1916;120:335.
13. Stertz G. Polymyositis. *Berl Klin Wochenshr.* 1916;53:489.
14. Levine SM. Cancer and myositis: new insights into an old association. *Curr Opin Rheumatol.* 2006;18(6):620–624.

15. Amato AA, et al. Unicorns, dragons, polymyositis, and other mythological beasts. [see comment]. *Neurology.* 2003;61(3):288–289.

16. van der Meulen MF, et al. Polymyositis: an overdiagnosed entity. [see comment]. *Neurology.* 2003;61(3):316–321.

17. Bohan A, Peter JB. Polymyositis and dermatomyositis (first of two parts). *N Engl J Med.* 1975;292(7):344–347.

18. Bohan A, Peter JB. Polymyositis and dermatomyositis (second of two parts). *N Engl J Med.* 1975;292(8):403–407.

19. Dalakas MC, et al. Polymyositis and dermatomyositis. [see comment]. *Lancet.* 2003;362(9388):971–982.

20. Hill CL, et al. Frequency of specific cancer types in dermatomyositis and polymyositis: a population-based study. [see comment]. *Lancet.* 2001;357(9250):96–100.

21. Callen J. Relationship of cancer to inflammatory muscle diseases. Dermatomyositis, polymyositis, and inclusion body myositis. *Rheum Dis Clin North Am.* 1994;20(4):943.

22. Walsh RJ, et al. Type I interferon-inducible gene expression in blood is present and reflects disease activity in dermatomyositis and polymyositis. *Arthritis Rheumat,* 2007;56(11):3784–3792.

23. Amato AA, et al. Treatment of idiopathic inflammatory myopathies. *Curr Opin Neurol.* 2003;16(5):569–575.

24. Dalakas MC. Controlled studies with high-dose intravenous immunoglobulin in the treatment of dermatomyositis, inclusion body myositis, and polymyositis. *Neurology.* 1998;51(6 Suppl 5):S37–S45.

25. Smestad C, et al. Amyloid myopathy presenting with distal atrophic weakness. *Muscle Nerve.* 2004;29(4):605–609.

26. Chapin JE, et al. Amyloid myopathy: characteristic features of a still underdiagnosed disease. *Muscle Nerve.* 2005;31(2):266–272.

27. Mandl LA, et al. Amyloid myopathy masquerading as polymyositis. *J Rheumatol.* 2000;27(4):949–952.

28. Spuler S, Emslie-Smith A, Engel AG. Amyloid myopathy: an underdiagnosed entity. *Ann Neurol.* 1998;43(6):719–728.

29. Amyloid myopathy (Chapter 15). In: George Karpati, Thomas P, Carpenter S, eds. *Structural and Molecular Basis of Skeletal Muscle Disease.* 2002:284–286.

30. al-Lozi MT, Pestronk A, Choksi R. A skeletal muscle-specific form of decorin is a target antigen for a serum IgM M-protein in a patient with a proximal myopathy. *Neurology.* 1997;49(6):1650–1654.

31. Herrmann DN, et al. Granulomatous myositis, primary biliary cirrhosis, pancytopenia, and thymoma. *Muscle Nerve.* 2000;23(7):1133–1136.

32. Batchelor TT, et al. Steroid myopathy in cancer patients. [see comment]. *Neurology.* 1997;48(5):1234–1238.

33. Kanda F, et al. Steroid myopathy: pathogenesis and effects of growth hormone and insulin-like growth factor-I administration. *Horm Res.* 2001;56(Suppl 1):24–28.

34. Kao K-L, Hung G-Y, Hwang B. Pyomyositis during induction chemotherapy for acute lymphoblastic leukemia. *J Chin Med Assoc.* 2006;69(4):184–188.

35. van Oosterhout AG, et al. Neurologic disorders in 203 consecutive patients with small cell lung cancer. Results of a longitudinal study. *Cancer.* 1996;77(8):1434–1441.

36. Argiles JM, et al. Molecular mechanisms involved in muscle wasting in cancer and ageing: cachexia versus sarcopenia. *Int J Biochem Cell Biol.* 2005;37(5):1084–1104.

37. Muscaritoli M, et al. Prevention and treatment of cancer cachexia: new insights into an old problem. *Eur J Cancer.* 2006;42(1):31–41.

38. Jackman RW, Kandarian SC. The molecular basis of skeletal muscle atrophy. *Am J Physiol Cell Physiol.* 2004;287(4):C834–C843.

39. Camps C, et al. Anorexia-Cachexia syndrome in cancer: implications of the ubiquitin-proteasome pathway. *Support Care Cancer.* 2006;14(12):1173–1183.

40. Acharyya S, et al. Dystrophin glycoprotein complex dysfunction: a regulatory link between muscular dystrophy and cancer cachexia.[see comment]. *Cancer Cell.* 2005;8(5):421–432.

41. Eley HL, Tisdale MJ. Skeletal muscle atrophy, a link between depression of protein synthesis and increase in degradation. *J Biol Chem.* 2007;282(10):7087–7097.

42. Khal J, et al. Increased expression of proteasome subunits in skeletal muscle of cancer patients with weight loss. *Int J Biochem Cell Biol.* 2005;37(10):2196–2206.

43. Levin, M.I., et al., Paraneoplastic neorotizing myopathy: clininical and pathological features. *Neurology,* 1998;50(3):764–767.

Motor Neuron Disease in Cancer

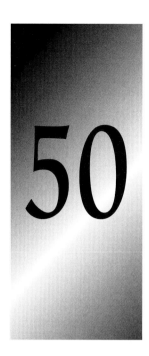

David S. Younger

Physicians involved in cancer and rehabilitation medicine should have a familiarity with motor neuron disease (MND) because it warrants a comprehensive orientation to diagnosis and treatment. The majority of cases of MND are amyotrophic lateral sclerosis (ALS) and are of the sporadic type, with only a minority of cases due to a known genetic or paraneoplastic basis. Although there is no known cure, amelioration of physical deficits associated with ALS and other forms of MND is possible in affected patients with a concerted program of occupational, physical therapy, orthotics, and other assistive devices. This chapter will focus on ALS as the paradigm of MND disorders.

DEFINITIONS

Amyotrophic lateral sclerosis was recognized as a distinct clinical and neuropathologic condition by Charcot and Joffroy (1). The clinical lower motor neuron (LMN) manifestations of weakness, wasting, and fasciculation are due to anterior horn cell degeneration and loss; those of the upper motor neuron (UMN) recognized by hyperreflexia, spasticity, clonus, and Hoffmann and Babinski signs are due to corticospinal tract degeneration.

ALS is part of a spectrum of diseases involving motor neuron loss termed motor neuron disease (MND). Lower motor neuron involvement of the brainstem and limbs without UMN signs is termed progressive spinal muscular atrophy (PSMA), while those with isolated bulbar involvement are termed progressive bulbar palsy (PBP) (2). Isolated UMN involvement is seen in primary lateral sclerosis (PLS) (3). Those with MND in a single limb have monomelic amyotrophy, while others with involvement of both arms is termed brachial amyotrophic diplegia, with either having a typically slower course than ALS.

The World Federation of Neurology El Escorial diagnostic criteria (4) provide a useful clinical classification of ALS. For classification purposes, LMN signs consist of weakness, atrophy, and fasciculation. UMN findings consist of overactive tendon reflexes, spasticity, Hoffmann and Babinski signs, and pseudobulbar features. The regions of the body are classified into bulbar, cervical, thoracic, and lumbosacral. Patients with *definite* ALS have UMN and LMN signs in three spinal regions or bulbar region and two spinal regions. Those with *probable* ALS have UMN and LMN signs in at least two regions. *Possible* ALS includes UMN and LMN signs in one region and UMN signs alone in two or more regions. *Suspected* ALS has LMN signs in two or more regions. While prognosis may not be clearly related to a particular clinical syndrome, long-term survival is best with PSMA or PLS, followed by ALS, and bulbar palsy, whereas survival is shortened in progressive bulbar palsy and bulbar-onset ALS.

The two main categories of inheritance in familial ALS (FALS) are autosomal dominant (AD) and autosomal recessive (AR) patterns, with further subdivision by known gene and chromosomal loci into eight recognized FALS syndromes, enumerated ALS1-7 as well as FALS with frontotemporal dementia (FTD); there is relatively little information about X-linked FALS.

The association of systemic cancer with ALS is usually coincidental, but two situations suggest a paraneoplastic pathogenesis. The first is when ALS occurs in the setting of a lymphoproliferative tumor, often with elevated cerebrospinal fluid protein content and pleocytosis. The second is when a well-characterized paraneoplastic antibody is detected, such as anti-Hu, which occurs with paraneoplastic encephalomyelitis and sensory neuronopathy in the setting of malignant small cell lung cancer.

With the exception of genetic and paraneoplastic forms of ALS, the remaining majority are of the sporadic type, which will be the emphasis of the discussion that follows.

CLINICAL PRESENTATION

The incidence of sporadic ALS is approximately 1–2 per 100,000 (range, 0.5–2.4 per 100,000) (5). The average age at onset is 56 and is more common in men than

women (1.5:1). It is less common below the age of 40. The average duration of illness is three to five years with a large variation in the duration of disease (6,7), with some patients expiring months after diagnosis and others surviving several decades. Most patients complain of weakness or some functional impairment that results from weakness, such as difficulty writing, buttoning, or holding onto objects indicative of involvement of the arms and frequent stumbling, tripping, and occasionally falls reflecting involvement of the legs. The weakness is usually asymmetric at onset, with progression from one limb to another, spreading relentlessly to cranial regions and to the remaining limbs.

DIAGNOSTIC TESTING

The singular role of testing in ALS is to establish the diagnosis and confidently eliminate other disorders that may bear clinical resemblance to it and identify other potentially serious and treatable disorders toward which therapy might also be directed. Clinically apparent or occult Hodgkin and non-Hodgkin lymphoma or macroglobulinemia may be the cause of a motor neuron syndrome resembling PSMA or ALS. Motor neuropathy may be clinically indistinguishable from PSMA. Patients with multifocal motor neuropathy resembling ALS-probable UMN signs, with or without GM1 antibodies, may have overactive or retained tendon reflexes despite weakness, wasting, and twitching (8,9). Those patients respond favorably to immunomodulatory therapy (10). Nonetheless, there is no reason to evaluate GM1 antibodies titers in patients with otherwise typical ALS (11).

Genetic testing is available for hereditary forms of ALS, including autosomal dominant FALS (13) and Kennedy syndrome (14). The latter occurs in men with perioral fasciculation, slowly progressive limb girdle and bulbar weakness, hypoactive deep tendon reflexes, and gynecomastia.

PROGNOSIS

The prognosis for an individual patient with ALS cannot be estimated from population studies. Rare patients have reversible syndromes (15). The onset of symptoms in ALS patients is assumed to occur when approximately 50%–80% of motor neurons are lost. According to Brooks et al. (16), 50% survival rate in patients with ALS is 36–48 months after onset. In this study, survival correlates more with changes in vital capacity and limb and axial functional tests, as well as falling, rather than directly with limb strength or use of gastrostomy, tracheotomy, or ventilators. Other studies found survival to correlate with age at first symptom, delay from the first symptom to first examination, rate of disease progression as measured by the Appel score (17), and rate of respiratory decline. Older patients and those with bulbar onset at any age have a poorer prognosis.

TREATMENT

Although there is no cure for ALS, the quality of life can be favorably altered by symptomatic therapy (Table 50.1) (18,19). Fatigue and insomnia are disabling symptoms at any time in the course of the illness. Nighttime use of noninvasive ventilatory support with intermittent positive pressure ventilation can be extremely helpful for those with incapacitating fatigue, respiratory muscle weakness, and carbon monoxide retention. Rapidly acting hypnotic medication can also safely facilitate sleep. Secretions can be controlled with anticholinergic medication, especially atropine. Cramps and fasciculation may be controlled with quinine sulfate and baclofen. Clinical depression, whether reactive or endogenous, should always be treated, including in those with bulbar palsy who may be prone to experi-

encing unrepressed emotional outbursts of depression. Rilutek (riluzole) is the first and only approved medication for the treatment of patients with ALS. Its action is to block the toxic effects of glutamate, leading to a slowing of disease progression in those with bulbar- but not limb-onset ALS (20) at a dose of 50 mg orally twice daily (21).

The possible contribution of oxidative stress to the degeneration of motor neurons in ALS (22) has led to its application in the promotion of high-dose vitamins known for their antioxidative properties, especially vitamin E (2,000 U/day), vitamin C (2,000 mg/day), and beta-carotene (25,000 U/day). Selegiline (Eldepryl), N-acetyl cysteine, and creatine, all neuroprotective agents, were ineffective in ALS (23–26). Promising results were obtained employing coenzyme Q10 in an animal model of ALS (27).

Recent studies have shown the importance of immune mechanisms and mediators of inflammation in the pathogenesis of motor neuron injury in ALS (28,29). Although there is no evidence to support the use of systemic immunosuppressants in sporadic ALS, selected patients may rationally choose an immunosuppressant regimen from among the available agents. These agents include azathioprine, cyclophosphamide, intravenous immunoglobulin, prednisone, cyclosporin, or plasmapheresis when there is evidence of a coexisting lymphoproliferative disorder, plasma cell dyscrasia, or connective tissue disorder. Calcium channel blockers have been shown to be ineffective in ALS (30). Minocycline, an antibiotic that slows the progression of ALS in a mouse model by crossing the blood–brain barrier and reducing inflammatory enzyme activation, is being studied in patients with ALS.

The excitotoxic theory pertaining to ALS (31–33) has led to the employment of the antiepileptic agents gabapentin (Neurontin) and topiramate (34), and the glutamate antagonist remacemide, both, however, without proven clinical benefit (35).

Investigations employing ciliary neurotrophic factor (CNF) (36), brain-derived nerve factor (BDNF), and insulin-like growth factor type 1 (IGF-1) showed conflicting or negative outcomes in ALS (37,38). A lentiviral vector expressing vascular endothelial growth factor (VEGF) injected in the muscles of a mouse model delayed onset and prolonged life expectancy without toxic effects, substantiating the role of this family of growth factors (39–44).

Molecular components of programmed cell death (PCD) have been implicated in the pathogenesis of ALS as a final common pathway leading to the death of motor neurons (45,46). Caspase and related cysteine proteases Bcl-, Bclx, Bax, Bad, and Bcl-xS are factors that have been shown to play a role in the enzymatic pathways leading to PCD in human and mouse models

TABLE 50.1
Symptomatic Therapeutic Interventions in ALS

Fatigue	SSRI, anticholinesterase drugs, amantadine, pemoline, rest, vitamins
Cramps	Magnesium, quinine sulphate, carbamazepine, phenytoin, calcium channel blockers, gabapentin, benzodiazepines
Spasticity	Baclofen, tizanidine, benzodiazepines, dantrolene, gabapentin, mobility assist devices
Sialorrhea, thick mucus	Amitriptyline, trihexyphenidyl, hyoscine patch, atropine, glycopyrrolate, propantheline, beta blockers, botulinum toxin
Dry mouth	Hydration, glycerin swabs, candy, humidifier
Respiratory therapy	Suction, nebulizers, cough machine, CPAP, BiPAP
Insomnia	Ambien, Sonata, avoid hypoventilation, diphenhydramine, amitriptyline
Depression/pathological laughing and crying	Amitriptyline, SSRI, lithium
Feeding	Food supplementation, PEG
Speech	Speech therapy, computer-based communication devices, alphabet chart
Skin care	Frequent turning/position changing, protective creams, hospital bed, air mattress
Urinary urgency	Oxybutynin, amitriptyline, propantheline, urological consultation
Palliative and family care	Discuss advance directive early, participation in ALS clinics

Abbreviations: BiPAP, bilevel positive airway pressure; CPAP, continuous positive airway pressure; PEG, SSRI, selective serotonin reuptake inhibitor.

of motor neuron PCD and potential therapeutic targets to prolong survival (47–51). Gene therapy and stem cell therapy are under exploration in ALS.

REHABILITATION

The diagnosis of ALS is usually established while the patient is ambulatory, allowing for the institution of physical and occupational therapy programs and orthotics. The goal should be to encourage independence of activities of daily living and safety in ambulation. Those with impaired leg strength and imbalance should be encouraged to first utilize a cane, walker, or crutch in conjunction with orthotics or bracing to avoid excessive tripping, and later a wheelchair for distances. Contractures almost never occur in ALS, but that should not dissuade affected patients from engaging in therapy to prevent musculotendinous shortening and to maintain normal ranges of passive joint movement. Although exercise has a limited role in the prognosis of weakened muscles, endurance training probably improves functional output of mildly weak muscles. Undernutrition can result from inability to feed oneself, swallowing impairments, shortness of breath, aspiration of food, presence of an indwelling tracheostomy, decreased appetite, and impairment of taste. Malnutrition can lead to a propensity for nerve entrapment around bony prominences due to loss of the protective fat pads, further impairing limb function.

Patients with pulmonary insufficiency due to respiratory muscle weakness should be monitored closely for insufficient cough and aspiration. Prior to loss of the ability to speak intelligibly, patients should be given an opportunity to use computerized speech augmentation devices so that there is a smooth transition to them when needed. In the terminal stages of ALS when there is little limb movement, the role of rehabilitation medicine becomes especially important in assuring comfort of the patient and in maintaining contact through eye-movement communication devices, signals, and letter boards. The decision of individual patients to maximize their life expectancy through life support casts further challenges upon the medical team.

References

1. Williams DB, Windenbank AJ. Motor neuron disease (amyotrophic lateral sclerosis). *Mayo Clinic Proc.* 1991;66:54–82.
2. Younger DS, Rowland LP, Latov N, et al. Motor neuron disease and amyotrophic lateral sclerosis: relation of high CSF protein content to paraproteinemia and clinical syndromes. *Neurology.* 1990;40:595–599.
3. Younger DS, Chou S, Hays AP, et al. Primary lateral sclerosis: a clinical diagnosis reemerges. *Ann Neurol.* 1988;45:1304–1307.
4. Brooks BR. El Escorial Workshop 1994; World Federation of Neurology criteria for the diagnosis of amyotrophic lateral sclerosis. *J Neurol Sci.* 1994;124(Suppl):96–107.
5. Kurtzke JF. Risk factors in amyotrophic lateral sclerosis. *Adv Neurol.* 1991;56:245–270.
6. Ringel SP, Murphy JR, Alderson MK, et al. The natural history of amyotrophic lateral sclerosis. *Neurology.* 1993;43:1316–1322.

7. Haverkamp L, Appel V, Appel SH. Natural history of ALS in a database population: validation of a scoring system and a model for survival prediction. *Brain*. 1995;118:707–719.

8. Lange DJ, Trojaborg WT, Latov N, Hays AP. Multifocal motor neuropathy with conduction block: a distinct clinical entity? *Neurology*. 1992;42:497–505.

9. Katz JS, Wolfe GI, Bryan WW, Jackson CE, Amato AA, Barohn RJ. Electrophysiologic findings in multifocal motor neuropathy. *Neurology*. 1997;48:700–707.

10. Nobile-Orazio E, Meucci N, Barbieri S, Carpo M, Scarlato G. High-dose intravenous immunoglobulin therapy in multifocal neuropathy. *Neurology*. 1993;43:537–544.

11. Kinsella LJ, Lange DJ, Trojaborg W, Sadiq SA, Younger DS, Latov N. The clinical and electrophysiological correlates of elevated ant-GM1 antibody titers. *Neurology*. 1994;44:1278–1282.

12. Kaufmann P, Pullman SL, Shungu DC, et al. Objective tests for upper motor neuron involvement in amyotrophic lateral sclerosis (ALS). *Neurology*. 2004;62(10):1753–1757.

13. Younger DS, Brown RH Jr. Familial amyotrophic lateral sclerosis. In DS Younger, ed. *Motor Disorders*, Chapter 41, 2nd ed. Lippincott, Williams and Wilkins, Philadelphia; 2005:501–506.

14. Amato AA, Prior TW, Barohn RJ, et al. Kennedy's disease: a clinicopathologic correlation with mutations in the androgen receptor gene. *Neurology*. 1993;43:791–794.

15. Tucker T, Layzer RB, Miller RG, Chad D. Subacute reversible motor neuron disease. *Neurology*. 1991;41:1541–1544.

16. Brooks BR, Sanjak M, Belden D, et al. Natural history of amyotrophic lateral sclerosis—impairment, disability, handicap. In: Martin Dunitz, Brown RH, Meininger V, and Swash M, eds. *Amyotrophic Lateral Sclerosis*. London: Martin Dunitz Ltd. 2000:31–58.

17. Appel V, Stewart SS, Smith G, Appel SH. A rating scale for amyotrophic lateral sclerosis: description and preliminary experience. *Ann Neurol*. 1987;22(3):328–333.

18. Forshew DA, Bromberg MB. A survey of clinicians' practice in the symptomatic treatment of ALS. *Amyotroph Lateral Scler Other Motor Neuron Disord*. 2003;4:258–263.

19. Lange DJ, Murphy PL, Maxfield RA, Skarvala AM, Reidel G. Management of patients with amyotrophic lateral sclerosis. *J Neuro Rehab*. 1994;8:75–82.

20. Bensimmon G, Lacomblez L, Meininger V, ALS/Riluzole Study Group I. A controlled trial of riluzole in amyotrophic lateral sclerosis. *N Engl J Med*. 1994;330:585–591.

21. Lacomblez L, Bensimon G, Leigh PN, Guillet P, Meininger V. Dose-ranging study of riluzole in amyotrophic lateral sclerosis/ Riluzole Study Group II. *Lancet*. 1996;347:1425–1431.

22. Simpson EP, Yen AA, and Appel SH. Oxidative stress: a common denominator in the pathogenesis of amyotrophic lateral sclerosis. *Curr Op Rheumat*. 2003;15:730–736.

23. Lange DJ, Murphy PS, Diamond B, et al. selegiline is ineffective in a collaborative double-blind, placebo-controlled trial for treatment of amyotrophic lateral sclerosis. *Arch Neurol*. 1998;55:93–96.

24. Louwerse ES, Weverling GJ, Bossuyt PM, Meyjes FE, de Jong JM. Randomized, double-blind, controlled trial of acetylcysteine in amyotrophic lateral sclerosis. *Arch Neurol*. 1995;52:559–564.

25. Mazzini L, Testa D, Balzarini C, Mora G. An open-randomized clinical trial of selegiline in amyotrophic lateral sclerosis. *J Neurol*. 1994;241:223–227.

26. Groeneveld GJ, Veldink JH, van der Tweel I, et al. A randomized sequential trial of creatine in amyotrophic lateral sclerosis. *Ann Neurol*. 2003;53(4):437–445.

27. Beal MF. Coenzyme Q10 as a possible treatment for neurodegenerative diseases. *Free Radic Res*. 2002;36(4):455–460.

28. Henkel JS, Engelhardt JI, Siklos L, et al. Presence of Dendritic Cells, MCP-1, and Activated Microglia/Macrophages in ALS Spinal Cord Tissue. *Ann. Neurol*. 2004;55:221–235.

29. Smith RG, Hamilton S, Hoffman F, et al. Serum antibodies to L-type calcium channels in patients with amyotrophic lateral sclerosis. *N Engl J Med*. 1992;327:1721–1728.

30. Miller RG, Smith SA, Murphy JR, et al. Verapamil does not slow the progressive weakness of amyotrophic lateral sclerosis. *Muscle Nerve*. 1996;19:511–515.

31. Rothstein JD. Excitotoxicity and neurodegeneration in amyotrophic lateral sclerosis. *Clin Neurosci*. 1996;3:348–359.

32. Plaitakis A, Coroscio JT. Abnormal glutamate metabolism in amyotrophic lateral sclerosis. *Ann Neurol*. 1987;22:575–579.

33. Rothstein JD, Martin LJ, Kuncl RW. Decreased glutamate transport by the brain and spinal cord in amyotrophic lateral sclerosis. *N Engl J Med*. 1992;326:1464–1468.

34. Miller RG, Moore DH 2nd, Gelinas DF, et al. Phase III randomized trial of gabapentin in patients with amyotrophic lateral sclerosis. *Neurology*. 2001;56(7):843–848.

35. Cudkowicz ME, Shefner JM, Schoenfeld DA, et al. A randomized, placebo-controlled trial of topiramate in amyotrophic lateral sclerosis. *Neurology*. 2003;61(4):456–464.

36. Miller RG, Armon C, Barohn RJ, et al. A placebo controlled trial of recombinant human ciliary neurotrophic factor (rhCNTF) in amyotrophic lateral sclerosis. *Ann Neurol*. 1996;39:256–260.

37. Lai EC, Felice KJ, Festoff BW, et al. Effect of recombinant human insulin-like growth factor-I on progression of ALS. A placebo-controlled study. The North America ALS/IGF-I Study Group. *Neurology*. 1997;49:1621–1630.

38. Borasio GC, Lange DJ, Lai EC, et al. A double blind placebo-controlled therapeutic trial to assess the efficacy of recombinant human insulin-like growth factor in the treatment of ALS: a multi-center, double-blind, placebo-controlled clinical study [abstract]. Sixth International Symposium on ALS/MND, Dublin, Ireland, 1995.

39. Schwartzberger P, et al. Favorable effect of VEGF gene transfer on ischemic peripheral neuropathy. *Nat Med*. 2000;6: 405–413.

40. Jin KL, Mao XO, Greenberg DA. Vascular endothelial growth factor: direct neuroprotective effect in in vitro ischemia. *Proc Natl Acad Sci*. 2000;97:10242–10247.

41. Oosthuyse B, et al. Deletion of the hypoxia-response element in the vascular endothelial growth factor promoter causes motor neuron degeneration. *Nat Genet*. 2001;28:131–138.

42. Lambrechts D, et al. VEGF is a modifier of amyotrophic lateral sclerosis in mice and humans and protects motoneurons against ischemic death. *Nat Genet*. 2003;34:383–394.

43. Azzouz M, Ralph SG, Storkenbaum E, et al. VEGF delivery retrogradely transported lentivector prolongs survival in a mouse ALS model. *Nature*. 2004;429:413–417.

44. Lambrechts D, Storkenbaum E, Carmeliet P. VEGF: necessary to prevent motoneuron degeneration, sufficient to treat ALS? *Trends in Molecular Med*. 2004;10(6):275–282.

45. Martin LJ. Neuronal death in amyotrophic lateral sclerosis is apoptosis: possible contribution of a programmed cell death mechanism. *J Neuropathol Exp Neurol*. 1999;58:459–471.

46. Guegan C, Przedborski S. Programmed cell death in amyotrophic lateral sclerosis. *J Clin Invest*. 2003;111:153–161.

47. Kostic V, Jackson-Lewis V, DeBilbao F, et al. Prolonging life in a transgenic mouse model of amyotrophic lateral sclerosis. *Science*. 1997;277:559–562.

48. Li M, Ona VO, Guegan C, et al. Functional role of caspase-1 and caspase-3 in ALS transgenic mouse model. *Science*. 2000;288:335–339.

49. Friedlander RM, Brown RH, Gagliardini V, et al. Inhibition of ICE slow ALS in mice. *Nature*. 1997;388:31.

50. Zhou S, Stavrovskaya I, Drozda M, et al. Minocycline inhibit cytochrome c release and delays progression of amyotrophic lateral sclerosis in mice. *Nature*. 2002;417:74–78.

51. Gordon PH, Miller RG, Moore DH, et al. Placebo controlled phase II studies of minocycline in amyotrophic lateral sclerosis. *Neurology*. 2003;60(Suppl 1):A136.

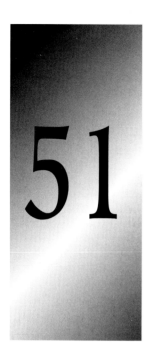

Autonomic Dysfunction in Cancer

51

Paul Magda
David S. Younger

Cancer can affect the autonomic nervous system in a variety of ways: direct tumor compression or infiltration, treatment effects (irradiation, chemotherapy), indirect effects (eg, malabsorption, malnutrition, organ failure, metabolic abnormalities), and paraneoplastic/autoimmune effects (1). In most cases, either the autonomic dysfunction is not a major part of the clinical picture or the cause of the dysautonomia is apparent with appropriate routine assessment; treatment is symptomatic and usually focuses on the prevention of symptomatic orthostatic hypotension. This chapter will focus on a diagnostic approach and treatment of cancer patients with dysautonomia, with an emphasis on immune-mediated autonomic dysfunction, a rare but potentially highly treatable cause of dysautonomia.

BACKGROUND CONSIDERATIONS

Because control of circulation is a major function of the autonomic nervous system and since orthostatic hypotension is frequently the cardinal symptom in patients with dysautonomia, it is important to briefly review the fluid shifts that occur with standing and mechanisms responsible for orthostatic tolerance. Within seconds of the erect posture, up to 1 liter of

blood shifts passively below the level of the diaphragm into the splanchnic and muscle capacitance vessels. After an additional 5–10 minutes of standing, 10%–20% of plasma is lost from the central blood volume due to filtration into the interstitial compartment. The result is a decrease in venous return to the heart and of cardiac output by up to 20% (2).

Orthostatic hypotension and syncope are prevented mainly by the following mechanisms: the baroreflex, skeletal-muscle pump, and venoarterioral reflex (2). The baroreflex maintains control of moment-to-moment fluctuations in blood pressure, and is the single most important component in the maintenance of normotension. Upon standing, mechanoreceptors in the carotid bulb sense a decline in blood pressure (BP) and send bilateral afferents via cranial nerve (CN) IX to the nucleus tractus solitarius (NTS) of the dorsolateral medulla. The NTS inhibits the nucleus ambiguus (NA) of CN X (vagus nerve), which results in cardioacceleration. The NTS also stimulates the rostral ventrolateral medulla (VLM) and the hypothalamic paraventricular nucleus (PVN), structures involved in maintenance of sympathetic tone. The net result is an increase in sympathetic output to splanchnic and muscle arterioles and the heart, resulting in increased peripheral vascular resistance and cardioacceleration (3).

KEY POINTS

- Cancer can affect the autonomic nervous system in a variety of ways: direct tumor compression or infiltration, treatment effects (irradiation, chemotherapy), indirect effects (eg, malabsorption, malnutrition, organ failure, metabolic abnormalities), and paraneoplastic/autoimmune effects.
- Orthostatic hypotension and syncope are prevented mainly by the following mechanisms: the baroreflex, skeletal-muscle pump, and venoarterioral reflex.
- Autonomic dysfunction can be divided into non-neurogenic (medical) and neurogenic (primary or secondary) causes.
- Symptoms of orthostatic intolerance include light-headedness, presyncope, actual syncope, cognitive and visual disturbances, palpitations, weakness, and neck and shoulder muscle aches (coat hanger syndrome) that are exacerbated by position changes, prolonged standing, warm temperatures, exercise, or meal ingestion.
- Conditions encountered in the cancer setting that are associated with autonomic dysfunction include Lambert-Eaton myasthenic syndrome (LEMS), anti-Hu antibody syndrome, collapsin response-mediator protein 5 (CRMP-5) , subacute autonomic neuropathy (SAN), neuromyotonia (Isaac syndrome), and intestinal pseudo-obstruction.
- Fludrocortisone (Florinef) is a synthetic adrenocortical steroid possessing potent mineralocorticoid and minimal glucocorticoid activity. It increases Na+ reabsorption (and K+ depletion) and raises extracellular fluid volume and blood pressure.

- Midodrine (ProAmatine) is a pure alpha adrenergic agonist that results in peripheral vasoconstriction and increased total peripheral resistance without cardioacceleration.
- Pyridostigmine (Mestinon) is a cholinesterase inhibitor that increases acetylcholine in sympathetic and parasympathetic ganglia. It was shown to be significantly effective in improving neurogenic orthostatic hypotension.
- Leg crossing results in a sustained increase in mean blood pressure (BP) of 13 mmHg in patients with dysautonomia, a relatively mild increase but similar in magnitude to treatment with fludrocortisone, erythropoietin, or midodrine.
- Regular submaximal exercise increases plasma volume, muscle mass, and tone (improving skeletal-muscle pump function) and reduces overall cardiovascular risk.
- Supplementation of water and salt increases plasma and blood volume, which decreased orthostatic intolerance and baroreceptor sensitivity in a double-blind, placebo-controlled study.
- Other important interventions or orthostasis include raising the head of the bed (6–12-inch blocks at head of bed or 45° in hospital bed), avoiding hot ambient temperatures and alcohol (which result in vasodilatation), compressive garments, smaller low-carbohydrate and more frequent meals for postprandial hypotension, and a high-fiber diet to prevent syncope with straining due to constipation.

The skeletal-muscle pump is considered "the second heart" of the body, and can partly compensate for dysfunction of the neural system (4). During the upright posture, approximately 80% of the blood pooled in the legs sits in the thigh and buttock musculature (2). Voluntary contraction of these muscles is effective at expelling this blood (eg, 30% expelled with a single maximal contraction). Reduced intramuscular pressure is associated with orthostatic dysfunction even in healthy individuals. Postural maneuvers designed to utilize the pump to expel blood from the thighs and buttocks have been shown to effectively delay or prevent orthostatic hypotension (2).

The venoarterioral reflex occurs locally at the level of the skin and subcutaneous tissue vasculature. An increase of the leg capacitance vessels' pressure to above 25 mmHg results in a reflexive increase in the peripheral vascular resistance of the local arterioles that can reduce lower extremity blood flow by up to 50% (5).

Chronic BP control is maintained by the neurohumoral system involving the renin-angiotensin-aldosterone and vasopressin hormones. This system is involved with chronic BP stability and with hypovolemic orthostatic stress, acting in concert with aortic arch baroreceptors (4,6).

DIAGNOSTIC APPROACH

Autonomic dysfunction can be divided into non-neurogenic (medical) and neurogenic (primary or secondary) causes (7). Primary neurogenic dysautonomia includes conditions where the autonomic nervous system dysfunction itself represents the disease state (eg, Shy-Drager syndrome), and secondary neurogenic causes include nonautonomic neurologic diseases that can affect the autonomic nervous system (eg, Parkinson disease, brain tumors, multiple sclerosis, epilepsy, diabetic neuropathy). In non-neurogenic disorders, a systemic condition causes dysfunction of the autonomic nervous system (eg, age/deconditioning/cachexia, medication adverse effects, volume depletion, anemia, pheochromocytoma, adrenal insufficiency).

Autonomic control is ubiquitous to the body, and a full listing of possible symptoms is beyond the scope of this chapter. For the sake of simplicity, one may focus on the symptoms most likely to bring the patient to medical attention and that are most amenable to treatment and objective testing, namely those that relate to orthostatic, gastrointestinal, and sudomotor function. Symptoms of orthostatic intolerance include lightheadedness, presyncope or actual syncope, cognitive and visual disturbances, palpitations, weakness, and neck and shoulder muscle aches (coat hanger syndrome) that are exacerbated by position changes, prolonged standing, warm temperatures, exercise, or meal ingestion (8). Sweating abnormalities may include hypo- or hyperhidrosis and heat intolerance. Gastrointestinal symptoms include severe constipation, alternating constipation and diarrhea, and nausea and vomiting (8).

The autonomic testing battery includes sudomotor, vasomotor, and cardiovagal function testing and objectively defines the severity and extent of dysautonomia. The Quantitative Sudomotor Axon Reflex Test (QSART) involves iontophoresis of acetylcholine across the skin to cause an axon reflex-mediated sweat response (5,9). The test assesses sympathetic postganglionic cholinergic fiber function. Tilt table and the Valsalva tests assess primarily sympathetic function. Multiple tilting protocols are described in the literature utilizing variable tilt angles and durations (range: 5–60 minutes), with or without pharmacologic challenge. Increasing tilt duration and administration of sympathomimetic or vasoactive medications can result in increased sensitivity, but also increases the possibility of false-positive results. One recent study found that a nonpharmacologic tilt for three to five minutes at 80° was able to fully characterize the orthostatic dysfunction and predict the patients who were likely to progress to syncope (10). This protocol is particularly useful given its brevity, increased patient tolerance, and decreased chance of false-positive responses. The Valsalva maneuver BP curve results from the patient exhaling through a mouthpiece connected to a sphygmomanometer with an expiratory pressure of 40 mmHg for 15 seconds. The BP curve has four phases, each of which has been pharmacologically dissected (11); phases II and IV are clinically most relevant and are associated with alpha and beta adrenergic functions, respectively. The sharp rise in BP in phase IV (overshoot) is directly responsible for the bradycardia observed during this time, which results in a calculated

Valsalva ratio (maximal heart rate [HR] during the end of phase III divided by the minimal HR during phase IV), an indirect measure of cardiovagal tone. The speed of blood pressure recovery following phase III, another measure of alpha adrenergic function, has also been evaluated (12); latency of >5 ms is felt to be abnormal (Low, PA, private communication). HRDB evaluates the parasympathetic (vagal) innervation of the heart. Rhythmic deep breathing results in HR variability that peaks as maximal inspiration is approached and is minimal toward the end of maximal expiration. The difference between the maximal and minimal HR of each cycle is a measure of vagal tone. The physiological basis of this reflex is complex and involves several reflex arcs (5). A systemic evaluation should also be undertaken, a description of which is beyond the scope of this chapter (7,13).

PARANEOPLASTIC SYNDROMES ASSOCIATED WITH DYSAUTONOMIA

Paraneoplastic syndromes occur in 1%–7% of all cancer patients, and can be divided into dermatologic, hematologic, endocrine, rheumatologic, and neurologic groups (14). Autoimmune responses play an important role in neurologic paraneoplastic syndromes (14). Onconeuronal antibodies associated with dysautonomia include ANNA-1 (Hu), ANNA-2, CRMP-5, P/Q VGCC, nicotinic ganglionic or muscle ACHR, VGKC, Purkinje cell cytoplasmic antibody-type 2 (PCA-2), and CV-2 (15). Evidence suggests significant overlap of paraneoplastic antibodies, which often coexist and predict an underlying cancer (most commonly small cell lung cancer [SCLC] and thymoma), but not a specific syndrome (8). Paraneoplastic causes should be considered if autonomic presentation is subacute, even when onconeuronal antibodies are not present (16). Treatment of the underlying malignancy and/or immunotherapy can prevent irreversible neurologic damage (14).

LAMBERT-EATON MYASTHENIC SYNDROME (LEMS)

LEMS is an IgG-mediated presynaptic disorder that affects the neuromuscular junction and autonomic targets. Subacute weakness is the most common presenting symptom. The most common autonomic symptoms are dry mouth (77%) and impotence (45% of men) (17). Electrodiagnosis reveals low-amplitude compound muscle action potentials (CMAPs); repetitive stimulation reveals a decremental response, as in myasthenia gravis; CMAP amplitudes increase above

100% of baseline postexercise. P/Q voltage-gated calcium channel (VGCC) antibodies are found in 95% of patients. The most common dysfunction on autonomic testing is sudomotor (83%) and cardiovagal (75%), with less frequent adrenergic dysfunction (37%). Composite autonomic scoring scale (CASS) results are abnormal in 93% of patients (severe: 20%; moderate: 17%; and mild: 63% of patients) (17). SCLC is found in 50%–60% of LEMS (17,18). SCLC expresses three of the major high-voltage–activated Ca++ channels that have been found in neurons (N, P/Q, and L). Immune responses to these tumor proteins are presumed to generate antibodies that bind to prejunctional Ca++ channels at muscle and autonomic synapses.

ANTI-HU ANTIBODY SYNDROME

Anti-Hu (ANNA-1) are antibodies directed against RNA-associated proteins produced by tumor cells and central, peripheral, and enteric neurons (8). The antibody is highly associated with SCLC (70%–90% of patients) (14). An unrelated primary coexisted with SCLC in 13% of patients. Presentation is subacute (<6 months) in approximately 80% of patients. The syndrome usually precedes cancer diagnosis by 8–11 months (19). The most common neurologic presentation is neuropathy (66%–80% of patients), followed by a cerebellar syndrome (3%–18% of patients), limbic encephalitis (7%–10% of patients), and Lambert-Eaton myasthenic syndrome (5% of patients). Cranial neuropathy (especially CN VIII), brachial plexopathy, myopathy, myalgias, and aphasia occur in 1%–2% of patients, respectively (19). Gastrointestinal dysmotility, most commonly gastroparesis, is the initial presentation in 12% of patients (19). Rarely, patients may present with dysautonomia (20); up to 27% of patients eventually develop autonomic neuropathy (19). In most patients, symptoms and signs are multifocal (19). It is unclear if anti-Hu antibodies themselves are pathogenic; nicotinic ganglionic ACHR (20) or other antibodies may be associated and pathogenic.

CBMP-5 Autoantibodies

The antigen is a neuronal cytoplasmic protein, 62kD in size, which is a member of the collapsin response-mediator protein (CRMP) family. Its presence is highly associated with SCLC (77% of patients) and rarely with thymoma (6% of patients) or other neoplasms (8% of patients). Antibodies bind to central nervous system and enteric neurons. In one study, 31% of patients with the antibody had dysautonomia (67% of which had isolated gastrointestinal [GI] dysmotility). Other clinical presentations include cortical, 40%

(dementia, seizures, confusion); basal ganglia, 14% (chorea); cerebellum, 26%; and cranial nerves, 17% (especially optic and olfaction/taste). In the majority of patients, signs and symptoms are multifocal (15).

SUBACUTE AUTONOMIC NEUROPATHY (SAN)

An assay to test for antinicotinic ganglionic acetylcholine receptor (ACHR) antibody was first developed in 1998 by Vernino et al. (21). This receptor differs from the skeletal-muscle ACHR only by the presence of an [alpha]3 subunit rather than [alpha]1 subunit. The antibodies are found in 42%–50% of patients with subacute autonomic neuropathy, 12% of LEMS, 50% of Isaac syndrome, and 3% of miscellaneous paraneoplastic disorders. Antibodies are absent in patients with other neurologic disorders, myasthenia gravis (MG), thymoma without MG, other autonomic disorders, and in healthy controls (21). In patients with SAN, gastrointestinal dysmotility is a prominent and initial symptom in 33% of patients (21). Cancer is found in 58% of patients with the antibodies (nearly 60% have SCLC). High levels of the antibodies are found to correlate with worse dysautonomia, and levels decreased or became undetectable with improvement of symptoms, suggesting that the antibodies are pathogenic. Characteristic clinical features are a subacute onset, severe gastrointestinal dysmotility, and an abnormal pupillary response to light and accommodation. Interestingly, this pupillary abnormality is the clinical feature that most reliably predicts seropositivity for the antibodies, and is consistent with the prominent mydriasis found in mutant mice lacking the (alpha)3 subunit of the ganglionic acetylcholine receptor (22). Some patients may be seronegative, given that the condition is monophasic; thus, transient seropositivity may be missed; or that the neuronal antigens may differ among patients; or nonimmune mechanisms may be responsible in some cases (22). Treatment includes intravenous immunoglobulin (IVIG), plasma exchange, immunosuppressant therapy, acetylcholinesterase inhibitors, and tumor-directed therapy (21).

NEUROMYOTONIA (ISAAC SYNDROME)

This condition is characterized by continuous muscle fiber activity of peripheral nerve origin (23) that is sometimes associated with thymoma, SCLC, or lymphoma (21,23), with increasing risk of cancer with age over 40 (24). Voltage-gated potassium channel (VGKC) antibodies result in hyperexcitable motor nerves, with an increase in acetylcholine release and prolonged action potentials (24). This translates into the clinical symptoms of muscle twitching or rippling (90%), often painful cramping (70%), muscle stiffness (often severe enough as to hinder physical activity and affect breathing), muscle hypertrophy (eg, calves), pseudomyotonia (eg, poor relaxation after hand grip without percussion myotonia), and mild muscle weakness (23). Associated autonomic changes may result in cardiac arrhythmias, constipation, increased sweating, and salivation (24). Antibodies to VGKC are found in 40% of patients (80% in patients with thymoma) and are a marker for the syndrome (23). Nicotinic ganglionic ACHR antibodies are found in 50% of patients (21). Treatment options include immunomodulant therapy with plasma exchange, azathioprine, or IVIG, as well as symptomatic therapy with phenytoin, carbamazepine, valproate, lamotrigine, or acetazolamide (23).

INTESTINAL PSEUDO-OBSTRUCTION

The enteric nervous system may be considered a "second brain," with an estimated 100 million neurons, similar in number to the spinal cord (25). There are two plexuses: myenteric (Auerbach) and submucosal (Meissner). The myenteric plexus is involved with contractility of the external musculature of the gut, and the submucosal plexus controls the secretory and absorptive activities of the mucosa and the tone of submucosal arterioles (25). The hallmark of intestinal pseudo-obstruction is an invasive inflammatory lymphocytic infiltrate of the myenteric plexus. Symptoms are those referable to dysregulation of motility: acute/subacute progressive constipation, abdominal pain, and vomiting. Causative antibodies include Hu, nicotinic ganglionic ACHR, N-type VGCC, and PCA-2 (8). In patients with anti-Hu antibodies, gastrointestinal dysmotility was the initial presentation in 12% (19). Laboratory evidence suggests that anti-Hu antibodies may be pathogenic (8).

TREATMENT OF ORTHOSTATIC HYPOTENSION

Pharmacologic Therapies

Fludrocortisone (Florinef) is a synthetic adrenocortical steroid possessing potent mineralocorticoid and minimal glucocorticoid activity (26). It increases Na+ reabsorption (and K+ depletion) and raises extracellular fluid volume and blood pressure. The starting dose is 0.1 mg once or twice daily (7 AM and 2 PM), with increases as needed to 0.3 mg once or twice daily. In severe orthostatic hypotension with normal cardiac

function, one can start at 0.5–1.0 mg twice daily for two to three days followed by maintenance of 0.2 mg once or twice daily. Peak plasma levels are reached within 45 minutes and elimination half-life in 7 hours (26). Full benefit requires a high dietary salt and fluid intake. Persistent supine blood pressure above 180/110 mmHg should be avoided, using head-up tilt sleeping and/or short-acting antihypertensive medications (sublingual nitroglycerine). Adverse effects include congestive heart failure, hypokalemia, and severe supine hypertension (7).

Midodrine (ProAmatine) is a pure alpha adrenergic agonist (7,27,28) that results in peripheral vasoconstriction and increased total peripheral resistance without cardioacceleration. It does not cross the blood–brain barrier and therefore has no central adverse effects (28). It was demonstrated in a placebo-controlled study to improve neurogenic orthostatic hypotension (28) and dramatically improves post-submaximal exercise blood pressure recovery and, therefore, exercise tolerance in patients with autonomic failure (by 25 mmHg at five minutes postexercise after a single 10-mg dose in comparison to controls) (27). Its duration of action is four hours. Dosing is begun at 2.5–5 mg, one to two tablets every three hours (40 mg/day max). Adverse effects include supine hypertension (25%), piloerection (13%), scalp pruritus (10%), paresthesias of body or scalp (9%), urinary retention (6%) (28), weight loss, tachyphylaxis, and increased urinary Na+ losses (7,26). The drug should not be given after 6 PM to avoid supine hypertension.

Pyridostigmine (Mestinon) is a cholinesterase inhibitor that increases acetylcholine in sympathetic and parasympathetic ganglia (29). It was shown to be significantly effective in improving neurogenic orthostatic hypotension at a dose of 60 mg without worsening supine hypertension in a double-blind randomized study (29), with similar efficacy for pre- and postganglionic disorders. It has only a modest effect on blood pressure (BP decline 27.6 mmHg vs 34 mmHg with placebo) and may be combined with low-dose midodrine (5 mg) for a more potent and sustained response (29).

Dihydroxyphenylserine (L-DOPS) is a synthetic amino acid that in the presence of L-aromatic amino acid decarboxylase (L-AADC) is converted to L-norepinephrine, bypassing the rate-limiting step of beta-hydroxylation in the normal formation of norepinephrine from dopamine. It is the ideal treatment for the rare disorder dopamine beta-hydroxylase deficiency (30). It was also found to be effective in patients with orthostatic hypotension and nicotinic acetylcholine receptor antibodies refractory to midodrine, fludrocortisone, erythropoietin, vasopressin, and salt and fluid loading (30). Duration of action is six hours. The effective dose is 200–400 mg once daily (7,26). No major side effects were reported in six studies (26).

Octreotide (Sandostatin) is a somatostatin analogue that inhibits gastrointestinal peptides, some of which have vasodilatory properties. The drug is administered subcutaneously starting at 25–50 µg. It has been found effective in postural, postprandial, and exertion-induced hypotension, in both peripheral and central autonomic disorders. It does not induce supine hypertension (26).

IVIG and plasma exchange are immunomodulating therapies effective in suspected cases of autoimmune dysautonomia (31–33). A detailed description of these treatments is beyond the scope of this chapter.

NONPHARMACOLOGIC THERAPIES

Activation of the skeletal-muscle pump: Leg crossing results in a sustained increase in mean BP of 13 mmHg in patients with dysautonomia, a relatively mild increase, but similar in magnitude to treatment with fludrocortisone, erythropoietin, or midodrine (34). Effect is largely due to the translocation of pooled blood into the chest cavity (35), and is immediate, additive with other therapies, and easy to perform for most patients (34).

Reconditioning exercises: Regular submaximal exercise increases plasma volume, muscle mass, and tone (improving skeletal-muscle pump function), and reduces overall cardiovascular risks (27).

Increasing water and salt intake: Supplementation increases plasma and blood volume, which decreases orthostatic intolerance and baroreceptor sensitivity in a double-blind, placebo-controlled study (36). Typical regimen is 2 liters of water and 175 mEq–250 mEq salt tablets daily (7). Patients who respond to salt intake have a 24-hour urinary Na+ excretion of <170 mmol (36).

Other important interventions include raising the head of the bed (6–12-inch blocks at head of bed or 45° in hospital bed), avoiding hot ambient temperatures and alcohol (7,26) (which result in vasodilatation), compressive garments (7), smaller low-carbohydrate and more frequent meals for postprandial hypotension (7,26), and a high-fiber diet to prevent syncope with straining due to constipation (7).

CONCLUSIONS

Patients with cancer and autonomic dysfunction can pose a difficult diagnostic challenge. In addition to common associated systemic disorders and effects of cancer or cancer treatments, one must also consider autoimmune-associated autonomic dysfunction, especially if symptom onset is subacute. Proper diagnosis can lead to directed treatment and improved outcome for the patient.

References

1. Pourmand R. Paraneoplastic peripheral neuropathies. In: Brown WF, Bolton CF, Aminoff MJ, eds. *Neuromuscular Function and Disease*. Philadelphia: W.B. Saunders Company; 2002:1221.
2. Smit A, Hallliwill JR, Low PA, Wieling W. Pathophysiological basis of orthostatic hypotension in autonomic failure. *J Physiol*. 1999;519:1–10.
3. Benarroch E. The central autonomic network. In: Low PA, ed. *Clinical Autonomic Disorders*. Philadelphia: Lippincott-Raven; 1997:17–23.
4. Wieling W, van Lieshout JJ. Maintenance of postural normotension in humans. In: Low PA, ed. *Clinical Autonomic Disorders*. Philadelphia: Lippincott-Raven; 1997:73–82.
5. Roy Freeman. Autonomic testing. In: Neuromuscular Function and Disease;. W.B. Saunders Company 2002: 483-500.
6. Zochodne DW. Overview of the autonomic nervous system: anatomy and physiology. In: Brown WF, Bolton CF, Aminoff MJ, eds. *Neuromuscular Function and Disease*. Philadelphia: W.B. Saunders Company; 2002:501–512.
7. Fealey RD, Robertson D. Management of orthostatic hypotension. In: Low PA, ed. *Clinical Autonomic Disorders*, 2nd ed. Philadelphia: Lippincott-Raven Publishers; 1997:763–775.
8. Etienne M, Weimer LH. Immune-mediated autonomic neuropathies. *Curr Neurol Neurosci Rep*. 2006;6:57–64.
9. Gibbons C, Freeman R. The evaluation of small fiber function-autonomic and quantitative sensory testing. *Neurol Clin*. 2004;22:683–702.
10. Gehrking JA, Hines SM, Benrud-Larson L, Opher-Gehrking T, Low PA. What is the minimum duration of head-up tilt necessary to detect orthostatic hypotension? *Clin Auton Res*. 2005;15:71–75.
11. Sandroni P, Benarroch EE, Low PA. Pharmacological dissection of components of the Valsalva maneuver in adrenergic failure. *J Appl Physiol*. 1991;71:1563–1567.
12. Vogel ER, Sandroni P, Low PA. Blood pressure recovery from Valsalva maneuver in patients with autonomic failure. *Neurology*. 2005;65:1533–1537.
13. Rees JH, Johnson MR, Hughes RA. The role of [(18)F]fluoro-2-deoxyglucose-PET scanning in the diagnosis of paraneoplastic neurological syndromes. *Brain*. 2004;127:2331.
14. Baijens LWJ, Manni JJ. Paraneoplastic syndromes in patients with primary malignancies of the head and neck. Four cases and a review of the literature. *Eur Arch Otorhinolaryngol*. 2006;263:32–36.
15. Yu Zhiya, Kryzer TJ, Griesmann GE, Kim K, Benarroch E, Lennon VA. CRMP-5 neuronal autoantibody: marker of lung cancer and thymoma-related autoimmunity. *Ann Neurol*. 2001;49:146–154.
16. Antoine J-C, Mosnier J-F, Absi L, Convers P, Honnorat J, Michel D. Carcinoma associated paraneoplastic peripheral neuropathies in patients with and without anti-onconeural antibodies. *Neurol Neurosurg Psych*. 1999;67:7–14.
17. O'Suilleabhain P, Low PA, Lennon VA. Autonomic dysfunction in the Lambert-Eaton myasthenic syndrome: serologic and clinical correlates. *Neurology*. 1998;50:88–93.
18. Nakao YK, Motomura M, Fukudome T, et al. Seronegative Lambert-Eaton myasthenic syndrome: study of 110 Japanese patients. *Neurology*. 2002;59:1773–1775.
19. Luccchinetti CF, Kimmel DW, Lennon VA. Paraneoplastic and oncologic profiles of patients seropositive for type 1 antineuronal nuclear autoantibodies. *Neurology*. 1998;50:652–657.
20. Winkler A-S, Dean A, Hu M, Gregson N, Chaudhuri KR. Phenotypic and neuropathologic heterogeneity of anti-Hu

antibody-related paraneoplastic syndrome presenting with progressive dysautonomia: report of two cases. *Clin Auton Res.* 2001;11:115–118.

21. Vernino S, Adamski J, Kryzer TJ, Fealey RD, Lennon VA. Neuronal nicotinic ACH receptor antibody in subacute autonomic neuropathy and cancer-related syndromes. *Neurology.* 1998;50:1806–1813.

22. Vernino S, Low PA, Fealey RD, Stewart JD, Farrugia G, Lennon VA. Autoantibodies to ganglionic acetylcholine receptors in autoimmune autonomic neuropathies. *N Eng J Med.* 2000;343:847–855.

23. Maddison P. Neuromyotonia. *Clin Neurophys.* 2006;117:2118–2127.

24. Rudnicki SA, Dalmau J. Paraneoplastic syndromes of the peripheral nerves. *Curr Opin Neurol.* 2005;18:598–603.

25. Sharkey KA, Lomax AE. Structure and function of the enteric nervous system: neurological disease and its consequences for neuromuscular function in the gastrointestinal tract. In: Brown WF, Bolton CF, Aminoff MJ, eds. *Neuromuscular Function and Disease.* Philadelphia: W.B. Saunders Company; 2002:527–555.

26. Lahrmann H, Cortelli P, Mathias CJ, Struhal W, Tassinari M. EFNS guidelines on the diagnosis and management of orthostatic hypotension. *Eur J Neurol.* 2006;13:930–936.

27. Schrage WG, Eisenach JH, Dinenno FA, et al. Effects of midodrine on exercise-induced hypotension and blood pressure recovery in autonomic failure. *J Appl Physiol.* 2004;97:1978–1984.

28. Low PA, Gilden JL, Freeman R, Sheng K-N, McElligott MA. Efficacy of midodrine in neurogenic orthostatic hypotension: a randomized, double-blind multicenter study. *JAMA.* 1997;277:1046–1051.

29. Singer W, Sandroni P, Opfer-Gehrking T, et al. Pyridostigmine treatment trial in neurogenic orthostatic hypotension. *Arch Neurol.* 2006;63:513–518.

30. Gibbons CH, Vernino SA, Kaufmann H, Freeman R. L-DOPS therapy for refractory orthostatic hypotension in autoimmune autonomic neuropathy. *Neurology.* 2005;65:1104–1106.

31. Adrianus S, Vermeulen M, Koelman J, Wieling W. Unusual recovery from acute panautonomic neuropathy after immunoglobulin therapy. *Mayo Clin Proc.* 1997;72:333–335.

32. Heafield MTE, Gammage MD, Nightingale S, Williams AC. Idiopathic dysautonomia treated with intravenous gamma-globulin. *Lancet.* 1996;347:28–29.

33. Schroeder C, Vernino S, Birkenfeld AL, et al. Brief report: plasma exchange for primary autoimmune autonomic failure. *N Eng J Med.* 2005;353:1585–1590.

34. Harkel TADJ, van Lieshout JJ, Wieling W. Effects of leg muscle pumping and tensing on orthostatic arterial pressure: a study in normal subjects and patients with autonomic failure. *Clin Sci.* 1994;87:553–558.

35. Krediet PCT, van Dijk N, Linzer M, van Lieshout JJ, Wieling W. Management of vasovagal syncope: controlling or aborting faints by leg crossing and muscle tensing. *Circulation.* 2002;106:1684–1689.

36. El-Sayed H, Hainsworth R. Salt supplement increases plasma volume and orthostatic tolerance in patients with unexplained syncope. *Heart.* 1996;75:134–140.

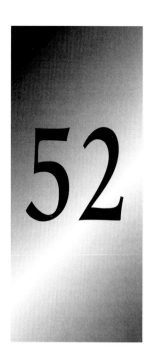

Electrodiagnosis in Cancer

Christian M. Custodio

As methods of early detection of cancer improve, and as cancer treatments evolve and become more effective, patients are living longer and the number of cancer survivors is increasing. As a result, more secondary complications due to cancer and its treatments are being recognized. Neuromuscular complications related to the underlying cancer itself or due to associated treatments such as surgery, chemotherapy, and radiation therapy are common but likely are underreported.

Neuromuscular abnormalities have been clinically detected in 2.5%–5.5% of patients with lung or breast cancer and in 28.5% of patients with various neoplasms using electrodiagnostic studies (1). Classification of these abnormalities can be organized on either an anatomical level or by etiology. Cancer can directly affect the peripheral nervous system at any level via numerous mechanisms. These include direct compression or infiltration, hematogenous spread, lymphatic spread, meningeal dissemination, or perineural spread. Peripheral nervous system involvement can also be caused by paraneoplastic syndromes or from common secondary effects related to cancer, such as malnutrition, weight loss, or infection. Finally, acquired neuropathies can result from side effects of the cancer treatments themselves, including surgery, chemotherapy, radiation therapy, hematopoietic stem cell transplantation, or immunologic therapy. Patients may also have preexisting neurologic conditions, such as diabetic polyneuropathy, that can be exacerbated by cancer or its related treatments. Often, a combination of etiologies can be recognized in individual patients.

Involvement can occur at any level of the peripheral nervous system, including the anterior horn cells, nerve roots, sensory ganglia, brachial or lumbosacral plexus, single or multiple peripheral nerves, neuromuscular junction, and the muscle. Anatomical levels are a convenient method of categorizing neuromuscular diagnoses in cancer. Often multiple levels are involved. Neural damage at the cellular level may take place at the cell body, axon, myelin, or a combination of all of these.

Electrodiagnostic tools, such as nerve conduction studies (NCS) and needle electromyography (EMG), are invaluable in assessing the function of the peripheral nervous system in cancer patients. Electrodiagnostic studies are an extension of the clinical examination, and the expected clinical and electrodiagnostic findings are dependent on the location, distribution, and pathophysiology of the neurologic lesion. NCS and needle EMG are uniquely suited to assess the function of all components of the peripheral nervous system, including sensory nerves, lower motor neurons, peripheral axons, the neuromuscular junction, and muscle fibers. There are many indications for performing electrodiagnostic studies. These studies can confirm a suspected neuropathic lesion as well as rule out other likely possibilities. Electrodiagnosis can help with localizing lesions, determining chronicity and severity, and detecting subclinical neuropathic/myopathic processes.

KEY POINTS

- Cancer can directly affect the peripheral nervous system via direct compression or infiltration, hematogenous spread, lymphatic spread, meningeal dissemination, or perineural spread. Indirect involvement can occur from paraneoplastic syndromes or secondary effects, such as malnutrition, weight loss, or infection.
- Any level of the peripheral nervous system can be affected, including the anterior horn cells, nerve roots, sensory ganglia, brachial or lumbosacral plexus, single or multiple peripheral nerves, neuromuscular junction, and the muscle.
- The indications for performing electrodiagnostic studies include confirming a suspected neuropathic lesion, ruling out other likely possibilities, localizing lesions, determining chronicity and severity, and detecting subclinical neuropathic/myopathic processes. Information regarding pathophysiology and assessing prognosis for neurologic recovery can be achieved with electrodiagnosis.
- Information obtained with nerve conduction studies (NCS) and needle electromyography (EMG) in the cancer patient can often assist in chemotherapy or radiation therapy decision making.
- One important caveat in performing and interpreting electrodiagnostic studies in the cancer patient is that these patients often present with a combination of neuromuscular disorders, both cancer-related and non-cancer–related, and this often adds an additional level of diagnostic complexity.
- A neuropathic injury may be classified as acute, subacute, or chronic. In addition, the underlying pathophysiology of a neuropathy may be primarily axonal, demyelinating, or mixed.
- Sensory responses should be normal in radiculopathy, as the location of injury is proximal to the dorsal root ganglion, thereby making the segment of nerve tested metabolically intact.
- A pattern of clinical and electrophysiologic involvement resembling mononeuritis multiplex may represent a paraneoplastic vasculitic neuropathy.
- While platinum toxicity can result in a distal, symmetric sensorimotor polyneuropathy, there also appears to be preferential damage to the dorsal root ganglia, causing a sensory neuronopathy with clinical and electrodiagnostic features, including sensory ataxia and upper extremity sensory nerve action potentials (SNAPs) being more affected than in the lower extremities.
- The presence of myokymic discharges and fasciculation potentials strongly suggests a radiation-induced contribution to plexus injury. However, the absence of myokymic discharges does not exclude radiation damage.

Information regarding pathophysiology and assessing prognosis for neurologic recovery can be achieved with electrodiagnosis. Objective information about peripheral nervous system function can be obtained in patients who are unable to cooperate, such as the sedated and intubated patient found in the intensive care unit. Finally, information obtained with NCS and needle EMG in the cancer patient can often assist in chemotherapy or radiation therapy decision making.

NERVE CONDUCTION STUDIES

Nerve conduction studies are typically divided into sensory NCS and motor NCS. Extensions of motor NCS commonly performed include late responses and repetitive stimulation. Motor and sensory NCS help assess the function of distal segments of the peripheral nervous system. Common parameters of NCS include amplitude of the response, measured in millivolts for motor responses or microvolts for sensory responses; latency of the response, measured in milliseconds; and conduction velocity, measured in meters per second.

Orthodromic stimulation of a motor or mixed nerve while recording over distal muscle fibers innervated by that nerve results in a compound muscle action potential (CMAP) (Fig. 52.1). A recording electrode is placed over the muscle to be studied, while a reference electrode is placed over an electrophysiologically neutral site, such as the distal musculotendinous junction of that muscle. A ground electrode is placed, usually between the recording site and stimulation site. The nerve is supramaximally stimulated at distal and proximal sites along the nerve, generating a CMAP. The amplitude and area of the CMAP are directly related to the number and size of muscle fibers in the muscle group and indirectly related to the number of intact motor units. Changes in the parameters of CMAPs, using both proximal and distal sites of stimulation, can identify and localize focal sites of nerve injury, characterize pathophysiology of nerve injury (ie, neurapraxia versus axonotmetic injury), and define severity in both focal and diffuse disorders.

Selection of nerves for testing is based on the clinical hypothesis and any anticipated technical difficulties. While CMAPs can be recorded over any muscle, recordings made over the smaller muscles of the hands and feet are usually more reliable and reproducible. This is due to ease of stimulation and minimal associated movement with stimulation. In addition, the

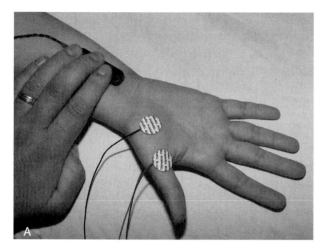

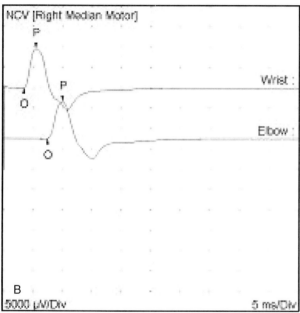

FIGURE 52.1

A: Median motor nerve conduction study recording over the abductor pollicis brevis and stimulating at the wrist. B: Median compound muscle action potentials.

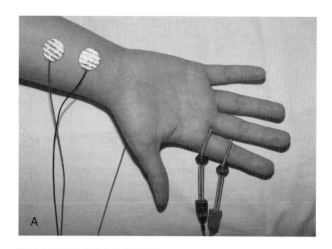

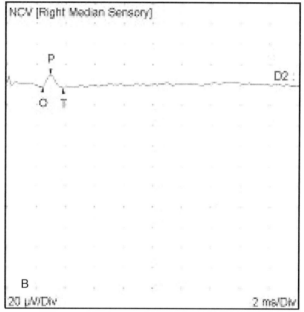

FIGURE 52.2

A: Orthodromic median sensory nerve conduction study recording over the median nerve at the wrist and stimulating at the second digit. B: Median sensory nerve action potential.

nerves involved in these motor studies (median, ulnar, peroneal, tibial) are commonly affected by a large number of neuropathic conditions. Recordings over proximal muscles should be performed as clinically indicated. Individual techniques regarding recommended placement of recording electrodes, sites of stimulation, and standard distances between stimulation and recording electrodes will vary from institution to institution, and is beyond the scope of this chapter.

Stimulation of a peripheral sensory nerve while recording over another site along that nerve generates a sensory nerve action potential (SNAP) (Fig. 52.2). Unlike orthodromic motor stimulation/recording, sen-

sory stimulation and recording can be performed either orthodromically or antidromically, which allows for greater range and variability of testing. The SNAP represents the summated action potentials of individual nerve fibers. SNAP amplitudes are generally much smaller than CMAP amplitudes, which makes assessment of sensory NCS more technically challenging. However, SNAPs are generally more sensitive than CMAPs in the evaluation of generalized and focused peripheral nervous system disorders (2). As with motor NCS, the sensory nerves selected for testing will be dependent on the clinical hypothesis generated during history and physical examination. In addition, any anticipated technical difficulties will determine the selection of nerves tested. As with motor NCS, certain sensory nerves are more easily stimulated and accessible, and thus more reliable and useful for routine studies.

Stimulation of a motor nerve often activates delayed responses following the generation of a CMAP. Whereas motor and sensory NCS provide information about the distal segments of peripheral nerves, these late responses, consisting of F-waves, A-waves, and H-reflexes, help assess the proximal portions of the peripheral nervous system. F-waves are small CMAPs recorded over distal muscles following distal motor nerve stimulation. When a nerve is stimulated, the generated action potential travels both orthodromically and antidromically. The signal traveling orthodromically will result in a standard CMAP. The action potential traveling antidromically will eventually reach the level of the anterior horn cell, whereupon it will cause adjacent anterior horn cells to depolarize. The action potentials in these adjacent anterior horn cells will then travel orthodromically until they reach the recorded muscle, typically generating a CMAP of much smaller amplitude. This smaller CMAP is the F-wave (Fig. 52.3). Thus, recording the F-wave latency incorporates the time it takes for an action potential to travel

antidromically to the anterior horn cells in the spinal cord and back orthodromically to activate fibers in the muscle being recorded. F-waves provide information regarding the conduction of proximal segments of the peripheral nervous system. F-waves are variable in size and latency, and are more reliably measured by recording 8 to 10 responses from a given nerve. Generally, the fastest latency is recorded. Prolonged F-wave latency may be seen in polyradiculopathy, plexopathy, and most neuropathies, and may be abnormal when the standard motor and sensory NCSs were normal.

In contrast to F-waves, A-waves are constant in latency, amplitude, and morphology (Fig. 52.4). The A-wave latency lies between the distal CMAP latency and the F-wave latency. A-waves result from antidromic action potentials, but are mediated by a collateral branch from the primary axon. Therefore, the presence of A-waves is electrophysiologic evidence of collateral branching or sprouting, which is commonly seen in the recovery of peripheral nerve disorders.

The H-reflex is a monosynaptic reflex response resulting from the electrical stimulation of 1A muscle spindle afferents. It is most commonly recorded over the soleus muscle following stimulation of the tibial nerve, although one can record an H-reflex over forearm flexors following median nerve stimulation. In the lower extremity, the H-reflex is similar to the Achilles tendon reflex. The H-reflex can be delayed in a

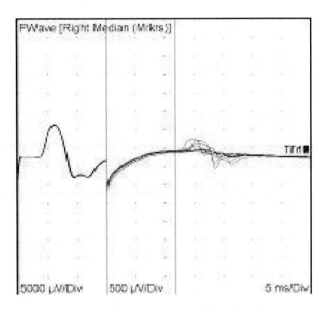

FIGURE 52.3

A normal series of F-waves recorded from the right median nerve. Approximately 10 tracings are superimposed to facilitate marking the onset of the fastest F-wave latency (right vertical line). Note the vertical line on the left indicating a change in gain from the M-waves (left of the line) recorded at 5000 uV/Div compared to the much smaller F-waves (right of the line) recorded at 500 uV/Div.

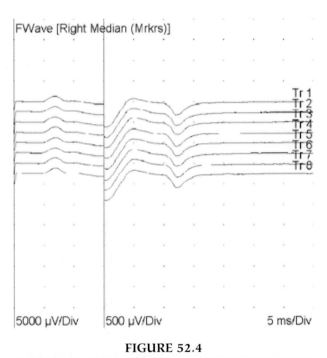

FIGURE 52.4

A-waves (right of vertical line indicating a split in gain) recorded from the right median nerve. Note that the A-waves are identical in morphology. No F-wave is present in this abnormal tracing.

number of peripheral nervous system disorders, but its main application is in identifying subclinical slowing of motor or sensory axons in an S1 radiculopathy in patients with normal reflexes on clinical examination. This study is not usually performed in the electrodiagnostic evaluation of the cancer patient, given its relative lack of clinical utility in this patient population.

Repetitive stimulation is a specialized technique used in assessing the function of the neuromuscular junction. Sequential stimulation of a peripheral motor nerve generates a series of identical CMAPs in normal subjects. In patients with disorders of neuromuscular transmission in addition to other select nerve and muscle disorders, a decremental change in CMAP amplitude and area can be seen with slow-frequency repetitive stimulation. With more rapid frequency stimulation or slow-frequency stimulation immediately following a short period of isometric exercise, postsynaptic disorders of neuromuscular transmission will demonstrate a repair of the decremental CMAP amplitude response, while presynaptic disorders will exhibit a marked increase or facilitation of CMAP amplitude.

NEEDLE ELECTROMYOGRAPHY

Electromyography is the recording of the electrical activity of muscle fibers in motor units in muscle. A single motor unit is defined as a single motor neuron, its axon and its branches, and all of the muscle fibers it innervates. A large number of neuromuscular diseases result in alteration of the motor unit. In addition to intramuscular needle EMG studies, there are other specialized forms of EMG, such as single-fiber EMG used in the more refined evaluation of neuromuscular junction disorders, or surface EMG used in the evaluation of central nervous system movement disorders. Description and explanation of these types of EMG testing is beyond the scope of this chapter. However, standard intramuscular needle EMG, using either concentric or monopolar needles, is at the core of the electrodiagnostic evaluation of peripheral nervous system disorders.

Needle EMG can be used to distinguish between lower motor neuron, peripheral nerve, neuromuscular junction, and muscle disease. The information obtained through needle EMG is complementary to the data collected through NCS, and one portion of the electrodiagnostic examination is rarely performed without the other. Although recognized to be a somewhat uncomfortable test, needle EMG is generally well tolerated, and a skilled electromyographer can minimize patient discomfort while quickly and efficiently obtaining the necessary electrophysiologic information.

EMG signals are analyzed while the muscle is at rest, followed by volitional contraction of the muscle being examined. The needle electrode records and generates both visible waveform and auditory signals. The electromyographer is trained to recognize the complex patterns comprising EMG signals, and through auditory recognition, one can distinguish between normal and abnormal electromyographic activity and can often analyze several waveforms simultaneously.

Muscle fibers are normally under neuronal control and fire only when volitionally activated. At rest, the muscle fibers should be electrophysiologically silent outside of the end-plate region. Normal needle insertional activity results in a short burst of electrical activity associated with the mechanical movement of the needle through the muscle. Normal spontaneous discharges noted around the end-plate region include miniature end-plate potentials and end-plate spikes. Miniature end-plate potentials, also called end-plate noise, occur randomly, with a characteristic "seashell" sound, and are associated with the random release of quanta of acetylcholine into the neuromuscular junction. End-plate spikes, firing irregularly and rapidly, sound characteristically like "bacon frying." These are spontaneous action potentials of muscle fibers due to the mechanical activation of a nerve terminal.

Volitional muscle activity is recorded as motor unit potentials (MUPs). The MUP is the summation of the potentials of muscle fibers innervated by a single anterior horn cell in the recording area of the needle electrode. Normal motor unit potentials have a characteristic semirhythmic firing pattern and stable waveform morphology. The firing pattern is also characterized by recruitment, which is the initiation of firing of additional motor units as the frequency of an active MUP increases. Parameters of MUP morphology include stability, duration, amplitude, and number of phases and turns. Normal parameters vary with a number of physiologic and technical factors, including patient age, the muscle being studied, the location of the needle within the muscle, the temperature of the muscle, and the type of recording needle used. Changes in insertional activity, presence of abnormal spontaneous discharges, changes in recruitment patterns, and changes in MUP morphology can all indicate the existence of a neuromuscular disorder, as well as provide information regarding the severity, chronicity, and pathophysiology of the disorder.

Neuromuscular diseases are best described by the pattern and distribution of abnormalities present on clinical and electrophysiologic examination. Localization of neuropathic lesions requires an intimate working knowledge of peripheral nervous system anatomy. On needle EMG, one may detect the presence of abnormal spontaneous discharges, abnormal MUPs, or both. A list of normal and abnormal spontaneous discharges is seen in Table 52.1. Two of the most common types of abnormal spontaneous activity—fibrillation potentials

TABLE 52.1

Spontaneous Discharges Noted on Needle Electromyography

Normal
  Needle movement
  End-plate noise
  End-plate spikes
Benign
  Fasciculations
  Cramps
  Tremors
Artifact
  Needle coating
  Pacemaker
  TENS/pumps
  60 Hz
  Cautery
  Loose connection
Abnormal
  Fibrillations
  Positive sharp waves
  Fasciculations
  Complex repetitive discharges
  Doublets, triplets
  Myokymia
  Myotonia
  Neuromyotonia
  Cramps
  Tremors
  Synkinesis

Abbreviation: TENS, transcutaneous electrical nerve stimulation.

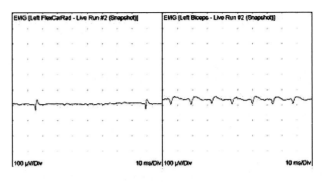

FIGURE 52.5

Fibrillation potentials (*left*) and positive sharp waves (*right*) are the most commonly seen abnormal spontaneous activity on needle electromyography. Their presence is most often associated with denervation from any cause, although they can also be seen in certain myopathies.

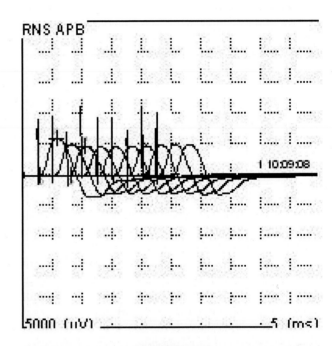

FIGURE 52.6

Typical decrement on repetitive stimulation of the abductor pollicis brevis muscle in a patient with myasthenia gravis.

and positive sharp waves—are demonstrated in Figure 52.5. It is important to note that some discharges can be seen in both benign and pathologic conditions, while other discharges are associated with certain diseases. A change in the recruitment pattern of MUPs is an early finding in neuropathic and myopathic disorders. Abnormal MUPs may vary in size, have an abnormal duration or amplitude, or have an abnormally high number of phases and turns (Fig. 52.6). Recognizing the pattern of abnormalities seen with NCS and needle EMG, taken in the appropriate clinical context, is the key to identifying and characterizing any potential peripheral nervous system disorder in the cancer patient. One important caveat in performing and interpreting electrodiagnostic studies in the cancer patient is that these patients often present with a combination of neuromuscular disorders, both cancer-related and non-cancer–related, and this often adds an additional level of diagnostic complexity.

CHRONICITY AND PATHOPHYSIOLOGY CORRELATES ON ELECTRODIAGNOSTIC TESTING

A neuropathic injury may be classified as acute, subacute, or chronic. In addition, the underlying pathophysiology of a neuropathy may be primarily axonal, demyelinating, or mixed. The natural evolution of a nervous system injury and recovery correlates with the timing of findings noted on NCS and needle EMG, and should correlate with the clinical scenario in which the neuropathic insult occurs.

An acute axonal process will present initially with reduced recruitment on needle EMG. Because Wallerian degeneration does not occur for 7–14 days, abnormal insertional activity indicative of muscle denervation, such as fibrillation potentials or positive sharp waves, will not be present in an acute injury. Thus, the presence of fibrillation potentials in a suspected neuropathic injury indicates either a subacute or chronic injury. Motor unit remodeling following injury, either in the form of axonal regrowth or collateral sprouting, does not occur until two to three months after injury. During remodeling, the MUP becomes unstable, increases in amplitude and duration, and becomes more complex with increased turns and phases. After recovery, the MUP stabilizes and fibrillation potentials disappear; however, the increased size of the MUP persists.

In an acute focal axonal nerve lesion, the segment distal to the site of injury will remain electrophysiologically functional for up to five days. Following that, as Wallerian degeneration occurs, the segment ceases to conduct. This phenomenon can be illustrated on serial motor NCS, with stimulation proximal and distal to the level of the lesion. Initially, with a focal axonal injury, stimulation distal to the site of injury will produce a normal CMAP response, while stimulation proximally will result in a reduced amplitude response, due to the axonal damage and the inability of the evoked action potential to propagate past the lesion. After five days, the distal segment is no longer as metabolically active. Stimulation of the distal segment will then result in a low-amplitude response. As the nerve recovers through axonal regrowth and collateral sprouting, both the distal and proximal CMAP amplitudes recover and increase. With a diffuse, chronic, axonal process, one would expect to see diffusely reduced SNAPs and CMAPs, with chronic MUP changes noted on needle EMG. Distal, symmetric neuropathies are just that, displaying electrodiagnostic findings in a distal-to-proximal gradient. A pattern of mononeuritis multiplex will be demonstrated on electrodiagnosis with asymmetrical, yet diffuse, findings.

With an acute focal demyelinating lesion, the hallmark electrodiagnostic finding is conduction block. Clinically, this correlates to the finding of weakness without atrophy. Stimulating a nerve proximal and distal to a given lesion immediately after injury onset will result in findings similar to those of an acute axonal injury—namely, reduced proximal CMAP amplitude and normal distal CMAP amplitude. After five days, however, the axon is still structurally and metabolically intact with a demyelinating injury. Thus, when repeating motor NCS, there is no drop in distal CMAP

amplitude. An additional finding in a focal demyelinating neuropathy is focal slowing of conduction velocity across the level of the lesion. If the lesion occurs at a distal site, as in the wrist in carpal tunnel syndrome, then the focal slowing will be manifest as a prolonged distal latency. Multifocal demyelinating neuropathies, such as one seen in Guillain-Barré syndrome, will demonstrate multiple areas of focal slowing and conduction block, often at signs not typical for nerve compression. A uniform demyelinating neuropathy, such as one seen in hereditary sensorimotor neuropathy type I (Charcot-Marie-Tooth disease), will demonstrate slowed conduction velocities and prolonged distal latencies uniformly, without areas of focal slowing or conduction block. A chronic demyelinating neuropathy, either uniform or multifocal, will demonstrate markedly slowed conduction velocities and distal latencies.

Localization of a neuropathic lesion requires an intimate knowledge of peripheral neuroanatomy. Understanding a given muscle's innervation and tracing it through its contribution from roots, segments of plexus, and its individual peripheral nerve allows the electromyographer to best select which combination of nerves and muscles to examine in order to properly test their clinical hypothesis. Tables 52.2 through 52.5 provide anatomical reference.

ELECTRODIAGNOSTIC FINDINGS IN CANCER

Radiculopathy

A single-level radiculopathy is defined as an axonal or demyelinating lesion affecting the nerve fibers of a single nerve root. A polyradiculopathy affects multiple nerve roots. Radiculopathies can be caused by compressive and noncompressive etiologies (Table 52.6). After disc disease and spinal stenosis, tumors involving the spine and spinal cord are the most common causes of radiculopathy (3). It is important to remember that any patient with a history of cancer who presents with unremitting back pain, radicular symptoms, and signs on physical examination warrants further evaluation with magnetic resonance imaging (MRI) to exclude a malignant etiology. An MRI of the total spine, not solely of the affected area, is subsequently obtained to determine extent of disease in instances where a neoplastic radiculopathy is identified. Single- or multilevel radiculopathies due to malignancy can result from primary or epidural metastatic tumor extension into the neural foramina. All tumor types can metastasize to the spine, although the most common primary malignancies that do so include breast, lung, prostate, colon, thyroid, and kidney. Common primary malignant

TABLE 52.2
Innervation of Select Upper Extremity Muscles

MUSCLE	NERVE	ROOTS	TRUNK	CORD
Levator scapulae	C3, 4 and dorsal scapular	C3, 4, 5		
Rhomboids	Dorsal scapular	C4, 5		
Supraspinatus	Suprascapular	C5, 6	Upper	
Infraspinatus	Suprascapular	C5, 6	Upper	
Deltoid	Axillary	C5, 6	Upper	Posterior
Biceps brachii	Musculocutaneous	C5, 6	Upper	Lateral
Brachioradialis	Radial	C5, 6	Upper	Posterior
Supinator	Radial	C5, 6	Upper	Posterior
Flexor carpi radialis	Median	C6, 7	Upper/middle	Lateral
Pronator teres	Median	C6, 7	Upper/middle	Lateral
Serratus anterior	Long thoracic	C5, 6, 7		
Latissimus dorsi	Thoracodorsal	C6, 7, 8	Upper/middle/lower	Posterior
Pectoralis major	Lateral pectoral	C5, 6, 7	Upper/middle	
Clavicular				
Sternal	Medial pectoral	C6, 7, 8; T1	Middle/lower	
Triceps brachii	Radial	C6, 7, 8	Upper/middle/lower	Posterior
Extensor carpi radialis longus	Radial	C6, 7	Upper/middle	Posterior
Extensor indicis proprius	Radial	C7, 8	Middle/lower	Posterior
Extensor digitorum	Radial	C7, 8	Middle/lower	Posterior
Extensor capri ulnaris	Radial	C7, 8	Middle/lower	Posterior
Palmaris longus	Median	C7, 8; T1	Middle/lower	Medial
Flexor pollicis longus	Median	C7, 8; T1	Middle/lower	Medial
Flexor carpi ulnaris	Ulnar	C7, 8; T1	Middle/lower	Medial
Flexor digitorum sublimis	Median	C7, 8	Middle/lower	Medial
Flexor digitorum profundus	Median/Ulnar	C7, 8; T1	Middle/lower	Medial
Abductor pollicis brevis	Median	C8; T1	Lower	Medial
First dorsal interosseous	Ulnar	C8; T1	Lower	Medial
Hypothenar group	Ulnar	C8; T1	Lower	Medial
Anconeus	Radial	C7, 8	Middle/lower	Posterior

spinal tumors include multiple myeloma, plasmacytoma, and Ewing and osteogenic sarcoma.

On clinical examination, patients with radiculopathy will often complain of a combination of neck or back pain, limb pain, sensory disturbance, and weakness in a given dermatome or myotome. On NCS, sensory responses should be normal, as the location of injury is proximal to the dorsal root ganglion, thereby making the segment of nerve tested metabolically intact. Motor responses will be normal or reduced in amplitude, depending on the severity of the radiculopathy and the myotomes involved. Needle EMG is the most sensitive electrodiagnostic test for evaluation of a radiculopathy. One would expect to see abnormalities in at least two muscles innervated by different peripheral nerves but sharing the same root innervation, including increased insertional activity, fibrillation potentials, reduced recruitment, and large, polyphasic MUPs. Because the paraspinal muscles

are innervated by the dorsal primary rami, branching directly off of the nerve root, abnormal EMG findings noted in the paraspinals further support the diagnosis of radiculopathy.

Leptomeningeal Metastases

Leptomeningeal disease is due to metastatic involvement of the leptomeninges from infiltrating cancer cells. The incidence of leptomeningeal metastasis ranges from 4%–15% and is felt to be increasing (4). The most common associated primary cancers are breast, lung, gastric, melanoma, and lymphomas (5). Of the leukemias, leptomeningeal disease is most commonly seen in acute lymphocytic leukemia (6). Patients can present with an asymmetric array of symptoms resulting from polyradicular involvement, including focal and radicular pain, areflexia, paresthesias, and lower motor neuron weakness. There may be associated find-

TABLE 52.3
Innervation of Select Lower Extremity Muscles

Muscle	Nerve	Roots
Iliopsoas	Femoral	L2, 3, 4
Adductor longus	Obturator	L2, 3, 4
Gracilis	Obturator	L2, 3, 4
Rectus femoris	Femoral	L2, 3, 4
Anterior tibial	Deep peroneal	L4, 5
Extensor hallucis longus	Deep peroneal	L4, 5
Extensor digitorum brevis	Deep peroneal	L4, 5; S1
Peroneus longus	Superficial peroneal	L5; S1
Peroneus tertius	Deep peroneal	L5; S1
Int. hamstrings (semimembranous, semitendinosus)	Sciatic	L4, 5; S 1
Ext. hamstrings (biceps femoris - short head)	Sciatic-peroneal div.	L5
Ext. hamstrings (biceps femoris - long head)	Sciatic-tibial div.	L5; S1
Gluteus medius	Superior gluteal	L4, 5; S1
Tensor fascia lata	Superior gluteal	L4, 5; S1
Gluteus maximus	Inferior gluteal	L5; S1, 2
Posterior tibial	Tibial	L5; S1
Flexor digitorum longus	Tibial	L5; S1
Abductor hallucis	Tibial (medial plantar)	L5; S1, 2
Abductor digiti quinti pedis	Tibial (lateral plantar)	S1, 2
Gastrocnemius lateral	Tibial	L5; S1, 2
Gastrocnemius medial	Tibial	S1, 2
Soleus	Tibial	S2

TABLE 52.4
Course of Select Upper Extremity Sensory Nerves

Nerve	Roots	Trunk	Cord
Lateral antebrachial cutaneous (branch of musculocutaneous)	C5, 6	Upper	Lateral
Median (first digit)	C6	Upper	Lateral
Median (second digit)	C6, 7	Upper/middle	Lateral
Median (third digit)	C7	Middle	Lateral
Radial	C6, 7	Upper/middle	Posterior
Ulnar	C8	Lower	Medial
Dorsal ulnar cutaneous	C8	Lower	Medial
Medial antebrachial cutaneous	C8; T1	Lower	Medial

TABLE 52.5
Course of Select Lower Extremity Sensory Nerves

Nerve	Roots	Plexus
Lateral femoral cutaneous	L2, 3	Lumbar
Saphenous	L4	Lumbar
Superficial peroneal	L5	Lumbosacral trunk
Sural	S1	Sacral

TABLE 52.6

Compressive and Noncompressive Causes of Radiculopathies

Compressive
Degenerative
  Disk herniation
  Facet joint hypertrophy
  Ligamentum flavum hypertrophy
  Postsurgical fibrosis
Tumors
  Epidural
  Intradural
    Leptomeningeal disease
  Intramedullary
Subdural bleed
Infection
Epidural abscess

Noncompressive
Toxic/metabolic
  Diabetes
    Diabetic amyotrophy
  Arachnoiditis
    Contrast agents
    Bloody spinal tap
    Anesthetics and corticosteroids
    Spinal surgery
  Chemotherapy
Autoimmune
  Guillain-Barré syndrome
    AIDP
    AMAN/AMSAN
    CIDP
  Infectious
    Mycobacterium tuberculosis
    Cryptococcus neoformans
    Lyme disease
    Syphilis
    HIV
  Ischemic
    Leptomeningeal disease
    Sarcoidosis

Abbreviations: AIDP, acute inflammatory demyelinating polyradiculoneuropathy; AMAN, acute motor axonal neuropathy; AMSAN, acute motor and sensory axonal neuropathy; CIDP, chronic inflammatory demyelinating polyradiculoneuropathy; HIV, human immunodeficiency virus.

MRI with gadolinium of the spine and brain should be performed initially in all suspected cases. Nodular enhancement of the leptomeninges is almost pathognomonic. The diagnosis is confirmed with the presence of malignant cells on cerebrospinal fluid (CSF) cytology. However, there is a high initial false-negative rate on CSF studies of 40%–50% (4). Repeat CSF studies following an initial negative result improves the diagnostic yield to 90% (7). Electrodiagnostic studies are consistent with a polyradiculopathy; however, underlying findings of an axonal, sensorimotor polyneuropathy, due to prior chemotherapy treatment, can often be noted and can confuse the issue. Absent F-waves or prolonged F-wave latencies on NCS are felt to be an early indicator of nerve root involvement, but are not specific for leptomeningeal disease (8).

Plexopathy

Brachial plexopathies from neoplasms are usually the result of metastatic disease, with breast and lung being the most common primary sources (9). In cancer patients, the frequency of neoplastic brachial plexopathy is 0.43% (10). If a patient has a history of prior radiation therapy to the axillary or supraclavicular lymph nodes, secondary radiation-induced neoplasms, such as sarcomas, should also be considered. Symptoms include pain, paresthesias, numbness, and weakness in the distribution of plexus involvement. Metastases can involve any portion of the brachial plexus, but usually involve the lower trunk, due to its proximity to axillary lymph nodes and the superior sulcus of the lung.

The pattern of motor and sensory nerve conduction abnormalities is important in the localization of both brachial and lumbosacral plexopathies. A more extensive evaluation of the sensory nerves than is done on most standard electrophysiological studies is extremely important, as each sensory nerve has a relatively consistent course through the plexus and abnormalities may be instrumental in determining which specific plexus structures are involved (Tables 52.4 and 52.5). For instance, upper extremity NCS in a lower trunk brachial plexopathy will demonstrate a characteristic pattern of normal median SNAP amplitudes, reduced ulnar SNAP amplitudes, and reduced median and ulnar CMAP amplitudes. Abnormalities will also be noted in the medial antebrachial cutaneous SNAP. Findings on needle EMG will demonstrate fibrillation potentials, reduced recruitment, and large, polyphasic motor unit potentials within the distribution of involvement. Assessment of C8–T1 fibers with needle EMG is essential and can help guide further imaging studies (11). Needle EMG of the paraspinal muscles is usually normal in a plexopathy. The Pancoast syndrome is a distinct clinical presentation, resulting from a superior pulmonary sulcus tumor and presenting with findings

ings of nuchal rigidity, as well as upper motor neuron signs, especially if there is concomitant brain involvement. Cranial nerves are often involved as well, with the oculomotor, facial, and auditory nerves most commonly affected.

of a lower trunk brachial plexopathy and a unilateral Horner syndrome (12).

Neoplastic lumbosacral plexopathies can result from metastatic disease, but are much more likely to be caused by direct extension of local tumor or perineural spread (13). Common tumors involved include colon, gynecologic tumors, lymphomas, and sarcomas. As in brachial plexopathies, neuropathic symptoms and abnormal needle EMG findings will be in the distribution of involvement. Sensory abnormalities will be present on sural and superficial peroneal sensory NCS, and MRI of the lumbosacral plexus is helpful in the diagnosis.

Neuropathy

As mentioned, neuropathies can be classified as focal or diffuse. Focal mononeuropathies directly related to cancer most often result from the external compression or invasion from tumor, such as an isolated radial neuropathy caused by a primary osteogenic sarcoma or a bone metastasis involving the spiral groove of the humerus. Malignant nerve sheath tumors are rare and usually arise from plexiform neurofibromas (11). There is a high association with neurofibromatosis type 1. The clinical presentation depends on the individual nerve involved, but severe pain and rapidly growing tumors suggest malignant transformation (14). Sarcomas compressing or infiltrating nervous system structures resulting from previous radiation therapy need to be evaluated for. NCS and needle EMG should demonstrate abnormalities solely in the distribution of the individual nerve.

Diffuse peripheral nerve infiltration from cancer, either in a diffuse symmetric pattern or in a mononeuritis multiplex pattern, is rare, but has been reported in hematologic malignancies, such as non-Hodgkin lymphoma and chronic lymphocytic leukemia (15,16). Amyloid deposition in systemic amyloidosis and multiple myeloma can also result in diffuse polyneuropathy (17).

Myopathy

Focal myopathies from tumor involvement are rare and usually result from direct infiltration from underlying bony metastases or local lymph node involvement rather than from hematogenous spread. A more proximal myopathy associated with macroglossia and muscle pseudohypertrophy is an uncommon manifestation of primary amyloidosis. Muscle biopsy is diagnostic and demonstrates amyloid deposition surrounding muscle fibers and blood vessels. NCSs are usually normal. Needle EMG findings in amyloid myopathy show rapid recruitment of short-duration, small-amplitude, polyphasic MUPs or a mixture of large and small MUPs,

with fibrillation potentials noted primarily in proximal muscles (18). The selection of muscle to biopsy can be guided by electrodiagnostic findings. A needle EMG evaluation for myopathy will usually be limited to one side, with the electrodiagnostic report offering guidance to biopsy the corresponding contralateral muscle with the most involvement. There is a concern that needle trauma from the EMG may make reading the biopsy difficult.

PARANEOPLASTIC SYNDROMES

Neuromuscular paraneoplastic syndromes cause damage to the peripheral nervous system as a result of remote effects from a malignant neoplasm or its metastases (19). Although rare, it is important to recognize these syndromes. The clinical presentation is usually more rapidly progressive and severe than what would normally be expected in a noncancerous etiology. They often precede the diagnosis of cancer, and early recognition may increase survival. Treatment of the underlying malignancy usually results in improvement of neurologic symptoms. In some disorders, neuronal antigens expressed by the tumor result in an autoimmune response against both the tumor as well as healthy neural tissue, and identification of these markers can help facilitate the workup of diagnosis of a primary tumor. Although some syndromes are associated with an identifiable neuro-oncologic autoantibody, frequently no such marker is detected.

Almost all tumor types have been associated with paraneoplastic syndromes, and any part of the nervous system can be affected. There are, however, certain tumors that have a higher association with paraneoplastic syndromes, with neuroblastoma most often seen in children and small cell lung cancer most often seen in adults. Paraneoplastic opsoclonus-myoclonus occurs in 2%–3% of children with neuroblastoma. One percent to 3 percent of patients with small cell lung cancer develop Lambert-Eaton myasthenic syndrome (LEMS) or some other paraneoplastic syndrome (20).

Sensory Neuronopathy

Paraneoplastic sensory neuronopathy or ganglionopathy presents with either an acute or insidious onset of pain and sensory loss. Clinical findings of sensory ataxia and pseudoathetosis are often present at various levels of severity. Both the clinical and electrodiagnostic findings can be diffuse, but are commonly more severe in the upper extremities and may be asymmetric. Motor dysfunction is usually absent; however, sensory neuronopathy can sometimes be seen along with more a diffuse paraneoplastic neurologic syndrome involving encephalomyelitis, autonomic neuropathy, and motor neuronopathy (19). A pattern of more severe sensory abnormalities on nerve conduction studies in the upper extremities compared to the lower extremities helps distinguish this entity from a length-dependent sensory neuropathy. Needle EMG is usually normal, although poor volitional activation of MUPs may be noted due to the severity of sensory abnormalities. The most common associated neoplasm is small cell lung cancer; however, breast, renal, chondrosarcoma, and lymphoma have also been implicated. The presence of anti-Hu antibodies helps support the diagnosis of paraneoplastic sensory neuronopathy.

Sensorimotor Polyneuropathy

The diagnosis of a true paraneoplastic distal, symmetric, sensorimotor polyneuropathy is difficult to confirm, as there are many more likely known etiologies that can cause this pattern of involvement, including diabetes mellitus, nutritional deficiencies, and toxic exposure such as chemotherapy. A subacute, sensorimotor polyneuropathy as a paraneoplastic syndrome is, therefore, a diagnosis of exclusion. Symptoms include pain, paresthesias, numbness, and weakness in a stocking-glove distribution, along with hyporeflexia. A more rapidly progressive course may be the only distinguishing factor differentiating a paraneoplastic syndrome from an idiopathic or diabetic etiology. Electrodiagnostic findings are consistent with an axonal process rather than demyelinating. This syndrome has been associated with lung and breast cancer (21).

Vasculitic Neuropathy

A pattern of clinical and electrophysiologic involvement resembling mononeuritis multiplex may represent a paraneoplastic vasculitic neuropathy. This syndrome has been most commonly reported in association with small cell lung cancer and lymphoma (22). Further support for vasculitis includes an elevated erythrocyte sedimentation rate and an elevated cerebrospinal fluid protein level. The anti-Hu antibody has been also been associated with this syndrome (23). Biopsy of the sural nerve confirms microvascular involvement. In addition to treating any underlying malignancy, the neuropathic symptoms may respond to immunosuppressive therapy directed against the vasculitis.

Lambert-Eaton Myasthenic Syndrome

LEMS is a presynaptic disorder of neuromuscular transmission, and is perhaps the best understood paraneoplastic neuromuscular syndrome. Clinically, patients present with fatigue, proximal weakness, hyporeflexia, and autonomic dysfunction. Repetitive strength testing may reveal a "warming-up" phenomenon, where one can display an initial increase in strength with repetition followed by eventual fatigue. Bulbar involvement is rare. LEMS tends to affect adults greater than 40 years of age, and has a male predominance. It can occur independently from cancer, but up to 40%–60% of cases have been shown to be associated with small cell lung cancer (9). LEMS has also been reported to be associated with lymphoma, breast, ovarian, pancreatic, and renal malignancies.

Electrodiagnostic studies are invaluable in the diagnosis of LEMS. Motor responses are reduced in amplitude at baseline. Sensory responses are normal. Repetitive stimulation of motor nerves at low frequency (2–3 Hz) demonstrates a further decrement in amplitude. Following brief isometric exercise, facilitation occurs and CMAP amplitudes show at least a 100% increase (24). This finding is almost pathognomonic for LEMS. Needle EMG findings are usually normal, except for the presence of varying, unstable MUPs. Antibodies directed against the P/Q-type voltage-gated calcium channels are seen in up to 92% of LEMS patients (9). Management involves administration of 3,4-diaminopyridine and treatment of any underlying malignancy.

Myasthenia Gravis

Myasthenia gravis (MG) is a postsynaptic disorder of neuromuscular transmission, and its relationship with benign thymomas is widely recognized. MG occurs in 30% of patients with thymoma, and 15% of patients with MG are found to have thymoma on further radiographic evaluation (21). Patients present with fatigue and proximal weakness, most notably in ocular and bulbar muscles. Electrodiagnostic studies demonstrate a decremental response in compound muscle potential amplitude with 2–3 Hz repetitive stimulation (Fig. 52.7). Unlike LEMS, baseline motor amplitudes are normal in MG, except in severe cases. Immediately following brief exercise, a repair of the decrement is noted. Postactivation exhaustion, with return of the decremental response, is noted two to four minutes after exercise. Patients under 60 years of age with generalized weakness, or patients with a documented thymoma, are treated via thymectomy (25). Treatment can also involve the use of cholinesterase inhibitors or immunosuppressive agents. Table 52.7 outlines the major clinical and electrophysiologic differences between LEMS and MG (26).

Syndromes of Neuromuscular Hyperactivity

Hyperactivity syndromes, such as stiff person syndrome or neuromyotonia (Isaac syndrome), are rare but have

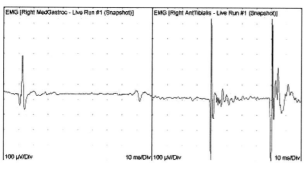

FIGURE 52.7

Normal (*left*) and abnormal (*right*) motor units. Note that both the abnormal motor units on the right demonstrate increased amplitude, increased duration, and marked polyphasia, all indicating a neuropathic process with subsequent motor unit remodeling.

been associated with malignancies, including small cell lung cancer, breast cancer, lymphoma, and invasive thymoma (27–29). Stiff person syndrome is a disorder characterized by muscle rigidity and worsening of symptoms with exposure to certain triggers, such as loud noise or startle. Continuous motor unit activity is the hallmark finding noted on needle EMG. Otherwise, electrodiagnostic findings are unremarkable. Antibodies to glutamic acid decarboxylase are present in up to 60% of patients, and in some instances, there is an association with antibodies against the presynaptic cell membrane protein amphiphysin. Isaac syndrome is an autoimmune channelopathy that has been reported in association with Hodgkin lymphoma as well as plasmacytoma (30,31). Antibodies to voltage-gated potassium channels are present in 50% of patients. Continuous motor unit activity is again noted on needle EMG; however, unlike stiff person syndrome, the symptoms and findings persist during sleep. Neurotonic discharges may also be present.

Myopathy

The findings of a symmetric, proximal myopathy on clinical examination and electrodiagnostic testing can also lead to the discovery of an undiagnosed cancer. Myopathy findings on needle EMG include fibrillation potentials and rapid recruitment of small-amplitude, short-duration, polyphasic MUPs. Findings are usually more pronounced in proximal versus distal muscles. NCSs are usually normal. Although their classification as a true paraneoplastic syndrome is controversial, polymyositis and especially dermatomyositis are associated with an increased incidence of malignancy compared with the general population (32). Breast,

lung, and gynecologic malignancies are most frequently implicated. Paraneoplastic necrotizing myopathy (33) and carcinoid myopathy are syndromes distinct from polymyositis/dermatomyositis. Carcinoid tumors may be associated with a progressive myopathy that has its onset years after the carcinoid syndrome (21).

Motor Neuron Disease

Sensory NCS in patients with motor neuron disease are normal. Motor responses will be either normal or reduced in amplitude. Needle EMG will demonstrate fibrillation and fasciculation potentials, reduced recruitment, and large, polyphasic, varying MUPs diffusely. With regard to motor neuron disease syndromes, as mentioned, the anti-Hu–associated paraneoplastic encephalomyelitis/sensory neuronopathy/motor neuropathy syndrome has a strong link with small cell lung cancer. Subacute motor neuropathy and primary lateral sclerosis have been associated with lymphoma and breast cancer, respectively (34). There is no known association between cancer and amyotrophic lateral sclerosis; however, in newly diagnosed motor neuron disease, a screening for cancer is usually part of the exclusionary diagnostic workup.

INDIRECT NEUROMUSCULAR EFFECTS OF CANCER

Immunocompromised patients are at risk for multiple infections, but with regard to the peripheral nervous system, the main pathogen is herpes zoster varicella. Reactivation of herpes zoster leading to shingles has been reported to occur in up to 34% of leukemia patients (35), with resulting radicular pain and potential postherpetic neuralgia. Sepsis with multisystem organ failure is a serious complication of cancer and reason for intensive care admission. In this setting, critical illness polyneuropathy and critical illness myopathy are often diagnosed (36). Other acute weakness syndromes, such as MG, LEMS, and steroid myopathies, must be excluded.

Weight loss is a common symptom of malignancy, and there is a higher risk of compression neuropathy, especially the peroneal nerve at the level of the fibular head. This is because the nerve is no longer protected by soft tissue and is more easily compressed against bony structures. Conduction block across the fibular head on peroneal motor NCS is a characteristic finding. A history of habitual leg crossing is sometimes elicited. There may be additional predisposition to injury given exposure to neurotoxic chemotherapy, which will be discussed later in the chapter. In addition to complications associated with weight loss, malnutrition can be

TABLE 52.7

Differentiating Characteristics of Myasthenia Gravis and Lambert-Eaton Myasthenic Syndrome

CHARACTERISTICS	MG	LEMS
Clinical Findings		
Limb weakness	Proximal	Proximal, diffuse
Bulbar weakness	Common	Uncommon
Repeated strength testing	Fatigable	Potentiation
Sensory	Normal	May be abnormal
Reflexes	Normal	Reduced
Autonomic dysfunction	Absent	Present
Pathophysiology		
Location	Postsynaptic	Presynaptic
Antibody	Acetylcholine receptor	P/Q-type voltage-gated calcium channel
Repetitive Nerve Stimulation		
Baseline CMAP	Normal	Reduced amplitude
At rest	Decrement if moderate or severe, no decrement if mild	Decrement
After brief exercise (10 s)	Repair if decrement at rest	Facilitation
After prolonged exercise (1 min)	Repair if decrement at rest	May miss facilitation
2–5 min post-exercise	Postexercise exhaustion	Postexercise exhaustion
Needle EMG		
Fibrillation potentials	Rare	Rare
MUPs	Varying, occasionally myopathic	Varying, occasionally myopathic

Abbreviations: MG, myasthenia gravis; LEMS, Lambert–Eaton myasthenic syndrome; CMAP, compound muscle action potential; EMG, electromyography; MUPs, motor unit action potentials.

Source: From Ref. 26.

further associated with a sensory neuropathy secondary to vitamin B12 deficiency. Renal failure from myeloma or amyloid involvement can result in a uremic neuropathy with axonal features. Cachexia and related metabolic proximal myopathies affecting primarily type 2 muscle fibers are also seen.

ELECTRODIAGNOSIS OF NEUROMUSCULAR COMPLICATIONS OF CANCER TREATMENTS

Surgery

Although uncommon, damage to the peripheral nervous system during the perioperative period can occur in both the cancer and noncancer patient. Because the nature of surgical procedures for the cancer patient is likely to be more complex, it is felt that the likelihood

of complications is greater. There are no studies, however, comparing the incidence of unintentional nerve injury in the cancer surgery population to that in the general population. In addition, peripheral nerves are sometimes intentionally sacrificed in the cancer surgery patient in order to obtain local disease control. The pattern and extent of neurologic involvement following surgery depends on the location of the tumor, patient positioning during surgery, and the patient's overall preoperative status and propensity to nerve injury (37). For example, through mechanisms mentioned previously, a cancer patient having undergone a significant amount of weight loss prior to treatment may be more susceptible to a perioperative peroneal neuropathy at the fibular head resulting from positioning following a prolonged surgery and postoperative recovery period.

Perioperative neurapraxic injuries resulting from compression of peripheral nerves are well-recognized phenomena. It is felt that these injuries result from the patient's position during anesthesia or during the immediate postsurgical recovery period (38). Common sites of injury and associated surgical procedures include brachial plexus injury during thoracotomy or mastectomy, given the abducted position of the involved upper extremity. Abduction of the upper extremity greater than 90 degrees during anesthesia will cause the humeral head to sublux inferiorly, resulting in compression and traction of the brachial plexus. Upon awakening, patients report varying degrees of pain, weakness, and numbness in both the upper and lower trunk distribution. Complete spontaneous recovery within weeks is common, even in cases of severe plegia. Ulnar neuropathies at the elbow, resulting from arm boards used to secure intravenous lines, and radial neuropathies at the spiral groove, resulting from prolonged time in the lateral decubitus position, are also noted following thoracic surgery.

Compression of the femoral nerve or lumbar plexus can result from traction during pelvic surgery. Patients undergoing hip arthroplasty or acetabular reconstruction are prone to injury, with the peroneal division of the sciatic nerve being the most commonly affected nerve. Injuries to the superior gluteal, obturator, and femoral nerves have also been reported (39). Cadaveric studies demonstrate that the lithotomy position, with the lower limbs placed in greater than 30 degrees of abduction, causes excessive traction on the obturator nerve. This strain is relieved, however, with concomitant hip flexion (40). Finally, delayed postoperative hemorrhages and hematomas should be excluded in all patients who develop new neuropathic symptoms 24–48 hours after surgery.

The spinal accessory nerve is often sacrificed during radical or modified radical neck dissection for head and neck cancers. The branch to the trapezius is usually more affected than the branch innervating the sternocleidomastoid. A resulting drooped shoulder and lateral scapular winging can lead to chronic shoulder pain. Motor NCS performed on the spinal accessory nerve while recording over the trapezius will demonstrate low-amplitude CMAP. Needle EMG will demonstrate a combination of fibrillation potentials, reduced recruitment, and large, polyphasic motor unit potentials in the trapezius, with sparing of the sternocleidomastoid.

Damage to lower extremity nerves is uncommon during abdominal or pelvic surgery, unless a tumor has already infiltrated nervous system structures. The rates of unintentional or planned nerve sacrifice are high in limb-sparing procedures for extremity sarcomas due to the need to achieve adequate tumor-free surgical margins. Electrodiagnostic studies performed immediately after surgery and two to three weeks afterward can help prognosticate neurologic recovery (41).

Chemotherapy

Peripheral neuropathy is a common adverse effect of medications in general; however, when these medicines are used to treat life-threatening illnesses such as cancer, it becomes challenging to balance the disabling limiting side effects with the obvious benefits of chemotherapy. Side effects tend to be dose-dependent, although it is important to recognize preexisting subclinical neuropathies or a family history of neuropathy, such as in the case of the hereditary sensory and motor neuropathies. The neurotoxic effects of chemotherapy in these patients can occur earlier than expected in the treatment course, and symptoms can be devastating and disabling (42–44). Although almost all agents have been associated with neuropathies, a select number of chemotherapeutics are especially prone to causing neuropathy. Chemotherapy-induced neuropathy generally is characterized by axonal loss via Wallerian degeneration, and presents with a subacute, length-dependent, sensory greater than motor polyneuropathy. NCS reveals normal or low-amplitude CMAPs and low-amplitude or absent SNAPs. Needle EMG may demonstrate fibrillation potentials, reduced recruitment, and large, polyphasic MUPs in distal limb muscles. The prognosis for neurologic recovery upon discontinuation of the offending agent is generally favorable, but depends on the severity of symptoms.

Two classes of chemotherapeutic agents in prevalent use are the vinca alkaloids and the taxanes. The vinca alkaloids, such as vincristine, vinblastine, and vinorelbine, are used in the treatment of solid tumors, lymphomas, and leukemias. They are usually given in combination with other chemotherapeutic agents. The mechanism of action with the vinca alkaloids is to arrest dividing cells in metaphase by binding tubulin and preventing its polymerization into microtubules. This is also the proposed mechanism of inducing neuropathy—by inhibiting anterograde and retrograde transport and causing axonal degeneration. Clinical features are those of a distal, symmetric, sensorimotor axonal polyneuropathy, affecting both large and small fibers. Taxanes, such as paclitaxel and docetaxel, are also used to treat solid tumors, such as breast and ovarian cancer. As in the vinca alkaloids, the taxane-induced neuropathy is a length-dependent, sensorimotor polyneuropathy resulting from damage to the axonal microtubule system (45). Similar agents generally resulting in a length-dependent, axonal neuropathy affecting sensory greater than motor fibers include thalidomide and bortezomib, both used in the treatment of multiple myeloma.

Platinum-based compounds are used in the treatment of solid tumors, such as ovarian, testicular, and bladder cancer. They include agents such as cisplatin, carboplatin, and oxaliplatin. While platinum toxicity can also result in a distal, symmetric, sensorimotor polyneuropathy, there also appears to be preferential damage to the dorsal root ganglia, causing a sensory neuronopathy with clinical and electrodiagnostic features, including sensory ataxia and upper extremity SNAPs being more affected than in the lower extremities. A "coasting phenomenon" may be noted, where symptoms can progress for months following discontinuation of the platinum compound. Prognosis for recovery in a sensory ganglionopathy is poor.

Cytarabine is used in the treatment of hematologic cancers. There have been reports of severe sensorimotor polyneuropathy, resembling Guillain-Barré syndrome, with high-dose administration of cytarabine (46). Electrophysiologic studies demonstrate a mixed axonal and multifocal demyelinating process.

Hand-foot syndrome is an unusual complication of several chemotherapeutic agents, including 5-fluorouracil, capecitabine, doxorubicin, docetaxel, and cytarabine. Clinical features include painful desquamation and discoloration of the palms and soles of the hands and feet. The pain is frequently described as burning in character. Clinical findings include reduced pain and temperature sensation, with preserved reflexes, proprioception, and strength. Electrodiagnostic studies are usually normal, as electrodiagnostic testing is limited to the evaluation of large fibers. Intraepidermal nerve fiber density evaluation demonstrates decreased numbers of small fibers, both proximally and distally, suggestive of a painful small-fiber neuropathy (47).

Glucocorticosteroids are perhaps the most frequently used medications in the oncology patient. The primary use of corticosteroids in cancer patients is to control brain and spinal cord edema, but they are also used in the treatment of cancers such as lymphoma. They are also helpful in treating pain, improving appetite, and managing nausea and vomiting caused by other chemotherapeutic agents. The major neuromuscular complication associated with corticosteroid use is steroid-induced myopathy. Patients present clinically with proximal weakness and myalgias and without sensory abnormalities. Muscle biopsies demonstrate type 2 muscle-fiber atrophy. Needle EMG findings are unremarkable, as type 1 muscle fibers are preferentially tested with electrodiagnosis. Prolonged high-dose use of corticosteroids can cause steroid-induced diabetes, which can lead to all of the associated secondary complications of diabetes, including distal, symmetric, axonal, peripheral neuropathy, or diabetic radiculoplexus neuropathies.

Radiation Therapy

Approximately 50% of all cancer patients will undergo radiation therapy at some point during the course of their disease, and radiation therapy is involved in approximately one-quarter of all cancer cures (48). As patients are living longer following cancer treatments, physicians are becoming more aware of late neuromuscular complications of therapy, especially radiation therapy. Side effects are essentially related to the dose of radiation and the volume of normal tissue that receives radiation (49). Despite numerous advances with dose-fractionation schedules, beam conformation technology, and the advent of intensity-modulated/image-guided radiation therapy, it is still necessary to include normal tissue within the treatment field, much like a successful surgery requires adequate negative margins in order to achieve local disease control.

Radiation causes tissue injury primarily by the induction of apoptosis due to free radial-mediated DNA damage. Rapidly dividing cells, such as neoplastic cells, are particularly susceptible. Normal cells are also affected but to a lesser extent. In addition, radiation causes direct and indirect tissue injury that is mediated by a combination of chemokines, cytokines, and other growth factors. This includes activation of the coagulation system, inflammation, epithelial regeneration, and tissue remodeling. Although the exact pathophysiologic mechanism is not entirely understood, it is felt that this damage to the vascular endothelial system, causing abnormal collagen deposition and fibrosis in the perivascular and extracellular matrix, is the primary method resulting in damage to the underlying neuromuscular structures (48).

The clinical effects of radiation on peripheral nerves have been well documented. Any structure in the nervous system, both centrally and peripherally, is susceptible to radiation toxicity, including brain, spinal cord, and the nerve roots. However, the majority of studies and articles examining the phenomenon of radiation-induced damage to the peripheral nervous systems focus on radiation-induced plexopathy, specifically brachial plexopathy.

The primary differential diagnostic concern in a cancer patient with brachial plexopathy is distinguishing between a neoplastic and radiation-induced etiology. Occasionally, the two conditions can coexist. Classically, radiation-induced plexopathy is delayed in onset, pain is less common than in neoplastic plexopathy, and symptoms of weakness and paresthesias are usually progressive (50,51). There is also more likely to be associated lymphedema in the involved limb. It has been reported that neoplastic plexopathy tends to preferentially affect the lower trunk and radiation plexopathy the upper portion of the plexus; however, further studies suggest that plexus involvement may be more diffuse and with more overlap in both etiologies than previously suspected (52). The presence of myokymic discharges and fasciculation potentials strongly suggests a radiation-induced contribution to plexus injury (51). However, the absence of myokymic discharges does not exclude radiation damage. Even in the setting of classic EMG findings, follow-up imaging of the brachial plexus with MRI is indicated to exclude a concomitant compressive or infiltrating lesion, which could be due to local recurrence, new metastases, or radiation-induced secondary tumors such as sarcomas.

Originally thought to be relatively radioresistant, it is becoming more apparent that skeletal muscle is also susceptible to late-onset effects of radiation therapy. The direct effect of radiation on muscle results in fibrosis and contracture (53). There have been multiple reports of a late dropped-head syndrome in patients who have received mantle field radiation therapy in the distant past as part of their treatment for Hodgkin lymphoma (54,55). Clinical features include slowly progressive atrophy of neck and shoulder girdle musculature. Neck flexor and extensor muscles are markedly weak, with remarkably preserved motor function in the shoulder girdle and upper extremities. Affected muscles have a firm, fibrotic character on palpation. The head tends to be in a forward-flexed position, with a secondary kyphotic spinal posture, due to anterior cervical muscle contracture. Secondary musculoskeletal complications related to impaired posture, such as rotator cuff impingement syndromes, are seen. Needle EMG demonstrates low-amplitude, short-duration, polyphasic motor unit potentials in affected muscles, with normal or decreased insertional activity and rare, if any, fibrillation potentials. There may also be findings of a concomitant brachial plexopathy (56). Creatinine kinase levels and inflammatory markers are normal. Muscle biopsy in one patient demonstrated nemaline rod depositions in affected muscles, while biopsy results from unaffected muscles were normal (56).

Hematopoietic Stem Cell Transplant

Hematopoietic stem cell transplantation is performed as part of the treatment for hematologic malignancies, such as leukemias, lymphomas, and multiple myeloma, as well as for select solid tumors and nonmalignant diseases. These patients will frequently receive additional chemotherapy and/or radiation therapy as part of their treatment regimen and are susceptible to related neurotoxic effects, as described earlier. Common neurotoxic chemotherapeutic agents used in the setting of stem cell transplantation include cisplatin, paclitaxel, docetaxel, etoposide, thalidomide, and cytarabine. The chronic immunosuppressed state of these patients also makes them more prone to opportunistic infections and secondary peripheral neuropathies, such as herpes varicella zoster. Metabolic derangements, such as steroid-induced diabetes and malabsorption syndromes, are also common following transplantation and can

likewise result in secondary peripheral nervous system dysfunction.

Chronic graft-versus-host disease (GVHD) is the primary late-term complication associated with transplant. The graft, containing immunologically competent cells, reacts to host tissue antigens and carries out an autoimmune response against the transplant recipient. Forty percent of patients having survived greater than 100 days after transplant will develop GVHD (57). There is a high association with chronic GVHD and autoimmune neuromuscular disorders, including inflammatory myopathies, myasthenia gravis, and both acute and chronic polyneuropathies.

Polymyositis, and to a lesser degree dermatomyositis, are well recognized but uncommon complications of chronic GVHD. The incidence of polymyositis in the GVHD population is greater than that of the general population (58). The clinical presentation, electrodiagnostic findings, and pathologic findings in GVHD-associated polymyositis are identical to idiopathic polymyositis. Differentiating an inflammatory myopathy from a steroid-induced myopathy is of obvious clinical importance.

MG in the setting of chronic GVHD usually develops between two and five years after transplantation during tapering of immunosuppressive drug therapy (59). Clinically and electrophysiologically, the findings are similar to typical autoimmune MG; treatment regimens are likewise similar, with equal efficacy. Acetylcholine receptor antibodies may or may not be present. There has not been a reported association with thymoma in patients with GVHD-associated MG.

Autoimmune neuropathies have also been associated with GVHD, and can present as either a distal symmetric sensorimotor polyneuropathy with characteristic electrodiagnostic findings or as a syndrome with features similar to Guillain-Barré syndrome (60,61).

CONCLUSION

With numerous advancements in early detection and multimodal therapy, cancer has become a chronic disease. As the number of cancer survivors continues to increase, physiatrists and other neuromuscular disease specialists are more likely to encounter individuals with residual impairments, disabilities, and/or handicaps resulting from cancer or related treatments. The cancer patient is especially prone to injury directed at the peripheral nervous system at multiple levels. Tumors can directly compress or infiltrate vital nervous system structures or can cause severe neuromuscular disorders through a paraneoplastic process. Immunocompromised cancer patients are susceptible to indirect neurologic insult through secondary mechanisms such as infection or metabolic disorders. Cancer treatments themselves, including surgery, chemotherapy, radiation therapy, and hematopoietic stem cell transplant, can result in devastating neuromuscular complications. Recognition of associated neuromuscular complications of cancer and cancer treatments can be challenging due to the wide multifactorial array of potential etiologies, and electrodiagnostic testing, through NCS and needle EMG, is an invaluable tool in the evaluation of neuromuscular disorders in this patient population. Detection of these cancer- and noncancer–related disorders is important in designing specific, individualized rehabilitation treatments to the oncologic patient and survivor.

References

1. Hughes R, Sharrack B, Rubens R. Carcinoma and the peripheral nervous system. *J Neurol*. 1996;243:371–376.
2. Sorenson EJ. Nerve action potentials. In: Daube JR, ed. *Clinical Neurophysiology*, 2nd ed. New York, NY: Oxford University Press; 2002:169–180.
3. Shelerud RA, Paynter KS. Rarer causes of radiculopathy: spinal tumors, infections, and other unusual causes. *Phys Med Rehabil Clin N Am*. 2002;13:646–696.
4. Taillibert S, Laigle-Donadey F, Chodkiewicz C, et al. Leptomeningeal metastases from solid malignancy: a review. *J Neurooncol*. 2005;75:85–99.
5. Stubgen JP. Neuromuscular disorders in systemic malignancy and its treatment. *Muscle Nerve*. 1995;18:636–648.
6. Demopoulous A, DeAngelis LM. Neurologic complications of leukemia. *Curr Opin Neurol*. 2002;15:691–699.
7. Wasserstrom WR, Glass P, Posner JB. Diagnosis and treatment of leptomeningeal metastasis from solid tumors: experience with 90 patients. *Cancer*. 1982;49:759–772.
8. Argov Z, Siegal T. Leptomeningeal metastases: peripheral nerve and root involvement—clinical and electrophysiologic study. *Ann Neurol*. 1985;17:593–596.
9. Breinberg HR, Amato AA. Neuromuscular complications of cancer. *Neurol Clin N Am*. 2003;21:141–165.
10. Jaeckle KA. Neurological manifestations of neoplastic and radiation-induced plexopathies. *Semin Neurol*. 2004;24:385–393.
11. Ferrante MA. Brachial plexopathies: classification, causes, and consequences. *Muscle Nerve*. 2004;30:547–568.
12. Pancoast HK. Superior pulmonary sulcus tumor. *JAMA*. 1932;99:1391–1396.
13. Ladha SS, Spinner RJ, Suarez GA, et al. Neoplastic lumbosacral radiculoplexopathy in prostate cancer by direct perineural spread: an unusual entity. *Muscle Nerve*. 2006;34:659–665.
14. Antoine J-C, Camdessanche J-P. Peripheral nervous system involvement in patients with cancer. *Lancet Neurol*. 2007;6:75–86.
15. Kelly JJ, Karcher DS. Lymphoma and peripheral neuropathy: a clinical review. *Muscle Nerve*. 2005;31:301–313.
16. Amato AA, Dumitru D. Acquired neuropathies. In: Dumitru D, Amato AA, Zwarts MD, eds. *Electrodiagnostic Medicine*, 2nd ed. Philadelphia, PA: Hanley and Blefus; 2002:937–1041.
17. Kelly JJ, Kyle RA, Miles JM, et al. The spectrum of peripheral neuropathy in myeloma. *Neurology*. 1981;31:24–31.
18. Rubin DI, Hermann RC. Electrophysiologic findings in amyloid myopathy. *Muscle Nerve*. 1999;22:355–359.
19. Darnell RB, Posner JB. Paraneoplastic syndromes involving the nervous system. *N Engl J Med*. 2003;349:1543–1554.
20. Dropcho EJ. Neurologic paraneoplastic syndromes. *Curr Oncol Rep*. 2004;6:26–31.
21. Posner JB. Paraneoplastic syndromes. In: Posner JB, ed. *Neurologic Complications of Cancer*, 1st ed. Philadelphia PA: F.A. Davis; 1995:353–385.
22. Oh SJ. Paraneoplastic vasculitis of the peripheral nervous system. *Neurol Clin*. 1997;15:849–863.
23. Younger D, Dalmau J, Inghirami G, et al. Anti-Hu-associated peripheral nerve and muscle microvasculitis. *Neurology*. 1994;44:181–183.
24. Stubblefield MD, Custodio CM, Franklin DJ. Cardiopulmonary rehabilitation and cancer rehabilitation. 3. Cancer rehabilitation. *Arch Phys Med Rehabil*. 2006;87(3 Suppl 1):S65–S71.
25. Keesey JC. Clinical evaluation and management of myasthenia gravis. *Muscle Nerve*. 2004;29:484–505.
26. Strommen JA, Johns JS, Kim C-T, Williams FH, Weiss LD, Weiss JM, Rashbaum IG. Neuromuscular rehabilitation and electrodiagnosis. 3. Diseases of muscles and neuromuscular junction. *Arch Phys Med Rehabil*. 2005;86(3 Suppl 1):S18–S27.
27. Bateman DE, Weller RD, Kennedy P. Stiffman syndrome: a rare paraneoplastic disorder? *J Neurol Neurosurg Psychiatry*. 1995;53:695–696.
28. Rosin L, DeCamilli P, Butler M, et al. Stiff-man syndrome in a woman with breast cancer: an uncommon central nervous system paraneoplastic syndrome. *Neurology*. 1998;50:84–88.
29. Hagiwara H, Enomoto-Nakatani S, Sakai K, et al. Stiff-person syndrome associated with invasive thymoma: a case report. *J Neurol Sci*. 2001;193:59–62.
30. Caress JB, Abend WK, Preston DC, et al. A case of Hodgkin's lymphoma producing neuromyotonia. *Neurology*. 1997;49:258–259.
31. Zifko U, Drlicek M, Machacek E, et al. Syndrome of continuous muscle fiber activity and plasmacytoma with IgM paraproteinemia. *Neurology*. 1994;44:560–561.
32. Yazici Y, Kagen LJ. The association of malignancy with myositis. *Curr Opin Rheumatol*. 2000;12:498–500.
33. Levin MI, Mozaffar T, Taher Al-Lozi M, et al. Paraneoplastic necrotizing myopathy: clinical and pathologic features. *Neurology*. 1998;50:764–767.
34. Younger DS. Motor neuron disease and malignancy. *Muscle Nerve*. 2000;23;658–660.
35. Poulsen A, Schmiegelow K, Yssing M. Varicella zoster infections in children with acute lymphoblastic leukemia. *Pediatr Hematol Oncol*. 1996;13:231–238.
36. Sliwa JA. Acute weakness syndromes in the critically ill patient. *Arch Phys Med Rehabil*. 2000;81(3 Suppl):S45–S52.
37. Posner JB. Neurotoxicity of surgical and diagnostic procedures. In: Posner JB, ed. *Neurologic Complications of Cancer*, 1st ed. Philadelphia PA: F.A. Davis; 1995:338–352.
38. Dawson DM, Krarup C. Perioperative nerve lesions. *Arch Neurol*. 1989;46:1355–1360.
39. DeHart MM, Riley LH Jr. Nerve injuries in total hip arthroplasty. *J Am Acad Orthop Surg*. 1999;7:101–111.
40. Litwiller JP, Wells RE Jr, Halliwill JR, et al. Effect on lithotomy positions on strain of the obturator and lateral femoral cutaneous nerves. *Clin Anat*. 2004;17:45–49.
41. Custodio CM. Barriers to rehabilitation of patients with extremity sarcomas. *J Surg Oncol*. 2007;95:393–399.
42. Graf WD, Chance PF, Lensch MW, et al. Severe vincristine neuropathy in Charcot-Marie-Tooth disease type 1A. *Cancer*. 1996;77:1356–1362.
43. Chauvenet AR, Shashi V, Selsky C, et al. Vincristine-induced neuropathy as the initial presentation of Charcot-Marie-Tooth disease in acute lymphoblastic leukemia: a Pediatric Oncology Group study. *J Pediatr Hematol Oncol*. 2003;25:316–320.
44. Chaudhry V, Chaudhry M, Crawford TO, et al. Toxic neuropathy in patients with pre-existing neuropathy. *Neurology*. 2003;60:337–340.
45. Peltier AC, Russell JW. Recent advances in drug-induced neuropathies. *Curr Opin Neurol*. 2002;15:633–638.
46. Openshaw H, Slatkin NE, Stein AS, et al. Acute polyneuropathy after high-dose cytosine arabinoside in patients with leukemia. *Cancer*. 1996;78:1899–1905.
47. Stubblefield MS, Custodio CM, Kaufmann P, et al. Small-fiber neuropathy associated with capecitabine (Xeloda)-induced hand-foot syndrome: a case report. *J Clin Neuromusc Dis*. 2006;7:128–132.

48. Hauer-Jensen M, Fink LM, Wang J. Radiation injury and the protein C pathway. *Crit Care Med.* 2004;32(5 Suppl):S325–S330.

49. Pan CC, Hayman JA. Recent advances in radiation oncology. *J Neuro-Opthalmol.* 2004;24:251–257.

50. Kori SH, Foley KM, Posner JB. Brachial plexus lesions in patients with cancer: 100 cases. *Neurology.* 1981;31:45–50.

51. Harper CM, Thomas JE, Cascino TL, et al. Distinction between neoplastic and radiation-induced brachial plexopathy, with emphasis on the role of EMG. *Neurology.* 1989;39:502–506.

52. Boyaciyan A, Oge AE, Yazici J, et al. Electrophysiological findings in patients who received radiation therapy over the brachial plexus: a magnetic stimulation study. *Electroencephalogr Clin Neurophysiol.* 1996;101:483–490.

53. Vissink A, Jansma J, Spijkervet FK, et al. Oral sequelae of head and neck radiotherapy. *Crit Rev Oral Biol Med.* 2003;14:199–212.

54. Portlock CS, Boland P, Hays AP, et al. Nemaline myopathy: a possible late complication of Hodgkin's disease therapy. *Hum Pathol.* 2003;34:816–818.

55. Rowin J, Cheng G, Lewis SL, et al. Late appearance of dropped head syndrome after radiotherapy for Hodgkin's disease. *Muscle Nerve.* 2006;34:666–669.

56. Okereke LI, Custodio CM, Stubblefield MD. Bilateral lower-trunk brachial plexopathy and proximal myopathy 19 years after mantle field radiation for Hodgkin's disease: a case report. *Arch Phys Med Rehabil.* 2004;85:e23–e24.

57. Beredjiklian PK, Drummond DS, Dormans JP, et al. Orthopedic manifestations of chronic graft-versus-host disease. *J Pediatr Orthop.* 1998;18:572–575.

58. Stevens AM, Sullivan KM, Nelson JL. Polymyositis as a manifestation of chronic graft-versus-host disease. *Rheumatology (Oxford).* 2003;42:34–39.

59. Krouwer HGJ, Wijdicks EFM. Neurologic complications of bone marrow transplantation. *Neurol Clin N Am.* 2003;21:319–352.

60. Amato AA, Barohn RJ, Sahenk Z, et al. Polyneuropathy complicating bone marrow and solid organ transplantation. *Neurology.* 1993;43:1513–1518.

61. Wen PY, Alyea EP, Simon D, et al. Guillain-Barré syndrome following allogenic bone marrow transplantation. *Neurology.* 1997;49:1711–1714.

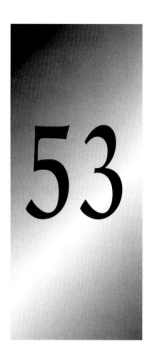

Intraoperative Neurophysiologic Monitoring in Cancer

53

Edward K. Avila
Sonia K. Sandhu

Intraoperative neurophysiologic monitoring (IONM) has become the standard of care for many neurosurgical, orthopedic, otolaryngology, and vascular surgeries. Initially, IONM was a research tool. However, as techniques became more sophisticated, applicability for clinical medicine was evident. The application of IONM has become crucial for the clarification of anatomy and testing of nervous system physiology, especially in situations where the normal anatomical arrangement has been disrupted. The purpose of IONM is to reduce neurologic damage during surgery. This is possible through the observation that the anatomical continuity and/or function of neural structures can change with surgical manipulation. When identified, these changes can be reversed by altering the surgical technique, whereas failure to act can result in permanent neural damage (1).

The clinical neurophysiologist must be familiar with a variety of surgical procedures for which IONM is requested in order to provide the best type of monitoring for the neurologic structure at risk. They must be adept in all aspects of neurophysiology and be able to interact and function within the "hostile environment" of the operating room. An array of potential sources of electrical interference exists in today's operating rooms, and eliminating sources of "noise" becomes a primary concern while performing

IONM. Knowledge of the different anesthetic regimens (eg, muscle relaxants, inhalants, injectable anesthetics) and their effect on neurophysiologic signals is vital to the interpretation of IONM. During a surgical procedure, the clinical neurophysiologist must coordinate care with the surgeon, anesthesiologist, and nurses in the operating room. IONM requires a close working relationship between the clinical neurophysiologist and the surgeon. Mutual respect and trust between both parties is essential for interpretation and application of the information garnered from IONM. The surgeon should be informed as much as possible in "real time" of any changes in recordings in order to assess if the changes are due to surgical technique or perhaps a false-positive result.

Injury to neural structures can occur from many sources, such as thermal, stretch (mechanical), and ischemia. All of these sources may be encountered during a typical operation. A spectrum of injury is believed to exist where initially a change in neural function can be recorded, which may correlate with partial or reversible injury. At the other end of the spectrum is a complete loss of neural function, which may correlate with irreversible injury.

The basic principles of IONM are threefold: (1) electrical potentials are reproducible and recorded in response to a stimulus, (2) these potentials change in a

KEY POINTS

- Intraoperative neurophysiologic monitoring (IONM) has become the standard of care for many neurosurgical, orthopedic, otolaryngology, and vascular surgeries.
- The purpose of IONM is to reduce neurologic damage during surgery, which can occur from thermal, stretch (mechanical), and ischemic injuries.
- The basic principles of IONM are threefold: (1) electrical potentials are reproducible and recorded in response to a stimulus, (2) these potentials change in a noticeable way as a result of surgically induced changes in function at a time when they are still reversible, and (3) proper surgical intervention, such as reversal of the surgical manipulation that caused the change, will prevent neural injury.
- IONM techniques can be applied to almost any level of the neural axis, including the cerebrum, skull base, brainstem, spine, and peripheral nerve.
- Somatosensory evoked potentials (SSEPs) are used to assess the neurophysiologic status of somatosensory pathways during surgical procedures involving
- peripheral nerves or plexus, spinal cord (eg, deformity correction, tumor removal), brainstem (posterior fossa mass removal), and midbrain (aneurysm repair).
- Acceptable criteria for alerting the surgeon are an SSEP amplitude drop of 50% or more and/or a greater than 10% increase in latency.
- Motor evoked potentials (MEPs) are compound muscle action potentials (CMAPs) elicited from muscles after either an electrical or magnetic stimulus has been delivered to the motor structures of the brain or spinal cord.
- Mapping of peripheral nerves is an important aid, especially when dealing with tumors involving the brachial plexus and cauda equina.
- Anesthetic effects accounted for many poor SSEP and MEP recordings in the past, but improved anesthetic regimens and increased communication between the anesthesiologist and the neurophysiologist have established adequate protocols to optimize intraoperative recordings.

noticeable way as a result of surgically induced changes in function at a time when they are still reversible, and (3) proper surgical intervention, such as reversal of the surgical manipulation that caused the change, will prevent neural injury (2).

TECHNIQUES

IONM techniques can be applied to almost any level of the neural axis. Surgeries involving the cerebrum, skull base, brainstem, spine, and peripheral nerve are amenable to monitoring with IONM. Modalities such as brainstem auditory evoked potentials (BAEPs), somatosensory evoked potentials (SSEPs), motor evoked potentials (MEPS), electromyography (EMG), compound muscle action potentials, electroencephalography, and electrocorticography are used to identify and monitor neural structures at risk.

Supratentorial surgeries for removal of tumors near eloquent cortex benefit greatly from IONM. Using somatosensory evoked potential phase-reversal identification, one can identify sensorimotor cortex. This type of monitoring, in addition to the use of electrocorticography and cortical stimulation, provides a neurophysiologic adjunct to other mapping techniques, such as functional magnetic resonance imaging (3). Skull base surgeries pose a risk for postoperative deficits,

as many lower cranial nerves are in close proximity to each other. IONM in this setting uses continuous electromyography as well as eliciting compound muscle action potentials for the confirmation of neurophysiologic function of the motor portion of a cranial nerve. In addition to anatomical visualization of cranial nerves during surgery, the use of IONM has decreased postoperative facial nerve deficits (4).

BAEPs have been shown to be useful for surgeries, particularly those that involve the cerebellopontine angle. There have been many published studies confirming their predictability and reproducibility intraoperatively, as well as their response to various anesthetic regimens (5–7).

Extensive literature has been devoted to intraoperative monitoring for spine surgeries. SSEPs initially found applicability for scoliosis correction surgeries, but have since been applied to a range of spine surgeries for degenerative disease and, more importantly, for tumor removal (8–10). Interpretation of changes for SSEPs has not always been predictive for postoperative motor deficits. Therefore, an additional method of monitoring was developed exclusively for the motor system via transcranial MEPs. MEPs are elicited by either transcranial magnetic or electrical stimulation. They have been shown to be safe, with few adverse effects when patients are carefully selected and appropriate safety measures are implemented (11).

EMG provides an additional modality for surgeries of the spine or peripheral nerve. Irritation of a nerve root may result in a neurotonic discharge, which is seen as a continuous "train" or intermittent "burst" of high-frequency motor unit potentials in the muscle being recorded (12). A neurotonic discharge indicates possible harm to the nerve in question and alerts the surgeon to change the surgical approach in order to prevent postoperative deficits. Although useful, free-run EMG monitoring does not confirm functional integrity of the structure. Eliciting a compound muscle action potential (triggered or stimulus-evoked EMG) can confirm the physiological integrity of the nerve distal to the site of stimulation monitored via the corresponding myotome.

BRAINSTEM AUDITORY EVOKED POTENTIALS

Evoked potentials are electrical responses arising from sensory stimulation. The generators of evoked potentials consist of two types: nerve bundles and nuclei. Nerve fiber bundles include peripheral nerves as well as central tracts.

Brainstem auditory evoked potentials generated from auditory stimulation are farfield potentials recorded from the afferent nerve volley in the eighth cranial nerve and the potentials produced by tracts and nuclei in the brainstem. BAEPs are used to monitor the integrity of the brainstem auditory pathway in the brain.

Five vertex-positive waveforms are present in the BAEP waveform (Fig. 53.1). They are numbered I through V, and represent different sequential activity in the peripheral component of the eighth cranial nerve (wave I), the cochlear nucleus (with a contribution from the peripheral component of the eighth cranial nerve) (wave II), the superior olivary nucleus (wave III), the lateral lemniscus (wave IV), and the inferior colliculus (wave V). Waveform absolute latencies, interpeak latencies, and amplitudes are measured. In the outpatient setting, these values are compared to normative data adjusted for age and gender. The values are expressed as a mean plus or minus 2.5–3.0 standard deviations. Latencies are considered abnormal if greater than 2.5–3.0 standard deviations from the mean.

In the operative setting, BAEPs are used commonly in posterior fossa, cerebellopontine angle, and brainstem surgeries in which the eighth cranial nerve is at risk of neural injury. Stimulating earplugs are placed in the ears, and usually a click stimulation is applied to the ipsilateral ear, with a masking stimulus (usually 25 dB less than the click stimulation) applied to the contralateral ear. The ideal stimulus for reproducible waveforms consists of 65–70 dB above the click hearing threshold, with an ideal repetition rate of 11.1/sec and a pulse duration of 100 μs. Recording electrodes are placed near both earlobes (left ear-A1, right ear-A2) and at the skull vertex (Cz).

Intraoperatively, the BAEP responses are averaged and comparisons are made during the surgical procedure to the patient's baseline operative BAEP (before surgical incision). Waveform latency prolongation and/or amplitude attenuation suggest damage to the nerve and can be localized along its anatomical pathway (Table 53.1). Commonly used alarm criteria for intraoperative BAEPs consist of waveform prolongation of 1.0 ms and a greater than 50% decrease in amplitude of wave V (13–15). James and Husain, however, have suggested that these criteria should vary, depending on the type of surgery performed (16). They suggest that during noncerebellopontine angle surgery, hearing loss is unlikely unless wave V becomes absent, so the criteria to alert the surgeon should be the point just before loss of wave V. For cerebellopontine angle surgery, the accepted alarm criteria threshold (1.0 ms latency delay, 50% amplitude drop) should be lowered and subtle waveform changes be communicated to the surgeon since hearing loss occurs more frequently in these cases.

Intraoperative changes can be reversible or irreversible based on the mechanism (eg, patient hypothermia, extreme anesthetic changes, problems with technical recordings, surgical drilling causing acoustic masking of the signals, vascular ischemia/infarction, mechanical forces [traction, compression], and thermal injury) (17).

BAEPs are mostly insensitive to anesthetic agents compared to other intraoperative neurophysiologic techniques (18). It has been observed that patient body

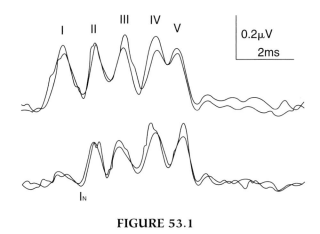

FIGURE 53.1

Normal BAEP in response to stimulation of the right ear. Response from the right is on top; response from the left is on the bottom. Note the absence of wave I in the contralateral recording. (From Ref. 89.)

TABLE 53.1
Interpretation of BAEP Findings

FINDING	INTERPRETATION
Increased wave I latency	Lesion of distal portion of acoustic nerve
Increased I–III interpeak interval	Lesion of pathway from proximal cranial VIII to pons, either in the nerve or in the brainstem (eg, acoustic neuroma)
Increased III–V interpeak interval	Lesion between caudal pons and midbrain
Increased I–III and III–V interpeak intervals	Lesion affecting brainstem above caudal pons plus either the caudal pons or acoustic nerve
Absence of wave I with normal III and V	Peripheral hearing disorder; conduction in the caudal pons cannot be evaluated
Absence of wave III with normal I and VI	Normal study
Absence of wave V with normal I and III	Lesion above the caudal pons; considered an extreme of wave III–V interpeak interval prolongation
Absence of all waves	Severe hearing loss

Source: From Ref. 36.

temperature has significant effects on the BAEP latency. Stockard et al. noted that latency shifts occur in the BAEP waveform when body temperature drops below 35.0°C (19).

SOMATOSENSORY EVOKED POTENTIALS

Introduction and Physiology

Somatosensory evoked potentials (SSEPs) have been used for more than 20 years for spinal surgery and remain the gold standard for spinal cord monitoring, although MEPs are rapidly changing this view (20). Specifically, SSEPs for scoliosis correction surgeries have been shown to lower postoperative deficits and have become the standard of care for patients requiring spinal deformity correction (8).

SSEPs are used to assess the neurophysiologic status of somatosensory pathways during surgical procedures involving peripheral nerves or plexus, spinal cord (eg, deformity correction, tumor removal), brainstem (posterior fossa mass removal), and midbrain (aneurysm repair) (21). Improved anesthesia and techniques that are more refined have made this procedure even more sensitive. They are relatively easy to do, provide important data, and are highly sensitive.

SSEPs monitor only afferent pathways in the spinal cord, specifically the dorsal columns, which are large-fiber sensory tracts. The recordings obtained are either farfield (potentials recorded from electrodes placed at remote locations distant to the nerve or the nuclei that are the source of the potential) or nearfield (potentials recorded by placing a recording electrode

directly on a nerve, a nucleus, or a muscle that generates a potential) (2). The recordings allow nearfield somatosensory cortical potentials, farfield brainstem and cervical potentials, as well as lumbar potentials. The cortical nearfield recordings are less affected by muscle artifact and movement artifact, but are sensitive to anesthetic effects. Conversely, farfield recordings at the cervical level are less affected by anesthetic, but are susceptible to muscle artifact; a combination is optimal (22).

Recordings are typically made over the scalp vertex approximating the postcentral cortical gyrus. For scalp recording, subdermal needle electrodes are preferred and stimulating surface electrodes distally. A ground electrode is also required. Commonly, the posterior tibial nerve, posterior to the medial malleolus, or the median nerve at the wrist, is used for lower and upper SSEPs, respectively (Figs. 53.2 and 53.3) (23). Alternatively, the ulnar, femoral, peroneal, and sciatic nerves may be used. If surgically possible, recordings are also made over the lumbar and cervical regions (ie, peripheral potentials). Peripheral potentials are used for SSEP recordings and may serve as controls. Controls are typically sites not involved in the surgical procedure and may differentiate SSEP changes from anesthetic effect, technical difficulties, and blood pressure fluctuations (24,25).

Stimuli are usually applied at 5 stimuli per second for optimal amplitude of the recorded potential (22). The recordings, however, are not real-time. The data obtained are the result of averaged responses, typically requiring up to 1,000 sweeps to obtain an average. However, some authors have suggested that SSEPs could be averaged for less time, possibly only 50–100 sweeps rather than 1,000, so that more immediate feedback can

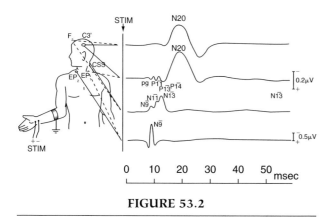

FIGURE 53.2

Median somatosensory evoked potentials. Stimulation at the median nerve with peripheral Erb point response (N9) and cortical response (N20). The cortical N20 response is used for phase-reversal identification. (From Ref. 90.)

be given to the surgeon (26). SSEP stimuli are alternated so that bilateral SSEPs can be monitored simultaneously and independently. Baselines are recorded and comparisons are made, not only from population normals, but also, more importantly, from the intraoperative baselines obtained from the patient.

Alarm Criteria for Somatosensory Evoked Potentials

Acceptable criteria for alerting the surgeon are an SSEP amplitude drop of 50% or more and/or a greater than 10% increase in latency. A study by Nuwer (1995) suggested that SSEP monitoring was effective in scoliosis surgery, leading to a 50% neurological injury reduction rate (8). The rate of false negatives was 0.127% and false positives was 1.51%. Alarm criteria for this study were 50% reduction in SSEP amplitude and 10% change in latencies. SSEP monitoring, however, does not monitor the descending corticospinal (motor) tracts in the anterior portions of the spinal cord, is affected by anesthetic changes, and does not offer real-time feedback to the surgeon. Criteria for alarm are not always uniform from center to center. In practicality, the limitation of "false-alarms," or false-positives that cause an interruption in surgery and possible loss of confidence in neuromonitoring, is ideal, and guidelines to this measure have yet to be defined. Intraoperative monitoring should only be requested for patients in whom the results of monitoring will change the surgeon's procedure and presumably the outcome.

Physiological Variables Affecting Somatosensory Evoked Potentials

Temperature can affect evoked potential amplitude and latencies. Core body temperature may drop by

greater than 1°C, with limb temperature usually dropping by several degrees. Nerve conduction velocities are temperature-dependent, and low limb temperature increases response latencies. It has been suggested that even with core body and limb temperature remaining constant, spinal cord temperature upon surgical exposure also may diminish SSEP amplitudes and increase latencies (27).

Hypotension can also affect SSEPs by decreasing amplitudes and prolonging latencies (22,28).

Advantages and Disadvantages of Intraoperative Somatosensory Evoked Potentials

Advantages to SSEP recordings are measurable and definable latencies and amplitudes. In addition, they can evaluate function over a long distance from peripheral nerve to somatosensory cortex. Not only can many levels of the nervous system be tested, but also any nerve with sensory fibers can be used.

Disadvantages include the observation that SSEPs are sensitive to various anesthetics, as well as physiological parameters, such as body temperature and blood pressure (28). Electrical interference from other devices used in the operating room, as well as 60 Hz artifact, can make SSEPs difficult to obtain. In addition, SSEPs are poor for use in evaluating the nerve root level and do not directly monitor motor pathways.

Improved techniques, more effective anesthetic regimens, and communication in the operating room continue to improve SSEP recordings. Because SSEPs may have false-negative readings, the addition of motor evoked potential monitoring has proved to be useful as an adjunctive monitoring tool (9–11). MEPs combined with SSEPs provide additional monitoring capabilities, allowing for anterior pathway monitoring and real-time recordings (26,29). The use of combined SSEPs and MEPS has made the Stagnara wake-up test nearly obsolete, especially since IONM provides intraoperative feedback compared to the wake-up test, which only provides information after the procedure has been completed (29,30). Because fixation or correction is completed, it becomes difficult to identify the precise moment when the injury occurred (31). The wake-up test, however, should still be done in the event of technical failure or persistent suppression or loss of SSEPs or MEPS with no identifiable cause.

MOTOR EVOKED POTENTIALS

Introduction and Physiology

Although SSEPs are useful, methods to monitor motor pathways better assess risk of motor deficits

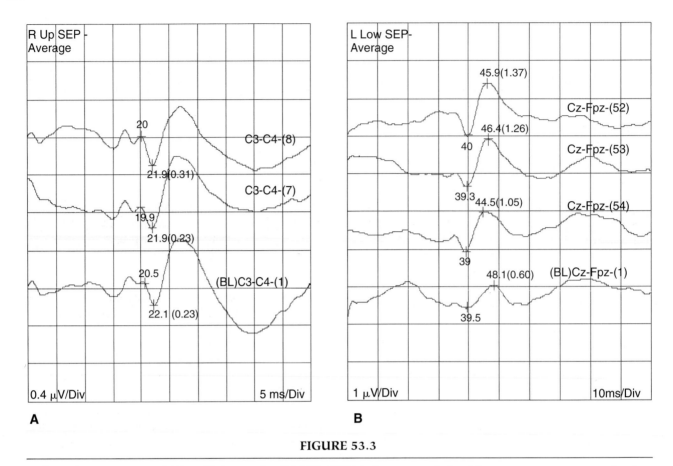

FIGURE 53.3

Right median nerve control (A) and left posterior tibial (B) SSEP during a thoracic-level bone aneurysm cyst resection in a 15-year-old child. First negative peak for the median is the cortical N20, and the first positive peak for left lower extremity is the cortical P37. *Abbreviation*: BL, baseline.

intraoperatively. There are currently three methods to assess motor activity of the spinal cord: (1) transcranial magnetic stimulation (TCMS), (2) transcranial electrical stimulation (TEMS), and (3) direct or indirect stimulation of the spinal cord itself.

MEPs were introduced by Levy in the 1980s (32). Motor cortex is stimulated via transcranial electrical or magnetic stimulation. MEPs are CMAPs elicited from muscles after either an electrical or magnetic stimulus has been delivered to the motor structures of the brain or spinal cord (33). MEPs are the most common way to assess the central motor pathways in the operating room. Recent Food and Drug Administration (FDA) approval has made MEPs even more popular. Responses are obtained from high-intensity, high-rate trains of transcranial electrical or magnetic pulses; three to seven pulses at 300–500 Hz. The resulting descending volley is recorded from the spinal surface through epidural or subdural electrodes or from limb muscles.

TEMS with between 250 and 450 volts produces a D (direct) wave and I (indirect) waves. These waves

represent microelectrode recordings of anterior horn cell depolarization in response to cortical stimulation (33). The initial large wave is the D wave, and the series of smaller depolarization waves are I waves. Stimulating electrodes are placed, with the anode over the scalp vertex and the cathode lateral to the anode at approximately 7 cm. Recording electrodes are placed in multiple limb muscles or specific muscles of clinical concern. Selection of appropriate muscles also requires knowledge of the surgical procedure in order to select muscles that can be identified without voluntary contraction, as is the case in an anesthetized patient (Fig. 53.4).

TCMS was first described in the 1980s by Barker et al. (34). It is a technique in which current flow is induced in the underlying tissue by an electrically induced pulse of the magnetic field. Typically, an intense pulse of current is delivered by an external coil that induces a magnetic field, which transmits through skin and bone and causes axonal or neuronal depolarization in brain tissue, which descends as action potentials in the corticospinal pathways (23). Recording

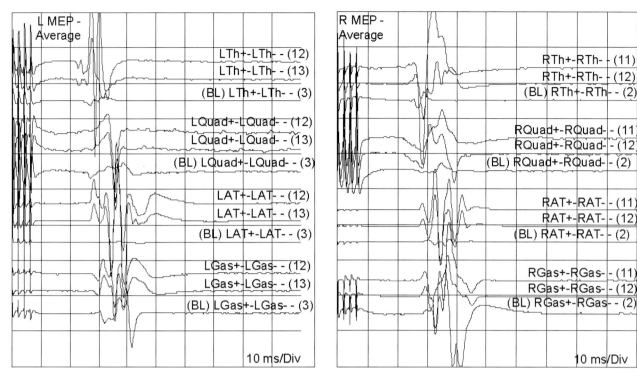

FIGURE 53.4

Multipulse motor evoked potentials in bilateral lower extremities for a thoracic-level tumor resection (multiple trials). *Abbreviations*: L MEP, left lower extremity MEP; R MEP, right lower extremity MEP; BL, baseline; Th, thenar eminence; Quad, quadriceps muscle; AT, anterior tibialis muscle; Gas, gastrocnemius muscle.

electrodes are placed in peripheral muscles. TCMS is more difficult to perform than transcranial electrical stimulation, and the CMAP responses are generally not supramaximal, which occurs more often with electrical motor cortex stimulation. Additionally, TCMS is impractical for IONM because minimal levels of anesthesia are required for adequate responses (35).

Alarm Criteria for Motor Evoked Potentials

Alarm criteria for MEP monitoring have been varied in the past. Some centers have informed the surgeon of changes with a decrease in 50% of the amplitude or a change in the latency of the response (36). Amplitude changes greater than 50% can be associated with a postoperative deficit, whereas amplitude changes equal to or less than 50% can be associated with no postoperative deficit or a rapid recovery. Amplitude changes as low as 20%–30% of baseline can also be associated with a postoperative deficit and, therefore, should be taken into consideration (37). Interestingly, one series reported that decreases in amplitude of up to 80% of baseline might not be associated with a

postoperative deficit (38). Alternatively, another criterion has been the use of threshold-level responses. Calancie et al. reported patients in whom thresholds for eliciting a CMAP increased by 100 V and remained so for one hour emerged from anesthesia with an increase in postoperative weakness (39).

Criteria for MEPs include a complete loss of signals, percentage loss of amplitude signals, or a change in threshold parameters for obtaining a response.

Advantages and Disadvantages of Intraoperative Motor Evoked Potentials

Motor pathway monitoring measures pyramidal tract function and is theoretically more advantageous than monitoring somatosensory pathways, as paraplegia is the most devastating neurological complication during spinal surgery. This can be especially useful for anterior spinal artery ischemia, since only the anterior portion of the cord is injured and SSEP recordings do not assess corticospinal pathways.

There are many potential complications to using MEPs during spinal surgery, such as kindling, seizures, stimulation-induced bite injuries resulting from patient movement (eg, jaw fractures), and epidural complications. There have been case reports of several of these complications; however, they are rare (40).

The theory of kindling, increasing the incidence of precipitating a seizure, has not been shown in patients selected without a prior history of seizures (39,40). As a precaution when using multipulse or trains of stimuli, some groups have advocated the use of a time interval between trains in their protocols (eg, 30 seconds, 1 minute, 5 seconds) (39,41,42).

Seizures are rare with low-frequency (<0.5 Hz) pulses or brief (<0.03 second) high-frequency pulse trains. A recent study evaluated several different publications involving 2,915 anesthetized patients without a history of seizures, in which no seizures were reported in 1,201 patients undergoing low-frequency single-pulse or 1,714 undergoing brief high-frequency pulse train (43).

Tongue laceration and bites are the most common adverse events that occur with MEP monitoring, occurring due to forceful contractions of facial muscles during MEP stimulation. An MEP stimulator device manufacturer, Digitimer Ltd., identified 27 known incidents of tongue or lip laceration in more than 10,000 cases using the Digitimer D185. The company distributes caution labels to its customers and advises the use of soft bite blocks (44). In addition, there was one report of a mandible fracture in a young man undergoing MEP monitoring for laminectomy and laminoplasty where a bite block was not used (45).

Patient movement is another consideration during MEP monitoring due to the stimulus delivered and the subsequent muscle contraction. In order to prevent injuries, the surgeon may need to be forewarned while the stimulus is delivered. This movement, in addition to the anesthetic requirements, necessitates coordination between the intraoperative monitoring team, the anesthesiologist, and the surgeon in order to prevent any adverse outcomes during the surgery. It should be noted that movement is often negligible when using threshold-level transcranial electrical stimulation and a Mayfield head holder (39).

There are several contraindications to performing transcranial electric MEP, including patients with a history of seizures or a lowered seizure threshold, skull defects, head injury, or implanted mechanical or electrical devices (eg, pacemakers, vascular clips, bullet fragments, bone plates, cochlear implants, or deep brain stimulators).

In spite of the possible adverse effects mentioned, it should be noted that there are few occurrences of published adverse events (43). At this time, with the current data available, the benefit of preventing neurological complications outweighs the minimal risk encountered during MEP monitoring. MEP monitoring is safe and effective when performed by an experienced neurophysiologist with adherence to safety protocols.

INTRAOPERATIVE ELECTROMYOGRAPHY

Introduction and Physiology

The use of continuously running EMG (or free-run EMG) for the detection of neurotonic discharges can be applied to monitoring any nerve in which its corresponding myotome can be accurately accessed. Monitoring and mapping (stimulus evoked EMG) of peripheral nerves for cervical and lumbar spine surgeries, as well as monitoring of the motor portions of cranial nerves, are examples of important applications of intraoperative EMG. Mapping of peripheral nerves is an important aid, especially when dealing with tumors involving the brachial plexus and cauda equina (46,47).

Free-run EMG evaluates interference patterns that are seen as motor unit potential firing at rates of 30–100 Hz (48). This type of firing is termed a neurotonic discharge when it relates to the irritation of a motor axon. Furthermore, the presence of a neurotonic discharge is subdivided into "bursts" and "trains." Neurotonic discharges may be elicited by tactile stimulation, thermal activity, or mechanical traction of the nerve and axon. When this type of activity is self-limited and associated with a specific surgical maneuver, it is considered benign and simply a warning sign. However, when the discharges are seen in trains and persist after surgical manipulation, they are considered pathological and may be associated with a postoperative deficit.

It should be noted that monitoring only free-run EMG is not sufficient to determine nerve/nerve root integrity, as there can be false-positives and false-negatives (49). Axonal integrity can be tested by stimulating a nerve in the surgical field and recording a CMAP from one or more distal muscles that the nerve innervates. This allows the surgeon to distinguish tumor from nerve and to assess the integrity of the nerve. Recordings are made using surface or, more often, intramuscular needle electrodes. Stimulation is performed using either a handheld monopolar or bipolar stimulator. The use of a rectangular pulse of approximately 100 μsec in duration from either a constant voltage or constant current stimulator is routinely used (2,50).

Cranial Nerve EMG

Multimodality recording allows the clinical neurophysiologist to continuously monitor several cranial nerves simultaneously.

Prior to the introduction of facial nerve IONM, there was a significant percentage of patients who developed postoperative facial nerve paresis or palsy, especially for large tumors in the cerebellopontine angle. The use of free-run EMG, in addition to recording a CMAP, has increased facial nerve preservation during cerebellopontine angle surgery over the last decade (12,51–53). Recordings are usually made by selecting muscles from different branches of the facial nerve (eg, orbicularis oculi, orbicularis oris) and using a bipolar montage. Stimulating the intracranial portion of the nerve at risk at regular intervals during the surgical dissection gives an accurate picture of functional loss that may occur (48). A stimulation threshold of 0.05–0.1 mA has been correlated with good prognosis for facial function postoperatively (Fig. 53.5) (1,53).

Monitoring of the lower cranial nerves (IX, X, XII) has not been studied as rigorously as facial nerve IONM. However, several reports suggest that this type of monitoring is useful, especially when dealing with surgeries at the skull base, including the jugular foramen, the foramen magnum, and the petroclival region (54,55). The glossopharyngeal nerve can be monitored by placing bipolar needle electrodes into the lateral aspect of the soft palate ipsilateral to the tumor (or the operative side). The vagus nerve can be monitored

indirectly using a special endotracheal tube, with bipolar surface electrodes exposed at the level of the vocal cords. The vagus nerve can also be directly monitored by placing bipolar needle electrodes into the vocalis muscle, but this technique may be associated with vocal cord edema secondary to trauma. The spinal accessory nerve is most commonly monitored via bipolar needle electrodes in the trapezius muscle. Lastly, the hypoglossal nerve can be monitored by placing bipolar needle electrodes in the lateral aspect of the tongue (genioglossus muscle) (49).

EMG for Head and Neck Surgery

A brief mention should be made regarding the monitoring of the extracranial portion of the facial nerve and the recurrent laryngeal nerve. The extracranial portions of cranial nerves VII and X (recurrent laryngeal nerve) are at risk during resection of tumors involving the parotid, thyroid, and parathyroid glands. There were two large uncontrolled studies of resection of recurrent parotid tumors and IONM of the facial nerve. A 0%–4% risk of permanent facial paralysis was reported

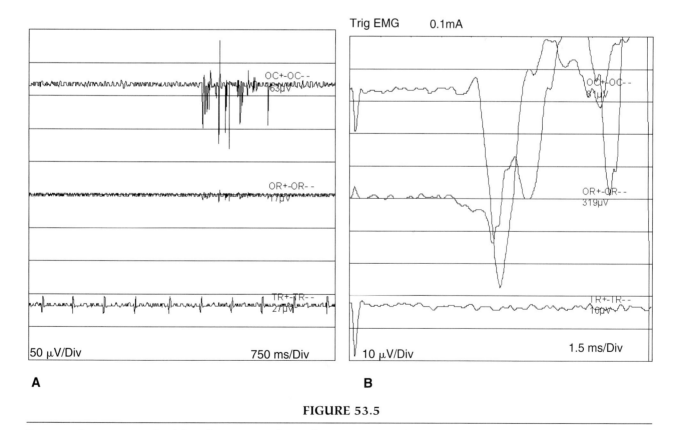

A

B

FIGURE 53.5

Free-run electromyography (A) and a compound muscle action potential (B) in the orbicularis oculi and orbicularis oris muscles supplied by the seventh cranial nerve during resection for a cerebellopontine angle tumor. The trapezius is used as a control. Note that in (A) there is a burst of neurotonic activity in the orbicularis oculi muscle. *Abbreviations*: OC, orbicularis oculi; OR, orbicularis oris; TR, trapezius.

(56,57). While this type of monitoring helps distinguish facial nerve from fibrous tissue, it has not been proven to reduce postoperative damage, and larger controlled studies are needed. Monitoring of the recurrent laryngeal nerve has been shown to be useful; however, there is a dearth of evidence regarding the prognostic or predictive value of this technique (58).

Peripheral Nerve EMG

Free-run EMG, as well as stimulus evoked or triggered EMG, are helpful with pedicle screw placement with spinal instrumentation as well as tethered cord release surgeries (59). Drilling may perforate the cortical bone, exposing or impinging on nerve roots, resulting in pain and radiculopathy. Perforation causes a low impedance to nerve root stimulation, resulting in a lower current intensity required to depolarize the nerve root to generate a CMAP. Hole and screw thresholds are measured, and average values may vary from center to center. At Johns Hopkins Medical Center, for example, using a monopolar stimulator with a constant current pulse of 0.2 ms duration, hole thresholds over 7 mA, and screw thresholds greater than 10 mA, was likely to rule out perforation and suggest that the screw is placed entirely in the pedicle (60). Other centers also use a stimulus threshold of 10 mA (hole and screw) to warn the surgeon of a possible nerve root injury and the need for possible corrective measures. However, chronically compressed nerve roots may require higher stimulus thresholds (up to 20 mA) and, therefore, these cases should use the nerve itself as a control (61). The utility of pedicle screw stimulation is seen in comparative computed tomography (CT) studies of pedicle screw placement, with and without stimulation, where the use of intraoperative stimulation was 93%–98% sensitive, whereas intraoperative radiographic guidance only provided 63%–83% sensitivity (62–64).

Several disadvantages of EMG are that preexisting nerve injury may not make EMG monitoring useful and motor nerve transection may mimic a burst of polyphasic activity then silence (65). In addition, ischemic nerve injury would theoretically not be evident, as with conduction block. It must be understood that continuous EMG monitoring is not monitoring the functional integrity of a pathway, but rather it is the observation of random injury-evoked activity. Lastly, the absence of said activity may not necessarily indicate the absence of injury (59).

Warning Criteria

Warning signs for possible injury to nerve axons are in the form of neurotonic discharges. At any point in the surgical procedure, a neurotonic discharge should be relayed to the surgeons so that they may evaluate

location of neural structures. If this is unclear, a CMAP should be obtained to confirm the presence or absence of a nerve or to differentiate surrounding tissue from neural structures (66–68).

SOMATOSENSORY EVOKED POTENTIAL PHASE-REVERSAL IDENTIFICATION, ELECTROCORTICOGRAPHY, AND CORTICAL STIMULATION

During intracranial surgery for brain tumors and epilepsy, several neurophysiologic techniques have been developed and refined to identify anatomical cortical areas, such as the central sulcus, the primary motor and sensory areas, and the areas related to language (frontal and temporal) (69–76). SSEP phase-reversal identification, electrocorticography (ECoG), and cortical stimulation can assist in defining cortical anatomical areas, determining epileptogenic areas, and guiding the limits of lesion resection and the completeness of the excision.

Somatosensory Evoked Potential Phase-Reversal Identification

Median nerve SSEPs are used for localizing the central sulcus by identifying the primary motor and sensory area transition (69,70). The contralateral median nerve is stimulated and a median SSEP recorded from the primary sensory cortex (Fig. 53.2). A subdural strip electrode is placed so that contacts are located anterior and posterior to the central sulcus (or proposed location of the central sulcus). A mirror-image waveform can be elicited on the motor cortex region. The electrode contact or contacts in which the polarity inversion (phase reversal) of the waveform occurs identifies the central sulcus region (Fig. 53.6). Although this technique is useful in identifying the central sulcus, it fails to localize descending subcortical motor and sensory white matter tracts, thus requiring the adjunctive use of cortical stimulation with ECoG.

Electrocorticography

Electrocorticography is used to monitor brain electrical activity recorded over the brain cortex, just as electroencephalography (EEG) is used to monitor brain activity recorded over the cranium. Over the past 50 years, ECoG has been used in epilepsy surgery to define epileptogenic areas of the brain prior to resection of an epileptogenic focus (77). A recording subdural electrode strip or grid is placed directly on the brain and referenced to an electrode placed in the proximity of the recording (referential recording). Bipolar recording may also be performed. Baseline ECoG is recorded, with notation made regarding any areas of intrinsic

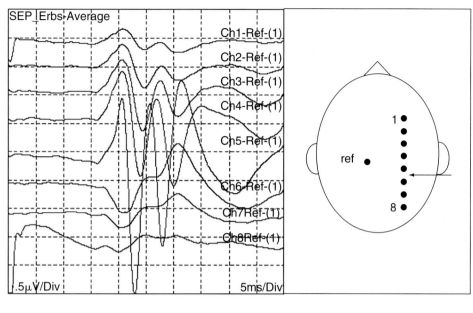

FIGURE 53.6

Median SSEP to identify sensorimotor cortex and identification of central sulcus. Note the phase reversal between contacts 5 and 6.

cortical dysfunction (Fig. 53.7). ECoG is also useful in the detection of the afterdischarge threshold to establish adequate stimulation intensities for functional mapping in brain tumor or epilepsy surgery, as described next.

Cortical Stimulation

Cortical stimulation in conjunction with ECoG can help to localize motor and language areas prior to lesion resection, particularly in eloquent cortex and along subcortical motor pathways.

With cortical stimulation, a handheld bipolar stimulator is used by the surgeon in conjunction with a constant current stimulator device generating biphasic square wave pulses at a rate of 60 Hz, a pulse duration of 0.5–1.5 ms, with varying intensities recorded in milliamperes (mA) (78,79). Cortical stimulation thresholds may vary according to the anesthetic condition of the patient, with lower currents needed under "awake" conditions (80).

Typically, the patient is kept awake during language mapping and asleep during motor mapping. The presence of positive (eg, speech preservation, hand flexion) or negative responses (eg, speech arrest) are recorded. Not only can motor responses be visually observed, but sensitivity also is increased with the use of electromyographic recordings of representative muscle groups, oftentimes requiring lower stimulation intensities (81).

Simultaneous observation of the ECoG defines any areas of change in baseline ECoG, such as after-

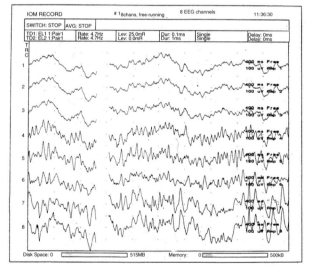

FIGURE 53.7

Baseline normal electrocorticography.

discharges or electrographic seizure activity (Fig. 53.8). Afterdischarges are waveform morphologies that differ from the baseline ECoG that exhibit variable morphology and often appear repetitive (77). After discharges may also appear as single spikes or sharp waves and suggest areas of cortical dysfunction or an electrographic ictal focus (77). Ice-cold lactated Ringer's solution should be available and applied to the cortex if seizure activity develops. This has been demonstrated

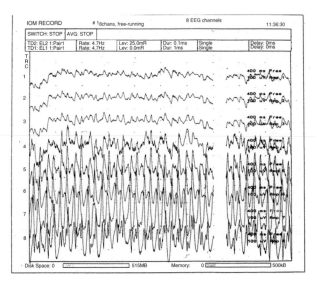

FIGURE 53.8

Electrocorticography with ictal activity.

to rapidly abort focal seizure activity during cortical stimulation (71).

Because functional motor, sensory, or language tissue may reside within macroscopically identified tumor tissue and surrounding infiltrated brain, phase-reversal identification, cortical stimulation, and ECoG aid to map functional cortex in order to diminish neurological deficit while maximizing lesion resection (82).

ANESTHESIA AND IONM

Electromyography

Neuromuscular blockade should be minimized during EMG and for the purpose of recording motor nerve conductions. It has been shown that neuromuscular blockade less than 80% reliably produces nerve root thresholds that are similar to thresholds without blockade (44). Partial neuromuscular blockade can be used, but with continuous titration in order to assess muscle twitch. The amplitude of a single twitch response maintained at 20%–50% of baseline using a closed-loop infusion system facilitates a level of neuromuscular blockade that allows adequate operating conditions during spinal surgery, yet maintains sufficient CMAP amplitude at a peripheral muscle (eg, tibialis anterior) (38,83). In general, the omission of neuromuscular blockade during the intraoperative period where EMG is being monitored is preferred.

Evoked Potentials (SSEPs and MEPs)

Anesthetic effects accounted for many poor recordings in the past, but improved anesthetic regimens and increased communication between the anesthesiologist and the neurophysiologist have established adequate protocols to optimize intraoperative recordings.

Halogenated agents, such as isoflurane, enflurane, desflurane, and sevoflurane, can produce a dose-related increase in latency and a reduction in amplitude of cortically recorded potentials (SSEPs) (84). Most protocols suggest 0.5% minimal alveolar concentrations of halogenated agents for optimal SSEPs. MEPs appear to be most easily abolished by halogenated agents (85).

Other agents that have been shown to reduce or abolish MEP amplitudes are propofol combined with nitrous oxide, especially at levels above 50% for nitrous oxide (86). Combinations of nitrous oxide and other inhalational anesthetic agents may also produce synergistic amplitude attenuation of the SSEP than either agent alone (18).

Total intravenous anesthesia has been shown to be optimal for recording SSEPs and MEPs. Combinations including intravenous opioids (eg, alfentanil, fentanyl, remifentanil), intravenous sedatives (eg, benzodiazepines, etomidate), and ketamine have been shown to be effective in obtaining and maintaining responses intraoperatively (87).

Propofol continues to be used in combination with opioid anesthetics because its rapid metabolism allows for rapid titration to control depth of anesthesia (88). Continuous infusions of propofol (nonbolused) do not have a profound effect on SSEPs (84).

CONCLUSION

Intraoperative neurophysiological testing is an important tool for decision making and outcome prediction in surgeries in which the integrity of the nervous system is at risk. It has become the standard of care for many surgical procedures, including spine and skull base tumor surgery. Since its inception more than years ago, intraoperative neurophysiologic monitoring has become an indispensable tool to combat the risk of iatrogenic insult to the central nervous system. During the surgical procedure, the intraoperative monitoring team must identify waveforms and label pertinent peaks, evaluate amplitude and latency calculations, review change in waveform morphology, and give feedback to the surgeon. There is great utility in electrophysiological monitoring, and many of its applications are appropriate for surgery in which neural structures are at risk.

References

1. Grundy BL. Intraoperative monitoring of sensory evoked potentials. *Anesthesiol.* 1983;58:72–87.
2. Moller A. *Intraoperative Neurophysiologic Monitoring*, 1st ed. Luxembourg: Harwood Academic Publishers GmbH; 1995.

3. Gasser T, Ganslandt O, Sandalcioglu E, Stolke D, Fahlbusch R, Nimsky C. Intraoperative functional MRI: implementation and preliminary experience. *Neuroimag.* 2005;26:685–693.

4. Romstock J, Strauss C, Fahlbusch R. Continuous electromyography monitoring of motor cranial nerves during cerebellopontine angle surgery. *J Neurosurg.* 2000;93:586–593.

5. Moller A, Jannetta P. Monitoring auditory nerve potentials during operations in the cerebellopontine angle. *Otolaryngol Head Neck Surg.* 1985;92:434–439.

6. Glassock III ME, Hays JW, Minor LB, Haynes DS, Carrasco VN. Preservation of hearing in surgery for acoustic neuromas. *J Neurosurg.* 1993;78:864–870.

7. Grundy BL, Janetta PJ, Procopio PT, Lina A, Boston R, Doyle E. Intraoperative monitoring of brainstem auditory evoked potentials. *J Neurosurg.* 1982;57:674–681.

8. Nuwer MR, Dawson EG, Carlson LG, Kanim LE, Sherman JE. Somatosensory evoked potential spinal cord monitoring reduces neurologic deficits after scoliosis surgery: results of a large multicenter survey. *Electroencephalogr Clin Neurophysiol.* 1995;96:6–11.

9. Deletis V, Sala F. Intraoperative neurophysiological monitoring during spine surgery: an update. *Curr Opin Ortho.* 2004;15:154–158.

10. Hilibrand AS, Schwartz DM, Sethuraman V, Vaccaro AR, Albert TJ. Comparison of transcranial electric motor and somatosensory evoked potential monitoring during cervical spine surgery. *J Bone Joint Surg Am.* 2004;86(6):1248–1253.

11. Sala F, Lanteri P, Bricolo A. Motor evoked potential monitoring for spinal cord and brain stem surgery. *Adv Tech Stand Neurosurg.* 2004;29:133–169.

12. Harner SG, Daube JR, Ebersold MJ, Beatty CW. Improved preservation of facial nerve function with the use of electrical monitoring during removal of acoustic neuromas. *Mayo Clin Proc.* 1987;69:92–102.

13. Radtke RA, Erwin CW, Wilkins RH. Intraoperative brainstem auditory evoked potentials: significant decrease in postoperative morbidity. *Neurology.* 1989;39:187–191.

14. Raudzens PA, Shetter AG. Intraoperative monitoring of brainstem auditory evoked potentials. *J Neurosurg.* 1982;57:341–348.

15. Watanabe E, Schramm J, Strauss C, Fahlbusch R. Neurophysiologic monitoring in posterior fossa surgery. II. BAEPwaves I and V and preservation of hearing. *Acta Neurochir.* 1989;98:118–128.

16. James ML, Husain AM. Brainstem auditory evoked potential monitoring: when is a change in wave V significant? *Neurology.* 2005;65:1551–1555.

17. Legatt A. Mechanisms of intraoperative brainstem auditory evoked potential changes. *J Clin Neurophysiol.* 2002;19(5):396–408.

18. Sloan TB, Rogers J, Rogers J, Sloan H. MAC fractions of nitrous oxide and isoflurane are not electrophysiologically additive in the ketamine anesthetized baboon. *J Neurosurg Anesth.* 1995;7:314.

19. Stockard JJ, Sharbrough F, Tinker J. Effects of hypothermia on the human brainstem auditory response. *Ann Neurol.* 1978;3:368–370.

20. Nash CL Jr, Lorig RA, Schatzinger LA, Brown RH. Spinal cord monitoring during operative treatment of the spine. *Clin Orthop Relat Res.* 1977;126:100–105.

21. Toleikis, JR. ASNM, position statement, intraoperative monitoring using somatosensony evoked potentials. [Journal of Clinical Monitoring and Computing. *ASNM, Position Statement, Intraoperative Monitoring Using Somatosensory Evoked Potentials.* June 2005;19(3): 241–258.

22. Nuwer MR. Spinal cord monitoring. *Muscle Nerve.* 1999;22:1620–1630.

23. Padberg A, Bridwell K. Spinal cord monitoring. *Orthoped Clin N Am.* 1999;30:407–433.

24. Owen JH, Bridwell KH, Grubb R, et al. The clinical application of neurogenic motor evoked potentials to monitor spinal cord function during surgery. *Spine.* 1991;16:S385–S390.

25. Schwartz DM, Sestokas AK, Turner LA. Neurophysiological identification of iatrogenic neural injury during complex spinal surgery. *Semin Spine Surg.* 1998;10:242–251.

26. MacDonald D, Zayed Z, Khoudeir I, Stigsby B. Monitoring scoliosis surgery with combined multiple pulse transcranial electric motor and cortical somatosensory-evoked potentials from the lower and upper extremities. *Spine.* 2003;28:194–203.

27. Seyal M, Mull B. Mechanisms of signal change during intraoperative somatosensory evoked potential monitoring of the spinal cord. *J Clin Neurophysiol.* 2002;19:409–415.

28. Wiedemayer H, Fauser B, Sandalcioglu IE, Schafer H, Stolke D. The impact of neurophysiological intraoperative monitoring on surgical decisions: a critical analysis of 423 cases. *J Neurosurg.* 2002;96:255–262.

29. Pelosi L, Lamb J, Grevitt M, Mehdian SM, Webb JK, Blumhardt LD. Combined monitoring of motor and somatosensory evoked potentials in orthopaedic spinal surgery. *Clin Neurophysiol.* 2002;113:1082–1091.

30. Vauzelle C, Stagnara P, Jouvinroux P. Functional monitoring of spinal cord activity during spinal surgery. *Clin Orthop Relat Res.* 1973;93:173–178.

31. Epstein NE. Intraoperative evoked potential monitoring. In: Benzel EC, ed. *Spine Surgery: Techniques, Complication Avoidance and Management.* New York: Churchill Livingstone; 1999:1249–1257.

32. Levy W, York D, McCaffrey M, Tanzer F. Motor evoked potentials form transcranial stimulation of the motor cortex in humans. *Neurosurgery.* 1984;15:287–302.

33. Daube J. *Clinical Neurophysiology,* 2nd ed. New York: Oxford University Press; 2002.

34. Barker AT, Jalinous R, Freeston IL. Non-invasive magnetic stimulation of human motor cortex. *Lancet.* 1985;1:1106–1107.

35. Gugino LD, Aglio LS, Seyal ME, et al. Use of transcranial magnetic stimulation for monitoring spinal cord motor pathways. *Semin Spine Surg.* 1997;9:315–336.

36. Morota N, Deletis V, Constantini S, Kofler M, Cohen H, Epstein F. The role of motor evoked potentials during surgery for intramedullary spinal cord tumors. *Neurosurgery.* 1997;41:1327–1336.

37. Burke D, Hicks R, Stephen J, Woodforth I, Crawford M. Trial-to-trial variability of corticospinal volleys in human subjects. *Electroenc Clin Neurophys.* 1995;97:231–237.

38. Lang EW, Beutler AS, Chesnut RM, et al. Myogenic motorevoked potential monitoring using partial neuromuscular blockade in surgery of the spine. *Spine.* 1996;21:1676–1686.

39. Calancie B, Harris W, Broton J, Alexeeva N, Green B. "Threshold-level" multipulse transcranial electrical stimulation of motor cortex for intraoperative monitoring of spinal motor tracts: description of method and comparison to somatosensory evoked potential monitoring. *J Neurosurg.* 1998;88: 457–470.

40. Isley M, Balzer J, Pearlman R, et al. Intraoperative motor evoked potentials. *Am J END Technol.* 2001;41:266–338.

41. Jones SJ, Harrison R, Koh KF, Mendoza N, Crockard HA. Motor evoked potential monitoring during spinal surgery: responses of distal limb muscles to transcranial cortical stimulation with pulse trains. *Electroencep Clin Neurophy.* 1996;100:375–383.

42. Ubags L, Kalkman C, Been H, Drummond J. The use of a circumferential cathode improves amplitude of intraoperative electrical transcranial myogenic motor evoked responses. *Anesth Analg.* 1996;82:1011–1014.

43. MacDonald D. Safety of intraoperative transcranial electrical stimulation motor evoked potential monitoring. *J Clin Neurophys.* 2002;19:416–429.

44. *Digitimer Ltd Multipulse Stimulator Model D185 Operator's Manual.* Welwyn Garden City, UK: Digitimer Ltd.; 2002.

45. Calancie B, Harris W, Brindle, F, Green B, Landy H. Threshold-level repetitive transcranial electrical stimulation for intraoperative monitoring of central motor conduction. *J Neurosurg (Spine 1).* 2001;95:161–168.

46. Kothbauer K, Schmid U, Seiler RW, Eisner W. Intraoperative motor and sensory monitoring of the cauda equina. *Neurosurgery.* 1994;34:702–707.

47. Legatt AD, Schroeder CE, Gill B, Goodrich JT. Electrical stimulation and multichannel EMG recording for identification of

functional neural tissue during cauda equina surgery. *Childs Nerv Syst.* 1992;8:185–189.

48. Harper CM. Intraoperative cranial nerve monitoring. *Muscle Nerve.* 2004;29:339–351.

49. Schlake H, Goldbrunner RH, Milewski C, et al. Intra-operative electromyographic monitoring of the lower cranial motor nerves (LCN IX-XII) in skull base surgery. *Clin Neur Neurosurg.* 2001;103:72–82.

50. Chiappa K. *Evoked Potentials in Clinical Medicine.* Lippincott-Raven; Philadelphia. 1997.

51. Esses BA, LaRouere MJ, Graham MD. Facial nerve outcome in acoustic tumor surgery. *Am J Otol.* 1994;15:810–812.

52. Grey PL, Moffat DA, Palmer CR, Hardy DG, Baguley DM. Factors which influence the facial nerve outcome in vestibular schwannoma surgery. *Clin Otolaryngol.* 1996;21:409–413.

53. Selesnick SH, Carew JF, Victor JD, Heise CW, Levine J. Predictive value of facial nerve electrophysiologic stimulation thresholds in cerebellopontine-angle surgery. *Laryngoscope.* 1996;106:633–638.

54. Schlake H, Goldbrunner R, Milewski C, et al. Technical developments in intraoperative monitoring for the preservation of cranial motor nerves and hearing in skull base surgery. *Neuro Res.* 1999;21:11–24.

55. Mann WJ, Maurer J, Marangos N. Neural conservation in skull base surgery. *Otolaryngol Clin N Am.* 2002;35:411–424.

56. Brennan J, Moore EJ, Shuler KJ. Prospective analysis of the efficacy of continuous intraoperative nerve monitoring during thyroidectomy, parathyroidectomy, and parotidectomy. *Otolaryngol Head Neck Surg.* 2001;124:537–543.

57. Dulguerov P, Marchal F, Lehmann W. Post-parotidectomy Facial nerve paralysis: Possible etiologic factors and results with routine facial nerve monitoring. *Laryngoscope.* 1999;109:754–762.

58. Snyder SK, Hendricks JC. Intraoperative neurophysiology testing of the recurrent laryngeal nerve: plaudits and pitfalls. *Surgery.* 2005;138:1183–1191; discussion 1191–1192.

59. Kothbauer K, Novak K. Intraoperative monitoring for tethered cord surgery: an update. *Neurosurg Focus.* 2004;16:1–5.

60. Minahan RE, Riley LH 3rd, Lukaczyk T, Cohen DB, Kostuik JP. The effect of neuromuscular blockade on pedicle screw stimulation thresholds. *Spine.* 2000;25:2526–2530.

61. Holland N. Intraoperative electromyography during thoracolumbar spinal surgery. *Spine.* 1998;23:1915–1922.

62. Glassman S, Dimar J, Puno R, Johnson JR, Shields CB, Linden RD. A prospective analysis of intraoperative electromyographic monitoring of pedicle screw placement with computed tomographic scan confirmation. *Spine.* 1995;20:1375–1379.

63. Maguire J, Wallace S, Madiga R, Leppanen R, Draper V. Evaluation of intrapedicular screw position using intraoperative evoked electromyography. *Spine.* 1995;20:1068–1074.

64. Ferrick M, Kowalski J, Simmons E. Reliability of roentgenogram evaluation of pedicle screw position. *Spine.* 1997;22:1249–1253.

65. Nelson KR, Vasconez HC. Nerve transection without neurotonic discharges during intraoperative electromyographic monitoring. *Muscle Nerve.* 1995;18:236–238.

66. Nakao Y, Piccirillo E, Falconi M, Taibah A, Kobayashi T, Sanna M. Electromyographic evaluation of facial nerve damage in acoustic neuroma surgery. *Otol Neurootol.* 2001;22:554–557.

67. Grayeli AB, Kalamarides M, Fraysse B, et al. Comparison between intraoperative observations and electromyographic monitoring data for facial nerve outcome after vestibular schwannoma surgery. *Acta Oto-Laryng.* 2005;125:1069–1074.

68. Isaacson B, Kileny PR, El-Kashlan H. Intraoperative monitoring and facial nerve outcomes after vestibular schwannoma resection. *Otol Neurootol.* 2003;24:812–817.

69. Wood CC, Spencer DD, Allison T, McCarthy G, Williamson PD, Goff WR. Localization of human sensorimotor cortex during surgery by cortical surface recording of somatosensory evoked potentials. *J Neurosurg.* 1988;68:99–111.

70. Cedzich C, Taniguchi M, Schafer S, Schramm J. Somatosensory evoked potential phase reversal and direct motor cortex stimulation during surgery in and around the central region. *Neurosurgery.* 1996;38:962–970.

71. Sartorius CJ, Berger MS. Rapid termination of intraoperative stimulation-evoked seizures with application of cold Ringer's lactate to the cortex. Technical note. *J Neurosurg.* 1998;88:349–351.

72. Kombos T, Suess O, Funk T, Kern BC, Brock M. Intra-operative mapping of the motor cortex during surgery in and around the motor cortex. *Acta Neurochir.* 2000;142:263–268.

73. Haglund MM, Berger MS, Shamseldin M, Lettich E, Ojemann GA. Cortical localization of temporal lobe language sites in patients with gliomas. *Neurosurgery.* 1994;34(4):567–576.

74. Herholz H, Reulen HJ, von Stockhausen HM, et al. Preoperative activation and intraoperative stimulation of language-related areas in patients with glioma. *Neurosurgery.* 1997;41:1253–1262.

75. Ojemann G, Ojemann J, Lettich E, Berger M. Cortical language localization in left, dominant hemisphere: an electrical stimulation mapping investigation in 117 patients. *J Neurosurg.* 1989;71:316–326.

76. Sartorius CJ, Wright G. Intraoperative brain mapping in a community setting. Technical considerations. *Surg Neurol.* 1997;47:380–388.

77. Penfield W, Jasper H. *Epilepsy and the Functional Anatomy of the Human Brain.* Boston: Little, Brown; 1954.

78. Berger MS, Ojemann GA. Techniques for functional brain mapping during glioma surgery. In: Berger MS, Wilson CB, eds. *The Gliomas.* Philadelphia: Saunders; 1999:421–435.

79. Ojemann GA. Intraoperative electrocorticography and functional mapping. In: Wyler AR, Hermann BP, eds. *The Surgical Management of Epilepsy.* Boston: Butterworth-Heineman 1994:189–198.

80. Berger MS. The impact of technical adjuncts in the surgical management of cerebral hemispheric low-grade gliomas of childhood. *J Neurooncol.* 1996;28:129–155.

81. Yingling CD, Ojemann S, Dodson B, Harrington MJ, Berger MS. Identification of motor pathways during tumor surgery facilitated by multichannel electromyographic recording. *J Neurosurg.* 1999;91:922–927.

82. Skirboll SS, Ojemann GA, Berger MS, Lettich E, Winn HR. Functional cortex and subcortical white matter located within gliomas. *Neurosurgery.* 1996;38(4):678–685.

83. Lotto M, Banoub M, Schubert A. Effects of anesthetic and physiologic changes on intraoperative motor evoked potentials. *J Neurosurg Anesthesiol.* 2004;16:32–42.

84. Sloan TB. Anesthetic effects on electrophysiologic recordings. *J Clin Neurophysiol.* 1998;15:217–226.

85. Haghighi SS, Green KD, Oro JJ, Drake RK, Kracke GR. Depressive effect of isoflurane anesthesia on motor evoked potentials. *Neurosurgery.* 1990;26:993–997.

86. Jellinek D, Platt M, Jewkes D, Symon L. Effects of nitrous oxide on motor evoked potentials recorded from skeletal muscle in patients under total anesthesia intravenously administered propofol. *Neurosurgery.* 1991;29:558–562.

87. Sihle-Wissel, M, Scholz, M, Cunitz G. Transcranial magnetic-evoked potentials under total intravenous anesthesia and nitrous oxide. *Br J Anesth.* 2000;85:465–467.

88. Pechstein U, Nadstawek J, Zentner J, Schramm J. Isoflurane plus nitrous oxide versus propofol for recording of motor evoked potentials after high frequency repetitive electrical stimulation. *Electroenc Clin Neurophys.* 1998;108:175–181.

89. Misulis KE, Head TC. *Essentials of Clinical Neurophysiology,* 3rd ed. Elsevier Science (USA); 2003.

90. Spehlmann R. *Evoked Potential Primer.* Boston: Butterworth-Heineman Ltd; Philadelphia. 1985.

VI

MUSCULOSKELETAL COMPLICATIONS OF CANCER

Spine Disorders in Cancer

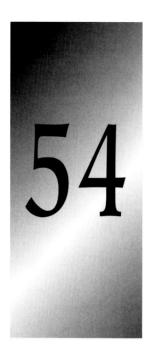

54

Christian M. Custodio
Michael D. Stubblefield

Back pain is a common symptom for both the cancer patient and noncancer patient alike. Up to 25% of the population will have low back pain in any given year, and most people will experience an episode of back pain at some point in their lifetime (1). In most patients, with or without a history of cancer, the underlying cause of spinal pain can be traced to a benign condition. Nonmalignant causes of back pain are much more prevalent than etiologies that are more serious. Back pain is typically caused by degenerative changes or by mild, repetitive trauma. With conservative management, up to 90% of patients with this type of back pain will improve significantly within four weeks (2).

Following degenerative disorders, such as disc disease and spinal stenosis, tumors of the spine, spinal cord, and spinal axis infections are the most common causes of back pain and radiculopathy (3). Although serious causes of back pain, such as malignancy or infection, are generally rare, the clinical impact of these conditions cannot be overstated. In approximately 10% of patients with cancer, symptomatic spinal metastases may be the initial presentation (4). Pain is the most common complaint in the patient with primary or metastatic spine tumors or spinal infections. Back pain is the presenting symptom in 90% of patients with spinal tumors (5). Spinal metastases and associated nerve root and spinal cord compression is a well-recognized

complication of cancer, and can occur in 5%–10% of patients with systemic disease (6).

The spine is the most common skeletal site of metastasis. The malignancies most likely to metastasize to the spine include breast, lung, prostate, colon, thyroid, and renal cancers. Common primary benign spinal tumors include hemangioma, osteoid osteoma, osteoblastoma, osteochondroma, and giant cell tumor. The most common primary malignancies involving the spine are multiple myeloma, Ewing sarcoma, osteosarcoma, chondrosarcoma, and chordoma. Early diagnosis of these conditions is essential in improving morbidity, mortality, and preserving neurologic function. And while survival has improved for many tumor histologies, treatments such as surgery, chemotherapy, and radiation therapy, and their associated complications, can have an additional impact on the functional outcomes of cancer patients with back pain.

EVALUATION

History

A careful and thorough history and physical examination are the cornerstones to determining if a patient's back pain is due to a benign process or a more serious

KEY POINTS

- Back pain is a common symptom in the general population. In most patients, with or without a history of cancer, the underlying cause of spinal pain can be traced to a benign condition.
- Pain is the most common complaint in the patient with metastatic spine disease, primary spine tumors, and spinal infections. Back pain is the initial presenting symptom in 90% of patients with spinal tumors.

- A prior history of cancer has very high specificity, such that these patients who present with back pain should be considered to have recurrence and spinal involvement until proven otherwise.
- Magnetic resonance imaging (MRI) is considered the gold-standard imaging modality in the assessment for neoplastic spinal disease, especially in patients with a history of cancer.

condition. Frequently, a specific cause to a patient's spine pain cannot be identified. Therefore, it is often fruitful to focus the history and physical on determining whether a patient's back pain is due to a systemic condition and whether there is neurologic compromise that would prompt intervention from neurosurgery or radiation oncology.

Nonmalignant back pain is often described as aching in character, waxes and wanes, and is often exacerbated by movements such as lumbar flexion, transitional movements (such as arising from a seated position), lifting, or with maneuvers that increase intradiscal/intra-abdominal pressure, such as coughing, straining, or sneezing. The pain is localized to the back, most commonly at the lumbosacral junction, and does not usually radiate. Weight gain is a common feature of benign back pain due to immobility. The pain is usually alleviated with rest, recumbency, nonsteroidal anti-inflammatory medications, and physical therapy.

Back pain associated with cancer on the other hand, is not relieved with rest or with lying down. The thoracic spine is a more common location for metastases than the lumbosacral spine due to its relative volume. The pain is frequently worse at night, and may awaken the patient from sleep. Increasing pain despite conservative management and any symptoms suggesting a progressive neurologic deficit warrant further prompt diagnostic investigation. Other important historical factors in the evaluation of the malignant spine are patient age and a prior or current history of cancer. A prior history of cancer has very high specificity, such that these patients with back pain should be considered to have recurrence and spinal involvement until proven otherwise (7). Metastases to the spine and multiple myeloma have their peak incidence in the fifth and sixth decades (3). A history of fevers, chills, weight loss, and night sweats should raise concern for a possible abscess or spinal infection in addition to the presence of malignancy. The pain associated with diskitis/osteomyelitis of the spine is often severe and debilitating. Infection should also be suspected in patients who are

immunocompromised or have a recent history of spinal procedures. A history of changes in bowel, bladder, or sexual function should be elicited.

Physical Examination

The physical examination should focus on the spine and neurologic system. Inspection may reveal a kyphosis or scoliosis related to compression fracture. Range of motion may be limited secondary to pain. Palpation of the spine can sometimes reveal a mass. Vertebral tenderness to percussion is surprisingly absent in 70% of patients with a spinal tumor (5).

The pain associated with metastatic spine disease can present in a number of ways. Correct classification of pain has both prognostic and therapeutic implications in regards to treatment choices, including medications, injections, etc. Pain can be described as either nociceptive or non-nociceptive. Nociceptive pain results from noxious stimulation and activation of nociceptors, mediated by A-delta and unmyelinated-C nerve fibers. Spinal nociceptive somatic pain originates from nociceptor stimulation from somatic tissues in the spinal column, such as bone, joint, discs or ligaments, or muscle. Nociceptive visceral pain originates from a visceral organ, and can sometimes refer to the back. Examples of nociceptive visceral pain resulting in back pain include pain related to pelvic disorders (prostatitis, endometriosis), renal disorders (nephrolithiasis, pyelonephritis), vascular disorders (abdominal aortic aneurysm), or gastrointestinal disorders (pancreatitis, cholecystitis, bowel perforation).

Neuropathic pain can be caused by direct compression of nervous system structures from tumor or degenerative changes, fibrosis related to prior surgery or radiation, paraneoplastic effects, or as a complication of neurotoxic chemotherapy (8). Neuropathic pain is usually described as burning, shooting, stabbing, lancinating, or electrical in character. Often, a combination of nociceptive pain and neuropathic pain exists in the same patient.

When evaluating back pain, it is important to recognize that a variety of tissues and structures within the vertebral column can contribute to pain. Pain-sensitive structures within the spinal column include the periosteum, intervertebral discs, ligaments, neural structures, muscles, and fascia. It is also important to note that the marrow of the vertebral body is generally pain-insensitive, so a metastatic or primary lesion confined to the marrow will not generate pain (Fig. 54.1). Approximately 5%–36% of patients with spinal tumors will present without back pain, and in these cases, the tumors are usually confined within the vertebral body marrow (3).

The pattern of back pain in a patient with possible spinal tumors can also help guide diagnosis and treatment. Localized spinal pain is just that—pain that is confined to a specific spinal area or segment affected by tumor. It usually is caused by an expanding tumor, originally confined to the vertebral body marrow, that has begun to infiltrate or irritate the periosteum and initiates a local inflammatory response. This pain usually responds to corticosteroid administration (9) or palliative radiation therapy. Radicular pain may be caused by tumor compression of a spinal nerve root, resulting in neuropathic pain in a dermatomal distribution. The radicular pain may be accompanied by additional neurologic findings of paresthesias, weakness, or muscle stretch reflex changes. Mechanical instability pain results when the spinal motion segment is disrupted. Pain is aggravated with movement and activity, especially with movements resulting in increased axial loading, such as sitting or standing. Mechanical pain is not usually responsive to corticosteroids.

It should be noted that disorders seemingly unrelated to spinal pathology can be directly or indirectly related to it. An example is when damage to the C5 or C6 cervical nerve roots (or upper brachial plexus) causes weakness of the rotator cuff musculature and referred pain to the lateral shoulder and arm. If rotator cuff weakness perturbs shoulder motion and allows for anterior translation of the humerus within the glenoid fossa, then impingement of the rotator cuff tendons may develop with subsequent rotator cuff tendonitis, adhesive capsulitis, and pain. This may be important clinically, as it is often shoulder dysfunction and not spinal pathology that limits rehabilitation efforts in patients with spinal malignancy.

A thorough neurologic examination is paramount in the evaluation of back pain in the cancer patient because of concerns regarding possible epidural spinal cord compression or nerve root compression. Physicians must be aware of the usual progression of epidural spinal cord compression. Patients will initially present with back pain, followed by radicular pain, lower extremity weakness, sensory loss, and finally, loss of sphincter control (10). Early recognition of cord compression allows for prompt intervention and improved prognosis for restoration or preservation of function.

The second most common presenting complaint of patients with spinal metastases is weakness. It is estimated that 60%–85% of these patients are weak on initial presentation (11). Patients whose weakness is caused by radiculopathy will present with weakness within a myotomal distribution. Those whose weakness is caused by compressive myelopathy will present with an upper motor neuron pattern of weakness. Often, a combination of radiculopathy and myelopathy is present and may involve multiple levels (Fig. 54.2). Among those patients with epidural spinal cord compression, those who present with severe deficits or rapid progression of deficits have a much poorer prognosis for functional recovery. Those who are diagnosed early and retain the ability to ambulate are more likely to remain ambulatory following treatment (12).

Sensory abnormalities typically correlate with the presence of motor abnormalities. Evaluation of the extent and degree of deficits in pain, temperature, light touch, and proprioception modalities should

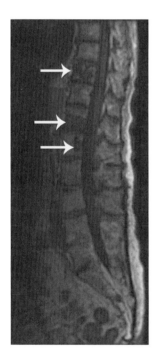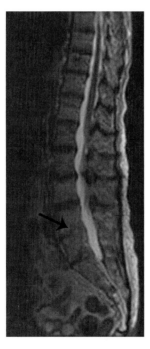

FIGURE 54.1

Sagittal T1 (A) and T2 (B) MRIs demonstrating multiple breast cancer metastases (white arrows) in the thoracic spine. Note the marked degenerative changes and the presence of a partial fusion of the L4–L5 disk space from a prior surgery (black arrow). This patient's metastases are asymptomatic and not contributing to her chronic low back pain and radiculopathy.

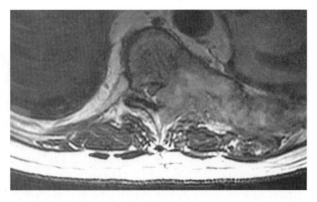

FIGURE 54.2

Axial T2 MRI demonstrating spinal cord and nerve root compression in a patient with metastatic renal cell cancer.

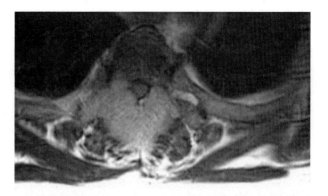

FIGURE 54.3

Axial T2 MRI demonstrating posterior epidural spinal cord compression at the T3 level in a patient with metastatic prostate cancer. This patient suffered from a profound loss of proprioception (likely due to damage to the paired posterior spinal arteries) and marked difficulties with gait despite relatively preserved motor strength.

be undertaken. Assessment of joint position sensory loss is important, since a profound lower extremity proprioceptive loss due to involvement of the dorsal columns of the spinal cord by epidural compression is not uncommon in the cancer setting (Fig. 54.3). Similarly, damage to the ascending spinocerebellar tracts can result in intractable ataxia. Such deficits can be a significant barrier in the successful rehabilitation of cancer patients despite the retention of normal lower extremity strength.

Diagnostic Testing

Diagnostic testing of back pain is performed to identify and/or exclude possibly serious systemic etiologies. Early identification and treatment can prevent or delay complications, such as worsening pain, pathological fracture, weakness, paralysis, or loss of bowel and bladder function. According to Deyo and Diehl, in the primary care patient population, the four clinical findings most likely to predict a cancerous etiology in someone presenting with back pain (assuming no other red flags such as cauda equina syndrome, systemic infection, fracture, etc.) were (1) a prior history of cancer, (2) age of 50 years or older, (3) failure to improve with conservative therapy, and (4) unexplained weight loss of more than 10 pounds in six months (13).

If cancer is suspected in the primary care setting, initial testing should include a complete blood cell count, erythrocyte sedimentation rate (ESR), C-reactive protein level, urinalysis, prostate-specific antigen level, and fecal occult blood testing. Normal results are usually reassuring that the likelihood of an occult malignancy is low. The ESR and C-reactive protein level are generally elevated in the setting of systemic cancer. Although plain x-rays are usually obtained as a first imaging study, spinal tumors are not well visualized on radiographs until significant destruction has occurred (14). X-rays are indicated in the evaluation of patients with spinal hardware, as hardware failure cannot be demonstrated on MRI or computed tomography (CT) (Fig. 54.4).

Nuclear scintigraphy, or bone scanning, is better than plain x-rays at detecting tumors, except for purely lytic lesions, as can be seen in processes like myeloma. Bone scanning, however, has low specificity, as a positive bone scan can be seen in processes like inflammation, infection, or productive osteoarthritis. In addition, the resolution of bone scans is poor, and often a follow-up imaging study, such as CT scanning or MRI, is required to exclude benign processes or to better define the lesion and local anatomy in order to better plan treatment intervention with surgery and/or radiation therapy (15).

MRI is considered the gold-standard imaging modality in the assessment for neoplastic spinal disease (4) MRI best displays the status of the bone marrow and has excellent contrast resolution in soft tissue. Bone marrow infiltrated by tumor demonstrates decreased signal on T1 weighted imaging and high signal on T2 weighted imaging. Enhancement after administration of gadolinium further delineates neoplastic tissue from normal tissue and is important in characterizing and grading tumors (16). CT scans are excellent in defining osseous anatomy, and are best used when a fracture is suspected. When used in conjunction with myelography, it provides an accurate view of compressed neural elements. CT scans are also performed in patients in whom obtaining an MRI is not feasible, such as those with metallic implants or who are claustrophobic.

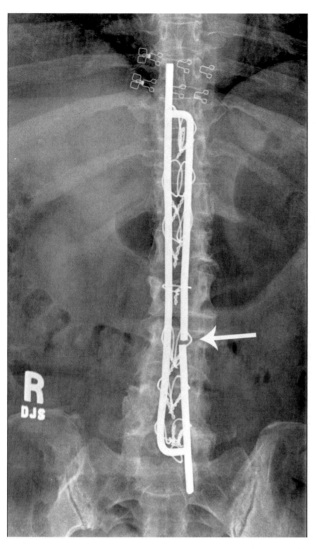

FIGURE 54.4

X-ray demonstrating broken spinal hardware in a patient treated with decompression and stabilization of a papillary thyroid cancer metastasis several years earlier. This patient presented with excruciating back pain due to spinal instability, which resolved completely with surgical repair of the hardware. This defect would not have been readily identified on MRI or CT.

Joines et al. conducted a decision analysis to compare diagnostic strategies, based on the clinical findings described by Deyo and Diehl (17). Eleven diagnostic strategy algorithms were examined, using a combination of clinical findings, ESR, plain spine radiographs, and imaging (bone scan or MRI) +/− percutaneous biopsy. Cost effectiveness was also analyzed, with the understanding that the optimal choice of strategy involves a trade-off between sensitivity, specificity, and cost. The authors found that the most sensitive detection method, as well as the most expensive, is to obtain an MRI for every patient. The most specific strategy was that of obtaining an ESR and x-rays, followed by MRI if both x-rays and ESR were positive. This particular strategy was inexpensive, but demonstrated poor sensitivity. Fewer than 50% of cancer cases were found utilizing this strategy, even with repeat biopsy. The most balanced diagnostic strategy, in their analysis, was to obtain an MRI in patients with a history of cancer or if either the plain x-ray or the ESR were positive.

Diagnostic accuracy and specificity is tremendously important to the successful identification and treatment of pain in patients with spinal malignancies. The importance of a thorough clinical assessment, particularly history and physical examination, cannot be overstated. The clinician should not rely solely on imaging to determine a cause of pain, as it is often misleading. There should be congruence between the patient's history, physical examination, and imaging. For instance, a patient with lateral shoulder pain and epidural tumor at T2 is unlikely to have their shoulder pain relieved by treatment of the tumor, as they are not anatomically congruent and likely unrelated to one another. A patient with epidural disease at C5 and shoulder pain, however, is likely to benefit symptomatically from treatment of the cervical metastases, as the lesion is in exactly the location expected to cause radicular pain to the lateral shoulder and potentially shoulder girdle dysfunction.

ETIOLOGY

A partial list of the numerous noncancerous causes of back pain is listed in Table 54.1. A full discussion of the broad differential diagnosis of nonmalignant spinal and back pain is beyond the scope of this chapter. Nevertheless, it bears repeating that nonmalignant causes of back pain are much more likely to be the source of pain in any given patient, whether or not there is a history of cancer. Although these are not felt to be sinister causes of back pain, an evaluation to exclude neurologic compromise is still indicated in the evaluation of these conditions. A list of neoplastic and more serious systemic causes of spine pain is seen in Table 54.2.

Primary Benign Tumors

Primary benign tumors of the spine include hemangiomas, giant cell tumors, aneurysmal bone cysts, eosinophilic granulomas, osteoblastomas, osteoid osteomas, and osteochondromas. Most are asymptomatic; however, they can be slow-growing and may cause pain if they begin to compress on a pain-sensitive structure. Generally seen in children and young adults, they may cause pain and/or vertebral body collapse in

TABLE 54.1
Differential Diagnosis of Back Pain (Nonmalignant)

Muscle strain
Ligament sprain
Degenerative disease
    Degenerative disc disease
    Degenerative facet arthritis
Failed back syndrome
Fracture
    Traumatic
    Osteoporotic
Spondylolysis (pars interarticularis fracture)
Spondylolisthesis
Spinal stenosis
Scoliosis
Myofascial pain
Fibromyalgia
Visceral pain
    Vascular
    Solid organ
Benign tumors
    Hemangioma
    Osteoblastoma
    Osteoid osteoma
    Osteochondroma
    Giant cell tumor
    Aneurysmal bone cyst
    Eosinophilic granuloma

TABLE 54.2
Differential Diagnosis of Back Pain (Malignant and Systemic Conditions)

Primary spine tumors
    Multiple myeloma/plasmacytoma
    Ewing sarcoma
    Osteogenic sarcoma
    Chordoma
    Lymphoma
Metastatic spine tumors
Radiation-induced spinal tumors (ie, sarcomas)
Infection
    Osteomyelitis
    Discitis
    Epidural/paraspinal abscess
    Tuberculosis
    Herpes zoster
Inflammatory arthritis
    Ankylosing spondylitis
    Psoriatic arthritis
    Reiter syndrome
    Inflammatory bowel disease
Epidural hematoma
Broken spinal instrumentation hardware

some cases (18). Benign lesions are usually observed, unless pain becomes disabling or progressive neurologic deficit is detected. An exception is osteoblastoma, which accounts for 3% of all bone tumors. Pain starts insidiously and progresses due to a relatively more rapid increase in size over time. Osteoblastomas are most likely to be located in the lumbosacral spine and involve the posterior spinal elements. Cord compression is more likely to occur because of its larger size. Radicular pain is present in 33% of patients (19).

Giant cell tumors are most common in the sacrum and represent one-fifth of all benign tumors of bone, 10% of which involve the spine, most commonly the sacrum. They can be locally aggressive, but generally do not metastasize, although malignant transformation has been reported to occur. They often mimic a sacral radiculopathy in presentation (20).

Primary Malignant Tumors

Primary malignant tumors of the spine are less common compared with metastatic disease. The more common primary malignancies include multiple myeloma, Ewing sarcoma, chondrosarcoma, and chordoma. Details regarding multiple myeloma, sarcomas, and primary malignancies that frequently metastasize to bone can be found in their respective chapters. Although rare, it is important to recognize the possibility of a secondary radiation-induced sarcoma within a prior field of radiation to the spine. Overall, mortality is poor, thought to be due to a delay in diagnosis, lack of effective adjuvant treatment, and that these lesions are often large and unresectable (21).

Infection

Spinal infection is a serious condition that commonly presents with back pain. Infections can present indolently or can rapidly progress, resulting in severe vertebral destruction (Fig. 54.5) (22). A high index of suspicion is necessary so as not to overlook a potentially serious infection with possible neurologic deterioration. The difficulty in diagnosis is that often, early infection presents similarly to nonspecific low back pain. Any primary source of infection can lead to a spinal infection, including urinary tract infections, pneumonias, carditis, and cellulitis. *Staphylococcus aureus* is the most common organism identified (23). Patients at increased risk include the elderly, immunocompromised persons, people with diabetes, those who have a history of recent infection, and those who have undergone recent invasive procedures.

Examination early in the presentation can mimic that of idiopathic, focal back pain. As pain progresses, it is exacerbated with movement and weight bearing,

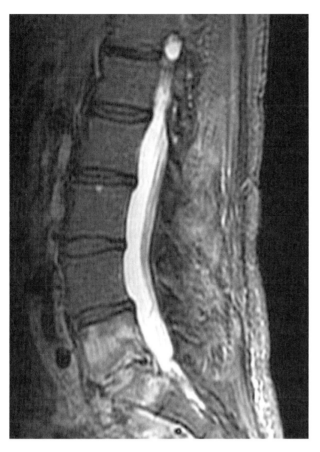

FIGURE 54.5

Sagittal short tau inversion recovery (STIR) MRI demonstrating L5–S1 diskitis/osteomyelitis with bony destruction in a patient with severe lumbar pain and radiculopathy.

and patients often have difficulty finding a comfortable position. There may be pain with vertebral body percussion and overlying muscle spasm and limitation of movement. Fever is only present in approximately one-third of patients (24). Laboratory findings may reveal an elevated ESR, which is the most sensitive test for infection. Forty percent of patients will have a normal white blood cell count (25). MRI can help differentiate between infection and neoplastic disease, although CT scanning may be better at demonstrating the extent of bony involvement. It is important to note that epidural abscess occurs in 10% of spinal infections and that half of the patients are misdiagnosed on their initial evaluation (26). However, primary spinal epidural abscess without a recent history of vertebral osteomyelitis is rare (27).

Fractures

Spinal fractures in the cancer population may be due to malignancy, osteoporosis, trauma, infection, or underlying metabolic disorders. Often, the fractures are asymptomatic. The frail, elderly cancer patient often receives corticosteroids as part of their cancer therapy, and anyone with this profile who presents with back pain should be evaluated for compression fractures (7). There is usually no or minimal history of trauma. If symptomatic, patients present with a stooped, kyphotic posture. Pain is worse with weight bearing, especially with activities that forward-flex the spine, such as sitting or bending. There is usually pain with palpation or percussion over the involved vertebrae. Neurologic testing is usually normal. Plain x-rays may demonstrate loss of vertebral body height and an exaggerated thoracic kyphosis; however, an acute fracture may appear normal on x-rays. An MRI better demonstrates new focal vertebral-body edema in an acute fracture (Fig. 54.6).

SUMMARY

Most cancer and noncancer patients who present to the clinician with back pain will likely have a benign condition causing their symptoms. However, it is important for the physician to be aware and identify spinal conditions that are more serious, including metastatic disease, primary malignancies, serious infections, and

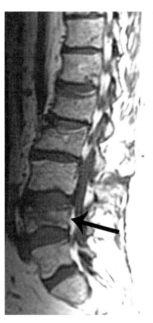 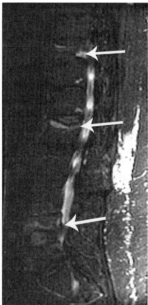

FIGURE 54.6

Sagittal T1 (A) and infrared (B) MRIs demonstrating acute to subacute osteoporotic compression fractures at T10, L1, L2, and L4. The L4 vertebral body is most severely affected (black arrow), with at least 50% loss of vertebral body height centrally. Note also the presence of increased signal on the IR images, suggesting the presence of edema and the acute-to-subacute natures of these fractures.

fractures. A physical examination evaluating for potential neurologic compromise is paramount in early recognition and intervention in order to reduce pain and preserve and restore neurologic function.

References

1. Atlas SJ, Nardin RA. Evaluation and treatment of low back pain: an evidenced-based approach to clinical care. *Muscle Nerve.* 2003;27:265–284.

2. Pengel LH, Herbert RD, Maher CG, Refshauge KM. Acute back pain: systematic review of its prognosis. *BMJ.* 2003;327:323–325.

3. Shelerud RA, Paynter KS. Rarer causes of radiculopathy: spinal tumors, infections, and other unusual causes. *Phys Med Rehabil Clin N Am.* 2002;13:645–696.

4. Sciubba DM, Gokaslan ZL. Diagnosis and management of metastatic spine disease. *Surg Oncol.* 2006;15:141–151.

5. Gilbert RW, Kim JH, Posner JB. Epidural spinal cord compression from metastatic tumor: diagnosis and treatment. *Ann Neurol.* 1978;3:40–51.

6. Plotkin SR, Wen PY. Neurologic complications of cancer therapy. *Neurol Clin.* 2003;21:279–318.

7. Deyo RA, Rainville J, Kent DL. What can the history and physical examination tell us about low back pain? *JAMA.* 1992;268:760–765.

8. Stubblefield MD, Bilsky MH. Barriers to rehabilitation of the neurosurgical spine cancer patient. *J Surg Oncol.* 2007;95:419–426.

9. Gokaslan ZL. Spine surgery for cancer. *Curr Op Oncol.* 1996;8:178–181.

10. O'Connor MI, Currier BL. Metastatic disease of the spine. *Orthop.* 1992;15:611–620.

11. Helweg-Larsen S, Sorensen PS. Symptoms and signs in metastatic spinal cord compression: a study from first symptom until diagnosis in 153 patients. *Europ J Cancer.* 1994;30A:396–398.

12. Portnoy RK, Lipton RB, Foley KM. Back pain in the cancer patient: an algorithm for evaluation and management. *Neurology.* 1987;37:134–138.

13. Deyo RA, Diehl AK. Cancer as a cause of back pain: frequency, clinical presentation, and diagnostic strategies. *J Gen Intern Med.* 1988;3:230–238.

14. Edelstyn GA, Gillespie PJ, Grebbel FS. The radiological demonstration of osseous metastases. Experimental observations. *Clin Radiol.* 1967;18:158–162.

15. Moore KR. Radiology of metastatic spine cancer. *Neurosurg Clin N Am.* 2004;15:381–389.

16. Runge VM, Lee C, Iten AL, Williams NM. Contrast-enhanced magnetic resonance imaging in a spinal epidural tumor model. *Invest Radiol.* 1997;32:589–595.

17. Joines JD, McNutt RA, Carey TS, Deyo RA, Rouhani R. Finding cancer in primary care outpatients with low back pain: a comparison of diagnostic strategies. *J Gen Intern Med.* 2001;16:14–23.

18. Mohan V, Gupta SK, Tuli SM. Symptomatic vertebral hemangiomas. *Clin Radiol.* 1980;31:575–579.

19. Nemoto O, Moser RP, Van Dam BE. Osteoblastoma of the spine: a review of 75 cases. *Spine.* 1990;15:1272–1280.

20. Keplinger JE, Bucy PC. Giant-cell tumors of the spine. *Ann Surg.* 1961;154:648–660.

21. Smith J. Radiation-induced sarcoma of bone: clinical and radiographic findings in 43 patients irradiated for soft-tissue neoplasms. *Clin Radiol.* 1982;33:205–221.

22. Carragee EJ. Pyogenic vertebral osteomyelitis. *J Bone Joint Surg Am.* 1997;79:874–880.

23. Eismont FJ, Bohlman HH, Soni PL. Pyogenic and fungal osteomyelitis with paralysis. *Clin Orthop.* 1991;269:142–150.

24. Malawski SK, Lukawski S. Pyogenic infection of the spine. *Clin Orthop.* 1991;272:58–66.

25. Digby JM, Kersley JB. Pyogenic non-tuberculous spinal infection: an analysis of thirty cases. *J Bone Joint Surg Br.* 1979;61:47–55.

26. Kaufman DM, Kaplan JG, Litman N. Infectious agents in spinal epidural abscesses. *Neurology.* 1980;30:844–850.

27. Siemionow K, Steinmetz M, Bell G, Ilaslan H, McLain RF. Identifying serious causes of back pain: cancer, infection, fracture. *Cleve Clin J Med.* 2008;75:557–565.

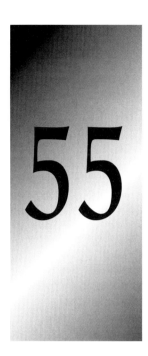

55

Upper Extremity Disorders in Cancer

Justin C. Riutta

Upper extremity pain disorders in the cancer population can be a great source of distress and lead to significant functional impairments. Breast, melanoma, and lung cancer patients are the most frequently affected population with upper extremity pain disorders. In the breast cancer population, seven out of every eight patients will develop a pain syndrome in the upper extremity after diagnosis (1). Pain disorders in the upper extremity may be related directly to malignancy, its treatment, or a variety of unrelated etiologies. One of the major challenges faced by the physiatrist is to determine the cause of upper extremity pain and clarify the interrelationship between benign, malignant, and treatment-related etiologies. The objective of this chapter is to describe the common upper extremity pain disorders most commonly seen in the cancer population. A systemic approach will provide a construct for thorough assessment and accurate diagnosis so that comprehensive and effective treatment geared toward functional restoration can be initiated.

EVALUATION

The evaluation of upper extremity pain disorders includes cancer history, pain history, and functional assessment. The cancer history is imperative in patients with a history of malignancy. It should include date and means of diagnosis. In addition, staging and grade of tumor helps to identify initial prognosis and spread.

The surgical procedures and complications from surgery can identify common postoperative pain processes. Adjuvant treatment, such as chemotherapy, radiation therapy, and hormonal therapy, should be clarified. Details regarding chemotherapeutic agent, dose, and treatment complications can identify risk for neuropathy. Radiation therapy dose and location may help identify risk for lymphedema and plexopathy. Hormonal therapies may be associated with polyarthralgia and myalgia, and may be correlated with onset of these symptoms. Identifying constitutional symptoms as they relate to pain complaints may be a red flag for recurrence. In addition, cancer surveillance should be addressed.

The pain history is obtained to help clarify the pain generator. The onset and location of pain usually begins the interview. Severity, duration, and temporal course help to clarify trends in pain symptoms. Referral patterns and underlying neurological deficits may clarify neurologically mediated pain symptoms. The character of symptoms, including descriptors such as burning, stabbing, aching, lancinating, and throbbing, may help identify the system involved with the pain. Assessing prior workup during history may help with diagnosis and guide further diagnostic testing that may be required. Investigation into prior management trials may help with diagnosis and improve therapeutic efficiency.

The final component of the history is the functional assessment. The importance of the functional assessment

KEY POINTS

- Upper extremity pain disorders in the cancer patient may be caused by the primary malignancy, treatment (including surgery, chemotherapy, and radiation therapy), or benign degenerative causes.
- One of the challenges of the physiatrist is determining whether pain is cancer-related.
- The evaluation of upper extremity pain disorders includes cancer history, pain history, and functional assessment.
- Management of upper extremity pain disorders includes diagnosis, pain control, functional restoration, and return to prior activity.
- While pain may not be seen with all upper extremity bony metastases, when present, the pain is usually localized, severe, insidious, and unremitting.
- Rotator cuff dysfunction is common in cancer patients with chest wall procedures such as breast cancer, melanoma, and post-thoracotomy patients.

- Frozen shoulder is common in the cancer population and is defined as loss of range of motion in all planes, with abduction, forward flexion, and external rotation most affected.
- The most common cause of radiculopathy is impingement of the nerve root as it exits the neuroforamen secondary to degenerative changes; however, prior chemotherapy, radiation therapy, and disorders associated with vasculitis cause noncompressive radiculopathy.
- In cancer patients, the brachial plexus is most commonly affected by direct infiltration of the plexus by tumor or by the effects of radiation therapy.
- Mononeuropathies of the upper extremity are defined by focal injury to a peripheral nerve. They are important to establish in the cancer population, not only because they are common, but also to avoid the unnecessary discontinuation of chemotherapy because of presumed neurotoxicity.

is to identify barriers to normal daily activities as it relates to pain. Frequently, these barriers are the focus for management along with symptom control. In the upper extremity identifying sleep disruption, activity of daily living capacity, shoulder function, prehensile activities, and fine motor coordination may clarify a patient's functional status. Within the allowances of pain, each of these activities can be augmented through judicious use of therapy and assistive devices.

The physical exam in upper extremity pain disorders focuses on identifying recurrence, neurological compromise, and evaluating the musculoskeletal system. The most common areas for recurrence affecting the upper extremity include local lymph nodes, chest wall, and skeleton. A careful examination of the skin, supraclavicular and infraclavicular fossa, and bone palpation can help identify recurrent tumor. The neurological examination should start with identification of central versus peripheral nervous system pathology. Localizing the pain generator to the brain, spinal cord, nerve root, plexus, or peripheral nerve helps to streamline the workup and may ultimately provide the diagnosis. The musculoskeletal exam begins at midline, with cervical and thoracic spine examinations; identification of tenderness over the posterior spinous processes and abnormal range of motion may be clues to local pathology. Dural tension signs may identify underlying nerve root compression. The palpation of areas of muscle pain can identify myofascial nodules or focal tendinopathy. The clinical exam should identify loss of range of motion, impingement signs, and gross weakness in

the shoulder girdle. The humerus should be evaluated for point tenderness, as this may be a clue to underlying skeletal disruption. The elbow should be evaluated for abnormal mechanics and tendonopathies at the medial and lateral epicondyle. The wrist and hand examination should identify areas of pain with palpation and loss of range of motion. Disorder-specific tests, such as the Finkelstein test, Phalen maneuver, and Tinel sign, can identify common causes of wrist and hand pain, such as De Quervain tenosynovitis and carpal tunnel syndrome. The final component of the examination of the upper extremity is the functional assessment. This should include assessment of prehensile activities along with power and fine motor function in the hand. The key to the functional exam is identifying any limiting factors, such as pain, range-of-motion restriction, or neurological compromise.

Diagnostic imaging studies in the cancer rehabilitation setting are typically performed for two reasons: to confirm the diagnosis and to exclude malignancy. Plain radiographs are inexpensive, fast, and easily accessible, but provide only limited information in regard to skeletal abnormalities and are poorly sensitive in identifying metastatic disease to the bone. For identification of bone metastases, the triple-phase bone scan is often the initial test of choice due to its high sensitivity and capacity to assess the entire skeleton. Computed tomography is frequently used in skeletal lesions to localize the lesion and for surgical planning. Magnetic resonance imaging (MRI) is commonly utilized, especially in the evaluation of specific anatomical locations, such as the shoulder or cervical spine, as it allows for the assessment of soft tissues as well as bone. Gadolinium enhancement can be used to differentiate tumor (which tends to be hypervascular relative to normal tissues) from scar or tissues with similar signal, such as the brain and spinal cord. MRI is frequently used to image the cervical spine, brachial plexus, shoulder, and soft tissues of the upper extremity to identify anatomical pathology that may correlate with clinical findings to help establish the diagnosis. Duplex ultrasonography is used as a noninvasive means to assess the vascular system and can identify arterial or venous occlusive disease. Electrodiagnostic studies are utilized to establish peripheral nervous system pathology. The most common diagnoses include cervical radiculopathy, brachial plexopathy, mononeuropathies, and polyneuropathies.

MANAGEMENT

Management of upper extremity pain disorders includes diagnosis, pain control, functional restoration, and return to prior activity. The approach to diagnosis is outlined previously and is the most critical step in determining management. Pain management is typically diagnosis-specific, but certain general principles can be followed, and the reader is referred to other pain management sections of this book. For those with acute onset of pain symptoms, judicious use of anti-inflammatories can blunt the inflammatory process. As pain progresses and the severity increases, the use of short-acting opioids is indicated. As the use of short-acting opioids increases to 24-hour use to maintain pain control, a transition to long-acting opioids should be considered. For those with neurogenic pain, anticonvulsants and tricyclic antidepressants may be beneficial. Interventional procedures may be used to establish a diagnosis, diminish local pain, and blunt inflammatory responses. For those with severe, unremitting pain, intrathecal administration of opioids may be used. Functional restoration in the event of an upper extremity pain disorder is focused on obtaining normal joint kinetics, followed by strength training, endurance training, and return to activity. Frequently, the final phases of rehabilitation will require the assistance of a skilled physical or occupational therapist.

MUSCULOSKELETAL PAIN DISORDERS

Malignant Bone Disease

Malignant bone disease is one of the most feared causes of upper extremity pain in patients carrying a cancer diagnosis. Metastatic disease to bone is commonly associated with breast, prostate, thyroid, lung, and renal cell malignancies (Tables 55.1 and 55.2). On autopsy, 50%–85% of breast and prostate cancer patients will have metastatic bone disease (2). Based on the protracted survival time in breast and prostate cancer, early management is imperative to avoid functional loss (3,4). Less commonly seen tumors such as multiple myeloma and lymphoma are associated with high degrees of morbidity secondary to the primary lytic lesions. Though only 10%–15% of metastatic bone disease is identified in the upper extremity, pain and functional loss can lead to high levels of morbidity (5). The vast majority of metastatic bone disease to the upper extremity occurs in the humerus, although metastases to the scapula and clavicle are also seen. Rarely, lung and renal cell carcinomas can metastasize to the forearm and hands (acrometastases) (6,7).

The clinical presentation of patients with metastatic bone disease to the upper extremity is typically associated with pain. While pain may not be seen with all upper extremity bony metastases, when present, the pain is usually localized, severe, insidious, and unremitting (8). The disease may be associated with functional loss in the upper extremity. The pain itself may limit volitional use of the extremity, with secondary loss of strength, adhesive capsulitis, and other disor-

TABLE 55.1
Incidence of Primary Tumor and Bone Metastases on Autopsy

Breast 73%
Prostate 68%
Thyroid 42%
Lung 36%
Renal cell 35%
Gastrointestinal 5%

Source: From Ref. 1.

TABLE 55.2
Cancer-Related Brachial Plexopathy

	Neoplastic	Radiation-Induced
Onset	Acute	Delayed/gradual
Pain	Severe	Minimal to none
Trunk involved	Lower	Upper
Associated factors	Vascular compromise	Lymphedema
Electrodiagnosis	Denervation	Myokymic potentials

ders. In 25% of patients, lesions may be asymptomatic and will be identified incidentally on routine imaging studies (8).

The evaluation process for metastatic lesions requires a detailed history, including constitutional symptoms, functional deficits, malignancy history, risk factors, and family history. Laboratory evaluation should include complete blood count, calcium, serum protein electrophoresis, and urinalysis and comprehensive metabolic panel to exclude systemic disease. Imaging studies are required to identify the extent of the lesion and for systemic evaluation for disease. The triple-phase bone scan has high sensitivity and is an excellent means to screen the entire body and requires only 10% cortical destruction to identify metastatic disease (9,10). A caveat to bone scan is that primarily lytic lesions, such as those seen in myeloma and lymphoma, may go unrecognized secondary to lack of osteoblastic activity required for bone scan identification (10). Radiographs are less beneficial because 40%–50% of cortical destruction must occur before abnormalities are identified (9). Advanced imaging, such as computed tomography (CT) or MRI, is utilized for surgical or radiation therapy planning and may give tremendous insight into whether a given bony metastases is responsible for the pain disorder under evaluation. Mirels scoring system identifies the site, nature, size, and symptoms of metastatic bone deposits and can guide clinicians in regard to surgical referral (11). Since the upper extremity is a nonweight-bearing component of the skeleton, higher levels of cortical destruction (up to 75%) may be tolerated without risk of fracture (12). In most cases, referral of the patient to a surgeon is appropriate for evaluation of fracture risk. In addition, for smaller lesions, referral to a radiation oncologist may be appropriate.

The treatment of metastatic bone disease requires an established diagnosis of the primary tumor. This typically requires systemic cancer screening for a primary tumor and is usually undertaken by a medical oncologist. In addition, biopsy may be necessary to identify the underlying malignancy. Fracture identification is important as a guide to treatment. Most patients without a high fracture risk can respond to local radiation therapy for palliation of pain (12). Radiation therapy has been shown to decrease tumor size and decrease local chemical mediators of pain (10). The majority of patients respond to radiation, but only 50% obtain complete relief of pain symptoms (13). Systemic treatment with hormonal therapy can be beneficial in cases of breast, prostate, and endometrial malignancies (10). Systemic chemotherapy has not resulted in a clear decrease in pain and bone morbidity (10).

Surgical referral is appropriate in most cases with metastatic bone disease to assess for fracture risk and treat identified fractures. In those with primarily lytic tumors (myeloma, lymphoma), a high risk for fracture usually requires surgical assessment. Surgical management can include local fixation, endoprosthetic management, and humeral head replacement, depending on the location of the tumor. Local fixation is used for shaft fractures and results in pain relief and functional restoration in 90% of patients (12). Endoprosthetic management is seen more frequently in primary tumors and large shaft lesions (12). Humeral head replacement for proximal lesions is an excellent means of pain control, but commonly results in restriction with above-head activities (12).

Pharmaceutical pain management of metastatic bone disease includes analgesics and bisphosphonates. Analgesic use consists primarily of nonsteroidal anti-inflammatories (NSAIDs) and opioids according to the World Health Organization pyramid for pain control. NSAIDS are effective in controlling local bone edema and diminishing the periosteal reaction (10). NSAIDS should be used first line and in synergy with opioids for pain control. Drug holidays and close monitoring for gastritis, renal dysfunction, and bleeding disorders are imperative to prevent systemic complications (10). Opioids should be used judicially and are dosed to effect or side effect. In those patients with systemic side effects, interventional procedures, such as nerve blocks and morphine pump placement, can be used for pain control. The use of bisphosphonates in malignant bone disease decreases osteoclastic activity and has been shown to decrease bone morbidity and bone events (10). Dosing of bisphosphonates is usually on a monthly basis, intravenously, and can be used to prevent and treat bone disease. Radioisotope administration has been used to decrease bone morbidity in advanced disease. The major risk includes myelosuppression.

The rehabilitation principles of upper extremity metastatic bone disease consist of pain control, protection, range of motion, and functional restoration. Pain control should be the initial primary focus of treatment. Pain control and protection of the extremity can be obtained with orthotic utilization and activity modification. In those with a lytic tumor and high fracture risk, weight bearing and lifting activities should be restricted. Once bone stability is established, whether through radiation therapy, systemic therapy, or surgery, preserving and restoring range of motion becomes imperative. Active range of motion in a pain-free arc should be initiated first. Identifying glenohumeral or scapulohumeral restriction can guide therapy orders. Functional restoration includes an assessment of employment, vocational, and recreational activities. Identifying goals of treatment helps to guide successful return to premorbid activities. The initial objective is to obtain independence with basic and advanced activities of daily living. The goals of rehabilitation should always take into account the state of underlying malignancy and current treatments to identify other factors that may affect functional recovery.

Soft Tissue Metastases

Soft tissue metastases are a rare occurrence, with only 1 case for every 37 cases of primary soft tissue sarcoma (14). Multiple reasons have been provided for the rarity of metastatic disease to muscle even in areas over bone. The most common factor seems to be the inconsistent delivery of nutrients to muscle that varies based on metabolic activity of the muscle groups (15). The most common presentation for soft tissue metastases is as an occult malignancy (15). The most common tumors associated with soft tissue extension include lung, kidney, and colon (15). Upper extremity metastases are seen less frequently than in the psoas, intra-abdominal, and paraspinal muscle groups (16). Clinically, patients present with a painful soft tissue mass. This contrasts with soft tissue sarcomas that are typically painless (15). In addition, patients frequently will have redness and warmth over the tumor site. Diagnosis typically requires biopsy, but soft tissue imaging (MRI) can aid in diagnosing malignant characteristics and extent of tumor involvement.

Management of soft tissue metastases is challenging, and the presentation is associated with a poor prognosis. Management includes observation, local radiation therapy, systemic chemotherapy, and surgical resection (15). The goal of treatment is typically palliation. The location and primary tumor depict the overall management. Rehabilitation management includes pain control, modification of activity, orthotics when indicated, and functional restoration in those with resection.

Rotator Cuff Dysfunction

Rotator cuff dysfunction is common in the general population, affecting 1 in 50 adults (17). It is also frequently seen in cancer patients with chest wall procedures such as breast cancer, melanoma, and post-thoracotomy patients. The rotator cuff is a dynamic stabilizer of the glenohumeral joint, maintaining congruity of the humeral head in the glenoid fossa during active range-of-motion activities (18). The function of the rotator cuff is dependent on the normal range and synchrony of the scapulothoracic and glenohumeral articulations. Abnormal mechanics leads to excessive loads on the musculotendinous complex and can ultimately lead to clinical symptoms. Rotator cuff abnormalities have been classically attributed to extrinsic

or intrinsic causes (19). Intrinsic causes are related to degeneration or tears in the tendons. Extrinsic factors result in impingement of the tendon complex secondary to bony changes in the subacromial space. Other identified causes include excessive stretch on the rotator cuff tendons, hypovascularity of the tendons, glenohumeral instability, and loss of scapular mobility.

In patients undergoing chest wall or axillary procedures, such as breast surgery or thoracotomies, rotator cuff dysfunction is increased. A specific factor has not been identified, but immobilization and abnormal movement patterns seem to be the primary issues. Immobilization until the surgical site heals can result in decreased muscle tension generation and excessive loads on the tendon complex. In addition, pain in the chest wall and axilla can result in abnormal movement patterns and excessive rotator cuff loads. In breast cancer patients, tightness in the pectoralis minor can result in depression of the scapula and alter scapulothoracic mobility. In post-thoracotomy patients, transection of the serratus anterior and latissimus dorsi can lead to abnormal scapular mechanics and glenohumeral instability. The effects associated with external beam radiation can further significantly affect normal shoulder function.

Weakness of the rotator cuff muscles from a C5 or C6 radiculopathy or upper trunk brachial plexopathy is a common cause of rotator cuff dysfunction in the cancer setting. These neural structures can be damaged from radiation, chemotherapy, local recurrence, or degenerative changes, and result in rotator cuff weakness and neuropathic pain referred to the lateral arm. Rotator cuff weakness perturbs glenohumeral motion and in the setting of relatively strong pectoral muscles may cause anterior migration of the humerus within the glenoid and subsequent repetitive impingement of the rotator cuff tendons beneath the acromion. This, in turn, will lead to rotator cuff tendonitis.

Patients with rotator cuff dysfunction present with pain deep in the shoulder that refers to the deltoid insertion (18,20). The symptoms of shoulder pain are worsened with above-head activities and excessive loads on an abducted or forward-flexed glenohumeral joint. The physical examination may reveal diminished active and passive range of motion of the shoulder. Active range-of-motion assessment should include evaluation of movement at the scapulothoracic and glenohumeral articulations to identify restrictions and abnormal synchrony. In addition, impingement of the supraspinatus tendon may be identified with Hawkin test or Neer impingement test (21). Weakness of the rotator cuff is most common in the supraspinatus and is identified by weakness with resisted abduction in the scapular plane. Evaluation of the other rotator cuff musculature is carried out by checking internal and external rotation strength. The drop arm test is used to identify full-thickness tears of the supraspinatus and can guide the clinician in regard to advanced imaging (21). A complete neurological examination is performed to exclude concurrent nerve injury resulting in rotator cuff pathology. Evaluation for cervical radiculopathy, upper trunk plexopathy, suprascapular nerve injury, and serratus anterior dysfunction from long thoracic nerve injury should be included in a complete upper extremity neurological exam. The final aspect of the clinical exam is identifying functional restrictions related to the rotator cuff dysfunction.

Diagnostic testing may be required in select instances of rotator cuff dysfunction. Imaging studies, includingplain radiographs, are utilized to identify degenerative changes and extrinsic causes of rotator cuff dysfunction. Magnetic resonance imaging is the test of choice for identifying rotator cuff tears. Electrodiagnostic testing can be complementary in cases of suspected nerve injury.

The treatment of rotator cuff dysfunction initiates with activity modification to reduce risk of further shoulder injury. Local injections and systemic anti-inflammatories can be utilized to control pain (18). Opioids are rarely required, but can be useful for severe symptoms. Thermal modalities, such as cryotherapy or ultrasound, are effective for diminishing pain and may assist with joint mobility. The first step in rehabilitation is attaining pain-free range of motion (18). Typically, this requires a range-of-motion regimen targeting the glenohumeral joint, scapulothoracic articulation, and muscle-based restrictions (pectoralis and latissimus). Once pain-free range of motion is obtained, normalization of scapulohumeral rhythm is initiated. Scapulohumeral training may require the utilization of a trained therapist. The final phase of rehabilitation includes strengthening of the rotator cuff musculature and activity-specific training (22).

Adhesive Capsulitis

Frozen shoulder (adhesive capsulitis) is frequently encountered in the cancer population. This is common in the breast, melanoma, and post-thoracotomy population. Frozen shoulder is defined as loss of range of motion in all planes, with abduction, forward flexion, and external rotation most affected (23,24). Risk factors for frozen shoulder include diabetes mellitus, cervical spinal cord pathology, prolonged immobilization, and thyroid disease (24). Frozen shoulder is defined by three phases: a painful freezing stage, a pain-free adhesive phase, and a resolution phase (24). Patients present with painful shoulder restriction that affects all movements. Pain is exacerbated by end range of motion and lying on the affected side at night. Clinical evaluation includes identifying restriction in range of

motion. Identifying contributing factors, such as rotator cuff dysfunction, immobilization, and underlying neurological compromise, is paramount. In rare cases, acute frozen shoulder may be seen with malignant transformation of the glenohumeral joint and may require aspiration. Imaging studies include bone scan, arthrography, and MRI, but are rarely needed in a clear clinical setting. Patient education is an important aspect of management. Most patients return to full function, but a protracted convalescent phase is typical (25). Treatment includes pain control with NSAIDs and judicious use of injections (24). Opioids can be used for severe cases that disrupt sleep. Initial range of motion should be gentle and performed in a pain-free arc. Once the pain resolves, more aggressive means of ranging, including manipulation under anesthesia and surgical release, may be considered. Once full pain-free range of motion is obtained, strength training and task-specific training concludes the rehabilitation process (26).

Myofascial Pain

Myofascial pain is defined as localized muscle pain with trigger points and specific referral patterns (27). Trigger points consist of small areas of hyperirritability with tautlike bands. The most common upper extremity muscles affected include the trapezius, levator scapulae, and the infraspinatus (27). Cancer patients frequently encounter myofascial pain, and this has been related to immobility and fatigue in the aforementioned muscle groups. Diagnosis is based on local deep palpation of the muscle group, with reproduction of pain in the same location and referral pattern of the presenting symptoms. The clinical exam should identify any underlying pathology that contributes to overload of the muscle groups, such as sleep disruption, local muscle pathology, and neurogenic causes. Treatment consists of routine, regular stretching of the affected muscle groups. In addition, normalization of mechanics is necessary to reduce recurrence. Local injections with lidocaine or botulinum toxin have been used with varying degrees of success (28,29). Physical therapy with the use of modalities and myofascial release may assist with symptom control.

Lateral Epicondylitis

Lateral epicondylitis, commonly referred to as tennis elbow, is pain generated at the extensor complex of the elbow. The pain is common in those with repetitive hand occupations and in those with underlying restriction in shoulder function (30). It is seen 10 times more frequently than medial epicondylitis and is located in the dominant arm in 75% of cases (31). Though referred to as tennis elbow, 95% of cases occur in nontennis players (30). The pathogenesis is excessive repetitive loads on the wrist extensor complex, resulting in overload of the tendon and enthesitis, with irritation of Sharpey fibers as they insert into the periosteum. The most commonly implicated tendon insertions are the extensor carpi radialis brevis, extensor carpi radialis longus, and the extensor communis. Though called epicondylitis, it is rarely inflammatory and is more frequently referred to as a tendinosis (21). The clinical presentation is of local lateral elbow pain worse with gripping and resisted wrist extension (21). The diagnosis is clinical and requires evaluation for underlying kinetic chain abnormalities, including cervical radiculopathy, shoulder restriction (in particular, external rotation), rotator cuff weakness, and abnormalities in elbow range of motion. Identifying offending activities is important in combating symptoms, and a workplace or recreational history is required. The management of lateral epicondylitis consists of relative rest to avoid painful activities that can aggravate symptoms. In severe cases, a cock-up wrist splint can be used. Oral and topical anti-inflammatories are beneficial in both the short and long term. Corticosteroid injections are beneficial in the short term, but may lead to early recurrence and long-term detriment (32). The rehabilitation of lateral epicondylitis consists of improving flexibility of the shoulder, elbow, and wrist in all planes. Improving flexibility is followed by strengthening with isometric followed by concentric and then eccentric resistance training. The final phase of rehabilitation is return to activity; counterforce bracing and activity modification may reduce risk of recurrence.

Medial Epicondylitis

Medial epicondylitis is defined as pain at the origin of the flexor compartment of the forearm, and is often referred to as golfer's elbow. The pain is most commonly associated with activities requiring repetitive wrist flexion and pronation (21). The implicated muscle groups are the pronator teres and flexor communis. Diagnosis is clinical and requires exclusion of proximal deficits, such as cervical radiculopathy, lower trunk or medial cord plexopathy, and shoulder restriction. The management consists of relative rest and anti-inflammatories. Oral and topical anti-inflammatories have been shown to be beneficial. Local injections are not recommended secondary to the proximity of the ulnar nerve. Rehabilitation consists of normalizing range of motion within the kinetic chain. After attaining pain-free range of motion, strengthening of wrist flexors, wrist extensors, pronators, and supinators is undertaken utilizing progressive resistance exercises. Return to activity is predicated on pain-free function and may require modification of activity.

De Quervain Tenosynovitis

De Quervain tenosynovitis is inflammation of the first dorsal compartment of the thumb. The tendons primarily involved are the extensor pollicis brevis and abductor pollicis longus. The history consists of pain localized to the radial side of the wrist. It is felt to be a result of overload of the tendons secondary to repetitive ulnar deviation at the wrist. The patient's clinical examination reveals focal tenderness over the radial side of the wrist reproduced with ulnar deviation of the wrist with the thumb flexed into the palm: Finkelstein test. On clinical exam, one must rule out concurrent neurological deficits, as the superficial radial nerve and C6 nerve root have a similar distribution. Management includes rest via activity modification and use of a thumb spica splint. Local anti-inflammation with cryotherapy or topical NSAIDs is effective. Local steroid injections are used for refractory cases. Rehabilitation consists of evaluating and addressing abnormalities in the kinetic chain that resulted in the tendon overload (shoulder dysfunction, lateral epicondylitis). A trained therapist can perform local thermal modalities combined with range of motion within the kinetic chain. Return to activity is the final component of the rehabilitation process.

Hemiplegic Shoulder

Shoulder pain is a common complication of hemiplegia and may be seen frequently with primary central nervous system (CNS) malignancies, brain metastases, and cerebrovascular disease as a sequelae of cancer treatment. Hemiplegic shoulder occurs in 72% of patients followed over an 11-month period after neurological impairment (33). The etiology of hemiplegic shoulder pain is most commonly related to weakness/subluxation, spasticity, adhesive capsulitis, rotator cuff dysfunction, or complex regional pain syndrome (CRPS) (34). Referred pain must always be considered in the differential and can include cervical radicular pain, plexopathy, intra-abdominal referred pain, and central thalamic pain (35).

The clinical presentation of hemiplegic shoulder pain coincides with the primary etiology. Subluxation of the shoulder, though controversial as a cause of pain, results from weakness of the supporting muscle groups of the shoulder girdle. Symptoms are primarily related to pain when the elbow and shoulder are unsupported. The pain can be relieved with support and relocation of the humeral head within the glenoid fossa. This is typically accomplished with shoulder slings or lap trays. Spasticity-mediated pain is common, occurring in up to 85% of stroke survivors (33). Spasticity-mediated pain is velocity-dependent and is more prevalent at end range of motion (34). The management includes daily stretching, proper positioning, and pharmacological management, with Lioresal, tizanidine, and dantrolene sodium being the most commonly used agents. Adhesive capsulitis is seen as pain with loss of range of motion in all planes, with abduction and external rotation being the most limited. Paralysis, spasticity, complex regional pain syndrome, and synergy movement patterns have all been implicated as causes of hemiplegic frozen shoulder. Clinically, patients present with pain that is worse at end range of motion and lying on the affected side at night. Management includes gentle pain-free range of motion, positioning, and anti-inflammatories when warranted (34). Rotator cuff dysfunction and pain manifests itself when loads are placed on the arm when abducted or forward-flexed. Hemiplegic patients are predisposed to rotator cuff dysfunction because of weakness in the muscle groups and increased rate of impingement of the supraspinatus tendon under the acromion. Pain and weakness with above-head activities is the hallmark of rotator cuff dysfunction. Management includes normalizing range of motion and scapulohumeral mechanics followed by strengthening. Anti-inflammatories via oral, topical, or injectable routes can be beneficial in cases of tendonitis.

Complex regional pain syndrome results in hypersensitivity, allodynia, and vasomotor changes of the extremity. Patients typically present with shoulder pain, loss of range of motion, and concurrent hand pain with metacarpalgia. The diagnosis is clinical, but can be corroborated by an abnormal bone scan. Management options include oral steroids, Lioresal, neuropathic pain agents, range-of-motion exercises, and desensitization techniques. Referred pain must be considered when the pain complaints and evaluation do not correlate with those outlined previously or do not respond to appropriate therapy.

NEUROGENIC UPPER EXTREMITY PAIN DISORDERS

Central Pain

Central pain is associated with a central nervous system lesion. Though previously referred to as thalamic pain syndrome, lesions in the spinal cord and brain can both lead to central pain syndromes (36). Traumatic spinal cord injury and vascular brain pathology are the most commonly identified causes of central pain. Neoplastic lesions can result in central pain at both locations and, therefore, must be considered in the differential of upper extremity pain. The pathophysiology of central pain is felt to be secondary to hyperexcitability of

central nociceptors (36). This central sensitization is caused by continuous firing of unmyelinated C fibers, resulting in amplification of central nervous system responses (37). The neurotransmitter felt to play the most prevalent role are the NMDA receptors (37). Lesions located in the thalamus have been identified as playing a role in central hypersensitivity. Ectopic activity within the ascending spinothalamic tracts (funicular pain) may also be a common cause of central pain in the cancer setting.

Central pain is very difficult to diagnose and treat. Patients can present with a wide array of symptoms that vary on a day-to-day basis. The classical presentation is poorly localized pain with sensations of dysesthesias, hyperpathia, allodynia, and lancinating pain (36). The clinical assessment initiates with attempts to identify a peripheral nociceptor or central lesion contributing to the onset or amplification of pain responses. Lesions in the spinal cord, brain, peripheral spasticity, and persistent peripheral nociceptor stimulation should be identified. The physical examination should identify the type of neurogenic pain that is present and include a complete neuromuscular assessment. Imaging studies should include magnetic resonance imaging of the brain and cervical spine with gadolinium in patients with suspected central upper extremity pain. Electrodiagnostic testing may aggravate hyperpathia symptoms and should be used judiciously.

Management of central pain is equally challenging. The most effective agents such as intravenous (IV) lidocaine and IV morphine have limited clinical utility (36). Oral regimens with mexiletine, amitriptyline, lamotrigine, and gabapentin have had mixed results, with no one agent proven to be maximally beneficial and dosing usually leading to unwanted side effects (36,37). Oral opioids have also been effective but limited by side effects. Treatment of peripheral nociceptors helps to attenuate symptoms. The most common agents include NSAIDs and antispasticity medications. Newer treatment options, such as intrathecal administration of pharmaceuticals, deep brain stimulation, and gamma knife procedures, are potentially effective management methods that may be used more regularly in the future (36).

Cervical Radiculopathy

Cervical radiculopathy is a neurological condition resulting from irritation of a cervical nerve root that commonly refers pain into the upper extremity and can cause weakness in a myotomal distribution. Cervical radiculopathy is a common cause of pain in both the general and cancer populations. In the cancer population, cervical radiculopathy symptoms are more likely to be due to degenerative causes than malignancy, but a neoplastic cause should always be considered and excluded. When cervical radiculopathy is related to malignancy, most patients are known to have widespread metastatic disease; however, a solitary metastases affecting the neural foramen can also cause significant pain and dysfunction. In addition, prior chemotherapy, radiation therapy, and disorders associated with vasculitis such as multiple myeloma and lymphomas can cause noncompressive radiculopathy or contribute to more significant dysfunction in compressive radiculopathy.

The most common cause of radiculopathy is impingement of the nerve root as it exits the neuroforamen secondary to degenerative changes in the zygapophyseal and uncovertebral joints (38,39). Disc herniation and the ensuing inflammatory process have also been implicated as a direct result of nerve root irritation. The sixth and seventh cervical nerve roots are implicated in 90% of cervical radiculopathies, with C7 predominating. (C8) e (T1) level radiculopathiesare relatively rare and require careful consideration for alternative diagnoses, such as metastatic disease and lower trunk plexopathy.

The clinical presentation of radiculopathy in most patients includes arm pain with associated neurological deficits, such as weakness and sensory abnormalities. Pain is usually aggravated with traction on the affected arm and extension of the neck. Alternatively, symptoms may be relieved by tilting the head away from the affected arm or resting the affected hand on top of the head. Patients may identify a specific distribution of sensory loss or pain that correlates with a dermatome. The clinical examination includes evaluation of the cervical spine for paraspinal spasm, range of motion, and provocative maneuvers, such as Spurling maneuver and the dural stretch test. The neurological examination should include strength, reflex, and sensory testing to identify a nerve root distribution. It is imperative to perform a full neurological evaluation to exclude central nervous system processes such as myelopathy and intracranial pathology. The diagnostic test of choice to define cervical anatomy is magnetic resonance imaging. Electrodiagnostic testing is very sensitive and specific for nerve root dysfunction, and can be beneficial in excluding other peripheral causes of neurogenic symptoms, such as plexopathy, mononeuropathy, and polyneuropathy. The management of cervical radiculopathy is multimodal and includes anti-inflammatories, judicious use of opioids, physical therapy with cervical traction, interventional procedures, and surgery in those with refractory cases or progressive neurological compromise. For those with metastatic disease, radiation therapy may be a palliative option for symptom control.

Brachial Plexopathy

The brachial plexus in cancer patients is most commonly affected by direct infiltration of the plexus by tumor or by the effects of radiation therapy. Each etiology has a unique clinical presentation with some overlap (Table 55.2). Radiation effects to the brachial plexus are most commonly seen in breast cancer patients, but also may be seen in local treatment for other malignancies. The breast cancer population has been the most studied, and it has been identified that total dose and dose per session of radiation therapy affect the risk for radiation therapy. Dose per session less than 2.5 Gy and total doses less than 40 Gy are associated with much less risk than doses above this level (40). Higher doses up to 4 Gy and 44 Gy of cobalt radiation have been associated with rates of 92% for brachial plexus injury (41).

The presentation of patients with radiation-induced brachial plexopathy is that of painless weakness with initial impact on the upper trunk (42). Most commonly, there is a delay in onset greater than six months after radiation therapy. An acute, transient brachial plexopathy has been reported, with primary sensory symptoms during radiation therapy, which typically resolves without sequelae. Radiation effects to the plexus usually progress insidiously and may involve the entire plexus. A flaccid, nonfunctional arm with profound lymphedema is characteristic of radiation-induced brachial plexopathy. The diagnosis of radiation-induced plexopathy is usually clinical, based on onset, progression, and identification of concurrent lymphedema. The physical exam will identify primary shoulder girdle weakness with involvement of the whole plexus as the disorder progresses. The diagnosis may be corroborated by magnetic resonance imaging and electrodiagnostic studies. A clear association between myokymic discharges on electrodiagnostic studies and radiation-induced plexopathy has been reported (42). It should be noted that the presence of myokymia, while highly supportive of a radiation injury, does not exclude a tumor recurrence. The management of radiation-induced brachial plexopathy is primarily supportive. Patients can derive a great deal of benefit from management and control of lymphedema. Initial management is focused on stabilizing and maintaining the function of the shoulder girdle. Balanced forearm orthoses may be used to assist in activities of daily living when shoulder function is lost. Shoulder support to avoid subluxation and overload of the shoulder girdle may benefit patients. Patients losing hand function may benefit from orthotic devices or modification of utensils to maintain hand function.

Malignant involvement of the brachial plexus has unique features and is most commonly associated with breast, lung (Pancoast tumor), melanoma, and sarcoma.

The clinical presentation is that of sensory loss followed by pain that initiates in the lower trunk distribution and progresses to involve the entire plexus. The severity of pain and onset of symptoms in the absence of lymphedema helps to distinguish this from radiation-induced brachial plexopathy. Sensory loss is the earliest symptom and is identified in the medial arm, medial forearm, and fourth and fifth digits (43). The differential diagnosis early on includes cervical radiculopathy, intercostobrachial neuropathy, and ulnar neuropathy. The progression of symptoms, with increased pain, hand-intrinsic weakness, and radial nerve involvement, are further clues to malignant involvement of the plexus (43). An ipsilateral Horner syndrome (ptosis, miosis, anhydrosis) may be seen secondary to involvement of the sympathetic ganglion. The evaluation of patients with lower trunk brachial plexopathy should include a chest radiograph, magnetic resonance imaging, and electrodiagnostic studies. The primary treatment is directed to the underlying malignancy. Radiation therapy and chemotherapy are frequently instituted for the primary tumor and may help with pain symptoms. Pain control with neuropathic pain agents and opiates is frequently required. Interventional procedures, including intrathecal pain pumps, and dorsal cordotomy may be used in severe incapacitating pain as palliative measures for pain relief. The rehabilitation principles are primarily related to maintaining hand function. This may be accomplished early on with an ulnar bar to stabilize the metacarpophalangeal joints. Dynamic wrist splints may be used when radial nerve involvement limits wrist extension. Modification of utensils may help to maintain independence as hand function diminishes. Overall, the prognosis without effective treatment of the underlying tumor is poor and the focus becomes palliation of pain.

Chemotherapy-Induced Polyneuropathy

Chemotherapy-induced polyneuropathy (CIPN) is a commonly encountered in cancer patients and is often seen with the taxanes, vinca alkaloids, and platinum-based compounds. In patients receiving these agents, almost 100% will develop symptoms of nerve dysfunction (44). Up to 33% will have functional loss as a result of treatment (44). Many new agents with neurotoxicity are becoming widely used clinically, and older agents, such as thalidomide, are finding new indications.

The taxanes (paclitaxel, docetaxel) are frequently used in the treatment of breast, lung, and ovarian carcinomas. The pathogenesis of taxane and vinca alkaloid-induced CIPN is felt to be secondary to microtubule dysfunction with perturbation of axoplasmic flow and thus axonal housekeeping. This results in an axonal degradation and a "dying back" distal symmetric axonal neuropathy of both the motor and sensory nerves, with the longest nerves affected first (44). Clinically, the sensory fibers seem more affected, as the motor fibers are somewhat more resilient due to their larger size and capacity for regeneration. The onset of symptoms is cumulative and temporally related to chemotherapy administration.

The platinum-based agents cause direct damage to DNA and have their primary clinical neurotoxicity at the dorsal root ganglion. This causes a sensory ganglionopathy characterized clinically by numbness, sensory ataxia, dysesthesias, and occasionally allodynia. Higher doses of platinum agents can result in anterior horn cell damage and weakness. The platinum drugs are unique in their ability to continue to cause progressive nerve dysfunction long after the drug has been discontinued. This phenomenon, known as "coasting," results from progressive DNA damage. As opposed to the neuropathy encountered with the tubulin inhibitors, such as the taxanes and vinca alkaloids, the neuropathy from platinum drugs is nonlength-dependent.

The evaluation of a patient with suspected CIPN should include a complete history of symptom onset, location, and association with neurotoxic chemotherapeutic agents. The clinical exam should identify extent of sensory loss and any evidence of motor loss. Focal neurological deficits should be identified to exclude other causes of neuropathic symptoms, such as radiculopathy, mononeuropathy, and plexopathy. Long tract signs should be identified to rule out central nervous system processes. Functional assessment includes assessment of fine motor coordination and gait. In addition, history of disruption of daily routine identifies level of disability and can be a focus for treatment. Laboratory workup to identify other reversible causes for peripheral neuropathy includes complete blood count (CBC), electrolytes, glucose, serum protein electrophoresis, rheumatoid factor, antinuclear antibodies, vitamin B_{12}, and folate levels. Electrodiagnostic testing may be used to clarify the diagnosis and in equivocal cases can be used to exclude other etiologies. This is important because neuropathic symptoms are frequently associated with discontinuation of chemotherapy and an established diagnosis of CIPN may affect treatment. Imaging studies are used to identify CNS lesions in those whose clinical exam warrants further investigation.

The treatment of CIPN begins with discontinuation of the offending agent when possible. Unfortunately, the clinical efficacy of most chemotherapeutics is as dose-dependent as the neurotoxicity, making the decision to terminate the use of a drug prematurely a difficult one. The use of neuroprotective agents (glutamate and glutamine) has not been clearly identified as effective. Neuropathic pain agents are primarily utilized when pain disrupts sleep or leads to limitation in mobility.

The rehabilitation of CIPN includes early education about gait instability. The use of assisted devices can reduce the risk of falls. In addition, patients need to be counseled about loss of fine motor coordination in the hands. Orthotic devices for eating, hygiene, and dressing can be helpful. A course of occupational therapy to maintain and augment upper extremity function may be beneficial. Overall, patients will show recovery of neurological impairment after chemotherapy is discontinued, but recovery is typically incomplete and may result in residual functional loss.

Paraneoplastic Neuropathy

Paraneoplastic syndromes are a remote effect of cancer related to antibody formation by the primary tumor that results in neuromuscular dysfunction. Paraneoplastic processes are rare and can precede the diagnosis of cancer by years. The most common primary malignancy associated with paraneoplastic syndromes is small cell lung cancer, accounting for 50%–75% of cases (45). The identification of paraneoplastic processes is imperative because it may improve survival and affect the continuation of treatment. The paraneoplastic syndromes most relevant to upper extremity pain disorders include subacute sensory neuropathy, sensorimotor neuropathy, and demyelinating neuropathy.

Subacute sensory neuropathy is a syndrome of dysesthetic pain and numbness that frequently begins in the upper extremity and progresses in a short time period (days to weeks) (45–47). The neuropathy is associated with small cell lung cancer in 67% of patients and may be identified by the presence of anti-Hu antibodies (47). The onset of symptoms precedes the diagnosis of the primary malignancy in 71%–88% of patients (45). The clinical findings include loss of proprioception, touch, temperature, and pain sense, absent reflexes without motor impairment (45,46). The hallmark of the disease process is the rapid onset. Diagnosis is clinical and can be supported by anti-Hu antibodies and electrodiagnostic studies. Electrodiagnostic studies frequently identify sensory abnormalities on nerve conduction studies without motor study abnormalities. Treatment of the primary tumor is the primary means of management. Supportive care, including education and symptom control, are secondary means of management.

The subacute sensorimotor paraneoplastic syndrome is a rapid onset (days to weeks) syndrome that involves both the sensory and motor systems. Small cell lung cancer is the most common primary malignancy, and anti-Hu antibodies are found in 25% of cases. Patients present with rapid onset of sensory and motor impairment that may be asymmetrical or monomelic (45). The diagnosis is established by excluding other possible causes, including diabetes mellitus, alcoholic neuropathy, B_{12} deficiency, nutritional deficiencies, and vincristine neuropathy (47). Treatment is supportive. The demyelinating paraneoplastic syndrome is rare and is frequently associated with lymphomas. The clinical presentation is similar to that of acute inflammatory demyelinating polyneuropathy with rapid onset of weakness, absent reflexes, and evidence of demyelination on electrodiagnostic studies.

Mononeuropathy

Mononeuropathies of the upper extremity are defined by focal injury to a peripheral nerve. They are important to establish in the cancer population, not only because they are common, but also to avoid the unnecessary discontinuation of chemotherapy because of presumed neurotoxicity. They may occur in isolation or as a component of a systemic process resulting in multiple focal nerve injuries (mononeuropathy multiplex). The diagnosis is clinical and is identified by neurological impairment in the distribution of a single peripheral nerve. The clinical exam can be augmented by electrodiagnostic studies identifying the focal nerve lesion on nerve conduction studies.

The most common nerves associated with mononeuropathy in the upper extremity include the median, ulnar, and radial nerves. The median nerve may be impacted at any point along its course, but most commonly is affected in the carpal tunnel (carpal tunnel syndrome or CTS). CTS is identified by numbness and tingling affecting the first four digits, typically worse at night and with repetitive hand motion, with sparing of palmar sensation. The diagnosis is clinical, but is strongly supported by slowing on nerve conduction studies across the carpal tunnel space. The median nerve may also be compressed above the elbow, between the two heads of the pronator teres, and in the flexor digitorum superficialis. Each of these areas of compression results in unique clinical findings that may be verified by electrodiagnostic studies.

The ulnar nerve is most commonly affected at the elbow. The resulting clinical abnormalities include numbness in the fourth and fifth digits and ulnar surface of the palm with sparing of the forearm. Weakness may be found in the ulnar innervated hand intrinsics. The ulnar nerve may also be compressed at the wrist and in the palm, with unique clinical deficits and sparing of sensory loss in the distribution of the dorsal ulnar cutaneous nerve. In cancer patients, excluding lower trunk brachial plexopathy and cervical radiculopathy with ulnar nerve distribution symptoms is imperative.

The radial nerve is frequently damaged at the spiral groove in the proximal forearm and in the wrist. The spiral-groove–level injury results in the classic "Saturday night palsy" with wrist drop and sparing of elbow extension. The elbow-level lesions may result in posterior interosseous nerve syndrome with no sensory loss and partial weakness to wrist extension with absent finger extension. The superficial radial nerve may be compressed at the radial side of the wrist, resulting in sensory loss in the radial side of the hand—a condition called cheiralgia paresthetica. The diagnosis of mononeuropathies is clinical and can be supported by electrodiagnostic studies identifying focal slowing or loss of amplitude across the affected segment. The management of mononeuropathies is typically education, splinting, and physical therapy, and in severe cases surgical repair. The diagnosis can be beneficial in that it reduces the likelihood of unnecessarily stopping chemotherapy due to suspected neurotoxicity.

CIRCULATORY DISORDERS

Arterial Claudication

Arterial claudication is associated with malignancies because of physiological changes in the hemodynamics and secondary to treatment. Arterial claudication presents with symptoms of exertional pain and fatigue. The pain is usually diffuse in nature and is associated with pallor, paresthesias, coolness, and diminished pulses. In cancer patients, the proximal vascular supply above the axillary artery is most frequently implicated. Possible etiologies include direct tumor invasion, thrombophilia, radiation-induced claudication, and idiopathic. A high index of suspicion is required to identify the disorder. The clinical exam should identify a diminished pulse or blood pressure on the affected side. Palpating for masses and venous engorgement may identify tumor invasion. Assessing warmth, neurological status, and level of discomfort may alert the clinician as to the urgency of the situation. Surgical consultation should not be delayed in patients with suspected ischemia. Arterial duplex ultrasonography and magnetic resonance angiography may assist with diagnosis. Ultimately, surgical procedures are utilized to restore normal vascular supply.

Venous Thromboembolic Disease

Venous thromboembolic disease is a common cause of pain and swelling in the cancer population. Rates of deep venous thrombosis (DVT) are increased 4.1 times the general population in cancer patients (48). Malignancies most commonly associated with DVT include mucin-producing tumors, such as pancreas, lung, stomach, and some adenocarcinomas. The management of malignancies may also contribute to DVT, with increased rates associated with hormonal therapy, chemotherapy, antiangiogenesis agents, and catheters (49). For those presenting with initial DVT and no underlying history of malignancy, chest radiograph, blood work, and clinical examination will exclude 90% of malignancies (50).

The presentation of upper extremity DVT is typically an acute onset of swelling with associated erythema and warmth. The clinical exam will identify pitting edema, enlarged venous collaterals, and improvement of swelling and erythema with elevation of the arm. Diagnostic studies include venous duplex ultrasound and magnetic resonance venous imaging in equivocal cases or with suspected proximal DVT. A hypercoagulable workup may be warranted in those without active malignancy and no clear etiology. Management of DVT consists of sustained anticoagulation. The standard treatment has been long-term use of warfarin. A recent study has identified decreased complication and recurrence rates with the use of low molecular weight heparin (51). For those with acute DVT activity, modification may be warranted until stable anticoagulation is obtained. For those with large proximal clots, a surgical evaluation may be warranted for stenting procedures or clot removal.

Lymphedema

The lymphatic system is a component of the circulatory system designed to mobilize fat globules, proteins, infectious complexes, and breakdown products of metabolism (52). The objective is to transport these particles to local and regional lymph nodes for degradation and than returning the fluid to the central vasculature. The peripheral lymphatic system is divided into superficial and deep lymphatics (52). The superficial lymphatics are weblike and course directly under the skin. The deeper lymphatics run in concert with the vascular system. In the upper extremity, the lymphatic system mobilizes fluid slowly via muscle contraction and respiration toward the centrally located lymph nodes in the axilla and supraclavicular regions. For surgical purposes, the lymph nodes are divided into three stations and the supraclavicular region. After lymph node processing, the fluid drains to the lymphatic ducts and central vasculature.

Lymphedema is a disorder of lymphatic fluid accumulation resulting in swelling, typically in an extremity. The most common malignancies associated with lymphedema include breast, melanoma, and lymphoma. Breast cancer and melanoma are associated with lymphedema primarily because staging and treatment of these malignancies includes axillary lymph node dissection. In breast cancer, a full axillary dissection typically involves removal of station 1 and 2 lymph nodes, whereas in melanoma, station 1–3 lymph nodes are removed (52). The sentinel lymph node dissection, which includes sampling of lymph nodes that drain directly from the site of the tumor, leads to smaller numbers of lymph nodes being removed and may reduce rates of lymphedema. Lymphoma is associated with lymphedema secondary to direct invasion of lymph nodes with malignancy. In the breast cancer population, lymphedema rates approximate 25% and are associated with risk factors of axillary lymph node dissection, metastatic involvement of lymph nodes, radiation therapy, obesity, and increasing age (53).

Lymphedema presents as painless, colorless swelling, usually of gradual onset with heaviness and loss of arm contour. In patients presenting with rapid onset of swelling with pain or erythema, metastatic seeding (malignant lymphedema), infection, and thromboembolic disease must be excluded. Two types of presentation are seen in patients with lymphedema. The first type is those who have gradual onset of fluid accumulation after lymph node removal secondary to overload of the lymphatic system with normal daily fluid production (normal-output lymphedema). The second presentation is those patients who have an acute increase in lymphatic fluid that overwhelms the compromised system (high-output lymphedema). Common causes of high-output lymphedema include cellulitis, lymphangitis, trauma, thermal burns, and increased metabolism in the at-risk extremity. Lymphedema progresses in stages. The first stage is a primarily fluid stage in which arm volumes diminish with elevation and compression garments. As lymphatic fluid accumulates in the extremity, an inflammatory reaction ensues that results in subcutaneous fibrosis and hardening of tissue—this is considered the hallmark for stage 2 lymphedema. Stage 2 lymphedema does not resolve with elevation and compression garments. Stage 3 lymphedema is identified by cutaneous fibrosis and verrucous hyperplastic changes of the skin, and is rarely seen in the upper extremity (52). As lymphedema progresses, pain develops secondary to constriction of underlying soft tissue structure and overload of the supporting structures of the shoulder (54).

The clinical evaluation of lymphedema should include a history of the primary malignancy and the aspects of treatment that have affected the lymphatic system. The onset, duration, and progression of lymphatic swelling should be identified. In addition, identifying attempted management methods is important. Identification of functional restrictions related to lymphedema (loss of shoulder or hand function) should be inquired. The physical exam should include a full musculoskeletal and neurological exam to identify any underlying restriction or neurological deficits related to the arm swelling. The skin examination should focus on soft tissue restriction of the proximal lymphatics, with a focus on surgical and irradiated sites. In addition, identification of cellulitis or lymphangitis is paramount to halt processes that may contribute to worsening lymphedema. The lymphatic evaluation includes palpation of all lymphatic territories. The arm examination should include volume measurements via tape measure or volumetric displacement. A comparison to the opposite unaffected extremity is beneficial (55).

The management of lymphedema is performed to maintain function and decrease risk of recurrent infection. Complex decongestive therapy (CDT) is the most effective means to decongest the lymphedematous extremity (56). CDT consists of proximal lymphatic clearance via manual lymphatic drainage, a massage technique promoting fluid motility to unaffected lymphatic territories. Skin care to reduce risk of infection is important and should be combined with stretching and soft tissue mobilization techniques to the proximal upper extremity, helping to reduce stasis of the lymphatic system. Wrapping the extremity with short stretch bandages to promote fluid motility out of the arm is the next phase, and can be augmented by use of high-tensile foam to break up fibrosis. The final phase is exercises with wrappings in place to use the physiological muscle pump to propel fluid to the proximal lymphatics. CDT is typically divided into a decongestive phase, which consists of 24-hour-per-day compression, usually under the guidance of a trained physical or occupational therapist, and a maintenance phase consisting of wrapping at night (performed by the patient or caregiver) and compressive garments during the day. In the maintenance phase, regular surveillance by a physician should be performed to assure volume reduction is maintained.

Axillary Cording

Axillary cording, also known as axillary web syndrome, is a common side effect of axillary lymph node removal. It starts in the midaxillary line and can extend to the medial arm, antecubital fossa, and thumb (57). In rare cases, the cording may extend back into the area of the breast. The cord feels like a piano wire under the skin and may be comprised of multiple cords bound together like a web. The cording has a delayed onset usually greater than one week after surgery. It is associated with lymph node removal and is more prevalent in dissections that are more extensive (58). In addition, cording can be more pronounced after radiation therapy to the axilla. The composition of the cords on biopsy is that of sclerosed and thrombosed lymphatics.

The major clinical implication of cording is the restriction in forward flexion and abduction in the ipsilateral shoulder (57). Though cording is worrisome for patients, it is typically self-limiting and resolves within two to three months (59). The primary aspect of assessment includes evaluation of the entire lymphatic drainage territory of the arm and excluding concurrent lymphangitis. It is also important to exclude allodynia secondary to neurological compromise. Management includes reassurance, education, soft tissue mobilization techniques for the cord, and gentle range-of-motion techniques for the shoulder. Patients should be alerted to the fact that a cord can actually have an audible snap and result in immediate resolution of the shoulder restriction. Over time, patients can be assured that the cord will resolve and they should have progressive return of range of motion with the aforementioned techniques. Refractory, recurrent, or protracted courses of axillary cording require further investigation.

INTEGUMENTARY DISORDERS

Infection

Infections of the upper extremity are common sequelae of malignancy and have a particularly high prevalence in patients with axillary lymph node removal secondary to inadequate lymphatic clearance of pathogens. The types of infection most frequently encountered include cellulitis and lymphangitis. Cellulitis is considered an acute pyogenic inflammation of the dermis and subcutaneous tissues (60). Cellulitis typically presents with a tender, warm, erythematous, and swollen arm with poor demarcation of the affected area (60). Lymphangitis is an infection of the lymphatic drainage territories and results in streaking erythema and tenderness along the volar forearm and medial arm. The primary etiologies for the underlying infections include trauma, skin breakdown, venous stasis, and lymphostasis. The primary pathogen is Gram-positive cocci and specifically group B *Streptococcus*. The major implication in patients with lymphostasis is the infection not only increases lymphatic fluid production, but also results in damage to the superficial lymphatics secondary to infiltration by the pathogen (61). Hence, those at risk for lymphedema who develop an infection require prompt treatment to reduce risk of recurrent infections.

The clinical evaluation attempts to identify systemic systems, such as fever, chills, or general malaise. Hemodynamic stability should be assessed through vital signs to exclude evidence of systemic infection. The clinical examination includes attempts to identify the source and the extent of the infection. Basic laboratory assessment, including a complete blood count, is warranted. Management depends on risk factors and extent of infection. For those with systemic infections and in immunocompromised individuals, treatment with intravenous antibiotics is appropriate. The most common agents include cefazolin, ceftriaxone, nafcillin, levofloxacin, and in methicillin-resistant *Staphylococcus aureus* (MRSA) patients, vancomycin (60). For less complicated infections, oral regimens with amoxicillin, amoxicillin/clavulanic acid, cefuroxime, cefadroxil, and Levaquin are frequently used. Caution should be used with cephalexin in patients on acid-reducing medications because this may reduce the gastric absorption and diminish eradication rates (62). Patients with concurrent fungal infections require topical antifungals to reduce risk of skin compromise and recurrent infections. Additional measures for management include elevation, support stockings, and hygiene of the affected extremity (60).

DISEASE-SPECIFIC DISORDERS

Postmastectomy Pain Syndrome

Postmastectomy pain syndrome (PMPS) is defined as a chronic pain condition that can occur following surgery to the breast (63). PMPS can occur with any breast procedure, including mastectomy, lumpectomy, axillary lymph node dissection, reconstruction, and augmentation. PMPS has long-term implications for approximately 40% of patients and is more common in younger patients, patients with increased postoperative pain, surgery that is more extensive, and higher levels of anxiety (64–67).

The causes of PMPS include phantom breast pain, incisional pain, intercostobrachial neuralgia, and neuroma pain (68). Phantom breast pain consists of painful sensations in the area of the removed breast and may affect 23% of patients (69). Incisional pain can be from local adherence of the incision to the chest wall or hypersensitivity. Typically, the clinical presentation is that of hypersensitivity and decreased mobility of the incision. The intercostobrachial nerve is the lateral cutaneous nerve of the second thoracic root. The nerve courses along the axillary vein and then provides sensation to the medial and posterior portion of the arm, the axilla, and the lateral portion of the chest wall. The intercostobrachial nerve is frequently affected by axillary lymph node dissections and is a common cause of PMPS. Symptoms can include absent sensation, abnormal sensation, and allodynia. Neuroma pain is identified by a focal area of hypersensitivity most commonly seen along the borders of the incision. This must be distinguished from incisional hypersensitivity, which can be seen after chest wall procedures. The local pain and identifying a small soft tissue mass are helpful in clarifying the diagnosis. If a soft tissue mass is identified, excluding recurrence is important before initiating treatment.

The clinical exam for PMPS should focus on identifying the etiology of pain and excluding other etiologies (Table 55.3). General inspection should evaluate for muscle wasting, asymmetry, and gross masses. The musculoskeletal exam should focus on shoulder range, costovertebral, costochondral, and rib integrity. The incision should be evaluated for adherence, fibrosis, neuromas, infections, and local recurrence. The neurological exam should focus on the motor testing, focusing on muscles of the shoulder girdle innervated by nerves potentially affected by breast surgery (thoracodorsal, long thoracic, medial, and lateral pectoral). Sensory testing should include all dermatomes in the chest wall and upper extremity. Special attention should be paid to the posterior thorax area, as sensory loss can be a clue to spinal pathology. The sensory exam of the axilla should identify the distribution, severity, and type of sensory abnormality. Diagnostic studies may be utilized to confirm a diagnosis and exclude other causes of pain. Mammogram, MRI, and position emission tomography (PET) scan can be utilized to exclude recurrence. If suspected, MRI of the thoracic spine is warranted to exclude other causes for neuropathic pain in the breast dermatomes, such as radiculopathy. Electrodiagnosis can be helpful to exclude motor nerve abnormalities and plexopathy.

The management of PMPS commences perioperatively. This includes minimizing dissection, nerve-sparing procedures, and early pain control. Early pain control is imperative because severe early pain is one of the most consistent factors in PMPS (67). Early postoperative pain control is typically accomplished with anesthetic pump procedures and judicious use of NSAIDs and opioids. Early desensitization techniques can limit neuropathic pain symptoms and can be initiated once the incision is healed. A massage technique of gentle incision mobility and soft tissue massage extending from the axilla to the chest wall is recommended. For those with uncontrolled pain resulting in sleep disruption and functional loss, neuropathic pain agents may be instituted. Long-acting opioids can be utilized

when the aforementioned agents fail to control pain. The rehabilitation of PMPS patients requires the identification of functional limitations. Shoulder restriction is a major factor in functional loss in PMPS. The management includes pain control followed by active and passive range of motion. The pectoralis major, pectoralis minor, and latissimus dorsi should be targeted muscles for stretching. Once full pain-free shoulder mobility with normal scapulohumeral mechanics is obtained, strengthening and task-specific function become the targets of rehabilitation.

Post-Thoracotomy Pain Syndrome

Post-thoracotomy pain syndrome (PTPS) is defined as pain that persists at the incision site or in the distribution of an incised intercostal nerve for greater than two months after thoracotomy (70). The thoracotomy is utilized to access intrathoracic contents most commonly for tumor resection. The classic thoracotomy consists of a posterolateral incision of the thorax, bisecting the latissimus dorsi and serratus anterior, separation of the ribs, disruption of the intercostal nerves, and a pleural incision. The procedure is noted to be one of the most painful. Generally, 40% of patients will have chronic postoperative pain (71,72). Approximately 50% of patients will have long-term disruption in capacity to perform daily tasks. Sleep disruption occurs in 25%–30% of patients. Fortunately, only 3%–5% of patients develop severe disabling pain. Predictive factors for PTPS include pain level at 24 hours postoperative, female gender, preoperative opioid use, and radiation therapy (72,73).

The most common etiology for PTPS is intercostal neuralgia. This typically presents with allodynia, dysesthesias, and lancinating pain in the distribution of the affected intercostal nerves (70,72). The symptoms are aggravated by direct impact to the ribcage or extremes of shoulder range of motion. The disruption of the latissimus dorsi and serratus anterior predisposes to muscle-based pain and abnormal scapulohumeral mechanics. Subsequently, shoulder dysfunction and myofascial pain are commonly encountered in the PTPS patient and are the primary etiology for functional loss after thoracotomy (74). The symptoms of myofascial pain include palpatory tenderness of the affected muscles. Shoulder dysfunction can result in painful, restricted shoulder range of motion, and the potential for adhesive capsulitis exists. Other etiologies for pain that should be considered include pleuritic pain that is usually sharp, poorly localized, and worsens with deep respiratory excursion. In addition, costochondral dislocation and costochondritis can present with localized musculoskeletal pain that worsens with compression and movement of the ribcage. The possibility of malignant

TABLE 55.3
Postmastectomy Pain Syndrome Differential Diagnosis

Tumor recurrence
Paraneoplastic neuropathy
Chemotherapy-induced neuropathy
Plexopathy
Rib fracture
Intraparenchymal lung pathology
Thoracic nerve root impingement
Intercostal neuralgia
Zoster/postherpetic neuralgia
Postsurgical scar/adhesions

invasion of the ribcage and intrathoracic region should be considered in cases of progressive refractory pain symptoms. Spinal column pain should be considered in those that present with referred pain from midline; typical etiologies include thoracic radiculopathy and vertebral collapse. Intrathoracic pathology, such as cardiac ischemia, aortic dissection, pneumonia, and pleural effusion, are other sources of chest wall pain that should be considered.

The clinical evaluation of PTPS is performed to exclude other causes of pain (Table 55.4). It should include inspection of the chest wall and incision site. Viewing patients during deep respiratory excursion can help to identify abnormal chest wall movements and may reproduce pleuritic pain. Palpation over the incision site is performed to identify scar adherence, hypersensitivity, or intercostal nerve pain. The ribcage should be evaluated in its entirety to exclude fractures, costochondral avulsions, and costochondritis. Assessment of regional musculature for postoperative disruption, atrophy, and myofascial pain is important. Adhesive capsulitis and shoulder girdle dysfunction should be assessed through active and passive range of motion and provocative maneuvers for scapular dysfunction (such as a wall push-up for scapular winging). The neurological examination includes motor testing of both extremities, assessment of all thoracic dermatomes, and evaluation for scapular winging. The gait and functional assessment should include movement pattern; assessment of basic activities of daily living; and a general screen for lifting capacity, fine motor coordination, and balance. Diagnostic testing for PTPS can include baseline radiographs of the ribcage or chest wall to identify bone disruption, fracture, or intrathoracic pathology. In equivocal cases, CT scanning can be used to better define the bone and intrathoracic structures. MRI may be relevant in those suspected to have thoracic radiculopathy. An intercostal nerve block can be used for diagnosis or treatment.

TABLE 55.4
Factors Associated with Post-Thoracotomy Pain

Intercostal neuroma
Rib fracture
Adhesive capsulitis
Infection
Pleurisy
Costochondral dislocation
Costochondritis
Local tumor recurrence
Myofascial pain
Vertebral collapse

Source: From Refs. 1 and 4.

The management of PTPS includes early aggressive pain management. Preemptive analgesia is used to diminish postoperative pain by blocking pain pathways before surgery via thoracic epidural anesthesia, intercostal nerve blockade, opiates, and NSAIDs (70). This has been shown to diminish postoperative pain from 50% to 9.9% (71,72). The surgical approach, with the advent of muscle-sparing procedures and smaller incisions, may lead to less postoperative pain and dysfunction. Postoperative pain immediately after surgery is best controlled with the combination of anesthesia, opiates, and NSAIDs (75). Once wound healing has occurred, early scar mobilization and gentle stimulation of the incision and intercostal nerve distribution can diminish long-term pain. Pharmacological management for persistent pain may include intercostal nerve blockade, topical lidocaine, neuropathic pain agents, oral opiates, or in those with severe pain, intrathecal opiates (71,76).

The rehabilitation of PTPS commences preoperatively with nutritional assessment. Pulmonary rehabilitation consisting of breathing techniques, energy conservation, secretion management, assisted cough, and aerobic conditioning can reduce postoperative breathing restrictions, retention of secretions, atelectasis, and pneumonia (77). After wound healing, scar mobilization via soft tissue massage should be initiated to reduce pain and increase chest wall mobility. Shoulder dysfunction affects 33% of post-thoracotomy patients and can be secondary to muscle disruption, chest wall pain with arm movement, and myofascial pain. The focus should be on normalizing glenohumeral and scapulohumeral mechanics. With disruption of the serratus anterior, scapular fixation and shoulder abduction are impaired. This is identified by restriction in abduction when upright that resolves when supine, with the thorax fixed against a hard surface. Fixing the scapula mechanically with taping, bracing, or through physical therapy can help to normalize scapular mechanics. In rare case, surgical fixation may be required. Latissimus disruption can lead to weakness in adduction. More commonly, patients develop restriction to forward flexion and abduction secondary to latissimus tightness. Latissimus tightness is usually addressed with soft tissue techniques and forward-flexion wall walking. Once normal range of motion is obtained, scapulohumeral rhythm and strengthening of the shoulder commence. Strengthening and normalization of movement may take up to one year in patients with shoulder dysfunction. In certain cases, physical therapy may benefit patients for scapular stabilization techniques. The final phase of rehabilitation is return to vocational and recreational activity. This should be addressed while keeping in mind the status of the underlying disease process. In those with significant underlying pulmonary compromise, concurrent pulmonary rehabilitation may be beneficial.

CONCLUSION

Upper extremity pain disorders in the cancer population can be distressing and result in severe functional loss. An understanding of the underlying malignancy and treatment can clarify common etiologies of cancer pain. For those with an unclear etiology, a systematic approach is required to exclude recurrent malignancy and establish a clear diagnosis. An established diagnosis can be a great relief to the patient and may avoid unnecessary delays in cancer treatment. Once the diagnosis is established, pain control and functional restoration become the focus of treatment.

References

1. Stubblefield MD, Custodio CM. Upper extremity pain disorders in breast cancer. *Arch Phys Med Rehabil.* 2006;87(3 Suppl 1):S96–S99.
2. Buckwalter JA, Brandser EA. Metastatic disease of the skeleton. *Am Fam Physician.* 1997;55:1761–1768.
3. Coleman RE. Clinical features of metastatic bone disease and risk of skeletal morbidity. *Clin Cancer Res.* 2006;12(20 Suppl):6243s–649s.
4. Fang K, Peng C. Predicting the probability of bone metastases through histological grading of prostate carcinoma: a retrospective correlative analysis of 81 autopsy cases with ante-mortem transurethral resection specimens. *J Urol.* 1983;57:715–720.
5. Abrams HL. Metastases in carcinoma. *Cancer.* 1950;3:74–85.
6. Healey JH, Turnbull ADM, et al. Acrometastases: a study of 29 patients with osseous involvement of the hands and feet. *J Bone Joint Surg Am.* 1986;68:743–746.
7. Libson E, Bloom RA, et al. Metastatic tumors of the bones of the hand and foot: A comparative review of and report of 43 additional cases. *Skeletal Rad.* 1987;16:387.
8. Hage WD, et al. Orthopedic management of metastatic disease. Incidence, location, and diagnostic evaluation of metastatic bone disease. *Ortho Clin North Am.* 2000;31(4):515–528.
9. Brage ME, Simon MA. Metastatic bone disease. Evaluation, prognosis and medical treatment considerations of metastatic bone tumors. *Orthopedics.* 1992;15:589–596.
10. Mercadante S. Malignant bone pain: pathophysiology and treatment. *Pain.* 1997;69:1–18.
11. Mirels H. Metastatic disease in the long bones. A proposed scoring system for diagnosing impending pathological fractures. *Clin Orthopedics.* 1989;249:256–264.
12. Frassica FJ, Frassica DA. Evaluation and treatment of metastases to the humerus. *Clin Orth Related Res .*2003;415S:S212–S218.
13. Needham PR, Hoskin PJ. Radiotherapy for painful bone metastases. *Palliat Med.* 1994;8:95–104.
14. Sudo A, et al. Intramuscular metastases of carcinoma. *Clin Ortho.* 1993;296:213–217.
15. Damron TA, Heiner J. Orthopedic management of metastatic disease. Management of metastatic disease to soft tissue. *Ortho Clin North Am.* 2000;31(14).
16. Willis RA. Secondary tumors in sundry unusual locations. The Spread of Tumours in the Body. *Butterworths.* 1973;282–300.
17. Van der Windt DA, et al. Shoulder disorders in general practice. Incidence, patient characteristics and management. *Ann Rheum Dis.* 1995;54:959–964.
18. Gomoll AH, et al. Rotator cuff disorders. Recognition and management among patients with shoulder pain. *Arthritis Rheum.* 2004;50(12):3751–3761.
19. Uhthoff HK. Classification and definition of tendonopathies. *Clin Sports Med.* 1991;10:693–705.
20. Nadler SF, Schuler S, Nadler JS. Cumulative trauma disorders. In: *Physical Medicine and Rehabilitation Principles and Practice,* 4th ed. 2005:620–621.
21. Wilson JJ, Best TM. Common overuse tendon problems. A review and recommendations for treatment. *Am Fam Physician.* 2005;72:811–818.
22. Barr KP. Rotator cuff disorders. *Phys Med Rehabil Clin N Am.* 2004;15:475–491.
23. Klaiman MD, Fink K. Upper extremity soft tissue injuries. In: *Physical Medicine and Rehabilitation Principles and Practice,* 4th ed. 2005:835.
24. Dias R, et al. Frozen shoulder. *BMJ.* 2005;331:1453–1456.
25. Reeves B. The natural history of frozen shoulder. *Scand J Rheumatism.* 1976;4:193–196.
26. Harrast MA, Rao AG. The stiff shoulder. *Phys Med Rehabil Clin N Am.* 2004;15:557–573.
27. Walsh NE, Dumitru D, et al. Treatment of the patient with chronic pain. In: *Physical Medicine and Rehabilitation Principles and Practice,* 4th ed. 2005:519–520.
28. Ready LB, Kozody R, Barsa JE, Murphy TM. Trigger point injection versus jet injection in the treatment of myofascial pain. *Pain.* 1983;15:201–206.
29. Chesire WP, et al. Botulinum toxin in the treatment of chronic myofascial pain. *Pain.* 1994;59:65–69.
30. Klaiman MD, Fink K. Upper extremity soft tissue injuries. In: *Physical Medicine and Rehabilitation Principles and Practice,* 4th ed. 2005:837–838.
31. Leach RE, Miller JK. Lateral and medial epicondylitis of the elbow. *Clin Sports Med.* 1987;6:259–272.
32. Bissett L, et al. Mobilization with movement and exercise, corticosteroid injection, or wait and see for tennis elbow. A randomized controlled trial. *BMJ.* 2006;333:939–945.
33. Van Ouwenaller. Painful shoulder in hemiplegia. *Arch Phys Med Rehabil.* 1986;67:2326.
34. Yu D. Hemiplegic shoulder. *Phys Med Rehabil Clin N Am.* 2004;15(3):683–697.
35. Snels IAK, et al. Treating patients with hemiplegic shoulder pain. *Am J Phys Med Rehabil.* 2002;81:150–160.
36. Nicholson BD. Evaluation and treatment of central pain syndromes. *Neurology.* 2004;62(Supp 2):S30–S36.
37. Schwartzman RJ, et al. Neuropathic central pain epidemiology, etiology and treatment. *Arch Neurol.* 2001;58(10):1547–1550.
38. Carette S, Phil M, Fehlings MG. Cervical radiculopathy. *NEJM.* 2005;353:392–399.
39. Rao R. Neck pain, cervical radiculopathy and cervical myelopathy. Pathophysiology, natural history and clinical evaluation. *J Bone Joint Surg Am.* 2002;84:1872–1884.
40. Galecki J, et al. Radiation induced brachial plexopathy and hypofractionated regimens in adjuvant irradiation of patients with breast cancer. A review. *Acta Oncologica.* 2006;45:280–284.
41. Johannson S. Radiation induced brachial plexopathies. *Acta Oncologica.* 2006;45:253–257.
42. Posner JB. Neurologic complications of cancer. *Contemp Neurol Ser.* 45:330–332.
43. Posner JB. Neurologic complications of cancer. *Contemp Neurol Ser.* 45:185–190.
44. Hausheer FH, et al. Diagnosis, management and evaluation of chemotherapy-induced peripheral neuropathy. *Semin Oncol.* 2005;33:15–49.
45. Spies JM, Macleod JG. Paraneoplastic neuropathy. In: Dyck PJ, Thomas PK, eds. *Peripheral Neuropathy,* Vol. 4. 2005:2471–2485.
46. Amato AA, Dumitru D. Acquired neuropathies. Neuropathies associated with malignancy. In: *Electrodiagnostic Medicine,* 2nd ed. 2002:989–990.

47. Posner JB. Neurologic complications of cancer. *Contemp Neurol Ser.* 45:353–385.

48. Heit JA, et al. Risk factors for deep vein thrombosis and pulmonary embolism. A 25-year population based study. *Arch Int Med.* 1998;158:585–593.

49. Lee AYY, Levine MN. Venous thromboembolism and cancer: risks and outcomes. *Circulation.* 2003;107:I17–I21.

50. Cormuz J, et al. Importance of the initial evaluation for cancer in patients with symptomatic idiopathic deep venous thrombosis. *Ann Int Med.* 1996;125:785–793.

51. Lee AYY, et al. Low molecular weight heparin versus Coumadin for the prevention of venous thromboembolism in cancer. *NEJM.* 2003;349:146–153.

52. Morrell RM, et al. Breast Cancer-Related Lymphedema. *Mayo Clin Proc.* 2005;80(11):1480–1484.

53. Herd-Smith A, et al. Prognostic factors for lymphedema after primary treatment of breast carcinoma. *Cancer.* 2001;92:1783–1787.

54. Stubblefield MD, Custodio CM. Rotator cuff tendonitis in lymphedema: a retrospective case series. *Arch Phys Med Rehabil.* 2004;85(12):1939–1942.

55. Petrek JA, et al. Lymphedema: current issues in research and management. *CA Cancer J Clin.* 2000;50:292–237.

56. Erickson VS, Pearson ML, et al. Arm edema in breast cancer patients. *J Natl Cancer Inst.* 2001;93:96–111.

57. Moskovitz AH. Axillary web syndrome after axillary dissection. *Am J Surg.* 2001;181:434–439.

58. Leidenius M, et al. Motion restriction and axillary web syndrome after sentinel node biopsy and axillary clearance in breast cancer. *Am J Surg.* 2003;185(2):127–130.

59. Rezende LF, Franco RL, Gugel MSC. Axillary web syndrome practical implications. *Breast J.* 2005;11(6):531.

60. Swartz MN. Cellulitis. *NEJM.* 2004;350:904–912.

61. Woo PCY, et al. Cellulitis complicating lymphedema. *Eur J Clin Microbiol Inf Dis.* 2000;19:294–297.

62. Madaras-Kelly KJ, Arbograst R. Increased therapeutic failure of cephalexin versus comparator antibiotics in the treatment of uncomplicated outpatient cellulitis. *Pharmacotherapy.* 2000;20(2):199–205.

63. Macdonald L, et al. Long-term follow-up of breast cancer survivors with post-mastectomy pain syndrome. *Br J Cancer.* 2005;92(2):225–230.

64. Schulze T, et al. Long-term morbidity of patients with early breast cancer after sentinel lymph node biopsy compared to axillary lymph node dissection. *J Surg Oncol.* 2006;93(2):109–119.

65. Smith WC, et al. A retrospective cohort study of post-mastectomy pain syndrome. *Pain.* 1999;83:91–95.

66. Tasmuth, et al. Pain and other symptoms after different treatment modalities of breast cancer. *Ann Oncol.* 1995;6:453–459.

67. Katz J, et al. Risk factors for acute pain and its persistence following breast cancer surgery. *Pain.* 2005;119(1–3):16–25.

68. Jung BF, et al. Neuropathic pain following breast cancer surgery: proposed classification and research update. *Pain.* 2003;104(1–2):1–13.

69. Rothenmund Y, et al. Phantom phenomena in mastectomized patients and their relation to chronic and acute pre-mastectomy syndrome. *Pain.* 2004;107(1–2):140–146.

70. Hazelrigg SR, et al. Acute and chronic pain syndromes after thoracic surgery. *Surg Clinics North Am.* 2002;82:849–865.

71. Erdek M, Staats PS. Chronic pain after thoracic surgery. *Thoracic Surg Clin.* 2005;15(1):123–130.

72. Karmakar M, Ho A. Post-thoracotomy pain syndrome. *Thoracic Surg Clin.* 2004;14(3):345–352.

73. Gotoba Y, et al. The morbidity, time course and predictive factors for persistent post-thoracotomy pain. *Eur J Pain.* 2001;5:89–96.

74. Li W, Lee T, Yim A. Shoulder function after thoracic surgery. *Thoracic Surg Clin.* 2004;14(3):331–343.

75. Richardson J, et al. Post-thoracotomy neuralgia. *Pain Clin.* 1994;7(2):87–97.

76. Merskey H. Classification of chronic pain: description of chronic pain syndromes and definitions of pain terms. *Pain.* 1986;3:S138–S139.

77. Yegin A, et al. Early post-operative pain after thoracic surgery: pre- and post-operative versus post-operative analgesia: a randomized study. *Eur J Cardiothoracic Surg.* 2003;24(3):420–424.

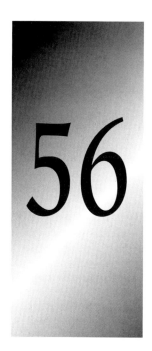

Lower Extremity Disorders in Cancer

56

Robert W. DePompolo
Julia F. Boysen
Mary J. Scherbring
David Martin Strick

Cancer and its treatment can result in various lower extremity musculoskeletal complications that may negatively influence a patient's function. This may be from underlying skeletal complications or from muscular, vascular, neuropathic, or systemic causes. Articular problems from noncancer origin, such as osteoarthritis, can occur in patients with cancer. In addition, many other musculoskeletal conditions likely coexist in patients with cancer. It is incumbent on those who care for patients with cancer to be familiar with these various complications and underlying conditions and how they may present. By the timely diagnosis and effective treatment of these problems, we can limit lower extremity pain that would otherwise limit the mobility and independence of patients with cancer and thereby improve the person's overall quality of life. This chapter will discuss the causes, evaluation, and treatment of common lower extremity musculoskeletal complications and conditions likely to occur in patients with cancer.

ETIOLOGY

Pain is common in patients with cancer. It is estimated that one-third of patients receiving active treatment have pain, with many more cases of pain in patients with advanced disease (1). The causes of lower extremity pain in patients with cancer are numerous. The pain may be from muscle, joint, or bone disorders. In addi-

tion, there are neurologic, vascular, and systemic causes that should be considered. Pain may result from the direct effects of tumor or be related to treatments such as surgery, chemotherapy, or radiation. It is important to remember that pain is often unrelated to the cancer or its treatment. When a patient with cancer presents with lower extremity pain, one must have a well-thought-out approach to discover its cause so that optimal treatment can be provided.

MUSCULOSKELETAL CAUSES

Bone Metastases

Lower extremity pain in the general population is often caused by musculoskeletal problems. In patients with cancer, nonmalignant (degenerative or traumatic) disorders of muscle and bone are also common causes of lower extremity pain. However, malignant causes need to be considered. If the pain has mechanical features, bone metastasis should be considered present until proven otherwise. Mechanical features include increased pain with weight bearing, joint range of motion, resisted forces during muscle testing, and/or other mechanical loading, such as torque, bending, or axial loading. Tumors likely to metastasize to bone, especially the pelvis, spine, and proximal long bones, include breast, prostate, and lung cancers (2). Plain radiographs (x-rays) of the painful area are an

KEY POINTS

- In addition to the effects of cancer and its treatments, such as surgery, chemotherapy, and radiation therapy, lower extremity pain in patients with cancer may result from muscle, joint, or bone problems as well as neurologic, vascular, and systemic causes.
- If lower extremity pain has mechanical features, bone metastasis should be considered present until proven otherwise.
- Overall bone density may be indirectly affected by cancer and its treatments, and could contribute significantly to the potential for insufficiency fractures.
- Point tenderness over the lateral hip (greater trochanter bursa) and medial knee (pes anserine bursa) may suggest bursitis, which may respond to corticosteroid injection.
- The majority of the arthritis seen in the cancer setting is due to osteoarthritis.
- Sprains are not infrequent in hospitalized or debilitated cancer patients, but may not be readily recognized, as the patient may not always recount the injurious event. Signs of trauma such as pain, swelling, erythema, and warmth may follow the injury by several hours and prompt investigation of other disorders, such as thromboembolism or cellulitis.
- Leptomeningeal carcinomatosis may affect a single nerve root (monoradiculopathy), but frequently involves multiple nerve roots, resulting in a polyradicular syndrome that often mimics sensorimotor polyneuropathy.
- The most common cause of cancer-associated neuropathies is related to the administration of antineoplastic neurotoxic agents.
- It has long been recognized that persons with a diagnosis of cancer are at increased risk for development of deep vein thromboses (DVTs).
- A thorough yet focused history ascertaining the character, location, onset, and duration of the patient's pain is important in establishing a differential diagnosis for the cancer patient's lower extremity pain complaints.

inexpensive and simple first step in excluding metastasis as a cause of pain. However, significant cortical destruction must occur before radiographic abnormalities are apparent. If any irregularities are noted, or if clinical suspicion is high, magnetic resonance imaging (MRI) or computed tomography (CT) is indicated to better define pathology in the area of interest.

Insufficiency Fractures

In addition to the direct impact on the bone by tumor, overall bone density may be indirectly affected by cancer and its treatments and contribute significantly to the potential for insufficiency fractures. Immobility due to prolonged illness can cause osteopenia, as can poor nutrition from anorexia. Chemotherapeutic agents, such as methotrexate and doxorubicin, may contribute to bone loss both directly and indirectly. Steroids are commonly used in the cancer setting and are perhaps the most common pharmacologic cause of bone density deterioration in oncology patients. Radiation therapy has also been linked to osteopenia and can cause radio-osteonecrosis (3,4). Besides possible insufficiency fracture, avascular necrosis of the femoral head and other bones can occur from steroid use and/or radiation therapy. It is, therefore, imperative to consider bony pathology as the cause of lower extremity pain in patients with cancer.

Soft Tissue Tumors

Soft tissue metastases are a relatively rare cause of lower extremity pain, but should be considered in the differential diagnosis of cancer patients presenting with leg, pelvic, or buttock pain. Carcinomas, lymphomas, sarcomas, schwannomas, multiple myelomas, and melanomas are tumors that can cause limb pain by their impact on surrounding structures. Often, these soft tissue tumors present as a painful mass in patients without prior history of cancer (5,6). However, non-neoplastic conditions, such as myositis ossificans, ganglion cyst, abscess, and bursitis, can also present as a painful soft tissue mass in the leg (7).

Bursitis

While lower extremity and hip pain with weight bearing may represent bone cancer, point tenderness over the pelvis and hip may suggest bursitis. Ischiogluteal bursitis causing back and leg pain has been reported in patients with cancer and can mimic soft tissue metastasis (8,9). Likewise, greater trochanteric bursitis over the hip and pes anserine bursitis of the medial knee may cause limb pain in patients with cancer. These conditions can nicely respond to corticosteroid injections and physical modalities. Therefore, after metastatic disease has been excluded, these soft tissue pains need to be considered, as the pain can be readily controlled, allowing the patient better mobility and function.

Myofascial Pain

Buttock and leg pain may also be from myofascial pain syndromes. Underlying bone or neurologic disorders may result in secondary muscle tightness and spasm, with subsequent soft tissue shortening, contractures, microischemia, and inflammation all resulting in myofascial pain. Gluteal and pyriformis muscles can become painful from back and radicular pain or from underlying bone lesions or hip joint pain. The hamstrings and gastrocsoleus muscles can become contracted from prolonged immobilization precipitated by illness or due to underlying bone pain from tumor. Regardless of whether the pain is primarily myofascial or secondarily by myofascial from underlying disease, it often responds to heat, cold, diathermy, massage, and stretching. The pain may also respond to nonsteroidal anti-inflammatory drugs (NSAIDs), muscle relaxants, and nerve stabilizers (pregabalin, gabapentin, nortriptyline). Trigger point injections with local anesthetics (lidocaine, bupivacaine) may also provide significant relief for as long as four weeks in some patients. Identifying its existence is, therefore, useful for improving pain control and patient function. Even if the underlying disease causing the myofascial pain is untreatable, the myofascial pain can be better controlled, reducing pain and often eliminating a barrier to walking or sitting. Interestingly, widespread and regional body pain in the general population seems to be associated with an increased risk of cancer and reduced cancer survival after diagnosis (10).

Arthritis

If the lower extremity pain is isolated to a joint, such as hip, knee, ankle, or foot, it may be due to an inflammatory or noninflammatory arthritis. Given that many patients with cancer are immunosuppressed and thrombopenic, joint sepsis or hemarthrosis should be considered if the joint shows evidence of inflammation, such as increased warmth, erythema, and/or marked swelling. Other possible causes of monoarticular inflammatory arthritis include gout and pseudogout, both of which can be precipitated by cancer treatment. A joint aspiration may be helpful in diagnosis.

The majority of the arthritis seen in the cancer setting is due to osteoarthritis. The treatment approach in the cancer population is similar to that of the general public and may include, as appropriate, education, weight loss, physical therapy, gait aids, NSAIDs and other pain medications, and injections with corticosteroids or viscosupplementation. It should be noted that in patients with a poor overall prognosis who suffer from mono- or oligoarticular arthritis that limits their function and quality of life, steroid injections, when effective, can be given more frequently than in other patients, as the long-term integrity of the joint is not a concern. The risk of infection and adrenal suppression, however, should be weighed against the risk of further functional decline.

Plantar Fasciitis

Lower extremity pain that is more isolated to the foot may be plantar fasciitis. The deconditioning and weakness that occurs with cancer may cause patients to load their foot and ankle improperly, stressing the plantar fascia. In addition, the plantar fascia may be tightened by prolonged immobility during treatment or flare of the disease. As the patient becomes active again, they may aggravate the plantar fascia, causing inflammation and pain over the bottom of the foot. Findings may include plantar surface foot pain with walking that is decreased with rest, heat, and cold. Palpation of the plantar surface of the foot is painful, as is stretch to the plantar fascia. Plantar fasciitis can be treated with heat, cold, stretches, proper shoe orthotics to support the arch, and nonsteroidal anti-inflammatory drugs. Improving any underlying abnormal gait mechanics is important to achieving a durable therapeutic response and preventing plantar fasciitis from returning.

Sprains

Generalized weakness can result in poor gait mechanics, transfer technique, joint loading, and susceptibility to falls, all of which can result in joint sprains. Weakness also leads to immobility, further contributing to contractures and tightening of supporting soft tissue structures. This lack of mobility and flexibility makes joints more prone to injury when subjected to trauma. Sprains are not infrequent in hospitalized or debilitated cancer patients, but may not be readily recognized, as the patient may not always recount the injurious event and signs of trauma such as pain, swelling, erythema, and warmth may follow the injury by several hours and prompt investigation of other disorders, such as thromboembolism or cellulitis.

Following acute injury, protecting the injured joint with bracing may be required. The use of superficial cold, compression, elevation, and nonsteroidal anti-inflammatory drugs can be helpful with pain management. Once pain control is achieved, restoring joint range of motion and strengthening associated muscle groups are important goals of rehabilitation. Finally, improving any aberrant gait or transfer mechanics is essential to avoid further injury to the joint involved or other trauma to soft tissue or bone.

NEUROPATHIC CAUSES

Neuropathic lower extremity pain may occur from damage to any part of the neural axis, including the thalamus, ascending spinothalamic tracts, nerve root, lumbosacral plexus, and peripheral nerves. Peripheral nerve damage may be part of a generalized large-fiber neuropathy, a small-fiber neuropathy, a mononeuropathy multiplex, or a mononeuropathy.

Central Pain

Primary spinal tumors can be classified according to location: extradural or intradural. Intradural tumors either arise within the spinal cord (intramedullary) or outside of it (extramedullary). Approximately 70% of intradural tumors are extramedullary and 30% are intramedullary. Of the primary intradural tumors, intradural extramedullary schwannoma (neurilemmoma) and meningioma are the most common and are attached to sensory nerve roots and to dura, respectively. Of the intramedullary tumors, 40% are ependymomas, with the next most common being astrocytomas (11).

Spinal tumors can cause pain by bone destruction with subsequent instability or by compressing spinal tracts or exiting nerve roots. The dermatomal distribution of radicular pain is well known to most clinicians. Central pain (also known as funicular pain), however, is not as well understood, but is believed to be caused by disruption of the ascending spinothalamic tracts or posterior columns. Funicular pain generally exhibits the qualities of other neuropathic pain disorders in that it is characterized by deep, ill-defined, and painful dysesthesias, burning, or stinging. Lhermitte phenomenon (lightninglike sensations down the back with neck flexion) may be present. Funicular pain may affect any part of the body, including the face, trunk, and extremities, but does not follow radicular distributions and is not useful in lesion localization.

Radiculopathy

Spinal nerve roots may be affected by meningeal infiltration from various cancers (12). Leptomeningeal carcinomatosis may affect a single nerve root (monoradiculopathy), but frequently involves multiple nerve roots, resulting in a polyradicular syndrome that often mimics sensorimotor polyneuropathy (13). Injury to nerve roots occurs as a result of altered blood supply and metabolism as tumor invades the roots by travers-

ing the subarachnoid space (12,14). Clinically, there is radicular pain, dermatomal sensory loss, areflexia, and lower motor neuron weakness (15,16).

Primary spinal nerve root tumors are rare and include neurofibromas and schwannomas. These tumors present insidiously with progressive radiculopathy and/or myeloradiculopathy. The most common symptom is gradual and progressive pain in the radicular distribution of the corresponding dermatome of the affected nerve root. Hypesthesia, tingling, numbness, and burning are also frequently associated. Weakness is the second most common symptom and may be associated with myelopathy or lower motor neuron weakness (17).

Plexopathy

Radiation

The lumbosacral plexus is vulnerable to radiation because of its close proximity to commonly radiated areas. However, this complication of irradiation for pelvic or lower abdominal cancer (uterus, ovary, testis, rectum, or lymphoma) is far less common than brachial plexopathy (18). Signs and symptoms of radiation-induced plexopathy, including pelvic pain and bilateral lower extremity weakness, may rarely occur acutely. Early-delayed lumbosacral plexopathy is generally transient and begins a few months (median four months) after radiation therapy. Typically, there are bilateral distal paresthesias of the lower extremities. Clinical examination is normal in most cases and improvement follows within three to six months. Late-delayed lumbosacral plexopathy follows radiation therapy by 1–30 years (median 5 years) (19–23). There is usually little or no pain initially, although this may develop or worsen over time (21). Tingling, itching, burning, or numbness may be present in up to 30% of patients (15,23). The clinical course is characterized by slow, progressive, usually asymmetric and bilateral motor deficits associated with less marked sensory deficits. Lower extremity weakness is the earliest manifestation of radiation-induced lumbosacral plexopathy in more than 60% of patients (15). The upper part of the lower plexus (L4–S1) is most frequently involved (15). The patient may stabilize after several months or years (21). Alternatively, the weakness may progress and result in significant function impairment, depending on the neural structures involved.

The risk of developing a lumbosacral plexopathy is greater if the total dose and fraction sizes are higher. Damage to the lumbosacral plexus can occur following local total doses exceeding 4000–6000 cGy (21,24,25). Vascular endothelial cells and Schwann cells are the most affected by radiation, as they have the highest rate of cell turnover. The pathogenesis of postirradiation plexopathy involves radiation-induced vasculopathy, nerve fibrosis, and subsequent Wallerian degeneration (15,23).

Radiation-induced lumbosacral plexopathies usually cannot be differentiated from malignant plexopathies based on anatomical involvement. L5/S1 distribution signs and symptoms are common for both. Lumbosacral radiation injury usually presents with unilateral lower extremity weakness, reduced reflexes, paresthesias, and pain in less than 25% of patients (23). Of note, radiation-induced pain tends to be much less severe than pain produced by tumor invasion (22,23).

Metastatic

The lumbosacral plexus is in close proximity to the colon and rectum, prostate, uterus and ovaries, pelvic, and abdominal lymph nodes. Any tumor invading these structures can invade the plexus (26,27). However, metastatic plexopathy has been reported to occur from extra-abdominal tumors, including breast, lung, thyroid, and stomach as well as melanoma (26). Neoplastic lumbosacral plexopathy is recognizable by pain and sensorimotor deficits in the lower extremities extending outside the territory of a single root or nerve. The symptoms and signs are often unilateral (15). The interval between development of malignancy and diagnosis of plexopathy is usually within one to three years (22,26,27). In approximately 15% of patients, plexopathy was the presenting sign of cancer (22).

Pain is usually the first symptom of metastatic lumbosacral plexopathy (22,23) and it can be the only sign of plexopathy (22). The character of the pain can be cramping (15), aching, pressurelike, stabbing, or burning (26). The lumbosacral plexus is situated within the substance of the psoas muscle and is divided into an upper part (L1–L4) and a lower part (L4/L5–S4). The upper plexus is involved 31% of the time in malignancy (26). Involvement of the upper plexus results in pain at the costovertebral angle. Pain is felt in the groin, anterolateral, or anteromedial thigh and hip. Pain may be referred to the flank or iliac crest (15,22).

The lower lumbar and sacral plexus is involved 51% of the time (26) and produces pain in the buttocks and perineum. Pain extends into the posterolateral thigh, leg, sole, and/or dorsum of the foot (15,22,23). Pain may also be referred to the hip and ankle (22). Panplexopathy (L1–S3) occurs in 18% of patients (26). In this condition, there is pain in the lumbosacral area and referred pain is variable (22). The pain is usually continuous in nature and commonly exacerbated by sudden movement or hip extension (ie, stretching of the iliopsoas muscle).

Within weeks to months after the onset of pain, leg weakness, numbness, or paresthesias may develop. When the upper plexus is involved, weakness of the iliopsoas, adductor, quadriceps, and sometimes anterior tibialis (L4) muscles occurs with loss of the patellar reflex. Sensory changes are not as pronounced, but there may be decreased sensation on the anterior, medial and lateral thigh, and medial leg (15,22,23). Metastasis to the lower lumbar and sacral plexus causes weakness of the glutei, hamstrings, tibialis anterior and posterior, peronei, and gastrocnemius. There is loss of the heel cord reflex, and numbness may be present in the posterior thigh and sole (22,23). Sensory loss occurs in the foot, lateral ankle, and lateral and posterior leg (15). Primary intra-abdominal tumors are more often associated with upper plexopathy or panplexopathy, while metastatic tumors are more often associated with lower plexopathy because of metastasis to the sacrum (22).

Neuropathy

There are three main mechanisms of peripheral neuropathy: (1) Neuronal degeneration (neuronopathy) in which nerve cell bodies are the primary site of malignancy; (2) Axonal degeneration (axonopathy) in which distal axonal breakdown is usually due to a systemic metabolic disorder or toxicity. The process may extend to the myelin sheath of affected axons, start distally, and usually progresses back to the nerve cell body (a "dying-back neuropathy"). This type of neuropathy is manifested clinically as a symmetrical, distal loss of sensory and motor functions beginning in the legs (28). This is the most common neuropathy. (3) Immune-mediated segmental demyelination with relative sparing of axons in peripheral nerves (16).

Compression

Lower extremity peripheral nerve compression can occur from primary pelvic tumors (colon, bladder, prostate, or cervical) that compress nerves as they exit the lumbar or sacral plexus by posterior growth. Compression can also occur as a result of metastatic tumor to adjacent soft tissue or in bone (29). The site of compression is more often in the pelvis than the limb (22).

Nerve compression can be painful, with the pain being radicular in nature and accompanied by severe local aching. The mechanism by which compression causes nerve dysfunction is not entirely known, but direct pressure and ischemia probably both participate. The first pathologic change appears to be demyelination with relative preservation of the axon. Focal demyelinating neuropathies are often asymmetric with depressed deep tendon reflexes and prominent weakness with minimal atrophy (15). Later, axon loss occurs, suggesting ischemia of the nerve (22,29). Axonal polyneuropathy tends to be a distal, symmetrical sensorimotor neuropathy with impairment of distal deep tendon reflexes with distal atrophy in chronic cases (15).

Neuropathies associated with cancer can be distinguished by their time course, affected modality, and underlying pathology. Peripheral neuropathy is present in all cancer patients by the time they have lost 15%–40% of their body weight, and its severity correlates with increasing percentage of weight loss (30).

Mononeuropathy usually occurs in the setting of widespread metastatic tumor. Acute onset of neuropathy is often suggestive of an inflammatory, immunologic, or vascular etiology (15). However, there are reports of individuals with limited disease in whom mononeuropathy was the presenting sign of malignancy. Obturator neuropathy has been reported to signal pelvic cancer (31), obturator nerve and genitofemoral nerve impingement indicative of cervical cancer (32), inferior gluteal and posterior femoral cutaneous nerve demonstrative for colorectal cancer (33), and sciatic neuropathy from gluteal metastasis.

Chemotherapy

The most common cause of cancer-associated neuropathies is related to the administration of antineoplastic neurotoxic agents (15). Pain produced by chemotherapy agents is usually due to injury of the peripheral nerve. In most cases, this is length-dependent, sensorimotor axonal polyneuropathy. Chemotherapy-induced neuropathies usually present initially as burning and tingling, beginning at the toes, and can rapidly be followed by muscle weakness (17). In most cases, the neuropathy is dose-dependent (15) and self-limiting, with the symptoms resolving if the drug dose is reduced or the drug is stopped (15,17). However, recovery may be incomplete. Symptomatic relief of neuropathic pain is often obtained with adjuvant analgesics (17).

Some of the most frequently encountered neuropathies have been reported to be associated with the use of vinca alkaloids, such as vincristine; platinum-based compounds, such as cisplatin; and taxanes, such as paclitaxel (15). Vincristine is an essential component of most regimens for lymphoproliferative diseases. Peripheral neuropathy is observed at conventional doses. Vincristine exerts its antineoplastic effect by inhibiting microtubule dynamics in mitotic spindles and preventing cell division (34). The effect on microtubules causes damage to axons and disrupts axonal transport. These effects account for paresthesias, dysesthesias, and hyperalgesia that often start at the toes (and fingers), the areas innervated by the longest sensory neurons and presum-

ably the most sensitive to disrupted axonal transport (35). Motor weakness can develop within days, may be severe, and is the dose-limiting effect (36).

Paclitaxel (Taxol) exerts its antineoplastic activity on the microtubule system of cells. Paclitaxel binds to the B-subunit of tubulin and inhibits microtubule depolymerization, inducing cell cycle arrest (16). The interference with microtubule-based axonal transport results in axonal degeneration and neuropathy (37). Approximately 70% of patients who receive paclitaxel develop signs or symptoms of neuropathy (38). A predominantly large-fiber sensory polyneuropathy invariably occurs at doses >200 mg/m^2. Symptoms include paresthesias, numbness, and/or burning pain in a stocking/glove distribution. They are usually symmetrical, but unilateral involvement may occur at the beginning and can develop as early as 72 hours after the initiation of therapy. Motor neuropathy, autonomic neuropathy, central nervous system (CNS) toxicity, myalgias, and arthralgias may also occur (39). Neuromuscular toxicity is the principal dose-limiting toxicity.

Cisplatin has been a major component of most combination regimens to treat advanced ovarian cancer. The primary target of this drug may be the dorsal root ganglion (40). The resulting neuropathy is purely sensory (16) and involves predominantly large-diameter, myelinated sensory fibers, affecting vibration and position sense. Progression of symptoms may occur for several (three to eight) weeks and even after discontinuation of the drug (41). Neuropathy has become the major dose-limiting toxicity (42,43).

Paraneoplastic Neuropathies

A neuropathy that cannot be attributed to any of the previously mentioned cancers or cancer-treatment-related causes, or that is related to specific cancer-related immunological mechanisms, is termed paraneoplastic. Paraneoplastic neurologic disorders may affect any part of the central and peripheral nervous systems, and may mimic any other neurologic complications of cancer. A paraneoplastic disorder usually develops before the presence of cancer is known (44). Symptoms may present in a subacute or acute fashion and are usually progressive, although some patients have relapsing and remitting symptoms (45). The most common presentation of paraneoplastic neuropathies is a distal, symmetrical, sensorimotor polyneuropathy (15).

PARANEOPLASTIC SENSORY NEUROPATHY. A rare paraneoplastic syndrome of purely sensory polyneuropathy has been described in cancer patients (15,46). The neuropathy usually develops over weeks and months and may be slowly progressive or stable

(47,48). It may present as numbness, paresthesias, or pain in the hands and feet. Proprioception may be severely impaired, resulting in severe gait ataxia and pseudoathetoid movements of the limbs (20,49). Muscle strength tends to be preserved despite some muscle wasting. Autonomic dysfunction is common and can be fatal (15). Paraneoplastic sensory neuropathy in most patients is associated with small lung cell carcinoma, but can be in association with breast, gynecological, and gastrointestinal cancer (15,46,50–54). There is also an association with the presence of type 1 antineuronal nuclear antibodies (anti-Hu antibodies) (46,51). More than 90% of patients with small cell lung cancer and purely sensory neuropathy have significantly elevated titers of anti-Hu antibodies in their sera and CSF (55). Sensory neuropathy has been reported to precede cancer diagnosis by six months to six years (56,57).

PARANEOPLASTIC SENSORIMOTOR NEUROPATHY. Sensorimotor neuropathy is more common than purely sensory neuropathy and occurs most commonly with lung carcinoma, but also with tumors of the stomach, breast, colon, rectum, pancreas, uterus, cervix, thyroid, kidney, prostate, or testis (58). This type of neuropathy may be acute, subacute, or chronic remitting. The acute peripheral neuropathy resembles Guillain-Barré syndrome with acute onset of respiratory symptoms (59). The neuropathy may be demyelinating, but axonal features are more frequent. Subacute neuropathy may present prior to or after cancer diagnosis and is predominately axonal in nature, affecting the distal regions of the extremities. It may be associated with severe weight loss and cachexia (60). Chronic relapsing and remitting sensorimotor neuropathy is less commonly associated with lung cancer (45). This neuropathy is progressive, initially asymmetric and painful, and may precede by up to 29 months the discovery of malignancy.

Mononeuropathy/Mononeuropathy Multiplex

Mononeuropathy or mononeuropathy multiplex may occur as neoplastic neuropathies resulting from direct or metastatic infiltration of peripheral nerves (15,31,61); however, this is extremely rare. The pathogenesis appears to involve infiltration of the nerves by malignant cells or ischemia of the nerve fibers secondary to occlusion of small blood vessels and vasa nervorum with tumor cells (15). The diagnosis is often confirmed by positive CSF cytology or demonstration of infiltration of the nerve(s) by malignant cells by nerve biopsy. Occasionally, neoplastic neuropathies improve after treatment with steroids and plasma-

pheresis. Mononeuropathy may also occur, as in the case of peroneal mononeuropathy that results from compression of the nerve against the fibular head. This entrapment neuropathy has been described in patients with systemic cancer and has been attributed to weight loss (62).

VASCULAR DISORDERS

The most common arterial-based problems encountered in the cancer population involve cerebral arteries and not peripheral arteries. In fact, arterial occlusions affecting the lower extremity are rare in this patient group. Venous complications, however, are common and should be considered when a patient presents with unilateral lower extremity pain. It has long been recognized that persons with a diagnosis of cancer are at increased risk for development of deep vein thromboses (DVTs). The presence of lower extremity edema is not uncommon in the cancer setting, and further studies to better define DVT screening assessment criteria may be valuable (63).

Known risk factors for DVT include the frequent use of vascular access devices; patient immobility, which often results at various points along the cancer trajectory; the hypercoagulable state, which is generally created by the existence of an active malignancy (64); the use of various drugs, including chemotherapy, which may increase a person's risk of DVT development; and the presence of other comorbid conditions that increase the risk of DVT development, including advancing age. In addition, there is currently research into other possible cancer-mediated pathways of DVT development.

There is wide variability in the degree to which patients with cancer experience symptoms such as pain or impairment in the use of their lower extremity upon development of a DVT. Once the diagnosis has been made and treatment initiated, mobility and edema management issues should be addressed. Generally, this includes the use of compression with garments or compression wraps, as well as elevation to slowly reduce edema. Decisions about custom-made versus standard-sized stockings, as well as the type of compression wrap (low stretch vs high stretch) are best made by the treating therapist in collaboration with the patient. Among the factors that influence this decision are the patient's motivation and ability to manage these interventions. The management of any other associated symptoms is also indicated. Facilitating the patient's mobility with the use of appropriate compensatory strategies, which may include a gait aid, should also occur early in the course of treatment.

INTEGUMENTARY/SYSTEMIC DISORDERS

Persons with a diagnosis of cancer may develop a variety of skin disorders as a complication or manifestation of the primary tumor, as a treatment-induced side effect, or as a result of a metastatic process from a large number of solid and hematologic tumors. The skin of the lower extremity is among the sites where cutaneous changes may manifest themselves; therefore, impairment in function may accompany these skin changes. Malignant melanoma, while not the most common skin cancer, may create significant impairments in skin integrity with accompanying functional deficits. Treatment-related skin changes can occur with a large number of chemotherapy agents that are used (65), although the newer biologic or targeted drugs appear less likely to cause this type of problem except on the skin of the face. The use of radiation therapy also creates skin changes, some of which are more immediate, and others which may occur months to years after treatment. In addition, various infectious processes may occur in any cutaneous tissues. It should also be mentioned that cutaneous paraneoplastic processes, such as acanthosis nigricans, are another complication of cancer (66). The nature of the skin problem must be assessed and treated. Concurrent attention to any functional deficit will allow the patient to have the best chance for maximizing their recovery and maintaining previous function.

Particularly in the elderly, who often have a variety of diffuse musculoskeletal concerns, malignancy can be found to present itself in a number of less common ways. Among this group of problems is included amyloid arthritis, carcinomatosis polyarthritis, dermatomyositis/polymyositis, hypertrophic pulmonary osteoarthropathy, Raynaud phenomenon, secondary gout, and vasculitis. It is noteworthy that lower extremity involvement is more commonly seen with carcinomatosis arthritis than upper extremity involvement. The clinical management and response of the patient's malignancy is likely to be closely associated with any response in the musculoskeletal symptoms that the patient presented with (67).

Infections

Due to the high rate of compromised immunity among cancer patients, infections, including both systemic but especially those localized to an area or a joint, should be among the differential diagnoses considered in evaluating patients with lower extremity complaints. The presentation of this problem may be atypical (less localizing symptoms, a white blood cell count that is not grossly elevated) due to the host's inability to mount an effective immune response. Diagnostic tests, including cultures of the affected area, may not always reveal a distinct microorganism. Empiric use of antibiotics is not uncommon, and often results in rapid improvement in patient symptoms. Early intervention by a physical therapist to promote ambulation is likely to enhance the patient's recovery.

Myositis/Polymyositis

There is a lack of data about this complication in cancer patients, including both tumor or treatment-related. Inflammatory myopathies generally present with myalgias and weakness more prominent in proximal musculature. In the general population, there is some evidence of benefit with mild exercise, but more data are needed (68). It was recently hypothesized that there may be a paraneoplastic process involving expression of autoantigens involved in creating a cancer-associated myositis (69).

LOWER EXTREMITY EVALUATION

Obtaining a thorough medical history is as important as the physical examination. This is especially critical when obtained from a patient who has not been formally diagnosed with cancer and is being seen by the clinician for "musculoskeletal pain." Cancer can present with many varying symptoms. Pain is a common complaint for cancer patients, with approximately 70% of patients stating that they have experienced severe pain at some time during the course of the illness (70). There are situations wherein referred pain is radiated into the lower extremities. Referred pain is pain that is perceived in a body part that is not innervated by the true source of the pain.

HISTORY, SYSTEMS REVIEW, DIAGNOSTIC TESTING

A thorough yet focused history ascertaining the character, location, onset, and duration of the patient's pain is important in establishing a differential diagnosis for the cancer patient's lower extremity pain complaints. Identifying exacerbating and remitting factors can help guide management. Sometimes it is helpful to create a symptom map, if applicable. It is imperative that the clinician review the medical record and recent health screening information before performing a review of systems.

MUSCULOSKELETAL PHYSICAL EXAMINATION

The examination should take a systematic approach to aid in proper diagnosis. The following is an example:

> Inspection of extremities and spine
> Palpation
> Joint range of motion (ROM)
> Neurologic:
> > Mental status
> > Cranial nerves
> > Muscle strength
> > Reflexes
> > Sensation
> > Balance/coordination
> Functional assessment
> > Gait/station
> > Ability to transfer
> > Bed mobility
> > Toileting/bathing
> > Activities of daily living

MANAGEMENT

The management of lower extremity pain and dysfunction is dependent on the underlying causative factors and is influenced by the patient's underlying cancer process. If the patient has stable disease, restoration efforts will tend to be more aggressive then if the patient were at end of life and receiving hospice and/or palliative care services. There are a variety of treatment options to consider in addition to the use of pharmacologic agents for pain control.

MODALITIES AND EXERCISE

Nonpharmacologic modalities can be advantageous to the cancer patient to avoid unnecessary drug interactions and decrease the likelihood of adverse drug reactions and side effects. Transcutaneous electrical nerve stimulation (TENS) can be beneficial for neuropathic, visceral, musculoskeletal, or postsurgical pain control. Application of ice packs or ice massage can ease musculoskeletal pain, and use of superficial heat can reduce muscle spasms and promote muscle relaxation. Exercise for the cancer patients includes flexibility, strengthening, conditioning, and aerobic exercises. Submaximal strengthening should be the only strengthening program for a hospital-based program for several reasons, but the main concern in cancer patients undergoing chemotherapy or radiation is platelet counts. Platelets

should be monitored daily for inpatients when an exercise program is first established. Patients and families should be educated on safe strengthening measures to ensure understanding.

ASSISTIVE DEVICES AND BRACING FOR THE LOWER EXTREMITY

The best gait aid for the patient in need of an assistive device is based on several factors: the age of the patient, history of falls, inconsistent strength, numbness, reduced proprioception, neuropathy, endurance, pain, or weight-bearing limitations. Options include single-point canes, quad canes/hemiwalkers, front-wheeled walkers, four-wheeled walkers with hand brakes and a seat, axillary crutches, forearm crutches, and if upper extremities are involved, platform attachments. Braces can be used to help with gait stability, safety, and to prevent falls. There are over-the-counter ankle-foot orthoses that are appropriate for short time periods as long as the patient has good sensation and the brace fits well. When over-the counter orthoses are insufficient, an orthotist can make a custom-molded orthosis to offer better joint protection, reduce pressure points, and improve gait dynamics and stability.

DURABLE MEDICAL EQUIPMENT

Equipment needs are based on the patient's functional ability and level of pain. Gait aids can help to reduce weight bearing through the affected lower extremity, thereby reducing pain. Gait aids also help to improve stability and safety during ambulation and transfers. Bathroom aids, such as raised toilet seat, shower chairs, tub benches, and grab bars, can allow the patient to independently and safely transfer from the toilet or bathtub. Hospital beds are helpful for position changes to assist with skin integrity and pain reduction. There are many options for equipment in order to maximize function and independence. The American Cancer Society (ACS) is an excellent reference for local resources available to cancer patients. Services provided through ACS include advocacy, assistance, information and referral services, medical equipment and supplies, prostheses and accessories, support groups, and transportation (71).

GOALS

Goals should be determined based on patient's age, type and stage of cancer, and comorbidities, and should be established with the patient and family. As caregivers, we formulate goals and ideas of what the patient should be able to do; however, the patient and family need to have "buy in" to ensure that the goals are achievable. Past experiences related to the cancer treatment may play a role in the patient's thoughts and perceptions related to their own function. A perceived loss of control can affect how motivated the patient will be to regain independence. Family members can also hinder progression toward goals if they do not allow the patient to independently perform functional activities that the patient is capable of performing.

The goals of rehabilitation are to promote and assist the patient to achieve maximal physical and social functioning, to allow the patient to return to a level of premorbid functional status in mobility and activities of daily living, and to provide adaptive equipment to maximize independence and to assist family members with caring for the cancer patient (72).

CONCLUSION

The most recent data available regarding cancer continue to create a picture of improved survival. Jemal et al. report a 66% five-year survival rate for all races and all cancers in the United States (73). This data compel all clinicians involved in the care of cancer patients to consider what the needs of those patients, beyond the acute diagnosis and treatment stage, are likely to be. This subject has been gaining attention over the last several years, and the Institutes of Medicine report published in 2006 titled *From Cancer Patient to Cancer Survivor* (74) has added momentum to this initiative. Among the many suggestions that are coming forth are some that are specific to those health care providers whose focus is physical medicine and rehabilitation. For example, the authors suggest four essential components of survivorship care, with number 3 being "Intervention for consequences of cancer and its treatment, for example: medical problems such as lymphedema and sexual dysfunction; symptoms, including pain and fatigue; psychological distress experienced by cancer survivors and their caregivers; and concerns related to employment, insurance, and disability." (p. 3) The report is broad and comprehensive, with suggestions that address everything from the education of health care providers, to the development of evidence-based systems and models of care, to reimbursement for all phases of cancer care. What is quite striking throughout is the tremendous potential for addressing and improving the many aspects of care that are commonly the focus of physical medicine and rehabilitation practitioners, including eliminating barriers to activity such as leg pain.

DEDICATION

This chapter is dedicated to the memory of Mary Scherbring, RN, CNS. Mary was a beloved oncology clinical nurse specialist at Mayo Clinic when she was diagnosed with a rare form of lymphoma in February 2007. Throughout her career, she devoted much of her time and energy to serving patients with cancer. Although Mary was undergoing intense chemotherapy and radiation therapy during the writing of this chapter, she diligently continued to research and assist with completion of the project. She felt strongly about ensuring that patients with cancer had optimum quality of life, and that passion gave Mary the persistence to see this chapter to fruition. We completed this chapter in May. Mary passed away in June 2007.

References

1. Foley KM. Support care and quality of life. In: DeVita VT, Hellman S, Rosenberg SA, eds. *Cancer: Principles & Practice of Oncology*, 7th ed. Philadelphia: Lippincott Williams & Wilkins; 2005:2615.
2. Catala E, Martinez J. Bisphosphonates. In: de Leon-Casasola OA, ed. *Cancer Pain: Pharmacologic, Interventional, and Palliative Approaches*, 1st ed. Philadelphia: Saunders Elsevier; 2006:337–347.
3. Croarkin E. Osteopenia in the patient with cancer. *Phys Ther.* 1999;79:196–201.
4. Hamilton SA, Pecaut MJ, Gridley DS, et al. A murine model for bone los from therapeutic and space-relevant sources of radiation. *J Appl Physiol.* 2006;101:789–793.
5. Damron TA, Heiner J. Distant soft tissue metastases: a series of 30 new patients and 91 cases from the literature. *Ann Surg Oncol.* 2000;7(7):526–534.
6. Ball AB, Serpell JW, Fisher C, Thomas JM. Primary soft tissue tumors of the pelvis causing referred pain in the leg. *J Surg Oncol.* 1991;47(1):17–20.
7. Crundwell N, O'Donnell P, Saifuddin A. Non-neoplastic conditions presenting as soft-tissue tumours. *Clin Radiol.* 2007;62(1):18–27.
8. Mill GM, Baethge BA. Ischiogluteal bursitis in cancer patients: an infrequently recognized cause of pain. *Am J Clin Oncol.* 1993;16(3):229–231.
9. Volk M, Gmeinwieser J, Hanika H, Manke C, Strotzer M. Ischiogluteal bursitis mimicking soft-tissue metastasis from a renal cell carcinoma. *Eur Radiol.* 1998;8(7):1140–1141.
10. McBeth J, Silman, AJ, Macfarlane GJ. Association of widespread body pain with an increased risk of cancer and reduced cancer survival. *Arthritis Rheum.* 2003;48(6):1686–1692.
11. Stieber VW, Tatter SB, Shaffrey ME, Shaw EG. Primary spinal tumors. In: Schiff D, O'Neill BP, eds. *Principles of Neuro-Oncology.* New York: McGraw-Hill Companies, Inc.; 2005:501–531.
12. Olson ME, Chernik NL, Posner JB. Infiltration of the leptomeninges systemic cancer. A clinical and pathologic study. *Arch Neurol.* 1974;30(2):122–137.
13. Allanore Y, Hilliquin P, Zuber M., Renoux M, Menkes CJ, Kahan A. A leptomeningeal metastasis revealed by sciatica. *Rev Rheum Engl Ed.* 1999;66(4):232–234.
14. Grossman SA, Krabak MJ. Leptomeningeal carcinomatosis. *Cancer Treat Rev.* 1999;25(2):103–119.
15. Selim M, Chad DA, Recht LD. Neuromuscular disease and its complications. In: Schiff D, Wen PY, Schiff D, Wen PY, eds. *Cancer Neurology in Clinical Practice.* Totowa, NJ: Humana Press, Inc.; 2003:121–134.

16. Balmaceda C, Korkin E. Cancer and cancer treatment-related neuromuscular disease. In: Schiff D, Wen PY, eds. *Cancer Neurology in Clinical Practice*. Totowa, NJ: Humana Press, Inc.; 2003:193–213.

17. Bhattacharyya AK, Guha A. Spinal root and peripheral nerve tumors. In: Schiff D, O'Neill BP, eds. *Principles of Neuro-Oncology*. New York: McGraw-Hill Companies, Inc.; 2005:533–549.

18. Schiodt AV, Kristensen O. Neurologic complications after irradiation of malignant tumor of the testis. *Acta Radiol Oncol Radiat Phys Biol*. 1978;17(5):369–378.

19. Béhin A, Delattre J-Y. Neurologic sequelae of radiotherapy on the nervous system. In: Schiff D, Wen PY, eds. *Cancer Neurology in Clinical Practice*. Totowa, NJ: Humana Press, Inc.; 2003:173–191.

20. Glass JP, Pettigrew LC, Maor M. Plexopathy induced by radiation therapy. *Neurology*. 1985;35(8):1261.

21. Thomas JE, Cascino TL, Earle JD. Differential diagnosis between radiation and tumor plexopathy of the pelvis. *Neurology*. 1985;35(1):1–7.

22. Sripathi N, Rogers LR. Cancer metastasis to the peripheral nervous system. In: Schiff D, O'Neill BP, eds. *Principles of Neuro-Oncology*. New York: McGraw-Hill Companies, Inc.; 2005:629–646.

23. Hammack JE. Cancer and cancer treatment-related neuromuscular disease. In: Schiff D, Wen PY, eds. *Cancer Neurology in Clinical Practice*. Totowa, NJ: Humana Press, Inc.; 2003:57–70.

24. Bowen J, Gregory R, Squier M, Donaghy M. The post-irradiation lower motor neuron syndrome: neuronopathy or radiculopathy? *Brain*. 1996;119(5):1429–1439.

25. Ashenhurst E, Quartey GR, Starrevald A. Lumbo-sacral radiculopathy induced by radiation. *Can J Neurol Sci*. 1977;4(4):259–263.

26. Jaeckle KA, Young DF, Foley, KM. The natural history of lumbosacral plexopathy in cancer. *Neurology*. 1985;35(1):8–15.

27. Taylor BV, Kimmel DW, Krecke KN, Cascino TL. Magnetic resonance imaging in cancer-related lumbosacral plexopathy. *Mayo Clin Proc*. 1997;72(9):823–829.

28. Redmond JM, McKenna MJ. Quantitative sensory testing. *Muscle Nerve*. 1996;19(3):403–404.

29. Posner JB. Pathophysiology of metastases to the nervous system. In: DeAngelis LM, Posner JB eds. *Neurologic Complications of Cancer*. Philadelphia: FA Davis Company; 1995:15–36.

30. Hawley R, Cohen M, Saini N, Armbrustmacher VW. The carcinomatous neuromyopathy of oat cell lung cancer. *Ann Neurol*. 1980;7(1):65–72.

31. Rogers LR, Borkowski GP, Albers JW, Levin KH, Barohn RJ, Mitsumoto H. Obturator mononeuropathy caused by pelvic cancer: six cases. *Neurology*. 1993;43(8):1489–1492.

32. Saphner T, Gallion HH, Van Nagell JR, Kryscio R, Patchell RA. Neurologic complications of cervical cancer. A review of 2261 cases. *Cancer*. 1989;64(5):1147–1151.

33. LaBan MM, Meerschaert JR, Taylor RS. Electromyographic evidence of isolated inferior gluteal nerve compromise: an early representation of recurrent colon carcinoma. *Arch Phys Med Rehabil*. 1982;63(1):33–35.

34. Tanner KD, Levine JD, Topp KS. Microtubule disorientation and axonal swelling in unmyelinated sensory axons during vincristine-induced painful neuropathy in rat. *J Comp Neurol*. 1998;395(4):481–492.

35. Tanner KD, Reichling DB, Levine JD. Nociceptor hyper-responsiveness during vincristine-induced painful peripheral neuropathy in the rat. *J Neurosci*. 1998;18(6):6480–6491.

36. Rosenthal S, Kaufman S, Vincristine neurotoxicity. *Ann Int Med*. 1974;80(6):733–737.

37. Rowinsky EK, Chaudhry V, Cornblath DR, Donehower RC. Neurotoxicity of Taxol. *Monogr Natl Cancer Inst*. 1993;15:107–115.

38. Campana WM, Eskeland N, Calcutt NA, Misasi R, Myers RR, O'Brien JS. Prosaptide prevents paclitaxel neurotoxicity. *Neurotoxicology*. 1998;19(2):237–244.

39. RS, Rowinsky EK. Patient care issues: the management of paclitaxel-related toxicities. *Ann Pharmacother*. 1994;28 (5 suppl):S27–S30.

40. ter Laak MP, Hamers FP, Kirk CJ, Gispen WH. rhGCF2 protects against cisplatin-induced neuropathy in the rat. *J Neurosci Res*. 2000;60(2):237–244.

41. Mollman JE, Hogan WM, Glover DJ, McCluskey LF. Unusual presentation of cis-platinum neuropathy. *Neurology*. 1988;38(3):488–490.

42. Roelofs RI, Hrushesky W, Rogin J, Rosenberg L. Peripheral sensory neuropathy and cisplatin chemotherapy. *Neurology*. 1984;34(7):934–938.

43. van der Hoop RG, van der Burg ME, ten Bokkel Huinink WW, van Houwelingen C, Neijt JP. Incidence of neuropathy in 395 patients with ovarian cancer treated with or without cisplatin. *Cancer*. 1990;66(8):1697–1702.

44. Roenfeld MR, Dalmau J. Paraneoplastic syndromes of the nervous system. In: Schiff D, Wen PY, Schiff D, Wen PY, eds. *Cancer Neurology in Clinical Practice*. Totowa, NJ: Humana Press, Inc.; 2003:159–169.

45. Croft PB, Urich H, Wilkinson M. Peripheral neuropathy of sensorimotor type associated with malignant disease. *Brain*. 1967;90(1):31–66.

46. Pourmand R, Maybury BG. AAEM case report #31: paraneoplastic sensory neuronopathy. *Muscle Nerve*. 1996;19(12):1517–1522.

47. Dropcho EJ. Neurologic paraneoplastic syndromes. *J Neurol Sci*. 1998;153(2):264–278.

48. Graus F, Bonaventura I, Uchuya M, et al. Indolent anti-Hu-associated paraneoplastic sensory neuropathy. *Neurology*. 1994;44(12):2258–2261.

49. Sterman AB, Schaumburg HH, Asbury AK. The acute sensory neuropathy syndrome: a distinct clinical entity. *Ann Neurol*. 1980;7(4):354–358.

50. Stübgen JP. Neuromuscular disorders in systemic malignancy and its treatment. *Muscle Nerve*. 1995;18(6):636–648.

51. Hughes R, Sharrack B, Rubens R. Carcinoma and the peripheral nervous system. *J Neurol*. 1996;243(5):371–376.

52. Amato AA, Collins MP. Neuropathies associated with malignancy. *Semin Neurol*. 1998;18(1):125–l44.

53. Croft PB, Wilkinson M. Carcinomatous neuromyopathy: its incidence in patients with carcinoma of the lung and carcinoma of the breast. *Lancet*. 1963;1:184–188.

54. Riva M, Brioschi AM, Marazzi R, Donato MF, Ferrante E. Immunological and endocrinological abnormalities in paraneoplastic disorders with involvement of the autonomic system. *Ital J Neurol Sci*. 1997;18(3):157–161.

55. Dalmau J, Graus F, Rosenblum MK, Posner JB. Anti-Hu associated paraneoplastic encephalomyelitis/sensory neuropathy: a clinical study of 71 patients. *Medicine (Baltimore)*. 1992;71(2):59–72.

56. Chalk CH, Windebank AJ, Kimmel DW, McManis PG. The distinctive clinical features of paraneoplastic sensory neuronopathy. *Can J Neurol Sci*. 1992;19(3):346–351.

57. Chalk CH, Lennon VA, Stevens JC, Windebank AJ. Seronegativity for type 1 antineuronal nuclear antibodies ("anti-Hu") in subacute sensory neuronopathy patients without cancer. *Neurology*. 1993;43(11):2209–2211.

58. Fisher CM, Williams HW, Wing ES Jr. Combined encephalopathy and neuropathy with carcinoma. *J Neuropathol Exp Neurol*. 1961;20:535–547.

59. Klingon GH. The Guillain Barré Syndrome associated with cancer. *Cancer*. 1965;18:157–163.

60. Croft PB, Wilkinson M. The course and the prognosis in some types of carcinomatous neuromyopathy. *Brain*. 1969;92(1):1–8.

61. Barron KD, Rowland LP, Zimmerman HM. Neuropathy with malignant tumor metastases. *J Nerv Ment Dis*. 1960;131:10–31.

62. Rubin DI, Kimmel DW, Cascino TL. Outcome of peroneal neuropathies in patients with systemic malignant disease. *Cancer*. 1998;83(8):1602–1606.

63. Kirkova J, Oneschuk D, Hanson J. Deep vein thrombosis (DVT) in advanced cancer patients with lower extremity edema referred for assessment. *Am J Hosp Palliat Med.* 2004;22:2,145–148.

64. Naschutz JE, Yeshurun d, Eldar S, Lev LM. Diagnosis of cancer-associated vascular disorders. *Cancer.* 1996;77:9,1759–1767.

65. Gallagher J. Management of cutaneous symptoms. *Semin Oncol Nurs.* 1995;11:4,239–247.

66. Crosby DL. Treatment and tumor-related skin disorders. In: Berger A, Portenoy RK, Weissman DE, eds. *Principles and Practice of Supportive Oncology.* Philadelphia: Lippincott-Raven; 1998:251–264.

67. Erkan D, Yazici Y, Paget S. Inflammatory musculoskeletal diseases in the elderly—Part 2. *Journal of Musculoskeletal Medicine.* 2002;19:320–329.

68. Iverson MD, Liang MH, Fincksh A. Major inflammatory and non-inflammatory arthritides. In: Frontera WR., Slovik DM, Dawson DM, eds. *Exercise in Rehabilitation Medicine,* 2nd ed. Champaign: Human Kinetics; 2006:157–179.

69. Levine SM. Cancer and myositis: new insights in an old association. *Curr Opin Rheumatol.* 2006;18(6):620–624.

70. Rubin P. *Clinical Oncology,* 8th ed. Philadelphia, Pennsylvania: Saunders Company; 2001.

71. American Cancer Society. (Accessed March 13, 2007, at http://www.cancer.org/docroot/home)

72. Cheville A. Cancer rehabilitation. *Semin Oncol.* 2005;32: 219–224.

73. Jemal A, Siegel R, Ward E, Murray T, Xu J, Thun MJ. Cancer statistics 2007. *CA Cancer J Clin.* 2007;57:1,43–66.

74. Institute of Medicine and National Research Council of the National Academies. From Cancer Patient to Cancer Survivor Lost in Transition. Washington DC: National Academies Press; 2006.

Radiation Fibrosis Syndrome

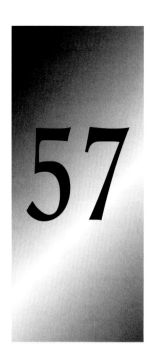

57

Michael D. Stubblefield

Cancer-related morbidity results not only from the direct and indirect effects of disease, but as importantly, from treatments such as surgery, chemotherapy, and radiotherapy (1). These treatments may result in neuromuscular and musculoskeletal complications, including pain, muscle spasm, spasticity, contracture, loss of sensation, weakness, and loss of limb (2). In addition, dysfunction of any visceral organ, including the heart, lungs, genitourinary, and gastrointestinal tract, may occur. Radiation-induced toxicity is a major cause of long-term disability following cancer treatment. This chapter will discuss radiation fibrosis syndrome (RFS), the term used to describe the myriad clinical manifestations of progressive fibrotic sclerosis that can result from radiation treatment. The long-term neuromuscular and musculoskeletal complications of radiation therapy will be emphasized, as visceral complications are discussed elsewhere in this textbook. While this chapter is primarily concerned with the long-term effects of radiation, the reader should note that patients treated for cancer rarely receive radiation in isolation and that surgery, chemotherapy, and degenerative disorders associated with aging and other processes may significantly contribute to the morbidity in a given patient.

PATHOPHYSIOLOGY

Radiation is essentially packets of energy that may include photons or particles such as protons, neutrons, and electrons. Penetration of tissue by these energy packets produces ionizations that can cause direct (ie, to DNA) or indirect tissue damage by the production of hydroxyl radicals (OH-). The anticancer strategy of radiation therapy is to use high-energy radiation to kill rapidly proliferating tumor cells with relative sparing of the surrounding and typically less active normal cells. The two basic modes of radiation delivery include external beam radiation (EBRT), where radiation is delivered from outside the body, and brachytherapy, where radiation is delivered from within the body. A variety of advanced dose-sculpting techniques have been developed to deliver extremely high doses of radiation to the targeted tissues with minimal exposure of the adjacent normal tissues. Dose-sculpting techniques include intensity-modulated radiotherapy (IMRT) and image-guided radiotherapy (IGRT) (3). Radiation can be used either for intent to cure or palliatively, with the intention of prolonging life, prolonging function, or decreasing pain (4,5). Radiation is often used adjuvantly with surgery or chemotherapy to maximize the potential benefit (6,7).

The primary effect of radiation on tissues is the induction of apoptosis or mitotic cell death via free radical-mediated DNA damage. A variety of other secondary effects occur that are mediated by cytokines, chemokines, and growth factors. These secondary effects include activation of the coagulation system, inflammation, epithelial regeneration, and tissue remodeling that is mediated by interacting molecular signals that include

KEY POINTS

- Radiation fibrosis syndrome (RFS) is the term used to describe the myriad clinical manifestations of progressive fibrotic sclerosis that can result from radiation treatment.
- It is the abnormal accumulation of thrombin in both the intravascular and extravascular compartments that is responsible for the progressive fibrotic tissue sclerosis that characterizes radiation fibrosis and underlies the RFS.
- Radiation fibrosis can affect any tissue type, including skin, muscle, ligament, tendon, nerve, viscera, and bone.
- The size of the radiation field, the type and susceptibility of underlying tissues to radiation, as well as the patient's individual resistance to the effects of radiation largely determine the potential morbidity of radiation treatment.
- The mantle field (MF) radiation port used to treat Hodgkin lymphoma (HL) includes all lymph nodes in the mediastinum, neck (cervical supraclavicular, infraclavicular), and axilla.
- At the Memorial Sloan-Kettering Cancer Center (MSKCC), we name the neuromuscular component of RFS based on the structures known to be involved. For instance, an HL survivor who received MF radiation and presents with lower extremity spasticity (from myelopathy) and peripheral nerve findings affecting the root, plexus, and nerves within the

radiation field, as well as local myopathy, would be diagnosed as having a "myelo-radiculo-plexo-neuro-myopathy."
- No group of cancer survivors better typifies the potential for long-term radiation complications than those treated for Hodgkin lymphoma.
- A variety of medications, including pentoxifylline (Trental) and tocopherol (vitamin E), as well as hyperbaric oxygen and anticoagulation, have been touted has having a role in stabilizing or even reversing radiation fibrosis. In our clinical experience, these treatment modalities have been disappointingly ineffective.
- The fact that the progressive fibrotic sclerosis of the microvasculature that underlies RFS cannot be affected at this point in time does not mean that there is no treatment of RFS.
- The basic principles that underlie all other disciplines within rehabilitation medicine are applicable to and effective for cancer survivors with RFS.
- No single modality is more important in the successful treatment of RFS than physical and occupational therapy.
- We have found botulinum toxin injection to be of potential benefit in several specific complications of RFS, including radiation-induced cervical dystonia, trismus, painful paraspinal muscle spasms, and focal neuropathic pain disorders.

cytokines, chemokines, and growth factors. Radiation causes endothelial cell apoptosis, increased endothelial permeability, expression of chemokines, and expression of adhesion molecules with the subsequent loss of vascular thromboresistance. The loss of vascular thromboresistance is a result of decreased fibrinolysis, increased expression of tissue factor and von Willebrand factor, and decreased expression of prostacyclin and thrombomodulin. Due to increased vascular permeability, this increased expression of tissue factors and increased local thrombin formation occurs intravascularly, in the perivascular areas, and within the extracellular matrix. It is the abnormal accumulation of thrombin in both the intravascular and extravascular compartments that is responsible for the progressive fibrotic tissue sclerosis that characterizes radiation fibrosis and underlies the RFS (8) (Fig. 57.1).

Radiation fibrosis can affect any tissue type, including skin, muscle, ligament, tendon, nerve, viscera, and bone (9–11) (Table 57.1). The effects of radiation can be acute (occurring during or immediately after treatment), early-delayed (up to three months after

completion of treatment), or late-delayed (occurring more than three months following completion of treatment) (12). Radiation fibrosis is generally a late complication of radiation therapy, which may not manifest clinically for years after treatment. When it does manifest, it may progress insidiously or rapidly and is not reversible (13,14). The progression of RFS is a moving target that can change day to day, month to month, year to year, or even decade to decade. A problem such as severe pain that takes considerable time and effort to control may suddenly and inexplicably resolve only to be replaced by weakness or other surprise symptoms. This phenomenon is unfortunately more likely to be due to demise of an affected neuromuscular structure than to a process of healing.

RADIATION FIELDS

RFS can result locally from radiation treatment to any part of the body (15). The size of the radiation field, the type and susceptibility of underlying tissues

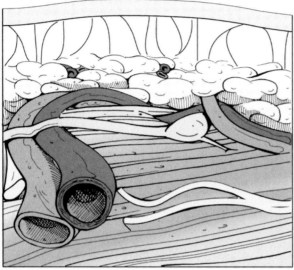

Normal tissue

A

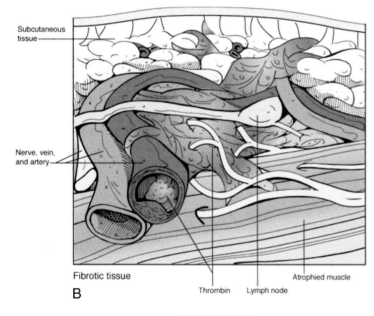

Subcutaneous tissue

Nerve, vein, and artery

Fibrotic tissue

Atrophied muscle

B

Thrombin   Lymph node

FIGURE 57.1

Normal tissue (A) and tissue affected by radiation fibrosis (B). (*See color insert following page 736*)

TABLE 57.1	
Select Tissue Effects of Radiation	
Skin	Dermatitis
	Ulceration
	Infection
Fat	Necrosis
Muscle	Myopathy
Tendon	Rupture
Ligament	Rupture
Bone	Radio-osteonecrosis
Brain	Necrosis
	Infarct
	Encephalopathy
Spinal cord	Necrosis
	Infarct
	Myelopathy
Nerve roots	Radiculopathy
Plexus	Plexopathy
Peripheral nerves	Neuropathy
Blood vessels	Atherosclerosis
	Thromboembolism
	Obliterative endarteritis
	Occlusion
Lymphatics	Lymphedema
	Lymphangitis
Pulmonary	Pneumonitis
	Bronchiolitis obliterans with organizing pneumonia (BOOP)
	Fibrosis
	Pneumothorax
Oral	Stomatitis
	Trismus
	Ulceration
	Candidiasis
	Osteoradionecrosis
	Xerostomia
Cardiac	Pericarditis
	Pericardial effusion
	Coronary artery disease
	Constrictive pericarditis
	Cardiomyopathy
	Valvular heart disease
	Conduction abnormalities
Gastrointestinal	Nausea
	Vomiting
	Gastroenteritis
	Perforation
	Dysmotility
	Malabsorption
	Volvulus
	Intussusception
Bladder	Cystitis
	Fistula
Reproductive organs	Ovarian failure
	Gonadial failure
	Vaginitis
	Vaginal stenosis

to radiation, as well as the patient's individual resistance to the effects of radiation largely determine the potential morbidity of radiation treatment. Some radiation fields are quite extensive, as in the mantle field (MF) radiation port used to treat Hodgkin lymphoma (HL), which involves all lymph nodes in the mediastinum, neck (cervical supraclavicular, infraclavicular), and axilla (Fig. 57.2). Such broad

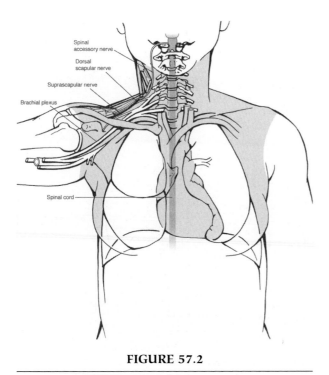

FIGURE 57.2

Mantle field radiation port (shaded area). Note the presence of numerous important and radiosensitive structures within the radiation field.

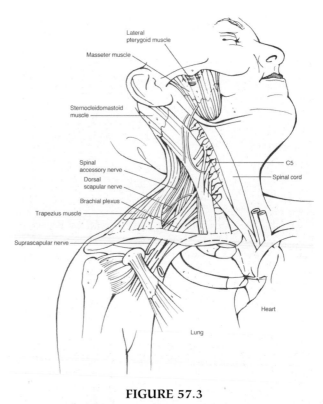

FIGURE 57.3

Patients treated with radiation for head and neck cancers are at particular risk for radiation fibrosis syndrome due to the close proximity of multiple important structures within the head and neck.

radiation fields can result in widespread sequelae of RFS (16). The radiation field can be focal, as when treating isolated vertebral metastases, an extremity sarcoma, a local breast cancer recurrence in the chest wall, or a neoplasm of the head or neck (17,18). Patients radiated for head and neck cancer (HNC) are likely to develop RFS due to the high doses of radiation needed for tumor control and the close proximity of many vital tissues (Fig. 57.3). Understanding the radiation field used to treat a given patient may be instrumental in determining if their signs, symptoms, and functional deficits can be attributable to the radiation (Fig. 57.4). In general, for a structure to be considered affected by RFS, it must either be within the radiation field or, more importantly, receive neural or vascular innervation that traverses the field. Similarly, drainage of lymphatics or veins into the field can result in swelling due to lymphedema or venous insufficiency.

NEUROMUSCULAR AND MUSCULOSKELETAL COMPLICATIONS

The neuromuscular and musculoskeletal complications of RFS stem from both direct and indirect effects

of progressive fibrosis on nerve, muscle, tendons, ligaments, bone, skin, lymphatics, blood vessels, and other tissues.

Nerve

Any level of the nervous system can be affected in RFS (19) (Fig. 57.5). Peripheral nervous system dysfunction can result from ischemia due to fibrosis and stenosis of the vaso vasorum, from external compressive fibrosis of soft tissues, or both (20,21). The primary clinical effects of RFS-induced nerve dysfunction are pain, sensory loss, and weakness, any of which can contribute to functional deficits and decreased quality of life. Autonomic sequelae resulting from damage to autonomic nerves, though rarer, can be extremely disabling and may include orthostatic hypotension, bowel and bladder dysfunction, or sexual dysfunction.

Neuropathic pain is common in RFS. The basic pathophysiology underlying neuropathic pain is the generation of abnormal ectopic activity in neural structures, with the subsequent transmission of those signals into the spinal cord, thalamus, and ultimately

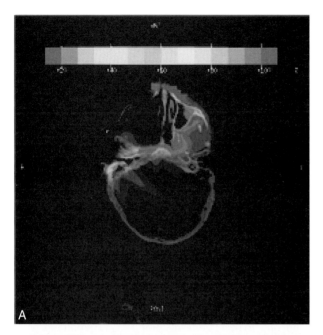

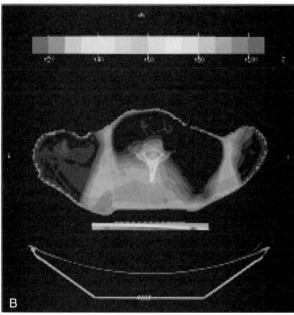

FIGURE 57.4

The 100% isodose curves for radiation treatment planning are depicted overlying a computed tomography scan: planned treatment for a parotid malignancy (A) and treatment planning for a nasopharyngeal cancer (B). (*See color insert following page 736*)

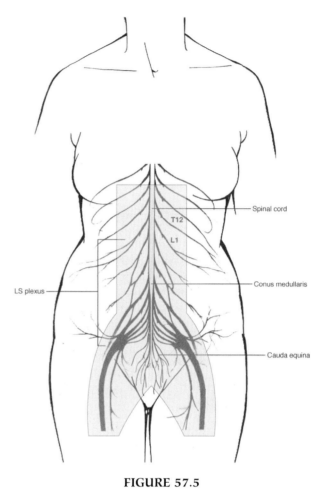

FIGURE 57.5

Neural structures that would be involved by inverted-Y radiation. Note that the spinal cord, conus medullaris, cauda equina, nerve roots, plexus, and peripheral nerves are all within the field and potentially subject to damage.

brain, where they are perceived as painful (22). Because neuropathic pain is not physiologically generated, the experience of pain can be severe and markedly out of proportion to the perceived pathology. Radiation-induced ectopic activity can develop in any affected neural structure, including the brain, spinal cord, nerve root, plexus, and peripheral nerve. The damage generating the signal can be compressive and/or ischemic with subsequent demyelination and/or axonal loss. Ephaptic cross-talk between demyelinated neurons may also result in self-propagating pain signals and is also the process that underlies myokymia.

When the ascending spinal thalamic tracts of the spinal cord are the primary generator of pain signals, the resulting pain can be perceived as both excruciating and nebulous. This is known as funicular pain (23). Funicular pain can be difficult to diagnose because it does not follow dermatomal and other patterns of nerve pain referral familiar to most clinicians. Radiation damage to the funiculi of the cervical spinal cord, for instance, can cause pain perceived in any body part caudal to the area of injury. This may result in pain in the thorax, abdomen, or lower extremities that mimics the pain of radiculopathy, plexopathy, polyneuropathy, mononeuropathy multiplex, or mononeuropathy. More than one area of the body, unilaterally or bilaterally, may be affected. The culprit lesion cannot be localized based on the symptoms of patients with funicular pain. The incidence of funicular pain in patients with RFS is not known, as the disorder is rarely recognized or diagnosed by most clinicians.

More commonly, the neuropathic pain of RFS results from damage to the nerve root, plexus, and/or peripheral nerve. The neural structures involved are largely determined by the location and dose of radiation; however, preexisting or emerging disorders, such as diabetes or spinal degeneration, can affect the nerve root, leaving it more susceptible to the damage caused by RFS. Multiple neural structures may be involved simultaneously. For instance, a patient radiated for nasopharyngeal cancer may demonstrate clinically evident damage to the C5 and C6 nerve roots, upper trunk of the brachial plexus, and spinal accessory nerve. Similarly, a patient with an upper extremity sarcoma may receive damage to the median, ulnar, and/or radial nerves.

It is important to remember that neuropathic pain is generally perceived as referred distal to the lesion. In the case of funicular pain, the pattern of referral has no clinically discoverable bearing on the location of the culprit lesion, save that it is caudal to the lesion. In lesions of the peripheral nervous system, however, the pattern of pain referral is extremely useful for anatomical location. An in-depth understanding of these sensory distributions is critical so that the clinician can determine if a given pain complaint is anatomically congruent with the area of known radiation and thus consistent with RFS. The reader should familiarize themselves with the sensory distributions of the various dermatomes, plexus structures, and peripheral nerves discussed extensively in Chapter 35 on the approach to evaluation of pain disorders.

Neuropathic pain is often accompanied by loss of sensory modalities. Sensory loss from RFS can, however, exist without pain. The primary modalities affected include light touch, pain perception, thermoperception, vibratory sensation, and proprioception. Loss of sensation may render the patient more susceptible to injury and have profound effects on gait and the ability to perform basic activities of daily living, such as buttoning shirts.

Like neuropathic pain in RFS, weakness can be caused by damage to any structure, including the spinal cord, nerve root, plexus, or peripheral nerve. Direct radiation effects on muscle can also be a significant cause of weakness.

Myelopathy is a potential complication any time radiation involves the spinal cord. Patients with myelopathy present with progressive spastic paraparesis or quadriparesis, depending on the level (or levels) of spinal cord irradiated. While symptoms can progress insidiously, they may be punctuated by periods of rapid progression with the potential to result in complete plegia.

Damage to the nerve roots causes weakness in a myotomal pattern. Often, multiple nerve roots are involved. The upper cervical (C1–C6) nerve roots are commonly involved in patients treated for HNC, which can have significant clinical implications as the shoulder girdle (rhomboids, rotator cuff muscles, deltoid, and biceps) are innervated by the C5 and C6 nerve roots. Patients who have received radiation to the conus medullaris and/or cauda equina can present with cauda equina syndrome, a type of polyradiculopathy. We have found subacute and slowly progressive cauda equina syndrome to be a late-term complication in patients with HL who have received periaortic or inverted-Y radiation.

Damage to the brachial and lumbosacral plexus is perhaps the best-known cause of weakness to result from prior radiation. Brachial plexus damage is most common and can be profound with resultant weakness and pain. The upper plexus may be more prone to damage, as its superior location puts it within the field of many head and neck radiation ports and because the pyramidal shape of the chest provides less protective tissue around the upper plexus (24). As with C5 or C6 cervical radiculopathy, damage to the upper trunk of the brachial plexus can weaken the rotator cuff muscles, biceps, and deltoid, with sparing of the rhomboid, as it is innervated before the formation of the plexus. In many cases of RFS, it is difficult to distinguish an upper trunk brachial plexopathy from an upper cervical radiculopathy, both clinically and electrophysiologically, as they are so commonly seen together.

Peripheral nerve dysfunction may be obvious when the radiation involved an extremity, as for sarcoma. It may be less obvious when it keeps company with a variety of other peripheral nerve disorders. For instance, Hodgkin survivors may have a combination of radiculopathy, plexopathy, and mononeuropathies affecting nerves within the radiation field. Commonly affected nerves include the dorsal scapular nerve (C5 before plexus) innervating the rhomboid muscles and the suprascapular nerve (C5, C6, upper trunk of brachial plexus) innervating the supraspinatus and infraspinatus muscles. The summation of radiation damage to nerve pathways at multiple points (C5, C6, brachial plexus) prior to the origination of these peripheral nerves greatly compounds the clinical effects of the mononeuropathies themselves, and is likely an important contributor to the profound muscle weakness and atrophy that can be seen in these muscles in Hodgkin survivors.

Though alluded previously, the concept of neuronal predisposition should be expressly stated, as it can have profound clinical effects in RFS patients. Any preexisting or emerging nerve disorder, at any level of the neural axis from the brain to the distal extremities, can predispose the patient to developing signs and symptoms of nerve dysfunction when challenged with another neural insult along the course of the same nerve (25). For instance, a patient with a brachial plexopathy who requires neurotoxic chemotherapy, develops diabetic neuropathy, or experiences a cervical disk herniation at a level anatomically congruent with their plexus lesion is likely to develop more signs and symptoms than they would have had the lesions not been present together.

Muscle

Progressive fibrosis in muscle fibers within the radiation field can cause focal myopathy that is associated with the formation of nemaline rods (10). These myopathic muscles are weak relative to normal muscle and prone to painful spasms. Progressive damage to the cervical paraspinal muscles combined with damage to neural structures (nerve roots and the posterior primary rami) likely causes the progressive neck weakness and head drop often seen in HL and HNC survivors.

The muscle spasms seen in RFS may also result from direct radiation damage to the muscle. However, just as neuropathic pain arises from the afferent transmission of painful neural activity to the brain, muscle cramps can arise from spontaneous discharges of the motor nerve, sending volleys of neural activity to and across the neuromuscular junction (26). This process has tremendous clinical implications, depending on the nerve or nerves involved. For instance, the ectopic activity in the spinal accessory nerve may be causally related to the spasms of the sternocleidomastoid muscle and trapezius that often characterize radiation-induced cervical dystonia (27). The spinal accessory nerve is involved in the radiation field of many HNCs because it receives a large contribution of fibers from upper cervical nerve roots and the cervical plexus (28). Similarly, radiation damage to the nerve roots can cause painful focal paraspinal or extremity muscle spasms.

The pain associated with muscle spasms is likely similar in many ways to that associated with myofascial trigger points (MTPs) and often occurs in the similar anatomical regions, such as the midtrapezius and rhomboid muscles. Increased activity at the motor endplate (due to ectopic activity in the motor nerve) results in excessive local acetylcholine production and sarcomere shortening. This continuous focal muscle contraction requires high levels of energy and thus oxy-

gen to be maintained, resulting in a decreased local pH. This continuous muscle contraction also results in constriction of local blood supply with subsequent tissue hypoxia. Focal hypoxia and acidification result in the release of inflammatory mediators, neuropeptides, catecholamines, and cytokines with subsequent sensitization of nociceptive nerve fibers. The sensitization of these local pain neurons results in the generation of localized muscle pain (29).

As discussed previously, it is often the case that a patient with RFS will have dysfunction at many levels of the neuromuscular axis. It is important to recognize this component of RFS clinically and describe it appropriately. At the Memorial Sloan-Kettering Cancer Center (MSKCC), we name the neuromuscular component of RFS based on the structures known to be involved. For instance, an HL survivor who received MF radiation and presents with lower extremity spasticity (from myelopathy) and peripheral nerve findings affecting the root, plexus, and nerves within the radiation field, as well as local myopathy, would be diagnosed as having a "myelo-radiculo-plexo-neuro-myopathy." Similarly, if no clinically evident myelopathy was seen but all other levels of the neuromuscular axis were affected, the patient would be deemed to have a "radiculo-plexo-neuro-myopathy."

Tendons and Ligaments

The clinical effect of radiation on tendons and ligaments is one of progressive fibrosis with subsequent loss of elasticity, shortening, and contracture. This is most evident when a mobile joint is involved in the field. Radiation that involves the neck, shoulder, elbow, wrist, hip, knee, ankle, or digits can cause progressive and often marked loss of range of motion and function. The effects of radiation on tendons and ligaments may not occur directly. Indirect effects can occur due to compromise of neuromuscular structures. For instance, weakness of the rotator cuff from radiation affecting the neck with damage to C5, C6, and/or the upper plexus may cause perturbation of normal shoulder motion and is causally related to the development of rotator cuff tendonitis and adhesive capsulitis (30).

Bone

Radiation can contribute to abnormal growth, scoliosis, accelerated osteoporosis, and osteonecrosis (including osteoradionecrosis, avascular necrosis, and aseptic osteonecrosis). Abnormal bone growth is a potential issue for children treated with radiation for sarcoma or other malignancies of the long bones or spine, as the bones may not mature normally if the growth plate is affected (18). Abnormal bone growth is likely due to a combination of direct radiation effects on bone as well as endocrine abnormalities, particularly if radiation involved the cranium (31). Osteoporosis is clinically silent, but may leave patients more susceptible to osteoporotic fractures later in life and should be monitored. Osteonecrosis in survivors of childhood cancers most commonly affects the hip, shoulder, knee, ankle, jaw, elbow, and spine (32).

Skin

Radiation-induced dermatitis is a major acute complication of radiation therapy and usually improves with time. Chronic skin changes include progressive fibrosis, sclerosis, and induration with tenacious and often intractable adherence to underlying tissues. Ulceration of the skin and fistula formation is a particularly unfortunate complication and is most commonly seen in patients treated at or above the tissue tolerance levels for radiation due to recurrent malignancies. Such ulcerations may never heal regardless of treatment (Fig. 57.6).

Lymphatics

Lymphedema is a common complication of cancer and may result from radiation, surgery, or progressive disease. While the lymphatics are fragile and susceptible to radiation injury, it is often difficult to determine the relative contribution of radiation therapy to the development of lymphedema, as radiation therapy is so often accompanied by surgical dissection and/or progressive cancer. Lymphedema can affect any part of the body, including the face, neck, trunk, breast, abdomen, genitalia, and extremities. Most commonly, lymphedema complicates radiation therapy for breast cancer. Treatment of other malignancies, particularly in the pelvis or extremities, can be complicated by lymphedema. Lymphedema is discussed at length in Chapter 79.

Blood Vessels

Microvascular thrombosis is pathogenic in RFS. This thrombosis can affect the arteries, capillaries, and veins. Medium and large blood vessels can also be involved. Occlusion of arteries can be from accelerated atherosclerosis or obliterative endarteritis, as in the cardiac disease associated with MF and other types of radiation affecting the heart. Similarly, peripheral vascular disease can occur in arteries involved in periaortic or inverted-Y radiation fields. Veno-occlusive disease and thromboembolism are also potential complications of RFS. Swelling and postphlebitic syndrome may occur as a result of radiation-induced venous insufficiency.

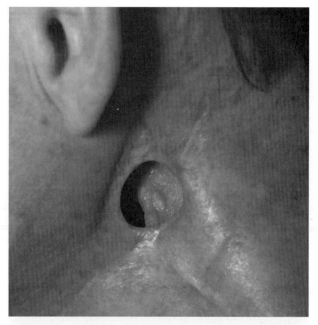

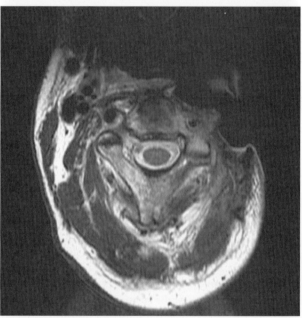

FIGURE 57.6

Photograph (A) and T2 weighted MRI (B) demonstrating a severe radiation-induced ulcer with fistula in a patient treated with multiple resections and three courses of radiation therapy for a head and neck cancer.

RISK FACTORS

The risk of RFS depends on the structures involved in the radiation field, the dose and type of radiation given, and, more importantly, factors intrinsic to the patient, such as preexisting medical conditions (33). For instance, patients radiated for a nasopharyngeal carcinoma may have relatively circumscribed symptoms compared to a patient who has received MF radiation. Though confined to a relatively small area, the manifestations of head and neck radiation for the nasopharyngeal carcinoma may also develop and progress more rapidly than those of the MF radiation given for HL due to the higher doses of radiation used and the proximity of structures within the field. The age and comorbidities of the patient can also have a tremendous impact. HL, for instance, is more likely to affect younger patients than HNC is. These younger patients may be more resilient to the effects of radiation, at least while they are young. As these patients age, not only do the tissue changes of radiation fibrosis tend to progress, but degenerative processes and diseases such as diabetes also may emerge and precipitate the development of symptoms at least partially referable to their past radiation. Similarly, the older patients that comprise the group at risk for HNC are likely to have preexisting cervical degenerative changes prior to their treatment that can predispose them to the effects of radiation.

The effects of radiation are cumulative, and patients radiated more than once at the same location for recurrent disease can be expected to develop worse radiation fibrosis. Patients given higher-than-normal doses of radiation are more likely to develop complications. It is likely that certain patients are more prone to the effects of radiation based on a variety of genetic, environmental, and other as yet uncharacterized factors (34).

DIAGNOSIS-SPECIFIC SEQUELAE

Hodgkin Lymphoma

No group of cancer survivors better typifies the potential for long-term radiation complications than those treated for HL. An in-depth understanding of the pathophysiology responsible for the pain and functional deficits in HL will equip the reader to understand the disorders encountered in survivors of other malignancies treated with radiation. HL is named for Thomas Hodgkin who first described the clinical history and postmortem finding in six patients with massive enlargement of the lymph nodes and spleens (35). In the early 1900s, the first reports that x-rays could shrink the enlarged lymph nodes associated with HL emerged (36). Radiation techniques continued to progress, and the first evidence that limited-stage HL could be cured with high-dose, fractionated radiation therapy was presented in 1950 by Peters, who reported 5-year and 10-year survival rates of 88% and 79%, respectively (37). The concept that early-stage HL could be cured by radiation therapy was not generally accepted until the 1960s. Before then, most patients with lim-

ited HL were either not treated at all or were treated with small doses of radiation (38). Up until the 1990s, patients treated for HL were generally treated using radiation as a single modality and with radiation fields, dose, and technology that are now obsolete. Known as "radical RT" or "total lymphoid irradiation," this approach radiated all involved and uninvolved lymph nodes as well as the spleen to 4400 cGy—a dose near the tissue tolerance level. The advent of treatment combining chemotherapy and radiation allowed for more targeted "involved-field RT" and "involved node RT" with subsequent radiation dose reduction from 4400 to 3000 cGy or even 2000 cGy (39). This approach has allowed for a decrease in morbidity without compromising survival. The common radiation ports used in HL are depicted in Figure 57.7.

HL has an age-related and bimodal incidence, with the largest peak in the third decade and a much smaller peak after age 50 (40). This means that the majority of patients present with HL in their 20s and that the initial survivors of this disease were treated in the 1960s. These initial survivors would now be more than 40 years post-treatment and in their 60s. This fits with our clinical experience and is consistent with the steady stream of 10-, 20-, 30-, and 40-plus-year survivors seen in the MSKCC rehabilitation clinic.

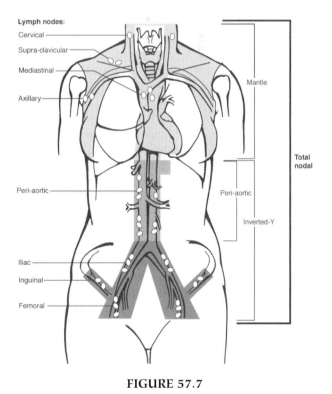

FIGURE 57.7

Common radiation ports used in the treatment of Hodgkin lymphoma include the mantle, periaortic, and inverted-Y fields. When all of these ports are radiated, it is termed "total nodal" irradiation.

Many of these long-term HL survivors have lived rich, full lives. However, most, if not all, have medical issues directly related to their radiation history (41). Psychosocial morbidity is also extremely common in Hodgkin survivors (42). Moreover, many of these survivors express a great deal of dissatisfaction with the medical community at large and describe frequent encounters with clinicians who either fail to recognize or deny that their medical ailments are related to their distant radiation history. The Internet has allowed online support groups to develop and link together cancer survivors from all over the globe. For instance, the Association of Cancer Online Resourses (www.acor.org) has an excellent list-serve dedicated to long-term cancer survivors, many of whom have survived HL. Such resourses have allowed not only the sharing of personal stories, many concerning disappointing interactions with the medical community, but, just as importantly, also the sharing of basic medical information concerning complications and practitioners skilled in the identification and treatment of these maladies.

The late complications experienced by Hodgkin disease (HD) survivors are many, complicated, and interrelated. While most are the result of radiation, many are due to toxic chemotherapeutics, such as doxorubicin, which can cause cardiomyopathy. Less toxic chemotherapeutic regimens have evolved in recent years. Visceral complications of HD treatment include but are by no means limited to heart disease (cardiomyopathy, constrictive pericarditis, pericardial effusion, valvular heart disease, accelerated coronary artery disease, conduction abnormalities), lung disease (pulmonary fibrosis, pulmonary hypertension), vascular disease (carotid stenosis, carotid barrow receptor dysfunction), endocrine dysfunction (hypothyroidism), as well as a variety of gastrointestinal, genitourinary, and sexual disorders (infertility, impotence). Along with cardiac disease, secondary malignancies are perhaps the most ominous late complication of HL and significant causes of mortality (43) (Fig. 57.8). The clinician who evaluates and treats radiation complications should be acutely aware of the vast potential for individual variation in the presenting symptoms and the underlying pathophysiology of disease in Hodgkin survivors. In our clinic, it is not uncommon to encounter surprising and previously undescribed complications of RFS. For instance, one disorder seen in several of our HD survivors is detrusor sphincter dyssynergia (DSD). Commonly seen in patients with multiple sclerosis or spinal cord injury, this disorder in HD survivors may be related to a subacute demyelinating myelopathy. We have also encountered several patients with electrophysiologically documented cauda equina syndrome from distant radiation to periaortic and inverted-Y fields. Electrodiagnostic testing in these patients confirmed polyradiculopathy, as would be expected in cauda

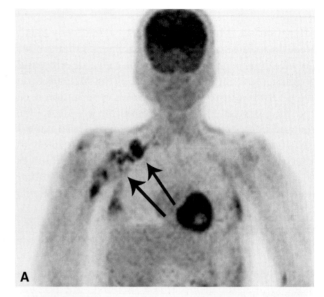

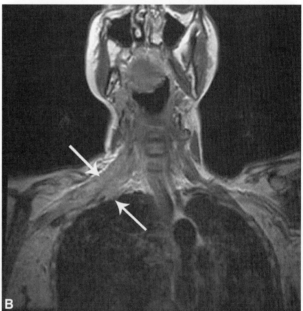

FIGURE 57.8

Positron emission tomography (PET) scan (A) depicting a spindle cell sarcoma in the right brachial plexus of a Hodgkin lymphoma survivor treated with mantle field radiation (arrows). B: Gadolinium-enhanced T1 weighted MRI depicting a malignant peripheral nerve sheath tumor (MPNST) in the right brachial plexus of another HL survivor treated with MF radiation (arrows). Unfortunately, these radiation-induced secondary malignancies are common in this population of patients and represent a significant cause of morbidity and mortality.

equina without evidence for lumbosacral plexopathy. Magnetic resonance imaging (MRI) of their spines did not show central spinal stenosis, disk herniation, or other abnormalities to explain the severity and distribution of clinical and electrophysiologic findings.

Myelopathy

Subacute myelopathy is estimated to occur in as many as 15% of patients treated with MF irradiation for HD (19). In our experience, the myelopathy encountered in HD survivors rarely results in complete paraplegia or quadriplegia. The spinal cord dysfunction is generally more subtle and difficult to fully characterize. DSD as described previously is one manifestation. Other clinical manifestations may include bowel dysfunction, lower extremity spasticity, weakness, sensory abnormalities, ataxia, disordered gait, and funicular pain. Myelopathy is a likely contributing factor to the fatigue seen in many HD survivors.

Myelopathy in HD rarely occurs in isolation and is usually part of a myelo-radiculo-plexo-neuro-myopathy. MRI of the spinal cord rarely demonstrates parenchymal abnormalities, although degenerative changes are often seen in older patients. While there is no definitive test to prove the presence of myelopathy in HD survivors, somatosensory evoked potentials (SSEPs) elicited from the lower extremities may have utility in patients treated only with MF irradiation. Patients with significant peripheral nervous system dysfunction, as from peripheral neuropathy or radiation-induced cauda equina syndrome, cannot be reliably evaluated with SSEPs, as damage to the peripheral nervous system would preclude isolation of deficits to the central nervous system.

Radiculopathy

Radiculopathy in HD survivors is often part of a myelo-radiculo-plexo-neuro-myopathy, but it is more commonly seen without clinically obvious myelopathy. It may be seen rarely in isolation or more commonly as part of a radiculo-plexopathy or a radiculo-plexo-neuro-myopathy. Neuronal predisposition from preexisting or emergent degenerative spine disease is likely an extremity important as an etiologic factor in the development of radiculopathy. Patients treated with MF irradiation generally develop radiculopathy in the upper (C5, C6) levels, but may have more widespread involvement. Patients treated with periaortic or inverted-Y radiation may develop radiculopathy at any lumbosacral segment, but the L5 or S1 levels are most frequently involved, likely due to their coexistence with degenerative changes such as disk herniations and central or neuroforaminal spinal stenosis. A diffuse polyradiculopathy is also seen. As noted previously, polyradiculopathy is consistent with a radiation-induced cauda equina syndrome when no degenerative or other changes (as evidenced by MRI) are present to explain the nerve root dysfunction documented clinically and on electrophysiologic testing.

Electrophysiologically, the radiculopathy associated with radiation is similar, if not identical, to the pattern seen from other causes. In cauda equina syndrome, the findings are more widespread and involve the distribution of more nerve roots. The typical pattern on nerve conduction studies is one of low-amplitude compound muscle action potentials (CMAPs) with normal sensory nerve action potentials (SNAPs). This pattern, however, is only useful for evaluation of C8 or T1 radiculopathies in the upper extremities and L5 or S1 radiculopathies in the lower extremities due to intrinsic limitations of how the test is performed. Electromyography (EMG) may demonstrate widespread spontaneous activity distally, proximally, and in the paraspinal muscles, as well as evidence of motor unit remodeling. Myokymia may or may not be present, and its absence does not exclude radiation as an etiologic contributor. Electrophysiological assessment is greatly complicated when radiculopathy coexists with other disorders of the peripheral nervous system, specifically the plexopathy, neuropathy, and myopathy commonly seen together in HD survivors treated with radiation.

Plexopathy

In our clinical experience, plexopathy is less common in HD survivors than radiculopathy. Plexopathy from MF irradiation is more common than plexopathy from periaortic or inverted-Y irradiation. Brachial plexopathy is rarely seen without a component of radiculopathy, neuropathy of the nerves within the radiation field, and localized myopathy. One possible reason for plexopathy being somewhat less common than radiculopathy is that degenerative changes do not affect the plexus directly. Plexopathy from MF irradiation generally affects the upper brachial plexus more severely than the rest of the plexus, but a panplexopathy can be seen. The pyramidal shape of the thorax provides less tissue to protect the upper plexus, and this may be part of the reason for selective involvement of the upper brachial plexus. Lumbosacral plexopathy from periaortic and inverted-Y radiation is relatively uncommon, but may be seen, usually in combination with the polyradiculopathy of cauda equina syndrome. Electrophysiological assessment of radiation-induced plexopathy in HD is usually complicated by the presence of radiculopathy, focal mononeuropathies, and myopathy.

Neuropathy

The neuropathy associated with MF radiation affects only proximal nerves confined within the field. A polyneuropathy from prior treatment with neurotoxic chemotherapy or other causes, such as diabetes, may be present, but is usually obvious based on history. These polyneuropathies are not due to radiation, but may predispose the patient to the peripheral nervous system dysfunction caused by radiation. Radiation-induced mononeuropathy from MF radiation affects nerves arising directly from the brachial plexus. Nerves originating from the proximal and superior plexus are most commonly involved and include the dorsal scapular nerve to the rhomboids and the suprascapular nerve to the supraspinatus and infraspinatus. Other proximal nerves, including the long thoracic nerve to the serratus anterior, the intercostal nerves, and even the phrenic nerve, can be affected. Nerves originating from the more distal brachial plexus, such as the pectoral nerves, are rarely involved clinically. While it is likely that nerves originating from the lumbosacral plexus (ie, femoral nerve, lateral femoral cutaneous nerve) can be affected by local radiation, we have yet to identify any clinical complications arising from their involvement in HD survivors. As with brachial plexopathy, the electrophysiological assessment of focal mononeuropathies in HD survivors treated with MF radiation is usually complicated by the presence of coexistent pathology, such as radiculopathy, plexopathy, and focal myopathy.

Myopathy

Myopathy is a common complication of MF radiation and is a major contributor to disability in these patients, particularly neck drop. As previously discussed, this nemaline rod myopathy is localized and only affects muscle fibers within the radiation field, such as the cervical and thoracic paraspinal, rhomboid, supraspinatus, and infraspinatus muscles (Fig. 57.9). Patients who have been biopsied for myopathy in muscles outside the radiation field (ie, deltoid) should demonstrate normal muscle tissue. We do not routinely biopsy HD survivors; however, electrophysiological testing is standardly performed, and needle EMG generally demonstrates clearly myopathic motor units in affected muscles (Fig. 57.10). These myopathic units are often interspersed with neuropathic units reflecting the multifac-

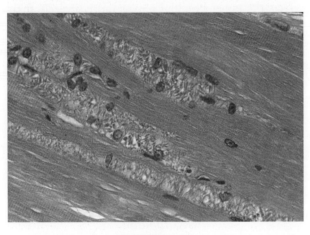

FIGURE 57.9

Trapezius muscle biopsy from a patient with Hodgkin lymphoma treated with mantle field radiation. Note the numerous nemaline rods within the muscle fibers. (From Ref. 10, with permission.) (*See color insert following page 736*)

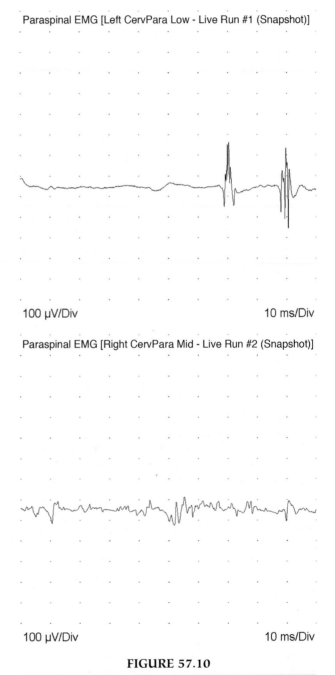

Paraspinal EMG [Left CervPara Low - Live Run #1 (Snapshot)]

100 µV/Div   10 ms/Div

Paraspinal EMG [Right CervPara Mid - Live Run #2 (Snapshot)]

100 µV/Div   10 ms/Div

FIGURE 57.10

Myopathic motor units as seen on needle electromyogram from the cervical paraspinal muscles of a patient treated with mantle field radiation for Hodgkin lymphoma.

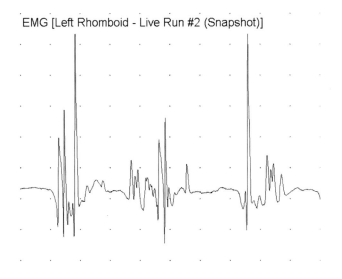

EMG [Left Rhomboid - Live Run #2 (Snapshot)]

100 µV/Div   10 ms/Div

FIGURE 57.11

Neuropathic motor units from the left rhomboid of the same patient in Figure 57.7. Note that these units are neuropathic in nature as opposed to myopathic. Myopathic motor units may also be seen in the rhomboids of patients treated with mantle field radiation.

torial and multilevel nature of neuromuscular dysfunction in RFS patients (Fig. 57.11).

Neck Drop

One of the most common, obvious, and disabling disorders afflicting HD survivors is neck atrophy and weakness (Fig. 57.12). At its worst, this usually painful condition can progress to complete neck drop with inability to maintain the head in a normal upright posture. The atrophy of cervical musculature that precedes neck weakness is essentially universal in HD survivors treated with MF radiation. The underlying pathophysiology is the myelo-radiculo-plexo-neuro-myopathy described previously. Why the neck is so affected in these patients is not entirely clear, but is likely related to the way MF radiation was previously delivered. The pyramidal shape of the neck likely resulted in higher relative doses compared with tissues surrounded by more tissue, as no dose sculpting was used.

While there is no way to reverse the cervical atrophy resulting from MF radiation, the function and quality of life of such patients can be meaningfully improved with physical therapy to improve core as well as neck strength, posture, body mechanics, and endurance. Emphasis on a lifelong home exercise program

is paramount if a durable benefit is to be achieved. In more advanced cases, the use of a cervical collar to assist elevation of the chin is recommended. We find that most patients prefer the Headmaster Cervical Collarmanufactured by Symmetric Designs in Salt Spring Island, British Columbia, as it is generally smaller, lighter, and more adjustable than other collars (Fig. 57.13). Some patients, however, do prefer other cervical collar (ie, the Miami J) designs, and their preferences should be accommodated whenever possible. The cervical collar is not generally intended to be used at all times. It is intended for use as an energy conservation device. We encourage patients who experience pain due to muscular overload or who develop fatigue and inability to elevate their head as the day progresses

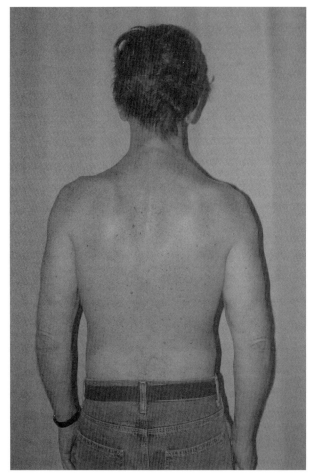

FIGURE 57.12

Muscle atrophy in a patient previously treated with mantle field radiation for Hodgkin lymphoma. Note the prominence of the spinous processes, which extend from the neck to the midback, as well as the scooped-out appearance of the rotator cuff musculature and rhomboids. The deltoids, triceps, and other distal upper extremity muscles are preserved.

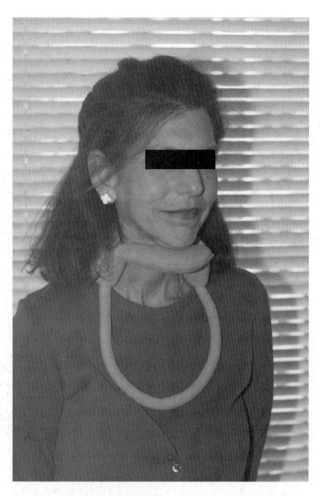

FIGURE 57.13

A Hodgkin lymphoma survivor with neck extensor weakness using a Headmaster Cervical Collar. This design of cervical collar is generally smaller, lighter, and more adjustable than other collars, making it more comfortable and better accepted by most long-term cancer survivors with neck drop.

to use the collar whenever possible and convenient. Activities amenable to use of the collar might include housework, meals, time spent in front of the computer, watching television, reading, etc. Use of the collar during such activities may rest the neck muscles so the patient can tolerate and enjoy activities that occur later in the day without using the collar. For instance, using the collar during work might make it possible to go to dinner with friends after work comfortably without the aid of the collar. It should be noted that the collar is *not* a substitute for a lifelong home exercise program.

Shoulder Pain and Dysfunction

Shoulder pain and dysfunction are common presenting complaints of HL survivors and are usually causally related to their radiation treatment. While much of the shoulder is outside of the direct effects of the radiation field, many of the nerves and muscles that actuate the shoulder are not. The directly radiated structures include the cervical nerve roots, brachial plexus, the rotator cuff muscles, and the peripheral nerves that innervate the rotator cuff. Any damage to the C5 or C6 cervical nerve roots (or upper brachial plexus) causes further weakness of the rotator cuff muscles and referred neuropathic pain to the lateral shoulder and arm. If rotator cuff weakness results in perturbed shoulder motion and allows for anterior translation of the humerus within the glenoid, impingement of the rotator cuff (RTC) tendons may develop and cause a secondary rotator cuff tendonitis and potentially a tertiary adhesive capsulitis due to the local inflammation within the shoulder capsule (44,45).

RTC tendonitis may cause pain at rest that is aggravated by motion. Its diagnosis is generally made on clinical grounds. Diagnostic maneuvers include the Hawkin impingement test, Neer impingement test, and the supraspinatus test (aka empty can test). The Hawkin impingement test is performed by forward-flexing the patient's shoulder to 90°, flexing the elbow to 90?, and forcibly internally rotating the shoulder. This movement pushes the supraspinatus tendon against the anterior surface of the coracoacromial ligament. Pain indicates a positive test for rotator cuff tendonitis (46,47).

This test has a sensitivity of 87%–89% and specificity of 60% for predicting rotator cuff pathology (48,49). To perform the Neer impingement test, forcibly elevate the patient's arm through forward flexion while depressing the scapula. This causes compression of the greater tuberosity against the anteroinferior acromial surface, and discomfort indicates a positive test result (50). The sensitivity of this test for rotator cuff pathology is 89% (49). To perform the supraspinatus test, abduct the patient's shoulder to 90° with neutral rotation and provide resistance to abduction. The shoulder is then medially rotated and angled forward 30° so that the patient's thumb points toward the floor. Resistance to abduction is given while examining for weakness or pain indicating a positive result (46). This test has a sensitivity of 84%–89% and a specificity of 50%–58% for diagnosing rotator cuff tendonitis (47,48). Varying degrees of RTC tearing are often present and can be assessed with the drop arm test. The patient is asked to fully abduct the arm and then slowly lower it. If a tear of the RTC is present, the arm will drop quickly to the patient's side when it reaches approximately 90% of abduction. Adhesive capsulitis is evidenced clinically by restricted shoulder range of motion (particularly external rotation), both actively and passively.

Imaging of the RTC is only done only if clinical assessment, including physical examination, is not

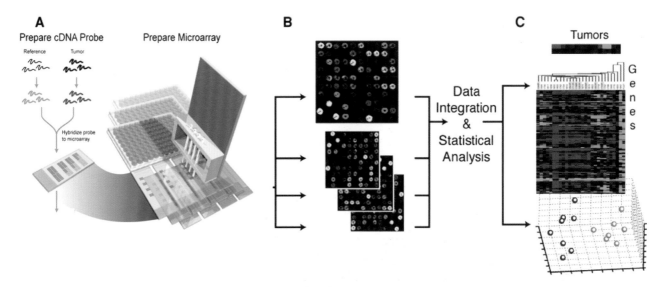

FIGURE 2.1

Gene expression profiling technology. (A) Total RNA from the reference source and the tumor is fluorescently labeled with either Cye-3 or Cye-5-dUTP using a single round of reverse transcription. The fluorescently labeled cDNAs are pooled and allowed to hybridize to the clones on the array. (B) The slide is then scanned with a confocal laser–scanning microscope to measure the fluorescence pattern, monochrome images from the scanner are imported into specialized software, and the images are colored and merged for each hybridization with RNA from the tumor and reference cells. (C) Several statistical methods are used to visualize the expression patterns between tumor samples.

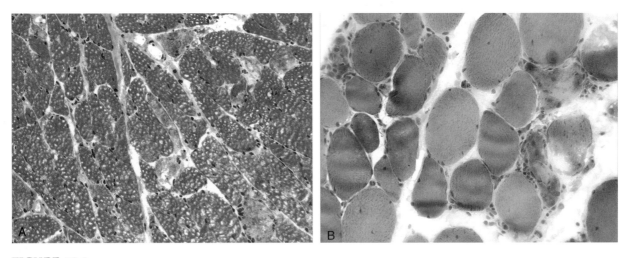

FIGURE 49.2

Paraneoplastic necrotizing myopathy. Scattered necrotic myofibers are present, but there is no accompanying inflammatory infiltrate.

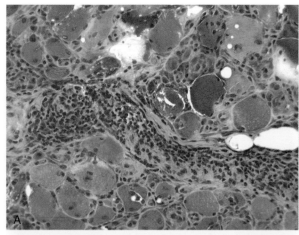

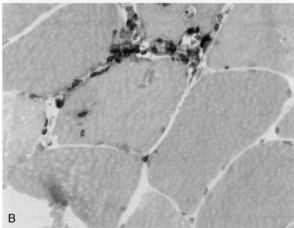

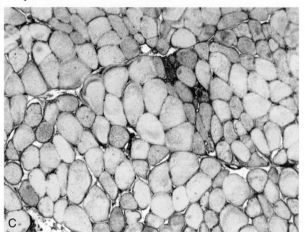

FIGURE 49.3

Polymositis. Marked chronic inflammation, necrosis, and regeneration of muscle fibers (A). Autoaggresive inflammation in polymyositis. T cells attacking an intact muscle fiber (B). Diffuse de novo membraneous MHC-1 expression in muscle fibers (C).

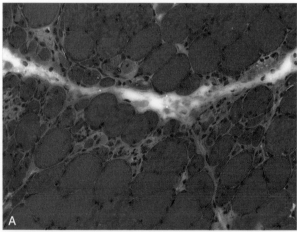

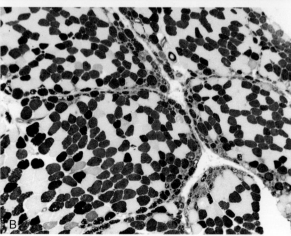

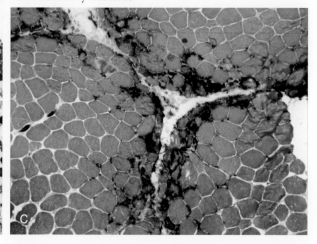

FIGURE 49.4

Paraneoplastic necrotizing myopathy. Scattered necrotic myofibers are present, but there is no accompanying inflammatory infiltrate.

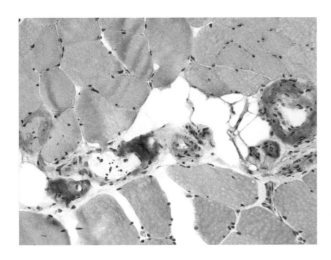

FIGURE 49.5

Amyloid myopathy. Amyloid deposits (arrow) surrounding a muscle fiber, and as intramural/perivascular deposits in the perimysial fibroadipose tissue.

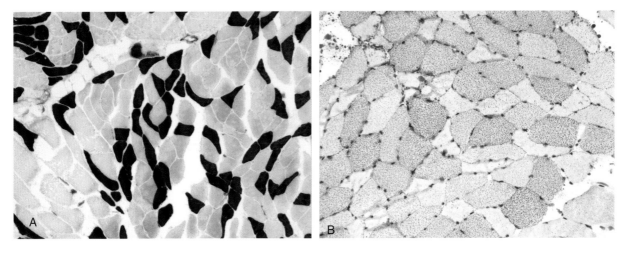

FIGURE 49.6

Steroid myopathy. Selective atrophy of type 1 fibers (A). Type 1 myofibers have increased lipid content (B).

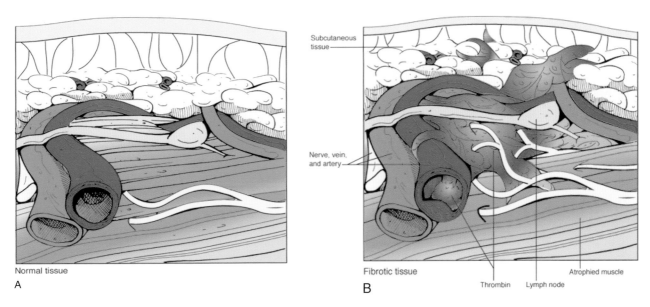

FIGURE 57.1

Normal tissue (A) and tissue affected by radiation fibrosis (B).

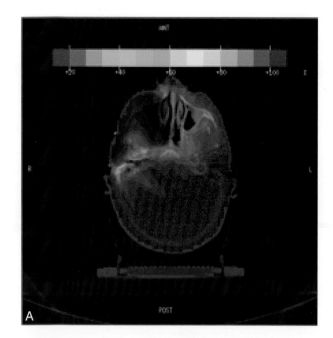
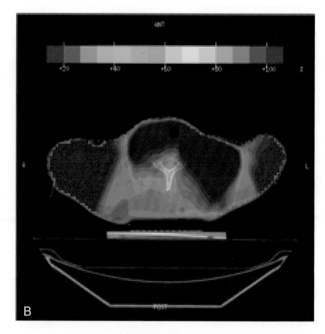

FIGURE 57.4

The 100% isodose curves for radiation treatment planning are depicted overlying a computed tomography scan: planned treatment for a parotid malignancy (A) and treatment planning for a nasopharyngeal cancer (B).

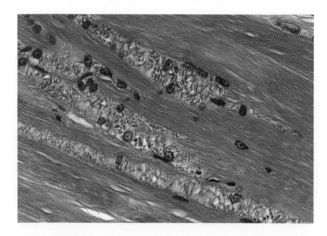

FIGURE 57.9

Trapezius muscle biopsy from a patient with Hodgkin lymphoma treated with mantle field radiation. Note the numerous nemaline rods within the muscle fibers. (From Ref. 10, with permission.)

consistent with what is expected. For instance, MRI would be performed if a palpable mass is present or the pain elicited is atypical (ie, sharply localized to the spine of the scapula suggesting malignancy or fracture). Alternatively, imaging might be indicated if a patient has not responded to initial treatment measures and surgical intervention is contemplated. Generally, shoulder surgery should be avoided in RFS patients, as it is unlikely to affect the marked and progressive neuromuscular disorders that precipitated and will continue to drive the shoulder pathology. Conservative measures are the mainstay of treatment for shoulder pathology. Physical therapy is the primary modality and the only treatment to confer a durable benefit. Therapy should address, among other disorders, rotator cuff weakness and tightness of the pectoral girdle, with the goal of restoring the normal anatomical alignment of the shoulder and thus the rotator cuff tendons within the coracoacromial arch. Anti-inflammatory and/or neuromodulatory medications are often indicated. Subacromial injection, while not curative, may facilitate physical therapy efforts.

HEAD AND NECK CANCER

Head and neck cancers are second only to HL in the number of radiation-related disorders that can be anticipated. As would be expected, sequelae predominantly affect the head and neck region and/or, as in HL, nerves, blood vessels, and lymphatics that traverse the radiation field. Visceral structures outside of the field, such as the heart and lungs, are not affected, but the carotid arteries, thyroid, etc. can be severely affected. The manifestations experienced by a given patient largely depend on the location and size of the radiation field, as well as the dose or doses given (many patients require repeat radiation for recurrence). Manifestations will also depend on preexisting disorders and factors intrinsic to the patient and may range from subclinical to life-threatening.

Disorders including myelopathy, radiculopathy, plexopathy, neuropathy, myopathy, neck drop, and shoulder pain/dysfunction, as discussed previously for HL survivors, are common in HNC survivors and have the same basic pathophysiology and treatment (Fig. 57.14). Neuromuscular and musculoskeletal disorders more likely to be seen in HNC than HL include radiation-induced cervical dystonia and trismus. Radiation-induced trigeminal and anterior cervical neuralgia are also seen. Dysphagia, dysarthria, esophageal stenosis, xerostomia, and other disorders more appropriately addressed by speech and swallowing specialists commonly affect this population and are discussed in Chapter 74.

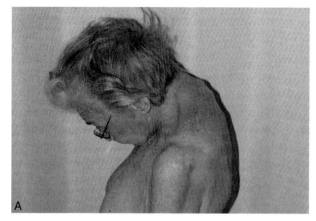

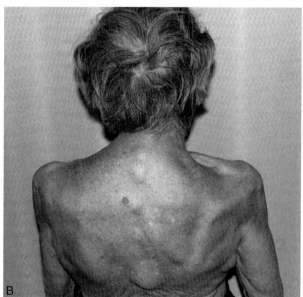

FIGURE 57.14

RFS in an elderly woman five years following treatment of a right-sided nasopharyngeal carcinoma with external beam radiation. Note the severe head drop (A). Marked atrophy of the right rotator cuff muscles, trapezius, and rhomboid (B) is due to radiculo-plexo-neuro-myopathy and results in significant shoulder dysfunction and pain. Though an extreme example, these findings are typical and illustrative of those seen in RFS. This patient was likely treated with a radiation port similar to that seen in Figure 57.4B but lateralized to the right side.

Cervical Dystonia

Cervical dystonia (CD) is a common manifestation of RFS and is termed radiation-induced cervical dystonia when seen as a complication of radiation. CD can result not only from the treatment of HNC, but also from treatment of any tumor where radiation involves the occiput, cervical spine, or upper thoracic spine (51). This includes metastatic disease from any cancer type, sarcomas, HL, thyroid cancer, etc.

Idiopathic cervical dystonia is broadly defined as a movement disorder characterized by involuntary contractions of the head and shoulders, which may be twisted into aberrant positions, including torticollis, laterocollis, retrocollis, and anterocollis (52). In radiation-induced cervical dystonia, progressive radiation fibrosis likely causes ectopic activity in the spinal accessory nerve, cervical nerve roots, and cervical plexus, with subsequent spasms of the trapezius, sternocleidomastoid, scalene, and other neck muscles. Direct radiation effects on muscle may also contribute to muscle spasms. Uncontrollable cervical muscle spasms can cause symmetric or asymmetric positioning of the head and neck.

As radiation fibrosis progresses, fixed contractures develop. Contracture is likely multifactorial from the radiation effects on muscle, nerve, and all involved connective tissues. Muscle spasms may place the head and/or neck in postures that allow for shortening of the tendons and ligaments. The radiation effects on connective tissues also cause progressive fibrosis with subsequent induration, loss of elasticity, and shortening transmurally through affected tissues. The net effect is one of progressive and potentially severe neck tightness and pain. Inability to position the head due to progressive fibrosis can affect swallowing, phonation, and activities of daily living, such as driving and work-related tasks.

Trismus

Radiation-induced trismus is a complication of RFS and may coexist with radiation-induced trigeminal neuralgia, cervical dystonia, or other disorders such as dysphagia or dysarthria. Radiation-induced ectopic activity in trigeminal nerve motor fibers results in spasm and pain, particularly in the masseter and pterygoids. Direct radiation effects on muscle likely contribute to the spasms. If left unchecked, persistent spasms of the masseter can contribute to fixed contracture and ultimately the inability to open the jaw. This phenomenon is almost certainly aided by the adverse effects of radiation on local connective tissues, including the ligaments and tendons. Patients with severe trismus and jaw contracture may have difficulty speaking, eating, drinking, performing oral hygiene, etc. Moreover, the lack of ability to open one's mouth may also affect other social activities and intimacy.

Prevention and early recognition are of paramount importance in trismus, as it can be extremely difficult to improve once it has developed. At MSKCC, we have developed a protocol for identification and early intervention for patients with trismus (Fig. 57.15). In the first six months following treatment, the patients are generally followed by the speech and swallowing service and a Therabite trismus system is employed

Prevention and Management of Trismus

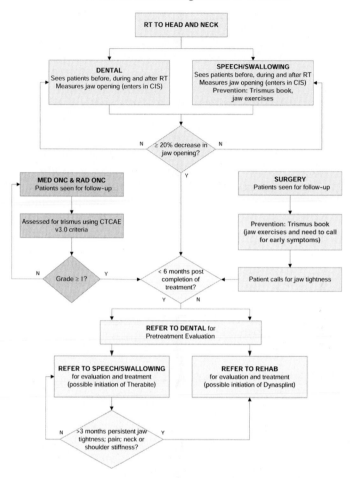

FIGURE 57.15

The Memorial Sloan-Kettering Cancer Center Prevention and Management of Trismus Protocol.

(Fig. 57.16). If the patient's deficits are rapidly progressive, severe, or accompanied by other neuromuscular or musculoskeletal complications, the patients are referred to the rehabilitation medicine service for further assessment.

Once evaluated by a rehabilitation physician, a Dynasplint trismus system is generally ordered (Fig. 57.17). The Dynasplint uses the principle of low-load prolonged stretch, which we have found to be a much more physiologic and effective way to stretch radiated tissue (53). The bite plate of the device is customized by a specialized physical therapist, who will train the patient on the use of the device and individualize a therapy program emphasizing core stabilization, neck range of motion, and ultimately jaw mobilization through deep tissue massage coupled with relaxation and stretching techniques. Any neuromuscular and musculoskeletal complications are treated in conjunction with trismus. A home exercise program

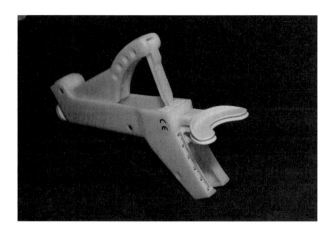

FIGURE 57.16

The Therabite trismus system. This device is generally used for treatment of acute radiation-induced trismus (<6 months post-primary treatment).

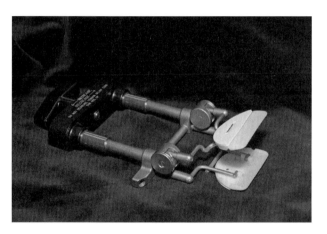

FIGURE 57.17

The Dynasplint trismus system. This device is generally used for treatment of chronic radiation-induced trismus (>6 months post-primary treatment).

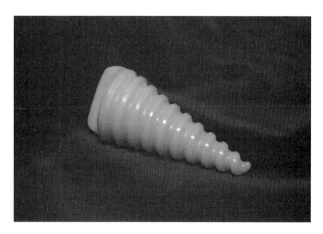

FIGURE 57.18

A corkscrew trismus device. This device is ineffective and should not be used in the management of trismus.

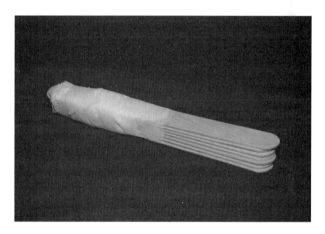

FIGURE 57.19

Tongue depressors are generally ineffective and should not be used in the management of trismus.

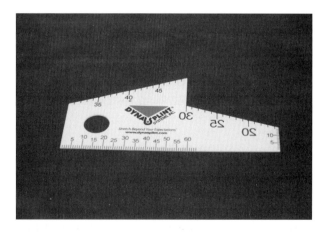

FIGURE 57.20

Jaw-opening measurement device supplied by Dynasplint. This simple and inexpensive plastic device is an effective way to objectively measure and follow the patient's jaw opening and response to therapy for trismus.

is of paramount importance and will not only involve therapeutic exercises, but also use of the Dynasplint for 30 minutes three times per day. We no longer use corkscrew jaw-opening devices or tongue depressors, as we have found these devices to be ineffective (Figs. 57.18 and 57.19). Jaw opening is measured objectively using a simple plastic measuring device obtained from Dynasplint (Fig. 57.20).

The rehabilitation medicine physician will evaluate and treat pain, spasm, and any other disorders that interfere with the successful rehabilitation of the patient. Botulinum toxin injections are often used to decrease the pain and spasm of the masticatory muscles, particularly the masseter. It should be noted that botulinum toxin injections are ineffective at improving jaw opening when used in isolation; a jaw-stretching device must also be employed.

Trigeminal and Anterior Cervical Neuralgia

Radiation-induced trigeminal and anterior cervical neuralgia are common complications of radiation for HNC. Extensive surgical resections are often used with radiation and may significantly contribute to damage of one or more branches of the trigeminal nerve or cervical plexus. The symptoms of trigeminal neuralgia may be in any trigeminal nerve distribution, with V2 and V3 being the most common. Symptoms are generally ipsilateral to the side of the tumor, but can be bilateral. The pathophysiology is likely ectopic activity in the affected sensory nerve due to radiation and or postsurgical scarring. The neuralgic pain experienced by some patients can be extremely severe and disabling. Treatment generally includes nerve-stabilizing medications, opioids, and occasionally botulinum toxin injection.

Breast Cancer

While breast cancer is commonly treated with local radiation therapy, neuromuscular and musculoskeletal sequelae are relatively uncommon as compared with distant survivors of HL or HNC. Lymphedema is the most common long-term complication of primary breast cancer treatment and can result not only from radiation, but also from surgery, and is more likely to manifest if both modalities are used together (54).

Shoulder dysfunction, most commonly adhesive capsulitis, can occur from axillary radiation for breast cancer. Adhesive capsulitis is more likely to be an acute phenomenon more related to localized pain and inflammation of the skin and soft tissues, with reluctance to voluntarily move the arm. Significant neuromuscular damage is unlikely in this setting. Patients treated with radiation for local (chest wall or axilla) breast cancer recurrence, however, can have significant neuromuscular and musculoskeletal dysfunction. Radiation fibrosis may be contributory in this setting, but the effects of locally progressive tumor on the plexus and other neural structures are as or more likely to be the cause of dysfunction.

Extremity Tumors

Extremity tumors, including sarcomas or metastatic disease, are often treated with radiation, with the subsequent development of RFS (55). Common neuromuscular and musculoskeletal complications of radiation and surgical treatment in patients with extremity tumors include mononeuropathy and contracture (Fig. 57.21). The focal myopathy and soft tissue fibrosis that accom-

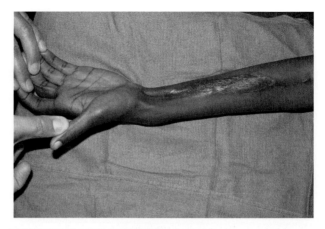

FIGURE 57.21

Wrist flexion contracture with median and ulnar mononeuropathies resulting from resection and radiation of an extremity sarcoma.

pany radiation to other parts of the body are no less of an issue in the extremity.

Mononeuropathy can occur in any nerve within the radiation field. Often, multiple nerves are involved when they are located within close proximity, such as the median, ulnar, and radial nerves of the arm or the peroneal and tibial nerves of the leg. Radiation-induced mononeuropathies are often extremely painful, with marked neuropathic pain resulting from abnormal ectopic activity in the affected nerves. Similarly, spasm of the muscles innervated by the affected nerve or nerves is common. Progressive weakness occurs when motor fibers are involved and can progress to complete plegia with subsequent atrophy of muscles distal to the area of insult.

Contracture and loss of range of motion can result when radiation involves a joint or the muscles actuating a joint. This may result in an inability to extend the elbow or knee, flex the wrist, close the fingers, etc. In most instances, contracture is an unwanted complication and must be addressed aggressively. We have seen resolution of foot drop due to radiation-induced peroneal mononeuropathy. This likely resulted from progressive fibrosis and shortening of the foot dorsiflexors and near fixed contracture at the ankle, obviating the need for an ankle-foot orthosis without a return of strength or function (56).

Spinal Tumors

Tumors affecting the spinal axis are often treated with surgical resection and stabilization, radiotherapy, or a combination of both modalities. The net effect of tumor, radiation, and surgery can result in severe localized pain and spasm. The mechanism of pain and spasm is often attributable, at least in part, to ectopic activity in spinal and intercostal nerves. While not purely RFS, these disorders deserve mention in this chapter, as the treatments employed, specifically botulinum toxin injections and other medications, overlap the treatment of other manifestations of radiation fibrosis syndrome.

CLINICAL EVALUATION

History

The diagnosis of radiation fibrosis syndrome is not always straightforward. Symptoms should be referable to and anatomically consistent with a history of prior radiation therapy. A complete history should include all preexisting medical conditions, particularly neuromuscular and musculoskeletal conditions, such as rotator cuff tendonitis, cervical radiculopathy, neuropathy, etc. The importance of preexisting or emerging neuromuscular and musculoskeletal conditions should not be underestimated, as these can affect greatly the development of symptoms in the setting of radiation.

A complete oncologic history should be detailed from diagnosis to presentation. All oncologic therapies given, such as surgeries, chemotherapy, and radiotherapy, should be documented and include the specifics of type, dosing, duration, and location. The time course of the development of symptoms should be understood and carefully documented, as they may give clues to comorbid disorders that are contributing to symptoms and dysfunction and may be of prognostic importance.

Symptoms of radiation fibrosis can develop during radiation or years later. More rapidly progressive symptoms generally, but not always, indicate a worse prognosis. In some cases, the radiation fibrosis is relatively static and the development of symptoms is due to a new and otherwise unrelated disorder, such as an acute cervical radiculopathy from a disk herniation. Ruling out superimposed disorders is extremely important as they are likely to change your treatment strategy.

The details of the patient's pain, tightness, spasm, and the language they use to describe their symptoms are important. Patients often describe constant or frequent muscle spasms in or outside the radiation field. Symptoms may be nonspecific, but are often described as "tight," "pulling," or "cramping." Neuropathic terms, such as "burning," "stabbing," "searing," etc., may be used to describe the pain associated with nerve injury. The practitioner should make every effort to differentiate symptoms associated with muscle spasms from those associated with neuropathic pain.

The patient's description of symptoms should be anatomically congruent to the radiation field. That is, they should occur either directly within the radiation field or within the myotomal, dermatomal, or peripheral nerve, vascular, or lymphatic distribution of the field. If the patient's symptoms are not anatomically congruent, other diagnostic possibilities other than RFS should be strongly considered.

Physical Examination

Physical evaluation is of paramount importance in understanding, evaluating, and treating the clinical manifestations of RFS. While a full accounting of a comprehensive neuromuscular and musculoskeletal examination is beyond the scope of this chapter, the reader is encouraged to review Chapter 35, an approach to evaluation of pain disorders, and Stanley Hoppenfeld's famous work on physical examination of the spine and extremities (57).

DIFFERENTIAL DIAGNOSIS

As was discussed extensively, the diagnosis of RFS necessitates that the signs and symptoms referable to the disorder be either within the radiation field or within the distribution of neural, vascular, or lymphatic structures that traverse the field. It is important to recognize the contribution of superimposed degenerative and other disorders to the signs and symptoms in a given patient treated with radiation and subject to RFS. While the pathophysiology underlying many of the neuromuscular and musculoskeletal disorders in RFS is different from other causes of such disorders, their evaluation is generally identical.

ADDITIONAL INVESTIGATIONS

Imaging

Imaging is often useful in the evaluation of RFS. Imaging should generally only be ordered if it is likely to change your management of the patient. A baseline MRI of the total spine in patients with RFS from HL treatment and of the cervical spine in HNC patients is often indicated on their initial visit to exclude degenerative processes of the spine or secondary malignancies.

MRI is the test of choice for evaluating the spine, soft tissues of the head, and joints such as the shoulder. The addition of gadolinium contrast is needed when a brain metastasis, intramedullary spinal tumor, or leptomeningeal disease are diagnostic possibilities. Gadolinium is also required when a postoperative or previously irradiated site is being evaluated to facilitate differentiation of tumor from a background of scar or fibrotic tissue. A computed tomogram (CT) with contrast is usually the test of choice to evaluate the viscera of the chest, abdomen, and pelvis for metastatic or progressive disease. CT may also be used when MRI is contraindicated (pacemaker, aneurism clips, breast tissue expanders). A CT myelogram is indicated when metallic hardware, such as from previous spinal instrumentation, causes excessive artifact that precludes adequate visualization of the spinal canal. A bone scan is useful for identification of most bony metastases, but does not generally provide adequate anatomical information since the soft tissues are not visualized. X-rays are useful when evaluating spinal stabilization hardware or joint replacement prostheses for loosening or failure.

Electrodiagnostic Testing

Electrodiagnostic evaluation is useful to identify, localize, confirm, and differentiate radiculopathy, plexopathy, neuropathy, or myopathy in patients with RFS. Needle EMG can confirm muscle denervation and may identify myokymia, fasciculations, and muscle spasm. Understanding and clarifying the multiple overlapping disorders present on electrodiagnostic testing is, at best, difficult in RFS. It is highly recommended that practitioners referring patients for electrodiagnostic testing seek out electromyographers who are board-certified by the American Board of Electrodiagnostic Medicine and who have considerable experience in the evaluation of complex neuromuscular disorders. A thorough discussion of electrodiagnosis in cancer can be found in Chapter 52.

TREATMENT

There is no cure for the progressive fibrotic sclerosis that occurs as a result of radiation treatment and thus no cure for RFS. A variety of medications, including pentoxifylline (Trental) and tocopherol (vitamin E), as well as hyperbaric oxygen and anticoagulation, have been touted as having a role in stabilizing or even reversing radiation fibrosis. In our clinical experience, these treatment modalities have been disappointingly ineffective.

The fact that the progressive fibrotic sclerosis of the microvasculature that underlies RFS cannot be affected at this point in time does not mean that there is no treatment of RFS. Quite the contrary, we have enjoyed tremendous success in relieving pain and improving the function and quality of life of cancer survivors with RFS. There is no magic in these successes. The basic principles that underlie all other disciplines within rehabilitation medicine are applicable to and effective for cancer survivors with RFS.

Education

Education is of paramount importance to cancer survivors with RFS. All too often, these patients have been forced to negotiate a medical system that does not understand and is unresponsive to their unique needs. They are commonly told that they should be grateful that they are cured of their original cancer, that their current issues are unrelated to their cancer treatment, or worse, that nothing can be done for them. We find that patients are, in general, extremely grateful when they find a practitioner who will listen to and try to understand their complaints. They become hopeful when the basic pathophysiology and interrelationship of their disorders are understood and explained to them. It is this understanding, both on the part of the clinician and the patient, that forms the cornerstone of successful treatment.

While the progressive fibrotic sclerosis of RFS cannot be reversed, individual disorders, such as the pain of a cervical radiculopathy, the debility resulting from a frozen shoulder, and the social isolation that results from severe head drop, often can. It is the realization that the specific diagnoses that form the components of the RFS can be identified and treated that will result in successful treatment of a population of patients that has often been regarded as untreatable.

Physical and Occupational Therapy

No single modality is more important in the successful treatment of RFS than physical and occupational therapy. The principles of physical and occupational therapy in cancer, the use of therapeutic modalities, and the use of therapeutic exercise are discussed extensively in Chapters 61, 62, and 63], respectively. While the basic principles of successful therapy in RFS are similar to those in other cancer disorders, there are several important concepts that should be emphasized.

Consistency is of paramount importance in successful treatment of RFS. RFS will continue to progress for the life of the patent and is no more reversible than growing older. It is much easier to lose function than to gain it. As such, it should be made clear to patients that their exercise program should be considered a lifelong effort. The therapist's role is to design, individualize, help initiate, and progress a program that addresses the neuromuscular and musculoskeletal deficits of a given patient. The patient will ultimately be discharged from therapy. It falls to the patient to incorporate these activities into their life with the goal of diminishing the progressive impact of RFS.

Fibrotic tissue can generally be stretched, but not nearly as easily as normal tissue. The principle of applying a low-load, prolonged stretch maximizing total end range time is tremendously important in RFS. It is the tenacity of the patient in terms of consistency and not their ability to tolerate discomfort (from overstretching) that is more likely to result in functional gain.

The value of a strong and stable core cannot be overstated. This is as important in a patient with RFS and trismus as it is in a HL survivor with head drop. Failure to meet therapeutic goals may result from failure to recognize the importance of core strength and proceeding directly and entirely to deficits that are more obvious.

Orthotics

The role of orthotics in the management of RFS follows the same basic principles of orthotic use in other neuromuscular and musculoskeletal disorders. The various designs of cervical orthotics to control neck extensor weakness are discussed previously. Upper extremity orthotics are rarely used, but may be appropriate in select situations to improve function in patients with severe radiculopathy or plexopathy. These are discussed more extensively in Chapter 78 on activities of daily living.

In general, lower extremity orthotics, such as ankle-foot orthoses (AFO), may be used for patients with dorsiflexion weakness from any cause, including myelopathy, radiculopathy (usually L5), plexopathy (lumbosacral trunk), or neuropathy (sciatic, common peroneal, deep peroneal). We generally prefer to use poster-leaf-spring (PLSO)–type AFOs, as they are small, light, and provide good functional benefit in most cases. A custom-molded AFO can be fabricated when off-the-shelf versions are inadequately stable or fit poorly. When plantar flexion weakness and inability to control the ankle is present, a more ridged custom design, such as a modified AFO or a hinged AFO, may be used. A solid AFO is only appropriate when severe spasticity must be controlled, and this is rarely the situation in RFS survivors, as deficits most commonly affect the peripheral nervous system. Control of the knee to prevent buckling is sometimes indicated. Most patients with reasonable vigor can ambulate well with weakness of knee extension by positioning their center of gravity in front of the knee, thus generating a posteriorly directed force at the knee and forcing it into extension. This may, however, result in knee pain and degeneration. Older patients and patients with weakness affecting multiple joints may benefit from a knee immobilizer. Several designs are available, but in general, we prefer a custom-made device with drop or other locks that will allow the patient to easily bend the knee to sit (58). If knee extension weakness and difficulty with dorsiflexion are present, a knee immobilizer can often be fabricated to fit in a modular fashion over

an AFO. We find this to generally be more acceptable and easier to don and doff for the patient than a knee-ankle-foot-orthosis (KAFO).

Medications

Medications are often needed to control pain and muscle spasms in RFS. While the assessment and management of pain in the cancer patient and in cancer survivor are discussed extensively in other sections of this textbook, there are several important considerations for patients with RFS. The most important determination for effective pain management is to differentiate neuropathic pain from musculoskeletal (somatic) pain. In many patients, both neuropathic and somatic pain are present together.

In patients with neuropathic pain, treatment with a nerve stabilizer is indicated as first-line treatment. Our preference is to start with pregabalin (Lyrica) in most patients, as the medication is highly effective for neuropathic pain and to some degree muscle spasms, works quickly, and has low potential for drug-drug interactions (59). Gabapentin (Neurontin) has the same mechanism of action as pregabalin, but is generally less efficacious, is poorly absorbed, and takes considerably longer to titrate. In patients who do not respond to pregabalin, duloxetine (Cymbalta) can be considered (60). It has a different mechanism of action (serotonin and norepinephrine reuptake inhibition) and can be used in conjunction with pregabalin. The clinician should be aware that duloxetine can interact adversely with other drugs that affect serotonin reuptake, including tricyclic antidepressants (TCAs), tramadol, and triptans, among others. Duloxetine also takes considerably longer to take effect. TCAs can be used in some patients, but their potential for arrhythmias, orthostatic hypotension, and other anticholinergic side effects such as urinary retention and constipation limit their usefulness in RFS. Opioids are often added to either or both pregabalin and duloxetine when needed.

Somatic pain from inflammation of the rotator cuff, adhesive capsulitis, and underlying degenerative changes is often present in RFS and will not respond adequately to nerve stabilization medications. A trial of a nonsteroidal anti-inflammatory drug (NSAID) is generally indicated when inflammation or pain from degenerative changes is diagnosed. Positive results are generally evident within a few days of their institution. If an NSAID is effective, it may control only part of the patient's pain syndrome. For instance, the patient may have less shoulder pain but continue to experience radicular pain. In such cases, the NSAID should be combined with nerve-stabilizing agents. If an NSAID is not effective, it should be discontinued for fear of long-term side effects, such as gastrointestinal ulceration or elevated blood pressure, with subsequent increased cardiovascular infarction risk. Patients with cardiac issues from prior radiation or other causes or renal insufficiency should be monitored closely while on NSAIDs. Opioids are often used when NSIDS are ineffective or contraindicated to control somatic pain.

Muscle relaxants, including baclofen, tizanidine (Zanaflex), and various benzodiazepines may help relieve the pain associated with muscle spasms and are often worth a short trial. They should be discontinued if they are ineffective.

Injections

The role of therapeutic injection in cancer pain management is discussed in Chapter 41 on interventional pain management in the cancer patient. Two types of procedures deserve special attention as they are of particular benefit in specific conditions associated with RFS. These include trigger-point injections and botulinum toxin injections.

Trigger-point injection is simply the injection of a local anesthetic into the area of a painful muscle spasm. They may be of tremendous benefit to patients with painful muscle spasms in the trapezius, rhomboids, cervical paraspinal, and other muscles. The risk of injection is minimal in experienced hands. Usually, 2–5 cc of 0.25% bupivacaine is used per location, up to a maximum of 20 cc divided between one and eight sites. The injection temporarily inhibits the ability of the motor endplate to respond to abnormal ectopic activity in the motor nerve, resulting in local muscle relaxation, reperfusion, and decreased pain. The benefit of the injection may last anywhere from a few hours to several days, and injections are often repeated at monthly intervals.

Botulinum toxin injection has emerged as both primary and adjunctive treatment for musculoskeletal pain, muscle spasms, spasticity, migraines, neuropathic pain, and a variety of other disorders (61). Specific cancer-related indications for which botulinum toxin injections have been studied include chronic and neuropathic pain following neck dissection, muscle spasms following radiation therapy to the head and neck, and radiation-induced trismus (62–66). We have found botulinum toxin injection to be of potential benefit in several specific complications of RFS, including radiation-induced cervical dystonia, trismus, painful paraspinal muscle spasms, and focal neuropathic pain disorders (67). Only practitioners skilled in the use of botulinum toxin injections in other disorders should attempt its use in cancer patients, as the potential for complications including worsening neck drop and dysphagia is relatively high. A comprehensive discussion of the use of botulinum toxin in RFS is available (27).

FOLLOW-UP AND SURVEILLANCE

RFS is a serious and lifelong disorder. While the various complications of RFS are usually treatable, they require vigilance on the part of the clinician and patient. This is because disorders not only are often easier to treat when identified early, but also because they will often keep company with an ominous risk for secondary malignancies, cardiovascular dysfunction, and other directly related medical issues. An understanding of the basic pathophysiology of progressive fibrotic tissue sclerosis that results from radiation treatment and how radiation fibrosis manifests clinically will allow the clinician to effectively evaluate and treat the various disorders that comprise RFS.

References

1. Plotkin SR, Wen PY. Neurologic complications of cancer therapy. *Neurol Clin.* 2003;21:279–318.
2. Falah M, Schiff D, Burns TM. Neuromuscular complications of cancer diagnosis and treatment. *J Support Oncol.* 2005;3:271–282.
3. Chou WW, Puri DR, Lee NY. Intensity-modulated radiation therapy for head and neck cancer. *Expert Rev Anticancer Ther.* 2005;5:515–521.
4. Saarto T, Janes R, Tenhunen, Kouri M. Palliate radiotherapy in the treatment of skeletal metastases. *Eur J Pain.* 2002;6;323–330.
5. Chow E, Wu J, Loblaw A, Perez CA. Radiotherapeutic approaches to metastatic disease. *World J Urol.* 2003;21:229–242.
6. O'Meara WP, Lee N. Advances in nasopharyngeal carcinoma. *Curr Opin Oncol.* 2005;17:225–230.
7. Tannock IF. Combined modality treatment with radiotherapy and chemotherapy. *Radiother Oncol.* 1989;16:83–101.
8. Hauer-Jensen M, Fink LM, Wang J. Radiation injury and the protein C pathway. *Crit Care Med.* 2004;32(Suppl.):S325–S330.
9. Libshitz HI, DuBrow RA, Loyer EM, Charnsangavej C. Radiation change in normal organs: an overview of body imaging. *Eur Radiol.* 1996:6;786–795.
10. Portlock CS, Boland P, Hays AP, Antonescu CR, Rosenblum MK. Nemaline myopathy: a possible late complication of Hodgkin's disease therapy. *Hum Pathol.* 2003;34:816–818.
11. Johansson S, Svensson H, Larsson L, Denekamp J. Brachial plexopathy after postoperative radiotherapy of breast cancer patients: a long-term follow-up. *Acta Oncologica.* 2000;39:373–382.
12. New P. Radiation injury to the nervous system. *Curr Opin Neurol.* 2001;14:725–734.
13. Johansson S. Svensson H, Denekamp J. Dose response and the latency for radiation-induced fibrosis, edema, and neuropathy in breast cancer patients. *Int J Radiation Oncology Biol Phys.* 2002;52:1207–1219.
14. Johansson S, Svensson H, Denekamp J. Timescale of evolution of late radiation injury after postoperative radiotherapy of breast cancer patients. *Int J Radiation Oncol Biol Phys.* 2000;48:745–750.
15. Stone HB, Coleman CN, Anscher MS, McBride WH. Effects of radiation on normal tissue: consequences and mechanisms. *Lancet Oncol.* 2004;4:529–536.
16. Lund MD, Kongerud J, Boe J, et al. Late complications after treatment of Hodgkin's disease [Article in Norwegian]. *Tidsskr Nor Laegeforen.* 1999;10:933–937.
17. Falkmer U, Järhult J, Wersäll P, Cavallin-Ståhl A. A systematic overview of radiation therapy effects in skeletal metastases. *Acta Oncologica.* 2003;42:620–633.

18. Paulino AC. Late effects of radiotherapy for pediatric extremity sarcomas. *Int J Radiation Oncology Biol Phys.* 2004;60: 265–274.

19. Cross NE, Glantz MJ. Neurologic complications of radiation therapy. *Neurol Clin N Am.* 2003;21;249–277.

20. Gillette EL, Mahler PA, Powers BE, Gillette SM, Vujaskovic Z. Late radiation injury to muscle and peripheral nerves. *Int J Radiation Oncology Biol Phys.* 1995;31:1309–1318.

21. Greenfield MM, Stark GM. Post-irradiation neuropathy. *AJR Am J Roentgenol.* 1948;60:617–622.

22. Zimmermann M. Pathobiology of neuropathic pain. *Eur J Pharmacol.* 2001;429:23–37.

23. Posner JB. Spinal metastases In: Posner JB. *Neurologic Complications of Cancer.* Philadelphia, PA: F.A. Davis Company; 1995:120.

24. Jaeckle KA. Neurological manifestations of neoplastic and radiation-induced plexopathies. *Semin Neurol.* 2004;24:385–393.

25. Stubblefield MD, Slovin S, MacGregor-Cortelli B, et al. An electrodiagnostic evaluation of the impact of pre-existing peripheral nervous system disorders in patients treated with the novel proteasome inhibitor bortezomib. *Clin Oncol.* 2006;18: 410–418.

26. Miller TM, Layzer RB. Muscle cramps. *Muscle Nerve.* 2005;32:431–442.

27. Stubblefield MD. Radiation fibrosis syndrome. In: Cooper G, ed. *Therapeutic Uses of Botulinum Toxin.* Totowa, NJ: Humana Press; 2007:19–38.

28. Karuman PN, Soo KC. Motor innervation of the trapezius muscle: a histochemical study. *Head and Neck.* 1996;18:254–258.

29. *Shah JP, Danoff JV, Desai MJ, Parikh S, Nakamura LY, Phillips TM, Gerber LH. Biochemicals associated with pain and inflammation are elevated in sites near to and remote from active myofascial trigger points. Arch Phys Med Rehabil.* 2008;89:16–23.

30. Tytherleigh-Strong G, Hirahara A, Miniaci A. Rotator cuff disease. *Curr Opin Rheumatol.* 2001;13:135–145.

31. Spoudeas HA. Growth and endocrine function after chemotherapy and radiotherapy in childhood. *Eur J Cancer.* 2002;38:1748–1759.

32. Kadan-Lottick NS, Dinu I, Wasilewski-Masker K, et al. Osteonecrosis in adult survivors of childhood cancer: a report from the childhood cancer survivor study. *J Clin Oncol.* 2008;26: 3038–3045.

33. Zackrisson B, Mercke C, Strander H, Wennerberg J, Cavallin-Ståhl E. A systematic overview of radiation therapy effects in head and neck cancer. *Acta Oncologica.* 2003;42: 443–461.

34. Jung H, Beck-Bornholdt H, Svoboda V, Alberti W, Herrmann T. Quantification of late complications after radiation therapy. *Radiother Oncol.* 2001;61:233–246.

35. Hodgkin T. On some morbid appearances of the absorbent glands and spleen. *Medico-Chirugical Trans.* 1832;17:68.

36. Pusey W. Cases of sarcoma and of Hodgkin's disease treated by exposures to X-rays: a preliminary report. *JAMA.* 1902;38:166.

37. Peters M. A study of survivals in Hodgkin's disease treated radiologically. *Am J Roentgenol.* 1950;63:299.

38. Volker D, Re D, Harris NL, Mauch PM. Hodgkin lymphoma. In: DeVita, Hellman, Rosenberg, eds. *Cancer: Principles & Practice of Oncology.* Philadelphia, PA: Lippincott Williams & Wilkins; 2008:2183.

39. Brennan S, Hann LE, Yahalom J, Oeffinger KC, Rademaker J. Imaging of late complications from mantle field radiation in lymphoma patients. *Radiol Clin N Am.* 2008;46:419–430.

40. MacMahon B. Epidemiological evidence of the nature of Hodgkin's disease. *Cancer.* 1957;10:1045.

41. Matasar MJ, Butos JN, McCallen LN, et al. Prevalence of late morbidity in survivors of Hodgkin's lymphoma (HL) treated during adulthood. *J Clin Oncol.* 2008;26:abstr 9589.

42. Ford JS, Schwartz LN, McCallen LN, et al. Psychosocial functioning in survivors of Hodgkin lymphoma (HL) treated during adulthood. *J Clin Oncol.* 2008;26:abstr 9592.

43. Aleman BM, van den Belt-Dusebout AW, Klokman WJ, Van't Veer MB, Bartelink H, Van Leeuwen FE. Long-term cause-specific mortality of patients treated for Hodgkin's disease. *J Clin Oncol.* 2003;21:3431–3439.

44. Herrera JE, Stubblefield MD. Rotator cuff tendonitis in lymphedema: a retrospective case series. *Arch Phys Med Rehabil.* 2004;85:1939–1942.

45. Stubblefield MD, Custodio CM. Upper-extremity pain disorders in breast cancer. *Arch Phys Med Rehabil.* 2006;87(3 Suppl. 1): S96–S99.

46. Magee DJ. *Orthopedic Physical Assessment,* 3rd ed. Philadelphia: Saunders, 1997:90–142.

47. Greene W, ed. *Essentials of Musculoskeletal Care,* 2nd ed. Rosemont, IL: American Academy of Orthopedic Surgeons; 2001:113,136–138.

48. Itoi E, Kido T, Samo A, Urayama M, Sato K. Which is more useful, the "full can test" or the "empty can test," in detecting the torn supraspinatus tendon? *Am J Sports Med.* 1999;27:65–68.

49. MacDonald PB, Clark P, Sutherland K. An analysis of the diagnostic accuracy of the Hawkins and Neer subacromial impingement signs. *J Shoulder Elbow Surg.* 2000;9:299–301.

50. Almekinders LC. Overuse injuries in the upper extremity: impingement syndrome. *Clin Sports Med.* 2001;20(3):491–503.

51. Astudillo L, Hollington L, Game X, et al. Cervical dystonia mimicking dropped-head syndrome after radiotherapy for laryngeal carcinoma. *Clin Neurol Neurosurg.* 2003;106:41–43.

52. Costa J, Espirito-Santo C, Borges A, et al. Botulinum toxin type A therapy for cervical dystonia. *Cochrane Database Syst Rev.* 2005;25:CD003633.

53. Flowers KR, LaStayo P. Effect of total end range time on improving passive range of motion. *J Hand Ther.* 1994;7: 150–157.

54. Sakorafas GH, Peros G, Cataliotti L, Vlastos G. Lymphedema following axillary lymph node dissection for breast cancer. *Surg Oncol.* 2006;15:153–165.

55. Custodio CM. Barriers to rehabilitation of patients with extremity sarcomas. *J Surg Oncol.* 2007;95:393–399.

56. Farrell A, Stubblefield MD. Resolution of foot drop as a result of radiation-induced fibrosis: a case report [poster]. American Academy of Physical Medicine and Rehabilitation, 64th Annual Assembly, Chicago, Illinois, October 9–12, 2003.

57. Hoppenfeld S. *Physical Examination of the Spine & Extremities.* East Norwalk: Appleton & Lange; 1976.

58. Jones VA, Stubblefield MD. The role of knee immobilizers in cancer patients with femoral neuropathy. *Arch Phys Med Rehabil.* 2004;85:303–307.

59. Stacey BR, Swift JN. Pregabalin for neuropathic pain based on recent clinical trials. *Curr Pain Headache Rep.* 2006;10: 179–184.

60. Sultan A, Gaskell H, Derry S, Moore RA. Duloxetine for painful diabetic neuropathy and fibromyalgia pain: systematic review of randomized trials. *BMC Neurol.* 2008;8:29.

61. Royal MA. The use of botulinum toxins in the management of pain and headache. *Phys Med Rehabil Clin N Am.* 2003;14;805–820.

62. Lou JS, Pleninger P, Kurlan R. Botulinum toxin A is effective in treating trismus associated with postradiation myokymia and muscle spasms. *Mov Disord.* 1995;10:680–681.

63. Van Daele DJ, Finnegan EM, Rodnitzky RL, Zhen W, McCullock TM, Hoffman HT. Head and neck muscle spasms after radiotherapy. Management with botulinum toxin A injection. *Arch Otolaryngol Had Neck Surg.* 2002;128:956–959.

64. Wittekindt C, Liu WC, Klaussmann JP, Guntinas-Lichius O. Botulinum toxin type A for the treatment of chronic neck pain after neck dissection. *Head Neck.* 2004;26:39–45.

65. Okereke LI, Stubblefield MD, Custodio CM. Botulinum toxin type A for radiation-induced trismus and facial pain: a case report. *Arch Phys Med Rehabil.* 2004;85:E37.

66. Wittekindt C, Liu WC, Preuss SF, Guntinas-Lichius O. Botulinum toxin A for neuropathic pain after neck dissection: a dose-finding study. *Laryngoscope.* 2006;116:1168–1171.

67. Stubblefield MD, Levine A, Custodio CM, Fitzpatrick T. The role of botulinum toxin type A in the radiation fibrosis syndrome: a preliminary report. *Arch Phys Med Rehabil.* 2008;89:417–421.

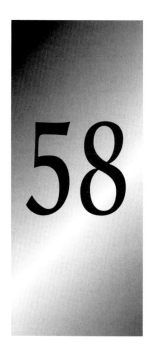

Graft-Versus-Host Disease

Lynn H. Gerber
Amanda Molnar

Graft-versus-host disease (GVHD) is a complication of allogeneic hematopoietic stem cell transplantation that may affect many organ systems. In one of the early descriptions of the syndrome (1) in which the organ systems most likely to be involved were described, there was mention of the observation that the Karnofsky Performance Status Scale was the best measure of the overall severity of the disease. This signaled some of the concerns that oncologists had, and continue to have, about GVHD, including issues of performance and function.

Twenty-five years later, the National Institutes of Health Consensus Development Project on Criteria in Chronic Graft-versus-Host Disease published a series of papers outlining agreed-upon project criteria for future collaborative efforts to help define, diagnose, assess, and study the disease (2–7). Participants agreed to use a core set of assessment tools to try to accomplish aspects of this ambitious task. In particular, the criteria for ancillary therapy and supportive care acknowledged and identified specific areas relevant to rehabilitation needs of patients with acute and chronic GVHD. These collaborative efforts are likely to result in a better understanding of the disease and its natural history. This new knowledge is likely to lead to early warning signs for illness and functional abnormalities and to identify targets for treatment.

DEFINITION OF GVHD

GVHD is a widespread immune response of donor tissue to host that is thought to be T-cell–mediated. It has features of immune dysregulation with sequelae similar to autoimmune and immunodeficiency disorders. Chronic GVHD (cGVHD) develops after the third month following transplantation and accounts for 54% of nonrelapse deaths (8). A good discussion of the protean nature of cGVHD, its multisystem involvement, and a practical treatment approach is available (9). In this paper, Vogelsang mentions the value of physical and occupation therapy in maintaining and increasing strength, range of motion, and mobility, as well as maximizing function, all of which may be compromised by cGVHD. The recommendations for evaluation and treatment have been based primarily on her professional experience treating many with cGVHD. Each patient is unique in the biological, psychological, and sociocultural sense. Each may also have unique needs and desires with respect to life activities. This creates an extremely complex evaluation matrix to assess patients and devise a comprehensive treatment plan to meet their needs.

One approach that can be used to evaluate and treat this chronic problem is to apply the rehabilitation model to this process. The model provides a useful and

KEY POINTS

- Graft-versus-host disease (GVHD) is a complication of allogeneic hematopoietic stem cell transplantation that may affect multiple organ systems via a widespread immune response of donor tissue to host that is thought to be T-cell–mediated.
- The rehabilitation model for GVHD involves assessment of three domains: (1) impairments, (2) physical activity and functional status, and (3) participation in chosen roles.
- Rehabilitation issues associated with chronic GVHD are frequently musculoskeletal in nature and include muscle atrophy from disuse, steroid use, or as a result of myositis or neuropathy, limb edema, arthralgias, and avascular necrosis.
- As a result of GVHD and its treatments, patients are often subjected to prolonged periods of immobilization and bed rest, leading to decreased strength, decreased endurance, and even changes in mood and mental status.

- Changes can occur in both the peripheral and central nervous systems in patients with graft-versus-host disease primarily due to the toxic effects of chemotherapy, immunosuppressive agents, and other drugs.
- Pulmonary complications, including pneumonia, pulmonary edema, and bronchiolitis obliterans, can occur in as many as 40%–60% of patients following an allogeneic transplant.
- Acute GVHD occurs within the first three months following allogeneic transplantation and can affect multiple systems simultaneously.
- GVHD is considered chronic three months following allogeneic transplant, and the patient is usually managed as an outpatient, except for acute medical problems that may arise.
- Patients with graft-versus-host disease can benefit greatly from rehabilitation services, and a variety of intervention strategies are used to combat the many complications and deficits that occur.

systematic scheme for analyzing the problems encountered in cGVHD. The World Health Organization has supported this in its effort to expand the concept of health as being more than the absence of disease (10). It espoused the view that health includes physical, mental, and social well-being of the whole person, and we must strive to manage disease and its consequences. The rehabilitation model is an attempt to be inclusive of these ideas and provides a schema for assessing three domains: (1) impairments, the abnormalities of anatomy structure and physiology at the level of the body; (2) physical activity and functional status of an individual (disability), which measures the degree to which a person can perform daily activities; and (3) participation in chosen roles without limitation, which occurs at the level of society. Each domain can also be categorized in terms of the organ/system, the whole person, or the societal level, each with its own assessments and outcome measures. In the WHO nomenclature of the International Classification of Functioning, Disability, and Health, (www.who.int/classifications/icf/en), this includes impairments, activity, and participation. This approach, when used consistently, may help manage this particularly complex, chronic process (Table 58.1).

APPLYING THE REHABILITATION MODEL

GVHD (acute and chronic) is typically characterized by the following organ system involvement, not all of which is associated with functional impact or disabil-

TABLE 58.1
Domains of the Rehabilitation Model

IMPAIRMENT (BODY)	ACTIVITY (INDIVIDUAL)	PARTICIPATION (SOCIETY)
Physiology Anatomy Structures	Performance Activity Function Disability	Participation Societal limitation Environmental factors

ity. Nonetheless, these are frequently associated with symptoms that may cause individuals discomfort or concern; hence, they should be assessed with respect to their potential impact on overall functional status (Table 58.2).

Successful management of the disease process of cGVHD is highly dependent upon a number of factors thought to be related to mortality. Several series have shown that these usually include: (a) the presentation of GVHD in the progressive form, (b) diffuse skin involvement, (c) low platelet count, (d) poor performance (usually measured by the Karnofsky Performance Status Scale), and (e) hyperbilirubinemia (11,12). Treatment for extensive or severe cGVHD is immunosuppression of the graft, typically using cyclosporine A and prednisone (13). Newer agents have been tried with some success and include thalidomide (14), tacrolimus (15), and psoralen ultraviolet treatment (PUVA) with extracorporeal photopheresis (16).

TABLE 58.2
Areas Affected, Symptoms, and Impact of GVHD

ORGAN/SYSTEM	CLINICAL FINDINGS	SYMPTOM/IMPACT
Skin/nails/hair	Rash, onycholysis, alopecia	Pruritus/pain/cosmesis
Eyes	Sicca, injection, abrasion	Pain, burning
Mouth/teeth	Sicca, ulceration, fungal infection, carries	Pain, difficulty eating and chewing
Sinus	Infection, discharge	Sinus headache
Pulmonary	Bronchiolitis, abnormal FEV_1, D_{LCO}	Dyspnea, cough
Gastrointestinal	Decreased motility, diarrhea	Weight loss
Liver	Elevated liver enzymes	Fatigue
Musculoskeletal	Myositis, fasciitis, arthritis, osteoporosis, avascular necrosis, joint contractures, limb edema	Weakness, loss of range of motion, mobility problems, pain, decreased stamina, dependence in self-care, fatigue
Hematopoietic	Anemia, thrombocytopenia	Fatigue, bleeding
Immune status	Autoimmunity, immunodeficient	Arthritis
Metabolic status	Hyperglycemic, insulin resistance, obesity	Fatigue, muscle atrophy, neuropathic pain, decreased stamina

Abbreviations: D_{LCO}, diffusing capacity of lung for carbon monoxide; FEV_1, forced expiratory volume in the first second of expiration.

The impact of cGVHD or its treatments is a challenge to the rehabilitation team because it presents a chronic, complex, and ever-changing series of impairments, functional limitations, and disabilities (Table 58.2). Specifically, the rehabilitation problems associated with cGVHD are most frequently those involving the musculoskeletal system. Contractures may result from muscle atrophy from disuse, steroid use, or as a result of myositis or neuropathy, limb edema, arthralgias, and avascular necrosis. They are often associated with a reduction in mobility and physical activity. The impact of lower respiratory infection and/or the pulmonary fibrosis and bronchiolitis obliterans that may accompany the immunological abnormalities seen in cGVHD may result in a reduction in stamina and physical performance. The need for chronic steroids to suppress the GVHD and its inflammatory sequelae produces metabolic changes often associated with abnormalities of glucose uptake, fat metabolism, and energy production. These changes are frequently associated with fatigue. In short, the combinations of impairments and symptoms seen in cGVHD have a substantial affect on function and life activities. The rehabilitation approach depends upon performing a careful and comprehensive neuromusculoskeletal assessment; measures of function and performance; and patient self-reports of symptoms, well-being, and quality of life (Table 58.3) (17). Once this is completed, a treatment plan can be developed to reverse the functional loss.

Recommendations for measuring outcomes for patients with GVHD reflect the types of impairments, functional limitations, performance problems, and well-being and quality-of-life changes typically seen.

In general, the assessments should not take longer than 45 minutes to complete, and the questionnaires should be limited to 15 minutes in the outpatient setting. All of these instruments are validated and have been used in the cancer population, although not all have been validated for those who have received bone marrow transplantation (17). The basic evaluation set should include a strength measure, a measure of range of motion, a pain scale, a fatigue measure, a measure of activities of daily living (ADL) and mobility, a health status instrument/quality-of-life measure, and possibly a measure of mood and sexual function when appropriate. These can be used as evaluation tools and outcome measures, and provide reliable information for treatment planning.

Rehabilitation in the Acute Transplant Phase

Acute GVHD occurs within the first three months following allogeneic transplantation and can affect multiple systems simultaneously (18). Rehabilitation goals during this phase are addressed within an inpatient, acute care setting. Patients with no or minimal deficits can benefit from rehabilitative services to provide recommendations and programs to prevent future complications and impairments throughout the body. It is even beneficial for patients and families to be introduced to such programs prior to transplantation so that they are familiar with the expected level of participation (19). Once impairments and limitations are evident, a combination of medical management and rehabilitative efforts are used to restore loss of function.

TABLE 58.3 Recommended Measurements for Patients with GVHD

FINDING/SYMPTOM	IMPAIRMENT MEASURE	FUNCTIONAL/PERFORMANCE MEASURE	WELL-BEING/ QUALITY OF LIFE
Weakness	Manual/isokinetic muscle testing, grip strength	ADL, mobility (walk time), up and go, sickness impact profile	FACIT-F, SF36, sexual function
Fatigue	Strength test, pulmonary function, cardiac output, endocrine status, glucose	ADL, mobility (walk time), human activity profile, sickness impact profile	FACIT-F, sleep index, CES-D, sexual function
Contracture	ROM, VAS pain	ADL, mobility	SF36
Edema	ROM, MMT, limb volume	ADL, mobility	SF36, EURoQOL
Arthritis/arthralgia	ROM, MMT, VAS pain	ADL, mobility, up and go	FACIT-F, SF36, sleep, sexual function
Fasciitis	VAS pain, limb volume, ROM	ADL, mobility	

Abbreviations: ADL, activities of daily living; CES-D, Center for Epidemiologic Studies Depression; EURoQOL, European Quality of Life scale; FACIT-F, Functional Assessment of Chronic Illness Therapy-Fatigue; MMT, manual muscle test; ROM, range of motion; SF36, Medical Outcomes Study; VAS, Visual analog scale.

Skin Involvement

The integumentary system is often the first and most common system affected by acute graft-versus-host disease. Due to the inflammatory and fibrotic changes, skin integrity can easily become impaired (20). The histological changes to skin tissue in combination with patients' increased immobility can lead to skin and joint contractures or skin breakdown. A variety of treatment approaches can be used to prevent or restore skin integrity, with the goal of allowing the patient to remain as functional as possible.

Range of motion (ROM) and stretching techniques are used to promote full, functional range and prevent or reduce contractures. Manual stretching or passive range of motion (PROM) can be provided by the physical or occupational therapist. The patient can become more involved with techniques such as active or active assistive range of motion (AROM or AAROM) or other stretching techniques such as contract-relax-contract.

Splinting or bracing is another technique to prevent or restore range-of-motion complications based on the joint affected. For preventative purposes, a splint or brace can be worn to maintain the existing range of motion at a joint. Once loss of range of motion has occurred and is limiting a patient functionally, more aggressive splinting or bracing measures may need to be taken. Dynamic splinting or serial casting may be required to restore range of motion within functional limits (21).

One of the key components of rehabilitative efforts involving skin integrity is patient education. Patients and families need to play an active role to ensure an optimal outcome. Patients must demon-strate a good understanding and follow through with ROM, stretching, and home exercise programs (HEPs). Patients should be educated on performing skin checks to assess skin integrity, especially if wearing splints or braces. Lastly, patients with decreased skin integrity or who are immobile should be educated regarding turning schedules and weight shifting. Patients, either independently or with assistance, should be able to alternate positions in bed every two hours or weight shift when seated out of bed to avoid sustained pressure or friction on one area of the body. If patients are unable to consistently follow through, specialized mattresses or cushions may need to be provided.

Musculoskeletal Involvement

As a result of GVHD and its treatments, patients are often subjected to prolonged periods of immobilization and bed rest. Immobility can lead to decreased strength, decreased endurance, and even changes in mood and mental status. Muscle atrophy can occur, with a decrease of as much as 1% per day of bed rest. Corticosteroids can cause steroid-induced myopathy, and while lower extremity weight-bearing muscles and postural muscles are often most affected, changes can occur throughout the entire body (19,21). Bone strength can also diminish due to immunosuppressive and corticosteroid treatments, leading to complications such as osteoporosis and necrosis of the bone. Both preventative and restorative measures are necessary to combat these complications.

Therapeutic exercise is a key component in assisting patients to maintain and build strength and endurance. There is evidence that exercise during this phase hastens discharge and rapid return of hematological indices (22–24). Before beginning an exercise program, it is important to remember to take into consideration a patient's age, previous activity level, and current condition in order to determine the appropriate intensity, duration, and frequency of exercise. Patients should be encouraged to ambulate frequently, not just during physical therapy sessions, but also throughout the day. For patients who are on isolation precautions due to immunosuppression, this may require them to wear gowns, gloves, and masks before leaving their room. For patients who are not permitted to leave their room because of severe immunosuppression, alternatives must be used. Patients who must remain in their hospital room can be instructed to use an in-room ergometer or small stationary bicycle, if available (22). Lastly, patients should also be instructed in a progressive resistance exercise program. Patients may initially have difficulty performing exercise with resistance, but can be progressed to low levels of resistance using gravity-resistive positions or resistive bands.

With decreasing strength and endurance, patients are likely to have a decline in functional activities and can benefit greatly from functional training. Patients may need assistance and retraining for activities such as self-care, bed mobility, transfers, and ambulation. Along with functional training, patients who suffer from fatigue can benefit from energy conservation techniques. Higher-functioning patients may be independent completing activities, but may fatigue quickly. These patients benefit from learning energy conservation techniques, maintaining daily energy logs, and utilizing assistive devices and adaptive equipment to minimize energy expenditure. In addition to adaptive techniques, aerobic conditioning should be used to increase patients' endurance levels.

Neurological Involvement

Changes can occur in both the peripheral and central nervous systems in patients with graft-versus-host disease. Nervous system dysfunction primarily occurs due to the toxic effects of chemotherapy, immunosuppressive agents, and other drugs. However, patients with a decreased immune response may develop infections, which can also lead to neurologic dysfunction. Some of the most common neurological impairments include neuropathies and changes in mood and mental status.

Treatment approaches to neurological dysfunction vary greatly, depending on what area of the nervous system is affected and what deficits are present. Patients experiencing neuropathies may experience decreased sensation, ROM, and strength. Splinting, bracing, and orthoses are used to provide adequate and functional positioning, while therapeutic exercise is used to build strength. Assistive devices and adaptive equipment can also be used to improve patient safety and functioning. However, patients with mood and mental status changes require a completely different treatment approach. Cognitive retraining activities, such as memory aids, lists, visual and auditory reminders, sequencing, and problem solving exercises, can be used to assist the patient in achieving the highest level of cognition.

Other Considerations

Pulmonary complications can occur in as many as 40%–60% of patients following an allogeneic transplant. Complications such as pneumonia, pulmonary edema, and bronchiolitis obliterans (BO) can arise. Patients experiencing these complications can benefit greatly from pulmonary hygiene, including ventilatory muscle strengthening, cough and airway clearance techniques, thoracic mobility, and percussion/vibration techniques (25). During treatment sessions, respiratory status should always be checked by monitoring vital signs.

Patients may also experience hematopoietic changes following an allogeneic transplant. Anemia, thrombocytopenia, and neutropenia are all complications that may arise as a result of transplantation, graft-versus-host disease, or immunosuppressive therapy. Patients' lab values, vital signs, and symptoms should be closely monitored before, during, and after treatment sessions. Intensity, duration, and level of resistance may need to be modified accordingly in order to prevent additional complications from a rehab session.

Postacute Transplant Phase

After the first three months following allogeneic transplant, the process is called cGVHD and the patient is usually managed as an outpatient, except for acute medical problems that may arise. Rehabilitation goals are generally addressed in a home or outpatient setting. Once a patient is discharged home, he or she may be expected to remain within the home due to an impaired immune system. If a continuation or progression of impairments from the acute phase occurs, any or all of the treatment approaches previously discussed can be used. While structured rehab sessions continue to address goals, an emphasis on an HEP is important with these patients in order to build a maximum level of functioning. This usually consists of inspection of skin to make sure that prevention of ulceration and/or its early treatment can be initiated. Contractures are usually treated with a heat and stretch program, whereas fasciitis or arthralgia is frequently treated with ice or a wrap made of a bag of frozen peas. Limb edema is monitored closely using limb volumetric measures in order to provide compression garments and, if necessary, manual lymph drainage. It is thought that the lymph itself may be inflammatory and contribute to fasciitis.

The combination of steroid myopathy, pulmonary involvement from BO, and restricted activity because of immunosuppressive therapy often contributes to deconditioning. It is imperative that these patients exercise. Aerobic conditioning has significant impact on function. The inactive, steroid-dependent person is likely to be overweight, have hyperglycemia, and also abnormalities of lipid metabolism, which may progress to cardiac disease. This condition requires significant attention be paid to the maintenance of fitness as part of the routine treatment planning. All patients should be encouraged to participate in physical activity and return to work (26). It is imperative that patients and families demonstrate a good understanding of the HEP.

SUMMARY

Patients with graft-versus-host disease can benefit greatly from rehabilitation services, and a variety of intervention strategies are used to combat the many complications and deficits that occur. When working with this patient population, it is important to remember that many modifications may need to be made to both treatment sessions and goals. Throughout all phases of transplant and stages of graft-versus-host disease, patients should be encouraged to reach maximal functional potential.

*R*eferences

1. Shulman HM, Sullivan KM, Weiden PL, et al. Chronic graft-versus-host syndrome in man: a long term clinico-pathological study of 20 Seattle patients. *Am J Med.* 1980;69:204–217.
2. Filipovich AH, Weisdorf D, Pavletic S, et al. National Institutes of Health consensus development project on criteria for clinical trials in chronic graft-versus-host disease: I. Diagnosis and staging working group report. *Biol Blood Marrow Transplant.* December 2005;11(12):945–956.
3. Shulman HM, Kleiner D, Lee SJ, et al. Histopathologic diagnosis of chronic graft-versus-host disease: National Institutes of Health Consensus Development Project on Criteria for Clinical Trials in Chronic Graft-versus-Host Disease: II. Pathology Working Group Report. *Biol Blood Marrow Transplant.* 2006;12:31–47.
4. Schultz KR, Miklos DB, Dowler D, et al. Toward biomarkers for chronic graft-versus-host disease: National Institutes of Health consensus development project on criteria for clinical trials in chronic graft-versus-host disease: III. Biomarker Working Group Report. *Biol Blood Marrow Transplant.* 2006;12:126–137.
5. Pavletic SZ, Martin P, Lee SJ, et al. Measuring therapeutic response in chronic graft-versus-host disease: National Institutes of Health Consensus Development Project on Criteria for Clinical Trials in Chronic Graft-versus-Host Disease: IV. Response Criteria Working Group Report. *Biol Blood Marrow Transplant.* 2006;12:252–266.
6. Couriel D, Caprenter PA, Cutler C, et al. Ancillary therapy and supportive care of chronic graft. *Biol Blood Marrow Transplant.* 2006;12:375–396.
7. Martin PJ, Weisdorf D, Przepiorka D, et al. National Institutes of Health Consensus Development Project on criteria for clinical trials in chronic graft-versus-host disease: VI. Design of Clinical Trials Working Group report. *Biol Blood Marrow Transplant.* May 2006;12(5):491–505.
8. Socie G, Stone JV, Wingard JR, et al. Long term survival and late deaths after allogeneic bone marrow transplantation. *NEJM.* 1999;341:14–21.
9. Vogelsang G. How I treat chronic graft-versus-host disease. *Blood.* 2001;97:1196–1201.
10. WHO Constitution, Basic Documents, Geneva, 1948. Available at www.who.int/governance/eb/constitution/en/index.html.
11. Lee SJ, Vogelsang G, Flowers ME. Chronic graft-versus-host disease. *Biol Blood Marrow Transplant.* 2003;9:215–233.
12. Wingard J, Piantadosi S, Vogelsang G, et al. Predictors of death from chronic graft versus host disease after bone marrow transplantation. *Blood.* 1989;74:1428–1435.
13. Lonnquist N, Aschan J, Ljungman P, et al. Long-term cyclosporine therapy may decrease the risk of chronic graft-versus-host disease. *Br J Hematol.* 1990;74:547–548.
14. Vogelsang GB, Farmer ER, Hess AD, et al. Thalidomide for the treatment of chronic graft-versus-host disease. *N Engl J Med.* April 16, 1992;326(16):1055–1058.
15. Tzakis AG, Abu-Elmagd K, Fung JJ, et al. FK 506 rescue in chronic graft-versus-host-disease after bone marrow transplantation. *Transplant Proc.* December 1991;23(6):3225–3227.
16. Greinix HT, Volc-Platzer B, Rabitsch W, et al. Successful use of extracorporeal photochemotherapy in the treatment of severe acute and chronic graft-versus-host disease. *Blood.* November 1, 1998;92(9):3098–3104.
17. McDowell I, Newell C. *Measuring Health: A Guide to Rating Scales and Questionnaires,* 2nd ed. New York: Oxford University Press; 1996.
18. Couriel D, Caldera H, Champlin R, et al. Acute graft-versus-host disease: pathophysiology, clinical manifestations, and management. *Cancer.* 2004;101:1936.
19. Gillis TA, Donovan ES. Rehabilitation following bone marrow transplantation. *CANCER Suppl.* 2001;92:998–1007.
20. Kohler S, Hendrickson MR, Chao NJ, et al. Value of skin biopsies in assessing prognosis and progression of acute graft-versus-host disease. *Am J Surg Pathol.* 1997;21:988.
21. Grant J, Young MA, Pidcock FS, et al. Physical medicine & rehabilitation management of chronic graft vs. host disease. *Rehabilitation Oncology.* 1997;15:13–15.
22. Dimeo FC, Stieglitz RD, Novelli-Fischer U, Fetscher S, Keul J. Effects of physical activity on the fatigue and psychologic status of cancer patients during chemotherapy. *Cancer.* May 15, 1999;85(10):2273–2277.
23. Dimeo F, Bertz H, Finke J, Fetscher S, Mertelsmann R, Keul J. An aerobic exercise program for patients with haematological malignancies after bone marrow transplantation. *Bone Marrow Transplant.* December 1996;18(6):1157–1160.
24. Mello M, Tanaka C, Dulley FL. Effects of an exercise program on muscle performance in patients undergoing allogeneic bone marrow transplantation. *Bone Marrow Transplant.* October 2003;32(7):723–728.
25. Epler GR. Bronchiolitis obliterans and airways obstruction associated with graft-versus-host disease. *Clin Chest Med.* 1988;9:551.
26. Hunt JL. Organ transplantation. In: Paz JC, West MP, eds. *Acute Care Handbook for Physical Therapists,* 2nd ed. Boston, MA: Butterworth-Heinemann; 2002:733–743.

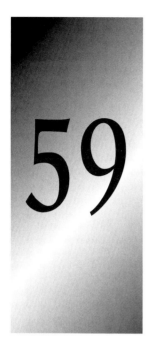

Osteoporosis in Cancer

Azeez Farooki
Hanna Chua Rimner

This chapter aims to provide clinically relevant information and discusses diagnostic evaluation and management of the cancer patient with osteoporosis. Although this information is relevant to any patient with bone loss, issues of specific relevance to oncologic patients are emphasized.

PATHOPHYSIOLOGY AND DEFINITION

Bone tissue is 5% cellular, 25% organic proteins (90% Type I collagen), and 70% inorganic mineral components (hydroxyapatite). Many biochemical markers of bone turnover (measurable in urine and/or serum) are breakdown products of type I collagen (amino and carboxy terminal telopeptides). Bone turnover or bone remodeling can be defined as the physiological process whereby older bone is replaced by newer bone. Bone resorption (removal of bone by osteoblast-produced proteases and osteoclast-mediated acid decalcification and proteolytic digestion) is synchronized with immediate bone formation (the production of bone matrix and subsequent calcification). In adults, approximately 3% of cortical bone and 25% of trabecular bone are resorbed and replaced every year. A net loss of bone mineral density is due to an imbalance in the bone turnover process favoring bone loss. Microarchitectural deterioration of horizontal trabeculae or "struts" (Fig. 59.1), decreased cortical thickness, and increased cortical porosity all contribute to bone loss and propensity to fracture.

Osteoporosis is a disease characterized by compromised bone strength, leading to bone fragility and an increased risk for fractures, especially of the hip, spine, and wrist (1). Bone strength reflects both bone density and "bone quality." Bone quality determinants include bone microarchitecture, bone turnover, damage accumulation (microfractures), and mineralization (1). Currently, noninvasive tools to measure bone quality are limited. Dual-energy x-ray absorptiometry (DXA) is the gold-standard technique to measure bone mineral density (BMD). BMD is determined by peak bone mass minus net amount of bone loss over that time. Therefore, osteoporosis may result from low peak bone mass, subsequent bone loss, or both factors. In general, humans accrue bone mass until approximately age 30; bone mass plateaus for a variable time and is followed by mild bone loss of 0.5%–1.0% per year until approximately age 50 (the time of menopause). Thereafter it is lost at increased rates of 1%–2% per year for an "accelerated phase" possibly lasting 5–10 years, followed by lesser age-related bone loss. For men, assuming normal gonadal function, there is no accelerated phase.

CLINICAL MANIFESTATIONS

Osteoporosis has no clinical manifestations or symptoms until there is a fracture, analogous to asymptomatic hypertension increasing risk for a subsequent myocardial infarction or stroke. The majority of patients

KEY POINTS

- Osteoporosis is a disease characterized by compromised bone strength, leading to bone fragility and an increased risk for fractures, especially of the hip, spine, and wrist.
- Dual-energy x-ray absorptiometry (DXA) is the gold-standard technique to measure bone mineral density (BMD).
- Osteoporosis has no clinical manifestations or symptoms until there is a fracture.
- Ten million people in the United States have osteoporosis, and 34 million people have low bone mass, or osteopenia.
- The widely accepted World Health Organization definition of osteoporotic bone mineral density is a T-score of minus 2.5 and below.
- The point of screening patients for osteoporosis is to be able to intervene clinically before the first fracture occurs.

- Modifiable risk factors for osteoporotic fracture include low vitamin D and calcium intake, smoking, imbibing greater than two alcoholic drinks per day, a sedentary lifestyle devoid of weight-bearing exercise, and household fall hazards such as loose rugs.
- The currently recommended total calcium intake from all sources is 1200 mg per day in divided doses.
- A comprehensive physical therapy program should incorporate weight-bearing and resistance exercises to preserve or increase bone strength, as well as balance training and multidisciplinary fall prevention strategies to minimize fall and fracture risk.

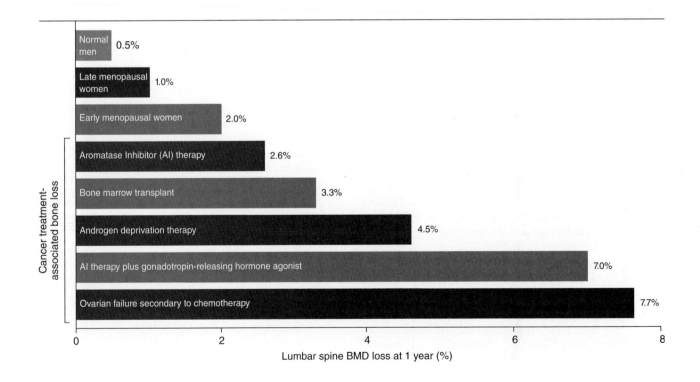

FIGURE 59.1

Bone loss associated with various cancer therapies. Reproduced with permission Ref. 114.

with osteoporotic fractures do not receive evaluation or treatment for underlying osteoporosis.

Vertebral Fracture

Vertebral fracture is the most common clinical manifestation of osteoporosis. Two-thirds of these fractures are asymptomatic and therefore many remain undiagnosed; an imaging technique that visualizes the lateral spine is required for diagnosis (Fig. 59.2). Findings on physical exam that suggest vertebral fractures with kyphosis are inability to touch the occiput to the wall and the presence of a gap of less than three fingerbreadths between the costal margin and the iliac crest (2). Findings such as these and/or documented height loss of greater than 2 cm (0.75 inches) should prompt evaluation for occult vertebral fractures. Any prior vertebral, wrist, or hip fracture increases the risk of subsequent fractures at all of these three most common sites for fragility fractures (3).

Vertebral fractures may be triggered by forward flexion associated with normal activities, without trauma. Severe, acute back pain may radiate laterally to the flanks and anteriorly. Multiple fractures can lead to height loss and exaggerated dorsal kyphosis, the "dowager's hump." Some patients with severe thoracic kyphosis due to vertebral fractures have many complaints, such as neck pain due to constant extension required

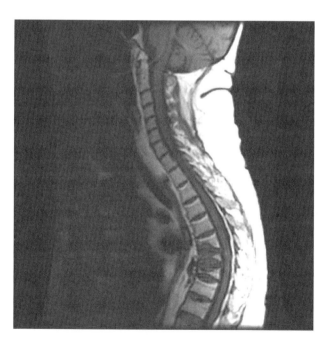

FIGURE 59.2

Sagittal magnetic resonance imaging (MRI) (T1) of vertebral compression fractures (T6, T7, T8) in a patient with osteoporosis.

to look forward, early satiety due to compression of abdominal contents, and dyspnea due to restrictive lung disease. Vertebral fractures due to osteoporosis in vertebrae above T7 are rare—malignancy should be suspected in such cases (4).

Hip Fracture

Hip fractures are a potentially lethal manifestation of osteoporosis, affecting 15% of women and 5% of men by 80 years of age. Mortality in the year following a hip fracture has been reported to be 24%–33%, depending on the population studied (5,6). Quality of life can be severely affected: At six months, just 15% of hip fracture patients can walk across a room unaided. Long-term care, with its associated economic and psychological burdens, is required in 20% of previously ambulatory patients. Long-term nursing care was described by participants in one study as less desirable than death (7). Osteoporotic hip fractures usually follow a low-energy fall and cause pain and inability to bear weight. The affected extremity is often shortened and externally rotated. Failure to diagnose and treat osteoporosis following a hip fracture is still quite common.

PSYCHOLOGICAL ISSUES

Loss of self-esteem and depression may occur as a result of changes in body habitus such as loss of height and kyphosis (8). Kyphoscoliosis may limit mobility and independence. Intractable, chronic pain from vertebral compression fractures (VCFs) can also lead to depression.

EPIDEMIOLOGY AND IMPORTANCE

Ten million people in the United States have osteoporosis, and 34 million people have low bone mass, or osteopenia. The incidence of osteoporotic fractures in the United States per year is 1.5 million (9). In comparison, there are fewer than 200,000 cases per year of breast cancer and about 513,000 heart attacks per year. A 50-year-old white woman has an 18% lifetime chance of suffering a hip fracture (10). In 2001, about 315,000 Americans age 45 and over were admitted to hospitals with hip fractures. As the number of women with osteopenic BMD (roughly half the adult female population) far outnumbers that with osteoporotic BMD, more than half of fragility fractures occur in women with T-scores at the total hip less than 2.5 (11). The estimated national direct care expenditures for osteoporotic fractures are more than $18 billion per year.

EVALUATION

Bone Densitometry

Bone mineral density (BMD) is calculated as [bone mineral content (grams)/bone area (cm^2)]. Therefore, BMD measures a two-dimensional area and does not provide a true volumetric bone density. DXA of the axial skeleton (spine, hip, and sometimes the radius) is the gold-standard technique used to measure BMD, follow treatment, and thereby help assess fracture risk. Note that a disease such as osteomalacia, which results from deficiencies in calcium and phosphorus, two important components of mineral contained in bone matrix, might lower the bone mineral density into the "osteoporotic" range. This is of high clinical relevance since the treatment of osteomalacia is different from that of osteoporosis. Two other limitations of DXA are (1) vertebral compression fracture may increase the BMD of the affected vertebra (since the areal BMD is being measured rather than the volumetric BMD), possibly creating false confidence in the current management and (2) extraneous calcifications (aortic, etc.) in the path of the x-rays may cause measurement artifact. The lumbar spine value is generally represented as an average of the first through the fourth (L1–L4) vertebrae; deformed vertebrae should not be included in the analysis, and at least two usable vertebrae are needed to compute a value.

The widely accepted World Health Organization definition of osteoporotic bone mineral density is a T-score of –2.5 and below (12). BMD is given a corresponding T-score, which is the number of standard deviations (SDs) from the mean BMD of a healthy, sex-matched young adult between age 25 and 30 years old. A normal value is within 1 SD of a young adult, or greater than –1 SD. Low bone mass, or osteopenia, is defined as a T-score between –1.0 and –2.5 (Table 59.1). A Z-score represents the number of SDs from the mean value for normal subjects of the *same* age, sex, and ethnicity. Z-scores, not T-scores, should be used in premenopausal women (especially those less than 30 years old who may not yet have achieved peak bone mass).

The point of screening patients for osteoporosis is to be able to intervene clinically before the first fracture occurs. A history of fragility fracture (defined as a fracture resulting from a fall from standing height or a fracture without trauma) warrants a diagnosis of osteoporosis, regardless of bone mineral density. Vertebral fracture assessment (VFA) is a lateral view of the spine available through software on most DXA machines that allows visualization of otherwise occult vertebral fractures; a lateral thoracolumbar x-ray serves the same purpose.

BMD cutoffs have been proposed by various organizations concerning when to start treatment for low BMD. The National Osteoporosis Foundation (NOF) recommends initiating therapy in patients with (1) T-scores below -2.0 by central DEXA with no risk factors, (2) T-scores below –1.5 with one or more risk factors (see the following section), (3) a prior vertebral or hip fracture. Note that a history of fragility fracture warrants the diagnosis of osteoporosis and subsequent treatment, regardless of BMD.

Monitoring Response to Treatment

DXA readings from different manufacturers are not directly comparable due to differences in calibration. Therefore, serial measurements should be done at the same center using a densitometer of a given make. Serial comparisons should be made using BMD rather than T-scores. When comparing serial DXA readings done at a given center, it is important to take the precision error of measurement into account. At a given testing center, the precision errors of measurement at each anatomical site should be calculated and, subsequently, the BMD values necessary for a "least significant change" at each respective anatomical site determined. Precision error rates are estimated at <1% for the anterior-posterior spine and 1%–2% for the hip (13). The least significant change is calculated as 2.77 multiplied by the precision error at a given site. Then, serial measurements may be interpreted in light of significant versus nonsignificant changes in BMD. For example, if the least significant change at the spine is equal to 3% and an individual "lost" 1.5% of their BMD over two years, in reality, there has been no significant change. Repeat testing should be done when the expected change in BMD equals or exceeds the least significant change. In conditions predisposing to rapid loss in BMD, such as glucocorticoid use, DXA may be repeated in six-month intervals, whereas two to three years is acceptable given "age-related" bone loss of 1% per year.

TABLE 59.1
World Health Organization Classification of Bone Mineral Density

CLASSIFICATION	T-SCORE
Normal	–1.0 or greater
Osteopenia	Less than –1.0 and greater than –2.5
Osteoporosis	–2.5 or less
Severe osteoporosis	–2.5 or less with a fragility fracture

Source: From Ref. 125.

Overly frequent monitoring of BMD by DXA may cause unnecessary confusion and anxiety about the test results. A statistical phenomenon called regression to the mean may occur with frequent monitoring of BMD by DXA. An analysis of an alendronate trial of postmenopausal women with at least one vertebral fracture found a high degree of variability in BMD when tested after one year of treatment. This variability in response after the first year normalized in the second year (regression to the mean) (14). A second analysis showed that when women were divided into eight groups, the group with the greatest increase in BMD in the first year (10.4%) also had the greatest decrease (1.0%) in year 2. Conversely, the group with the greatest decrease in year 1 (6.6%) had the greatest increase in year 2 (4.8%). The variability in response among the eight groups was approximately 17% (+10.4% to −6.6%) in year 1 and narrowed to a 6% difference after two years of BMD data were available (15,16).

Evidence has demonstrated that an individual need not gain BMD on treatment to still obtain some degree of fracture protection efficacy. However, statistically significant decreases in BMD are not desirable and should prompt evaluation for secondary causes of bone loss. Another related point is that changes in bone mineral density explain less than half of the vertebral antifracture efficacy of antiresorptive agents; changes in bone turnover, which occur earlier and in temporal association with fracture protection, appear to explain much of the rest. In large clinical trials, alendronate and risedronate both reduce vertebral fractures by about 50%. Although alendronate produces a greater increase in bone mineral density, this has not translated into greater antifracture efficacy. Antiresorptive treatments typically reduce systemic bone resorption markers [serum C-telopeptide of type 1 collagen (CTx) and N-telopeptide of type 1 collagen (NTx)] by 40%–70% and bone formation markers [bone-specific alkaline phosphatase, osteocalcin, and serum amino-terminal propeptide of type 1 procollagen (P1NP)] by 30%–50%. These commercially available tests offer an early method to confirm biological effect and medical compliance vis-a-vis antiresorptive therapies.

Risk Factors for Fracture

A thorough history and physical exam should be performed to identify risk factors for fragility fracture. Modifiable risk factors include low vitamin D and calcium intake, smoking, imbibing greater than two alcoholic drinks per day, a sedentary lifestyle devoid of weight-bearing exercise, and household fall hazards such as loose rugs. A World Health Organization (WHO) task force will shortly be producing an absolute

fracture risk equation, which will provide a 10-year fracture risk on every bone densitometry report; each country will need to determine the risk threshold where treatment is deemed worthwhile.

Low bone density correlates with increased fracture risk in postmenopausal women. For each standard deviation decrease in BMD (one T-score unit), fracture risk increases by 1.5- to 3.0-fold, depending on the site assessed (17–19). The T-score cutoff of −2.5 standard deviations below mean-peak BMD was chosen since it produced a 17% prevalence of osteoporosis in the femoral neck that was similar to the estimated 15% lifetime risk of hip fracture for 50-year-old white women in the United States (20). Many factors must be taken into account when determining overall fracture risk—the decision to treat a patient should not be based solely on BMD. In the author's opinion, some patients need to be educated and/or reassured (to decrease their anxiety) that low bone mineral density alone does not necessarily put them at high risk for fracture. Age is a powerful predictor of fracture risk, independent of BMD (21). A 50-year-old female with a T-score of −2.5 and no other risk factors for fragility fracture has a 10-year fracture risk of 5%, whereas this risk goes up to 20% at the age of 65 (22). This may be due to microarchitectural deterioration (loss of horizontal trabeculae) and increased fall risk with age. Another extremely important risk factor for fracture independent of BMD is a history of prior fragility fracture (23); a fragility fracture at a given site increases risk for future fragility fractures *at all sites*. Detection of vertebral fractures by lateral thoracolumbar x-ray or by DXA with VFA (see the previous section "Bone Densitometry") may therefore be the key in determining need for treatment. See Table 59.2 for some independent risk factors for vertebral and hip fractures.

Levels of biochemical markers of bone resorption and formation above a premenopausal range have been shown to be independent risk factors for fracture and add synergistically to low BMD to predict fracture risk (24). However, studies evaluating the ability of these markers to predict bone loss in individual patients have yielded mixed results, probably due to marked diurnal variation and substantial intrapatient variability (25). There may be a subset of patients with osteopenia whom elevated markers of bone turnover can cost-effectively select for treatment, but no definite conclusions can be drawn at this point (26).

History and Physical Examination

The initial history and physical exam should seek evidence for medical conditions (secondary causes) associated with bone loss as well as conditions and/

TABLE 59.2

Risk Factors Besides Low BMD that Increase Fracture Risk in Postmenopausal Women

RELATIVE RISK (HIP/ VERTEBRAL FRACTURE)	RISK FACTOR
2–4	Current corticosteroid use
2–3	White race vs black or Hispanic
2–2.5	Poor health (frailty)
1.5–2/1.5	Fragility fracture as adult
1.5–2/4	Vertebral fracture on spine radiograph
2/1.5	Older age (per 10-yr increase)
2/2–2.5	Rheumatoid arthritis
2/1.5	Parental history of hip fracture
1.5–2/1.5–2	Current smoking (vs never or past)
2.0/?	Elevated bone turnover (N-telopeptide)
1.7/?	Increased body sway

Source: Adapted from Ref. 20.

or medications that increase the risk of fracture due to nonskeletal reasons, such as poor balance. Drugs with anticholinergic side effects as well as sedative hypnotics may predispose to poor balance and falls. The initial history should assess chronicity of the condition and rate of change in BMD relative to the least significant statistical change; a sharp decline in BMD may raise suspicion for development of a secondary cause. Current and historical dietary calcium intake should be assessed. Weight loss, extremely common in cancer patients, is also a risk factor for bone loss and fracture. Reproductive history, including age of menarche, any amenorrhea, and age of menopause, also should be assessed, as hypoestrogenemia will affect bone density. Symptoms of hypogonadism (fatigue, decreased libido) should be sought in men. Exercise history is also assessed, as a sedentary lifestyle contributes to bone loss. Signs or symptoms of thyroid disease, Cushing syndrome, hepatic or gastrointestinal disease, and disorders predisposing to poor balance should be sought out. The patient should be questioned about excess use of alcohol (more than two drinks a day), tobacco, and caffeine. Taking an accurate height is important—a historical loss of height of 1.5 inches or a documented loss of height of 0.75 inches should raise suspicion for vertebral fracture. Orthostatic vitals signs should be performed on any patient with complaints of dizziness, as this may increase fall risk. A neurological examination to assess gait and balance is also important given the significant contribution of these variables

to hip fracture risk. For more detailed fall prevention strategies, please refer to the section Fall Prevention Measures below.

Secondary Causes of Bone Loss

Laboratory Testing

The Institute for Clinical Systems Improvement (ICSI) has issued recommendations for laboratory testing in patients with newly diagnosed osteoporosis (Table 59.3). Note that additional tests are suggested if the patient's Z-score is below –1.0 or the patient has a history of premature osteoporotic fracture, since these patients are at higher risk of having secondary causes of osteoporosis. Although bone turnover markers are not included in the ICSI guidelines, in patients treated with antiresorptive agents, they are a useful method to assess both medical compliance and whether an undiagnosed secondary cause is confounding treatment efforts, since suppression of these markers is expected on antiresorptive medications. The urinary N-telopeptide cross-links (NTX) should be done as a second morning void or on a 24-hour urine sample; serologic markers should be done in a fasting state. In renal insufficiency, serum markers are preferred.

In men, a secondary cause of osteoporosis can be found in 30%–60% of cases (hypogonadism, glucocorticoid use, and alcoholism are the most common) (27). In postmenopausal women, Tannenbaum et al. (28) have found the prevalence of undetected disorders of bone and mineral metabolism, with osteoporosis to be 32%; however, the definition of vitamin D deficiency used in this study, 12.5 ng/mL, is overly conservative by current practice standards. In a subsequent study, using a cutoff of 30 ng/mL, Holick et al. (29) reported inadequate serum 25-hydroxyvitamin D (25-OHD) levels in 52% of 1,536 postmenopausal women under treatment for osteoporosis. The 25-OHD level is the best measure of nutritional vitamin D status; the optimum level is debatable, but is probably between 30 and 80 ng/mL. Achieving a 25-OHD level above 30 ng/mL eliminates secondary hyperparathyroidism and optimizes calcium absorption (30,31). Using this definition of adequacy, vitamin D insufficiency is probably the most common secondary contributor to bone loss. A useful caveat regarding secondary hyperparathyroidism is that the upper limit of the age-appropriate reference range for parathyroid hormone in people less than age 45 is approximately 45 pg/mL, whereas in people older than 45 years, the laboratory reference range upper limits may be used. In any patient with persistent hyperparathyroidism after vitamin D levels are replete, the glomerular filtration rate (GFR) should be calculated to rule out chronic kidney disease (CKD),

TABLE 59.3

ICSI Guidelines for Laboratory Testing in Patients with Newly Diagnosed Osteoporosis

LABORATORY TEST	RATIONALE
Z-score above –1.0 (patients less likely to have secondary causes of osteoporosis)	
Serum creatinine and calculated GFR	Renal failure (GFR <60) may be associated with secondary hyperparathyroidism
Liver function tests	Intrinsic liver diseases and cholestatic disorders are associated with multifactorial causes of osteoporosis
Serum calcium	Increased in patients with hyperparathyroidism and decreased in those with malabsorption or vitamin D deficiency
Alkaline phosphatase	Increased in patients with Paget disease of bone, prolonged immobilization, acute fractures, and other bone diseases
Serum phosphorus	Decreased in patients with osteomalacia, elevated in chronic renal failure
Thyroid studies (TSH and free T4)	Hyperthyroidism-associated bone loss
Sedimentation rate or bone loss	May indicate an inflammatory process or monoclonal gammopathy associated with C-reactive Protein
Complete blood cell count	To evaluate for bone marrow malignancy, infiltrative processes (anemia, low WBC, or low platelets), or malabsorption (anemia, microcytosis, or macrocytosis)
Urinary calcium excretion	24-h urinary calcium excretion on a optimal calcium intake diet screens for: (1) malabsorption (low 24-h urinary calcium excretion suggests vitamin D deficiency, osteomalacia, or malabsorption due to small bowel disease such as celiac sprue) or, (2) hypercalciuria (a correctable cause of bone loss)
Serum 25-OHD	To identify vitamin D insufficiency or deficiency
Serum intact (whole-molecule) PTH	Screening for primary or secondary hyperparathyroidism
Z-score below –1.0 or premature osteoporotic fracture (patients at higher risk of having secondary causes of osteoporosis)	
All the above tests, plus the following additional tests:	
Serum testosterone (total and free)	Screening for hypogonadism in men; if abnormal, LH, FSH, and prolactin measurements may be indicated to determine the cause of the hypogonadism
Serum estradiol	Screening for hypogonadism in premenopausal or perimenopausal women; if abnormal, LH, FSH, and prolactin measurements may be indicated to determine the cause of the hypogonadism
Tissue transglutaminase antibodies	If gluten enteropathy (celiac sprue) is suspected clinically
24-h urinary free cortisol and/or 1mg dexamethasone suppression	If hypercortisolemia is suspected
Serum and urine protein electrophoresis	If monoclonal gammopathy is suspected (with immunoelectrophoresis as indicated)

Abbreviations: FSH, follicle-stimulating hormone; GFR, glomerular filtration rate; ICSI, Institute for Clinical Systems Improvement; LH, luteinizing hormone; PTH, parathyroid hormone; serum 25-OHD, 25-hydroxy vitamin D; WBC, white blood cell count; TSH, thyroid stimulating hormone.

Adapted from Ref. 4.

which can cause elevations in parathyroid hormone when the GFR falls below 60 mL/min per 1.73 m². Renal osteodystrophy, or the new term "CKD-mineral and bone disorder," (32) may raise fracture risk and contribute to bone loss through multiple mechanisms; appropriate management should be instituted.

A 24-hour calcium collection may be performed in cases suspicious for a secondary cause. Calcium excretion is low in calcium malabsorption states, such as that resulting from vitamin D deficiency. Celiac disease may cause both calcium and vitamin D malabsorption. Patients with low BMD and weight loss should be screened for celiac disease, even if they do not have gastrointestinal symptoms (33). Weight loss (common in cancer patients) without an organic cause warrants referral to a nutritionist for improvement of caloric intake. If there is a history of renal stones, 24-hour urine calcium should be performed. Idiopathic hypercalciuria and primary hyperparathyroidism may cause bone loss, hypercalciuria, and elevations in parathyroid hormone levels. In idiopathic hypercalciuria, the serum calcium tends to be low-normal—this condition is treated with a thiazide diuretic.

Multiple myeloma and other lymphoproliferative malignancies may cause diffuse bone loss or vertebral compression fractures similar to osteoporosis; the authors suggest a low threshold for laboratory evaluation to rule out these disorders.

Medications

Another common secondary cause of bone loss is medications: Glucocorticoids, antiepileptics (largely due to perturbations of vitamin D metabolism), immunosuppressive agents, long-term heparin, total parenteral nutrition, cytotoxic drugs, and medications given to induce a hypogonadal state (aromatase inhibitors and luteinizing hormone-releasing hormone agonists) all may contribute.

TREATMENT

Nonpharmacologic Therapy

Calcium and Vitamin D

The currently recommended total calcium intake from all sources is 1200 mg per day in divided doses (5). Calcium citrate is the preferred calcium formulation for patients who have low gastric acidity, such as those taking proton pump inhibitors (PPIs). A recent study associating PPI use with increased risk for hip fracture has underlined this point (34). The U.S. recommended daily allowance (RDA) for vitamin D appears to be inadequate for optimum bone health (35). Additionally, vitamin D repletion may prevent falls and improve muscle function (36). Hypothetically, optimizing vitamin D status may benefit cancer patients, in particular due to antiproliferative and proapoptotic effects of the activated form (37). As mentioned, we routinely measure serum 25-OHD and replete nutritional vitamin D stores to achieve a level greater than 30 ng/mL. When 25-OHD levels are between 10 and 20 ng/mL, we pre-

TABLE 59.4
Vitamin D Repletion Based on 25-Hydroxy-D Level with Goal >30 ng/mL

CURRENT 25-OHD SERUM LEVEL (NG/ML)	TREATMENT
<10	Long-term ergocalciferol 50,000 IU weekly
10–20	Ergocalciferol 50,000 IU weekly × 8 wks followed by maintenance: If > age 65: 50,000 IU every 2 wks If < age 65: 50,000 IU every 3 wks
20–30	[30 – (current level)] × 100 = extra daily IU over-the-counter vitamin D₃ cholecalciferol
>30	Continue current practice

Abbreviations: IU: international unit; serum 25-OHD, 25-hydroxy vitamin D.

scribe ergocalciferol (vitamin D₂), 50,000 IU weekly for eight weeks, followed by a maintenance regimen (Table 59.4). Using pharmacologic vitamin D repletion is safe, provided there is no evidence of granulomatous disease such as sarcoidosis and no evidence of primary hyperparathyroidism with elevated serum calcium. Vitamin D levels less than 10 ng/mL associated with secondary elevations in parathyroid hormone and alkaline phosphatase suggest osteomalacia—long-term calcium and high-dose vitamin D therapy should be employed with the aid of endocrinology evaluation.

Physical Therapy Interventions

Despite the high prevalence of osteopenia and osteoporosis in the general and oncologic population, there is a lack of knowledge among rehabilitation professionals and the public with regard to safe and effective therapy interventions. A comprehensive physical therapy program should incorporate weight-bearing and resistance exercises to preserve or increase bone strength, as well as balance training and multidisciplinary fall prevention strategies to minimize fall and fracture risk. A strong emphasis should also be placed on postural retraining to correct or prevent hyperkyphotic posture and associated postural malalignments, such as forward-head posture. Body mechanics, positioning, and activity counseling tailored to the osteoporotic patient are equally essential to prevent repeated excessive loading of the vertebral bodies during activities of daily living (ADLs). Excellent resources include the NOF publications "Health Professional's Guide to Rehabilitation of the Patient with Osteoporosis" (38) and "Boning Up on Osteoporosis" (39), as well as physical therapist

Sara Meeks' book *Walk Tall* (40), which is also suitable for patients.

WEIGHT-BEARING AND RESISTIVE EXERCISE. Weight-bearing exercise may decrease fracture risk by improving of BMD (41) and reducing fall risk (42). Increase in bone mineral content following exercise intervention is greatest in early puberty or before menarche (2%–5% per year in the L-spine and femoral neck) (43,44). For this reason, jumping activities (45) and other high- and variable-impact activities, such as soccer, racquet sports, volleyball, gymnastics, and step aerobics (46,47), should be encouraged during childhood to optimize peak bone mass. In postmenopausal women, exercise appears to preserve rather than significantly increase BMD, yielding a BMD net gain of only 1%–3% (48,49). This may be at least partially attributable to a decrease in estrogen receptors (50) and the reduced ability to engage in an exercise program with high-magnitude loading (47) without overloading already compromised bone. On an encouraging note, animal studies suggest that modest BMD gains are accompanied by large improvements in structural properties of bone in response to mechanical loading (51). Since these properties contribute to 20%–30% of bone strength (47,52), optimazation of this component of bone strength may reduce fracture risk.

Optimal bone loading should be dynamic and direct weight-bearing forces through the sites most susceptible to fracture (ie, the axial skeleton and hips). Therefore, walking is an excellent initial choice of weight-bearing exercise for cancer patients and survivors. Unlike muscle, bone does not appear to respond to exercise in a linear fashion. Animal studies have demonstrated that short bouts of dynamic exercise separated by rest periods of several hours are more effective osteogenic stimuli than a single sustained session. This is thought to be due to the rapid desensitization of mechanoreceptors (50,51). Therefore, weight-bearing exercise prescription for patients with low bone density should entail daily or alternate daily walking sessions of 30 minutes in one to three bouts (49). Because customary mechanical loading makes bone cells less responsive to routine loading signals, weight-bearing exercise should aim to create a novel strain distribution to effect changes in bone density and architecture (50). One suggested loading strategy is to "surprise the bones" by dancing or walking over varied terrain at different speeds, with varying step lengths, and in different patterns (sideways, backwards) (40).

The addition of Nordic walking poles (modified cross-country poles) to walking has several well-substantiated benefits for the osteoporotic patient. It encourages a more upright posture and decreases the stress on spine and knees (53). Using walking poles as an assistive device also improves gait mechanics as compared to walking with a walker or cane. Due to the active involvement of the upper extremities, it may even increase cardiovascular work without increasing subjective exertion (54).

Because the largest physiological load on a bone result from muscle contraction (55,56), a walking program should be complemented by progressive resistive training two to three times per week. Resistive exercise has been shown to increase BMD, in particular, at the hip (41) and radius, and can be done using one's body weight (eg, wall push-ups), free weights, elastic tubing, or gym equipment. It should incorporate both eccentric and concentric muscle contractions and involve moderate-to-high loading and low repetitions (three to eight repetitions) (38,57). Initial instruction is recommended to ensure proper alignment form, and proper progression of resistance (57).

WHOLE BODY VIBRATION (WBV). Since vigorous weight-bearing and strength training regimens tend to be associated with low compliance rates and with risk of injury in the frail and elderly, there is a need to explore safe alternative strategies to enhance BMD and reduce fractures in this population. Animal-based studies have demonstrated dramatic increases in weight-bearing trabecular bone after WBV (58), and an increasing number of randomized controlled trials has investigated the effects of WBV in humans. WBV delivered via vibrating platforms have been associated with positive outcomes, including increased hip BMD, balance (59), and muscle strength (60). High compliance rates decreased fall risk and increased health-related quality of life have been reported in nursing home residents (61). In children with mobility disabilities, low-magnitude, high-frequency WBV has produced volumetric trabecular BMD net gains in the order of 17% in the proximal tibia as compared to controls (62). To date, no vibration-related side effects, such as back disorders, have been reported after therapeutic use of WBV when performed with correct posture. Unfortunately, most studies are limited by small sample sizes and were conducted with young and healthy study participants. As a result, the possibility of long-term side effects in the elderly population still warrants further investigation (63). Further research is also required to determine the optimal dose and frequency for this promising modality, as well as the optimal parameters of a combined vibration and resistance program (63). Of note, the largest amount of clinical data lies with the vibrating platforms manufactured by Juvent Medical, Inc. Unlike other vibrating platforms now commonly found in gyms, the Juvent device features the osteogenic parameters pioneered by Rubin (58) and is significantly more expensive. Currently, WBV therapy or dynamic motion therapy (DMT) via the Juvent machine is approved for clinical treatment of osteopenia and osteoporosis in Canada, but not yet in the United States.

FALL PREVENTION MEASURES. Falls have a complex etiology and precede the majority of hip and other appendicular fractures, as well as a substantial proportion of VCFs (64). Therefore, it is paramount to identify any medical condition or medication that may predispose a person to fall, timely referral to relevant services, including physiatry, neurology, physical, and occupational therapy is essential. In conjunction with an environmental modifications as indicated by an occupational home assessment, recurrent fall risk can be reduced significantly (57). Physical therapy-mediated interventions can effectively counter the consequences of age-associated sarcopenia and balance deficits (65–67). Fall-directed interventions include transfer and gait training, including the prescription of assistive devices, proprioceptive dynamic posture training (68), and progressive hip, quadriceps, and ankle muscle strengthening. Numerous studies have also credited Tai Chi with improving balance and reducing falls in older adults by up to 40% (69–71). Furthermore, health care professionals should encourage an active lifestyle, as inactivity is a well-documented risk factor for falls in the geriatric population. A prospective cohort study by Gregg and colleagues demonstrated a substantially lower incidence of hip fracture in older women (>65 years of age) who engaged in walking, gardening, or social dancing for at least one hour/week versus no activity, and those who sat less than 6 hours/day versus >9 hours/day (72). Hip protectors represent another preventative measure for institutionalized elderly prone to falls, even though issues surrounding adherence have limited studies attempting to demonstrate effectiveness (73,74).

POSTURAL RETRAINING. An exaggerated thoracic kyphosis is commonly observed in this population and warrants treatment, as it (1) augments the flexion moment on the vertebral bodies (75), thus rendering them more vulnerable to VCF (76), which, in turn, may further worsen kyphosis (77); (2) places the erector spinae at a mechanical disadvantage to counteract the increased thoracic flexion moment; (3) alters the alignment of the body, thus frequently leading to postural pain syndromes; and (4) increases the propensity for falls due to a forward shift in the center of gravity (78).

Several studies suggest that the negative sequelae of hyperkyphosis are amenable to physical therapy interventions. Sinaki and colleagues demonstrated

a significant decrease in the incidence of VCFs with improved erector spinae strength, without an increase in spinal BMD (79). Since the majority of VCFs occurs in the lower thoracic and upper lumbar spine, strengthening of the corresponding portion of the erector spinae in the supine and prone position is recommended (79,80). Improvements in trunk strength with exercise have even been demonstrated in older women (mean age = 80) (81). A recent study by Katzman et al. suggested that significant improvements in the angle of kyphosis and spinal extension strength in community-dwelling women with kyphosis are achievable with a three-month group exercise intervention with emphasis on progressive spinal extension and scapular strengthening, core stability, and postural alignment training (82). Furthermore, a four-week home-based exercise program developed by Sinaki et al. using a weighted kypho-orthosis (WKO) or postural training support (PTS) was effective in improving balance, gait, and risk of falls in patients with moderate kyphosis. Use of this inexpensive and user-friendly spinal orthosis also improved subjective back pain and back extensor strength. Subjects were instructed to wear the WKO daily for 90 minutes in the morning and afternoon during ambulatory activities and while performing once-daily spinal extension exercises (10 repetitions). In addition, they engaged in a twice-daily 10-minute proprioceptive balance program (83). There is some evidence that therapeutic taping can decrease the angle of kyphosis, but has not been shown to have an effect on the activation of trunk muscles as measured by trunk electromyography (EMG) (84). One case study utilized neurodevelopmental techniques (NDT) with remarkable improvement in angle of kyphosis, balance, and posture (85).

PRECAUTIONS. Despite the importance of erector spinae strengthening, the amount of spinal extension must be carefully monitored if comorbidities such as spondylolisthesis and spinal stenosis are present. In many cases, a short psoas muscle can contribute to the aforementioned pathologies by causing excessive lumbar lordosis via its attachment to the anterior lumbar vertebral bodies. In these cases, mobilization of the psoas muscle, which is preferably done when lying on the side (80), can make a certain amount of spinal extension safe and symptom-free.

In addition, individuals with low spinal bone density should avoid spinal flexion exercises, particularly abdominal crunches, as this exercise increases compression on the vertebral bodies.

This recommendation is based on the biomechanical consideration that spinal flexion exerts increased compression forces on the anterior part of the vertebral body.

Moreover, sit-ups mainly target the rectus abdominis muscle, which contributes little to the stability of the low back and the improvement of low back pain. Instead, emphasis should be placed on lower abdominal muscles (transversus abdominis and internal/external oblique muscles) strengthening in a neutral spine position (86). Gym, yoga, or Pilates exercises involving spinal flexion should therefore be avoided or done cautiously with an elongated spine under the supervision of instructors knowledgeable in the aforementioned precautions (57).

PATIENT EDUCATION. VCFs can also result from repeated stresses of everyday life activites (87,88). Therefore, patients should be instructed to maintain a normal lumbar lordosis in sitting and sleeping positions, as well as during transitional movements (eg, getting up from a chair or in and out of bed). Training patients to hip-hinge during ADLs as an alternative to forward bending with lifting is likewise crucial, as the latter can increase the compressive load on the spine by up to eight times (89,90). For patients with severe hip or knee limitations, adaptive aids such as a long-handled reacher, shoe horn, and bath brush may be indicated to avoid repeated spinal flexion during ADLs.

Patient education on the principles of safe versus unsafe bone loading activities is likewise important. While high-impact activities, such as high-impact aerobics and jumping, are beneficial for osteogenesis in the healthy, premenopausal population (91), such activities may overload an osteopenic or osteoporotic spine and predispose to VCFs. For the same reason, activities that emphasize spinal flexion, loaded rotation, and side-bending, such as golfing and bowling, should be avoided in individuals with low spinal bone density (80,92). Swimming (breast and backstroke), by contrast, should be safe and may be beneficial for posture and pain control, as it promotes thoracic spinal extension. Modified yoga training may have beneficial effects as well (93).

PHYSICAL THERAPY CONSIDERATIONS AFTER ACUTE COMPRESSION FRACTURES. For patients with severe pain, early referral to pain management should be considered. Physical therapy should also be initiated for patients with acute vertebral compression fractures to restore function. Because of the well-known deleterious effects of prolonged bed rest, including a loss of about 1% of bone per week (94), partial bed rest with periodic bouts of ambulation is recommended. A rolling walker can facilitate safe mobility and a more erect posture, and is preferred over a standard walker, which requires lifting for advancement (95). For the duration of the acute phase, prolonged sitting, especially with slumped posture, should be avoided, as this places high loads on the healing vertebral fracture (90). The authors recommend supported upright or reclined sitting (96) (eg, in a reclining wheelchair) using a towel roll as a lumbar support. When in bed, patients should be encouraged to lie as close to full supine as possible with their knees bent for 15-minute intervals several times a day and to initiate the "re-alignment routine" as outlined by Meeks (40,80). This positioning and isometric exercise should unload the vertebral bodies and may facilitate healing of VCFs (80). Alternative resting positions are side lying or the semi-Fowler 30°–30° position with emphasis on the bed bending at the level of the hips and not the spine (97). Since patients with VCFs are at an increased risk for further compression fractures (98), guidelines for safe movement during ADLs should be reviewed (see Ref. 57 for detailed and illustrated guidelines), including lifting restrictions of approximately 10 lb. After the acute phase, most patients can benefit from a slowly progressive exercise program in supported positions to avoid high loads on the vertebrae (57). In cases of intractable pain despite conservative management, vertebroplastly or kyphoplasty may be considered. These procedures, however, are no substitute for rehabilitative measures after fracture, since recurrent fracture risk persists.

Individuals with osteoporosis who cannot refrain from bending or lifting due to occupational demands, such as caring for young children, may benefit from bracing. Use of rigid braces for VCFs has been limited by discomfort due to restricted motion and respiration, poor fit secondary to short stature, unappealing aesthetic appearance, and atrophy of trunk muscles, leading to low compliance (99,100). Alternatives include a recently developed spinal orthosis (*Spinomed*), which consists of a moldable aluminum back piece and an abdominal pad. It can be worn like a backpack under clothing and is well tolerated in individuals with mild to moderate scoliosis due to the flexibility of its back piece. The proposed mechanism of action of this brace is via the principle of biofeedback. A recent prospective randomized controlled trial investigated the effectiveness of this orthosis in community-dwelling postmenopausal women with VCFs due to osteoporosis. Wearing the brace two hours a day for six months showed a 90% compliance rate and significant improvements in pain and function. Back extensor strength improved by 73%, and the angle of kyphosis was reduced by 11%. In addition, a decrease in body sway of 25% was observed, which may also decrease the risk for falls (101). These results are promising, even though the study was limited by a small sample size ($n = 62$).

SPECIAL THERAPY CONSIDERATIONS FOR CANCER PATIENTS. Many oncologic patients are at risk for bone loss due to medications (See "Scenarios Unique to Oncology Patients"), decreased mobility, and weight loss. Even if a patient has active disease, physical therapy interventions, as tolerated, may serve to increase quality of life and prevent the rapid bone loss associated with low physical activity and cancer treatments, such as stem cell transplantation, chemotherapy-induced ovarian failure, long-term corticosteroid use, aromatase inhibitor, and gonadotropin-releasing hormone agonist therapy. Written guidelines to promote an active lifestyle and fall prevention, as well as illustrated exercises to encourage osteogenic weight bearing, resistance, and postural exercises are recommended.

Ambulatory cancer survivors with osteopenia and osteoporosis may benefit from enrollment in a multi-disciplinary osteoporosis group program comprised of weekly physical therapy-led exercise sessions complemented by weekly education components with cancer-specific precautions mediated by physiatry, physical therapy, endocrinology, and dietetics. In the authors' experience, a five-week program may be a cost-effective way to improve disease management skills and exercise compliance, as well as balance, posture, and body mechanics. Prior to enrollment, a physical therapy examination aimed at assessing the severity of postural change, functional, and cognitive status is recommended to ensure suitability for group therapy. Likewise, a thorough review of comorbidities is indicated to ensure exercise is modified to accommodate musculoskeletal and cancer-specific precautions. Common example include spinal stenosis, spondylolisthesis, total hip replacements, lymphedema, bone metastases, avascular necrosis post-radiation, and aspiration-risk postesophagectomy precluding a completely supine position.

Pharmacologic Therapy

See Table 59.5 for clinically relevant information on FDA approved therapies for treatment of postmenopausal osteoporosis.

Bisphosphonates

These agents inhibit osteoclastic bone resorption and increase BMD through secondary mineralization; they are considered antiresorptives. Bisphosphonates have a

TABLE 59.5

Major Therapeutic Options in the Treatment of Postmenopausal Osteoporosis

	DOSING	MECHANISM/ CLASS	ANTI-FRACTURE EFFICACY	SELECTED CAVEATS
Risedronate	35 mg orally weekly or 150 mg monthly	Antiresorptive/ bisphosphonate	Vertebral+ nonvertebral	For optimal efficacy and safety, must follow administration instructions precisely
Alendronate	70 mg orally weekly	Antiresorptive/ bisphosphonate	Vertebral+ nonvertebral	For optimal efficacy and safety, must follow administration instructions precisely
Ibandronate	150 mg orally monthly or 3 mg IV push every 3 mo	Antiresorptive/ bisphosphonate	Vertebral	For optimal efficacy and safety, must follow administration instructions precisely
Zoledronate	5 mg IV yearly (over 15 min)	Antiresorptive/ bisphosphonate	Vertebral+ nonvertebral	(1) Get baseline and follow-up dental exams (2) Self-limited "flulike" reaction common in up to 44% after first dose
Raloxifene	60 mg orally daily	Antiresorptive/ selective estrogen receptor modulator	Vertebral	Avoid if: (1) history of venous thrombosis or (2) recently completed 5 yrs of tamoxifen or (3) currently on aromatase inhibitor
Teriparatide (recombinant parathyroid hormone)	20 mg subcutaneous daily	Anabolic/stimulates osteoblastic bone formation	Vertebral+ nonvertebral	(1) Black box warning (2) Contraindicated with history of radiation therapy (3) Try to avoid use in any patient with history of cancer (see text)

low bioavailability and consequently must be taken in a fasting state with 8 ounces of nonmineral water (no other liquid), without subsequent food or drink for at least 30 minutes (60 minutes for ibandronate) in order to be absorbed. To avoid pill esophagitis, patients must remain upright at least for this duration. Risedronate and alendronate are oral bisphosphonates administered with weekly dosing that have been proven to reduce the risk for vertebral and nonvertebral fractures. Alendronate and risedronate increase lumbar spine BMD by 5%–7% and hip BMD by 3%–6% when used for approximately three years (102,103). Formulations of alendronate with extra vitamin D are available, which contain the equivalent of 400 and 800 IU of vitamin D_3 per day, respectively. An oral bisphosphonate that is administered monthly, ibandronate has been shown to prevent spine fractures but has not been shown to prevent hip fractures thus far. Zoledronic acid is a potent intravenous bisphosphonate recently Food and Drug Administration (FDA)-approved at a dose of 5 mg yearly for postmenopausal osteoporosis. Bisphosphonates as a class have long half-lives in bone. Therefore, after five years of use, the author considers drug "holidays" of up to five years, depending on the trend in bone turnover markers off of drug, and with the exception of those patients who are at high risk for fracture (104).

Contraindications to bisphosphonate use include pregnancy, hypersensitivity, inability to stand or sit upright for at least 30 minutes after ingestion, hypocalcemia, any medical problem that delays esophageal emptying such as esophageal stricture or achalasia (since prolonged contact with the drug will irritate the esophagus), and end-stage renal disease with adynamic bone disease. Precautions include chronic renal failure and a history of severe upper gastrointestinal (GI) disease. Adequate vitamin D and calcium intake should be ensured and vitamin D stores replete before starting these drugs. The drug should be discontinued if an esophageal reaction (eg, dysphagia, odynophagia, retrosternal pain, worsening heartburn) occurs.

SELECTED ADVERSE EVENTS. A transient flulike illness may occur following administration (particularly intravenous bisphosphonates). On post-hoc analysis, oral bisphosphonates appear to be safe (no deterioration in renal function) and effective at preventing fracture in chronic renal failure patients with glomerular filtration rates as low as 15 mL/min (105). Renal deterioration with intravenous bisphosphonates appears to be infusion-duration-dependent, and any patient with a GFR less than 30 mL/min should probably have their infusion time increased. Adynamic bone disease, which occurs almost entirely in patients with end-stage renal disease (GFR<15 mL/min), is a contraindication to bisphosphonate use.

Cases of osteonecrosis of the jaw have been reported in osteoporosis patients treated with oral bisphosphonates; a rough guess at the incidence is 1/100,000, though the background population incidence is not currently known (106). Since two-thirds of cases are associated with invasive dental procedures, a prudent approach is to have dental problems identified and treated before beginning the drugs. This complication is much more common in patients with skeletal metastases or multiple myeloma being treated with monthly intravenous bisphosphonates.

In large clinical trials, the incidence of upper gastrointestinal problems in women receiving alendronate or risedronate was not different from those receiving placebo.

Raloxifene

This is a selective estrogen receptor modulator (SERM) that acts as an estrogen agonist in some tissues (bone, liver) and as an estrogen antagonist in breast tissue. Like estrogen, it is an antiresorptive. In postmenopausal osteoporotic women, it has been shown to prevent vertebral fractures but not hip fractures, perhaps due to less potent bone turnover suppression than bisphosphonates.

When considering this agent for treatment of postmenopausal patients with hormone-receptor-positive, early-stage breast cancer and bone loss, a few caveats should be noted. In patients with estrogen-receptor-positive breast cancer, either tamoxifen (a first-generation SERM) or a selective aromatase inhibitor is the standard of care for adjuvant hormonal therapy. Prolonging treatment duration beyond five years of adjuvant tamoxifen may be associated with worse outcomes (107,108). Also, the oncologic role of additional tamoxifen in women who have received an aromatase inhibitor for five years is unknown. Worse outcomes were associated with tamoxifen use for more than five years; the safety of using another SERM, raloxifene, immediately after a woman has completed five years of tamoxifen has not been established and is best avoided. A final question is whether to use raloxifene as bone prophylaxis in the setting of aromatase inhibitor use. No oncologic benefit was shown by combining tamoxifen with the aromatase inhibitor anastrozole (109), while a tamoxifen-letrozole combination decreased letrozole levels. Since raloxifene is a less potent antiresorptive compared to bisphosphonates, the author suggests using it in patients receiving aromatase inhibitors only if oral or intravenous (IV) bisphosphonates are not options.

Raloxifene has been associated with an increased risk of fatal stroke (hazard ratio [HR] 1.49; absolute risk increase 0.7 per 1,000), and venous thromboembolism (HR 1.44; absolute risk increase 1.3 per 1,000) in the Raloxifene Use for the Heart (RUTH) trial of postmenopausal women with a history of coronary artery disease and/or risk factors (110). A decreased risk of invasive breast cancer was shown in the RUTH trial, confirming previous findings from an osteoporosis treatment trial (111) and also from a trial of postmenopausal women at high risk for breast cancer (112). The latter trial demonstrated that raloxifene reduced the incidence of invasive breast cancers with equal efficacy to tamoxifen and that raloxifene carried a lower risk of deep venous thrombosis, pulmonary embolus, and cataracts versus tamoxifen. Hot flushes, leg cramps, peripheral edema ,and gallbladder disease are more common with raloxifene than with placebo.

Teriparatide

Recombinant parathyroid hormone is the first anabolic agent approved for treatment of postmenopausal osteoporosis. It has been shown to reduce the incidence of spine and nonvertebral fractures with similar efficacy to the oral bisphosphonates, while increases of spine BMD are of greater magnitude. It is the most expensive treatment option and is administered with a daily subcutaneous injection for two years, after which bisphosphonate therapy must promptly be given to consolidate the newly formed bone. A black box warning accompanies the drug due to an increased incidence of osteosarcoma in rats that was dependent on both dose and duration. It is contraindicated in patients with increased baseline risk of osteosarcoma, such as those with Paget disease of bone, open epiphyses, or prior radiation therapy involving the skeleton.

Although no data in cancer patients exist, teriparatide is best avoided in patients with a history of malignancy prone to metastasize to bone. The drug works to stimulate bone formation and markedly increases bone turnover—a high turnover state may be favorable to propagation of microscopic bone metastases. Additionally, the pathophysiology of cancer metastases to bone involves tumor-produced parathyroid hormone-related peptide (PTHrP) and a vicious cycle of bone turnover creating bone-derived cytokine release. However, in cases of severe osteoporosis with fractures occurring on bisphosphonate therapy, the benefits may outweigh these theoretical risks. In such patients with a remote history of cancer, teriparatide could be considered.

Calcitonin

Calcitonin nasal spray is an antiresorptive medication approved for the treatment of osteoporosis in women at least five years postmenopause. It produces minimal increases in BMD and reduces the risk of vertebral fractures; the effect on hip and nonvertebral fractures is not known (113). It is probably the least potent treatment option and therefore is seldom used.

Scenarios Unique to Oncology Patients

Many cancer treatments may result in rapid and severe bone loss (Fig. 59.1). Commonly, this bone loss is due to iatrogenic induction of a hypogonadal state (prostate cancer and breast cancer). This subject has recently been reviewed (114). Bone marrow transplant (115), chronic corticosteroid treatment, supraphysiologic thyroid hormone suppression therapy, and chemotherapy-induced bone cell toxicity are other situations that may lead to bone loss in cancer patients. All such patients should have laboratory tests done to look for secondary causes (see "Secondary Causes of Bone Loss") and should be counseled on proper nutrition and exercise. Phosphaturia and changes in bone turnover markers are newly detected effects of the tyrosine kinase inhibitor imatinib—the impact on BMD and fracture risk remains to be seen. Bone loss in breast cancer and prostate cancer patients will be addressed herein.

Breast Cancer

Breast cancer patients with node-negative disease have 15-year survival rates in the range of 60%–70%. Therefore, efforts to optimize bone health and decrease morbidity and mortality from bone loss are increasingly more important. In women with newly diagnosed breast cancer without clinical evidence of skeletal metastases, the incidence of new vertebral fracture over the next three years was about fivefold higher than in the normal population; in women with recurrent breast cancer and no evidence of skeletal metastases, the risk of vertebral fracture was 20-fold greater (116). Therefore, clinical suspicion for occult vertebral fracture in breast cancer patients should be high. Among breast cancer patients, chemotherapy-induced ovarian failure and aromatase inhibitor treatment are two major clinical scenarios that predispose to rapid bone loss. Regarding the former, Shapiro et al. reported a striking 7.7% decrease in BMD at the spine and a 4.6% decrease at the femoral neck one year after chemotherapy-induced ovarian failure (117). One-year results from a trial of women with breast cancer (up to eight years post-chemotherapy-induced menopause) has shown that weekly risedronate increased BMD to a small extent versus placebo and decreased bone turnover markers by 20%–30% (118). In contrast to the previously reported dramatic drop in BMD at one year post-chemotherapy-induced menopause, the placebo arm of this more variable population of women showed no significant change in BMD

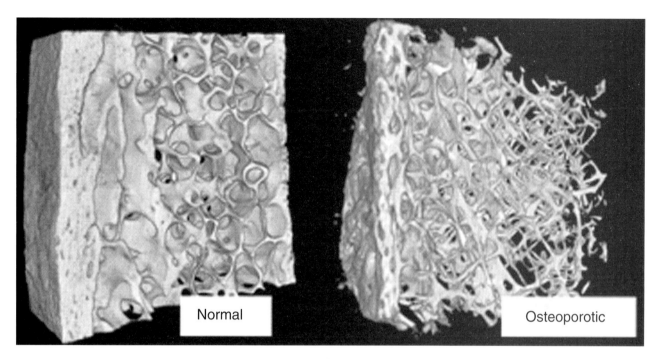

FIGURE 59.3

Human iliac crest biopsies.

over one year at the spine and a small but significant decrease of 0.8 ± 0.3% at the total hip.

Aromatase inhibitors have emerged as first-line adjuvant therapies over tamoxifen in the treatment of estrogen-receptor-positive early breast cancer. Tamoxifen has estrogen agonist activity on bone, whereas aromatase inhibitors lower estrogen to profoundly low levels. Aromatase inhibitors have been shown to elevate bone turnover markers, cause bone loss, and increase fracture risk, both in head-to-head comparison with and subsequent to tamoxifen use (119). Early data suggesting that exemestane has the least harmful profile on bone has not been confirmed. A prospective, randomized study has compared whether empirical administration of zoledronic acid 4 mg every six months made a difference in BMD versus initiating treatment when the T-score declined to less than −2 standard deviations. A substantial BMD benefit at the lumbar spine and total hip with the empirical treatment strategy was demonstrated (120,121). In the delayed group, more patients progressed from mild or moderate to severe osteopenia compared with the upfront group (12 patients [14.8%] vs 1 patient [1.4%], respectively). Eight patients in the delayed group with osteopenia at baseline improved to a normal BMD of the lumbar spine by month 12. Only two of these patients received zoledronic acid at month 6. There were no cases of osteonecrosis of the jaw. Similarly, in premenopausal women, dramatic loss of BMD due to treatment with anastrozole/goserelin (mean T-score reduction, −2.6) or lesser reductions due to tamoxifen/goserelin (mean T-score reduction, −1.1) was prevented in zoledronic acid-treated patients (stable BMD) (121).

Published guidelines regarding bisphosphonate use issued by the American Society of Clinical Oncology in 2003 are relatively conservative in recommending which patients to treat (T-score ≤−2.5), but do mention that the decision to treat osteopenic patients should be made on an individual basis. In the author's opinion, any patient with osteopenic or worse BMD who has undergone premature menopause within the last three years should be prophylaxed with a bisphosphonate. It is not clear if any agent is superior. In patients with normal BMD but other strong risk factors for fracture, treatment may also be prudent. In patients receiving aromatase inhibitors (without concomitant medical ovarian ablation), the magnitude of potential bone loss may be less, and a year of watchful waiting in those patients with osteopenic BMD at relatively low risk for fracture is acceptable. It is the author's practice to measure biochemical markers of bone turnover, since "normal" (midpremenopausal range) or "very high" levels may help predict changes in BMD. Even if a given patient currently is at relatively low risk for fracture, prophylactic prevention of anticipated bone loss can be justified, since once bone loss occurs, the patient's risk will increase. Most patients who demonstrate significant bone loss over one year should be treated with bisphosphonate therapy.

Prostate Cancer

Locally advanced prostate cancer is often treated with gonadotropin-releasing hormone (GnRH) agonists. The discussion here concerns patients without bone metastases. GnRH agonists induce a hypogonadal state, cause loss of BMD, and increase fracture risk (122). The intravenous bisphosphonates and raloxifene have each been studied in this context, respectively. Although zoledronic acid produced impressive BMD gains compared to placebo with every-three-month dosing, the author advises dosing less frequently (every six months to one year) since effective suppression of bone turnover can be achieved with less frequent dosing and more frequent (monthly) dosing of intravenous bisphosphonates in oncologic patients with bone metastases appears to be associated with higher risk for osteonecrosis of the jaw. Regarding raloxifene, a small prospective study showed BMD gains and reduction in bone turnover markers (123). This agent was investigated, since estrogens have an important role not only in female, but also male skeletal health.

Glucocorticoid Use

Even physiologic or replacement doses of glucocorticoids can cause bone loss. Any patient receiving prednisone (or another steroid at equivalent dose) 5 mg or more for at least three months is at risk for bone loss in a dose-dependent manner. We concur with published guidelines for prevention of glucocorticoid-induced bone loss and fractures (124). Salient points include (1) calcium and vitamin D supplementation (1500 mg/day and 800 IU/day, respectively); (2) bisphosphonate therapy (in premenopausal women, contraception counseling is necessary); (3) replacement of gonadal steroids in men if deficient; (4) a trial of nasal calcitonin at a dose of 200 IU/day for pain relief from fractures. Also, we suggest that an exercise program of 30 minutes daily weight bearing (according to the guidelines outlined in the therapy section previously) be initiated. In addition, proximal muscle strengthening should help prevent steroid-induced myopathy and the possible increased risk of falls and fractures accompanying it. The 24-hour urinary calcium excretion should be measured, as glucocorticoids cause hypercalciuria. Urine calcium values above 300 mg/day should be treated with a thiazide diuretic and a sodium-restricted diet.

Monitoring Treatment

Yearly DXA is indicated in cancer patients at high risk for bone loss. We also prefer to monitor treatment efficacy in such oncologic patients, as discussed, with the aid of biochemical markers of bone turnover.

Given the lack of data in these patient populations who are prone to high rates of bone loss, confirming the efficacy of antiresorptive treatment seems prudent. The author's opinion concerning treatment with zoledronic acid at more than yearly intervals is to consider tailoring treatment frequency to the results of bone turnover markers in order to avoid theoretical risks associated with unnecessarily frequent dosing. In general, bone turnover markers near the lower limit of detection (below the premenopausal range) while on bisphosphonate therapy may warrant withholding therapy until they rise.

References

1. Osteoporosis prevention, diagnosis, and therapy. JAMA. 2001;285:785–795.
2. Green AD, Colon-Emeric CS, Bastian L, Drake MT, Lyles KW. Does this woman have osteoporosis? JAMA. 2004;292:2890–2900.
3. Klotzbuecher CM, Ross PD, Landsman PB, Abbott TA, 3rd, Berger M. Patients with prior fractures have an increased risk of future fractures: a summary of the literature and statistical synthesis. J Bone Miner Res. 2000;15:721–739.
4. De Smet AA, Robinson RG, Johnson BE, Lukert BP. Spinal compression fractures in osteoporotic women: patterns and relationship to hyperkyphosis. Radiology. 1988;166:497–500.
5. Physician's Guide to Prevention and Treatment of Osteoporosis. Washington, DC: National Osteoporosis Foundation; 2003.
6. Keene GS, Parker MJ, Pryor GA. Mortality and morbidity after hip fractures. BMJ (Clinical research ed). 1993;307:1248–1250.
7. Salkeld G, Cameron ID, Cumming RG, et al. Quality of life related to fear of falling and hip fracture in older women: a time trade off study. BMJ (Clinical research ed). 2000;320:341–346.
8. Silverman SL, Shen W, Minshall ME, Xie S, Moses KH. Prevalence of depressive symptoms in postmenopausal women with low bone mineral density and/or prevalent vertebral fracture: results from the Multiple Outcomes of Raloxifene Evaluation (MORE) study. J Rheum. 2007;34:140–144.
9. Riggs BL, Melton LJ, 3rd. The worldwide problem of osteoporosis: insights afforded by epidemiology. Bone. 1995;17:505S–511S.
10. Kanis JA. Osteoporosis. London: Blackwell-Healthcare Communications Ltd; 1997.
11. Wainwright SA, Marshall LM, Ensrud KE, et al. Hip fracture in women without osteoporosis. J Clin Endocrinol Metab. 2005;90:2787–2793.
12. Kanis JA, Melton LJ, 3rd, Christiansen C, Johnston CC, Khaltaev N. The diagnosis of osteoporosis. J Bone Miner Res. 1994;9:1137–1141.
13. Mazess R, Chesnut CH, 3rd, McClung M, Genant H. Enhanced precision with dual-energy X-ray absorptiometry. Calcif Tissue Int. 1992;51:14–17.
14. Bonnick SL. Monitoring osteoporosis therapy with bone densitometry: a vital tool or regression toward mediocrity? J Clin Endocrinol Metab. 2000;85:3493–3495.
15. Cummings SR, Palermo L, Browner W, et al. Monitoring osteoporosis therapy with bone densitometry: misleading changes and regression to the mean. Fracture Intervention Trial Research Group. JAMA. 2000;283:1318–1321.
16. Hochberg MC, Ross PD, Black D, et al. Larger increases in bone mineral density during alendronate therapy are associated with a lower risk of new vertebral fractures in women with postmenopausal osteoporosis. Fracture Intervention Trial Research Group. Arthritis Rheum. 1999;42:1246–1254.

17. Cummings SR, Nevitt MC, Browner WS, et al. Risk factors for hip fracture in white women. Study of Osteoporotic Fractures Research Group. *N Engl J Med.* 1995;332:767–773.

18. Silman AJ. Risk factors for Colles' fracture in men and women: results from the European Prospective Osteoporosis Study. *Osteoporos Int.* 2003;14:213–218.

19. Schuit SC, van der Klift M, Weel AE, et al. Fracture incidence and association with bone mineral density in elderly men and women: the Rotterdam Study. *Bone.* 2004;34:195–202.

20. Cummings SR. A 55-year-old woman with osteopenia. *JAMA.* 2006;296:2601–2610.

21. Cummings SR, Bates D, Black DM. Clinical use of bone densitometry: scientific review. *JAMA.* 2002;288:1889–1897.

22. Raisz LG. Clinical practice. Screening for osteoporosis. *N Engl J Med.* 2005;353:164–171.

23. Sambrook P, Cooper C. Osteoporosis. *Lancet.* 2006;367:2010–2018.

24. Garnero P, Hausherr E, Chapuy MC, et al. Markers of bone resorption predict hip fracture in elderly women: the EPIDOS Prospective Study. *J Bone Miner Res.* 1996;11:1531–1538.

25. Garnero P, Mulleman D, Munoz F, Sornay-Rendu E, Delmas PD. Long-term variability of markers of bone turnover in postmenopausal women and implications for their clinical use: the OFELY study. *J Bone Miner Res.* 2003;18:1789–1794.

26. Schousboe JT, Bauer DC, Nyman JA, Kane RL, Melton LJ, Ensrud KE. Potential for bone turnover markers to cost-effectively identify and select post-menopausal osteopenic women at high risk of fracture for bisphosphonate therapy. *Osteoporos Int.* 2007;18:201–210.

27. Mauck KF, Clarke BL. Diagnosis, screening, prevention, and treatment of osteoporosis. *Mayo Clin Proc.* 2006;81:662–672.

28. Tannenbaum C, Clark J, Schwartzman K, et al. Yield of laboratory testing to identify secondary contributors to osteoporosis in otherwise healthy women. *J Clin Endocrinol Metab.* 2002;87:4431–4437.

29. Holick MF, Siris ES, Binkley N, et al. Prevalence of Vitamin D inadequacy among postmenopausal North American women receiving osteoporosis therapy. *J Clin Endocrinol Metab.* 2005;90:3215–324.

30. Chapuy MC, Preziosi P, Maamer M, et al. Prevalence of vitamin D insufficiency in an adult normal population. *Osteoporos Int.* 1997;7:439–443.

31. Heaney RP, Dowell MS, Hale CA, Bendich A. Calcium absorption varies within the reference range for serum 25-hydroxyvitamin D. *J Am Coll Nutr.* 2003;22:142–146.

32. Sprague SM. Renal function and risk of hip and vertebral fractures in older women: is it always osteoporosis? *Arch Intern Med.* 2007;167:115–116.

33. Stenson WF, Newberry R, Lorenz R, Baldus C, Civitelli R. Increased prevalence of celiac disease and need for routine screening among patients with osteoporosis. *Arch Intern Med.* 2005;165:393–399.

34. Yang YX, Lewis JD, Epstein S, Metz DC. Long-term proton pump inhibitor therapy and risk of hip fracture. *JAMA.* 2006;296:2947–2953.

35. Vieth R, Bischoff-Ferrari H, Boucher BJ, et al. The urgent need to recommend an intake of vitamin D that is effective. *Am J Clin Nutr.* 2007;85:649–650.

36. Janssen HC, Samson MM, Verhaar HJ. Vitamin D deficiency, muscle function, and falls in elderly people. *Am J Clin Nutr.* 2002;75:611–615.

37. Beer TM, Myrthue A. Calcitriol in the treatment of prostate cancer. *Anticancer Res.* 2006;26:2647–2651.

38. *Health Professional's Guide to Rehabilitation of the Patient with Osteoporosis.* Washington, DC: National Osteoporosis Foundation; 2003.

39. *Boning Up on Osteoporosis—A Guide to Prevention and Treatment.* National Osteoporosis Foundation; 2005.

40. Meeks S. *Walk Tall: An Exercise Program for the Prevention and Treatment of Osteoporosis.* Gainesville, FL: Triad Publishing Company; 1999.

41. Kerr D, Ackland T, Maslen B, Morton A, Prince R. Resistance training over 2 years increases bone mass in calcium-replete postmenopausal women. *J Bone Miner Res.* 2001;16:175–181.

42. Feskanich D, Willett W, Colditz G. Walking and leisure-time activity and risk of hip fracture in postmenopausal women. *JAMA.* 2002;288:2300–2306.

43. Linden C, Ahlborg HG, Besjakov J, Gardsell P, Karlsson MK. A school curriculum-based exercise program increases bone mineral accrual and bone size in prepubertal girls: two-year data from the pediatric osteoporosis prevention (POP) study. *J Bone Miner Res.* 2006;21:829–835.

44. Fuchs RK, Bauer JJ, Snow CM. Jumping improves hip and lumbar spine bone mass in prepubescent children: a randomized controlled trial. *J Bone Miner Res.* 2001;16:148–156.

45. MacKelvie KJ, Khan KM, Petit MA, Janssen PA, McKay HA. A school-based exercise intervention elicits substantial bone health benefits: a 2-year randomized controlled trial in girls. *Pediatrics.* 2003;112:e447.

46. Nikander R, Sievanen H, Heinonen A, Kannus P. Femoral neck structure in adult female athletes subjected to different loading modalities. *J Bone Miner Res.* 2005;20:520–528.

47. Jiang Y, Zhao J, Rosen C, Geusens P, Genant HK. Perspectives on bone mechanical properties and adaptive response to mechanical challenge. *J Clin Densitom.* 1999;2:423–433.

48. Bonaiuti D, Shea B, Iovine R, et al. Exercise for preventing and treating osteoporosis in postmenopausal women. *Cochrane Database Syst Rev.* 2002;3:CD000333.

49. Asikainen TM, Kukkonen-Harjula K, Miilunpalo S. Exercise for health for early postmenopausal women: a systematic review of randomised controlled trials. *Sports Med.* 2004;34:753–778.

50. Lanyon L, Skerry T. Postmenopausal osteoporosis as a failure of bone's adaptation to functional loading: a hypothesis. *J Bone Miner Res.* 2001;16:1937–1947.

51. Robling AG, Hinant FM, Burr DB, Turner CH. Improved bone structure and strength after long-term mechanical loading is greatest if loading is separated into short bouts. *J Bone Miner Res.* 2002;17:1545–1554.

52. Felsenberg D, Boonen S. The bone quality framework: determinants of bone strength and their interrelationships, and implications for osteoporosis management. *Clin Ther.* 2005;27:1–11.

53. Bohne M, Abendroth-Smith J. Effects of hiking downhill using trekking poles while carrying external loads. *Med Sci Sports Exerc.* 2007;39:177–183.

54. Rodgers CD, VanHeest JL, Schachter CL. Energy expenditure during submaximal walking with Exerstriders. *Med Sci Sports Exerc.* 1995;27:607–611.

55. Lu TW, Taylor SJ, O'Connor JJ, Walker PS. Influence of muscle activity on the forces in the femur: an in vivo study. *J Biomech.* 1997;30:1101–1106.

56. Bassey EJ, Littlewood JJ, Taylor SJ. Relations between compressive axial forces in an instrumented massive femoral implant, ground reaction forces, and integrated electromyographs from vastus lateralis during various "osteogenic" exercises. *J Biomech.* 1997;30:213–223.

57. Bonner FJ, Jr., Sinaki M, Grabois M, et al. Health professional's guide to rehabilitation of the patient with osteoporosis. *Osteoporos Int.* 2003;14(Suppl 2):S1–S22.

58. Rubin C, Turner AS, Bain S, Mallinckrodt C, McLeod K. Anabolism. Low mechanical signals strengthen long bones. *Nature.* 2001;412:603–604.

59. Gusi N, Raimundo A, Leal A. Low-frequency vibratory exercise reduces the risk of bone fracture more than walking: a randomized controlled trial. *BMC Musculoskelet Disord.* 2006;7:92.

60. Verschueren SM, Roelants M, Delecluse C, Swinnen S, Vanderschueren D, Boonen S. Effect of 6-month whole body vibration training on hip density, muscle strength, and postural control in postmenopausal women: a randomized controlled pilot study. *J Bone Miner Res.* 2004;19:352–359.

61. Bruyere O, Wuidart MA, Di Palma E, et al. Controlled whole body vibration to decrease fall risk and improve health-related quality of life of nursing home residents. *Arch Phys Med Rehabil.* 2005;86:303–307.

62. Ward K, Alsop C, Caulton J, Rubin C, Adams J, Mughal Z. Low magnitude mechanical loading is osteogenic in children with disabling conditions. *J Bone Miner Res.* 2004;19:360–369.

63. Cardinale M, Rittweger J. Vibration exercise makes your muscles and bones stronger: fact or fiction? *J Br Menopause Soc.* 2006;12:12–18.

64. Bouxsein ML, Myers ER, Hayes WC. Biomechanics of age-related fractures. In: Marcus R, Feldman D, Kelsey J, eds. *Osteoporosis.* New York: Academic Press; 1996:373–393.

65. Frontera WR, Hughes VA, Fielding RA, Fiatarone MA, Evans WJ, Roubenoff R. Aging of skeletal muscle: a 12-yr longitudinal study. *J Appl Physiol.* 2000;88:1321–1326.

66. Fiatarone MA, Marks EC, Ryan ND, Meredith CN, Lipsitz LA, Evans WJ. High-intensity strength training in nonagenarians. Effects on skeletal muscle. *JAMA.* 1990;263:3029–3034.

67. Buchner DM, Cress ME, de Lateur BJ, et al. The effect of strength and endurance training on gait, balance, fall risk, and health services use in community-living older adults. *J Gerontol A Biol Sci Med Sci.* 1997;52:M218–M224.

68. Sinaki M, Lynn SG. Reducing the risk of falls through proprioceptive dynamic posture training in osteoporotic women with kyphotic posturing: a randomized pilot study. *Am J Phys Med Rehabil.* 2002;81:241–246.

69. Li F, Harmer P, Fisher KJ, McAuley E. Tai Chi: improving functional balance and predicting subsequent falls in older persons. *Med Sci Sports Exerc.* 2004;36:2046–2052.

70. Li F, Harmer P, Fisher KJ, et al. Tai Chi and fall reductions in older adults: a randomized controlled trial. *J Gerontol A Biol Sci Med Sci.* 2005;60:187–194.

71. Wolf SL, Barnhart HX, Kutner NG, McNeely E, Coogler C, Xu T. Reducing frailty and falls in older persons: an investigation of Tai Chi and computerized balance training. Atlanta FICSIT Group. Frailty and Injuries: Cooperative Studies of Intervention Techniques. *J Am Geriatr Soc.* 1996;44:489–497.

72. Gregg EW, Cauley JA, Seeley DG, Ensrud KE, Bauer DC. Physical activity and osteoporotic fracture risk in older women. Study of Osteoporotic Fractures Research Group. *Ann Intern Med.* 1998;129:81–88.

73. Parker MJ, Gillespie WJ, Gillespie LD. Effectiveness of hip protectors for preventing hip fractures in elderly people: systematic review. *BMJ.* 2006;332:571–574.

74. van Schoor NM, Smit JH, Bouter LM, Veenings B, Asma GB, Lips P. Maximum potential preventive effect of hip protectors. *J Am Geriatr Soc.* 2007;55:507–510.

75. Briggs AM, van Dieen JH, Wrigley TV, et al. Thoracic kyphosis affects spinal loads and trunk muscle force. *Phys Ther.* 2007;87:595–607.

76. Huang MH, Barrett-Connor E, Greendale GA, Kado DM. Hyperkyphotic posture and risk of future osteoporotic fractures: the Rancho Bernardo study. *J Bone Miner Res.* 2006;21:419–423.

77. White AAI, Panjabi MM. *Clinical Biomechanics of the Spine,* 2nd ed. Philadelphia: J.B. Lippincott Company; 1990.

78. Lynn SG, Sinaki M, Westerlind KC. Balance characteristics of persons with osteoporosis. *Arch Phys Med Rehabil.* 1997;78:273–277.

79. Sinaki M, Itoi E, Wahner HW, et al. Stronger back muscles reduce the incidence of vertebral fractures: a prospective 10 year follow-up of postmenopausal women. *Bone.* 2002;30:836–841.

80. Meeks S. The role of the physical therapist in the recognition, assessment, and exercise intervention in persons with, or at risk for, osteoporosis. *Topics in Geriatric Rehabilitation.* 2005;21(1):42–56.

81. Gold DT, Shipp KM, Pieper CF, Duncan PW, Martinez S, Lyles KW. Group treatment improves trunk strength and psychological status in older women with vertebral fractures: results of a randomized, clinical trial. *J Am Geriatr Soc.* 2004;52:1471–1478.

82. Katzman WB, Sellmeyer DE, Stewart AL, Wanek L, Hamel KA. Changes in flexed posture, musculoskeletal impairments, and physical performance after group exercise in community-dwelling older women. *Arch Phys Med Rehabil.* 2007;88:192–199.

83. Sinaki M, Brey RH, Hughes CA, et al. Significant reduction in risk of falls and back pain in osteoporotic-kyphotic women through a Spinal Proprioceptive Extension Exercise Dynamic (SPEED) program. Balance disorder and increased risk of falls in osteoporosis and kyphosis: significance of kyphotic posture and muscle strength. *Mayo Clin Proc.* 2005;80:849–855.

84. Greig AM, Bennell KL, Briggs AM, Hodges PW. Postural taping decreases thoracic kyphosis but does not influence trunk muscle electromyographic activity or balance in women with osteoporosis. *Man Ther.* 2007;11:11.

85. Roehrig SM. Use of neurodevelopmental treatment techniques in a client with kyphosis: a case report. *Physiother Theory Pract.* 2006;22:337–343.

86. Richardson CA TR. A initial evaluation of eight abdominal exercises. *Aust J Physiother.* 1990;36:6–11.

87. Cummings SR, Melton LJ. Epidemiology and outcomes of osteoporotic fractures. *Lancet.* 2002;359:1761–1767.

88. Keller TS, Harrison DE, Colloca CJ, Harrison DD, Janik TJ. Prediction of osteoporotic spinal deformity. *Spine.* 2003;28:455–462.

89. Bouxsein ML, Melton LJ, 3rd, Riggs BL, et al. Age- and sex-specific differences in the factor of risk for vertebral fracture: a population-based study using QCT. *J Bone Miner Res.* 2006;21:1475–1482.

90. Nachemson A, Morris JM. In vivo measurements of intradiscal pressure. Discometry, a method for the determination of pressure in the lower lumbar discs. *J Bone Joint Surg Am.* 1964;46:1077–1092.

91. Vainionpaa A, Korpelainen R, Leppaluoto J, Jamsa T. Effects of high-impact exercise on bone mineral density: a randomized controlled trial in premenopausal women. *Osteoporos Int.* 2005;16:191–197.

92. Schultz AB, Andersson GB, Haderspeck K, Ortengren R, Nordin M, Bjork R. Analysis and measurement of lumbar trunk loads in tasks involving bends and twists. *J Biomech.* 1982;15:669–675.

93. Greendale GA, McDivit A, Carpenter A, Seeger L, Huang MH. Yoga for women with hyperkyphosis: results of a pilot study. *Am J Public Health.* 2002;92:1611–1614.

94. Krolner B, Toft B. Vertebral bone loss: an unheeded side effect of therapeutic bed rest. *Clin Sci (Lond).* 1983;64:537–540.

95. Wu SS, Lachmann E, Nagler W. Current medical, rehabilitation, and surgical management of vertebral compression fractures. *J Women's Health (Larchmt).* 2003;12:17–26.

96. Nachemson A. Towards a better understanding of low-back pain: a review of the mechanics of the lumbar disc. *Rheumatol Rehabil.* 1975;14:129–143.

97. Defloor T. The effect of position and mattress on interface pressure. *Appl Nurs Res.* 2000;13:2–11.

98. Lindsay R, Silverman SL, Cooper C, et al. Risk of new vertebral fracture in the year following a fracture. *JAMA.* 2001;285:320–323.

99. Kaplan RS, Sinaki M. Posture Training Support: preliminary report on a series of patients with diminished symptomatic complications of osteoporosis. *Mayo Clin Proc.* 1993;68:1171–1176.

100. Patwardhan AG, Li SP, Gavin T, Lorenz M, Meade KP, Zindrick M. Orthotic stabilization of thoracolumbar injuries. A biomechanical analysis of the Jewett hyperextension orthosis. *Spine.* 1990;15:654–661.

101. Pfeifer M, Begerow B, Minne HW. Effects of a new spinal orthosis on posture, trunk strength, and quality of life in women with postmenopausal osteoporosis: a randomized trial. *Am J Phys Med Rehabil.* 2004;83:177–186.

102. Cranney A, Tugwell P, Adachi J, et al. Meta-analyses of therapies for postmenopausal osteoporosis. III. Meta-analysis of risedronate for the treatment of postmenopausal osteoporosis. *Endocr Rev.* 2002;23:517–523.

103. Cranney A, Wells G, Willan A, et al. Meta-analyses of therapies for postmenopausal osteoporosis. II. Meta-analysis of alendronate for the treatment of postmenopausal women. *Endocr Rev.* 2002;23:508–516.

104. Black DM, Schwartz AV, Ensrud KE, et al. Effects of continuing or stopping alendronate after 5 years of treatment: the Fracture Intervention Trial Long-term Extension (FLEX): a randomized trial. *JAMA.* 2006;296:2927–2938.

105. Miller PD. Efficacy and safety of long-term bisphosphonates in postmenopausal osteoporosis. *Expert Opin Pharmacother.* 2003;4:2253–2258.

106. Bilezikian JP. Osteonecrosis of the jaw—do bisphosphonates pose a risk? *N Engl J Med.* 2006;355:2278–2281.

107. Stewart HJ, Forrest AP, Everington D, et al. Randomised comparison of 5 years of adjuvant tamoxifen with continuous therapy for operable breast cancer. The Scottish Cancer Trials Breast Group. *Br J Cancer.* 1996;74:297–299.

108. Fisher B, Dignam J, Bryant J, Wolmark N. Five versus more than five years of tamoxifen for lymph node-negative breast cancer: updated findings from the National Surgical Adjuvant Breast and Bowel Project B-14 randomized trial. *J Natl Cancer Inst.* 2001;93:684–690.

109. Baum M, Buzdar A, Cuzick J, et al. Anastrozole alone or in combination with tamoxifen versus tamoxifen alone for adjuvant treatment of postmenopausal women with early-stage breast cancer: results of the ATAC (Arimidex, Tamoxifen Alone or in Combination) trial efficacy and safety update analyses. *Cancer.* 2003;98:1802–1810.

110. Barrett-Connor E, Mosca L, Collins P, et al. Effects of raloxifene on cardiovascular events and breast cancer in postmenopausal women. *N Engl J Med.* 2006;355:125–137.

111. Martino S, Cauley JA, Barrett-Connor E, et al. Continuing outcomes relevant to Evista: breast cancer incidence in postmenopausal osteoporotic women in a randomized trial of raloxifene. *J Natl Cancer Inst.* 2004;96:1751–1761.

112. Vogel VG, Costantino JP, Wickerham DL, et al. Effects of tamoxifen vs raloxifene on the risk of developing invasive breast cancer and other disease outcomes: the NSABP Study of Tamoxifen and Raloxifene (STAR) P-2 trial. *JAMA.* 2006;295:2727–2741.

113. Chesnut CH, 3rd, Silverman S, Andriano K, et al. A randomized trial of nasal spray salmon calcitonin in postmenopausal women with established osteoporosis: the prevent recurrence of osteoporotic fractures study. PROOF Study Group. *Am J Med.* 2000;109:267–276.

114. Guise TA. Bone loss and fracture risk associated with cancer therapy. *Oncologist.* 2006;11:1121–1131.

115. Tauchmanova L, Colao A, Lombardi G, Rotoli B, Selleri C. REVIEW: bone loss and its management in long-term survivors from allogeneic stem cell transplantation. *J Clin Endocrinol Metabol.* 2007;92:4536–4545.

116. Kanis JA, McCloskey EV, Powles T, Paterson AH, Ashley S, Spector T. A high incidence of vertebral fracture in women with breast cancer. *Br J Cancer.* 1999;79:1179–1181.

117. Shapiro CL, Manola J, Leboff M. Ovarian failure after adjuvant chemotherapy is associated with rapid bone loss in women with early-stage breast cancer. *J Clin Oncol.* 2001;19:3306–3311.

118. Greenspan SL, Bhattacharya RK, Sereika SM, Brufsky A, Vogel VG. Prevention of bone loss in survivors of breast cancer: a randomized, double-blind, placebo-controlled clinical trial. *J Clin Endocrinol Metabol.* 2007;92:131–136.

119. Chien AJ, Goss PE. Aromatase inhibitors and bone health in women with breast cancer. *J Clin Oncol.* 2006;24:5305–5312.

120. Brufsky A, Harker WG, Beck JT, et al. Zoledronic acid inhibits adjuvant letrozole-induced bone loss in postmenopausal women with early breast cancer. *J Clin Oncol.* 2007;25:829–836.

121. Gnant MF, Mlineritsch B, Luschin-Ebengreuth G, et al. Zoledronic acid prevents cancer treatment-induced bone loss in premenopausal women receiving adjuvant endocrine therapy for hormone-responsive breast cancer: a report from the Austrian Breast and Colorectal Cancer Study Group. *J Clin Oncol.* 2007;25:820–828.

122. Smith MR. Treatment-related osteoporosis in men with prostate cancer. *Clin Cancer Res.* 2006;12:6315s–6319s.

123. Smith MR, Fallon MA, Lee H, Finkelstein JS. Raloxifene to prevent gonadotropin-releasing hormone agonist-induced bone loss in men with prostate cancer: a randomized controlled trial. *J Clin Endocrinol Metabol.* 2004;89:3841–3846.

124. American College of Rheumatology Ad Hoc Committee on Glucocorticoid-Induced Osteoporosis. Recommendations for the prevention and treatment of glucocorticoid-induced osteoporosis: 2001 update. *Arthritis Rheum.* 2001;44:1496–1503.

125. WHO Study Group on Assessment of Fracture Risk and Its Application to Screening for Postmenopausal Osteoporosis. Assessment of fracture risk and its application to screening for postmenopausal osteoporosis. World Health Organization. Technical report series 843, Geneva 1994.

Bone Metastasis

60

Gary C. O'Toole
Patrick J. Boland
Maryann Herklotz

The American Cancer Society estimated that 1.37 million cases of cancer (excluding basal cell and squamous cell cancers of skin) were diagnosed in the United States in 2007 (1). Since more than 60% of patients with cancer are over 65 years of age and with increasing longevity in the population, the incidence of cancers and metastases are likely to rise dramatically in the next few decades unless a cure is found. Approximately 50% of the aforementioned 1.37 million cases are tumors of the breast, prostate, lung, kidney, and thyroid. These tumors commonly metastasize to bone and account for 80% of all skeletal metastases (2). The high incidence of metastatic bone disease compares to an estimated 2,570 cases of primary malignant bone tumors that will be diagnosed annually. These figures emphasize the importance of being able to recognize, investigate, manage, and intervene appropriately in the course of metastatic disease to preserve function and quality of life while minimizing complications.

As the skeleton is one of the most common sites of distant metastases (1) and tumor involvement of the bone is the most common cause of cancer pain (2), metastasis is the main differential diagnosis that must be considered in patients with a known history of cancer reporting localized bone pain (3). The suspicion should be even stronger if several sites within the skeleton are involved (4). The most common site of bone metastases is in the axial skeleton (1,5). Other common sites include the humerus, femur, skull, ribs, and pelvis (1,3,5).

The earliest evidence of skeletal metastases dates back to 400 BC (4). The term *metastasis* was first used by Hippocratic physicians. It is of Greek origin and means "change in the seat of the disease." Throughout the nineteenth century, the mechanism of metastases was scrutinized. This era gave rise to the "seed and soil" theory, suggesting that tissues receiving tumor cells could be either congenial or hostile (3). Others explained metastases on a purely stochastic basis (5,6). It is now accepted that both methods occur. Approximately 60% of metastatic sites can be predicted on a purely hematologic and/or lymphatic route basis. The remainder of metastases involves intricate interactions between the tumor and host sites at the cellular and molecular levels.

Hematologic metastases result from the leakage of cells from an established primary tumor into the circulation. The capacity to enter the circulation requires that neoplastic cells must have intrinsic properties that facilitate this process. The tumor must have the ability to induce neovascularization and be capable of crossing from the tumor stroma to the vasculature by invading the basement membrane of the vascular endothelium (7). This process is facilitated by cell adhesion molecules (CAMs). Several categories of CAMs exist, including intercellular adhesion molecules (ICAMs), selectins, and cadherins.

Tumor cells have an innate capacity to modulate the expression of their CAMs. CAMs mediate tumor cell adhesion to themselves, host cells, and extracellular

KEY POINTS

- The most common site of bone metastases is in the axial skeleton. Other common sites include the humerus, femur, skull, ribs, and pelvis.
- Metastasis is the main differential diagnosis that must be considered in patients with a known history of cancer reporting localized bone pain.
- Although bone metastases are frequently asymptomatic, the vast majority of patients will develop symptoms during the course of their disease. Clinical features include pain, loss of function, hypercalcemia, and depression, resulting in significant reduction in quality of life and performance status.
- Bone destruction will result in altered mechanical strength and this, in turn, will cause pain by stimulating periosteal receptors and may lead to complete fractures in both the bones of the appendicular and axial skeletons.
- Nonoperative treatments aimed at halting progression of a metastatic lesion and preventing fractures include use of systemic hormones, chemotherapy, radiation therapy, protected weight bearing, and external immobilization.
- Radiation therapy is the treatment of choice for most symptomatic bone metastases.
- In situations where an impending pathological fracture exists, prophylactic surgical fixation is desirable, since it is less traumatic than suffering a fracture and undergoing emergency surgery.
- With the exception of lymphoma and some metastatic germ cell tumors of the testes, treatment is usually palliative. The aims of treatment include (1) relief of pain, (2) prevention of fractures, (3) maintenance or restoration of function, (4) prolongation of survival, and (5) improvement of quality of life.
- It is the responsibility of the physical therapist to help ensure that the patient with bony metastasis is maintaining their functional mobility within reasonable limits.
- Therapists must be aware of the risk of pathological fracture in patients with bony metastasis.
- When performing physical therapy interventions, precautions may include but are not limited to obtaining weight-bearing restrictions, following range-of-motion restrictions, avoidance of resistance exercise, positioning recommendations and/or restrictions, and the use of assistive devices.

matrices. Therefore, CAM expression must be lacking for tumor cells to detach from the primary site, and it has been shown that overexpression of E-selectin in highly invasive cancer cells significantly diminishes their invasiveness. Conversely, the expression of CAMs is required later for the accumulation of tumor cells at the site of malignancy (8,9).

Once in the circulation, the embolization of the tumor cell is facilitated by adhesion to P- and L-selectins, located on platelets and leucocytes, respectively. Adhesion to the endothelium of the metastatic tissue is mediated via E-selectin. Upon adhesion, an integrin-signaling pathway is initiated, the net result of which is up-regulation of both the antiapoptotic machinery and proteolytic activity in the microenvironment, thus facilitating the extravasation of tumor cells out of the circulation and their invasion into the host tissue (9,10). Lymphatic metastases remain a key prognostic indicator for many tumors. Debate exists as to whether lymphatic drainage channels exist within tumors or whether lymphangiogenic cytokines stimulate proliferation of peritumoral vessels aiding dissemination (11). Once in the lymphatics, tumor cells are carried to the subcapsular sinus of the draining node, where they may succumb to the host defenses or leave via the efferent lymphatic channels. It is postulated that the ability of a tumor cell to generate lymphatic metastases is dependent on expression of CD44 variant adhesion molecules (12,13).

The preference of metastatic tumor cells for certain tissue types remains enigmatic. It is accepted that the process involves balanced interactions between metastatic-promoting molecules, such as chemotactic growth factors (eg, bone sialoprotein), local growth factors (eg, epidermal growth factor receptor), local environmental modifying agents (eg, parathyroid hormone-related protein), and metastatic inhibitory influences (eg, tissue inhibitors of matrix metalloproteinase and suppressor genes) (14–17).

While our understanding of the molecular mechanisms of metastases has improved significantly since the earliest observations of Billroth (18), we remain ignorant of the intricacies of metastases. Selective therapeutic agents targeted exclusively at metastatic cells have yet to be developed (19), and much remains to be discovered about the critical determinants of metastatic process. However, the accelerated advances in the fields of molecular biology and genetics auger well for the future.

CLINICAL FEATURES

Although bone metastases are frequently asymptomatic, the vast majority of patients will develop symptoms during the course of their disease. Clinical features include pain, loss of function, hypercalcemia, and depression, resulting in significant reduction in quality of life and performance status. Medical oncologists use performance status in assessing a patient's suitability for receiving chemotherapy.

Pain may be severe, and as patient surveys suggest, it is the cancer complication patients fear most (20). Since there are many possible causes of pain, careful evaluation is essential in order to properly manage the problem. Bone pain in a patient with a history of cancer should be considered secondary to metastasis until otherwise proven. The mechanism of pain production in patients with intraosseus tumors is complex and includes mechanical factors such as increased marrow pressure distorting the periosteum and medullary blood vessels. Chemical mediators produced by the metastatic process include cytokines, histamine, and substance P, which cause pain by stimulating nociceptors. Bone destruction will result in altered mechanical strength and this, in turn, will cause pain by stimulating periosteal receptors and may lead to complete fractures in both the bones of the appendicular and axial skeletons. When complete fractures occur, severe pain usually results, often requiring internal or external stabilization. Pathological fractures are serious complications and often require admission to hospital for treatment that frequently includes major surgery. Non-operative treatments aimed at halting progression of a metastatic lesion and preventing fractures include use of systemic hormones, chemotherapy, radiation therapy, protected weight bearing, and external immobilization. In situations where an impending pathological fracture exists, prophylactic surgical fixation is desirable, since it is less traumatic than suffering a fracture and undergoing emergency surgery. Prophylactic surgery can be done on a semielective basis, which allows us to optimize the patient's condition for surgery. This is not always possible when emergency surgery is necessary.

IMPENDING PATHOLOGICAL FRACTURES

Unfortunately, making a diagnosis of an impending fracture in the appendicular skeleton is difficult. Several authors have proffered guidelines based mainly on retrospective studies. Factors include the anatomical site of involvement, the severity of pain, the origin of the primary tumor, the amount of bony destruction, and whether the lesion is lytic or blastic (21–23). Pain

that is caused by contracting muscles around a lesion is known as "functional pain" and is often an indication of an impending fracture. Inability to actively straight-leg raise due to pain in the groin may indicate an impending pathological fracture of the hip. For humeral lesions, Sim recommends internal fixation for lytic lesions measuring 3 cm in diameter. When 50% of the cortex is destroyed, or if there is persistent pain following radiation therapy (regardless of the radiographic appearance) (22), Harrington recommends prophylactic fixation for lytic lesions of the femur with measurements greater than 2.5 cm in diameter, lytic destruction lesions involving greater than 50% of the cortex, and persistent pain with weight bearing despite radiation therapy (23). Lytic destruction and/or pathological avulsion fractures of the lesser trochanter are frequently cited as an indication for prophylactic fixation of a painful hip.

Based on a retrospective study, Mirels proposed a weighted scoring system with a view to quantify the risk of sustaining a fracture (Table 60.1) (24). Parameters include the anatomical location of the lesion, the severity of pain, and radiographic features including the size of the lesion relative to the diameter of the bone and whether the lesion is lytic or blastic. Each parameter is assigned a score from 1 to 3, with a maximum possible score of 12. Based on his observation, the higher the score, the greater the risk of fracture. He recommends prophylactic fixation for patients with scores greater than 9.

Subsequent studies by other authors have validated the accuracy of this system, while others have not (25). Most clinicians, however, find it helpful in evaluating indications for surgery. Bunting and Shea highlight problems in using many of these features as predictive factors, such as the fact that destructive lesions are not static and may increase in size without treatment, sometimes at a rapid rate (26). None of the studies mentioned takes into consideration the stress that is applied to the bone involved. It is likely that a heavy, active patient is more apt to apply more deforming forces on a weakened bone than a light, debilitated

	TABLE 60.1 *Mirels Scoring System for Fracture Risk*		
VARIABLE	**SCORE**		
	1	2	3
Site	Upper limb	Lower limb	Peritrochanter
Pain	Mild	Moderate	Functional
Lesion	Blastic	Mixed	Lytic
Size	<1/3	1/3–2/3	>2/3

patient is. Activities such as climbing stairs greatly increase the amount of stress on the hip and proximal femur (27). Methods of reducing these stresses must be implemented by physical therapists when managing these patients to prevent fractures from occurring. A prospective study was performed on 54 patients with bony metastases undergoing inpatient rehabilitation to assess the risk of physical therapy causing the fracture. None of the patients had findings suggestive of impending fractures on skeletal surveys. During the treatment period, 16 fractures occurred in 12 patients. Only one, a vertebral fracture, occurred while the patient was participating in rehabilitation activities. Sex fractures (three of them humeral fractures and one a humeral fracture) occurred while the patients were in bed. This clearly indicates that bed rest does not prevent pathological fractures. The authors of this study also point out that younger patients and those with the greatest number of sites of bony involvement suffered the highest incidence of fractures (28).

EVALUATION OF PATIENTS WITH BONE METASTASES

Assessment of patients with bone metastasis begins with a detailed history and physical examination. A careful evaluation of the general condition of the patient is essential when planning treatment and will help with prognostication. While pain may be due to benign conditions, patients with a history of visceral carcinoma should be regarded as having metastatic disease until proven otherwise. Unless specifically asked, patients may fail to report a history of past primary cancer, especially if there has been a long, disease-free interval from the time of initial diagnosis. The characteristics of the type of pain, including factors that aggravate and relieve it, may help in identifying the precise cause of the pain. For example, groin pain aggravated by active flexion of the hip may point to an impending pathological fracture of the hip or proximal femur. Back pain associated with radiculopathy may indicate root compression secondary to epidural tumor extension, while back pain aggravated by movement favors vertebral fractures and spinal instabilities. Disturbance of bowel and bladder function are important indicators of the onset of myelopathy. It is important to assess the patient for anxiety and depression, which are common and frequently overlooked.

Radiographic evaluation includes plain x-rays of the portion of the skeleton involved and a chest x-ray. It should be borne in mind that 50% of bone mass must be destroyed before it is apparent on a plain x-ray. Yet 80% of patients have an abnormal plain radiograph at the time of presentation. The radiographic nature of the lesion may help with diagnosis. For instance, sclerotic lesions favor a metastatic prostate in a male patient, while several punched out lytic lesions are highly suggestive of multiple myeloma.

A technetium-labeled methyl-diphosphonate bone scan is usually positive in patients with bone tumors, and multiple areas of increased uptake are highly suggestive of metastatic disease. Single focus of uptake favors a diagnosis of primary bone lesions. Since increased uptake is a reflection of reactive osteogenesis, cancers that are largely osteolytic—such as multiple myeloma and some aggressive lung and kidney metastases—may have false-negative bone scans.

Computed axial tomography is useful in examining cortical bone integrity and is usually more useful than magnetic resonance imaging (MRI) in assessing lesions at risk of causing fracture. An MRI scan with gadolinium is most useful in assessing spinal metastases. A scan of the entire spine should be done in patients with suspected spinal disease. This examination outlines the extent of the bony involvement and demonstrates epidural and perivertebral tumor extension. The extent of disease in both the shin and long bones has important implications, whether the physician is fitting an orthosis or planning surgery. Surgical or external orthotic stabilization must extend beyond the limits of tumor involvement, if possible, in order to prevent failure and fractures above or below the diseased and weakened bone not protected. MRI with and without gadolinium is the imaging modality of choice for demonstrating intradural and leptomeningeal disease. MRI scans are contraindicated in patients with intracranial metal clips and in those with cardiac pacemakers. The presence of rods, screws, and plates used in spinal reconstruction is not contraindicated in MRI scans.

Laboratory analysis includes complete blood count, electrolytes, and liver function tests. Patients with lytic bone lesions should have serum protein electrophoresis as well as serum and urine immunofixation. Indications for biopsy include (1) appearance of possible metastatic lesion known to have cancer, (2) any suspicious lesion in a patient without a history of cancer, (3) patients with a history of more than one primary tumor.

METASTATIC BONE DISEASE WITH AN UNKNOWN PRIMARY

The evaluation of patients with metastases from unknown primaries deserves special mention. Rougraff (29) found that 3%–4% of patients with metastatic disease had unknown primary sites. A thorough history and detailed physical examination may reveal the diagnosis or suggest special investigations that would lead to a diagnosis. For example, a patient with difficulty swallowing or alteration of bowel habits should undergo endoscopy, a test that would not normally be carried out when investigating an unknown primary. Serious consideration should be given to the possibility of lung cancer in a patient with a lytic lesion and a strong history of smoking.

While breast and prostate cancers are the most common primary sources of bone metastases, Rougraff and others found that metastases from unknown primaries are more likely to originate in the lung or kidney and are rarely from the breast. Investigations in these patients after the history and physical should include chest x-ray; computed tomography (CT) scan of chest, abdomen, and pelvis; bone scan; serum protein electrophoresis; serum and urine immunofixation; and prostate-specific antigen. Positron emission tomography (PET) is only occasionally helpful in identifying the primary site. Finally, a biopsy should be done. The most accessible lesion should be biopsied. If the biopsy creates a significant defect in the cortex of a weight-bearing bone, this should be protected following the biopsy to prevent fracture.

TREATMENT OF PATIENTS WITH METASTATIC BONE DISEASE

With the exception of lymphoma and some metastatic germ cell tumors of the testes, treatment is usually palliative. The aims of treatment include (1) relief of pain, (2) prevention of fractures, (3) maintenance or restoration of function, (4) prolongation of survival, and (5) improvement of quality of life.

Many patients have asymptomatic bone lesions and are successfully managed with systemic treatment, including hormonal manipulation, where appropriate, or chemotherapy. Metastases from sensitive tumors such as breast and lymphoma may disappear with such treatment. During treatment, consideration should be given to the institution of weight-bearing precautions in larger lesions, especially those in lower limbs. Patients with symptomatic bone metastases usually require management by a multidisciplinary team, including pain and palliative care, rehabilitation medicine, medical oncology, and orthopedic and neurologic surgery services. Pain relief may be accomplished by using simple measures such as a sling for a painful upper limb lesion or a nondisplaced pathological fracture of the humerus. For mild pain, oral non-narcotic analgesics and non-steroidal anti-inflammatories are usually effective. For moderate to severe pain, both long- and short-acting opioids should be used (30). Opioids may be administered orally or by injection or by transdermal patch (fentanyl). Tricyclic antidepressants, such as amitrip-

tyline, often potentiate the opioids in neuropathic pain. Anticonvulsants, such as gabapentin, are being used increasingly for the management of neuropathic pain. Corticosteroids may have multiple benefits, including elevation of mood, appetite stimulation, and reduction of inflammation. They are routinely used as part of the management of the spinal cord and root compression. Bisphosphonates are also being used increasingly in patients with metastatic bone disease, especially those with breast cancer and multiple myeloma. Studies have demonstrated significant pain relief and reduction of skeletal complications, at least in the short term, in both the axial and appendicular skeletons (31).

Hypercalcemia is commonly associated with bone metastases, and if left untreated, may lead to death. The symptoms of hypercalcemia include confusion, which may be attributed to the use of narcotics. Administration of bisphosphonates combined with hydration is now the treatment of choice for this condition. Patients in whom hypercalcemia occurs while they are on bisphosphonates are considered to have a poor prognosis.

RADIATION THERAPY

Radiation therapy is the treatment of choice for most symptomatic bone metastases. Gainor demonstrated that the healing of pathological fractures would occur if they were immobilized and radiation doses less than 3000 cGy were used. Fracture healing depended on the primary pathology and the length of patient survival. Patients with multiple myeloma had the highest rate of healing, while no patient with lung cancer healed. A life expectancy longer than six months was the primary factor determining osseous healing in all patients (32). External beam radiation is the most commonly used modality. The aim of treatment is to relieve pain, improve ambulation, restore function, and prevent pathological fractures. External beam radiation is the most common treatment and remains the cornerstone of palliative treatment. Hundreds of thousands of patients undergo this form of treatment in the United States annually. Radiotherapy for bone metastases attempts to exploit the radiosensitivity characteristics inherent to tumor cells, such as significant vascularization, high proliferation, and nondifferentiation (33). The exact mechanism of radiation therapy, however, remains speculative.

Clinically, several choices exist regarding the use of radiation therapy. Opinions differ on the best regimen for each patient, the most suitable radiation dose, timing, and the best delivery mechanism. The Radiation Therapy Oncology Group (RTOG) conducted a prospective randomized trial (RTOG 74-02). Patients with solitary metastases randomized to receive 2000 cGy using 400-cGy fractions delivered over a short five-day period or 4050 cGy delivered using 2.7-Gy fractions over a three-week period. There was no difference in the outcome as measured by pain relief. Similar results were seen in patients with multiple metastases who were randomized to receive 300 cGy in 10 fractions over two weeks, 1500 cGy in 5 fractions over one week, 2000 cGy in 5 fractions over one week, or 2500 cGy in 5 fractions over one week (34).

Since the RTOG trial, there have been several trials evaluating dose-fractionation schemes (35,36), with no schedule or dose demonstrating significantly better outcome.

Single-fraction radiation therapy has been advocated as a cost-effective way to palliate bony metastases, especially in debilitated patients who have difficulty traveling to and from radiation therapy units. A single dose of 8 Gy has been shown to have improved response rates when compared to a single dose for 4 Gy (37). When a single-dose regimen was compared to a multifraction regimen of 20 Gy and 5 fractions or 30 Gy and 10 fractions, no difference was noted in the time to symptomatic improvement, time to relief of pain, or first relapse of pain up to 12 months post-treatment (38).

It is now accepted that an accelerated regimen may be appropriate in clinical situations where there is a short life expectancy or where social circumstances decree that a patient cannot return on a daily basis. A protracted course may be more appropriate where the disease is more indolent or where the patient has good performance status with a long life expectancy (37).

Modern techniques, including image-guided, intensity-modulated radiation therapy or stereotactic radiosurgery, have now been increasingly employed in order to accurately deliver larger doses to tumors while sparing adjacent normal tissue. Administration of systemic radioisotopes may also be useful in the management of certain painful bone metastases. Iodine-131 is effective in treating metastatic thyroid cancer. Strontium-89 or samarium-153 can be effective in the management of severe pain due to bone-producing metastases, as those that occur in prostate cancer. The beneficial effects of strongium-89 or samarium-153 rarely last more than six months and may result in bone marrow suppression, so use of these agents is usually reserved for patients with recalcitrant pain and limited life expectancy.

NONSURGICAL ORTHOPEDIC MANAGEMENT

In common with all other forms of treatment, the goals of nonsurgical orthopedic treatment are relief of pain,

prevention of fracture, and maintenance or restoration of mobility. As mentioned, many metastatic lesions (even with fractures) will heal with nonsurgical methods, including those on systemic therapies or treated with radiation therapy (32). Many lesions, however, may fracture or are painful if they are not immobilized. Debilitated patients may not be surgical candidates, and certain pathological fractures may not be amenable to surgical fixation. The majority of these patients, however, will require some form of external immobilization until pain disappears and healing occurs. In the upper limb, simple slings often provide significant pain relief to lesions in the proximal humerus or clavicle. Lesions of the humeral diaphysis can be managed using cast braces, while lesions around the elbow or forearm can be treated with hinge braces. Satisfactory bracing of the upper limb may be particularly difficult in patients with symptomatic lower limb disease. In these cases, use of two-handed devices such as a walker may not be possible. This situation often constitutes a relative indication for surgical stabilization of the humerus. In cases where this not possible, a hemi-walker or wheelchair may be required for ambulation.

Pelvic lesions, including fractures of the sacrum iliac bone and pubic bones, are best managed with radiation therapy and protected weight bearing while symptomatic. Surgery is rarely indicated in management of these lesions. Fractures of the hip and femur are extremely difficult to manage conservatively. In moribund patients with these fractures, abduction pillows used in bed may relieve pain and facilitate perineal care. Distal femoral and proximal tibial lesions can be managed with a long hinge brace. Cast braces may be applied to tibial diaphysial lesions, while bony pathological lesions of the foot are managed with special wooden rocker-bottom shoes.

For painful lesions of the cervical spine, immobilization can be achieved with a soft collar or a more rigid one. Special care must be exercised in order to avoid pressure on the chin or occiput. Symptomatic lesions of the lower cervical and upper thoracic spine are best managed with rigid neck orthoses. For lumbosacral lesions, immobilization may be achieved with a three-point fixation device such as a Jewett brace. Prefabricated, custom-molded orthoses afford better immobilization. They are, however, difficult to apply and are often uncomfortable, especially in debilitated patients.

SURGERY

The aims of surgical treatment for metastases of the axial and appendicular skeletons are (1) relief of pain, (2) achievement of stability such that immediate weight bearing can be allowed without the need for brace, and (3) preservation or restoration of function.

The decision to operate on these patients will depend on their estimated length of survival. This is determined by factors such as the general medical condition of the patient, the histology of the primary tumor, and the extent of bone and visceral metastases. The estimated time may also determine the extent of surgery performed and the durability of prosthesis used. Obviously, the survival time should be greater than the estimated time of recovery from the surgical procedure. To date, no satisfactory method for assessment of estimated survival time has been devised (39).

Surgical fixation should not rely on bone healing in these patients. For this reason, rigid fixation is achieved by using rigid rods and methyl methacrylate in diaphysial areas of bones. Resection of bone and replacement with mega prosthesis are favored for lesions close to joints. These principles apply to lesions both in the upper and lower limbs (Fig. 60.1). Rigid fixation of spinal fractures is indicated in order to allow immediate ambulation without the need for a brace (40,41).

In rare cases where pain relief in the appendicular skeleton cannot be achieved by the methods already described, amputation may be an option.

THERAPY IMPLICATIONS

A physical therapist has a role in the care of the patient with cancer throughout the patient's course, from the time of diagnosis to after surgery or any other palliative medical treatment interventions that the patient may experience. An important goal of treatment is to preserve patients' functional independence and maintain their quality of life (42).

Any physical therapist is likely to encounter patients with bony metastasis throughout their career, whether these lesions are diagnosed or undiagnosed at the time of the patient visit. For this reason, it is important to know the red flag signs that are associated with bony metastasis. Typically, the onset of bone pain is gradual and intermittent, increasing at night and relieved by activity. As the lesion progresses, the pain

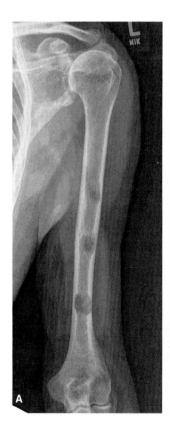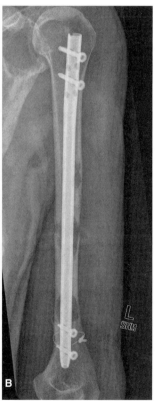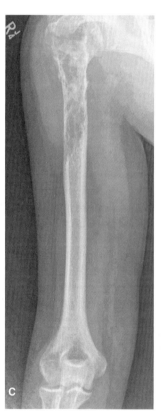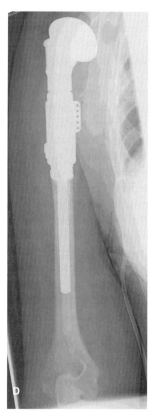

FIGURE 60.1

Different fixation methods for metastases of the humerus. A and B: Pre- and postoperative x-rays of a 71-year-old male with painful metastatic lesions secondary to renal cell carcinoma. The humerus was stabilized using a locked intramedullary nail with a prophylactic distal cerclage wire. Excellent pain relief was achieved. C and D: X-rays showing the pre- and postoperative status of a 40-year-old female with painful metastatic breast carcinoma. The painful lesion was excised and replaced with an endoprostheses. Good symptomatic relief was achieved.

becomes more constant (42). When pain is located in the back, if the pain is exacerbated when assuming a recumbent position, and is progressive and unremitting despite rest and conservative treatment, one should suspect a structural lesion (43).

It is the responsibility of the physical therapist to ensure that the patient with bony metastasis is maintaining their functional mobility within reasonable limits. The goals are preventing the patient from becoming bed-bound and helping them to maintain as much independence as possible. Safety and prevention of further comorbidity of their disease is to be maintained. Treatment sessions should address training the patient how to use their residual function, developing compensatory techniques, training in the use of assistive equipment, and educating the patient and the family to help them adjust to the altered way of life (26).

Therapists must be aware of the risk of pathological fracture in patients with bony metastasis. Known bony metastasis should trigger the treating therapist to follow specific precautions. The typical physical therapy assessment may be modified based on the patient's subjective history and findings documented in the medical chart. Manual muscle testing is not performed on an involved limb, nor is passive or active-assisted range of motion (26). Only active movement is assessed, as this is likely to be limited by pain.

When performing physical therapy interventions, precautions may include but are not limited to obtaining weight-bearing restrictions, following range-of-motion restrictions, avoiding resistance exercise, positioning recommendations and/or restrictions, and using assistive devices.

Weight-bearing and range-of-motion restrictions must be determined by the patient's physician. As mentioned earlier in the chapter, several factors may guide a physician's decision to allow weight bearing through a bone with a metastatic lesion.

When a surgical approach is not indicated in a patient, the establishment of a decreased weight-bearing status is a new way of life for these patients. Therapy is based on maintaining mobility and preventing fractures. Establishment of weight-bearing status for patients with impending or existing pathological fractures helps the therapist to achieve these goals safely. Assistive devices are necessary for patients with lower extremity lesions to maintain decreased weight bearing during transfers and ambulation. Stair climbing techniques can be taught to patients with metastasis in the lower extremity with the use of crutches and handrails to maintain a decreased weight-bearing status when it is appropriate. Patients with bony lesions in the upper extremity that are being treated conservatively usually benefit from the provision of a sling and education regarding avoidance of weight bearing on that

extremity during transfers. Occupational therapists can educate patients on how to perform one-handed activities (26).

For patients who have a surgical fixation, weight bearing and early mobilization can usually begin immediately after surgery. Provision of assistive devices such as canes, crutches, or walkers may be provided to the patients to decrease postoperative pain and allow the patient to regain confidence in his or her ability to bear weight on the affected limb (26).

When considering chest physical therapy treatment, rib metastasis must be ruled out prior to performing chest percussion and vibration to these patients (26). When rib metastases are present, deep breathing exercises, postural drainage, and an effective cough technique are educated to the patient to clear their secretions and improve their lung aeration.

Although cancer is responsible for less than 1% of back pain in the general population, 98% of patients with cancer who present with back pain have underlying metastasis in their vertebra (44). Up to one-third of patients dying of cancer develop metastasis to the spine at some time during their illness (43). The thoracic spine is the most common site of the spine to develop metastasis (43). Carcinomas of the prostate or colon are known to more commonly affect the lumbosacral region (43). Vertebral metastases, with or without spinal cord compression, cause pain that is often more prominent in the lying position and sometimes relieved by sitting up (43). Pain that is present when the patient is immobile and cannot be relieved by positional manipulation may be the symptoms of a serious condition, such as malignancy (43). Severe back pain, inability to walk, and/or sensory problems may indicate the presence of spinal cord compression (42).

Patients with spinal metastasis benefit from physical therapy interventions. Treatment is focused on instruction of back-sparing maneuvers for bed mobility and transfers and the use of assistive devices for ambulation. Spinal precautions should be taught to these patients with known lesions to the vertebral column. Spinal precautions include the avoidance of any excessive flexion, extension, rotation, or side bending.

Transfers are an important focus for all patients at this late stage of disease. The focus is on safety of the patient and caregiver. When metastases are in the long bones of the lower extremity, assistive devices such as a cane, crutches, or walker are provided to the patient to maintain decreased weight bearing on that extremity. For patients who require the assistance of another person, the caregiver must be educated on how to assist the patient while maintaining precautions to prevent pathological fracture. Guarding and assistance should not be given over the thorax for a patient with lesions in the rib cage. Spinal precautions must be maintained throughout the transfer for patients with metastasis in the spine. Consideration of precautions must be kept in mind for patients who are dependent or nearly dependent. Some total-lift devices may be inappropriate for patients with spinal metastasis, as these devices may position the patient in too much flexion, thus increasing their risk for fracturing at the site of their lesions.

For the patient who already has bony metastasis, the therapist may be concerned about future development of bony metastasis in other locations. Subjective reports by the patient regarding any new symptoms must be addressed. These subjective comments by the patient, along with any new objective findings, must be relayed to the physician in a timely manner to allow for quick diagnosis of any new metastases or malignancies.

Although there are risks associated with mobilizing a patient with bony metastases, the alternative is not a better approach. Education is a key part of physical therapy intervention. The patient and family must be aware that there are many risks associated with bed rest. Such risks include muscle contractures, weakness and atrophy, osteoporosis, orthostatic hypotension, pressure sores, pneumonia, confusion and disorientation, and increased risk of a thromboembolic event (26).

In the acute care setting, careful consideration must be given in regard to the discharge plan of the patient. For patients who may have been living alone or who have stairs in the home, having a newly diagnosed metastatic lesion is something that may prevent them from returning to their previous setting. Communication with discharge planners early on is important for setting up the appropriate discharge plan for the patient when assistance is needed in the home or if the patient will benefit more from an alternate discharge setting, such as an inpatient rehabilitation facility, nursing home, or hospice.

Treatment of a patient with bony metastasis should be a multidisciplinary approach (45). Communication between the doctor, nurse practitioner, case manager, social worker, and primary caregiver(s) of the patient is necessary throughout the course of care.

References

1. American Cancer Society. *Cancer Facts and Figures, 2007.* Atlanta, GA: American Cancer Society; 2007.
2. Buckwalter JA, Brandser EA. Metastatic disease of the skeleton. *Am Fam Physician.* April 1997;55(5):1761–1768.
3. Paget S. The distribution of secondary growths in cancer of the breast. *Lancet.* 1889;133:571–573.
4. Urteaga O, Pack GT. On the antiquity of melanoma. *Cancer.* May 1966;19(5):607–610.
5. Ewing J. *Neoplastic Diseases: A Textbook on Tumors.* Philadelphia and London: WB Saunders; 1919.
6. Batson OV. The function of the vertebral veins and their role in the spread of metastases. *Ann Surg.* July 1940;112(1):138–149.
7. Liotta LA, Kohn E. Cancer invasion and metastases. *JAMA.* February 23, 1990;263(8):1123–1126.
8. Mundy GR. Mechanisms of bone metastasis. *Cancer.* October 15, 1997;80(8 Suppl):1546–1556.
9. Mareel MM, Behrens J, Birchmeier W, et al. Down-regulation of E-cadherin expression in Madin Darby canine kidney (MDCK) cells inside tumors of nude mice. *Int J Cancer.* April 1, 1991;47(6):922–928.
10. Orr FW, Wang HH, Lafrenie RM, Scherbarth S, Nance DM. Interactions between cancer cells and the endothelium in metastasis. *J Pathol.* February 2000;190(3):310–329.
11. Chambers AF, Naumov GN, Varghese HJ, Nadkarni KV, MacDonald IC, Groom AC. Critical steps in hematogenous metastasis: an overview. *Surg Oncol Clin N Am.* April 2001;10(2):243–255, vii.
12. Eccles SA. Cell biology of lymphatic metastasis. The potential role of c-erbB oncogene signalling. *Recent Results Cancer Res.* 2000;157:41–54.
13. Kainz C, Tempfer C, Kohlberger P, et al. Immunohistochemical detection of adhesion molecule CD44 splice variants in lymph node metastases of cervical cancer. *Int J Cancer.* June 21, 1996;69(3):170–173.
14. Radinsky R. Paracrine growth regulation of human colon carcinoma organ-specific metastasis. *Cancer Metastasis Rev.* September 1993;12(3–4):345–361.
15. Iguchi H, Tanaka S, Ozawa Y, et al. An experimental model of bone metastasis by human lung cancer cells: the role of parathyroid hormone-related protein in bone metastasis. *Cancer Res.* September 1, 1996;56(17):4040–4043.
16. Bar-Yehuda S, Barer F, Volfsson L, Fishman P. Resistance of muscle to tumor metastases: a role for a3 adenosine receptor agonists. *Neoplasia.* March–April 2001;3(2):125–131.
17. Yoshida BA, Sokoloff MM, Welch DR, Rinker-Schaeffer CW. Metastasis-suppressor genes: a review and perspective on an emerging field. *J Natl Cancer Inst.* November 1, 2000;92(21):1717–1730.
18. Billroth T. *General Surgical Pathology and Therapeutics in Fifty Lectures.* Translated by Hackley CE. New York: Appleton and Company; 1871:233–243.
19. Freije JM, Lawrence JA, Hollingshead MG, et al. Identification of compounds with preferential inhibitory activity against low-Nm23-expressing human breast carcinoma and melanoma cell lines. *Nat Med.* April 1997;3(4):395–401.
20. Levin DN, Cleeland CS, Dar R. Public attitudes toward cancer pain. *Cancer.* November 1, 1985;56(9):2337–2339.
21. Beals RK, Lawton GD, Snell WE. Prophylactic internal fixation of the femur in metastatic breast cancer. *Cancer.* November 1971;28(5):1350–1354.
22. Sim FH, Pritchard DJ. Metastatic disease in the upper extremity. *Clin Orthop Relat Res.* September 1982(169):83–94.
23. Harrington KD, Sim FH, Enis JE, Johnston JO, Diok HM, Gristina AG. Methylmethacrylate as an adjunct in internal fixation of pathological fractures. Experience with three hundred and seventy-five cases. *J Bone Joint Surg Am.* December 1976;58(8):1047–1055.
24. Mirels H. Metastatic disease in long bones: a proposed scoring system for diagnosing impending pathologic fractures. 1989. *Clin Orthop Relat Res.* October 2003(415 Suppl):S4–S13.
25. Damron TA, Morgan H, Prakash D, Grant W, Aronowitz J, Heiner J. Critical evaluation of Mirels' rating system for impending pathologic fractures. *Clin Orthop Relat Res.* October 2003(415 Suppl):S201–S207.
26. Bunting RW, Shea B. Bone metastasis and rehabilitation. *Cancer.* August 15, 2001;92(4 Suppl):1020–1028.
27. Hipp JA, Springfield DS, Hayes WC. Predicting pathologic fracture risk in the management of metastatic bone defects. *Clin Orthop Relat Res.* March 1995(312):120–135.
28. Bunting R, Lamont-Havers W, Schweon D, Kliman A. Pathologic fracture risk in rehabilitation of patients with bony metastases. *Clin Orthop Relat Res.* January–February 1985;192:222–227.

29. Rougraff BT. Evaluation of the patient with carcinoma of unknown origin metastatic to bone. *Clin Orthop Relat Res.* October 2003;415(Suppl):S105–S109.

30. World Health Organization. *Cancer Pain Relief: With a Guide to Opioid Availability, Ed. 2.* Geneva, Switzerland: World Health Organization; 1996.

31. Hortobagyi GN, Theriault RL, Lipton A, et al. Long-term prevention of skeletal complications of metastatic breast cancer with pamidronate. Protocol 19 Aredia Breast Cancer Study Group. *J Clin Oncol.* June 1998;16(6):2038–2044.

32. Gainor BJ, Buchert P. Fracture healing in metastatic bone disease. *Clin Orthop Relat Res.* September 1983;178:297–302.

33. Goblirsch M, Lynch C, Mathews W, Manivel JC, Mantyh PW, Clohisy DR.Radiation treatment decreases bone cancer pain through direct effect on tumor cells. *Radiat Res.* October 2005;164(4 Pt 1):400–408.

34. Tong D, Gillick L, Hendrickson FR. The palliation of symptomatic osseous metastases: final results of the Study by the Radiation Therapy Oncology Group. *Cancer.* September 1, 1982;50(5):893–899.

35. Okawa T, Kita M, Goto M, Nishijima H, Miyaji N. Randomized prospective clinical study of small, large and twice-a-day fraction radiotherapy for painful bone metastases. *Radiother Oncol.* October 1988;13(2):99–104.

36. Niewald M, Tkocz HJ, Abel U, et al. Rapid course radiation therapy vs. more standard treatment: a randomized trial for bone metastases. *Int J Radiat Oncol Biol Phys.* December 1, 1996;36(5):1085–1089.

37. Jeremic B, Shibamoto Y, Acimovic L, et al. A randomized trial of three single-dose radiation therapy regimens in the treatment of metastatic bone pain. *Int J Radiat Oncol Biol Phys.* August 1, 1998;42(1):161–167.

38. Yarnold JR. 8 Gy single fraction radiotherapy for the treatment of metastatic skeletal pain: randomised comparison with a multifraction schedule over 12 months of patient follow-up. Bone Pain Trial Working Party. *Radiother Oncol.* August 1999;52(2):111–121.

39. Nathan SS, Healey JH, Mellano D, et al. Survival in patients operated on for pathologic fracture: implications for end-of-life orthopedic care. *J Clin Oncol.* September 1, 2005;23(25):6072–6082.

40. Boland PJ, Lane JM, Sundaresan N. Metastatic disease of the spine. *Clin Orthop Relat Res.* September 1982;169:95–102.

41. Bilsky MH, Lis E, Raizer J, Lee H, Boland P. The diagnosis and treatment of metastatic spinal tumor. *Oncologist.* 1999;4(6):459–469.

42. Kinnane N. The burden of bone disease. *Eur J Oncol Nurs.* 2007;10:1016.

43. Posner JB. Back pain and epidural spinal cord compression. *Med Clin N Am.* 1987;71(2):185–205.

44. Deyo RA, Diehl AK. Cancer as a cause of back pain: frequency, clinical presentation, and diagnostic strategies. *J Gen Intern Med.* 1988;3:230.

45. Sharma H, Bhagat S, McCaul J, et al. Intermedullary nailing for pathological femoral fractures. *J Orthop Surg.* 2007;15(3):291–294.

VII

GENERAL TOPICS IN CANCER REHABILITATION

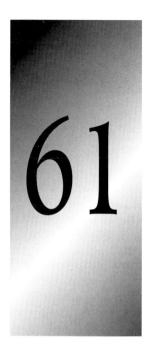

Principles of Physical and Occupational Therapy in Cancer

61

Teresa W. Fitzpatrick

Advances in early detection, diagnosis, and treatment have resulted in survival for many people with cancer. More than 50% of all newly diagnosed cancer patients will survive for more than five years (1), and many with early-stage disease can look forward to a normal life expectancy. Therapy for people who are actively undergoing cancer treatments and for cancer survivors requires both a holistic and systematic approach. Many cancers and their treatments affect every body system, so management needs to focus on the whole person. Understanding of the basic disease histology and the stage of that disease at diagnosis is crucial to ensure a safe and effective assessment and treatment strategy, whether it is for physical, occupational, or speech therapy. In addition, the patient's current status along the continuum of cancer care will significantly affect goal setting and intensity with which the therapist can push the patient toward his goals. A cancer survivor who has completed all treatments will often tolerate a much more aggressive rehabilitation program than someone who is actively receiving treatments to fight their cancer. A person who is seen pretreatment will likely tolerate an aggressive program, while a person whose cancer has spread to other parts of the body—metastatic disease—will require a carefully crafted program that allows for fluctuations in activity tolerance and functional abilities.

This chapter illustrates the importance of understanding disease process and staging, patient status along the continuum of cancer care, and the short- and long-term effects some cancer treatments can have on a person's ability to perform well in therapy. According to Dietz (2), goal setting and treatment planning for cancer patients can be separated into four broad categories: preventative, restorative, supportive, and palliative. The role of physical and occupational therapy in each of these categories will be discussed in detail. In addition, the reader will gain insight into some of the general and specific precautions and contraindications that guide therapy assessment and treatment strategies for cancer patients. Guidelines, as opposed to protocols, provide therapists with the knowledge and expertise to evaluate each patient's unique situation, weigh the pros and cons of treatment versus no treatment, and make an appropriate decision about a patient's care at any unique moment in time.

Direct access to physical therapy services is available to the majority of Americans today. This means that a patient doesn't need to see a physician for a prescription before they can be assessed and treated by a physical therapist. Of course, with this independence comes the responsibility of ensuring that all differential diagnoses are explored when establishing a treatment diagnosis. Whether a therapist is practicing as a consultant under direct access or in a more traditional physician referral system, knowledge of the red flags, or cardinal symptoms that could indicate a cancerous process, is critically important. This chapter will provide some red flags therapists should keep in mind and offer suggestions regarding next steps when red flags are recognized.

KEY POINTS

- Therapy for people who are actively undergoing cancer treatments and for cancer survivors requires both a holistic and systematic approach.
- Goal setting and treatment planning for cancer patients can be separated into four broad categories: preventative, restorative, supportive, and palliative.
- Knowledge of the "red flags," or cardinal symptoms that could indicate a cancerous process, is critically important.
- When an adverse response to treatment is recognized, or when the patient comes in with an unexplainable and seemingly unrelated symptom, the therapist needs to determine whether a change in the patient's treatment plan is necessary, the patient needs to be referred back to the referring physician for a medical evaluation, or both are necessary.

- The long-term sequelae of radiation are largely due to the accumulation of abnormal proteins within the microscopic vasculature and interstitium, with subsequent tissue ischemia and dysfunction. This process is known as radiation fibrosis and the sequelae as the radiation fibrosis syndrome.
- Chemotherapy dosing schedules will significantly affect a physical or occupational therapy program, especially if the drugs carry a highly toxic footprint.
- Before laying hands on a new patient, a thorough understanding of the patient's chief complaints, present illness, course of treatment, planned future treatments, past medical history, level of functioning at home and work, and goals for the therapeutic experience should be obtained.

DISEASE PROCESS AND STAGING

Understanding disease status is critical when establishing a physical or occupational therapy treatment plan for a cancer patient. The size of the tumor at diagnosis, whether the disease process is benign or malignant, whether it is progressing slowly or quickly, and whether it has spread to other parts of the body are all factors the therapist will consider when determining an appropriate course of action for physical or occupational therapy. A diagnosis of "brain tumor" illustrates this point well. If the brain tumor is benign and resectable, like a meningioma, for example, the prognosis and treatment planning will be significantly different than if the brain tumor is a malignant glioblastoma multiforme, which carries a poorer prognosis and frequently requires a long course of multimodal cancer treatments.

A patient's status along the continuum of cancer care will not only affect the therapist's assessment, but will also significantly affect the goals and treatment plan. Duration and frequency of treatment will also depend on the patient's status along this continuum. When planning therapy, the therapist can look at the continuum of care, as the following steps:

- Pretreatment: Recently diagnosed, but no treatment initiated.
- Active care: Actively receiving treatment, with the intent to cure the disease. May be initial treatment or treatment for a relapse.
- Maintenance: Receiving long-term maintenance chemotherapy, hormonal, or other antineoplastic

therapy to keep a disease in remission or under tight control.
- Postcare/remission: Finished with all cancer treatments and considered disease-free.
- Palliative: Receiving palliative treatment for an incurable form of cancer.

Although each patient will respond differently to cancer treatments, Table 61.1 offers basic guidelines regarding what to expect during the assessment, how to establish an effective treatment plan, and how to establish a reasonable frequency and duration for treatment at each step in the continuum.

Whether the patient is in remission or is actively receiving cancer treatments and what type of treatment interventions the patient is facing are valuable data when establishing a therapeutic treatment plan. Ideally, a pretreatment evaluation by a physical and/or occupational therapist can help to prepare for anticipated functional limitations and to provide education about the required posttreatment rehabilitation interventions (3); however, today's health care market makes this a challenging effort. Ganz et al. suggest that posttreatment morbidity can be reduced by taking a preventive approach rather than by waiting until problems become severe and more difficult to manage (3). More research is needed, however, to convince most insurance companies of the benefits of pretreatment therapeutic assessments. A patient that has completed all, or at least the most intense, steps in their cancer treatment will typically have few, if any, restrictions and precautions. A patient whose cancer is being actively treated with chemotherapy or radiation therapy

TABLE 61.1 Therapy Throughout the Continuum of Cancer Care

	ASSESSMENT	TREATMENT PLANNING	FREQUENCY AND DURATION
Pretreatment	Should tolerate a full assessment. Document all pretreatment function that may be affected by the impending cancer treatments.	Education regarding general conditioning and strength pretreatment. Prepare the patient for typical functional problems they may encounter after treatment begins.	Usually only one to two visits to prepare the patient for cancer treatments.
Active care	Must assess all systems, especially if the patient is receiving any radiation or chemotherapy. Will require an efficient assessment, since fatigue is common. Brief impairment-specific assessments should be completed as needed to document any changes that have occurred since initiation of care. May require more than one session to complete.	Treatment sessions should focus initially on functional disabilities and education. General conditioning should be addressed, when possible, to prevent deconditioning.	Frequency and duration will vary greatly, depending on the intensity of other treatments and their effect on the patient's status. Duration ranges from 10–20 wks and frequency ranges from 1–2 sessions per week.
Maintenance	Must assess all systems, since general deconditioning is often an underlying cause of more specific complaints. Pay particular attention to surgical/radiation sites for signs of restriction and sensation/proprioception assessed, since many long-term treatments affect them. Compare current impairments with previous assessments, when available.	Treatment sessions should focus on general conditioning and specific complaints equally. Often, patients in this stage will have specific complaints, which are exacerbated by underlying core weakness or poor posture.	Frequency ranges from one to three sessions weekly, depending on the person's ability to perform a home program. Duration is usually four to six wks.
Postcare	Must assess all systems, since general deconditioning is often an underlying cause of more specific complaints. Pay particular attention to surgical/radiation sites for signs of restriction and sensation/proprioception assessed, since many long-term treatments affect them. Compare current impairments with previous assessments, when available.	Treatment sessions should focus on general conditioning and specific complaints equally. Often, patients in this stage will have specific complaints, which are exacerbated by underlying core weakness or poor posture.	Frequency is usually two to three sessions weekly. Duration is usually two to six wks, depending on the person's ability to perform a home program.
Palliation	Assessments should focus on impairments and disabilities that have potential for improvement and potential to improve the patient and caregiver's quality of life.	Treatments should focus on maximizing strengths, offering training in the use of adaptive equipment to make ADLs easier, and maintaining a safe form of locomotion for the patient.	Frequency is usually one to two sessions per week. Duration is typically one to three wks to establish a home program and equipment training.

Abbreviation: ADL, activities of daily living.

concurrently with physical or occupational therapy will need to be monitored closely. Those patients who are actively receiving cancer treatments, those with complicated medical histories, and those with multiple disabilities offer a unique challenge to many outpatient physical and occupational therapy clinics. Cancer patients tend to require more individualized time with a licensed therapist who is trained to constantly reassess how the patient is responding to their treatments.

Frequently, on-the-spot adjustments to the program are necessary to maximize a cancer patient's benefit from each session. When an adverse response to treatment is recognized, or when the patient comes in with an unexplainable and seemingly unrelated symptom, the therapist needs to determine whether a change in the patient's treatment plan is necessary, the patient needs to be referred back to the referring physician for a medical evaluation, or both are necessary.

RADIATION THERAPY AND ITS EFFECTS ON TREATMENT PLANNING

Radiation therapy can be used for curative or palliative purposes, as a standalone treatment, or as a component of a multimodal treatment plan. The goal of radiation therapy is typically to eradicate as much of the tumor as possible with maximal preservation and minimal irradiation of surrounding normal tissue.

Reactions to radiation therapy are determined by the type, quantity, duration, and site of exposure. Effects may be immediate or may appear a number of months or years following treatment. Table 61.2 provides a list of common side effects associated with radiation therapy.

TABLE 61.2
Radiation Therapy Side Effects

Myelosuppression (ie, bone marrow depression), particularly leukopenia.
Fatigue and decreased endurance.
Erythema, mild burning or tanning, pigmentation of the skin.
Moist or dry desquamation, ulcerations of skin and mucous membranes, mucositis.
Pneumonitis from external irradiation of lungs followed by fibrosis. Radioactive implants in lungs may cause blood-tinged secretions.
Fibrosis and atrophy in soft tissue, causing decreased range of motion.
Decreased vascularity and lymphedema, causing delayed healing and decreased ability to disseminate heat and cold from irradiated tissues.
Alopecia (hair loss).
CNS effects: CNS tissue is more radiosensitive than peripheral nerves.
Radiation myelitis, or inflammation of the spinal cord, may occur as a delayed reaction and will be manifested by paresis or plegia.
Radiation sickness: systemic illness usually caused by abdominal irradiation and often manifested by anorexia, nausea and vomiting, and weakness.
Bone and joint necrosis, delayed or impaired growth in immature bone (infrequent).
Radiation-induced neoplasia in the irradiated area (rare).
Emotional reactions, including:
   Fear of pain or of being burned
   Negative body image caused by alopecia, skin changes, and visible dye markings.
   Depression and withdrawal behavior caused by disruption in lifestyle, economic hardship, or physical changes and discomfort.

Source: Reprinted from Memorial Sloan-Kettering Cancer Center's Radiation Guidelines.
Abbreviation: CNS, central nervous system.

Radiation can be administered through different methods:

1. External beam radiation: Radiation delivered from outside the body. It focuses on the region of the tumor and the surrounding tissue.
2. Brachytherapy: Radioactive seeds inserted into the tumor bed.

External Beam Radiation Therapy Considerations

When treating a patient while they are actively receiving radiation therapy, there are a few things to consider. In addition to achieving each patient's goals, therapists should concern themselves with the skin integrity in the radiated area. Skin can become red, tender, and even blistered. This is known as dry desquamation. Special care should be taken to avoid the area while the skin is in this fragile state. Treatment in the radiated area is typically limited to active and active-assistive range of motion, gentle strengthening, and functional mobility. If, at any time, wet desquamation, or open blisters/lesions, develops, all therapy to the radiated area should cease. While bones are actively receiving radiation, they can become weaker and can be at risk for fracture. Care should be taken to minimize heavy resistance on bones while they are being irradiated. Occasionally, depending on the fragility of the bone being irradiated, a patient's weight-bearing status will be changed to protect the bone. An appropriate assistive device should be evaluated and fitted by the physical therapist and training should be completed to ensure the patient can adhere to his weight-bearing restrictions.

Brachytherapy Therapy Considerations

There are two basic types of brachytherapy: permanent and temporary. If a person receives permanent brachytherapy in the form of radioactive seeds, the radiation slowly dissipates over time until the patient is no longer radioactive. Typically, the radiation a person emits as a result of seed placement is low, but some basic precautions are encouraged. Treatment can be provided as usual, but the therapist is recommended to avoid placing their hands directly over the radiation site for long periods. When treating a patient who has brachytherapy in place, the therapist should approach the patient with a treatment plan that will minimize the therapist's exposure to the patient. Radioactive seeds are used often to treat prostate and lung cancers. If a patient sleeps with a bed partner, they should be encouraged to avoid prolonged periods of close contact between the irradiated body parts/areas and the bed partner.

Temporary brachytherapy is used to treat soft tissue sarcomas and thyroid cancers. Thyroid cancer patients drink radioactive iodine, which goes directly to the thyroid and destroys it. A person who is being treated with radioactive iodine is usually isolated for three days and then follows exposure guidelines for approximately one month after administration. All therapy services should be planned before or after radioactive iodine administration whenever possible.

Another form of temporary brachytherapy is seed placement into the center of a tumor bed through removable catheters. These seeds are left in place for three to seven days, and the patient remains in isolation during that time. When the seeds are removed, the patient is immediately radiation-free. Patients who are scheduled for temporary brachytherapy should receive a physical therapy (PT) consult prior to having the brachytherapy seeds loaded to ensure independence with in-room mobility. An occupational therapy (OT) consult may be necessary to make sure the patient can perform all activities of daily living (ADLs) in a safe and independent manner while they are isolated. Radiation shields should be used and contact should be kept as brief as possible when entering the room of a patient receiving this form of brachytherapy.

Radiation-Induced Fibrosis Therapy Considerations

The development of radiation-induced fibrosis (RIF) is influenced by multiple factors, including the radiation dose and volume, fractionation schedule, previous or concurrent treatments, genetic susceptibility, and comorbidities such as diabetes mellitus. RIF can occur at any time after radiation is completed, but symptoms will typically manifest six months to five years after radiation treatment is completed and can progress indefinitely. Although RIF originally was thought to be a slow, irreversible process, more recent studies suggest that RIF is not necessarily an unalterable process (4). In patients thought to be at high risk for RIF, early initiation of active and passive physical therapy measures is helpful. For example, in a patient with early signs or symptoms of trismus, forced mouth opening is recommended (5). If a patient has a history of radiation treatment, the treating therapist should assess the pliability of the skin and joints around the radiated area. In addition, the therapist should evaluate for any asymmetries in muscle bulk, strength, and coordination. Many patients who experience radiation fibrosis will benefit from soft tissue mobilization of the radiated area and the areas around the radiated area. Once blood flow to the area is maximized through massage and mobilization of the soft tissue, stretching and strengthening exercises should be incorporated. Muscle damaged by radiation will not respond normally to stretching or strengthening, but with patience and careful attention to recruitment of the remaining healthy muscle fibers, muscle length can approach normal and strength can improve. As muscle/skin pliability improves and muscle strength increases, therapists should attend closely to movement quality. Neuromuscular reeducation is frequently necessary to assist patients with gaining coordinated and efficient movement quality in the area affected. Shoulder dysfunction following breast cancer treatment provides a common example of this scenario. Often, the first step is assessing and treating the soft tissue and joint restrictions resulting from surgical incisions and radiation treatment. Once the patient can bring their neck and shoulder into adequate alignment, muscle strengthening can begin. Often, patients require education focused on breaking maladaptive movement patterns and adapting healthy ones.

CHEMOTHERAPY AND ITS EFFECTS ON TREATMENT PLANNING

Antineoplastic chemotherapeutics, either alone or in combination, have become an integral part in the control of cancer. Table 61.3 provides a list of common toxic side effects that can affect a patient's participation in therapy, as well as the agents responsible for the toxicity. Chemotherapy dosing schedules will significantly affect a physical or occupational therapy program, especially if the drugs carry a highly toxic footprint. Therapists need to understand each patient's chemotherapy schedule and establish their treatment plan accordingly. Vital signs, lab values, and peripheral sensation should be monitored before, during, and after each session to ensure patient safety during exercise and recovery. Signs of myelosuppression, cardiac and pulmonary toxicities, and peripheral neuropathies should be discussed with the oncologist or physiatrist immediately. Knowledge of the potential side effects is critical. A therapist's frequent contact with his patients, often two to three times per week, puts him in a unique position to recognize when toxicity levels should be brought to the oncologist's attention.

SURGERY AND ITS EFFECTS ON TREATMENT PLANNING

Physical and occupational therapy following cancer surgery is similar to therapy following any surgical procedure; however, every cancer surgery is customized to the patient's needs. Since limb salvage procedures for osteosarcoma in children are undertaken to remove the tumor and preserve as much function as possible, each

TABLE 61.3
Chemotherapy Side Effects and Guidelines

1. Myelosuppression (ie, bone marrow depression). Since the bone marrow is one of the main blood-forming organs, this depression results in decreased production of all the blood components. It is important to obtain a complete blood count (WBC, platelets, Hct, or Hgb) before each rehabilitation session, since vigorous resistive exercise or activities requiring sharp tools may be contraindicated if blood counts are low.

2. Thrombocytopenia (low platelet count)
   Therapy with various platelet levels:
   Normal value: 200,000–5,000,000 per cu.mm.
   Between 30,000 and 50,000 per cu.mm.: A resistive exercise or ambulation program should be changed to active exercises without resistance due to risk of internal hemorrhage.
   Below 30,000 per cu.mm.: Gentle exercise at bedside can be performed.
   Below 20,000 per cu.mm.: Patients should be limited to minimal exercise.

   Keep in mind that the treatment limitations for the aforementioned platelet values are not absolute. The activity level of different patients with the same platelet count may vary, depending on such factors as acute versus chronic thrombocytopenia or a stable versus hemorrhagic condition.

3. Leukopenia (low white blood cell count): Normal value: 5,000–10,000 per cu. M.M.
   Since leukopenic patients are extremely susceptible to infections, contact with other persons should be limited and strict hygiene procedures should be observed.

4. Anemia

Normal Values:	Male	Female
Hct. (packed cell volume)	45%–47%	40%–42%
Hgb. (gm, per 100 mL)	13.8–17.2	12.1–15.1
RBC (million/cu, M.M.)	5.0	4.5

   Anemic patients may have an elevated heart and respiration rate due to the body's effort to maintain an adequate oxygen supply. Therapists should carefully monitor pulse and blood pressure before, during, and after an exercise or activity. Patients may also be easily fatigued with minimal exertion. If this is the case, a maintenance, bedside exercise program is recommended. Although patient responses to anemia will vary, many patients will experience symptoms when their Hgb reaches 8 gm/mL or lower. Treatment plans are frequently altered at this point, and the patient's status is discussed with the referring clinician.

5. Cardiac toxicity. Adriamycin or daunomycin may cause irreversible cardiac damage. Complications such as congestive heart failure can develop, so vital signs should be checked frequently.

6. Pulmonary fibrosis. Bleomycin may cause this side effect, with resulting restrictive lung disease and impaired gas exchange.

7. Peripheral neuropathy. Vincristine, in particular, may cause weakness and paresthesias. This typically affects the distal more than proximal muscles. This may result in wrist drop, foot drop, a loss of strength in the intrinsic muscles, or a combination of these. Splints, dorsiflexion-assist orthotics, and strengthening exercises may be indicated.

8. Fibrosis. If infiltration of an intravenously administered drug occurs, cellulitis may develop. This results in hard edema and fibrotic tissue, which may limit a patient's range of motion. These patients may require splinting and range-of-motion exercises to prevent contractures. If fibrosis develops in lung tissue, patients may have difficulty breathing. Vital signs need to be checked frequently.

9. Gastrointestinal toxicity. Moderate to severe nausea, vomiting, diarrhea, and ulceration of the mucosal lining may occur. Therapy to maintain strength and endurance should be continued if a patient can tolerate it.

10. Alopecia (hair loss). This is a temporary side effect of certain drugs. Although the texture and color may be slightly altered, regrowth of the hair always occurs either during or after chemotherapy treatment.

11. Psychosocial issues. Any of the previously listed side effects may cause a variety of emotional reactions, such as depression, anxiety, withdrawal, and hostility. Emotional reactions are also direct side effects of certain drugs.

Additional Chemtherapeutic Agents and Common Side Effects
Vinblastine: neutropenia, thrombocytopenia, anemia, nausea, vomiting, constipation
Cisplatin: renal insufficiency, ototoxicity (tinnitus, hearing loss), peripheral neuropathy
Carboplatin: nausea, vomiting, electrolyte changes, renal insufficiency
Ifosfamide: hemorrhagic cystitis, confusion, depressive psychosis
Taxol: heart block, bradycardia, respiratory distress

Source: Reprinted from Memorial Sloan-Kettering Cancer Center Chemotherapy Guidelines.
Abbreviations: Hct, hematocrit; Hgb, hemoglobin; RBC, red blood cell; WBC, white blood cell.

procedure will result in a different functional prognosis. Some factors that affect functional prognosis include:

- How much bone was removed
- What kind of hardware was used to stabilize the area
- Which muscles and nerves were removed
- Which muscles were detached and reattached elsewhere to maintain some functional movement

The therapist should review the surgical report and speak to the surgeon, if necessary, to ensure a clear understanding of functional potential following surgery. As with any postsurgical patient, unless otherwise indicated by the surgeon, cancer patients are encouraged to begin walking postoperative day one. Pulmonary status should be monitored closely and chest physical therapy initiated early, if necessary. Immediate postoperative care, as with any surgical patient, is focused on functional mobility and surgical site protection to allow for adequate healing. Once surgical sites are healed, some cancer patients will require outpatient therapy services to assist in the recovery of function and strength following surgery.

THERAPY ASSESSMENT

Before laying hands on a new patient, a thorough understanding of the patient's chief complaints, present illness, course of treatment, planned future treatments, past medical history, level of functioning at home and work, and goals for the therapeutic experience should be obtained. When gathering information regarding course of treatment, detail is critical. The initial intake interview should include a review of surgical reports and x-rays whenever possible. Radiation therapy dosages and locations should be noted and a follow-up evaluation of the skin, muscle, and nerve function in the radiated area should be completed. Chemotherapy regimens, including the type of drug used and the common side effects experienced by the patient, should be noted. Remember that any single cancer treatment (or combination of treatments) can lead to a few general problems, including fatigue, generalized weakness (especially core weakness), and poor posture. In a study of 189 women who had survived at least 18 months after treatment for ovarian cancer, chronic fatigue and anxiety were present, both in those who had relapsed and in those who were disease-free following their initial cancer management (6). Armed with a thorough understanding of the patient and their situation, the therapist can determine whether any special precautions will be required to complete the assessment and where they may want to focus the assessment.

Physical and occupational therapists who specialize in the care of cancer patients utilize the same assessment techniques and standardized tests and measures that are used in any setting. The method used to complete the assessment, however, may change based on the information acquired in the intake interview. Despite similar diagnoses, cancer patients may receive different curative treatments and each will respond uniquely to those treatments. Henceforth, therapists should be familiar with a variety of tests and measures. Choosing the tests and measures that will provide the most valuable representation of a patient's deficits will highlight patient progress in future reassessments. Since cancer affects people of all ages, knowledge and understanding of normal development across the lifespan is important. The elderly population is a group in which cancer is being diagnosed and treated more aggressively, so functional impairment from cancer and its treatment is particularly important (7). In addition, the effects of cancer and its treatment on functional limitations may be of particular concern for the elderly because of other age-related conditions, such as diabetes or high blood pressure, which also make them susceptible to a decline in physical function (8).

ESTABLISHING GOALS AND TREATMENT PLANS

Goal setting with cancer patients and survivors should be a collaborative process between the therapist, the patient, the patient's caregivers, and the referring clinician. When establishing therapy goals, the therapist should talk to the patient about what they hope to accomplish in physical or occupational therapy. Encourage each patient to offer concrete examples of his ultimate goal, such as, "I want to be able to get on and off the floor easily so I can play with my grandchildren," "I want to be able to walk across the stage to receive my high school diploma without crutches or a limp," or "I want to run a marathon." Once the therapist knows what the patient really hopes to accomplish, they can establish short-term goals and treatment strategies that will move the patient closer toward their ultimate goal. The key to a successful rehabilitation program is the patient's active participation. Physical medication and rehabilitation (PM&R) teams can achieve that by setting up reasonable rehabilitation goals, considering patients' associated symptoms and privileging their comfort (9).

Therapists frequently face challenges regarding a patient's ability to be realistic about their goals. It is this author's opinion that a patient should never be told to forget about their ultimate goal because it is unattainable. Instead, make an effort to respect the patient's ultimate goal and work with the patient to help them set more realistic short-term goals that will improve their function immediately. Frequent assurance that any goal designed to improve a patient's function today will move that person a step closer to their ultimate goal may provide comfort to the patient.

J. Herbert Dietz, Jr. categorized goal setting and treatment planning into four basic categories, which can be followed today (2).

Preventive Interventions

Preventive (or "preventative") interventions lessen the effect of expected disabilities and emphasize patient education. For example, preoperative education and training provided to prepare a patient for postoperative weight-bearing restrictions will enhance a patient's preparedness for his deficits after surgery, minimize the time the patient is immobile after surgery, and provide for safe, efficient mobility training while maintaining precautions. Preoperative training is not affected by normal postop pain and/or postanesthesia symptoms. Preventive measures also include approaches to improving a patient's physical functioning and general health status. Memorial Sloan-Kettering Cancer Center offers a five-week, multidisciplinary osteoporosis education and exercise program, which focuses on providing patients with the knowledge and skill to reduce their risk for developing osteoporosis after their cancer treatments.

Restorative Interventions

Restorative interventions are procedures that attempt to return patients to previous levels of physical, psychological, social, and vocational functioning. Postoperative range-of-motion (ROM) exercises for patients undergoing mastectomy or head and neck resection are examples of interventions included in this category. Acute physical therapy, including basic mobility training and pulmonary conditioning after surgery, is another example of restorative care.

Supportive Interventions

Supportive rehabilitation focuses on teaching patients ways to accommodate for existing disabilities. In addition, supportive rehabilitation attempts to minimize debilitating changes from ongoing disease. Occupational therapists' interventions during this category of management may include teaching patients how to use devices and procedures that assist in self-management, self-care abilities, and independent functioning. Following brain tumor resection, patients often receive supportive interventions by occupational therapists, including techniques to help improve memory and complex cognitive processing. Education and training regard-

ing prosthetic devices after amputation is an example of physical therapy's role during this phase of care.

Palliative Interventions

The goal of palliative care is the achievement of the best possible quality of life for patients and their families (10). During the rehabilitation of terminally ill patients, maintaining a balance between optimal function and comfort becomes a key issue. In patients with advanced disease, fatigue, pain, and generalized weakness are the most commonly reported symptoms (11), while progressive debility, caretaker dependency, thoughts of uncontrolled pain and isolation, and loss of autonomy are among the most distressing concerns (12). Physical strength, hours spent in recumbency, and the ability to do what one wants are ranked highly by patients and their spouses with respect to overall quality of life (13). Therefore, therapists should work closely with each patient to determine their functional goals and provide treatment that will help maintain strength and function for as long as possible. When increasing disability and advanced disease process may be present, interventions and goals focus on minimizing or eliminating complications and providing comfort and support. Palliative goals should be constantly revised and adjusted, taking into consideration the stage of the disease; the patient's medical status, cognition, and prognosis; and the site of planned discharge (14). Therapy goals typically include pain control, prevention of contractures and pressure sores, prevention of unnecessary deterioration from inactivity, and energy conservation. A balance must be found between increasing rest to alleviate asthenia and promoting deconditioning (15). Caregiver training in the use of adaptive equipment, such as patient lifts, to aid in the care of a patient is of paramount importance during this phase of care.

GENERAL PRECAUTIONS

In addition to the surgery-specific precautions/restrictions and radiation-specific restrictions that were discussed in the surgery and radiation treatment planning sections previously, there are some general precautions that therapists should be cognizant of when treating cancer patients.

METASTATIC DISEASE

Bone

Metastatic spread of a cancer from one part of the body to another can drastically change a therapist's approach to a patient's care. For example, metastasis to any bone requires that a therapist understand exactly which bones are affected by the disease and to what extent those bones are affected. Since many variables affect fracture risk, an orthopedic surgeon should be asked to determine whether someone is at risk for fracture. If information from an orthopedic surgeon is not available, open communication with the referring clinician to determine a safe weight-bearing status for the affected limb is critical. Since it is not possible to precisely determine which patients with metastatic bone disease will go on to fracture a bone, some general guidelines for treating these patients have evolved, mostly based on common sense (16). The typical therapy assessment should be modified in consideration of fracture risk. Manual muscle testing or passive or active-assisted range of motion should be deferred on an involved limb. Only active range of motion should be assessed, as this will likely be limited by pain. Resistive exercise involving an affected area is generally contraindicated. Likewise, provision of chest percussion and vibration over rib metastases is typically avoided (16). In case of lesions of the lower extremity in which partial weight bearing is permitted, the therapist should be aware of the condition of patients' upper extremities because lesions in these areas may preclude use of walking aids, bed trapezes, etc. Therapy goals, when working with a patient with metastatic bone disease, should include strengthening of the muscles that surround the affected bone and education regarding weight-bearing restrictions and body mechanics that will protect the bone from damage.

Spinal Cord Compression

Spinal cord compression of nontraumatic origin accounts for 33%–79% of all spinal cord injury rehabilitation admissions (17). Spinal cord compression can present as a sudden onset of weakness, with or without pain, but it can also come on more slowly. Motor abnormalities usually precede sensory deficits due to epidural extension preferentially affecting the anterior spinal cord, and recovery usually occurs in the reverse order. Rapidly progressive paresis or plegia rarely reverses. Loss of bowel and bladder function is a poor prognostic sign and is usually irreversible (18). If spinal cord compression is suspected, it should be treated as a medical emergency and the referring professional should be contacted immediately. Recovery of spinal cord function after compression is directly associated with the extent of compression and the amount of time the spinal cord was compromised; thus, prompt diagnosis and immediate treatment are critically important. Rehabilitation of patients with spinal cord tumors focuses on relief of symptoms, quality-of-life improvement, functional independence, and prevention of further complications (18).

Brain

Brain tumors comprise some of the most challenging cancer diagnoses requiring rehabilitation. The spectrum of cognitive, communication, behavioral, and physical deficits substantially complicates the medical and psychological issues inherent in any cancer diagnosis (19,20). Cerebral metastases make up about half of all intracranial tumors (18). The most common source of brain metastases is lung cancer; however, breast, melanoma, renal, and testicular cancers will metastasize. The management of cerebral metastasis is mostly palliative, and even with optimal treatment the median survival is less than one year (21). A therapist working with a patient who has brain metastasis should continually monitor the patient's cognitive status for any changes. Therapy instructions and home programs may need to be modified to ensure adequate comprehension and safety. Occupational therapy is particularly skilled in the area of cognitive assessment and safety awareness, and should be involved in the care of these patients. Brain metastasis is often treated with whole-brain radiation, which will affect a patient's cognition also. Physical and occupational therapists who treat patients while they are receiving whole-brain radiation, or in the few days after radiation, should monitor patients for fluctuations in cognition and arousal, as these changes could indicate a change in intracranial pressure. Changes in intracranial pressure are typically treated with corticosteroids. During and after whole-brain radiation and surgery, patients may need to maintain the head of their bed at 30° elevation. Therapy should preclude any activities like quadruped or Trendelenburg positions, which require the head to be in a dependent position.

Pulmonary

Lung tissue is the most common site for metastatic disease because of the intense venous drainage to the area. Any patient with a cancer history who experiences atypical shortness of breath, shortness of breath after activity that does not resolve as expected, hemoptysis, or a dry persistent cough should be referred back to his primary physician for medical follow-up. Vital signs, including heart rate, respiratory rate, and O_2 saturations, should be monitored closely in any patient with known pulmonary disease.

Myelosuppression

Some chemotherapy can cause extreme fluctuations in normal blood chemistry levels. Some of these fluctuations will have a significant impact on a patient's ability to participate in a physical or occupational therapy program safely. Table 61.3 describes relative norms, signs and symptoms associated with alterations in these norms, and the implications to therapy. Typically, therapists monitor lab values for patients who are acutely hospitalized, but they don't often track them in their outpatient population. When providing physical or occupational therapy for cancer patients, it is important to monitor lab values for anyone actively receiving chemotherapy and for anyone who recently completed chemotherapy. Lab values that are observed most closely in cancer patients because of their tendency to fluctuate are hemoglobin/hematocrit, platelet levels, white blood cell counts, and international normalized ratio (INR). Although Table 61.3 provides guidelines for treatment with altered blood levels, it is not a protocol or standard of care. These guidelines are meant to give therapists a place from which to begin critical decision making regarding the benefits and risks associated with planned therapeutic interventions. Some factors to consider when deciding whether to treat and what kind of treatment to provide include:

- Is the value in question chronically low or high? If so, the best clinical decision is to determine what therapy can be provided to the patient safely, given their compromised blood levels. Even a minimal amount of activity can offset the negative effects of bed rest on overall strength and function. Extra safety measures should be employed to eliminate the risk of falling. It may be necessary to discuss your plans to work with this patient with the referring clinician.
- Is this an acute change that warrants further medical investigation? In this case, it would be advisable to wait until more information is available to make a decision.

Cancer patients experience a higher prevalence of deep vein thrombosis (DVT) and pulmonary embolism (PE). Once again, it is difficult to create a protocol or standard of care to address the complicated needs of cancer patients. Memorial Sloan-Kettering Cancer Center's guidelines for the management of DVT and PE are presented in Table 61.4. When treating a cancer patient who has a DVT, or is at high risk for developing a DVT, utilize the guidelines along with the patient's individual case information to make a clinically safe decision about the most beneficial type of intervention.

GENERAL CANCER SIGNS AND SYMPTOMS

The American Cancer Society has published a list of general (nonspecific) signs and symptoms associated with cancer, which are important for therapists to keep in mind while assessing and educating their patients (22):

Unexplained Weight Loss: An unexplained (unintentional) weight loss of 10 pounds or more may be the first sign of cancer, particularly cancers of the pancreas, stomach, esophagus, or lung. Weight loss should be addressed in a therapist's initial assessment of each patient.
Fever: Fever is common with cancer, but is more often seen in advanced disease. Almost all patients with cancer will have fever at some time, especially if the cancer or its treatment affects the immune system and makes it harder for the body to fight infection. Less often, fever may be an early sign of cancer, such as with leukemia or lymphoma.
Fatigue: Fatigue may be an important symptom as cancer progresses. However, it may happen early in cancers such as leukemia, or if the cancer is causing an ongoing loss of blood, as in some colon or stomach cancers.
Pain: Pain may be an early symptom with some cancers, such as bone cancers or testicular cancer, but most often, pain is a symptom of advanced disease.
Skin Changes: Along with cancers of the skin, some internal cancers can cause visible skin signs. These changes include the skin looking darker (hyperpigmentation), yellow (jaundice), or red (erythema); itching; or excessive hair growth.

SPECIFIC CANCER SIGNS AND SYMPTOMS

Along with the aforementioned general symptoms, therapists should discuss with their patients and watch for the following common symptoms, which could be an indication of cancer. There may be other causes for each of these, but it is important to bring them to a doctor's attention as soon as possible so that they can be investigated.

Change in bowel habits or bladder function: Long-term constipation, diarrhea, or a change in the size of the stool may be a sign of colon cancer. Pain with urination, blood in the urine, or a change in bladder function (such as more frequent or less frequent urination) could be related to bladder or prostate cancer. Any reported changes in bladder or bowel function should be reported to a patient's doctor.
Nonhealing Skin Lesions: Skin cancers may bleed and look like sores that do not heal. A long-lasting sore in the mouth could be an oral cancer and should be dealt with right away, especially in patients who smoke, chew tobacco, or frequently drink alcohol. Sores on the penis or vagina may either be signs of infection or an early cancer, and should not be overlooked.
Unusual Bleeding or Discharge: Unusual bleeding can happen in either early or advanced cancer. Blood in the

---

TABLE 61.4
DVT/PE Prophylaxis and Rehabilitation Therapy Guidelines

Lower Extremities

1. For patients with acute lower extremity deep vein thrombosis (DVT), with or without pulmonary embolism (PE), and no inferior vena cava (IVC) filter, therapy (including physical, occupational, and lymphedema with bandaging and manual lymphatic drainage [MLD]) can be initiated once they are *therapeutic* on an anticoagulant:

   Low molecular weight heparin (LMWH) preparations are preferred, as they are therapeutic immediately following the first injection. Monitoring is not required. Common preparations include enoxaparin (Lovenox), dalteparin (Fragmin), and tinzaparin (Innohep).

   Unfractionated heparin may take one to two days to become therapeutic and is more prone to bleeding complications than LMWH. The adjusted partial thromboplastin time (APTT) should be monitored, and therapy can begin when it is between 50 and 70.

   Warfarin (Coumadin) may take several days to become therapeutic. The international normalized ratio (INR) should be monitored, and therapy can begin when it is between 2 and 3.

2. For patients with acute lower extremity DVT (with or without PE) and an IVC filter, therapy can be initiated *immediately*, regardless of their anticoagulation status.

3. For patients with acute lower extremity DVT who cannot be anticoagulated and an IVC filter cannot be placed, therapy *should not* be done except with palliative intent, as such patients are at very high risk for PE and death. Any planned therapy interventions should be discussed with the patient's primary attending or the rehabilitation medicine attending prior to initiation.

Upper Extremities

1. Upper extremity DVT is more likely to embolize secondary to a lack of valves between the upper extremity (UE) and lungs. Filters are not protective. Therapy involving upper extremity resistance or compression should not be started until the patient has been *therapeutic for at least three days* on an anticoagulant to give the thrombus time to mature. Activity of daily living (ADL) training supervised by an occupational therapist is appropriate. (See anticoagulation guidelines).

2. Therapy involving upper extremity resistance or compression should *not* be performed on patients who cannot be anticoagulated. ADL training supervised by an occupational therapist is appropriate.

Reprinted from Memorial Sloan-Kettering Cancer Center Rehabilitation Service Policy and Procedure Manual.

---

sputum (phlegm) may be a sign of lung cancer. Blood in the stool (or a dark or black stool) could be a sign of colon or rectal cancer. Cancer of the cervix or the endometrium (lining of the uterus) can cause vaginal bleeding. Blood in the urine may be a sign of bladder or kidney cancer. A bloody discharge from the nipple may be a sign of breast cancer.

Thickening or Lump in Breast or Other Parts of the Body: Many cancers can be felt through the skin, mostly in the breast, testicle, lymph nodes (glands), and the soft tissues of the body. A lump or thickening may be an early or late sign of cancer. Patients should be encouraged to report any lump or thickening to their doctor, especially if they have just discovered it or noticed it has grown in size.

Indigestion or Trouble Swallowing: While they commonly have other causes, indigestion or swallowing problems may be a sign of cancer of the esophagus, stomach, or pharynx (throat).

Recent Change in a Wart or Mole: Patients should be encouraged to monitor warts, moles, and freckles and report any changes in color, size, or shape. In addition, a mole, wart, or freckle that loses its definite borders should be reported to a doctor immediately. The skin lesion may be a melanoma, which, if diagnosed early, can be treated successfully.

Nagging Cough or Hoarseness: A cough that does not go away may be a sign of lung cancer. Hoarseness can be a sign of cancer of the larynx (voice box) or thyroid.

While the signs and symptoms listed here are the more common ones seen with cancer, many others are less common and are not listed here. If any of these signs are noticed or mentioned during a therapy session, the patient should be encouraged to see his physician. If it has nothing to do with cancer, the doctor can investigate it and treat it, if needed. If it is cancer, the patient has the opportunity to have it treated early, when treatment is most likely to be effective (22).

CONCLUSION

Physical and occupational therapy are valuable and often underutilized tools in the management of cancer and the sequelae of its treatments. A survey of 500 patients with colorectal, lung, and prostate cancer who, on average, had been living with the disease for more than three years found that greater than 80% reported problems related to mobility (difficulty walking, bending, lifting) and more than 50% of those people reported their problem as severe. Forty-one percent of colorectal cancer, 69% of lung cancer and 40% of prostate cancer patients reported difficulty with activities of daily living. These functional problems occurred in a relatively "functional" sample whose average Karnofsky Performance Status Scale scores were greater than 80% and 40% had no sign of active disease at the time of the survey (3). This study highlights the insensitivity of performance status scales like Karnofsky in the assessment of functional status. Thus, physicians should obtain the advice and consultation of a physical and/or occupational therapist when difficulties of mobility or activities of daily living are suspected.

Physical and occupational therapy for cancer patients can occur in the home, an outpatient clinic, an inpatient rehabilitation center, or in an acute care hospital. As medical treatments develop, changing the prognosis and survival for many patients afflicted with cancer, the focus of physical and occupational therapy interventions must evolve and change as well. As more and more people who develop cancer become survivors, they are beginning to demand resources that can help them regain their previous quality of life, or even improve upon it. Rehabilitation specialists, such as physical and occupational therapists, are uniquely positioned and skilled to help cancer survivors achieve their goals. In most cases, improved survival rates are directly proportional to advances in multimodal therapies, which enhance the employment of more toxic cancer treatments safely. Physical and occupational therapists who understand the complexities of oncology rehabilitative care can have a huge impact on cancer patients' ability to tolerate such toxic treatments by working with them to maintain their strength and function.

References

1. Cole P, Rodu B. Declining cancer mortality in the United States. *Cancer.* 1996;78:2045.
2. Dietz JH Jr. *Rehabilitation Oncology.* Somerset, NJ: John Wiley & Sons; 1981:23–31.
3. Ganz PA, Coscarelli A. Cancer rehabilitation. In: Haskell CM, ed., *Cancer Treatment,* 5th ed. Philadelphia: WB Saunders; 1995:381–391.
4. Weiss E, Chung T. In: www.uptodate.com, Kavanagh B, Ross M, eds. Clinical manifestations and treatment of radiation-induced fibrosis. Last review for revision January 31, 2008.
5. Sciubba JJ, Goldenberg D. Oral complications of radiotherapy. *Lancet Oncol.* 2006;7:175.
6. Liavaag AH, Dorum A, Fossa SD, et al. Controlled study of fatigue, quality of life and somatic and mental morbidity in epithelial ovarian cancer survivors: how lucky are the lucky ones? *J Clin Oncol.* 2007;25(15): 2049–2056.
7. Sweeney C, Schmitz KH, Lazovich D, et al. Functional limitations in elderly female cancer survivors. *J Natl Cancer Inst.* 2006;98:521.
8. Guaralnik JM, LaCroix AZ, Abbott RD, et al. Maintaining mobility in late life. I. Demographic characteristics and chronic conditions. *Am J Epidemiol.* 1993;137:845–857.
9. Fattal C, Gault D, Leblond C, et al. Metastatic paraplegia: care management characteristics within a rehabilitation center. *Spinal Cord.* 2009;47(2):115–121.
10. Report of the WHO Expert Committee on Cancer Pain Relief and Active Supportive Care. Cancer pain relief with a guide to opioid availability. Technical Report Series 804. Geneva: World Health Organization; 1996.
11. Coyle N, Adelhart J, Foley KM, et al. Character of terminal illness in the advanced cancer patient: pain and other symptoms during the last four weeks of life. *J Pain Symptom Manag.* 1991;6:408–410.
12. Brietbart W, Chochinov H, Passik S. Psychiatric aspects of palliative care. In: Doyle D, Hanks G, Macdonald N, eds. *Oxford Textbook of Palliative Medicine.* New York: Oxford University Press; 1998:933–954.
13. Axelsson B, Sjoden PO. Quality of life of cancer patients and their spouses in palliative home care. *Palliat Med.* 1998;12: 29–39.
14. Santiago-Palma J, Payne R. Palliative care and rehabilitation. *Cancer Supplement: Cancer Rehabilitation in the New Millennium.* August 15, 2001;92(4):1049–1052.
15. Watanabe S, Bruera E. Anorexia and cachexia, asthenia and lethargy. *Med Clin North Am.* 1996;10:189–206.
16. Bunting RW, Shea B. Bone metastasis and rehabilitation. *Cancer Supplement: Cancer Rehabilitation in the New Millennium.* August 15, 2001;92(4):1020–1028.
17. McKinley WO, Seel RT, Hardman JT. Nontraumatic spinal cord injury: incidence epidemiology and functional outcome. *Arch Phys Med Rehabil.* 1999;80:619–623.
18. Kirshblum S, O'Dell MW, Ho C, Barr K. Rehabilitation of persons with central nervous system tumors. *Cancer Supplement: Cancer Rehabilitation in the New Millennium.* August 15, 2001;92(4):1029–1038.
19. Bell KR, O'Dell MW, Barr K, Yablon SA. Rehabilitation of the patient with brain tumor. *Arch Phys Med Rehabil.* 1998;79:S37–S46.
20. Mellette SJ, Blunk KL. Cancer rehabilitation. *Semin Oncol.* 1994;21:779–782.
21. Greenberg MS. *Handbook of Neurosurgery.* Vol. 1. Lakeland, FL: Greenberg Graphics; 1997:240–322.
22. American Cancer Society. *Signs and Symptoms of Cancer.* Atlanta GA, lasted revised November 30, 2007.

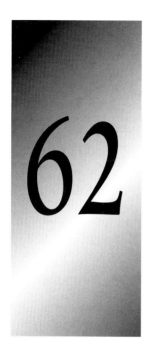

Therapeutic Modalities in Cancer

Jill R. Wing

The use of physical agents and mechanical and electro-therapeutic modalities is a well-accepted practice across a variety of rehabilitation settings and is indicated for a range of diagnoses. In fact, the use of physical agents has been a traditional treatment technique in medicine for centuries and has been used widely across many cultures. Clinicians may balk at the use of physical agents and modalities for patients with cancer, but when all aspects of clinical presentation are closely considered, physical agents and modalities may be applied safely.

To appropriately apply physical agents and modalities to patients with cancer, it is important to have a good understanding of the physiological principles of cancer occurrence and metastasis. The presence of a tumor in the body does not completely negate the use of physical agents or modalities. Rehabilitation clinicians treating patients with cancer should recognize the general signs and symptoms of cancer occurrence as described by the American Cancer Society: unintentional weight loss, fever, fatigue, pain, and skin changes. More specifically, signs and symptoms may include changes in bowel and bladder function, non-healing sores, unusual bleeding, thickening of tissue or presence of a lump, difficulty swallowing, changes in a wart or mole, or nagging cough or hoarseness (1). Throughout the course of rehabilitation, including during and after the application of physical agents and modalities, the clinician must recognize signs and symptoms of cancer occurrence or recurrence and respond accordingly with treatment alterations and notification of the medical team.

Pain is an unfortunate side effect for many patients with cancer. This may be a direct result from tumor growth in a specific area, metastatic spread, or treatments such as surgery, chemotherapy, radiation, or biological therapies. Untreated, pain can lead to fatigue, inability to perform activities of daily living, inability to perform job and household responsibilities, and limitations in functional mobility. Physical dysfunction may also be a result of oncology treatments such as surgical resection or reconstruction, chemotherapy, or radiation. Patients with cancer may have damage to their skin, joints, muscles, or nerves as a result of their treatment, and this can lead to functional deficits in range of motion, strength, balance, coordination, and mobility. Certainly, there are many indications for the rehabilitation professional to use physical agents and mechanical and electrotherapeutic modalities for patients with cancer as an intervention that may reverse these negative impairments.

PHYSICAL AGENTS

Physical agents are various forms of energy and materials that are applied to tissues in a systematic manner (2,3). Physical agents are indicated to increase tissue extensibility, increase rate of wound healing, modulate

KEY POINTS

- The use of physical agents has been a traditional treatment technique in medicine for centuries and has been used widely across many cultures. When all aspects of clinical presentation are closely considered, physical agents and modalities may be applied safely in cancer patients.
- Physical agents are indicated to increase tissue extensibility, increase rate of wound healing, modulate pain, reduce or eliminate soft tissue swelling or inflammation, remodel scar tissue, or treat skin conditions.
- Mechanical modalities may be used to improve circulation, increase range of motion, modulate pain, decrease and control edema, or stabilize an area that requires temporary support.
- Electrotherapeutic modalities may include biofeedback, iontophoresis, and electrical stimulation,

- including electrical muscle stimulation (EMS), functional electrical stimulation (FES), neuromuscular electrical stimulation (NMES), or transcutaneous electrical nerve stimulation (TENS).
- Understandably, there are several physiological considerations when applying physical agents and modalities to patients with malignancy.
- Although this is of particular concern with ultrasound, which has been shown to increase blood flow and tumor spread when tested on mice, there is no current evidence from human trials to support the development of micrometastases with use of thermal or electrotherapeutic modalities.
- Physical agents, including superficial heat and deep heat, should never be applied directly over an area of active tumor.

pain, reduce or eliminate soft tissue swelling or inflammation, remodel scar tissue, or treat skin conditions (2). Physical agents may include cryotherapy (cold packs, ice massage, vapocoolant spray), hydrotherapy (contrast baths, pools, whirlpool tanks), light agents (infrared, laser, ultraviolet), sound agents (phonophoresis, ultrasound), and thermotherapy (dry heat, hot packs, paraffin) (2). Physical agents are frequently used in conjunction with other therapeutic interventions, such as functional training, manual therapy, and therapeutic exercise (3).

MECHANICAL MODALITIES

Mechanical modalities are a group of devices that apply mechanical force on the body in the way of approximation, compression, or distraction (2,3). Mechanical modalities may be used to improve circulation, increase range of motion, modulate pain, decrease and control edema, or stabilize an area that requires temporary support (2). Mechanical modalities may be further classified into compression therapies (compression bandaging, compression garments, taping, vasopneumatic compression devices), gravity-assisted compression devices (standing frame, tilt table), continuous passive motion devices (CPM), and traction devices (intermittent, positional, sustained) (2).

ELECTROTHERAPEUTIC MODALITIES

Electrotherapeutic modalities are a broad group of devices that apply electrical current to tissue. Electrotherapeutic modalities are indicated to assist functional training; assist muscle force generation and contraction; decrease unwanted muscular activity; increase the rate of healing of open wounds and soft tissue; maintain strength after injury or surgery; modulate or decrease pain; or reduce or eliminate soft tissue swelling, inflammation, or restriction (2). Electrotherapeutic modalities may include biofeedback, iontophoresis, and electrical stimulation, including electrical muscle stimulation (EMS), functional electrical stimulation (FES), neuromuscular electrical stimulation (NMES), or transcutaneous electrical nerve stimulation (TENS) (2).

According to the American Physical Therapy Association's *Guide to Physical Therapist Practice*, Second Edition, a physical therapist may use physical agents and modalities "to decrease neural compression; decrease pain and swelling; decrease soft tissue and circulatory disorders; enhance airway clearance; enhance movement performance; enhance or maintain physical performance; improve joint mobility; improve tissue perfusion; prevent or remediate impairments, functional limitations, or disabilities to improve physical function; reduce edema; or reduce risk factors and complications" (2). Similarly, electrotherapeutic modalities may be used to "decrease edema and swelling; enhance activity and task performance; enhance health, wellness, or fitness; enhance or maintain physical performance; enhance wound healing; increase joint mobility, muscle performance, and neuromuscular performance; increase tissue perfusion; prevent or remediate impairments, functional limitations, or disabilities to improve physical function; or reduce risk factors and complications" (2).

INDICATIONS FOR THERAPEUTIC MODALITIES

As described, the clinician may decide to use a physical agent or mechanical or electrotherapeutic modality for a patient with cancer for a variety of reasons. All general indications are applicable to patients, regardless of their cancer history. In addition, there are several indications for the use of physical agents and electrotherapeutic modalities that are unique to the oncology population.

Cryotherapy may be used to minimize alopecia for patients undergoing chemotherapy. Creating scalp hypothermia by application of cooling caps or cooling gel may decrease the amount of hair loss experienced by the patient during a chemotherapy cycle. Although clinically effective in some cases, evidence supporting this technique is inconclusive and elicits the question of development of subsequent scalp metastases (4,5). Cryotherapy is also used as a technique to reduce the severity of oral mucositis for patients undergoing chemotherapy. Studies have shown reduced mucositis ratings on patient-centered surveys as well as clinical exams completed by doctors and nurses (6,7).

There is some research to suggest that TENS may be an effective antiemetic for patients undergoing chemotherapy. TENS electrodes or an electrical stimulation band is placed over acupuncture points (Pc5, Pc6) to reduce the incidence and severity of nausea and vomiting during and immediately following the delivery of chemotherapy (8). Again, quality evidence supporting this technique is limited.

CONTRAINDICATIONS FOR THERAPEUTIC MODALITIES

With use of any physical agent or mechanical or electrotherapeutic modality, general contraindications apply to all patients. Rehabilitation textbooks often describe a contraindication for use of such agents and modalities for patients with an active malignancy. This contraindication would exclude the use of any agent or modality when working with the oncology population. However, precautions and contraindications should be examined further to determine safety with the use of physical agents and modalities for patients with cancer.

Understandably, there are several physiological considerations when applying physical agents and modalities to patients with malignancy. Physical agents and electrotherapeutic modalities have the potential to break down cell membrane barriers or change transmembrane potentials, thus stimulating growth of abnormal tissue. Agents and modalities, by design, may increase blood flow to tissue, bringing essential nutrients and oxygen to the treatment area. The resulting negative impact is that this may also potentially enhance tumor growth by supplying the tumor with necessary nutrients and encouraging development of metastatic spread via tumor angiogenesis. There is a concern that using electrical and thermal modalities may enhance micrometastases even when used in an area distant from the primary malignancy. Although this is of particular concern with ultrasound, which has been shown to increase blood flow and tumor spread when tested on mice, there is no current evidence from human trials to support the development of micrometastases with use of thermal or electrotherapeutic modalities. Lastly, there is a concern that physical agents may enhance the treatment effect of patients who are actively undergoing radiation treatment or chemotherapy. Specifically, the concern is that application of a thermal modality may enhance the radiation treatment effect or increase blood flow and delivery of chemotherapy to tissue (9).

In light of these general concerns, it is important to describe absolute contraindications for the use of physical agents and modalities in patients with cancer. Each patient must be carefully considered on an individual basis.

Physical agents, including superficial heat and deep heat, should never be applied directly over an area of active tumor. As previously described, thermal modalities may enhance blood flow and increase local metabolism, thus potentially feeding the malignancy with essential nutrients and oxygen. In addition, increased blood flow will assist with the transport of waste materials away from the tumor, contributing to more efficient growth. Mechanical modalities, such as traction, should also be avoided in the area of malignancy. Tumor may cause structural instability to an anatomical area, and adding mechanical force may put the patient at risk for fracture. Electrotherapeutic modalities have the potential to change transmembrane potentials and cell membrane barriers, thus encouraging the cells to allow abnormal or uncontrolled growth of the tumor.

Physical agents should not be used in an area of dysvascular tissue (9). Again, superficial and deep heating agents, as well as cryotherapy techniques, are aimed to affect the amount of local blood flow. If the blood supply to this area has been damaged or is impaired from the effects of radiation, the modality will be taxing a system that is already compromised. In addition, the nerves in the treatment area will not be well nourished with blood and may demonstrate impairments of sensory deficit. Applying physical agents to an area of dysvascular tissue sets the patient up for risk of tissue injury.

Physical agents and modalities should not be used in an area at risk for potential bleeding or hemorrhage (9). Patients with cancer may be receiving high doses of chemotherapy, which could diminish the ability to adequately coagulate blood, leading to a risk for bleeding. Similarly, patients with cancer may be placed on long-term corticosteroids, which also increase the risk for hemorrhage. Using a thermal agent for these patients would further increase the potential or severity of bleeding.

Physical agents and modalities should not be used in an area of damaged or regenerating nerves. Generally, physical agents and electrotherapeutic modalities should not be applied to any patient with sensory impairments. Patients with cancer are at particular risk because chemotherapeutic agents and/or radiation can cause damage to nerve tissue. Therefore, any patient who has received chemotherapy or radiation should have a detailed assessment of sensory integrity prior to the application of physical agents or modalities. Patients who demonstrate a deficit in sensory exam are at risk for potential burns or injury from the use of modalities.

Physical agents and modalities should not be used over an area where an implanted device has been placed (9). In general, modalities should be avoided for patients with pacemakers or defibrillators, joint prosthetics, or plastic or cement components that often comprise orthopedic reconstruction. Due to the atypical nature of tumor formation, patients with cancer who have completed orthopedic resection and reconstruction may have an unusual assortment of prosthetic components to restructure their frame. Detailed assessment of the surgical procedure for patients with cancer is recommended so that an understanding of presence and placement of these components can be obtained. There are several other instances when patients may have implanted devices. Patients with breast cancer may have a resection followed by reconstruction with tissue expanders or breast implants. Patients with a hepatopancreatobiliary type of cancer may have a

hepatic pump placed. Patients with severe chronic pain or those in a palliative phase of treatment may have a morphine pump implanted. These are clinical examples, but by no means an inclusive list. The use of physical agents or mechanical or electrotherapeutic modalities in an area of any type of implanted device is contraindicated.

Mechanical and electrotherapeutic modalities should not be used in an area that is deemed to be at risk for potential pathological fracture. The presence of primary or metastatic tumor in a bone compromises the integrity of the structure to provide stability. Placing mechanical force, whether by approximation, compression, or distraction, on an area that is unstable increases the chance that the structure will fracture. Electrotherapeutic modalities, including electrical stimulation and TENS, create electrical impulses that are delivered to the tissue. The vibration of such impulses on an unstable area will also increase the risk for the bone to fracture.

SPECIAL CONSIDERATIONS

With an understanding of absolute contraindications in place, the clinician must consider that there are special circumstances for which there are exceptions to the rule. Primarily, these cases are those in which the benefit to the patient outweighs the risk of increasing tumor growth. In an acute phase of treatment, in which the patient has been newly diagnosed with cancer and is actively undergoing treatment, or in a subacute phase, immediately following treatment (generally 6–12 months), adherence to precautions and contraindications as previously described is important. However, in a chronic, curative, or palliative stage, there are no rules that apply for all situations (9). The presentation of each patient should be considered on an individual basis, with emphasis on communication between all members of the medical team.

In a chronic stage of management, roughly the first five years after treatment, the patient is at a progressively decreasing risk for developing recurrence. When the patient has been deemed by the medical oncologist to be free of signs or symptoms of cancer and/or has had recent negative scans, the use of physical agents and modalities is indicated within the guidelines of general precautions and contraindications (9). There is a low risk that a physical agent or modality used at this stage will affect the oncologic health of the patient. However, in light of the patient's past oncologic history, the clinician should maintain awareness for all signs and symptoms of new cancer occurrence or recurrence.

In a curative stage of management, or greater than five years after treatment by most standards, with the absence of clinical signs and symptoms of cancer, the use of physical agents and modalities can be applied following guidelines for general precautions and contraindications. The risk for negative impact from the use of physical agents and modalities at this stage is comparable to that of the general population (9).

In a palliative stage of management, caution should be applied with the use of any physical agent or modality in any treatment area of the body. At this stage, a serious discussion between representatives of the medical team is warranted. There are circumstances when palliation is the primary goal and the rehabilitation professional can apply techniques using physical agents and mechanical or electrotherapeutic modalities that would provide symptom relief. It is likely that these techniques would contribute, however minimally, to the advancement of tumor growth and progression of disease. However, if the benefit of palliation outweighs the relative risk of tumor growth, the collaborative team may decide that application of physical agents or modalities is justified and acceptable.

SUMMARY

The presence of a malignancy in the body does not negate the use of physical agents or modalities. There are many factors to consider when choosing and applying a physical agent or mechanical or electrotherapeutic modality to a patient with cancer. Careful consideration should be given to oncologic treatment history, treatment-related deficits, presence of active disease,

and placement of the modality. When these elements have been thoughtfully considered and discussed with members of the medical team, physical agents and modalities may be applied safely. In all phases of oncologic medical management, physical agents and mechanical and electrotherapeutic modalities can be effective tools for the rehabilitation professional to use in order to improve function and quality of life for the patient.

References

1. American Cancer Society. *Detailed Guide: Cancer (General Information)*. November 13, 2007. Available at: http://www.cancer.org. Accessed August 4, 2008.
2. *Guide to Physical Therapist Practice*, Second Edition. Phys Ther. 2001;81:9–744.
3. Cameron MH. *Physical Agents in Rehabilitation from Research to Practice*. Philadelphia, PA: W.B. Saunders Company; 1999.
4. Tierney AJ. Preventing chemotherapy-induced alopecia in cancer patients: is scalp cooling worthwhile. *J Adv Nurs*. 1987;12(3):303–310.
5. Door VJ. A practitioner's guide to cancer-related alopecia. *Semin Oncol*. 1998;25(5):562–570.
6. Karagozoglu S, Ulusoy MF. Chemotherapy: the effect of oral cryotherapy on the development of mucositis. *J Clin Nurs*. 2005;14(6):754–765.
7. Nikoletti S, Hyde S, Shaw T, et al. Comparison of plain ice and flavoured ice for preventing oral mucositis associated with the use of 5 fluorouracil. *J Clin Nurs*. 2005;14(6):750–753.
8. Pearl ML, Fischer M, McCauley DL, et al. Transcutaneous electrical nerve stimulation as an adjunct for controlling chemotherapy-induced nausea and vomiting in gynecologic oncology patients. *Cancer Nurs*. 1999;22(4):307–311.
9. Goodman CC, Boissonnault WG, Fuller KS. *Pathology: Implications for the Physical Therapist*, 2nd ed. Philadelphia, PA: Saunders; 2003.

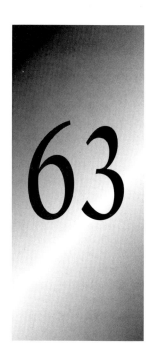

Therapeutic Exercise in Cancer

Noel G. Espiritu

Recent trends showing increased survival rates (1) and the growing emphasis on quality of life and healthier lifestyle in persons with cancer highlight the importance of therapeutic exercise as more than an adjunct treatment in cancer management. Exercise is associated with a reduction in risk of cardiovascular disease and decreased incidence of obesity and type 2 diabetes, colorectal and breast cancer, and osteoporosis in the general population (2–5), while in patients with cancer, it has been cited for its role in reducing fatigue, depression, anxiety, improving the quality of life, and even reducing the risk of mortality (6–14).

Therapeutic exercise, as defined by the American Physical Therapy Association, is the "systematic performance or execution of planned physical movements, postures, or activities intended to enable the patient/client to remediate or prevent impairments, enhance function, reduce risk, optimize overall health, and enhance fitness and well-being." In oncologic rehabilitation, improvement in well-being and quality of life is achieved by preventing and reducing impairments brought about by cancer and its treatment, maximizing function and promoting independence with activities of daily living throughout the cancer continuum. Therapeutic exercise encompasses different techniques, such as resistance training, aerobic exercise, stretching, balance, and coordination training, to improve safety and mobility. It is a natural, noninvasive, nonpharmaceutical, relatively risk-free and safe intervention when performed with proper guidance by competent personnel.

PRINCIPLES OF THERAPEUTIC EXERCISE IN ONCOLOGY

Goals of Therapeutic Exercise

The following goals for therapentic exercise coincide with the overall goals of rehabilitation as described by H.J. Dietz (6):

1. "Preventive—When treatment before development of a potential disability can be expected to lessen its severity or shorten its duration
2. Restorative—When the patient can be expected to become able to return to premorbid status without essential handicap or known residual disease, and where return to gainful occupation can be planned
3. Supportive—When ongoing disease is able to be controlled and the patient may remain active and to some degree productive, but with known residual disease and possibly slowly progressive handicap; and where increased tolerance and circumvention of residual disability can be expected from adequate supportive training and care
4. Palliative—When increasing disability is to be expected from relentless progression of disease, but where appropriate program provision will prevent or reduce some of the complications that might otherwise develop"

Therapeutic exercise plays a positive role in oncologic management throughout the entire cancer

803

KEY POINTS

- Exercise is associated with a reduction in risk of cardiovascular disease and decreased incidence of obesity and type 2 diabetes, colorectal and breast cancer, and osteoporosis in the general population, while in patients with cancer, it has been cited for its role in reducing fatigue, depression, and anxiety; improving the quality of life; and even reducing the risk of mortality.
- Therapeutic exercise, as defined by the American Physical Therapy Association, is the "systematic performance or execution of planned physical movements, postures, or activities intended to enable the patient/client to remediate or prevent impairments, enhance function, reduce risk, optimize overall health, and enhance fitness and well-being."

- Therapists need to continuously assess the patient to ensure that all goals are relevant and realistic.
- When the benefits of therapeutic exercise potentially outweigh the risks involved (eg, exercise and gait training for a debilitated patient with low hemoglobin), a decision to proceed with exercise, although cautiously, can be made.
- Radiation, surgery, chemotherapy, and medications all have side effects that could interfere with the safe performance of exercises.
- Communication between the physician, physical therapists, occupational therapists, nurses, and other health care providers is necessary to ensure that information regarding conditions that may preclude performance of therapeutic exercise is appropriately disseminated.

continuum (7–9,15,16). During the early diagnosis and pretreatment phase, goals for therapeutic exercise are mostly preventive, aimed at maximizing cardiopulmonary status, strength, and function in order to build up physiological reserves needed to offset the side effects of chemotherapy, radiation, or surgery. For the duration of cancer treatment and at its conclusion, therapeutic exercise is used to restore independent function to prepare for return to community life. Patients with permanent disability, those in the advance stage of the disease, or those with fair prognosis may continue to benefit from therapeutic exercise with supportive goals that enable them to continue regular functioning, albeit with certain restrictions, required adaptations, and precautions in certain areas. During cancer survivorship, in the absence of any carryover disability and acute medical condition, therapeutic exercise should ideally approach normal age-adjusted level of intensity. The focus at this point is to get the same benefits from exercise as would be obtained by the general population. This is important, as cancer survivors are at high risk for chronic diseases such as osteoporosis, obesity, diabetes, and cardiovascular disease (10). Patients with poor prognosis and severe debility will continue to need therapeutic exercise to facilitate mobility for comfort, that is, general strengthening and conditioning to enable ease of turning in bed for positioning and prevention of pressure ulcers and to improve transfers and ambulation.

Goals established for a patient can change during the course of treatment, and it is not uncommon for physical and occupational therapists to upgrade

or downgrade a patient's goals depending on current medical condition and prognosis. Therapists need to continuously assess the patient to ensure that all goals are relevant and realistic.

Common Impairments Addressed by Therapeutic Exercise

Cancer and its treatments have neurological, musculoskeletal, and cardiopulmonary complications that result in impairment and functional decline. Examples of impairments in cancer and the conditions that cause them are:

1. Decreased strength—Seen in steroid myopathy, neuropathy, prolonged bed rest (eg, post surgery), sedentary individuals, in critical illness, spinal cord compression, brain tumors, and lymphedema.
2. Decreased range of motion—Seen in patients with pain, muscle guarding and spasms, radiation fibrosis (eg, trismus), cervical contracture, frozen shoulder, in neuropathy, graft-versus-host disease (GVHD), lymphedema, osteoporosis, weakness, and after surgery or immobilization due to fractures.
3. Decreased endurance—Seen after radiation, chemotherapy or surgery (especially to the lungs), during prolonged bed rest, in mechanically ventilated patients, and in sedentary or geriatric patients with poor functional reserve.
4. Impaired coordination, balance, and gait—seen in patients with brain tumors, leptomeningeal disease, spinal cord compression, neuropathy,

after prolonged immobilization, and in orthopedic surgeries (eg, hemipelvectomy, amputation, rotationplasty, and sacrectomies).

THERAPEUTIC EXERCISE

Strengthening Exercise

Progressive resistance exercise (PRE) to improve strength is based on the principle of muscle overload and adaptation. Muscle tension is augmented by increasing the amount of resistance and number of repetitions used in the exercise. High-load, low-repetition exercise increases strength, while low-load, high-repetition exercise improves muscle endurance. The amount of resistance uesd varies, depending on the technique used (11). In Delorme's method, resistance is given at 50%, 75%, and 100% of 10 repetition maximum (RM), each for a set of 10 repetitions (10 RM being the amount of weight one person can lift 10 times before muscle failure), while the reverse is true using Oxford's (11). Resistance can be provided with the use of weight machines, dumbbells, Thera-Bands, and pulleys. Resistance training is associated with a decrease in the risk of coronary artery disease (CAD), hypertension, and improved glycemic control (12). A study on cancer survivors performing supervised exercise at 65%–80% of 1 RM for 2 sets of 10 repetitions for 12 weeks (followed by 8 weeks of muscle endurance exercise) in combination with cycling found resistive exercise to be feasible while also improving muscle strength, cardiopulmonary function, and quality of life (13). Other studies also show that a supervised resistive exercise program can counteract many of its side effects, including fatigue, weakness, and decreased function during cancer treatment (14,15).

In the presence of an acute medical condition, when vigorous exercise is contraindicated or when the patient is unable to tolerate RM assessment, graded resistance can be provided based on the patient's symptom presentation, rating of perceived exertion (RPE), and vital signs (16). Functional exercises (eg, marching during sitting, chair rises, ambulation), shown to improve strength in disabled elderly patients (17), can take the place of PREs until the patient develops increased tolerance to exercise.

Aerobic Exercise

Aerobic exercise involves the continuous repeated contraction of the large muscle groups and is linked to improved cardiovascular conditioning. It is associated with improved quality of life, reduction of fatigue, decreased insulin levels, and hip circumference among cancer survivors and those concluding cancer treatment (15,18,19). It is also a key component in rehabilitation before and after lung cancer surgery (20–22). Intensity for this exercise is usually from low to moderate (65%–85% of age-adjusted heart rate (HR) and rate of perceived exertion (RPE) of 12–13 "somewhat hard") (18), while the minimum effective duration is 20–30 minutes. Treadmills, stationary bicycles, and stepping machines can be used in the gym, while walking, swimming, and riding the bicycle can be encouraged to be performed in the community. The patient should be given the most enjoyable form of exercise, as aerobic exercise is time-intensive. In severely debilitated and lower functioning patients, Restorator exercise in sitting, exercise to promote sitting or standing tolerance, and progressive ambulation can facilitate contraction of the large postural muscles and contribute to increasing endurance.

Range of Motion and Flexibility

Range of motion (ROM) and flexibility—Alteration in the mechanical properties of soft tissues crossing a joint results in contractures (23,24). Reduced ROM frequently leads to decreased function and difficulties with activities of daily living, such as dressing, bathing, and ambulation.

Prolonged stretching induces fibroblast formation and remodeling in the soft tissues (24). In general, low-torque, high-duration stretching is more effective than high-torque, low-duration stretching in increasing ROM (23). However, reports on the exact ideal duration for stretching have been varied, from 30 seconds (25) to at least 20 minutes (24). Because of the time-intensive nature of this technique, orthotics that provide extended stretching should be considered whenever possible. Functional stretch (eg, ambulation and weight-bearing exercise for ankle plantar flexion contractures) can also be performed to supplement stretching done during therapy.

Chest Physical Therapy (CPT)

CPT is employed for patients who are at risk for pulmonary complications, especially before and after thoracic, abdominal, and head and neck surgery; after lung cancer radiation; for patients with steroid myopathy; and those that are mechanically ventilated, bed-bound, immobilized, nonambulatory, or severely debilitated. Exercise is an important component of CPT along with postural drainage, percussion, vibration, and suctioning. The overall goals are to mobilize secretions, improve airway ventilation, and facilitate efficient cough. Patients are instructed on diaphragmatic, costal and segmental, and pursed lip breathing as well as coughing and huffing.

Coordination and Balance Training

Coordination exercise entails repetitive performance of certain tasks in order to improve overall functional performance. Emphasis is placed on accurate control, timing, and sequence of muscle movements. Balance training involves exercises aimed at increasing the ability of the patient to return to the center of gravity (COG) after any perturbation. Weight-shifting exercise is performed in front of the mirror or using a Balance Master for feedback when necessary. Resistive exercise to strengthen upper extremity and postural muscles is helpful in providing stability during standing and ambulation.

THERAPEUTIC EXERCISE CONSIDERATIONS

Fatigue

The incidence of cancer-related fatigue (CRF) is high, occurring in about 70%–100% of patients with cancer (26). CRF is usually increased during the cancer treatment phase (27,28), when the need for therapeutic exercise to counter side effects is greatest. CRF is multifactorial and is correlated to pain, emotional distress, sleep disturbance, anemia, nutritional deficiencies, deconditioning, and comorbidities (26). While there have been several studies showing the contribution of exercise in reducing fatigue (9,29,30), rest is usually prescribed to the patient, potentially leading to further weakness, deconditioning, and thus, more fatigue. The multidisciplinary health care team, especially the physicians, needs to set a tone that conveys the importance of physical activity and exercise to the patient. Physical and occupational therapists can coordinate with the patient to schedule treatment during the time when the patient has the most energy to maximize treatment quality. The patient should be referred to the appropriate health care professional (eg, nutritionist or psychiatrist) when a need is identified by the team.

Pain

Pain can be from any tumor-related injury, cancer treatments, or from unrelated sources (31). It is one of the symptoms that patients dread most, significantly affecting their comfort, function, and quality of life (31,32). Pain is often managed with medications; however, a closer look at some pain etiologies may indicate a more active role for therapeutic exercise in its prevention and management. In patients after surgery, early intervention with exercise and mobilization may help prevent complications that could potentially produce pain, such as joint contractures and pressure ulcers (31). Exercise to improve gait technique or training to decrease weight bearing to a painful extremity using an assistive device can alleviate pain during ambulation. Stretching contracted and irradiated areas (eg, cervical, shoulder, and anterior chest muscles for breast or head and neck cancer) can reduce shoulder, cervical, and upper thoracic pain, improving function and increasing independence when performing activities of daily living (ADLs). Core strengthening and stretching for patients with posture-related back pain (eg, after spine, abdominal, head and neck, or breast surgery) promotes increased back support and alignment, decreasing pain.

It is important to continuously and accurately assess pain to determine progress made with therapeutic exercise. Therapists need to encourage patients to report pain and to take their pain medications when needed. Therapeutic exercises need to be timed when pain medication has taken effect. Therapists need to monitor patients for side effects of pain medications, such as nausea, cognitive dysfunction, or any respiratory distress.

PRECAUTIONS AND CONTRAINDICATIONS

Precautions and contraindications for therapeutic exercise in oncology sometimes vary according to an institution's or clinician's preference. Regardless of the difference, the principal precept of *primum non nocere* is observed. In certain instances, however, especially in an acute care setting when the benefits of therapeutic exercise potentially outweigh the risks involved (eg, exercise and gait training for a debilitated patient with low hemoglobin), a decision to proceed with exercise, although cautiously, can be made. This decision should only be undertaken if it is carefully reviewed with the health care team, starting with the physician and the patient. It is recommended that the clinician consult the institution's ethics committee when in doubt.

A comprehensive physical examination and assessment of patient history is important before initiating therapeutic exercise. Radiation, surgery, chemotherapy, and medications all have side effects that could interfere with the safe performance of exercises. Patients' complaints of pain and shortness of breath should be investigated thoroughly. Communication between the physician, physical therapists, occupational therapists, nurses, and other health care providers is necessary to ensure that information regarding conditions that may preclude performance of therapeutic exercise is appropriately disseminated. Therapists need to ensure safety by monitoring patients' lab values and checking vital signs before and after treatment or whenever necessary. Exercise should be provided by a qualified individual at all times.

Beyond the regular precautions for exercise, such as chest pain, lightheadedness, dizziness, nausea, palpitation, and so on., some exercise precautions common to patients with cancer include:

Hematologic: The hematologic guidelines for exercise observed by Memorial Sloan-Kettering Cancer Center (MSKCC) is found in Chapter 61.

Venous thromboembolism (VTE): VTEs in patients with cancer are associated with higher mortality rates (33–35). Solid tumors, advancing age, infection, and leucopenia increase the risk for deep venous thrombosis (DVT) (34). Hospitalization, cancer therapies such as chemotherapy, radiation, surgery, immobilization, and central venous catheter placement also raise the risk for VTEs (33,35,36).

Postsurgical: Precautions for postsurgical cancer patients are broader because of the complexity of some of these surgeries and the higher risk of complications. Weight bearing is frequently limited in patients after lower extremity orthopedic surgeries, sarcoma resections, skin lesion excisions, or fibular resections for mandibular grafting. Range of motion is usually restricted in a joint near an area with tissue grafts or flaps until healing occurs. Exercise needs to be executed gently when performed close to an incision to avoid wound dehiscence. Positioning for exercise in full supine is often avoided in patients after craniotomies, thoracotomies, abdominal, and esophageal surgeries for various reasons, including to prevent increase in intracranial pressure or to prevent aspiration or reflux. In addition, patients with craniotomies are instructed to avoid performing isometric exercises and taught not to perform the Valsalva maneuver during exercises.

Exercise with heavy weights, spinal rotation, and flexion is contraindicated in patients with recent spinal surgeries (ie, vertebral resections).

In all cases, it is important for the physical and occupational therapists and any clinicians involved with the care of the patient to get clear directions from the surgical team to avoid causing harm to the patient and damage to the surgery.

Cardiac: Certain cancer treatments, such as cyclophosphamide and doxorubicin (anthracycline) used for acute lymphoblastic leukemia (ALL) and radiotherapy to the mediastinum for lymphoma, are toxic to myocardial cells (37–40). Children and adolescent survivors of these therapies are especially vulnerable to cardiomyopathy-associated heart failure (40,41). Cardiac status of survivors needs to be evaluated by the physician before recommending exercise and during the course of the program (39). RPE and vital signs

should be monitored throughout the therapeutic exercise session. Aerobic exercise that is of low to moderate intensity is preferred over isometric and heavy isotonic exercise (39).

Orthostatic hypotension: Patients with orthostatic hypotension have a higher risk for falls and should be closely observed for lightheadedness and syncope during standing and ambulating (42). Regular monitoring of any drop in systolic blood pressure of at least 20 mmHg or diastolic pressure of at least 10 mmHg should be performed immediately and within three minutes after standing and during the rest of the standing activity.

Posttreatment: Literature is lacking on how much time immediately after radiation or chemotherapy is safe before any exercise can be initiated. Recommendations have been made that two hours is needed, as anything less tends to increase treatment side effects (16).

THERAPEUTIC EXERCISE FOR SPECIFIC CANCER CONDITIONS

Steroid Myopathy

Myopathy is a debilitating condition seen in patients receiving steroids as treatment for cancer. Particularly affected are patients receiving high-dose steroids to decrease brain and spinal edema (43,44) and in bone marrow transplant as treatment of graft-versus-host disease (45). The onset can be insidious or rapid, occurring as early as 15 days after initiation of steroids (43). Functional impairment may be mild to severe, depending on the extent of muscle weakness. Patients experience proximal upper and lower extremity weakness, especially in the quadriceps muscles (46), resulting in difficulty ambulating, climbing stairs, and getting up from the chair. Dyspnea may be present because of weakness in the respiratory muscles (43).

Patients benefit from therapeutic exercise programs that result in improved general body strength and conditioning. Assisted range-of-motion exercise, bed mobility, and transfer training may be needed for those who have significant weakness. Severely debilitated patients are given appropriate assistive devices, such as walkers, to assist with ambulation, enhance safety, and increase function. Patients are instructed on how to use the incentive spirometer and perform breathing exercises. Aerobic exercise using the treadmill or stationary bicycle helps improve overall endurance. Exercises with steps and stairs are important for lower extremity strengthening and improving function. Limited data exists on the effectiveness of strengthening exercises that target the myopathic muscles themselves in patients with cancer. A study on heart transplant patients on steroids for immunosuppression indicated increased skeletal muscle strength after six months of resistive exercises (47). Another study recommends moderate-intensity exercise after an experiment with rats with steroid myopathy yielded muscle atrophy after being subjected to intensive exercises (48). In any case, resistive exercise to affected muscles should be performed to tolerance, avoiding severe muscle fatigue.

Osteoporosis

Diminished bone mass in osteoporosis increases the risk of falls and fractures (49,50). Exercise to prevent falls include posture, strength, balance, and flexibility training (51). Postural training with weighted orthosis and back extensor strengthening have been found to improve balance and gait in kyphotic patients (52). Resistive exercise using dumbbells, ankle weights and Thera-Bands helps to increase upper and lower extremity strength. Upper extremity strength is needed in compensatory mechanisms to prevent falls in the elderly (53), while knee extensor strength promotes static and dynamic balance in women with osteoporosis (54).

Strengthening the back extensors improves posture and lessens the risk of vertebral fractures in osteoporosis (55,56). Resisted trunk extension exercises while prone are effective at increasing back strength, even at a reduced level and intensity (15% of the maximal isometric back extensor force) (55,57). Patients who are frail and unable to lie prone can perform isometric back extension exercise in supine with pillow support. Trunk exercises in flexion, heavy weights, and excessive trunk rotation may cause vertebral fracture and are avoided (58). Bone mass can be increased by applying overloading forces to the bone through weight-bearing and resistive exercise (49).

Radiation Fibrosis

Radiation fibrosis is a late-occurring, irreversible complication of radiotherapy that often becomes evident several years after treatment (59). Damage to tissues such as skin, muscles, nerve, fascia, and bone happens due to direct injury to the cells by radiation, ischemia, or constriction by fibrotic tissues (59,60). Remote effects are seen when neural tissues are involved (61). Patients who received high-energy radiation for sarcoma, breast, and head and neck cancer are frequently affected (59,62,63). Debility ensues when tissue damage causes pain, weakness, sensory deficits, and decreased ROM. Connective tissues lose their elasticity (eg, around the temporomandibular joint, cervical spine, and shoulders) after head and neck radiation. Similarly, the cervical and thoracic spine, anterior chest, and shoulders are affected after radiation for breast cancer.

The goals of therapeutic exercise include increasing ROM and facilitating realignment of contracted irradiated soft tissues (using myofascial technique, scar release massage, joint mobilization, contract relax, and static stretching) and strengthening the weaker muscles. In patients irradiated for head and neck or breast cancer where the anterior muscles are usually affected, stretching should be in the direction of cervical and shoulder external rotation retraction and spine extension. Affected shoulders typically need to be stretched in flexion, abduction, and external rotation.

Neuropathy

Neuropathy occurs as a side effect of surgery, chemotherapy, and radiation (64–68). The extent of disability depends on the degree of nerve damage. Femoral neuropathy is a complication of pelvic surgery resulting from nerve stretching or compression with the blades of a retractor (65). Quadriceps muscle weakness develops and is usually characterized by falling when the patient attempts to ambulate after surgery. Patients are usually referred to physical therapy for assisted range of motion, balance exercise, knee orthotic fitting, and gait training. Graded quadriceps strengthening is performed, avoiding overtaxing of the muscle.

Neck dissection, even with spinal accessory nerve preservation, can result in nerve damage, causing shoulder impairment and dysfunction (69). The trapezius muscle is affected, leading to shoulder girdle instability and difficulty and pain with arm abduction (69,70). Frozen shoulder usually develops with shoulder drooping, scapular protraction, and scapular winging. Therapeutic exercise, such as active assistive range of motion and stretching to abduction and external rotation, is performed to maintain or increase flexibility. Care must be taken to avoid impingement of the rotator cuff during flexion and abduction exercises. Stretching of tight pectoral and anterior chest muscles is usually indicated. Strengthening of the shoulder girdle muscles, including the rhomboids and the levator scapula, is important for stability. Shoulder shrugs can be performed with weights to increase upper trapezius muscle strength.

Some chemotherapy agents are toxic to neural cells and can cause sensory and motor neuropathies (71). Platinum compounds produce sensory neuropathies that may worsen months after treatment is finished (71,72). Distal numbness and loss of proprioception lead to sensory ataxia and difficulty with ambulation. Vincristine can cause sensory and motor polyneuropathy with distal weakness, paresthesias, and loss of muscle stretch reflex (72). Numbness and decreased grip strength leads to difficulty with activities such as writing and buttoning (73). Grip strengthening with Theraputty, fine motor coordination, and dexterity exercises help improve upper extremity function. Ankle dorsiflexion weakness results in instability and in some cases, foot drop (67). Stretching of the stronger antagonist muscle, such as the gastrocnemius, may be necessary to maintain normal muscle alignment in weaker muscles. Resistive exercise to distal lower extremity with ankle weights and Thera-Bands can be employed to increase muscle strength. Closed chain exercises, squats, and single leg standing with vestibular and wobble boards and foams help improve ankle strength and stability, proprioception, and postural reactions and prevent ankle sprains. Balance exercises in standing and during ambulation, heel and toe walking, and tandem walking also enhances gait stability. General conditioning and aerobic exercises are useful in improving cardiovascular fitness and increasing muscle endurance (67).

Critical Illness

Muscular weakness and atrophy is a complication of critical illness that delays recovery and hinders weaning the patient from mechanical ventilation (74,75). Muscle dysfunction in the intensive care unit (ICU) is associated with multiple organ failure, steroids, neuromuscular blocking agents, mechanical ventilation, antibiotics, and immobility (74–76). Critical illness polyneuropathy and myopathy are separate nosological entities that produce respiratory and general muscle weakness with consequent impairment in mobility and function. Entrapment neuropathies, such as peroneal nerve palsy, leads to foot drop (77). Prolonged bed rest results in contractures, especially when extremities are rested in positions of comfort. Therapeutic exercise in the ICU focuses on preventing complications due to immobility; maintaining joint range of motion; improving strength, respiratory, and cardiovascular status; and maximizing function. Assisted to active range of motion is performed followed by stretching to structures susceptible to tightness, such as the hamstrings and heel cord. Resistive exercises provided manually or with Thera-Bands tied to bed rails are given to increase strength. Functional training in bed mobility, such as rolling and transfers, improves endurance and strength. Chest physical therapy to assist in expectoration of sputum and breathing exercises that strengthen inspiratory muscles are particularly beneficial. Endurance can be improved with aerobic activities, such as pedaling a Restorator. Patients should be progressed to balance training in sitting and standing to ambulation when possible.

Hematopoietic Stem Cell Transplantation

Preparative regimens for patients undergoing hematopoietic stem cell transplantation (HSCT), such as chemotherapy, radiation, and corticosteroids, have side effects that cause pulmonary morbidity, skeletal muscle weakness, and functional decline (78,79). Mobility is further decreased due to fatigue, anemia, neutropenia, and thrombocytopenia associated with high-dose chemotherapy.

Several studies have emphasized the benefits of exercise for patients throughout the HSCT regimen in increasing quality of life, physical performance, and reduction of fatigue (19,80–82). Moderate-intensity aerobic and resistive exercise have been mentioned as promoting physical fitness related to quality of life (82). Any exercise program is preferably initiated in an outpatient setting prior to beginning treatment, with the goal of increasing the patient's functional reserve.

During HSCT, patients need to continue daily aerobic and strengthening exercises under the direction of the physical and occupational therapist using treadmills, stationary bicycles, Thera-Bands, and weights. For those who are frail or have significant weakness and disability, range of motion and functional exercise, such as rolling in bed, transfer training, balance exercise, and short-distance ambulation, may be sufficient. Incentive spirometry, diaphragmatic, and resistive breathing exercises are introduced to improve respiratory function. Laboratory values must be checked on a daily basis to make sure that hemoglobin and platelet counts are adequate for the exercises. Patients with chronically low hemoglobin and platelet levels may continue to perform therapeutic exercises with supervision when there is a critical need to increase strength and endurance for mobilization. Lower hemoglobin and platelet parameters may be set by physicians when necessary. Therapists need to provide creative treatments and consistently monitor patients for unwanted symptoms before, during, and after treatment. Communication between physicians, nurses, therapists, and patients is essential to ensure that exercise is carried out in a safe and appropriate manner. Patients should be instructed on how to measure heart rate and perform home exercise programs accurately.

Chronic Graft-Versus-Host Disease

Chronic GVHD is a late complication of allogeneic HSCT (occurring after 100 days) that has a significant impact on the patient's function and quality of life (46,83). It is distinguished by sclerodermatous skin changes from collagen deposition (84,85), resulting in skin tightness, reduced range of motion, joint contractures, and postural changes. Patients typically present with fibrotic, thickened skin with diminished elasticity, flexed posture, and occasionally, difficulty with balance.

Surgery is mentioned in literature as a possible intervention for lengthening soft tissues, with varying success (84,85). Conservative treatments include bracing and physical and occupational therapy. Goals for therapeutic exercise are to improve posture, regain skin and muscle length and range of motion, and increase function. Deep friction massage to the skin, joint mobilization, and stretching the trunk and extremity flexors are indicated to increase flexibility and range of motion. Strengthening of the hip and knee extensors is needed to improve posture, balance, and ambulation. Patients should be educated on appropriate skin care, range of motion, and self-stretch exercises.

Palliative Care

Therapeutic exercise is not contraindicated in patients receiving palliative care. Even in cases where life expectancy is expected to be only a few months, therapeutic exercise can help improve quality of life and function. Patients receiving palliative care are still willing to participate in an exercise program (86), and this may be because of the value and dignity placed in functional independence. During the advanced stage of the disease when there is severe disability, therapeutic exercise can help the patient maintain a level of strength required for minimum mobility, comfort, and prevention of complications from bed rest, such as pressure ulcers and painful contractures.

BARRIERS

Individuals respond differently to the various challenges presented by cancer and its treatment. Different barriers may exist that prevent patients from participating effectively in an exercise program. Several authors have described pain, nausea, fatigue, lack of time and social support, and the demands of life's responsibilities as common barriers (31,87–89). Perceptions of the existence of barriers and negative affect can also influence a patient's attitude toward exercise (90). An awareness of the different barriers that hinder full patient participation in exercise is important, as much of the success of the program depends on the patient's internal motivation. Barriers need to be addressed as soon as they are identified. Patients who report lack of time, priority, or other job and family responsibilities may be given more home exercise programs so that fewer visits to outpatient therapy is required, or they may be referred to social work for time management or child/parent care advice.

Barriers may also depend on the type of cancer and treatments, as well as the timing of therapeutic exercise (diagnosis, pretreatment, treatment, or post-treatment). Cognitive deficits, fatigue, and nausea (87) may be more pronounced during treatment (eg, chemotherapy). Pain may be more prominent during advanced cancer (32).

Depression and age-related sensory and motor deficits, such as hearing loss and decline in visual acuity, can affect geriatric patients' response to therapeutic exercise. In multicultural societies, language can be a barrier for members of minority groups.

SUMMARY

The diagnosis of cancer is a life-altering event. Control and cure become the main priority, as physical activity is reduced once cancer treatment is initiated. However, focus on exercise and improving quality of life in persons with cancer has been growing. This is fortunate because therapeutic exercise has plenty to offer in terms of reducing cancer symptoms such as pain and fatigue and, equally important, in restoring a person's function and independence in ADLs. Successful implementation of therapeutic exercise in patients with cancer requires knowledge of the disease process, the side effects of cancer and its treatments, precautions, contraindications, and barriers to treatment. Assessments need to be continuous and comprehensive, while treatments should be individualized and creative. Goals must be clearly defined and realistic. As the science and art of therapeutic exercise in rehabilitation oncology continues to evolve, more research is needed in order to provide answers to the current challenges being faced by persons with cancer.

References

1. Espey DKDK, Wu XCX-C, Swan JJ, et al. Annual report to the nation on the status of cancer, 1975–2004, featuring cancer in American Indians and Alaska Natives. *Cancer.* 2007;110(10):2119–2152.
2. Kesaniemi YYK, Danforth EE, Jensen MMD, Kopelman PPG, Lefèbvre PP, Reeder BBA. Dose-response issues concerning physical activity and health: an evidence-based symposium. *Med Sci Sports Exerc.* 2001;33(6 Suppl):8.
3. Howard RA, Freedman DM, Park Y, Hollenbeck A, Schatzkin A, Leitzmann MF. Physical activity, sedentary behavior, and the risk of colon and rectal cancer in the NIH-AARP Diet and Health Study. *Cancer Causes Control.* 2008;19(9):953.
4. Kruk JJ. Lifetime physical activity and the risk of breast cancer: a case-control study. *Cancer Detect Prev.* 2007;31(1):18–28.
5. Haskell WLWL, Lee IMIM, Pate RRRR, et al. Physical activity and public health: updated recommendation for adults from the American College of Sports Medicine and the American Heart Association. *Med Sci Sports Exerc.* 2007;39(8):1423–1434.
6. Dietz, JH, ed. *Rehabilitation Oncology.* 1st ed. New York: John Wiley & Sons, Inc.; 1981.
7. Kelm JJ, Ahlhelm FF, Weissenbach PP, et al. Physical training during intrahepatic chemotherapy. *Arch Phys Med Rehabil.* 2003;84(5):687–690.

8. Dimeo FF, Schwartz SS, Fietz TT, Wanjura TT, Böning DD, Thiel EE. Effects of endurance training on the physical performance of patients with hematological malignancies during chemotherapy. *Support Care Cancer*. 2003;11(10):623–628.

9. Monga UU, Garber SLSL, Thornby JJ, et al. Exercise prevents fatigue and improves quality of life in prostate cancer patients undergoing radiotherapy. *Arch Phys Med Rehabil*. 2007;88(11):1416–1422.

10. Demark-Wahnefried W, Aziz NM, Rowland JH, Pinto BM. Riding the crest of the teachable moment: promoting long-term health after the diagnosis of cancer. *J Clin Oncol*. 2005;23(24):5814–5830.

11. Fish DEDE, Krabak BJBJ, Johnson-Greene DD, DeLateur BJBJ. Optimal resistance training: comparison of DeLorme with Oxford techniques. *Am J Phys Med Rehabil*. 2003;82(12):903–909.

12. Tanasescu MM, Leitzmann MFMF, Rimm EBEB, Willett WCWC, Stampfer MJMJ, Hu FBFB. Exercise type and intensity in relation to coronary heart disease in men. *JAMA*. 2002;288(16):1994–2000.

13. De Backer ICIC, Van Breda EE, Vreugdenhil AA, Nijziel MRMR, Kester ADAD, Schep GG. High-intensity strength training improves quality of life in cancer survivors. *Acta Oncol*. 2007;46(8):1143–1151.

14. Galvão DADA, Nosaka KK, Taaffe DRDR, et al. Resistance training and reduction of treatment side effects in prostate cancer patients. *Med Sci Sports Exerc*. 2006;38(12):2045–2052.

15. Dimeo F, Schwartz S, Wesel N, Voigt A, Thiel E. Effects of an endurance and resistance exercise program on persistent cancer-related fatigue after treatment. *Ann Oncol*. 2008;19(8):1495–1499.

16. Drouin JSJS, Beeler JJ. Exercise and urologic cancers. *Urol Oncol*. 2008;26(2):205–212.

17. Krebs DEDE, Scarborough DMDM, McGibbon CACA. Functional vs. strength training in disabled elderly outpatients. *Am J Phys Med Rehabil*. 2007;86(2):93–103.

18. Daley AJAJ, Crank HH, Saxton JMJM, Mutrie NN, Coleman RR, Roalfe AA. Randomized trial of exercise therapy in women treated for breast cancer. *J Clin Oncol*. 2007;25(13):1713–1721.

19. Dimeo FF, Fetscher SS, Lange WW, Mertelsmann RR, Keul JJ. Effects of aerobic exercise on the physical performance and incidence of treatment-related complications after high-dose chemotherapy. *Blood*. 1997;90(9):3390–3394.

20. Jones LWLW, Peddle CJCJ, Eves NDND, et al. Effects of pre-surgical exercise training on cardiorespiratory fitness among patients undergoing thoracic surgery for malignant lung lesions. *Cancer*. 2007;110(3):590–598.

21. Cesario AA, Ferri LL, Galetta DD, et al. Post-operative respiratory rehabilitation after lung resection for non-small cell lung cancer. *Lung Cancer*. 2007;57(2):175–180.

22. Spruit MAMA, Janssen PPPP, Willemsen SCSCP, Hochstenbag MMMMH, Wouters EFEFM. Exercise capacity before and after an 8-week multidisciplinary inpatient rehabilitation program in lung cancer patients: a pilot study. *Lung Cancer*. 2006;52(2):257–260.

23. Usuba M, Akai M, Shirasaki Y, Miyakawa S. Experimental joint contracture correction with low torque—long duration repeated stretching. *Clin Orthop Relat Res*. 2007;456:70–78.

24. Harvey LLA, Herbert RRD. Muscle stretching for treatment and prevention of contracture in people with spinal cord injury. *Spinal Cord*. 2002;40(1):1–9.

25. Bandy WWD, Irion JJM. The effect of time on static stretch on the flexibility of the hamstring muscles. *Phys Ther*. 1994;74(9):845–850; discussion 50.

26. Mock VV, Atkinson AA, Barsevick AA, et al. NCCN practice guidelines for cancer-related fatigue. *Oncology*. 2000;14(11A):151–161.

27. de Jong NN, Candel MMJJM, Schouten HHC, Abu-Saad HHHH, Courtens AAM. Prevalence and course of fatigue in breast cancer patients receiving adjuvant chemotherapy. *Ann Oncol*. 2004;15(6):896–905.

28. Jereczek-Fossa BABA, Marsiglia HRHR, Orecchia RR. Radiotherapy-related fatigue. *Crit Rev Oncol Hematol*. 2002;41(3):317–325.

29. Dimeo FFC, Stieglitz RRD, Novelli-Fischer UU, Fetscher SS, Keul JJ. Effects of physical activity on the fatigue and psychologic status of cancer patients during chemotherapy. *Cancer*. 1999;85(10):2273–2277.

30. Schwartz AAL, Mori MM, Gao RR, Nail LLM, King MME. Exercise reduces daily fatigue in women with breast cancer receiving chemotherapy. *Med Sci Sports Exerc*. 2001;33(5):718–723.

31. Silver JJ, Mayer RSRS. Barriers to pain management in the rehabilitation of the surgical oncology patient. *J Surg Oncol*. 2007;95(5):427–435.

32. Benedetti CC, Brock CC, Cleeland CC, et al. NCCN practice guidelines for cancer pain. *Oncology*. 2000;14(11A):135–150.

33. Geerts WHWH, Pineo GFGF, Heit JAJA, et al. Prevention of venous thromboembolism: the Seventh ACCP Conference on Antithrombotic and Thrombolytic Therapy. *Chest*. 2004;126(3 Suppl):338S–400S.

34. Lin JJ, Wakefield TWTW, Henke PKPK. Risk factors associated with venous thromboembolic events in patients with malignancy. *Blood Coagul Fibrinolysis*. 2006;17(4):265–270.

35. Tagalakis VV, Levi DD, Agulnik JSJS, Cohen VV, Kasymjanova GG, Small DD. High risk of deep vein thrombosis in patients with non-small cell lung cancer: a cohort study of 493 patients. *J Thorac Oncol*. 2007;2(8):729–734.

36. Falanga AA, Zacharski LL. Deep vein thrombosis in cancer: the scale of the problem and approaches to management. *Ann Oncol*. 2005;16(5):696–701.

37. Lipshultz SESE. Exposure to anthracyclines during childhood causes cardiac injury. *Semin Oncol*. 2006;33(3 Suppl 8):14.

38. Simbre VCVC, Duffy SASA, Dadlani GHGH, Miller TLTL, Lipshultz SESE. Cardiotoxicity of cancer chemotherapy: implications for children. *Paediatr Drugs*. 2005;7(3):187–202.

39. Adams MJMJ, Lipshultz SESE. Pathophysiology of anthracycline- and radiation-associated cardiomyopathies: implications for screening and prevention. *Pediatr Blood Cancer*. 2005;44(7):600–606.

40. von der Weid NXNX. Adult life after surviving lymphoma in childhood. *Support Care Cancer*. 2008;16(4):339–345.

41. Lipshultz SESE. Heart failure in childhood cancer survivors. *Nat Clin Pract Oncol*. 2007;4(6):334–335.

42. Karvinen KHKH, Courneya KSKS, North SS, Venner PP. Associations between exercise and quality of life in bladder cancer survivors: a population-based study. *Cancer Epidemiol Biomarkers Prev*. 2007;16(5):984–990.

43. Batchelor TTT, Taylor LLP, Thaler HHT, Posner JJB, DeAngelis LLM. Steroid myopathy in cancer patients. *Neurology*. 1997;48(5):1234–1238.

44. Hempen CC, Weiss EE, Hess CFCF. Dexamethasone treatment in patients with brain metastases and primary brain tumors: do the benefits outweigh the side-effects? *Support Care Cancer*. 2002;10(4):322–328.

45. Lee HHJ, Oran BB, Saliba RRM, et al. Steroid myopathy in patients with acute graft-versus-host disease treated with high-dose steroid therapy. *Bone Marrow Transplant*. 2006;38(4):299–303.

46. Jones LWLW, Demark-Wahnefried WW. Diet, exercise, and complementary therapies after primary treatment for cancer. *Lancet Oncol*. 2006;7(12):1017–1026.

47. Braith RRW, Welsch MMA, Mills RRM, Keller JJW, Pollock MML. Resistance exercise prevents glucocorticoid-induced myopathy in heart transplant recipients. *Med Sci Sports Exerc*. 1998;30(4):483–489.

48. Uchikawa KK, Takahashi HH, Hase KK, Masakado YY, Liu MM. Strenuous exercise-induced alterations of muscle fiber cross-sectional area and fiber-type distribution in steroid myopathy rats. *Am J Phys Med Rehabil*. 2008;87(2):126–133.

49. Kohrt WMWM, Bloomfield SASA, Little KDKD, Nelson MEME, Yingling VRVR. American College of Sports Medicine Position Stand: physical activity and bone health. *Med Sci Sports Exerc*. 2004;36(11):1985–1996.

50. Englund UU, Littbrand HH, Sondell AA, Pettersson UU, Bucht GG. A 1-year combined weight-bearing training program is

beneficial for bone mineral density and neuromuscular function in older women. *Osteoporos Int.* 2005;16(9):1117–1123.

51. Sinaki MM, Brey RHRH, Hughes CACA, Larson DRDR, Kaufman KRKR. Balance disorder and increased risk of falls in osteoporosis and kyphosis: significance of kyphotic posture and muscle strength. *Osteoporos Int.* 2005;16(8):1004–1010.

52. Sinaki MM, Lynn SGSG. Reducing the risk of falls through proprioceptive dynamic posture training in osteoporotic women with kyphotic posturing: a randomized pilot study. *Am J Phys Med Rehabil.* 2002;81(4):241–246.

53. Tang PPF, Woollacott MMH. Inefficient postural responses to unexpected slips during walking in older adults. *J Gerontol A Biol Sci Med Sci.* 1998;53(6):80.

54. Carter NDND, Khan KMKM, Mallinson AA, et al. Knee extension strength is a significant determinant of static and dynamic balance as well as quality of life in older community-dwelling women with osteoporosis. *Gerontology.* 2002;48(6):360–368.

55. Hongo MM, Itoi EE, Sinaki MM, et al. Effect of low-intensity back exercise on quality of life and back extensor strength in patients with osteoporosis: a randomized controlled trial. *Osteoporos Int.* 2007;18(10):1389–1395.

56. Sinaki MM, Itoi EE, Wahner HHW, et al. Stronger back muscles reduce the incidence of vertebral fractures: a prospective 10 year follow-up of postmenopausal women. *Bone.* 2002;30(6): 836–841.

57. Hongo MM, Itoi EE, Sinaki MM, Shimada YY, Miyakoshi NN, Okada KK. Effects of reducing resistance, repetitions, and frequency of back-strengthening exercise in healthy young women: a pilot study. *Arch Phys Med Rehabil.* 2005;86(7): 1299–1303.

58. Lin JTJT, Lane JMJM. Nonpharmacologic management of osteoporosis to minimize fracture risk. *Nat Clin Pract Rheumatol.* 2008;4(1):20–25.

59. Johansson SS, Svensson HH, Larsson LLG, Denekamp JJ. Brachial plexopathy after postoperative radiotherapy of breast cancer patients—a long-term follow-up. *Acta Oncol.* 2000;39(3):373–382.

60. Davis AMAM, Dische SS, Gerber LL, Saunders MM, Leung SFSF, O'Sullivan BB. Measuring postirradiation subcutaneous soft-tissue fibrosis: state-of-the-art and future directions. *Semin Radiat Oncol.* 2003;13(3):203–213.

61. Stubblefield MDMD, Levine AA, Custodio CMCM, Fitzpatrick TT. The role of botulinum toxin type A in the radiation fibrosis syndrome: a preliminary report. *Arch Phys Med Rehabil.* 2008;89(3):417–421.

62. Davis AMAM, O'Sullivan BB, Turcotte RR, et al. Late radiation morbidity following randomization to preoperative versus postoperative radiotherapy in extremity soft tissue sarcoma. *Radiother Oncol.* 2005;75(1):48–53.

63. Jensen KK. Measuring side effects after radiotherapy for pharynx cancer. *Acta Oncol.* 2007;46(8):1051–1063.

64. Fanning JJ, Carol TT, Miller DD, Flora RR. Postoperative femoral motor neuropathy: diagnosis and treatment without neurologic consultation or testing. *J Reprod Med.* 2007;52(4):285–288.

65. Corbu CC, Campodonico FF, Traverso PP, Carmignani GG. Femoral nerve palsy caused by a self-retaining polyretractor during major pelvic surgery. *Urol Int.* 2002;68(1):66–68.

66. Polomano RCRC, Farrar JTJT. Pain and neuropathy in cancer survivors. Surgery, radiation, and chemotherapy can cause pain; research could improve its detection and treatment. *Am J Nurs.* 2006;106(3 Suppl):39–47.

67. Carter GTGT. Rehabilitation management of peripheral neuropathy. *Semin Neurol.* 2005;25(2):229–237.

68. Argyriou AA, Polychronopoulos P, Iconomou G, Chroni E, Kalofonos HP. A review on oxaliplatin-induced peripheral nerve damage. *Cancer Treat Rev.* 2008;16(3):231–237.

69. Lloyd SS. Accessory nerve: anatomy and surgical identification. *J Laryngol Otol.* 2007;121(12):1118–1125.

70. Chaukar DDA, Pai AA, D'Cruz AAK. A technique to identify and preserve the spinal accessory nerve during neck dissection. *J Laryngol Otol.* 2006;120(6):494–496.

71. Windebank AJAJ, Grisold WW. Chemotherapy-induced neuropathy. *J Peripher Nerv Syst.* 2008;13(1):27–46.

72. Dropcho EJEJ. Neurotoxicity of cancer chemotherapy. *Semin Neurol.* 2004;24(4):419–426.

73. Verstappen CCCP, Koeppen SS, Heimans JJJ, et al. Dose-related vincristine-induced peripheral neuropathy with unexpected off-therapy worsening. *Neurology.* 2005;64(6):1076–1077.

74. Winkelman CC. Inactivity and inflammation: selected cytokines as biologic mediators in muscle dysfunction during critical illness. *AACN Clin Issues.* 2004;15(1):74–82.

75. Schweickert WDWD, Hall JJ. ICU-acquired weakness. *Chest.* 2007;131(5):1541–1549.

76. Latronico NN, Shehu II, Seghelini EE. Neuromuscular sequelae of critical illness. *Curr Opin Crit Care.* 2005;11(4):381–390.

77. Herridge MSMS. Long-term outcomes after critical illness: past, present, future. *Curr Opin Crit Care.* 2007;13(5):473–475.

78. White ACAC, Terrin NN, Miller KBKB, Ryan HFHF. Impaired respiratory and skeletal muscle strength in patients prior to hematopoietic stem-cell transplantation. *Chest.* 2005;128(1):145–152.

79. Soubani AAO, Miller KKB, Hassoun PPM. Pulmonary complications of bone marrow transplantation. *Chest.* 1996;109(4):1066–1077.

80. Carlson LLE, Smith DD, Russell JJ, Fibich CC, Whittaker TT. Individualized exercise program for the treatment of severe fatigue in patients after allogeneic hematopoietic stem-cell transplant: a pilot study. *Bone Marrow Transplant.* 2006;37(10):945–954.

81. Dimeo F, Schwartz S, Fietz T, Wanjura T, Boning D, Thiel E. Effects of endurance training on the physical performance of patients with hematological malignancies during chemotherapy. *Support Care Cancer.* 2003;11(10):623–638.

82. Hayes SS, Davies PPSW, Parker TT, Bashford JJ, Newman BB. Quality of life changes following peripheral blood stem cell transplantation and participation in a mixed-type, moderate-intensity, exercise program. *Bone Marrow Transplant.* 2004;33(5):553–558.

83. Fraser CJ, Bhatia S, Ness K, et al. Impact of chronic graft-versus-host disease on the health status of hematopoietic cell transplantation survivors: a report from the Bone Marrow Transplant Survivor Study. *Blood.* 2006;108(8):2867–2873.

84. Kim JB, Liakopoulou E, Watson JS. Successful treatment of refractory joint contractures caused by sclerodermatous graft versus host disease. *J Plast Reconstr Aesthet Surg.* 2007;61(10):1235–1238.

85. Beredjiklian PPK, Drummond DDS, Dormans JJP, Davidson RRS, Brock GGT, August CC. Orthopaedic manifestations of chronic graft-versus-host disease. *J Pediatr Orthop.* 1998;18(5):572–575.

86. Oldervoll LMLM, Loge JHJH, Paltiel HH, et al. Are palliative cancer patients willing and able to participate in a physical exercise program? *Palliat Support Care.* 2005;3(4):281–287.

87. Rogers LLQ, Courneya KKS, Shah PP, Dunnington GG, Hopkins-Price PP. Exercise stage of change, barriers, expectations, values and preferences among breast cancer patients during treatment: a pilot study. *Eur J Cancer Care.* 2007;16(1):55–66.

88. Custodio CMCM. Barriers to rehabilitation of patients with extremity sarcomas. *J Surg Oncol.* 2007;95(5):393–399.

89. Stubblefield MDMD, Bilsky MHMH. Barriers to rehabilitation of the neurosurgical spine cancer patient. *J Surg Oncol.* 2007;95(5):419–426.

90. Perna FMFM, Craft LL, Carver CSCS, Antoni MHMH. Negative affect and barriers to exercise among early stage breast cancer patients. *Health Psychol.* 2008;27(2):275–279.

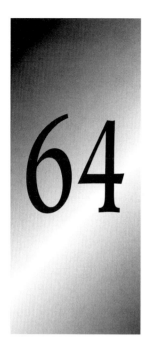

Postsurgical Rehabilitation in Cancer

Sharlynn M. Tuohy
Annelise Savodnik

This chapter focuses on the rehabilitation implications for several surgeries specific to the oncology setting. The goal is to guide physical and occupational therapists in the safe and effective restoration of function and quality of life in these unique and complex patients. The topics to be addressed include breast surgery, sacrectomy, neck dissection, and total pelvic exenteration.

While it is important to maintain strict surgical precautions immediately after surgery, rehabilitative efforts should continue to focus on safely returning the patient to full function as soon as possible, as immobility can lead to negative sequelae, including progressively impaired function, decreased mobility, and susceptibility to complication.

BREAST SURGERY

Rehabilitation plays a vital role in an individual's recovery from breast surgeries, including lumpectomy, mastectomy, axillary lymph node dissection, and reconstruction. Effective rehabilitation consists of patient education and the development of a therapeutic exercise program based on the procedure performed and the individual's health care status and needs. Patient education and rehabilitation can be accomplished on an individual basis with a physical therapist or in a group setting. The group class can be presented before or immediately following breast surgery.

Mobilizing the shoulder and upper extremity immediately postoperatively may decrease the morbidity associated with breast surgery (1). There is, however, conflicting evidence in the literature regarding early versus delayed initiation of arm exercises, with no significant advantage reported with delayed exercise initiation (2). At Memorial Sloan-Kettering Cancer Center (MSKCC), we encourage arm exercises to be initiated on postoperatively day one. We believe this strategy maximizes the return of normal upper extremity function and functional independence while minimizing complications.

The goals of early patient rehabilitation are to educate individuals about the sensations they may experience following surgery, define lymphedema, discuss lymphedema precautions for those patients at risk (ie, individuals with axillary lymph node dissection), and instruct and perform upper extremity and shoulder exercises. Written booklets should be provided to reinforce information presented during the patient education sessions. A description of content that should be covered in a patient education session is as follows.

SENSATIONS

Patients may experience various sensations after breast surgery. There are three types of sensations we teach patients about after surgery: incisional sensation, referred sensation, and phantom sensation.

KEY POINTS

- While it is important to maintain strict surgical precautions immediately after surgery, rehabilitative efforts should continue to focus on safely returning the patient to full function as soon as possible, as immobility can lead to negative sequelae, including progressively impaired function, decreased mobility, and susceptibility to complication.
- Mobilizing the shoulder and upper extremity immediately postoperatively may decrease the morbidity associated with breast surgery.
- The goals of early patient rehabilitation after mastectomies are to educate individuals about the sensations they may experience following surgery, define lymphedema, discuss lymphedema precautions for those patients at risk (ie, individuals with axillary lymph node dissection), and instruct and perform upper extremity and shoulder exercises.
- Individuals who require axillary lymph node dissection (ALND) for locoregional control of breast cancer have lifetime susceptibility to lymphedema.

- Postsurgical restrictions protect the integrity of the healing skin incisions, vascular flaps, and other affected tissues as well as cosmesis following reconstruction.
- Potential postoperative complications of partial and total sacrectomy include deep venous thrombosis (DVT), pneumonia, decreased lower extremity strength, sensory loss, bowel and bladder dysfunction, sexual dysfunction, blood loss, and wound infection.
- Sequelae of neck dissection include reduced neck range of motion, reduced strength in the shoulder and trapezius muscles, disfigurement, pain, and inability to perform activities of daily living or occupational duties.
- Total pelvic exenteration for gynecological cancer is an ultraradical surgical procedure consisting of extensive resection resulting in significant functional mobility changes, including the inability to sit for several weeks and changes in a woman's bowel, bladder, and sexual function.

Incisional sensations are described as a feeling of pulling directly over the incision during the act of lifting the arm. Patients are instructed to stop lifting at any sign of pulling while the incision is healing, even during their exercise routine. If the patient experiences this pulling during an activity, instructing the patient to cease the exercise and perform deep breathing exercises can be helpful in alleviating the pulling. If the pulling diminishes, it is safe to continue to perform the particular exercise or activity. However, if the patient continues to experience pulling despite deep breathing efforts, the patient must limit that particular movement to a pain-free range of motion.

Referred sensations are described as an odd or unusual type of feeling that may occur in or around the shoulder, lateral trunk on the same side as surgery, or anywhere along the arm on the same side of surgery. Patients are instructed that referred sensations are normal after surgery and not to be alarmed if they experience them. Stress, fatigue, and feeling cold can individually or together contribute to increasing the magnitude of these sensations. Referred sensations generally dissipate after six months; however, they can last up to one year.

Phantom sensation describes the feeling of the breast or nipple that was removed as still present. A mastectomy is an amputation of the breast; therefore, it is not surprising that patients would experience a phantom sensation similar to an arm or leg being amputated. Patients who choose to have their breast or breasts reconstructed rarely describe phantom sensations. Again, this sensation typically subsides six months postoperatively; however, it can also last up to one year, or even longer. Patients are provided with techniques in physical or occupational therapy to aid with diminishing this sensation.

LYMPHEDEMA

Individuals who require axillary lymph node dissection (ALND) for locoregional control of breast cancer have lifetime susceptibility to lymphedema (3). People who receive a sentinel lymph node biopsy have a significantly lower risk of developing lymphedema compared to people undergoing an ALND (4). In contrast, patients with ALND have a higher chance of developing lymphedema, with reports ranging from 2%–56% (5). When ALND and radiation are combined, they have a synergistic effect on the development of lymphedema associated with an 8–10 times greater risk than ALND alone (5).

Since the patient education class is often the first time that women are introduced to information on the lifelong precautions for lymphedema, they may become frustrated, fearful, or angry about this condition. As health care professionals, the physical and occupational therapists can reassure individuals that lymphedema is not a universal sequela to ALND and that prevention or early identification and treatment are effective for alleviating lymphedema conditions. Physicians are encouraged to discuss lymphedema precautions with patients prior to surgery.

ACTIVITY RESTRICTIONS FOR BREAST RECONSTRUCTION SURGERY

Patients receiving mastectomies without reconstruction have no formal restrictions to activity after surgery. These patients are only subject to limitations of pain or incisional pulling during post-op activity and exercises. Oftentimes, women chose to have a reconstruction procedure of their breast or breasts after a mastectomy. Women may opt to undergo reconstruction immediately after a mastectomy or at a later time.

Postsurgical restrictions protect the integrity of the healing skin incisions, vascular flaps, and other affected tissues as well as cosmesis following reconstruction. The precautions utilized at MSKCC by procedure type are listed in Table 64.1. Restrictions may vary from patient to patient; therefore, it is vital to check with the breast surgeon and plastic surgeon to clarify any restrictions.

All patients are provided with instructions and begin exercises post-op day one. The exercise prescription varies according to the type of surgery the patient receives. Patients are instructed to perform exercises to promote decreased morbidity of the arm and to return to their prior level of function as quickly as possible. These restrictions are reviewed with the patients prior to the initiation of exercise. It is necessary for patients to perform their exercises within the range of motion (ROM) restriction guidelines set forth by the physician.

- Refer to Table 64.1 for the ROM restrictions for each surgery. Following all types of surgery, there are no restrictions for elbow ROM; therefore, individuals may perform activities of daily living such as washing, grooming and styling their hair, or placing a hat or wig on their head.
- For six weeks, individuals should not lift anything weighing more than 5 pounds on the operative side.
- For six weeks, individuals should not perform any activities that will bounce or jar the operative area. This translates to no running, no dancing, and no vigorous sexual activity. Riding a stationary bike and walking are encouraged after surgery.

SHOULDER EXERCISES FOLLOWING BREAST RECONSTRUCTION SURGERY

Seven exercises form the postoperative rehabilitation program following breast reconstruction surgery. Table 64.2 lists the exercises and identifies at which point in the recovery phase patients begin a particular exercise, based upon the type of reconstructive procedure performed. Upper extremity exercises are demonstrated in Figure 64.1.

TABLE 64.1
Procedure and Restrictions

Surgery Description	Shoulder ROM Restriction Sagittal and Coronal Planes (two wks)	Lifting Restriction of 5 lbs on Surgical Side (six wks)	No Bouncing or Jarring of Chest Wall (six wks)
Breast surgery without reconstruction	No restriction	NO	NO
Tissue expander	90°	YES	YES
Pedicle flap TRAM	90°	YES	YES
Free flap TRAM (internal mammary artery)	90°	YES	YES
Free flap TRAM (thoracodorsal artery)	45°	YES	YES
Myocutaneous latissimus flap	60°	YES	YES

TABLE 64.2
Exercises After Surgery

EXERCISE	No RECONSTRUCTION	TISSUE EXPANDER	LATISSIMUS FLAP	TRAM PEDICLE FLAP	TRAM FREE FLAP
1. Deep breathing	Post-op day 1	Post-op day 1	Post-op day 1	Post-op day 1	Post-op day 1
2. Shoulder circles	Post-op day 1	Post-op day 1	Post-op day 1	Post-op day 1	Post-op day 1
3. Wings	Post-op day 1	Post-op day 1	Post-op day 1	Post-op day 1	Post-op day 1
4. Arm circles	Post-op day 1	Post-op day 1	Post-op day 1	Post-op day 1	Post-op day 1
5. Internal rotation stretch	Post-op day 1	Post-op day 1	1 wk post-op	Post-op day 1	2 wks post-op
6. Wall crawl flexion	Post-op day 1	2 wks post-op	2 wks post-op	2 wks post-op	2 wks post-op
7. Clasped hands behind head	Post-op day 1	1 mo	1 mo	1 mo	1 mo

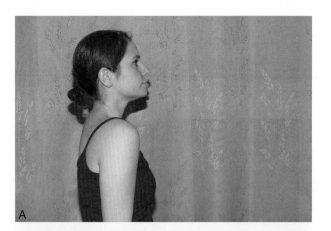
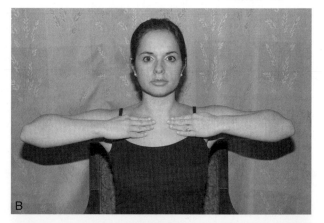
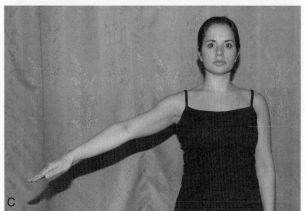
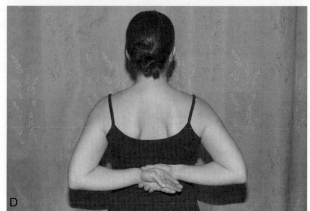

FIGURE 64.1 A–D

Upper extremity exercises performed following breast reconstruction surgery include (A) shoulder circles, the shoulders are rolled in both clockwise and counterclockwise directions; (B) wings, the arms are abducted from the sides with hands on the clavicle; (C) arm circles, clockwise and counterclockwise shoulder circles performed with straight elbows and without trunk rotation; (D) internal rotation stretch, the hands are clasped together behind the back and lifted towards the middle back.

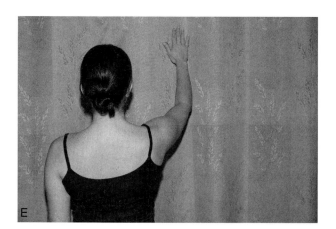
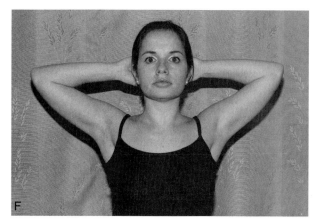

FIGURE 64.1 E AND F

(E) wall crawl (note that the patient needs to be symmetrical in order to gain appropriate ROM), standing approximately one foot from and facing the wall, lift the affected hand to touch wall and slowly climb the wall with that hand until a pull or stretch is felt through the chest wall or shoulder; (F) clasped hands behind head, clasping the hands together and moving them behind the head and once settled there, gently open the elbows away from each other.

TISSUE EXPANDERS AND PEDICLE FLAPS

Exercises 1–5 are performed up to 90° of motion at the shoulder joint during the first two weeks after surgery. Once the incision has healed, usually within 14 days after surgery, the remaining exercises are added to the program. At this time, the 90° restriction is removed.

FREE TRAM FLAPS

Exercises 1–4 are performed during the first two weeks after surgery following the appropriate ROM restriction guidelines. Patients with free transverse rectus abdominis myocutaneous (TRAM) flaps are instructed to stay forward-flexed at their thoracic and lumbar spines in order to prevent pulling of the muscle and incisions. After the surgical incisions are healed, usually within 14 days after surgery, the remaining exercises, without restrictions, are added to the program.

All exercises are done five times daily with 10 repetitions each. The number of sets and repetitions is adjusted based on the individual's pain tolerance as well as tissue healing progress. Normal shoulder range of motion should be achieved within six weeks after surgery. If limitation in range of motion persists, women are instructed to notify their physician, who may prescribe physical or occupational therapy to regain full ROM and function.

SACRECTOMY

A sacrectomy involves removing a portion, or complete removal, of the sacrum to effectively remove or debulk tumors of the sacrum and its surrounding structures. A partial sacrectomy involves removal of only a portion of the bony structure of the sacrum and potentially nerves associated with the tumor. A complete sacrectomy involves removing the entire sacrum and its nerves. The type of tumor and extent of disease dictates the degree of surgery required to effectively remove or debulk the tumor. The surgery can be straightforward initially; however, due to its complex nature, long-term complications can persist. The nerves that control bowel and bladder function run through the sacrum; therefore, patients may experience permanent incontinence. Cure rates for these patients, like most patients undergoing surgery or other treatment for cancer, are dependent on the stage or grade of tumor at time of diagnosis, the ability to obtain clear margins if the patient requires surgery, and obtaining a positive response to adjuvant treatment with either chemotherapy or radiation (6).

Surgery may be curative to remove a primary tumor, or palliative to decrease the symptoms caused by a metastatic lesion. Total sacrectomy (Fig. 64.2) is rare and may require spinopelvic reconstruction (7,8). A total sacrectomy is performed in a two-stage process, including an anterior and posterior surgical approach to expose the tumor, identify and ligate the main tumor vessels, and perform an anterior partial sacrectomy (9). To close the wound defect, a rectus abdominus muscle flap is harvested and a posterior sacrectomy is performed and closed using the myocutaneous flap (8).

Research suggests that reconstruction of the lumbosacral junction after sacrectomy may allow for earlier mobilization of patients after surgery (9). Spinopelvic reconstruction can include the use of surgical plates,

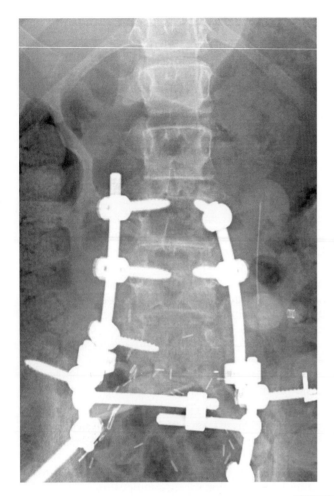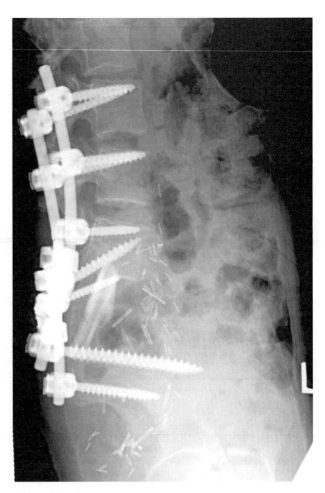

FIGURE 64.2

X-ray demonstrating reconstruction hardware in a patient with osteogenic sarcoma following total sacrectomy.

which are placed between the iliac wings to fix oppos-ing bones to each other. It can also include spinal instrumentation to support the spinal column and bone grafts to promote fusion between the iliac wings (9).

COMPLICATIONS

Potential postoperative complications include DVT, pneumonia, decreased lower extremity strength, sensory loss, bowel and bladder dysfunction, sexual dysfunc-tion, blood loss, and wound infection (6). Bowel and bladder dysfunction may require self-catheterization, self-disimpaction, or possibly colostomy. Sphincter function can be preserved if the resection is performed below the S3 vertebrae. Resection of bilateral S2–S4 nerve roots would lead to urinary and fecal incon-tinence and impotence for men; however, unilateral preservation of the S2 nerve roots can maintain bowel continence (6).

POSTOPERATIVE CARE/ REHABILITATION

Depending on the extent of surgery, patients may be placed on bed rest for one to five days postsurgery. These patients are placed on special airflow mattresses to aid in prevention of pressure ulcers and to optimize healing at the surgical site, especially if a myocutane-ous flap is used. Many patients have difficulty with bed mobility in this type of hospital bed, as the soft and fluid surfaces make it difficult to move and reposition in bed. A trapeze above the patient's bed is highly rec-ommended to facilitate bed mobility. It is important to initiate bed mobility training early to further decrease the chance of skin breakdown, beginning with rolling. A pillow may be placed between the patient's knees to allow for joint approximation at the hip for both comfort and decreased pull at the surgical site. The physician should prescribe a turning schedule for the patient, and this schedule should be reinforced with the nursing staff and the patient in order to promote healing and healthy skin integrity.

One of the most common precautions for these patients is that they may not sit immediately after surgery for two reasons: Sitting may cause a shearing force at the suture site; and if a muscle flap is used, maintaining viability of that flap is crucial for optimal healing. Therefore, when patients are allowed out of bed, it is important that the physical therapist is the first to initiate this transfer for safety and education with all caregivers with these patients.

After surgery, patients typically have multiple lines and tubes that can complicate transfers out of bed. With a sitting restriction, the risk of DVT and pneumonia are high; therefore, a strict pulmonary toilet program is initiated. This pulmonary program consists of percussion and vibration as indicated, incentive spirometry, and deep breathing exercises. Ambulation resumes once the patient is medically cleared. This can become problematic for patients, especially if they have been on bed rest for a number of days. Issues of orthostasis may arise. The physical therapist can be instrumental in educating the patient and all staff involved with caring for that patient in safe transfer techniques out of bed to ensure wound and/or flap integrity, balance for the patient, and safe body mechanics.

Transfers from supine or side-lying to standing often bypass sitting due to the location of the incision. Sometimes, the plastic surgeon and orthopedic surgeon will agree to allow very brief periods of sitting, no more than 30 seconds, on the edge of bed solely for the purpose of transferring to standing. After the patient is transferred from the side-lying to standing position and can maintain that standing position with normal vital signs and without complaints of dizziness, pregait activities, such as stepping or marching in place, may begin. If after 5–10 minutes in the upright position there are no signs of orthostasis, the physical therapist may initiate gait training or ambulation. We recommend limiting ambulation to short distances initially in case the patient needs to stop and will not be able to sit if they feel lightheaded. Ambulation distances should be progressed daily as tolerated by the patient with stable vital signs.

Gentle therapeutic exercises are also initiated for patients on the first day of physical therapy. In bed, patients can perform active range of motion (AROM) exercises for the ankles, knees, and hips as long as any ROM restrictions imposed by the surgeon are followed.

It is important for these patients to optimize upper extremity strength with resistive bands or dumbbells, in addition to their lower extremity strength, as they may not be allowed to sit for up to six to eight weeks after surgery. As the patient can tolerate increased time out of bed, standing exercises may begin.

As previously stated, patients status post-sacrectomies are not allowed to sit during the initial phase of healing. Generally, this precaution is put in place to protect shearing forces over the incisional site. On some occasions, depending on the direction of closure at the sacrectomy site (and surgeon-dependent), patients are allowed to sit in a high hip chair for no more than 30 minutes. The reason for the short amount of time is to allow for the benefits of the upright position for cardiopulmonary health, postural muscle endurance, and eating and drinking without subjecting the patient to excessive shearing forces or pressure at the surgical site.

For most of these patients, achieving goals of minimal assistance with bed mobility, primarily with returning to bed, ambulation, and even stair climbing, is reached within two to three weeks after surgery. The most difficult problem that may remain is that patients are either bowel- and/or bladder-incontinent. Physicians should explore the role of rehabilitation in bowel and bladder retraining in the acute care setting, as these patients generally do not go to an inpatient rehabilitation center after sacrectomies. Secondary issues related to bowel and bladder function can become permanent and may require incontinence training that can last up to one year. This can be performed by physical therapists that are trained in incontinence rehabilitation.

NECK DISSECTION

Patients with head and neck cancers also have unique considerations postsurgery. These patients undergo various levels of neck dissections. A significant population of patients report shoulder pain after neck dissections (19). These complaints range from reduced range of motion, reduced strength in the shoulder and trapezius muscles, disfigurement, pain, and inability to perform necessary activities of daily living or occupational duties. Many patients who experience pain have spinal accessory nerve involvement due to either resection or damage of the nerve. This can include decreased blood supply or a nerve stretch injury due to retraction of the nerve during surgery. Innervation by the cervical plexus may possibly contribute to motor function when the spinal accessory nerve is damaged, depending on how many branches of the plexus are preserved (11).

Immediately postoperatively patients are generally hospitalized for 7–14 days. Some patients have reconstruction; therefore, their flaps require monitoring. Many of the patients cannot eat and require nutritional support via tube feedings. Almost all patients receive a tracheostomy and require teaching for suctioning. Aggressive pulmonary toileting is required and performed along with frequent suctioning as part of the postoperative regimen. Patients undergoing head and neck surgery usually are ambulatory shortly after surgery. In cases where the fibula is utilized for reconstruction of the mandible, weight-bearing restrictions are prescribed place after surgery, which require a physical therapist to provide gait training to the patient. Cervical ROM restrictions for the first two weeks are in place to avoid pulling at the incisions and the structures within the head and neck region. After two weeks, patients can begin gentle AROM exercises to regain neck mobility. Patients should also be instructed in postural exercises and in good postural habits to promote normal alignment and effective breathing patterns.

Patients who are to undergo postoperative radiation should be evaluated preoperatively for temporomandibular joint (TMJ) dysfunction and mouth-opening measurements. Once radiation begins, any patient who experiences a decline in their ROM should be fitted for a device, such as a Dynasplint or Therabite, to prevent further ROM losses and curb the possibility of losing the ability to open their mouth, which can lead to the inability to masticate, perform oral hygiene, and, in worse cases, the inability to even use a straw. If trismus sets in, it is extremely difficult to treat, even with physical therapy. Unfortunately, these patients are often referred to physical therapy only after they have a significant decline in their ability to open their mouth. Careful monitoring of these patients should be a priority in any setting that provides radiation therapy to the head and neck region. Physical therapists play a valuable and necessary role in treating these patients by incorporating a variety of soft tissue mobilization techniques, joint mobilizations, modalities, and exercises. Botulinum toxin injections may help relax the muscle and allow the physical therapist to better facilitate mouth opening. These patients benefit from a thorough head and neck evaluation by physical therapists that are trained in assessing the muscles of the head, face and jaw. In addition, the entire upper quadrant, as well as postural alignment, cannot be ignored. Early education and careful monitoring before and during radiation therapy or surgery are imperative to ameliorate symptoms of trismus.

Other sequelae that can occur after neck dissection surgeries are cervical dysfunction, postural dysfunction, shoulder dysfunction, and neuropraxia of the shoulder girdle due to spinal accessory nerve injury or resection (12). Spinal accessory nerve injuries affect the trapezius muscle, which is a major scapula stabilizer. The trapezius elevates, rotates, and retracts the scapula, contributing to scapulohumeral rhythm. If the spinal accessory nerve is damaged, the scapulohumeral rhythm is compromised and the shoulder girdle becomes unstable. This leads to pain, as well as disablement and disfigurement. Because the scapula translates laterally and downwardly rotates, the shoulder droops and the scapula wings. Oftentimes, these patients do not have the kinesthetic awareness of the position of their scapula.

To improve ROM or joint mobility, physical therapy techniques of passive or active assistive ROM may be utilized. Patients may also require mobilization of the shoulder joint, cervical spine, or clavicle. Of course, the patient must be assessed carefully in order to not mobilize a hypermobile or lax joint. Physical therapy intervention is necessary in these patients in order to facilitate strengthening, provide neuromuscular reeducation, and pain relieving modalities as indicated. Strengthening must focus not on the upper trapezius as much as the middle and lower portions of the trapezius muscle. Scapular retraction and scapular depression exercises are important to teach in gravity-eliminated positions, progressing as able. Exercises may include supine retraction, side-lying proprioceptive neuromuscular facilitation (PNF) patterns, prone clocks, or prone lying with scapular retraction. The physical therapist plays an important role because of their skillful monitoring and facilitation of the proper alignment and position of the scapula, shoulder joint, and overall posture until the patient is able to maintain these positions independently.

Patients with neurapraxia are quite challenging to rehabilitate due to their decreased kinesthetic awareness of the position of their scapula. Neuromuscular reeducation techniques are an important part of the rehabilitation intervention. Some of these techniques can include taping, PNF, Bodyblade exercises, visual feedback using a mirror, and manual facilitation of movements. Postural education and repetition are also of utmost importance when rehabilitating these patients.

Ideally, any patient undergoing head and neck cancer treatment, whether radiation or surgery, should be evaluated thoroughly prior to treatment and followed during their treatments. These patients are often treated successfully as far as reducing or eliminating the cancer; however, they suffer significant declines in their quality of life due to physical, emotional, and social declines. Early education, monitoring, and follow-up can obviate the need for prolonged rehabilitation interventions and mitigate the effects of radiation fibrosis. Physicians should advocate early on in their patients' treatments and incorporate physical therapists in their rehabilitation programs in order to maximize the quality of life for patients and survivors.

TOTAL PELVIC EXENTERATION

Total pelvic exenteration for gynecological cancer is an ultraradical surgical procedure consisting of resection of the uterus, fallopian tubes, ovaries, parametrium, bladder, rectum or rectal segment, vagina, urethra, and a portion of the levator muscles. The approach, either anterior or posterior, is decided by the surgeon based on the location of the cancer, presence of radiation fibrosis, patient's anatomy, and postoperative expectations. At times, an adjuvant approach, the perineal phase, is necessary to resect the anus, urethra, and portions of the vulva.

This drastic procedure is rare; there are only approximately 10 cases at MSKCC performed annually. The five-year survival rate for women with advanced gynecologic cancer confined to the pelvis is 50% (13,14). Pelvic exenteration is ultimately performed when other treatment options have failed or cannot be used. The surgical procedure's design is complete resection of the cancer with adequate margins. Therefore, the gynecologic cancer in question must be confined to the pelvis. Exenterative surgery is most commonly considered for advanced cervical cancer because it spreads through invasion of local tissue in its later stages. Ovarian and endometrial cancers both have the propensity to spread beyond the pelvis much earlier via the lymphatic, blood, or peritoneal vessels, causing women afflicted with these cancers to be poor candidates for this procedure. The five-year survival rate after pelvic exenteration is only 20%–40% (15,16). A limited role exists for exenterative surgery for women diagnosed with advanced vulvar cancer; however, radiation and chemotherapy alone are proven to adequately treat these patients (17,18). Exenteration has been used to treat vaginal carcinomas, rhabdomyosarcomas, and other gynecologic cancers. Ultimately, whenever conservative therapies have failed, total pelvic exenteration can be considered for treatment of gynecologic cancers.

Patient Selection

Patient selection is based upon both psychological and medical examination. A woman must be prepared to accept significant changes in her body image. She must be aware of the possibility of caring for two new stomas, a colostomy and an ileal conduit, as well as a change in her sexual function. Probability of a prolonged hospital course, including time in the intensive care unit, is also likely, and must be discussed with the patient. The patient must be aware of the possibility of aborting the procedure intraoperatively secondary to discovery of unresectable disease. It is often recommended that the prospective surgical candidate have extended conversations with other women who have undergone this surgery to further gain insight into its magnitude.

Medical examination is necessary to confirm the presence of cancer and to find evidence of unresectable or metastatic disease. The surgeon first reviews the met-

astatic triad of symptoms. This includes unilateral leg edema, ipsilateral sciatic pain, and hydronephrosis—all symptoms indicative of metastatic disease to the posterolateral pelvic sidewall. Women demonstrating one or two of these symptoms are likely to have metastatic disease, making them unsuitable candidates for pelvic exenteration.

Overall, a woman's general medical condition should be adequate to withstand prolonged operation, extensive fluid shifts, transfusions, and nutritional support. On physical examination, the surgeon investigates presence of cachexia, inguinal and supraclavicular lymphadenopathy, hepatomegaly, or intra-abdominal masses. Palpable lymph nodes are biopsied and examined for presence of metastatic disease.

Imaging studies, such as the computed tomography-positron emission tomography (CT-PET) scans of the abdomen, pelvis, and chest, are performed to evaluate presence of metastatic disease. Another laboratory exam, diagnostic laparoscopy, includes lymph node sampling, aspiration of peritoneal fluid, and biopsy, all aiding in the detection of metastatic disease (19,20). Cytoscopy and sigmoidoscopy procedures are completed if there are plans to preserve either the bladder or rectum.

Preoperative Preparation

If a woman is an appropriate candidate and chooses to undergo the exenteration, preoperative preparations must be made. Central lines and mediports are placed for postoperative fluid management. Total parenteral nutrition (TPN) may be used preoperatively and postoperatively, since the patient may remain unable to take anything by mouth for several days to weeks after surgery. Prophylactic antibiotics are prescribed to reduce risk of infection. If time permits, the surgeon treats anemia, beginning iron replacement therapy to raise hemoglobin to 11 g/dL. The sites of the stomas are marked the morning of surgery, the ostomy team taking care to avoid skin creases and sites where the patient wears her belt or waistband. Finally, the patient is instructed on incentive spirometer to be used postoperatively to reduce the risks of atelectasis and pneumonia.

Operative Procedure

The patient is placed in a low-dorsal lithotomy position with stirrups supporting the hips, thighs, and knees. This optimal position allows simultaneous abdominal-pelvic examination and resectability, particularly with the perineal phase and for myocutaneous graft reconstruction. A midline incision is made, extending upward as needed, to explore both the upper and lower abdomen. The surgeon inspects abdominal organs, including diaphragm, liver, gallbladder, stomach, spleen, omentum, large and small bowel, abdominal and pelvic peritoneum, for metastatic disease. Abnormal findings are biopsied, and a frozen section is sent to pathology. The next stage is to clear the pelvic nodes and para-aortic nodes of any metastatic disease. If both areas are found to be clear of cancer, the pelvic exploration ensues.

The exenteration may be anterior, posterior, or total with a perineal phase. The anterior exenteration includes removal of the bladder, urethra, and anterior vagina with sparing of the posterior vagina and rectum. Anterior exenteration is the preferred approach for tumors confined to the cervix and upper vagina. Posterior exenterations are performed to treat primary stage IV cervical cancer with invasion of the rectum. In a posterior exenteration, the bladder and urethra are spared. The total exenteration with perineal phase, including resection of the anus, urethra, and portions of the vulva, leave a significant pelvic defect that is often replaced with large myocutaneous flap of either the gracilis or rectus abdominis muscles. On occasion, the surgeon may opt to fill the pelvis with a large pelvic pack made of nylon.

Depending on the type of exenteration performed, the vagina may need to be reconstructed. It is most successful when a significant portion of the vaginal mucosa is spared. Large myocutaneous flaps, such as the gracilis and rectus abdominis muscles, best serve as grafts for the neovagina, especially when a perineal phase is performed.

Results of urinary function postoperatively have been encouraging; most women maintain continence by catheterizing through their stoma regularly. Postoperative complications involving the urinary structures are greater than 50%, especially for those patients status postradiation. However, complications such as stricture, stones, fistulae, leakage, and infection have been treated without additional operation (21–23).

Postoperative Care

With postoperative care, fluid balance is essential, particularly for those women with large pelvic defects. This population will weep serum in significant amounts. Lab values, including hematocrit, prothrombin time, and serum protein levels, are all monitored closely.

These patients are on bed rest for several days after surgery, particularly with pelvic reconstruction. Women with pelvic packs are kept on bed rest until the packs are removed 72–96 hours postoperatively. Those women with reconstruction with myocutaneous flaps, including the neovagina, are on bed rest for several days after surgery; out-of-bed mobility ensues with clearance from the plastic surgeon. These patients sleep on a specialized pressure-relief bed to maintain skin and myocutaneous flap integrity throughout their acute care course. Sitting is not permitted for these patients on average 4–6 weeks postoperatively.

Aggressive pulmonary toileting is imperative immediately after surgery secondary to prolonged bed rest. Physical therapy, respiratory therapy, and nursing all participate in pulmonary hygiene for this patient population. Pulmonary toileting includes regularly monitoring pulse oximetry and respiratory rate with rest and physical activity; auscultation of both lung fields; positioning; deep breathing exercises, including incentive spirometry, percussion, and vibration; as well as both patient and caregiver education to decrease postoperative pulmonary complications.

When the patient is medically cleared for out-of-bed mobility, physical therapy assists with initial mobility. The physical therapist evaluates each patient's strength and functional mobility, taking into consideration all lines, tubes, and drains. The patient must be educated on the proper technique for transferring into and out of bed, since sitting is generally not permitted for several weeks. Because of several days of bed rest and probable fluid imbalance, the patient may demonstrate orthostatic hypotension when initially transferring out of bed. The physical therapist must monitor the patient's blood pressure closely with initial standing and report any symptoms of orthostatic hypotension to the surgical team.

A general lower extremity exercise regimen may be utilized in physical therapy. It is recommended to educate the patient on gentle active or active assistive range of motion to increase strength and flexibility. Passive range of motion of the lower extremities should be deferred, particularly with myocutaneous flap reconstruction. The patient may benefit from an assistive device to decrease discomfort with ambulation, ultimately improving the patient's balance and safety. Progression of all physical activity after the acute care hospital course must be cleared by plastic surgery.

CONCLUSION

This chapter identifies the rehabilitation implications of several types of surgeries that can negatively affect the quality of a person's life if proper education and intervention do not occur. Although this chapter focuses on the rehabilitation implications for special postoperative conditions, early intervention and monitoring can ameliorate the negative effects of these symptoms. Regardless of the type of treatment a patient has for a cancer diagnosis, the treatment, or combination of treatments affect a person physically, mentally, and emotionally. Health care professionals have a duty to examine the patient as a whole and have the ability to provide a patient with an improved overall outcome by paying attention to all of the factors that affect their health. Identifying possible outcomes that will negatively affect a person's quality of life and referring patients appropriately to rehabilitation services will facilitate overall better outcomes, with improved patient satisfaction and, most importantly, quality of life.

References

1. Box RC, Reul-Hirche HM, Bullock-Saxton JE. Results of a randomized controlled study of postoperative physiotherapy. *Breast Cancer Res Treat.* September 2002;35–50.
2. Shamley DR, Barker K, Simonite V. Delayed versus immediate exercises following surgery for breast cancer: a systematic review. *Breast Cancer Res Treat.* April 2005;90(3):263–271.
3. Otto S. *Nursing Oncology.* St. Louis MO: Mosby, Inc.; 2001:137–139.
4. *Francis, W, Abghari P, Du W, Rymal C, Suna M, Kosir M.* Improving surgical outcomes: standardizing the reporting of incidence and severity of acute lymphedema after sentinel lymph node biopsy and axillary lymph node dissection. Am J Surg. November 2006;192(5):636–639.
5. Sakorafas, G, Peros, G, Cataliotti, L, Vlastos, G. Lymphedema following axillary lymph node dissection for breast cancer. *Surg Oncol.* November 2006;12(3):153–165.
6. Malawer M, Sugarbaker P. Musculoskeletal cancer surgery: treatment of sarcomas and allied diseases. Kluwer Academic Publishers; 2001:Chapter 27.
7. Zileli M, Hoscoskun C, Brastianos P, Sabah D. Surgical treatment of primary sacral tumors: complications associated with sacrectomy. *Neurosurg Focus.* 2003;15:1–8.
8. Zhang HY, Thongtrangan I, Balabhadra RS, Murovic JA, Kim DH. Surgical techniques for total sacrectomy and spinopelvic reconstruction. *Neurosurg Focus.* August 15, 2003;15(2):E5.
9. Doita M, Harada T, Iguchi T, et al. Total sacrectomy and reconstruction for sacral tumors. *Spine.* 2003;28(15):296–301.
10. *van Wilgen C, Dijkstra P, van der Laan B, Plukker J, Roodenburg J.* Shoulder and neck morbidity in quality of life after surgery for head and neck cancer. Head Neck. October 2004;26(10):839–844.
11. *Cappiello J, Piazza C, Nicolai P.* The spinal accessory nerve in head and neck surgery. Curr Opin Otolaryngol Head Neck Surg. April 2007;15(2):107–111.
12. *Parliament M, Courneya K, Seikaly H, Jha N, Scrimger R, Hanson J.* A pilot study of a randomized controlled trial to evaluate the effects of progressive resistance exercise training on shoulder dysfunction caused by spinal accessory neuropraxia/ neurectomy in head and neck cancer survivors. Head Neck. June 2004;26(6):518–530.
13. Berek JS, Howe C, Lagasse LD, Hacker NF. Pelvic exenteration for recurrent gynecologic malignancy; survival and morbidity of the 45-year experience at UCLA. *Gynecol Oncol.* 2005;99:153.
14. Goldberg GL, Sukumvancih P, Einstien MH, et al. Total pelvic exenteration: the Albert Einstein College of Medicine/Montefiore Medical Center Experience (1987 to 2003). *Gynecol Oncol.* 2006;101:261.
15. Morris M, Alvarez RD Kinney WK, Wilson TO. Treatment of recurrent adenocarcinoma of the endometrium with pelvic exenteration. *Gynecol Oncol.* 1996;60:288.
16. Barakat RR, Goldman NA, Patel DA, et al. Pelvic exenteration for recurrent endometrial cancer. *Gynecol Oncol.* 1999;75:99.
17. Phillips B, Buchsabaum Hj, Lifshitz S. Pelvic exenteration for vulvovaginal carcinoma. *Am J Obstet Gynecol.* 1981;141:1038.
18. Boronow RC, Hickman BT, Reagan MT, Smith RA. Combined therapy as an alternative to exenteration for locally advanced vulvovaginal cancer. II. Results, complications, and dosimetric and surgical considerations. *Am J Clin Oncol.* 1987;10:171.
19. Kohler C, Tozzi R, Possover M, Schneider A. Explorative laparoscopy prior to exenterative surgery. *Gynecol Oncol.* 2002;86:311.
20. Plante M, Roy M. Operative laparoscopy prior to a pelvic exenteration in patients with recurrent cervical cancer. *Gynecol Oncol.* 1998;69:94.
21. Houvenaeghel G, Moutardier V, Karsenty G, et al. Major complications of urinary diversion after pelvic exenteration for gynecologic malignancies: an 89-patient series. *Gynecol Oncol.* 2003;89:155.
22. Ramirez PT, Modesitt SC, Morris M, et al. Functional outcomes and complications of continent urinary diversions in patients with gynecologic malignancies. *Gynecol Oncol.* 2002;85:285.
23. Karsenty G, Moutardier V, Lelong B, et al. Long-term follow-up of continent urinary diversion after pelvic exenteration for gynecologic malignancies. *Gynecol Oncol.* 2005;97:524.

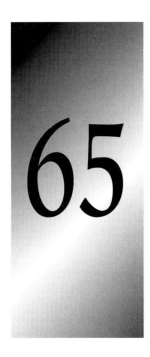

Nutritional Care of the Cancer Patient

Veronica McLymont

Nutrition is an integral component in the management of patients with cancer (1). The nutritional status of a patient with malignant disease may be affected by the tumor, the therapy directed against the tumor, or associated complications (2). Treatments including major surgery, chemotherapy, and radiation therapy often impede a cancer patient's ability and desire to eat (3).

CANCER TREATMENT AND NUTRITIONAL IMPLICATIONS

Chemotherapy

Adverse effects of chemotherapy that may alter a patient's nutritional status include nausea, vomiting, anorexia, mucositis, esophagitis, fatigue, and alterations in bowel habits, such as constipation, bloating, or diarrhea. Normal gut function may also be affected because of damage to the cells lining the gastrointestinal tract. This results in changes in digestion and absorption that can further compromise nutritional status (4). Antineoplastic agents, such as cisplatin, doxorubicin, and fluorouracil, can indirectly affect food intake or absorption by inducing severe gastrointestinal symptoms, such as nausea, vomiting, anorexia, abdominal pain, diarrhea, fever, stomatitis, mucositis, and food aversions (5).

Radiation

Patients undergoing radiation therapy to the head and neck, chest, abdomen, or pelvis are at increased risk for nutritional compromise (6). For example, radiation therapy to the head and neck causes mucositis of the treated area, which usually begins during the second week of treatment. This side effect continues throughout treatment and then gradually disappears. Most patients with head and neck cancer experience xerostomia (dry mouth), odynophagia (feeling of burning when swallowing), and ageusia (absence of taste sensation) during the second or third week of treatment (7–10). In addition, radiation to the oral cavity can decrease the production of saliva. This lack of saliva causes dry mouth, decreased taste acuity, and impaired swallowing (11).

Surgery

Many individuals experience fatigue, pain, and loss of appetite following surgery and are unable to consume a regular diet. Surgery may also cause mechanical or physiological barriers to consuming adequate nutrition. For example, patients undergoing bowel resection may experience malabsorption (12).

KEY POINTS

- Nutrition is an integral component in the management of patients with cancer.
- The nutritional status of a patient with malignant disease may be affected by the tumor, the therapy directed against the tumor, or associated complications.
- Treatments including major surgery, chemotherapy, and radiation therapy often impede a cancer patient's ability and desire to eat.
- Adverse effects of chemotherapy that may alter a patient's nutritional status include nausea, vomiting, anorexia, mucositis, esophagitis, fatigue, and alterations in bowel habits, such as constipation, bloating, or diarrhea. Normal gut function may also be affected because of damage to the cells lining the gastrointestinal tract.
- Patients undergoing radiation therapy to the head and neck, chest, abdomen, or pelvis are at increased risk for nutritional compromise.
- Many individuals experience fatigue, pain, and loss of appetite following surgery and are unable to consume a regular diet.
- A nutrition screening is essential to identify risk of malnutrition and is generally followed by a nutrition assessment to make a nutrition diagnosis, determine appropriate intervention, and monitor and evaluate nutritional care outcomes.
- Nutritional management of the patient with cancer includes oral dietary therapy, enteral nutrition, and parenteral nutrition.
- The registered dietitian should review the nutrition-related problems reported by the patient, such as anorexia, taste changes, fatigue, dry mouth, or nausea, and discuss treatment options.
- The concurrent use of supplements, especially high-dose antioxidants or complex botanical agents, during chemotherapy or radiation therapy can be problematic due to drug-supplement interaction.

NUTRITION ASSESSMENT

Nutritional care of the cancer patient should be individualized (13). A nutrition screening is essential to identify risk of malnutrition (14). Screening is followed by a nutrition assessment, which is the first step of the nutritional care process, and is used to make a nutrition diagnosis, determine appropriate intervention, and monitor and evaluate nutritional care outcomes (13). The registered dietitian should obtain the following patient/client information to identify nutrition-related problems and their causes:

Food/nutrition history: Food and nutrient intake, patient/client's nutrition-related knowledge
Biochemical data, medical tests: Laboratory data, for example, electrolytes, lipid panel, glucose
Anthropometric measurements: Height, weight, body mass index
Physical examination findings: Oral health, physical appearance, muscle wasting
Client history: Medications, supplements, medical and social family histories (13,15)

The Patient-Generated Subjective Global Assessment (PG-SGA) is a quick, inexpensive, and noninvasive method that may be used to prioritize patients for nutrition intervention, referrals, and assessing nutritional status (16). The PG-SGA is completed by the patient and contains questions concerning weight changes, food intake, symptoms, and functional ability. The patient's answers are rated from 0 to 4 and then summed for a rating total. A high total indicates malnutrition (12).

NUTRITIONAL THERAPIES

Nutritional management of the patient with cancer includes oral dietary therapy, enteral nutrition, and parenteral nutrition (17).

Oral Dietary Therapy

Oral dietary therapy can improve nutrition in patients who are able to eat but require special diets because of impairments in the gastrointestinal tract (18). Lack of appetite, taste changes due to medications, and the timing of meals are among the reasons for poor food intake among hospitalized cancer patients. The conventional meal delivery system provides menu selections 24 hours in advance of each meal. However, a "room service" meal delivery system that provides meals on demand has been shown to improve overall food intake and patient satisfaction (19).

Enteral Nutrition

Enteral nutrition therapy is critical in preventing and treating malnutrition associated with cancer. The placement of feeding tubes into the stomach or small intestine can overcome some of the most common causes of impaired food intake in patients with cancer. For example, enteral nutrition can provide optimal nutrition to patients with obstructions or defects in the oropharynx, esophagus, stomach, or duodenum (17).

Parenteral Nutrition

Parenteral nutrition is intravenous feeding consisting of an admixture of protein, carbohydrates, fat, vitamins, minerals, and other nutrients. It is reserved for conditions in which enteral nutrition is contraindicated, unsuccessful, or inadequate (20). For example, parenteral nutrition may be indicated if a patient's gastrointestinal tract malfunctions (21). When total parenteral nutrition (TPN) was investigated in randomized studies, only a "select subgroup" of patients receiving cancer treatment was shown to benefit (17).

NUTRITIONAL MANAGEMENT OF SYMPTOMS

Dysphagia

Patients with moderate to severe dysphagia or poor oral-phase abilities require supervision with meals. Puréed and pudding-like foods are allowed, while coarse textures, raw fruits or vegetables, and nuts are eliminated. When chewing ability is present, puréed foods are advanced to more solid textures, and mechanically altered foods, such as chopped or ground foods, are added (22,23).

Anorexia and Cachexia

Anorexia and cachexia are common causes of malnutrition among cancer patients. Anorexia (the loss of appetite or desire to eat) is a common symptom among people with cancer. Cachexia is a wasting syndrome that causes weakness and a loss of weight, fat, and muscle (24). Both the cancer and its various therapeutic modalities contribute to cachexia (18). Patients with cancer-induced anorexia/weight loss syndrome may benefit from appetite stimulants such as corticosteroids and progestational agents. However, appetite stimulants may be contraindicated if a patient refuses (25).

Constipation

Constipation is a common issue among cancer patients and thought to be among the top 10 adverse drug reactions of cancer treatments (27). Factors that may contribute to constipation include pain medications, decreased physical activity, and poor nutrition, such as inadequate intake of fluids or foods containing fiber (26). Although constipation frequently occurs, predicting and preventing its incidence varies among patients (27).

Diarrhea

Oral food intake can be reduced significantly due to the discomfort associated with diarrhea and abdominal cramping. Some factors that may contribute to diarrhea include antibiotic treatment, stress, or anxiety (28). Dehydration, electrolyte imbalances, and weight loss can result if the diarrhea is not resolved or if these losses are not replaced (29).

Nausea and Vomiting

Patients may also experience nausea without vomiting, or vomiting that is not associated with nausea. A wide range of medications are used as antiemetics. Dietary management of nausea and vomiting may not eliminate the problem, but manipulation of the patient's oral intake can often successfully reduce the severity of the symptoms (6).

PATIENT EDUCATION

The registered dietitian should discuss the nutrition-related problems reported by the patient, such as anorexia, taste changes, fatigue, dry mouth, or nausea. Encourage the patient to relax at mealtime. The patient should be counseled on the importance of eating foods that are easily tolerated and preferred (12).

Table 65.1 shows nutrition-related side effects and recommendations for patients.

Dietary Supplements and Herbal Remedies

The use of biologically based complementary and alternative therapies, such as herbs and other dietary supplements, is popular among cancer patients (30–32).

The concurrent use of supplements, especially high-dose antioxidants or complex botanical agents, during chemotherapy or radiation therapy can be problematic due to drug-supplement interaction (33,34). Patients undergoing active treatment should be told to stop using herbal remedies because some herbs cause interactions with chemotherapeutic agents, sensitization of the skin to radiation therapy, dangerous blood pressure swings, and other unwanted interactions with anesthetics during surgery (35).

TABLE 65.1
Nutrition-Related Problems

Nutrition-Related Side Effects	Nutrition Recommendation To Patients
Taste change/loss	Choose foods with strong flavors.
	Try tart or spicy foods. Avoid these if mouth or throat becomes sore.
	Use plastic silverware to reduce metallic taste.
Thick saliva/dry mouth	Use salt and soda mouthwash (1 tsp salt and 1 tsp baking soda to 1 qt water) before meals and snacks, and during the day.
	Add gravy to starchy foods, such as rice, noodles, bread, and potatoes.
	Soften breads, crackers, and biscuits by dipping in coffee, milk, or soup.
	Try sour foods, such as lemons or limes, to increase saliva.
	Avoid these if mouth or throat becomes sore.
	Take sips of water often.
Diarrhea	Eat smaller portions of food, but eat more often.
	Avoid high-fiber foods, such as whole grain breads and cereals, raw vegetables, beans, nuts, and fruits.
	Avoid fried, greasy, or spicy foods.
	Avoid milk and milk products if they cause diarrhea.
	Drink plenty of clear fluids, such as apple juice, water, weak tea, clear broth, or ginger ale.
	For mild diarrhea, try the BRAT (bananas, rice, applesauce, and toast) diet to help lessen the occurrence of bowel movements.
Nausea and vomiting	Eat small amounts of food frequently over the course of the day.
	Drink liquids at least an hour before or after mealtime instead of with meals.
	Chew food well.
	Eat and drink slowly.
	Avoid sugary, fried, or fatty foods.
	Eat foods cold or at room temperature to avoid strong smells.
	Avoid strong odors, such as cooking smells, smoke, or perfume.
	If nausea is a problem in the morning, try eating dry foods, such as cereal, toast, or crackers, before getting up. Avoid these if mouth or throat becomes sore.
	Antiemetics may be prescribed by the physician as necessary.
Constipation	Drink plenty of warm fluids.
	Eat high-fiber foods, such as whole grain breads and cereals, raw vegetables, beans, nuts, and fruits.
	Increase physical activity.
Oral and esophageal mucositis	Eat nonacidic and bland or mildly seasoned foods, such as custard, puddings, cream soups, ice cream, and milk shakes.
	Eats foods with a smooth consistency.
	Vary diet to minimize taste fatigue.
Dysphagia	Add gravy or sauces to foods to increase moisture.
	Eat blended or commercially prepared baby foods.

(Continued)

TABLE 65.1
Nutrition-Related Problems Continued

NUTRITION-RELATED SIDE EFFECTS	NUTRITION RECOMMENDATION TO PATIENTS
Fatigue	Include commercially prepared nutritional supplements and milkshakes for additional calories and protein.
	Eat iron-rich foods.
	Eat small, frequent meals/snacks every two to three hours to consume adequate amounts of calories and protein.
	Include commercially prepared nutritional supplements and milkshakes for additional calories and protein.
	For convenience, include ready-to-use foods that are canned, frozen, or otherwise commercially prepared, such as frozen meals.
	Order meals from restaurants.
	Have preportioned foods readily available.

CONCLUSION

For many patients, side effects of cancer and cancer treatments make it difficult to obtain the nutrients needed to maintain body weight, prevent body tissue from breaking down, rebuild tissue, and fight infections (24). Symptoms that interfere with eating include anorexia, nausea, vomiting, diarrhea, constipation, mouth sores, trouble with swallowing, and pain. Appetite, taste, smell, and the ability to eat enough food or absorb the nutrients from food may be affected (25). Poor nutritional status can result in a decreased quality of life, functional status, and response to therapy. Nutrition screening and assessment of cancer patients can identify those at risk for malnutrition. Nutritional intervention, in the form of specialized diets, oral supplements, and tube feeding, can affect patient outcomes (25).

*R*eferences

1. Cimino JE, McLymont V. Nutrition and cancer across the continuum. In: *Topics in Clinical Nutrition*. ASPEN Publishers, Inc; 2000:1.
2. Donaldson SS, Lenon RA. Alterations of nutritional status: impact of chemotherapy and radiation therapy. *Cancer.* 1979;43:2036–2052.
3. Ross BT. Cancer's impact on the nutrition status of patients. In: Bloch AS, ed. *Nutrition Management of the Cancer Patient.* Rockville, MD: Aspen Publishers 1990:11.
4. Chemotherapy and nutrition implications. In: Elliott L, Molseed LL, McCallum PD, Grant B, eds. *The Clinical Guide to Oncology Nutrition*, 2nd ed. Chicago, IL: American Dietetic Association; 2006:75.
5. Darbinian J, Coulston AM. Impact of chemotherapy on the nutrition status of the cancer patient. In: Bloch AS, ed. *Nutri-*

tion Management of the Cancer Patient. Rockville, MD: Aspen Publishers; 1990:161–169.
6. The current role of nutrition in patients with cancer. Minneapolis, MN: Novartis Nutrition Corporation; 2003:9.
7. *Xerostomia*. Chicago, IL: American Dietetic Association Nutrition Care Manual, 2008. (Accessed January 28, 2008, at *http://www.nutritioncaremanual.org/index.cfm?Page=Nutritional_Therapy&topic=17392&headingid=17426#17426*.)
8. *Swallowing Pain or Burning*. Bethesda, MD: Medline Plus, 2006. (Accessed January 31, 2008, at *http://www.nlm.nih.gov/medlineplus/ency/article/003116.htm*.)
9. *Taste and Smell Alterations*. Chicago, IL: American Dietetic Association Nutrition Care Manual, 2008. (Accessed January 28, 2008, at *http://www.nutritioncaremanual.org/index.cfm?Page=Nutritional_Therapy&topic=17389&headingid=17423#17423*.)
10. Kyle UG. The patient with head and neck cancer. In: Bloch AS, ed. *Nutrition Management of the Cancer Patient*. Rockville, MD: Aspen Publishers; 1990:57.
11. Bradford KL. Dysphagia and the cancer patient. In: Bloch AS, ed. *Nutrition Management of the Cancer Patient*. Rockville, MD: Aspen Publishers; 1990:68.
12. Capra S, Ferguson M, Reid K. Cancer: impact of nutrition intervention outcome- nutrition issues for patients. *Nutrition.* 2001;17:769–772.
13. International dietetics and nutrition terminology (IDNT) reference manual: standardized language for the nutrition care process. Chicago, IL: American Dietetic Association; 2007:8.
14. Erskine J, Perrett J. Prevalence of nutrition screening in ambulatory cancer patients and its relationship to nutrition intervention: a pilot study. *Oncol Nutr Conn.* 2006;14:1–6.
15. Lacey K, Pritchett E. Nutrition care process and model: ADA adopts road map to quality care and outcome management. *J Amer Diet Assoc.* 2003;103:1061–1072.
16. Thoresen L, Fjeldstad I, Krogstad K, Kaasa S, Falkmer UG. Nutritional status of patients with advanced cancer: the value of using the subjective global assessment of nutritional status as a screening tool. *Palliat Med.* 2002;16:33–42.
17. Shils ME, Shike M, Ross AC, Caballero B, Cousins RJ. *Modern Nutrition in Health and Disease*, 10th ed. Philadelphia, PA: Lippincott Williams and Wilkins; 2006:1297–1299.

18. Shike, M. Nutrition therapy for the cancer patient. *Hematol Oncol Clin North Am.* 1996;10:221–234.

19. McLymont V, Cox S, Stell F. Improving patient meal satisfaction with room service meal delivery. *J Nurs Care Qual.* 2003;18:27–37.

20. Escott-Stump S. *Nutrition and Diagnosis–Related Care*, 5th ed. Philadelphia, PA: Lippincott Williams & Wilkins; 2002:691.

21. Mercadante S. Parenteral verses enteral nutrition in cancer patients: indications and practice. *Support Cancer Care.* 1998;6:85–93.

22. American Dietetic Association. National dysphagia diet: standardization for optimal care. In: *National Dysphagia Diet Task Force.* Chicago, IL: American Dietetic Association; 2002:10–19.

23. American Dietetic Association. *Dysphagia.* Chicago, IL: American Dietetic Association Nutrition Care Manual, 2008. (Accessed January 28, 2008, at http://www.nutritioncaremanual.org/index.cfm?Page=Nutritional_Therapy&topic=17381&headingid=17415#17415.)

24. National Cancer Institute Overview of Nutrition in Cancer Care. Nutrition in Cancer Care (PDQ®). Bethesda, MD: National Cancer Institute, 2007. (Accessed January 15, 2008, at http://www.cancer.gov/cancertopics/pdq/supportivecare/nutrition/Patient.)

25. Jatoi A. Pharmacologic therapy for the cancer anorexia/weight loss syndrome: a data-driven, practical approach. *J Support Oncol.* 2006;4:499–502.

26. Constipation. American Cancer Society, 2007. (Accessed January 31, 2008, at http://www.cancer.org/docroot/MBC/content/MBC_2_3X_Constipation.asp.)

27. Lau PM, Stewart K, Dooley M. The ten most common adverse drug reactions (ADR's) in oncology patients: do they matter to you? *Support Care Cancer.* 2004;12:626–633.

28. *Gastrointestinal Complications: Diarrhea.* Bethesda, MD: National Cancer Institute, 2006. (Accessed January 15, 2008, at *http://www.cancer.gov/cancertopics/pdq/supportivecare/gastrointestinalcomplications/Patient/page6/print.*)

29. Shield J, Mullen MC. Patient education materials. In: *Supplement to the Manual of Clinical Dietetics*, 3rd ed. Chicago, IL: American Dietetic Association 2001:9.

30. Hyodo I, Amano N, Egushi K, et al. Nationwide survey on complementary and alternative medicine in cancer patients in Japan. *J Clin Oncol.* 2005;23:2645–2654.

31. Molassiotis A, Fernandez-Ortega P, Pud D, et al. Use of complementary and alternative medicine in cancer patients: a European survey. *Ann Oncol.* 2005;16:655–663.

32. Kumar NB, Hopkins K, Allen K, et al. Use of complementary/integrative nutritional therapies during cancer treatment: implications in clinical practice. *Cancer Control.* 2002;9:236–243.

33. Labriola D, Livingston R. Possible interactions between dietary antioxidants and chemotherapy. *Oncology (Williston Park).* 1999;13:1003–1008; discussion 1008, 1011–1012.

34. Seifried HE, McDonald SS, Anderson DE, et al. The antioxidant conundrum in cancer. *Cancer Res.* 2003;63:4295–4298.

35. Cheng B, Hung CT, Chiu W. Herbal medicine and anaesthesia. *Hong Kong Med J.* 2002;8:123–130.

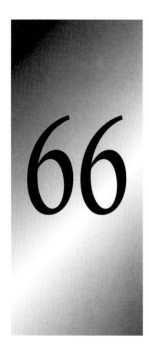

Sexuality Issues in Cancer Rehabilitation

66

Don S. Dizon
Michael Krychman

According to the American Cancer Society, more than 1.3 million new cases of cancer are diagnosed annually (1). Fortunately, increased technological advancements and medical breakthroughs in treatment and diagnosis have resulted in an increase in the population of patients surviving cancer. Approximately 62% of cancer survivors are expected to live at least five years after their original diagnosis, and as of 2000, close to 10 million cancer survivors were alive in the United States (2). As such, recognition of the sequelae of diagnosis and treatments, which can last far longer than the end of treatment, has spurred on a new research and therapeutic interest in cancer survivorship. No longer is it appropriate to assume that a patient can resume a "normal" precancer existence. Although many do achieve a new sense of normalcy at the end of treatment, many issues remain, and important among these is sexuality and sexual dysfunction, defined by disturbances in sexual desire and/or in the physiological changes that comprise the sexual response (3).

Although patients with any cancer are susceptible to sexual side effects from diagnosis and/or treatment, the majority of what we have learned about sexual dysfunction comes from work done with patients diagnosed with prostate and bladder cancer in men, and breast and gynecologic cancers in women. In this chapter, we will review the issue of sexual dysfunction and discuss evaluation strategies, therapeutic options, and discuss sexual rehabilitation.

HUMAN SEXUALITY: AN INTRODUCTION

In order to discuss sexual dysfunction, a primer on human sexuality is essential. Human sexuality is not a static concept, but one that is dynamic and multi-dimensional. It is a product of interpersonal, biological, psychological, and cultural mechanisms that help formulate an individual's personal view of sexuality, something Andersen and colleagues have termed a sexual self-schema, a way to understand and identify an individual's personal view of his or her own sexuality (4,5). As each individual has a personal and unique sexual schema, it is not possible to impose a singular approach and view on sexuality that will apply uniformly across races, sexes, and ages.

Much of what we understand about normal sexual function is based on the work performed by Masters and Johnson, who are credited with characterizing the physiological changes that comprise the sexual response: arousal, plateau, orgasm, and resolution (6). An alternate model incorporated desire as a prelude to arousal in order to construct a model that is applicable to both men and women, although it could be argued that not all women will experience all phases (7). This work became the frame set used to classify diagnoses related to sexual dysfunction adopted by the American Psychiatric Association and the World Health Organization (3,8).

So who is at risk for sexual dysfunction? In a substudy of the National Health and Social Life Survey,

KEY POINTS

- Human sexuality is not a static concept, but one that is dynamic, multidimensional, and a product of interpersonal, biological, psychological, and cultural mechanisms that help formulate an individual's personal view of sexuality.
- Although we often consider sexual dysfunction as a side effect of cancer therapy, it is important to recognize that it is often present at diagnosis.
- This sudden loss of estrogen from oophorectomy induces menopausal symptoms, vaginal thinning and dryness, and, psychologically, can interfere with a self-view from the loss of reproductive capacity.
- Urinary incontinence and erectile dysfunction are reported to occur in 30%–98% of men following radical prostatectomy, and radiotherapy for prostate cancer can cause erectile dysfunction in as many as 70% of men.
- Both men and women are susceptible to the effects of chemotherapy, and almost any agent can cause nausea, diarrhea, fatigue, or weakness, all of which can contribute to a lack of interest and loss of libido.
- Patients may experience sadness, melancholy, or depressive symptoms concerning body image, fear of recurrence, and sexual problems even after they are successfully treated for their cancers and have been free of disease.
- Many health care providers wrongly assume that their cancer patients are involved in heterosexual relationships. Bisexual and same-sex relationships can also be affected by cancer, and sexuality is as important to this group of people as to those in more traditional relationships.
- It is not enough to assume that assessing sexuality is "someone else's responsibility." It is also not sufficient to assume that a patient experiencing a sexual problem will freely bring it to their provider's attention.
- If sexual concerns are discovered and the physician is unsure what to do, referral to a sexual medicine clinic, sexual psychiatrist or psychologist, or other specialized profession for both initial evaluations and follow-up surveillance should be considered.
- The approach to the evaluation for sexual dysfunction must be tailored to the individual, but begins with a detailed medical history, a comprehensive general physical and genital examination, and a psychological as well as psychosexual examination.
- Patients with sexual complaints are always encouraged to make lifestyle modifications and changes in their behavior that will enhance and improve quality of life.
- It is important for the single cancer survivor to understand that not all potential partners will be supportive and understanding; some may be unable to handle such disclosure and will reject becoming more intimate, but by no means should this be considered a foregone conclusion.

Laumann et al. identified emotional distress, social status, and traumatic sexual experiences as major risks for sexual dysfunction, defined in this study as low desire, sexual pain, or an arousal disorder (9). Although we often consider sexual dysfunction as a side effect of cancer therapy, it is important to recognize that it is often present at diagnosis. Using a postal survey of men completing treatment for locally advanced prostate cancer, Schover estimated that up to 36% of men have erectile dysfunction at the time of diagnosis (10). In women, the figure was even higher; Anderson reported that distressing sexual complaints occur in up to 90% of women who have been diagnosed with cancer.

SURGICAL THERAPY AND SEXUAL DYSFUNCTION

For both men and women, operative procedures can directly affect sexual function, though for men and women, the etiologies may be quite different.

Radical prostatectomy has been demonstrated to be effective in producing long-term cancer control, but research in men with prostate cancer has also demonstrated it can cause a high degree of morbidity, including urinary incontinence and erectile dysfunction; the latter has been reported in 30%–98% of men undergoing this procedure (11–13). The pathophysiology involves direct or indirect injury to the neurovascular bundle and/or the injury of internal and accessory pudendal arteries. In addition, long-term sequelae from radical prostatectomy can arise, including atrophy and fibrosis of the penile smooth muscle and neural degeneration, contributing to or exacerbating sexual difficulties. In these circumstances, erectile dysfunction is due to disruption of important anatomical and neurovascular structures. Fortunately, surgical procedures that spare the prostate or involve a posterior bladder dissection, which spares the seminal vesicle plane, have successfully preserved sexual function (14–16). It is imperative that only patients with early disease confined to the bladder be selected for such procedures.

For women, removal of pelvic organs causes both physiological and psychological injury, which can directly interfere with sexual function. Premenopausal women who have undergone an oophorectomy also undergo irreversible menopause almost immediately. This sudden loss of estrogen induces menopausal symptoms, vaginal thinning and dryness, and, psychologically, can interfere with a self-view from the loss of reproductive capacity. Work has demonstrated that such changes in the hormonal milieu affecting both estrogen and testosterone are a likely etiology of women's sexual side effects (17). For women with early ovarian cancer followed out to two years, estimates are that more than 50% feel that their sex life was negatively affected and up to 75% feel that their sex life is no better than "adequate" (18). Of greater concern is that more than a third report a moderate or great sense of loss regarding the loss of sexuality. Similar findings occur in women who have undergone hysterectomy. Women undergoing surgical treatment for cervical, vaginal, or vulvar cancers also experience anatomical changes that may induce dyspareunia (painful intercourse) by shortening the vaginal length or inducing surgical scarring and fibrosis, with attendant effects on mobility. As a result, avoidance of vaginal penetration can occur as finding a comfortable sexual position may become difficult and challenging.

Surgery for breast cancer can also result in sexual dysfunction, and both lumpectomy and mastectomy have been associated with changes in sexuality. The reasons range from the psychological, including significant changes in body image and self-esteem, or anatomical, resulting from loss of feeling or hyperesthesia in the area treated surgically. Lymphedema, which can be a complication of surgery, can also affect comfort during sexual activity and may make sexual intimacy difficult or even painful. Taken together, it can cause larger problems beyond sexual function, also affecting partner relationships.

RADIATION THERAPY

The effects of radiation therapy on the sexual self have been well described. For men receiving radiotherapy for prostate cancer, estimates of erectile dysfunction can be as high as 70%. Fortunately, tailored and localized therapeutic approaches, such as brachytherapy, have the potential to reduce severe side effects. For women with breast cancer, radiotherapy can result in skin changes that can cause thickening, contractures, changes in texture and color, or, in some cases, chronic breast pain. Radiotherapy to the breast can also result in changes, including fibrosis, skin thickening, and sometimes mastalgia, any of which can affect

a woman's desire or ability to enjoy sexual function. For women who undergo pelvic radiation, vaginal fibrosis, with stiffening and hardening of a shortened vaginal vault, can be caused by direct radiation to the vagina, which can seriously affect a woman's capacity for penetrative intercourse as well as affect her genital pelvic and clitoral sensitivity during sexual activity. In one study, women with cervical cancer who were treated with surgery, radiation, or combined surgery and radiation were evaluated (19). The results showed that less than 1% who underwent surgery had complaints consistent with vaginal shortening. However, nearly 80% of women who had received radiotherapy reported sexual changes related to their vagina. These changes also tend to persist; sexual dysfunction has been reported out to five years of follow-up in women with cervical cancer (20). Finally, sexual sensation or orgasms may be diminished or less intense than before, resulting in a diminished intensity of sexual activity such that it may take longer to reach the same level of excitement and arousal.

CHEMOTHERAPY

Both men and women are susceptible to the effects of chemotherapy, and almost any agent can cause nausea, diarrhea, fatigue, or weakness, all of which can contribute to a lack of interest and loss of libido. For premenstrual women, chemotherapy has the capacity to induce ovarian failure, leading to an acute and sudden loss of estrogen. This, in turn, has multiple effects, including thinning of the vaginal membrane, with attendant dryness, premature menopausal symptoms, and lack of interest. Due to these changes, a woman may experience dyspareunia and chafing during penetration, which can sometimes result in bleeding. Near-total alopecia due to some agents, such as the anthracyclines and taxanes, can affect one's perception of sexual attractiveness. We have even published a case of vaginal erythrodysesthesia related to liposomal doxorubicin, demonstrating that chemotherapy side effects of the skin can also affect mucous membranes, including the vaginal mucosa and rectal membranes (21).

Endocrine Therapy

Both breast and prostate cancers are often treated by disrupting hormonal secretions. In men, androgen ablation either chemically or surgically has a proven role in treating prostate cancer. Unfortunately, it is almost certain to cause profound changes in sexuality, both by causing impotence and by reducing libido. In one study, more than 80% of men experienced these issues one year after initiation of androgen blockade (12).

The aromatase inhibitors (letrozole, anastrozole, and exemestane) and the selective estrogen receptor modulators (tamoxifen) block the conversion of testosterone to estrogen and significantly lower levels of circulating estradiol. This often is the objective for breast cancer therapy; however, it can aggravate menopausal symptomatology and can cause osteopenia and osteoporosis. Research that has examined the effects of tamoxifen on sexual functioning in women is conflicting and inconclusive. The Breast Cancer Prevention Trial states that minor differences in sexual functioning were observed among tamoxifen users versus those not on the medication (22). In contrast, Mortimer demonstrated no changes in any phase of the sexual response cycle for women on tamoxifen (23). More scientific trials are needed in order to specifically address the sexual ramifications of the aromatase inhibitors.

SEXUALITY AT THE END
OF TREATMENT

Patients may experience sadness, melancholy, or depressive symptoms concerning body image, fear of recurrence, and sexual problems even after they are successfully treated for their cancers and have been free of disease.

For men, surveys have shown an increase in sexuality-related symptoms following treatment for prostate cancer; however, few men surveyed sought assistance or further evaluation (24). Estimates place the incidence of men with sexual dysfunction after treatment for prostate cancer at more than 60% and as high as 80% in those treated surgically (25).

A longitudinal study to characterize the incidence of sexual problems in gynecologic cancer survivors was conducted by Andersen (26). She conducted a series of interviews with 47 women survivors of early disease and compared them to 18 women previously diagnosed with benign disease and 57 healthy women who served as controls. At one-year follow-up, approximately 50% of women cancer survivors were diagnosed with at least one sexual problem, and all sexual problems (inhibition of desire, problems with excitement, lack of orgasm, or dyspareunia) were significantly higher in this group compared to the other two. Others have reported posttreatment sexual dysfunction incidences ranging from 30%–100%. Most women report lowered desire and painful intercourse (dyspareunia). Nearly one-quarter of those who survived leukemia or Hodgkin disease have distressing sexual dysfunction. In one survey of women surviving early-stage cervical cancer, partner relations was among the significant predictors of sexual dysfunction (27).

The importance of including the partner in any plan for sexual rehabilitation cannot be underestimated. Often, the relationship dynamics change at the point one has been diagnosed with cancer. The partner may have their role reversed—he or she may become the caregiver or primary wage earner—and that person may have difficulty adjusting to such an alteration in familial roles. Marital and financial tension can also be a source of great stress. Other concerns, such as the threat of disease recurrence, early death, and bodily disfigurement, as well as economic, employment, and insurance concerns, all continue to play out, even during cancer therapy.

EVALUATION OF PATIENTS FOR
SEXUAL DYSFUNCTION

Many health care providers wrongly assume that their cancer patients are involved in heterosexual relationships. Bisexual and same-sex relationships can also be affected by cancer, and sexuality is as important to this group of people as to those in more traditional relationships. Health care providers should be sensitive to the sexual issues that gay men and lesbian women may be experiencing; intake office forms should be generic and unassuming. The health care provider should also be culturally aware and accepting of men and women of differing sexual orientations.

One of the difficulties with addressing sexual dysfunction is the lack of recognition that it is a problem. Too often, cure and control are the only goals of the oncologist, and in the context of a busy practice, other issues, such as sexuality, fertility, and routine medical follow-up, are relegated to other providers, such as social workers or primary care providers. Without an explicit understanding of how the care of the cancer survivor is coordinated, issues such as sexuality are often left unattended. In fact, a global survey designed to assess the importance of sexuality and intimacy across 29 countries was conducted, enrolling 26,000 men and women between 40 and 80 years (28). It found that sexuality and intimacy was not discussed by physicians, and this was indeed a global phenomenon. Within the United States, only 14% reported that a physician had asked about their sexual concerns within the past three years. Therefore, it is not enough to assume that assessing sexuality is "someone else's responsibility." It is also not sufficient to assume that a patient experiencing a sexual problem will freely bring it to their provider's attention. One opinion poll surveyed 500 adults 25 years and older to assess the frequency and reasons patients were reluctant to bring sexual concerns to their doctors (29). Fear that their concern would be dismissed was a finding in 71%, that their physicians would be uncomfortable with talking about this was reported by 68%, and the lack of treatment options by 76%. Lending further credence to this "don't ask, don't tell" communication style between health care providers and patients, Bachmann et al. reported that without direct questioning, only 3% of patients reported issues spontaneously (30). With direct questioning, by contrast, this figure was closer to 20%. For practitioners, the demands of practice oftentimes make it impossible to review for symptoms aside from those directly related to cancer or its immediate side effects (ie, those related to chemotherapy). In a survey performed on gynecologic oncologists in practice in New England, less than half made it a practice to take a sexual history in new patients and 80% did not feel there was sufficient time to devote to exploring sexual issues (31). Only 20% felt they had sufficient time to speak to their patients about these issues, which was the sentiment of both male (85%) and female (73%) respondents.

The approach to the evaluation for sexual dysfunction must be tailored to the individual, but begins with a detailed medical history, a comprehensive general physical and genital examination, and a psychological as well as psychosexual examination. For women, this also includes a comprehensive and detailed gynecologic evaluation. Many patients often have other underlying medical conditions and illnesses that directly affect sexual health and the sexual response cycle. Chronic illnesses, such as uncontrolled hypertension, hypercholesterolemia, anemia, or an underlying thyroid dysfunction, should be identified and treated. Arthritis may affect mobility and limit comfortable sexual positioning. Uncontrolled diabetes may impede neural and/or vascular function in the genital pelvic region and may affect blood flow and vasocongestion and pelvic engorgement or excitement. Underlying genital infections, such as *Candida* (yeast), bacterial vaginosis, and trichomoniasis, should be treated. Screening complete blood profile examinations, including complete blood count, to rule out underlying anemia and chronic fatigue, and complete lipid profiles as well as prolactin levels can be helpful. Most drug classes can affect the female sexual response cycle and cause sexual problems. Many antidepressants and antihypertensive medications can change sexual desire, arousal, and orgasm.

The incorporation of several screening questions will allow the patient to feel safe and protected about revealing personal, and what may be felt to be embarrassing, information. Open-ended questions are a good strategy for eliciting complaints of sexuality, from "Is there anything else you want to talk about?" to more specific questions on sexuality, such as, "Are you having any problems in arousal, desire, or orgasm?" are all appropriate. Inclusion of questions on a general intake form is another way to offer the opportunity for patients to bring up these topics.

If sexual concerns are discovered and physicians are unsure what to do, referral to a sexual medicine clinic,

sexual psychiatrist or psychologist, or other specialized profession for both initial evaluations and follow-up surveillance should be considered. Since the etiology of sexual dysfunction is often complex and multidimensional, treatment schemas should involve a multimodal approach, which frequently includes the partner.

TREATMENT OPTIONS FOR SEXUAL DYSFUNCTION

Patients with sexual complaints are always encouraged to make lifestyle modifications and changes in their behavior that will enhance and improve quality of life. A well-balanced, nutritious diet combined with an active aerobic exercise plan, stopping the use of tobacco and illicit drugs, and minimizing alcohol consumption are all encouraged. If fatigue is a problem, frequent naps and plans for sexual intimacy scheduled around times when one is well rested can be helpful.

The end of treatment can result in a much different appearance than when one was first diagnosed. Alopecia, weight loss or weight gain, and surgical sequelae all can affect the way a patient views him- or herself. This can have a negative impact on one's view of him- or herself as a sexual person and can result in withdrawal or depression, which may take a toll on both the patient and his or her partner. Although much less recognized in men, body image may be as much a problem and warrants the attention of health care providers.

For women, the "Look good … Feel better" program is a free service provided for women with cancer where they can learn new and innovative ways to restore body image and cope with the changes in appearance that cancer may have caused. The program is a joint venture between the American Cancer Society, the Cosmetic, Toiletry and Fragrance Association Foundation, and the National Cosmetology Association, and makes available certified beauty consultants, skin and nail care specialists, and professional make-up artists who are available to the cancer survivor to teach new techniques to enhance their physical image.

For patients with ostomies, the visual appearance of their bag and concerns regarding foul odors and spillage may be distressing and affect one's self esteem and inner spirit, and limit their ability to pursue new friendships and sexual relationships. Acceptance that an ostomy may be permanent is the first step in overcoming these challenges. Preparing for social events by changing the bag frequently may alleviate some of the fear of accidents, and the use of specially designed odor-controlling tablets that can be placed within the bag can help to minimize offensive odors. For intimate encounters, pouch covers are available to mask the bag itself. Dietary modifications may help reduce flatus and

TABLE 66.1
Dietary Modifications for Patients With Ostomies

PROBLEM	FOODS ASSOCIATED WITH INCREASED RISK
Obstruction/ileus	Celery, coconut, corn, coleslaw, dried fruits, grapefruit, nuts, peas, popcorn, rice
Gas production/ odors	Legumes, cabbage, Brussels sprouts, avocados, artichokes, asparagus, broccoli, spinach, melons, apples, prunes, cheese, fish, eggs, carbonated drinks
Diarrhea	Cabbage, green beans, buttermilk, applesauce, tapioca, boiled rice, milk, yogurt

orders (Table 66.1). Finally, choosing sexual positions that are comfortable and have minimal pressure on ostomy bags is encouraged.

Men: Erectile Dysfunction

For men who have undergone radical prostatectomy, options do exist. Unfortunately, compliance is generally reported to be poor, with almost 50% discontinuation at one year (32). Suggestions range from patient education to penile prosthesis. Perhaps the most important message that patients have to receive is to not expect immediate recovery of erectile dysfunction. Following radical prostatectomy, studies suggest that maximal recovery is not seen until approximately 18 months after surgery (33). Penile rehabilitation programs have been developed to help in recovery of erectile function. The mainstay of therapy is the use of vasoactive agents, either as oral phosphodiesterase type 5 (PDE5) inhibitors (Table 66.2), with or without intracavernosal injections of other vasodilatory agents. Initiation of treatment early in the postoperative course and lasting up to nine months may be required (34,35).

Sufficient data are available to support the use of rehabilitation programs such as these. Mulhall conducted a study of oral sildenafil in men who underwent radical prostatectomy (36). Nonresponders were then given intracavernosal injection, and both groups were compared to a placebo arm. Pharmacologic therapy was shown to improve outcomes, including the proportion achieving recovery of spontaneous erections. Vacuum erection devices provide yet another nonpharmacologic option for men with erectile dysfunction (ED), and in patients who are compliant with therapy, effectiveness is more than 50%. Use with PDE5 inhibitors has been

shown to increase sexual satisfaction to 77% (37). Stephenson et al. also reported on the use and treatment outcomes using Surveillance, Epidemiology, and End Results (SEER) data (38). In their survey of more than 1,900 men treated with surgery or radiation for localized prostate cancer, more than 50% of respondents reported use of ED treatments. Penile prostheses were used rarely, but for those who did, more than 50% felt it helped them. In contrast, sildenafil was reported to help significantly in only 12% of those taking it.

Women: Arousal Disorders

Women are often uneducated about sexual responsiveness and their own genital anatomy and may not realize there is a normal physiological response to sexual stimuli and arousal. To this end, literature is an important means of self-awareness and consists of many take-home items, such as pamphlets, books, videos, and other visual aids, which provide educational reinforcement and serve as a future reference. Erotic reading lists may also be given to patients, and multiple resources are available, including from the Women's Sexual Health Foundation, The International Society for the Study of Women's Sexual Health (ISSWSH), North American Menopause Society (NAMS), and the American College of Obstetricians and Gynecologists (ACOG).

For women, there is a device approved by the Food and Drug Administration (FDA) for the treatment of sexual complaints that can be prescribed. This device, known as the Eros Clitoral Stimulation Device (CSD), is battery-operated and has a vacuum suction that attaches to the clitoral area. It is presumed to help facilitate vasocongestion in the clitoral tissue. In a pilot trial of 13 women treated for cervical cancer, Schroder demonstrated that at three months, there were statistically significant improvements in sexual function compared to baseline, as measured with the Female Sexual Function Index (39). These improvements were associated with improvements in mucosal color and moisture of the vagina and with decreased bleeding and ulceration. Still, the Eros-CSD remains a costly maneuver, and thus far, there have been no randomized controlled studies comparing it to handheld self-stimulators.

Women: Dyspareunia

Estrogen is one of many hormones necessary for sexual function in females. Estrogen replacement is the key in the management of female sexual arousal and relief of dyspareunia. Central arousal, peripheral sexual response, and pelvic sexual response are dependent on estrogen and in some instances testosterone levels. Estrogen has effects on the urogenital system and not

TABLE 66.2
PDE5 Inhibitors

	SILDENAFIL (*VIAGRA*)	VARDENAFIL (*LEVITRA*)	TADALAFIL (*CIALIS*)
Initial dose	50 mg	10 mg	10 mg
Frequency	Once daily	Once daily	Once daily
Half-life	4 h	4 h	17.5 h
Duration of action	Up to 4 h	Up to 4 h	Up to 36 h

Abbreviation: GMP, guanosine monophosphate.

Mechanism: Inhibition of *phosphodiesterase* type 5–induced degradation of *cyclic GMP* in the *smooth muscle* cells lining the blood vessels supplying the *corpus cavernosum* of the *penis*

only promotes epithelial maturation and proliferation and increased vascularity and blood flow, but also stimulates glandular secretions. A decrease of estrogen causes decreased vasocongestion, increased atrophic vaginitis, and leads to dyspareunia and possibly lowered desire as a secondary consequence. Despite this, decisions regarding estrogen replacement must be discussed in the context of cancer therapy. This is particularly true in patients with estrogen-receptor-positive breast cancers, in whom antiestrogen therapy remains a mainstay of cancer therapy. In addition, the risk to cardiovascular health must be taken into account, particularly in light of data from the Women's Health Initiative showing that estrogen did not exert a cardioprotective effect and was associated with an increased incidence on thromboembolic disease (40–42).

Still, for the woman suffering from sexual dysfunction, estrogen therapy may provide the most effective treatment. The use of local vaginal estrogen is effective for vaginal atrophy, and many products are minimally absorbed systemically. Many sexual health care providers prescribe a vaginal tablet preparation of 17?-estradiol, which patients report are easier to use, less messy than cream preparations, and technically easier to insert than estrogen rings.

In addition to pharmacologic aides, the liberal use of local nonmedicated, nonhormonal vaginal moisturizers can provide alternative relief for the symptoms of vaginal atrophy. One application commonly used is Replens, which can last up to 72 hours or longer and comes in a convenient, single-dose applicator. It has a pH of 3.0, which can closely resemble the normal healthy vaginal environment. A placebo-controlled trial completed by the North Central Cancer Treatment Group evaluated Replens for the management of vaginal atrophy and found it to be effective (43). Replens is available without a prescription, does not harm condoms, and can help maintain the elasticity and pliability of the vaginal mucosal lining. Vitamin E

oil can also be used as a vaginal moisturizer. Patients should be instructed to wear a light pad when using vitamin E suppositories because it may stain undergarments. Some women are sensitive to these vaginal moisturizers, and a complete evaluation should be instituted if increased vaginal complaints develop after beginning these products.

For women with vaginal dryness and atrophy, the use of water-based vaginal lubricants is encouraged with intercourse. Those lubricants that contain microbicides, perfumes, coloration, and flavors should not be used, as these additives may irritate an already sensitive vaginal mucosa. Similarly, household products, such as petroleum jelly, baby oil, or olive oil, should be avoided since they can upset the natural balance of the vaginal flora.

Women: Vaginismus

Patients who have undergone pelvic surgery may suffer from vaginal shortening, vaginal narrowing, and scar tissue formation that can impede penetration and cause vaginal pain and pelvic discomfort, prompting avoidant sexual behavior. One solution is to educate the couple about alternative sexual positioning, such as the side-to-side and female-superior position. Patients should limit deep pelvic thrusting to help minimize vaginal discomfort during penetration. If movement and mobility is an issue, pillows or down comforters can help facilitate a comfortable sexual situation.

Vaginal dilators may be prescribed as part of a sexual rehabilitation program to facilitate lengthening and widening the vagina. These dilators are graded vaginal inserts that come in a variety of sizes and are usually made of plastic or silicone. They should be used with water-based lubricants. Suggested schedules include once daily for 10–15 minutes or at least three times weekly in the morning hours just before starting the day to facilitate compliance.

Men/Women: Low Sexual Desire

Replacement of testosterone in females remains controversial due to confusing and conflicted data, and its use following cancer therapy is not routinely recommended, given the lack of safety data, especially as it relates to recurrence-free survival. There is concern that the testosterone can be converted or aromatized to estrogen, which may reactivate, promote, or stimulate tumor growth. In addition, testosterone products carry the risk of several potentially serious side effects, including increased facial and body hair growth (hirsutism), weight gain, clitoromegaly, hair loss (alopecia), changes in lipid profiles, and liver or hematologic changes. Women who have taken testosterone supplements have also reported emotional changes. At time of this publication, there is no FDA-approved androgen product available for women.

THE ROLE OF THE SEX THERAPIST

Since the etiology of sexual complaints in women is a complex phenomenon and situational issues are a fundamental part of the diagnosis, a comprehensive treatment regimen would not be complete without appropriate sexual counseling and therapy. Sexual complaints are best treated by a certified sexual therapist who is educated and trained to deal with patients with sexual complaints. These specialists are qualified to deal with psychosexual issues, including body image and changes in intimacy, sexuality, self-esteem, and mood, as well as the ramifications of cancer and its therapy. Patients may also benefit from marital, individual, couple, and group therapy, depending on the need and specific complaint. In general, most patients can benefit from brief psychosexual interventions, including education, counseling/support, and symptom management. Psychotherapists and psychologists can be extremely effective when vaginal dilators are prescribed for the treatment of vaginismus. Close surveillance and contact with the medical clinician and the psychosexual therapist can help improve compliance and assist progress with sexual symptoms.

Referral for an evaluation by a subspecialist may be appropriate for certain clinical conditions. Consultants may include oncologists, social services providers, nutritionists, exercise therapists, and psychiatrists. A list of clinicians and ancillary staff who are sensitive to sexual issues should be readily available for patients who take part in sexual rehabilitation programs. Providers need to reassure patients and their partners that even at the end of life, when intercourse may not be feasible, intimacy and emotional closeness is possible. The giving and receiving of sexual pleasure can be accomplished with sensual massage, oral and digital, and noncoital stimulation with gentle caressing.

Sexual complaints are often complex and require the joint treatment efforts of a medical professional and a psychotherapist who are both trained in the field of sexual medicine. Intimacy and sexual function are often vital aspects of quality of life and as such should be a major concern for the clinician. The goal of a comprehensive sexual health evaluation and the resulting therapy is to promote sexual health by fostering open communication, provide anticipatory guidance, and validate normalcy with respect to sexual thoughts and feelings. Individual treatment plans are created and implemented by the sexual health care professional team to educate patients so they can enjoy fulfilling sexual lifestyle defined by their own beliefs and value systems.

Local and national support organizations; the American Association for Sex Education, Counseling and Treatment (AASECT; www.aasect.org); and the Association of Reproductive Health Professionals (ARHP) can provide further information and support to help patients achieve greater comfort with these issues, both within their relationships and families and within themselves.

SEXUALITY AND THE SINGLE SURVIVOR

Cancer survivors want to have productive, healthy relationships with the opposite sex or same sex and want intimate and emotional connections. One of the most difficult issues facing a single cancer survivor is the area of disclosure; when is it appropriate to discuss one's illness with a potential partner? When is it the "right time" to mention that you only have one breast, for women, and when should one discuss possible infertility or decreased longevity? It is important to know that there is no right or wrong time to discuss this, and it often depends on the individual and one's level of comfort with this new partner. It is important to understand that not all potential partners will be supportive and understanding; some may be unable to handle such disclosure and will reject becoming more intimate, but by no means should this be considered a foregone conclusion.

With more and more cancer survivors dating, issues regarding safer sex maintain their relevance. It is always important to discuss issues of birth control and sexually transmitted diseases. Regarding birth control, many options are available, including hormonal contraception, the use of condoms and spermicides, and vaginal dams. The bottom line is to maintain good sense when it comes to protecting oneself from other illnesses, and these include reducing risk to hepatitis

C, human immunodeficiency virus (HIV), and other sexually transmitted diseases (STDs).

CONCLUSION

Sexual health is an integral and fundamental part of being human. A cancer diagnosis does not negate this, and patients should not be left to assume that wanting to maintain a sexual life is no longer part of their reality. Consideration and careful attention to patients on issues of survivorship is important, and sexuality should not be considered a luxury, but a right. Sexuality is a complex, multidimensional phenomenon and warrants a detailed comprehensive evaluation and treatment plan by a knowledgeable sexual health care provider; the treatment often involves both biological and psychological interventions, which can be successful and improve quality-of-life concerns for the cancer survivor.

References

1. http://www.cancer.org/downloads/STT/282, 2006 Estimated US Cancer Cases; accessed 4/7/2007.
2. Ganz PA. A teachable moment for oncologists: cancer survivors, 10 million strong and growing! *J Clin Oncol.* 2005;23(24): 5458–5460.
3. Basson R, Berman J, Burnett A, et al. Report of the international consensus development conference on female sexual dysfunction: definitions and classifications. *J Urol.* 2000;163(3): 888–893.
4. Hordern A. Intimacy and sexuality for the woman with breast cancer. *Cancer Nurs.* 2000;23(3):230–236.
5. Andersen BL. Surviving cancer: the importance of sexual self-concept. *Med Pediatr Oncol.* 1999;33(1):15–23.
6. Masters WH, Johnson VE. *Human Sexual Response.* Boston: Little Brown & Co.; 1966.
7. Kaplan HS. *Disorders of Sexual Desire and Other New Concepts and Techniques in Sex Therapy.* New York: Brunner/Mazel Publications; 1979.
8. World Health Organization. *ICD 10: Internal Statistical Classification of Disease and Related Health Problems.* Geneva: World Health Organization; 1992.
9. Laumann EO, Paik A, Rosen RC. Sexual dysfunction in the United States: prevalence and predictors. *JAMA.* 1999;281(6):537–544.
10. Schover LR, Fouladi RT, Warneke CL, et al. Defining sexual outcomes after treatment for localized prostate carcinoma. *Cancer.* 2002;95(8):1773–1785.
11. Bianco FJ, Jr., Scardino PT, Eastham JA. Radical prostatectomy: long-term cancer control and recovery of sexual and urinary function ("trifecta"). *Urology.* 2005;66(5 Suppl):83–94.
12. Katz A. What happened? Sexual consequences of prostate cancer and its treatment. *Canadian Family Physician Medecin de Famille Canadien.* 2005;51:977–982.
13. Schover LR, Fouladi RT, Warneke CL, et al. The use of treatments for erectile dysfunction among survivors of prostate carcinoma. *Cancer.* 2002;95(11):2397–2407.
14. Colombo R, Bertini R, Salonia A, et al. Overall clinical outcomes after nerve and seminal sparing radical cystectomy for the treatment of organ confined bladder cancer. *J Urol.* 2004;171(5):1819–1822; discussion 1822.
15. Muto G, Bardari F, D'Urso L, Giona C. Seminal sparing cystectomy and ileocapsuloplasty: long-term followup results. *J Urol.* 2004;172(1):76–80.
16. Rozet F, Harmon J, Arroyo C, Cathelineau X, Barret E, Vallancien G. Benefits of laparoscopic prostate-sparing radical cystectomy. *Expert Rev Anticancer Ther.* 2006;6(1):21–26.
17. Judd HL, Judd GE, Lucas WE, Yen SS. Endocrine function of the postmenopausal ovary: concentration of androgens and estrogens in ovarian and peripheral vein blood. *J Clin Endocrinol Metab.* 1974;39(6):1020–1024.
18. Stewart DE, Wong F, Duff S, Melancon CH, Cheung AM. What doesn't kill you makes you stronger: an ovarian cancer survivor survey. *Gynecol Oncol.* 2001;83(3):537–542.
19. Abitbol MM, Davenport JH. Sexual dysfunction after therapy for cervical carcinoma. *Am J Obstet Gynecol.* 1974;119(2): 181–189.
20. Bergmark K, Avall-Lundqvist E, Dickman PW, Henningsohn L, Steineck G. Vaginal changes and sexuality in women with a history of cervical cancer. *N Engl J Med.* 1999;340(18): 1383–1389.
21. Krychman ML, Carter J, Aghajanian CA, Dizon DS, Castiel M. Chemotherapy-induced dyspareunia: a case study of vaginal mucositis and pegylated liposomal doxorubicin injection in advanced stage ovarian carcinoma. *Gynecol Oncol.* 2004;93(2):561–563.
22. Day R, Ganz PA, Costantino JP, Cronin WM, Wickerham DL, Fisher B. Health-related quality of life and tamoxifen in breast cancer prevention: a report from the National Surgical Adjuvant Breast and Bowel Project P-1 Study. *J Clin Oncol.* 1999;17(9):2659–2669.
23. Mortimer JE, Boucher L, Baty J, Knapp DL, Ryan E, Rowland JH. Effect of tamoxifen on sexual functioning in patients with breast cancer. *J Clin Oncol.* 1999;17(5):1488–1492.
24. Galbraith ME, Arechiga A, Ramirez J, Pedro LW. Prostate cancer survivors' and partners' self-reports of health-related quality of life, treatment symptoms, and marital satisfaction 2.5–5.5 years after treatment. *Oncol Nurs Forum.* 2005;32(2):E30–E41.
25. Heinrhich-Rynning T. Prostate cancer treatments and their effects on sexual functioning. *Oncol Nurs Forum.* 1987;14(6):37–41.
26. Andersen BL, Anderson B, deProsse C. Controlled prospective longitudinal study of women with cancer: I. Sexual functioning outcomes. *J Consult Clin Psychol.* 1989;57(6):683–691.
27. Donovan KA, Taliaferro LA, Alvarez EM, Jacobsen PB, Roetzheim RG, Wenham RM. Sexual health in women treated for cervical cancer: characteristics and correlates. *Gynecol Oncol.* 2007;104(2):428–434.
28. The Pfizer Global Study of Sexual Attitudes and Behaviors. Available at: http://www.pfizerglobalstudy.com/study/study-results.asp. Accessed 5/7/2007.
29. Marwick C. Survey says patients expect little physician help on sex. *JAMA.* 1999;281(23):2173–2174.
30. Bachmann GA, Leiblum SR, Grill J. Brief sexual inquiry in gynecologic practice. *Obstet Gynecol.* 1989;73(3 Pt 1):425–427.
31. Wiggins DL, Wood R, Granai CO, Dizon DS. Intimacy and the gynecologic oncologist: survey results of the New England Association of Gynecologic Oncologists (NEAGO). *J Psychosoc Oncol.* 2007;25(4):61–70.
32. Zippe CD, Raina R, Thukral M, Lakin MM, Klein EA, Agarwal A. Management of erectile dysfunction following radical prostatectomy. *Curr Urol Rep.* 2001;2(6):495–503.
33. Walsh PC. Nerve grafts are rarely necessary and are unlikely to improve sexual function in men undergoing anatomic radical prostatectomy. *Urology.* 2001;57(6):1020–1024.
34. Montorsi F, Althof SE, Sweeney M, Menchini-Fabris F, Sasso F, Giuliano F. Treatment satisfaction in patients with erectile dysfunction switching from prostaglandin E(1) intracavernosal injection therapy to oral sildenafil citrate. *Int J Impot Res.* 2003;15(6):444–449.
35. Padma-Nathan H, McCullough AR, Giuliano F, et al. Postoperative nightly administration of sildenafil citrate significantly improves the return of normal spontaneous erectile function

after bilateral nerve-sparing radical prostatectomy. *J Urol.* 2003;169(Suppl): 75; (abstract 1,402).

36. Mulhall J, Land S, Parker M, Waters WB, Flanigan RC. The use of an erectogenic pharmacotherapy regimen following radical prostatectomy improves recovery of spontaneous erectile function. *J Sex Med.* 2005;2(4):532–540; discussion 40–42.

37. Raina R, Lakin MM, Agarwal A, Ausmundson S, Montague DK, Zippe CD. Long-term intracavernous therapy responders can potentially switch to sildenafil citrate after radical prostatectomy. *Urology.* 2004;63(3):532–537; discussion 8.

38. Stephenson RA, Mori M, Hsieh YC, et al. Treatment of erectile dysfunction following therapy for clinically localized prostate cancer: patient reported use and outcomes from the Surveillance, Epidemiology, and End Results Prostate Cancer Outcomes Study. *J Urol.* 2005;174(2):646–650; discussion 50.

39. Schroder M, Mell LK, Hurteau JA, et al. Clitoral therapy device for treatment of sexual dysfunction in irradiated cervical can-cer patients. *Int J Radiat Oncol Biol Phys.* 2005;61(4):1078–1086.

40. Rossouw JE, Anderson GL, Prentice RL, et al. Risks and benefits of estrogen plus progestin in healthy postmenopausal women: principal results From the Women's Health Initiative randomized controlled trial. *JAMA.* 2002;288(3):321–333.

41. Hsia J, Criqui MH, Rodabough RJ, et al. Estrogen plus progestin and the risk of peripheral arterial disease: the Women's Health Initiative. *Circulation.* 2004;109(5):620–626.

42. Anderson GL, Limacher M, Assaf AR, et al. Effects of conjugated equine estrogen in postmenopausal women with hysterectomy: the Women's Health Initiative randomized controlled trial. *JAMA.* 2004;291(14):1701–1712.

43. Nachtigall LE. Comparative study: Replens versus local estrogen in menopausal women. *Fertil Steril.* 1994;61(1):178–180.

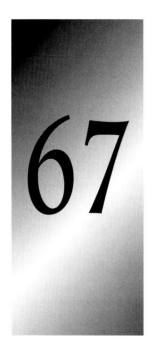

Depression, Anxiety, and Psychosocial Dysfunction in the Cancer Patient

Jimmie C. Holland
Talia R. Weiss
Jessica Stiles

The most central issue for patients is "getting back to normal" after a cancer diagnosis. This translates into the return to normal function in the domains of living that count most: physical, psychological, work, social, and sexual. This area has become more important as patient-centered medicine has evolved and health-related quality of life (HRQOL) has been better appreciated. It is of interest that rehabilitation oncology has been slow to develop, given this central desire of patients. Similarly, the psychological aspects of oncology were neglected until approximately the last 30 years, when the subspecialty of psycho-oncology has developed as an integral area of patient care (1). This historical picture relates in part to the fact that cancer was regarded for so long as a death sentence that rehabilitation was not recognized as an important option after treatment. The assumption was that all patients would die, and rapidly. Mid-twentieth century, patients could not receive a prosthesis after a limb amputation until one year of survival after treatment. The emotional stress of cancer was equally stigmatized—patients were not to ask questions about diagnosis and prognosis—and the concept of asking for psychological help was considered a sign of moral weakness. Today, these issues are managed better, but rehabilitation and psychosocial care remain "weak sisters" to the more robustly funded and highly regarded traditional treat-ment modalities in oncology, despite their importance to patients and families.

Rehabilitation oncology is a growing and expand-ing discipline today. There is likely no area of cancer treatment that is more dependent upon the patient's motivation and cooperation. Psychiatric disorders and psychological and social problems are common rea-sons for patients not meeting the full rehabilitation goals to get them "back to normal." The physiatrist today must be aware of the prevalence of the com-mon problems anxiety and depression, how to man-age them, and when to refer for more specialized help (2,3). This chapter describes clinical practice guidelines established by the National Cancer Centers Network (NCCN), which have been developed to better inte-grate psychosocial care into routine clinical oncology treatment (4). The first principle of these guidelines is the use of a brief screening tool to rapidly identify patients who are distressed and who are in need of psy-chosocial intervention. The screen gives an algorithm for when a referral to a mental health professional, social worker, or clergy member is appropriate. And the chapter outlines the clinical practice guidelines for management of anxiety, depression, and psychoso-cial dysfunction related to personality disorders and traits that complicate all aspects of cancer care, but particularly rehabilitation.

KEY POINTS

- The most central issue for patients is "getting back to normal" after a cancer diagnosis. This translates into the return to as near normal function as possible in the domains of living that count most: physical, psychological, work, social, and sexual.
- Psychiatric disorders and psychological and social problems are common reasons for patients not meeting the full rehabilitation goals to get them "back to normal."
- To assist the physiatrist in routinely taking the common anxiety and depressive symptoms into account and treating the "whole patient," the National Cancer Centers Network (NCCN) established a multidisciplinary Panel on Management of Distress in Cancer, which has developed consensus and evidence-based clinical practice guidelines.
- For the physiatrist in a busy rehabilitation ambulatory practice, a common problem is to quickly determine: "Is this patient's level of distress 'normal' or 'not normal' and should it be treated?"
- A large survey of almost 5,000 patients with cancer showed that, overall, 35% of patients were experiencing significant distress.
- When patients are unable to follow rehabilitation recommendations due to psychological factors, it is crucial to determine the cause and to correct it, since achieving adequate functional return may depend on it.
- Anxiety is the commonest form of distress seen in patients at all stages of disease.
- It is important to recognize that a medical problem or a medication may be producing the patient's anxiety. It is unwise to assume it is "psychological" until all medical factors have been ruled out.
- Pain is the most common cause of anxiety.
- The challenge for the physiatrist who is initially evaluating a patient for rehabilitation is to determine if and when the normal sadness that accompanies a life-threatening illness like cancer has reached a level that is deserving of a full psychiatric evaluation and treatment.
- In contrast to anxiety and depression, for which there are clear interventions and treatment, personality disorders (eg, angry, dramatic, anxious, dependent) represent longstanding traits and ways of responding that are highly resistant to change.

SCREENING FOR DISTRESS

For the physiatrist in a busy rehabilitation ambulatory practice, a common problem is to quickly determine: "Is this patient's level of distress 'normal' or 'not normal' and should it be treated?" A large survey of almost 5,000 patients with cancer showed that, overall, 35% of patients were experiencing significant distress (3). The percentage was even greater in patients with brain, pancreas, and lung cancer. Yet experience in most cancer centers is that less than 10% of outpatients are evaluated and treated for distress.

To assist the physiatrist in routinely taking the common anxiety and depressive symptoms into account and treating the "whole patient," the NCCN established a multidisciplinary Panel on Management of Distress in Cancer in 1997 (5). This panel has developed consensus- and evidence-based clinical practice guidelines, which have been updated annually. The American Psychosocial Oncology Society adopted these guidelines to provide the basis for its handbook "Quick Reference for Oncology Clinicians: The Psychiatric and Psychological Dimensions of Cancer Symptom Management" (6). The handbook provides a rapid "psych curbside consult" in a small handbook suitable for use in the

clinic and on hospital rounds (6). It may be ordered online at www.apos-society.org.

The guidelines were developed to provide a way to rapidly screen for level of distress in busy oncology and rehabilitation clinics, thereby assuring that the psychological domain is considered as a part of a routine visit, with guidelines for management by the oncologist or physiatrist and recommendations for triage of the patient to the appropriate psychosocial discipline when more extensive evaluation and treatment is needed.

The NCCN panel first determined that the terms "psychological" and "psychiatric" are strongly disliked by patients, who fear being "labeled" as "psychiatric." The word "distress" was chosen as an acceptable, normal, and nonstigmatizing term that covers the range of psychological, social, and spiritual problems patients experience in coping with life-threatening illness. The rehabilitation team, particularly the physiatrist and rehabilitation clinic nurse, are the "front line" of psychological care for all patients and the cornerstone of good psychosocial care. Most clinics have a social worker available, but one is not usually available to see every patient. To adequately manage this front line, the physiatrist must be able to identify the common symptoms of distress, be empathetic to the patient's

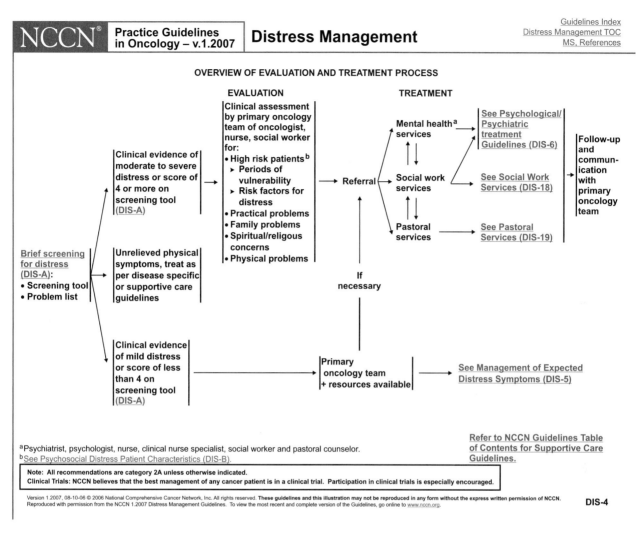

FIGURE 67.1

Symptoms, interventions, and reevaluation in distress management. Reprinted with permission from Ref. 27.

functional loss, and be able to express concern and caring in the context of a trusting relationship. Figure 67.1 (NCCN DIS-5) outlines the common and expected distress symptoms and the evaluation and interventions the team should be aware of, recognizing the patient should be re-evaluated at the next visit and referred to a social worker or mental health professional if not improved (7). Figure 67.2 (8) (NCCN DIS-B) outlines patients who are at increased risk for distress and the points in illness when they are most vulnerable (8).

The NCCN guidelines strongly endorse the screening of all new patients for level of distress using the same paradigm, which has remarkably improved pain management in the United States. The question used now for asking about pain is, "How is your pain on a scale of 0–10?" Patients understand this scale and

accurately report their subjective pain level. Similarly, NCCN distress guidelines recommend using the Distress Thermometer, which is a graphic "thermometer" of a 0–10 scale, asking "What is the level of your distress, 0–10?" It can be presented to the patient in the waiting room on a touch screen or paper and pencil (Fig. 67.3 [NCCN DIS-A]) (9). This single-item scale serves as a "broad-stroke" approach to be followed by questions that are more specific, usually by the oncology nurse, if the patient scores 4 or above on the scale. The oncology nurse is often the person who asks the additional psychosocial questions. There is a set of free online lectures for nurses about screening for distress on the APOS Web site at www.apos-society.org.

Early validation studies showed 5 to be the clinically appropriate cutoff, compared to the score for

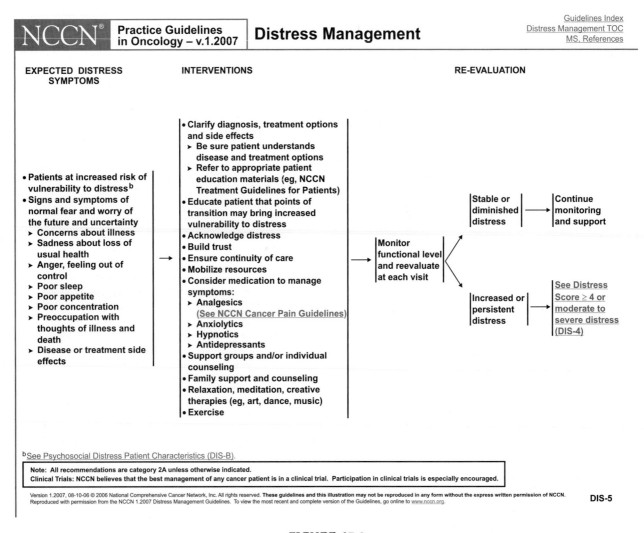

FIGURE 67.2

Psychosocial patient characteristics in distress management. Reprinted with permission from Ref. 27.

clinical "caseness" on the Hospital Anxiety Depression Scale; however, later studies have identified 4 as more accurate (10–13). The Problem List, which is on the same page with the Distress Thermometer, asks the patient to check off the reasons for their distress (eg, practical problems, family, emotional, spiritual or religious concerns). A list of physical symptoms helps to identify problems the patient might not mention to the physician. The nature of the problems checked on the Problem List determines whether referral should be to a social worker (for practical and psychosocial needs), a mental health professional (for a serious psychiatric disorder, particularly if medication may be needed), or a clergy member (when a spiritual crisis is present, since many patients look to a clergy member for their

key psychological support). Figure 67.4 (NCCN DIS-4) (14) gives an algorithm for the use of the brief screening tool, noting how the cutoff score ($\geq$–4) for distress assists in determining patients who should be referred for more extensive psychological evaluation and those who should continue to be managed by the rehabilitation team and community resources (14).

These guidelines assure that the psychosocial aspects are a part of total care from the initial visit, when baseline screening should be done, and repeated as clinically appropriate or when there are transitions in treatment (eg, curative to palliative). When patients are unable to follow rehabilitation recommendations due to psychological factors, it is crucial to determine the cause and to correct it, since achieving adequate

NCCN® | **Practice Guidelines in Oncology – v.1.2007** | **Distress Management**

SCREENING TOOLS FOR MEASURING DISTRESS

Instructions: First please circle the number (0-10) that best describes how much distress you have been experiencing in the past week including today.

Extreme distress — 10

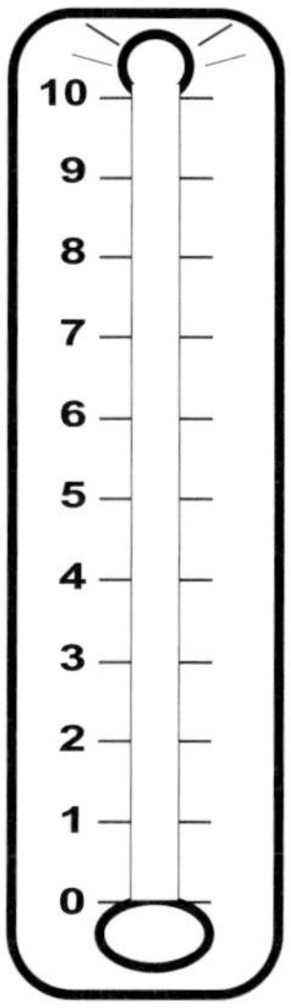

9

8

7

6

5

4

3

2

1

No distress — 0

Second, please indicate if any of the following has been a problem for you in the past week including today. Be sure to check YES or NO for each.

YES NO Practical Problems
- ☐ ☐ Child care
- ☐ ☐ Housing
- ☐ ☐ Insurance/financial
- ☐ ☐ Transportation
- ☐ ☐ Work/school

Family Problems
- ☐ ☐ Dealing with children
- ☐ ☐ Dealing with partner

Emotional Problems
- ☐ ☐ Depression
- ☐ ☐ Fears
- ☐ ☐ Nervousness
- ☐ ☐ Sadness
- ☐ ☐ Worry
- ☐ ☐ Loss of interest in usual activities

- ☐ ☐ **Spiritual/religious concerns**

YES NO Physical Problems
- ☐ ☐ Appearance
- ☐ ☐ Bathing/dressing
- ☐ ☐ Breathing
- ☐ ☐ Changes in urination
- ☐ ☐ Constipation
- ☐ ☐ Diarrhea
- ☐ ☐ Eating
- ☐ ☐ Fatigue
- ☐ ☐ Feeling Swollen
- ☐ ☐ Fevers
- ☐ ☐ Getting around
- ☐ ☐ Indigestion
- ☐ ☐ Memory/concentration
- ☐ ☐ Mouth sores
- ☐ ☐ Nausea
- ☐ ☐ Nose dry/congested
- ☐ ☐ Pain
- ☐ ☐ Sexual
- ☐ ☐ Skin dry/itchy
- ☐ ☐ Sleep
- ☐ ☐ Tingling in hands/feet

Other Problems: _____

_____

DIS-A

FIGURE 67.3

The Distress Thermometer and rapid screening for distress. Reprinted with permission from Ref. 27.

functional return may depend on it. The most common symptoms of distress encountered by the physiatrist are anxiety and depression. Either or both may interfere with treatment. Their management is outlined in the following section.

ANXIETY DISORDERS

Anxiety is the commonest form of distress seen in patients at all stages of disease. It is often mild and managed by reassurance, but more significant levels require evaluation to identify the etiology and treatment. The NCCN guidelines for management of anxiety disorder provide a useful framework from which to con-

sider recognition, differential diagnosis, and treatment (Fig. 67.5 [NCCN DIS-14]) (15). It outlines the common signs of anxiety, which may be occurring from fears of illness, but may also have a medical or medication etiology.

Symptoms may be largely physical (tachycardia, diaphoresis, restlessness, pacing, tremor, insomnia, dry mouth) or psychological (fears, worry about specific problems of illness, treatment, or an impending procedure). When the basis is response to illness, it is usually situationally related and is referred to as an adjustment disorder with anxiety. The first caveat is to recognize that a medical problem or a medication may be producing the patient's anxiety. It is unwise to assume it is "psychological" until all medical factors have been

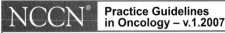

Practice Guidelines in Oncology – v.1.2007 | **Distress Management**

PSYCHOSOCIAL DISTRESS PATIENT CHARACTERISTICS[c]

PATIENTS AT INCREASED RISK FOR DISTRESS[d]

- History of psychiatric disorder/substance abuse
- History of depression/suicide attempt
- Cognitive impairment
- Communication barriers[e]
- Severe comorbid illnesses
- Social problems
  - Family/caregiver conflicts
  - Inadequate social support
  - Living alone
  - Financial problems
  - Limited access to medical care
  - Young or dependent children
  - Younger age; woman
  - Other stressors

PERIODS OF INCREASED VULNERABILITY

- Finding a suspicious symptom
- During workup
- Finding out the diagnosis
- Awaiting treatment
- Change in treatment modality
- End of treatment
- Discharge from hospital following treatment
- Stresses of survivorship
- Medical follow-up and surveillance
- Treatment failure
- Recurrence/progression
- Advanced cancer
- End of life

---

[c]For site-specific symptoms with major psychosocial consequences, see Holland, JC, Greenberg, DB, Hughes, MD, et al. Quick Reference for Oncology Clinicians: The Psychiatric and Psychological Dimensions of Cancer Symptom Management. (Based on NCCN Distress Management Guidelines). IPOS Press, 2006. Available at www.apos-society.org.
[d]From the NCCN Palliative Care Clinical Practice Guidelines in Oncology. Available at www.nccn.org.
[e]Communication barriers include language, literacy, and physical barriers.

Note: All recommendations are category 2A unless otherwise indicated.
Clinical Trials: NCCN believes that the best management of any cancer patient is in a clinical trial. Participation in clinical trials is especially encouraged.

DIS-B

FIGURE 67.4

Overview of evaluation and treatment process. Reprinted with permission from Ref. 27.

ruled out. Pain is the most common cause of anxiety. It diminishes with adequate pain control. Table 67.1 outlines the range of frequent medical problems and medications that may produce anxiety. Also, an early symptom of alcohol or opioid withdrawal may be acute anxiety and tremulousness. One should also take a history as to whether anxiety existed prior to illness, which may be generalized anxiety disorder, panic or phobic disorder (PTSD), chemotherapy-conditioned response (nausea and vomiting with anxiety), or obsessive-compulsive disorder (OCD). Patients who have chronic anxiety disorders often experience an exacerbation of their symptoms in the context of illness. Patients with OCD are particularly likely to be compromised in their rehabilitation by an inability to make a decision or commitment to a program, and they are anxious and fearful about any new procedure or medication.

The treatment of anxiety is psychopharmacologic and psychological. The medications ordinarily used are benzodiazepines, selective serotonin reuptake inhibitors (SSRIs), and low-dose antipsychotics. Benzodiazepines are useful because of the immediate relief they produce and are often given initially with an SSRI, which is slower (up to two to three weeks) to produce an antianxiety effect. Table 67.2 outlines the commonly used drugs and their dosage. Patients are often fearful of addiction to benzodiazepines and must be encouraged to use them and reassured that they will be monitored to prevent addiction, though it is an unrealistic fear in patients with no prior history of addiction.

In terms of nonpharmacologic interventions, several forms of psychotherapy and counseling are useful:

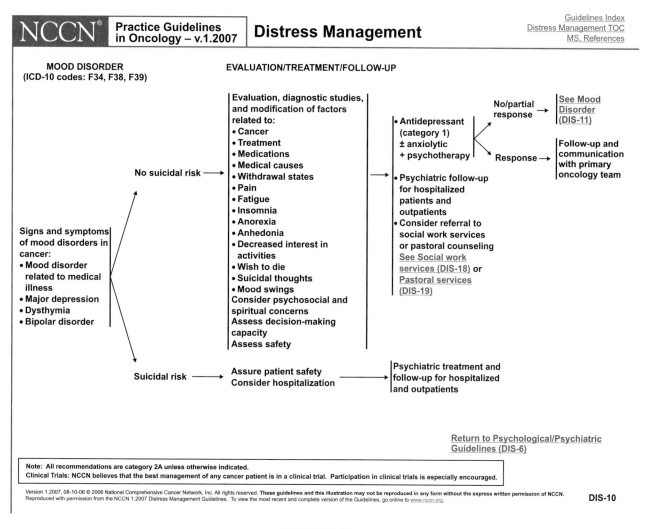

FIGURE 67.5

Evaluation, treatment, and follow-up of anxiety disorder. Reprinted with permission from Ref. 27.

- Support and reassurance from the rehabilitation team with attention to control of troublesome symptoms (eg, insomnia)
- Referral to a social worker or mental health professional for supportive psychotherapy, given either individually or in groups
- Cognitive behavioral therapy to help patients through cognitive reframing of symptoms, guided imagery, relaxation, and meditation
- The Internet, chat rooms, and virtual groups are emerging as easily accessible, but they are largely unsupervised
- Complementary therapies (see Chapter 42)

Supportive and behavioral intervention randomized controlled trials have been conducted at all stages of disease. Evidence from meta-analyses in the United States and Australia support inclusion of psychotherapy as an evidence-based intervention in clinical practice guidelines (16,17). While the rehabilitation team treats most situational anxiety well, when the etiology is a preexisting anxiety disorder, referral to a mental health professional will be useful. OCD and generalized anxiety disorders are often resistant to treatment, and both can significantly complicate the management of cancer therapy and rehabilitation.

DEPRESSION (MOOD DISORDERS)

The challenge for the physiatrist who is initially evaluating a patient for rehabilitation is to determine if and when the normal sadness that accompanies a life-threatening illness like cancer has reached a level that

TABLE 67.1
Medical and Medication-Related Causes of Anxiety

Metabolic	Hyperkalemia
	Hyperthermia
	Hypoglycemia
	Hyponatremia
Tumor-related	Delirium (restlessness, agitation)
	Pain
	Central nervous system neoplasms
	Carcinoid syndrome
	Paraneoplastic disorders
Endocrine	Adrenal
	Thyroid
	Parathyroid
	Pituitary
	Pheochromocytoma
Cardiovascular	Arrhythmia
	Congestive heart failure
	Myocardial infarction
	Angina pectoris
	Valvular disease
Pulmonary	Pulmonary embolism
	Asthma
	Chronic obstructive pulmonary disease
	Pneumothorax
	Pulmonary edema
Medications	Corticosteroids
	Neuroleptics used as antiemetics (akathesias)
	Sympathomimetic agents
	Antibiotics (cephalosporins, acyclovir, isoniazid)
Withdrawal states	Alcohol, opioids, sedatives-hypnotics, caffeine

is deserving of a full psychiatric evaluation and treatment. Similar to anxiety, there are medical factors and medications that may cause depression. A workup must consider a wide range of potential correctable causes in the differential diagnosis. It is important that significant depressive symptoms not be dismissed on the presumption of being part of the normal response to cancer. Equally difficult is the fact that physical symptoms of cancer and somatic symptoms of depression are similar (eg, insomnia, fatigue, poor concentration). When the depressed mood begins to interfere with coping, or when insomnia, fatigue, or distress become significant, this represents the most common depressive disorder: situational depression, called adjustment disorder with depressive symptoms. Most of these patients are handled well by the rehabilitation team with reassurance and medications to target their specific symptoms (eg, insomnia, fatigue).

However, persistent and more severe symptoms require a thoughtful workup, since there are many medical causes for depressive symptoms. These depressive symptoms in their moderate levels are called subsyndromal depression, indicating that they are distressing but do not reach criteria for a major depressive disorder (characterized by dysphoria; anhedonia; hopelessness; guilt; change in sleep, appetite, concentration; feeling life is not worth living; and suicidal ideation). Major depression is seen less often than the subsyndromal disorders, but it causes the greatest risk of suicidal behavior. Mania is unusual in cancer patients, but is seen most often in response to medication or in a patient with preexisting bipolar disorder.

The NCCN guidelines for recognition and management of mood disorders (Fig. 67.6 [NCCN DIS-10 and NCCN DIS-11]) (18,19) outline the common mood

TABLE 67.2
Medications Commonly Used to Treat Anxiety

DRUG	BRAND NAME	STARTING DOSE (MG)	MAINTENANCE DOSE (MG)
SSRIs: Selective serotonin reuptake inhibitors			
Escitalopram[a]	Lexapro	10–20	10–20
Fluoxetine[a]	Prozac	10–20 (qAM)	20–60
Paroxetine[a]	Paxil	20 (qAM)	20–60
Sertraline[a]	Zoloft	20–25 (qAM)	50–150
Benzodiazepines			
Alprazolam	Xanax	0.25–1.0	PO q 6–24h
Clonazepam	Klonopin	1.5–2.0	PO q 6–24h
Diazepam	Valium	2–10	PO/IV q 6–24h
Lorazepam	Ativan	0.5–2.0	PO/IM/IVP/IVPB q 4–12h

Abbreviations: IM, intramuscular; IVP, IV push; IVPB, IV piggyback; PO, oral.
Source: Ref. 6.

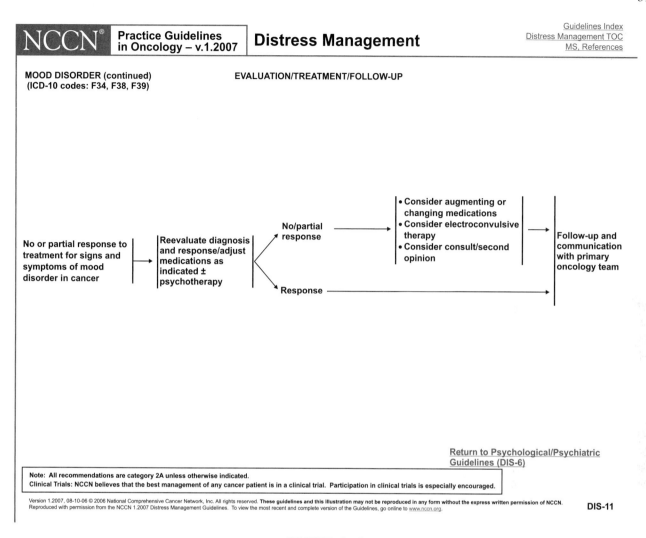

FIGURE 67.6

Evaluation, treatment, and follow-up of mood disorder. Reprinted with permission from Ref. 27.

disorders and the evaluation of the symptoms and factors that may contribute to depression. After establishing the cause, treatment is directed toward correcting the medical problem or stopping the medication, when possible (eg, interferon). Often, the offending agent cannot be removed and treatment must be instituted for the depression. Suicidal-risk patients should be immediately referred.

Table 67.3 outlines the common medical causes for depression. Most common and most likely to produce suicidal thoughts is unrelenting and unrelieved pain. Medications, chemotherapy agents, metabolic derangement, and some sites of cancer are associated with greater depression. The role of proinflammatory cytokines is becoming more clear in producing symptoms of depression, fatigue, anxiety, and poor concentration (20,21). This may account for the asso-

ciation of pancreatic cancer, for example, with greater depression.

Assessment of Suicide Risk

Any patient who is significantly depressed should be asked about suicidal ideation. Contrary to beliefs about this, asking about it does not increase risk; in fact, it decreases risk. A question such as, "Do you ever have thoughts that life isn't worth living?" can be followed with more direct questions if the answer is affirmative. Most patients admit to "thinking about it" and express "I would do it if things get bad enough." However, suicide attempts and suicide are relatively uncommon in patients with cancer. Patients who should be considered at higher risk (and more carefully monitored) are those who have unrelieved pain, advanced

TABLE 67.3
Medical Causes of Depressive Symptoms

Unrelieved pain	Significant cause of depression, as well as fear of unrelieved pain. A major variable in physician-assisted suicide requests.
Medications	Corticosteroids may cause marked mood change Opioids, analgesics, interferon alpha, and interleukin-2 are particularly related Vinca alkaloids, L-asparaginase, procarbazine.
Metabolic	Electrolyte abnormalities, particularly sodium, thyroid, and parathyroid function.
Cancer	Pancreatic, occult, brain tumors, and CNS lymphomas.

Abbreviation: CNS, central nervous system.
Source: Modified from Ref. 6.

disease, prior depression, or alcohol or substance abuse. Patients who have delirium are at greater risk to poorer impulse control in the context of their depressed mood and sometimes make suicide attempts that are poorly planned.

Management

Depression is treated by psychological and psychopharmacologic interventions. Psychological support from the rehabilitation team is critical. Referral for supportive or cognitive behavior psychotherapy is supported by meta-analyses of clinical trials that show a significant evidence base (22). In Australia and the United States, evidence-based clinical practice guidelines include psychotherapeutic interventions similar to findings in other medical illnesses (17,22).

Patients with mood disorders are treated by antidepressants largely, but also by psychostimulants, which rapidly improve alertness and may reduce fatigue. Table 67.4 outlines the commonly used medications.

TABLE 67.4
Medications Commonly Used to Treat Depression

SSRIs: Selective Serotonin Reuptake Inhibitors				
Fluoxetine[a]	Prozac	5–10	5–40	Varying degrees of gastrointestinal distress, nausea, headache, insomnia, increased anxiety, sexual dysfunction; sertraline, citalopram, and escitalopram produce the least P450 system interactions
Sertraline[a]	Zoloft	25–50	25–200	
Paroxetine[a]	Paxil	5–10	5–40	
Citalopram[a]	Celexa	10–20	10–40	
Escitalopram[a]	Lexapro	5–10	5–20	
Newer antidepressants				
Bupropione	Wellbutrin Wellbutrin SR, and Wellbutrin XL	75	75–300	Activating, seizures if predisposed; no sexual dysfunction
Venlafaxine	Effexor and Effexor XR	18.75	18.75–225	Activating, nausea, anxiety, sedation, sweating, hypertension
Duloxetine	Cymbalta	20–30	20–60	Activating, nausea, anxiety
Mirtazapine	Remeron	7.5–15	7.5–45	Sedation, weight gain; dissolvable tablet form available
Stimulants and wakefulness-promoting agents				
Dextroamphetamine	Dexedrine	2.5	5–30	Possible cardiac complications; agitation, anxiety, nausea
Methylphenidate	Ritalin	2.5	5–10 twice a day	
Modafinil	Provigil	50	50–200	Activating nausea, cardiac adverse effects; usually well treated

[a]Available in liquid form.
Source: From Ref. 23.

While there are few controlled trials in cancer for psychotropic drugs, the few that have been done, when reviewed in the meta-analyses, support their efficacy and inclusion in guidelines (17,22).

PERSONALITY DISORDERS AND PSYCHOSOCIAL DYSFUNCTION

The most common and troublesome cause of psychosocial dysfunction is a personality disorder. In contrast to anxiety and depression, for which there are clear interventions and treatment, personality disorders represent longstanding traits and ways of responding that are highly resistant to change. The type of personality disorder and its severity determines the management principles. The overanxious, manipulative, angry, suspicious, or paranoid person can be particularly vexing to the team. It is helpful with such a difficult patient to be sure that all team members are aware of the issues and that the team presents a shared common front to the patient.

The *Diagnostic and Statistical Manual of Mental Disorders* (Fourth Edition) (DSM-IV) categorizes the 10 major personality disorders (Table 67.5) for types and key components (6).

Kahana and Birbring were the first to describe the management of these personality disorders in a medical setting. These disorders are difficult to diagnose, especially in the presence of significant depression or anxiety. However, they often significantly affect adherence to treatments, leading to noncompliance, even to cancer treatment or clinical rehabilitation for best results (24). Patients with personality disorders often lack the control and persistence required in rehabilitation. They often create animosity in physicians, who become understandably annoyed and angry with these difficult, uncooperative patients. It is important to be aware of these feelings and share them with the team (who are feeling the same). Borderline patients are particularly annoying because of their acting-out behavior (eg, suicidal threats, outbursts toward treating staff, and intermittent substance abuse). Table 67.6 outlines how to identify and evaluate for personality disorder (6).

Figure 67.7 (NCCN DIS-17) outlines the NCCN guidelines for the management of patients with personality disorders (25). Management principles are several: set limits on behavior and inform team members of the nature of the difficult or manipulative behavior. These patients often try to "split" the staff by manipulative means: "You are great, but Dr. X is terrible." Make a plan for management to which the team members agree. It may be necessary to write a behavioral con-

TABLE 67.5 *Types of Personality Disorders and Their Key Components*	
Paranoid	Suspicious of others
	Perceives attacks by others quickly
	Categorizes people as an enemy or friend
	Rarely confides in others
	Unforgiving
Schizoid	Flat affect
	Tends to be solitary in nature
	Indifferent to criticism and praise
	Marked absence of close friends or relationships
Schizotypal	Has magical thinking or odd beliefs
	Exhibits anxiety in social situations
	Paranoid ideation
	Experiences unusual perceptions
Antisocial	Lacks conformity to laws
	Ignores obligations
	Impulsive
	Irritable and aggressive
Borderline	Fears abandonment
	Suicidal behavior
	Mood instability
	Chronic feelings of emptiness
Histrionic	Easily influenced
	Rapidly shifting emotions
	Theatrical emotions
	Provocative or sexual behavior
Narcissistic	Belief in being "special"
	Lacks empathy
	Arrogant
	Sense of entitlement
Avoidant	Views self as inferior
	Inhibited in new relationships
	Tries to avoid embarrassment
	Fear of rejection in social situations
Dependent	Fears being left alone
	Lack of self-confidence
	Requires reassurance when making decisions
	Unlikely to express disagreement for fear of rejection
Obsessive-compulsive	Preoccupied with details
	Tendency for perfectionism
	Inflexible and stubborn
	Unable to discard worthless objects
Personality disorder not otherwise specified	Reserved for disorders that do not fit any of the other categories
	Can also describe people who exhibit features of several personality disorders without meeting full criteria for any one disorder

Source: From Ref. 6.

TABLE 67.6
Personality Disorder Screening and Evaluation

Taking a psychological history	Be straightforward in assessing a taboo subject. Those with a history of psychological distress or personality disorders are more likely to suffer from both in the future. Personality disorders are difficult to diagnose. Significant comorbidity exists among personality disorders. Comorbidity leads to difficulty in identifying a primary personality diagnosis. Axis I disorders will complicate the identification of personality disorders.
The physician's perspective	The clinician with the personality-disordered patient does not need to make the diagnosis to be successful, but he or she must respond to the behavior. Avoid stereotyping patients. Be aware of your own feelings towards your patients, especially those who cause you to have emotional reactions.
Make a referral to a mental health provider, social worker, psychologist, or psychiatrist, depending on what is available in your community/organization.[a]	Cancer patients utilize mental health professionals more often than the general public (7.2% vs 5.7%). When a patient is challenging the resources of the physician and staff, it is a wise decision to enroll the aid of a mental health provider.

[a]It is always useful to establish a relationship in your practice with mental health providers. They should have an understanding of and respect for the challenges of dealing with cancer patients who also have a comorbid personality disorder. Frequent feedback and discussion of the patient's status is helpful to all involved.
Source: From Ref. 6.

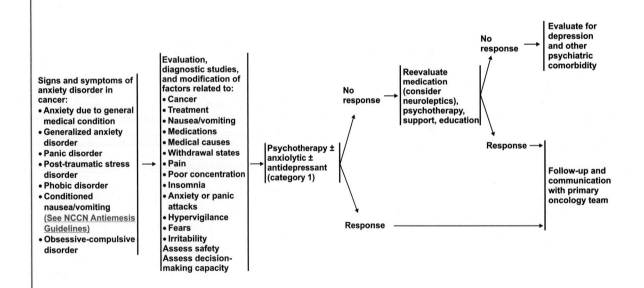

FIGURE 67.7

Evaluation, treatment, and follow-up of personality disorder. Reprinted with permission from Ref. 27.

tract with the patient so that when the patient fails to adhere to the rules agreed upon, it then becomes the basis for refusal to continue treatment (26).

SUMMARY

Psychiatric and psychological aspects are being increasingly incorporated in routine cancer care and rehabilitation. This is a needed step in rehabilitation, and it can be facilitated by the use of the NCCN guidelines. Control of distress is often central to a patient's well-being and ability to carry on communication with others, a normal family life, and to comply with treatment and achieve full rehabilitation. Severe and acute forms of distress (often depression and anxiety occur together) and personality disorders interfere with cancer treatment and rehabilitation; they can become central reasons for nonadherence to treatment. The availability today of evidence-based clinical practice guidelines has been a major step forward. Indicators for quality of psychosocial care are being developed that will permit the first opportunity for establishing accountability in terms of how well a rehabilitation center or service adheres to guidelines for management of psychosocial aspects of patient care.

References

1. Holland J. History of psycho-oncology: overcoming attitudinal and conceptual barriers. *Psychosom Med.* 2002;64:206–221.
2. Holland JC; Boettger S. Depression and anxiety. In: *Handbook of Supportive Care in Oncology.* Manhasset, NY: CMP Healthcare Media, Oncology Publishing Group; 2005.
3. Zabora J, BrintzenhofeSzoc K, Curbow B, et al. The prevalence of psychological distress by cancer site. *Psycho-Oncology.* 2001;10:9–28.
4. Holland JC, Anderson B, Breitbart W, et al. The NCCN distress management clinical practice guidelines in oncology. *J NCCN.* 2007;5:66–98.
5. Holland JC, Anderson B, Breitbart W, et al. The NCCN distress management clinical practice guidelines in oncology. *J NCCN.* 2007;5:66–98.
6. APOS Institute for Research and Education. *Quick Reference for Oncology Clinicians: The Psychiatric and Psychological Dimensions of Cancer Symptom Management.* Charlottesville, VA: IPOS Press; 2006.
7. Expected Distress Symptoms, Interventions, Re-Evaluation (DIS-5). Reproduced with permission from the NCCN. v.1. 2007. *The Complete Library of NCCN Clinical Practice Guidelines in Oncology,* v.1.2007 Distress Management. Jenkintown, Pennsylvania: National Comprehensive Cancer Network.
8. Psychosocial Distress Patient Characteristics (DIS-B). Reproduced with permission from the NCCN. v.1. 2007. *The Complete Library of NCCN Clinical Practice Guidelines in Oncology,* v.1.2007 Distress Management. Jenkintown, Pennsylvania: National Comprehensive Cancer Network.
9. Screening Tools for Measuring Distress (DIS-A). Reproduced with permission from the NCCN. v.1. 2007. *The Complete Library of NCCN Clinical Practice Guidelines in Oncology,*

v.1.2007 Distress Management. Jenkintown, Pennsylvania: National Comprehensive Cancer Network.
10. Hoffman B, Zevon M, D'arrigo M, Cecchini T. Screening for distress in cancer patients: the NCCN rapid-screening measure. *Psycho-oncology.* 2004;13:792–799.
11. Akizuki Y, Akechi T, Nakano T, Uchitomi Y. Development of an impact thermometer for use in combination with the distress thermometer as a brief screening tool for adjustment disorders and/or major depression in cancer patients. *J Pain Symptom Manage.* 2005;29(1):91–99.
12. Jacobsen P, Donovan K, Trask P, et al. Screening for psychologic distress in ambulatory cancer patients. *Cancer.* 2004;103(7):1494–1502.
13. Ransom S, Jacobsen P, Booth-Jones M. Validation of the distress thermometer with bone marrow transplant patients. *Psycho-Oncology.* 2006;15(7):604–612.
14. Overview of Evaluation and Treatment Process (DIS-4). Reproduced with permission from the NCCN. v.1. 2007. *The Complete Library of NCCN Clinical Practice Guidelines in Oncology,* v.1.2007 Distress Management. Jenkintown, Pennsylvania: National Comprehensive Cancer Network.
15. Anxiety Disorder (DIS-14). Reproduced with permission from the NCCN. v.1. 2007. *The Complete Library of NCCN Clinical Practice Guidelines in Oncology,* v.1.2007 Distress Management. Jenkintown, Pennsylvania: National Comprehensive Cancer Network.
16. Fricchione G. Clinical practice. Generalized anxiety disorder. *N Engl J Med.* 2004;351(7):675–682.
17. National Breast Cancer Centre and National Cancer Control Initiative. *Clinical Practice Guidelines for the Psychosocial Care of Adults with Cancer.* National Breast Cancer Centre, Camperdown, NSW; 2003.
18. Mood Disorder (DIS-10). Reproduced with permission from the NCCN. v.1. 2007. *The Complete Library of NCCN Clinical Practice Guidelines in Oncology,* v.1.2007 Distress Management. Jenkintown, Pennsylvania: National Comprehensive Cancer Network.
19. Mood Disorder (DIS-11). Reproduced with permission from the NCCN. v.1. 2007. *The Complete Library of NCCN Clinical Practice Guidelines in Oncology,* v.1.2007 Distress Management. Jenkintown, Pennsylvania: National Comprehensive Cancer Network.
20. Cleeland CC, Bennet GJ, Dantzer R, et al. Are the symptoms of cancer and cancer treatment due to a shared biologic mechanism? A cytokine-immunologic model of cancer. *Cancer.* 2003;97:2919–2925.
21. Musselman DL, Miller AH, Porter MR.Higher than normal plasma interleukin-6 concentrations in cancer patients with depression: preliminary findings. *Am J Psychiatry.* 2001;158:1252–1257.
22. Jacobsen P, Donovan Z, Swaine Z, Watson I. Management of anxiety and depression in adult cancer patients: toward an evidence-based approach. In: *Oncology: An Evidence-based Approach.* New York, NY: Springer-Verlag; 2006.
23. Holland J, Alici Evcimen, Y. Common psychiatric problems in elderly patients with cancer. *American Society of Clinical Oncology Educational Book.* 2007:307–311.
24. Feinstein R. Personality traits and disorders. In: Blumenfield MS, ed. *Psychosomatic Medicine.* Philadelphia: Lippincott Williams & Wilkins; 2006:843–865.
25. Management of Personality Disorders (DIS-17). Reproduced with permission from the NCCN. v.1. 2007. *The Complete Library of NCCN Clinical Practice Guidelines in Oncology,* v.1.2007 Distress Management. Jenkintown, Pennsylvania: National Comprehensive Cancer Network.
26. Muskin P. Personality disorders. In: Holland J, ed. *Psycho-Oncology.* New York: Oxford University Press; 1998: 619–629.
27. The National Comprehensive Cancer Network. *Distress Management Clinical Practice Guidelines in Oncology.* NCCN Dis-5. Vol. 1; 2008: Available at http://nccn.org.

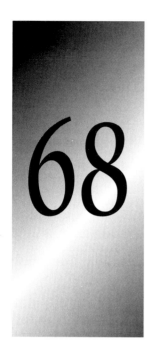

Rehabilitation of the Pediatric Cancer Patient

David William Pruitt
Rajaram Nagarajan

Childhood malignancy accounts for approximately 1% of all cancers diagnosed in the United States each year. Despite the rarity of childhood cancer, approximately 12,400 children and adolescents younger than 20 years will be diagnosed with cancer in the United States (8,700 cases among children 0–14 years of age and 3,800 cases among 15- to 19-year-olds) (1). The incidence of specific cancer diagnoses in the pediatric population varies by age (Fig. 68.1). In children less than 15 years of age, acute lymphoblastic leukemia (ALL) and acute myeloid leukemia (AML) account for 31% of all cancer diagnoses followed by central nervous system (CNS) cancers, which account for 20% of all diagnoses. Together, leukemia and CNS cancers account for one-half of all cancer diagnoses in children less than 15 years of age. In adolescents 15–19 years of age, the distribution of cancer diagnoses is significantly different, with lymphomas (25%), germ cell and gonadal tumors (14%) and carcinomas, and other epithelial tumors (20%) being the most frequently diagnosed cancers.

The overall likelihood of a person developing cancer by the age of 20 is approximately 1 in 300 (1). Survival rates for children 0–14 years of age have improved dramatically since the 1960s, when the overall five-year survival rate after a cancer diagnosis was estimated at 28% (2). Improvements in survival rates continue to improve, with three-year survival rates exceeding 80% and five-year survival rates exceeding 75% for children and adolescents diagnosed with cancer in the 1990s (3). It is estimated that 45,000 long-term survi-

vors exist today; one in 1,000 individuals is a cancer survivor (4,5). However, despite these improvements, childhood cancer remains one of the top four leading causes of disease-related mortality among children (Fig. 68.2) (6).

The type and aggressiveness of the treatment for childhood cancer varies and can include any combination of chemotherapy, surgery, radiation, and biological therapies. Morbidities affecting impairment, activity, or participation can occur as a result of these treatments and location of the cancer. Pediatric rehabilitation is an important component in minimizing the adverse effects and maximizing the return of independence and function in these children and young adults. Specific impairments from different types of cancer and its treatment may have an impact on the child's age-appropriate activity affecting mobility, self-care, communication, cognition, and/or psychological and social function (Table 68.1) (7–9). Goals of pediatric disability management include minimizing the impairment and maximizing activity in age-appropriate life roles of school, recreation, and work. Efforts are directed toward achieving maximum independence despite the disorder, primarily through six categories of intervention strategies to help mitigate disability (10). These include (1) preventing or correcting additional secondary disability, (2) enhancing function in the affected system, (3) enhancing function in unaffected systems, (4) using adaptive equipment to promote function, (5) modifying the social and vocational environment, and

KEY POINTS

- Survival rates for children 0–14 years of age have improved from a five-year 28% rate in the 1960s to more than 75% in the 1990s.
- The most common rehabilitation problems associated with the treatment of acute lymphocytic leukemia (ALL) are peripheral neuropathies and myopathies.
- Moderately vigorous exercise is acceptable when platelet counts are at least 30,000 and low-impact aerobic exercise (but not resistive activities) with counts of 10,000–20,000, but exercise is not recommended with platelet counts less than 10,000.
- For the child in rehabilitation during radiation and/or chemotherapy, the team should monitor for pain, nausea, anorexia, constipation, somnolence, and poor endurance, which can affect rehabilitation prescription and prognosis.

- Hearing loss is associated with cisplatin, with a higher risk in the setting of previous or concomitant cranial irradiation, preexisting hearing loss, decreased renal function, faster infusion rate, use of other ototoxic medications, very young age, and higher cumulative dose, in addition to individual susceptibility.
- Amputation has traditionally been a primary treatment with bone sarcomas, but over time, limb-sparing surgeries were developed, and as a result, amputations are currently performed in only 5%–15% of all cases.
- Among patients with pediatric cancers, the 30-year cumulative incidence of having at least one chronic condition is 73.4%, 39.2% for having more than two chronic conditions, and 42.4% for having a severe or life-threatening condition.

(6) using psychological techniques to enhance patient performance and patient/family education. In pediatric rehabilitation, prescriptions for therapy programs, adaptive equipment, orthoses, and prostheses must be appropriate to the age and the developmental level of the child and include considerations related to ongoing growth and development.

SPECIFIC CHILDHOOD CANCERS AND REHABILITATION ISSUES

Leukemia

Pediatric leukemias are the most common malignancy in childhood, accounting for nearly 30% of diagnoses.

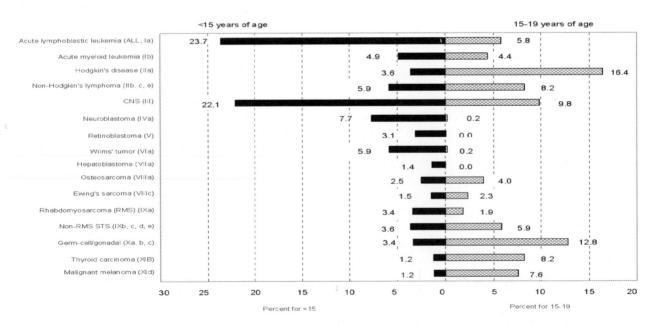

FIGURE 68.1

Distribution of specific cancer diagnoses for children (0 to 14 years) and adolescents (15 to 19 years), 1992 to 2001. Percent distribution by International Classification of Childhood Cancer diagnostic groups and subgroups for younger than 15 years and 15 to 19 years of age (all races and both sexes). CNS, central nervous system; RMS, rhabdomyosarcoma; STS, soft tissue sarcoma. (Incidence date are from the Surveillance, Epidemiology and End Results program, National Cancer Institute. From Ref 3 with permission)

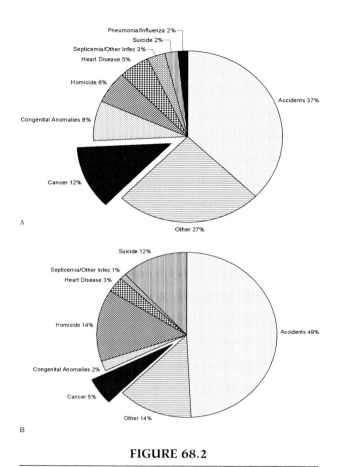

FIGURE 68.2

Leading cause of death in children in the United States, 2001. Causes of death among (A) children 1 to 14 years and (B) adolescents 15 to 19 years of age. (Death data are from the National Center for Health Statistics public use file. From Ref 3 with permission).

Of the two types of leukemia, ALL and AML, ALL is more common (85%). Pediatric ALL is often cited as one of the true success stories of modern medicine, with the cure rate improving from virtually zero prior to the advent of modern chemotherapy (in the 1950s) to current event-free survival rates of approximately 80% (11). In these patients, attention to both short-term and long-term complications from the leukemia and its treatment need to be monitored by the rehabilitation team.

The most common rehabilitation issues developing during ALL therapy relate to peripheral neuropathies and myopathies. Corticosteroid treatment is common during the entire treatment. During certain portions of treatment, corticosteroids are given for a prolonged period (induction and delayed intensification), while during other periods of treatment, patients receive bursts of steroids. Some children may experience resulting symptoms of proximal muscle weakness that is painless and symmetrical in nature. The child may complain of difficulty rising from a chair or ascending stairs due to lower extremity weakness and difficulty

with overhead activities as a result of upper extremity weakness. An electrodiagnostic examination is unlikely to reveal significant abnormalities due to the preferential atrophy of type II fibers that are not evaluated by electromyography (12). The myopathy is usually reversible if the drug is withdrawn or the dose reduced (13). There is no current evidence supporting certain dosages of steroids leading to myopathy, nor is there information related to gene polymorphisms increasing the risk of development of myopathy. Strengthening and endurance exercise can lessen but not eliminate glucocorticoid-induced muscle atrophy and weakness (14). An exercise program should emphasize passive stretching and proper positioning of proximal muscle joints.

The use of vincristine is integral to ALL therapy and is used throughout treatment. It can cause an axonal, sensorimotor polyneuropathy with symptomatology including loss of distal muscle stretch reflexes and paresthesias prior to the onset of focal distal weakness. The weakness may progress to more proximal limbs, but generally recovers with dose reduction or cessation (13). Pain management typically includes neuropathic pain agents, such as gabapentin, initially at a dose of 5 mg/kg/dose and gradually increased to three times per day dosing at 8–35 mg/kg/day (15). Therapy should focus on passive stretching of affected musculature and use of appropriate orthotics to address functional deficits. If the weakness causes foot drop, a custom-molded ankle-foot orthosis should be recommended. A thorough musculoskeletal and neurologic examination is essential in the diagnosis of steroid-induced myopathy and vincristine neuropathy, and communication with the pediatric oncologist is important to see if dose modifications are necessary.

Hematologic abnormalities are frequently seen during the treatment of ALL and can affect the patient's endurance and ability to perform exercise. Pancytopenia can often occur during or shortly following a course of treatment, and monitoring certain indices is important in the management of the child in a therapy program. In general, moderately vigorous exercise can be pursued when platelet counts are at least 30,000–50,000, and low-impact aerobic, but not resistive, activities can be considered with counts of 10,000–20,000 (16). Exercise is not recommended for those with platelet counts lower than 10,000 (17). It has also been suggested that exercise be discontinued with a hemoglobin less than 7.5 g (16). Additionally, one must be mindful of a patient's susceptibility to infection due to the leukemia and leukopenia from treatment.

Cardiotoxicity of antineoplastic agents, such as the anthracyclines, and cardiac irradiation can also impair functional performance of the child and affect rehabilitative plans. Acute cardiac toxicity is rarely

TABLE 68.1

Impact of Anticancer Therapies on Function

TREATMENT	PATHOPHYSIOLOGY	IMPAIRMENT	DISABILITY	QUALIFIERS
Surgical resection	Unclear	Deficits dependent on location and extent of surgery, age, and tumor type	Functional limitations related to areas of deficit	
Posterior fossa surgery	Unclear	Cerebellar mutism. May see high-level linguistic and cognitive deficits	Limited verbal communication, may affect social skills and school performance	
Cranial irradiation	Neural/glial degeneration. Gliosis. Proliferative/sclerosing angiopathy. Demyelination	Cognitive dysfunction: learning disabilities; ↓ memory; attention problems; language deficits; ↓ executive function; ↓ verbal and performance IQ	↓ academic potential. ↓ communication skills: language disorder/delay; may affect behavior, social competence, and vocational potential	Impact related to dose and volume of CNS irradiated and inversely related to age of child at time of exposure. Effects potentiated by IT or high-dose intravenous methotrexate
	Ischemic events related to cerebral vasculopathy. Progressive, necrotizing leukoencephalopathy	Functional deficits related to location and extent of ischemia	Potential for marked functional impairments in all affected areas, including dementia, dysarthria, ataxia and/or spasticity	Rehabilitation managed as in stroke. Usually seen when treatment has included methotrexate
	Negative impact on GHRH when posterior fossa involved	Short stature	May affect self-image, social competence	Cosmesis included in problem list for adolescents
Spinal irradiation	May cause radiation myelitis	Spastic quadriplegia or paraplegia	Functional impairments in mobility and ADLs dependent on level of injury	Management as in spinal cord injury
		Neurogenic bowel and bladder	May require special program for evacuation of bladder and bowel	Cosmesis of particular psycho-social impact for adolescents
	Failure of vertebral growth	Short stature, increased risk of scoliosis or kyphosis	Potential altered self-image and ↓ social competence	

(Continued)

TABLE 68.1

Impact of Anticancer Therapies on Function Continued

TREATMENT	PATHOPHYSIOLOGY	IMPAIRMENT	DISABILITY	QUALIFIERS
Mediastinal irradiation	Vascular damage, fibrosis	Pulmonary fibrosis Pneumonitis	Disability dependent on degree of restrictive lung changes and can significantly limit ADLs, exercise tolerance when severe	Decrease in radiation-induced late pulmonary toxicity seen over last decade due to refinements in radiation therapy
	In very young, possible interference with both lung and chest wall growth	Decreases in lung volume, compliance, and CO_2 diffusing capacity		
	Fibrosis of the parietal pericardium (most common), intimal proliferation of myofibroblasts, collagen, and lipid accumulation	Constrictive pericarditis, myocardial damage (rare), conduction system defects, coronary artery disease	Functional limitations related to degree of cardiac dysfunction	
Methotrexate	Neurotoxicity, including acute, strokelike encephalopathy, chronic leukoencephalopathy (progressive demyelinating encephalopathy)	Cognitive impairment, developmental delay, learning problems, potential motor impairment with deficits in coordination and high-level skills	May affect school performance, ↓ age-appropriate ADL independence; may limit participation in athletics, team sports; affect self-esteem and social competence	Neurotoxicity potentiated by cranial irradiation Alert parents to monitor for school problems developing in upper grades when ↑ independence and efficiency required
	Osteopathy	With intrathecal dosing, can see ascending radiculopathy, similar to GBS	Loss of motor function with consequent mobility and ADL deficits dependent on extent of weakness	
		Osteoporosis/ increased risk of pathologic fractures, bone pain	Limitations in mobility and ADLs related to areas involved	Toxicity cumulative
Corticosteroids	Preferential atrophy of type 2 muscle fibers	Myopathy	Decreased mobility related to proximal muscle weakness Increased risk of pathological fracture	Reversible when drug withdrawn or dose reduced
		Osteoporosis avascular necrosis Growth failure	Hip pain, gait abnormality Affects self-esteem and social competence	↑ risk for osteonecrosis of weight bearing joints in children when ↑ doses used

(Continued)

VII GENERAL TOPICS IN CANCER REHABILITATION

TABLE 68.1

Impact of Anticancer Therapies on Function Continued

TREATMENT	PATHOPHYSIOLOGY	IMPAIRMENT	DISABILITY	QUALIFIERS
Vincristine/vinblastine	Axonal sensorimotor polyneuropathy		Paresthesias, neuritic pain, distal weakness, which may impair hand function and cause foot drop and walking difficulty	Neurotoxicty more prominent in presence of CMT Usually recovers with end of therapy or ↓ dose Neurotoxicity usually minimal with vinblastine
	Impairment of efferent and afferent pathways from the sacral spinal cord, autonomic neuropathy	Impaired rectal emptying	Constipation, which may alter ADLs and comfort	
Anthracycline (doxorubicin, daunorubicin)		Can cause arrhythmias, conduction abnormalities, decreased left ventricular function, chronic cardiomyopathy	Diminished capacity to perform age-appropriate ADLs, decreased endurance, decreased exercise tolerance, limited ability to participate in sports, may affect self-esteem and social competence	Potentiates radiation reactions Increased toxicity with lower age
Cisplatin	Injury to hair cells of the organ of Corti	High-frequency sensorineural hearing loss Tinnitis	Affects communication skills and potentially speech/language development in the young child; may affect social competence	Ototoxic and neurotoxic effects are cumulative
		Reversible sensory peripheral neuropathy	Paresthesias/neuritic pain may interfere with ADLs, comfort	Symptoms may progress after discontinuation
Carboplatin	Minor or absent loss of hair cells of the organ of Corti	High-frequency sensorineural hearing loss	Affects communication skills and potentially speech/language development in the young child; may affect social competence	Effects are cumulative Ototoxicity and nephrotoxicity milder than cisplatin
Cyclophosphamide/ Ifosfamide		Reversible neurotoxicity with somnolence, disorientation, lethargy, hallucinations	Negative impact on ability to perform age-appropriate ADLs	Risk of neurotoxicity increased with prior use of high-dose cisplatin. Reversible or preventable with methylene blue
	Can cause hemorrhagic cystitis secondary to urotoxic metabolite acrolein	Potential loss of renal function		Occurrence decreased by use of MESNA

Abbreviations: ADLs, activities of daily living; CMT, Charcot-Marie-Tooth Disease; GBS, Guillain-Barrè syndrome; GHRH, growth hormone releasing hormone; IT, intrathecal.
Source: From Ref. 9, with permission.

seen. Most cardiotoxicity is seen late and is dependent on multiple factors, such as age at exposure and the amount of exposure. Children receiving cardiotoxic treatments will have a baseline echocardiogram and will have regularly scheduled cardiac follow-up. Knowledge of any cardiac issues is important in recommending safe exercise precautions (18). Echocardiogram and electrocardiogram (ECG) recommendations are made based on anthracycline exposure, radiation exposure, and the age at exposure. If the echocardiogram demonstrates low ejection fraction, recommendations for only low aerobic exercise activity have been recommended (19). If there is presence of recent premature ventricular contractions, atrial or ventricular arrhythmias, or any evidence or concern for ischemic patterns, exercise should be avoided and consultation with a pediatric cardiologist for further recommendations on the exercise program should be pursued (19,20).

There are short-term and long-term effects of childhood ALL treatment on the skeletal system, which can include osteopenia, osteoporosis, avascular necrosis (AVN), and spinal deformities. These may be caused by steroids, methotrexate, and craniospinal irradiation. Some data suggest that bone density may increase one year following treatment of ALL but that the risk of fracture remains high, suggesting that changes in bone architecture not accessible by dual energy x-ray absorptiometry (DEXA) scans may be relevant (21). AVN, with an incidence of 5% in childhood ALL, is part of the spectrum of decreased bone density and usually develops during therapy, although it has a latency period as long as 13 years after treatment. The treatment risk factors leading to AVN are corticosteroid treatment and radiation therapy. The incidence in retrospective studies has revealed a higher incidence in older children (10–20 years) and in females (22–24). Dexamethasone appears to have both a more potent antileukemic effect and more bone toxicity than equivalent doses of prednisone (25). Increased cumulative exposure conveys increased risk (26). AVN may be asymptomatic, but may also cause severe pain, joint swelling, limited range of motion, and ultimately joint damage and articulate collapse (23,27). AVN most commonly affects the femoral heads, where it may be accompanied by slipped capital femoral epiphysis, but it can occur in many joints and is typically multifocal. Evaluation of AVN should include participation of a pediatric orthopedic surgeon to determine necessity of surgical intervention, as potential for collapse of femoral head must be considered. Nonoperative treatments include nonsteroidal anti-inflammatory medications and physical therapy services (28).

The prevalence of obesity after therapy for ALL is 16%–56% and is caused by cranial irradiation, steroid therapy, physical inactivity, and increased dietary intake (29). Other risk factors are age of less than four years at treatment, female gender, and associated medical conditions, including hypothyroidism and familial dyslipidemias (30). In adult survivors of childhood ALL, cranial irradiation at >20 Gy has been associated with obesity, particularly in girls who were treated at 0–4 years of age (31). Chemotherapy without cranial irradiation may also lead to obesity in survivors of childhood ALL. Obesity developing during adolescence or young adulthood is strongly related with several common adult health problems, including adult-onset diabetes mellitus, hypertension, dyslipidemia, and cardiovascular disease (30). Initiation and maintenance of participation in activity-based leisure activities and exercise programs throughout and following treatments can assist in weight loss and associated comorbidities.

With regard to neurocognitive late effects of antileukemic therapy, the greatest risk occurs in those children who receive CNS irradiation or intrathecal (IT) chemotherapy. Despite early reports suggesting that CNS preventive therapy with lower-dose cranial irradiation and IT chemotherapy was devoid of significant side effects, a large body of evidence indicates that this treatment may produce abnormal brain scans, impaired intellectual and psychomotor functions, and neuroendocrine abnormalities (32–34). The incidence of these abnormalities appears to correlate with the intensity of CNS preventive therapy (34). The observation that computed tomography (CT) scan lesions may first appear as late as seven to nine years after initiation of therapy emphasizes the importance of long-term follow-up. This should include neuropsychological testing to permit early identification of deficits and allow for therapeutic intervention. Involvement of speech and language pathology therapists and occupational therapists is essential in assisting the child or adolescent with strategies to improve cognitive function in those with deficits found through testing. In addition, school reentry personnel should be available to assist the child, parents, and educators in coordinating an Individualized Education Plan to provide an optimal educational environment.

CENTRAL NERVOUS SYSTEM TUMORS

Intracranial tumors represent the second most common type of childhood cancer. During the first two years of life, supratentorial tumors predominate, whereas infratentorial lesions are more common through the rest of the decade. Supratentorial tumors again predominate in late adolescence and into adulthood. There are certain tumors of embryonal histology, including medulloblastoma and supratentorial primitive neuroectodermal tumors, that occur almost exclusively in children and young adults. High-grade gliomas, including glioblastoma multiforme, are much less common in children than adults (35).

For most childhood brain tumors, treatment modalities typically involve surgical resection, which is then followed by radiation and/or chemotherapy, depending on the diagnosis and extent of surgical resection. Each treatment modality may be associated with both transient and long-term effects, which may have an effect on duration of survival, functional outcome, and quality of life (36) (Table 68.1). Despite the significantly decreased surgical morbidity due to improvements in surgery, anesthesia, and postoperative care, surgical resections may be associated with significant neurological morbidity related to the age and preoperative clinical status of the child, type of tumor, location, and extent of resection (37).

Although the introduction of radiation therapy has made significant improvements in the duration of survival in a number of CNS tumors, it has significant morbidity as well. The extent of radiation-induced injury or leukoencephalopathy is directly related to the site, dose, and volume of the CNS irradiated, as well as the age of the child. Histologic changes in the brain following cranial irradiation may include neuronal dropout, gliosis, and proliferative and sclerosing angiopathy (38). Children treated before four or five years of age are at a higher risk for cognitive impairment in comparison to older children (39). The deleterious effects can have a major impact on intellectual and academic performance, social competence, behavior, and vocational potential (9). A mean IQ loss of 27 points has been demonstrated two years following cranial irradiation in children less than seven years old, while no significant difference was seen in the performance of older children at reevaluation (40). Deficits have included significant impairment in verbal and performance IQ, perceptual motor skills, language development, and attention/executive skills in those children who received cranial irradiation compared to nonirradiated children (41). In addition, radiation myelitis with spastic paraplegia or quadriplegia may result from spinal cord irradiation. Scoliosis and kyphosis can result from radiation to the vertebrae in young children. Delayed effects from chemotherapy, including peripheral neuropathies, myopathies, and hearing loss, in addition to leukoencephalopathy, are all areas of focus that the pediatric rehabilitation medicine specialist can address.

For the child who is receiving rehabilitation services while undergoing radiation and/or chemotherapy, attention must be paid to treatment-related symptoms, such as pain, nausea, anorexia, constipation, somnolence, and poor endurance, which can affect rehabilitation prescription and prognosis. Strategies to assist in these symptoms, including medications, counseling, and relaxation techniques, when appropriate, may be facilitated through recommendations from the rehabilitation specialist.

Motor deficits are common in CNS tumors as a result of tumor location and its treatment. Common sequelae from treatment include peripheral neuropathies, resulting in focal motor deficits such as foot drop from a peroneal neuropathy, commonly seen with vincristine therapy. Proximal motor weakness resulting from steroid myopathy is also commonly seen in this population. Delays in attaining or regressing from age-appropriate gross or fine motor milestones may be the first insight into treatment sequelae or late effects from chemotherapy in children who are diagnosed and treated at a very young age. Communication with the neuro-oncologist when these diagnoses are suspected is essential in the treatment decision process and may include modifications of therapy. Physical or occupational therapy assessments and recommendations are also important to address strengthening, mobility, and fine motor deficits. Communication with the therapists during treatment is essential in optimization of the treatment plan and recognition of any new symptomatology. Recommendations for orthotic fitting to address gait impairment and reduction of difficulties with mobility and endurance deficits are also initiated by the rehabilitation specialist.

Sensory deficits, including visual impairment and hearing deficits, may also be an issue due to a combination of tumor location, as well as due to medical interventions. Thorough ophthalmologic assessment should be completed and visual function monitored as part of the rehabilitation plan. Visual loss, visual field deficits, gaze palsies, and involuntary ocular movements may all impair vision and result in functional impairment. Elevation in intracranial pressure may affect visual function as well, and thus visual changes may be the presenting symptom of the disease itself or of disease progression in CNS tumors. The occupational therapist can address compensatory strategies for visual deficits in addition to addressing visual-motor and visual-perceptual deficits. A low-vision specialist should also be consulted as part of the rehabilitation plan when visual impairments are affecting function. School services, including provisions to an Individualized Education Plan, need to be implemented to ensure successful academic functioning.

Hearing loss due to chemotherapeutic agents, most commonly cisplatin and carboplatin, must also be monitored by the rehabilitation team. Factors associated with a higher risk of cisplatin toxicity include previous or concomitant cranial irradiation, preexisting hearing loss, decreased renal function, faster infusion rate, use of other ototoxic medications, very young age, and higher cumulative dose, in addition to individual susceptibility (42). Irradiation is associated with a relatively late, pronounced, typically unilateral sensorineural hearing loss that occurs in 10%–15% of children after doses of more than 50–54 Gy (35). Baseline audiologic evaluations need to be obtained prior to initiation of chemotherapy, and regular reevaluation should occur at intervals determined by the treatment plan. Interventions such as a hearing aid, use of an auditory trainer, or instruction in sign language can assist with improved independent functioning.

Oral motor dysfunction, seen in posterior fossa tumors, is a result of involvement of the lower cranial nerves. Clinical evaluation of the swallowing mechanism through bedside swallow examination or in a videofluoroscopic evaluation when warranted by a speech pathologist is recommended to ensure that the child can be fed safely. It is critical to recognize that silent aspiration is a common finding with bulbar dysfunction, especially in the presence of pharyngeal sensory deficits (9).

Cognitive deficits, related to cranial irradiation as well as to tumor location, especially in hemispheric and supratentorial midline tumors, must also be monitored as part of the rehabilitation plan. Neuropsychological testing as well as interventional school specialists should be instituted so that an optimal education plan can be instituted. Children younger than three years of age should be enrolled into an early intervention program to evaluate and encourage developmental milestone achievements through appropriate therapies and parental education. Educational interventions have been associated with improvements in spelling and reading, particularly when written feedback was provided to parents and schools, even years after therapy (43). Vocational services to address the transition from secondary school services are also an important intervention to assist with the transition to further education or employment opportunities.

BONE SARCOMAS

Bone sarcomas account for 6% of all pediatric cancers. This represents about 650–700 new cases per year in children under the age of 21, with the most common bone sarcoma diagnoses being osteosarcoma (60%) and Ewing sarcoma (33%). The majority of bone sarcomas are diagnosed during adolescence, with a peak age of 15 years, but the age of peak incidence varies by gender. In males, the peak incidence occurs between 15 and 17 years, and for females, the peak age is 13 years. This corresponds to the gender-specific adolescent growth spurts. In terms of site of disease, the most common are the distal femur, proximal tibia, and

proximal humerus. Overall, two-thirds of the patients have the primary lesion in the lower extremity and pelvis (2,44).

The therapy for bone sarcomas is rather extensive and is dependent on the type of bone sarcoma and stage of disease, so it is important to establish an accurate diagnosis. Generally, this is made by a bone biopsy. Once the diagnosis is established and staging complete, therapy can begin. For the most common types of bone sarcoma in children, neoadjuvant chemotherapy is used for approximately two to three months, followed by local control surgery with removal of the primary site of disease. Following surgery, postoperative chemotherapy is given. Depending on the diagnosis and site of disease, additional surgeries and sometimes radiation therapy are needed if there are other sites of disease (44,45).

Local surgical control is an integral part of the treatment of bone sarcomas, but it can carry with it a significant impact on the patient. In the past, amputation was the treatment of choice, as the majority of tumors occurred most frequently in the lower extremity. Tumors at other sites involved a wide resection. Over time, limb-sparing surgeries were developed under the premise that patients with a limb-sparing surgery would have improved function and quality of life. As a result, amputations are currently performed in only 5%–15% of all cases. Limb-sparing surgery technique varies, depending on the clinical scenario, surgeon's expertise, size and site of the reconstruction, and patient's age. The variations of limb-sparing surgery include an endoprosthetic reconstruction, allograft reconstruction, a composite endoprosthetic allograft reconstruction, and arthrodesis (44). Physical maturity is an important consideration in deciding the type of surgical procedure, especially if the sarcoma involves a growth plate. If there is significant growth potential, the surgical options include an expanding endoprostheses, rotationplasty reconstruction, or an amputation.

Following surgery, activity restrictions exist and vary by surgeon and the type and size of the reconstruction. After surgery, it is important for the patient to start appropriate rehabilitation and physical therapy, after orthopedic approval, in order to develop and maintain function, strength, and range of motion. The concerns for poor muscle strength and eventual contracture development and subsequent extremity disuse and impaired mobility are issues that the rehabilitation team must be involved in. Appropriate pain control, both acute and chronic, also needs to be addressed, as this can hinder the survivor's participation and compliance with treatment plans.

Rehabilitation management following amputation includes initial skin management and eventual soft dressings for the promotion of wound healing and edema control. Therapies initially focus on preprosthetic training, with goals of maintenance of range of motion in joints proximal to the amputation, strengthening the gluteus medius and maximus, as well as mobility and transfer training using a mobility device if needed prior to prosthetic fit. Following prosthetic fitting, gait and balance training with the prosthesis on all surfaces and training on proper donning and doffing of prosthesis, as well as skin care, is important. Monitoring for complications of amputations, including bony overgrowth, leg length discrepancy, and prosthetic device malfunction, in addition to skin breakdown related to prosthetic wear, is an important role of the rehabilitation team.

Rehabilitation following limb-sparing procedures is more difficult than that following amputation and is dependent on the type of procedure and size and extent of the surgery. Early and more aggressive rehabilitation programs result in better outcomes (46). Exercise regimens can often start one to –two days postoperatively (46,47). Standing may be appropriate within a week after endoprosthetic replacement surgery, unless a muscle flap was performed (47). Gradual weight bearing using two crutches may be possible two weeks after surgery, with progression to full weight bearing after a few months (46). For patients with total or proximal femur replacements, bed rest with hip abduction for two to four weeks, followed by hip abduction bracing for three months, may be recommended (48). Children and adolescents who undergo allograft reconstruction typically have prolonged non-weight-bearing restrictions to assure optimal healing of the donor allograft and native bone. Often, the surgeon may wait months before partial weight bearing in the affected extremity is allowed.

Almost 50% of children who have resection of primary bone tumors with expandable endoprosthetic replacement will not require use of an orthosis or gait assistive device (47). Unassisted ambulation is more likely if the quadriceps mechanism is preserved, either following expandable endoprosthetic replacement or after prosthetic knee replacement following distal femur bone tumor resection (47,49). Rehabilitative needs of children who undergo limb-sparing surgery or amputation include early mobilization, gait training, and continued monitoring to ensure active participation.

Complications following limb-sparing surgery do occur and are problematic (50). Complications are divided into two periods: early and late. Early complications are most often related to wound healing and are seen after both amputations and limb-sparing procedures. Late complications vary between amputations (residual limb problems, phantom pain, bony overgrowth, etc.) and different types of limb-sparing

surgery (nonunion, implant breakage, infection, etc.). Complications can lead to delays in chemotherapy, multiple surgical revisions or replacements over time, and chronic pain. The frequency of complications is reported to be higher following limb-sparing surgery, particularly in the long-term, but as techniques and materials improve, the frequency is likely to decrease. Given the longer expected life spans of childhood cancer survivors and the incidence of surgical complications following limb-sparing surgery, it is important that appropriate rehabilitative services are available to assess and make recommendations on these additional issues that arise following the initial surgery.

The chemotherapy involved in bone sarcomas is extensive and can have long-term side-effects in the survivors. These late effects of therapy are varied and include cardiac dysfunction, secondary malignancies, and fertility issues (Table 68.1). The development of these late effects is often variable and is dependent on treatment-related factors (type and schedule of chemotherapies), disease-related factors (site and size of the sarcoma), and host genetic predisposition (e.g., how a patient metabolizes chemotherapy). Acute complications (nausea, fatigue, neuropathies, anemia) also occur and can lead to decreased physical activity. These, in combination with any bed rest or non-weight-bearing requirements due to the surgery, can lead to rapid deconditioning and impairments in activities of daily life. Therefore, the child's clinician must be watchful for opportunities to intervene to improve conditioning, strength, and range of motion.

Several studies from the Childhood Cancer Survivor Study (CCSS) have looked at the long-term outcomes of childhood cancer survivors. The CCSS is the largest cohort of childhood cancer survivors assembled, with more than 14,000 members. Participants are five or more years from diagnosis (>1,000 with a bone sarcoma) diagnosed between 1970 and 1986 at one of 26 collaborating institutions (51). In particular, one study looked at chronic health conditions as graded by the Common Terminology Criteria for Adverse Events (version 3). The estimated 30-year cumulative incidence of having at least one chronic condition was 73.4%, 39.2% for having more than two chronic conditions, and 42.4% for having a severe or life-threatening condition. Overall, bone tumor survivors were among the highest at risk (including brain tumor and Hodgkin survivors) for developing a chronic health condition and multiple conditions (52). They were also at elevated risk for having a severe condition, but this may be due to the relatively high number of amputations performed during the treatment timeframe. Another study from the CCSS assessed the health status of childhood cancer survivors, including general health, mental health, functional impairment, activity limitations, pain, and anxiety. Bone sarcoma survivors were more likely to report adverse health outcomes in all domains, except mental health, when compared to leukemia survivors. Functional limitations, activity status, and pain as a result of cancer or its treatment were most affected (52). A third study focused primarily on physical performance and daily activities and found that one-third of survivors of bone sarcomas reported physical limitations and 11% reported that poor health restricted their ability to attend work or school. Overall, bone sarcoma survivors were again among the most likely to report performance limitations, restricted ability to do routine activities, and restricted ability to attend work or school (53). Of note, a fourth study looked at self-reported quality of life and function of survivors of a lower extremity or pelvic bone sarcoma and had relatively good quality of life and function, but certain subgroups were at risk (54). Although the bone sarcoma survivors were treated in an earlier era, which may not reflect current management and surgical techniques, these studies are important in demonstrating the need for long-term assessments to assist with maximizing functional outcome.

OTHER SOLID TUMORS

Other common solid tumors in the pediatric population include neuroblastoma (7%) and rhabdomyosarcoma (3%) (55,56). Neuroblastomas demonstrate a spectrum of biological behavior, from spontaneous regression to tumor activity requiring substantial amounts of therapy, including chemotherapy, radiation therapy, surgery, and bone marrow transplant. Unfortunately, the majority of patients with neuroblastoma present with high-risk disease and require extensive treatment. Although neuroblastoma primarily presents in the abdomen, it can present anywhere within the sympathetic nervous system and can be widely metastatic. Rhabdomyosarcoma can also require substantial therapy, including chemotherapy, radiation therapy, and surgery. It is most commonly found in the connective tissue and muscle, with the most common sites being the extremities, head and neck, and genitourinary tracts. As with other cancers, the acute effects of chemotherapy used for both neuroblastoma and rhabdomyosarcoma can be significant and lead to deconditioning and neuropathies. Surgery- and radiation-related impairments are also possible, but vary depending on the site of intervention (abdomen and bladder/prostate surgery and reconstruction, head and neck irradiation). Individualized evaluation of impairment and disability as a result of tumor or treatment is essential in the care of these patients, and long-term follow-up is essential for maximizing functional outcomes.

CONCLUSION

The involvement of pediatric rehabilitation medicine in the care of patients with oncological diagnosis is important, both acutely, during the treatment phases of most diagnoses, and during long-term follow-up in order to assist in the diagnosis of treatment-related complications that affect areas of independent functioning in the home, school, or work environment. Appropriate assessment of these patients, including evaluations in the areas of impairment, subsequent disability, and levels of participation, is the focus of the pediatric rehabilitation medicine specialist. The role of the pediatric rehabilitation medicine specialist can include identification of appropriate treatment modalities, such as exercise recommendations and precautions, referrals to therapy, and neuropsychological testing, in addition to working with school intervention coordinators towards achieving appropriate educational services. Optimal independent functioning in areas of mobility, activities of daily living, communication, cognition, and participation throughout and following treatment is the overall goal of pediatric rehabilitation.

References

1. Ries LA, Percy CL, Bunin GR. Introduction-SEER pediatric monograph. In: Ries LA, Smith M, Gurney JG, et al., eds. *Cancer Incidence and Survival among Children and Adolescents: United States SEER Program 1975–1995*. Bethesda, MD: National Cancer Institute, SEER Program, NIH; 1999:1–15.
2. Ries LA, Smith M, Gurney JG, et al., eds. *Cancer Incidence and Survival among Children and Adolescents: United States SEER Program 1975–1995*. Bethesda, MD: National Cancer Institute, SEER Program, NIH; 1999.
3. Gurney JG, Bondy ML. Epidemiology of childhood cancer. In: Pizzo PA, Poplack DG, eds. *Principles and Practice of Pediatric Oncology*. Philadelphia: Lippincott Williams and Wilkins; 2006:1–13.
4. Herold AH, Roetzheim RG. Cancer survivors. *Prim Care: Clinics in Office Practice*. 1992;19(4):779–791.
5. Peckham VC. Learning disabilities in long-term survivors of childhood cancer: concerns for parents and teachers. *Int Disabil Stud*. 1991;13(4):141–145.
6. Minino AM, Heron MP, Smith BL. *Deaths: Preliminary Data for 2004*. National Center for Health Statistics 2006;Vital Health Stat Series No. 19(54).
7. Balis FM, Holcenberg JS, Blaney SM. General principles of chemotherapy. In: Pizzo PA, Poplack DG, eds. *Principles and Practice of Pediatric Oncology*, 4th ed. Philadelphia: Lippincott Williams & Wilkins; 2002:237–308.
8. Dreyer ZE, Blatt J, Bleyer A. Late effects of childhood cancer and its treatment. In: Pizzo PA, Poplack DG, eds. *Principles and Practice of Pediatric Oncology*, 4th ed. Philadelphia: Lippincott Williams & Wilkins; 2002:1431–1461.
9. Michaud LJ. Ried SR, McMahon MA, Pruitt DW. Rehabilitation of the child with cancer. In: Pizzo PA, Poplack DG, eds. *Principles and Practice of Pediatric Oncology*, 5th ed. Philadelphia: Lippincott Williams & Wilkins; 2006:1399–1413.
10. Delisa JA, Currie DM, Martin GM. Rehabilitation medicine: past, present, and future. In: Delisa JA, Gans B, eds. *Rehabilita-

tion Medicine: Principles and Practice. Philadelphia: Lippincott-Raven; 1998:3–32.

11. Margolin JF, Steuber CP, Poplack DG. Acute lymphoblastic leukemia. In: Pizzo PA, Poplack DG, eds. *Principles and Practice of Pediatric Oncology*, 5th ed. Philadelphia: Lippincott Williams & Wilkins; 2006:538–590.

12. Dumitru D. *Electrodiagnostic Medicine*. Philadelphia: Hanley & Belfus; 1995.

13. Stubgen JP. Neuromuscular disorders in systemic malignancy and its treatment. *Muscle Nerve*. 1995;18(6):636–648.

14. Sliwa JA. Acute weakness syndromes in the critically ill patient. *Arch Phys Med Rehabil*. 2000;81(3 Suppl 1):S45–S52.

15. Galloway KS, Yaster M. Pain and symptom control in terminally ill children. *Pediatr Clin North Am*. 2000;47(3):711–746.

16. Gerber LH, Vargo M. Rehabilitation for patients with cancer diagnoses. In: Delisa JA, Gans B, eds. *Rehabilitation Medicine: Principles and Practice*, 3rd ed. Philadelphia: Lippincott-Raven; 1998:1293–1317.

17. James MC. Physical therapy for patients after bone marrow transplantation. *Phys Ther*. 1987;67(6):946–952.

18. Dickerman JD. The late effects of childhood cancer therapy. *Pediatrics*. 2007;119(3):554–568.

19. Gerber L. Rehabilitation of the cancer patient. In: Devita H, Hellman S, Rosenberg SA, eds. *Cancer: Principles and Practice of Oncology*. Philadelphia: Lippincott-Raven Publishers; 1997.

20. Nori SL, Magill D. Rehabilitation. In: Keating RF, Goodrich JT, Packer RJ, eds. *Tumors of the Pediatric Central Nervous System*. New York: Thieme Medical Publishers; 2001:502–510.

21. van der Sluis IM, de Muinck Keizer-Schrama SM, van den Heuvel-Eibrink MM. Bone mineral density in childhood acute lymphoblastic leukemia (ALL) during and after treatment. *Pediatr Blood Cancer*. 2004;43(2):182–183; discussion 4.

22. Arico M, Boccalatte MF, Silvestri D, et al. Osteonecrosis: an emerging complication of intensive chemotherapy for childhood acute lymphoblastic leukemia. *Haematologica*. 2003;88(7):747–753.

23. Burger B, Beier R, Zimmermann M, Beck JD, Reiter A, Schrappe M. Osteonecrosis: a treatment related toxicity in childhood acute lymphoblastic leukemia (ALL)—experiences from trial ALL-BFM 95. *Pediatr Blood Cancer*. 2005;44(3):220–225.

24. Mattano LA, Jr., Sather HN, Trigg ME, Nachman JB. Osteonecrosis as a complication of treating acute lymphoblastic leukemia in children: a report from the Children's Cancer Group. *J Clin Oncol*. 2000;18(18):3262–3272.

25. Ito C, Evans WE, McNinch L, et al. Comparative cytotoxicity of dexamethasone and prednisolone in childhood acute lymphoblastic leukemia. *J Clin Oncol*. 1996;14(8):2370–2376.

26. Halton JM, Wu B, Atkinson SA, et al. Comparative skeletal toxicity of dexamethasone and prednisone in childhood acute lymphoblastic leukemia. *J Pediatr Hematol Oncol*. 2000; 22(369).

27. Ojala AE, Paakko E, Lanning FP, Lanning M. Osteonecrosis during the treatment of childhood acute lymphoblastic leukemia: a prospective MRI study. *Med Pediatr Oncol*. 1999;32(1):11–17.

28. Crawford A. Orthopedics. In: Rudolph CD, Rudolph AM, Hostetter MK, Lister GE, Siegel NJ., eds. *Rudolph's Pediatrics*. 21st ed. New York: McGraw-Hill; 2003:2419–2458.

29. Gregory JW, Reilly JJ. Body composition and obesity. In: Wallace WH, Green DM, eds. *Late Effects of Childhood Cancer*. London, United Kingdom: Arnold; 2004:147–161.

30. Bhatia S, Landier W, Robison L. Late effects of childhood cancer therapy. In: DeVita V, Hellman S, Rosenberg S, eds. *Progress in Oncology 2002*. Sudbury, MA: Jones and Bartlett Publications; 2003:171–201.

31. Oeffinger KC, Mertens AC, Sklar CA, et al. Obesity in adult survivors of childhood acute lymphoblastic leukemia: a report from the Childhood Cancer Survivor Study. *J Clin Oncol*. 2003;21:1359–1365.

32. Brouwers P, Riccardi R, Fedio P, Poplack DG. Long-term neuropsychologic sequelae of childhood leukemia: correlation with CT brain scan abnormalities. *J Pediatr*. 1985;106(5):723–728.

33. Ochs J. Neurotoxicity due to central nervous system therapy for childhood leukemia. *Am J Pediatr Hematol Oncol*. 1989;11:93–105.

34. Ochs J, Mulhern R, Fairclough D, et al. Comparison of neuropsychological functioning and clinical indicators of neurotoxicity in long-term survivors of childhood leukemia given cranial radiation or parenteral methotrexate: a prospective study. *J Clin Oncol*. 1991;9:145–151.

35. Blaney SM, Kun LE, Hunter J et al. Tumors of the central nervous system. In: Pizzo PA, Poplack DG, eds. *Principles and Practice of Pediatric Oncology*, 5th ed. Philadelphia: Lippincott Williams & Wilkins; 2006:786–864.

36. Siffert J, Greenleaf M, Mannis R, Allen J. Pediatric brain tumors. *Child Adolesc Psychiatr Clin N Am*. 1999;8(4):879–903.

37. Packer RJ. Childhood medulloblastoma: progress and future challenges. *Brain Dev*. 1999;21(2):75–81.

38. Poussaint TY, Siffert J, Barnes PD, et al. Hemorrhagic vasculopathy after treatment of central nervous system neoplasia in childhood: diagnosis and follow-up. *Am J Neuroradiol*. 1995;16(4):693–699.

39. Duffner PK, Cohen ME, Anderson SW, et al. Long-term effects of treatment on endocrine function in children with brain tumors. *Ann Neurol*. 1983;14(5):528–532.

40. Radcliffe J, Packer RJ, Atkins TE, et al. Three- and four-year cognitive outcome in children with noncortical brain tumors treated with whole-brain radiotherapy. *Ann Neurol*. 1992;32(4):551–554.

41. Copeland DR, deMoor C, Moore BD, 3rd, Ater JL. Neurocognitive development of children after a cerebellar tumor in infancy: a longitudinal study. *J Clin Oncol*. 1999;17(11):3476–3486.

42. Freilich RJ, Kraus DH, Budnick AS, Bayer LA, Finlay JL. Hearing loss in children with brain tumors treated with cisplatin and carboplatin-based high-dose chemotherapy with autologous bone marrow rescue. *Med Pediatr Oncol*. 1996;26(2):95–100.

43. Anderson VA, Godber T, Smibert E, Weiskop S, Ekert H. Cognitive and academic outcome following cranial irradiation and chemotherapy in children: a longitudinal study. *Br J Cancer*. 2000;82(2):255–262.

44. Link M, Gebhardt M, Meyers P. Osteosarcoma. In: Pizzo PA, Poplack DG, eds. *Principles and Practice of Pediatric Oncology*, 4th ed. Philadelphia: Lipincott Williams & Wilkins; 2002:1051–1089.

45. Ginsberg S, Woo S, Johnson M, Hicks M, Horowitz M. Ewing's sarcoma family of tumors: Ewing's sarcoma of bone and soft tissue and the peripheral primitive neuroectodermal tumors. In: Pizzo PA, Poplack DG, eds. *Principles and Practice of Pediatric Oncology*, 4th ed. Philadelphia: Lipincott Williams & Wilkins; 2002:973–1016.

46. Ham SJ, Schraffordt Koops H, Veth RP, van Horn JR, Molenaar WM, Hoekstra HJ. Limb salvage surgery for primary bone sarcoma of the lower extremities: long-term consequences of endoprosthetic reconstructions. *Ann Surg Oncol*. 1998;5(5):423–436.

47. Frieden RA, Ryniker D, Kenan S, Lewis MM. Assessment of patient function after limb-sparing surgery. *Arch Phys Med Rehabil*. 1993;74(1):38–43.

48. Eckardt JJ, Kabo JM, Kelley CM, et al. Expandable endoprosthesis reconstruction in skeletally immature patients with tumors. *Clin Orthop Relat Res*. 2000(373):51–61.

49. Kawai A, Muschler GF, Lane JM, Otis JC, Healey JH. Prosthetic knee replacement after resection of a malignant tumor of the distal part of the femur. Medium to long-term results. *J Bone Joint Surg Am*. 1998;80(5):636–647.

50. Nagarajan R, Neglia JP, Clohisy DR, Robison LL. Limb Salvage and amputation in survivors of pediatric lower-extremity bone tumors: what are the long-term implications? *J Clin Oncol*. 2002;20(22):4493–4501.

51. Robison LL, Mertens AC, Boice JD, et al. Study design and cohort characteristics of the Childhood Cancer Survivor Study: a multi-institutional collaborative project. *Med Pediatr Oncol*. 2002;38(4):229–239.

52. Hudson MM, Mertens AC, Yasui Y, et al. Health status of adult long-term survivors of childhood cancer: a report from the Childhood Cancer Survivor Study [see comment]. *JAMA.* 2003;290(12):1583–1592.

53. Ness KK, Mertens AC, Hudson MM, et al. Limitations on physical performance and daily activities among long-term survivors of childhood cancer [summary for patients in *Ann Intern Med.* November 1, 2005;143(9):I30; PMID: 16263881]. *Ann Intern Med.* 2005;143(9):639–647.

54. Nagarajan R, Clohisy DR, Neglia JP, et al. Function and quality-of-life of survivors of pelvic and lower extremity osteosarcoma and Ewing's sarcoma: the Childhood Cancer Survivor Study. *Br J Cancer.* 2004;91(11):1858–1865.

55. Brodeur GM, Maris JM. Neuroblastoma. In: Pizzo PA, Poplack DG, eds. *Principles and Practice of Pediatric Oncology,* 5th ed. Philadelphia: Lippincott Williams & Wilkins; 2006:933–970.

56. Wexler LH, Meyer WH, Helman L. Rhabdomyosarcoma and the undifferentiated sarcomas. In: Pizzo PA, Poplack DG, eds. *Principles and Practice of Pediatric Oncology,* 5th ed. Philadelphia: Lippincott Williams & Wilkins; 2006:971–1001.

Geriatric Issues in Cancer Rehabilitation

Taryn Y. Lee
Sandy B. Ganz

As Americans live longer, it is expected that by the year 2030, individuals over the age of 65 will increase from 36 million to 72 million and represent 20% of the U. S. population (1). It is estimated that 9.6 million will be over the age of 85. Cancer incidence increases with age; 60% of all malignancies occur in those aged 65 and older (2). Many of these individuals will have rehabilitation needs as they prepare for or recover from various treatment protocols. Of community-dwelling Medicare recipients, 27% of those over 65 and 35% of those over 80 have difficulty performing at least one basic activity of daily living (BADL), such as toileting, transferring, feeding, grooming, bathing, and dressing (3). In the oncologic geriatric patient, this number may be as high as 50%. In addition, 75% of these patients may require help with one or more instrumental activity of daily living (IADL), such as the ability to use a telephone, travel, shop, prepare meals, perform household chores, take medications, and manage finances (4). Regardless of whether a patient is undergoing a curative or palliative care regimen, rehabilitation in the management of elderly patients with a diagnosis of cancer has been shown to improve physiological, physical, and psychological well-being (5–10).

The geriatric population is a heterogeneous group of patients with varying levels of baseline functional ability. Cancer may coexist with other chronic diseases and add to the complexity of the care of the older patient. A geriatric assessment includes an evaluation of the medical, cognitive, psychosocial, and functional status of the older patient. In both geriatric and reha-

bilitation medicine, an interdisciplinary team approach to care is emphasized, with the primary goal of maximizing a patient's function.

This chapter will highlight some of the common problems that may impact upon the rehabilitation of the older cancer patient and discuss a geriatric approach to addressing these issues.

FRAILTY

Aging is accompanied by physiological changes that include impaired metabolism, decreased renal function, increased fat stores, reduced albumin levels, and decreased muscle mass (11). These alterations may result in the older patient having less overall bodily reserve to maintain homeostasis when an organ system sustains an insult. Diminishment of social and economic resources also adds to the vulnerability of the geriatric cancer patient to any life stressors. Geriatric patients at risk for frailty are often older than 85 years of age, require assistance in at least one activity of daily living (ADL), have a serious comorbid condition, or exhibit at least one geriatric syndrome such as dementia, delirium, or depression (11).

DEMENTIA

Dementia is defined as an acquired loss of memory sufficient to impair normal functioning in an alert patient.

KEY POINTS

- It is expected that by the year 2030, individuals over the age of 65 will increase from 36 million to 72 million and represent 20% of the United States population.
- Of community-dwelling Medicare recipients, 27% of those over 65 and 35% of those over 80 have difficulty performing at least one basic activity of daily living (BADL), such as toileting, transferring, feeding, grooming, bathing, and dressing.
- Cancer may coexist with other chronic diseases and add to the complexity of the care of the older patient.
- Aging is accompanied by physiological changes that include impaired metabolism, decreased renal function, increased fat stores, reduced albumin levels, and decreased muscle mass, which may result in the older patient having less overall physiological reserve to maintain homeostasis when an organ system sustains an insult.
- Of the people over 85 years of age, 50% may have some cognitive impairment.
- Delirium is present in 14%–55 % of hospitalized cancer patients and 38% of older cancer patients.
- Pain should be aggressively treated in the older cancer patient.

- Depression is prevalent in the geriatric population and may be as high as 50% in the older oncologic patient population.
- Sleep disorders are prevalent in the older patient and can affect energy level during rehabilitation efforts.
- The medication regimen of older patients should be reviewed and attempts made to minimize polypharmacy and possible drug-related adverse events such as falls.
- Poor nutritional status may result from underlying malignancy, poor appetite, dementia (forgetting to eat), financial instability, inability to access food due to physical or environmental barriers, inability to swallow, inadequate dentition, medication effects causing changed taste perception, depression, and pain.
- Assessment tools used to obtain objective measures of physical function in the older patient include the Tinetti Gait and Balance Tool, functional reach test, timed up and go, and six-minute walk test.
- The geriatric approach to care must be individually tailored, taking into consideration not just a patient's medical and functional status, but also the financial, psychosocial, and environmental circumstances.

Its prevalence increases with age. Of the people over 85 years of age, 50% may have some cognitive impairment (11). Flood et al. noted that 27% of individuals admitted to a geriatrics oncology unit were found to have memory impairment (4).

The most common cause of memory loss is Alzheimer disease. However, vascular dementia is common, and often a patient may have a mixed (both Alzheimer and vascular) form of dementia (12). The Folstein Mini-Mental State Examination (MMSE) is often used to screen for memory impairment (13). A score of 24 or less is suggestive of a memory problem. However, depending on the individual's level of education, the cut-off score may vary (14). More in-depth testing can be performed by a neuropsychologist to further evaluate for cognitive impairment.

Currently, there is no cure for dementia. Acetylcholinesterase inhibitors such as donepezil may be tried (15). These medications may cause gastrointestinal side effects. Another agent, memantine, an N-methyl-D-aspartate receptor antagonist, has also been developed for patients with moderate to severe dementia (16). However, neither class of medication will reverse memory loss. These agents, at best, will prevent worsening of

memory and may control some of the behavioral problems, such as agitation, that accompany dementia (17).

Memory deficits affect care because patients must be compliant with treatment recommendations, whether it requires taking medications, going to chemotherapy or radiation sessions, or following posthospitalization discharge instructions. It also affects overall treatment and rehabilitation goals. In the severely demented patient, families may choose to forgo aggressive treatment plans that have high risk and choose more palliative options.

DELIRIUM

Delirium is defined as a disturbance of consciousness, attention, and cognition that develops in a short time with a potentially fluctuating pattern. It is present in 14%–55% of hospitalized cancer patients (18). In older cancer patients, the prevalence is 38% (18), and the rate increases further in those that are at the end of life. The delirious patient is unable to participate in physical or occupational therapy and thus, overall recovery time from an illness may take longer. Due to age, advanced illness, comorbidities, and underlying cognitive impairment, older patients are especially prone to delirium (19).

A patient's altered mental status may signal an acute medical change, such as infection, myocardial infarction, urinary retention, fecal impaction, bleeding, or other metabolic derangement. In the cancer patient, medical developments associated with an acute onset of confusion may include hepatic or renal failure, hypoxia, paraneoplastic syndrome, hypercalcemia, hyper/hyponatremia, and cranial irradiation (20).

The addition of any new medication can result in delirium. Medications may have a different pharmacokinetic profile in the older patient due to changes in absorption, distribution, metabolism, and excretion ability (21). In oncology patients, interferon, interleukin-2, methotrexate, fluorouracil, bleomycin, carmustine, cisplatinum, ifosfamide, steroids, antiemetics, benzodiazepines, and opioids may cause confusion (18). Failure to continue a longstanding drug (ie, benzodiazepines, alcohol, opioids, steroids), or failure to give adequate doses of a medication (ie, pain medication) can result in delirium. In addition, polypharmacy or interactions between medications may cause delirium.

Delirium can be difficult to diagnose, especially when it appears in the more common hypoactive form (22). Patients who are lethargic or quiet are less likely to draw attention to themselves and less likely to cause concern to health professionals, especially if they are not well known to the staff. The loud, agitated patient that is pulling out catheters and taking off her oxygen will be more likely to get noticed. Every effort should be made to determine if there is a new medical development. The Confusion Assessment Method (CAM) developed by Inouye et al. (Fig. 69.1) can be used to detect delirium (23). Delirious patients have higher morbidity, mortality, and longer hospital and nursing home stays (22). Even when the underlying medical problem is discovered and addressed, delirium may take weeks to months to resolve (24).

While the underlying cause of delirium is investigated, there may be the immediate need to control a delirious patient's agitation and interference with necessary tests and treatment. Low-dose antipsychotics (ie, haloperidol 0.5 mg, olanzapine 2.5 mg, risperidone 0.25 mg) can be tried (25). Olanzapine also exists as a wafer formulation that can easily dissolve in the mouth. In patients with parkinsonian symptoms, quetiapine is less likely to have extrapyramidal side effects (26). Low-dose benzodiazepine use (lorazepam 0.5 mg oral or intravenous) may be necessary in those who cannot tolerate an antipsychotic (25). However, efforts should be made to minimize chemical sedative and physical restraints, as they can worsen agitation and confusion.

CONFUSION ASSESSMENT METHOD

Feature 1. Acute Onset and Fluctuating Course
This feature is usually obtained from a family member or nurse and is shown by
positive responses to the following questions:
Is there evidence of an acute change in mental status from the patient's baseline? Did the (abnormal) behavior fluctuate during the day, that is, tend to come and go, or increase and decrease in severity?

Feature 2. Inattention
This feature is shown by a positive response to the following question:
Did the patient have difficulty focusing attention, for example, being easily distractible or having difficulty keeping track of what was being said?

Feature 3. Disorganized Thinking
This feature is shown by a positive response to the following question:
Was the patient's thinking disorganized or incoherent, such as rambling or irrelevant conversation, unclear or illogical flow of ideas, or unpredictable switching from subject to subject?

Feature 4. Altered Level of Consciousness
This feature is shown by any answer other than "alert" to the following question:
Overall, how would you rate this patient's level of consciousness? Alert (normal), vigilant (hyperalert), lethargic (drowsy, easily aroused), stupor (difficult to arouse), or coma (unarousable)

FIGURE 69.1

Confusion Assessment Method. Diagnosis of delirium requires the presence of Features 1 and 2, and either 3 or 4. (From Ref. 23, with permission.)

Nonpharmacologic means to address agitation should be utilized whenever possible (19). Having an individual stay with the patient for continuous one-on-one observation to ensure safety is preferred to ordering a medicine or restraint that can result in unwanted adverse consequences. Efforts should be made to minimize further stimulation from loud noises. Invasive devices, such as a urinary catheter or intravenous lines, should be discontinued if not needed. Sensory deficits should be optimized with glasses, hearing aids, or amplifiers to lessen chances of confusion (27). A room with a window and the presence of a clock or calendar can help to reorient the patient to time. Regular, structured activities such as radiation therapy, physical therapy, and recreational therapy that occur at predictable times daily will help to minimize confusion (28).

Encouraging frequent family and friend visitors will help to reassure and reorient the patient at high risk for developing delirium.

PAIN MANAGEMENT

Pain is a common complaint in many oncology patients and affects a patient's ability to achieve optimal function. Pain should be aggressively treated in the older cancer patient. In patients with memory impairment, it may be difficult to assess for pain. A thorough physical exam is especially important in these patients to detect a potential pain source. In patients with advanced dementia, behavioral cues, such as facial grimacing, groaning, guarding, crying, refusing to eat, combativeness, rigid body, and increased confusion, can provide clues to possible pain being experienced (29). Family and caregivers can provide important history about what treatments in the past helped to reduce pain. A picture scale (facial expressions) or a numerical rating scale ("On a scale from 0 to 10, 0 meaning no pain and 10 meaning the worst pain you can imagine, how much pain are you having now?") can be used to assess for pain in those patients without advanced dementia (30).

For patients with mild to moderate levels of pain (and without significant hepatic dysfunction), acetaminophen is the preferred agent. As long as the dose does not exceed 3,000–4,000 mg per day, this medication is safe to use in older patients. Nonsteroidal anti-inflammatory drugs (NSAIDs) should be avoided in patients with congestive heart failure, peptic ulcer disease, bleeding tendency, or renal insufficiency. Tramadol (Ultram), a weak μ-receptor binder, also inhibits reuptake of norepinephrine and serotonin. As a result, tramadol can cause confusion, seizures, and serotonin syndrome (21). A local anesthetic patch such as Lidoderm may be tried for musculoskeletal or neuropathic pain to try to minimize the need for systemic oral medications. Corticosteroids may have psychiatric adverse effects. Tricyclic antidepressants used for neuropathic pain should be used with caution in the older patient, as they can cause confusion, orthostatic hypotension, urinary retention, and cardiac arrhythmias. Anticonvulsant medications, such as gabapentin and pregabalin, may also cause excessive sedation or confusion in the geriatric patient.

Narcotics are generally well tolerated as long as opioids are titrated appropriately for each patient. When starting opioids, it should be kept in mind that these medications may have a prolonged half-life in older patients, making them more sensitive to their effects than younger patients (31). Side effects such as

respiratory depression, drowsiness, and confusion may develop, especially in the beginning or if the opioid is titrated up too quickly. After a few days, tolerance to these adverse effects develops (31). However, tolerance does not develop to constipation, and this side effect should be aggressively treated. If possible, fluids should be increased and mobility encouraged. Natural remedies such as prune juice may help. Prior to the use of stronger laxatives, patients should be assessed for fecal impaction and obstruction. If there are no contraindications, manual disimpaction and enema treatments may be necessary prior to the use of oral agents to relieve constipation. A regular bowel regimen treatment plan that includes a stool softener and stimulant (senna, bisacodyl) or osmotic laxatives (sorbitol, lactulose) should always coincide with the initiation of opioids. In some patients, regular use of enemas may be required to ensure effective bowel evacuation.

Propoxyphene (Darvocet) is not more potent than acetaminophen, has a long half-life, and produces metabolites that can cause ataxia and dizziness (32). Codeine is also a weak opioid and ineffective in those individuals who lack the enzyme to metabolize this medication (11). Meperidine (Demerol) has active metabolites that can accumulate (especially in patients with renal failure) and cause anxiety, tremors, and seizures (31). Opioids with mixed agonist and antagonist receptor activity such as pentazocine (Talwin) can lead to reversal of analgesia and withdrawal symptoms in those patients already on full agonist opioids such as morphine. Because of its long half-life, methadone should be used with caution in the elderly (32). The transdermal fentanyl patch should never be used in an opioid-naïve patient or in those patients just begun on opioids. Because the drug's reservoir is the skin and not the patch, the half-life is at least 72 hours and removal of the patch will be ineffective in stopping further drug delivery (31). This medication should be used only in those patients already on high-dose narcotics (at least 60 mg oral morphine/day or its equivalent) and who are able to tolerate this dosage for more than just a few days.

Although older patients may have an increased sensitivity to opioids, morphine, hydromorphone, oxycodone, and fentanyl are well tolerated if used judiciously. In patients with renal failure, it may be less preferable to use morphine, as neurotoxins may accumulate (21). As in any other cancer patient experiencing severe pain, once the older patient has been on opioids at adequate doses for an extended time, doses may be increased appropriately to titrate for pain control. However, in the opioid-naïve older patient, only the short-acting formulations should be started and titrated to avoid side effects.

DEPRESSION

Depression is prevalent in the geriatric population and may be as high as 50% in the older oncologic patient population (4). Detection and treatment is important, as depression can affect a patient's motivation level to participate effectively in rehabilitation therapy. Chemotherapeutic agents, such as interferon, interleukin-2, vincristine, vinblastine, procarbazine, and asparaginase, can cause depression (33). Hypothyroidism, inadequate pain control, and cancer itself may contribute to depression. The Geriatric Depression Scale (Fig. 69.2) is often used to screen for depression (34,35). Or just the simple question "Do you often feel sad or depressed?" may be a quicker route to detecting depression.

Psychotherapy and cognitive behavioral therapy is used to manage depression. When medications are added, the recommendation of, "start low, go slow" is often followed in beginning and titrating doses. Serotonin reuptake inhibitors are generally safe to use in patients. The most common adverse effect may involve gastrointestinal side effects. Atypical agents include mirtazapine, bupropion, and venlafaxine (36). Mirtazapine may be selected for its sedating and appetite-stimulating properties. Bupropion has stimulant properties and should be avoided in patients with seizure disorders. Venlafaxine may cause hypertension. A new antidepressant, duloxetine, may help to treat neuropathic pain (33). Tricyclic antidepressants can cause arrhythmias and anticholinergic side effects (dry mouth, constipation, urinary retention, sedation, confusion, and orthostatic hypotension). The most preferable agent in this class is nortriptyline, as its side effect profile is less. Due to their potential adverse effects and drug interactions, monoamine oxidase inhibitors should only be prescribed in those patients that are followed closely by a psychiatrist. Electroconvulsive therapy may be considered in severely depressed patients who do not have evidence of an intracranial tumor. Its main side effect is short-term memory loss.

SLEEP

Sleep disorders are prevalent in the older patient and can affect energy level during rehabilitation efforts.

GERIATRIC DEPRESSION SCALE (SHORT FORM)

Choose the best answer for how you felt over the past week.

1. Are you basically satisfied with your life?	Yes/**No**
2. Have you dropped many of your activities and interests?	**Yes**/No
3. Do you feel that your life is empty?	**Yes**/No
4. Do you often get bored?	**Yes**/No
5. Are you in good spirits most of the time?	Yes/**No**
6. Are you afraid that something bad is going to happen to you?	**Yes**/No
7. Do you feel happy most of the time?	Yes/**No**
8. Do you often feel helpless?	**Yes**/No
9. Do you prefer to stay at home, rather than going out and doing new things?	**Yes**/No
10. Do you feel you have more problems with memory than most?	**Yes**/No
11. Do you think it is wonderful to be alive?	Yes/**No**
12. Do you feel pretty worthless the way you are now?	**Yes**/No
13. Do you feel full of energy?	Yes/**No**
14. Do you feel that your situation is hopeless?	**Yes**/No
15. Do you think that most people are better off than you are?	**Yes**/No

Score 1 point for each bolded answer. Score above 5 suggests depression.

FIGURE 69.2

Geriatric Depression Scale. (From Ref. 34, 35, with permission)

If a mood disorder is present, simply treating the psychiatric condition may improve sleep without requiring an additional sedating medication. Poor sleep may be due to medications, pain, shortness of breath, and frequent urination. Efforts should be made to address these possible contributing factors. Nonpharmacologic methods, such as a warm drink, relaxation tapes, or massage, may be tried, especially in patients prone to delirium (27). If a patient is already on a sedative that is effective and not causing any adverse effects, it may be continued with caution. Unfortunately, all sleeping pills can cause confusion, oversedation, daytime drowsiness, and potential dependence. In those patients requesting a sleeping medication, the antidepressant trazodone at low doses 25–100 mg can be tried for its sedating properties as a nonaddictive sleeping agent (36).

POLYPHARMACY

The medication regimen should be reviewed and attempts made to minimize polypharmacy and possible drug-related adverse events such as falls. Anticholinergics, such as diphenhydramine, should be avoided if possible, as they can cause confusion. Benzodiazepines should be prescribed with caution. If necessary to treat anxiety, nausea, or agitation, a shorter-acting agent (ie, lorazepam) at the lowest possible dose should be tried (36). If a patient is on digoxin, the drug level should be monitored (especially in patients with renal insufficiency) to make sure toxicity does not result. All medications should be renally dosed, especially antibiotics. Caution is recommended in prescribing any new medication. Efforts should be made to start only one new medication at a time so that it can be discontinued immediately should an adverse reaction occur. Medications in noncombination formulations are preferred for cleaner titration of doses. Pain medication should be administered 30 minutes prior to expected physical activity to minimize side effects and maximize therapy benefit for the patient.

NUTRITION

Poor nutritional status may result from underlying malignancy, poor appetite, dementia (forgetting to eat), financial instability, inability to access food due to physical or environmental barriers, inability to swallow, inadequate dentition, medication effects causing changed taste perception, depression, and pain (11). Malnutrition affects ability to recover from surgery and treatment. It also affects future treatment options, as it contributes to the overall functional status of the older individual. The Mini Nutritional Assessment tool may be used to screen for poor nutritional status (37). Mucositis and pain should be aggressively treated. Therapists trained in swallowing assessments (ie, occupational and/or speech therapists) can assist in both the diagnosis and treatment of swallowing dysfunction. Diets should be liberalized and families encouraged to supplement meals with patients' favorite foods. Vitamins and nutritional supplements can be offered. Medications should be reviewed to see if any changes may help to encourage food intake. Patients may need physical assistance to eat. Dentures should be utilized or diets altered to mechanical soft or pureed consistency as necessary.

DISCHARGE PLANNING AFTER HOSPITALIZATION

After a hospitalization, the older cancer patient has several discharge options. They may go home with no services if they are doing well medically, physically, and functionally. They may go home with home care services if some assistance is necessary. They may go to a skilled nursing facility, such as a nursing home, for short-term rehabilitation or long-term custodial care if a safe discharge plan to home cannot be formulated. Or they may qualify for rehabilitation at an acute rehabilitation facility. In addition, another discharge option is to a hospice program, either inpatient or to home with hospice home care services.

Medicare will cover care a stay at a rehabilitation facility if the patient meets specific criteria. For an acute inpatient rehabilitation stay, the patient must be able to tolerate, at a minimum, three hours of therapy daily and have a qualifying diagnosis. Medicare will also pay for a brief inpatient stay at a nursing home (100% of the first 20 days, then 80% of the next 80 days) if the patient has had a three-day hospital admission, requires therapy, or has a Medicare-qualifying skilled need. After the first 100 days, if the patient needs continued care at a nursing home level, the patient is financially responsible for their stay. If the patient has long-term care insurance, it may cover some of these costs. If the patient has Medicaid, this will cover the remaining nursing home stay.

Medicare also covers home care services, which will provide a visiting nurse, physical therapy, occupational therapy, speech therapy services, and possibly a few hours of home attendant assistance several days each week. Referral for home care services can be initiated from both the outpatient and inpatient setting. However, these services are only temporary and cease when the patient no longer demonstrates a skilled need or reaches a plateau in their rehabilitation progress.

Patients may continue their rehabilitation by participating in outpatient physical therapy, occupational therapy, and speech therapy several times a week. Again, Medicare will cover an outpatient rehabilitation treatment plan ordered by a physician as long as the patient continues to show improvement.

Hospice patients are also covered under Medicare. These patients can continue to receive rehabilitation services, whether they are at home or in the inpatient setting, as long as they are able to participate in therapy and show a positive benefit.

If a patient has managed Medicare insurance, the insurance company may limit the amount of coverage for any of the aforementioned discharge rehabilitation options.

HOME VISIT EVALUATION

For patients receiving therapy at home, the home visit provides the health professional with a great opportunity to assess economical, physical, and environmental barriers to medical and functional recovery. This is often referred to as a home safety evaluation and may be performed by a nurse or physical or occupational therapist.

An examination of the kitchen and refrigerator, bathroom, bedroom setup, medication bottles, floor coverings, and general tidiness of the home provides abundant information about how a patient lives and their possible needs. A home safety evaluation may result in the addition of grab bars, raised toilet seats, a shower bench, a Hoyer lift, and a bedside commode.

A referral to a social worker may be initiated to improve assistance for a patient. Referrals may be made to Meals on Wheels, Friendly Visitor Program, community aid agency services, and physicians that make house calls. Applications for transportation ambulette services can be initiated, and patients may be counseled and assisted in financial and long-term care planning.

MOBILITY AND FALLS

Older cancer patients may exhibit a myriad of functional impairments and limitations before, during, and after initiating various treatment regimens. These individuals may have functional activity intolerance, leading to deconditioning and fatigue; loss of muscle mass, resulting in functional strength deficits; and lowered aerobic capacity (38,39). It is not uncommon for these impairments to lead to functional dependence, creating a financial and caregiver burden to families. Increased disability in the elderly is associated with a decrease in functional performance, and referral for physical

and/or occupational therapy services are necessary to establish a baseline in function (40).

The following tests described can be done in any setting and require no special equipment other than a stopwatch and ruler. Specific performance-based measures commonly utilized in geriatrics to obtain objective measures of baseline physical function are Tinetti Gait and Balance Tool (TGTB), functional reach test (FR), timed up and go test (TUG), and six-minute walk test (6MW).

Tinetti Gait and Balance Tool

The Tinetti Gait and Balance Scale was described by Tinetti in 1986 and uses an ordinal scale to rate a patient's ability to perform gait and balance maneuvers statically and dynamically (41). There are two sections. The first is balance, consisting of 16 points. In this section, eight areas are addressed: sitting balance, arising from a chair, immediate and prolonged standing balance, withstanding a sternal nudge from standing position, standing with eyes closed, and balance while completing a turn during walking, and sitting down. The second section is gait and is comprised of 12 points. The patient walks with or without a device and the following is observed: initiation of gait, step height, step length, step continuity, step symmetry, gait path deviation, trunk sway, walking stance, and turning while walking. Both sections are scored on a scale of 0 to 2. A 0 is given if the patient is unable to complete the task. A score of 2 is given if the task is completed. The maximum score is 28/28. It takes between 5 and 10 minutes to perform. Criterion, construct, face, content, and predictive validity have been tested in multiple clinical settings. It has been shown to be a reliable instrument with good sensitivity (41,42) (Fig. 69.3). As an objective measure of fall risk, a score of less than 19 indicates a high fall risk, 19–23 indicates an increased risk for falls, and greater than 23 is indicative of a low risk of falls (41).

Functional Reach Test

The functional reach test, developed by Duncan in 1990, is a clinical test of balance addressing limits of postural stability (43). It is the measurement of the maximal distance one can reach forward beyond arm's length (in the horizontal plane) while maintaining a fixed base of support in the standing position. Reliability, criterion, concurrent construct, and predictive validity of the functional reach have been established. The functional reach test correlates well with other measures of balance, mobility, activities of daily living, and risk of falls. A reach performed at less than 6 inches is a high risk for falls. A reach performed at greater than 10 inches without external support is normal (43).

Tinetti Balance Scale

Item	# of Points
1. Sitting Balance	____
a. Leans or slides in chair = 0	
b. Steady, safe = 1	
2. Arises	____
a. Unable without help = 0	
b. Able, uses arms to help = 1	
c. Able, without using arms = 2	
3. Attempts to arise	____
a. Unable without help = 0	
b. Able, requires > 1 attempt = 1	
c. Able to rise, 1 attempt = 2	
4. Immediate standing balance (first 5 seconds)	____
a. Unsteady (swaggers, moves feet, trunk sways) = 0	
b. Steady but uses cane or other support = 1	
c. Steady without walker or other support = 2	
5. Standing Balance	____
a. Unsteady = 0	
b. Steady but wide stance (medial heels > 4" apart)	
and uses cane or other support = 1	
c. Narrow stance without support = 2	
6. Nudged (subject at max position with feet as close as possible, examiner pushes three with palm on subjects sternum)	____
a. Begins to fall = 0	
b. Staggers, grabs, catches self = 1	
c. Steady = 2	
7. Eyes closed (same as position 6)	____
a. Unsteady = 0	
b. Steady = 1	
8. Turning 360 degrees	____
a. Discontinuous Steps = 0	
b. Continuous = 1	
a. Unsteady (grabs, staggers) = 0	____
b. Steady = 1	
9. Sitting Down	____
a. Unsafe (misjudged distance, falls into chair) = 0	
b. Uses arms or not a smooth motion = 1	
c. Safe, smooth motion = 2	
BALANCE TOTAL	/16

FIGURE 69.3

TINETTI GAIT SCALE

10. Initiation of Gait (immediate initiation)   ____
    a. Any hesitancy or multiple attempts to start = 0
    b. No hesitancy = 1

11. Step Length and height   ____
    a. Right Swing Foot
        Does not pass left stance foot with step = 0
        Passes left stance foot = 1

        Right foot does not clear floor = 0   ____
        Right foot completely clears floor = 1

    b. Left Swing Foot   ____
        Does not pass right stance foot with step = 0
        Passes right stance foot = 1

        Left foot does not clear floor = 0   ____
        Left foot completely clears floor = 1

12. Step Symmetry   ____
    a. Right and left step length not equal (estimate) = 0
    b. Right and left step length appear equal = 1

13. Step Continuity   ____
    a. Stopping or discontinuity between steps = 0
    b. Steps appear continuous = 1

14. Path (estimate 12 inch floor tiles over 10 feet)   ____
    a. Marked deviation = 0
    b. Mild/moderate deviation or uses walking aid = 1
    c. Straight without walking aid = 2

15. Trunk   ____
    a. Marked sway or uses walking aid = 0
    b. No sway but flexion of knees or back or spreads arms = 1
    c. No sway, no flexion, no use of arms or aid = 2

16. Walking time   ____
    a. Heels apart = 0
    b. Heels almost touching while walking = 1
GAIT TOTAL   /12
BALANCE TOTAL   /16
TOTAL SCORE   /28

FIGURE 69.3

Tinetti Gait and Balance Scales. (From Ref. 41, with permission.)

Timed Up and Go

The timed up and go test, described by Podsiadlo in 1991, measures mobility, balance, and locomotor performance in patients with rheumatoid arthritis, osteoarthritis, and deconditioned elderly people (44).

The patient rises from a standard armchair (46-cm seat height to ground) walks 3 m at a comfortable pace, turns, and walks back to the chair and sits down. The test takes two to three minutes to complete. Inter-rater reliability, criterion, and construct validity are high, correlating well with laboratory and clinical measures of gait and balance. A score of <10 seconds is normal. A score of >30 seconds indicates assisted mobility and risk for falls (44).

Six-Minute Walk Test

The six minute walk test was originally developed to assess exercise tolerance among individuals with respiratory disease (45). Content, criterion, and construct validity have been established in the community-dwelling elderly, individuals with fibromyalgia, and patients who have undergone total hip arthroplasty. It is used to measure the maximum distance that a person can walk in six minutes. Normative data for the 6MWT distance reported by Enright was 576 m (1,889 ft) for men (median age 59.5) and 494 m (1,620 ft) for women (median age 62.0) (46).

THERAPY IMPLICATIONS

Following the physical therapy evaluation, baseline data is documented for comparison and a treatment plan is established with concomitant treatment goals. The physical therapy plan of care is based on the disablement model, which addresses pathology, impairment, functional limitation, and disability (Table 69.1) (40). Each patient's treatment plan is individualized and may be accomplished through a variety of treatment techniques, such as therapeutic exercise, physical modalities, functional activities, and patient education.

When describing physical therapy implications for the treatment of geriatric cancer patients, the physical therapy management of these patients falls into two main categories: (1) physical therapy treatment that is restorative in nature, and significant improvement will occur in a short and predictable period; and (2) physical therapy treatment is performed to maintain function, and improvement is unlikely to occur. The treatment goal is the same for both categories, which is to provide the patient with the highest quality of care during whatever treatment intervention is performed.

For patients with a poor rehabilitation prognosis in which improvement in physical function is unlikely, the plan of care is more palliative in nature and the treatment is to provide the patient with the appropriate intervention for comfort. This may include appropriate seating and positioning in a standard wheelchair, reclining wheelchair, or tilt-in-space chair. The type of chair is determined by the patient's trunk stability. For those patients who are bedbound, various types of positioning and positioning devices to prevent pressure ulcers from occurring may be the principal physical therapy treatment. Regardless of whether the patient is bed-bound or wheelchair-bound, an important aspect of management is therapeutic exercise in the form of range of motion (ROM). The primary goal of ROM is to prevent contractures and joint stiffness. The more mobile the joints, the easier it is for the patient and/or caregiver to perform activities of daily living, such as hygiene, bathing, and toileting.

Physical therapists treating patients who are likely to make significant progress will be challenged with the continuous change in the plan of care as the patient's condition gets better. This may entail progression of exercises as strength improves or advancement from one assistive device to another, such as walker to cane.

In both categories of patients, physical therapists must be cognizant of the geriatric cancer patient's prognosis. The plan of care continually needs to be modified as the patient declines and as the patient improves, concomitantly maintaining the highest possible quality of life. Modification of the plan of care applies to all patients, regardless of age or diagnosis, as they improve or decline. It is not uncommon for these patients to demonstrate a fluctuation in their ability to transfer, ambulate, and perform activities of daily living throughout the course of their cancer treatment.

TABLE 69.1
Disablement Model

PATHOLOGY	IMPAIRMENT	FUNCTIONAL LIMITATIONS	DISABILITY
Cancer	Increased pain	Bed mobility	Leisure activities
	Functional strength deficit	Transferring	
	Functional activity	Ambulation	
	intolerance	Stair climbing	Work
		ADLs	Social function
		IADL	

Abbreviations: ADLs, activities of daily living; IADLs, instrumental activities of daily living.

It is imperative for physical therapists, occupational therapists, physicians, social workers, and nursing staff to work together as a cohesive interdisciplinary team to tailor the patient's plan of care with improvements or declines in physical function.

CONCLUSION

Because every geriatric oncology patient is potentially at risk for frailty, social workers, physicians, nurses, and therapists involved in their care ideally should work together to detect, prevent, maintain, and improve upon each patient's unique set of problems. Little research exists in the rehabilitation literature about the treatment of the older cancer patient. Therefore, the geriatric approach to care must be individually tailored, taking into consideration not just a patient's medical and functional status, but also the financial, psychosocial, and environmental circumstances.

Spirituality and advance directives should be discussed to help determine the overall goals of care. Sometimes, the patient may be socially isolated, having outlived most of their friends. Or bitter family conflicts may exist when there are multiple relatives wanting to be involved. Usually, only one or two main caregivers (spouse or adult child) take on most of the responsibility of directly caring for the patient. Besides focusing on comfort for the older patient, attention and support must also be given to the caregivers involved, especially during end-of-life care.

When a patient has a shortened life expectancy, rehabilitation goals must be carefully constructed to ensure that the benefits of treatment outweigh the burden. The treatment plan for the geriatric cancer patient will vary, depending on the medical therapy, nature of the malignancy, underlying cognitive impairments, comorbid medical conditions, and patient resources. The quality of an individual's social support network may determine what treatments the patient can successfully undergo and benefit from. The goals of rehabilitation in the management of the older cancer patient include providing geriatric-sensitive care, symptom management, and maximizing functional ability and comfort to enhance quality of life while providing patient and caregiver safety.

References

1. Rao A, Cohen H. Symptom management in the elderly cancer patient: fatigue, pain, and depression. *J Natl Cancer Inst Monogr.* 2004;32:150–157.
2. Yancik R, Ries L. Cancer in older persons: magnitude of the problem—how do we apply what we know? *Cancer.* 1994;74:1995–2003.
3. Goodwin J, Coleman E, Shaw J. Short functional dependence scale: development and pilot test in older adults with cancer. *Cancer Nurs.* 2006;29(1):73–81.
4. Flood K, Carroll M, CV L, Ball L, Esker D, Carr D. Geriatric syndromes in elderly patients admitted to an oncology-acute care for elders unit. *J Clin Oncol.* 2006;24:2298–2303.
5. Oldervoll L, Kaasa S, Hjermstad M, Lund J, Loge J. Physical exercise results in the improved subjective well-being of a few or is effective rehabilitation for all cancer patients? *Eur J Cancer.* 2004;40:951–962.
6. Oldervoll L, Loge J, Paltie H, et al. The effect of a physical exercise program in palliative care: a phase II study. *J Pain Symptom Manage.* 2006;31(5):421–430.
7. Penedo F, Schneiderman N, Dahn J, Gonzalez J. Physical activity intervention in the elderly: cancer and comorbidity. *Cancer Invest.* 2004;22(1):51–67.
8. Young-McCaughan S, Mays M, Arzola S, et al. Change in exercise tolerance, activity and sleep patterns and quality of life in patients with cancer participating in a structured exercise program. *Oncol Nurs Forum.* 2003;30(3):441–454.
9. Scialla S, Cole R, Scialla T, Bednarz L, Scheerer J. Rehabilitation for elderly patients with cancer asthenia: making a transition to palliative care. *Palliat Med.* 2000;14:121–127.
10. Galvao D, Newton R. Review of exercise intervention studies in cancer patients. *J Clin Oncol.* 2005;23:899–909.
11. Balducci L, Beghe C. The application of the principles of geriatrics to the management of the older person with cancer. *Crit Rev Oncol Hematol.* 2000;35:147–154.
12. Chertkow H BH[N117], Schipper HM, Gauthier S, Bouchard R, Fontaine S, Clarfield AM. Assessment of suspected dementia. *Can J Neurol Sci.* 2001;28(Suppl 1):S28–S41.
13. Folstein M, Folstein S, McHugh P. "Mini-Mental State" a practical method for grading the cognitive state of patients for the clinician. *J Psychiatr Res.* 1975;12:189–198.
14. Boustani M, Peterson B, Hanson L, Harris R, Lohr KN. Screening for dementia in primary care: a summary of the evidence for the U.S. Preventive Services Task Force. *Ann Intern Med.* 2003;138:927–937.
15. Group AC. Long-term donepezil treatment in 565 patients with Alzheimer's disease (AD2000): randomized double-blind trial. *Lancet.* 2004;363:2105–2115.
16. Tariot P, Farlow M, Grossberg G, Graham S, McDonald S, Gergel I. Memantine treatment in patients with moderate to severe Alzheimer disease already receiving donepezil: a randomized controlled trial. *J Am Med Assoc.* 2004;291:317–324.
17. Cummings J. Alzheimer's disease. *NEJM.* 2004;351:56–67.
18. Bond S, Neelon V, Belyea M. Delirium in hospitalized older patients with cancer. *Oncol Nurs Forum.* 2006;33:1075–1083.
19. Weinrich S, Sarna L. Delirium in the older person with cancer. *Cancer.* 1994;74:2079–2091.
20. Boyle D. Delirium in older adults with cancer: implications for practice and research. *Oncol Nurs Forum.* 2006;33:61–78.
21. Dworkin RH GB, Cohen RI. Pharmacologic treatment of chronic pain in the elderly. *Supplement to Annals of Long-Term Care and Clinical Geriatrics.* 2004;12:S1–S10.
22. Inouye SK. Delirium in older persons. *NEJM.* 2006;354:1157–1165.
23. Inouye SK, Van Dyck C, Alessi C, Balkin S, Siegal A, Horwitz R. Clarifying confusion: the confusion assessment method, a new method for detection of delirium. *Ann Int Med.* 1990;113:941–948.
24. Gleason O. Delirium. *Am Fam Phys.* 2003;67:1027–1034.
25. Kindermann S, Dolder C, Bailey A, Katz I, Jeste D. Pharmacological treatment of psychosis and agitation in elderly patients with dementia. *Drugs Aging.* 2002;19:257–276.
26. Alexopoulos G, Streim J, Carpenter D, Docherty J. Using antipsychotic agents in older patients. *J Clin Psychiatry.* 2004;65(Suppl 2):1–20.
27. Inouye.SK, Bogardus S, Chapentier P, et al. A multi-component intervention to prevent delirium in hospitalized older patients. *NEJM.* 1999;340:669–676.

28. Gray K. Managing agitation and difficult behavior in dementia. *Clin Geriatr Med.* 2004;20:69–82.

29. Panel on persistent pain in older persons A. The management of persistent pain in older persons. *J Am Geriatr Soc.* 2002;2002:S205–S24[N118].

30. Herr K. Pain assessment in cognitively impaired older adults. *Am J Nurs.* 2002;102:65–68.

31. Gloth F. Pain management in older adults, prevention and treatment. *J Am Geriatr Soc.* 2001;49:188–199.

32. AGS CPC. *Guidelines Abstracted from the American Academy of Neurology's Dementia Guideline for Early Detection, Diagnosis, and Management of Dementia.* 2003[N119].

33. Winell J, Roth A. Psychiatric assessment and symptom management in elderly cancer patients. *Oncology.* 2005;October:479.

34. Yesavage J, Brink T, Rose T, et al. Geriatric Depression Scale (GDS) recent evidence and development of a shorter version. *J Psychiatr Res.* 1983;17(1):37–49.

35. Seikh J, Yesavage J. Geriatric Depression Scale (GDS) recent evidence and development of a shorter version. *Clin Gerontol.* 1986;5:165–173.

36. Roth A, Modi R. Psychiatric issues in older cancer patients. *Crit Rev Oncol Hematol.* 2003;48:185–197.

37. Sheirlinkx K, Nicholas A, Nourhashemi F, Vellas B, Albaredem J, Garry P. The MNA score in successfully aging persons. In Mini Nutritional Assessment (MNA): research and practice in elderly. In: B. [N120]Vellas PG, Guigoz Y, eds. *Nestle Clinical and Performance Nutrition Workshop Series.* Philadelphia: Lippincott-Raven; 1998:61–66.

38. Burnham T, Wilcox A. Effects of exercise on physiological and psychological variables in cancer survivors. *Med Sci Sports Exerc.* 2002;34(12):1863–1867.

39. Evans W, Lambert C. Physiological basis of fatigue. *Am J Phys Med Rehabil.* 2007;86(1):S29–S46.

40. Guide to physical therapist practice. *Phys Ther.* 2001;77:1163–1650[N121].

41. Tinetti ME. Performance-oriented assessment of mobility problems in elderly patients. *J Am Geriatr Soc.* 1986;34(2):119–126.

42. Tinetti ME, Ginter SF. Identifying mobility dysfunctions in elderly patients. Standard neuromuscular examination or direct assessment? *JAMA.* 1988;259(8):1190–1193.

43. Duncan PW, Weiner DK, Chandler J, Studenski S. Functional reach: a new clinical measure of balance. *J Gerontol.* 1990;45(6):M192–M197.

44. Podsiadlo D, Richardson S. The timed "Up & Go": a test of basic functional mobility for frail elderly persons. *J Am Geriatr Soc.* 1991;39(2):142–148.

45. Guyatt G, Sullivan MJ, Thompson PJ, et al. The 6-minute walk: a new measure of exercise capacity in patients with chronic heart failure. *Can Med Assoc J.* 1985;132:919–923.

46. Enright P. The six-minute walk test. *Respir Care.* 2003;48:783–785.

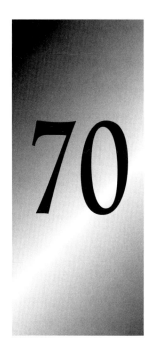

Palliative Care of the Cancer Patient

70

Desiree A. Pardi
Golda B. Widawski
Dory Hottensen
Elizabeth Schack

"All the work of the profession team … is to enable the dying person to live until he dies, at his own maximum potential performing to the limit of his physical and mental capacity with control and independence whenever possible."

—*Dame Cecily Saunders* (196)

Palliative care is interdisciplinary care that anticipates and prevents suffering in order to ensure maximal quality of life. Palliative care does this by focusing on expert management of physical symptoms, functionality, and psychological and spiritual health, as well as social issues. It is care that is provided to all patients and their families throughout the course of any serious illness, irrespective of the presence of a "terminal" diagnosis, and in conjunction with all other appropriate medical therapies. As stated in the clinical practice guidelines for quality palliative care, "palliative care goes beyond traditional disease-model medical management to include the goals of enhancing quality of life for patient and family, optimizing function, helping with decision-making and providing opportunities for individual personal growth" (1). Expert palliative care can increase tolerability of treatments, decrease the need for hospitalization, and increase patient and family satisfaction (2).

REHABILITATION AND PALLIATIVE CARE

Inherently, one may think that palliative care and rehabilitation are at opposite ends of the spectrum; however, upon further examination, the two disciplines can be quite complementary. Both look to support life and to relieve discomfort (3). Additionally, palliative care medicine and rehabilitation are both symptom-oriented and utilize a multidisciplinary approach to care in order to improve a patient's quality of life (4). Assisting our patients to maintain their independence and quality of life, as they define and interpret it, is one of the greatest gifts we as health care professionals can provide as patients move through the course of their illness. Indeed, when it is no longer realistic to expect a cure, reversal of disease progression, or return to a prior level of physical functioning or independence, rehabilitation can take on different forms that can add an important dimension of being human as one approaches life's end. In palliative care, rehabilitation focuses on respect for each individual patient and is grounded in concern for preserving hope, human dignity, and autonomy. The overall goal of rehabilitation at the end of life is to assist patients and families to make the most out of each day in the context of their own disease course (5).

KEY POINTS

- Routine assessment of symptoms has been demonstrated to allow for identification of often overlooked or underreported symptoms, which then allows for more effective management.
- Simple interventions that may be helpful in controlling nausea include eating before parenteral medication, frequent small meals to avoid abdominal distension and emptiness, massage, relaxation therapy, hypnosis, guided imagery, and acupuncture/acupressure.
- Studies have shown a "dose-response" relationship between increasing physical activity and depres-

sion, and that low-moderate levels of physical activity may be helpful in preventing depressive symptoms.
- When asked, most but not all patients want to know their prognosis, though they may not always want full disclosure. For those patients who do not wish to know the prognosis, it is helpful to ask if there is someone whom they would like the medical team to talk with.
- Superficial heat and ice, transcutaneous electrical nerve stimulation (TENS), massage, and relaxation can be used to help control pain and discomfort.

Throughout this chapter, we will follow the case of Mr. T. as he transitions through the various phases of his cancer in order to illustrate how the palliative care team can work in conjunction with rehabilitation services to provide optimal care to a patient.

THE CASE OF MR. T.

Mr. T. is a 44-year-old man who, aside from the removal of a small melanoma from his back two years ago, has been otherwise healthy. Two months ago, during an evaluation of low back pain that had failed conservative management, multiple metastases of melanoma were discovered in the lumbar vertebrae, liver, and lungs. Shortly after his diagnosis, Mr. T. began chemotherapy. However, he has had significant difficulty tolerating the treatments secondary to severe nausea, which has caused multiple delays throughout the two cycles. The nausea has also contributed to anorexia, resulting in significant weight loss. Additionally, as the sole financial provider in the family, he has been trying to continue working, and as a result of severe fatigue has often had to decide between chemotherapy and going to work, further delaying his treatment. Given the difficulty Mr. T. is having tolerating chemotherapy secondary to multiple symptoms, his oncologist refers him to an outpatient palliative care specialist team.

CASE DISCUSSION

Symptom Assessment

Routine assessment of symptoms has been demonstrated to allow for identification of often overlooked or underreported symptoms, which then allows for

more effective management (6). Expert symptom management is associated with greater patient and family satisfaction and quality of life (7). In the case of Mr. T., on meeting first with the palliative care team nurse practitioner, the Modified Edmonton Symptom Assessment Scale (MESAS) was utilized (8). This scale, a commonly used scale in palliative care, has been validated in the cancer population, and has been shown to be short, sensitive, responsive to change, and easily self-completed without being significantly burdensome to the patients, even at the end of life (8). Currently, multiple Web sites provide useful assessment instruments as well as other tools and information pertinent to palliative care. One such site is the Center to Advance Palliative Care (www.capc.org).

Biopsychosocial Assessment

Comprehensive and culturally competent social work assessment in the context of palliative care includes relevant past and current health issues affecting the patient and family. Some of these health issues include pain, depression, anxiety, and decreased mobility. Part of the assessment includes exploring financial resources and insurance coverage. Family structures and roles, as well as patterns and styles of communication, are also important components of the biopsychosocial assessment (9).

CASE CONTINUES

Subsequent to meeting with both the palliative care nurse practitioner and social worker, Mr. T. meets with the palliative care physician. After speaking with and examining Mr. T., the physician determines that though Mr. T. is miserable due to the side effects of the chemotherapy, his major source of distress is related to his inability to continue on schedule with the treatment prescribed by his oncologist. The palliative care physician explains to Mr. T. that as it is clear that Mr. T.'s current goal is to continue with chemotherapy, the primary goal of the palliative treatment plan will be to help improve his ability to tolerate his treatments on schedule. The physician then meets with the nurse practitioner and social worker to devise an appropriate palliative treatment plan, which will incorporate physical therapy (PT) in accordance with Mr. T.'s current goals for his care.

CASE DISCUSSION

Nausea and Vomiting

Nausea and vomiting, whether acutely related to chemotherapy or chronic, can be a significant source of suffering and poor quality of life. Indeed, many patients say that they would rather suffer from chronic pain than chronic nausea (10). As in the case of Mr. T., severe nausea and vomiting can have effects beyond simple physical distress. It can interfere with important, life-prolonging or palliative treatments (11); result in anorexia, which itself can result in dehydration and severe cachexia; and can also result in significant psychological suffering (12).

Causes

Vomiting Center

In emetogenesis, all roads lead to the vomiting center (VC). Located in an area of the medulla known as the nucleus tractus solitarius, the vomiting center is the final common pathway in emesis, receiving input from the gastrointestinal (GI) tract, the vestibular system, the chemoreceptor trigger zone (CTZ), and the cortex. The vomiting center is rich in histamine (H1), dopamine (D2), and neurokinin-1 (NK1) receptors (13,14).

Gastrointestinal Tract

Input from the GI tract can result from multiple mechanisms. GI mucosal irritation or inflammation, such as from esophageal reflux, nonsteroidal anti-inflammatory drugs (NSAIDs), irradiation, and infection, can cause nausea and vomiting. GI paresis as seen in "squashed stomach syndrome" (when the viscera are enlarged as a result of tumor, for example, thereby "squashing" the stomach), poorly controlled diabetes, or resulting from opioids (and other medications) can also result in nausea and vomiting. GI obstruction, often from the primary tumor or peritoneal metastases, can cause severe nausea and vomiting. Emesis related to these mechanisms involves the actions of acetylcholine, histamine, serotonin, and substance P, which trigger nausea and

vomiting via activation of both the parasympathetic and sympathetic nervous systems. In addition to acetylcholine and histamine receptors, multiple serotonin receptor subtypes (15) can be found in abundance in the GI tract. Besides stimulating nausea, acetylcholine is also involved in the secretory and motility functions of the GI tract. Substance P has agonistic actions at NK1 receptors in the VC (16).

Vestibular Apparatus

The vestibular apparatus is rich in acetylcholine and histamine receptors, though the role of histamine in vestibular-induced emesis is thought to result from its central cholinergic actions (17). As the vestibular apparatus is involved in motion and proprioception, it is due to stimulation of this system that one may find themselves vomiting over the side of a boat in seasickness. Irritation or dysfunction of the vestibular apparatus also can occur on initiation of morphine or due to cerebellar or skull metastases, for example.

Chemoreceptor Trigger Zone

The CTZ is located in the area postrema in the floor of the fourth ventricle and contains copious serotonin (5HT3) and dopamine (D2) receptors, as well as muscarinic acetylcholine (mACh) and gamma aminobutyric acid (GABA) receptors (18). The CTZ is stimulated by toxins, drugs, and metabolic disturbances such as hypercalcemia and uremia (13,14).

Cortex

The mechanism involved in the contribution of cortical factors in nausea and vomiting is unclear. However, aside from the nausea and vomiting that result from cerebral edema, it appears to be important in nausea and vomiting related to the memory of a prior event, as occurs in anticipatory nausea and vomiting.

MANAGEMENT OF NAUSEA AND VOMITING

Rational treatment necessitates knowledge of the vomiting pathway and its associated neurotransmitter receptors, combined with the knowledge of the most likely mechanisms involved. In palliative care, the cause is most often multifactorial. However, with a careful history, physical exam, and, if appropriate within the context of the goals of care, diagnostic tests, one can often arrive at a hypothesis regarding the most predominant mechanism. Often, management requires a multimodal approach (Table 70.1).

TABLE 70.1
Antiemetics

PREDOMINANT CAUSE	MEDICATION	MECHANISM	SPECIAL CONSIDERATIONS
GI mucosal irritation	Sucralfate Bismuth solutions	Coating agent	
	Cimetidine Ranitidine Famotidine Nizatidine	H2 receptor antagonists	
	Aluminum/magnesium hydroxide Calcium carbonate	Neutralizes gastric acid	
	Omeprazole Lansoprazole Rabeprozole Pantoprozole Esomeprazole	PPI	Expensive
	Ondansetron Granisetron	Antagonize 5HT3 receptors in GI tract and CTZ	Useful for nausea and vomiting associated with abdominal irradiation (24) May slow GI transit Can cause diarrhea, which can limit use
	Misoprostol	Cytoprotective agent	
Medications (eg, chemotherapy, opioids, etc.) metabolic disturbances and/or inflammation (24-26)	Ondansetron Granisetron	Antagonize 5HT3 receptors in CTZ and GI tract	May slow GI transit
	Aprepitant	Antagonizes NK1 receptors in the VC	Expensive, FDA-approved for delayed nausea induced by certain chemotherapies (16)

	Phenothiazines and butyrophenones[a]
	  Promethazine
	  Chlorpromazine
	  Prochlorperazine
	  Haloperidol
		Antagonizes D2 receptors in the CTZ and VC	Little effect on GI transit (22)
			All but haloperidol have significant anticholinergic and antihistamine effects

	Substituted benzamides Metoclopramide		Prokinetic effects on upper GI tract Least potent D2 antagonist (27)
	Diphenhydramine Meclizine Hydroxyzine	Antagonizes H1 receptors in the VC	Nonsedating, not effective, as they do not cross the blood–brain barrier
	Benzodiazepines	Antagonists at GABA receptors in the CTZ	
	Dronabinol	Act at CNS cannabinoid-1 receptors (18)	Can cause or worsen delirium NNT (28) for nausea = 6 NNT for vomiting = 8 NNH = 11

(Continued)

TABLE 70.1
Antiemetics Continued

Predominant Cause	Medication	Mechanism	Special Considerations
GI Paresis (eg, ileus)[b]	Substituted benzamides Metoclopramide	Acts at gut 5HT4 receptors to stimulate acetylcholine release	Prokinetic effects on smooth muscle of upper GI tract Prokinetic effects are antagonized by co-administration of medications with anticholinergic properties (eg, diphenhydramine, tricyclic antidepressants) (29) Higher doses required for D2 receptor antagonism Avoid in mechanical obstruction
	Erythromycin	Agonist at gut motilin receptors	Increases gastric and duodenal motility Nausea and vomiting are common side effects Avoid in mechanical obstruction
Mechanical obstruction	Scopolamine	Antagonizes mACh receptors in GI tract to decrease GI secretion; antagonizes mACh receptors in the VC	Relaxes GI smooth muscle Helpful in reducing painful cramping
	Octreotide (30)	Acts at somatostatin receptors to inhibit GI secretion	Requires SQ injection at least twice a day May prevent complete bowel obstruction (31)
	Corticosteroids	? decreases GI edema	May reverse malignant bowel obstruction (32)
	Phenothiazines and butyrophenones[a] Promethazine Chlorpromazine Prochlorperazine Haloperidol	Antagonizes D2 receptors in the CTZ and VC	Little effect on GI transit (22) All but haloperidol have significant anticholinergic and antihistamine effects
	Diphenhydramine Meclizine Hydroxyzine	Antagonizes H1 receptors in the VC	Can slow GI transit
Vestibular irritation	Scopolamine	Antagonizes mACh receptors in the vestibular apparatus and VC	
	Diphenhydramine Meclizine Hydroxyzine	May act via central anticholinergic effects (17)	
Brain metastases or meningeal irritation	Corticosteroids	Decreases cerebral edema	
	Phenothiazines and butyrophenones[a] Promethazine Chlorpromazine	Antagonizes D2 receptors in the VC	Haloperidol and chlorpromazine can decrease the seizure threshold

(Continued)

TABLE 70.1
Antiemetics Continued

PREDOMINANT CAUSE	MEDICATION	MECHANISM	SPECIAL CONSIDERATIONS
	Prochlorperazine Haloperidol Substituted benzamides Metoclopramide		
	Diphenhydramine Meclizine Hydroxyzine	Antagonizes H1 receptors in the VC	Can cause or worsen delirium
Peritoneal/GI metastases	Corticosteroids	? Decreases GI edema	
	Phenothiazines and butyrophenones[a] Promethazine Chlorpromazine Prochlorperazine Haloperidol Substituted benzamides Metoclopramide	Antagonizes D2 receptors in the VC	
	Diphenhydramine Meclizine Hydroxyzine	Antagonizes H1 receptors in the VC	
Anxiety/pain or anticipatory nausea	Corticosteroids	Unknown mechanism	May worsen anxiety
	Benzodiazepines	Acts at GABA receptors in the CTZ	

[a]Listed in order of potency of binding D2 receptors (30).
[b]Excluding mechanical obstruction.

Abbreviations: 5HT4, CNS, central nervous system; CTZ, chemoreceptor trigger zone; FDA, Food and Drug Administration; GABA, gamma-aminobutyric acid; GI, gastrointestinal; H1, histamine; mACh, muscarinic acetylcholine; NK1, neurokinin receptor 1; NNH, number needed to harm; NNT, number needed to treat; PPI, proton pump inhibitor; SQ, subcutaneous; VC, vomiting center.

Nonpharmacologic

Simple interventions can often be helpful, particularly when combined with pharmacotherapy. If the history points toward medication as a possible culprit and withdrawing the drug is not an option, often merely having the patient take the medication with food may solve the problem. Parenteral medication can also stimulate nausea and vomiting that may be relieved by having the patient eat prior to its administration. Frequent small meals to avoid both extremes of abdominal distension and emptiness can be helpful, as can a bland diet, avoiding spicy food or foods with a strong odor. Complementary methods, such as massage (19), relaxation therapy, hypnosis, guided imagery, and acupuncture/acupressure, may also provide benefit (20,21). Surgical intervention, such as percutaneous gastrostomy, diverting colostomy, intestinal bypass, and laparotomy, may be useful in relieving nausea and vomiting caused by mechanical obstruction. Given the lack of adequate evidence for or against surgical intervention for mechanical obstruction in palliative care (22), it is necessary to consider risks and benefits within the framework of overall goals of care for each individual patient. Less invasive procedures, such as endoscopic placement of a stent at the site of an obstruction (23), may be a viable alternative for those unwilling or who are not candidates for surgery.

Pharmacologic

Anorexia and Cachexia

Anorexia, or loss of appetite, is one of the most common symptoms in cancer patients receiving palliative care (33,34). The associated cachexia, or weight loss, occurring in up to 80% of patients with advanced cancer and associated with poor prognosis (35,36), often compounds the degree of suffering caused by anorexia (37). The management of these symptoms, even by palliative care specialists, is hindered by the current lack of effective treatment. While the pathogenesis underlying cachexia is still unclear, it appears to involve an interaction between cytokines (mainly interleukin-1, interleukin-6, and tumor necrosis factor alpha [TNFα]); hormones, including testosterone and insulin growth factor-1; and disease-related factors (38). The presence of proinflammatory cytokines, inducing catabolism, may explain the inability of artificial feeding techniques to improve the cachexia associated with terminal illness (39).

In the evaluation of anorexia and cachexia, it is necessary to first assess for reversible causes of anorexia or factors that may be interfering with appetite or the ability to eat (Table 70.2). Determination, particularly in patients who are at the end of life, of whether a lack

TABLE 70.2
Reversible Causes of Anorexia

POSSIBLE CAUSE	HISTORY AND PHYSICAL EXAMINATION	TREATMENT
Unrelieved pain	Pain Visual Analog Scale scores	Aggressive treatment of pain
Nausea and vomiting		Aggressive management of nausea and vomiting
Dysphagia	Food gets "stuck" Regurgitation Coughing and/or choking during swallowing Pain on swallowing Oral thrush	Workup and treatment for specific causes of dysphagia Pureed diet Occupational therapy
Poorly fitting dentures	Extensive weight loss Oral ulcers or excoriations along gum line	New dentures Pureed diet
Dysguesia	Food has metallic taste Food "no longer tastes good" Low serum zinc level	Assess for sinusitis Zinc replacement
Depression	Anhedonia Depressed mood Hopelessness Helplessness	Treat depression (see section on management of depression)
Xerostomia	Patient taking medication known to cause xerostomia History of radiation to head and neck Dry lips and mucous membranes	Reduce or discontinue medication if possible Change to alternate medication if possible Pilocarpine Saliva substitute Sugar-free gum or sour hard candies Increase oral liquid intake if possible Meticulous oral hygiene Avoidance of glycerin swabs or lemon juice
Constipation/slowed GI transit	Patient taking medications known to cause constipation/slow GI transit Infrequent or hard stools Early satiety Nausea	Treat constipation (see section on management of constipation) Prokinetic agents
Oral candidiasis	Painful swallowing Oral thrush	Nystatin suspension Clotrimazole troches Ketoconazole Diflucan
Stress and tension	Family members continuously expressing concern regarding patient's food intake or weight loss Family members attempting to force-feed patient	Patient and family education Involve patient in meal planning Provide calm environment

Source: Adapted from Ref. 197.
Abbreviation: GI, gastrointestinal.

of appetite is bothersome may be necessary. Often, the patient is unconcerned while the family is greatly distressed (37). In fact, it may be that the greatest source of angst attributable to this symptom is due to patient anxiety related to family members' actions and reactions (40,41). Discovery of the true source of suffering related to this symptom can allow for tremendous quality-of-life improvement via provision of patient and family education.

MANAGEMENT OF ANOREXIA/CACHEXIA

Nonpharmacologic

Anorexia and cachexia that only partially or does not respond to treatment of a reversible cause requires a multimodal approach to management. While the evidence for efficacy of nutritional counseling is lacking (42), an evaluation should be included as part of the initial workup for most patients, even if only for the effects the evaluation may have on decreasing anxiety in the patient and/or family. The importance of a renewed sense of control for the patient and/or family should not be understated (43). As with any evaluation or treatment, the risks and benefits should be thoroughly discussed. Though the evidence for efficacy of nutritional supplementation via parenteral or enteral routes in the cancer population is mostly lacking, an evaluation of the appropriateness of such therapy should be considered in select patients (44,45).

Patient and family education can be a valuable tool that is often underutilized. As many patients and families grappling with end-of-life issues believe that cachexia in cancer is related to caloric intake, it is often helpful to explain that anorexia and cachexia is a natural part of the advancement of the disease. It is, therefore, an irreversible physiological process, and thus the patient is not "starving to death" (46). Consequently, whether the patient's caloric intake increases or not will not change the timing nor the ultimate outcome of death (44). Furthermore, it should be explained that studies have demonstrated that terminally ill cancer patients rarely complain of hunger or thirst. Indeed, even if they do, offering small amounts of food or sips of water is often enough to relieve the symptoms (47).

As the symptom of anorexia may fluctuate throughout the day, it may be helpful to plan meals around the patient's appetite rather than having set meal times. Arranging for the largest meal to occur earlier in the day when the patient is likely to be least fatigued also may be helpful. Furthermore, rather than force-feeding the patient, providing favorite foods or foods with a variety of textures may be beneficial. For those patients in whom anorexia is a troubling symptom, the use of nutritional supplements or medications may be worthwhile.

Pharmacologic Fatigue

Cancer-related fatigue (CRF) is the most common symptom experienced by patients with cancer. It is defined by the National Comprehensive Cancer Network (NCCN) as "a distressing, persistent, subjective sense of tiredness or exhaustion related to cancer or cancer treatment that is not proportional to recent activity and interferes with usual functioning" (67). It reportedly affects 70% or more of patients with cancer and has been attributed to the disease itself, as well as its treatments (68,69). While CRF can affect patients during treatment (chemotherapy, radiation, and/or surgery), it may also continue after treatment has been completed (70–72).

CRF is thought to be a subjective state, which may affect many aspects of a person's life, including the ability to perform activities of daily living, thereby affecting their quality of life (69). Symptoms of CRF can include physical, psychological, and cognitive symptoms (73). Factors that contribute to fatigue include pain, emotional distress (depression and/or anxiety), sleep disturbance, anemia, decreased or poor nutrition, deconditioning, and comorbidities (70,74) (Tables 70.3 and 70.4). Attentional fatigue, which influences concentration, memory, and information processing, is also felt to be a factor in CRF (73,75).

The NCCN recommends screening for CRF at each patient encounter. The screening, which is best initiated by the oncology care team for the patient, should assess the presence and severity of fatigue (67,68,70). Since CRF is a subjective state, it is best assessed through patient self-report and a comprehensive assessment that includes a thorough review of systems, medications, comorbidities, nutritional status, and functional/activity status (67,68,70,72). A number of assessment tools are available to evaluate CRF, including the Linear Analog Scale Assessment (68,70) (see Chapter 73 for further discussion and management options).

Depression

Psychological suffering is practically a universal experience for patients at the end of life. Block suggests that suffering exists on a continuum and that it has many sources: grief about current and anticipated losses, fear and uncertainty about the future, unresolved issues from the past, and concerns about loved ones (76).

TABLE 70.3

Pharmacologic Management of Anorexia

Drug	Suggested Dosing	Side Effects	Important Considerations
Corticosteroids (48–51)	eg, Dexamethasone (or equivalent) 2–4 mg in the morning	Short term: anxiety, tremor, insomnia, mood swings, water retention, hypertension, gastritis or peptic ulcer disease, increased serum glucose, and increased risk of infection Long term: myopathy, osteoporosis, adrenal suppression	Improves appetite, mood, sense of well-being, quality of life No effect on weight No effect on mortality; effects wane after 4–8 wks 1-wk trial should be initiated with continuation on symptomatic improvement
Megestrol acetate (50–55)	Begin 160 mg/d and titrate to max 800 mg/d in divided doses Optimal: 480–800 mg/d	Increased liver enzymes, increased risk of thromboembolism, adrenal suppression	Improves appetite, fatigue, quality of life Results in weight gain (mainly fat); can take several weeks to see increases in weight No effect on mortality As an orexigenic, is equivalent to corticosteroids Discontinue via tapering if no effect on appetite after 2 wks at maximal dose
Dronabinol (56,57)	2.5–5 mg/d	Sedation, delirium, tachycardia	Improves appetite No effect on weight No effect on mortality Less effective than megestrol acetate

TABLE 70.4

Other Potentially Useful Pharmacologic Agents in the Management of Anorexia

Drug	Important Considerations
Androgens (58)	Useful in management of anorexia/cachexia in HIV/AIDS Further studies required in management of cancer-related anorexia/cachexia
Thalidomide (59–61)	Potent inhibitor of TNFa production In a preliminary report, doses of 100 mg/d were shown to improve appetite and feelings of well-being in patients with cancer Improves lean body mass in patients with advanced cancer No effect on mortality Sedation, reportedly transient, can be problematic Teratogenic
Antiserotonergic agents (62,63) (eg, cyproheptadine and ondansetron)	Mildly improves appetite No effect on weight loss
Melatonin (64,65)	Doses of 18–20 mg at bedtime May result in appetite maintenance with minimization of cachexia compared to placebo Recent pilot study suggested enhanced effect when combined with fish oil
Fish oil (eicosapentaenoic acid) (51,66)	Promotes weight gain and lean body mass in patients with adult respiratory distress syndrome Improved 28-d mortality No effect on appetite, weight, or mortality in advanced cancer Number of pills required to achieve effective dose may be considered burdensome in palliative care population

Abbreviations: HIV, human immunodeficiency virus; TNFα, tumor necrosis factor alpha.

Preexisting and new psychiatric disorders like depression can only intensify suffering. In order to alleviate psychological suffering related to depression, health care providers caring for palliative care and dying patients must be experts in assessing, managing, and treating this source of suffering. No patient should suffer from a potentially treatable symptom such as depression (see Chapter 67 for further discussion and management options).

REHABILITATIVE MANAGEMENT OF DEPRESSION

While medication is the most utilized treatment for depression, exercise has been shown to have a beneficial effect on its management as well. Studies have shown a "dose-response" relationship between increasing physical activity and depression, and that low-moderate levels of physical activity may be helpful in preventing depressive symptoms (77). Both aerobic and anaerobic (resistance) exercise have demonstrated antidepressant effects among patients with mild to moderate depression, with the benefits often outlasting the period of exercise. Additionally, higher energy expenditure exercise appears to be more effective in decreasing depressive symptoms than lower energy expenditure exercise, though some antidepressive effects were seen with lower energy expenditure as well. It has also been observed that while patients need to continue exercising to see ongoing benefits, many of the patients in the studies who used exercise to assist in management of their depression continued to exercise once the study was completed. It is noteworthy that these benefits are seen in both younger and elderly patients. Another study suggested that group aerobic exercise may also be useful in treating depression, often as effective as medication, though medication appears to have a quicker response time. It was additionally suggested that the social interaction of the group exercise might have contributed to the beneficial effects (78–81).

Why exercise has an antidepressive effect is not fully understood, though several hypotheses have been put forth. The mechanisms suggested are physiological, psychological/social, and biological changes that occur with exercise. Physiologically, the increased circulation of beta-endorphins and monoamines, as well as the increase in body temperature and fitness level that are seen with exercise, are believed to contribute, and the role of the hypothalamic-pituitary-adrenal axis is also being explored (78–81). Biological changes include the relief of somatic symptoms, which leads to better physical functioning and improved quality of life. Psychosocial changes are seen with short amounts of training and affect change in mood by improving self-esteem,

self-efficacy, self-image, and self-worth; decreasing social isolation and reducing dysfunctional or negative thought patterns; and distracting from negative emotion (78–81). Research is still needed to determine "dosage" (intensity, frequency, amount, type) of exercise recommended in order to achieve these antidepressant effects.

Exercise has similarly been shown to have beneficial effects in cancer patients, including improving quality of life and decreasing depression. Many of the studies related to this topic have focused on patients with breast cancer, though other cancers are being researched as well. Courneya provides a comprehensive review of research in cancer survivors, looking at the effect of exercise on patients with breast cancer and with other cancers both during and after treatment (surgery, radiation, chemotherapy) (82). In general, all the populations studied tended to show improvements in fatigue, physical well-being, self-esteem, mood, depression, anxiety, and overall quality of life.

Other studies, looking specifically at the effects of exercise on depression in patients with cancer, have shown similar results. After participation in 12 weeks of supervised exercise, breast cancer patients demonstrated improved physical and psychological functioning when compared to a control group, and these benefits were maintained at a six-month follow-up. It is theorized that exercise classes appear to help through the exercise itself, the group experience, or a combination of both (83). A study of patients with testicular cancer found that depression was higher in physically inactive patients as compared to active patients, and the more physically active the patient, the less likely he was to have depression. In this study, this effect was more evident with older patients than younger ones (84). Badger and colleagues studied women with breast cancer and their partners. They noted that women with depression and anxiety may experience more physical side effects of treatment and have more difficulty managing them, as well as decreased overall quality of life (QOL), and that partner/caregiver depression/anxiety may be higher than in the patient. They found that even telephone-monitored exercise could assist with decreasing the depression and/or anxiety (85). Another study looking at breast cancer survivors found that mild to moderate aerobic exercise may be therapeutic with respect to depressive and anxiety symptoms. They also found that physician recommendation to exercise may have a positive effect on having a patient exercise as well (86). One study looked specifically at patients receiving chemotherapy and found that exercise may have a beneficial effect on psychological distress in patients with cancer (87).

Overall, the documented antidepressive benefits of exercise that are seen in the general population appear to be similar in cancer patients as well. Before initiating an exercise program, it is recommended that patients see their physician for any specific guidelines or precautions they need to follow as related to their cancer diagnosis or comorbid conditions. Considerations before initiating an exercise program may include effects of lower blood counts (neutropenic patients may want to avoid busy times at the gym, ensure good hand washing; thrombocytopenic patients may need to tconsider amount of resistance used with exercise), stage in disease process (depending on patient's status, aggressiveness of an exercise program can be adjusted), and side effects from treatment (ie, peripheral neuropathy, cardiomyopathy, nausea). Rehabilitation professionals can assist patients in initiating a comprehensive exercise program as well.

CASE CONTINUES

Mr. T. is much improved by the interventions made by the palliative care team and PT. His mood and appetite begin to improve, and he is now better able to consistently tolerate chemotherapy. Now that Mr. T.'s symptoms are under control, the palliative care team meets with Mr. T. and his wife to discuss the goals for his care.

CASE DISCUSSION

Goals-of-Care Discussions

Knowing the goals a patient has for their care allows for a context in which all other medical decisions can be made. For example, if a patient had expressed a desire to die peacefully without any further surgery or other invasive treatments but was admitted with an acute bowel obstruction, one would not call surgery to evaluate, but would instead ensure excellent pain and symptom management. As goals of care tend to be dynamic (88), they should be addressed at the time of diagnosis of any chronic or terminal illness and then at multiple times throughout the course of the disease, particularly at those points when the patient's health status changes. Guidelines have been developed for establishing goals of care (89).

It is important to begin by getting an idea of the patient's own understanding of their illness and its course. This can often be quite different from the medical team's understanding. For instance, many cancer patients receiving *palliative* chemotherapy believe that they are receiving curative treatment (90). As one can imagine, it is difficult to discuss issues such as patient thoughts on hospice if the patient believes they are not likely to die from the illness. Indeed, patients who

overestimate their life expectancy or the life-prolonging ability of treatments are more likely to choose life-prolonging therapy rather than comfort care (91).

Before sharing any information, it is important to discover whether the patient would like to know the information. When asked, most patients, but not all, want to know their prognosis (92), though they may not always want full disclosure (93). Therefore, making patients aware that they can signal the clinician to stop at any time with a raise of a hand, for example, can provide comfort and a sense of control to many patients. For those patients who do not wish to know the prognosis, it is helpful to ask if there is someone whom they would like the medical team to talk with. It is also important to find out whether the patient would like this person to make medical decisions for them despite the patient having capacity to make their own decisions with regard to medical care. This information must be documented in the medical record.

In sharing information, the aim is to "get everyone on the same page," so to speak, so that realistic goals can be elicited, discussed, and decided upon. The determination of realistic goals then allows for a context in which to make decisions regarding appropriate therapies and advanced directives, including preferences for cardiopulmonary resuscitation (94). This is especially important in terminal cancer, when treatments are more likely to be associated with burden rather than benefit (95). Indeed, while some patients prefer life-prolongation at any cost, most seriously ill patients prefer treatments aimed at pain control and those promoting preparation for death (96) (Table 70.5).

CASE CONTINUES

It has been a year since Mr. T. was diagnosed. Unfortunately, he begins to have trouble walking secondary to lower extremity weakness, along with some paresthesias in his right lower extremity associated with worsening lower back pain. He is admitted to the hospital for testing and symptom management. It is discovered that Mr. T. has epidural disease, causing some spinal cord compression at L3, L4, and L5, for which he receives opioid therapy, steroids, and undergoes radiation treatment for pain control and to help relieve the compression on his spinal cord. The medical team is hoping these treatments will reverse some of the neurological symptoms as well. However, though his pain is controlled, he is severely constipated from the opioids. While the team is addressing his pain and other medical issues, he has been referred to physical and occupational therapies (OT) to assess his current functional status, to initiate a rehabilitation plan, and for discharge recommendations.

TABLE 70.5
Goals-of-Care Discussions

What is patient's understanding of their disease?	"Can you tell me what is your understanding of what is going on with your health right now?"
What has the patient been told?	"What have the doctors told you about your illness?"
What does the patient want to know?	"I have some more information that I would like to share with you, but I would like to ask you how much you want to know." "Is there someone else you would like me to talk with?"
Share information	1. State of patient's illness at current time 2. Prognosis (likely course from this point on)
Respond to emotions	"I know this must be very difficult for you to hear." "I hate having to tell patients/families this kind of information."
Explore the patient's goals for their future based on aforementioned information	"What concerns you most about the future?" "What are your biggest fears?" "How do you see your future?" "What is most important to you as you move forward in your illness?"

Source: Adapted from Ref. 89.

Given that Mr. T.'s medical condition has changed since the prior discussion, the primary medical team, along with the palliative care team meets with Mr. T. and his wife to readdress goals of care. Mr. T. elects to enter acute rehabilitation followed by a trial with an experimental treatment for his cancer rather than hospice at this time. Given that his symptoms are improved, Mr. T, his wife, and his medical team are in agreement with this plan and referral to rehabilitation medicine is made. Mr. T. is accepted to a rehabilitation unit at the hospital and is transferred there to complete his radiation therapy and to begin a more aggressive rehabilitation program. Once he is discharged home from the rehab unit, Mr. T. receives home PT and OT, and then progresses to outpatient rehab to continue his recovery.

CASE DISCUSSION

Assessment and Management of Pain

Given that approximately 80% of patients with cancer experience pain, one can see why entire textbooks have been devoted to cancer pain management. As the types, assessment, and management of pain have been covered elsewhere in this textbook, we will not review aspects of pain management here, except those related to rehabilitative interventions for pain management. Instead, we will briefly discuss psychological pain, as this type of pain is often undetected and therefore left untreated (97,98). The importance of accurate detection and treatment of psychological pain should not be underestimated, given its effects on patient well-being, perception of other symptoms, amount of medical services utilized, length of hospital stay, costs of medical services, and possibly even effects on survival (99,100).

Psychological pain has been defined as pain in response to "noxious psychological stimuli," which can be considered analogous to physical pain in response to "noxious physical stimuli" (101). Others have defined psychological pain as a "unique, discomforting, emotional state experienced by an individual in response to a specific stressor or demand that results in harm, either temporary or permanent, to the person" (102). These "noxious psychological stimuli" or "stressors" can include serious illness such as cancer. Using functional magnetic resonance imaging, it has been suggested that psychological pain may activate many of the same pain pathways within the central nervous system (CNS) as physical pain (17). Psychological pain is thought to run along a continuum, with normal transient feelings of fear, apprehension, worry, and depressed mood to highly clinically significant constant feelings of fear, hopelessness, spiritual concerns, meaninglessness, and thoughts of suicide that interfere with daily functioning (99,101).

Psychological pain is often present in varying degrees in many patients with cancer and is particularly prominent in palliative care (99,103). Psychological pain can be expressed as physical or spiritual pain (104), anxiety, or depression (105). Existential distress, described as meaninglessness, hopelessness, or loss of control or of dignity (106), may also be expressed as psychological pain and is associated with desire for hastened death in terminally ill cancer patients (107).

Given that many patients with cancer experience some degree of psychological pain, whether manifested as physical pain or not, pain assessment should include methods to evaluate for the presence of psychological pain. This is particularly important given that less than 25% of cancer patients will offer this information independently despite the fact that, at least in one study, 100% want to discuss these issues (108). In general, a clue to the presence of psychological pain is physical pain that appears poorly managed despite optimal medical management (109). Other clues include nonverbal behaviors such as lack of or excessive movement, flat affect, a flat or distressed tone of voice, and a dejected or unkempt appearance (110). Answers to questions that directly assess for depression, anhedonia, hopelessness, dignity, meaninglessness, guilt, religious or spiritual concerns, fear, impairments in social functioning, and coping ability may provide considerable evidence for the presence of psychological pain. The use of self-completed quality-of-life questionnaires (111) or patient question/concern prompt sheets (112) may also be valuable in the detection of the presence of psychological pain. Additionally, a single-item screening tool developed by the NCCN, a Distress Thermometer, designed to assess physical, psychological, social, and spiritual concerns, has been validated in the cancer population (113,114).

Just as with physical pain, clinically significant psychological pain often requires aggressive management, which should include spiritual and psychological counseling (115), often in combination with medical management. Clinical guidelines designed to address the various components of psychological distress observed in palliative care patients have been developed by the NCCN and are available on the Web (http://www.nccn.org). Others have proposed various strategies to aid in the management of specific facets of existential distress (116). It is important to stress to patients that treatment of their psychological pain is only one aspect of their care and does not mean that "it is all in their head" (117).

REHABILITATIVE MANAGEMENT OF PAIN IN PALLIATIVE CARE

In addition to the use of medication, rehabilitation professionals, physiatrists, and physical and occupational therapists can all assist in managing a patient's pain. Nonpharmacologic techniques may include bracing, use of assistive devices and adaptive equipment, exercise, use of modalities (including ice and heat), distraction, relaxation training, massage (positive mental), imagery, cutaneous stimulation through a variety of sources (eg, transcutaneous electrical nerve stimulation [TENS] or massage), as well as other complimentary interventions (118–120). The rehabilitation approach to pain management tends to look at both the underlying cause of the pain and the functional limitations related to the pain (121).

When a patient may benefit from bracing, either for an extremity or for the spine, it is imperative to involve an orthotist who can fit a patient with the most appropriate brace and properly fit the brace to the patient. A brace may be used to help unload a painful joint, provide external stability, and help compensate for weak muscles (121). Likewise, assistive devices, including walkers and wheelchairs, need to be ordered and adjusted appropriately for each patient.

A number of modalities have been found useful in helping to manage pain as well. Superficial heat and ice can be used to decrease postoperative pain, pain related to inflammation, and alleviate stiffness associated with pain and immobility (120). Deeper heating modalities, such as ultrasound, are often contraindicated. TENS provides mild electrical stimulation to affected areas and is thought to disrupt the pain pathway through sensory nerve stimulation. The use of TENS for patients with cancer has been controversial, though is not contraindicated (122). It should not be used in patients with pacemakers, over the anterior neck/carotid sinus, internally, over the anterior chest wall in patients with cardiac problems, or with incompetent patients who would not be able to manage the device appropriately (119,122). Massage can be beneficial as well through promotion of warmth and relaxation, as well as in assisting with decreasing muscle tension/stiffness (118,120).

A variety of complimentary therapies/techniques have also been shown to be useful adjunctive therapies in managing pain and cancer-related pain. These may include mind–body techniques such as relaxation, meditation, guided imagery, hypnosis, biofeedback, cognitive behavioral therapy, and psychoeducational approaches (ie, supportive group therapy). In addition to assisting in pain management, these interventions may have a role in improving mood, quality of life, and coping (118,123). Interventions such as acupuncture, therapeutic touch, and qigong, as well as other traditional Chinese medicine techniques, reiki, and yoga are also valuable in managing cancer-related pain (120).

REHABILITATION MANAGEMENT OF NEUROLOGICAL SYMPTOMS

Involving rehabilitation professionals, especially physical and occupational therapists, is important at this stage. A thorough evaluation will look specifically at patients' prior and current level of functioning. This will include obtaining a thorough history and a complete assessment of transfers, ambulation and gait, activities of daily living (ADLs), balance in both sitting and standing, range of motion, strength, posture, cognitive status, and fine motor skills, in addition to special tests if indicated (ie, vestibular assessment). Therapists will take into consideration location of disease, including metastases (especially to bone), stage of disease, and patient/family/caregiver goals (124,125). All of this information is compiled to establish an ideal treatment program and plan for the patient. Patients with neurological symptoms, whether from spinal cord compression, as with Mr. T., leptomeningeal disease, or brain metastases or tumor, may be treated by rehabilitation professionals in the acute hospital, inpatient rehabilitation, home, or outpatient settings.

While the patient's disease and overall status needs to be considered, rehabilitation interventions utilized with this patient population are the same as with someone who presents with a spinal cord injury (traumatic or nontraumatic), a stroke, or any other noncancerous neurological diagnosis (124). An individualized treatment program is established incorporating therapist findings with patient/family/caregiver goals (125). Patients' functional deficits are addressed through standard therapy techniques and may include transfer training, body mechanics training (patient and family), therapeutic exercises, gait training, wheelchair skill/management training if indicated, family education, ADL training, and assessment for assistive device and other adaptive equipment as indicated (124). Additionally, as part of the interdisciplinary team, rehabilitation professionals, physiatry, and therapists may assist in determining bracing needs for patients (ie, back brace for additional trunk support if patient has compression fractures (thoracic lumbosacral orthosis [TLSO], etc.) or ankle foot orthosis (AFO) if the patient has weakened dorsiflexors) (126).

Constipation

Constipation can generally be defined as the slow movement of feces through the large intestine (127), resulting in hard, dry stool that may be difficult to expel. Despite this clear medical definition, constipation has different meanings for different people (128). Patients may report constipation if feces are hard and dry; if there is difficulty, straining, or discomfort in expelling stool; or if stools are less frequent than normal for them. The estimated incidence of constipation in the general population is 5%–20% (129,130). Research shows that in persons with advanced cancer and other terminal illness, the prevalence of constipation ranges

from 23%–55% (131–134). In general, constipation is uncomfortable and must be treated quickly and aggressively.

Normal bowel function involves communication between many body systems to break down food, permit proper absorption and transport of fluids and nutritional elements, and propel the remaining food residue through the gastrointestinal tract to form stool for excretion (129,130). Any alteration in this process can negatively affect normal bowel function and cause complications such as constipation (135). Knowledge of possible underlying etiology of constipation can be helpful in both prophylaxis and treatment. The most important of these are immobility, poor fluid and dietary intake, fecal impaction, and medications, particularly opioids.

There are many causes of constipation. Constipation can be caused by cancer-related complications such as hypercalcemia, intra-abdominal or pelvic disease, spinal cord compression, cauda equina syndrome, or depression (135,136). Debility is frequently associated with constipation. Resulting effects of debility can include weakness, inactivity or bed rest, poor nutrition and fluid intake, confusion, and an inability to reach the toilet (135,136). Pharmaceutical treatments of other illnesses may also cause constipation, including opioids, antiemetics, anticholinergics, aluminum salts, and nonsteroidal anti-inflammatory drugs (136,137). Other concurrent disorders that can result in constipation are hemorrhoids, anal fissure, fecal impaction, and endocrine dysfunction (136).

Constipation is identified based on a patient's report of infrequent or absent bowel movements; decrease in bowel movement volume; difficulty or pain with defecation; incomplete defecation; abdominal distention; oozing liquid stool; or hard, dry stool (129,130). In addition, patients may also present with the following associated symptoms: abdominal pain, bloating or change in gas pattern, nausea, vomiting, rectal fullness or pressure, confusion, restlessness, anxiety, or urinary retention (129,130). In all cases, it is important for the clinician to determine the patient's definition of constipation and normal bowel habits. The history and physical examination should include the following: general assessment, history related to the complaint of constipation, gastrointestinal assessment, rectal examination, and psychoemotional assessment. Simple disimpaction of retained feces may alleviate patient symptoms and avoid the use of concurrent medications. Bowel obstruction must be ruled out prior to any further intervention.

Frequently, despite use of prophylactic interventions, patients with terminal illness require laxatives to both treat and prevent constipation (137). Interventions and treatment of constipation extend beyond just laxative therapy. Particular attention should be paid to patient symptoms (especially pain), diet, fluid intake, mobility, and toileting, as all these items contribute to an effective outcome.

Laxatives, however, do remain the mainstay of therapeutic options. The goal of laxative treatment is to achieve a comfortable defecation experience, rather than a particular frequency of bowel movements. The choice of laxative depends on the cause of the constipation, the nature of the stools, and acceptability to the patient (135). Laxatives can be subdivided into three groups. The first group contains predominantly softening agents: surfactants (eg, sodium docusate), osmotic laxatives (eg, Lactulose), bulking agents (eg, methyl cellulose), saline laxatives (eg, magnesium sulfate), and lubricants (eg, liquid paraffin). The second group includes predominantly peristalsis-stimulating agents: anthracenes (eg, senna) and polyphenolics (eg, bisacodyl). The final group includes a combination of the previous two (135). When selecting the appropriate laxative, it is helpful to know the primary mechanism of action.

Treatment should not be limited to medications, but should be focused on etiologies of constipation. When treating patients at the end of their life, a distended colon or rectum can be a potent cause of agitation and pain. It is important to attempt to relieve the constipation, which may provide complete relief of pain and agitation. The use of opioids to treat the pain of constipation may only make the constipation, and ultimately the pain, worse, thus creating a vicious cycle.

CASE CONTINUES

After discharge from the rehabilitation unit, Mr. T. returns to the palliative care clinic for follow-up. Since his discharge, Mr. T. has been undergoing treatment with an experimental chemotherapy, which he has been tolerating well with few side effects. However, the palliative care nurse practitioner learns that his pain has begun to increase again over the past week and a magnetic resonance imaging (MRI) performed the day before revealed further progression of the disease in his spine. The nurse practitioner discusses the advantages of entering hospice and suggests that he meet again with the palliative care social worker to evaluate the different options.

The palliative care social worker speaks with Mr. T. and his wife and explains the philosophy of hospice. If Mr. T. chooses to no longer pursue curative treatment, hospice is an option for care. Hospice provides aggressive symptom management and focus on comfort and relief from suffering. This suffering can

be physical, emotional, or spiritual. A multidisciplinary team, including a nurse, social worker, and chaplain, will be available to meet the needs of the Mr. T. and his wife and children. The hospice plan of care includes counseling for Mr. T. as well as for his wife and children and visits from the chaplain. Home hospice programs provide a home health aide for 20 hours per week to help with personal care. Most home hospice programs are flexible about how these hours are distributed. Physical therapy and other rehabilitative services can also be a part of the hospice treatment plan. Hospice can be provided at home or in an inpatient unit. While hospice is a home-based program, there are times that both patients and families have need for an inpatient hospice. If a patient on a home hospice program requires more intensive symptom management, the patient can be transferred to the inpatient hospice unit. Hospice can provide blood transfusions, intravenous (IV) hydration, and patient-controlled analgesic pumps if necessary for optimal symptom management. Inpatient facilities are available for family members of patients on home programs who may require caregiving respite. Most inpatient hospices allow families to visit 24 hours a day if necessary and often have accommodations and amenities available for families. Some skilled nursing and other long-term care facilities provide hospice care.

The social worker also explains that while the hospice plan of care is not curative, sometimes, palliative chemotherapy and radiation are indicated for maximum symptom management and can be provided. Some hospice programs do not require that a patient agree to a do not resuscitate (DNR) order, which means that if Mr. T. decided that he wanted to be resuscitated, the family could call 911 and he would be transferred to a hospital. Mr. T. reiterates that he would like to have a DNR order placed in his home to ensure that an attempt at resuscitation not be made. It is decided that Mr. T. will enter a home hospice program to help ensure that his goals of dying peacefully at home without machines, with his family present, will be met when the time comes.

CASE DISCUSSION

Physical Therapy in Hospice

Involving a physical (and/or occupational) therapist when a patient enters hospice can be beneficial. As the patient's physical and functional status declines, the therapist may provide the caregiver(s) with education on body mechanics, guarding techniques, and optimal positioning for comfort and breathing (137). Recommendations for additional adaptive equipment, such as a hospital bed, bedside commode, elevated toilet seat, tub bench, grab rail by the bed, seat cushion, etc., may also be helpful in caring for a patient at home.

Physical therapy, or more specifically, rehabilitation professionals, do have a role in the hospice setting, whether inpatient or at home. While there may be limited financial resources available in hospice, physical therapy has been shown to be effective in this setting in terms of maximizing patients' functional status within the limitations imposed by their disease process, as well as improving quality of life. Therapy involvement at this stage is indicated if it is what the patient wants, and it is imperative that all members of the hospice team work together in this light (137).

CASE CONTINUES

Over the next three months, Mr. T. thrives in hospice and is able to travel to many parts of the country he had always wished to see and also to spend a great deal of time with his family. He has worked with the hospice social worker to get his financial affairs in order and feels confident that he has prevented a burden from being placed on his wife when he dies. He has spent many hours with the chaplain and feels at peace with God and his impending death, and has even organized his own memorial service, which will include a self-made slide show of himself and his family during happier times. He has spent several hours composing letters and video messages for his wife and children to be read and played at various events in their lives.

CASE DISCUSSION

Spiritual Issues and Search for Meaning

Spiritual pain: Spiritual care is an integral part of hospice and palliative care programs. At the end of life, being at peace with God ranks only marginally below the desire to ease physical pain (138). At the end of life, patients may return to the roots of their early religious experience or develop a new set of values, which brings them a sense of meaning. In order to ascertain how to better intervene to assist in relieving spiritual pain, it is essential to ask specific questions. First, it is important to determine the patient's faith or belief. Second, the importance of that belief must be assessed. What role does that belief play in determining the end of life and belief in the afterlife? It is also important to determine whether the patient is supported by a faith community and the role of the community in providing spiritual and emotional support. Finally, it is important to determine how the health care team can support the

patient's spirituality (139). Hospital or hospice chaplains are available for religious rituals and for patients who have questions about theology. Patient needs may range from religious rituals such as prayers, anointing, scripture reading, or using Sabbath candles to discussion of more existential issues.

Based on the British model of hospice pioneered by Dame Cicely Saunders, the American model more broadly focuses on respecting the rights of the individual, which encompasses diverse spiritual practices (140). Spirituality may be expressed as a relationship with God, but it can also be defined more broadly. Spirituality can also be about art, music, family, nature, or whatever values and beliefs give a person a sense of meaning and purpose (139). Interventions can involve listening and encouraging patients to articulate their stories and struggles. It is not uncommon for patients to articulate a new sense of what is important in life.

As patients struggle with physical pain at the end of life, they also may focus on an inward search for meaning. Common existential issues for patients at the end of life may include hopelessness, futility, meaninglessness, disappointment, remorse, death anxiety, and disruption of personal identity (77). Like physical pain, spiritual pain is fluid and requires ongoing assessment (141). Those caring for the dying must be attentive to nurturing a supportive environment where these issues can be articulated, explored, and affirmed. It is important for those providing spiritual care to be comfortable with their own spiritual practice in order to create an open and nonjudgmental atmosphere (142).

Finding meaning can mean leaving a legacy for children or other loved ones. Sometimes, letters, videos, or other means of communication can provide comfort and peace to the dying patient. The knowledge that some part of the patient will live on in the lives of others will assure continuity (143).

CASE CONCLUDES

Mr. T.'s pain begins to increase markedly, and his opioid doses are raised quickly to ensure adequate pain control. Mr. T. has stopped eating and drinking and sleeps most of the day. The hospice nurse explains that Mr. T. is entering the dying phase and explains to the family what they might expect to encounter over the next few days to weeks. His pain appears well controlled, and the family helps to relieve Mr. T.'s dry mouth with ice chips and small sips of water as he tolerates.

As the days pass, Mr. T. becomes increasingly short of breath, for which the hospice nurse orders oxygen and opioids and places a fan on a table near Mr. T.'s face. He has also become increasingly confused and will often speak of seeing angels or dead family members around his bed. The hospice nurse explains to the family that she feels the end is near. She tells them to continue to speak to him and touch him, as touch and hearing are the last two senses to be lost as people die. The hospice social worker spends time with Mr. T's wife and children to provide support during this time. Two days later, Mr. T becomes unconscious and dies peacefully several hours later at home with his family at his side. The hospice social worker is available to help the family with bereavement. Bereavement programs are mandated by hospice and continue for 13 months following the death of the patient, recognizing the fact that families often have a difficult time with the first anniversary date of the death of a loved one. Mr. T's family writes letters to the oncologist, palliative care team, physical and occupational therapists, and the hospice team thanking everyone for all of their hard work in ensuring that Mr. T. lived as well and as fully as he could when he was alive and was as comfortable as he could be when he died.

CASE DISCUSSION

The Dying Process

Guidelines for quality palliative care have endorsed educating patients and families regarding what to expect during the terminal phase of an illness (144). Interestingly, physicians are notorious for overestimating survival (145) and often do not recognize the symptoms and signs of impending death or may instead attribute them to the same or another disease process (146). This lack or delay in recognition of the terminal phase on the part of the physician can result in a "missed opportunity" to provide this important patient and family education.

Usually, one of the first signs that death is near is social withdrawal (147). The person becomes less interested first in the world around them, with a gradual decrease in interest in the news/newspaper, television, and/or radio. Also during this time, the patient and/or family may notice a decreased interest in food as the need for nourishment decreases while the body begins to shut down. This may actually improve patient well-being, as it has been suggested that the resulting ketosis may diminish discomfort (148). This effect of ketoacids has even led to the suggested use of β-hydroxybutyrate, the principal ketoacid formed, as a therapeutic agent in end-of-life care (149). The patient and family will often report that the person has required less to drink and may even stop drinking altogether. Families and health care workers alike may be concerned that the patient will become dehydrated and thereby uncom-

fortable. However, many experts believe that terminal dehydration may also promote comfort due the resulting rise in endorphins, which contributes to a sense of well-being (150). There may also be a fear that the patient will suffer thirst and would therefore benefit from intravenous fluids. However, the evidence has repeatedly demonstrated that the sensation of thirst is not related to fluid balance in dying patients and that the administration of intravenous fluids does not relieve thirst (148,151,152). Instead, in the majority, thirst is related to the sensation of dry mouth and can be controlled with local measures such as ice chips, small sips of water (family can give drops of water with a medicine dropper or gentle mists with a small spray bottle), moistened sponge sticks, petrolatum application to the lips, and meticulous oral hygiene (148,153). In addition, health care workers need to be aware that a decreased pulse or blood pressure in a dying patient is part of the dying process and is not due to dehydration and therefore not an indication for intravenous fluid therapy (148). Taking the time to explain to the family that loss of the need for nourishment or drink is all a natural part of the dying process, rather than that the patient is "starving to death" or "dying of thirst," can go a long way toward providing comfort for both the patient and family during this difficult time.

As a result of changes in the body's metabolism in response to disease progression, the dying person will also begin to spend more time sleeping (144). Eventually, most patients become unconscious altogether (148). As hearing is the last of the five senses to be lost, one can encourage the family to continue to speak to the patient as if they were still conscious. Encouraging family members to utilize this time to ensure that they tell the patient all of the things they would want the patient to know before death, such as "goodbye," "I forgive you," and "I love you," can provide significant comfort to the family.

With decreasing consciousness and declining neurological function comes impairment in swallowing ability. Once this occurs, family members should be cautioned about continuing oral intake, as this may lead to aspiration. An associated decrease in the gag reflex results in pooling of normal naso-oropharyngeal secretions in the posterior oropharynx, which may result in a gurgling sound during breathing, sometimes termed "death rattle." In the majority of patients, the appearance of the "death rattle" is associated with death within 48 hours (154). While this pooling is not considered a source of distress for the dying patient, it may be so for the family. Oropharyngeal suctioning is not recommended in this setting and is considered ineffective and uncomfortable. The use of antimuscarinic medications, by decreasing secretions, can be effective in this situation, though they will not have an effect on secretions that have already accumulated (39). Disorientation to date, time, and persons around them, particularly as death approaches, may occur. The dying person may speak of seeing angels, family members and friends who have already died, or other hallucinations. As this can be distressing to family members, it should be explained that as long as these "visions" are not concerning to the patient, it is most beneficial not to argue with or correct the patient, though the person can be gently reoriented if that is the patient's wish (144). Occasionally, disorientation may be associated with acute onset of restlessness and agitation, with the patient attempting to get out of bed or pulling or picking at bed sheets. This may suggest the presence of terminal delirium (see section on delirium).

Particular physical changes are associated with the dying process. Vital sign changes include decreasing blood pressure, tachycardia or bradycardia, and fluctuations in body temperature (144). Fever is common and should be treated symptomatically with acetaminophen and cold packs. Changes in the breathing pattern, thought to represent severe neurological compromise, can occur such that periods of apnea or Cheyne-Stokes respirations may occur. Agonal breathing or gasping breaths are associated with use of accessory muscles of respiration and may cause concern for suffocation or breathlessness. Families should be assured that unconscious patients are not experiencing these sensations. When appropriate, opioids or benzodiazepines can be used to manage any perception of dyspnea (148). As a result of a decrease in cardiac output and resultant decreased peripheral perfusion, the extremities will become cool and cyanotic, possibly with mottling of the skin and venous pooling. As perfusion of the kidneys decreases, oliguria or anuria will also occur.

Dyspnea

Dyspnea, defined as difficulty breathing, occurring in up to 70% of patients with cancer in some studies (155) and in up to 90% of patients seen by palliative care teams (156), is reportedly one of the most troublesome symptoms in palliative care patients and is associated with a large negative impact on quality of life (157). Mechanisms involved in causing dyspnea are: (1) stimulation of peripheral or central chemoreceptors, (2) stimulation of intrapulmonary receptors, (3) stimulation of respiratory muscle mechanoreceptors, and (4) increased motor command or increased sensation of effort required to breathe (158). Most often, there is an overlap in mechanisms.

Dyspnea, distinct from tachypnea in that it is associated with discomfort, is, like pain, a subjective sensation and as such, the only reliable measure is patient self-report. Patients often describe dyspnea as

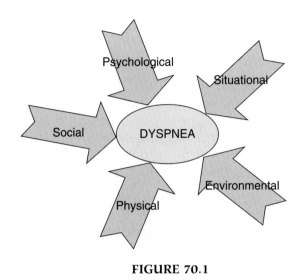

FIGURE 70.1

Multiple factors affecting the perception of dyspnea.

a feeling of breathlessness, shortness of breath, inability to pull enough air into the lungs, or a feeling of being smothered or of suffocating. The experience of dyspnea results from multiple factors acting in concert (Fig. 70.1). This explains the hypoxemic or tachypneic patient who denies any dyspnea, as well as the patient with severe dyspnea who has a normal arterial partial pressure of oxygen (PaO_2) or respiratory rate (RR). Therefore, as a guide to management, it is important to consider the interaction of these factors when assessing dyspnea.

Many different scales have been used in various populations to assess the degree of distress or the intensity of dyspnea (159). Although none of these scales has been evaluated or validated in the palliative care population, a recent study evaluating the different scales has demonstrated that the majority of critically ill patients, those who are likely the most similar to palliative care patients, preferred an analog scale similar to that used for the assessment of pain (160). This is a 0–10-point numerical scale, with 0 representing the absence of dyspnea and 10 representing the greatest amount imaginable. When asking patients about dyspnea, it is important to ask about their levels at rest *and* with activity, as many patients curb their activities as a result of dyspnea.

MANAGEMENT OF DYSPNEA

The initial step in the management of dyspnea is to assess, within the confines of the established goals of care, for a treatable or reversible etiology. In patients with congestive heart failure, chronic obstructive pulmonary disease, or asthma, optimization of disease-specific treatment may be all that is required. Antibiotics for infection, thoracentesis or placement of a pleuro-peritoneal catheter or pleurodesis in pleural effusion, placement of a chest tube for treatment of a pneumothorax, paracentesis or semipermanent drainage catheter placement in ascites, and blood transfusion in anemia may all provide relief of dyspnea related to a specific etiology.

Regardless of whether one is assessing for a reversible cause, symptomatic relief can be provided utilizing a host of nonpharmacologic and pharmacologic treatments. Simple interventions, such as providing reassurance, elevating the head of the bed, opening a window, or providing a small fan, can be helpful (89). A cool breeze through an open window or from a fan is thought to reduce dyspnea as a result of stimulation of upper airway receptors mediated by the trigeminal nerve (159). Though most studies are performed in patients with chronic obstructive pulmonary disease, complementary treatments such as relaxation exercises (161) or acupressure/acupuncture (162) may also prove beneficial. Pulmonary rehabilitation may also be useful in some instances (163). As always, patient and family education can go a long way toward decreasing distress levels.

Oxygen

Oxygen, a potent symbol of medical care, can provide relief in patients, regardless of the presence of hypoxemia (165). Oxygen itself acts on chemoreceptors to decrease ventilation, and the flow itself also stimulates nasal receptors and thereby the trigeminal nerve, both of which may be beneficial in relieving dyspnea (159). Face masks can worsen the sensation of suffocation/dyspnea and should be avoided if possible (159).

Opioids

Opioids remain at the core of treatment for dyspnea, especially in the terminally ill. Despite the fact that prescribing opioids for the palliation of dyspnea is consistent with good medical practice, as well as the wide availability of dosing guidelines, there is still hesitancy on the part of many clinicians to prescribe opioids for the management of dyspnea (89). Though there is debate as to whether it even applies to the use of opioids and sedatives in palliative care (165), when one faces hesitation such as this, it is often helpful to remind oneself of the doctrine of double effect. This ethical construct applies whenever one is using a treatment for an ethical, intended positive effect, knowing that there may also be secondary adverse effects, including death. As long as the intent in using the treatment is for its beneficial effects according to best practice, one cannot be held morally, ethically, or legally responsible if the known dire adverse effects occur. This construct also applies, though is often forgotten, when an oncologist prescribes chemotherapy, medications whose known side effects can include death.

Opioids are thought to act via both peripheral and central mechanisms to decrease the perception of dyspnea and to decrease respiratory drive (159). A recent systematic review of the use of opioids for the management of dyspnea demonstrated a highly significant effect of oral and intravenously administered opioids on the sensation of dyspnea. Despite the known presence of pulmonary opioid receptors, a subgroup analysis failed to show a similar effect of inhaled opioids (166). Interestingly, in this systematic review, which included studies in patients with chronic obstructive pulmonary disease (COPD), there was no evidence for deleterious effects of opioids on arterial oxygen (PaO_2) and carbon dioxide ($PaCO_2$) tensions or on oxygen saturation. Another study, this one involving patients in a palliative care unit, excluding those with COPD, demonstrated a lack of effect of the equivalent of 10 mg of intravenous morphine on $PaCO_2$ levels or on oxygen saturation, despite a significant reduction in respiratory rate (167). As the risk of respiratory depression increases with rapidly rising blood levels, more important than absolute opioid dose is the rate of opioid titration (28). Thus, the dictum "start low and go slow," often proscribed for prescribing medications in the elderly, is also useful in initiating opioids in the management of dyspnea. Given that each opioid has a different potency, when using opioids, whether for the management of dyspnea or pain, it is important to use the opioid equianalgesic table whenever changing route of administration or between opioids (see Part IV on pain management).

Miscellaneous

Though there is little evidence for a role of anxiolytics in the management of dyspnea, when anxiety is thought to be a significant factor or when dyspnea does not resolve with opioids alone, a trial of benzodiazepines or buspirone is not unreasonable (168,169). In the case of dyspnea related to carcinomatous lymphangitis or radiation pneumonitis, corticosteroids may be of benefit (170).

Delirium

The *Diagnostic and Statistical Manual of Mental Disorders*, Fourth Edition (DSM-IV), defines delirium based upon disordered attention (arousal) and cognitive disturbance (170). Without careful clinical assessment, delirium can easily be mistaken for other primary psychiatric conditions because of its neuropsychiatric symptoms that are also commonly seen in other disorders, such as dementia, depression, and psychosis (169,171). Unfortunately, delirium is a common and often distressing medical complication in the patient with advanced illness (172,173). Depending on the population studied and criteria used, it is estimated that delirium occurs in 28%–85% of patients who are reaching the end of their life (172,174,175). In hospitalized adult patients, it is associated with significant morbidity and mortality along with lengthy hospital stays and nursing home placement (176).

CLINICAL ASSESSMENT

Delirium is not a disease, but a complex syndrome, typically with an acute onset (usually over hours to days) and a fluctuating course (169,177). The clinical features of delirium may include prodromal symptoms (restlessness, anxiety, sleep disturbance, irritability); rapidly fluctuating course; reduced attention; altered arousal; increased or decreased psychomotor activity; disturbance of the sleep-wake cycle; affective symptoms (emotional lability, sadness, anger, euphoria); altered perceptions (misperceptions, illusions, poorly formed delusions, hallucinations); disorganized thinking and incoherent speech; disorientation to time, place, or person; and memory impairment (171). Neurological features that may be present during delirium include motor abnormalities (tremor, asterixis, myoclonus, reflex or tone changes), and cortical abnormalities (dysgraphia, constructional apraxia, dysnomic aphasia) (171).

There are three clinically described subtypes of delirium that are classified according to arousal disturbance and psychomotor behavior (178). The subtypes are hyperactive, hypoactive, and mixed (170). With the hyperactive subtype, patients may be agitated, disoriented, delusional, and may experience hallucinations (170). As a result, this presentation can be mistaken for agitated dementia, schizophrenia, or a psychotic disorder (170,176). In patients with the hypoactive subtype of delirium, they typically present lethargic, quietly confused, disoriented, and apathetic (170). Hypoactive delirium may be confused with depression or dementia (177,179). The mixed subtype of delirium is characterized by a presentation that fluctuates between both the hyperactive and hypoactive subtypes (177).

Delirium is frequently misdiagnosed and under- or inappropriately treated, especially in patients with advanced disease and in the terminally ill (179). Moaning, groaning, and grimacing by actively dying patients is often interpreted by families and health care workers to signal physical pain, but may, in fact, represent delirium. It is a myth that pain, if not previously a problem, will suddenly arise at the end of life (148).

In fact, morphine may worsen delirium, as metabolites accumulate in these patients secondary to poor renal clearance. While a trial of opioids may be appropriate if agitation is not relieved or worsens, management of delirium is required. If delirium is poorly managed or unmanaged, the family will likely remember a terrible death in which their loved one "died in pain," regardless of the excellence of all previous care (148).

Particularly in the context of advanced disease, it is helpful for the clinician to evaluate disturbances in consciousness, cognition, and onset. In identifying and distinguishing delirium from other disorders, screening and diagnostic tools are valuable to a clinician's evaluation. Many screening tools are available to assist clinicians in identifying delirium. The most commonly used and familiar tool is the Folstein Mini-Mental State Examination (MMSE) (180). The MMSE is a cognitive impairment screening tool that assists clinicians in identifying delirium symptoms, but it cannot be used for diagnostic purposes. It can also be used for monitoring the improvement or decline of a patient's cognitive function (181).

Two examples of delirium diagnostic instruments to be used in conjunction with a clinical examination are the Confusion Assessment Method (CAM) (182), and the Delirium Rating Scale (DRS) (183). Both the DRS and CAM were developed to be used by a clinician to first identify delirium and then reliably distinguish it from dementia and other neuropsychiatric disorders (171,179). A useful tool that assesses the severity of delirium in patients with advanced disease is the Memorial Delirium Assessment Scale (MDAS) (184).

MANAGEMENT OF DELIRIUM

Management options include identification and treatment of potential underlying causes, with correction, if possible, of the identified contributing factors as well as symptomatic treatment with both nonpharmacologic and pharmacologic (Table 70.6) interventions.

Delirium can have numerous potential causes that can be simultaneously contributing to the state of delirium. The most common known causes of delirium include drugs, metabolic abnormalities, infection, CNS pathology, and drug/alcohol withdrawal (171,179). Based upon the evidence, a full clinical diagnostic workup and physical exam is indicated to evaluate the potentially reversible causes of delirium.

In the terminally ill or dying patient who develops delirium in their last days of life (terminal delirium), the medical management is unique and can present many dilemmas for clinicians, other health care providers involved in care, patients, and families. An ongoing debate continues to exist about the appropriate

TABLE 70.6
Pharmacologic Management of Delirium

Drug/Class (Suggested Dosing)	Side Effects (Not Exhaustive)	Important Considerations
Butyrophenones: Haloperidol (186,187) (1–5 mg orally/IV/SQ every 30 min until calm. Max dose 30 mg/24 h)	Extrapyramidal effects Dystonic reactions Akathesia QT interval prolongation	First-line agent, except in alcohol withdrawal and anticholinergic excess Can lower seizure threshold Reorienting Not very sedating Co-administer with a benzodiazepine to increase sedation Contraindicated in Parkinson disease
Phenothiazines: Chlorpromazine (188,189) (25 mg IV/SQ/orally every 1–2h until calm. This dose then divided every 6h. Max dose 300 mg/24 h)	Hypotension (with rapid intravenous administration) Extrapyramidal effects Sedation Akathesia Agranulocytosis	Most sedating Useful in agitated/terminal delirium More likely to lower seizure threshold Contraindicated in Parkinson disease
Atypical neuroleptics (190,191): Olanzapine Quetiapine Risperidone	Possible small increase in risk of adverse cerebrovascular events Sedation Extrapyramidal effects (much less likely than butyrophenones and phenothiazines	Helpful in confusional states Not considered first-line treatments for delirium Can be used in Parkinson disease Olanzapine and quetiapine are sedating and may be useful in agitated delirium Expensive
Barbiturates (192): Phenobarbital (30 mg subcutaneously (SQ) every 4h)	Sedation Hypotension Agranulocytosis Respiratory depression (with rapid intravascular administration)	Useful in agitated delirium No decrease in seizure threshold Can be used in Parkinson disease and Lewy body disease
Benzodiazapines (193,194): Lorazepam Midazolam	Sedation Respiratory depression	Monotherapy should be avoided, except in cases of alcohol or sedative withdrawal Can worsen restlessness and/or cognitive impairment Midazolam has short half-life

extent of diagnostic evaluation and workup that should be pursued in a dying patient with terminal delirium (133,173). Ultimately, the desired clinical outcome may be altered by the natural course of the dying process. Most palliative care clinicians determine the degree of workup based on understanding of the disease trajectory and established goals of care. The pursuit usually includes interventions that carry minimal burden or risk of inducing further distress and suffering.

Nonpharmacologic interventions can help manage delirium and often assist in its prevention. The key items are to provide support and orientation, a comfortable environment, and maintain competency as long as possible (195). Measures that may help to reduce anxiety and disorientation include a quiet,

well-lit room with familiar objects, a visible clock or calendar, and the presence of family and friends. It is important to keep the patient safe by adequate supervision with avoidance of restraint use whenever possible. Delirium can be a frightening experience for both the patient and family. It is important to use education as a tool to reassure both that the patient is not going crazy, the delirium may be reversible, and the symptoms can be managed (196).

References

1. *Clinical Practice Guidelines for Quality Palliative Care.* Brooklyn (NY): National Consensus Project for Quality Palliative Care; 2004:. 67 p.

2. Hearn J, Higginson IJ. Do specialist palliative care teams improve outcomes for cancer patients? A systematic review. *Palliat Med.* 1998;12:317–322.

3. Yoshioka H. Rehabilitation for the terminal cancer patient. *Am J Phys Med Rehabil.* 1994;73:199–206.

4. Cheville AL. Cancer rehabilitation and palliative care. In: *Handbook from CME Course June 4–5, 1999: Cancer Rehabilitation in the New Millennium: Opportunities and Challenges.* New York, NY: Memorial Sloan Kettering Cancer Center; 125–128.

5. Michael K. A case for rehabilitation in palliative care. *Rehabil Nurs.* 2001;26(3):84, 113.

6. Manfredi PL, Morrison RS, Morris J, Goldhirsch SL, Carter JM, Meier DE. Palliative care consultations: how do they impact the care of hospitalized patients? *J Pain Symptom Manage.* 2000;20:166–173.

7. Morrison RS, Meier DE. Palliative care. *NEJM.* 2004;350:2582–2590.

8. Chang VT, Hwang SS, Feuerman M. Validation of the Edmonton symptom assessment scale. *Cancer.* 2000;88:2164–2171.

9. National Association of Social Workers. *NASW Standards for Palliative and End of Life Care.* Washington, DC, 2004.

10. Griffin AM, Butow PN, Coates AS, et al. On the receiving end V: patient perceptions of the side effects of cancer chemotherapy in 1993. *Ann Oncol.* 1996;7:189–195.

11. Scwartzberg LS. Chemotherapy-induced nausea and vomiting: clinician and patient perspectives. *J Support Oncol.* 2007;5:S5–S12.

12. Bergkvist K, Wengstrom Y. Symptom experiences during chemotherapy treatment-with focus on nausea and vomiting. *Eur J Oncol Nurs.* 2006;10:21–29.

13. Andrews PLR. Physiology of nausea and vomiting. *Br J Anaesth.* 1992;69:2S–19S.

14. Clayton BD, Frye CB. Nausea and vomiting. In: Herfinal ET, Gourley DR, eds. *Textbook of Therapeutics: Drug and Disease Management.* Baltimore, MD: Williams and Wilkins; 1996:503–515.

15. Neal KB, Bornstein JC. Serotonergic receptors in therapeutic approaches to gastrointestinal disorders. *Curr Opin Pharmacol.* 2006;6:547–552.

16. Prommer E. Aprepitant (EMEND): the role of substance P in nausea and vomiting. *J Pain Palliat Care Pharmacother.* 2005;19:31–39.

17. Zajonc TP, Roland PS. Vertigo and motion sickness. Part II: pharmacologic treatment. *Ear Nose Throat J.* 2006;85:25–35.

18. Hornby PJ. Central neurocircuitry associated with emesis. *Am J Med.* 2001;111:106S–112S.

19. Billhult A, Bergbom I, Stener-victorin E. Massage relieves nausea in women with breast cancer who are undergoing chemotherapy. *J Alt Comp Med.* 2007;13:53–57.

20. Molassiotis A, Helin AM, Dabbour R, Hummerston S. The effects of p6 acupressure in the prophylaxis of chemotherapy-related nausea and vomiting in breast cancer patients. *Complem Ther Med.* 2007;15:3–12.

21. Mansky PJ, Wallerstedt DB. Complementary medicine in palliative care and cancer symptom management. *Cancer J.* 2006;12:425–431.

22. Dalal S, DelFabbro E, Bruera E. Symptom control in palliative care-part I: oncology as a paradigmatic example. *J Pall Med.* 2006;9:391–408.

23. Kaw M, Singh S, Gagneja H, Azad P. Role of self-expandable stents in the palliation of malignant duodenal obstruction. *Surg Endosc.* 2003;17:646–650.

24. Priestman TJ, Lucraft H, Collis CH, Adams M, Upadhyaya BK, Priestman S. Results of a randomized, double-blind comparative study of ondansetron and metoclopramide in the prevention of nausea and vomiting following high-dose upper abdominal irradiation. *Clin Oncol (R Coll Radiol).* 1990;2:71–75.

25. Neal KB, Bornstein JC. Serotonergic receptors in therapeutic approaches to gastrointestinal disorders. *Curr Opin Pharmacol.* 2006;6:547–552.

26. Roberts JT, Priestman TJ. A review of ondansetron in the management of radiotherapy-induced emesis. *Oncology.* 1993;50:173–179.

27. Peroutka SJ, Snyder SH. Antiemetics: neurotransmitter receptor binding predicts therapeutic actions. *Lancet.* 1982;1:658–659.

28. Tramer MR, Carroll D, Campbell FA, Reynolds DJM, Moore RA, McQuay HJ. Cannabinoids for control of chemotherapy induced nausea and vomiting: quantitative systematic review. *BMJ.* 2001;323:16–21.

29. Hallenbeck JL. *Palliative Care Perspectives.* New York, NY: Oxford University Press, Inc.; 2003.

30. Mercandante S. The role of octreotide in palliative care. *J Pain Symptom Manage.* 1994;9:406–411.

31. Mercandante S, Kargar J, Nicolosi G. Octreotide may prevent definitive intestinal obstruction. *J Pain Symptom Manage.* 1997;13:325–326.

32. Feuer DJ, Braodley KE. Corticosteroids for the resolution of malignant bowel obstruction in advanced gynaecological and gastrointestinal cancer. *Cochrane Database Syst Rev.* 2000;2:CD001219.

33. Donnelly S, Walsh D. The symptoms of advanced cancer. *Semin Oncol.* 1995;22:67–72.

34. Shragge JE, Wismer WV, Olson KL, Baracos VE. The management of anorexia by patients with advanced cancer: a critical review of the literature. *Palliat Med* 2006;20:623–629.

35. Ma G, Alexander HR. Prevalence and pathophysiology of cancer cachexia. In Bruera E, Portenoy RK, eds. *Topics in Palliative Care.* New York: Oxford University Press; 1998:91–129.

36. DeWys WD, Begg D, Lavin PT. Prognostic effect of weight loss prior to chemotherapy in cancer patients. *Am J Med.* 1980;69:491–499.

37. Poole K, Froggatt K. Loss of weight and loss of appetite in advanced cancer: a problem for the patient, the carer or the health professional? *Palliat Med.* 2002;16:499–506.

38. Morley JE, Thomas DR, Wilson MG. Cachexia: pathophysiology and clinical relevance. *Am J Clin Nutr.* 2006;83:735–743.

39. Plonk WM, Arnold RM. Terminal care: the last weeks of life. *J Pall Med.* 2005;8:1042–1054.

40. Strasser F, Binswanger J, Cerny T, Kesselring A. Fighting a losing battle: eating-related distress of men with advanced cancer and their female partners. A mixed-methods study. *Pall Med.* 2007;21:129–137.

41. McClement SE, Degner LF. Family responses to declining intake and weight loss in a terminally ill relative. Part 1: fighting back. *J Pall Care.* 2004;20:93–100.

42. Ovesen L, Aliingstrup L, Hannibal L, Mortensen EL, Hansen OP. Effects of dietary counseling on food intake, body weight, response rate, survival and quality of life in cancer patients undergoing chemotherapy: a prospective randomized study. *J Clin Oncol.* 1993;11:2043–2049.

43. Marin-Caro MM, Laviano A, Pichard C. Nutritional intervention and quality of life in adult oncology patients. *Clin Nutr.* 2007;26(3):289–301.

44. Hallenbeck J. Fast facts and concepts #11 To feed or not to feed. August 2005, 2nd ed. End-of-Life Physician Education Resource Center www.eperc.mcw.edu.

45. Mirhosseini N, Fainsinger RL, Baracos V. Parenteral nutrition in advanced cancer: indications and clinical practice guidelines. *J Pall Med.* 2005;8:914–918.

46. MacDonald N, Easson AM, Mazurak VC, Dunn GP, Baracos VE. Understanding and managing cancer cachexia. *J Am Coll Surg.* 2003;197:143–161.

47. McCann RM, Hall WJ, Groth-Juncker A. Comfort care for terminally ill patients. The appropriate use of nutrition and hydration. *JAMA.* 1994;272:1263–1266.

48. Popiela T, Lucchi R, Giongo F. Methylprednisolone as an appetite stimulant in patients with cancer. *Eur J Cancer Clin Oncol.* 1989;25:1823–1829.

49. Moertel CG, Schutt AJ, Reitemeier RJ, Hahn RG. Corticosteroid therapy of preterminal gastrointestinal cancer. *Cancer.* 1974;33:1607–1609.

50. Yavuzsen T, Davis MP, Walsh D, LeGrand S, Lagman R. Systematic review of the treatment of cancer-associated anorexia and weight loss. *J Clin Oncol.* 2005;23:8500–8511.

51. Elamin EM, Glass M, Camporesi E. Pharmacological approaches to ameliorating catabolic conditions. *Curr Opin Clin Nutr Metab Care.* 2006;9:449–454.

52. Kornblith AB, Hollis DR, Zuckerman E, et al. Effect of megestrol acetate on quality of life in a dose-response trial in women with advanced breast cancer. *J Clin Oncol.* 1993;11:2081–2089.

53. Lopez AP, Figuls MR, Cuchi GU, et al. Systematic review of megestrol acetate in the treatment of anorexia-cachexia syndrome. *J Pain Symptom Manage.* 2004;27:360–369.

54. Loprinzi CL, Kugler JW, Sloan JA, et al. Randomized comparison of megestrol acetate versus dexamethasone versus fluoxymesterone for the treatment of cancer anorexia cachexia. *J Clin Oncol.* 1999;17:3299–3306.

55. Del Fabbro E, Dalal S, Bruera E. Symptom control in palliative care-part II: cachexia/anorexia and fatigue. *J Pall Med.* 2006;9:409–421.

56. Walsh D, Nelson KA, Mahmoud FA. Established and potential therapeutic applications of cannabinoids in oncology. *Support Care Cancer.* 2003;11:137–143.

57. Jatoi A, Windschitl HE, Loprinzi CL, et al. Dronabinol versus megestrol acetate versus combination therapy for cancer-associated anorexia: a north central cancer treatment group study. *J Clin Oncol.* 2002;20:567–573.

58. Loprinzi CL, Jatoi A. Pharmacologic management of cancer anorexia/cachexia. In: *UpToDate,* Rose BD, ed. Waltham, MA: UpToDate, 2007.

59. Bruera E, Neumann CM, Pituskin E, Calder K, Ball G, Hanson J. Thalidomide in patients with cachexia due to terminal cancer: preliminary report. *Ann Oncol.* 1999;10:857–859.

60. Gordon JN, Trebble TM, Ellis RD, Duncan HD, Johns T, Goggin PM. Thalidomide in the treatment of cancer cachexia: a randomized placebo controlled trial. *Gut.* 2005;54:540–545.

61. Khan ZH, Simpson EJ, Cole AT. Esophageal cancer and cachexia: the effect of short-term treatment with thalidomide on weight loss and lean body mass. *Aliment Pharmacol Ther.* 2003;17:677–682.

62. Kardinal CG, Loprinzi CL, Schaid DJ, et al. A controlled trial of cyproheptadine in cancer patients with anorexia and/or cachexia. *Cancer.* 1990;65:2657–2662.

63. Edelman MJ, Gandara DR, Meyers FJ, et al. Serotonergic blockade in the treatment of cancer anorexia-cachexia syndrome. *Cancer.* 1999;86:684–688.

64. Lissoni P. Is there a role for melatonin in supportive care? *Support Care Cancer.* 2002;10:110–116.

65. Persson C, Glimelius B, Ronalid J, Nygren P. Impact of fish oil and melatonin on cachexia in patients with advanced gastrointestinal cancer: a randomized pilot study. *Nutrition.* 2005;21:170–178.

66. Bruera E, Strasser F, Palmer JL, Willey J, Calder K, Amyotte, Baracos V. Effect of fish oil on appetite and other symptoms in patients with advanced cancer and anorexia/cachexia: a double-blind, placebo-controlled study. *J Clin Oncol.* 2003;21:129–134.

67. National Comprehensive Cancer Network Practice Guidelines in Oncology. Cancer-Related Fatigue, v.2.2007. National Comprehensive Cancer Network. Retrieved April 12, 2007 from the World Wide Web: http://www.nccn.org/professionals/physician_gls/PDF/fatigue.pdf or http://www.nccn.org.

68. Fatigue Section from Cancer Symptoms.org. Retrieved April 12, 2007, from the World Wide Web: http://www.cancersymptoms.org/fatigue/index/shtml or http://www.cancersymptoms.org.

69. Packel L, Claghorn KVB, Dekerlegand J. Cancer-related fatigue and deconditioning: a program evaluation. *Rehabil Oncol.* 2006;24(2):3–8.

70. Madden J, Newton S. Why am I so tired all the time? Understanding cancer-related fatigue. *Clin J Oncol Nurs.* 2006;10(5):659–661.

71. Graydon JE, Bubela N, Irvine D, Vincent L. Fatigue-reducing strategies used by patients receiving treatment for cancer. *Cancer Nurs.* 1995;18(1):23–28.

72. Manzullo EF, Escalante CP. Research into fatigue. *Hematol Oncol Clin N Am.* 2002;16:619–628.

73. Nail LM, Winningham ML. Fatigue and weakness in cancer patients: the symptom experience. *Semin Oncol Nurs.* 1995;11(4):272–278.

74. Mock V. Evidence-based treatment for cancer-related fatigue. *J Natl Cancer Inst Monogr.* 2004;32:112–118.

75. Winningham ML. Strategies for managing cancer-related fatigue syndrome: a rehabilitation approach. *Cancer (Supplement).* 2001;92(4):988–997.

76. Block SD. Psychological issues in end-of-life care. *J Palliat Med.* 2006;9:751–772.

77. Brown WJ, Ford JH, Burton NW, Marshall AL, Dobson AJ. Prospective study of physical activity and depressive symptoms in middle-aged women. *Am J Prev Med.* 2005;29(4):265–272.

78. Sjosten N, Kivela SL. The effects of physical exercise on depressive symptoms among the aged: a systematic review. *Int J Geriatr Psychiatry.* 2006;21:410–418.

79. Barbour KA, Blumenthal JA. Exercise training and depression in older adults. *Neurobiol Aging.* 2005;26S:119–123.

80. Blumenthal JA, Babyak MA, Moore KA, et al. Effects of exercise training on older patients with major depression. *Arch Intern Med.* 1999;159:2349–2356.

81. Wise LA, Adams-Campbell LL, Palmer JR, Rosenberg L. Leisure time physical activity in relation to depressive symptoms in the Black Women's Health Study. *Ann Behav Med.* 2006;32(1):68–76.

82. Courneya KS. Exercise in cancer survivors: an overview of research. *Med Sci Sports Exerc.* 2003;35:1846–1852.

83. Mutrie N, Campbell AM, Whyte F, et al. Benefits of supervised group exercise programme for women being treated for early stage breast cancer: pragmatic randomized controlled trial. *BMJ.* 2007;1074.

84. Thorsen L, Nystad W, Stigum H, et al. The association between self-reported physical activity and prevalence of depression and anxiety disorder in long-term survivors of testicular cancer and men in a general population sample. *Support Care Cancer.* 2005;13:637–646.

85. Badger T, Segrin C, Dorros SM, Meek P, Lopez AM. Depression and anxiety in women with breast cancer and their partners. *Nurs Res.* 2007;56(1):44–53.

86. Segar ML, Katch VL, Roth RS, et al. The effect of aerobic exercise on self-esteem and depressive and anxiety symptoms among breast cancer survivors. *Oncol Nurs Forum.* 1998;25(1):107–113.

87. Midtgaard J, Rorth M, Stelter R, et al. The impact of a multidimensional exercise program on self-reported anxiety and depression in cancer patients undergoing chemotherapy: a phase II study. *Palliat Support Care.* 2005;3(3):197–208.

88. Burns CM, Broom DH, Smith WT, Dear K, Craft PS. Fluctuating awareness of treatment goals among patients and their caregivers: a longitudinal study of a dynamic process. *Support Care Cancer.* 2007;15:187–196.

89. The EPEC Project: Education on palliative and end-of-life care. Accessed at http://www.epec.net112.

90. Craft PS, Burns CM, Smith WT, Broom DH. Knowledge of treatment intent among patients with advanced cancer: a longitudinal study. *Eur J Cancer Care.* 2005;14:417–425.

91. Weeks JC, Cook EF, O'Day SJ, et al. Relationship between cancer patients' predictions of prognosis and their treatment preferences. *JAMA.* 1998;279:1709–1714.

92. Gaston CM, Mitchell G. Information giving and decision-making in patients with advanced cancer: a systematic review. *Soc Sci Med.* 2005;61:2252–2264.

93. Christakis NA, Lamont EB. Extent and determinants of error in doctors' prognoses in terminally ill patients: a prospective cohort study. *BMJ.* 2000;320:469–472.

94. Phillips RS, Wenger NS, Teno J, et al. Choices of seriously ill patients about cardiopulmonary resuscitation: correlated and outcomes. *Am J Med.* 1996;100:128–137.

95. Morrison RS, Meier DE. Palliative care. *NEJM.* 2004;350:2582–2590.

96. Steinhauser KE, Christakis NA, Clipp EC, McNeilly M, McIntyre L, Tulsky JA. Factors considered important at the end of life by patients, family, physicians and other care providers. *JAMA.* 2000;284:2476–2482.

97. Fallowfield L, Ratcliffe D, Jenkins V, Saul J. Psychiatric morbidity and its recognition by doctors in patients with cancer. *Br J Cancer.* 2001;84:1011–1015.

98. Sanson-Fisher R, Girgis A, Boyes A, Bonevski B, Burton L, Cook P. The unmet supportive care needs of patients with cancer. *Cancer.* 2000;88:226–237.

99. Ryan H, Schofield P, Cockburn J, et al. How to recognize and manage psychological distress in cancer patients. *Eur J Cancer Care.* 2005;14:7–15.

100. Spiegel D, Bloom JR, Kraemer HC, Gottheil E. Effect of psychological treatment on survival of patients with metastatic breast cancer. *Lancet.* 1989;2:888–891.

101 Mee S, Bunney BG, Reist C, Potkin SG, Bunney WE. Psychological pain: a review of evidence. *J Psych Res.* 2006;40:680–690.

102. Ridner SH. Psychological distress: concept analysis. *J Adv Nurs.* 2004;45:536–545.

103. Kelly B, McClement S, Chochinov HM. Measurement of psychological distress in palliative care. *Pall Med.* 2006;20:779–789.

104. Satterly L. Guilt, shame and religious and spiritual pain. *Holist Nurs Pract.* 2001;15:30–39.

105. Mystakidou K, Tsilika E, Parpa E, Katsouda E, Galanos A, Vlahos L. Psychological distress of patients with advanced cancer. Influence and contribution of pain severity and pain interference. *Cancer Nurs.* 2006;29:400–405.

106. Bolmsjo I. Existential issues in palliative care—interviews with cancer patients. *J Pall Care.* 2000;16:20–24.

107. Breitbart W, Rosenfeld B, Pessin H, et al. Depression, hopelessness and desire for hastened death in terminally ill patients with cancer. *JAMA.* 2000;284:2907–2911.

108. Maguire P. Improving the detection of psychiatric problems in cancer patients. *Soc Sci Med.* 1985;20:819–823.

109. Strasser F, Walker P, Bruera E. Palliative pain management: when both pain and suffering hurt. *J Palliat Care.* 2005;21:69–79.

110. Davenport S, Goldberg D, Millar T. How psychiatric disorders are missed during medical consultations. *Lancet.* 1987;2:439–441.

111. Detmar SB, Aaronson NK. Quality of life assessment in daily clinical oncology practice: a feasibility study. *Eur J Cancer.* 1998;34:1181–1186.

112. Brown RF, Butow PN, Dunn SM, Tattersall MHN. Promoting patient participation and shortening cancer consultations: a randomized trial. *Br J Cancer.* 2001;85:1273–1279.

113. Holland J. NCCN practical guidelines for the management of psychosocial distress. *Oncology.* 1999;13:113–147.

114. Ransom S, Jacobsen PB, Booth-Jones M. Validation of the distress thermometer in bone marrow transplant patients. *Psychooncology.* 2006;15:739–747.

115. Moorey S, Greer S. *Cognitive Behaviour Therapy for People with Cancer.* Oxford: Oxford University Press; 2002.

116. Morita T, Kawa M, Honke Y, et al. Existential concerns of terminally ill cancer patients receiving specialized palliative care in Japan. *Support Care Cancer.* 2004;12:137–140.

117. Cathcart F. Psychological distress in patients with advanced cancer. *Clin Med.* 2006;6:148–150.

118. U.S. Department of Health and Human Services. *Clinical Practice Guideline (Number 9): Management of Cancer Pain* (AHCPR Publication No. 94-0592). Rockville, MD: 1994:75–87.

119. Mannheimer JS, Lampe GN. *Clinical Transcutaneous Electrical Nerve Stimulation.* Philadelphia, PA: F.A. Davis Company; 1984:57–58, 456–457.

120. Menefee LA, Monti DA. Nonpharmacologic and complementary approaches to cancer pain management. *JAOA Suppl 5.* 2005;105(11):515–520.

121. Bloch R. Rehabilitation medicine approach to cancer pain. *Cancer Invest.* 2004;22(6):944–948.

122. Watson T. Lecture posted online: The Use of TENS in Cancer and Palliative Care—ACPOCP May 2003.

123. Astin JA, Shapiro SL, Eisenberg DM, Forys KL. Mind-body medicine: state of the science, implications for practice. *JABFP.* 2003;16(2):131–147.

124. Kirshblum S. Neurorehabilitation in spinal cord cancer. In: *Handbook from CME Course June 4–5, 1999: Cancer Rehabilitation In the New Millennium: Opportunities and Challenges.* New York, NY: Sponsored by Memorial Sloan Kettering Cancer Center; 83–86.

125. Gerber LH, Hicks JE. *Functional Preservation Throughout the Trajectory of Malignant Disease. From Lecture Notes and Handbook from CME Course June 4–5, 1999: Cancer Rehabilitation In the New Millennium: Opportunities and Challenges.* New York, NY: Sponsored by Memorial Sloan Kettering Cancer Center; 161–162.

126. Bunting RW. *Rehabilitation of the Patient with Bone Metastases. From Lecture Notes and Handbook from CME Course June 4–5, 1999: Cancer Rehabilitation In the New Millennium: Opportunities and Challenges.* New York, NY: Sponsored by Memorial Sloan Kettering Cancer Center; 177–179.

127. Guyton AC, Hall JE. Physiology of gastrointestinal disorders. In: Guyton AC, Hall JE, eds. *Textbook of Medical Physiology,* 9th ed. Philadelphia: W.B. Saunders; 1996:845–851.

128. Mercadante S. Diarrhea, malabsorption, and constipation. In: Berger A, Portenoy RK, Weissman DE, eds. *Principles and Practice of Supportive Oncology.* Philadelphia: Lippincott-Raven; 1998:191–205.

129. Heidrich DE. Constipation. In: Kuebler KK, Berry PH, Heidrich DE, eds. *End of Life Care: Clinical Practice Guidelines.* Philadelphia: Saunders; 2002:221–233.

130. Conill C, Verger E, Henriquez I, et al. Symptom prevalence in the last week of life. *J Pain Symptom Manage.* 1997;14(6):328–331.

131. Curtis E, Krech R, Walsh TD. Common symptoms in patients with advanced cancer. *J Palliat Care.* 1991;7(2):25–29.

132. Lichter I, Hunt E. The last 24 hours of life. *J Palliat Care.* 1990;6(4):7–15.

133. Vainio A, Auvinen A. Prevalence of symptoms among patients with advanced cancer: an international collaborative study. *J Pain Symptom Manage.* 1996;12(1):3–10.

134. Basta S, Anderson DL. Mechanisms and management of constipation in the cancer patient. *J Pharm Care Pain Symptom Control.* 1998;6(3):21–40.

135. Fallon M, O'Neill B. ABC of palliative care: constipation and diarrhea. *Br Med J.,* 1997;315:1293–1296.

136. Sykes NP. Constipation and diarrhea. In: Doyle D, Hanks GWC, MacDonald N, eds. *Oxford Textbook of Palliative Medicine,* 2nd ed. New York: Oxford University Press; 1998:513–526.

137. Santiago-Palma J, Payne R. Palliative care and rehabilitation. *Cancer Suppl.* 2001;92(4):1049–1052.

138. Szabo, Liz. Health system struggles with spiritual care. *USA Today,* 2/15/07.

139. Puchalski, Christina, & Romer, Anna L. Taking a spiritual history allows clinicians to understand patients more fully. *J Palliat Med.* 2000;3(1):129–137.

140. Conrad, Nancy L. Spiritual support for the dying. *Nurs Clin N Am.* 1985;20(2):415–426.

141. O'Connor, Patrice. The role of spiritual care in hospice. *Am J Hosp Care.* 1988;July/August:31–37.

142. Carr, Elizabeth W, Morris, Thomas. Spirituality and patients with advanced cancer: a social work response. *J Psychosoc Oncol.* 1996;14(1):71–81.

143. Erikson, Eric. *Identity and the Life Cycle.* New York, NY: WW Norton; 1991.

144. Clinical Practice Guidelines for Quality Palliative Care, National Consensus Project on Quality Palliative Care, 2004. www.nationalconcensusproject.org

145. Christakis NA, Lamont EB. Extent and determinants of error in doctors' prognoses in terminally ill patients: a prospective cohort study. *BMJ.* 2000;320:469–472.

146. Glare P, Virik K, Jones M, et al. A systematic review of physicians' survival predictions in terminally ill cancer patients. *BMJ.* 2003;327:195–198.
147. von Gunten CF. Fast fact and concept #149 Teaching the family what to expect when the patient is dying. February, 2006. End-of-life physician education resource center www.eperc.mcw.edu
148. Ferris FD, von Gunten CF, Emanuel LL. Competency in end-of-life care: last hours of life. *J Pall Med.* 2003;6:605–613.
149. Cahill GF, Veech RL. Ketoacids? Good medicine? *Trans Am Clin Climatol Assoc.* 2003;114:149–161.
150. Musgrave CF. Terminal dehydration: to give or not to give intravenous fluids? *Cancer Nurs.* 1990;13:62–66.
151. Ellershaw JE, Sutcliffe JM, Saunders CM. Dehydration and the dying patient. *J Pain Symptom Manage.* 1995;10:192–197.
152. Musgrave CF, Bartal N, Opstad J. The sensation of thirst in dying patients receiving i.v. hydration. *J Palliat Care.* 1995;11:17–21.
153. Billings JA. Comfort measures for the terminally ill: is dehydration painful? *J Am Geriatr Soc.* 1985;33:808–810.
154. Wildiers H, Menten J. Death rattle: prevalence, prevention, and treatment. *J Pain Symptom Manage.* 2002;23:310–317.
155. Reuben DB, Mor V. Dyspnea in terminally ill cancer patients. *Chest.* 1986;89:234–236.
156. Rousseau P. Non-pain symptom management in terminal care. *Clin Geriatr Med.* 1996;12:313–327.
157. Tanaka K, Akechi T, Okuyama T, Nishiwaki Y, Uchitomi Y. Prevalence and screening of dyspnea interfering with daily life activities in ambulatory patients with advanced lung cancer. *J Pain Symptom Manage.* 2002;23:484–489.
158. Spector N, Klein D. Chronic critically ill dyspneic patients: mechanisms and clinical measurement. *AACN Clin Issues.* 2001;12:197–201.
159. Spector N, Connolly MA, Carlson KK. Dyspnea: applying research to bedside practice. *AACN Adv Crit Care.* 2007;18:45–60.
160. Powers J, Bennett SJ. Measurement of dyspnea in patients treated with mechanical ventilation. *Am J Crit Care.* 1999;8:254–261.
161. Gift A, Moore T, Soeken K. Relaxation to reduce dyspnea and anxiety in COPD patients. *Nurs Res.* 1992;41:242–246.
162. Pan CX, Morrison R, Ness J, Fugh-Berman A, Leipzig RM. Complementary and alternative medicine in the management of pain, dyspnea, and nausea and vomiting near the end of life: a systematic review. *J Pain Symptom Manage.* 2000;20:374–387.
163. Kim Ae Kyung RN, DNSC, Patricia A Chin RN, DNS. The effect of a pulmonary rehabilitation programme on older patients with chronic pulmonary disease.*J Clin Nurs (OnlineEarly Articles).* doi:10.1111/j.1365-2702.2006.01712.x.
164. Dudgeon D. Dyspnea, cough and death rattle. In: Ferrell BR, Coyle N, eds. *Textbook of Palliative Nursing.* New York: Oxford University Press; 2001:164–174.
165. Sykes N, Thorns A. The use of opioids and sedatives at the end of life. *Lancet.* 2003;4:312–318.
166. Jennings AL, Davies AN, Higgins JPT, Gibbs JSR, Broadley KE. A systematic review of the use of opioids in the management of dyspnea. *Thorax.* 2002;57:939–944.
167. Clemens KE, Klaschik E. Symptomatic therapy of dyspnea with strong opioids and its effect on ventilation in palliative care patients. *J Pain Symptom Manage.* 2007;33:473–481.
168. Tice MA. Managing breathlessness: providing comfort at the end of life. *Home Healthc Nurse.* 2006;24:207–210.
169. DelFabbro E, Dalal S, Bruera E. Symptom control in palliative care—part III: dyspnea and delirium. *J Palliat Med.* 2006;9:422–433.
170. American Psychiatric Association. *Diagnostic and Statistical Manual of Mental Disorders,* 4th ed. Washington, DC: Author; 1994.
171. Friedlander MM, Brayman Y, Breitbart WS. Delirium in palliative care. *Oncology.* 2004;18(12):1541–1549.
172. Bruera E, Miller L, McCallion J, Macmillan K, Krefting L, Hanson J. Cognitive failure in patients with terminal cancer: a prospective study. *J Pain Symptom Manage.* 1992;7(4):192–195.
173. Breitbart W, Bruera E, Chochinov H, Lynch M. Neuropsychiatric syndromes and psychological symptoms in patients with advanced cancer. *J Pain Symptom Manage.* 1995;10:131–141.
174. Breitbart W, Marotta R, Platt M. A double-blind comparison trial of haloperidol, chlorpromazine, and lorazepam in the treatment of delirium in hospitalized AIDS patients. *Am J Psychiatry.* 1996;153, 231–237.
175. Fainsinger R, Young C. Cognitive failure in a terminally ill patient. *J Pain Symptom Manage.* 1991;6:492–494.
176. Samuels SC, Evers MM. Delirium: pragmatic guidance for managing a common, confounding and sometimes lethal condition. *Geriatrics.* 2002;57:33–38.
177. Gleason OC. Delirium. *Am Fam Phys.* 2003;65(5):1027–1034.
178. Lawlor PG, Fainsinger RL, Bruera ED. Delirium at the end of life: critical issues in clinical practice and research. *J Am Med Assoc.* 2000;284(19):2427–2429.
179. Breitbart W, Strout, D. Death and dying: delirium in the terminally ill. *Clin Geriatric Med.* 2000;16(2).
180. Folstein MF, Folstein SE, McHugh PR. "Mini-mental state." A practical method for grading the cognitive state of patients for the clinician. *J Psychiatr Res.* 1975;12(3):189–198.
181. Chan D, Brennan NJ. Delirium: making the diagnosis, improving the prognosis. *Geriatrics.* 1999;54(3):28–42.
182. Inouye SK, Van Dyck CH, Alessi CA, Balkin S, Siegal AP, Horwitz RI. Clarifying confusion: the Confusion Assessment Method. *Ann Intern Med.* 1990;113:941–948.
183. Trzepacz PT, Baker RW, Greenhouse J. A symptom rating scale for delirium. *Psychiatr Res.* 1988;1:89–97.
184. Breitbart W, Rosenfeld B, Roth A, et. al. The memorial delirium assessment scale. *J Pain Symptom Manage.* 1997;13:128–137.
185. Ingham JM, Caraceni AT. Delirium. In: Berger AM, Portenoy RK, Weissman DE, eds. *Principles and Practice of Supportive Oncology.* Philadelphia: Lippincott-Raven; 1998:477–495.
186. Breitbart W, Cohen KR. Delirium. In: Holland JC, ed. *Psychooncology.* New York: Oxford University Press; 1998:564–575.
187. McIver B, Walsh D, Nelson K. (1994). The use of chlorpromazine for symptom control in dying cancer patients. *J Pain Symptom Manage.* 1994;9:341–345.
188. Twycross R. *Symptom Management in Advanced Cancer,* 2nd ed. Oxon, UK: Radcliffe Medical Press; 1997.
189. Sipahimalani A, Massand PS. Olanzapine in the treatment of delirium. *Psychosomatics.* 1998;39:422–430.
190. Sipahimalani A, Sime RM, Massand PS. Treatment of delirium with risperidone. *Int J Geriatr Psychopharmacol.* 1997;1:24–26.
191. Cheng C, Roemer-Becuwe C, Pereira J. When midazolam fails. *J Pain Symptom Manage.* 2002;23:256–265.
192. American Psychiatric Association. Practice guidelines for the treatment of patients with delirium. *Am J Psychiatry.* 1999;156(Suppl 5):1–20.
193. Waller A, Caroline NL. *Handbook of Palliative Care in Cancer,* 2nd ed. Boston: Butterworth-Heinemann; 2000.
194. Meagher DJ. Delirium: optimizing management. *Br Med J.* 2001;322:146.
195. Kuebler KK, Heidrich DE. Constipation. In: Kuebler KK, Berry PH, Heidrich DE, eds. *End of Life Care: Clinical Practice Guidelines.* Philadelphia: Saunders; 2002:253–267.
196. Saunders C. Foreword. In: Doyle D, Hanks G, MacDonald N, eds. *Oxford Textbook of Palliative Medicine.* New York, NY: Oxford University Press; 1998:v–ix.
197. Storey P, Knight CF. UNIPAC Four: Management of selected non-pain symptoms in the terminally ill. New York: Mary Ann Liebert, Inc.; 2003:22–28.

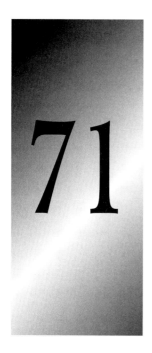

Complementary Therapies in Cancer Rehabilitation

71

Barrie R. Cassileth
Robin C. Hindery
Jyothirmai Gubili

Cancer patients experience a range of symptoms that often span the course of the disease, treatment, and survivorship. These include problems such as pain, the enduring results of muscle and nerve damage, mood disturbance, and more. Increasing numbers of cancer patients turn to complementary therapies to help alleviate and manage their symptoms, and in the past decade, progressively more scientific effort has been expended to evaluate the efficacy of complementary modalities.

The term *complementary and alternative medicine* (CAM) has been used to describe these therapies. However, this terminology is problematic, as it encompasses both viable, evidence-based complementary therapies, as well as those that have been disproved or remain unproven. The latter, so-called "alternative," therapies include ineffective or potentially harmful interventions often billed as legitimate substitutes for mainstream care.

This chapter will focus on "complementary therapies" that are used as adjuncts to mainstream treatment and rehabilitation. These therapies do not cure or treat disease. Instead, they provide noninvasive means of symptom control as part of the broader effort to ease the physical, psychosocial, and spiritual distress commonly associated with cancer and other chronic illnesses.

Dozens of international surveys indicate that up to 85% of cancer patients use complementary or alternative therapies. A study surveying more than 1,400 Canadian women with breast cancer found that the percentage of women who had used a CAM product or therapy or visited a CAM practitioner increased from 66.7% in 1998 to 81.9% in 2005 (1). Prevalence of CAM use varies substantially, depending on surveyor definitions or respondent interpretations of the terminology. These therapies are sought to combat depression, anxiety, and insomnia, as well as for medical problems and symptoms associated with cancer treatment. Patients surveyed all but unanimously tend to believe that these therapies improve their quality of life by helping them cope with stress, decreasing symptoms, and offering them some control over their treatment and well-being.

The National Center for Complementary and Alternative Medicine (NCCAM) groups CAM therapies into four basic categories: mind–body medicine, including meditation and hypnotherapy; biologically based practices, including dietary supplements and herbal products; manipulative and body-based practices, including massage and "energy therapies," such as reiki; and "therapeutic touch," which involves no touch.

The NCCAM also recognizes whole medical systems that cross these multiple categories, including ayurveda, the traditional system of India, and traditional Chinese medicine. Both encompass mind–body practices, manipulative techniques, and herbal treatments; traditional Chinese medicine also includes acupuncture.

Today, complementary therapies are a multibillion dollar business in the United States. They are increasingly

KEY POINTS

- Increasing numbers of cancer patients turn to complementary therapies to help alleviate and manage their symptoms.
- Complementary and alternative medicine encompasses both viable, evidence-based complementary therapies, as well as those that have been disproved or remain unproven. The latter, so-called "alternative," therapies include ineffective or potentially harmful interventions often billed as legitimate substitutes for mainstream care.
- Up to 85% of cancer patients use complementary or alternative therapies.
- Massage therapy appears to be effective in treating cancer-related pain, fatigue, nausea, anxiety, and depression.
- Studies have found that acupuncture can successfully reduce nausea and vomiting, and may be useful in treating depression, xerostomia, sensory morbidity, and other symptoms associated with contemporary cancer treatments.
- Hypnosis is effective in reducing anxiety, depression, pain, nausea, and vomiting, and it has a particularly favorable risk–benefit ratio.
- Exercise has been shown in many studies to improve quality of life following cancer diagnosis.
- Anxiety, which often increases as cancer advances, may cause patients to overestimate the risks associated with treatment and the likelihood of poor outcome.
- Massage therapy, mind–body relaxation therapies, yoga, or acupuncture often alleviate transient depression.

available not only on a private basis, but also through clinics as a standard component of symptom control. While the overall number of randomized controlled trials (RCTs) of CAM therapies remains somewhat small and further in-depth research is essential, sufficient promising evidence exists to merit professional and public attention.

Following an overview and brief description of major complementary modalities, this chapter notes appropriate use of these therapies according to common symptoms experienced by cancer patients.

OVERVIEW OF COMPLEMENTARY MODALITIES

Massage Therapy

Massage therapy appears to be effective in treating cancer-related pain, fatigue, nausea, anxiety, and depression. In an analysis of 1,290 Memorial Sloan-Kettering Cancer Center patients, reports of symptom severity before and after massage therapy, ratings of pain, fatigue, anxiety, nausea, depression, and "other" fell by approximately 50% across presenting symptoms, even among patients reporting high baseline scores (2).

Massage therapy involves various manipulative techniques, such as strokes, rubs, and varying pressure, applied to the muscles and soft tissues. There are many different forms of massage, including Swedish, deep tissue, shiatsu, and very light-touch massage that is especially appropriate for frail or terminally ill patients. The therapy is tailored to each patient's clinical status, with

the goal of reducing tension and discomfort, improving circulation, and promoting relaxation.

Acupuncture

Another complementary therapy with multiple perceived benefits for cancer patients is acupuncture. Originally a component of traditional Chinese medicine, acupuncture is based on the ancient concept that the body's energy, or "qi," flows through hypothesized channels, termed "meridians." Acupuncture points are located at specific points along those channels. When an individual's energy is blocked, the theory states, illness ensues. It is believed that the stimulation of acupuncture points with needles or pressure will restore the flow of life energy and, with it, health.

There is currently no verifiable anatomical or histologic basis for the existence of meridians. Instead, there is evidence that peripheral nerve beds are involved in mediating acupuncture's well-documented analgesic properties. The electrical impedance of the skin is lower at many classical acupuncture points, and many of these points correlate with the locations of cutaneous nerve beds. In addition to pain, studies have found that acupuncture can successfully reduce nausea and vomiting, and may be useful in treating depression, xerostomia, sensory morbidity, and other symptoms associated with contemporary cancer treatments.

Hypnosis

Studies show that hypnosis is effective in reducing anxiety, depression, pain, nausea, and vomiting, and it has a particularly favorable risk–benefit ratio. Hypnosis is a state between wakefulness and sleep, a deepened meditative state and one in which the subject is more open and responsive to suggestion. Ideally, hypnotherapy enables patients to gain more control over their behavior, thoughts, or well-being. Hypnosis can be administered by a trained therapist or self-administered, although some research has found the latter to be less effective for symptom management. Children are especially good candidates for hypnotherapy treatment.

Fitness

Fitness, including proper nutritional intake and exercise, is an essential aspect of rehabilitation for cancer patients. The problems associated with obesity are well documented: Obesity and weight gain were shown to increase the risk of breast carcinoma (3), and weight gain following a diagnosis of breast cancer was associated with increased risk of recurrence and death (4–6). Exercise has been shown in many studies to improve quality of life following cancer diagnosis. In a study of breast and colorectal cancer patients, brisk walking for 20 minutes each day conferred a major survival benefit (7). Data from another prospective study of breast cancer survivors showed a 50% risk reduction in active women compared to those who were inactive following diagnosis (8).

Other complementary therapies, including meditation and music therapy, are less well documented when it comes to treating cancer symptoms, but they show promise, especially in reducing stress.

The remainder of this chapter will examine some common symptoms affecting cancer patients today and present the evidence for use of complementary therapies to combat those symptoms.

FATIGUE

Fatigue is a serious problem, especially during chemotherapy and radiotherapy. Eighty percent to ninety-six percent of patients undergoing chemotherapy and 60%–93% of those undergoing radiation therapy report significant fatigue (9). Fatigue may also be caused or exacerbated by tumor-related factors or stress. Treatment-induced fatigue has few reliable treatments in patients when it does not occur as the result of a correctable condition, such as anemia.

Acupuncture

Acupuncture may have an important role for some cancer patients. A phase 2 pilot study of acupuncture for postchemotherapy fatigue randomly assigned 37 patients at Memorial Sloan-Kettering Cancer Cen-

ter to once- or twice-weekly treatments for six weeks and four weeks, respectively (10). The patients, all of whom had completed cytotoxic chemotherapy, showed a mean improvement of 31.1% upon completion of acupuncture treatment. There was no significant difference in improvement between once- versus twice-weekly treatment.

Massage Therapy

A massage study randomized cancer patients scheduled to undergo bone marrow transplantation to either massage therapy or standard care (11). The massage therapy consisted of 20-minute sessions of shoulder, head, neck, and facial massage an average of three times a week during the patients' three-week hospital stay. Patients in the massage group experienced statistically significant reduction in fatigue compared to the control group when symptoms were measured seven days into treatment.

Relaxation Therapies

A small, randomized pilot trial combined physical and relaxation breathing exercises to examine their effect on allogenic hemopoietic stem cell transplantation patients suffering from fatigue (12). Thirty-five patients were randomly assigned to an exercise group or a control group receiving standard care. The exercise intervention lasted for 30 minutes every day for six weeks, and consisted of a 10-minute warm-up of physical exercise, followed by 10 minutes of deep abdominal breathing, and then 10 minutes of self-massage and stretching. Participants in the exercise group had markedly reduced levels of fatigue at the end of the six weeks compared with the control group.

Meditation

A study of 63 cancer outpatients examined the effects of an eight-week Mindfulness-Based Stress Reduction (MBSR) program on sleep, mood, stress, and fatigue (13). MBSR combines meditation with yoga to help patients cope with stress, pain, and illness by promoting moment-to-moment awareness. Participants in the outpatient study reported significant reductions in fatigue at the end of the course.

A larger mind–body study with chemotherapy patients involved massage and healing touch, an energy therapy that involves the placement of the practitioner's hands above and on the patient's body (14). This randomized crossover study of 230 patients compared the effects of therapeutic massage and healing touch with presence alone and also with standard care in promoting relaxation and alleviating other symptoms. Each intervention was administered once a week for four weeks. Compared with standard care, healing touch was associated with lowered fatigue.

ANXIETY

Anxiety, which often increases as cancer advances, may cause patients to overestimate the risks associated with treatment and the likelihood of poor outcome. It may also heighten their perception of physical symptoms. A number of complementary therapies may help reduce anxiety. Patient choice should be encouraged.

Massage Therapy

In the same randomized crossover study that examined the effects of massage on fatigue in 230 chemotherapy patients, massage therapy was found to reduce anxiety compared with standard care or presence alone (14). Patients were assigned to one of four groups—massage therapy, healing touch, standard care, or presence alone. After treatment weekly for four weeks, researchers examined effects on relaxation, anxiety, fatigue, nausea, and total mood disturbance.

A 288-patient RCT involving aromatherapy massage also found improvements in self-reported anxiety (15). One group of patients received four weekly sessions of massage, while another group received standard care. Those receiving massage had significantly reduced anxiety levels compared to the control group up to two weeks after the end of the intervention. Aromatherapy massage is preferred by some patients, but others may experience nausea from the fragrance. Patients always should be asked before aroma is added to massage therapy.

Mind-Body Therapies

Numerous studies have found hypnosis effective in relieving anxiety in pediatric cancer patients undergoing painful medical procedures. In a randomized trial of pediatric cancer patients undergoing lumbar puncture, 80 children between the ages of 6 and 16 were assigned to one of four groups: hypnosis through direct suggestion, hypnosis through indirect suggestion, an attention control group, or standard care alone (16). Hypnosis groups experienced significantly less anxiety than those in the other two groups.

In a randomized trial of 50 adult, terminally ill cancer patients, those who received four weekly hypnotherapy sessions had lower levels of anxiety at the end of the intervention than a control group receiving standard care (17).

A randomized trial of 181 women with breast cancer assigned patients to either a 12-week regimen of standard group support or a 12-week intervention in which participants were taught the use of meditation, affirmation, imagery, and ritual (18). Both interventions were significantly effective in decreasing anxiety.

Music Therapy

Controlled trials indicate that music therapy produces emotional and physiological benefits, including anxiety reduction. In a trial involving 64 patients undergoing flexible sigmoidoscopy, subjects were randomly assigned to a control condition of standard care or to a procedural condition of music therapy during the examination (19). Subjects in the music group reported less anxiety than subjects in the control group.

DEPRESSION

Depression is common and normal after a diagnosis of cancer. Enduring depression requires referral to a psychiatrist, and often prescription medication is needed. Fatigue, nausea, and pain may exacerbate or be exacerbated by depression. Massage therapy, mind–body relaxation therapies, yoga, or acupuncture often alleviate transient depression.

Massage Therapy

A multicenter RCT of 288 cancer patients in the United Kingdom found that aromatherapy massage appears to provide clinically important benefit for up to two weeks to patients suffering from depression (15). Patients were assigned to receive aromatherapy massage or standard care alone, and the massage group had significant improvement in depression compared to the control group at six weeks postrandomization.

Another RCT of 34 women with stage I or II breast cancer also examined the effects of aromatherapy massage on depression (20). The massage group received three 30-minute massages per week for five weeks, while a control group received standard care. Both after the first treatment and over the course of the intervention, the massage group showed significant improvement in depression over the standard-care controls.

Acupuncture

Several studies tested the efficacy of acupuncture for depression in cancer-free patients, and their results were sufficiently promising to merit further studies of cancer-related depression. Acupuncture, as is the case for all complementary modalities, is free of negative side effects associated with pharmacologic therapies.

A randomized trial of 151 patients with major depressive disorder assessed the efficacy of acupuncture in symptom management over an eight-week intervention period (21). One group of patients received 12 sessions of acupuncture for depression, while a control group received acupuncture at a comparable number of points not specifically targeted to depressive symptoms. A second control group waited without intervention for the eight-week period. Groups receiving acupuncture improved more than wait-list patients, but no evidence of differential efficacy emerged for the depression-specific versus nonspecific acupoint placement. Results fail to support the efficacy of acupuncture as a monotherapy for major depressive disorder.

Mind-Body Therapies

A trial of 50 terminally ill cancer patients randomized subjects to four weekly sessions of hypnotherapy or standard care (17). At the end of the intervention, patients in the hypnosis group had significantly lower levels of depression than controls.

Similar results were found in an RCT that examined the effects of an MBSR program on 90 cancer outpatients suffering from stress and mood disturbance (22). Patients in the treatment group participated in a weekly, 90-minute group meditation session for seven weeks in addition to home meditation practice. After the intervention, patients in the treatment group had significantly lower scores on total mood disturbance and a subscale of depression than the control group. Overall reduction in total mood disturbance for the treatment group was 65%.

NAUSEA AND VOMITING

Acupuncture

Numerous studies have found that acupuncture significantly reduces nausea as well as the number of vomiting episodes among chemotherapy patients. In 1997, a National Institutes of Health Consensus Panel concluded there was "clear evidence" to support the use of acupuncture for adult postoperative and chemotherapy-induced nausea and vomiting (23). A systematic Cochrane review of nine trials from 1987 to 2003 found that acupuncture reduced the incidence of acute vomiting by 22% compared to 31% for controls (24).

One of the earliest studies of acupuncture's antiemetic properties involved patients with a previous history of nausea and vomiting as a result of cisplatin-containing chemotherapeutic agents (25). One group

of patients received electroacupuncture, while a control group received acupuncture at a sham position on the elbow expected to deliver no physical benefit. All patients receiving real acupuncture reported complete or partial symptom relief, while 10% of the patients reported benefit from the sham acupuncture.

Another study of cisplatin-induced nausea was performed in Italy with a group of 26 breast cancer patients (26). This pilot study compared the benefit of acupuncture for dexamethasone-, metoclopramide-, and diphenhydramine-produced nausea. Each patient received needle acupuncture during chemotherapy infusion. In addition, a permanent needle was implanted for patients to self-stimulate acupoints at home in the event of recurring symptoms. In comparison to controls who received an identical antiemetic regimen in the same setting before enrollment in the study, the acupuncture group had a significant increase in complete protection from nausea and a decrease in the intensity and duration of nausea and vomiting.

In one of the most comprehensive studies to date, the effectiveness of acupuncture in treating high-dose chemotherapy-related emesis was investigated in a three-arm RCT. This involved 104 women with high-risk breast cancer undergoing myeloablative chemotherapy who were randomly assigned to electroacupuncture, placebo acupuncture, or traditional antiemetics without acupuncture. The number of emesis episodes during the subsequent five days was recorded for each patient. The electroacupuncture group averaged 5 emesis episodes, while the placebo acupuncture group had 10 episodes, and the no-intervention group had 15 episodes. No differences among the three groups remained at nine-days follow-up (27).

Massage Therapy

A crossover RCT of massage among 87 cancer patients found that nausea decreased significantly after each of two 10-minute foot massages administered on two separate days, while it did not decrease significantly on a third day when no massage was given (28).

Mind-Body Therapies

Hypnotherapy reduced chemotherapy-related nausea and vomiting in a study of 54 pediatric cancer patients (29). After baseline levels of chemotherapy-related distress were measured, subjects were randomly assigned to receive hypnosis, nonhypnotic distraction/relaxation, or attention placebo (control) during their next course of chemotherapy. Hypnosis was more effective than both cognitive distraction/relaxation and placebo in reducing anticipatory and postchemotherapy nausea and vomiting.

A randomized controlled trial of 50 noncancer patients undergoing breast reduction surgery revealed less postoperative vomiting in the group receiving preoperative hypnosis (39% experienced that symptom) versus the control group receiving standard care (68% experienced vomiting) (30). Nausea within the hypnosis group was also reduced.

In a study of 16 adult cancer patients affected by chemotherapy-induced anticipatory nausea and vomiting, hypnosis was administered to each patient prior to chemotherapy (31). All patients experienced a complete remission of anticipatory nausea and vomiting, and most also demonstrated significantly reduced chemotherapy-induced emesis.

PAIN

For a thorough discussion of complementary therapies in pain management, see Chapter 42.

CONCLUSION

Cancer patients face a range of physical and psychological symptoms that can be successfully ameliorated with noninvasive complementary therapies. These pleasant, side effect–free, cost-effective modalities have an important role in cancer rehabilitation. They also offer patients the opportunity to select and participate in their own recovery from cancer and the benefit of facilitating active coping behavior. Complementary therapies give patients the ability to take decisive action on their own behalf and counteract the common sense of hopelessness in the face of serious chronic illness.

Although herbs and other botanicals are under study internationally for their potential role in cancer rehabilitation, many of these agents can interact with prescription medications, altering their pharmacokinetic characteristics and leading to clinically significant interactions, including death. Herbal supplements taken in combination with pharmaceutical agents can affect their absorption, distribution, metabolism, and excretion, including chemotherapeutic drugs. Therefore, herbal and other over-the-counter remedies should be avoided by patients on active cancer treatment or on other prescription pharmaceuticals (32).

References

1. Boon HS, Olatunde F, Zick SM. Trends in complementary/alternative medicine use by breast cancer survivors: comparing survey data from 1998 and 2005. BMC Women's Health. 2007;7(1):4.
2. Cassileth BR, Vickers AJ. Massage therapy for symptom control: outcome study at a major cancer center. J Pain Symptom Manage. 2004;28(3):244–249.
3. Oguma Y, Sesso HD, Paffenbarger RS, Jr., Lee IM. Physical activity and all cause mortality in women: a review of the evidence. Br J Sports Med. 2002;36(3):162–172.
4. Friedenreich CM, Orenstein MR.Physical activity and cancer prevention: etiologic evidence and biological mechanisms. J Nutr. 2002;132(11 Suppl):3456S–3464S.
5. Friedenreich CM. Physical activity and breast cancer risk: the effect of menopausal status. Exerc Sport Sci Rev. 2004;32(4):180–184.
6. Knowler WC, Barrett-Connor E, Fowler SE, et al. Reduction in the incidence of type 2 diabetes with lifestyle intervention or metformin. N Engl J Med. 2002;346(6):393–403.
7. Mutrie N, Campbell AM, Whyte F, et al. Benefits of supervised group exercise programme for women being treated for early stage breast cancer: pragmatic randomised controlled trial. BMJ. 2007;334(7592):517.
8. Holmes MD, Chen WY, Feskanich D, Kroenke CH, Colditz GA. Physical activity and survival after breast cancer diagnosis. JAMA. 2005;293(20):2479–2486.
9. Stasi R, Abriani L, Beccaglia P, Terzoli E, Amadori S. Cancer-related fatigue: evolving concepts in evaluation and treatment. Cancer. 2003;98(9):1786–1801.
10. Vickers AJ, Straus DJ, Fearon B, Cassileth BR. Acupuncture for postchemotherapy fatigue: a phase II study. J Clin Oncol. 2004;22(9):1731–1735.
11. Ahles TA, Tope DM, Pinkson B, et al. Massage therapy for patients undergoing autologous bone marrow transplantation. J Pain Symptom Manage. 1999;18(3):157–163.
12. Kim SD, Kim HS. Effects of a relaxation breathing exercise on fatigue in haemopoietic stem cell transplantation patients. J Clin Nurs. 2005;14(1):51–55.
13. Carlson LE, Garland SN. Impact of mindfulness-based stress reduction (MBSR) on sleep, mood, stress and fatigue symptoms in cancer outpatients. Int J Behav Med. 2005;12(4):278–285.
14. Post-White J, Kinney ME, Savik K, Gau JB, Wilcox C, Lerner I. Therapeutic massage and healing touch improve symptoms in cancer. Integr Cancer Ther. 2003;2(4):332–344.
15. Wilkinson SM, Love SB, Westcombe AM, et al. Effectiveness of aromatherapy massage in the management of anxiety and depression in patients with cancer: a multicenter randomized controlled trial. J Clin Oncol. 2007;25(5):532–539.
16. Liossi C, Hatira P. Clinical hypnosis in the alleviation of procedure-related pain in pediatric oncology patients. Int J Clin Exp Hypn. 2003;51(1):4–28.
17. Liossi C, White P. Efficacy of clinical hypnosis in the enhancement of quality of life of terminally ill cancer patients. Contemporary Hypnosis. 2001;18:145–150.
18. Targ EF, Levine EG. The efficacy of a mind-body-spirit group for women with breast cancer: a randomized controlled trial. Gen Hosp Psychiatry. 2002;24(4):238–248.
19. Chlan L, Evans D, Greenleaf M, Walker J. Effects of a single music therapy intervention on anxiety, discomfort, satisfaction, and compliance with screening guidelines in outpatients undergoing flexible sigmoidoscopy. Gastroenterol Nurs. 2000;23(4):148–156.
20. Hernandez-Reif M, Ironson G, Field T, et al. Breast cancer patients have improved immune and neuroendocrine functions following massage therapy. J Psychosom Res. 2004;57(1):45–52.
21. Allen JJ, Schnyer RN, Chambers AS, Hitt SK, Moreno FA, Manber R. Acupuncture for depression: a randomized controlled trial. J Clin Psychiatry. 2006;67(11):1665–1673.
22. Speca M, Carlson LE, Goodey E, Angen M. A randomized, wait-list controlled clinical trial: the effect of a mindfulness meditation-based stress reduction program on mood and symptoms of stress in cancer outpatients. Psychosom Med. 2000;62(5):613–622.
23. NIH. Acupuncture. NIH Consensus Statement. 1997;15(5):1–34.

24. Ezzo JM, Rickardson MA, Vickers A, et al. Acupuncture-point stimulation for chemotherapy-induced nausea or vomiting. *Cochrane Database Syst Rev.* 2006;(2):CD002285.

25. Dundee JW, Ghaly RG, Fitzpatrick KT, Lynch G, Abram P. Optimising antiemesis in cancer chemotherapy. *Br Med J (Clin Res Ed).* 1987;294(6565):179.

26. Aglietti L, Roila F, Tonato M, et al. A pilot study of metoclopramide, dexamethasone, diphenhydramine and acupuncture in women treated with cisplatin. *Cancer Chemother Pharmacol.* 1990;26(3):239–240.

27. Shen J, Wenger N, Glaspy J, et al. Electroacupuncture for control of myeloablative chemotherapy-induced emesis: a randomized controlled trial. *JAMA.* 2000;284(21):2755–2761.

28. Grealish L, Lomasney A, Whiteman B. Foot massage. A nursing intervention to modify the distressing symptoms of pain and nausea in patients hospitalized with cancer. *Cancer Nurs.* 2000;23(3):237–243.

29. Zeltzer LK, Dolgin MJ, LeBaron S, LeBaron C. A randomized, controlled study of behavioral intervention for chemotherapy distress in children with cancer. *Pediatrics.* 1991;88(1):34–42.

30. Enqvist B, Bjorklund C, Engman M, Jakobsson J. Preoperative hypnosis reduces postoperative vomiting after surgery of the breasts. A prospective, randomized and blinded study. *Acta Anaesthesiol Scand.* 1997;41(8):1028–1032.

31. Marchioro G, Azzarello G, Viviani F, et al. Hypnosis in the treatment of anticipatory nausea and vomiting in patients receiving cancer chemotherapy. *Oncology.* 2000;59(2):100–104.

32. AboutHerbs Web site (Accessed April 10, 2007, at http://www.mskcc.org/aboutherbs.)

VIII

SPECIFIC DIAGNOSES IN CANCER REHABILITATION

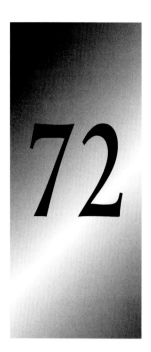

Balance and Gait Dysfunction in the Cancer Patient

72

Elizabeth M. Kilgore
Cynthia G. Pineda

Cancer and cancer treatments can cause significant impairments to multiple organs and systems (1). The neurologic and musculoskeletal systems, which provide the framework for movement, are particularly vulnerable, with impaired mobility cited as one of the most common functional impairments in the cancer population (2). Lehmann studied 805 patients at various cancer referral centers and found that 35% of patients had generalized weakness, 30% had impairment of activities of daily living, and 25% had difficulties with ambulation (3). Ganz et al. (4) surveyed 500 patients with colorectal, lung, and prostate cancer who had been living with cancer for more than one year and found that more than 80% reported gait problems, with 50% indicating that these problems were severe. In a study by Movsas (5), a Rehabilitation Needs Assessment identified that 58% of patients admitted to an inpatient medical oncology unit demonstrated impairments in mobility.

Mobility is such a critical functional determinant that performance tools such as Karnofsky and Eastern Cooperative Oncology Group (ECOG) use it as a measure of overall functional status and, in some cases, prognosis of the cancer itself (6,7). Gait limitations and abnormalities increase with age (8). Age-related changes in joint range of motion, soft tissue properties, and muscle strength may affect normal gait (9). On average, healthy older persons score 20%–40% lower on strength tests than young adults, and in nursing home residents, strength is even lower (10). Reasons include deconditioning due to prolonged bed rest, as well as cardiac, pulmonary, and other chronic conditions, including cancer. Aging is reported to increase postural sway, decrease gait velocity, decrease stride length and step height, prolong reaction time, and decrease visual acuity and depth perception. In the general population, at least 20% of noninstitutionalized older adults admit to difficulty with walking or require the assistance of another person or special equipment to walk (11,12). Gait disorders affect 20%–50% of elderly persons, and nearly 75% of nursing home residents require assistance with ambulation or cannot ambulate (10).

Gait disorders are important not only because of their prevalence, but also because of the increased risk for falls and injury (12,13). Gait and balance impairments have been shown to be significant risk factors for falls, associated with a four- and fivefold increase, respectively (10). Thus, gait and balance impairments are the most important immediate causes for and the most serious risk factors for falls (10,12,13).

Statistically, cancer is more often found in older patients who are already dealing with multiple comorbidities (14). Therefore, this places the elderly cancer patient at an even greater risk of having a gait abnormality at some phase during cancer treatment, recovery and survival. The impact of comorbidity in the patient with cancer cannot be understated. One study reported that in the older cancer survivor, regardless of duration following diagnosis, the presence of comorbidity rather than the history of cancer itself correlated most with

KEY POINTS

- Impaired mobility is cited as one of the most common functional impairments in the cancer population.
- Mobility is such a critical functional determinant that performance tools such as Karnofsky and Eastern Cooperative Oncology Group (ECOG) use it as a measure of overall functional status and, in some cases, prognosis of the cancer itself.
- Gait limitations and abnormalities increase with age and affect 20%–50% of elderly persons.
- Approximately 30% of people older than aged 65 suffer falls each year, and 10% of these falls result in injury, the most serious sequelae of balance or gait abnormality.
- Aging is reported to increase postural sway, decrease gait velocity, decrease stride length and step height, prolong reaction time, and decrease visual acuity and depth perception.
- In the older cancer survivor, regardless of duration following diagnosis, the presence of comorbidity rather than the history of cancer itself correlated most with impaired functional status.

- Patients with cancer are at increased risk of developing disorders of balance due to neurotoxic agents affecting the central, peripheral, or autonomic nervous systems.
- Evaluating and managing mobility disorders in the cancer population is dependent on the stage of cancer, the trajectory of the disease, the type of treatment the patient is receiving or has received, and their comorbidities.
- Cancer can affect nerves by direct infiltration or compression, neurotoxicity from chemotherapy, fibrosis from radiation therapy, or from paraneoplastic disorders.
- Five steps for developing a treatment plan for gait abnormality have been identified: (1) identify the gait abnormality; (2) determine the cause(s); (3) interpret the relationship between impairments and physical performance; (4) set appropriate goals; and (5) choose appropriate treatment strategies and techniques.

impaired functional status (15). Another study found that age older than 85, three or more chronic conditions, and the occurrence of stroke, hip fracture, or cancer predicted catastrophic loss of walking ability (12).

Approximately 30% of people older than aged 65 suffer falls each year, and 10% of these falls result in injury, the most serious sequelae of balance or gait abnormality (16). In the nursing home population, weakness and gait problems were the most common causes of falls, accounting for approximately 25% of reported cases (10). There is a correlation between lower extremity weakness and independent living. Some studies have reported lower extremity weakness in 48% of elderly persons living in the community, 57% of elderly persons living in intermediate care facilities, and nearly 80% of nursing home residents (17,18) More than two-thirds of persons who have fallen have substantial gait disorders, a prevalence 2.4–4.8 times higher than the prevalence among persons who have not fallen (17,18). The frequency of falls in hospices has not been as extensively studied as in the nursing home population. One study, however, reported that falls in hospices occur almost four times more frequently than in nursing homes (19).

Balance dysfunction predisposes a patient to falls, injuries, and loss of independence. Patients often develop a fear of falling, which may create a further cycle of weakness due to lack of exercise and activity.

Frail, high-risk elderly people living in institutions tend to have a higher incidence of falls caused by gait disorders, weakness, dizziness, and confusion (7,10,19). Dizziness is identified as the cause of falls in the elderly in 25% of reported nursing home falls (10). Dizziness is a vague term with diverse causes. True vertigo (a sensation of rotational movement) may indicate a disorder of the vestibular apparatus. Many patients describe a feeling of lightheadedness. An estimated 90 million Americans will experience dizziness at least once in their lifetime (20). Some patients develop permanent balance deficits with functional limitations. Patients with cancer are at increased risk of developing disorders of balance due to neurotoxic agents affecting the central, peripheral, or autonomic nervous systems.

Evaluating and managing mobility disorders in the cancer population is dependent on the stage of cancer, the trajectory of the disease, the type of treatment the patient is receiving or has received, and their comorbidities. The purpose of this chapter is to identify the more common causes of balance and gait disorders in the cancer population, to present an overview of basic rehabilitation terminology and definitions pertaining to balance and gait, to determine appropriate methods for assessing and diagnosing balance or gait dysfunction, and to review general rehabilitation treatments and interventions for managing impairments of balance or gait.

CAUSES OF BALANCE AND GAIT DISORDERS IN CANCER

The causes for balance and gait disorders in the cancer population are multifactorial. The functional status of the cancer patient may vary throughout the course of the cancer and cancer treatment(s). Because of this variability, it is difficult to determine the exact incidence and prevalence of balance and gait disorders in the cancer population.

Cancer and cancer treatments can produce both acute and chronic effects that make it important for the health care provider, as well as the patient, to be ever vigilant in monitoring functional changes, as early recognition can lead to prompt referral to rehabilitation and a more successful outcome (21).

Cancer and cancer treatments can cause neurologic, musculoskeletal, and/or systemic effects as discussed below:

Neurologic

Cancer can affect nerves by direct infiltration or compression by tumor, neurotoxicity from chemotherapy, fibrosis from radiation therapy, or from paraneoplastic disorders. An estimated 15%–20% of patients with cancer have symptomatic neurologic complications during the course of their illness (22). The most common complaints are back pain, mental status changes, headache, limb pain, and leg weakness. According to one study, motor symptoms, including gait disturbances, occurred in 24% of patients with brain metastasis from breast cancer (23,24).

Neurologic problems are second only to routine chemotherapy as reasons for hospitalization of patients with systemic cancer. As survival rates increase, it is expected that there will be more cancer survivors experiencing neurologic complications at some stage of their cancer care. Investigators at one oncology center reported that 46% of patients admitted to their solid tumor service over a three-month period required either evaluation or treatment of a neurologic problem (25). Another study found that approximately 30% of patients with small cell lung cancer had serious neurologic complications during the course of the disease (26).

Neurologic complications in patients with cancer can affect any level of the central and peripheral nervous system. The most frequently involved tumors are from lung, breast, colon, rectum, prostate, and head and neck, as well as tumors related to leukemia and lymphoma (22). Direct involvement of the nervous system includes brain metastasis, intramedullary spinal cord metastases, epidural spinal cord compression, and leptomeningeal metastases, in addition to cranial and peripheral neuropathies. Cranial neuropathies are most commonly caused by leptomeningeal metastases within the subarachnoid space (22,27–29). Nasopharyngeal carcinoma can present with cranial nerve palsies in 15%–30% of patients (22,30). Other base-of-skull tumors can also affect cranial nerves. Visual changes resulting from cranial nerve damage can affect balance and gait.

Spinal cord dysfunction is a devastating but relatively common complication of cancer with resultant balance and gait abnormalities (31). Spinal cord dysfunction in the setting of cancer can result from either metastatic or nonmetastatic causes. Metastatic lesions can further be classified into epidural, intradural, or intramedullary (32). Neoplastic epidural spinal cord compression (ESCC) is a common complication of cancer, and usually produces fairly symmetric lower extremity weakness that can progress from impaired gait to total paralysis (33). At the time of diagnosis, weakness may be present in 60%–85% of patients; it is usually preceded by pain. Gait ataxia in the setting of back pain in a cancer patient should raise the possibility of epidural spinal cord compression (34). Metastasis to the spinal cord parenchyma itself is classified as an intramedullary metastasis and occurs much less frequently than epidural metastases, which are most commonly seen in patients with widespread disease (31). The initial symptoms may be weakness (30%) and gait unsteadiness (5%), with only about 20% of patients capable of independent ambulation at diagnosis (31,35). Leptomeningeal disease affects the central nervous system at more than one site, causing multifocal signs and symptoms (32). Spinal symptoms and signs are the most common manifestation of leptomeningeal metastasis, which is characterized by absent deep tendon reflexes and a cauda equina syndrome with leg weakness, foot numbness, and bowel and bladder impairment (36). Gait abnormalities in leptomeningeal disease may be related to increased intracranial pressure, as well as gait apraxia or cerebellar dysfunction and lower motor neuron radicular involvement (32,36). Ambulation following spinal cord compression appears directly related to ambulatory ability on initial presentation. Ambulation after treatment was observed in 0%–25% of patients who presented with paraplegia, and 58%–100% of patients who were ambulatory on initial presentation were observed to be ambulatory posttreatment (48). Early recognition and treatment of spinal cord compression is critical to overall functional outcome (37,48).

Non-neoplastic causes of neurologic dysfunction include infections, vascular disorders, or treatment effects from radiation and/or chemotherapy (32). Radiation myelopathy is a complication that can occur several weeks or months after radiation to the spine or nearby structures. Early-delayed radiation myelopathy, which usually begins 12–20 weeks after radiation treatment, is generally characterized by paresthesias or electric shock sensations called Lhermitte's sign. Late-delayed radiation myelopathy can present as a progressive myelopathy with paraparesis or quadriparesis, or as motor neuron dysfunction or hemorrhagic myelopathy with leg weakness resulting in gait and balance dysfunction (31,32).

Brachial and lumbosacral plexopathies are often caused by infiltration or compression by tumor or progressive fibrosis from radiation or surgery. Lumbosacral plexopathy can result from direct extension of local tumor from colorectal, cervical, and prostate cancers. Brachial plexopathies can result from locally recurrent breast cancer, lung cancer (Pancoast tumors), and other primary and metastatic tumors to the plexus. Surgery involving retroperitoneal lymph node dissection can cause fibrosis and contribute to lumbosacral plexopathy. Radiation can also cause plexopathies that tend to progress slowly and insidiously, and share many clinical features with plexopathies caused by tumor.

Chemotherapy-induced peripheral neuropathies are common with neurotoxic agents including tubulin inhibitors such as vincristine (Oncovin) (38) and platinum-based compounds such as cisplatin (Platinol) (22,39,40). Peripheral neuropathies associated with chemotherapy vary between agents. Tubulin inhibitors such as vincristine and paclitaxel (Taxol) tend to cause a sensory more than motor axonal neuropathy in a length-dependent distal symmetric distribution. The platinum-based compounds directly affect the cell bodies in the sensory ganglion and, at more toxic doses, the motor neurons in the anterior horn of the spinal cord. Clinically, the platinum-based compounds cause a painful sensory neuropathy with sensory ataxia that may progress (coast) following discontinuation of the drug. The coasting effect results from progressive DNA damage within the sensory ganglion. After cessation of most chemotherapeutics, some of these deficits may resolve quickly, but others have a persistent peripheral polyneuropathy that can impact strength, balance, and function (41,42).

Paraneoplastic neurologic syndromes can affect any nervous system structure, including the cerebellum, brain, and peripheral nerves, with potentially devastating consequences (43,44). The Lambert-Eaton myasthenic syndrome (LEMS) is associated with the anti-HU antibodies. The syndrome preferentially affects the sensory ganglia and in severe cases, the motor cell bodies in the anterior horn cell and autonomic neurons, with subsequent sensory ataxia, weakness, and autonomic dysfunction (43). Paraneoplastic syndromes targeting the Purkinje cells of the cerebellum can result in severe cerebellar degeneration and ataxia.

Causes of vestibular lesions in patients with cancer could include infections, vascular insufficiency, tumor, trauma, metabolic disorders, and toxic drugs. Neoplasia can compromise vestibular function when it occurs near any part of the vestibular system. Schwannomas (acoustic neuromas) can damage the sheath of the vestibular nerve or extend into the pontocerebellar angle and cause symptoms similar to cerebellar lesions. Meningiomas can grow into the temporal lobe area, resulting in pressure to the vestibular apparatus. Surgical removal of tumors in these areas can cause a balance disturbance. Medications such as aminoglycoside antibiotics and antineoplastics (cisplatin, bleomycin, vincristine and vinblastine) are ototoxic and can cause damage to the vestibular hair cells (45). Carcinomatous sensory neuropathy involves the dorsal root ganglion cells and their axons, and can cause ataxia. It is characterized by paresthesias or dysesthesias, which can affect sensory feedback for balance and gait (46). Peripheral somatosensory loss in patients with cancer can occur after spinal cord injury, chemotherapy-induced neuropathy, and amputation.

Musculoskeletal

Musculoskeletal effects of cancer or cancer treatments often overlap with or are found to coexist with or be caused by neurologic dysfunction. Frequently encountered musculoskeletal disorders include contracture from prolonged bed rest, surgery, or radiation, with subsequent scar tissue formation and impaired range of motion. Graft-versus-host disease is particularly devastating to the soft tissues, causing nearly intractable contractures. Any solid or soft tissue tumors can directly or indirectly impact muscles, ligaments, tendons, and bones. Both radiation and chemotherapy can have an effect on muscle components, and can lead to atrophy and a decreased ability to generate force (42). In one study, women with breast cancer undergoing chemotherapy were noted to have a loss of lean body mass, primarily in the lower trunk and legs (42,47). Bony weakness due to pathologic changes or osteoporosis may be observed in the femur and humerus, which are the most frequent long bone sites affected by metastases (48). Osteoporosis, which can cause lead to fractures, can also result as a complication of immobility or due to medications used in cancer (particularly steroids). Compression fractures of the vertebrae can cause significant pain and affect functional mobility. Myopathies seen in the cancer population are often the result of steroid administration or critical illness. Myopathy associated with paraneoplastic syndrome often precedes the diagnosis of the cancer itself.

Systemic

Systemic effects in cancer can include side effects from chemotherapy, radiation, or surgery. Anemia, orthostatic hypotension, pain, fatigue, decreased endurance, electrolyte abnormalities, and cardiopulmonary effects are but a few systemic complications. Indirect effects of systemic cancer include vascular disorders, infections, metabolic abnormalities, and paraneoplastic syndromes. Patients with neurologic complications of systemic cancer can experience weakness, dementia, seizure activity, loss of ambulation, pain, and incontinence, which, either singly or in combination, can cause significant mobility disorders (22).

DEFINING GAIT AND BALANCE

Mobility is defined as the ability to move (49). Independent mobility requires an effective energy source and intact neurologic and musculoskeletal systems. Therefore, any condition that affects endurance, strength, sensation, or balance will affect mobility. From a rehabilitation standpoint, mobility is further classified into the most basic act of bed mobility, then progression to transfers and finally, to ambulation.

Bed mobility activities include rolling from side to side and rolling from a supine to a prone position and back. Transitional movements allow the individual to change from one level of mobility to another, such as going from supine to sitting, sitting to standing, and back again (49). Sitting is a basic functional skill that requires adequate trunk and neck stability or strength and ability to establish midline orientation. Midline orientation allows the patient to recognize normal upright body position. Good standing skills are required prior to functional ambulation. Independent standing requires adequate midline orientation, trunk stability, strength, and balance. Adequate bilateral leg stability and strength are also required. Walking involves the combination of multiple skills to include balance, strength, coordination, and midline orientation.

Gait or walking can be defined as a series of losses and recoveries of balance (50). Effective and safe gait requires the coordination of muscle contraction, joint movement, and sensory perception. The basic unit of walking is described as one gait cycle, or stride (51). It is the sequence of lower limb action from initial floor contact by one foot to the next instant of floor contact by the same foot. The gait cycle is divided into two periods: the period of floor contact (stance phase), which comprises about 60% of the cycle; and the period of midair limb advancement (swing phase), which comprises about 40% of the gait cycle (51,52).

Gait velocity is defined as the speed of walking. Stride and cadence determine the velocity of walking (46). Normal walking speed may vary. Factors that slow gait speed are considered contributors to gait disorders. Studies in the geriatric population have shown that speed of walking remains stable until about age 70,

then declines about 15% per decade for usual gait and 20% per decrease for maximal gait. Gait velocity has become a powerful assessment and outcome measure (53,54). It can be measured as part of a timed short-distance walk or in terms of distance walked over time, and has been used to predict disease activity, cardiopulmonary function, and mobility (54,55). Gait velocity has also been shown to be useful as an outcome measure in rehabilitation (53,54). In a study done with a group of patients requiring inpatient rehabilitation, a gait speed that was higher on admission predicted higher gait speed at the time of discharge and lower rates of institutionalization (54,56).

Cadence is defined as the rhythm of walking. The normal cadence is between 90 and 120 steps per minute (57). Cadence generally does not change with age. Each person has a preferred cadence, which is related to leg length and usually represents the most energy-efficient rhythm for the individual's body structure (58). Double-leg stance is that phase of gait in which parts of both feet are on the ground and is also referred to as double support (57). In normal gait, this occurs twice during the gait cycle and represents about 25% of the cycle. This has been found to increase with age from 18% in young adults to greater than 26% in healthy elderly persons (58). Elderly persons with a fear of falling increase their double stance time. Double stance time is a strong predictor of gait velocity and step length (58). Step length or gait length is defined as the distance between successive contact points on opposite feet (57).

Balance can be defined as the ability to maintain the center of body mass within stability limits largely determined by the base of support (46). Balance is the ability to control the center of gravity over the base of support in a given sensory environment (45). Balance is the ability to sit, stand, or walk safely without postural deviation, falling, or reaching for external support. Balance, like gait, is a coordinated response of the neuromuscular and musculoskeletal systems, incorporating visual and sensory perception. Balance depends on the interaction of the peripheral, nervous, proprioceptive, vestibular, cerebellar, and visual systems. The center of mass is located 2 cm in front of the second sacral vertebrae with the body in anatomic position. During walking, the center of mass moves in a sinusoidal path, with a mean of 5 cm of vertical and horizontal displacement. This displacement of the center of mass requires energy.

ASSESSING GAIT AND BALANCE IN PATIENTS WITH CANCER

Evaluation of a patient presenting with a chronically progressive or acute disorder of gait includes three

TABLE 72.1
Functional Physical Examination

Coordination
    Finger-to-nose testing
    Rapid alternating movements
    Rhythmic toe tap
    Thumb to alternating fingertips
Proprioception
    Great toe
Strength
    Finger flexors
    Elbow extensors
    Thumb-index finger pinch strength
ROM
    Active arm flexion and abduction of at least 135°
    each
Balance
    Dynamic sitting balance
    Single foot balance
Transfers
    Standing from seated position
Gait
    Reciprocal
    Tandem
    Heel walk

Source: From: Ref. 5.

TABLE 72.2
Physical Impairments that Can Influence Gait

MUSCULOSKELETAL	NEUROLOGICAL	CARDIOVASCULAR
Posture	Sensory perception; sensory interpretation	Aerobic capacity
Joint structure	Motor planning	Endurance
Joint alignment	Motor programming	Energy metabolism
Joint range of motion	Timing and coordination	Vascular integrity
Muscle length and flexibility	Sensory and motor integration	
Muscle strength and endurance	Pain	

Source: From Ref. 46.

steps: history, physical examination, and functional assessment of gait and balance. A careful history and systems review can uncover the factors contributing to the gait disorder. Therefore, it is important to know the patient's medications, pertinent laboratory data, type and stage of cancer, and past or current treatments. The function-based physical examination should include a neurologic, musculoskeletal, and mental status assessment, at minimum. Table 72.1 provides an example of a function-based physical examination (5).

The goal of a gait assessment is to evaluate walking in an effort to isolate dysfunction. Areas of impairment may include muscle weakness, loss of joint range, incoordination, or poor postural control. Table 72.2 describes the physical impairments that can influence gait and that should be assessed (46) Gait evaluations can range from the most basic in-office observation of any gait deviations to sophisticated, computerized gait analysis labs that assess motion, force platform data, and electromyography (53,54). In a simple gait assessment, the patient is observed during standing (static testing) and walking (dynamic testing). Initially, the patient is examined in the standing position to evaluate posture as well as bone and soft-tissue symmetry. The clinician evaluates the foot and ankle during standing to assess any deviation in the rear foot and forefoot. Step length and height should also be observed and measured, as well as cadence. The patient is then asked

to walk across the floor while the clinician evaluates the gait cycle. The clinician assesses joint range of motion, speed and quality of gait, as well as synchrony of all upper and lower extremity joints. The patient should be evaluated walking barefoot as well as while wearing normal walking shoes and observed walking from the back, front, and side and with their usual mobility device and/or orthotic.

Functional in-office assessment of gait should include proximal muscle testing, which is performed by asking the patient to arise from a chair without using his arms. Functional assessment of gait includes the use of timed walking tests to determine gait velocity, and is measured using a stop watch and a fixed distance (45). In patients with cancer, Simmonds found significant deficits on a number of physical performance measures, which includes the six-minute walk test and a forward reach test (59). The Get Up and Go test, which can also be used in balance assessment, was originally scored using levels of abnormal performance in rising from a chair, turning, walking, and returning to the chair (54,60). A modified timed version of this test has been developed (61). The Functional Ambulation Classification scale involves rating the use of an assistive device, degree of human assistance, distance the patient can walk, and the types of surfaces the patient can negotiate (62). Table 73.3 lists the more common gait impairment and functional gait assessment tests.

Analysis of balance is complex, and requires many systems to work at optimum levels. A comprehensive assessment of balance control also includes the evaluation of the efficacy of sensory, motor, and cognitive systems contributing to postural control. Any prob-

TABLE 72.3
Gait Impairment and Assessment Tests

GAIT IMPAIRMENT TESTS	FUNCTIONAL GAIT ASSESSMENTS
Automated up-timer	3 min walk test
Clinical gait assessments	5 min walk test
Functional ambulation profile	6 min walk test
Gait Abnormality Rating Scale (GARS)	12 min walk test

Source: From Ref. 45.

lem affecting strength, joint motion, vision, sensory perception, or vestibular systems can cause balance impairment. Balance, like gait, needs to be evaluated both statically and dynamically. A variety of tests have been used in patients with neurological problems to measure different aspects of postural control (45). These tests are observed during quiet standing, active standing, and using sensory manipulation, which can be useful in identifying impairments affecting balance. The goal of quiet standing (static) is to test the ability of the patient definition to hold still while in the standing position. Active standing (dynamic) tests are also performed with the patient in the standing position, but the movement being tested is the ability to voluntarily weight shift. The classic Romberg Test, Sharpened Romberg test (tandem Romberg),k and One-legged Stance test are static balance tests (63) The Functional Reach Scale was originally developed for use with the elderly to determine the risk of falls and is an example of an active standing or dynamic test (45,64). Functional balance, mobility, and gait scales are used to evaluate the performance of whole-body movement tasks such as sit-to-stand, walking, and stepping on objects; these scales can be used to identify disabilities. The Berg Balance Scale (65) Timed Get Up and Go (61), Modified Gait Assessment Rating Scale (m-GARS) (66) and Tinneti Balance and Gait Scale (also known as Performance-Mobility Assessment, or POMA) (67) are some of the functional scales more commonly used. Combinations of test batteries have also been used in balance assessment, as there is no single test that can give a complete picture of the multidimensional aspects of balance (45).

DIAGNOSING GAIT AND BALANCE DISORDERS

A gait disorder is defined as a slowing of gait speed or a deviation in smoothness, symmetry, or synchrony of body movement (58). Upon completion of the function-

based history and examination, including specific testing, the clinician needs to determine whether a disorder exists and the most likely cause in an effort to determine the most effective treatment plan.

In a study of 120 patients without cancer, the etiologies for gait dysfunction included sensory deficits (18.3%), myelopathy (16.7%), multiple infarcts (15%), parkinsonism (11.7%), cerebellar disease (6.7%), hydrocephalus (6.7%), and unknown etiology (14%) (8). There is no pathognomonic characteristic gait pattern seen in the patient with cancer. Functional limitations and gait patterns in these patients are, however, related to the extent of the disease, and may vary throughout the course of the disease and the system affected.

Gait disorders can be classified according to anatomic site, sensorimotor or descriptive gait patterns. From an anatomic standpoint, gait disorders can be broadly classified into the following nine categories: (1) frontal gait disorders, (2) cortical-subcortical gait disorders, (3) subcortical hypokinetic disorders, (4) subcortical hyperkinetic disorders, (5) subcortical disequilibrium, (6) pyramidal gait disorders, (7) cerebellar gait disorders, (8) neuropathic disorders, and (9) myopathic gait disorders (8).

Another useful way of classifying gait disorders is according to the sensorimotor level, which has been divided into low, middle, and high levels of dysfunction (12). This type of classification is especially helpful in patients with cancer, since the use of a neurologic sensory or motor level can be identified. Table 72.4 lists the sensorimotor levels and associated gait dysfunction (12). In the patient with cancer, low-level deficit causes include vestibular disorders, peripheral neuropathy, posterior column deficits, or visual ataxia. Peripheral motor deficits may be caused by arthritic, myopathic, or neuropathic conditions. If the gait disorder is limited to the low sensorimotor level and the central nervous system is intact, adaptation is generally good because the patient can compensate. Middle-level deficits are often due to spasticity from myelopathy or cerebellar ataxia. Initiation of gait may be normal but stepping patterns are abnormal. Circumduction and broad-based gait are frequently seen with this level of dysfunction. High-level deficits are characterized by impaired cognition and behavioral aspects such as fear of falling. These disorders are often more difficult to correct because the compensatory strategies may be lacking. Most patients have deficits at more than one level, but determining the primary level of deficit may help direct treatment more specifically.

Another clinically useful and practical approach to classifying gait disorders is through a descriptive pattern of pathology (57). Similarly, balance disorders can be defined as the impairment of one or more components in the balance equation. Symptoms often

TABLE 72.4
Gait Disorders Vary According to the Level of Sensorimotor Deficit

LEVEL	DEFICIT/CONDITION	GAIT CHARACTERISTICS
Low	Peripheral sensory ataxia: posterior column, peripheral nerves, vestibular and visual ataxia	Unsteady, uncoordinated (especially without visual input), tentative, "drunken
	Peripheral motor deficit due to arthritis (antalgic gait, joint deformity)	Avoids weight-bearing on affected side; shorter stance phase Painful hip may produce Trendelenburg gait (trunk shift over affected side) Painful knee is flexed Painful spine produces short, slow steps and decreased lumbar lordosis Nonantalgic features include contractures, deformity-limited motion, including Trendelenburg gait
	Peripheral motor deficit due to myopathic and neuropathic conditions (weakness)	Pelvic girdle weakness produces exaggerated lumbar lordosis and lateral trunk flexion (Trendelenburg and "waddling" gait) Proximal motor neuropathy produces waddling and foot slap Distal motor neuropathy produces distal weakness, especially ankle dorsiflexion and "foot drop", which may lead to exaggerated hip flexion, knee extension, foot lifting (steppage gait), and foot slap
Middle	Spasticity from hemiplegia, hemiparesis	Leg swings outward and in semi-circle from hip (circumduction); knee may hyperextend (genu recurvatum); ankle may show excessive plantar flexion and inversion (equinovarus); with less paresis, some may only lose arm swing and only drag or scrape the foot
	Spasticity from paraplegia, paresis	Circumduction of both legs; steps are short, shuffling and scraping; when sever, hip adducts so that knees cross in front of each other (scissoring)
	Parkinsonism	Small and shuffling steps, hesitation, acceleration (festination), falling forward (propulsion),falling backward (retropulsion), moving the whole body while turning (turning en bloc), no arm swinging
	Cerebellar ataxia	Wide-based gait with increase trunk sway, irregular stepping, staggering (especially on turns)
High	Cautious gait	Fear of falling with appropriate postural responses, normal to widened gait base, shortened stride, slower, turning en bloc
	Frontal-related or white-matter lesions: cerebrovascular lesions, normal-pressure hydrocephalus	Frontal gait disorder: difficulty initiating gait; short, shuffling gait, like parkinsonian, but with wider base, upright posture, arm swing, leg apraxia, and "freezing" when turning or when attention is diverted May also have cognitive, pyramidal, urinary disturbances

Source: From Ref. 12.

associated with disorders of balance include vertigo, dizziness, ataxia, apraxia, and dyscoordination. Balance is the result of interactions between the individual, the task the individual is performing, and the environment in which the task must be performed (45). Both sensory inputs and processing and motor planning and execution are required. Peripheral and central components are required in the cycle. In order to diagnose a balance disorder the clinician needs to understand the relationship between the vestibular system, sensory, and motor systems. From a practical standpoint, a balance disorder is determined if a patient is unable to perform tandem stance or single-leg stance for greater five seconds or longer (58). In a patient with cancer, disorder in balance may result from multiple factors and each of these parameters should be assessed to determine where the deficit may be occurring.

TREATMENT AND REHABILITATIVE INTERVENTIONS

Treatment of balance and gait disorders in the patient with cancer should incorporate both medical and rehabilitative interventions. Medical treatments may include medication adjustments such as limiting or changing chemotherapy, modifying dose radiation or areas being irradiated, treating underlying anemia, replacing electrolytes, and other medical management depending upon the cause of the problem. Rehabilitative interventions may include physiatry evaluations, physical therapy and/or occupational therapy, prescription of orthotics, adaptive equipment, mobility devices, and environmental modifications.

Five steps for developing a treatment plan for gait abnormality have been identified (46):

1. Identify the gait abnormality
2. Determine the cause(s)
3. Interpret the relationship between impairments and physical performance
4. Set appropriate goals
5. Choose appropriate treatment strategies and techniques

Most gait-training programs encompass some aspect of improving strength, endurance, or flexibility. Strengthening for gait training should emphasize the trunk muscles and proximal muscles with both isometric and resistance training. Endurance training incorporates use of aerobic exercises. Flexibility is encouraged using range-of-motion exercises especially for the ankles and hips. Some studies have reported that task-specific gait training with the use of body support and treadmill may be beneficial (12).

Various orthotics and mobility aids are used to improve safety during ambulation. Lower extremity orthoses are used to stabilize, protect, and support a limb joint and to aid in therapeutic standing and functional ambulation. The type of orthosis depends on the severity and location of weakness. Lower extremity orthoses include the hip-knee-ankle-foot (HKAFO), which is used in patients with thoracic or high lumbar spinal cord lesions or those with significant hip flexion weakness; the knee-ankle-foot (KAFO) is used in patients with weak quadriceps but intact thigh flexors, The ankle-foot (AFO) is used for those with good hip and thigh strength but weak ankle dorsi/plantar flexion due to peripheral nerve injuries, peripheral neuropathies, or distal lower limb weakness. Spinal orthoses are also used to provide additional stability and control truncal motion (68). Physical therapy can help determine the most appropriate assistive device and train the patient with that device (69).

In some patients with cancer, a gait abnormality may be transient, reversible, and temporary due to dose limiting side effects of medication as an example. The goals for therapeutic intervention in this case would be to provide an appropriate mobility device to ensure safety until the patient's gait returns to or near pretreatment level. At the other end of the spectrum, a patient with cancer could have a primary or metastatic brain lesion that is expected to worsen over time. The goals for therapeutic intervention are still safety based but the frequency, intensity, and duration of rehabilitation will vary greatly from someone with short-term impairment. The overall goal is always to maximize the capacity for safe ambulation, including stability, speed, endurance, and adaptability to the patient's lifestyle (46).

Balance has multiple dimensions, and improving any balance skill training should be carried out in a context-specific manner. It is felt that recurring exposure to specific postural and balancing activities needs to occur to ensure the acquisition of the skill. Generally, no one type of balance training has been found to be more effective than another. Masdeu (46) reported a review of 25 "balance training" studies performed with older adults. When all variables were taken into account, it appeared that ten (40%) of the studies resulted in no significant improvement in one or more balance outcome measures. Randomized control trials were equally represented within the improvement versus non-improvement categories. As a group, the studies with successful outcomes appeared to take a more intensive approach to training (46).

Vestibulo-ocular exercises have been used in individuals with vestibular hypofunction or with benign positional nystagmus. Spatial perception training has been reported as an effective strategy. In one study by Schaie and Willis (46,70) a brief period (five 1-hour sessions) of cognitive spatial retraining (mental rotation of figures) resulted in a significant reversal of decline in this function. Tai chi is a movement technique that directs attention to spatial and body interaction. In two studies, tai chi training resulted in improved balance and decreased falls risk in the elderly (71–74). Mental imagery increasing vestibular sensory inputs have also been used (46).

CONCLUSIONS

Cancer rehabilitation is the process by which the cancer survivor is enabled to live as fully and effectively as possible within the limitations of impairments resulting from their disease and its treatment (5). The goal of cancer rehabilitation is to enable a person with cancer obtain optimal physical, psychological, vocational, and social functioning, which supports the interdisciplinary approach to cancer rehabilitation (1,75). Functional limitations and rehabilitation needs of a patient with cancer are directly related to the extent of the disease at the time of the diagnosis and concomitant cancer treatment. Any of these problems can be devastating to functional ability and cause emotional and social distress to the patient as well as the caregiver(s) (76).

Balance and gait dysfunctions are commonly seen in patients with cancer. Balance and gait are interrelated, and it is challenging to isolate the independent contributions of each to the performance of activities of daily living. Since the causes of balance and gait disorders in a patient with cancer are multifactorial, a careful history and a comprehensive functional examination are recommended to assess the presence of impairments and determine the appropriate intervention. Physical function and independence should be maintained as long as possible to improve a patient's quality of life and reduce burden of care for caregivers (77). Patients with cancer should be encouraged to participate in exercise programs to increase or maintain strength and functional level and mobility with appropriate guidance and precautions based on the impairments that have resulted from cancer, comorbidities, and endurance level (78). Future research in cancer rehabilitation with focus on balance and gait dysfunction would be helpful in defining safe and appropriate interventions.

References

1. Fialka-Moser V, Crevenna R, Korpan M, Quittan M. Cancer rehabilitation: particularly with aspects on physical impairments. *J Rehabil Med.* 2003;35:153–162.
2. Gillis TA, Garden FH. Principles of cardiac rehabilitation. In: Braddom RL, ed. *Physical Medicine and Rehabilitation*, 2nd ed. Philadelphia, PA: Saunders, 2000:1305–1320.
3. Lehmann JF, DeLisa JA, Warren CG, DeLateur BJ, Sand Bryant PL, Nicholson CG. Cancer rehabilitation: assessment of need, development, and evaluation of a model of care. *Arch Phys Med Rehabil.* 1978;59:410–419.
4. Ganz PA, Coscarcelli Schag CA, Heinrich RL. Rehabilitation. In: Haskell CM, ed. *Cancer Treatment.* Philadelphia: WB Saunders; 1990:883–892.
5. Movsas SB, Chang VT, Tunkel RS, Shah VV, Ryan LS, Millis SR. Rehabilitation needs of an inpatient medical oncology unit. *Arch Phys Med Rehabil.* 2003;84:1642–1646.
6. Gerber LH, Vargo MM, Smith RG. Rehabilitation of the cancer patient. In: De Vita VT, Hellman S, Rosenberg SA, eds. *Cancer: Principles and Practice of Oncology*, 7th ed. Philadelphia, PA: Lippincott-Raven; 2005:2719–2746.
7. Yates JW. Comorbidity considerations in geriatric oncology research. *CA Cancer J Clin.* 2001;51:329–336.
8. Manek S, Lew M. Gait and balance dysfunction in adults. *Curr Treat Options Neur.* 2003;5:177–185.
9. Buckwalter JA, et al. Current concepts review, soft-tissue aging and musculoskeletal function. *J Bone Joint Surg.* 1993;75:1533–1548.
10. Rubenstein LZ, Josephson KR, Robbins AS. Falls in the nursing home. *Ann Intern Med.* 1994;121:442–451.

11. Ostchega Y, Harris TB, Hirsh R, Parsons VL, Kington R. The prevalence of functional limitations and disability in older persons in the US: data from the National Health and Nutrition Examination Survey III. *J Am Geriatr Soc.* 2000;49:1132–1135.
12. Alexander NB, Goldberg A. Gait disorders: search for multiple causes. *Cleve Clin J Med.* 2005;72:586–600.
13. Sudarsky L. Gait disorders: prevalence, morbidity, and etiology. *Adv Neurol.* 2001;87:111–117.
14. Nusbaum NJ. Rehabilitation of the older cancer patient. *Am J Med Sci.* 2004;327:86–90.
15. Garman KS, Pieper CF, Seo P, Cohen HJ. Function in elderly cancer survivors depends on comorbidities. *J Gerentol A Biol Sci Med Sci.* 2003;58:M119–M1124.
16. Sudarsky L. Geriatrics: gait disorders in the elderly. *N Engl J Med.* 1990;322:1441–1446.
17. Tinetti ME, Williams TF, Mayewski R. Fall risk index for elderly patients based on number of chronic disabilities. *Am J Med.* 1986;80:429–434.
18. Robbins AS, Rubenstein LZ, Josephson KR, Schulman BL, Osterweil D, Fine G. Predictors of falls among elderly people. Results of two population-based studies. *Arch Intern Med.* 1989;149:1628–1633.
19. Pearse H, Nicholson L, Bennett M. Falls in hospices: a cancer network observational study of fall rates and risk factors. *Palliat Med.* 2004;18:478–481.
20. Bauer CA. Vestibular rehabilitation, 2005. Accessed March 26, 2007, at http://www.emedicine.com/ent/topic666.htm Bauer.
21. Schwartz AL. Cancer. In: Durstine JL, Moore GE, eds. *ASCM's Exercise Management for Persons with Chronic Disabilities*, 2nd ed. Champaign, IL: Human Kinetics; 2003:166–172.
22. Newton HB. Neurologic complications of systemic cancer. *Am F Phys.* 1999;59:878–886
23. Chang EL, Lo S. Diagnosis and management of central nervous system metastasis from breast cancer. *Oncologist.* 2003;8:398–410.
24. Tsukada Y, Fouad A, Pickren JW, et al. Central nervous system metastasis from breast carcinoma. Autopsy study. *Cancer.* 1983;52:2349–2354.
25. Gilbert MR, Grossman SA. Incidence and nature of neurologic problems in patients with solid tumors. *Am J Med.* 1986;81:951–954.
26. Sculier JP, Feld R, Evans WK, De Boer G, et al. Neurologic disorders in patients with small cell lung cancer. *Cancer.* 1987;60:2275–2283.
27. Boogerd W, Hart AAM, van der Sande JJ, Engelsman E. Meningeal carcinomatosis in breast cancer. Prognostic factors and influence of treatment. *Cancer.* 1991;67:1685–1695.
28. Balm M, Hammack J. Leptomeningeal carcinomatics. Presenting features and prognostic factors. *Arch Neurol.* 1996;53:626–632.
29. Chad DA, Recht LD. Neuromuscular complication of systemic cancer. *Neurol Clin.* 1991;9:901–918.
30. Stillwagon GB, Lee DJ, Moses H, Kashima H, Harris A, Johns M. Response of cranial nerve abnormalities in nasopharyngeal carcinoma to radiation therapy. *Cancer.* 1986;57:2272–2274.
31. Schiff D. Spinal metastases. In: Schiff D, Wenn PY, eds. *Cancer Neurology in Clinical Practice.* Tottowa, New Jersey: Humana Press Inc.; 2003:93–106.
32. Posner JB. *Neurologic Complications of Cancer.* Philadelphia, PA: F.A. Davis Company; 1995;111–171.
33. Helweg-Larsen S, Sorensen PS. Symptom and signs of metastatic spinal cord compression: a study of progression from first symptom until diagnosis in 153 patients. *Eur J Cancer.* 1994;30A:396–398.
34. Hainline B, Tuszynski MH, Posner JB. Ataxia in epidural spinal cord compression. *Neurology.* 1992;42:2193–2195.
35. Schiff D, O'Neill BP. Intramedullary spinal cord metastases: clinical features and treatment outcome. *Neurology.* 1996;47:906–912.

36. Mason WP. Leptomeningeal metastases. In: Schiff D, Wen PY, eds. *Cancer Neurology in Clinical Practice*. Tottowa, New Jersey: Humana Press Inc; 2003:107–118.

37. Stubblefield MD, Bilsky MH. Barriers to rehabilitation of the neurosurgical spine cancer patient. *J Surg Oncol*. 2007;95:415–426.

38. Casey EB, Jellife AM, Le Quesne PM, Millet YL. Vincristine neuropathy: clinical and electrophysiological observations. *Brain*. 1973;96:69–86.

39. Siegal T, Haim N. Cisplatin-induced peripheral neuropathy. *Cancer*. 1990;66:1117–1123.

40. Cavaletti G, Marzorati L, Bogluin G, et al. Cisplatin induced peripheral neurotoxicity is dependent on total-dose intensity and single dose intensity. *Cancer*. 2002;94:2434–2440.

41. Visovsky C, Daly BJ. Clinical evaluation and patterns of chemotherapy-induced peripheral neuropathy. *J Am Acad Nurse Pract*. 2004;16(8):353–359.

42. Galantino ML, Machese V, Ness K, Gilchrist LS. Oncology physical therapy research: a need for collaboration and the quest for quality of life in cancer survivors. *Rehabil Oncol*. 2005;23:10–16.

43. Posner JB. Neoplastic disorders: nonmetastatic complications of cancer, 2006. Accessed April 4, 2006, at http://www.medscape.com/viewarticle/534598.

44. Dropocho EJ. Remote neurologic manifestations of cancer. *Neurol Clin*. 2002;20(1):85–122.

45. Umphred DA. *Neurological Rehabilitation*, 4th ed. St. Louis, MO: Mosby, Inc.; 2001:616–660.

46. Masdau JC, Sudarsky L, Wolfson L, eds. *Gait Disorders of Aging: Falls and Therapeutic Strategies*. Philadelphia, PA: Lippincott-Raven Publishers; 1997:1–443.

47. Denmark-Wahnfried W, Petersen BL, Winer EP, et al. Changes in weight body composition, and factors influencing energy balance among premenopausal breast cancer patient receiving adjurant chemotherapy. *J Clin Oncol*. 2001;19(9):2367–2369.

48. Heary RF, Filart R. Tumors of the spine and spinal cord. In: Kirshblum S, Campagnolo DI, Delisa JA, eds. *Spinal Cord Medicine*. Philadelphia, PA; Lippincott Williams and Wilkins; 2002:480–497.

49. McPeak LA. Physiatric history and examination. In: Braddom RL, ed. *Physical Medicine and Rehabilitation*, 2nd ed. Philadelphia, PA: Saunders; 2000:3–45.

50. Simoneau GG. Kinesilogy of walking. In: Neumann DA, ed. *Kinesiology of the Musculoskeletal System: Foundations for Physical Rehabilitation*. St. Louis, MO: Mosby, Inc.; 2002:523–569.

51. Esquenazi A, Talaty M. Gait analysis: technology and clinical applications. In: Braddom RL, ed. *Physical Medicine and Rehabilitation*, 2nd ed. Philadelphia, PA: Saunders; 2000:93–108.

52. Perry J. *Gait Analysis: Normal and PFunction*. New York, NY: McGraw-Hill, Inc.; 1992:3–16.

53. Hausdorff JM, Alexander MB, eds. *Gait Disorders: Evaluation and Management*. Boca Raton, FL: Taylor and Francis Group; 2005:1–408.

54. Alexander NB. Gait disorders in older adults. *Clin Geriatr*. 1999;7:1070–1389.

55. Guyatt GH, et al. The 6 minute walk: a new measure of exercise capacity in patients with chronic heart failure. *Can Med Assoc J*. 1985;132:919–923.

56. Friedman PJ, Richmond DE, Baskett JJ. A prospective trial of serial gait speed as a measure of rehabilitation in the elderly. *Age Aging*. 1988;17:227–235.

57. Magee DJ. *Orthopedic Physical Assessment*, 4th ed. St. Louis, MO: Saunders Elsevier; 2006:847–872.

58. Beers MH, ed. *The Merck Manual of Geriatrics*, 3rd ed. Whitehouse Station, NJ: Merck Research Laboratories; 2000:203–211.

59. Simmonds MJ. Physical function in patients with cancer: psychometric characteristics and clinical usefulness on a physical performance battery. *J Pain Symptom Manage*. 2002;24(2):404–414.

60. Mathias A, Nayak USL, Isaacs B. Balance in elderly patients: the "get up and go" test. *Arch Phys Med Rehabil*. 1986;67:387–389.

61. Posiadlo D. Richardson S. The timed "Up and Go": a test of basic functional mobility for frail elderly persons. *J Am Geriatr Soc*. 1991;39:142–148.

62. Holden, MK, Gill KM, Magliozzi MR.Gait assessment for neurologically impaired patients; standards for outcome assessment. *Phys Ther*. 1986;66:1530–1539.

63. Anemaet WK, Moffa-Trotter ME. Functional tools for assessing balance and gait impairments. *Top Geriatr Rehabil*. 1999;15(1):66–83.

64. Duncan PW, Weiner DK, Chandler J, Studenski S. Functional reach: a new clinical measure of balance. *J Gerontol*. 1990;45:M192–M197.

65. Berg K, et al. Measuring balance in the elderly: preliminary development of an instrument. *Physio Ther Can*. 1989;41(6):304–311.

66. Wolfson LI, Whipple R, Amerman P, Tobin JN. Gait assessment in the elderly: a gait abnormality rating scale and its relationship to falls. *J Gerontol*. 1990;45:M12–M19.

67. Tinetti ME, Williams TF, Mayewski R. Fall risk index for elderly patients based on number of chronic disabilities. *Am J Med*. 1986;80:429–434.

68. Smith RG, Vargo MM. Rehabilitative medicine. In: Berger AM, Shuster JL, Von Roenn JH, eds. *Palliative Care and Supportive Oncology*, 3rd ed. Philadelphia, PA: Lippincott Williams and Wilkins; 2007:765–776.

69. Van Hook FW, Demonbreun D, Weiss BD. Ambulatory devices for chronic gait disorders in the elderly. *Am F Physician*. 2003;67:1717–1724.

70. Schaie KW. The course of adult intellectual development. *Am Psychol*. 1994;49:301–313.

71. Wolfson L, et al. Training balance and strength in the elderly to improve function. *J Am Geriat Soc*. 1993;41:341–343.

72. Wolf S, Kutner N, Green R, McNeely E. Reducing frailty in elders: two exercise interventions at Emory University and Wesley Woods Geriatric Center. *J Am Geriat Soc*. 1993;41:329–332.

73. Wolfson L, et al. Balance and strength training in older adults: intervention gains and tai chi maintenance. *J Am Geriat Soc*. 1996;44:498–506.

74. Wolf S, et al. Reducing frailty and falls in older persons: an investigation of tai chi and computerized balance training. *J Am Geriat Soc*. 1996;44:489–497.

75. Cromes GF Jr. Implementation of interdisciplinary cancer rehabilitation. *Rehabil Counseling Bull*. 1978;21:230–237.

76. Van Weert E, Hoekstra-Weebers JEHM, Grol BMF, et al. Physical functioning and the quality of life after cancer rehabilitation. *Intern J Rehab Res*. 2004;27:27–35.

77. Santiago-Palma J, Payne R. Palliative care and rehabilitation. *Cancer*. 2001;94:1049–1052.

78. Hicks JE. Exercise for cancer patients. In: Basmajian JV, Wolf SL, eds. *Therapeutic Exercise*, 5th ed. Baltimore, MD: Williams and Wilkins; 1990:351–369.

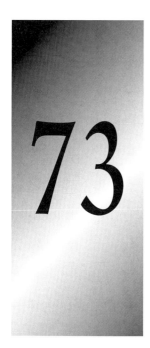

Cancer-Related Fatigue

Deborah Julie Franklin
Lora Packel

"It leaves you feeling knackered and shagged out—
and that's on a good day"

—*RJ, cancer survivor*

Cancer-related fatigue (CRF) is recognized as one of
the most prevalent symptoms experienced by oncology patients (1). A decade of research and discussion
has produced rational management protocols, but has
also revealed the need for ongoing efforts to improve
the efficacy of current treatment strategies. Fatigue is a
normal physiological response to exertion; it becomes
pathological when it occurs during routine activities,
persists for long periods, and does not respond to rest
(2,3). CRF is defined by the National Comprehensive
Cancer Network (NCCN) as a "distressing persistent,
subjective sense of tiredness or exhaustion related to
cancer or cancer treatment that is not proportional to
recent activity and interferes with usual functioning"
(4). CRF often leads to a reduction in daily activity
levels, which has further physical, psychological, social,
and economic impact on the well-being of the patient
and their family (5). Portenoy and Itri were among the
first to observe that in addition to diminished energy
and an increased need to rest, CRF is associated with
cognitive symptoms such as decreased concentration
and attention as well as perceived problems with
short-term memory. Decreased motivation or interest
in participating in usual activities may be coupled with
marked emotional reactivity (eg, sadness, frustration,
or irritability) to feeling fatigue. Insomnia as well as
hypersomnia are common and sleep is often experienced as un-refreshing or nonrestorative (6).

ASSESSMENT

Twenty years ago, fatigue was most commonly assessed
as one item contributing to an overall quality of life
or functional assessment score. More recently, specific
tools dedicated to the assessment of fatigue have been
introduced and validated. Maximum benefit is achieved
when patients are assessed regularly and consistently.
For this reason, the NCCN recommends screening
for the presence and severity of fatigue at the time of
diagnosis and at regular intervals—not just during
treatment, but as part of long-term follow-up care (7).
This approach allows early identification of CRF and
provides baseline data for evaluating the efficacy of
interventions.

Screening

CRF evaluation is best assessed using one of the objective, validated scales described below. Busy clinicians,
however, may need to resort to a mild/moderate/severe
designation using the 0–10 Likert-type scale. Patients
reporting fatigue intensity of 1–3 are considered as having mild CRF, 4–6 as moderate, and 7–10 as severe.

KEY POINTS

- Cancer-related fatigue (CRF) is one of the most common symptoms affecting oncology patients. Numerous studies in peer-reviewed journals consistently report prevalence rates between 60% and 90%.
- Fatigue is a normal physiological response to exertion, but becomes pathological when it occurs during routine activities, persists for long periods, and does not respond to rest.
- CRF is defined by the National Comprehensive Cancer Network (NCCN) as a "distressing persistent, subjective sense of tiredness or exhaustion related to cancer or cancer treatment that is not proportional to recent activity and interferes with usual functioning."
- The NCCN recommends screening for the presence and severity of fatigue at the time of diagnosis and at regular intervals, not just during treatment but as part of long-term follow-up care.
- The pathophysiology of CRF is remarkably complex. The profound question of whether CRF is a physiologically distinct mechanism or "a final common pathway to which many predisposing or etiologic factors contribute" continues to be addressed by basic scientists as well as clinical researchers.
- Clinical studies have identified a range of specific factors that are consistently associated with CRF, including pain, emotional distress, sleep disturbance, anemia, nutritional deficiencies, deconditioning, and comorbidities.
- Successful amelioration, if not elimination, of CRF often requires the coordinated collaboration of various clinicians to address the specific combination of etiologic factors affecting a specific patient. NCCN guidelines identify four categories of intervention: (1) education and counseling, (2) general strategies, (3) nonpharmacologic, and (4) pharmacologic.
- Mild to moderate aerobic as well as anaerobic exercise programs have been shown to ameliorate CRF in many oncology populations without evidence of adverse effects.

Patients with oncologic diagnoses who initially report no or mild fatigue should nonetheless receive education and counseling about CRF and will still require reevaluation at regular intervals. Objective information about the possibility of CRF during treatment helps prepare patients who might experience it, and prevents them from worrying that the appearance of this common symptom represents treatment failure or disease progression (8).

Measurement Tools

More than 10 instruments have been developed for the purpose of measuring fatigue; several of these were specifically designed for patients with cancer (Table 73.1). Panels of experts in CRF, however, have been unable to achieve a consensus in favor of one tool despite the recognition that this would greatly facilitate comparisons between studies (9). An additional issue with respect to measurement has been the construction of a case-definition basis that would create the ability to translate measurement results from any tool into a categoric identification of the presence or absence of clinically significant fatigue (10). In response to this need, David Cella and others have proposed criteria for identifying CRF based on a case definition or clinical syndrome approach (11) (Table 73.2). One impetus for promoting a standardized case definition approach has been to achieve inclusion of CRF in the International Classification of Diseases.

INCIDENCE, PREVALENCE, INTENSITY, AND DURATION

Significant obstacles have limited the collection of reliable epidemiological data describing the incidence and prevalence of CRF (Table 73.3). Despite these factors, stable patterns have emerged, with numerous studies in peer-reviewed journals consistently detecting prevalence rates between 60% and 90%. Efforts to correlate the occurrence of CRF with specific diagnoses, treatment protocols, and patient characteristics are reviewed below.

Most data has been collected on patients during or after treatment for cancer diagnoses, but Jacobsen's prospective study of 54 breast cancer patients and age-matched healthy controls showed statistically significant levels of fatigue in the cancer population prior to the initiation of chemotherapy (22). An earlier study by Irvine et al. did not detect increased levels of fatigue in patients prior to treatment when compared to healthy controls (23). Overall, the prevalence of CRF appears to be highest in patients undergoing active treatment and those with advanced disease, but levels over 30% have also been reported among disease-free survivors (24). Regardless of disease stage, CRF is known to persist after the completion of treatment. Even after applying the most rigorous definition of CRF, the Fatigue Coalition found that 37% of 379 survey participants who had completed cancer treatment between one and five years prior still reported at least a two-week period of fatigue during the preceding month (25). Comparable

TABLE 73.1
Select Fatigue Measurement Scales

SCALE (REF.)	DESCRIPTION
Profile of mood states (POMS) fatigue and vigor subscale (12)	Adjective checklist of 65 items scored with a 0–5 Likert-type scale shown to be a reliable measure of fatigue intensity but does not assess duration or impact on daily function
Functional assessment of cancer therapy-fatigue and anemia subscale (FACT-F) (13)	In addition to 27 questions that measure the physical, functional, emotional and social aspects of daily life, the fatigue subset includes 7 questions that address the need for sleep, feelings of tiredness and weakness as they relate to activity. Consistent test-retest scores suggest that the fatigue subscale can be used independently as a means of reducing the testing time and effort associated with the full FACT scale
Piper fatigue self-report scale (14)	42 self-reported items measure the temporal, sensory, and affective aspects of fatigue relying on a visual analog scale. Shown to correlate well with other objective measures but is cumbersome for patients to complete. Requirement that patients be presently experiencing fatigue precludes use as screening tool
Fatigue assessment instrument (15)	29 self reported items divided into categories: global fatigue severity (11 items), situation specificity (6 items), consequences of fatigue (3 items), responsiveness to rest/sleep (2 items) and 7 additional items using a 1–7 Likert type scale
Multidimensional fatigue inventory (MFI) (16)	20 items divided into five subscales assessing general fatigue, physical fatigue, mental fatigue, reduced motivation and reduced activity. Items include positively and negatively phrased questions so that some items require recoding. Five point Likert type scale is used with higher values indicating less fatigue
Fatigue symptom inventory (17)	Thirteen self-reported items designed to measure intensity and duration of fatigue and impact on quality of life
Brief fatigue inventory (18)	9 questions assess fatigue levels over the course of the last 24 h using a 10 point scale. It takes less than 10 min to administer and has been shown to correlate well with other more elaborate tools but is limited by the 24 h time frame and requires greater cross-cultural validation
Medical outcomes study 36-item short form health survey fatigue subscale (19)	The widely used SF-36 measures general quality of life including physical, emotional, and social-well-being. Four additional items are included in the fatigue subscale with the goal of assessing the impact of fatigue over the past week. Further validation studies are needed in the oncology population to show that the scale's sensitivity and statistical validity are maintained for this sub-group
EROTC fatigue subscale (20)	Three questions assessing symptom of fatigue over past week extracted from validated multidimensional quality of life instrument

TABLE 73.2
Proposed Diagnostic Criteria

Criterion A	2-wk period within preceding month during which significant fatigue or diminished energy was experienced each day, or almost every day, along with the experience of at least five of ten additional fatigue-related symptoms
Criterion B	the experience of fatigue results insignificant distress or impairment of functioning
Criterion C	clinical evidence suggesting that fatigue is a consequence of cancer or cancer therapy
Criterion D	Fatigue not be primarily a consequence of a concurrent psychiatric condition (eg, major depressive disorder)

Source: From Ref. 21.

TABLE 73.3
Barriers to Consistent Epidemiologic Data for Cancer-Related Fatigue

Subjective nature of cancer-related fatigue

Occurrence and recurrence at various stages of oncologic disease and treatment

Multiplicity of measurement tools

Changing pressures for under- and over-reporting
> Patient reluctance from fear of limiting treatment options
> Increased attention as pain and nausea have been better controlled

Synergistic association with other variables such as depression, anemia, and pain rates have been confirmed by other investigators studying CRF in specific populations. For example, 459 Swedish patients who had completed treatment for Hodgkin lymphoma reported 20% higher rate of fatigue than was found in the general population. Mean time since completion of treatment at the time of the study was 12 years (26).

PATHOPHYSIOLOGY

The pathophysiology of CRF is remarkably complex. The profound question of whether CRF is a physiologically distinct mechanism or "a final common pathway to which many predisposing or etiologic factors contribute" continues to be addressed by basic scientists as well as clinical researchers (27).

Exercise physiologists define physical fatigue as the reduction in force or muscle tension capacity with repeated stimulation. Factors that impair muscle function, including decreased oxygen delivery from anemia, loss of lung volume, or altered ventilation/perfusion ratios after chest irradiation, affect muscle fatigability. Skeletal muscle atrophy from bedrest, prostaglandin E production during inflammatory responses, and specific medications such as corticosteroids and cyclophosphamide, can compromise muscle performance. Disruption of the excitation-contraction (E-C) coupling response can result from exposure to ionizing radiation as well as to tumor necrosis factor (TNF) in patients with cancer (28). Increasing knowledge about the role of cytokines produced by low level activation of the immune system in cancer patients may provide greater understanding of CRF, as well as opportunities for biomodulation of this troubling symptom (29).

Other investigators, such as Smets et al., have investigated CRF within a broader psychosocial framework (30). Their hypothesis that fatigue is the result of a discrepancy between resources and demands was not supported in a study of patients undergoing radiation treatment. Resources were assessed based on physical condition, personality traits, social support, age, gender, and level of social support. Demands were related to prognosis, radiotherapy dose, and patients' perception of overall burden. Multidimensional Fatigue Inventory (MFI) scores correlated most closely with pretreatment physical condition. After treatment, physical condition and perceived burden were the most significant determinants. Demands did not add to the variance in fatigue explained by resources or vice versa.

CRF is frequently characterized as both a side effect of treatment and a biologic consequence of the actual oncologic process (31). Only one study, however has sought to determine the role of treatment versus disease. In one study, 127 patients with small cell lung cancer were assessed during the course of a randomized clinical trial comparing two chemotherapy regimens. Fatigue was the most common symptom throughout but, along with other symptoms, decreased over the course of the treatment. Results were interpreted as indicative of a high response to chemotherapy. Multivariate analysis attributed 43% of the variance in fatigue to disease alone and 35% to treatment toxicity (32).

Despite ongoing debates about the etiology of CRF, clinical studies have identified a range of specific factors that are consistently associated with CRF and are therefore postulated to precipitate it or intensify its impact. These associated factors include pain, emotional distress, sleep disturbance, anemia, nutritional deficiencies, deconditioning, and comorbidities (33). Consistent identification of a plurality of associated factors has supported the assumption that CRF is often multifactorial, but does not distinguish adequately between CRF occurring at different stages of disease and treatment where one or two etiologies may predominate. Clinicians adopting a multifactorial explanation of CRF must remember that only select etiologies will be meaningfully applicable to an individual patient at a given time. Identification of lead factors is essential for designing effective treatment strategies at each stage in the disease continuum.

Treatment-Associated Fatigue

CRF has been most frequently studied in populations undergoing active oncologic treatment such as chemotherapy or radiation. Jacobsen and colleagues used the Fatigue Scale from the Profile of Mood States (POMS-F) to compare fatigue in 54 women with stage I–III breast cancer prior to and during three cycles of chemotherapy with fatigue in age-matched controls (34). Prevalence began at 72% and increased to 94% during the third of four cycles of single or multidrug chemotherapy regimens consisting primarily of doxorubicin (Adriamycin) +/- cyclophosphamide (Cytoxan). Irvine reported a significant increase in fatigue in 47 patients 14 days after receiving chemotherapy for breast, lung, or ovarian cancer when compared to health controls (35). Estimated prevalence of CRF reached 58% in this group. Richardson's descriptive study of 109 patients receiving single or multi-regimen chemotherapy suggested that fatigue was greatest during the first four to five days following treatment and gradually improved until the nadir period around day 15, when increased fatigue was again observed (36). Eighty nine percent of patients documented fatigue at some point during treatment but variation was observed based on type of chemotherapy as well as disease site. Patients receiving weekly 5-fluorouracil as part of a single or multidrug regimen demonstrated the greatest fatigue.

CRF has also been associated with radiation treatment. A prospective study of 250 patients found that 46% reported being tired most of the time during their radiation treatment (37). Jerzek-Fossa and colleagues' review of the existing literature confirmed that fatigue is experienced by nearly 80% of patients during or shortly after a course of radiotherapy (38). Fatigue associated with radiation therapy has been found to increase during treatment reaching a plateau during the fourth week (approximately 17 fractionations) (39). Thirty percent of patients develop chronic fatigue after completing treatment (40,41). Fatigue is a common sequela of cranial irradiation and a major component of the somnolence syndrome that occurs frequently in patients following whole brain radiotherapy, particularly during the first months after treatment (42). In other groups, complications of radiotherapy, such as chronic dyspnea from pulmonary fibrosis, diarrhea from intestinal injury, or the effects of hormonal insufficiency, may contribute to the persistence of CRF long after completion of treatment.

Demographic Factors and Disease Specificity

Efforts are underway to correlate the occurrence of CRF with certain diagnoses, disease stages and other patient characteristics (43,44). Forlenza and colleagues made use of the extensive Swedish Twin Registry and the Swedish Cancer Registry to estimate the prevalence of CRF and its variability based on cancer site as well as gender (45). Fatigue was self-reported by respondents as prolonged, chronic (greater than six months), or chronic with impairment. Adjusted prevalence odds ratio (POR) for reporting all types of fatigue was 1.23 (95% CI 2.06–1.42) for persons listed in the cancer registry when compared to age, education, and gender-matched controls from the twin registry. Statistically significant associations were also detected for patients with lung cancer, prostate cancer, and cervical cancer. Patients with lung cancer had an adjusted POR of 3.21 for developing chronic fatigue and 3.71 for developing chronic fatigue with impairment. Men with prostate cancer had an adjusted POR of 2.24 for chronic fatigue and 2.57 for chronic fatigue with impairment. Women with cervical carcinoma had an adjusted POR of 1.22 for chronic fatigue and 1.27 for chronic fatigue with impairment. No significant associations occurred between chronic fatigue and malignant melanoma, colorectal, ovarian, or breast cancer. The latter findings were discussed by the authors, given the identification of fatigue in breast cancer patients in other studies. A plausible explanation may be based on the timing of fatigue in relation to both disease stage and treatment course. Thus, while women with breast cancer may experience fatigue during and for some time after treat-

ment, high rates of early detection and intervention with decreased progression to advanced disease may limit the prevalence of later fatigue in this population. Different treatment regimens may also account for the appearance of disease specific variation. Thus, while Irvine et al. found higher rates of fatigue in breast than in lung cancer patients receiving chemotherapy, Smets found greater fatigue in lung cancer rather than breast cancer patients following radiotherapy (46).

Forlenza's group and others have noted that linkage between gender and specific diagnoses, particularly breast, ovarian, and prostate, make it difficult to obtain statistically meaningful information about an independent relationship between gender and CRF (47). Nonetheless, at least two studies have detected increased levels of CRF in women when compared to men. Nine months after completion of radiotherapy, Smets and colleagues attributed a 5% variance in fatigue rates to gender with women reporting greater fatigue than men (48). The Fatigue Coalition's telephone survey of 419 patients who had completed radiation or chemotherapy also found that women reported more fatigue than men (49).

Most studies have shown that CRF is largely independent of age (50). Although medical co-morbidities are associated with increased CRF and occur more frequently in older populations, younger patients generally demonstrate higher rates of CRF when discrepancies are detected (51,52). This may reflect the choice, particularly in the past, of less aggressive treatment protocols for older persons. Others have suggested that younger patients are more likely to try to return to work and have greater family responsibilities, both of which may make fatigue a more burdensome symptom (53). Fatigue and resulting deconditioning from decreased activity, however, are of additional importance in older persons as they can increase fall risk (54). Almost no attention has been given to the prevalence and impact of fatigue in pediatric populations with cancer diagnoses.

Specific Comorbid Factors

Given and colleagues did find a correlation between the number of comorbidities and the prevalence of CRF in 841 patients older than aged 65 with newly diagnosed breast, prostate, lung, or colon cancer who were followed for one year (55). Other researchers have focused on specific comorbidities, as summarized below.

Anemia

Anemia occurs in over 50% of cancer patients and represents a significant reversible cause of fatigue (56). It may be the direct result of disease processes through blood loss, bone marrow infiltration, or hemolysis, but can also be a side effect of chemotherapy or radiation treatment. Platinum-derived drugs effect erythropoietin production due to renal toxicity, while other regimens may cause transient or prolonged anemia through stem cell damage, myelodysplasia, microangiopathic mechanisms, and immune-mediated cell destruction (57). In a validation study of the Functional Assessment of Cancer Therapy-Anemia (FACT-An) Scale involving 50 patients with a range of oncologic diagnoses, Cella found statistically significant difference in fatigue between patients with hemoglobin levels less than 12 g/dl and those with hemoglobin levels greater than 12 g/dl (58).

Electrolyte Imbalances and Nutritional Parameters

The NCCN recommends that patients with CRF should undergo a nutritional evaluation to assess changes in weight, barriers to adequate nutrition, and to address fluid and electrolyte imbalances. The syndrome of inappropriate antidiuretic hormone (SIADH), hypercalcemia, or hypophosphatemia can occur in specific sub-populations of patients treated for cancer, and may contribute to fatigue and reduced functional performance. Side effects of cancer and its treatment including mucositis, anorexia, nausea, diarrhea, and constipation may severely influence food and fluid intake. Dehydration is a well-known component of fatigue. A certain percentage of patients will develop cancer cachexia, comprehensively described elsewhere. Gutstein and others have hypothesized that energy imbalance, including deficient nutritional substrate or cytokine-induced metabolic derangement, may contribute to fatigue (59). Wang and colleagues were able to demonstrate a significant relationship between low albumin levels and CRF in patients being treated for leukemia and non-Hodgkin lymphoma (60). Other clinical studies, however, have been unable to correlate fatigue with weight loss or nutritional markers such as prealbumin (61,62). Nor have low albumin levels been shown to hinder functional gains during a comprehensive inpatient rehabilitation program (63).

Endocrine

The effect of cancer and its treatment on the hypothalamic-pituitary-adrenal axis as well as the endocrine perturbations associated with interferon (IFNα) and other treatments warrant laboratory evaluation in select patients. IFN-α can cause hypothyroidism, and possibly adrenal suppression (64). Whole-body radiation may lower testosterone levels, although no association was found between fatigue and mild Leydig cell dysfunction in survivors of hematologic malignancies (65).

Sleep Disruption

Savard and colleagues studied 300 Canadian women with mostly stage I and II breast cancer (66). Time since diagnosis ranged from two months to 30 years, with nearly half (48%) reporting impaired sleep and 28% using sleep medication. Expected prevalence of sleep disruption in the general population was between 9% and 12%. Thirty-three percent of patients with sleep difficulties reported onset at the time of diagnosis. A subset reported aggravation of existing sleep difficulties. The impact of cancer and its treatment on sleep has been attributed to numerous factors including anxiety, vasomotor symptoms associated with hormonal manipulation from tamoxifen or orchiectomy, and poor pain control. The intuitive relationship between sleep disruption and CRF was confirmed by a second Canadian study of 982 patients with median time since diagnosis of 34 months. Patients with insomnia were 2.5 times more likely to experience fatigue (67). Lee et al. reviewed the literature on impaired sleep in cancer patients and provide extensive disease specific information on this subject (68).

Pain

Although chronic pain is recognized as causing fatigue in patients with non-oncologic diagnoses, surprisingly little has been published about the relationship between pain and fatigue in cancer patients. One study of 368 adult oncology outpatients demonstrated a statistically significant correlation between pain intensity and fatigue using the POMS fatigue subscale (69). Pain-related sleep disruption as well as sedation from poorly selected analgesic regimens are other ways in which pain probably plays a significant but poorly described role in CRF.

Depression

A strong association between depression and fatigue has been documented in all disease stages. A prospective study of 104 patients receiving either chemotherapy or radiotherapy and 53 healthy controls found that the best predictors of fatigue were symptom distress and mood disturbance (70). Bower and colleagues' study of 1,957 disease-free survivors of stage 0, I, or II breast cancer found that depression and then pain were the best predictors of fatigue one to five years after completion of treatment (71). A study of 64 patients with advanced breast cancer also detected a significant correlation between depression and asthenia (defined as a combination of physical and mental fatigue) but none for nutritional status, anemia, or type of treatment (72). Tchekmedyian et al. showed that reduced fatigue in anemic lung cancer patients treated with dar-bepoetin alpha was associated with decreased anxiety and depression (73). The strong association between depression and CRF warrants further exploration, as it may be that a sense of fatigue is a symptom of depression. Dimeo, for instance, showed a high correlation between fatigue, depression, somatization, and anxiety in 78 cancer patients, but none between fatigue and maximal physical exertion (74). The same study, however, showed that poor physical performance, a possible result of fatigue, was an independent predictor of emotional distress, suggesting that while depression may contribute to fatigue, CRF and resulting impairment in physical performance may also precipitate depression.

COMPREHENSIVE EVALUATION AND TREATMENT

Once the presence of CRF has been established, a thorough search for contributing factors is a necessary prerequisite to designing an effective treatment plan. Reversible factors such as anemia, electrolyte imbalances, and endocrine dysfunction may be addressed by the treating oncologist, but it may fall to the physiatrist to point out the functional impact of borderline hemoglobin levels or hypercalcemia.

Interventions

Successful amelioration if not elimination of CRF often requires the coordinated collaboration of various clinicians to address the specific combination of etiologic factors affecting a specific patient. The National Comprehensive Cancer Network Guidelines identify four categories of intervention: (1) education and counseling, (2) general strategies, (3) nonpharmacologic, and (4) pharmacologic (75). Recognizing that CRF affects patients throughout the cancer continuum, the organization provides guidelines for three types of patients: patients on active treatment, patients on long-term follow-up, and patients at end of life (76).

Education

General education about the nature and management of CRF provides reassurance and leads to earlier recognition and mitigation of its effects. Concern that CRF reflects disease progression or treatment failure should be allayed. Simple techniques for self-monitoring of fatigue level help patients and clinicians work together to formulate appropriate programs as needed. Patient handouts, presentations to support groups, and discussion during office visits or treatment administrations are effective opportunities for providing needed educational information.

General Strategies

General strategies as opposed to cause-specific interventions are intended to minimize the impact and intensity of existing CRF after reversible causes have been addressed. Energy conservation strategies developed by rehabilitation professionals for pulmonary, cardiac, or otherwise debilitated patients are equally effective for patients with CRF (77). In an inpatient rehabilitation setting, these will be routinely addressed by physical and occupational therapists, but they should be integrated into the rehabilitation prescription for patients referred to outpatient facilities as well. The NCCN also recommends attention restoring therapy as a general strategy for CRF in all phases of the disease continuum. The efficacy of this intervention is predicated on the importance of attentional fatigue in CRF, defined as a decreased capacity to concentrate or direct attention.

The role of distracting activities such as games, music, and social interaction has been descriptively documented but remains poorly understood (78). The efficacy of distracting strategies may reflect the contribution of psychological factors such as anxiety and depression in an individual cancer patient's experience of CRF. One study identified increased CRF in women who relied on catastrophizing as a coping strategy (79). Such results should not incline practitioners to dismiss CRF as "all in the head," but rather promote the use of psychological interventions, including the introduction of adaptive coping strategies for patients with CRF who achieve significant scores on scales measuring emotional or psychological distress (80).

Nonpharmacologic Interventions

The NCCN's nonpharmacologic guidelines combine activity enhancement strategies including strengthening and endurance programs, psychosocial interventions, nutritional management, and sleep optimization. The effect of exercise and guidelines for exercise interventions for CRF are discussed separately.

The NCCN's recommendations for psychosocial interventions for CRF include stress management, relaxation, and support groups (81). Various complementary therapies, including acupuncture, yoga, massage therapy, and mindfulness-based stress reduction, effect CRF by combining physical and psychosocial modalities (82–84).

Nutritional assessment and ensuing interventions can mitigate CRF by reducing dehydration, energy imbalances and electrolyte disturbances. CRF patients with B12 deficiencies are among those who may benefit from vitamin or mineral repletion. Carnitine deficiency and supplementation with levocarnitine have been studied as means of addressing fatigue in patients receiving cisplatin or ifosfamide chemotherapy (85). Nutritionists as well as integrative medicine programs affiliated with cancer centers can be valuable resources for many persons with CRF.

The prevalence of disrupted sleep among persons with cancer diagnoses makes it one of the most common and intuitively obvious factors in CRF (86). Numerous cognitive and behavioral strategies exist for promoting restorative nighttime sleep and minimizing daytime sleepiness (87). Addressing underlying anxiety and depression often improves sleep, as does increasing physical activity. Sleep can also be addressed with judicious use of pharmacologic agents.

Pharmacologic Interventions

Anemia: Blood transfusions may be useful for more rapid correction of profound anemia, particularly in an inpatient rehabilitation setting following tumor resection or stem cell transplantation. Several large scale studies demonstrated the utility of erythropoietin for both increasing hemoglobin and reducing fatigue scores in patients with anemia associated with chemotherapy (88). However, the use of erythropoietin in cancer patients is being reassessed in light of recent data concerning increased risk of thrombotic events in dialysis patients receiving erythropoietin (89). Moreover, some studies have actually shown a decreased survival rate in cancer patients treated with erythropoietin that was not associated with thrombotic events (90). Current consensus appears to suggest that target hemoglobin levels of 12 g/dL can confer symptomatic benefit without increasing risk (91).

In addition to medical management of factors contributing to CRF, physicians may use a range of prescription medications to treat CRF directly. Psychostimulants such as methylphenidate (Ritalin) and modafinil (Provigil) have been used to treat CRF, but their efficacy has not been definitively established (92). Hanna et al. studied 37 disease-free patients with a history of breast cancer and moderate to severe fatigue, as measured with the BFI (93). Methylphenidate was started at 5 mg in the morning and at noon and increased to 10 mg during the second week if BFI remained greater than four. Fifty-four percent of patients responded with decreased scores of two points or greater, for an average decrement of 3.5 points. Bruera and colleagues did not find a difference when methylphenidate was compared to placebo during a shorter, one-week study (94). Corticosteroids have also been used to address symptoms including fatigue in patients with advanced cancer (95).

Physical Therapy Interventions for CRF

Numerous studies have explored the safety and efficacy of exercise interventions for patients with CRF (96–110). Meta-analyses have identified the greatest statistically significant impact in studies limited to a specific disease population such as breast cancer with less effect demonstrated when patients with heterogeneous diagnoses were recruited (111). Even when exercise interventions do not directly reduce fatigue scores, they nonetheless play an important role in the management of CRF by stemming the decline in functional performance that occurs as patients with CRF reduce their activity levels, often precipitating a cycle of deconditioning.

Mock and colleagues found that 23 women undergoing radiation treatment for breast cancer who maintained an individualized, self-paced, home-based walking exercise program experienced decreased CRF as well as improved sleep, a presumed etiological factor in CRF (112). Anna Schwartz and colleagues' study of 61 women with histologically documented breast cancer receiving adjuvant chemotherapy showed decreased rates of CRF among those who participated in an eight-week, home-based exercise program (113). Thirty-four oncology patients (stage I–IV) who had completed treatment at least three months prior to participating in a multimodal rehabilitation program including biweekly bicycle ergometry and resistance training, reported statistically significant reductions on the general fatigue, physical fatigue, and reduced motivation domains of the Multi-Fatigue index (114).

Once a patient has been screened by a physician for participation in a moderate intensity exercise program, they should be referred for an individualized program with ongoing monitoring, preferably by a physical therapist specializing in cancer rehabilitation. The recommendations below are based on a review of the literature, but it must be noted that the vast majority of studies were in the breast cancer population and excluded those with metastatic disease.

The physical therapy assessment should include a fatigue measure that is tracked over the course of the exercise program. Cancer history, including treatments, evidence of metastatic disease, comorbidities, medications, and recent laboratory and radiology findings should be recorded.

The aerobic component of the prescribed exercise program should designate frequency, intensity, duration, and mode. Most studies demonstrating efficacy have utilized a frequency of three to seven times per week. Breast cancer patients in Schwartz's study of a low to moderate home-based exercise program during three cycles of chemotherapy experienced decreased CRF symptoms on exercise days when compared to non-exercise days, suggesting a possible benefit from daily rather than every-other-day exercise patterns at this level of intensity (115).

The vast majority of studies prescribed moderate intensity aerobic exercise in the range of 65%–85% HR_{max} or 40%–60% of heart rate reserve (HRR). The recommendations for moderate intensity exercise from the American College of Sports Medicine are 64%–94% of HR_{max} or 40%–85% of HRR (116). The ACSM, however, does not presently have guidelines for patients undergoing cancer treatment or for cancer survivors. Mild to moderate intensity programs are advisable until more studies are published demonstrating safe and efficacious use of higher exercise intensities. The duration of aerobic training varied from 20 to 40 minutes. Dimeo et al. employed interval training when studying patients during and after bone marrow transplantation. In one study, subjects used a bed ergometer for a total of 30 minutes daily. The subjects biked at approximately 50% of the HRR for 15 one-minute intervals separated by a one-minute rest period. When compared to controls, the exercise group's fatigue reached a plateau, whereas the control group had greater increases in fatigue (117). Interval training as opposed to steady state protocols should be considered for patients undergoing intensive medical treatment, those who are significantly deconditioned, or those whose comorbidities led to reductions in physical capacity prior to their diagnosis of cancer.

In general, walking has been the most frequently used mode of exercise in studies assessing the effect of physical therapy interventions on CRF, although a recent study focused on high intensity training utilizing cycle ergometry (118). Published studies include a heterogenous mixture of home programs, as well as supervised exercise in a group setting. The group programs reported low drop-out rates and high levels of support among group exercisers, although this was not always monitored in an objective fashion. None of the studies reviewed reported any serious adverse events related to the prescribed exercise program.

Strength training has not been as well studied in oncology populations as aerobic exercise. Nonetheless, a randomized prospective study of 155 men with prostate cancer receiving androgen deprivation therapy demonstrated significant reduction in fatigue as measured with the FACT-F scale after participating in 12-week resistance exercise program (119). The thrice weekly supervised program include two sets of 8 to 12 repetitions of nine exercises performed at 60%–70% of one-repetition maximum. Resistance was increased by five lbs when 12 repetitions could be comfortably completed. Fatigue improved in patients who were being treated with curative as well as palliative intent.

Another recent study by Andersen et al. utilized high-intensity physical training as part of a multifaceted exercise program in a heterogeneous population undergoing chemotherapy (120). Subjects trained with five to eight repetitions at 85%–95% of a one-repetition maximum three times per week. The outcomes measured were fatigue, pain, appetite, constipation, myalgia, arthralgia, diarrhea, and an overall symptoms/side-effect score. The overall side-effect score significantly decreased over the course of the six-week study. Fatigue, defined as treatment-related fatigue, physical fatigue, and mental fatigue, showed a downward trend that fell short of statistical significance. No adverse events were reported for this high intensity strength training program, but it should be noted that patients with bone metastases were excluded from the study.

In fact, very few studies have included patients with late-stage disease or bone metastases. One study utilized a moderate intensity seated exercise intervention for women with stage IV breast cancer (121). In this quasi-experimental study, subjects watched a video and performed a seated exercise program three days per week. Fatigue and physical function scores were compared to a non-exercising control group. Over the course of four chemotherapy cycles, both groups demonstrated increased fatigue and decreased physical function. However, the intervention group declined at a slower rate than the control group. This study indicates that tailored moderate-intensity exercise can be tolerated by patients with advanced breast cancer and may help to diminish cancer-related fatigue in this population. However, larger more rigorous studies are needed before definitive recommendations are made.

Overall, moderate intensity aerobic exercise can help ameliorate CRF during and after treatment and minimize its effect on overall function and quality of life. Strength training is beginning to show positive effects as well for fatigue management although there are fewer studies supporting its role. Exercise interventions should be prescribed by clinicians who are have experience with oncologic patients and are familiar with relevant precautions and contraindications. Exercise studies targeting CRF in populations with comorbidities as well as metastatic disease are direly needed to elucidate the role of exercise interventions for these patients.

CONCLUSIONS

Effective management of CRF requires a holistic approach that is best achieved through an integrated, interdisciplinary team including physicians, oncology nurses, physical, occupational, and speech language therapists, nutritionists, and psychologists. The University of Texas M.D. Anderson Cancer Center pioneered a dedicated fatigue clinic and demonstrated high rates of patient satisfaction as well as some clinical improvement (122). Less formal CRF programs have been trialed elsewhere and are easily integrated into physiatric practices with well established access to interdisciplinary team members with oncologic experience. Additional research exploring the relative importance of specific etiologic factors in different oncologic populations will improve our ability to design maximally effective programs for individual patients.

References

1. Vogelzang NJ, Breitbart W, Cella D, et al. Patient, caregiver, and oncologist perceptions of cancer-related fatigue: results of a tripart assessment survey. *Semin Hematol.* 1997;34/S3:4–12.
2. Dimeo FC. Effects of exercise on cancer-related fatigue. *Cancer.* 2001;92:1689–1693.
3. Fukuda K, Straus SE, Hickie I, Sharpe MC, Dobbins JG, Komaroff A. The chronic fatigue syndrome: a comprehensive approach to its definition and study. *Ann Inten Med.* 1994;121:953–959.
4. National Comprehensive Cancer Network Practice Guidelines in Oncology: Cancer Related Fatigue 2007 Version 2: FT-1. Available at www.nccn.org.
5. Meyerowitz BE, Sparks FC, Spears IK. Adjuvant chemotherapy for breast carcinoma. *Cancer.* 1979;43:1613–1618.
6. Portenoy RK, Itri LM. Cancer-related fatigue: guidelines for evaluation and management. *Oncologist.* 1999;4:1–10.
7. National Comprehensive Cancer Network Practice Guidelines in Oncology: Cancer Related Fatigue 2007 Version 2: FT-1. Available at www.nccn.org.
8. Mock V. Fatigue management: evidence and guidelines for practice. *Cancer.* 2001;92:1699–1707.
9. Rieger PT. Assessment and epidemiologic issues related to fatigue. *Cancer.* 2001;92:1733–1736.
10. Andrykowski MA, Schmidt JE, Salsman JM, Beacham AO, Jacobsen PB. Use of a case definition approach to identify cancer-related fatigue in women undergoing adjuvant therapy for breast cancer. *J Clin Oncol.* 2005;23:6613–6622.
11. Cella D, Davis K, Breitbart W, Curt G. for the Fatigue Coalition. Cancer-related fatigue: prevalence of proposed diagnostic criteria in a United States sample of cancer survivors. *J Clin Oncol.* 2001;19:3385–3391.
12. McNair DM, Lorr M, Droppleman L. *Profile of Mood States,* 2nd ed. San Diego CA: Educational and Industrial Testing Service; 1992.
13. Yellen SB, Cella DF, Webster K, Blendowski C, Kaplan E. Measuring fatigue and other anemia-related symptoms with the Functional Assessment of Cancer Therapy (FACT) measurement system. *J Pain Symptom Manage.* 1997;13:63–74.
14. Piper BF, Dibble SL, Dodd MJ, Weiss MC. Slaughter RE, Paul SM. The revised Piper Fatigue Scale: psychometric evaluation in women with breast cancer. *Oncol Nurs Forum.* 1998;25:677–684.
15. Schwartz JE, Jandorf L, Krupp LB. The measurement of fatigue: a new instrument. *J Psychosom Res.* 1993;37:753–762.
16. Smets EM, Garssen B, Broke B, de Haes JC. The Multidimensional Fatigue Inventory (MFI): psychometric qualities of an instrument to assess fatigue. *J Psychosomatic Res.* 1995;39:315–325.
17. Hann, DM, Jabocbsen PB, Azzarello LM, et al. Measurement of fatigue in cancer patients: development and validation of the Fatigue Symptom Inventory. *Qual Life Res.* 1998;7:301–310.
18. Mendoza T, Wang XS, Cleeland CS, et al. The rapid assessment of fatigue severity in cancer patients. *Cancer.* 1999;85:1186–1196.
19. Ware JE, Sherbourne CD. The MOS 36 item sort-form health survery (SF-36). I. Conceptual framework and item selection. *Med Care.* 1992;30:473–483.
20. Pater JL, Zee B, Palmer M, Johnston D, Osoba D. Fatigue in patients with cancer: results with National Cancer Institute of Canada Clinical Trials Group Studies employing the EORTC QLC-C30. *Support Care Cancer.* 1997;5:410–413.
21. Cella D, Davis K, Breitbart W, Curt G for the Fatigue Coalition. Cancer-related fatigue: prevalence of proposed diagnostic criteria in a United States sample of cancer survivors. *J Clin Oncol.* 2001;19:3385–3391.
22. Jacobsen PB, Hann DM, Azzarello LM, Horton J, Balducci L, Lyman GH. Fatigue in women receiving adjuvant chemotherapy for breast cancer: characteristics, course, and correlates. *J Pain Symptom Manage.* 1999;18:233–242.
23. Irvine D, Vincent L, Graydon JE, Bubela N, Thompson L. The prevalence and correlates of fatigue in patients receiving treatment with chemotherapy and radiotherapy: a comparison with the fatigue experienced by healthy individuals. *Cancer Nurs.* 1994;17:367–378.
24. Bower JE, Ganz PA, Desmond KA, Rowland JH, Meyerowitz BE, Belin TR. Fatigue in breast cancer survivors: occurrence, correlates, and impact. *J Clin Oncol.* 2000;18:743–753.
25. Cella D, Kavis K, Breitbart W, Curt G for the Fatigue Coalition. Cancer-related fatige: prevalence of proposed diagnostic criteria in a United States sample of cancer survivors. *J Clin Oncol.* 2001;19:3385–3391.
26. Loge JH, Abrahamsen AF, Ekeberg O, Kaasa S. Hodgkin's disease survivors more fatigued than the general population. *J Clin Ocol.* 1999;17:253–261.
27. For the former view see Gutman HB. The biologic basis of fatigue. *Cancer.* 2001;92:1678–1683 for the latter Portenoy RK, Itri LM, Cancer-related fatigue: guidelines for evaluation and management. *Oncologist.* 1999;4:1–10.
28. Lucia A, Earnest C, Pérez M. Cancer-related fatigue: can exercise physiology assist oncologists? *Lancet Oncol.* 2003;4:616–625.
29. Marty M, Bedairia N, Laurence V, Espie M, Cottu P-H. Factors related to fatigue in cancer patients: the key to specific therapeutic approaches. In Marty M, Pecorelli S, eds. *Fatigue and Cancer.* New York: Elsevier Science; 2001:33–44.
30. Smets EMA, Visser MRM, Garssen B, Frijda NH, Ousterveld P, de Haes JCJM. Understanding the level of fatigue in cancer patients undergoing radiotherapy. *J Psychosom Res.* 1998;45:277–293.
31. Lawrence DP, Kupelnick B, Miller K, Devine D, Lau J. Evidence report on the occurrence, assessment, and treatment of fatigue in cancer patients. *J Natl Cancer Inst Monogr.* 2004;32:40–50.
32. Hurny C, Bernhard J, Joss R, et al. "Fatigue and malaise" as a quality-of-life indicator in small-cell lung cancer patients. *Support Care Cancer.* 1993;1:316–320.
33. NCCN Clinical Practice Guidelines in Oncology: Cancer-Related Fatigue. v.2.2007:FT-5-7. www.ncn.org.
34. Jacobsen PB, Hann DM, Azarello LM, Horton J, Balducci Ludovico, Lyman GH. Fatigue in women receiving adjuvant chemotherapy for breast cancer characteristics, course, and correlates. *J Pain Symptom Manage.* 1999;18:233–242.
35. Irvine D, Vincent L, Graydon, JE, Bubela N, Thompson L. The prevalence and correlates of fatigue in patients receiving treatment with chemotherapy and radiotherapy: a comparison with the fatigue experienced by healthy individuals. *Cancer Nurs.* 1994;17:367–378.
36. Richardson A, Ream E, Wilson-Barnett J. Fatigue in patients receiving chemotherapy: patterns of change. *Cancer Nurs.* 1998;21:17–30.
37. Smets EM, Visser MR, Willems-Groot AF, et al. Fatigue and radiotherapy: (A)Experience in patients undergoing treatment. *Br J Cancer* 1998;78:899–906.
38. Jereczek-Fossa BA, et al. Radiotherapy-related fatigue. *Crit Rev Oncol Hematol.* 2002;41:317–325.

39. Greenberg DB, Sawicka J, Eisenthal S, Ross D. Fatigue syndrome due to localized radiation. *J Pain Symptom Manage.* 1992;7:38–45.

40. Smets EM, Visser MR, Willems-Groot AF, et al. Fatigue and radiotherapy: (B)experience in patients 9 months following treatment. *Br J Cancer.* 1998;78:907–912.

41. Hickok JT, Morrow GR, McDonald S, Bellg AJ. Frequency and correlates of fatigue in lung cancer patients receiving radiation therapy: implications for management. *J Pain Symptom Manage.* 1996;11:370–377.

42. Faithful S, Brada M. Somnolence syndrome in adults following cranial irradiation for primary brain tumours. *Clin Oncol.* 1998;10:250–254.

43. Wang XS, Janjan NA, Guo H, et al. Fatigue during preoperative chemoradiation for resectable rectal cancer. *Cancer.* 2002;92:1725–1732.

44. Forlenza MJ, Hall P, Lichentenstein P, Evengard B, Sullivan PF. Epidemiology of cancer-related fatigue in the Swedish twin registry. *Cancer.* 2005;104:2022–2031.

45. Fordenza MJ, Hall P, Lichtenstein P, Evengard B, Sullivan PF. Epidemiology of cancer-related fatigue in the Swedish twin registry. *Cancer.* 2005;104:2022–2031.

46. Irvine D, Vincent L, Graydon, JE, Bubela N, Thompson L. The prevalence and correlates of fatigue in patients receiving treatment with chemotherapy and radiotherapy: a comparison with the fatigue experienced by healthy individuals. *Cancer Nurs.* 1994;17:367–78; Smets EM, Visser MR, Willems-Groot AF, et al. Fatigue and radiotherapy: (A)experience in patients undergoing treatment. *Br J Cancer.* 1998;78:899–906.

47. Pater JL, Zee B, Palmer M, Johnston D, Osoba D. Fatigue in patients with cancer: results with National Cancer Institute of Canada Clinical Trials Group studies employing the EORTC QLQ-C30. *Support Care Cancer.* 1997;5:410–413.

48. Smets EMA, Visser MRM, Willems-Groot AFMN, Garssen B, Schuster-Uitterhoeve ALJ, de Haes JCJM. Fatigue and radiotherapy: (B)experience in patients 9 months following treatment. *Br J Cancer.* 1998;78:907–912.

49. Vogelzang NJ, Breitbart W, Cella D, et al. Patient, caregiver, and oncologist perceptions of cancer-related fatigue: results of a tripart assessment survey. *Semin Hematol.* 1997;34/S3:4–12.

50. Patarca-Montero R. *Handbook of Cancer-Related Fatigue.* New York: Haworth Medical Press; 2004:25–29.

51. Vogelzang NJ, Breitbart W, Cella D, et al. Patient, caregiver, and oncologist perceptions of cancer-related fatigue: results of a tripart assessment survey. *Semin Hematol.* 1997;34/S3:4–12.

52. Bower JE, Ganz PA, Desmond KA, Rowland JH, Meyerowitz BE, Belin TR. Fatigue in breast cancer survivors: occurrence, correlates, and impact on quality of life. *J Clin Oncol.* 2000;18:743–753.

53. Woo B, Dibble SL, Piper BF, Keating SB, Weiss MC. Differences in fatigue by treatment methods in women with breast cancer. *Oncol Nurs Forum.* 1998;25:915–920.

54. Holley S. A look at the problem of falls among people with cancer. *Clin J Oncol Nurs.* 2002;6:193.

55. Given CW, Given B, Azzouz F, Kozachik S, Stommel M. Predictors of pain and fatigue in the year following diagnosis for elderly cancer patients. *J Pain Symptom Manage.* 2001;26:456–466.

56. Mercadante S, Gebbia V, Marrazzo A, Filosto S. Anaemia in cancer: pathophysiology and treatment. *Cancer Treat Rev.* 2000;26:303–311.

57. Bron D. Biological basis of cancer-related anaemia. In: Marty M, Pecorelli S, eds. *Fatigue and Cancer.* New York: Elsevier Science; 2001:45–50.

58. Cella D. The Functional Assessment of Cancer Therapy-Anemia (FACT-An) scale: a new tool for the assessment of outcomes in cancer anemia and fatigue. *Semin Hematol.* 1997;34:13–19.

59. Gutstein HB. The biologic basis of fatigue. *Cancer.* 2001;92:1678–1683.

60. Wang XS, Giralt SA, Mendoza TR, et al. Clinical factors associated with cancer related fatigue in patients being treated for leukemia and non-Hodgkin's lymphoma. *J Clin Oncol.* 2002;20:1319–1328.

61. Lawrence DP, Kupelnick B, Miller K, Devine D, Lau J. Evidence report on the occurrence, assessment, and treatment of fatigue in cancer patients. *J Natl Cancer Inst Monogr.* 2004;32:40–50.

62. Bruera E, Brenneis C, Michaud M, et al. Association between asthenia and nutritional status, lean body mass, anemia, psychological status, and tumor mass in patients with advanced breast cancer. *J Pain Symptom Manage.* 1989;4:59–63.

63. Guo Y, Palmer JL, Kaur Guddi, Hainley S, Young B, Bruera E. Nutritional status of cancer patients and its relationship to function in an inpatient rehabilitation setting. *Support Care Cancer.* 2005;13:169–175.

64. Malik UR, Makower DF, Wadler S. Interferon-mediated fatigue. *Cancer.* 2001;92:1664–1668.

65. Howell SJ, Radford JA, Smets EMA, Shalet SM. Fatigue, sexual function and mood following treatment for haematological malignancy: the impact of mild leydig cell dysfunction. *Br J Cancer.* 2000;82:789–793.

66. Savard J, Morin CM. Insomnia in the context of cancer: a review of a neglected problem. *J Clin Oncol.* 2001;19:895–908.

67. Davidson JR, Maclean AW, Brundage MD, Schulze K. Sleep disturbance in cancer patients. *Soc Sci Med.* 2002;54:1309–1321.

68. Lee K, Cho M, Miaskowski C, Dodd M. Impaired sleep and rhythms in persons with cancer. *Sleep Med Rev.* 2004;8:199–212.

69. Glover J, Dibble SL, Dodd MJ, Miaskowski C. Mood states of oncology outpatients: Does pain make a difference? *J Pain Symptom Manage.* 1995;10:120–128.

70. Irvine D, Vincent L, Graydon, JE, Bubela N, Thompson L. The prevalence and correlates of fatigue in patients receiving treatment with chemotherapy and radiotherapy: a comparison with the fatigue experienced by healthy individuals. *Cancer Nurs.* 1994;17:367–378.

71. Bower JE, Ganz PA, Desmond KA, Rowland JH, Meyerowitz BE, Belin TR. Fatigue in breast cancer survivors: occurrence, correlates, and impact on quality of life. *J Clin Oncol.* 2000;18:743–753.

72. Bruera E. Association between asthenia and nutritional status, lean body mass, anemia, psychological status and tumor mass in patients with advanced breast cancer. *J Pain Symptom Manage.* 1989;4:59.

73. Tcheckmedyian NS, Kallich J, McDermott A, Fayers P, Erder MH. The relationship between psychlogic distress and cancer-related fatigue. *Cancer.* 2003;98:198–203.

74. Dimeo F, Stieglitz RD, Novelli-Fischer U, Fetscher S, Metelsmann R, Keul J. Correlation between physical performance and fatigue in cancer patients. *Ann Oncol.* 1997;8:1251–1255.

75. NCCN Clinical Practice Guidelines in Oncology: Cancer-Related Fatigue. v.2.2007:FT-5-7. www.ncn.org.

76. NCCN Clinical Practice Guidelines in Oncology: Cancer-Related Fatigue. v.2.2007:FT-5-7. www.ncn.org .

77. Barsevick AM, Dudley W, Beck S, Sweeney C, Whitmer K, Nail L. A randomized clinical trial of energy conservation for patients with cancer-related fatigue. *Cancer.* 2004;100:1302–1310.

78. Graydon JE, Bubela N, Irvine D, et al. Fatigue-reducing strategies used by patients receiving treatment for cancer. *Cancer Nurs.* 1995;18:23–28,43.

79. Broekel JA, Jacobsen PB, Horton J, et al. Characteristics and correlates of fatigue after adjuvant chemotherapy for breast cancer. *J Clin Oncol.* 1998;16:1689–1696.

80. Jacobsen PB, Danette MH, Azzarello LM, Horton J, Balducci L, Lyman GH. Fatigue in women receiving adjuvant chemotherapy for breast cancer: characteristics, course, and correlates. *J Pain Symptom Manage.* 1999;18:233–242.

81. Jacobsen PB, Meade CK, Stein KD, Chirikos TN, Small BJ, Ruckdenschel JC. Efficacy and costs of two forms of stress management training for cancer patients undergoing chemotherapy. *J Clin Oncol.* 2002;20:2851–2862.

82. Cohen L, Warneke C, Fouladi RT, et al. Psychological adjustment and sleep quality in a randomized trial of the effects of a Tibetan yoga intervention in patients with lymphoma. *Cancer.* 2004;100:2253–2260.

83. Cassileth BR, Vickers AJ. Massage therapy for symptom control: outcome study at a major cancer center. *J Pain Symptom Manage.* 2004;2:332–344.
84. Vickers AJ, Strauss DJ, Fearon B, Cassileth BR. Acupuncture for postchemotherapy fatigue: a phase II study. *J Clin Oncol.* 2004;22:1731–1735.
85. Graziano F, Bisonni R, Catalano V, et al. Potential role of levocarnitine supplementation for the treatment of chemotherapy induced fatigue in non-anaemic cancer patients. *Br J Cancer.* 2002;86:1854–1857.
86. Lee K, Cho M, Miaskowski C, Dodd M. Impaired sleep and rhythms in persons with cancer. *Sleep Med Rev.* 2004;8:199–212.
87. Lee K, Cho M, Miaskowski C, Dodd M. Impaired sleep and rhythms in persons with cancer. *Sleep Med Rev.* 2004;8:199–212 .
88. Itri L. Epoeitin alpha intervention for anemia-related fatigue in cancer patients. In: Marty M, Pecorelli S, eds. *Fatigue and Cancer.* New York: Elsevier Science; 2001:129–144.
89. Lenzer J. FDA to review safety of erythropoietin. *BMJ.* 2007;334:495.
90. Leland-Jones B, Semiglazov V, Pawlicki M, et al. Maintaining normal hemoglobin levels with epoetin alfa in mainly nonanemic patients with metastatic breast cancer receiving first-line chemotherapy: a survival study. *J Clin Oncol.* 2005;23:5960–5972.
91. National Comprehensive Cancer Network: version 2:2006, www.nccn.org, Crawford J. Erythropoietin: high profile, high scrutiny. *J Clin Oncol.* 2007;25:1021–1023.
92. Bruera E, Driver L, Barnes E, et al. Patient-controlled methylphenidate for the management of fatigue in patients with advanced cancer: a preliminary report. *J Clin Oncol.* 2003;21:4439–4443; Morrow GR, Shelke AR, Roscoe JA, Hickok JT, Mustian K. Management of cancer-related fatigue. *Cancer Invest.* 2005;23:229–239.
93. Hanna A, Sledge G, Mayer ML, et al. A phase II study of methylphenidate for the treatment of fatigue. *Support Care Cancer.* 2006;14:210–215.
94. Bruera E, Valera V, Driver L, et al. Patient-controlled methylphenidate for cancer fatigue: a double-blind randomized, placebo-controlled trial. *J Clin Oncol.* 24:2073–2078.
95. Lunstrom SH, Furst CH. The use of corticosteroids in Swedish palliative care. *Acta Oncologica.* 2006;45:430–437.
96. Adamsen L, Andersen C, Quist M, Moeller T, Roerth M. Transforming the nature of fatigue through exercise: qualitative findings from a multidimensional exercise programme in cancer patients undergoing chemotherapy. *Eur J Cancer Care.* 2004;13:362–370.
97. Adamsen L, Quist M, Midtgaard J, et al. The effect of a multidimensional exercise intervention on physical capacity, well being and quality of life in cancer patients undergoing chemotherapy. *Support Care Cancer.* 2006;14:116–127.
98. Andersen C, Adamsen L, Moeller T, et al. The effects of a multidimensional exercise programme on symptoms and side-effects in cancer patients undergoing chemotherapy—the use of semi-structured diaries. *Eur J Oncol Nurs.* 2006;10:247–262.
99. Campbell A, Mutrie N, White F, McGuire F, Kearney N. A pilot study of a supervised group exercise programme as a rehabilitation treatment for women with breast cancer receiving adjuvant treatment. *Eur J Oncol Nurs.* 2005;9:56–63.
100. Dimeo F, Stieglitz R, Novelli-Fischer U, Fetscher S, Keul J. Effects of physical activity on the fatigue and psychologic status of cancer patients during chemotherapy. *Cancer.* 1999;85:2273–2277.
101. Dimeo F, Stieglitz R, Novelli-Fischer U, Fetscher S, Keul J. Effects of physical activity on the fatigue and psychologic status of cancer patients during chemotherapy. *Cancer.* 1999;85:2273–2277.
102. Dimeo F, Fetsher S, Lange W, Merelsmann R, Keul J. Effects of aerobic exercise on the physical performance and incidence of
103. Headley J, Ownby K, John L. The effect of seated exercise on fatigue and quality of life in women with advanced breast cancer. *ONF.* 2004;31:977–983.
104. Losito J, Murphy S, Thomas M. The effects of group exercise on fatigue and quality of life during cancer treatment. *ONF.* 2006;33:821–825.
105. Mock V, Frangakis C, Davidson N, et al. Exercise manages fatigue during breast cancer treatment: a randomized controlled trial. *Psycho-Oncology.* 2005;14:464–477.
106. Packel, L, Claghorn K, Dekerlegand J. Cancer-related fatigue and deconditioning: a program evaluation. *Rehabil Oncol.* 2006;24(2):3–8.
107. Ream E, Richardson A, Evison M. A feasibility study to evaluate a group intervention for people with cancer experiencing fatigue following treatment. *Clin Effectiveness in Nursing.* 2005;9:178–187.
108. Schwartz A. Fatigue mediates the effects of exercise on quality of life. *Qual Life Res.* 1999;8:529–538.
109. Segal RJ, Reid RD, Courneya KS, et al. Resistance exercise in men receiving androgen deprivation therapy for prostate cancer. *J Clin Oncol.* 2003;21:1653–1659.
110. Van Weert E, Hoekstra-Weebers JEHM, Grol BMF, et al. Physical functioning and quality of life after cancer rehabilitation. *Int J Rehabil Res.* 2004;27:27–35.
111. Stevinson C, Lawlor DA, Fox KR. Exercise interventions for cancer patients: systematic review of controlled trials. *Cancer Causes Control.* 2004;15:1035–1056.
112. Mock V, Dow KH, Meares CH, et al. Effects of exercise on fatigue, physical functioning and emotional distress during radiation therapy for breast cancer. *Oncol Nurs Forum.* 1997;24:991–1000.
113. Schwartz AL, Mor M, Gao Renlu, Nail LM, King ME. Exercise reduces daily fatigue in women with breast cancer receiving chemotherapy. *Med Sci Sports Exerc.* 2001;33: 717–723.
114. Van Weert E, Hoekstra-Weebers JEHM, Grol BMF, et al. Physical functioning and quality of life after cancer rehabilitation. *Int J Rehabil Res.* 2004;27:27–35.
115. Schwartz AL, Mor M, Gao Renlu, Nail LM, King ME. Exercise reduces daily fatigue in women with breast cancer receiving chemotherapy. *Med Sci Sports Exerc.* 2001;33;717–723.
116. *American College of Sports Medicine: Guidelines for Exercise Testing and Prescription,* 7th ed. Lippincott Williams & Wilkins; 2006:141.
117. Dimeo F, Fetscher S, Lange W, Mertelsmann R, Keul J. Effects of aerobic exercise on the physical performance and incidence of treatment-related complications after high-dose chemotherapy. *Blood.* 1997;90:3390–3394.
118. Andersen C, Adamsen A, Moeller T, et al. The effect of a multidimensional exercise programmed on symptoms and side-effects in cancer patients undergoing chemotherapy-the use of semi structured diaries. *Eur J Oncol Nurs.* 2006;10: 247–262.
119. Segal RJ, Reid RD, Courneya KS, et al. Resistance exercise in men receiving androgen deprivation therapy for prostate cancer. *J Clin Oncol.* 2003;21:1653–1659.
120. Andersen C, Adamsen L, Moeller T, et al. The effect of a multidimensional exercise programme on symptoms and side-effects in cancer patients undergoing chemotherapy-the use of semi-structured diaries. *Eur J Oncol Nurs.* 2006;10:247–262[N166].
121. Headley JA, Ownby KK, John LD. The effect of seated exercise on fatigue and quality of life in women with advanced breast cancer. *Oncol Nurs Forum.* 2004;31:977–983.
122. Escalante CP, Grove T, Johnosn BA, et al. A fatigue clinic in a comprehensive cancer center. *Cancer.* 2001;92:1708–1713.

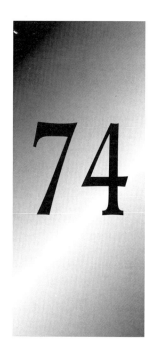

Communication and Swallowing Dysfunction in the Cancer Patient

Margaret L. Ho

Communication and swallowing are activities that not only serve vital physical functions, but also contribute to an individual's emotional health. As physicians and patients consider cancer treatment options, more attention is now given to the effects of the various treatments on the functions of swallowing, speech, voice, language, and hearing. These functions and other quality of life measures are increasingly recognized as integral aspects of cancer survivorship. This chapter will describe the changes in swallowing and communication that may occur with cancer and cancer treatment, and current approaches to evaluating and rehabilitating these functions.

NORMAL COMMUNICATION

Communication is comprised of both speech and language processes. Speech refers to the motor aspects of communication, while language encompasses the cognitive processing of auditory or written verbal stimuli and the formulation of thoughts into words and sentences. When an auditory speech stimulus is delivered, the individual needs to first receive and hear the stimulus, and then perceive it as either environmental or speech input. Once the receptive and perceptual processes have been performed, the auditory signal can be analyzed in the brain for the linguistic elements, and the message is then interpreted for its meaning (1). This processing of speech at the phonological, semantic, syntactic, and discourse levels appears to involve bilateral regions of the temporal lobe, including the superior and middle temporal regions, the temporal pole, Wernicke's area, and the supramarginal gyrus. The superior parietal region and parts of the frontal lobe also contribute to language processing (2). Language formulation is thought to occur in various parts of the frontal lobe, including Broca's area and the supplementary motor cortex (2), and the angular gyrus in the inferior parietal lobe, along with feedback from Wernicke's area in the left temporal lobe (3–5). A growing body of literature suggests that the cerebellum not only is involved in motor coordination but also in language formulation (2,6–10). However, the role of the cerebellum in naming and other linguistic functions is not well understood, and may relate to its contribution to executive functions such as memory and inhibition (11), a cerebrocerebellar signal pathway (6,10), or other hypotheses (12). After a formulated linguistic message is encoded in the parietal lobe, it is sent to Broca's area in the left frontal lobe, where motor speech commands are produced and sent to the appropriate speech muscles. At this point, the message is produced into audible speech by coordination and innervation of the muscles for respiration, phonation, resonation, and articulation (1).

NORMAL SWALLOWING

Sensory and motor functions of the central nervous system and cranial nerves are integral to the normal swallowing process (13). Swallowing is typically divided

KEY POINTS

- Communication is comprised of both speech and language processes. Speech refers to the motor aspects of communication, while language encompasses the cognitive processing of auditory or written verbal stimuli and the formulation of thoughts into words and sentences.
- Swallowing is typically divided into four phases: oral preparatory, oral, pharyngeal, and esophageal.
- It is important to remember that the mechanisms for cricopharyngeal opening are not limited to relaxation of the cricopharyngeus, but include intrabolus pressure generation at the level of the tongue base and hyolaryngeal excursion.
- Ototoxicity is a sequela of high doses of certain chemotherapy agents, most commonly the platinum-based agents, cisplatin and carboplatin.
- Dysphagia occurs frequently during and after radiation therapy, with or without chemotherapy.
- A major and chronic effect of radiotherapy with head and neck cancers is xerostomia (intraoral dryness).
- Patients with cancer in the head and neck region will frequently require or elect radiation to the neck lymph nodes. This means that the base of tongue, epiglottis, hypopharynx, larynx, and upper esophageal sphincter (UES) may be in the radiation field, even if the primary tumor is not in those regions.

- Following radiation therapy, stricture of the cervical esophagus and dysfunction of UES opening may be observed, warranting esophageal dilation.
- Pretreatment exercises have been found to improve post-treatment dysphagia related quality of life as well as post-treatment swallowing function.
- Trismus is another consequence of radiation induced fibrosis, which can occur early or late after treatment, and sometimes during treatment.
- Swallowing evaluation, in the form of clinical evaluation, videofluoroscopy (VFSS), flexible endoscopic evaluation of swallowing (FEES) or FEESST (FEES with sensory testing), is essential for many patients with cancer.
- Patients who undergo total laryngectomy should receive speech therapy to enable them to acquire one or more of the three main alaryngeal speech methods: (1) electrolarynx; (2) esophageal speech; or (3) tracheoesophageal puncture (TEP).
- Swallowing therapy for head and neck patients should be initiated soon after treatment, whether they receive surgery or chemoradiation.
- If trismus develops, assistive exercise or stretching devices such as the Therabite Jaw Mobilization device or the Dynasplint may be required for adequate restoration of mouth opening, along with manual physical therapy of the jaw and neck.

into four phases: oral preparatory, oral, pharyngeal, and esophageal (14).

In the oral preparatory phase, the main task is to accept, contain, and manipulate the food or liquid bolus within the oral cavity, and eventually to gather the bolus into a unit in preparation for the next phase. Activity during this phase includes forming a seal anteriorly at the lips, a posterior seal at the soft palate, manipulating the bolus for taste, mixing the bolus with saliva, masticating, and tensing the buccal musculature to prevent spillage of the bolus into the lateral oral sulci (14). Sensory input is important in this stage to activate the muscles of the face, lips cheeks, tongue, mandible, and soft palate for coordinated movements.

After the bolus has been gathered together, the oral phase begins, involving the transfer of the bolus to the posterior oral cavity and oropharynx. The tongue has the primary role in this phase as it presses against the hard palate and alveolar ridges in an anterior to posterior motion to propel the bolus. At the same time, the lip and buccal muscles contract (14).

Once the "head" (leading edge) of the bolus enters the oropharynx, the pharyngeal phase is initiated. When the bolus head reaches the region of the tongue base that is at the level of the inferior border of the mandible,

the pharyngeal swallow is elicited. In this phase, several movements need to occur for successful transport of the bolus through the pharynx to the esophagus. These include velopharyngeal port closure, contact of the base of tongue to the posterior pharyngeal wall, airway closure, superior and anterior movement of the hyoid bone and larynx, epiglottic inversion, and lastly, opening of the upper esophageal sphincter (UES) (14). The key role played by the base of tongue in the oropharyngeal swallow cannot be overemphasized. Not only is it important in propelling boluses into the pharynx, but it is instrumental in creating adequate bolus driving pressure. This pressure is one of the major mechanisms required for adequate upper esophageal sphincter opening (15,16) and pharyngeal clearance (16,17). The UES consists of three muscles: the cricopharyngeal muscle, the inferior pharyngeal constrictor muscle, and the upper esophageal muscle (18). Once the tongue base and the posterior pharyngeal wall meet, the pharyngeal constrictors contract in a superior to inferior sequence (19), narrowing the pharyngeal space (13), and adding further pressure to the bolus (14). These actions are highly coordinated and dependent on each other. For example, without adequate laryngeal elevation, UES relaxation, or bolus pressure, the opening of the UES will be compromised (15,20). During airway closure, the arytenoids medialize prior to vocal fold adduction (21), resulting in a temporary cessation of breathing (19,22). There is also anterior displacement of the arytenoids and approximation of the ventricular folds (13). The timing of the apneic period has been found to occur before the onset of laryngeal elevation (22), while UES relaxation occurred during laryngeal elevation, followed closely by the opening of the UES (20).

The esophageal phase is essentially involuntary in nature, (19) and as a consequence, is not amenable to therapeutic maneuvers (14). In the esophageal phase, the bolus is transported through the esophagus by a series of peristaltic waves until it reaches the lower esophageal sphincter (LES), which relaxes and allows the bolus to enter the stomach (23).

Although there is evidence that the cortex and subcortex may influence swallowing function, the specific mechanisms have not been well defined. Much of the evidence is based on observations of swallowing dysfunction following stroke or cerebral palsy, and on cortical stimulation studies of animals, which have demonstrated significant variation in results (24). More recently, investigators utilizing functional magnetic resonance imaging (fMRI) have added important new findings pertaining to brain function and swallowing. Most investigators agree that the primary motor (precentral) cortex appears to play a vital role in the oral movements needed for swallowing (13,24,25). Evidence has also been reported suggesting the importance of other cortical areas, such as the premotor cortex anterior to the motor cortex (also referred to as the lateral precentral cortex, including Brodmann's areas 4 and 6) (13,,24,26). The latter two regions are felt to exercise some control over the pharyngeal muscles during swallowing. It has also been postulated that hemispheric dominance for swallowing may exist (27,28), although bilateral representation has been reported (29). In addition, cortical processing of sensory input is considered to be crucial for normal swallowing function, and may proceed via fibers being sent to both the brainstem and the cortex (13). Functional magnetic resonance imaging (fMRI) has shown activation in the primary somatosensory cortex during normal swallowing tasks, suggesting an integrative role via connections to the primary motor cortex (25,29,30). The insula, thalamus (25), cerebellum, and basal ganglia (31,32) also showed activation during swallowing.

CANCER EFFECTS ON HEARING, SPEECH, VOICE, LANGUAGE, AND SWALLOWING

Impairments in hearing, speech, voice, language, and swallowing may occur as sequelae of cancer in the head and neck region, lungs, esophagus, central nervous system, and peripheral nervous system. The presence of the tumor itself prior to treatment can disrupt these functions. For example, in patients with nasopharyngeal carcinoma, destruction of the tensor palatini muscle by tumor invasion, and the displacement of the Eustachian tube, leads to effusion in the middle ear and mastoid cells (33,34). With tumor progression, dysarthria and dysphagia may also develop as a result of pressure on cranial nerves or the brainstem (35).

A mass in the tongue or nasopharynx will result in obvious speech deficits in the form of imprecise articulation and hypernasality, respectively. Individuals with glottic laryngeal cancer will exhibit vocal hoarseness and aspiration (36), and those with brain tumors may demonstrate dysarthria, aphasia, and dysphagia. A pharyngeal or esophageal mass can cause odynophagia and difficulty in swallowing due to stricture or obstruction, impeding the transport of liquid or food boluses through the pharynx or esophagus. More difficulty is usually experienced with solids than with liquids because of the narrowed passageway. Patients with esophageal cancer may also report early satiety, belching, and gastroesophageal reflux. In a small percentage of patients with intrathoracic esophageal carcinoma, vocal cord paralysis may be present, usually caused by a metastatic lymph node on the recurrent laryngeal nerve (37).

A pulmonary or mediastinal mass may press on the esophagus, resulting in esophageal phase dysphagia. Other effects of lung cancer on swallowing relate to the high incidence of brain metastases (38). Another common effect of lung cancer is unilateral vocal fold paralysis, caused by the tumor pressing on the recurrent laryngeal nerve branch of the vagus nerve. When unilateral vocal fold paralysis occurs, there is incomplete glottic closure and resultant breathy, hoarse voice. Aspiration and coughing with thin liquids are also commonly observed. Other cancer sites that may cause vocal cord paralysis or paresis (sometimes bilateral) include the skull base, central nervous system, leptomeninges, carotid body, larynx, pharynx, neck, thyroid, trachea, and esophagus (39).

Brain tumors in the cortex, subcortical regions, cerebellum, and brainstem can all cause dysarthria, aphasia, and dysphagia. Associated seizures may exacerbate speech, language, or swallowing deficits (40). Another etiology of speech, language, and swallowing dysfunction is the spread of cancer to the leptomeninges, most commonly from primary adenocarcinomas of the breast and lung non-Hodgkin lymphoma, and malignant melanoma (41). The pathophysiology of leptomeningeal metastatic effects on speech, language, and swallowing relates to hydrocephalus, intracranial pressure, cranial neuropathies, focal brain dysfunction, and meningeal inflammation from tumor invasion (41).

Paraneoplastic cerebellar degeneration, a rare complication of certain cancers (lung, gynecologic, Hodgkin) (42) appears to be an immune reaction that often causes significant dysarthria and swallowing difficulty (43). Skull base tumors can also result in cranial neuropathies, affecting both speech and swallowing functions. However, patients often compensate fairly well prior to surgery because of the gradual nature of the progression of cranial neuropathies (44).

TREATMENT EFFECTS ON HEARING, SPEECH, VOICE, LANGUAGE, AND SWALLOWING

Surgery

Surgical management of cancers of the head and neck, lung, mediastinum, esophagus, trachea, cervical spine, base of skull, and brain can all affect speech, language, hearing, voice, and swallowing. Surgeries of the head and neck include total laryngectomy, partial laryngectomy, glossectomy (total or partial), mandibulectomy, maxillectomy, and resections of various areas of the oral cavity, oropharynx, and hypopharynx, often involving composite resections and free flap reconstructions.

Perhaps the most obvious effect on voice occurs after a total laryngectomy, as the removal of both vocal cords renders the patient aphonic, in terms of traditional voice via vocal cord vibration (45). Swallowing after total laryngectomy is generally not a problem (45). However, in the immediate postoperative period, some patients may complain of food or liquid being lodged in the throat or regurgitated. This complaint is associated with increased pharyngeal resistance to bolus flow after total laryngectomy (46). In addition, stenosis of the proximal esophagus may occur as a late effect after total laryngectomy. Patients who have been irradiated, whether before or after total laryngectomy, appear to be at higher risk for stenosis (47). Other causes of dysphagia after total laryngectomy include benign stricture of the hypopharynx, cricopharyngeal dysfunction, and pseudoepiglottic fold formation (44). In the pharyngolaryngectomy population, etiology of dysphagia can be varied, including lymphedema, benign stricture, redundant jejunum, tumor recurrence, graft dysmotility, functional obstructions at the anastomosis, reduced lingual efficiency, and brainstem metastasis. Often it is a combination of several of these deficits that contribute to the dysphagia. Nasal and oral regurgitation can result from one or more of these deficits. Patients with tumor recurrence sometimes have previously complained of the sensation of swallowing obstruction that could not be identified at the time, either endoscopically or radiographically (48).

A partial laryngectomy refers to several types of resection, including supraglottic laryngectomy, hemilaryngectomy (vertical type), or supracricoid laryngectomy. Voice after a supraglottic laryngectomy is typically unaffected, as both true vocal folds remain, while the false vocal folds, epiglottis, and other structures superior to the glottis are removed. However, the pharyngeal phase of swallowing is significantly impaired as a result of the loss of airway protection normally provided by the epiglottis and false vocal folds. Aspiration is a common problem in these patients, requiring intensive swallowing evaluation and therapy to minimize aspiration episodes (14). These patients also exhibit reductions in tongue base retraction and laryngeal elevation (49).

A hemilaryngectomy involves the resection of one vertical half of the larynx, including one true vocal fold, one false vocal fold, one ventricle, and one-half of the thyroid cartilage, sparing one of the true vocal folds (14). These patients may be able to produce voice, though it is usually hoarse, if present. Videostroboscopic analysis after vertical partial laryngectomy revealed that phonation occurred most often by vibration of the remaining false vocal fold against the resected side, while vibration at the level of the arytenoid or true vocal fold was less frequent (50). In patients undergoing vertical frontolateral partial laryngectomy, voice quality and glottic closure improved with time and were better in those in which a glottic flap reconstruction was performed (51–54). Swallowing deficits may occur after hemilaryngectomy due to incomplete glottic closure and resultant risk for aspiration. However, with standard hemilaryngectomy, there is usually sufficient tissue on the reconstructed side, affording complete glottic closure and the development of a functional swallow (14). Furthermore, the remaining supraglottic structures (hyoid bone, epiglottis) protect the airway during the swallow. If the resection extends anteriorly (frontolateral laryngectomy), initial difficulty with aspiration is more frequent, but patients often improve. If the resection extends posteriorly to include the arytenoid cartilage, aspiration is more likely to persist (14).

Supracricoid laryngectomy (SCL) may be considered one approach to preserving the larynx (55) and natural voice, despite removal of the true vocal folds. It involves the resection of both true vocal folds, both false vocal folds, the entire thyroid, usually one arytenoid, and sometimes the epiglottis (56). If the epiglottis is removed, the reconstructive technique used is called cricohyoidopexy (CHP), in which the cricoid cartilage is attached to the hyoid bone and base of tongue. If the epiglottis is preserved, the closure technique is called cricohyoidoepiglottopexy (CHEP), involving pexy of the cricoid to the hyoid, base of tongue and epiglottis (57). Voice is produced by the close approximation of

management of these important functions. Further research is needed to continue to help patients maintain these functions longer. As cancer treatments become more successful and patients survive longer, our interventions for communication and swallowing are even more necessary.

ACKNOWLEDGMENTS

I thank Ms. Susan Weil, Manager, Media Services, Memorial Sloan-Kettering Cancer Center (MSKCC) for her expert assistance in generating the figures, and Ms. Amy Budnick, Director, Audiology, MSKCC, for her suggestions regarding audiology issues in patients with cancer.

References

1. Nation JE, Aram DM. *Diagnosis of Speech and Language Disorders.* St. Louis: CV Mosby; 1977.
2. Gernsbacher MA, Kaschak MP. Neuroimaging studies of language production and comprehension. *Annu Rev Psychol.* 2003;54:91–114.
3. Geschwind N. Disconnexion syndromes in animals and man. I. *Brain.* June 1965;88(2):237–294.
4. Geschwind N. Disconnexion syndromes in animals and man. II. *Brain.* September 1965;88(3):585–644.
5. Luria AR. *Higher Cortical Functions in Man.* New York: Basic Books; 1966.
6. *Murdoch BE, Whelan BM.* Language disorders subsequent to left cerebellar lesions: a case for bilateral cerebellar involvement in language? *Folia Phoniatr Logop.* 2007;59(4):184–189.
7. Gebhart AL, Petersen SE, Thach WT. Role of the posterolateral cerebellum in language. *Ann NY Acad Sci.* December 2002;978:318–333.
8. Marien P, Engelborghs S, Fabbro F, De Deyn PP. The lateralized linguistic cerebellum: a review and a new hypothesis. *Brain Lang.* December 2001;79(3):580–600.
9. Gasparini M, Di Piero V, Ciccarelli O, Cacioppo MM, Pantano P, Lenzi GL. Linguistic impairment after right cerebellar stroke: a case report. *Eur J Neurol.* May 1999;6(3):353–356.
10. Leiner HC, Leiner AL, Dow RS. The human cerebro-cerebellar system: its computing, cognitive, and language skills. *Behav Brain Res.* August 29, 1991;44(2):113–128.
11. Bellebaum C, Daum I. Cerebellar involvement in executive control. *Cerebellum.* 2007;6(3):184–192.
12. DeSmet HJ, Baillieux H, DeDeyn PP, Marien P, Paquier P. The cerebellum and language: the story so far. *Folia Phoniatr Logop.* 2007;59(4):165–179.
13. Miller AJ. *The Neuroscientific Principles of Swallowing and Dysphagia.* San Diego: Singular Publishing Group, Inc.; 1999.
14. Logemann JA. *Evaluation and Treatment of Swallowing Disorders,* 2nd ed. Austin: PRO-ED, Inc.; 1998.
15. *Cook IJ, Dodds WJ, Dantas RO, et al.* Opening mechanisms of the human upper esophageal sphincter. *Am J Physiol.* November 1989;257(5 Pt 1):G748–G759.
16. *Pauloski BR, Logemann JA.* Impact of tongue base and posterior pharyngeal wall biomechanics on pharyngeal clearance in irradiated postsurgical oral and oropharyngeal cancer patients. *Head Neck.* March 2000;22(2):120–131.
17. *Lazarus C.* Tongue strength and exercise in healthy individuals and in head and neck cancer patients. *Semin Speech Lang.* November 2006;27(4):260–267.
18. Mu L, Sanders I. Neuromuscular organization of the human upper esophageal sphincter. *Ann Otol Rhinol Laryngol.* May 1998;107(5 Pt 1):370–377.
19. Aviv JE. The normal swallow. In Carrau RL, Murray T, eds. *Comprehensive Management of Swallowing Disorders.* San Diego: Singular Publishing Group, Inc.; 1999:23–29.
20. Jacob P, Kahrilas PJ, Logemann JA, Shah V, Ha T. Upper esophageal sphincter opening and modulation during swallowing. *Gastroenterology.* December 1989;97(6):1469–1478.
21. Van Daele DJ, McCulloch TM, Palmer PM, Langmore SE. Timing of glottic closure during swallowing: a combined electromyographic and endoscopic analysis. *Ann Otol Rhinol Laryngol.* June 2005;114(6):478–487.
22. Martin BJ, Logemann JA, Shaker R, Dodds WJ. Coordination between respiration and swallowing: respiratory phase relationships and temporal integration. *J Appl Physiol.* February 1994;76(2):714–723.
23. Levy B, Young MA. Pathophysiology of swallowing and gastroesophageal reflux. In Carrau RL, Murray T, eds. *Comprehensive Management of Swallowing Disorders.* San Diego: Singular Publishing Group, Inc.; 1999:175–186.
24. Martin RE, Sessle BJ. The role of the cerebral cortex in swallowing. *Dysphagia.* 1993;8(3):195–202.
25. Mosier K, Patel R, Liu WC, Kalnin A, Maldjian J, Baredes S. Cortical representation of swallowing in normal adults: functional implications. *Laryngoscope.* September 1999;109(9):1417–1423.
26. *Hamdy S, Aziz Q, Rothwell JC,* et al. The cortical topography of human swallowing musculature in health and disease. *Nat Med.* November 1996;2(11):1190–1191.
27. Hamdy S, Aziz Q, Rothwell JC, et al. Explaining oropharyngeal dysphagia after unilateral hemispheric stroke. *Lancet.* September 6, 1997;350(9079):686–692.
28. Mosier KM, Liu WC, Maldjian JA, Shah R, Modi B. Lateralization of cortical function in swallowing: a functional MR imaging study. *Am J Neuroradiol.* 1999;20:1520–1526.
29. Kern MK, Jaradeh S. Arndorfer RC, Shaker R. Cerebral cortical representation of reflexive and volitional swallowing in humans. *Am J Physiol Gastrointest Liver Physiol.* March 2001;280:G354–G360.
30. Hamdy S, Mikulis DJ, Crawley A, et al. Cortical activation during human volitional swallowing: an event-related fMRI study. *Am J Physiol.* July 1999;277(1 Pt 1):G219–G225.
31. Suzuki M, Asada Y, Ito J, Hayashi K, Inoue H, Kitano H. Activation of cerebellum and basal ganglia on volitional swallowing detected by functional magnetic resonance imaging. *Dysphagia.* Spring 2003;18(2):71–77.
32. Mosier K, Bereznaya I. Parallel cortical networks for volitional control of swallowing in humans. *Exp Brain Res.* October 2001;140(3):280–289.
33. King AD, Kew J, Tong M, et al. Magnetic resonance imaging of the Eustachian tube in nasopharyngeal carcinoma: correlation of patterns of spread with middle ear effusion. *Am J Otol.* 1999;20(1):69–73.
34. Low WK, Lim TA, Fan YF, Balakrishnan A. Pathogenesis of middle-ear effusion in nasopharyngeal carcinoma: a new perspective. *J Laryngol Otol.* May 1997;111(5):431–434.
35. Bebin, J. Pathophysiology of acoustic tumors. In: House W, Luetje C, eds. *Acoustic Tumors. Vol. 1: Diagnosis.* Baltimore: University Park Press; 1979:45–83.
36. Stenson KM, McCracken E, List M, et al. Swallowing function in patients with head and neck cancer prior to treatment. *Arch Otolaryngol Head Neck Surg.* 2000;126:371–377.
37. Tachimori Y, Kato H, Watanabe H, Ishikawa T, Yamaguchi H. Vocal cord paralysis in patients with thoracic esophageal carcinoma. *J Surg Oncol.* August 1995;59(4):230–232.
38. Mackey CS, Ruckdeschel JC. Lung cancer. In: Sullivan PA, Guilford AM, eds. *Swallowing Intervention in Oncology.* San Diego: Singular Publishing Group, Inc.; 1999: 117–133.
39. Ridley MB. Effects of surgery for head and neck cancer. In: Sullivan PA, Guilford AM, eds. *Swallowing Intervention in Oncology.* San Diego: Singular Publishing Group, Inc.; 1999:77–97.

40. Gaziano JE, Kumar R. Primary brain tumors. In: Sullivan PA, Guilford AM, eds. *Swallowing Intervention in Oncology.* San Diego: Singular Publishing Group, Inc.; 1999:65–76.

41. Patchell, RA. Brain metastases and carcinomatous meningitis. In: Abeloff MD, Armitage JO, Lichter AS, Niederhuber JE, eds. *Clinical Oncology,* 2nd ed. Philadelphia: Churchill Livingstone; 2000:820–835.

42. Posner JB. Paraneoplastic cerebellar degeneration. *Can J Neurol Sci.* May 1993;20(Suppl 3):S117–S122.

43. Paslawski T, Duffy JR, Vernino S. Speech and language findings associated with paraneoplastic cerebellar degeneration. *Am J Speech Lang Pathol.* August 2005;14(3):200–207.

44. Kronenberger MB and Meyers AD. Dysphagia following head and neck cancer surgery. *Dysphagia.* 1994;9:236–244.

45. Casper JK, Colton RH. Medical/surgical examination, diagnosis, and treatment. In: Casper JK, Colton RH, eds. *Clinical Manual for Laryngectomy and Head/Neck Cancer Rehabilitation,* 2nd ed. San Diego: Singular Publishing Group, Inc.; 1998:11–34.

46. McConnel FM, Mendelsohn MS, Logemann JA. Examination of swallowing after total laryngectomy using manofluorography. *Head Neck Surg.* September–October 1986;9(1):3–12.

47. Vu KN, Day TA, Gillespie MB, et al. Proximal esophageal stenosis in head and neck cancer patients after total laryngectomy and radiation. *ORL J Otorhinolaryngol Relat Spec.* 2008;70(4):229–235.

48. Ward EC, Frisby J, O'Connor D. Assessment and management of dysphagia following pharyngolaryngectomy with free jejunal interposition: a series of eight case studies. *J Med Speech-Lang Pathol.* 2001;9(1):89–105.

49. Logemann JA, Gibbons P, Rademaker AW, et al. Mechanisms of recovery of swallow after supraglottic laryngectomy. *J Speech Hear Res.* October 1994;37(5):965–974.

50. Mandell DL, Woo P, Behin DS, et al. Videolaryngostroboscopy following vertical partial laryngectomy. *Ann Otol Rhinol Laryngol.* November 1999;108(11 Pt 1):1061–1067.

51. Kim CH, Lim YC, Kim YH, Choi HS, Kim KM, Choi EC. Vocal analysis after vertical partial laryngectomy. *Yonsei Med J.* December 30, 2003;44(6):1034–1039.

52. Biacabe B, Crevier-Buchman L, Hans S, Laccourreye O, Brasnu D. Vocal function after vertical partial laryngectomy with glottic reconstruction by false vocal fold flap: duration and frequency measures. *Laryngoscope.* May 1999;109(5):698–704.

53. Cruz WP, Dedivitis RA, Rapoport A, Guimaraes AV. Videolaryngostroboscopy following frontolateral laryngectomy with sternohyoid flap. *Ann Otol Rhinol Laryngol.* February 2004;113(2):124–127.

54. Biacabe B, Crevier-Buchman L, Hans S, Laccourreye O, Brasnu D. Phonatory mechanisms after vertical partial laryngectomy with glottic reconstruction by false vocal fold flap. *Ann Otol Rhinol Laryngol.* October 2001;110(10):935–940.

55. Holsinger FC. Swing of the pendulum: optimizing functional outcomes in larynx cancer. *Curr Oncol Rep.* March 2008;10(2):170–175.

56. Piquet JJ, Chevalier D. Subtotal laryngectomy with cricohyoido-epiglotto-pexy for the treatment of extended glottic carcinomas. *Am J Surg.* October 1991;162:357–361.

57. Zacharek MA, Pasha R, Meleca RJ, et al. Functional outcomes after supracricoid laryngectomy. *Laryngoscope.* September 2001;111:1558–1564.

58. Borggreven PA, Verdonck-de Leeuw I, Rinkel RN, et al. Swallowing after major surgery of the oral cavity or oropharynx: a prospective and longitudinal assessment of patients treated by microvascular soft tissue reconstruction. *Head Neck.* July 2007;29(7):638–647.

59. Schrag C, Chang Ym, Tsai CY, Wei FC. Complete rehabilitation of the mandible following segmental resection. *J Surg Oncol.* November 1, 2006;94(6):538–545.

60. Rieger J, Wolfaardt J, Seikaly H, Jha N. Speech outcomes in patients rehabilitated with maxillary obturator prostheses after maxillectomy: a prospective study. *Int J Prosthodont.* March–April 2002;15(2):139–144.

61. Seikaly H, Rieger J, Wolfaardt J, Moysa G, Harris J, Jha N. Functional outcomes after primary oropharyngeal cancer resection and reconstruction with the radial forearm free flap. *Laryngoscope.* May 2003;113(5):897–904.

62. McCombe D, Lyons B, Winkler R, Morrison W. Speech and swallowing following radial forearm flap reconstruction of major soft palate defects. *Br J Plast Surg.* 2005;58:306–311.

63. Chan WF and Lo CY. Pitfalls of intraoperative neuromonitoring for predicting postoperative recurrent laryngeal nerve function during thyroidectomy. *World J Surg.* May 2006;30(5):806–812.

64. Netto Ide P, Vartarian JG, Ferraz PR, et al. Vocal fold immobility alter thyroidectomy with intraoperative recurrent laryngeal nerve monitoring. *Sao Paulo Med J.* May 3, 2007;125(3):186–190.

65. Levine TM. Swallowing disorders following skull base surgery. *Otolaryngol Clin North Am.* November 1988;21(4):751–759.

66. Jennings KS, Siroky D, Jackson CG. Swallowing problems after excision of tumors of the skull base: diagnosis and management in 12 patients. *Dysphagia.* 1992;7(1):40–44.

67. Bielamowicz S, Gupta A, Sehar LN. Early artyenoid adduction for vagal paralysis after skull base surgery. *Laryngoscope.* March 2000;110(3 Pt 1):346–351.

68. Chiu ES, Kraus D, Bui DT, et al. Anterior and middle cranial fossa skull base reconstruction using microvascular free tissue techniques: surgical complications and functional outcomes. *Ann Plast Surg.* May 2008;60(5):514–520.

69. Kraus DH, Orlikoff RF, Rizk SS, Rosenberg DB. Arytenoid adduction as an adjunct to type I thyroplasty for unilateral vocal cord paralysis. *Head Neck.* January 1999;21(1):52–59.

70. Lam PK, Ho WK, Ng ML, Wei WI. Medialization thyroplasty for cancer-related unilateral vocal fold paralysis. *Otolaryngol Head Neck Surg.* March 2007;136(3):440–444.

71. Heitmiller RF and Jones B. Transient diminished airway protection after transhiatal esophagectomy. *Am J Surg.* 1991;162:442–446.

72. Lerut TE, van Lanschot JJ. Chronic symptoms alter subtotal or partial oesophagectomy: diagnosis and treatment. *Best Pract Res Clin Gastroenterol.* October 2004;18(5):901–915.

73. Donington JS. Functional conduit disorders after esophagectomy. *Thorac Surg Clin.* February 2006;16(1):53–62.

74. Kato H, Miyazaki T, Sakai M, et al. Videofluoroscopic evaluation in oropharyngeal swallowing after radical esophagectomy with lymphadenectomy for esophageal cancer. *Anticancer Res.* November–December 2007;27(6C):4249–4254.

75. Easterling CS, Bousamra M, Lang IM, et al. Pharyngeal dysphagia in postesophagectomy patients: correlation with deglutive biomechanics. *Ann Thoracic Surg.* April 2000;69(4):989–992.

76. Morgan AT, Sell D, Ryan M, Raynsford E, Hayward R. Pre and post-surgical dysphagia outcome associated with posterior fossa tumour in children. *J Neurooncol.* May 2008;87(3):347–354.

77. Newman LA, Boop FA, Sanford RA, Thompson JW, Temple CK, Duntsch CD. Postoperative swallowing function after posterior fossa tumor resection in pediatric patients. *Childs Nerv Syst.* October 2006;22(10):1296–1300.

78. Catsman-Berrevoets CE, Van Dongen HR, Mulder PG, Paz y Geuze D, Paquier PF, Lequin MH. Tumour type and size are high risk factors for the syndrome of "cerebellar" mutism and subsequent dysarthria. *J Neurol Neurosurg Psychiatry.* December 1999;67(6):755–757.

79. Huber JF, Bradley K, Spiegler BJ, Dennis M. Long-term effects of transient cerebellar mutism after cerebellar astrocytoma or medulloblastoma tumor resection in childhood. *Childs Nerv Syst.* February 2006;22(2):132–138.

80. Sherman JH, Sheehan JP, Elias WJ, Jane JA Sr. Cerebellar mutism in adults after posterior fossa surgery: a report of 2 cases. *Surg Neurol.* May 2005;63(5):476–479.

81. Akhaddar A, Belhachmi A, Elasri A, et al. Cerebellar mutism after removal of a vermian medulloblastoma in an adult. *Neurochirurgie.* August 2008;54(4):548–550.

82. Vitaz TW, Marx W, Victor JD, Gutin PH. Comparison of conscious sedation and general anesthesia for motor mapping and resection of tumors located near motor cortex. *Neurosurg Focus.* July 15, 2003;15(1):E8.

83. Hirsch J, Ruge MI, Kim KH, et al. An integrated functional magnetic resonance imaging procedure for preoperative mapping of cortical areas associated with tactile, motor, language, and visual functions. *Neurosurgery.* September 2000;47(3):711–721; discussion 721–722.

84. Lee NY, O'Meara W, Chan K, et al. Concurrent chemotherapy and intensity-modulated radiotherapy for locoregionally advanced laryngeal and hypopharyngeal cancers. *Int J Radiat Oncol Biol Phys.* October 1, 2007;69(2):459–468.

85. Logemann JA, Pauloski BR, Rademaker AW, et al. Swallowing disorders in the first year after radiation and chemoradiation. *Head Neck.* February 2008;30(2):148–158.

86. Kotz T, Costello R, Li Y, Posner MR.Swallowing dysfunction after chemoradiation for advanced squamous cell carcinoma of the head and neck. *Head Neck.* 2004;26:365–372.

87. Lazarus CL, Logemann JA, Pauloski BR, et al. Swallowing disorders in head and neck cancer patients treated with radiotherapy and adjuvant chemotherapy. *Laryngoscope.* 1996;106:1157–1166.

88. Rybak LP. Mechanisms of cisplatin ototoxicity and progress in otoprotection. *Curr Opin Otolaryngol Head Neck Surg.* October 2007;15(5):364–369.

89. *Weatherly RA, Owens JJ, Catlin FI, Mahoney DH.* cisplatinum ototoxicity in children. *Laryngoscope.* September 1991;101(9):917–924.

90. Rybak LP. Ototoxicity and antineoplastic drugs. Curr Opin Otolaryngol Head Neck Surg. 1999;7:239–243.

91. Knight KR, Kraemer DF, Neuwelt EA. Ototoxicity in children receiving platinum chemotherapy: underestimating a commonly occurring toxicity that may influence academic and social development. *J Clin Oncol.* December 1, 2005;23(34):8588–8596.

92. *Borg E, Edquist G, Reinholdson AC, Risberg A, McAllister B.* Speech and language development in a population of Swedish hearing-impaired pre-school children, a cross-sectional study. *Int J Pediatr Otorhinolaryngol.* July 2007;71(7):1061–1077.

93. Blamey PJ, Sarant JZ, Paatsch LE, et al. Relationships among speech perception, production, language, hearing loss, and age in children with impaired hearing. *J Speech Lang Hear Res.* April 2001;44(2):264–285.

94. Moeller MP, Hoover B, Putman C, et al. Vocalizations of infants with hearing loss compared with infants with normal hearing: Part I—phonetic development. *Ear Hear.* September 2007;28(5):605–627.

95. Moeller MP, Hoover B, Putman C, et al. Vocalizations of infants with hearing loss compared with infants with normal hearing: Part II—transition to words. *Ear Hear.* September 2007;28(5):628–642.

96. McGuckian M, Henry A. The grammatical morpheme deficit in moderate hearing impairment. *Int J Lang Commun Disord.* March 2007;42(Suppl 1):17–36.

97. Gilbert HR, Campbell MI. Speaking fundamental frequency in three groups of hearing-impaired individuals. J Commun Disord. May 1980;13(3):195–205.

98. Jagarlamudi R, Kumar L, Kochupillai V, Kapil A, Banerjee U, Thulkar S. Infections in acute leukemia: an analysis of 240 febrile episodes. *Med Oncol.* May 2000;17(2):111–116.

99. Buszman E, *Wrze;aasniok D, Matusi;aanski B.* Ototoxic drugs. I. Aminoglycoside antibiotics. Wiad Lek. 2003;56(5–6):254–259.

100. Selimoglu E. Aminoglycoside-induced ototoxicity. Curr Pharm Des. 2007;13(1):119–126.

101. Rizzi MD, Hirose K. Aminoglycoside ototoxicity. Curr Opin Otolaryngol Head Neck Surg. October 2007;15(5):352–357.

102. Choudry U. Esophageal carcinoma. In: Sullivan PA, Guilford AM, eds. *Swallowing Intervention in Oncology.* San Diego: Singular Publishing Group, Inc.; 1999:99–115.

103. Eisbruch A, Lyden T, Bradford CR, et al. Objective assessment of swallowing dysfunction and aspiration after radiation

104. Nguyen NP, Frank C, Moltz CC, et al. Aspiration rate following chemoradiation for head and neck cancer: an underreported occurrence. *Radiother Oncol.* September 2006;80(3):302–306.

105. Langerman A, MacCracken E, Kasza K, Haraf DJ, Vokes EE, Stenson KM. Aspiration in chemoradiated patients with head and neck cancer. *Arch Otolaryngol Head Neck Surg.* December 2007;133(12):1289–1295.

106. Rosenthal DI, Lewin JS, Eisbruch A. Prevention and treatment of dysphagia and aspiration after chemoradiation for head and neck cancer. *J Clin Oncol.* June 2006;24(17):2636–2643.

107. Berk LB, Shivnani AT, Small W. Pathophysiology and management of radation-induced xerostomia. *J Supportive Oncol.* May–June 2005;3(3):191–200.

108. Jedel E. Acupuncture in xerostomia—a systematic review. *J Oral Rehabil.* June 2005;32(6):392–396.

109. Cho JH, Chung WK, Kang W, Choi SM, Cho CK, Son CG. Manual acupuncture improved quality of life in cancer patients with radiation-induced xerostomia. *J Altern Complement Med.* June 2008;14(5):523–526.

110. Grégoire V, De Neve W, Eisbruch A, Lee N, Van den Weyngaert D, Van Gestel D. Intensity-modulated radiation therapy for head and neck carcinoma. *Oncologist.* May 2007;12(5):555–564.

111. *Nguyen NP, Moltz CC, Frank C, et al.* Impact of swallowing therapy on aspiration rate following treatment for locally advanced head and neck cancer. *Oral Oncol.* April 2007;43(4):352–357.

112. *Antonadou D, Pepelassi M, Synodinou M, Puglisi M, Throuvalas N.* Prophylactic use of amifostine to prevent radiochemotherapy-induced mucositis and xerostomia in head-and-neck cancer. *Int J Radiat Oncol Biol Phys.* March 1, 2002;52(3):739–747.

113. *Büntzel J, Glatzel M, Mücke R, Micke O, Bruns F.* Influence of amifostine on late radiation-toxicity in head and neck cancer—a follow-up study. *Anticancer Res.* July–August 2007;27(4A):1953–1956.

114. *Wasserman TH, Brizel DM, Henke M, et al.* Influence of intravenous amifostine on xerostomia, tumor control, and survival after radiotherapy for head-and- neck cancer: 2-year follow-up of a prospective, randomized, phase III trial. *Int J Radiat Oncol Biol Phys.* November 15, 2005;63(4):985–990.

115. Agarwala SS, Sbeitan I. Iatrogenic swallowing disorders: chemotherapy. In: Carrau RL, Murray T, eds. *Comprehensive Management of Swallowing Disorders.* San Diego: Singular Publishing Group, Inc.; 1999:125–129.

116. Abitbol AA, Friedland JL, Lewin AA, Rodrigues MA, Mishra V. Radiation therapy in oncologic management with special emphasis on head and neck carcinoma. In: Sullivan PA, Guilford AM, eds. *Swallowing Intervention in Oncology.* San Diego: Singular Publishing Group, Inc.; 1999:47–63.

117. Bahri S, Cano E. Iatrogenic swallowing disorders: radiotherapy. In: Carrau RL, Murray T, eds. *Comprehensive Management of Swallowing Disorders.* San Diego: Singular Publishing Group, Inc.; 1999:131–134.

118. *Jang WI, Wu HG, Park CI, et al.* Treatment of patients with clinically lymph node-negative squamous cell carcinoma of the oral cavity. Jpn J Clin Oncol. June 2008;38(6):395–401.

119. *Garden AS, Asper JA, Morrison WH, et al.* Is concurrent chemoradiation the treatment of choice for all patients with Stage III or IV head and neck carcinoma? *Cancer.* March 15, 2004;100(6):1171–1178.

120. Lim YC, Koo BS, Lee JS, Lim JY, Choi EC. Distributions of cervical lymph node metastases in oropharyngeal carcinoma: therapeutic implications for the neck N0 neck. *Laryngoscope.* July 2006;116(7):1148–1152.

121. Fung K, Yoo J, Leeper HA, et al. Vocal function following radiation for non-laryngeal versus laryngeal tumors of the head and neck. *Laryngoscope.* November 2001;111(11 Pt 1):1920–1924.

122. Lazarus CL. Effects of radiation therapy and voluntary maneuvers on swallow function in head and neck cancer patients. *Clin Commun Disord.* 1993;3:11–20.

123. Smith R, Kotz T, Beitler J, et al. Long-term swallowing problems after organ preservation therapy with concomitant radiation therapy and intravenous hydroxyurea: initial results. *Arch Otolaryngol Head Neck Surg.* 2000;126:384–389.

124. Eisele DW, Koch DG, Tarazi AE, Jones B. Aspiration from delayed radiation fibrosis of the neck. *Dysphagia.* 1991;6:120–122.

125. Lazarus CL, Logemann JA, Pauloski Br, et al. Swallowing disorders in head and neck cancer patients treated with radiotherapy and adjuvant chemotherapy. *Laryngoscope.* 1996;106:1157–1166.

126. Mittal BB, Pauloski BR, Haraf DJ, et al. Swallowing dysfunction—preventative and rehabilitation strategies in patients with head-and-neck cancer treated with surgery, radiotherapy, and chemotherapy: a critical review. *Int J Radiat Oncol Biol Phys.* 2003;57(5):1219–1230.

127. Gurtner GC, Werner S, Barrandon Y, Longaker MT. Wound repair and regeneration. *Nature.* May 15, 2008; 453(7193):314–321.

128. *Teguh DN, Levendag PC, Voet P, et al.* Trismus in patients with oropharyngeal cancer: relationship with dose in structures of mastication apparatus. *Head Neck.* May 2008;30(5):622–630.

129. Kent ML, Brennan MT, Noll JL, et al. Radiation-induced trismus in head and neck cancer patients. *Support Care Cancer.* March 2008;16(3):305–309.

130. Terpenning M. Geriatric oral health and pneumonia risk. *Clin Infect Dis.* June 15, 2005;40(12):1807–1810.

131. Azarpazhooh A, Leake JL. Systematic review of the association between respiratory diseases and oral health. *J Periodontol.* September 2006;77(9):1465–1482.

132. Paju S, Scannapieco FA. Oral biofilms, periodontitis, and pulmonary infections. *Oral Dis.* November 2007;13(6):508–512.

133. Scannapieco FA. Pneumonia in nonambulatory patients. The role of oral bacteria and oral hygiene. *J Am Dent Assoc.* October 2006;137(Suppl):21S–25S. Review. Erratum in: *J Am Dent Assoc.* March 2008;139(3):252.

134. Abe S, Ishihara K, Adachi M, Okuda K. Tongue-coating as risk indicator for aspiration pneumonia in edentate elderly. *Arch Gerontol Geriatr.* October 1, 2007;47(2):267–275.

135. American Speech-Language-Hearing Association: Guidelines for the audiologic management of individuals receiving cochleotoxic drug therapy. *ASHA.* 1994;36(suppl 12):11–19.

136. Knight KR, Kraemer DF, Winter C, Neuwelt EA. Early changes in auditory function as a result of platinum chemotherapy: use of extended high-frequency audiometry and evoked distortion product otoacoustic emissions. *J Clin Oncol.* April 1, 2007;25(10):1190–1195.

137. Stavroulaki P, Apostolopoulos N, Segas J, Tsakanikos M, Adamopoulos G. Evoked otoacoustic emissions—an approach for monitoring cisplatin induced ototoxicity in children. *Int J Pediatr Otorhinolaryngol.* May 31, 2001;59(1):47–57.

138. Coradini PP, *Cigana L, Selistre SG, Rosito LS, Brunetto AL.* Ototoxicity from cisplatin therapy in childhood cancer. *J Pediatr Hematol Oncol.* 2007;29(6):355–360.

139. Bertolini P, Lassalle M, Mercier G, et al. Platinum compound-related ototoxicity in children: long-term follow-up reveals continuous worsening of hearing loss. J Pediatr Hematol Oncol. October 2004;26(10):649–655.

140. Langmore SE, Aviv JE. Endoscopic procedures to evaluate oropharyngeal swallowing. In: Langmore SE, ed. *Endoscopic Evaluation and Treatment of Swallowing Disorders.* New York: Thieme Medical Publishers, Inc.; 2001:73–100.

141. Langmore SE. Interpretation of findings: a model of disordered swallowing. In: Langmore SE, ed. *Endoscopic Evaluation and Treatment of Swallowing Disorders.* New York: Thieme Medical Publishers, Inc.; 2001:144–155.

142. Donzelli J, Brady S, Wesling M, Craney M. Simultaneous modified Evans blue dye procedure and video nasal endoscopic evaluation of the swallow. *Laryngoscope.* October 2001;111(10):1746–1750.

143. O'Neil-Pirozzi TM, Lisiecki DJ, Jack Momose K, Connors JJ, Milliner MP. Simultaneous modified barium swallow and blue dye tests: a determination of the accuracy of blue dye test aspiration findings. *Dysphagia.* Winter 2003;18(1):32–38.

144. Leder SB, Sasaki CT. Use of FEES to assess and manage patients with tracheotomy. In: Langmore SE, ed. *Endoscopic Evaluation and Treatment of Swallowing Disorders.* New York: Thieme Medical Publishers, Inc.; 2001:188–200.

145. Low WK, Gopal K, Goh Lk, Fong KW. Cochlear implantation in postirradiated ears: outcomes and challenges. *Laryngoscope.* July 2006;116(7):1258–1262.

146. Adunka OF, Buchman CA. Cochlear implantation in the irradiated temporal bone. *J Laryngol Otol.* January 2007;121(1):83–86.

147. Wells-Friedman M. Care for the child with early onset of cancer. In: Sullivan PA, Guilford AM, eds. *Swallowing Intervention in Oncology.* San Diego: Singular Publishing Group, Inc.; 1999:257–267.

148. Arvedson JC, Rodgers BT. Pediatric swallowing and feeding disorders. *J Med Speech Lang Pathol.* 1993;1:203–221.

149. Arvedson JC. Management of swallowing problems. In: Arvedson JC, Brodsky L, eds. *Pediatric Swallowing and Feeding: Assessment and Management.* San Diego: Singular Publishing Group; 1993:327–387.

150. Morris SE. Development of oral-motor skills in the neurologically impaired child receiving non-oral feedings. *Dysphagia.* 1989;3:135–154.

151. Lundy DS, Casiano RR. Rehabilitation of speech and voice deficits following cancer treatments. In: Sullivan PA, Guilford AM, eds. *Swallowing Intervention in Oncology.* San Diego: Singular Publishing Group, Inc.; 1999:291–306.

152. Lof GL, Watson MM. A nationwide survey of nonspeech motor exercise use: implications for evidence-based practice. *Lang Speech Hear Serv Sch.* July 2008;39(3):392–407.

153. Netterville JL, Jackson CG, Civantos F. Thyroplasty in the functional rehabilitation of neurotologic skull base surgery patients. *Am J Otol.* September 1993;14(5):460–464.

154. Rosen CA. Vocal fold injection. In: Carrau RL, Murray T, eds. *Comprehensive Management of Swallowing Disorders.* San Diego: Singular Publishing Group, Inc.; 1999:285–290.

155. Rosen CA, Gartner-Schmidt J, Casiano R, et al. Vocal fold augmentation with calcium hydroxylapatite (CaHA). *Otolaryngol Head Neck Surg.* February 2007;136(2):198–204.

156. Bove MJ, Jabbour N, Krishna P, et al. Operating room versus office-based injection laryngoplasty: a comparative analysis of reimbursement. *Laryngoscope.* February 2007;117(2):226–230.

157. Lam PK, Ho WK, Ng ML, Wei WI. Medialization thyroplasty for cancer-related unilateral vocal fold paralysis. *Otolaryngol Head Neck Surg.* March 2007;136(3):440–444.

158. Lewin JS, Heber TM, Putnam JB Jr, DuBrow RA. Experience with the chin tuck maneuver in postesophagectomy aspirators. *Dysphagia.* Summer 2001;16(3):216–219.

159. Lerman JW. The artificial larynx. In: Salmon SJ, Mount KH, eds. *Alaryngeal Speech Rehabilitation for Clinicians by Clinicians.* Austin: Pro-Ed; 1991:27–45.

160. Duguay MJ. Esophageal speech training: the initial phase. In: Salmon SJ, Mount KH, eds. *Alaryngeal Speech Rehabilitation for Clinicians by Clinicians.* Austin: Pro-Ed; 1991:47–78.

161. Freeman SB, Hamaker RC. Tracheoesophageal voice restoration at time of laryngectomy. In: Blom ED, Singer MI, Hamaker RC, eds. *Tracheoesophageal Voice Restoration Following Total Laryngectomy.* San Diego: Singular Publishing Group, Inc.; 1998:19–25.

162. Singer MI, Gress CD. Secondary tracheoesophageal voice restoration. In: Blom ED, Singer MI, Hamaker RC, eds. *Tracheoesophageal Voice Restoration Following Total Laryngectomy.* San Diego: Singular Publishing Group, Inc.; 1998:27–32.

163. Leder SB, Blom ED. Tracheoesophageal voice prosthesis fittng and training. In: Blom ED, Singer MI, Hamaker RC, eds. *Tracheoesophageal Voice Restoration Following Total Laryngectomy*. San Diego: Singular Publishing Group, Inc.; 1998:57–65.

164. Cheng E, Ho M, Ganz C, et al. Outcomes of primary and secondary tracheoesophageal puncture: a 16-year retrospective analysis. *Ear Nose Throat J*. April 2006;85(4):262–267.

165. Blom ED, Remacle M. Tracheoesophageal voice restoration problems and solutions. In: Blom ED, Singer MI, Hamaker RC, eds. *Tracheoesophageal Voice Restoration Following Total Laryngectomy*. San Diego: Singular Publishing Group, Inc.; 1998:73–82.

166. Ameye D, Honraet K, Loose D, Vermeersch H, Nelis H, Remon JP. Effect of a buccal bioadhesive nystatin tablet on the lifetime of a Provox silicone tracheoesophageal voice prosthesis. *Acta Otolaryngol*. March 2005;125(3):304–306.

167. Seshamani M, Ruiz C, Kasper Schwartz S, Mirza N. Cymetra injections to treat leakage around a tracheoesophageal puncture. *ORL J Otorhinolaryngol Relat Spec*. 2006;68(3):146–148.

168. Mullan GP, Lee MT, Clarke PM. Botulinum neurotoxin for management of intractable central leakage through a voice prosthesis in surgical voice restoration. *J Laryngol Otol*. September 2006;120(9):789–792.

169. Leder SB, Acton LM, Kmiecik J, Ganz C, Blom ED. Voice restoration with the advantage tracheoesophageal voice prosthesis. *Otolaryngol Head Neck Surg*. November 2005;133(5):681–684.

170. Soolsma J, van den Brekel MW, Ackerstaff AH, Balm AJ, Tan B, Hilgers FJ. Long-term results of Provox ActiValve, solving the problem of frequent candida-and "underpressure"-related voice prosthesis replacements. *Laryngoscope*. February 2008;118(2):252–257.

171. Blom ED, Singer MI, Hamaker RC. Tracheostoma valve for post-laryngectomy voice rehabilitation. *Ann Otol Rhinol Laryngol*. 1982;91(6 pt 1):576–578.

172. Hilgers FJ, Ackerstaff AH, Balm AJ, Gregor RT. A new heat and moisture exchanger with speech valve (Provox Stomafilter). *Clin Otolaryngol*. 1996;21:414–418.

173. Ackerstaff AH, Hilger FJ, Aaronson NK, Balm AJ, Van Zandwijk N. Improvements in respiratory and psychosocial functioning following total laryngectomy by the use of a heat and moisture exchanger. *Ann Otol Rhinol Laryngol*. 1993;102:878–883.

174. Hilgers FJ, Ackerstaff AH. Development and evaluation of a novel tracheostoma button and fixation system (Provox LaryButton and LaryClip adhesive) to facilitate hands-free tracheoesophageal speech. *Acta Otolaryngol*. December 2006;126(11):1218–1224.

175. Blom ED. Tracheostoma valve fitting and instruction. In: Blom ED, Singer MI, Hamaker RC, eds. *Tracheoesophageal Voice Restoration Following Total Laryngectomy*. San Diego: Singular Publishing Group, Inc.; 1998:103–108.

176. Logemann JA, Kahrilas PJ, Kobara M, Vakil NB. The benefit of head rotation on pharyngoesophageal dysphagia. *Arch Phys Med Rehabil*. October 1989;70(10):767–771.

177. Lazarus C, Logemann JA, Song CW, Rademaker AW, Kahrilas PJ. Effects of voluntary maneuvers on tongue base function for swallowing. *Folia Phoniatr Logop*. July–August 2002;54(4):171–176.

178. Ohmae Y, Logemann JA, Kaiser P, Hanson DG, Kahrilas PJ. Timing of glottic closure during normal swallow. *Head Neck*. 1995;17:394–402.

179. Dworkin JP, Meleca RJ, Zacharek MA, et al. Voice and deglutition functions after the supracricoid and total laryngecotmy procedures for advanced stage laryngeal carcinoma. *Am Acad Otolaryngol Head Neck Surg*. October 2003;129(4):311–320.

180. Lewin JS, Hutcheson KA, Barringer DA, et al. Functional analysis of swallowing outcomes after supracricoid partial laryngectomy. *Head Neck*. May 2008;30(5):559–566.

181. Bohle G, Rieger J, Huryn J, Verbel D, Hwang F, Zlotolow I. Efficacy of speech aid prostheses for acquired defects of the soft palate and velopharyngeal inadequacy—clinical assessments and cephalometric analysis: a Memorial Sloan-Kettering study. *Head Neck*. March 2005;27(3):195–207.

182. Dettelbach MA, Gross RD, Mahlmann J, Eibling DE. Effect of the Passy-Muir Valve on aspiration in patients with tracheostomy. *Head Neck*. July–August 1995;17(4):297–302.

183. Mason MF. Vocal treatment strategies. In: Mason MF, ed. *Speech Pathology for Tracheostomized and Ventilator Dependent Patients*. Newport Beach: Voicing; 1993:336–381.

184. Kulbersh BD, Rosenthal EL, McGrew BM, et al. Pretreatment, preoperative swallowing exercises may improve dysphagia quality of life. *Laryngoscope*. June 2006;116(6):883–886.

185. *Carroll WR, Locher JL, Canon CL, Bohannon IA, McColloch NL, Magnuson JS. Pretreatment swallowing exercises improve swallow function after chemoradiation. Laryngoscope. January 2008;118(1):39–43.*

186. Fujiiu M, Logemann JA. Effect of a tongue holding maneuver on posterior pharyngeal wall movement during deglutition. *Am J Speech-Lang Pathol*. 1996;5:23–30.

187. Jordan K. Rehabilitation of the patients with dysphagia. *Ear Nose Throat J*. 1979;58:86–87.

188. Shaker R, Easterling C, Kern M, et al. Rehabilitation of swallowing by exercise in tube-fed patients with pharyngeal dysphagia secondary to abnormal UES opening. *Gastroenterology*. May 2002;122(5):1314–1321.

189. Pouderoux P, Kahrilas PJ. Deglutitive tongue force modulation by volition, volume and viscosity. *Gastroenterology*. 1995;108:1418–1426.

190. Lazarus C, Logemann JA, Gibbons P. Effects of maneuvers on swallow function in a dysphagic oral cancer patient. *Head Neck*. 1993;15:419–424.

191. Sullivan PA. Clinical dysphagia intervention. In: Sullivan PA, Guilford AM, eds. *Swallowing Intervention in Oncology*. San Diego: Singular Publishing Group, Inc.; 1999:307–327.

192. Cohen EG, Deschler DG, Walsh K, Hayden RE. Early use of a mechanical stretching device to improve mandibular mobility after composite resection: a pilot study. *Arch Phys Med Rehabil*. July 2005;86(7):1416–1419.

193. Shulman DH, Shipman B, Willis FB. Treating trismus with dynamic splinting: a cohort, case series. *Adv Ther*. January–February 2008;25(1):9–16.

194. Dijkstra PU, Kalk WW, Roodenburg JL. Trismus in head and neck oncology: a systematic review. *Oral Oncol*. October 2004;40(9):879–889.

195. Hartl DM, Cohen M, Julieron M, Marandas P, Janot F, Bourhis J. Botulinum toxin for radiation-induced facial pain and trismus. *OTL Head Neck Surg*. April 2008;138(4):459–463.

196. Stubblefield MD, Levine A, Custodio CM, Fitzpatrick T. The role of botulinum toxin type A in the radiation fibrosis syndrome: a preliminary report. *Arch Phys Med Rehabil*. March 2008;89(3):417–421.

197. Crary MA, Carnaby-Mann GD, Faunce A. Electrical stimulation therapy for dysphagia: descriptive results of two surveys. *Dysphagia*. July 2007;22(3):165–173.

198. Carnaby-Mann GD, Crary MA. Examining the evidence on neuromuscular electrical stiumulation for swallowing. *Arch OTL Head Neck Surg*. June 2007;133(6):564–571.

199. Ludlow CL, Humber I, Saxon K, Poletto C, Sonies B, Crujido L. Effects of surface electrical stimulation both at rest and during swallowing in chronic pharyngeal dysphagia. *Dysphagia*. January 2007;22(1):1–10.

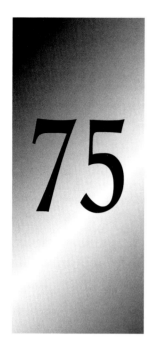

Bladder Dysfunction in the Cancer Patient

Todd A. Linsenmeyer
Georgi Guruli

With improvements in diagnosis and treatment of many types of cancer, overall cancer survival rates have increased (1). Cancer or its treatment may predispose patients to a variety of causes of urinary retention or incontinence. Unfortunately, there may be progression of the disease, and with this progression, changes in voiding. Therefore, it is important to not only accurately identify the specific voiding dysfunction, but also continue to assess and discuss various options. Working closely with the patient, family members, and cancer team will help alert the need for a possible change in bladder management.

The purpose of this chapter is twofold. The first is to review various strategies which may help in bladder management in those with cancer who may have a voiding disorder, including those with pelvic malignancies, where bladder may be affected during the treatment. The second is to review surgical treatments and postoperative care for patients with bladder cancer.

CAUSES OF VOIDING DYSFUNCTIONS FOLLOWING CANCER

There are a variety of causes of voiding dysfunctions following cancer. It is helpful to first characterize the problem as urinary incontinence or urinary retention or both. This can then be further characterized as a problem with the bladder or a problem with the out-

let/sphincter or not related to the bladder or sphincter. Treatment then can be accurately directed at the specific cause. Some of the more common causes of urinary incontinence and retention are listed in Tables 75.1 and 75.2.

TABLE 75.1
Possible Causes of Urinary Incontinence

Bladder	Genitourinary cancer (bladder, prostate), compression from pelvic tumors (uterine, GI cancers), neurogenic causes (spinal metastasis, inflammation of the bladder wall (urinary tract infection, radiation cystitis, cytoxan)
Outlet/ sphincter	Local nerve damage to pelvic nerves pre or post treatment (radical hysterectomy, radical prostectectomy), local cancer invasion into the sphincter (prostate and bladder cancer), chemotherapy (antiestrogens)
Other	Cognitive issues; medications such as diuretics (water pills), sleeping pills, or muscle relaxants; narcotics such as morphine, antihistamines, antidepressants, antipsychotic drugs, or calcium channel blockers; poor mobility; stool impaction (from poor diet, decreased mobility or medications); severe pain

KEY POINTS

- Patient history is particularly significant for evaluation of voiding dysfunction. Hand function, dressing skills, sitting balance, ability to perform transfers, and ability to ambulate are all important factors when developing bladder management strategies.
- When considering various types of bladder management, three important goals should be kept in mind: prevention of upper tract complications, prevention of lower tract complications, and establishing a program that will best fit into the individuals' lifestyle and allow them to be as independent as possible.
- Most behavioral techniques have been developed to manage those with urinary incontinence due to the bladder or sphincter and include fluid restriction, scheduled ("timed") voiding, and pelvic floor "Kegel" exercises with and without biofeedback and electrical stimulation. These strategies can

often be optimized with the addition of pharmacotherapy.
- Botulinum toxin type A injections into the detrusor have been shown to increase bladder capacity and to decrease detrusor overactivity. While botulinum toxin treatment may allow a person to discontinue oral medications, it does need to be repeated under anesthesia approximately every six months.
- Once a bladder is removed, urine can be diverted either into the intestine and through anal sphincter (ureterosigmoidostomy, rectal pouch, etc.), through the skin, or through the urethra (orthotopic neobladder).
- In most patients with invasive bladder cancer after cystectomy, the urethra can be spared, and an intestinal pouch can be anastomosed with urethra, creating a so-called neobladder, or orthotopic urinary diversion.

TABLE 75.2
Possible Causes of Urinary Retention

Bladder	GU and GI cancer, spinal metastasis (neurogenic bladder), local damage to pelvic nerves pre or post treatment
Outlet	Localized cancer, compression effects
Other	Cognitive issues, medications such as diuretics (water pills), sleeping pills, or muscle relaxants; narcotics such as morphine, antihistamines, antidepressants, antipsychotic drugs, or calcium channel blockers; poor mobility, stool impaction (from poor diet, decreased mobility or medications), severe pain

TABLE 75.3
Potential Reversible Causes of Urinary Incontinence or Retention

D	Delerium or other cognitive causes
I	Infection/inflammation of the urinary tract
A	Atropic vaginitis (elderly women and those of estrogen antagonists)
P	Pharmaceuticals
P	Pain
E	Endocrine (diabetes)
R	Restricted mobility
S	Stool impaction

EVALUATION OF VOIDING DISORDERS

Urologic History

The history plays an important role in developing a treatment strategy. However, it is important to note that it does not identify whether the problem is due to the bladder or sphincter, since both problems cause the same symptom. Therefore, if long-term treatment or surgical correction is being considered, a urodynamic evaluation is helpful. Urodynamics will objectively evaluate bladder and sphincter function.

A number of "reversible causes" or urinary retention or incontinence can be identified. A helpful pneumonic which can be used is DIAPPERS (2). A modifica-

tion to this pneumonic is seen in Table 75.3. While this pneumonic was not developed specifically for cancer patients, it is still applicable since a number of cancer treatments or the cancer itself may cause the "reversible causes" that are listed.

The physiatric history is particularly significant for voiding dysfunction. One should ask about hand function, dressing skills, sitting balance, ability to perform transfers, and ability to ambulate. These factors are important considerations when developing bladder management strategies.

Another important component of the history is the intake and output of a person with a voiding disorder. Many individuals with urinary incontinence have learned to restrict fluids. Care has to be taken that they do not have dehydration, especially in cancer patients undergoing chemotherapy with potentially nephrotoxic medications. An accurate assessment is best obtained using a 48–72 hour intake and output (I&O) sheet.

Urologic Physical Examination

The neurourologic physical examination should focus on the abdomen, external genitalia, and perineal skin. When performing the rectal examination, it is important to note that it is not the overall size of the prostate, but the amount of prostate growing inward that causes obstruction. Therefore, urodynamic study rather than rectal examination is needed to diagnose outflow obstruction objectively. In women, one should examine for the location of the urethral meatus, and whether or not there is a cystocele or rectocele. Anal sphincter tone also should be evaluated. Decreased or absent tone suggests a sacral or peripheral nerve lesion, whereas increased tone suggests a suprasacral lesion. Voluntary contraction of the anal sphincter tests sacral innervation, suprasacral integrity, and the ability to understand commands. The bulbocavernosus reflex has been reported as present only 70%–85% of the time in neurologically intact people (3). A false negative often is due to a person being nervous and already having their anal sphincter clamped down at the time of the examination.

Urologic Laboratory Evaluation

It is best to obtain a baseline urine for culture and sensitivity. A serum creatinine is not as helpful as a 24-hour creatinine clearance. This is because a significant amount of kidney damage must occur prior to the appearance of changes in the serum creatinine. Moreover, the serum creatinine may appear normal despite poor renal function in a person with advanced cancer because of significant loss of muscle mass. The serum creatinine is helpful particularly if elevated to monitor baseline changes.

Urologic Assessment of the Upper Urinary Tract

There are a variety of tests designed to evaluate the upper tracts (kidneys and ureters). Some tests are better at evaluating renal function and others at evaluating renal anatomy. Those that evaluate anatomy include an abdominal x-ray, an intravenous pyelogram (IVP), and renal ultrasound. More detailed imaging is obtained from an abdominal and pelvic computed tomography (CT) scan or magnetic resonance imaging (MRI). Tests which primarily evaluate renal function include a 24-hour urine creatinine clearance and quantitative 99mTc-mercaptoacetyltriglycine (MAG 3) renal scan

with effective renal plasma flow (ERPF) (4–7). The author finds a MAG 3 renal scan very helpful to screen for upper tract functional problems.

Urologic Assessment of the Lower Tract

Tests to evaluate the lower tracts include urodynamics, cystogram, and cystoscopy. Because each of these involve instrumentation, it is best to obtain a urine culture and sensitivity and give antibiotics if positive before the testing. Some indications for cystoscopy in those with voiding disorders include hematuria, recurrent symptomatic urinary tract infections, recurrent asymptomatic bacteriuria with a stone-forming organism (ie, *Proteus mirabilis*), an episode of genitourinary sepsis, urinary retention, incontinence, pieces of eggshell calculi obtained when irrigating a catheter, and long-term indwelling catheter. Cystoscopy also is indicated when removing an indwelling Foley catheter that has been in place two to four weeks and changing to a different type of management, such as intermittent catheterization (IC) or a balanced bladder. A cystoscopy is also indicated if sand or stones are noted on the catheter during a catheter change, since there is an 86% chance that there will be remaining stones within the bladder (8).

Urodynamic Evaluation

The physician's presence is important to help direct the urodynamics study. Typical decisions include how much water to put in the bladder, whether to repeat the study, and whether to have the patient sit or stand to void. Observing the patient during urodynamics also will help in getting an idea of factors that might influence the test, such as patient anxiety or inability to understand when told to void.

Evaluation of Bladder Filling (Storage Phase)

The bedside cystometrogram involves filling the bladder with water through a Foley catheter. It is often attached by means of a Y-connector to a manometer, which is used to measure the rise in water pressure. This test can be used to evaluate sensation, stability, and capacity. Major limitations to the bedside cystometrogram, in difficult to determine if small rises in the water column are due to intraabdominal pressure (ie, straining) or a bladder contraction and inability to evaluate the voiding phase.

Evaluation of Bladder Emptying (Voiding Phase)

One of the easiest screening tests to evaluate bladder emptying is a post-void residual (PVR); however, it should not be used to characterize the specific type of voiding dysfunction. A younger person should have no PVR; however, an elderly person with no voiding complaints may have a PVR of 100–150 mL. A normal PVR does not rule out a voiding problem. For example, a PVR may be normal despite significant outflow obstruction (eg, benign prostate hypertrophy, sphincter detrusor dyssynergia) due to compensatory increase in the strength of detrusor contractions, or increasing intraabdominal pressure (eg, Valsalva maneuver, Crede maneuver). Conversely, a large PVR may be due to not performing the test immediately after voiding, poor patient understanding, or an abnormal voiding situation (eg, given a bedpan at 3:00 AM).

Evaluation of Bladder Filling and Emptying

A water-fill pressure-flow urodynamic study is necessary to objectively measure both the filling and the emptying phase of micturition. The first is the filling (storage) phase during which water is infused into the bladder. The second portion of the study is the voiding (emptying) phase. The voiding phase is considered to begin when a person is told to void. More sophisticated urodynamic studies also may incorporate urethral pressure recordings, urethral sphincter or anal sphincter EMG, and videofluoroscopy.

URODYNAMIC FINDINGS/ TERMINOLOGY

The bladder may be described as overactive, underactive, or normal. The bladder is described as being overactive during the filling phase of urodynamics if the bladder has involuntary contractions (which may or may not cause incontinence depending on the sphincter activity). If this is due to a neurogenic cause, it is called neurogenic detrusor activity. If no cause is known, it is called idiopathic detrusor activity (9). During the voiding phase the bladder may be normal or abnormal. Abnormal bladder function can be further subdivided to detrusor underactivity (if there are weak contractions causing poor emptying) or an acontractile detrusor (no bladder contractions) (9). The sphincter during the filling phase is referred to as normal urethral closure mechanism or abnormal urethral closure mechanism (one that allows leakage in the absence of a bladder contraction). The point at which this occurs is known as the detrusor leak point pressure (9). The abnormal urethral closure mechanism may be due to anatomic urethral hypermobility, intrinsic sphincter damage (such as fibrosis from radiation, prolonged excessive stretching of the urethra with a Foley), or spinal cord (lower motor) injury.

The sphincter during the voiding phase may be described as normal or abnormal. Normal sphincter function refers to the sphincter relaxing before the bladder contraction and remaining open during voiding. Abnormal sphincter function refers to the sphincter not relaxing appropriately. In those with suprasacral spinal cord injury (SCI), detrusor sphincter dyssynergia is defined as a detrusor contraction concurrent with an involuntary contraction of the urethral and/or periurethral striated muscle. Those with lower motor injuries and those who are in pain or nervous may have a nonrelaxing sphincter.

VOIDING PHYSIOLOGY— VOIDING CENTERS

Facilitation and inhibition of voiding is under three main centers, the sacral micturition center, the pontine micturition center, and the higher centers (cerebral cortex, particularly the anterior cingulated gyrus). The sacral micturition center (S2–S4) is primarily a reflex center in which efferent parasympathetic impulses to the bladder cause a bladder contraction, and afferent impulses to the sacral micturition center provide feedback regarding bladder fullness. Damage to the sacral cord or roots generally results in a highly compliant acontractile bladder. In individuals with partial injuries, the areflexia may be accompanied by decreased bladder compliance resulting in increased intravesical pressure with filling. The exact mechanism by which sacral parasympathetic decentralization of the bladder causes decreased compliance is unknown (10).

The pontine micturition center is primarily responsible for coordinating relaxation of the urinary sphincter when the bladder contracts. Suprasacral SCI (below the pons) disrupts the signals from the pontine micturition center, which is why detrusor sphincter dyssynergia is common in those with suprasacral SCI. The net effect of the cerebral cortex on micturition is inhibitory to the sacral micturition center. Because suprasacral SCI also disrupts the inhibitory impulses from the cerebral cortex, those with suprasacral SCI frequently have small bladder capacities with involuntary (uninhibited) bladder contractions. In those with supra sacral injuries above the pons (higher centers), loss of inhibitory impulses causes detrusor overactivity; however, signals from the pons allow coordinated relaxation of the sphincter during the involuntary bladder contraction (10). There are a variety of voiding dysfunctions that can occur after SCI (Table 75.4).

TABLE 75.4
Predicted Voiding Pattern Bases on Level of Injury

Suprapontine (from cerebrovascular disease, hydrocephalus, intracranial neoplasms, traumatic brain injury, Parkinson disease, and multiple sclerosis)

Bladder	Detrusor overactivity
Sphincter	Sphincter synergy

Suprasacral SCI (from cervical SCI, cervical metastasis)

Bladder	Detrusor overactivity
Sphincter	Sphincter dyssynergia

Sacral SCI

Bladder	Detrusor—underactive or acontractile (sometimes poor bladder wall compliance)
Sphincter	Underactive

Abbreviation: SCI, spinal cord injury.

MANAGEMENT OF VOIDING DYSFUNCTIONS

Overview

When considering various types of bladder management, three important goals should be kept in mind. These are (1) prevention of upper tract complications (eg, deterioration of renal function, hydronephrosis, renal calculi, pyelonephritis); (2) prevention of lower tract complications (eg, cystitis, bladder stones, vesicoureteral reflux); and (3) a bladder management program that will best fit into the individuals' lifestyle and allow them to be as independent as possible. The first step in managing a voiding dysfunction in a person with cancer is to identify and treat "reversible" causes. A combination of treating "reversible" causes and behavioral strategies is often very effective in resolving the person's symptoms. Supportive measures with IC, diapers, or indwelling catheter, to circumvented the problem may also used. In those with a suspected neurogenic bladder (ie, spinal metastasis) or in those being considered for pharmacologic and surgical interventions, it is important to identify the type of voiding dysfunction with urodynamics. Empiric pharmacotherapy has a risk of potential side-effects of drugs that may have no benefit or make the problem worse. Even in a person for whom the problem is going to be circumvented with IC, diapers, or indwelling catheter, a follow urodynamic evaluation is helpful to see if the catheter is still needed.

The author has found it is best to wait one to three months before the urodynamic follow-up evaluation of a person with an indwelling catheter.

Behavioral Treatment Options in Those with Urinary Incontinence or Retention

Most behavioral changes have been developed to manage those with urinary incontinence due to the bladder or sphincter. Behavioral changes include, fluid restriction, scheduled "timed" voiding, and pelvic floor "Kegel" exercises with and without biofeedback and electrical stimulation. In the elderly, these modalities have had a mean reduction in incontinence of over 80% (11). These strategies can often be optimized with the addition of pharmacotherapy.

Fluid Restriction

One of the easiest behavioral interventions involves changes in fluid intake. A baseline I&O voiding diary is very helpful for advising of changes in fluid intake. Fluid restriction should be considered for those with fluid intake over 2,000 mL. It is also important to evaluate when a person is drinking fluids. Fluid often collects in the legs, particularly in those in wheelchairs. This fluid is then reabsorbed from the legs causing a diuresis at night. Elevating the legs during the day and limiting fluid intake after 5 PM is of the very helpful at reducing nocturia and urinary incontinence.

Scheduled (Timed) Voiding

Patients with incontinence due to poor cognition, aphasia, poor mobility, or significant pain but normal bladder function often are helped by being placed on a commode or offered a urinal at set intervals (ie, timed voiding). Patients who have uninhibited contractions also can have decreased incontinence by voiding by the clock rather waiting for a sense of fullness. Once they get a sense of fullness from the contraction it is often too late to prevent incontinence. The object of timed voiding in those with an underactive urethral sphincter mechanism but normal bladder is to prevent overflow incontinence.

In general, timed voiding is not helpful by itself for those with no bladder contractions. Timed voiding would need to be combined with increasing intravesical pressure either manually (ie, Crede maneuver) or through increased intraabdominal pressure (ie, Valsalva voiding) may help prevent bladder overdistention. Unfortunately, Crede and Valsalva maneuvers may cause exacerbation of hemorrhoids, rectal prolapse, or hernia. Therefore these maneuvers should be discouraged with the exception of individuals with decreased urethral sphincter activity, such as elderly women or SCI men with lower motor lesions and sphincterotomy. Timed voiding has not been reported as a successful method of treatment in patients with neurogenic sphincter detrusor dyssynergia. Increasing intraabdominal pressure in those with sphincter detrusor dyssynergia often worsens the dyssynergia (12). In patients with weak uninhibited bladder contractions, suprapubic bladder tapping may be used to trigger a contraction.

Kegel Exercises and Biofeedback

Kegel exercises and biofeedback can be effective in those with good cognition and mobility who have mild to moderate incontinence due to the bladder or sphincter (13). These techniques work by tightening the sphincter which reflexly inhibits the bladder from having a bladder contraction. A person is usually given a two-week trial of Kegel exercises. There is a great variation in the number of sets and repetitions described by various authors (14). If this is unsuccessful, then biofeedback can be undertaken. Patients have to be highly motivated, since improvement may not be seen for four to eight weeks. The effectiveness of biofeedback has not been reported in patients with neurogenic sphincter detrusor dyssynergia.

Supportive Treatment Options for Urinary Incontinence and Retention

Supportive treatment is often undertaken while behavioral management strategies or further evaluation for pharmacological or surgical interventions are underway. Supportive treatment includes diapers, external condom catheter for men, and intermittent or indwelling catheterization.

Diapers often are helpful either as primary management or as back-up to other managements in patients with overactive bladder or normal bladder function with incontinence due to mobility or cognitive factors. Custom-fit diapers are much more cosmetic than in the past. Major drawbacks include expense, patient embarrassment, difficulty getting them on and off, and potential skin breakdowns if not changed within two to four hours after getting wet. In addition, insurance companies frequently do not pay for diapers, so these can be an added expense to a patient and his/her family.

External condom catheters often are a good option for men. An advantage over diapers is that the condom catheter needs to be changed only once a day. Major drawbacks include wearing of a leg bag, potential for penile skin breakdown, condom catheter falling off,

and a possible increase in bladder infections. The risk of bladder infections increases in those with an elevated post-void residual urine.

Intermittent catheterization, is another effective way to manage patients who have urinary retention or have detrusor overactivity and incontinence. In those with detrusor overactivity, pharmacotherapy is usually needed to quiet the bladder to prevent incontinence between catheterizations. Lapides popularized clean intermittent catheterization (CIC). He emphasized that the key to preventing urinary tract infections and upper tract problems is to keep the bladder from getting over distended. He attributed the success of CIC to the ease of performing CIC compared to sterile technique so that patients were more likely to catheterize themselves and prevent bladder over distention than with sterile technique (15). Self-contained catheterization systems have made it much easier to perform sterile intermittent catheterization.

The important principles of IC are an adequate bladder capacity (greater than 200 mL), adequate hand function and dressing skills and anatomy to catheterize oneself, and high motivation to restrict fluids to 2 L a day and to catheterize frequently enough to keep the bladder from becoming over distended (less then 500 mL) (16). There are a number of reasons why not to consider intermittent catheterization. These are listed on Table 75.5.

An indwelling catheter is an effective method of bladder management in those with urinary retention who are unwilling or unable to perform intermittent catheterization. It is also a good option for those who do not want or cannot tolerate pharmacological or surgical intervention. Principles of management of an indwelling catheter are noted in Table 75.6.

Because there is no satisfactory external collecting device for women, an indwelling catheter may be a good option if diapers cannot be changed regularly

---

TABLE 75.5
Reasons Not to Consider Intermittent Catheterization

Not able to self-catheterize or be catheterized
Abnormal urethral anatomy, such as a false passage, significant urethral sphincter, or spasticity
Discomfort or an unwillingness to self-catheterize
Poor cognition
Poor motivation or are unwillingness to adhere to the catheterization time schedule or fluid restrictions
Require high fluid intake
Persistent urinary incontinence despite treatment

Source: Adapted from Ref. 16.

TABLE 75.6
Principles of Foley (Urethral) Catheter Management

Fluid intake of at least 2 L/day
In men, keep the catheter taped on the abdomen when lying down to help prevent stretching of the urethra (hypospadius)
Try to limit catheter size to 16 Fr to avoid stretching the urethra (especially in women)
Clean the urethral meatus of incrustations with soap and water twice a day
Prevent reflux of urine into the bladder by never raising the drainage bag above the level of the bladder
Use an anticholinergic is those with an overactive bladder
Change the Foley catheter every 2–4 wks

and they are unable to perform IC. An indwelling catheter also may be an option for men who are unable to wear a condom catheter or have contraindications to performing IC.

Because an indwelling catheter can irritate the bladder, causing increased uninhibited contractions, high intravesical pressure, and decreased drainage from the upper tracts, use of an anticholinergic should be strongly considered, particularly in someone with urodynamic evidence of an over active detrusor.

Before permanently removing an indwelling Foley catheter, the authors believe it is important to obtain urine C&S tests, and to treat with an appropriate antibiotic prior to catheter removal. This is to decrease the risk of bacteremia in cases where the patient is unable to void and gets an over distended bladder. If an indwelling catheter has been in place for two to four weeks prior to switching to IC, cystoscopy is recommended. This is to remove any eggshell calculi and debris that may have collected in the bladder which has the potential of becoming a nidus for the development of large bladder stones. Prophylactic antibiotics are not recommended for a patient with an indwelling catheter because of the risk of developing resistant organisms. Complications of an indwelling catheter include the development of the following: bladder stones, hematuria, bacteremia, especially if the catheter becomes obstructed, meatal erosions, penile scrotal fistulas, and epididymitis.

Interventions Based on Urodynamic Evaluations

If behavioral treatment has not been successful and pharmacological or surgical treatment is being completed, a urodynamic evaluation to determine the blad-

der and sphincter function and give direction on where to focus the treatment. The various options are divided into incontinence or retention due to the bladder or sphincter. When considering surgical options, careful consideration has to be given to the general health of the person with cancer and expected progression of the disease. Various pharmacological and treatment options for urinary incontinence and retention are noted in Tables 75.7 and 75.8.

Incontinence Due to the Bladder

Pharmacologic Treatment Options

Pharmacologic treatment often is needed in addition to timed voiding in patients with incontinence caused by an overactive bladder. There are a number of anticholinergic agents whose primary action is to block acetylcholine receptors competitively at the postganglionic autonomic receptor sites. There are various formulations allowing it to be given orally or with a patch. Oxybutynin is formulated to give orally. However intravesical instillations have been found to be effective which significantly reduces the systemic side effects. This is because oxybutynin not only has a localized smooth muscle antispasmodic effect distal to the cholinergic receptor site, but also a local anesthetic effect on the bladder wall. The major disadvantage to intravesical instillation is that it requires catheterization

TABLE 75.7
Examples of Pharmacologic and Surgical Treatment Options for Incontinence

Incontinence Due to the Bladder
Pharmacologic Treatment Options
Anticholinergic agents
Intravesical local anesthetics such as lidocaine and bupivacaine
Intravesical capsaicin and resiniferatoxin (afferent C fiber neurotoxin)-experimental
Botulinum toxin type A injections
Surgical Treatment Options
Augmentation cystoplasty
Neurostimulation Medtronic has an FDA-approved InterStim device
Incontinence Due to the Outlet or Sphincter
Pharmacologic Treatment Options
Alpha adrenergic agonists
Periurethral bulking agents
Incontinence Due to the Outlet or Sphincter
Surgical Treatment Options
Artificial urethral sphincter
Bladder neck suspension/sling
Urinary diversion with a catheterizable abdominal stoma with a suprapubic catheter

TABLE 75.8

Examples of Pharmacologic and Surgical Treatment Options for Retention

Retention Due to the Bladder
Pharmacologic Treatment Options
Bethanechol chloride
Surgical Treatment Options
Finetech-Brindley sacral afferent stimulator
Retention Due to the Outlet or Sphincter
Pharmacologic Treatment Options
Baclofen
Diazepam
Dantrolene
Surgical Treatment Options
Surgical ablation of the prostate stainless steel woven mesh stent (eg, UroLume endourethral wallstent, UroLume stent)
Transurethral sphincterotomy
Botulinum toxin

to instill the medication. It also requires the patient or family member to dissolve the medication in water or normal saline and then instill it. This route is therefore ideal for a person who is on intermittent catheterization or has an indwelling catheter. A commonly used dose is 10 mg of oxybutynin dissolved in 15–30 mL of saline and instilled through an intermittent or indwelling catheter three times a day (17,18).

A number of other agents have been reported or are being investigated to improve storage. Intravesical local anesthetics such as lidocaine and bupivacaine block the conduction of unmyelinated C fibers, which results in an increase of functional bladder capacity. Intravesical capsaicin and resiniferatoxin also affect the afferent C fiber innervation of the bladder, leading to a decrease in detrusor overactivity and also an increased bladder capacity (19,20). Botulinum toxin type A injections into the detrusor have been shown to increase bladder capacity and to decrease detrusor overactivity. While botulinum toxin treatment has the advantage of allowing a person to discontinue oral medications, it does need to be repeated under anesthesia approximately every 6 months (21,22).

Surgical Treatment Options

Surgical treatment to improve bladder capacity would not be expected to be a common treatment in those with cancer since patients are frequently debilitated and long-term prognosis may not be known.

The usual indications for surgical intervention are severe detrusor overactivity or poor bladder wall compliance, or continued upper tract deterioration despite aggressive pharmacotherapy and other types of

management. One technique to increase bladder capacity and lower intravesical pressures is an augmentation cystoplasty, in which a portion of the bladder is removed and a larger segment of bowel is attached to the remaining bladder (23).

Neurostimulation is used in the attempt to decrease uninhibited bladder contractions. Selective sacral root stimulation increases sphincter tone, which in turn suppresses detrusor activity. Medtronic has a U.S. Food and Drug Administration (FDA)-approved InterStim device that has been shown to be effective in able-bodied individuals with detrusor overactivity. There are no studies on its use in those with cancer (24).

Incontinence Due to the Outlet or Sphincter

Pharmacologic Treatment Options

Alpha adrenergic agonists may be useful at improving minimal to moderate stress incontinence due to the sphincter. Wyndaele has reported success at decreasing urinary leakage around the Foley catheter in incomplete SCI women with patulous urethras (25). Before using alpha adrenergic agonists, it is essential that detrusor overactivity or poor bladder compliance has been ruled out with urodynamics. Otherwise, increasing the urethral sphincter tone may increase intravesical pressures, which could result in poor drainage from the upper tracts.

Periurethral bulking agents such as collagen increase urethral resistance to the flow of urine. Appell reported that 80% of female patients treated by this method were continent after two treatments (26). This should also not be used in a person with forceful uninhibited bladder contractions, since obstructing the urethra could cause back pressure into the kidneys.

Surgical Treatment Options

In patients with a selective injury affecting just the sphincter mechanism, such as post-radical prostatectomy, surgical implantation of an artificial urethral sphincter may be considered. Surgery should be delayed at least six months to one year to make sure there is not going to be a return of sphincter function. Artificial sphincters are used infrequently in adults with neurogenic bladders, because they potentially can cause upper tract damage in those with detrusor overactivity and high intravesical pressure. In addition, there is an increased risk of prosthesis infection or erosion of the cuff in SCI patients because of frequent episodes of bacteriuria (27).

A variety of surgeries have been developed to anatomically improve the urethral support and treat position stress incontinence due to the sphincter, as well as intrinsic sphincter damage, such as from a long term indwelling catheter. These procedures are generally performed percutaneously or transvaginally, and even without surgical incisions. It should be noted that while there is a high initial success rate, five-year follow-up success rates have been reported to be 31%–69% (28,29).

A potential problem is that the operation works too well and causes retention. Patients therefore should be aware of the possibility of needing to perform post-operative IC. Other surgical options for those with intrinsic sphincter damage include surgical closure of the bladder neck, followed by urinary diversion with an abdominal stoma which can be catheterized or the insertion of a suprapubic tube.

Retention Due to the Bladder

Pharmacologic Treatment Options

Bethanechol chloride, which provides relatively selective stimulation of the bladder and bowel and is resistant to rapid hydrolysis by acetylcholinesterase, is often used to augment bladder contractions. A review of the literature shows that bethanechol is most useful in patients with bladder hypocontractility and coordinated sphincter function (30). Light and Scott reported that it failed to induce bladder contractions in SCI patients with detrusor areflexia (31). Sporer and associates found that bethanechol increased external sphincter pressures by 10–20 cm H_2O in SCI men (32). Therefore, it should not be used in those with sphincter detrusor dyssynergia. It also is contraindicated in patients with bladder outlet obstruction. Potential side effects and contraindications must be weighed against potential benefits when pharmacologic agents are used to improve emptying.

Surgical Treatment Options

Investigators continue to try to improve voiding through the use of neurostimulation. Techniques include placing electrodes on the bladder itself, the pelvic nerves, conus medullaris, sacral nerves and the sacral anterior roots. The largest experience is with a surgically implanted Finetech-Brindley sacral afferent stimulator. There have been an estimated 800 implants over 15 years (33). Prerequisites for successful neurostimulation include an intact sacral reflex arc and a detrusor capable of contracting. Stimulation of the sacral afferent nerves causes reflex activation of the efferent nerves to the sphincter. However, this reflex accommodates so that fatigue of the sphincter occurs and the pressure generated in the urethra is overcome by the bladder contraction. A posterior rhizotomy is often performed at the same time as the sacral implant. This is done to abolish uninhibited bladder contractions, abolish contractions of the sphincter, and improve bladder wall compliance. The disadvantage of the posterior rhizotomy is the loss of reflex erections and reflex ejaculations, loss of perineal sensation, and loss of reflex bladder contractions. Kerrebroeck and colleagues reviewed the world-wide experience with the Finetech-Brindley sacral stimulator. In 184 cases, of which 170 were using the stimulator, 95% had PVRS less than 60 ccs. There was no deterioration of the upper tracts. Two-thirds of men reported stimulated erections, however only one third used these for coitus (34).

Therapy for Retention Due to the Outlet or Sphincter

Pharmacologic Treatment Options

Placebo-controlled studies have shown both a clinical and statistically significant improvement in voiding in subjects taking alpha adrenergic blocking agents. They have been shown to be effective at improving bladder emptying in patients with outlet obstruction as well as those with suprasacral spinal cord injuries and sphincter detrusor dyssynergia (35,36). Three drugs that have been used for striated external sphincter relaxation are baclofen, diazepam, and dantrolene. In the author's experience, these agents are not as effective as alpha blocking agents and should not be used as the drugs of choice for external sphincter relaxation. Baclofen functions as an agonist for the inhibitory neurotransmitter gamma-aminobutyric acid (GABA), which blocks excitatory synaptic transmission, resulting in external sphincter relaxation. Diazepam is believed to cause external sphincter relaxation by increasing GABA inhibitory transmission in the spinal cord. Dantrolene acts peripherally by decreasing calcium release from the sarcoplasmic reticulum, thereby inhibiting excitation-contraction of the striated skeletal muscle fibers. Potential side effects and contraindications must be weighed against potential benefits when using pharmacologic agents to improve emptying (37,38).

Surgical Treatment Options

In men with bladder outlet obstruction due to the prostate, there are a variety of surgical treatments. Many techniques are minimally invasive. Since there are so many different alternatives, it is best to consult a urologist to review the various surgical methods and expected benefits, risks and alternatives. Another treatment of outlet obstruction is the stainless steel woven mesh stent (eg, Urolume Endourethral Wallstent, American

Medical Systems) that holds the prostate open. In a recent review of men who were catheter-dependent, 84% voided spontaneously after insertion of a UroLume stent and the improvement in symptoms was similar to that seen after transurethral prostate resection. However, 1 of 6 men needed the UroLume removed within a year because of complications. A total of 104 stents (16%) failed in 606 patients who were evaluable at one year. Migration was the most common cause of failure (38 stents or 37%). Most patients initially experienced perineal pain or irritative voiding symptoms following stent placement. Follow-up prevented conclusions on stent durability beyond one year. This review supports the recommendation that stents should be considered only in patients at high risk (39). Transurethral sphincterotomy is a well established treatment for SCI men with sphincter detrusor sphincter dyssynergia. Perkash reported an over 90% success rate at relief of dysreflexic symptoms, decrease in residual urine, decrease in infected urine, and significant radiologic improvement in those with hydronephrosis (40). The major concerns of most SCI patients are that the procedure is irreversible, it is a surgical procedure, and they will have to wear a leg bag. Longitudinal studies have shown a 25%–50% long term sphincterotomy failure rate (41).

Another method to decrease urethral sphincter pressure is botulism toxin. Dykstra and colleagues reported decreased detrusor dyssynergia in 10 of 11 men with suprasacral SCI with injection of botulism toxin into the sphincter (42). Since the initial use of botulinum toxin in men with SCI, others have expanded the use of botulinum toxin to treat pelvic floor spasticity and also to treat women. Prospective treatment was performed for voiding dysfunction in 8 men and 13 women aged 34–74 years old. The reasons for voiding dysfunction included neurogenic detrusor-sphincter dyssynergia in 12 cases, pelvic floor spasticity in eight and acontractile detrusor in one patient with multiple sclerosis who wished to void by the Valsalva maneuver. Of the 21 patients 14 (67%) reported significant subjective improvement in voiding. Follow up ranges from 3 to 16 months, with a maximum of three botulinum A injections in some patients (43).

FOLLOW-UP

It is helpful to follow up with inpatients approximately two weeks post-discharge. The main objectives of the visit are to make sure they are doing well with their bladder management program, tolerating their medications, and have adequate supplies (catheters, leg bags, etc.). If a person has an indwelling Foley catheter, the post-discharge visit is a good time to schedule their urodynamic evaluation. If a person is in urinary retention and has failed one or more trials of voiding as an inpatient, it has been the author's experience to wait approximately four to six weeks to allow the bladder to regain its bladder tone (by not being over distended) prior to a urodynamics test or another trial of voiding. Patients with spinal cord lesions are best evaluated three to six months after their initial urodynamics. If doing well, it is our practice to evaluate their lower tracts on a yearly basis. A baseline renal scan is also obtained and then repeated on a yearly basis to monitor renal function. A renal ultrasound, abdominal CT scan or MRI is done as needed (depending on the type of tumor) to evaluate renal anatomy.

REHABILITATION OF PATIENTS WITH BLADDER CANCER

Bladder cancer is one of the most common urologic tumors. More than 67,000 new cases of bladder cancer were predicted for 2007, with more than 13,700 of patients dying from this disease (44). Bladder cancer accounts for 7% of newly diagnosed cases in males, and 2.5%—in females (44). In addition, trends from 1974 indicate continuous increase in the incidence of bladder cancer. At the beginning of 2003, more than 372,000 persons were carrying the diagnosis of urinary bladder cancer in the United States (45).

Bladder cancer is virtually never found incidentally at autopsy (46,47), even though the means of its diagnosis—cystoscopic examination and biopsy—have remained almost unchanged since during the last several decades. Therefore, one cannot attribute the increased incidence of bladder cancer to technological innovations or changes in health care practice. That also means that bladder cancer almost always is symptomatic enough to be diagnosed during the life of the patient, and that preclinical latency period (time from the occurrence of disease to the development of symptoms) is relatively short.

Many compounds have been reported to be involved in the development of the bladder cancer, but not all of them were confirmed to be true carcinogens upon further studies (coffee, artificial sweeteners (48)). Occupational carcinogens include aniline dyes, combustion gases and soot from coal, and certain aldehydes such as acrolein used in chemical dyes (49). It has been estimated that occupational exposure accounts for roughly 20% of bladder cancer cases in the United States (50), with usually long latency periods (30–50 years).

Cigarette smokers have up to a fourfold higher incidence of bladder cancer than do people who have never smoked (48,51). It has been estimated that one-third of bladder cancer cases may be related to cigarette smoking (52). Chronic cystitis in the presence of indwelling catheters or calculi is associated with an increased risk of the bladder cancer as well, and the majority of patients will develop squamous cell carcinoma (53,54). Between 2% and 10% of paraplegics with long-term indwelling catheters develop bladder cancer. *Schistosoma haematobium* cystitis also appears to be one of the etiologic factors for bladder cancer. Cystitis-induced bladder cancer from all causes is usually associated with severe, long-term infections and the mechanisms of carcinogenesis are not entirely understood at this time.

Patients treated with cyclophosphamide have up to a ninefold increased risk of developing bladder cancer. A urinary metabolite of cyclophosphamide, acrolein is believed to be responsible for both hemorrhagic cystitis and bladder cancer (55). Studies suggest that the uroprotectant mesna (2-mercaptoethanesulfonic acid) may reduce the risk of bladder cancer (56). Radiotherapy for carcinoma of the uterine cervix or ovary in women results in twofold to fourfold increased risk of developing bladder cancer subsequently compared with women undergoing surgery only (57,58).

Urothelial carcinomas account for 90% of the primary bladder tumors in the United States. Squamous cell carcinomas account 3%–7% (however, in countries like Egypt, squamous cell carcinoma comprises 75% of all bladder cancers) and adenocarcinomas account for another 2%. Urinary bladder tumors can be classified by the level of differentiation as well. They can be described as papillary urothelial tumors of low malignant potential (well-differentiated), low-grade urothelial carcinomas (moderately differentiated), and high-grade urothelial carcinomas (poorly differentiated) (59). In the United States, 55%–60% of all newly diagnosed bladder cancers are well or moderately differentiated urothelial carcinomas confined to the urothelium or lamina propria (60). Forty to 45% of newly diagnosed tumors are high grade lesions, and half of them are usually muscle-invasive at the time of diagnosis (61). Five percent of the newly diagnosed patients have metastatic disease.

Cystoscopic examination and tumor biopsy is the main diagnostic method for bladder cancer. Usually, painless hematuria (microscopic or gross) is the most common presenting symptom that triggers cystoscopy. Transurethral resection of the bladder mass is usually performed next, to establish the depth of invasion (it can be therapeutic as well for the patients with tumors confined to the urothelium or lamina propria). For the staging purposes, computerized tomography scan, chest X-ray and other studies (ie, MRI, PET scan, bone scan—if needed) are performed as well.

Treatment of Superficial Bladder Tumors

The treatment for superficial and invasive bladder cancers is very different. If low-grade tumor is confined to the urothelium and lamina propria, radical transurethral excision is a real possibility, but in cases of high grade muscle invasive disease, cystectomy remains the gold standard of the treatment.

Transurethral resection of the bladder tumor (TURBT) is the main treatment option for patients with superficial bladder cancer. Though TURBT spares the bladder, it is accompanied with high recurrence rate (up to 70% (62)), and high rate of residual tumor (63). Therefore, additional treatment modalities have been developed to reduce the rate of recurrent disease, and postoperative intravesical treatment with BCG (attenuated live tuberculosis bacteria) became the standard of care for patients with superficial bladder cancer. Administration of BCG demonstrated the reduction of the recurrence rate by 30%–40% (64–66). Later studies, however, showed that this effect may be diminished over time (67,68).

Though most patients tolerate BCG therapy well, it may be accompanied with some side effects, requiring additional measures. Main side effects of the intravesical BCG therapy—increased frequency of micturition and burning during micturition—increased significantly with the frequency of the therapy, and at the end of therapy, 60% of patients reported to have side effects (69). In general, however, despite these side effects, patients expressed satisfaction with life, and their quality of life score was not much different from that of general population (69). These side effects usually can be easily treated with hydration, pyridium and anticholinergic medications. If infection is demonstrated, BCG should be withheld and antibiotics need to be used. If severe symptoms (fever, chills, dysuria) last longer that 48 hours, patients may require antituberculosis medications.

Treatment of Invasive Bladder Cancer

Virtually all patients with muscle-invasive locally confined bladder cancer, as well as some of the patients with high grade disease invading lamina propria, will require cystectomy as the major part of the radical treatment. Cystectomy offers the best chance for cure in these patients (70). Of the commonly performed urologic procedures, radical cystectomy is technically the most challenging, and is associated with the highest morbidity and mortality. Among 6,577 patients who underwent cystectomy during 1998–2002, there were 1,869 (28.4%) cases of complications and the mortality rate was 2.6% (71). Median total charge was $41,905 and median length of stay was nine days (71). However, the major problem seems to be not operation itself, but its consequences, and how to deal with them. Removal of the bladder poses a problem of urinary diversion, which requires major adjustments from the patient and may significantly alter his/her quality of life. Method of urinary diversion has a major impact on the rehabilitation of patients after radical cystectomy, and deterioration of the sexual function is another problem as well.

Urinary Diversion

Once bladder is removed, urine from the kidneys must be diverted somewhere. Urine can be diverted either into the intestine and through anal sphincter (ureterosigmoidostomy, rectal pouch, etc.), through the skin, or through the urethra (orthotopic neobladder). Ureterosigmoidostomy is the oldest method of urinary diversion and was used widely earlier, especially in children. It has been rarely used after radical cystectomy. The presence of the mix of the urine and feces in the ureterointestinal anastomosis area is associated with increased risk of infections and pyelonephritis. Ureterosigmoidostomy is associated with 6%–29% cancer development rate in the area of anastomosis after 10–20 years of latency period.

Metabolic Changes During Urinary Diversion

Before describing the individual methods of urinary diversion, it's important to discuss shortly the choice of intestinal segment, which needs to be incorporated into the urinary tract. Almost all segments of the bowel have been used for these purposes (Ileocecal or cecal, sigmoid, ileum, stomach). Use of any intestinal segment may result in metabolic disturbances, since intestinal segments, unlike the bladder wall, are permeable to urine. The advantage of using the stomach is that it's less permeable to urine solutes, acidifies the urine and produces less mucus. Stomach secrets chloride and protons, and its use in the urinary tract may result in hypochloremic, hypokalemic metabolic alkalosis— usually not a major problem, unless patient has renal failure with decreased bicarbonate excretion. In this case, omeprazol and acidification of the serum can be tried, but these measures are usually unsuccessful, and the stomach part in the urinary tract may need to be replaced. In case of jejunum, it secrets sodium and chloride and reabsorbs potassium and hydrogen, resulting in hyperkalemic, hyponatremic, hypochloremic meta-

bolic acidosis (27% of the cases). Treatment consists of rehydration with sodium chloride solution. Diuretics may be helpful (for hyperkalemia) as well. Since metabolic disturbances are pretty severe and common when jejunum is incorporated into the urinary tract, it is usually used when no other segment is available. Even in these cases, all attempts should be made to use as short a segment as possible. Use of ileal and colonic segments lead to the absorption of ammonium chloride in exchange for carbonic acid, resulting in hyperchloremic metabolic acidosis. In most cases it is mild, and can be treated with alkalizing agents, or blockers of chloride transport. Potassium replacement may be needed as well (72).

Ileal Conduit

Ileal conduit is the most common method of urinary diversion through the skin, and until recently was considered a "gold standard" of the urinary diversion after radical cystectomy. After an approximately 15 cm segment is isolated, the continuity of the intestinal tract is restored by ileoileal anastomosis. Bilateral ureteroileal anastomosis is performed with the proximal end of the isolated ileal conduit. The distal part of the conduit is brought through the rectus muscle and fascia in the right abdominal wall area. The area of urostomy is marked before operation, with patient in both standing and sitting position, so that stoma can fit under the clothes, below the beltline (Fig. 75.1A).

The proper management of permanent urostomy is the major part in the rehabilitation of bladder cancer patients after cystectomy. Effective containment of the urine and protection of the peristomal skin are essential for the acceptable quality of life. A number of pouching systems are available, which could be classified as one- or two-piece (Fig. 75.1B), flexible or rigid, and flat or convex (73). Management of the patients with urinary conduit is focused on the maintenance of the adequate fluid intake, nighttime management of the conduit, and strategies to minimize urinary odor, since most of the urinary pouches are odor-resistant rather than odor-proof.

Adequate fluid intake is critical to prevention of infection, since constant urine flow is the best protection against the colonization of the conduit. Patients must be taught to drink enough fluids (30 cc/kg/day), and to spread the consumption of the liquids throughout the day (73). Nighttime management of the urinary conduit can be a challenge. The patient either needs to get up at night several times to empty the pouch or to connect a pouch to a drainage system. They need to be taught to rinse night drainage unit daily.

Urostomy care must include the management of peristomal and stomal complications as well. Common peristomal complications include epithelial denudation, yeast dermatitis, and allergic dermatitis. For the management of epithelial denudation pouching system needs to be modified to eliminate contact between skin and drainage as much as possible. Yeast dermatitis is usually managed with the use of antifungal powder (nystatin). Systemic therapy with fluconazole can be administered as well. Management of allergic dermatitis depends mainly on eliminating the offending substance (73).

Common stomal complications include retraction, hernia formation, prolapse, and stenosis. Excessive bleeding may occur as well. Management of retraction involves the modification of the collection devise to match the surface contour. Peristomal hernias are usually managed conservatively, unless incarceration or strangulation occurs (both rare), in which case surgical intervention is needed. Conservative management of the stomal prolapse includes application of the hypertonic solution, to try and reduce stomal edema, so it can be reduced manually. Persistent or recurrent prolapse typically requires surgical intervention. Stomal stenosis, if mild, can be managed by gentle stomal dilation. However, most of these patients will require surgical intervention (73).

Continent Stoma

To avoid continuous leakage of the urine and urine collection device, continent urinary diversion can be performed with the construction of the intestinal pouch, which collects urine, and creation of the mechanism to prevent spontaneous urine leakage. This way, patient does not need to have a bag all the time, and he/she can catheterize and empty the pouch through continent stoma (so called "dry" stoma) at regular intervals (Fig. 75.1C). Continence mechanisms may use natural "valves" (ICV, UVJ, appendix), usually reinforced, or create artificial continence mechanism in the efferent limb of urinary diversion, which may be constructed using compression of tissue, peristalsis, equilibration of pressure and use of artificial valves. This type of diversion is usually used when urethra is affected by malignant process or by benign disease (ie, stricture) which makes it unusable.

Ileocecal valve (ICV) is one of the natural valves ready to be used for urinary continence mechanism. Continence is depended on ileocecal valve, an antiperistaltic length of ileum and small stoma. Earlier reports (74) stated a 94% continence rate. Later attempts were not as successful. Intraoperative examination of ICV showed complete continence in only 27% of patients, making clear the need for the enforcement of ICV in most cases (75). Surgeons used different means to enforce the continence of the ileocecal valve—tapering

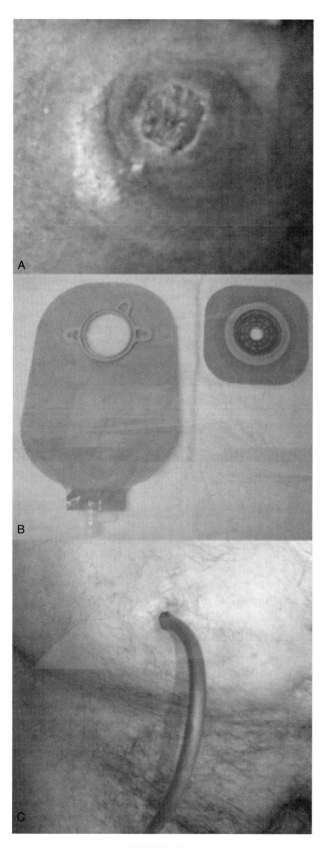

FIGURE 75.1

Stomas: Ileal conduit (A), two-piece urine collection device for urinary conduit (B), and continent catheterizable urostoma (C).

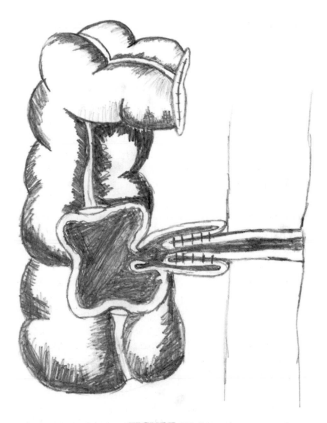

FIGURE 75.2

Intussuscepted ileocecal valve.

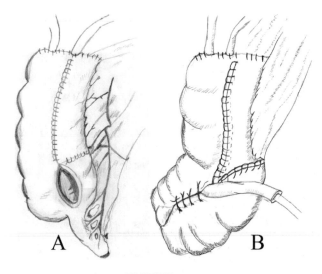

FIGURE 75.3

Appendix as a continent stoma. A: Submucosal space is created in the colon, as well as hole in the appendiceal mesentery. B: Pendix is rotated 180° and embedded into the created colonic pouch submucosally, creating catheterizable continent stoma. Small diameter of the appendix, compression of the appendix from the urine-filled reservoir, appendiceal peristalsis and valve all contribute to the continence (111).

of the efferent limb with staples and plication of the ileocecal valve (76,77), excisional plication of the ileocecal valve (78), and intussusception (Fig. 75.2) of the ileocecal valve (79). These modifications improved daytime continence rates from 90% to 100% (76,79).

The exclusion of the ileocecal valve from intestinal tract may interfere with the absorption of fats and bile salts, which are presented to the colon and result in diarrhea. Because of this, some surgeons try to avoid using ICV for urinary diversion, and prefer to construct the continence mechanism using the piece of ileum instead. Ileum can be intussuscepted (80,81), hydraulic valve can be constructed (82), or ileum can be plicated and embedded (75) to ensure continence. Using these techniques, continence rates can be achieved in more than 90% of the patients.

Appendix can be used as a continence mechanism as well, when available (83) (Fig. 75.3). Continence rate approaches 100% (84,85). Stomal stenosis was the most common late complication (10%–17%). If appendix is not available, ureter (86) or transverse ileopouchostomy (87) can be reliable alternatives.

To summarize, appendicostomy seems to be the best choice in cases of colon reservoirs. If appendix isn't available, or in the case of ileal reservoir, tapered or plicated ileum seems the next best choice.

Transverse ileostomy should have a serious consideration as well.

Orthotopic Urinary Diversion (Neobladder)

In most patients with invasive bladder cancer after cystectomy urethra can be spared, and intestinal pouch can be anastomosed with urethra, creating so called neobladder, or orthotopic urinary diversion. Technically, neobladder can be constructed in almost every patient after radical cystectomy if urethra is free of disease. In general, bladder cancer may recur in urethra in 10% of cases. There are no absolute contraindications for orthotopic diversion, if intraoperative frozen-section margins are negative, and urethra is free of disease. However, these patients need close postoperative monitoring for urethral recurrence.

Neobladder can be constructed using almost any part of the intestinal tract (except jejunum), but ileal (Fig. 75.4, Hautmann neobladder is described) and colonic reservoirs are the most common (88–92). Neobladder should have sufficient capacity to avoid reflux and incontinence due to high pressure in the reservoir. Since ileum and colon are readily available, the construction of low-pressure reservoir is not a problem. Ileal and colonic neobladders can achieve continence rates 75%–80%, while continence with sigmoid neobladder is around 50% and with gastric—33% (93).

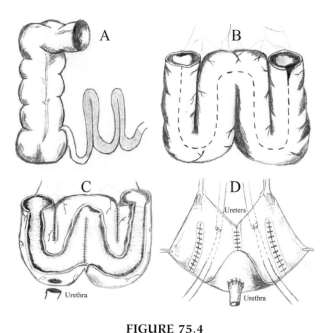

FIGURE 75.4

Construction of ileal neobladder. Most commonly used ileal segment (shaded), 45–60 cm (A); segment is isolated and ready for detubularization (B); detubularized ileal segment, with posterior wall stitched (C); final view of the ileal neobladder (D). (From Ref. 112.)

Compared with the other pouches, gastric and sigmoid reconstructions had the smallest capacity, were the least compliant, and were the most contractile. It needs to be noted that stomal reservoirs have the best continence rates (91%–100%) compared to neobladders. Day and night incontinence rates were nearly identical.

Continent urinary diversion requires the use of the larger intestinal segments (45–60 cm) compared to urinary conduit. Selection of the correct patient for continent urinary diversion cannot be overemphasized. The patient must be willing to comply with a regular lifelong followup and able to perform self-catheterization. An unwilling or hesitating patient should be offered an alternative method of urinary diversion (94).

Voiding training is one of the major parts of patient's rehabilitation after orthotopic diversion. A specially trained nurse needs to start teaching voiding techniques during hospitalization. Patients are advised to expect daytime continence in about three months and nighttime continence—in nine months. This process requires patient's active participation. Patients are instructed to void every two hours during the day and every three hours during the night. The nurse should explain to the patient that since there is no longer feedback between reservoir and brain, they should not expect a normal desire to void. Voiding occurs by relaxation of the pelvic floor and by slight abdominal straining, possibly helped with the slight hand-pressure

in the lower abdominal area and forward bending. Self-catheterization is performed every night to monitor the effectiveness of reservoir emptying. When the patient remains continent for the allocated period of time and not acidotic (determined by the serum bicarbonate levels), the voiding interval is gradually increases by half-hour increments. The goal is to maintain continence for at least 4 hours, and to create a low-pressure reservoir with the capacity of 500 mL. The functional outcome of the orthotopic urinary diversion depends on the method of reservoir construction, patient's age, and compliance with voiding instructions (95). During this process, special attention must be paid to the pelvic muscle rehabilitation with Kegel exercises (96,97). Sphincter training is taught by performing a digital rectal examination and asking patient to squeeze the anal sphincter only. Once patient knows how to perform the task, he is advised to do it at least 10 times every hour while awake, and keep contraction on for five to six seconds until continence is achieved.

Following catheter removal, the patient is at increased risk of metabolic disturbances. Since vast majority of neobladders are constructed by using ileum or colon, patient is at risk of developing metabolic acidosis, especially in the presence of residual urine or infection. The mechanism of hyperchloremic metabolic acidosis is the absorbtion of ammonium chloride across the lumen into the blood in exchange for carbonic acid (ie, CO_2 and water) (72,98). Symptoms include fatigue, weakness, lethargy, anorexia, nausea, vomiting, epigastric burning, and heartburn. Anorexia and dehydration lead to the rapid weight loss. Therefore, body weight monitoring is mandatory for these patients. They must be advised to consume 2–3 L of fluids per day and oral sodium bicarbonate (4 g/day) should be given (94). Potassium citrate, sodium citrate, and citric acid solution can be used as well (98). Meticulous lifelong monitoring is essential for oncological and functional reasons, to timely identify and prevent long-term complications. Use of large segment of ileum may lead to the vitamin B_{12} deficiency as well, therefore its levels need to be monitored and replacement given, when needed (98). Orthotopic urinary diversion is successful when patient has no infections, no incontinence, no acidosis, and no significant post-void residual urine.

Quality of Life

Cystectomy with urinary diversion is a major body image altering operation. Therefore, quality of life of these patients has been extensively assessed, to determine if their lifelong rehabilitation can be influenced by the method of urinary diversion. Radical cystectomy definitely affects the sexual function of the patients (99,100). Addressing this problem (in the form of nerve-sparing cystectomy when possible (100), insertion of penile prosthesis in younger patients (99), or vaginal reconstruction in females (101)) was associated with better sexual function in these patients. Interestingly, only 52% of patients with erectile dysfunction sought treatment after radical cystectomy (100).

Concerning the general quality of life (QOL), it seems to be the general feeling that continent urinary diversion offers better QOL in comparison to urinary conduit. In one study, only 25% of patients with "wet" stoma returned to preoperative activity, and one third of patients was willing to undergo another operation to get rid of urinary appliances, while vast majority of patients with continent diversion returned to preoperative activity (102). Other studies also confirmed improved overall patient satisfaction with continent urinary diversion when compared to a urinary conduit (103–106). Yoneda (107) also showed that there was essentially no difference in health related QOL between patients with a neobladder and age matched control population. However, several studies failed to demonstrate the advantage of continent urinary diversion over conduit (99,108–110). Patients seem to adjust well to their type of urinary diversion, and were satisfied with their conditions. As it was expected, long-term survivors of bladder cancer reported better quality of life (99).

CONCLUSIONS

In conclusion, majority of bladder cancer patients are able to achieve virtually full rehabilitation after cystectomy, especially if long-term control of the bladder cancer is achieved. It seems that continent urinary diversion with its better body image and better urinary control in comparison to conduit may be patient's best chance to fully return to their pre-disease activities.

References

1. Boring CC, Squires TS, Tong T, Montgomery S. Cancer statistics, 1994. *CA Cancer J Clin.* 1994;44:7–26.
2. Resnick NM. Geriatric incontinence. *Urol Clin North Am.* 1996;23:55–74.
3. Blaivas JG, Zayed AA, Labib KB. The bulbocavernosus reflex in urology: a prospective study of 299 patients. *J Urol.* 1981;126:197–199.
4. Rao KG, Hackler RH, Woodlief RM, Ozer MN, Fields WR. Real-time renal sonography in spinal cord injury patients: prospective comparison with excretory urography. *J Urol.* 1986;135:72–77.
5. Lloyd LK, Dubovsky EV, Bueschen AJ, et al. Comprehensive renal scintillation procedures in spinal cord injury: comparison with excretory urography. *J Urol.* 1981;126:10–13.
6. Bih LI, Changlai SP, Ho CC, Lee SP. Application of radioisotope renography with technetium-99m mercaptoacetyltriglycine on patients with spinal cord injuries. *Arch Phys Med Rehabil.* 1994;75:982–986.
7. Tempkin A, Sullivan G, Paldi J, Perkash I. Radioisotope renography in spinal cord injury. *J Urol.* 1985;133:228–230.
8. Linsenmeyer MA, Linsenmeyer TA. Accuracy of predicting bladder stones based on catheter encrustation in individuals with spinal cord injury. *J Spinal Cord Med.* 2006;29:402–405.
9. Abrams P, Cardozo L, Fall M, et al. The standardisation of terminology of lower urinary tract function: report from the Standardisation Sub-committee of the International Continence Society. *Neurourol Urodyn.* 2002;21:167–178.
10. Linsenmeyer TA, Stone JM. Neurogenic bladder and bowel dysfunction. In: DeLisa JA, Gans BM, eds. *Rehabilitation Medicine Principles and Practice*, 3rd ed. Philadelphia: Lippencott-Raven; 1998:1075–1079.
11. McDowell BJ, Burgio KL, Dombrowski M, Locher JL, Rodriguez E. An interdisciplinary approach to the assessment and behavioral treatment of urinary incontinence in geriatric outpatients. *J Am Geriatr Soc.* 1992;40:370–374.
12. Barbalias GA, Klauber GT, Blaivas JG. Critical evaluation of the Crede maneuver: a urodynamic study of 207 patients. *J Urol.* 1983;130:720–723.
13. Kegel AH. Progressive resistance exercises in the functional restoration of the perineal muscles. *Am J Obstet Gynecol.* 1948;56:238–248.
14. Wells TJ, Brink CA, Diokno AC, Wolfe R, Gillis GL. Pelvic muscle exercise for stress urinary incontinence in elderly women. *J Am Geriatr Soc.* 1991;39:785–791.
15. Lapides J, Diokno AC, Silber SJ, Lowe BS. Clean, intermittent self-catheterization in the treatment of urinary tract disease. *J Urol.* 1972;107:458–461.
16. SCI Consortium S. Bladder management for adults with spinal cord injury: a clinical practice guideline for health-care providers. *J Spinal Cord Med.* 2006;29:527–573.
17. Haferkamp A, Staehler G, Gerner HJ, Dorsam J. Dosage escalation of intravesical oxybutynin in the treatment of neurogenic bladder patients. *Spinal Cord.* 2000;38:250–254.
18. Guerrero K, Emery S, Owen L, Rowlands M. Intravesical oxybutynin: practicalities of clinical use. *J Obstet Gynaecol.* 2006;26:141–143.
19. Evans RJ. Intravesical therapy for overactive bladder. *Curr Urol Rep.* 2005;6:429–433.
20. Kim JH, Rivas DA, Shenot PJ, et al. Intravesical resiniferatoxin for refractory detrusor hyperreflexia: a multicenter, blinded, randomized, placebo-controlled trial. *J Spinal Cord Med.* 2003;26:358–363.
21. Leippold T, Reitz A, Schurch B. Botulinum toxin as a new therapy option for voiding disorders: current state of the art. *Eur Urol.* 2003;44:165–174.
22. Schurch B. Botulinum toxin for the management of bladder dysfunction. *Drugs.* 2006;66:1301–1318.
23. Chartier-Kastler EJ, Mongiat-Artus P, Bitker MO, Chancellor MB, Richard F, Denys P. Long-term results of augmentation cystoplasty in spinal cord injury patients. *Spinal Cord.* 2000;38:490–494.
24. Hussain Z, Harrison SC. Neuromodulation for lower urinary tract dysfunction—an update. *ScientificWorldJournal.* 2007;7:1036–1045.
25. Wyndaele JJ. Pharmacotherapy for urinary bladder dysfunction in spinal cord injury patients. *Paraplegia.* 1990;28:146–150.
26. Appell RA. Periurethral collagen injection for female incontinence. *Probl Urol.* 1991;5:134–140.
27. Light JK, Scott FB. Use of the artificial urinary sphincter in spinal cord injury patients. *J Urol.* 1983;130:1127–1129.
28. Reid SV, Parys BT. Long-term 5-year followup of the results of the vesica procedure. *J Urol.* 2005;173:1234–1236.
29. Gilja I. Tansvaginal needle suspension operation: the way we do it. Clinical and urodynamic study: long-term results. *Eur Urol.* 2000;37:325–330.
30. Finkbeiner AE. Is bethanechol chloride clinically effective in promoting bladder emptying? A literature review. *J Urol.* 1985;134:443–449.

31. Light JK, Scott FB. Bethanechol chloride and the traumatic cord bladder. *J Urol.* 1982;128:85–87.

32. Sporer A, Leyson JF, Martin BF. Effects of bethanechol chloride on the external urethral sphincter in spinal cord injury patients. *J Urol.* 1978;120:62–66.

33. Creasey GH, Bodner DR. Review of sacral electrical stimulation in the management of the neurogenic bladder. *Neuro Rehabil.* 1994;4:266–274.

34. Van Kerrebroeck PE, Koldewijn EL, Debruyne FM. Worldwide experience with the Finetech-Brindley sacral anterior root stimulator. *Neurourol Urodyn.* 1993;12:497–503.

35. Lepor H. Alpha blockers for the treatment of benign prostatic hypertrophy. *Probl Urol.* 1991;5:419–429.

36. Scott MB, Morrow JW. Phenoxybenzamine in neurogenic bladder dysfunction after spinal cord injury. I. Voiding dysfunction. *J Urol.* 1978;119:480–482.

37. Hoffman BB, Lefkowitz RJ. Adrenergic receptor antagonists. In: Gilman AG, Rall TW, Nies AS, Taylor J, eds. *Goodman and Gilman's the Pharmacological Basis of Therapeutics*, 8th ed. New York: Pergamon Press; 1990:221–243.

38. Cedarbaum JM, Schleifer LS. Drugs for Parkinson's disease, spasticity and acute muscle spasms. In: Gilman AG, Rall TW, Nies AS, Taylor J, eds. *Goodman and Gilman's the Pharmacological Basis of Therapeutics*, 8th ed. New York: Pergamon Press; 1990:463–484.

39. Armitage JN, Cathcart PJ, Rashidian A, De Nigris E, Emberton M, van der Meulen JH. Epithelializing stent for benign prostatic hyperplasia: a systematic review of the literature. *J Urol.* 2007;177:1619–1624.

40. Perkash I. Modified approach to sphincterotomy in spinal cord injury patients. Indications, technique and results in 32 patients. *Paraplegia.* 1976;13:247–260.

41. Yang CC, Mayo ME. External urethral sphincterotomy: long-term follow-up. *Neurourol Urodyn.* 1995;14:25–31.

42. Dykstra DD, Sidi AA, Scott AB, Pagel JM, Goldish GD. Effects of botulinum A toxin on detrusor-sphincter dyssynergia in spinal cord injury patients. *J Urol.* 1988;139:919–922.

43. Phelan MW, Franks M, Somogyi GT, et al. Botulinum toxin urethral sphincter injection to restore bladder emptying in men and women with voiding dysfunction. *J Urol.* 2001;165:1107–1110.

44. Jemal A, Siegel R, Ward E, Murray T, Xu J, Thun MJ. Cancer statistics, 2007. *CA Cancer J Clin.* 2007;57:43–66.

45. Hayat MJ, Howlader N, Reichman ME, Edwards BK. Cancer statistics, trends, and multiple primary cancer analyses from the Surveillance, Epidemiology, and End Results (SEER) Program. *Oncologist.* 2007;12:20–37.

46. Resseguie LJ, Nobrega FT, Farrow GM, Timmons JW, Worobec TG. Epidemiology of renal and ureteral cancer in Rochester, Minnesota, 1950–1974, with special reference to clinical and pathologic features. *Mayo Clin Proc.* 1978;53:503–510.

47. Kishi K, Hirota T, Matsumoto K, Kakizoe T, Murase T, Fujita J. Carcinoma of the bladder: a clinical and pathological analysis of 87 autopsy cases. *J Urol.* 1981;125:36–39.

48. Morrison AS. Advances in the etiology of urothelial cancer. *Urol Clin North Am.* 1984;11:557–566.

49. Messing EM. Urothelial tumors of the bladder. In: Wein AJ, Kavoussi LR, Novick AC, Partin AW, Peters CA, eds. *Campbell-Walsh Urology*, 9th ed. Philadelphia: Saunders; 2007:2407–2446.

50. Cole P, Hoover R, Friedell GH. Occupation and cancer of the lower urinary tract. *Cancer.* 1972;29:1250–1260.

51. Burch JD, Rohan TE, Howe GR, et al. Risk of bladder cancer by source and type of tobacco exposure: a case-control study. *Int J Cancer.* 1989;44:622–628.

52. Howe GR, Burch JD, Miller AB, et al. Tobacco use, occupation, coffee, various nutrients, and bladder cancer. *J Natl Cancer Inst.* 1980;64:701–713.

53. Kantor AF, Hartge P, Hoover RN, Narayana AS, Sullivan JW, Fraumeni JF, Jr. Urinary tract infection and risk of bladder cancer. *Am J Epidemiol.* 1984;119:510–515.

54. Locke JR, Hill DE, Walzer Y. Incidence of squamous cell carcinoma in patients with long-term catheter drainage. *J Urol.* 1985;133:1034–1035.

55. Cohen SM, Garland EM, St John M, Okamura T, Smith RA. Acrolein initiates rat urinary bladder carcinogenesis. *Cancer Res.* 1992;52:3577–3581.

56. Habs MR, Schmahl D. Prevention of urinary bladder tumors in cyclophosphamide-treated rats by additional medication with the uroprotectors sodium 2-mercaptoethane sulfonate (mesna) and disodium 2,2'-dithio-bis-ethane sulfonate (dimesna). *Cancer.* 1983;51:606–609.

57. Duncan RE, Bennett DW, Evans AT, Aron BS, Schellhas HF. Radiation-induced bladder tumors. *J Urol.* 1977;118:43–45.

58. Kaldor JM, Day NE, Kittelmann B, et al. Bladder tumours following chemotherapy and radiotherapy for ovarian cancer: a case-control study. *Int J Cancer.* 1995;63:1–6.

59. Epstein JI, Amin MB, Reuter VR, Mostofi FK. The World Health Organization/International Society of Urological Pathology consensus classification of urothelial (transitional cell) neoplasms of the urinary bladder. Bladder Consensus Conference Committee. *Am J Surg Pathol.* 1998;22:1435–1448.

60. Messing EM, Young TB, Hunt VB, et al. Comparison of bladder cancer outcome in men undergoing hematuria home screening versus those with standard clinical presentations. *Urology.* 1995;45:387–396.

61. Lutzeyer W, Rubben H, Dahm H. Prognostic parameters in superficial bladder cancer: an analysis of 315 cases. *J Urol.* 1982;127:250–252.

62. Kondylis FI, Demirci S, Ladaga L, Kolm P, Schellhammer PF. Outcomes after intravesical bacillus Calmette-Guerin are not affected by substaging of high grade T1 transitional cell carcinoma. *J Urol.* 2000;163:1120–1123.

63. Herr HW, Donat SM, Dalbagni G. Can restaging transurethral resection of T1 bladder cancer select patients for immediate cystectomy? *J Urol.* 2007;177:75–79.

64. Brosman SA. Experience with bacillus Calmette-Guerin in patients with superficial bladder carcinoma. *J Urol.* 1982;128:27–30.

65. Pagano F, Bassi P, Galetti TP, et al. Results of contemporary radical cystectomy for invasive bladder cancer: a clinicopathological study with an emphasis on the inadequacy of the tumor, nodes and metastases classification. *J Urol.* 1991;145:45–50.

66. Morales A, Nickel JC, Wilson JW. Dose-response of bacillus Calmette-Guerin in the treatment of superficial bladder cancer. *J Urol.* 1992;147:1256–1258.

67. Cookson MS, Herr HW, Zhang ZF, Soloway S, Sogani PC, Fair WR. The treated natural history of high risk superficial bladder cancer: 15-year outcome. *J Urol.* 1997;158:62–67.

68. Lerner SP, Tangen CM, Sucharew H, Wood D, Crawford ED. Patterns of recurrence and outcomes following induction bacillus Calmette-Guerin for high risk Ta, T1 bladder cancer. *J Urol.* 2007;177:1727–1731.

69. Bohle A, Balck F, von Weitersheim J, Jocham D. The quality of life during intravesical bacillus Calmette-Guerin therapy. [see comment]. *J Urol.* 1996;155:1221–1226.

70. Rivera I, Wajsman Z. Bladder-sparing treatment of invasive bladder cancer. *Cancer Control.* 2000;7:340–346.

71. Konety BR, Allareddy V. Influence of post-cystectomy complications on cost and subsequent outcome. *J Urol.* 2007;177:280–287.

72. Mills RD, Studer UE. Metabolic consequences of continent urinary diversion. *J Urol.* 1999;161:1057–1066.

73. Doughty D. Principles of ostomy management in the oncology patient. *J Support Oncol.* 2005;3:59–69.

74. Sullivan H, Gilchrist RK, Merricks JW. Ileocecal substitute bladder. Long-term followup. *J Urol.* 1973;109:43–45.

75. Gotsadze D, Pirtskhalaishvili G. Abdominal reservoirs for continent urinary diversion. *J Urol.* 1995;154:985–988.

76. Rowland RG, Kropp BP. Evolution of the Indiana continent urinary reservoir. *J Urol.* 1994;152:2247–2251.

77. Mannel RS, Manetta A, Buller RE, Braly PS, Walker JL, Archer JS. Use of ileocecal continent urinary reservoir in patients

with previous pelvic irradiation. *Gynecol Oncol.* 1995;59:376–378.

78. Smith AY, Borden T. Excisional plication of the ileocecal valve: a useful adjunct for the construction of continent urinary diversions. *J Urol.* 1996;156:1118–1119.

79. Thuroff JW, Alken P, Riedmiller H, Engelmann U, Jacobi GH, Hohenfellner R. The Mainz pouch (mixed augmentation ileum and cecum) for bladder augmentation and continent diversion. *J Urol.* 1986;136:17–26.

80. Kock NG. Intussuscepted ileal nipple valve—early experience. *Scand J Urol Nephrol Suppl.* 1992;142:59–63.

81. Boyd SD, Lieskovsky G, Skinner DG. Kock pouch bladder replacement. *Urol Clin North Am.* 1991;18:641–648.

82. Benchekroun A. Hydraulic valve for continence and antireflux. A 17-year experience of 210 cases. *Scand J Urol Nephrol Suppl.* 1992;142:66–70.

83. Mitrofanoff P. Trans-appendicular continent cystostomy in the management of the neurogenic bladder. *Chir Pediatr.* 1980;21:297–305.

84. Duckett JW, Lotfi AH. Appendicovesicostomy (and variations) in bladder reconstruction. *J Urol.* 1993;149:567–569.

85. Benge BN, Winslow BH. Use of the appendix in urologic reconstructive operation. *Surg Gynecol Obstet.* 1993;177:601–603.

86. Watson HS, Bauer SB, Peters CA, et al. Comparative urodynamics of appendiceal and ureteral Mitrofanoff conduits in children. *J Urol.* 1995;154:878–882.

87. Monti PR, Lara RC, Dutra MA, de Carvalho JR. New techniques for construction of efferent conduits based on the Mitrofanoff principle. *Urology.* 1997;49:112–115.

88. Lilien OM, Camey M. 25-year experience with replacement of the human bladder (Camey procedure). *J Urol.* 1984;132:886–891.

89. Light JK, Engelmann UH. Le bag: total replacement of the bladder using an ileocolonic pouch. *J Urol.* 1986;136:27–31.

90. Hautmann RE, Egghart G, Frohneberg D, Miller K. The ileal neobladder. *J Urol.* 1988;139:39–42.

91. Studer UE, Danuser H, Merz VW, Springer JP, Zingg EJ. Experience in 100 patients with an ileal low pressure bladder substitute combined with an afferent tubular isoperistaltic segment. *J Urol.* 1995;154:49–56.

92. Stein JP, Skinner DG. Orthotopic urinary diversion. In: Wein AJ, Kavoussi LR, Novick AC, Partin AW, Peters CA, eds. *Campbell-Walsh Urology,* 9th ed. Philadelphia: Saunders; 2007:2613–2648.

93. Santucci RA, Park CH, Mayo ME, Lange PH. Continence and urodynamic parameters of continent urinary reservoirs: comparison of gastric, ileal, ileocolic, right colon, and sigmoid segments. [Review] [21 refs]. *Urology.* 1999;54:252–257.

94. Perimenis P, Koliopanou E. Postoperative management and rehabilitation of patients receiving an ileal orthotopic bladder substitution. *Urol Nurs.* 2004;24:383–386.

95. Madersbacher S, Mohrle K, Burkhard F, Studer UE. Long-term voiding pattern of patients with ileal orthotopic bladder substitutes. *J Urol.* 2002;167:2052–2057.

96. Moul JW. Pelvic muscle rehabilitation in males following prostatectomy. *Urol Nurs.* 1998;18:296–301.

97. Kolcaba K, Dowd T, Winslow EH, Jacobson AF. Kegel exercises. Strengthening the weak pelvic floor muscles that cause urinary incontinence. *Am J Nurs.* 2000;100:59.

98. Dahl DM, McDougal WS. Use of intestinal segments in urinary diversion. In: Wein AJ, Kavoussi LR, Novick AC, Partin AW, Peters CA, eds. *Campbell-Walsh Urology,* 9th ed. Philadelphia: Saunders; 2007:2534–2578.

99. Hart S, Skinner EC, Meyerowitz BE, Boyd S, Lieskovsky G, Skinner DG. Quality of life after radical cystectomy for bladder cancer in patients with an ileal conduit, cutaneous or urethral kock pouch.[see comment]. *J Urol.* 1999;162:77–81.

100. Zippe CD, Raina R, Massanyi EZ, et al. Sexual function after male radical cystectomy in a sexually active population. *Urology.* 2004;64:682–685.

101. Gotsadze D, Charkviani L, Nemsadze G, Tsintsadze I, Pirtskhalaishvili G. Continent urinary diversion (Gotsadze Pouch) after pelvic exenteration for gynaecological malignancies. *Eur J Gynaecol Oncol.* 1994;15:369–371.

102. Gotsadze DT, Pirtskhalaishvili GG. The quality of life of patients after cystectomy for cancer. *Voprosy Onkologii.* 1992;38:489–493.

103. Yoneda T, Igawa M, Shiina H, Shigeno K, Urakami S. Postoperative morbidity, functional results and quality of life of patients following orthotopic neobladder reconstruction. *Int J Urol.* 2003;10:119–125.

104. Protogerou V, Moschou M, Antoniou N, Varkarakis J, Bamias A, Deliveliotis C. Modified S-pouch neobladder vs ileal conduit and a matched control population: a quality-of-life survey. *BJU Int.* 2004;94:350–354.

105. Burkhard FC, Kessler TM, Mills R, Studer UE. Continent urinary diversion. *Crit Rev Oncol Hematol.* 2006;57:255–264.

106. Henningsohn L. Quality of life after therapy for muscle-invasive bladder cancer. *Curr Opin Urol.* 2006;16:356–360.

107. Yoneda T, Adachi H, Urakami S, et al. Health related quality of life after orthotopic neobladder construction and its comparison with normative values in the Japanese population. *J Urol.* 2005;174:1944–1947.

108. Kitamura H, Miyao N, Yanase M, et al. Quality of life in patients having an ileal conduit, continent reservoir or orthotopic neobladder after cystectomy for bladder carcinoma. *Int J Urol.* 1999;6:393–399.

109. Gerharz EW, Mansson A, Hunt S, Skinner EC, Mansson W. Quality of life after cystectomy and urinary diversion: an evidence based analysis. *J Urol.* 2005;174:1729–1736.

110. Allareddy V, Kennedy J, West MM, Konety BR. Quality of life in long-term survivors of bladder cancer. *Cancer.* 2006;106:2355–2362.

111. Adapted from Duckett, J. W. and Snyder, H. M. The Mitrofanoff principle in continent urinary reservoirs. *Semin Urol.* 1987;5:55–62.

112. Adapted from Hautmann RE, Egghart G, Frohneberg D, Miller K. The ileal neobladder. *J Urol.* 1988;139:39–42.

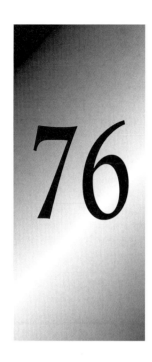

Bowel Dysfunction in the Cancer Patient

76

Susan V. Garstang

Patients with cancer often complain of adverse symptoms referable to the gastrointestinal (GI) tract. Up to 58% of patients with advanced cancer experience constipation as the most frequent GI symptom (1). However, other GI symptoms such as dry mouth, weight loss, early satiety, taste change, anorexia, bloating, nausea, abdominal pain, and vomiting occur not infrequently. Overall, constipation occurs in 25%–50% of patient with cancer, and is the most commonly occurring adverse effect of chronic opioid therapy in patients with advanced cancer (2,3).

There are many differing definitions of constipation. A consensus panel established criteria for the definition of constipation known as the Rome criteria. The Rome criteria state that in the past three months, patients with constipation should have straining, hard stools, incomplete evacuation, anorectal blockage needing disimpaction, and less than three bowel movements per week (4). In 1999, the criteria were modified to incorporate new knowledge gained, and they are now referred to as the Rome II criteria (5). The Rome II criteria for the diagnosis of chronic constipation incorporate two new symptoms to identify individuals with obstructed defecation: anal blockage, and needing manual maneuvers to defecate. In addition, the new criteria exclude subjects presenting with loose stool episodes and irritable bowel syndrome. Note that these criteria were not developed for use in patients with cancer.

Constipation in persons with cancer may be related to the patient's condition, a comorbid process, or it may

be secondary to medications (Table 76.1) Conditions seen in patients with cancer that may predispose to constipation include inactivity as well as dehydration or dietary alterations. Processes such as spinal cord or cauda equina compression (primary or metastatic), radiation myelopathy, or autonomic neuropathy may also cause bowel dysfunction and resultant constipation. Finally, medications may cause constipation; not only opioids but also antidepressants, antacids, anticholinergics, and diuretics (6). Deficiency states such as B12 deficiency may also cause myelopathy with resultant bowel dysfunction.

Symptoms of constipation include not only decreased frequency of bowel movements, but also bloating, abdominal fullness, nausea, vomiting, diarrhea, and abdominal pain. Initial history should include a review of bowel movement patterns, comorbid illnesses, and the patient's medications (past and current). Physical examination should focus on palpation of the abdomen for masses and a rectal examination looking for fecal impaction. An abdominal radiograph and routine electrolytes should complete the initial work-up. Transit time can be measured objectively using radio-opaque markers or radioactive substances that are ingested, followed by plain films or scintigraphy, respectively. Other tests for underlying conditions can be added as indicated (4).

Initial treatment of constipation should consist of increased fluid intake, increased physical activity, and changes in medications to try and reduce common

KEY POINTS

- Up to 58% of patients with advanced cancer have constipation, and more than 50% of opioid-treated patients have constipation, often despite appropriate laxative treatment.
- Constipation in persons with cancer may be related to the patient's condition, a comorbid process, or it may be secondary to medications.
- Initial treatment of constipation should consist of increased fluid intake, increased physical activity, and changes in medications to try and reduce common contributing factors.
- Strategies to treat opioid-induced bowel dysfunction include laxatives, opioid-agonists, and opioid rotation.
- Neurogenic bowel dysfunction is colonic dysfunction due to damage to the spinal cord, cauda equina, or peripheral nerves involved in innervation of the bowel, sphincters, or pelvic floor.
- Neurogenic bowel occurs in patients with cancer primarily as a result of tumor involvement of the spinal cord or cauda equina.

- Radiation can also cause spinal cord injury with resultant neurogenic bowel.
- Chemotherapeutic agents can cause bowel dysfunction, typically due to peripheral nerve damage or autonomic neuropathy from the agents, rather than spinal cord damage.
- Neurogenic bowel dysfunction can be divided into upper and lower motor neuron dysfunction, based on the location of damage to the nervous system.
- The steps for developing a bowel program in person with neurogenic bowel dysfunction are clearly outlined in the Clinical Practice Guidelines on Neurogenic Bowel Management in Adults with Spinal Cord Injury (Spinal Cord Medicine Consortium, 1998).
- There are a variety of medications used to treat bowel dysfunction, regardless of etiology. Major categories of these medications include bulk forming laxatives, osmotic laxatives, stimulant laxatives, lubricating agents, and others.

contributing factors. Placing patients on a regular bowel program is useful, and in the case of neurogenic bowel dysfunction, it is a key step in management. Most patients with cancer require an aggressive approach to constipation, with treatment targeted to the underlying exacerbating factors. In addition to common problems such as inactivity, constipating medications, and reduced fluid intake, issues seen in cancer patients that lead to severe constipation include opioid use, neurogenic bowel from cancer involving the spinal cord or cauda equina, and tumor-related dysmotility syndrome. This chapter will review normal bowel function, discuss

TABLE 76.1
Causes of Constipation in Persons With Cancer

NEUROLOGIC	METABOLIC	MEDICATIONS	OTHER
Myelopathy/Cauda Equina Syndrome: epidural spinal cord compression, leptomeningeal disease, intramedullary tumors, radiation	Hypercalcemia	Antihypertensives	Dietary alterations: poor oral fluid intake or dehydration, low fiber diet
	Hypokalemia	Anticonvulsants	
	Diabetes	Antihistamines	
	Hypothyroidism	Anticholinergics (includes antidepressants, antispasmodics, antipsychotics)	Unable to get to commode (impaired mobility)
Autonomic neuropathy: paraneoplastic neuropathy or chemotherapy toxicity	Cushing syndrome		
	Uremia	Opioids	Inactivity or lack of bowel routine
	B12 deficiency	Antacids	Hemorrhoids or anal fissures
		Diuretics	Obstruction by locally advanced abdominal or pelvic tumor
		Antiemetics	
		Contrast agents	

the pathophysiology and treatment of neurogenic bowel dysfunction, and review opioid-induced bowel dysfunction and tumor dysmotility syndrome. Management options for constipation in general and options specific to each condition will be discussed individually.

NORMAL BOWEL FUNCTION

Normal innervation to the large intestine and pelvic floor includes the somatic nervous system, the autonomic nervous system (both sympathetic and parasympathetic), and the enteric nervous system (Fig. 76.1).

The enteric nervous system includes an intramuscular plexus known as Auerbach's plexus, and a submucosal plexus known as Meissner's plexus (7). Auerbach's plexus consists of postganglionic parasympathetic cell bodies and unmyelinated fibers that coordinate peristalsis. Meissner's plexus in the submucosal layer relays local sensory and motor responses to Auerbach's plexus, which in turn relays these signals to the prevertebral ganglia and spinal cord (7). While the enteric nervous system acts under the control of the sympathetic and parasympathetic nervous systems, it can also function autonomously in the absence of normal bowel innervation (7). The resultant colonic

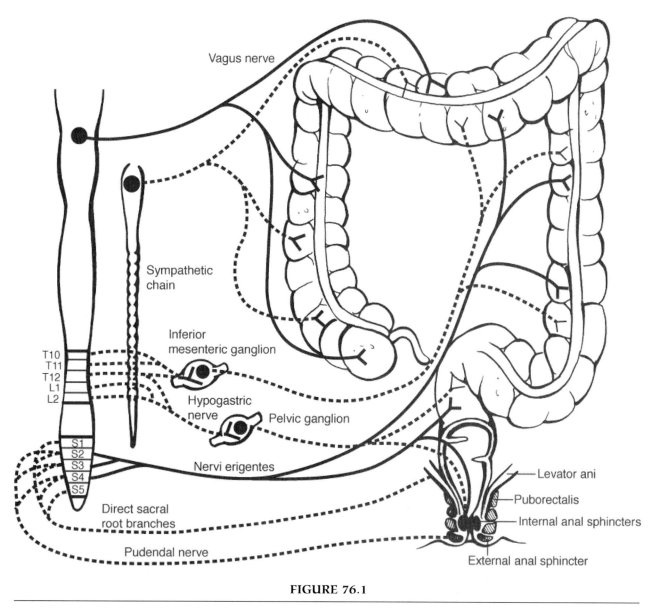

FIGURE 76.1

Innervation of large intestine and pelvic floor includes the somatic nervous system, the autonomic nervous system (both sympathetic and parasympathetic), and the enteric nervous system. (From Ref. 55)

motility relies on stretch or dilation to trigger muscle contractions, causing peristalsis to occur.

The parasympathetic nervous system innervates the small and large intestine via the vagus nerve, up to the splenic flexure of the colon. The descending colon and rectum receive parasympathetic innervation from the S2-4 segments of the spinal cord, via the pelvic nerve (also called the nervi erigentes or inferior splanchnic nerve) (8). The sympathetic nervous system provides innervation to the colon from the T5-L3 spinal segments. The mesenteric nerves (T5-L2) provide innervation to the small intestine and proximal colon via the superior mesenteric ganglion, while the hypogastric nerves (T12-L3) innervate the distal colon via the inferior mesenteric ganglion.

The somatic nervous system innervates the external anal sphincter and pelvic floor via the pudendal nerve, which also originates from the S2-4 spinal cord segments. The internal sphincter is a thickening of the colonic smooth muscle, and it is maintained in a tonically closed position by excitatory sympathetic discharges from the L1-2 levels of the spinal cord.

Normal defecation is a result of the combination of reflex and voluntary activities. Stool is propelled through the bowel by the functions of the autonomic nervous system. As the rectum distends, the internal sphincter relaxes and the distension of the rectum is sensed, which triggers a conscious urge to defecate. The external anal sphincter and pelvic floor contract tonically to retain stool (the holding reflex) (8). Anal dilation inhibits the tone of the internal sphincter (this is known as the rectoanal inhibitory reflex), as does digital stimulation (7). Defecation is primarily a voluntary process resulting from the relaxation of the external anal sphincter and pelvic floor, with contraction of the levator ani, external abdominals, and elevated intra-abdominal pressure via Valsalva to propel the stool out.

NEUROGENIC BOWEL DYSFUNCTION

Overview

Neurogenic bowel dysfunction is colonic dysfunction due to damage to the spinal cord, cauda equina, or peripheral nerves involved in innervation of the bowel, sphincters, or pelvic floor. While neurogenic bowel is not a common problem in patients with cancer, its management requires specialized knowledge to appropriately address the issues unique to this problem. Any patient whose tumor affects the spinal cord or cauda equina may develop neurogenic bowel dysfunction. In addition, radiation may affect the spinal cord or peripheral nerves and cause neurogenic bowel dysfunction. Finally, some chemotherapeutic medications can cause damage to either tracts in the spinal cord, the peripheral nerves, or the autonomic nervous system, again resulting in bowel dysfunction.

Spinal Cord Tumors

Neurogenic bowel occurs in patients with cancer primarily as a result of tumor involvement of the spinal cord or cauda equina. Tumors may be primary spinal cord tumors or represent metastatic spread. Tumors affecting the spinal cord can be categorized by location, and whether primary or secondary (Table 76.2). Nearly 70% of tumors affecting the spinal cord are spinal metastases, which are typically epidural and damage the cord by compression (9). Epidural disease from primary spine tumors such as chordoma can also cause spinal cord compression (10). Common causes of metastatic epidural spinal cord compression include breast, lung, prostate, renal, and gastrointestinal cancers as well as malignancies of the lymphoreticular system, sarcomas, and melanomas. In persons with cancer,

TABLE 76.2
Location and Etiology of Tumors Affecting the Spinal Cord

Location	Epidural (Extradural, Extramedullary)	Leptomeningeal (Intradural, Extramedullary)	Intramedullary (Intradural, Intramedullary)
Frequency	70%	20%	10%
Primary spinal tumor examples	Chordoma, sarcoma	Meningioma, schwannoma, neurofibroma	Astrocytoma, ependymoma
Metastatic tumor examples	Breast, lung, prostate, gastrointestinal, renal cancers, lymphoma	Melanoma, breast and lung cancer, leukemia, lymphoma	Lung, breast, gastrointestinal cancers, melanoma, lymphoma

between 5% and 30% will have spinal metastasis, and about 20% of these become symptomatic (11).

Leptomeningeal tumors are intradural but extramedullary, and account for 20% of tumors of the spinal cord (9). This category includes primary tumors, and so called "drop metastases" which are more common than primary tumors in this location. Intramedullary tumors are found in about 10% of cancer patients with spinal cord involvement (12). This includes primary spinal cord tumors such as astrocytoma and ependymoma, and secondary metastasis. Epidural tumors are most amenable to surgical intervention, while the intramedullary tumors are most difficult to resect (12).

Radiation Myelopathy

Radiation can also cause spinal cord injury, with resultant neurogenic bowel. Radiation-induced myelopathy can be transient, or progressive and permanent. Transient radiation-induced myelopathy is typically characterized by sensory symptoms, with Lhermitte's sign reported in cases of cervical spine irradiation (13). The pathogenesis is thought to be due to temporary demyelination of spinal neurons. This syndrome develops one to six months after radiation therapy, and gradually subsides over the next two to six months (14).

Delayed radiation myelopathy develops in segments of previously irradiated spinal cord and presents with neurologic symptoms referable to the spinal cord with no other justification to explain them (14). Delayed radiation myelopathy tends to be permanent, and progressive in nature. The resulting neurological symptoms from delayed radiation myelopathy are similar to those of spinal cord injury from other causes, including neurogenic bowel dysfunction. Thus, principles of bowel management do not differ from other etiologies of neurogenic bowel.

Chemotherapeutic Agents

Chemotherapeutic agents can cause bowel dysfunction, but this is typically due to peripheral nerve damage or autonomic neuropathy from the agents, rather than spinal cord damage. The vinca alkaloids, including vincristine (Oncovin), vinorelbine (Navelbine), and vinblastine (Velban), cause autonomic dysfunction in one-third of patients, which can include ileus, constipation, impotence, orthostasis, and urinary retention (15,16). The taxanes, including paclitaxel (Taxol) and docetaxel (Taxotere), can cause an autonomic neuropathy with bowel involvement, as well as CNS effects, seen predominantly with docetaxel (12). Bowel dys-

function associated with these neuropathies is most likely to be lower motor neuron, and should be managed accordingly.

Neurogenic Bowel Dysfunction

Neurogenic bowel dysfunction can be divided into upper and lower motor neuron dysfunction, based on the location of damage to the nervous system. Upper motor neuron bowel results from the interruption of innervation to the bowel above the conus medullaris. It is characterized by a spastic colon, with increased colonic and anal wall tone, and increased segmental peristalsis of the colon, but less propulsive peristalsis (7). Colonic transit time is diminished, with blunted post-prandial colonic response to food in the descending colon (17). In addition, spasticity of the external anal sphincter (EAS) and pelvic floor creates a hyperactive holding reflex (18). Thus, persons with spinal cord injury (SCI) resulting in upper motor neuron damage usually require a chemical or mechanical stimulus to trigger defecation.

Lower motor neuron bowel results from damage to the conus medullaris, cauda equina, or pelvic nerve. There is slowed peristalsis with decreased anal sphincter tone. The pelvic floor and EAS are functionally denervated and thus flaccid, resulting in risk of fecal incontinence. In both types of neurogenic bowel, voluntary control of defecation is gone. Management of neurogenic bowel includes control of the timing of defecation, improving the speed and completeness of defecation, and reducing the frequency of incontinent episodes.

Treatment of neurogenic bowel dysfunction relies on correctly diagnosing the type of bowel dysfunction into upper or lower motor neuron, and then applying the appropriate strategy based on both the type of dysfunction and results of treatment (7,19) Physical examination can be used to determine whether a patient has upper motor neuron or lower motor neuron dysfunction (20). Findings on neurological examination that are consistent with upper motor neuron damage include hyperreflexia, muscle spasticity with relatively preserved muscle bulk, and a spastic anal sphincter with preserved (or even augmented) reflex contraction. Lower motor neuron syndrome, conversely, is marked by the presence of hyporeflexia, flaccid muscle tone, muscle atrophy, decreased anal sphincter tone, and absent or weak sacral reflexes (such as bulbocavernosus or anal wink) (21).

Findings on imaging and historical information such as previous radiation to the spinal cord or known tumors that metastasize to the spinal cord should help to clarify the diagnosis if the physical examination is not clear. Autonomic dysfunction typically results in a lower motor neuron type bowel pattern, with clinical signs of abnormal autonomic nervous system functioning as well.

Establishing a Bowel Program for Neurogenic Bowel

The steps for developing a bowel program in persons with neurogenic bowel dysfunction are clearly outlined in the Clinical Practice Guidelines on Neurogenic Bowel Management in Adults with Spinal Cord Injury (Spinal Cord Medicine Consortium, 1998) (19). These recommendations are divided into the following sections: assessment of impairment and disability, assessment of function, designing a bowel program, nutrition, managing the neurogenic bowel at home or in the community, monitoring program effectiveness, managing complications of the neurogenic bowel, surgical and nonsurgical therapies, and education strategies for the neurogenic bowel. Readers are encouraged to read these guidelines in their entirety, but they will be summarized here.

The assessment should include a premorbid history including prior bowel habits, current symptoms, medications, and current bowel management. Physical examination should include examination of the abdomen, rectum, anal sphincter tone, and reflex integrity. Assessment of functional status should include cognition, strength, balance, mobility, spasticity, preserved function, and home environment and equipment needs.

The bowel program should be designed to provide predictable and effective elimination, and reduce problems associated with evacuation. Consideration should also be given to attendant care, schedules and role obligations, and quality of life. The determination of reflexic function guides the provider to develop a bowel program targeted to upper motor neuron (reflexic) or lower motor neuron (areflexic) bowel. Premorbid patterns of elimination can be used to guide optimal scheduling for the bowel program.

To establish a bowel program for those with upper motor neuron bowel function, follow these steps (as per the Clinical Practice Guidelines) (19):

1. Encourage appropriate fluids, diet, and activity.
2. Choose an appropriate rectal stimulant.
3. Provide rectal stimulation initially to trigger defecation daily.
4. Select optimal scheduling and positioning.
5. Select appropriate assistive techniques.
6. Evaluate medications that promote or inhibit bowel function.

Digital rectal stimulation causes left-sided colonic activity by increasing the frequency of peristaltic waves (during and after stimulation) in patients with intact sacral reflexes (22). However, patients with lower motor neuron bowel may need to maintain firmer stool to avoid incontinence than those with intact sacral reflexes and sphincter tone, and recommendations (2) and (3) above do not typically result in evacuation for patients with lower motor neuron bowel, due to lack of intact reflexes. Evacuation in these patients may require digital disimpaction or other mechanical assistance, such as large volume enemas or transanal irrigation. Pulsed irrigation evacuation has also been shown to be safe and effective in a wide variety of patients with chronic SCI, as an adjuvant to regular bowel care (23).

Once the bowel program is implemented, the program's effectiveness should be monitored, including frequency and duration of elimination and bowel care overall. Adverse reactions and unplanned evacuations should be noted and corrected. If the bowel program is not effective, a re-evaluation of the entire process should occur, including diet, fluid intake, level of activity, frequency of bowel care, position/assistive techniques, type of rectal stimulant, and oral medications. Adherence to treatment recommendations should be assessed. If changes are needed to the bowel program, these should be instituted one at a time, and three to five bowel care cycles should occur before any other change is made (19).

OPIOID-INDUCED BOWEL DYSFUNCTION

Opioids are commonly used to treat severe cancer-related pain, and while effective at managing pain, opioid use typically causes opioid-induced bowel dysfunction (OBD). Patients may develop tolerance to the analgesic effect of opioids, but tolerance does not develop to the gastrointestinal (GI) effects, especially the reduced GI motility caused by these drugs (24). Symptoms of OBD include gastric fullness, nausea, vomiting, hiccups, constipation (and overflow diarrhea), and impaction (25). More than 50% of opioid-treated patients have constipation, often despite appropriate laxative treatment (26). Opioids cause OBD by a variety of mechanisms, including decreased peristalsis and increased ileocecal and anal sphincter tone (24). In addition, liquid and electrolyte absorption is increased, and enterocyte secretion is decreased (3). The reduced gastric emptying is due to the action of the opioids on the mu-receptor in the stomach (27). The anti-secretory effect is due to the action of the opioids on the mu-receptor, which causes the release of serotonin from neurons in the myenteric plexus.

Assessment of patients on chronic opioid treatment includes inquiring about the frequency of evacuation, previous laxative use, medications that may affect bowel function, oral intake of liquids, and concomitant illnesses (28). Physical examination includes palpation of the abdomen, and a rectal examination to evaluate for impaction and assess sphincter tone. Radiologic assessment can determine the level of constipation by using established constipation scores, which are based on percentage of stool occupying each quadrant of the abdomen (29).

The mainstay of treatment of OBD is laxatives, which includes stool softeners and stimulant agents. Patients with OBD may take a combination of agents within these general categories to have an effect, and over half of patients on chronic opioid treatment require more than two types of treatment for constipation (24). Close to one-third of patients with OBD require medication rectally (24). There is no consensus regarding which laxative is best, and clinical efficacy should be considered along with cost effectiveness.

OBD is usually treated with a combination of stool softeners and stimulant laxatives; these agents will be discussed in detail in a later section of this chapter. However, specific to OBD is the use of opioid antagonists in treatment of more severe constipation. These agents have poor bioavailability, thus theoretically showing less antagonism in the CNS receptors (24). As a result, pain and opioid withdrawal symptoms can be minimized, while constipation and other GI side effects of opioids are reduced. These agents include naloxone (Narcan), which is currently available for clinical use, and methylnaltrexone (Relistor) and alvimopan (Entereg), which are still in clinical trials pending U.S. Food and Drug Administration (FDA) approval. Readers are referred to the comprehensive review by Becker and colleagues for a detailed discussion of the use of these agents in OBD (30).

Naloxone is the first opioid antagonist available and used for OBD. It is a mu-receptor-specific agent, with less than 2% bioavailability due to first pass hepatic metabolism into glucuronide, which is inactive (30). Naloxone has been shown to have laxative effects with minimal change in pain control, although some patients may have withdrawal symptoms with higher doses (31). Naloxone also decreases the number of days laxatives are needed (32). These studies also demonstrate that naloxone is effective in treating OBD, but has a very narrow therapeutic window before patients develop pain or opioid withdrawal. This is due to the fact that naloxone does cross the blood-brain barrier

and can thus reverse analgesia despite its low systemic bioavailability.

Two other opioid antagonists that do not cross the blood-brain barrier, methylnaltrexone and alvimopan, are currently in clinical trials (33). Both are quaternary opioid antagonists, which have relatively greater polarity and less lipid solubility, resulting in very little permeability at the blood-brain barrier (30).

Methylnaltrexone is a peripheral opioid receptor antagonist, which is a quaternary derivative of naltrexone. Because methylnaltrexone has a high affinity for peripheral mu-receptors, it does not cause opioid withdrawal or interfere with analgesia, even with subcutaneous or intravenous (i.v.) administration (24). Several studies demonstrated that i.v. methylnaltrexone administration significantly increases oralcecal transit times with no opioid withdrawal observed (34,35).

In addition, oral methylnaltrexone decreases the undesirable subjective effects associated with opioid medications, as well as completely preventing morphine-induced increases in oral-cecal transit time (36,37). Subcutaneous methylnaltrexone also antagonizes morphine-induced delay in oral-cecal transit time (38). More studies of methylnaltrexone are in large FDA phase III trials.

The other opioid antagonist that is in clinical trials is alvimopan (previously referred to as ADL 8-2698). Alvimopan is a mu-opioid receptor-selective antagonist, with a peripherally restricted site of action and minimal absorption (39). This drug has been shown to accelerate time to GI recovery, reduce postoperative hospital length of stay in phase III postoperative ileus clinical trials, and improve symptoms of OBD compared with placebo in phase II/III clinical trials (40). There is a developing body of literature discussing the effectiveness of alvimopan in postsurgical patients, in addition to studies in patients with OBD, because alvimopan is generally well tolerated and does not antagonize opioid analgesia (41).

In addition to the utilization of oral medications to counter the effects of opioids on bowel function, some authors suggest opioid rotation as a means of reducing constipation. Patients taking methadone rather than morphine or hydromorphone were found to have a lower laxative to opioid ratio, meaning smaller laxative doses were taken by patients whose pain was managed with methadone (42). Another study also found a reduction in constipation and laxative use in patients who were rotated to methadone (43). Patients converted from morphine to transdermal fentanyl had a significant decrease in the use of laxatives (although the number of patients with bowel movements did not change after the opioid switch) (44).

OTHER ETIOLOGIES OF BOWEL DYSFUNCTION

Tumor-Related Dysmotility

Patients with cancer may also have an alteration in bowel function due to paraneoplastic neuropathy, in addition to gastrointestinal dysmotility seen in cancer patients as a result of opioids or neurogenic bowel from spinal cord involvement. Paraneoplastic syndromes are often seen in association with malignant tumors of the lung, stomach, esophagus, and pancreas, and lymphoma (45). These paraneoplastic syndromes can include an autonomic neuropathy, or a visceral neuropathy (46). Paraneoplastic visceral neuropathy is associated primarily with small cell lung carcinoma, but can also been seen with other cancers such as breast cancer or bronchial carcinoid tumors. Patients may present with a variety of symptoms related to gut dysmotility, and often these symptoms precede the diagnosis of cancer (47). Histologically, a decrease in the number of neurons in the myenteric plexus is seen, with replacement of neurons by Schwann cells and collagen, and a plasma cell and lymphocytic infiltrate. Smooth muscle cells are not affected. Anti-enteric neuronal antibodies have been discovered, along with myenteric plexus degeneration, which has led to the hypothesis that the primary abnormality is autoimmune (48,49). This process affects the entire GI tract, and can include gastric dysmotility syndromes (50). There are also reports of motor neuron disease (MND) being associated with systemic cancer, with some patients having anti-Hu antibodies; thus a careful search for an underlying cancer is warranted in patients presenting with MND (51). The reader is referred to a comprehensive review of tumor-related dysmotility syndromes for other etiologies and further discussion (52). In most cases, bowel management will proceed based on the underlying reflexic function of the bowel, as per the section on management of neurogenic bowel.

MEDICATION MANAGEMENT OF BOWEL DYSFUNCTION

There are a variety of medications used to treat bowel dysfunction, regardless of etiology. These medications are primarily administered rectally and/or orally, although IV and subcutaneous routes are also being used for some medications, as mentioned above. The purpose of these medications, regardless of route of administration, is to alter stool consistency and improve motility and defection (7). Major categories of these medications include bulk-forming laxatives, osmotic laxatives, stimulant laxatives, lubricating agents, and others (see Table 76.3) (53).

Bulk formers are orally-administered, indigestible agents that serve to increase the water content and volume of stool. This increase in colonic residue stimu-

TABLE 76.3
Classes of Medications for Treatment of Constipation

Bulk-Forming	Osmotic	Stimulant	Lubricating	Other
Fiber (bran)	Saline laxatives: magnesium hydroxide (MOM); magnesium citrate; sodium phosphate (Fleet)	Peristaltic agents: anthraquinones (senna, cascara); diphenylmethane (Bisacodyl, sodium picosulfate)	Paraffin seed oils (flax) Mineral oil[a]	Softeners/surfactant (Docusate)[b]
Methylcellulose (Citrucel)	Poorly absorbed sugars: saccharine (lactulose)	Contact irritant (castor oil, glycerin)[c]		Rectal agents (fall into several classes in addition to local stretch)
Psyllium (Metamucil)	Sugar alcohols: sorbitol, mannitol	Prokinetic (bethanechol, chochicine, tegaserod)[d]		Opioid antagonists
Polycarbophil (Fibercon)	Polyethylene glycol (Miralax, macrogol)			

[a]some classify as stimulant
[b]may also have stimulant properties as contact irritant
[c]also an osmotic agent
[d]FDA-restricted use

lates peristalsis (28). The most common bulk-forming agents available include psyllium (Metamucil), calcium polycarbophyl (FiberCon), and methylcellulose (Citrucel), but many commercial formulations are available. Psyllium is a natural fiber that is degraded by bacteria in the bowel, which increases the risk of bloating and flatus with this agent. The other bulk-forming agents are synthetic or semi-synthetic and because they are resistant to bacterial degradation (which decreases bloating and flatus), these agents are better tolerated. All bulk-forming agents must be taken with adequate amounts of water. Some advocate avoidance of these medications in persons with cancer, as these patients have difficulty consuming enough water to make the bulk-forming agents effective.

Osmotic laxatives work by drawing water into the intestine along an osmotic gradient (28). This category includes saline laxatives, poorly absorbed sugars, and sugar alcohols. Saline laxatives are salts of magnesium, sodium, or potassium; examples are magnesium hydroxide (Milk of Magnesia), magnesium citrate, and sodium phosphate/biphosphate (Fleet's phosphosoda or Fleet's enema). Saline laxatives given orally act to draw fluid into the small intestine, which promotes colonic motility. Magnesium hydroxide also causes release of cholecystikinin, which may further stimulate motility (7). There is some absorption of magnesium in the small intestine, thus caution should be used in patients with renal disease (28). Sodium phosphate is a commonly used agent for bowel preparation before colonoscopy, but hyperphosphatemia can occur in patients with renal insufficiency.

Poorly absorbed sugars including lactulose, sorbitol, and polyethylene glycol (GoLYTELY or Miralax) are also hyperosmolar laxatives. These agents are converted to short-chain amino acids in the colon, which act osmotically to draw fluid intraluminally. These do not cause electrolyte imbalance or mucosal irritation. Lactulose is a synthetic disaccharide consisting of galactose and fructose, which is not absorbed but undergoes bacterial fermentation in the colon, causing gas and bloating as the most common side effects (28). The sugar alcohols such as sorbitol and mannitol are also poorly absorbed and undergo fermentation. Polyethylene glycol contains organic polymers that are not fermented by colonic bacteria. Miralax differs from GoLYTELY in that the former is packaged for regular use, and does not include electrolytes.

Stimulant laxatives include peristaltic stimulants, contact irritants, and stool softeners. Peristaltic stimulants include anthraquinone-containing substances such as Senna. Anthraquinones can be obtained from senna (Senokot), cascara, aloe, or rhubarb. Senna is a glycoside which is converted into an anthraquinone by the action of intestinal bacteria. It acts by generating increased propulsive activity by altering electrolyte

transport and increasing intraluminal fluid, as well as exerting a direct stimulant effect on the myenteric plexus which increases intestinal motility (7). An oral dose of senna takes 6–12 hours to act, and promotes emptying usually in concert with rectal stimulation (chemically or mechanically). Anthraquinones can cause melanosis coli, a benign condition with hyperpigmentation of the colon that is usually reversible within 12 months of stopping the medication, and not associated with colon cancer or myenteric nerve damage (28). Other stimulant laxatives include bisacodyl (Dulcolax), which is available in oral or rectal formulation, sodium picosulfate, and castor oil; these are all polyphenolic derivatives.

Stool softeners include docusate sodium (Colace) and potassium (Dialose). These are thought to act by lowering the surface tension of stool and allowing water and lipids to enter. They may also have an irritating action on the mucosa by stimulating the secretion of mucous, water, and electrolytes (54). Docusate may increase the uptake of other drugs, thereby increasing their toxicity. Other agents that act as stool softeners include liquid paraffin, mineral oil, and seed oils (such as flax seed, croton, or arachis oils). These agents act as lubricant laxatives, but can cause decreased absorption of fat-soluble vitamins.

Many different types of rectal agents, including enemas of varying composition and volume, are used in clinical practice. In general, enemas tend to act within two to six hours, but are messy and unpredictable, and may result in abdominal cramping (7). Glycerin suppositories act to stimulate rectal contraction by a direct irritating effect on the colonic mucosa and hyperosmolar action. Glycerin (soap suds) enemas act in a similar manner, but also increase colonic motility triggered by the increased fluid in the colon. Saline enemas act directly on the colonic mucosa to cause an influx of water and electrolytes, stimulating the distal colon and rectum. Therevac mini-enemas are small volume (4 mL) liquid enemas with contain docusate sodium in a base of glycerin and polyethylene glycol. These also come with benzocaine, which anesthetizes the rectal mucosa and may reduce autonomic dysreflexia in those who are prone. Therevac mini-enemas act within 15 minutes, and the mechanism of action is derived from the agents in the mini-enema. Bisacodyl also can be given in suppository form, where it maintains its peristaltic stimulant properties. The base used (ie, polyethylene glycol or vegetable oil) can affect the pharmacological properties of the delivery of medication.

CONCLUSIONS

Patients with cancer often have GI complications, with constipation being the most common adverse symptom referable to the GI tract in this population. Causes of constipation include neurologic involvement, metabolic or systemic illnesses, medications, and other factors such as dietary changes or immobility. Neurogenic bowel in persons with cancer should be classified as either upper or lower motor neuron, and treated accordingly. This dysfunction can be due to primary or metastatic tumor involvement, or the effects of radiation or chemotherapy. Tumor-related dysmotility syndromes also cause bowel dysfunction by affecting the autonomic or enteric nervous system. Opioid-induced bowel dysfunction is a common cause of constipation in persons with cancer who are treated with opioids. Treatments include standard laxative regimens as well as opioid antagonists. In summary, there are many causes of bowel dysfunction in the cancer patient, all which can be effectively managed with medications and principles of bowel care regimens taken from the neurogenic bowel population.

References

1. Komurcu S, Nelson KA, Walsh D, Ford RB, Rybicki LA. Gastrointestinal symptoms among inpatients with advanced cancer. *Am J Hosp Palliat Care.* September–October 2002;19(5): 351–355.
2. Fallon M, O'Neill B. ABC of palliative care. Constipation and diarrhoea. *BMJ.* November 15, 1997;315(7118):1293–1296.
3. Mancini I, Bruera E. Constipation in advanced cancer patients. *Support Care Cancer.* July 1998;6(4):356–364.
4. Lagman RL, Davis MP, LeGrand SB, Walsh D. Common symptoms in advanced cancer. *Surg Clin North Am.* April 2005;85(2):237–255.
5. Drossman DA. The functional gastrointestinal disorders and the Rome II process. *Gut.* September 1999;45(Suppl 2):II1–II5.
6. McNicol E, Horowicz-Mehler N, Fisk RA, et al. Management of opioid side effects in cancer-related and chronic noncancer pain: a systematic review. *J Pain.* June 2003;4(5):231–256.
7. Stiens SA, Bergman SB, Goetz LL. Neurogenic bowel dysfunction after spinal cord injury: clinical evaluation and rehabilitative management. *Arch Phys Med Rehabil.* March 1997;78(3 Suppl):S86–S102.
8. Craggs MD. Pelvic somato-visceral reflexes after spinal cord injury: measures of functional loss and partial preservation. *Prog Brain Res.* 2006;152:205–219.
9. Jacobs WB, Perrin RG. Evaluation and treatment of spinal metastases: an overview. *Neurosurg Focus.* December 15, 2001;11(6):e10.
10. Newton HB, Newton CL, Gatens C, Hebert R, Pack R. Spinal cord tumors: review of etiology, diagnosis, and multidisciplinary approach to treatment. *Cancer Pract.* July–August 1995;3(4):207–218.
11. Gabriel K, Schiff D. Metastatic spinal cord compression by solid tumors. *Semin Neurol.* December 2004;24(4):375–383.
12. St Clair WH, Arnold SM, Sloan AE, Regine WF. Spinal cord and peripheral nerve injury: current management and investigations. *Semin Radiat Oncol.* July 2003;13(3):322–332.
13. Thornton AF, Zimberg SH, Greenberg HS, Sullivan MJ. Protracted Lhermitte's sign following head and neck irradiation. *Arch Otolaryngol Head Neck Surg.* November 1991;117(11):1300–1303.
14. Rampling R, Symonds P. Radiation myelopathy. *Curr Opin Neurol.* December 1998;11(6):627–632.
15. Miller BR. Neurotoxicity and vincristine. *JAMA.* April 12, 1985;253(14):2045.
16. Pace A, Bove L, Nistico C, et al. Vinorelbine neurotoxicity: clinical and neurophysiological findings in 23 patients. *J Neurol Neurosurg Psychiatry.* October 1996;61(4):409–411.
17. Fajardo NR, Pasiliao RV, Modeste-Duncan R, Creasey G, Bauman WA, Korsten MA. Decreased colonic motility in persons with chronic spinal cord injury. *Am J Gastroenterol.* January 2003;98(1):128–134.
18. Holmes GM, Rogers RC, Bresnahan JC, Beattie MS. External anal sphincter hyperreflexia following spinal transection in the rat. *J Neurotrauma.* June 1998;15(6):451–457.
19. Clinical practice guidelines: Neurogenic bowel management in adults with spinal cord injury. Spinal Cord Medicine Consortium. *J Spinal Cord Med.* July 1998;21(3):248–293.
20. Mayer NH, Esquenazi A, Childers MK. Common patterns of clinical motor dysfunction. *Muscle Nerve Suppl.* 1997;6:S21–S35.
21. Sheean G. The pathophysiology of spasticity. *Eur J Neurol.* May 2002;9(Suppl 1):3–9; discussion 53–61.
22. Korsten MA, Singal AK, Monga A, et al. Anorectal stimulation causes increased colonic motor activity in subjects with spinal cord injury. *J Spinal Cord Med.* 2007;30(1):31–35.
23. Puet TA, Jackson H, Amy S. Use of pulsed irrigation evacuation in the management of the neuropathic bowel. *Spinal Cord.* October 1997;35(10):694–699.
24. Tamayo AC, Diaz-Zuluaga PA. Management of opioid-induced bowel dysfunction in cancer patients. *Support Care Cancer.* September 2004;12(9):613–618.
25. Pappagallo M. Incidence, prevalence, and management of opioid bowel dysfunction. *Am J Surg.* November 2001;182(5A Suppl):11S–18S.
26. Vanegas G, Ripamonti C, Sbanotto A, De Conno F. Side effects of morphine administration in cancer patients. *Cancer Nurs.* August 1998;21(4):289–297.
27. De Luca A, Coupar IM. Insights into opioid action in the intestinal tract. *Pharmacol Ther.* 1996;69(2):103–115.
28. Lembo A, Camilleri M. Chronic constipation. *N Engl J Med.* October 2, 2003;349(14):1360–1368.
29. Starreveld JS, Pols MA, Van Wijk HJ, Bogaard JW, Poen H, Smout AJ. The plain abdominal radiograph in the assessment of constipation. *Z Gastroenterol.* July 1990;28(7):335–338.
30. Becker G, Galandi D, Blum HE. Peripherally acting opioid antagonists in the treatment of opiate-related constipation: a systematic review. *J Pain Symptom Manage.* November 2007;34(5):547–565.
31. Latasch L, Zimmermann M, Eberhardt B, Jurna I. Treatment of morphine-induced constipation with oral naloxone. *Anaesthesist.* March 1997;46(3):191–194.
32. Meissner W, Schmidt U, Hartmann M, Kath R, Reinhart K. Oral naloxone reverses opioid-associated constipation. *Pain.* January 2000;84(1):105–109.
33. Foss JF. A review of the potential role of methylnaltrexone in opioid bowel dysfunction. *Am J Surg.* November 2001;182(5A Suppl):19S–26S.
34. Yuan CS, Foss JF, O'Connor M, et al. Methylnaltrexone for reversal of constipation due to chronic methadone use: a randomized controlled trial. *JAMA.* January 19, 2000;283(3):367–372.
35. Yuan CS, Foss JF, O'Connor M, Osinski J, Roizen MF, Moss J. Effects of intravenous methylnaltrexone on opioid-induced gut motility and transit time changes in subjects receiving chronic methadone therapy: a pilot study. *Pain.* December 1999;83(3):631–635.
36. Yuan CS, Foss JF, O'Connor M, Osinski J, Roizen MF, Moss J. Efficacy of orally administered methylnaltrexone in decreasing subjective effects after intravenous morphine. *Drug Alcohol Depend.* October 1, 1998;52(2):161–165.
37. Yuan CS, Foss JF, Osinski J, Toledano A, Roizen MF, Moss J. The safety and efficacy of oral methylnaltrexone in preventing morphine-induced delay in oral-cecal transit time. *Clin Pharmacol Ther.* April 1997;61(4):467–475.
38. Yuan CS, Wei G, Foss JF, O'Connor M, Karrison T, Osinski J. Effects of subcutaneous methylnaltrexone on morphine-

induced peripherally mediated side effects: a double-blind randomized placebo-controlled trial. *J Pharmacol Exp Ther.* January 2002;300(1):118–123.

39. Holzer P. Treatment of opioid-induced gut dysfunction. *Expert Opin Invest Drugs.* February 2007;16(2):181–194.

40. Leslie JB. Alvimopan: a peripherally acting mu-opioid receptor antagonist. *Drugs Today (Barc).* September 2007;43(9):611–625.

41. Paulson DM, Kennedy DT, Donovick RA, et al. Alvimopan: an oral, peripherally acting, mu-opioid receptor antagonist for the treatment of opioid-induced bowel dysfunction—a 21-day treatment-randomized clinical trial. *J Pain.* March 2005;6(3):184–192.

42. Mancini IL, Hanson J, Neumann CM, Bruera ED. Opioid type and other clinical predictors of laxative dose in advanced cancer patients: a retrospective study. *J Palliat Med.* Spring 2000;3(1):49–56.

43. Daeninck PJ, Bruera E. Reduction in constipation and laxative requirements following opioid rotation to methadone: a report of four cases. *J Pain Symptom Manage.* October 1999;18(4):303–309.

44. Radbruch L, Sabatowski R, Loick G, et al. Constipation and the use of laxatives: a comparison between transdermal fentanyl and oral morphine. *Palliat Med.* March 2000;14(2):111–119.

45. Stolinsky DC. Paraneoplastic syndromes. *West J Med.* March 1980;132(3):189–208.

46. Chinn JS, Schuffler MD. Paraneoplastic visceral neuropathy as a cause of severe gastrointestinal motor dysfunction. *Gastroenterology.* November 1988;95(5):1279–1286.

47. Schuffler MD, Baird HW, Fleming CR, et al. Intestinal pseudo-obstruction as the presenting manifestation of small-cell carcinoma of the lung. A paraneoplastic neuropathy of the gastrointestinal tract. *Ann Intern Med.* February 1983;98(2):129–134.

48. Lennon VA, Sas DF, Busk MF, et al. Enteric neuronal autoantibodies in pseudoobstruction with small-cell lung carcinoma. *Gastroenterology.* January 1991;100(1):137–142.

49. Condom E, Vidal A, Rota R, Graus F, Dalmau J, Ferrer I. Paraneoplastic intestinal pseudo-obstruction associated with high titres of Hu autoantibodies. *Virchows Arch A Pathol Anat Histopathol.* 1993;423(6):507–511.

50. Berghmans T, Musch W, Brenez D, Malarme M. Paraneoplastic gastroparesis. *Rev Med Brux.* November–December 1993;14(9–10):275–278.

51. Forsyth PA, Dalmau J, Graus F, Cwik V, Rosenblum MK, Posner JB. Motor neuron syndromes in cancer patients. *Ann Neurol.* June 1997;41(6):722–730.

52. DiBaise JK, Quigley EM. Tumor-related dysmotility: gastrointestinal dysmotility syndromes associated with tumors. *Dig Dis Sci.* July 1998;43(7):1369–1401.

53. Klaschik E, Nauck F, Ostgathe C. Constipation—modern laxative therapy. *Support Care Cancer.* November 2003;11(11):679–685.

54. Thomas J. Opioid-Induced Bowel Dysfunction. *J Pain Symptom Management.* 2008;35(1):103–113.

55. Adapted from Stiens SA, Bergman SB, Goetz LL. Neurogenic bowel dysfunction after spinal cord injury: clinical evaluation and rehabilitative management. *Arch Phys Med Rehabil.* March 1997;78(3 Suppl):S86–S102.

Cognitive Dysfunction in the Cancer Patient

Tracy L. Veramonti
Christina A. Meyers

Advances in cancer detection, treatment, and care have resulted in a steady increase in survival rates across all cancers combined over the past three decades. Current estimates suggest that there are over 10 million cancer survivors living in the United States in the early years of the 21st century, and this number is expected to rise as improvements in diagnosis, treatment delivery, and supportive care are realized. While many anti-cancer treatments confer an overall survival benefit, most unfortunately have the potential for unfavorable toxicities that give rise to adverse consequences for a patient's health and quality of life (QOL). Among some of the more common and distressing symptoms faced by patients with cancer is that of neurocognitive dysfunction.

CAUSES, ASSESSMENT, AND PATTERN OF NEUROCOGNITIVE DEFICITS

Causes of Neurocognitive Dysfunction

While neurocognitive symptoms are expected, and often herald the diagnosis, when cancer directly affects the brain, patients with extracerebral malignancies (eg, breast cancer, lung cancer, leukemia) frequently have multiple symptoms, including neurocognitive impairments, even before treatment is initiated (1–3). Additionally, while the success of many anti-cancer treatments has been achieved largely through multi-

modal, aggressive strategies that often combine surgery, radiation, chemotherapy and/or immunotherapy, many other cancer treatments are not highly specific and thus place normal cells and organs at risk. The central nervous system (CNS) may be particularly vulnerable to such treatments, leading to a worsening of neurocognitive symptoms and/or emergence of new symptoms after treatment commences. Furthermore, medications commonly prescribed to manage or control concurrent medical complications in patients with cancer (eg, corticosteroids, antiepileptic medications, immunosuppressive agents, antiemetics, and opioid narcotics) may also have cognitive side effects. In sum, neurocognitive dysfunction can be a primary symptom of cancer and a potential neurotoxicity of cancer treatment (4).

Neurocognitive complaints, including problems with memory, attention, processing speed, and/or difficulties multitasking, are commonly summarized broadly by patients with cancer as the experience of "chemobrain" or "chemofog." Sometimes, neurocognitive symptoms persist after treatment is completed, and even after patients (typically with extracerebral malignancies) are rendered "cured" or "disease-free." In these cases, patients may be embarrassed or even ashamed, feeling they should be thankful or relieved that their battle with cancer is over, as opposed to being distressed by a "memory problem" in the context of an otherwise successful outcome. However, the realization that many cancer treatments have potential neurotoxicities, and the importance of examining these long-term

KEY POINTS

- While neurocognitive symptoms are expected in cerebral tumors, patients with extracerebral malignancies (eg, breast cancer, lung cancer, leukemia) frequently have multiple symptoms, including neurocognitive impairments, even before treatment is initiated.
- Forgetfulness is described among patients with cancer as not recalling something they were told previously, confusing details of recent events, forgetting where items were placed, trouble sustaining attention on any one task for any length of time, or a problem dividing attention between multiple tasks at the same time (ie, multitasking).
- Neurocognitive assessment in oncology is useful for understanding cognitive problems from treatment, documenting how antineoplastic treatment regimens improve neurocognitive function, clarifying differential diagnostic possibilities (depression vs impaired executive or frontal lobe functions) and

- guiding therapeutic interventions, including pharmacologic and behavioral strategies.
- The cognitive problems in patients with brain tumors may be similar to traditional rehabilitation patients (eg, stroke or traumatic brain injury), but their disease status, recovery curve, prognosis, and need for ongoing medical treatments makes them distinctly unique.
- Stimulant therapy with methylphenidate has been associated with dramatic subjective and objective improvements in cognition and daily functioning, such as decreased fatigue, improved concentration, brighter mood, improved ambulation) in patients with brain tumors.
- Because patients with brain tumors experience predictable patterns of impairment, the possibility of intervening prior to the emergence of neurocognitive disabilities offers exciting possibilities for prophylactic behavioral rehabilitation, pharmacologic, and psychoeducational strategies.

or persisting effects of cancer and cancer treatment are underscored by numerous recent high-profile national reports addressing issues in cancer survivorship (5). The unfortunate truth is that neurocognitive symptoms may seriously compromise perceived QOL, lead to affective distress, diminish the ability to meet role-defined goals (including scholastic, vocational, and household roles), and result in reduced overall functioning and increased caregiver burden. Improved understanding of the onset, course, and persistence of neurocognitive symptoms has been an issue of critical importance, and will remain so, particularly given expected future growth in the number of cancer survivors and hence, in the number of individuals who understandably will continue to want to return to the many roles and activities they seamlessly engaged in prior to their diagnosis of cancer.

Assessment of Neurocognitive Dysfunction

Neuropsychologists working in the setting of oncology provide a quantitative assessment of the cognitive (eg, memory loss, inattention) and neurobehavioral symptoms that arise as a consequence of cancer, cancer treatment, and/or coexisting neurologic or psychological problems. One of the most frequent complaints brought to the attention of the neuropsychologist working in oncology, is that of forgetfulness. Patients with cancer may describe everyday difficulties recalling something they were told previously, forgetting or confusing details of recent events, forgetting to pass

on a message, forgetting where they have placed things in their home or office, or forgetting dates and times of appointments. Other common patient complaints include forgetting words or names of people and/or locations. In addition to these difficulties, patients may describe inefficiencies in attention, including trouble sustaining attention on any one task for any length of time or a problem dividing attention between multiple tasks at the same time (ie, multitasking). Patients often describe problems with organization or keeping up with conversations or occupational responsibilities due to slowed mental processing speed. Patients may describe their life in general as "no longer being on auto-pilot."

Neuropsychological evaluation to determine the nature and extent of a patient's cognitive impairment is a complex endeavor that requires knowledge, skill, and clinical sensitivity (6). While a memory problem or an attention problem sounds like a simple complaint, a comprehensive neuropsychological evaluation is necessary to examine the pattern of cognitive strengths and weaknesses and the likely etiology of the patient's difficulty. Brief screens of global neurocognitive dysfunction, such as those afforded by the Mini-Mental Status Examination (MMSE) (7) in this case are insensitive for documenting the kinds of cognitive disturbances most often seen in patients with cancer (8). In fact, reliance on "normal" MMSE scores as evidence for absence of cognitive dysfunction in patients with cancer may be outright dangerous (9). Additionally, simply relying on patient self-report of cognitive problems is likewise inappropriate. Because of their cognitive impairments, patients brain tumors in particular may have diminished insight into the nature, severity, or impact of cognitive problems on daily life (10). In other cancer populations, self-report of cognitive impairment has been shown to correlate more heavily with fatigue and mood disturbance than with objective evidence of cognitive dysfunction, as assessed by standardized neuropsychological tests (11–14). Thus, comprehensive neuropsychological assessment is necessary to clarify the differential diagnosis of cancer-related cognitive dysfunction and/or mood disturbance. Other differential diagnostic considerations include issues related to aging (older adults are at increased risk for having concurrent neurodegenerative diseases, such as Alzheimer disease, which may contribute to poor cognitive status), infection, and concurrent or chronic illnesses.

Neurocognitive assessment in oncology is useful for: (1) understanding what cognitive problems exist prior to initiation of treatment, both to intervene more proactively and to establish a baseline by which the neurotoxic effects of disease and treatment can be established; (2) appreciating the extent to which different antineoplastic treatment regimens improve neurocognitive function (due to better tumor control) or have short- or long-term neurotoxicities; (3) improving patient care by clarifying differential diagnostic possibilities (depression vs impaired executive or frontal lobe functions) and providing information to guide treatment decisions; and (4) guiding therapeutic interventions, to include pharmacologic and behavioral strategies aimed at reducing the functional disability associated with cancer and treatment-related cognitive dysfunction.

The feasibility and tolerability of neurocognitive assessment in patients with cancer has been well demonstrated, and neurocognitive outcomes are increasingly being incorporated into clinical trials of new antineoplastic agents (15). The utility of neuropsychological assessment is further noted by evidence demonstrating that the presence of neuropsychological impairment predicts survival better than clinical prognostic factors alone in patients with primary brain tumors, leptomeningeal disease, and parenchymal brain metastases (16–19).

Evolution and Pattern of Neuropsychological Impairment

Cognitive dysfunction has been associated with both intracerebral and systemic malignancies even prior to the induction of treatment. For example, Tucha and colleagues (20) reported cognitive dysfunction in 90% of patients with primary brain tumors, before intervention—

surgical or otherwise. Pretreatment cognitive impairment has also been described in patients with primary CNS lymphoma (21,22). However, observations of pretreatment cognitive deficits are not limited to patients with only CNS disease. Meyers and colleagues (2) reported impairments in memory, frontal lobe executive functions (eg, planning, multitasking), and motor coordination in a group of patients with small cell lung cancer before treatment. Subsequent studies have similarly documented pretreatment cognitive inefficiencies in patients with primary, nonmetastatic breast carcinoma (1), and in those with acute myelogenous leukemia and myelodysplastic syndrome (3). In sum, significant proportions of patients with various types of cancer have demonstrated that cancer itself may have adverse cognitive sequelae. Moreover, affective distress does not appear to be causally related to the presence of neurocognitive impairments prior to treatment (1).

While precise information regarding the nature, severity, and course of neurocognitive dysfunction in patients with cancer continues to emerge, a burgeoning body of literature suggests that learning and memory are among the most common neuropsychological impairments these patients face (4). This is not surprising, since learning and memory are thought to depend heavily on frontal subcortical networks in the brain, which have been shown to be preferentially disrupted as a consequence of numerous antineoplastic treatments against both intracerebral and systemic malignancies, including cranial irradiation, chemotherapy, endogenous administration of cytokines, and hormonal therapies (1,4,9,23,24). This frontal subcortical network dysfunction is reflected on objective neuropsychological testing as problems with learning efficiency (ie, acquisition) and memory retrieval in the context of relatively better memory consolidation processes. Frequently, there is concurrent evidence of additional cognitive difficulties commonly associated with frontal-subcortical white matter involvement, such as deficits in executive functions, verbal retrieval, cognitive processing speed, and bilateral speeded fine motor coordination.

For patients with brain tumors and those with intracerebral metastatic disease specifically, there may be focal or lateralizing neuropsychological findings caused by tumor impingement on critical neuroanatomic structures. For example, brain tumors in the left hemisphere may compromise language abilities and right-sided motor functioning, whereas tumors in the right hemisphere may lead to disturbances in visuospatial perception and construction and left-sided motor functioning (25). Although the nature of these focal deficits are typically less dramatic than those observed in patients with lesions of more acute onset (eg, secondary to a cerebrovascular accident) (26), certain additional symptoms, such as impaired frontal lobe executive functions (the capacity for intentional behavior, planning and organization skills, mental flexibility, abstraction, accurate self-awareness, personality), neurobehavioral slowing, and fatigue, are ubiquitous in patients with brain tumors.

Effect of Neurocognitive Symptoms on Functioning and QOL

For many patients with cancer, changes in cognition and personality may be the most feared symptoms to manage. For example, in a recent editorial highlighting patient perspectives on brain metastases in breast cancer one woman commented, "My first thought was not my brain! To me, that meant I would lose me. The threat of dying was not uppermost in my fears but losing my identity and becoming totally dependent on someone else for personal needs" (27).

The majority of individuals with primary brain tumors suffer from neurocognitive, emotional, and behavioral difficulties that compromise their independence and interfere with their academic, vocational, and/or social pursuits. Depending on the location of the brain tumor, there can be profound disturbances in personality, psychological well-being, and the ability to perform routine activities of daily living. Regarding work in particular, maintaining employment after diagnosis and treatment for a brain tumor is the exception, not the rule. In 1990, Fobair and colleagues documented that only 18% of patients return to work full-time and 10% return to work part-time after a brain tumor diagnosis and treatment (28). This finding was echoed in a recent survey conducted by the National Brain Tumor Foundation. Of 277 patients with brain tumors who responded to the online survey, 91% were employed prior to diagnosis, but only 33% were working post-diagnosis. Moreover, 62% of caregivers surveyed (*n* = 224) reported making work adjustments (eg, leave of absence, increased use of vacation time, decreased hours) and 16 % quit their jobs. Nearly half of all respondents (48%) reported downward shifts in household income (29). Prior research has demonstrated that, more often than not, it is neurocognitive difficulties, and not physical disabilities, that prevent patients with brain tumors from returning to work (30). Other diagnoses found to be particularly problematic for employment include stage IV blood and lymph malignancies and head and neck cancers(31) although the precise reasons for these latter findings have not yet been elucidated.

The impact of neurocognitive symptoms on a patient's functioning is often related to numerous individual, environmental, and sociocultural factors. Whether or not the patient was working at the time of diagnosis, the type of work he/she was doing, the pace of his/her normal work and leisure activities, availability of family and community supports, access to services, and other factors ultimately determine the degree to which a particular cognitive impairment impairs a patient's ability to function in daily life. For example, a young brain tumor patient with a severe verbal memory impairment will almost assuredly find that maintaining a typical college course load will be problematic, but the same individual may function much better if working in a well-established routine environment. At the same time, a high level business executive with an extracerebral malignancy suffering from cancer-related cognitive dysfunction (ie, "chemobrain") after undergoing aggressive medical treatment but who is otherwise considered disease-free may find even subtle inefficiencies in memory and attention to be quite frustrating and limiting in their historical work environment.

EVIDENCE-BASED COGNITIVE INTERVENTION STRATEGIES: PATIENTS WITH CEREBRAL VERSUS EXTRACEREBRAL MALIGNANCIES

Despite the often bleak prognosis and outlook associated with the diagnosis, many patients with brain tumors can enjoy improved levels of independence and functioning if provided appropriate assistance to manage the impact of cognitive symptoms on their daily life. In fact, interventions designed to minimize the adverse cognitive consequences of this disease and its treatment may represent one very important area in which there is a significant opportunity to improve the quality of a patient's life, regardless of the stage or extent of their illness. In 2000, the Brain Tumor Progress Review Group, cosponsored by the National Cancer Institute and the National Institute of Neurologic Disorders and Stroke, issued a specific call to review cognitive interventions used in other rehabilitation-related disciplines (eg, acquired brain injury, stroke) to determine whether evidenced-based interventions could be used successfully with patients with brain tumors (32). So far, answers to this call have remained limited.

Patients with brain tumors may represent a niche rehabilitation population; whereas the types of cognitive problems they experience may be similar to traditional rehabilitation patients (eg, stroke or traumatic brain injury), their disease status, recovery curve, prognosis, and need for ongoing medical treatments makes them unique. In this case, interventions focus on reducing disability in the context of an often severe, progressive medical condition. Under these circumstances, goals involve maximizing functioning, coping and QOL for the longest possible time through use of compensatory strategies, increased reliance on residual abilities, and caregiver cooperation. This approach is quite similar to that outlined in patients with progressive dementias (33) in which the underlying neuropathology is not the target of the intervention and cognitive deficits are managed and compensated for, rather than cured or rehabilitated in the traditional sense (ie, magnitude of gains tends to be less than what would be expected in individuals who experience a sudden neurologic insult, such as a stroke, followed by gradual recovery of functioning). Treatment goals, duration, and intensity must be extremely flexible in these cases to accommodate the changing needs of the patient and his/her family. For example, although not formally explored in the rehabilitation literature, our experience in working with lower functioning patients with the most severe cognitive impairments suggests that intervention efforts are most efficiently directed at acute compensatory interventions, such as making accommodations in the patient's home and hospital environment to increase structure, decrease demands for planning and decision making, and enhance orientation.

Other neurocognitive intervention candidates include patients with extracerebral disease, even those considered without evidence of active disease, who present with complaints of chemobrain or chemofog accompanied by neuropsychological evidence of associated cognitive sequelae. At either end of the spectrum, the adverse impact of cognitive symptoms on daily life may be lessened through practical, individualized, focused cognitive compensatory interventions (and in some specific cases, participation in a comprehensive, multidisciplinary program of rehabilitation). In patients with cancer, as in traditional rehabilitation populations, the specific goal of such interventions involves increasing "skill or knowledge, a change in behavior, and/or the use of a compensatory strategy that will increase or improve some aspect of independent functioning" (34).

Unfortunately, in comparison to physical symptoms, few if any specific treatments for patients with cancer target the cognitive impairments they experience—whether these cognitive impairments are mild and rather subtle (as is often the case in high functioning individuals suffering with cancer-associated cognitive symptoms secondary to neurotoxic side effects of disease and treatment) or frankly debilitating. In fact, primary cancer centers rarely offer cognitive rehabilitation services, even to patients with brain tumors, while traditional rehabilitation hospitals seldom target such individuals due to concerns about poor prognosis (30). The current state of affairs is rather surprising, given that neurologic rehabilitation disciplines focused on treating survivors of traumatic brain

injury and stroke have contributed a wealth of knowledge regarding effective behavioral practices against the cognitive impairments from which many of these patients suffer (35,36),

Comprehensive Rehabilitation Programs

A small body of literature regarding the effectiveness and generalizability of comprehensive rehabilitation programs (primarily designed for survivors of stroke or traumatic brain injury) has emerged for patients with brain tumors (Table 77.1). In the studies cited in Table 77.1, neurocognitive problems are treated in the context of an interdisciplinary rehabilitation program, which often includes a combination of care providers, including physicians, psychologists, neuropsychologists, physical, occupational, and speech/language therapists, and social workers. As can be observed in Table 77.1, studies emanating from such programs have generally revealed that: (1) persons with brain tumors who participate in a comprehensive, interdisciplinary inpatient rehabilitation program achieve significant gains in functional status; (2) participation in a postacute, outpatient, comprehensive, interdisciplinary treatment program leads to increased independence and productivity—and these gains are maintained post-discharge; (3) patients with brain tumors make gains in functional status that are comparable to other rehabilitation populations (eg, stroke, traumatic brain injury) often despite shorter length of stay, and thus lower overall cost of care; and (4) following discharge from an inpatient or outpatient rehabilitation program, patients with brain tumors enjoy improved QOL, even in the face of often progressive disease (37–41).

Goal-Focused Compensatory Interventions Against Specific Neurocognitive Symptoms

In patients with brain tumors and patients with cancer with extracerebral disease for whom comprehensive rehabilitation programs are not necessary or feasible, goal-focused compensatory interventions and behavioral strategies based on "best practices" from rehabilitation disciplines focusing on treating cognitive symptoms of noncancer populations (ie, traumatic brain injury, stroke, dementia) can often be quite helpful. As noted, while clinical experience suggests that these individualized approaches may be applied to patients with cancer-related cognitive dysfunction, there is a dearth of evidence from prospective, randomized, controlled experimental designs supporting their efficacy. In this section, we present examples from rehabilitation-related disciplines of some common, evidenced-based compensatory interventions that are applicable to patients with cancer-related

TABLE 77.1
Rehabilitation of Patients With Brain Tumors

STUDY	SUBJECTS	FINDINGS
Setting: Inpatient, interdisciplinary rehabilitation program		
Marciniak et al. (1996)	159 adults with cancer; 72 primary BT patients	BT patients made significant functional gains from admission to discharge; gains were comparable to patients with other cancer types (eg, breast, spinal cord, colon, lung). Concurrent radiation therapy or presence of metastatic disease (to brain or spinal cord in patients without BT) did not have a detrimental impact on outcome.
Huang et al. (1998)	63 adults with primary or metastatic BT; 63 CVA patients	BT and CVA patients matched according to age, sex, lesion location; admission functional status statistically similar across groups. Patients with BT made significant functional gains that were consistent with those made by CVA patients despite their shorter LOS (BT average 9 days less than CVA patients).
O'Dell et al. (1998)	40 adults with primary or metastatic BT; 40 TBI patients	BT and TBI patients matched according to age, gender, functional status at admission. Although TBI patients evidenced greater absolute functional gains at discharge, BT patients had shorter LOS (average 4 days less than TBI patients). After controlling for LOS, daily functional gains made by BT patients were statistically similar to those made by survivors of TBI.
Huang et al. (2001)	10 adults with primary BT	Patients evidenced significant improvement in total functional outcome between admission and discharge. There was no change in self-report QOL (FACT-BR) between admission and discharge; however, FACT-BR scores improved at 1- and 3-months post-discharge relative to admission. Functional outcome was not related to QOL at admission, discharge, 1- or 3-month follow-up.
Setting: Outpatient, interdisciplinary rehabilitation program		
Sherer et al. (1997)	13 primary BT patients with history of surgical resection, radiation, and chemotherapy	Two patients were discharged early due to medical complications. Six had increased independence and eight had increased productivity from start of rehab to discharge. Gains were maintained at follow up (average 8 months post-discharge). Average LOS for BT patients was approximately half as long as 150 TBI survivors treated during same time.

Abbreviations: BT, brain tumor; CVA, cerebrovascular accident/stroke; LOS, length of stay; TBI, traumatic brain injury.

cognitive dysfunction. Thus, this review will focus primarily on interventions designed to circumvent the impact of inefficiencies in learning and memory on daily life, since these are amongst the most common neuropsychological impairments patients with cancer face (4). While we also acknowledge that memory impairments do not typically occur in isolation, but rather are often accompanied by neuropsychological evidence of other frontal subcortical symptoms in patients with cancer-related cognitive dysfunction (ie, slowed information processing speed, inefficiencies in attention and executive functions), in working with these patients we have often observed that customized, practical interventions against a memory impairment involving implementa-

tion of an external aid can be helpful for managing other commonly associated deficits. In fact, as will be highlighted below, the popularity of external memory aids in traditional rehabilitation settings is secondary to their effectiveness in minimizing not only the impact of a memory problem but also deficits in attention and executive functioning (eg, planning, organization, time and goal management).

Neuropsychological interventions designed to minimize the interference of memory problems on everyday life come in diverse packages, and the reader is referred to recent reviews(36,42) for a more complete discussion of the evidence of various approaches. Of the available techniques, external memory aids (eg, checklists, planners or memory notebooks, wall calendars, and pagers) have been among the most widely used interventions for individuals with significant memory impairments following acquired brain injury (43). Their effectiveness has been well documented in the field of rehabilitation, leading one of the foremost researchers in the area to conclude that, "the literature is unequivocal in reporting that the use of external aids and compensation devices is useful for increasing the independence and functionality of people with memory impairments" (42). The Brain Injury Interdisciplinary Special Interest Group (BI-ISIG) of the American Congress of Rehabilitation Medicine for the cognitive rehabilitation of people with traumatic brain injury and stroke has further recommended compensatory memory strategy training (eg, through the use of a notebook or diary) as a practice standard for patients with memory impairment after traumatic brain injury or stroke (36).

In practice, external memory aids or cueing systems are customized specifically to meet the needs of the individual, taking into account their common activities, everyday vulnerabilities to memory failures (and thus targets for intervention), and neuropsychological strengths and weaknesses. Depending on these factors, external memory aids may vary in sophistication and reliance on technology (ie, simple wall calendar vs preprogrammed paging systems and computerized organizational media) as well as in generalizability (ie, to compensate for specific tasks or memory problems occurring across various tasks and settings). Depending on the individual patient's neurocognitive strengths and weaknesses, an external aid may be self-regulated (ie, self-directed use of a memory notebook or day planner) or the environment (ie, preprogrammed paging system) (44). Further, depending on targets for intervention, an external aid may be customized to address problems with both episodic (ie, memory for events) and prospective (ie, "remembering to remember," memory to act on future intentions) memory as well as deficits in executive functioning (eg, planning, organization, initiation of a task, and time estimation and management) (34). Systematic, explicit instruction involving supervised practice over multiple sessions has been recommended as a means of maximizing a patient's success with external aids (45–47).

As an example, if the target for intervention is solely to increase medication compliance, an external aid may involve instruction in use of a pill box to organize medications coupled with preprogrammed paging system alerts (or preprogrammed cell phone alerts) to remind a patient to take medications on time. More complicated intervention targets may involve compensation for difficulties with everyday memory failures, disorganization, and disturbances in planning com-

monly associated with memory and executive dysfunction identified on objective neuropsychological tests of cognition. This pattern of cognitive deficits often challenges patients' ability to be successful in work and personal endeavors and warrants a more sophisticated intervention plan that may involve use of a written or computerized day planner, which addresses the impact of neuropsychological difficulties across tasks and settings. In this case, intervention efforts would be directed towards systematic instruction and supervised practice in acquiring and refining the skills which facilitate use of the planner to compensate for deficits in planning and organization (eg, planning daily activities after considering the importance of tasks to be completed, time requirements associated with each task, and other conflicting responsibilities) as well as memory (eg, scheduling future appointments, recording notes of important events as they occur throughout the course of a day).

Thus, depending on their nature and scope and the needs of the patient in the context of their neuropsychological strengths and weaknesses, interventions involving implementation of an external aid against memory impairment may address not only a memory difficulty but the associated neuropsychological sequelae of executive system dysfunction commonly seen in patients with cancer-related cognitive deficits. Regardless of the specific system employed, external aids share in common the objective of limiting demands on the impaired cognitive system to help patients meet their everyday goals—whether the goal is planning and organizing a busy work schedule and reducing prospective memory failures, orienting patients to the date and time, or simply cueing patients to take medications on a specified schedule (45–54).

Although the precise nature of the interventions described above may differ in their target and scope, they all involve development of strategies to compensate for a cognitive deficit ("strategy training") rather than attempts to directly restore the underlying impaired cognitive function through repetitive practice or drills ("restitution training") (36). In fact, there has been no empirical support for the efficacy of drill-oriented approaches (eg, repetitive massed practice or general mental stimulation exercises) for restoring memory (42). As an example, Lowenstein and colleagues (55) compared instruction in the use of a memory notebook coupled with associated cognitive rehabilitation techniques to a mental stimulation condition which involved patients playing computer games such as matching pairs of letters or designs from memory, rearranging letters to generate the maximal number of words possible, and asking patients to spontaneously recall information from their recent or distant past. Patients included in this study had mild Alzheimer dementia and all received 24 individual training sessions lasting 45 minutes each. Results showed that patients who were instructed in the use of a memory notebook plus associated cognitive rehabilitation techniques improved in specific functional abilities, whereas those in the mental stimulation condition who played computer games did not. Similar findings, documenting the failure of mental stimulation exercises in restoring functioning to damaged neural circuits, have been reported in the attention rehabilitation literature as well (56). In short, there is no evidence that attempts to directly retrain damaged cognitive functions through repetitive practice on carefully selected exercises (commonly in the form of computer games) generalizes or transfers to tasks that differ considerably from those used in training. More specifically, while individuals may improve on a targeted outcome measure which is similar to that being trained (ie, from one computer game to a similar computer game) there is no support for the idea that improvement on a computer game will generalize or transfer to other tasks, and most importantly to the "real world" tasks patients with cancer are most vulnerable to err in, such as remembering when to pay bills, where one placed his/her wallet, recalling the times to take medications, or confusing events from the prior day.

Pharmacologic Management of Cognitive Impairment

As reviewed, the predilection for frontal lobe dysfunction in patients with brain tumors is secondary to adverse effects of both tumor and antineoplastic treatments. Frontal lobe dysfunction, including impairments in executive functioning manifested by apathy, diminished motivation and spontaneity together with neurobehavioral slowing and deficits in working memory, is likely secondary to disruption of the monoamine pathways of the frontal-brainstem reticular system. Additionally, catecholamines play an integral role in the modulation of attention and working memory. Stimulant therapy with methylphenidate hydrochloride, a mixed dopaminergic-noradrenergic agonist pharmacologically similar to amphetamines, has been associated with dramatic subjective and objective improvements in cognition and daily functioning (eg, decreased fatigue, improved concentration, brighter mood, improved ambulation) in patients with brain tumors (57). In a phase I trial of 30 patients with malignant glioma using a single treatment group, dose-escalating design (10, 20, 30 mg methylphenidate twice daily) patients with brain tumors demonstrated significant improvements in psychomotor speed, memory, visual-motor function, executive function, and bilateral motor speed without increased seizure activity and in conjunction

with reductions in glucocorticoid dosage (57). Adverse side effects (eg, irritability, tremors) were minimal and resolved immediately upon discontinuation of the drug. Moreover, the findings could not simply be attributed to improved mood and were particularly powerful given evidence of ongoing neurologic injury secondary to tumor progression and/or progressive radiation injury in 50% of study patients.

Lower and colleagues (58) presented preliminary data from a phase III, randomized placebo-controlled trial on the safety and efficacy of dexmethylphenidate (d-MPH, Focalin) for persistent fatigue and memory impairment in 132 adult patients with extracerebral malignancies (predominantly patients with breast cancer). Treatment with d-MPH (mean highest dose 27.7 mg/day) was associated with improvements in fatigue and in memory (as assessed by the High Sensitivity Cognitive Screen). Future studies, incorporating sensitive comprehensive neuropsychological assessment to capture the breadth and extent of cognitive impairment typically documented in patients with chemobrain are clearly warranted.

Modafinil, an oral wakefulness-promoting agent initially approved for use in narcolepsy, has also been investigated as an agent to alleviate fatigue and improve QOL in patients with brain tumors. In a small pilot study of 15 patients with primary brain tumor, Nasir (59) documented moderate to significant improvements in cancer-related fatigue in approximately two-thirds of patients after treatment with modafinil (200 mg daily, increased to 300 mg after four weeks in nonresponders). One patient had to discontinue treatment due to side effects of encephalopathy; otherwise side effects were mild (anxiety, dizziness) and did not necessitate discontinuation or drug dose reduction.

There has also been an interest in assessing the potential benefits of pharmacologic agents used in other neurologic disorders, such as Alzheimer disease, for patients with brain tumors. Shaw and colleagues (60) recently completed an open-label, Phase II clinical trial of donepezil, a acetylcholinesterase inhibitor commonly used in the treatment of Alzheimer-related dementia, in 35 patients who had undergone partial or whole-brain cranial irradiation for primary or metastatic brain tumors at least six months prior to enrollment. A 24-week course of donepezil (5 mg daily for six weeks, increased to 10 mg daily for 18 weeks) was associated with improvements in neurocognitive functioning (attention and memory) and brain-specific symptoms reflecting QOL (as measured by the Functional Assessment of Cancer Therapy—Brain Module). A phase III randomized, double-blind, placebo-controlled, multicenter trial of donepezil is being planned and investigation of other agents used in the treatment of dementia (eg, Memantine) are forthcoming.

Patients with nasopharyngeal carcinoma are particularly susceptible to temporal lobe radionecrosis after undergoing standard treatment with unilateral or bilateral temporal lobe radiation (61). The cognitive consequence of this unfortunate but common side effect primarily involves an impairment in memory. Recently, Chan and colleagues (62) examined the effect of megadose Vitamin E (1,000 IU, twice daily) using an open-label, nonrandomized, treatment versus control design, on cognitive functioning in patients with temporal lobe radionecrosis. After one year of dietary supplementation with megadose Vitamin E, patients in the treatment group demonstrated significant improvements in memory and executive functioning.

As our understanding of the pathogenesis of cognitive dysfunction in patients with cancer advances, targeted interventions based upon those mechanisms will be developed. For instance, there is growing evidence that cognitive impairment and other adverse cancer-related symptoms may be due in part to a cancer or cancer treatment-induced inflammatory response (ie, the induction of inflammatory cytokines) (3,63). Thus, modulating cytokines and their receptors may ameliorate or protect against the development of these symptoms. Research into the potential benefit of anti-inflammatory agents or specific cytokine antagonists in conjunction with standard rehabilitative approaches is just beginning and may hold great promise.

Prehabilitation Strategies: Considerations For A Preventive Model

Because patients with brain tumors often experience patterns of impairment that follow a somewhat predictable course based on tumor characteristics (eg, lesion location and size) and treatment plan (eg, surgery followed by chemotherapy and/or radiation), the possibility of intervening with patients and their caregivers prior to the emergence of neurocognitive disabilities offers exciting possibilities for prophylactic behavioral rehabilitation, pharmacologic, and psychoeducational strategies. Because of their focus on primary and secondary prevention of neurocognitive and emotional symptoms, such strategies may be considered *"prehabilitation"* as opposed to "rehabilitation." The goal of prehabilitative interventions in patients with brain tumors would be: (1) to protect the brain from further neurocognitive compromise associated with progression of disease and cancer treatment; (2) to implement compensatory behavioral strategies designed to circumvent probable problems before they progress to life-limiting disabilities; and (3) to decrease patient and caregiver distress by introducing supportive counseling and psychoeducational programs. Of note, the same "prehabilitation" model may be applied to individuals with extracerebral disease and fits particularly well with current plans for delivering quality cancer care in light of enhanced focus on issues of cancer survivorship (5).

Affective Distress and Fatigue

The National Comprehensive Cancer Network (NCCN) (64) defines distress as "a multifactorial unpleasant emotional experience of a psychological (cognitive, behavioral, emotional), social, and/or spiritual nature that may interfere with the ability to cope effectively with cancer, its physical symptoms and its treatment." A recent comprehensive review of the literature by Stanton (65) on psychological adjustment in individuals diagnosed with cancer yielded several broad conclusions: (1) individuals diagnosed with cancer are at risk for development of marked psychological distress and life disruption; (2) in patients with cancer, rates of clinically significant psychological disorder frequently exceed those of the general population; (3) for most individuals with cancer, distress remits during the first two years after diagnosis, though studies suggest that persistent psychological sequelae occur for a subset of survivors; and (4) many individuals extract positive meaning and benefit from their cancer experience.

Although a comprehensive review of the evidence supporting psychosocial interventions in patients with cancer is beyond the scope of this chapter, it is important to note that, beyond their obvious impact on quality of life, depression and other emotional disorders can affect ones' cognitive status. At one extreme are cases of pseudodementia, in which neuropsychological sequelae (eg, deficits in executive functions, psychomotor) are a consequence of depression in the absence of a coexisting dementia (66). In other cases, emotional distress can cause additional functional compromise in patients with cognitive impairment. Given that emotional distress frequently leads to excess cognitive disability and that many symptoms of affective disorders (including apathy, anhedonia, irritability) can impact one's motivation and effort to participate in treatment efforts, the emotional status of the patient must always be considered when constructing interventions against a neurocognitive problem (33). As an additional note, in patients with primary brain tumors, the site of the lesion may contribute to psychological symptoms. For example, tumors in the ventromedial frontal or parietal association areas may increase vulnerability to anxiety and irritability, while those in the dorsolateral frontal and somatosensory regions may be associated with emotional indifference or euphoria (10). Differentiating emotional and personality changes secondary to disease-based neurologic changes from those that are reactive or premorbid is important for informing treatment approaches (33).

Fatigue is the most common adverse symptom associated with cancer and cancer treatment. Cancer-related fatigue has been defined by the NCCN as "a distressing persistent, subjective sense of tiredness or exhaustion related to cancer or cancer treatment that is not proportional to recent activity and interferes with usual functioning" (67). In addition to physical tiredness, a cognitive aspect of fatigue, involving decreased concentration and reduced alertness, is being increasingly recognized as a component of cancer-related fatigue. Fatigue can have adverse effects on cognitive function and mood and impaired cognitive functioning and mood disorders may also cause fatigue (68). Comprehensive management of fatigue requires a multidimensional approach that recognizes the myriad of factors that may contribute to the fatigue experienced by patients with cancer, including anemia, coexisting medical problems (eg, infection, renal insufficiency, dehydration), hormonal disturbances, deconditioning, inadequate pain management, medication side effects, sleep disorders, underlying mood disorders, and cognitive symptoms (69).

Again, a comprehensive review of fatigue management strategies is outside of the scope of this chapter. Nonetheless, much like affective distress, fatigue can lead to excess cognitive disability and can impact one's motivation and effort to participate in neurocognitive and behavioral treatments and thus are of significant consideration when planning interventions. In addition to consultation from primary medical services to manage medically-related causes of fatigue, in setting targets for neurocognitive intervention with patients with cancer, behavioral or coping strategies to minimize the adverse impact of fatigue on functioning may often be incorporated. For example, one adaptive coping strategy to manage fatigue involves development of an "energy conservation plan" (70). First, patients are taught to take an inventory of their energy levels throughout the day, and then to schedule important activities at times when energy levels are greatest, rest when they are at their lowest, and delegate or delete non-essential tasks. In our experience, patients who use an external aid such as a day planner to compensate for a memory difficulty may additionally benefit from instruction in how to purposefully schedule activities throughout the day in such a way that they accomplish those cognitively demanding tasks which require maximal attention and energy when their fatigue levels are at their lowest. Patients may be further encouraged to take more frequent breaks to maximize attention and minimize frustration. Sometimes, alternative work schedules may be necessary. In addition to behavioral strategies, stimulants such as methylphenidate have been utilized to combat cancer-related fatigue (71).

CONCLUSIONS

It is generally recognized that patients with cancer may develop neurocognitive dysfunction as a direct result of cancer affecting the CNS, as an unfortunate consequence of therapeutic modalities (eg, radiotherapy, chemotherapy, bioimmunotherapy) used as primary or prophylactic treatment against cerebral and extracerebral malignancies, or as a side effect of adjuvant medications prescribed to prevent or limit medical complications (4). Evaluating the neurocognitive, behavioral and emotional sequelae that may occur in patients with cancer through objective neuropsychological assessment can assist in the identification of appropriate intervention strategies, thereby improving the quality of care, and ultimately the QOL, of patients, regardless of the nature or extent of their disease. In this chapter, we have discussed approaches for managing the neurocognitive dysfunction associated with cancer and cancer treatments. The various approaches have been somewhat artificially dichotomized (eg, behavioral vs pharmacologic strategies) to improve clarity. It should be stressed that for the majority of cases, however, a comprehensive, multimodal approach combining various therapies is often most effective for limiting the impact of neurocognitive dysfunction on everyday life. Empirical evaluation of behavioral interventions for managing neurocognitive dysfunction in patients with CNS and extracerebral malignancies and continued examination into the effectiveness of various pharmacologic approaches will hopefully continue in the future.

References

1. Wefel J, Lenzi R, Theriault R, Buzdar A, Cruickshank S, Meyers C. "Chemobrain" in breast carcinoma?: a prologue. *Cancer* 2004;101:466–475.
2. Meyers CA, Byrne KS, Komaki R. Cognitive deficits in patients with small cell lung cancer before and after chemotherapy. *Lung Cancer* 1995;12:231–235.
3. Meyers C, Albitar M, Estey E. Cognitive impairment, fatigue, and cytokine levels in patients with acute myelogenous leukemia or myelodysplastic syndrome. *Cancer* 2005;104:788–793.
4. Wefel JS, Kayl AE, Meyers CA. Neuropsychological dysfunction associated with cancer and cancer therapies: a conceptual review of an emerging target. *Br J Cancer.* 2004;90:1691–1696.
5. Rowland J, Hewitt M, Ganz P. Cancer survivorship: a new challenge in delivering quality cancer care. *J Clin Oncol.* 2006;24:5101–5104.
6. Vanderploeg RD. *Clinician's Guide to Neuropsychological Assessment.* Mahwah, NJ: Lawrence Erlbaum Associates, Inc., 2000.
7. Folstein MF, Folstein SE, McHugh PR. "Mini-mental state." A practical method for grading the cognitive state of patients for the clinician. *J Psychiatr Res.* 1975;12:189–198.
8. Meyers CA, Wefel JS. The use of the Mini-Mental State Examination to assess cognitive functioning in cancer trials: no ifs, ands, buts, or sensitivity. *J Clin Oncol.* 2003;21:3557–3558.

9. Meyers CA, Kudelka AP, Conrad CA, Gelke CK, Grove W, Pazdur R. Neurotoxicity of CI-980, a novel mitotic inhibitor. *Clin Cancer Res.* 1997;3:419–422.

10. Meyers CA. Issues of quality of life in neuro-oncology. In: Vecht CJ, ed. *Handbook of Clinical Neurology, Neuro-Oncology, Part I. Brain Tumors: Principles of Biology, Diagnosis and Therapy, Vol. 23.* Amsterdam: Elsevier Science B.V; 1997:389–409.

11. Cull A, Hay C, Love S, Mackie M, Smets E, Stewart M. What do patients with cancer mean when they complain of memory problems? *Br J Cancer.*1996;74:1674–1979.

12. Jenkins V, Shilling V, Deutsch G, et al. A 3-year prospective study of the effects of adjuvant treatments on cognition in women with early stage breast cancer. *Br J Cancer.*2006;94:828–834.

13. Castellon S, Ganz PA, Bower J, Petersen L, Abraham L, Greendale G. Neurocognitive performance in breast cancer survivors exposed to adjuvant chemotherapy and tamoxifen. *J Clin Exp Neuropsychol.* 2004;26:955–969.

14. Schagen S, Muller M, Boogerd W, van Dam F. Cognitive dysfunction and chemotherapy: neuropsychological findings in perspective. *Clin Breast Cancer.* Supplement 2002;3:S100–S108.

15. Meyers C, Brown P. Role and relevance of neurocognitive assessment in clinical trials of patients with CNS tumors. *J Clin Oncol.* 2006;24:1305–1309.

16. Meyers CA, Smith JA, Bezjak A, et al. Neurocognitive function and progression in patient with brain metastases treated with whole-brain radiation and motexafin gadolinium: results of a randomized phase III trial. *J Clin Oncol.* 2004;22:157–165.

17. Mehta MP, Shapiro WR, Glantz MJ, et al. Lead-in phase to randomized trial of motexafin gadolinium and whole-brain radiation for patients with brain metastases: centralized assessment of magnetic resonance imaging, neurocognitive, and neurologic end points. *J Clin Oncol.* 2002;20:3445–3453.

18. Meyers CA, Hess KR, Yung WKA, Levin VA. Cognitive function as a predictor of survival in patients with recurrent malignant glioma. *J Clin Oncol.* 2000;18:646–650.

19. Sherman AM, Jaeckle K, Meyers CA. Pretreatment cognitive performance predicts survival in patients with leptomeningeal disease. *Cancer* 2002;15:1311–1316.

20. Tucha O, Smely C, Preier M, Lange KW. Cognitive deficits before treatment among patients with brain tumors. *Neurosurgery* 2000;47:324–333.

21. Fleissbach K, Urbach H, Helstaedter C, et al. Cognitive performance and magnetic resonance imaging findings after high-dose systemic and intraventricular chemotherapy for primary central nervous system lymphoma. *Arch Neurol.* 2003;60:563–568.

22. Fleissbach K, Urbach H, Helmstaedter C, et al. Neuropsychological outcome after chemotherapy for primary CNS lymphoma: a prospective study. *Neurology* 2005;64:1184–1188.

23. Crossen JR, Garwood D, Glatstein E, Neuwalt EA. Neurobehavioral sequelae of cranial irradiation in adults: a review of radiation-induced encephalopathy. *J Clin Oncol.* 1994;12:627–642.

24. Meyers CA, Abbruzzese JL. Cognitive functioning in patients with cancer: effect of previous treatment. *Neurology* 1992;42:434–436.

25. Scheibel RS, Meyers CA, Levin VA. Cognitive dysfunction following surgery for intracerebral glioma: influence of histopathology, lesion location, and treatment. *J Neurooncol.* 1996;30:61–69.

26. Anderson SW, Damasio H, Tranel D. Neuropsychological impairments associated with lesions caused by tumor or stroke. *Arch Neurol.*1990;47:397–405.

27. Mayer M. A patient perspective on brain metastases in breast cancer. *Clin Cancer Res.* 2007;13:1623–1624.

28. Fobair P, Mackworth N, Varghese A, Prados M. Quality of life issues among 200 patients with brain tumors treated at the University of California in San Francisco, interviewed 1988. Brain Tumor Conference: A Living Resource Guide; 1990.

29. Patterson H. Nobody can afford a brain tumor...The financial impact of brain tumors on patients and families: a summary of findings. Report from the National Brain Tumor Foundation; 2007.

30. Meyers C, Boake C. Neurobehavioral disorders in patients with brain tumors: rehabilitation strategies. *Cancer Bull.* 1993;45:362–364.

31. Short P, JJ V, Tunceli K. Employment pathways in a large cohort of adult cancer survivors. *Cancer* 2005;103: 1292–1301.

32. Brain Tumor Progress Review Group. Report of the Brain Tumor Progress Review Group. NIH Publication No. 01–4902: National Cancer Institute and National Institute of Neurological Disorders and Stroke; 2000.

33. Attix D. An integrated model for geriatric neuropsychological intervention. In: Attix D, Welsh-Bomer K, eds. *Geriatric Neuropsychology Assessment and Intervention.* New York: Guilford Press; 2006:241–260.

34. Sohlberg M, Mateer C. *Cognitive Rehabilitation: An Integrative Neuropsychological Approach.* New York: Guilford Press; 2001.

35. Cicerone KD, Dahlberg C, Kalmar K, et al. Evidence-based cognitive rehabilitation: recommendations for clinical practice. *Arch Phys Med Rehabil.* 2000;81:1596–1615.

36. Cicerone KD, Dahlberg C, Malec JF, et al. Evidence-based cognitive rehabilitation: updated review of the literature from 1998 through 2002. *Arch Phys Med Rehabil.* 2005;86:1681–1692.

37. Marciniak CM, Sliwa JA, Spill G, Heinemann AW, Semik PE. Functional outcome following rehabilitation of the patient with cancer. *Arch Phys Med Rehabil.* 1996;77:54–57.

38. Huang ME, Cifu DX, Keyser-Marcus L. Functional outcome after brain tumor and acute stroke: a comparative analysis. *Arch Phys Med Rehabil.* 1998;79:1386–1390.

39. O'Dell MW, Barr K, Spanier D, Warnick RE. Functional outcome of inpatient rehabilitation in persons with brain tumors. *Arch Phys Med Rehabil.* 1998;79:1530–1534.

40. Huang ME, Wartella JE, Kreutzer JS. Functional outcomes and quality of life in patients with brain tumors: a preliminary report. *Arch Phys Med Rehabil.* 2001;82:1540–1546.

41. Sherer M, Meyers CA, Bergloff P. Efficacy of post acute brain injury rehabilitation for patients with primary malignant brain tumors. *Cancer.* 1997;80:250–257.

42. Sohlberg MM. External aids for management of memory impairment. In: High WM, Sander AM, Struchen MA, Hart KA, eds. *Rehabilitation for Traumatic Brain Injury.* New York: Oxford University Press; 2005.

43. Evans JJ, Wilson BA, Needham P, Brentnall S. Who makes good use of memory aids? Results of a survey of people with acquired brain injury. *J Int Neuropsychol Soc.* 2003;9:925–935.

44. Malec J, Cicerone K. Cognitive rehabilitation. In: Evans R, ed. *Neurology & Trauma.* New York: Oxford; 2005:238–261.

45. Sohlberg MM, Mateer CA. Training the use of compensatory memory books: a three stage behavioral approach. *J Clin Exp Neuropsychol.* 1989;11:871–891.

46. Donaghy S, Williams W. A new protocol for training severely impaired patients in the usage of memory journals. *Brain Inj.* 1998;12:1061–1070.

47. Schmitter-Edgecombe M, Fahy J, Whelan J, Long C. Memory remediation after severe closed head injury. Notebook training versus supportive therapy. *J Consult Clin Psychol.* 1995;63:484–489.

48. Ownsworth T, McFarland K. Memory remediation in long-term acquired brain injury: two approaches in diary training. *Brain Inj.* 1995;13:605–626.

49. Hart T, Hawkey K, Whyte J. Use of a portable voice organizer to remember therapy goals in traumatic brain injury rehabilitation: a within-subjects trial. *J Head Trauma Rehabil.* 2002;17:556–570.

50. van den Broek M, Downes J, Johnson Z, Dayus B, Hilton N. Evaluation of an electronic memory aid in the neuropsychological rehabilitation of prospective memory deficits. *Brain Inj.* 2000;14:455–462.

51. Wade T, Troy J. Mobile phones as a new memory aid: a preliminary investigation. *Brain Inj.* 2001;15:305–320.

52. Wilson B, Evans J, Emslie H, Malinek V. Evaluation of NeuroPage: a new memory aid. *J Neurol Neurosurg Psychiatry.* 1997;63:113–115.

53. Wilson B, Emslie H, Ouirk K, Evans J. Reducing everyday memory and planning problems by means of a paging system: a randomized control crossover study. *J Neurol Neurosurg Psychiatry*. 2001;70:477–482.

54. O'Connell M, Mateer C, Kerns K. Prosthetic systems for addressing problems with initiation: guidelines for selection, training, and measuring efficacy. *NeuroRehabilitation*. 2003;18:9–20.

55. Loewenstein D, Acevedo A, Czaja S, Duara R. Cognitive rehabilitation of mildly impaired Alzheimer's disease patients on cholinesterase inhibitors. *J Geriatric Psychiatry*. 2004;12:395–402.

56. Park N, Ingles J. Effectiveness of attention rehabilitation after an acquired brain injury: a meta-analysis. *Neuropsychology*. 2001;15:199–210.

57. Meyers CA, Weitzner MA, Valentine AD, Levin VA. Methylphenidate therapy improves cognition, mood, and function of patients with brain tumors. *J Clin Oncol*. 1998;16:2522–2527.

58. Lower E, Fleischman S, Cooper A, Zeldis J, Faleck H, Manning D. A phase III, randomized placebo-controlled trial of the safety and efficacy of d-MPH as new treatment of fatigue and "chemobrain" in adult patients with cancer. (Abstract). *J Clin Oncol*. 2005;23:8000.

59. Nasir S. Modafinil improves fatigue in primary patients with brain tumors (Abstract). *Society of Neuro Oncology*. 2003;5:335.

60. Shaw EG, Rosdahl R, D'Agostino RB, et al. Phase II study of Donepezil in irradiated patients with brain tumors: effect on cognitive function, mood, and quality of life. *J Clin Oncol*. 2006;24:1415–1420.

61. Cheung M, Chan AS, Law SC, Chan JH, Tse VK. Cognitive function of patients with nasopharyngeal carcinoma with and without temporal lobe radionecrosis. *Arch Neurol*. 2000;57:1347–1352.

62. Chan AS, Cheung M-C, Law SC, Chan JH. Phase II study of alpha-tocopherol in improving the cognitive function of patients with temporal lobe radionecrosis. *Cancer*. 2003;100:398–404.

63. Lee B, Dantzer R, Langley K, et al. A cytokine-based neuroimmunological mechanism of cancer-related symptoms. *Neuroimmunomodulation*. 2004;11:279–292.

64. National Comprehensive Cancer Network. 2007. Distress Management. NCCN Clinical Practice Guidelines in Oncology version 2.2007.

65. Stanton A. Psychosocial concerns and interventions for cancer survivors. *J Clin Oncol*. 2006;24:5132–5137.

66. Houston W, Bondi M. Potentially reversible cognitive symptoms in older adults. In: Attix K, Welsh-Bomer K, eds. *Geriatric Neuropsychology Assessment and Intervention*. New York: Guilford Press; 2006:103–131.

67. National Comprehensive Cancer Network. Cancer-Related Fatigue. NCCN Clinical Practice Guidelines in Oncology Version 2.2007: National Comprehensive Cancer Network; 2007.

68. Valentine AD, Meyers CA. Cognitive and mood disturbance as causes and symptoms of fatigue in patients with cancer. *Cancer*. 2001;92:1694–1698.

69. Franklin D, L P. Cancer-related fatigue. *Arch Phys Med Rehabil*. 2006;87:S91–S93.

70. Lovely MP. Symptom management of patients with brain tumors. *Semin Oncol Nurs*. 2004;20:273–283.

71. Sood A, Barton D, Loprinzi C. Use of methylphenidate in patients with cancer. *Amer J Hospice Palliative Med*. 2006;23:35–40.

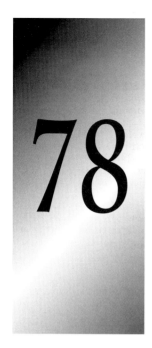

Activities of Daily Living in the Cancer Patient

78

Claudine Levy Campbell
Mackenzi Pergolotti

Activities of daily living (ADLs) include tasks that an individual completes on a daily basis to fulfill personal, social, and work-related roles. Self-care activities are the core of ADLs, and include overall mobility, getting in and out of bed, and moving or transferring from one surface to another (bed, chair, toilet, commode, shower, or tub), as well as grooming, feeding, dressing, bathing, toileting, and personal hygiene (1). Self-care activities are a major performance area that occupational therapists address when treating patients with cancer (2). Additionally, occupational therapists address instrumental activities of daily living (IADLs), which consist of activities that require the individual to interact with the physical and social environment. These activities include writing checks and paying bills, grocery shopping, meal preparation, medication management, light housework and home management, doing laundry, using transportation, caring for children, and leisure activities.

Patients with cancer are often susceptible to an overall decrease in activity secondary to multiple medical complications and repeated hospitalizations for treatment. The process of being diagnosed with cancer and receiving subsequent treatment can create various activity limitations with respect to ADLs, by affecting a patient's physical emotional, social, and cognitive capacities (3). Occupational therapists can provide restorative interventions or compensatory strategies to help patients with cancer achieve maximal physical, social, and psychological functioning within the parameters imposed by the disease and its treatment, and essentially maximize patients' participation in their ADLs (4).

It is imperative that patients with cancer remain active and willing participants in their ADL routines. By encouraging patients to care for themselves to the best of their abilities, patients maintain a sense of control and achievement. It is also important to consider what is most meaningful for patients with cancer to be able to achieve. Many patients who are going through the cancer process have strong desires to maintain their independence with basic everyday activities. ADLs can be modified to increase a patient's independence by using different techniques, altering body mechanics, taking extra time, or using adaptive equipment to reduce pain, fatigue, and strain (5). This chapter will describe how each component of self-care can be addressed when working with patients in a hospital or rehabilitation setting. Treatment principles are provided while the patient is in bed, seated at the edge of the bed, or sitting/standing out of bed.

TREATMENT PRINCIPLES

Grooming

Grooming tasks include oral care (brushing teeth/dentures), brushing or combing hair, shaving, applying makeup, and grooming nails. Given setup with items needed for these tasks (ie, toothbrush, toothpaste,

---

KEY POINTS

- Activities of daily living (ADLs) include tasks that an individual completes on a daily basis to fulfill personal, social, and work-related roles.
- Self-care activities are the core of ADLs, and include overall mobility, coming to a sitting position at the edge of the bed, getting in and out of bed, and moving or transferring from one surface to another (bed, chair, toilet, commode, shower, or tub), as well as grooming, feeding, dressing, bathing, toileting, and personal hygiene.
- Occupational therapists address instrumental activities of daily living (IADLs), which consist

- of activities that require the individual to interact with the physical and social environment such as writing checks and paying bills, grocery shopping, meal preparation, medication management, light housework and home management, doing laundry, using transportation, caring for children, and leisure activities.
- Patients with cancer are often susceptible to an overall decrease in activity secondary to multiple medical complications and repeated hospitalizations for treatment.

---

basin, etc.) the patient is able to perform tasks with a graded level of assistance with head of the bed raised, while seated in bed. At edge of the bed, the patient may require graded assistance to maintain sitting balance while applying makeup or completing oral care. In the bathroom, a patient may require balance assist, or a chair to alternate sitting with standing at the sink in order to complete shaving or oral care. A patient may also participate in higher-level tasks by retrieving the necessary items for grooming from a cabinet above the sink, turning light switches on/off, or opening and closing closet and room doors. Adaptive devices such as a universal cuff or built up foam handles for tooth or hair-brushes can improve completion of grooming tasks for patients with a weak grasp.

Feeding

Feeding includes opening containers, grasping utensils, bringing food to one's mouth, cutting food, and drinking from a cup. Graded tasks while in bed involve setup of all items on the patient's tray with the patient positioned appropriately. The patient may need the assistance of adapted or built up utensils, assistance with hand over hand assist, or verbal cues to successfully complete a feeding activity. The patient may require verbal instructions for swallowing, chewing, or biting food. While sitting at the edge of the bed, the patient may require assistance to set up the food on their tray, cut their food, open containers, manage finger food, or hold their posture while feeding in this unsupported position. While sitting in a chair at table height, the patient may only require instruction or graded assist with setup of their meal or adaptive devices to allow ease in setup or eating, such as dycem, a universal cuff, wide gripped fork, rocker knife, or scoop plate. A patient may require cues to use both hands function-

ally with feeding if one hand is weaker, or to learn how to use a one-handed technique.

Dressing the Upper Body

Positioned in bed, a patient may require assistance with donning a hospital gown or a shirt. The patient may need assistance with rolling and placing his/her arms in the proper sleeve. While sitting at the edge of bed the patient may need graded assistance with multiple types of clothing, as well as assistance with maintaining sitting balance during this dynamic task. The patient will need to be able to don and doff a pullover shirt or a garment with buttons or full zipper, brassiere and/or other undergarments, corset and/or brace, and hearing aide and/or eyeglasses. Patients in the acute care oncology setting may need assistance with donning and doffing specialized braces for the upper extremity. These patients may have restrictions with regard to upper extremity range of motion (ROM) or weight-bearing limitations. In these instances, the patient will need to learn compensatory strategies for upper body dressing, which may require the patient to use one-handed techniques or limit the use of one arm within certain parameters (5). The patient may also require special devices to maximize independence with upper body dressing, such as a long-handled reacher or button hook, or they may benefit from having their clothing adapted (3). In a standing position, the patient should have adequate dynamic standing balance in order to don and doff a jacket or robe, as well as adequate trunk rotation and shoulder ROM (external and internal rotation) to complete the task.

Dressing the Lower Body

While a patient may be bedridden or unable to get out of bed due to restricted activity/bed rest, they may still complete lower body dressing in bed with the provision of adapted equipment and instructions guided by the specific restrictions. The patient may also raise the head of their bed to better reach their lower extremities, or practice dressing in a long sitting position. While sitting at the edge of the bed, the patient will need dynamic sitting balance in order to successfully don and doff socks and shoes and shift weight forward. The patient may require graded assistance in sitting at the edge of the bed to don and doff undergarments, slacks, skirt, socks or stockings, shoes, any brace or prosthesis, and any fasteners included. Patients may benefit from using a combination sitting and standing when dressing their lower body to conserve energy and maintain safety. The patient may benefit from adaptive devices: long-handled reacher, dressing stick with shoe horn, sock aide, or button hook/zipper hook, to minimize flexion at the trunk and improve independence with lower body dressing despite physical limitations (5).

Bathing the Upper Body

While in bed, with the head of the bed raised, the patient may require setup to be able to perform upper body bathing of their face, hands, arms, and trunk with a basin of water, washcloth, and soap. The patient may require hand over hand assist, or some level of physical assistance to bathe under both arms if one arm is weaker, as well as rest breaks if their endurance level is low. In sitting, the patient may require assistance to sit at the edge of bed, or in a chair, with the setup of a basin of water, washcloth, and soap. The patient can also be provided with setup in a chair in front of the bathroom sink in order to complete upper-body sponge bathing in the bathroom. When the patient progresses, and has the ability and endurance to get in and out of a shower, the task can be graded using adaptive devices including a long-handled sponge, shower chair, and handheld showerhead. The task requires that the patient can rinse his/her face, arms, hands, and trunk with the handheld showerhead, and the ability to use a wash cloth to lather on soap and then rinse off the soap after the application. A patient may benefit from a bath mitt, which is strapped to the patient's hand. The bath mitt is beneficial for the patient who cannot grasp a washcloth, and does not have full use of both hands. The patient may have certain restrictions related to showering, specifically if they have just had surgery and have staples or stitches in place. The patient may also be affected by the steam/heat from the shower because of respiratory complications. Heat and humidity can increase shortness of breath and reduce a patient's aerobic capacity. Additionally, the patient may experience extreme fatigue because of the energy required to complete the task of showering. The patient may require adaptive devices, may need to take frequent rest periods and alter sitting with standing, or need to change the time of day to complete the showering activity to a time when energy levels are highest.

Bathing the Lower Body

Lower-body bathing includes bathing the groin area, upper and lower legs, feet, and buttocks. While supine with the head of the bed elevated, the patient may still perform lower-body bathing with appropriate positioning and adaptive mirrors or equipment. The patient may only be able to wash areas they can most easily reach, and may need physical assistance with their legs and feet. While sitting at the edge of the bed or in a chair, the patient may use a footstool to allow for greater reach to their lower legs and feet. As with lower-body dressing, the patient may benefit from a combination of sitting and standing to complete lower-body bathing, in addition to the use of adaptive devices such as a reacher or long-handled bath sponge. As with upper-body bathing, when the patient can tolerate transferring into the shower, they may use a shower seat to alternate sitting with standing in the shower in order to bathe the lower part of the body and conserve energy.

Toileting

The patient who is bed bound may not be able to get up in order to use a commode, and may therefore require assistance with rolling in order to use a bed pan. At this stage, the patient may require a lot of assistance with toileting, but can be encouraged to help by rolling, changing their position in bed, or managing clothing. Once the patient can transfer with assistance to a bedside commode or into the bathroom, the patient may need assistance with managing clothing during toileting due to weak grasp, while at the same time maintaining safe functional dynamic balance. The patient may require the use of adaptive devices such as a long-handled reacher or an inspection mirror (1). The patient may also need to alternate sitting with standing a few times in order to complete the toileting task safely and manage clothing (pulling up undergarments and pants) in a few stages.

Toilet Transfer

Once the patient is able to transfer out of bed with assistance, they can begin to practice commode transfers. The patient can be taught stand-pivot transfers to the commode with assistance, going toward the patient's stronger or weaker side. Eventually, the patient can learn to transfer to both the stronger and weaker sides independently. The patient may need to use a drop arm commode or a sliding board to the commode if there is lower extremity paralysis or weakness, and in this instance will benefit from transferring to the stronger side with family members, and until stronger and complete transfers to weaker side with the therapist only for practice. If the patient is using an ambulatory device, such as a rolling or standard walker, the patient can practice commode transfers with the device. Once the patient has the strength and endurance to be able to walk to the bathroom, they can practice functional mobility in and out of the bathroom in order to transfer on/off a standard or raised toilet. The patient can be instructed on how to use grab bars in the bathroom, or the commode frame can be placed over the toilet to increase patient safety and make the toilet transfer easier for the patient.

Shower Transfer

When the patient has the endurance to complete functional mobility into the bathroom, they can begin to practice getting in and out of a shower. The patient may need to use an ambulatory device such as a rolling walker, standard walker, crutches, or cane to perform functional mobility into the bathroom. Once the patient is in the bathroom, they may need instruction on how to safely step over the shower stall or tub and transfer into the shower. The patient may benefit from a shower seat and use of grab bars to make the shower transfer safe. The patient may need to sit on the shower seat first, and then pivot their body and legs into the shower, as opposed to stepping in. The patient may benefit from having family members trained on how to best assist them so that shower transfers can be safely performed in the home environment.

Bed Mobility

The ability to roll and sit at the edge of the bed are prerequisites for self-care activities. The patient may need to practice a modified rolling technique by using the side rails of the bed and/or the head of the bed raised. The patient may also need to use an overhead trapeze to pull himself/herself to a sitting position, and maneuver from supine to long sit. The patient who has had spine surgery or another surgery with precautions related to movement may need to learn how to log roll or complete supine to side-lying to sitting at the edge of the bed in one smooth motion. There are some surgeries that require a patient to refrain from sitting and putting pressure on the sacrum. In these instances, patients need to learn how to position themselves on their sides in bed at all times, and then go from side-lying to standing in one smooth motion, without sitting at the edge of the bed at all.

Energy Conservation and Body Mechanics

Most patients with cancer experience fatigue and impaired activity tolerance at some stage during their treatment course (4). Patients are often encouraged to alternate activity with rest in order to maximize activity tolerance without pushing themselves to the point of overwhelming fatigue (5). Adapting ADLs by using energy conservation principles and appropriate body mechanics can benefit patients who experience short-term or chronic fatigue and low endurance secondary to treatment. Some activities require higher levels of energy, so it is imperative that therapists working with cancer patients monitor their vital signs and oxygen saturation levels. Some energy conservation principles that can be useful for patients with cancer include minimizing the amount of bending with dressing and bathing by using long-handled devices and slip-on shoes instead of shoes that need to be tied, minimizing overexertion and taking frequent rest breaks, alternating sitting with standing during strenuous activities, organizing the environment to have all items necessary for an activity within reach, and using lightweight utensils or tools to prevent additional strain (5). In addition, patients can be taught deep-breathing exercises and regulated breathing.

Special Considerations

Patients on Isolation Precautions/Contact Isolation

Patients who receive bone marrow transplants (allogenic, syngeneic, or the patient's own, harvested bone marrow/peripheral blood) are often placed on isolation precautions. Before the transplantation procedure, these patients are given high doses of anticancer drugs and/ or radiation to destroy the cancer cells, which also kills healthy cells in the process. During this treatment phase and after the bone marrow transplant, these patients are very susceptible to infections. Patients are placed in protective isolation and cannot leave their hospital rooms. In addition, they are placed on restricted diets, which limit the intake of fresh fruits/vegetables and include thoroughly cooked foods to kill bacteria. These patients are often in the hospital for six weeks to upwards of a few months, and become deconditioned as a result of the cancer treatment and inactivity over a prolonged period of time. It is important for these patients to participate in ADLs as much as possible, and to have a routine of getting up in the morning to complete morning self-care routines. These patients may require adaptive equipment to make completing ADLs easier, and they may benefit from learning how to pace activities with energy conservation techniques. The primary ADL goal is to encourage participation in self-care activities in order to maintain activity tolerance and endurance levels.

Head and Neck Surgery/Facial Reconstruction

Patients with head and neck cancers often go through major facial reconstruction, which involves the removal of the identified lesions, involved surrounding structures and, at times, facial/cervical lymph nodes. During such procedures, these patients may have to be intubated for surgery and have tracheotomies or nasogastric tubes placed temporarily until they are healed enough to breathe and to swallow food independently. These patients may have to modify how they complete their ADLs. They may require the use of long-handled adaptive equipment for dressing and bathing, and they may need to modify how they shower/bathe. Likewise, they may need to sponge bathe temporarily due to restrictions with showering, or they may need to use a shower chair to conserve energy when showering.

Tikhoff-Linberg Procedure

The Tikhoff-Linberg procedure involves a total or partial scapulectomy with en-bloc removal of a portion of the humerus and preservation of neurovascular pedicle of the arm. This procedure preserves function of the elbow and hand, and has been used as a limb sparing surgery as opposed to the forequarter amputation. Therapists who work with patients who have had this type of procedure need to know which muscles were removed and which muscles were reconnected and attached to a new location. These patients will need to be taught how to dress, bathe, groom, and toilet themselves with one-handed techniques postoperatively, while the operated arm is being rehabilitated and regains some function. They may benefit from adapted clothing that has Velcro or snaps on the operated side, or they may need to wear button-down shirts and shoes with Velcro fasteners to maintain ease and independence with dressing. These patients will have to learn modified techniques for accomplishing self-care activities due to the loss of function of the operated arm.

Axillary and Sentinel Lymph Node Dissection

Patients who are status post an axillary lymph node dissection or sentinel lymph node dissection will have some ROM or movement restrictions following surgery (6). With regard to ADLs, these patients may need to be instructed in energy conservation and modified body mechanics techniques. They may be able to dress, bathe, and groom themselves independently by taking extra time to complete the tasks or using adaptive equipment, if needed. These patients may have lifting restrictions

put in place by their surgeons, so they will need to be instructed on how to safely perform ADLs once they return home from the hospital. Patient education can focus on using the non-operated arm for lifting and carrying items during home management or meal preparation tasks, and limiting the amount of strain placed on the operated arm until cleared by the surgeon (6).

Internal Hemipelvectomy

When an internal hemipelvectomy is performed, the leg is spared. It is imperative to review the surgeon's report to see which muscles and nerves were removed and which were likewise spared. Patients who have undergone this procedure are awaiting scar tissue to form in order to achieve joint stabilization. During the period when the muscles are scarring down, patients may have many restrictions in range of movement, specifically with hip flexion and abduction. Oftentimes, patients are fitted with hip abduction braces postoperatively. The hip abduction brace allows the surgeon to position the patient's hip in a protected position, so that the patient cannot freely flex, extend, abduct, or adduct the hip. These restrictions make lower-body care, transfers, and toileting more difficult.

Bathing and dressing need to be completed supine in bed. Long-handled reachers, dressing sticks, sock-aides, and long-handled bath sponges are required to maintain precautions. Long handled mirrors can be used for toileting and peri-care. Keep in mind that patients wearing a hip abduction brace may want to wear their clothes outside of the brace in order to toilet normally. If the patient wants to wear the brace on the outside of their clothing, they will require special pants and underwear that have a hole in the center of the garment (eg, a body suit with snaps at the bottom). For toileting, these patients must use a raised toilet seat to maintain their hip precautions. In addition, the toilet seat may need to be covered with extra padding or a cushion to allow for increased comfort when sitting.

External Hemipelvectomy

External hemipelvectomy involves the removal of the leg and half of the pelvis. Dressing and bathing is initially completed in bed with the use of reachers, dressing sticks, long-handled sponges, and sock aides. Long-handled mirrors may also assist with toileting. Immediate postoperative wound care is essential, as is flap are, if appropriate. Proper wound care is essential for healing to occur. Special adapted cushions maybe used to allow sitting for longer periods of time during the healing process. A scored cushion may be used to allow for pressure relief. Initially the cushion can be built up on the surgical side so that there is more support on that side, and less on the un-operated side. Then, once the wound heals, the cushion can be reversed to promote improved posture while sitting. For patients with whom a scored cushion will not provide adequate comfort, a gel insert into a foam cushion is used.

Sacrectomy

A sacrectomy is when the sacrum is removed. During the initial postoperative period, most patients are kept on a Clinitron Rite Height Air Fluidized Therapy Bed to allow for healing to occur (7). Once the patient is allowed out of bed, side-lying to stand is performed when getting out of bed to avoid any duration of sitting, and then stand to side-lying is performed in order to return to bed. Reachers, dressing sticks, sock aides and long-handled bath sponges are used to increase independence with dressing and bathing, which is completed first in bed. Once standing tolerance has improved, bathing and dressing can be completed in front of the sink. Standing tolerance activities should be progressively performed to increase the patient's endurance with ADLs and IADLs while standing. Additional activities that can be completed in standing include retrieving items from the refrigerator and cabinets, as well as performing a small meal task (eg, making a cup of tea). These tasks need to be performed and practiced to allow increased confidence with functional tasks before discharge home.

Craniotomy

A craniotomy is procedure when the skull is opened in order to remove brain lesions or tumors. Immediately after surgery, patients can be encouraged to participate in ADL tasks. An ADL and cognitive assessment can demonstrate how a patient might function at home with the onset of new neurological or physical deficits. During the first day of evaluation, tasks such as bed mobility, bedroom mobility (retrieving items from closets, drawers) and bathroom mobility are performed. ADL tasks include grooming at the sink, toileting, and upper- and lower-body dressing. All tasks should be completed without performing any excessive forward flexion (head below heart) or maintaining the head of the bed at a minimum 30 degrees. If the patient is doing well with the basic self-care activities, then utilizing more complex tasks with multistep commands can be added (eg, making a cup of coffee, making a sandwich, finding the pantry on the unit, and then returning to the patient's room). During ADL treatments, patients with cognitive deficits or mobility deficits may need simplified cueing or detailed instructions to complete the tasks successfully. These brain tumor patients may require similar therapeutic treatments as patients whose status is posttraumatic brain injury, stroke, aneurysm, or sub-

dural hematoma. Treatments such as neuromuscular re-education, transfer training, mobility training, ADL training, IADL training, and therapeutic activities can be adapted for this patient population (8). These patients may also require energy conservation instruction due to increased susceptibility to fatigue following surgery.

Forequarter Amputation

This procedure entails removal of the entire shoulder and ipsilateral arm. The immediate postoperative goals include getting out of bed and completing bathroom mobility. Due to the amputation, the patient's center of gravity has changed and balance is challenged. Basic ADLs need to be practiced in order to ensure independence with dressing and bathing, including education on how to perform these tasks with one-handed techniques. IADLs should be performed to problem solve through how to complete these tasks one-handed as well. Adaptive equipment such as a rocker knife, one-handed cutting board, or lip plate can be provided to increase independence with cutting food and eating without assistance. If interested, patients are offered a prosthetic shoulder orthosis to improve cosmesis.

Spinal Cord Compression/Compromise

Many patients acquire spinal cord compression due to metastatic disease to the spine or primary central nervous system lymphoma. These patients may have a shorter life span as compared to those with traumatic spinal cord injury. At the time of diagnosis, rehabilitation should include basic ADLs similar to traumatic injury, but with a palliative approach. Concentration on transfers and optimizing the patient's ability to complete basic self-care activities with or without family assistance/training is the primary goal. These patients may be receiving daily radiation treatments, and may need to be able to transfer in and out of a car. They may benefit from using long-handled reachers, dressing sticks, sock aides and long-handled bath sponges with dressing and bathing, in order to be able to do more for themselves. Drop-arm commodes, bathroom equipment, and appropriate wheelchair recommendations should be made for these patients to maximize their safety in their home environment.

Special Equipment/Orthotics/Adaptations

The use of custom-made devices and orthoses helps minimize dysfunction, maintain functional positions, and provide protection to various body parts (1). As a result, patients are able to resume normal daily activities and achieve independent mastery of life functions with or without assistance. The occupational therapy department at Memorial Sloan-Kettering Cancer Center has created several adaptive devices and modified already existing orthotics to enhance patients' abilities to participate in their daily routines, as well as improve their physical appearance and body image.

Adapted Slings

Slings can be adapted for patients with cancer so that their upper extremities can be more comfortable, or positioned according to specific orders from the medical team. Off the shelf shoulder immobilizers can be adapted by adding velcro to the straps, adding a waist strap, or adding a hand-based support if the patient has a flail wrist/hand. Slings can also be custom made with velfoam and strapping material to simulate a shoulder/arm support for patients with brachial plexopathy who need postural support, shoulder approximation, and hand support secondary to a flail arm and hand. Figure 78.1 demonstrates an example of a customized shoulder/hand support for a woman who was most comfortable with her hand positioned directly across her chest, and did not find a standard sling comfortable.

Adapted Glove

Patients with brachial plexopathy or tumor progression that is compressing the brachial plexus may present with atrophy and severe hand weakness. Gloves can be adapted so that these patients can hold objects with a modified technique. Gloves are modified so that patients can swing a golf club, hold a weight in order to strengthen forearm and elbow musculature, or grasp tools. Velcro strips and finger extensions are sewn onto an athletic glove to increase the security of a patient's functional grasp/composite fist with their daily activities (Fig. 78.2).

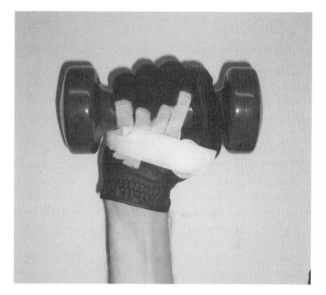

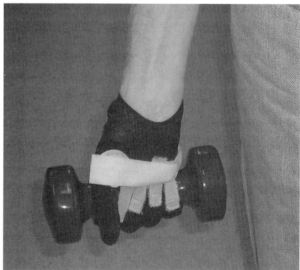

FIGURE 78.2

An adapted glove fabricated for a man diagnosed with Pancoast tumor and advanced brachial plexopathy. Note how the glove allows him to hold a weight securely. This same glove allowed the man to return to playing golf.

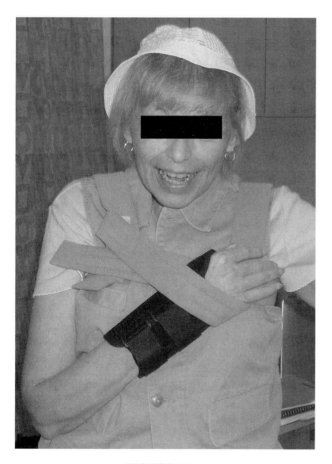

FIGURE 78.1

An adapted sling fabricated for a woman with advanced brachial plexopathy.

Chest Plate

The pediatric chest guard is designed for children who have had surgery in the thoracic region or a Medi-Port placed in their upper chest wall. As these children resume school and play activities, they require protection to prevent trauma to their chest, trunk, or Medi-Port site. Splinting material is molded to the patient's chest so that the end product contours to the patient's body while allowing the upper extremities freedom of movement. The anterior chest piece is held in place using riveted straps made from stockinette and Velcro strips. The chest guard allows children to safely return to their normal daily activities, which may include participation in gym classes, playing with friends, or engaging in extracurricular sports (Fig. 78.3).

Sarmiento Brace

The Sarmiento brace is a type of off the shelf shoulder abduction brace that limits shoulder abduction/adduc-

tion and immobilizes the patient's shoulder. Patients who have undergone orthopedic surgeries involving the shoulder joint, or have existing pathological fractures that cannot be surgically reduced, may be required to wear a Sarmiento brace to stabilize the glenohumeral joint. Therapists often have to modify the Sarmiento brace for individual patients by adjusting the straps, adding padding to the straps, or cutting portions of the upper arm support to improve the comfort and stability of the support.

Elbow Gutter Splint

The elbow gutter splint is often used with patients who have elbow contractures and cannot fully extend their elbows. This is often seen with patients who have graft versus host disease. The elbow gutter splint can be used as a serial splinting treatment technique to provide the patient with an elbow extension stretch over a prolonged period of time. Every one to two

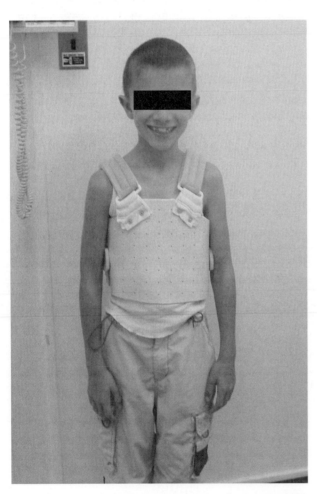
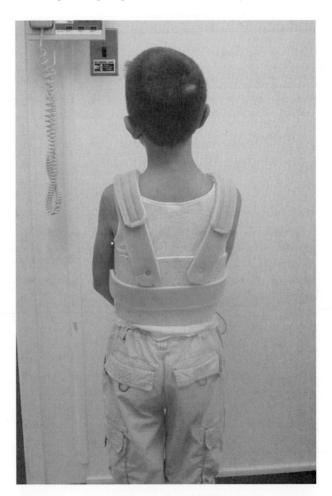

FIGURE 78.3

Anterior and posterior view of a pediatric chest plate fabricated for a boy in order to protect his chest MediPort during physical activity.

weeks, a new splint can be fabricated or the primary splint can be re-molded and adjusted to further increase the patient's elbow extension. This type of splint is beneficial for patients who have difficulty completing their self-ROM exercises consistently throughout the day. The end goal is to maximize the patient's elbow ROM in order to regain full function of the arm with ADLs and functional activities.

Commode Adaptations

Commodes often have to be adapted for patients who have undergone hip surgery, hemipelvectomy, or sacrectomy. Thick padding or a foam cushion can be applied to the commode seat and wrapped with a sanitary cover or lining to cushion the seat or add height. If patients have to maintain certain hip ROM precautions, and must sit without bending past a certain degree of hip flexion, more padding can be added to one side of the commode seat to accommodate that limitation.

Scrotal Supports

Scrotal supports are custom made for male patients who have edematous scrotums which can be painful, cause chafing, and make mobility uncomfortable and difficult. This swelling can result from various forms of cancer or cancer-related treatments. The scrotal supports function like a jock strap to elevate and give gentle compression to the scrotum, and to ultimately decrease pain and swelling. The supports are made with stockinette for a waistband and tubi-grip for the pouch. The patient is measured around the waist. Most patients also have abdomen swelling and their previous waist size can be inaccurate. After the waist is measured, the scrotum is measured for depth and width. With these measurements, a pouch is cut and sewn together with the tubi-grip material, which is then sewn to the waist strap. Velcro is sewn onto the waistband so that the patients can don and doff the supports easily. Some patients may require assistance with donning and doffing the support.

Head and Neck Forearm Flap Splint

When patients undergo head and neck surgery, the surgeons occasionally use forearm tissue/musculature for a free flap. Once this flap is taken, the surgeons request a custom-made forearm/hand splint. The purpose of the forearm splint is most often to immobilize the wrist and metacarpophalangeal (MP) joints so that the flap site can heal appropriately. The fingers and thumb are occasionally immobilized at the MP and proximal interphalangeal (PIP) joints. The surgeons usually have specific requirements for hand positioning, depending

on what structures of the forearm have been affected by the flap site. Oftentimes, the splints are custom made and need to be created with an open cut-out section to prevent pressure directly on the site, or to allow the surgeons to monitor the site and complete a venous ultrasound.

Cranial Prosthesis

Occasionally, patients who have had multiple craniotomies for removal of brain tumors develop infections. For the infection to heal, a portion of the skull may need to be removed. There are also circumstances in which a piece of skull must be removed to decrease intracranial pressure due to increased swelling in the brain. In these instances, surgeons request that patients wear a helmet to mobilize safely out of bed and protect the structures of the brain that are not covered by skull. A custom-made helmet can be made by an occupational therapist. These helmets are typically fabricated from thin splinting material and molded and contoured to the patient's head to offer a durable shield to the brain. The custom-made helmet can be worn inside a baseball hat or a knitted cap to allow patients to go into the community with a more aesthetically pleasing form of helmet, while maintaining adequate protection from injury.

Forequarter Amputation Prosthesis

Patients who have undergone a forequarter amputation may be provided with a prosthetic shoulder orthosis if they are interested. This orthosis is made to create the appearance of having bilateral and symmetrical shoulders. A molding is made with plastic splinting material of the remaining shoulder. Cotton fabric is used to cover the molding, and cotton padding is placed under the molding. A long strap is measured from the remaining portion of the clavicle where the prosthesis will sit on the patient's surgical side, to the contralateral trunk and under the axilla of the remaining arm. This strap is made like a bell curve to allow full coverage of the padded molding and to secure the prosthesis in place. Velcro is added to the two ends of the long strap and used to secure the prosthesis under the remaining arm. The prosthesis is applied to where the patient's shoulder joint previously was, and is worn under a shirt, to create symmetry and the effect of a full rounded shoulder.

Carpal Tunnel Splints/Resting Hand Splints

Some patients may have pain in their hands and wrists due to neuropathy, overuse, or carpal tunnel symptoms. Treatment for this includes the use of a prefabricated wrist support or a custom made wrist splint that can be fabricated by an occupational therapist. Patients with neuropathic or carpal tunnel symptoms may benefit from periods of wrist immobilization during the day and/or night to minimize their symptoms and optimize hand function with ADLs.

Adapted T-shirts

Patients who undergo surgeries of the scapula or shoulder may be required to limit their shoulder motion for a period of time with a shoulder immobilizer or sling. In order for patients to safely don and doff t-shirts, undershirts, or pullovers, these shirts may be adapted. A pullover shirt can be adapted by cutting a slit down the seam on the affected side, up through the sleeve. Then Velcro is sewn onto both sides to allow ease of closure. The shirt can be applied by placing the unaffected arm into the sleeve on that side first, pulling the shirt overhead, and then securing the sleeve on the operated side under the axilla and over the brace/sling by aligning the Velcro strips.

CONCLUSIONS

This chapter has reviewed ADLs pertaining to patients with cancer. In all stages of cancer rehabilitation, a patient's independence in performing ADLs may be compromised by weakness, fatigue, or loss of function. The occupational therapist's role in cancer rehabilitation is to enhance the patient's performance of ADLs, to provide education to maintain or increase daily living skills, and to make necessary adaptations to the environment or equipment to maximize safety and cosmesis (5).

References

1. Yadav R. Rehabilitation of surgical cancer patients at University of Texas M.D. Anderson Cancer Center. *J Surg Oncol.* 2007;95:361–369.
2. Soderback I, Paulsson EM. A needs assessment for referral to occupational therapy: nurses' judgment in acute cancer care. 1997;20(4):267–273.
3. Strong J. Occupational therapy and cancer rehabilitation. *Br J Occup Ther.* 1987;50(1):4–6.
4. Fialka-Moser V, Crevanna R, Korpan M, Quittan M. Cancer rehabilitation. *J Rehabil Med.* 2003;35(4):153–162.
5. Penfold SL. The role of the occupational therapist in oncology. *Cancer Treat Rev.* 1996;22:75–81.
6. Vockins H. Occupational therapy interventions with patients with breast cancer: a survey. *Eur J Cancer Care.* 2004;13:45–52.
7. Bauer K, Ghazinouri R. Rehabilitation after total sacrectomy. *Rehabil Oncol.* 2005;(2):9–13.
8. Mukand JA, Guilmette TJ, Tran M. Rehabilitation of patients with brain tumors. *Crit Rev Phys Rehabil Med.* 2003;15(2):99–111.

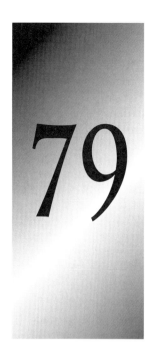

Lymphedema in the Cancer Patient

David Martin Strick
Gail Louise Gamble

Cancer as a diagnosis has attained the ranks of chronic disease (1,2). Although potential for recurrence is carefully monitored, other long-term and late effects may manifest (3). Many of these effects result in impaired function, and the condition of lymphedema is certainly among the potential issues facing cancer survivors. Managing the complex care related to lymphedema requires a thorough understanding of the anatomy, pathophysiology, risk factors, clinical presentation, diagnostic tests, and treatment options. Understanding the tissue level environment and accounting for individual risk factors and comorbidity allows the astute clinician to develop unique management strategies, thus optimizing a more successful edema control program for each patient.

STRUCTURE AND FUNCTION OF THE LYMPHATIC SYSTEM

The lymphatic system is a closed vascular system composed of endothelial-lined channels that parallel the arterial and venous systems. The lymphatics originate in the tissue interstitium as specialized capillaries. These capillaries are remarkably porous and readily permit the entry of even large macromolecules, including albumin. Lymphatic capillaries have also been observed to be intimately associated with fine strands of reticular fibers and collagen that are connected to surrounding tissues. These anchoring filaments provide a direct ana-

tomic connection between the lymphatic capillaries and the adjoining tissues (4). As interstitial fluid increases, the collagen fibers are pulled apart. This exerts traction on the lymphatic anchoring filaments and centrifugal pull on lymphatic capillaries that keeps the lumens patent, even in the presence of increasing interstitial pressure and interstitial edema. Beyond the lymphatic capillaries are the terminal lymphatic vessels. The walls of these vessels are devoid of any smooth muscle; however, intraluminal bicuspid valves are present. The valves partition the vessels into discrete contractile segments, termed lymphangions. Eventually, these vessels merge to form larger lymphatic collector vessels and lymphatic trunks that contain smooth muscle in their walls. Contraction of the smooth muscle propels the lymphatic fluid through the peripheral lymphatic vessels that eventually connect with the thoracic duct or right lymphatic duct. These latter lymphatic vessels join the venous system in the left and right cervical regions, respectively.

There is both a superficial and a deep collecting system of lymphatics in the extremities. Lymphatics from the skin and adjacent subcutaneous connective tissues drain into the superficial system. Lymph from the lymphatics in the fascial planes surrounding skeletal muscles drain predominantly into the deep lymphatic collecting system. The distribution of fluid between the blood vascular system and the tissues depends on the transcapillary balance between hydrostatic and protein osmotic pressure gradients. Normally, there

KEY POINTS

- Managing the complex care related to lymphedema requires a thorough understanding of anatomy, pathophysiology, risk factors, clinical presentation, diagnostic tests, and treatment options.
- A primary function of the lymphatic system is to return to the circulation not only fluid, but also large molecular weight substances such as protein and particulate matter that cannot reenter the blood capillaries directly.
- Interstitial fibrosis is often a significant complication of lymphedema. This phenomenon is often recognized as the brawny, nonpitting form of soft tissue swelling.
- Several postsurgical risk factors for lymphedema development have been reported. Among these are extent, location of the surgical intervention, radiation location, infection, weight gain, and age.
- When evaluating a patient with persistent limb swelling, possible systemic etiologies should be eliminated.
- Prevention of swelling and the protean complications of lymphedema is the ultimate goal of any treatment program.
- Exercise does not increase the risk for, or exacerbate the symptoms of lymphedema in breast cancer survivors.
- A specialized massage technique known as manual lymphatic drainage is now the standard of practice for lymphedema management.
- External compression is used for two purposes: (1) to try to reduce edema formation, and (2) to aid in removal of excess lymph already accumulated within the limb.
- Compression garments are constructed with graduated compression; they apply the greatest pressure distally and the least proximally, thus reducing the potential for a tourniquet effect.
- Generally, pharmacologic therapy has not played a significant role in lymphedema management.

is a slight hydrodynamic imbalance favoring a small, excess amount of fluid, salt, and macromolecules in the tissue spaces. This filtrate, or lymph, is collected by the lymphatics and returned to the venous system. Thus, a primary function of the lymphatic system is to return to the circulation not only fluid, but also large molecular weight substances such as protein and particulate matter that cannot reenter the blood capillaries directly. The lymphatic system also acts as a safety valve or buffer in the event of fluid overload, and therefore helps to prevent edema from forming. As interstitial fluid volume increases, interstitial fluid pressure increases. The result is a marked increase in local lymph flow (5). Unlike blood, which is pumped by the heart, lymph is propelled predominantly by spontaneous intrinsic contractions of the lymphangions and lymphatic trunks. Skeletal muscle contraction, active and passive range of motion, respiration, and blood vessel pulsation also aid significantly in the centripetal movement of lymph by external compression of lymphatic vessels.

PATHOPHYSIOLOGY OF LYMPHEDEMA

When lymphatic blockage occurs secondary to cancer infiltration of lymph nodes, lymphadenectomy, or radiation-induced lymph node fibrosis, blood capillary hemodynamic forces and permeability characteristics usually remain normal. Intralymphatic pressure distal to the site of the blockage increases. Lymphatic vessels dilate and their valves become incompetent. Increased intralymphatic pressure also dilates lymphatic capil-laries and results in incompetence in endothelial cellular junctions. These junctions normally serve as inlet valves, and their incompetence results in a reduction in lymph influx and an increase in tissue fluid volume.

Lymphedema may be categorized as either high-lymph-output failure or low-lymph-output failure. High-lymph-output failure results from an overproduction of capillary filtrate and leads to a greatly expanded extracellular fluid space. Examples of this state are decompensated heart failure, ascites from hepatic cirrhosis, and nephrotic syndrome. Low-lymph-output failure of the lymphatic circulation is characterized by a decreased rate of lymph absorption, and results from deficient or obliterated lymphatics. Chronic peripheral edema associated with lymphatic insufficiency is often attributed to the paucity of lymphatic trunks or obstruction of lymph flow. Interestingly, however, early laboratory studies directed at creating lymphedema in animals by lymphatic sclerosis or radical excision were highly unsuccessful (6–8). Because of the failure of these procedures to produce unremitting peripheral lymphedema, a theory developed that subclinical bacterial infection (lymphangitis) was necessary for the development of chronic lymphedema. Chronic, indolent, low-grade infection increases microvascular permeability to protein and contributes to progressive lymphatic obliteration and tissue scarring. Subsequent studies using lymphangiography showed that despite transient swelling, lymphatic regeneration and opening of lymphovenous shunts precluded the development of chronic lymphedema (6,9). When lymphedema did develop, it sometimes was not manifested for several years after the surgical destruction of lymphatics.

The long interval that can occur between the time of the experimental interruption of the lymphatic system and the development of persistent lymphedema, is characterized by progressive lymphatic obliteration, fusion of lymphatic vessels with surrounding tissues to form large vacuolar spaces, fibrosis of lymphatic vessel walls, and lymph stasis (10–12). Together, these alterations may help to explain the unpredictable occurrence of upper extremity lymphedema following breast surgery and treatment or the delayed onset of lower extremity lymphedema after radical groin or pelvic lymph node dissections.

Interstitial fibrosis is often a significant complication of lymphedema. This phenomenon is often recognized as the brawny, nonpitting form of soft tissue swelling. Although the exact mechanism of this scarring is unknown, there is a strong association between the high protein content of lymph and the proliferation of fibroconnective tissue. It has been postulated that fibrin or other specialized protein complexes dispersed throughout the interstitial matrix form an intricate lattice-template facilitating the deposition of collagen (13). Fibrosis may result also from the inability of local macrophages to digest the excessive protein load (14). The accumulation of protein promotes chronic inflammation and scar formation even under conditions of adequate lymphatic drainage and normal capillary permeability (15). Activation of tissue macrophages should enhance scavenger function and interrupt the cycle of progressive tissue protein accumulation and fibroplasias (16). The proteolysis of tissue macromolecules into component amino acids may result in lower molecular weight fragments being reabsorbed into the bloodstream (16), which relieves the load on the lymphatic system. Once the osmotic force created by the extravascular tissue protein is eliminated, excess salt and water diffuse back into the intravascular compartment. As the protein-rich tissue swelling regresses, the dynamic balance between collagen deposition and resorption shifts toward proteolysis and the fibrous tissue recedes.

Primary and Secondary Lymphedema

Primary, or idiopathic, lymphedema is due to a developmental abnormality in the lymphatic system (eg, aplasia, hypoplasia, or hyperplasia of lymphatic vessels), or fibrotic occlusion of lymphatic vessels or lymph nodes. Secondary lymphedema results from a well-defined disease process that causes obstruction or injury to the lymphatic system. In North America and Europe, the most frequent cause of secondary lymphedema is surgical excision and radiation treatment of axillary or inguinal lymph nodes for the treatment of an underlying malignancy, such as breast or prostate cancer, or malignant melanoma (17–19). The reported incidence of secondary lymphedemas is variable (20–25). Development of post-breast surgery upper extremity lymphedema has been reported to be approximately 25% (26). Other causes of secondary lymphedema include tumors invading the lymphatic vessels, such as those found in metastatic ovarian, testicular, colorectal, pancreatic, or liver cancers. Additional etiologies include bacterial and fungal infections, lymphoproliferative diseases, and trauma (27).

Risk Factors

Several postsurgical risk factors for lymphedema development have been reported (Table 79.1). Among these include extent, location of the surgical intervention (28), radiation location (29), infection (29), weight gain (26,30), and age (31). Of these, weight gain since surgery and one or more infections were the only significant factors documented in a 20-year follow-up study of 923 breast patients with cancer (26). Thus, in evaluating a postsurgical patient for risks, perioperative infections including drain site infections or infected postoperative seroma, obesity, extent of surgery including axillary dissection or complete lymphadenectomy, and extent and location of tumor resection should be considered.

Grades of Lymphedema

Regardless of the etiology, lymphedema has been classified as follows. Each grade may be sub-classified as mild, moderate, or severe.

Grade 0: Latent or subclinical condition wherein edema is not evident despite impaired lymph transport. It may exist months or years before overt edema occurs (32).

TABLE 79.1

Documented Risk Factors for Development of Secondary Lymphedema

Factor (Ref.)
Extent/location of surgery (28)
Radiation location (29)
Tumor obstruction
Infection (29)
Weight gain (76)
Age (31)
Trauma (77)
Chronic venous disease (78)

Grade 1: The edema pits in response to pressure and is reduced significantly by elevation. There is no clinical evidence of fibrosis.

Grade 2: Edema does not pit in response to pressure and is not reduced by elevation. Moderate to severe fibrosis is evident on clinical examination.

Grade 3: Lymphedema is irreversible and develops as a result of repeated inflammatory insults. Fibrosis and sclerosis of the skin and subcutaneous tissues is present. This stage of edema is known also as lymphostatic elephantiasis.

Lymphedema Diagnosis

The diagnosis of lymphedema is often made on the basis of clinical presentation. Patients with chronic lymphedema usually present with slowly progressive, painless swelling of the extremity. The edema is pitting in the early stages, but usually nonpitting in the chronic stage because of fibrotic changes that have occurred in the skin and subcutaneous tissues. The swelling characteristically starts at the distal end of the extremity and progresses proximally. In the lower extremities, the epidermal tissues over the proximal phalanges of the feet becomes thickened (positive Stemmer's sign) (33). In the early stages of lymphedema, the skin may have a pinkish-red color and mildly elevated temperature due to increased vascularity. In the chronic stage, the skin becomes thickened and exhibits areas of hyperkeratosis and a "peau d'orange" appearance. This reflects the reactive changes of the dermis and epidermis to chronic inflammation caused by lymph stasis (34). Recurrent chronic eczematous dermatitis or excoriation of the skin may occur. Unlike conditions of venous stasis, the skin maintains a higher degree of hydration and elasticity for a long time. Chronic lymph stasis, especially when it is accompanied by lymphatic hyperplasia and valvular incompetence, may result in the appearance of verrucae or small vesicles that drain clear lymph fluid frequently.

Objective criteria for diagnosing and/or quantifying lymphedema have included circumferential measurements made at standard points such as bony landmarks or at equi-distant intervals along a limb. The measurements have then been used to compute limb volumes (35). Alternatively, determining volume by water displacement can be accomplished by submerging the limb in a cylinder filled to a known level of water. However, the interrater reliability of these methods is not well documented. A possibly more reliable method for measuring limbs is the Juzo Perometer, an optoelectronic limb volumeter. This device consists of a square measuring frame containing rows of infrared light emitting diodes on two sides and corresponding light sensors on the opposite two sides of the frame. The limb is measured by moving the frame along the length of the limb causing shadows to be cast in two planes. The Perometer then calculates cross-sectional areas from serial segments 3 mm thick based on assumptions of circular or elliptical cross sections. Several studies comparing limb volumes calculated from measurements made by the Perometer to traditional methods of volume determination, such as water displacement and venous occlusion plethysmography, have shown the Perometer to be a valid and reliable measurement tool (36).

Lymphoscintigraphy is a reliable and reproducible method for confirming the clinical diagnosis of lymphedema. Lymphoscintigraphy is performed by injecting colloids with radioactive tracer into the interstitium of the distal regions of the extremities. A gamma camera is used to make sequential images of the extremities and proximal lymph nodes. In limbs with lymphedema, lymphoscintigrams may show abnormally slow or no uptake of the tracer from the injection site, the presence of a cutaneous or dermal backflow pattern, and/or reduced or no uptake in the lymph nodes of the axilla or groin (37–40). Computed tomography may be used to confirm or exclude any mass obstructing the lymphatic system, and may provide an anatomic definition of edema localization. Although expensive, it may also be used to monitor the response to therapy through serial measurements of the cross-sectional area and tissue density (41,42). Magnetic resonance imaging (MRI) is useful in illustrating nodal anatomy, as well as lymph nodes and larger lymphatic trunks in different tissue planes. At times, MRI is clinically useful in complementing findings observed by lymphoscintigraphy (43). Office ultrasound imaging may provide accurate measurement of clinical subcutaneous lymphedema in the future, but documentation of this modality by large clinical studies is lacking (44,45).

Differential Diagnosis

When evaluating a patient with persistent limb swelling, possible systemic etiologies should be eliminated. Cardiac diseases such as congestive heart failure, chronic constrictive pericarditis, and tricuspid regurgitation frequently cause pitting bilateral lower-extremity swelling. Hepatic or renal failure, hypoproteinemia, malnutrition, and endocrine disorders (myxedema) may also cause lower extremity swelling. Allergic reactions and angioedema are systemic causes that should be considered. Some drugs such as steroids, antihypertensives, and antiinflammatory agents may also cause swelling.

For acute or subacute unilateral edema, deep venous thrombosis must be considered. Because of increased incidence of DVT with some tumors, in nearly all cases of new onset unilateral edema in the cancer patient, occult deep venous thrombosis as an etiology must be excluded. Ultrasound is an efficient and cost-effective examination to rule out deep venous thrombosis as a cause of edema. Because of the related complication of pulmonary embolism and the fact that prompt treatment is indicated, this test should not be overlooked.

Simple venous edema is distinguished from lymphedema by its softness and easy refill of any pitting. It readily reduces with elevation overnight (although grade 1 lymphedema often reduces overnight, also). Varicose veins often are present. While a typical history, temporal association, and characteristic presentation most often suffice to establish the clinical diagnosis of lymphedema, additional tests are sometimes necessary to confirm the presence of impaired lymphatic flow and/or the actual pattern of impaired lymphatic flow within the tissues.

Chronic venous insufficiency is often characterized by the presence of varicosities, pigmentation, induration and possibly, venous ulcers. Chronic inflammation in subcutaneous tissues due to venous stasis may result in destruction of collecting lymph channels and lead to development of a mixed venous-lymphatic edema. While lymphedema usually is painless, venous disorders can produce pain and cramping that is commonly relieved with rest and elevation.

Lipedema is another form of edema that is primarily lower extremity focused and is characterized by deposition of large amounts of fatty tissue in the subcutaneous layers. Commonly, the fat deposition is localized to the lower half of the body (buttocks and lower extremities), but may involve the upper extremities. In its pure form, it rarely involves the feet or hands. It does not pit or have an elevated skin temperature. Evaluation of the lymphatic system with lymphoscintigraphy essentially is normal. Whether preexisting documented lipedema is a risk factor for cancer-related development of lymphedema is not known.

LYMPHEDEMA TREATMENT

Prevention of swelling and the protean complications of lymphedema is the ultimate goal of any treatment program. Efforts in this regard include an oncologic treatment plan utilizing surgical techniques, radiation, and pharmacologic interventions that reduce the risk of lymphedema. Following oncologic surgery, patient education regarding lymphedema and instructions for self care are critical, since delayed treatment can increase morbidity. When swelling does occur, therapy is focused on minimizing the lymphedema as well as reversing and restoring the functional and cosmetic nature of the affected region. Since infection of the affected limb or region can be a common and serious complication, efforts to minimize the risk of infection must be made.

The quality of the data regarding various treatment strategies employed to reduce edema is inconsistent. Nonetheless, there are three general management approaches to reducing lymphedema: rehabilitative, pharmacologic, and surgical.

Rehabilitative Treatment

Rehabilitative interventions have typically been employed by physical and occupational therapists. Combined manual therapy, often referred to as complex decongestive therapy (CDT), is considered by many to be the standard of care for lymphedema (46). CDT combines principles of elevation, skin care, exercise, a specialized massage technique (often referred to as manual lymphatic drainage) and application of external complex multilayered compression with low-stretch bandages (47,48).

Elevation

The mechanism of action of elevation may be through reduction of intravascular hydrostatic pressure, although this is unclear. While elevation of the limb is usually easily accomplished, compliance is untenable in the long term, as the position negatively impacts activities of daily living and sleep. Thus, the contribution of elevation to lymphedema reduction, though helpful, is impractical and cannot be considered the primary treatment intervention. It should, therefore, be considered an adjunct to other therapies.

Skin Hygiene

Skin hygiene is critical in the treatment of chronic lymphedema since patients are susceptible to infection, including cellulitis, an acute infection of the dermis and subcutaneous tissues typically resulting in pain, erythema, and warmth, and lymphangitis, an inflammation of the lymphatic vessels that occurs as a result of infection at a site distal to the vessels. The limbs should be washed regularly with soap and water, and while still moist, lubricated with an alcohol-free emollient cream that traps moisture. Patients with a history of trichophytosis should use a topical medication regularly. Clotrimazole cream 1% or miconazole nitrate cream 2% is sufficient for most patients. For rare refractory cases with associated recurrent episodes of cellulitis, systemic antifungal treatment may be required. Antibacterial agents should be used as appropriate for acute bacterial cellulitis. If treated early, penicillin or a first generation cephalosporin (cephalexin) will usually eradicate the infection. Rarely, intravenous antibiotic therapy is required.

Exercise

Exercise is an integral component of the rehabilitation program. It has been shown to enhance lymph flow and to improve protein resorption (49). It also strengthens muscles of the affected limb, thereby helping to avoid muscle atrophy. Despite a lack of evidence from prospective observational studies, occupational and leisure time physical activities have been feared to be possible risk factors for developing or exacerbating lymphedema. A recent study examined effects of supervised, twice-per-week, upper- and lower-body weight training over a period of six months on the incidence and symptoms of lymphedema. Results confirmed that exercise did not increase the risk for, or exacerbate, the symptoms of lymphedema in breast cancer survivors (50). Any exercise program, however, should be individualized to include combinations of flexibility, aerobic training, and strengthening, although the type, intensity, frequency, and exercise conditions have not been fully defined (51). Exercise is maximally effective when performed while the lymphedematous limb is bandaged or covered with a well-fitting compression garment to augment the compress in related fluid transport effects of muscles on lymphatic vessels. Whether exercise and compression alone are equal in efficacy to the standard comprehensive CDT program remains controversial. There is literature substantiating both views (52–59). This clinic has had excellent results with both methods. Patients for whom the treatment component with MDL is not financially, geographically or physically feasible, may indeed benefit from a reduction program of prescribed exercise and complex multilayered low-stretch compression wrapping program (Fig. 79.1).

Exercise and Cancer Management

Physical activity and exercise are not only important components of a lymphedema management program, but they may also be integral parts of cancer management. Patients with cancer often reduce their physical activity level after diagnosis and during treatment. With earlier detection, improved treatments and increasing survival, the patient's physical condition in the recovery period may amenable to resuming, or even beginning, an exercise program. Data from multiple studies regarding the potential physiologic benefits of exercise in patients with cancer have been summarized elsewhere (60,61) and may include increased aerobic capacity, weight loss and increased lean body mass, and increased strength and flexibility. Exercise may

also reduce the risk of death in patients with cancer. A prospective observational study based on responses of 2,987 women diagnosed with stage I, II, or III breast cancer was undertaken to examine the relationship between physical activity and risk of death (62). The study found that the adjusted relative risk of death was lower for women who walked at an average pace three to five hours per week, compared to those who exercised less.

Engaging in an exercise program may be challenging or difficult, however, for some patients with cancer. For example, radiation-induced brachial and lumbosacral plexopathies can be associated with pain, tingling, itching and burning, and muscle weakness (63). Painful neuropathies resulting from chemotherapy agents are often length-dependent sensorimotor axonal polyneuropathies that produce burning and tingling (63). These sequelae of cancer treatment may interfere with exercise performance and result in a reduction in activity from pre-diagnosis levels. This lack of physical activity may be shown in the future to have an overall effect on the development or management of cancer-related lymphedema, although current studies are lacking.

Specialized Massage

Traditional retrograde massage techniques probably produce a mild pressure gradient that serves to remove edema from the limb. However, a specialized massage technique known as manual lymphatic drainage (48) is now the standard of practice for lymphedema management. Manual lymphatic drainage massage incorporates regional massage with treatment of the affected limb. The body has a number of lymph drainage areas, called lymphotomes, with lymphatic watersheds or divisions between them. If the normal lymphatic drainage of one lymphotome is blocked, the lymph can drain into adjacent ones. Specialized manual lymphatic drainage massage techniques cause the collateral lymphatics of both superficial and deep networks that cross the watersheds to become dilated and reroute more lymph to the lymphotomes that drain normally. Massage also facilitates movement of tissue fluid and protein into lymphatic capillaries and along collecting lymphatics to the lymph nodes.

When deep lymphatic channels are blocked, there is considerable backflow of lymph from overloaded lymphatics into the network of superficial or dermal lymphatics. In these cases, massage is performed in a manner that promotes movement of fluid through these superficial lymphatic vessels to patent lymph nodes. This is possible because the superficial network of lymphatics is devoid of valves. Figure 79.2 shows the effect of complex decongestive therapy, including

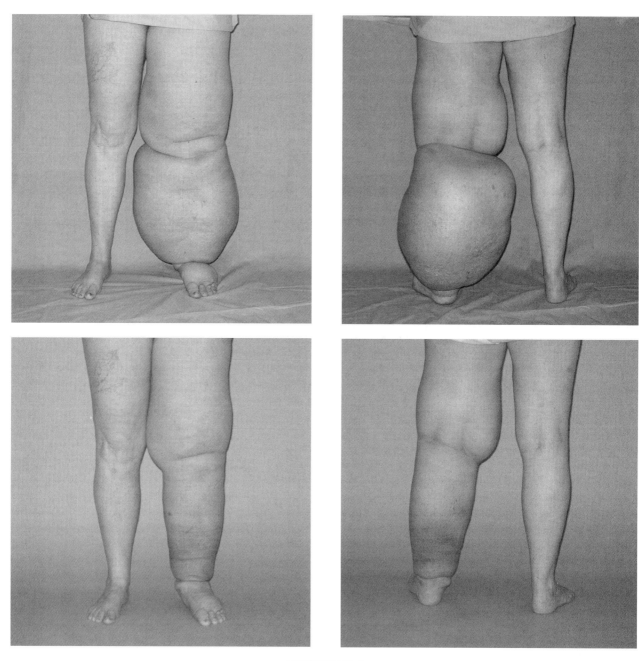

FIGURE 79.1

Severe lower extremity lymphedema developed in a 53-year-old woman after surgery and radiation treatment of cervical cancer. Note the dramatic lymphedema reduction that occurred in the same lower extremity after a program of low-stretch compression bandaging and exercise.

manual lymphatic drainage massage, on upper extremity lymphedema reduction.

Compression

External compression is used for two purposes: (1) to try to reduce edema formation and (2) to aid in removal of excess lymph already accumulated within the limb. Compression of an extremity causes an increase in total tissue pressure. This in turn decreases the hydrostatic pressure gradient from the blood to the tissues and increases the hydrostatic pressure gradient from the tissues to the initial lymphatics. The pressure gradient along the lymphatic trunks also is increased. Compression of lymphedematous limbs is necessary to support the tissues secondary to the loss of elastic fibers and to maintain reductions in swelling during and after treatment. Limbs may be compressed with either bandages

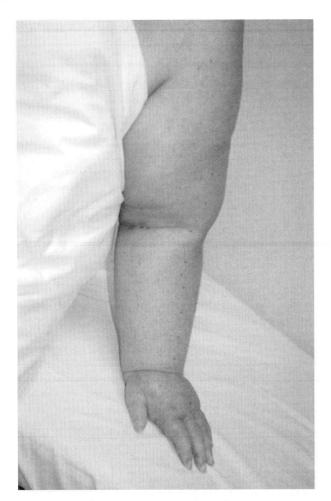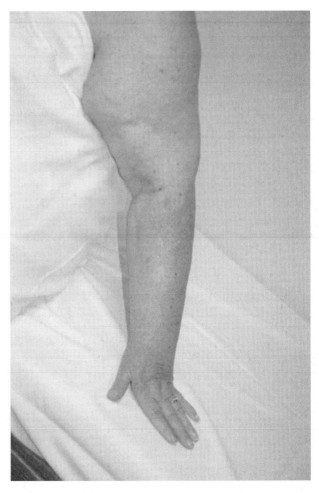

FIGURE 79.2

Left upper extremity lymphedema before and after a program of complex decongestive physiotherapy, including manual lymphatic drainage massage and low-stretch compression bandaging.

or garments. There are two basic types of compression bandages. Elastic or high-stretch compression bandages have a high resting pressure but a low working pressure. Usually they are mildly tight at rest and stretch in response to muscle contraction. Thus, total tissue pressure and lymphatic flow are raised minimally with muscle contraction. Low-elastic or low-stretch compression bandages have a low resting pressure and a high working pressure. They supply a comfortable amount of support to a relaxed limb but increase total tissue pressure when muscles contract. Lymphatic vessels are compressed between the muscles and the bandage(s), causing them to pump forward. Compression bandages are applied with a greater pressure at the distal end of the limb, and a gradually reduced pressure toward the proximal end. Compression bandages are used during the reduction phase of lymphedema management secondary to the more rigid nature of the bandages compared to compression garments. Bandages are also

better suited to reshaping a limb as various types of padding can be inserted beneath them and wrapping techniques can be modified to enhance specific pressure and flow patterns (Fig. 79.3).

Compression garments are constructed with graduated compression. That is, they apply the greatest pressure distally and the least proximally, thus reducing the potential for a tourniquet effect. Garments are available at various levels of compression. The level chosen depends upon how much compression is required to control the lymphedema. A Class I compression garment provides 20–30 mm Hg compression and typically is not used for lower extremity lymphedema, but may be used for mild varicose veins, combined venous and arterial insufficiency, or upper extremity lymphedema. For patients with mild to moderate lymphedema, a Class II compression garment that provides 30–40 mm Hg pressure may be more appropriate for either upper or lower extremity lymphedema. This

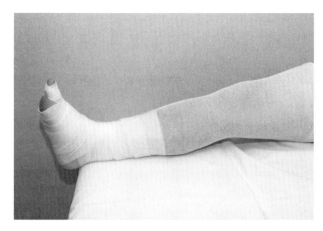

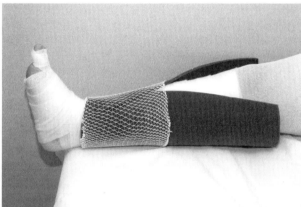

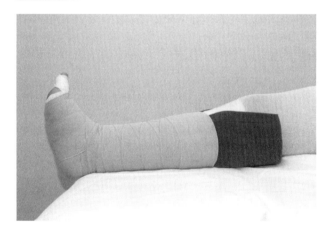

FIGURE 79.3

The basic elements of low-stretch compression bandaging of a lower extremity, including cotton padding for skin protection, foam for contouring of the limb, and nonelastic, low-stretch compression bandages.

may also be used for severe venous edema. A Class III compression garment (40–50 mm Hg) may be used for lymphedema of the leg. For severe lymphedema of the lower extremity, a Class IV compression garment (50–60 mm Hg) may be required. The lymphedema patient now benefits from expanded options in fabric weave, color, and more tailored sizing available from many different garment companies.

Intermittent Vasopneumatic Compression

Vasopneumatic compression had been the mainstay of lymphedema therapy for many years. However, there are no established guidelines regarding the use of multiple and varied compression pump options. Vasopneumatic compression therapy is administered by inserting the lymphedematous extremity or body part into a multi-air cell inflatable appliance (eg, sleeve, vest, boot, trouser) that is attached to an air compression pump. Sequential inflation and deflation of the air cells creates a distal to proximal compression wave that moves the water component, but not the excess protein component, of the lymph and interstitial fluid out of the affected territory (64). One study comparing the treatment of breast cancer-related upper extremity lymphedema with either manual lymphatic drainage massage or intermittent pneumatic compression found that both treatment methods significantly reduced limb volume, but did not find a statistically significant difference between the two methods (54). The use of intermittent compression as an adjunct to complex decongestive physiotherapy in the initial treatment of breast cancer-related upper extremity lymphedema has also been studied (53). This study found that combining complex decongestive physiotherapy with pneumatic compression resulted in greater mean limb volume reduction than complex decongestive physiotherapy alone.

Integral components of successful home management programs for lymphedema include the quality of the patient or caregiver-administered treatment(s) and patient compliance. Before the conclusion of initial, formal lymphedema therapy, patients are often taught self-administered manual lymphatic drainage massage techniques to use at home as part of the "maintenance" portion of the program. By nature, massage technique and quality may vary widely. Several studies have attempted to examine the potential benefit of using intermittent pneumatic compression on maintaining, or further reducing lymphedema, during the maintenance phase of management. The mechanical nature of pneumatic compression devices may provide more consistent, long-term treatment. One study found that when intermittent compression therapy was combined with self-administered manual lymphatic drainage massage, the effect on lymphedema reduction was significantly greater than with the massage alone (53). Another pilot study compared the response of cancer-related upper extremity lymphedema to treatment by self-administered massage and treatment with the Flexitouch, a device that is reported to mechanically simulate manual lymphatic drainage massage (65). The results of the study suggested that the Flexitouch was more effective in reducing lymphedema than self-administered massage alone. Further studies are needed to evaluate the potential contribution of vasopneumatic compression therapy as initial, or as adjunct intervention, in lymphedema treatment.

Pharmacologic Treatment

Generally, pharmacologic therapy has not played a significant role in lymphedema management. Many commonly used drugs have limited value. Since lymphedema is caused by stagnation of proteins in the interstitium (a high protein edema) and not by retention of sodium, diuretics should be used only to treat cases of generalized, low protein edema, and when total body sodium is elevated. When the effects of the diuretics cease, the colloid osmotic pressure exerted by the proteins will cause water to re-accumulate in the tissues.

Benzyopyrones such as coumarin and hydroxyethylrutin, and flavonoid derivatives such as diosmin have been tested in research studies (66–68). The mechanism of action of the drugs was thought to be the stimulation of tissue macrophage activity, resulting in a decrease in tissue protein concentration. The United States and Australia abandoned the use of oral coumarin due to liver toxicity and inconsistent efficacy (68).

Surgical Treatment

Excisional debulking or reduction surgery has sometimes been recommended for patients with significant functional impairment due to excessive lymphedema. This type of procedure may be appropriate to decrease the volume of the affected extremity when irreversible skin and subcutaneous tissue changes have occurred. Successful series of surgical reconstruction of obstructed lymphatics through procedures such as lymphatic grafting or lympholymphatic anastomoses (69,70) or lymphovenous anastomoses (71) have been reported. The effectiveness of these procedures is uncertain, as the long-term patency and function of such anastomoses is unknown. At present in the United States, these procedures are not considered first-line treatment for chronic lymphedema. Additionally, there is now a developing literature for liposuction as a useful procedure for tissue reduction in recalcitrant lymphedema (72). Literature regarding increased adipose tissue in mature lymphedema of the upper extremity has been reported (73). A free-flap graft has also been reported to be successful in restoring lymph flow (74,75). Further studies documenting the reproducibility of all of the above-mentioned surgical procedures are needed, and currently conservative medical management through

rehabilitative techniques remain the hallmark of treatment of this difficult clinical issue facing patients with cancer.

References

1. von Eschenbach AC. A vision for the National Cancer Program in the United States. *Nat Rev Cancer.* 2004;4(10):820–828.
2. von Eschenbach AC. Keynote speech: progress with a purpose. *Cancer.* 2005;104(12 Suppl):2903–2904.
3. Aziz N, Rowland J. Trends and advances in cancer survivorship research: challenge and opportunity. *Semin Radiat Oncol.* 2003;13(3):248–266.
4. Leak L. Electron microscopic observations on lymphatic capillaries and the structural components of the connective tissue lymph interface. *Microvasc Res.* 1970;2:361–391.
5. Guyton A, Taylor A, Granger H. *Circulatory Physiology II: Dynamics and Control of the Body Fluids.* Philadelphia, PA: WB Saunders; 1975.
6. Reichert F. The regeneration of the lymphatics. *Arch Surg.* 1926;13:871–881.
7. Danese C, Georgalas-Bertakis M, Morales L. A model of chronic postsurgical lymphedema in dogs' limbs. *Surgery.* 1968;64:814–880.
8. Olszewski W. On the pathomechanism of development of postsurgical lymphedema. *Lymphology.* 1973;6:35–52.
9. Blalock A, Robinson C, Cunningham R, et al. Experimental studies on lymphatic blockade. *Arch Surg.* 1937;34:1049–1055.
10. Edwards E. Recurrent febrile episodes and lymphedema. *JAMA.* 1963;184:102–110.
11. Homans J, Drinker C, Field M. Elephantiasis and clinical implications of its experimental reproduction in animals. *Ann Surg.* 1934;100:812–832.
12. Halsted WS. Replantation of entire limbs without suture of vessels, *Proc Natl Acad Sci. USA.* 1922;8(7):181–186.
13. Poslethwaite A, Keski-Oja J, Balian G, et al. Induction of fibroblast chemotaxis by fibronectin. *J Exp Med.* 1981;153:494–499.
14. Piller N. Lymphedema macrophages and benzopyrones. *Lymphology.* 1980;13:67–73.
15. Bolton T, Casley-Smith J. The in vitro demonstration of proteolysis by macrophages and its increase with coumarin. *Experientia.* 1975;31:271–273.
16. Casley-Smith J, Foldi-Borcsok E, Foldi M. Fine structural aspects of lymphedema in various tissues and the effects of treatment with coumarin and troxerutin. *Br J Exp Pathol.* 1974;55:88–93.
17. Lobb A, Harkins H. Postmastectomy swelling of the arm with note on effect of segmental resection of axillary vein at the time of radical mastectomy. *West J Surg.* 1949;57:550–555.
18. Veronesi U, Saccozzi R, Del Vecchio M, et al. Comparing radical mastectomy with quadrantectomy, axillary dissection, and radiotherapy in patients with small cancers of the breast. *N Engl J Med.* 1981;305(1):6–11.
19. Papachristou D, Fortner JG. Comparison of lymphedema following incontinuity and discontinuity groin dissection. *Ann Surg.* 1977;185(1):13–16.
20. Smith C. *The Pathophysiology of Lymphedema.* Tel Aviv, Israel: Immunology Research Foundation Inc; 1983.
21. Boris M, Weindorf S, Lasinski B, Boris G. Lymphedema reduction by noninvasive complex lymphedema therapy. *Oncology (Williston Park).* 1994;8(9):95–106; discussion 9–10.
22. Sener SF, Winchester DJ, Martz CH, et al. Lymphedema after sentinel lymphadenectomy for breast carcinoma. *Cancer.* 2001;92(4):748–752.
23. Cheville AL, Tchou J. Barriers to rehabilitation following surgery for primary breast cancer. *J Surg Oncol.* 2007;95(5):409–418.

24. Erickson VS, Pearson ML, Ganz PA, Adams J, Kahn KL. Arm edema in breast patients with cancer. *J Natl Cancer Inst.* 2001;93(2):96–111.

25. Petrek J, Presman P, et al. The American Cancer Society lymphedema: results from a workshop on breast cancer treatment-related lymphedema and lymphedema resource guide. *Cancer.* 1998;83:2775–2890.

26. Petrek J, Senie R, Peters M, Rosen P. Lymphedema in a cohort of breast carcinoma survivors 20 years after diagnosis. *Cancer.* 2001;92(6):1368–1377.

27. Smith RD, Spittell JA, Schirger A. Secondary lymphedema of the leg: its characteristics and diagnostic implications. *JAMA.* 1963;185:80–82.

28. Herd-Smith A, Russo A, Muraca MG, Del Turco MR, Cardona G. Prognostic factors for lymphedema after primary treatment of breast carcinoma. *Cancer.* 2001;92(7):1783–1787.

29. Segerstrom K, Bjerle P, Graffman S, Nystrom A. Factors that influence the incidence of brachial oedema after treatment of breast cancer. *Scand J Plast Reconstr Surg Hand Surg.* 1992;26(2):223–227.

30. Werner R, McCormick B, Petrek J, et al. Arm edema in conservatively managed breast cancer: obesity is a major predictive factor. *Radiology.* 1991;180(1):177–184.

31. Kocak Z, Overgaard J. Risk factors for arm lymphedema in breast cancer patients. *Acta oncologica.* 2000;39:389–392.

32. Consensus Document of the International Society of Lymphology. In: The diagnosis and treatment of peripheral lymphedema. *Lymphology.* 2003;36(2):84–91.

33. Stemmer R. Stemmer's sign—possibilities and limits of clinical diagnosis of lymphedema. *Wien Med Wochenschr.* 1999;149(2–4):85–86.

34. Schirger A. Lymphedema. *Cardiovasc Clin.* 1983;13(2):293–305.

35. Latchford S, Casley-Smith JR. Estimating limb volumes and alterations in peripheral edema from circumferences measured at different intervals. *Lymphology.* 1997;30(4):161–164.

36. Stanton AW, Northfield JW, Holroyd B, Mortimer PS, Levick JR. Validation of an optoelectronic limb volumeter (Perometer). *Lymphology.* 1997;30(2):77–97.

37. Weissleder H, Weissleder R. Lymphedema: evaluation of qualitative and quantitative lymphoscintigraphy in 238 patients. *Radiology.* 1988;167(3):729–735.

38. Vaqueiro M, Gloviczki P, Fisher J, Hollier LH, Schirger A, Wahner HW. Lymphoscintigraphy in lymphedema: an aid to microsurgery. *J Nucl Med.* 1986;27(7):1125–1130.

39. Collins PS, Villavicencio JL, Abreu SH, et al. Abnormalities of lymphatic drainage in lower extremities: a lymphoscintigraphic study. *J Vasc Surg.* 1989;9(1):145–152.

40. Gloviczki P, Calcagno D, Schirger A, et al. Noninvasive evaluation of the swollen extremity: experiences with 190 lymphoscintigraphic examinations. *J Vasc Surg.* 1989;9(5):683–689; discussion 90.

41. Hadjis NS, Carr DH, Banks L, Pflug JJ. The role of CT in the diagnosis of primary lymphedema of the lower limb. *AJR Am J Roentgenol.* 1985;144(2):361–364.

42. Monnin-Delhom ED, Gallix BP, Achard C, Bruel JM, Janbon C. High resolution unenhanced computed tomography in patients with swollen legs. *Lymphology.* 2002;35(3):121–128.

43. Lohrmann C, Foeldi E, Bartholomae JP, Langer M. Gadoteridol for MR imaging of lymphatic vessels in lymphoedematous patients: initial experience after intracutaneous injection. *Br J Radiol.* 2007;80(955):569–573.

44. Balzarini A, Milella M, Civelli E, Sigari C, De Conno F. Ultrasonography of arm edema after axillary dissection for breast cancer: a preliminary study. *Lymphology.* 2001;34(4):152–155.

45. Mellor RH, Bush NL, Stanton AW, Bamber JC, Levick JR, Mortimer PS. Dual-frequency ultrasound examination of skin and subcutis thickness in breast cancer-related lymphedema. *Breast J.* 2004;10(6):496–503.

46. Cheville AL MC, Petrek JA, Russo SA, Taylor ME, Thiadens SR. Lymphedema management. *Semin Radiat Oncol.* 2003;13(3):290–301.

47. Position Statement of the National Lymphedema Network: Exercise 2005. 2005. (Accessed March 1, 2009, at www.lymphnet.org/pdfDocs/nlntreatment.pdf)

48. The diagnosis and treatment of peripheral lymphedema. Consensus document of the International Society of Lymphology. *Lymphology.* 2003;36(2):84–91.

49. Leduc O, Peeters A, Bourgeois P. Bandages: scintigraphic demonstration of its efficacy on colloidal protein reabsorption during muscle activity; In: Nishi, ed. Progress in Lymphology. Amsterdam: Elsevier. 1990:421–423.

50. Ahmed RL, Thomas W, Yee D, Schmitz KH. Randomized controlled trial of weight training and lymphedema in breast cancer survivors. *J Clin Oncol.* 2006;24(18):2765–2772.

51. Position Statement of the National Lymphedema Network: Treatment 2006.

52. Johansson K, Albertsson M, Ingvar C, Ekdahl C. Effects of compression bandaging with or without manual lymph drainage treatment in patients with postoperative arm lymphedema. *Lymphology.* 1999;32(3):103–110.

53. Szuba A, Achalu R, Rockson S. Decongestive lymphatic therapy for patients with breast carcinoma-associated lymphedema. A randomized, prospective study of a role for adjunctive intermittent pneumatic compression. *Cancer.* 2002;95(11):2260–2267.

54. Johansson K, Lie E, Ekdahl C, Lindfeldt J. A randomized study comparing manual lymph drainage with sequential pneumatic compression for treatment of postoperative arm lymphedema. *Lymphology.* 1998;31(2):56–64.

55. McNeely ML, Magee DJ, Lees AW, Bagnall KM, Haykowsky M, Hanson J. The addition of manual lymph drainage to compression therapy for breast cancer related lymphedema: a randomized controlled trial. *Breast Cancer Res Treat.* 2004;86(2):95–106.

56. Andersen L, Hojris I, Erlandsen M, Andersen J. Treatment of breast-cancer-related lymphedema with or without manual lymphatic drainage—a randomized study. *Acta Oncol.* 2000;39(3):399–405.

57. Williams AF, Vadgama A, Franks PJ, Mortimer PS. A randomized controlled crossover study of manual lymphatic drainage therapy in women with breast cancer-related lymphoedema. *Eur J Cancer Care (Engl).* 2002;11(4):254–261.

58. Ko DS, Lerner R, Klose G, Cosimi AB. Effective treatment of lymphedema of the extremities. *Arch Surg.* 1998;133(4):452–458.

59. Szuba A CJ, Yousuf S, Rockson S. Decongestive lymphatic therapy for patients with cancer-related or primary lymphedema. *Am J Med.* 2000;109(4):296–300.

60. McTiernan A. Physical activity after cancer: physiologic outcomes. *Cancer Invest.* 2004;22(1):68–81.

61. Galvao DA, Newton RU. Review of exercise intervention studies in patients with cancer. *J Clin Oncol.* 2005;23(4):899–909.

62. Holmes MD, Chen WY, Feskanich D, Kroenke CH, Colditz GA. Physical activity and survival after breast cancer diagnosis. *JAMA.* 2005;293(20):2479–2486.

63. Hammack J. Cancer pain. In: Schiff D, Wen PY, eds. *Cancer Neurology in Clinical Practice.* Totowa, NJ: Humana Press, Inc.; 2003:57–70.

64. Miranda F, Jr., Perez MC, Castiglioni ML, et al. Effect of sequential intermittent pneumatic compression on both leg lymphedema volume and on lymph transport as semi-quantitatively evaluated by lymphoscintigraphy. *Lymphology.* 2001;34(3):135–141.

65. Wilburn O, Wilburn P, Rockson SG. A pilot, prospective evaluation of a novel alternative for maintenance therapy of breast cancer-associated lymphedema [ISRCTN76522412]. *BMC Cancer.* 2006;6:84.

66. Casley-Smith JR, Morgan RG, Piller NB. Treatment of lymphedema of the arms and legs with 5,6-benzo-[alpha]-pyrone. *N Engl J Med.* 1993;329(16):1158–1163.

67. Casley-Smith JR, Wang CT, Casley-Smith JR, Zi-hai C. Treatment of filarial lymphoedema and elephantiasis with 5,6-benzo-alpha-pyrone (coumarin). *BMJ.* 1993;307(6911):1037–1041.

68. Loprinzi CL, Kugler JW, Sloan JA, et al. Lack of effect of coumarin in women with lymphedema after treatment for breast cancer. *N Engl J Med.* 1999;340(5):346–350.

69. Baumeister RG, Siuda S, Bohmert H, Moser E. A microsurgical method for reconstruction of interrupted lymphatic pathways: autologous lymph-vessel transplantation for treatment of lymphedemas. *Scand J Plast Reconstr Surg.* 1986;20(1):141–146.

70. Baumeister RG, Siuda S. Treatment of lymphedemas by microsurgical lymphatic grafting: what is proved? *Plast Reconstr Surg.* 1990;85(1):64–74; discussion 5–6.

71. Campisi C, Boccardo F. Microsurgical techniques for lymphedema treatment: derivative lymphatic-venous microsurgery. *World J Surg.* 2004;28(6):609–613.

72. Brorson H. Liposuction in arm lymphedema treatment. *Scand J Surg.* 2003;92(4):287–295.

73. Brorson H, Ohlin K, Olsson G, Nilsson M. Adipose tissue dominates chronic arm lymphedema following breast cancer: an analysis using volume rendered CT images. *Lymphat Res Biol.* 2006;4(4):199–210.

74. Classen DA, Irvine L. Free muscle flap transfer as a lymphatic bridge for upper extremity lymphedema. *J Reconstr Microsurg.* 2005;21(2):93–99.

75. Slavin SA, Van den Abbeele AD, Losken A, Swartz MA, Jain RK. Return of lymphatic function after flap transfer for acute lymphedema. *Ann Surg.* 1999;229(3):421–427.

76. Werner RS, McCormick B, Petrek J, et al. Arm edema in conservatively managed breast cancer: obesity is a major predictive factor. *Radiology.* 1991;180(1):177–184.

77. Pavlotsky F, Amrani S, Trau H. Recurrent erysipelas: risk factors. *J Dtsch Dermatol Ges.* 2004;2(2):89–95.

78. Mortimer PS. Implications of the lymphatic system in CVI-associated edema. *Angiology.* 2000;51(1):3–7.

IX

SPECIAL TOPICS IN CANCER REHABILITATION

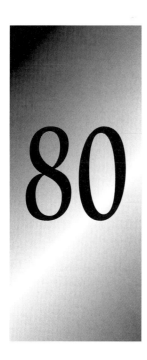

Metrics in Cancer Rehabilitation

Andrea L. Cheville

Function is vitally important to patients with cancer, whether they are receiving active treatment, free of disease, or in the far-advanced stages. Irrespective of patients' position on the disease continuum, they wish to retain and exercise their autonomy (1). Waning functional status and increasing dependency undermine patients' psychological well being and quality of life (QOL) (2). Patients' function also affects their utilization of health care resources as well as their caregivers' health (3). The importance of function has become increasingly appreciated by health care stakeholders. Function has been singled out by the Institute of Medicine, third party payers, and federal funding agencies as a principal clinical outcome (4). Future emphasis on functional outcomes can be safely anticipated in light of the increasing popularity of performance-based compensation.

Functional assessment is a distinguishing feature of rehabilitation medicine. Utilization of appropriate metrics will inevitably enhance judgments regarding patients' functional prognoses, needs, and treatment responsiveness. While poor measurement choices in an isolated clinician's practice may have less impact than those of an investigator conducting a major interventional trial, in an era of increased safety and quality awareness, the elimination of measurement error should be a priority for both. All measurement represents an effort to characterize variance that reliably associates with clinical phenomena. As such, both the simplest and

most intricate measurement techniques share commonalities which must be appreciated to minimize error.

Researchers and clinicians may harbor unexamined expectations of metrics, to their disadvantage. Frequent expectations include that metrics will be readily understood by patients, of undisputed clinical relevance, easy to administer, sensitive to the outcome of interest, insensitive to other factors, and responsive to change. When metrics produce differing scores, it is expected that these scores reflect "true" differences in patients. Further, researchers often take for granted that metrics are reliable, accurate, precise, and valid. These latter terms, defined in Table 80.1, have specific significance in relation to measurement. In short, metrics are expected to provide the clinician or researcher with the information they want unlimited by factors of lesser interest. Unfortunately, complexities confront would-be measurers with formidable pitfalls.

Metrics, like any common tool, have limited capabilities. However, metrics' failings are not always immediately obvious and may lead to erroneous investigative conclusions and clinical treatments. Few readers wish to be psychometricians, yet some awareness of measurement theory is needed for discriminating consumption of the medical literature, effective research, and savvy clinician judgments. The perfect metric does not exist. Selection of a metric, therefore, reflects a series of tradeoffs. This chapter aims to clarify some of the significant difficulties inherent in measuring function, particularly

KEY POINTS

- Function has been singled out by the Institute of Medicine and other health care stakeholders as a principal measure of clinical outcome.
- Functional assessment tools must be sensitive to the parameter of interest (eg, shoulder range of motion, gait stability) and, if used to track a trajectory of function over time, reasonable in terms of the burden of time and cost to administer.
- There are three general approaches to functional measurement: self report, clinician report, and objective testing, each with unique strengths, weaknesses, and costs.

- Clinicians should exercise caution when adding new questions to a standard instrument as this may substantially alter the validity of the tool.
- Weaknesses of clinician assessment include limited observations of proxy activities and relatively artificial testing circumstances in the clinic as opposed to those at home.
- A new approach to assessment is computer adaptive testing (CAT), wherein each test is individualized based on patients' responses to previous items, thus adjusting to the level of each patient and obviating the need to administer large numbers of potentially uninformative questions.

those pertaining to cancer patients, so that readers will be better equipped to make educated and conscious tradeoffs, and to appreciate the tradeoffs that others have made.

GOALS OF MEASUREMENT

In approaching functional measurement, a critical initial step is defining precisely what parameter should be measured in the population of interest. Common

reasons for measurement and questions that exemplify the need for each approach are listed in Table 80.2.

The goals of measurement to help prioritize the attributes of available metrics. For example, to assess the effects of a therapeutic intervention, a metric that is both sensitive to the clinical parameter of interest (eg, shoulder range of motion, gait stability) and, more importantly, responsive to change, should be selected. Other characteristics become somewhat less important, and a few undesirable attributes may be tolerated (eg, lack of validation in the population of interest) in a particularly responsive metric. On the other hand, to

TABLE 80.1
Terms Used to Describe Metrics

TERM (REF.)	DEFINITION
	A metric's capacity to:
Validity (28)	Allow the measurer to make confident inferences regarding the subject of measurement
Reliability (28)	Generate reproducible results under different conditions
Accuracy (46)	Represent what it is intended to represent without bias
Precision (46)	Generate exactly the same result each time under identical conditions
Sensitivity (47)	Yield a positive result when a condition is present (outcome classified as present or absent)
Specificity (47)	Yield a negative result when a condition is not present (outcome classified as present or absent)
Responsiveness (28)	Detect change when present

TABLE 80.2
Common Reasons for Function-Related Measurement

- To evaluate the effect of treatment: Does post-transplant aerobic conditioning improve mobility?
- To characterize a population: How well do elderly cancer survivors perform IADLs?
- To characterize change over time: What is the trajectory of disablement in advanced lung cancer?
- To define where an individual lies in relation to a larger population for prognostication and treatment determination: Is Patient X's emotional functioning poorer than other cancer patients?
- To estimate need: Will >30% of patients require manual wheelchairs following hip arthroplasty for bone metastases?
- To characterize the impact of a specific impairment: Do radiation-induced brachial plexopathies undermine ADL performance?
- To determine whether patients have crossed a critical threshold (high or low): Does Patient Y have sufficient oral excursion to eat normally?

characterize the trajectory of function over time, repeated assessments will be needed, and the priority becomes minimizing respondent burden and cost. In this case a short assessment instrument would be preferred and the downside of less comprehensive evaluation would be acceptable.

Clarification of metrics' performance parameters or "psychometric characteristics" is an essential step. The refereed medical literature provides an excellent starting point. There are journals devoted, to clinical measurement. Most QOL metrics in widespread use have numerous publications devoted to their psychometric performance in different clinical settings and research initiatives. The literature on functional metrics is less robust but worth searching. Often, the "Methods" section of papers dealing with particular research questions (eg, sexual function after cervical cancer treatment) will describe measurement approaches in considerable detail. Such descriptions can provide invaluable information about potential measurement tools as well as key references. An alternate approach is to question experienced clinicians or investigators in one's area of interest. Often, senior faculty will have insights regarding a metric that cannot be gleaned from the literature. Lastly, there is no substitute for piloting an instrument or measurement technique. No matter how extensively a metric has been described, one can never know exactly how it will perform in a unique setting, administered to specific patients by a particular investigator.

APPROACHES TO MEASURING FUNCTION

There are three basic approaches to functional measurement. They include self report, clinician report, and objective testing. Each approach has strengths and weaknesses that should be carefully considered—along with the depth of one's wallet, since their associated costs can vary considerably.

Self-Report

Self-reporting is the most common measurement approach in clinical research. This fact is manifest in the many instruments that have been developed for every imaginable parameter. Self-report measurement has at its root the conviction that patients are the best information source regarding their status. This is a compelling argument and, together with the many pros of this approach, listed in Table 80.3, accounts for its popularity.

There are essentially four options for self-report measurement of function in cancer cohorts: (1) function-oriented items from QOL instruments; (2) generic func-

tion instruments; (3) activity profiles; and (4) region- or domain-specific instruments. QOL instruments may be generic, such as Short Form-36 (SF-36) (5), or cancer-specific, such as Functional Assessment of Cancer Therapy (FACT) (6); Functional Living Index-Cancer (FLIC) (7); European Organization for Research and Treatment of Cancer Quality of Life Questionnaire (EORTC-QLQ) (8); and Cancer Rehabilitation Evaluation System (CARES) (9). Several of the cancer-specific metrics have been further tailored to address the unique features of specific cancer cohorts (eg, FACT-Breast). Since function is considered a critical QOL domain, each instrument includes function-specific items. The SF-36, for example, contains 10 functional items, which have been independently validated as the Physical Function-10 (PF-10) (10; Table 80.4). Because functional items are part of more extensive QOL instruments they are, of necessity, limited in scope and length. Hence, they may not cover areas deemed critical or cover them in a cursory manner. An up side to these instruments is the extensive support for their validity. The PF-10, for example, as part of the SF-36, has been validated in many clinical populations and languages.

Function-specific instruments may be preferable when greater depth of assessment is needed. These are more limited in number. Instruments generally encompass mobility, ADLs, and instrumental ADLs (IADLs) such as shopping meal preparation, etc. The Older Americans Resource Study (11) includes, for example, 14 items for ADL and IADL assessment. A major limitation of these instruments reflects their origins in assessment of the elderly and disabled. The items generally focus on basic activities and do not adequately assess the higher functional capacities required for independent living. A clinician or investigator may add non-validated questions, but in doing so, the investigator is rendered vulnerable to criticism regarding lack of validation, which some reviewers consider de rigueur.

Activity profiles query patients about how often they perform activities and assess the complex activities involved in leisure and vocational pursuits. The Baecke Physical Activity Questionnaire (12) and the Godin Leisure Time Exercise Questionnaire (13) (Table 80.5) are examples. The fact that these tools assess "high-level" activities can be a significant disadvantage when assessing cancer patients. Many patients may have ceased such activities and the activity profiles will not discriminate effectively. The Baecke Physical Activity Questionnaire, for example, includes questions about respondents' primary and secondary sports. These questions may be appropriate for the healthy young Dutch who participated in the initial validation study, but they are largely uninformative in cancer cohorts.

Region or activity-specific functional instruments are plentiful and utilized by many medical disciplines.

TABLE 80.3
Pros and Cons of General Approaches to Measuring Function

	SELF-REPORT	CLINICIAN REPORT	OBJECTIVE TESTING
Pros			
Wide range of available metrics	√		√
Closely reflects patients "true" experience ("from the horses mouth")	√		
Relatively inexpensive	√		
Many ways to administer (in person, via telephone, by mail, over the Internet)	√		
Can reflect patient's entire experience	√		
Facilitates reproducibility of other investigator's results	√		√
Use of sophisticated assessment techniques		√	√
Trained and experienced eye capable of subtle distinctions		√	
Common language of functional assessment		√	
Ability to quantify inter-rater reliability	√	√	√
Limited number of measurers relative to study sample		√	√
Generate parametric data			√
Minimize inter-rater inconsistencies			√
Cons			
Can be influenced by patient-based factors (e.g. mood, pain)	√		
Subject to social acceptability and other biases	√		
Clinician assessment biases		√	
Patients may lack a reference frame for certain questions (They do not have a job, caregiver, etc.)	√		
Patients may frankly misrepresent themselves	√		
Expensive		√	√
Limited to activities that can be performed at test site		√	√
Patients must travel to test site		√	√
Proxy for activity of interest		√	√

These instruments are focused in scope and query patients regarding specific activities or the use of a discreet body region. Swallowing, elimination, and sexual function questionnaires are examples of the former, while the Disability of Shoulder, Arm, and Hand (DASH) (14) is an example of the latter. Such specialized metrics are capable of detecting signals that would be lost to metrics of broader scope.

The overarching problem with self-reporting is that patients' responses may not accurately reflect their "true" functional status for a number of reasons. Patients may deliberately dissemble, as has been reported in some elderly patients who fear being stripped of their autonomy. Cancer patients may similarly fear being deemed ineligible for promising treatments if they report poor functioning. Patients may also satisfice. Satisficing refers to the practice of rapidly completing questionnaires without giving questions adequate consideration, so that answers do not reflect respondents'

"true" state or experience. Conversely, the efforts of many patients who sincerely try to represent themselves accurately may be undermined by other factors. Factors relevant to cancer cohorts include depression, denial, inaccurate self-assessment, and failure to appreciate their dependence on caregiver assistance. Such sources of inaccuracy are one of the most compelling arguments for clinician report metrics.

Clinician Report

Clinician report offers the opportunity to circumvent patient-based measurement problems. While clinicians are certainly not bias free, ideally they have a highly trained and experienced eye capable of rendering accurate assessments. The benefits of assessment by a skilled professional must be weighed against the considerable cost. An additional downside to clinician-report is the requirement for patients to travel to the

---

TABLE 80.4

The Physical Function-10 (PF-10) Questionnaire

The following questions are about activities you might do during a typical day. Does your health now limit you in these activities? If so, how much? **(Please circle one number on each line.)**

	Yes, Limited A Lot	Yes, Limited A Little	Yes, Limited At All
3(a) **Vigorous activities**, such as running, lifting heavy objects, participating in strenuous sports	1	2	3
3(b) **Moderate activities**, such as moving, a table, pushing a vacuum cleaner, bowling, or playing golf	1	2	3
3(c) Lifting or carrying groceries	1	2	3
3(d) Climbing **several** flights of stairs	1	2	3
3(e) Climbing **one** flight of stairs	1	2	3
3(f) Bending, kneeling, or stooping	1	2	3
3(g) Waling **more than a mile**	1	2	3
3(h) Walking **several blocks**	1	2	3
3(i) Walking **one blocks**	1	2	3
3(j) Bathing or dressing yourself	1	2	3

TABLE 80.5

Godin Leisure-Time Exercise Questionnaire

1. During a typical 7-day period (a week), how many times on the average do you do the following kinds of exercise for more than 15 minutes during your free time (write on each line the appropriate number).
   a. Strenuous Exercise (heart beats rapidly) (e.g. running, jogging, hockey, football, soccer, squash, basketball, cross country skiing, judo, roller skating, vigorous swimming, vigorous long distance bicycling). Times per week_____
   b. Moderate Exercise (not exhausting) (e.g. fast walking, baseball, tennis, easy bicycling, volleyball, badminton, easy swimming, alpine skiing, popular and folk dancing). Times per week_____
   c. Mild Exercies (minimal effort) (e.g. yoga, archery, fishing from river bank, bowling, horseshoes, golf, snow-mobiling, easy walking). Times per week_____
2. During a typical 7-day period (a week), in your leisure time, how often do you engage in any regular activity long enough to work up a sweat (heart beats rapidly)?
   a. Often
   b. Sometimes
   c. Never/rarely

assessment site, which may become challenging as cancer progresses and renders patients increasingly disabled. A related limitation is the fact that evaluations must be restricted to activities that can be performed at the assessment site. For basic mobility and self-care activities this is not problematic; however, in the absence of specialized equipment, many higher level activities cannot be assessed.

Most clinician report instruments are composite tools including multiple items that cover one or more functional domains. Examples include the Functional Independence Measure (15) (Table 80.6), the Barthel Mobility Index (16), and the Tinetti Balance Scale (17). All require the clinician to observe patients as they perform discrete activities, to make trained assessments, and to rate their performance, generally on ordinal scales. Individual items are then tallied to produce a summary score. A downside of this approach is that multiple functional domains (eg, mobility, self-care) may be collapsed to generate a single score and Important information may be lost in this manner.

Clinician-rated scales are well known in routine oncology practice. The Karnofsky Performance Scale (KPS) (18) and the Eastern Cooperative Oncology Group (ECOG) Scale (19) are both clinician-rated, ordinal scales that rate patients' global performance status. In contrast to the clinician-rated tools commonly used in rehabilitation settings, the KPS and ECOG scales do not require direct clinician observation of specific

TABLE 80.6
The Functional Independence Measure (FIM)

	ADMISSION	DISCHARGE	FOLLOW-UP
Self-care			
Eating			
Grooming			
Bathing			
Dressing: upper body			
Dressing: lower body			
Toileting			
Sphincter control			
Bladder management			
Bowel management			
Transfers			
Bed, chair, wheelchair			
Toilet			
Tub, shower			
Locomotion			
Walk/wheelchair			
Stairs			
Motor subtotal score			
Communication			
Comprehension			
Expression			
Social cognition			
Social interaction			
Problem solving			
Memory			
Cognitive subtotal score			
TOTAL FIM score			

LEVELS

Independent: no helper required
7 complete independence (timely, safely)
6 modified independence (device)

Modified dependence: requires helper
5 supervision (subject = 100%+)
4 minimal assist (subject = 75%+)
3 moderate assist (subject = 50%+)

Complete dependence: requires helper
2 maximal assist (subject = 25%+)
1 total assist (subject = less than 25%)

Note: Leave no blanks. Enter 1 if patient is not testable due to risk.

functional tasks. Rather, assessments are based on clinicians' general impressions of patients' overall performance. The potential for rater bias is considerable, since oncologists have unique knowledge of patients' disease status from serological and imaging studies, as well as their cancer treatment histories.

An important consideration of clinician rated tools is the fact that they are based on limited observation of proxy activities. That is to say, clinicians observe patients performing an activity once, or at most a very few times. From this limited sample, clinicians generalize to the patient's "true" ability to perform the activity. The observed activity (eg, a functional transfer) becomes the proxy for all the times a patient must perform the activity under different conditions and with varying levels of pain, fatigue, and support. As any statistician will confirm, generalizing from a limited sample can be hazardous. If the consequences of error are small and pose no danger to the patient, the hazard may be acceptable. However, in functional assessment this is not always the case. Clinician judgments determine what equipment insurers will pay for, whether patients are safe to drive, if a potentially toxic medication is effective, and so forth. Because weighty decisions are based on the outcome of clinician-rated assessments, it is critical that scores reflect an adequate and representative sample of patients' functional capabilities.

Objective Testing

Objective testing minimizes clinician subjectivity. Objective tests produce interval or ratio data in the form of time, number of missteps, distance, and so forth. They include such metrics as the six-minute walk (20), timed up-and-go (21), sit-to-stand (22), and box and blocks (23) tests. In their ideal form, objective measures can be administered by anyone and yield identical results. This characteristic underlies two of their principal advantages over clinician-rated measures. First, their use need not be restricted to highly trained and experienced personnel. Second, inter- and intra-rater reliability can be maximized and easily quantified. Since a primary goal of measurement is the reduction of unexplained variance, objective measures have great appeal. A downside is their potential requirement for specialized equipment, which may be prohibitively expensive and limitedly available. Additionally, objective testing requires patients to travel to the assessment site.

The limitations of proxy assessment may become particularly problematic.

In contrast to clinician rating approaches in which activities such as stair climbing or toileting are observed in toto, objective measures generally asses a single parameter (eg, required time, distance walked) of an activity. This parameter becomes a proxy assessment of patients' capacity to perform the entire activity. By extracting a single or very limited number of attributes from a complex task, critical information may be lost. For example, a patient may perform the Timed Up and Go very quickly but demonstrate gross instability. The patient's score, based solely on time to complete, is an imperfect reflection of their ability to move safely. The scoring of some tests addresses this deficiency by lowering scores for missteps or other flaws in execution.

The limitations of proxy assessment highlight the need for validation processes. As Landy asserts, "Validation processes are . . . directed toward the integrity of the . . . inferences that can be made about the attributes of the people who have produced . . . test scores" (24). If a patient performs well on the timed up-and-go, how certain can the clinician be that the patient has few mobility limitations? The degree to which a test's validity has been established will determine how confidently investigators can make inferences regarding the activity of interest. Often, scientific papers cite prior validation studies for the outcome measures. Tests that have been extensively validated are popular because investigators can justify their inferences on the basis of prior experience.

MEASUREMENT PITFALLS

Inconsistent Discrimination

Metrics are generally not equally sensitive across their entire range of measurement. An instrument may differentiate extremely well at low levels of function but poorly at higher levels, or vice versa. The presence of inconsistent discrimination may cause scores to cluster where discrimination is poor. This partially accounts for "floor" and "ceiling" effects, wherein scores clump at the top and bottom of a scale, respectively. Figure 80.1 displays a scatter plot of PF-10 and FIM mobility subscale scores from a cohort of patients with metastatic breast cancer (25). FIM mobility subscale scores are disproportionately clustered at and just below the maximal score of 35, even in patients with PF-10 scores less than 20. A clear ceiling effect is present. In theory, clustering can occur at any point along the continuum being measured. It is critical to bear in mind that clustering may also be a function of the population under study.

Low Sensitivity to the Parameter of Interest

Clinical measurement is an effort to distinguish signal from noise. A given variable is seldom only noise or only signal, and one investigator's noise may be another's signal. The likelihood of detecting signal increases as

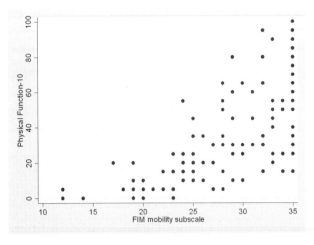

FIGURE 80.1

Scatter plot of PF-10 and FIM mobility subscale scores illustrating a *"ceiling effect"* at the maximal FIM mobility subscale score of 35.

noise is minimized. One way to reduce noise is by selecting a metric that is limitedly influenced by factors other than the outcome of interest. For example, if the goal is to measure function, then administering an entire QOL instrument and utilized scors summed across multiple subscales will produce data contaminated with considerable noise (e.g. psychological status) relative to the signal of interest. A researcher's goal should be to measure only what he wants to measure and *nothing* more, at least with the primary outcome measure. This may sound elementary, yet it is a common source of beta error in rehabilitation research.

Low Responsiveness to Change

Responsiveness to change is unfortunately not an attribute of all valid and reliable metrics. Instruments may discriminate well when administered in cross sectional surveys, yet fail to detect change when administered repeatedly in longitudinal studies. This failure has been documented for some of the most widely utilized QOL instruments (26). The solution of simply asking patients if they have changed (eg, "Compared to six months ago, how well are you able to go up stairs?") has not been embraced, since patients' recollection is unreliable. An investigation found that 42% of patients did not recall their hospitalizations one year after the event (27). A comprehensive discussion of why instruments with excellent discriminative capacity are poorly responsive is beyond the scope of this chapter. Readers are referred to Streiner and Norman's treatment of the subject, in *Health Measurement Scales, A Practical Guide to Their Development and Use* (28). Suffice it to say that if one's goal is detection of change, particularly

when the effect is subtle, ensuring the responsiveness of a metric is essential through literature review and, ideally, collection of pilot data.

Score Affected by Alternate Factors

A concern with self-report metrics is the possibility that the patient's recollection and evaluation of their abilities will be influenced by other factors such as pain, anxiety, and depression (29). It is easy to imagine how a patient might consider functional tasks more difficult to perform when depressed relative to when their mood is elevated. The impact of patients' psychoemotional state is a critical consideration in cancer cohorts. Approximately two-thirds of patients develop reactive depression after receiving a cancer diagnosis, and half of these patients experience sustained clinical depression (30). Furthermore, pain and other symptoms can influence the way that patients perceive their functional status. In one study, 11% of the variance in patients' PF-10 scores was explained by their Brief Pain Inventory scores (25).

The influence of factors other than patients' "true" functional status is inescapable in self report. The degree of influence clearly varies depending on the study population and instrument. In certain clinical populations, investigators have found no discrepancy between self- and clinician-rated measurement (31). Fortunately, a relatively straightforward solution presents itself: Measure any factors suspected of "polluting" self-report function scores and adjust for them statistically.

NOVEL APPROACHES TO FUNCTIONAL MEASUREMENT

The majority of functional metrics discriminate well across limited performance ranges. For example, the capacity to perform ADLs does not deteriorate until a patient's functional status has become moderately compromised. Therefore, ADL-based metrics discriminate well only late in the disablement process (32–34). In fact, the inability to perform even single ADL in patients with metastatic breast cancer indicates a significant level of generalized disability (25). Since most prospective studies evaluating function in patients with cancer have relied on ADL-based measures, little is known about instigating and sustaining factors in their early disablement (35,36).

Past investigators have utilized ADL-based measures because of the challenges inherent in comprehensive assessment. "Functional status" is a broad, multidimensional construct. Accurate functional assessment across a broad range of performance therefore requires lengthy self-report questionnaires (37). Investigators must balance the competing constraints of limited functional assessment and respondent burden (38).

Computer adaptive testing (CAT) may offer a solution to this quandary. CAT is an increasingly utilized measurement approach that permits comprehensive and precise measurement of patient outcomes with a lessened respondent burden (39–41). The approach is "adaptive" in that each test is individualized based on patients' responses to previous items, thus adjusting to the level of each patient and avoiding the need to administer large numbers of potentially uninformative questions. CATs are commonly used by profersional licensure and accred totion boards. The utility of CAT in the rehabilitation setting has been suggested by empirical simulations conducted using previously collected data to replicate CAT sessions.

The Activity Measure for Post-Acute Care (AM-PAC-CAT) is currently the only functional metric available in a CAT platform that has been validated and shown to discriminate across a broad range of functional abilities (42,43). The measure includes three domains (applied cognition, personal care and instrumental activities, and physical and movement activities), each of which requires less than two minutes to score in its CAT form. The AM-PAC-CAT minimizes respondent burden and allows repeated administration for longitudinal assessment. No floor and minimal ceiling effects were detected in a convenience sample of 1,815 patients receiving rehabilitation services (44). The instrument holds great promise for the assessment of cancer populations, particularly those with advanced disease who are intolerant to excessive respondent burden.

CONCLUSIONS

The functional measurement of patients with cancer is challenging but highly rewarding. Function remains one of patients' greatest priorities. In the words of Cecily Saunders, the cancer patient wishes "to live . . . at his own maximum potential performing to the limit of his physical . . . capacity with control and independence whenever possible" (45). Without the ability to measure patients' functional ability clinicians can never discover their potential, let alone help them to achieve it.

References

1. Yoshioka H. Rehabilitation for the terminal cancer patient. *Am J Phys Med Rehabil.* June 1994;73(3):199–206.
2. Stanton AL, Krishnan L, Collins CA. Form or function? Part 1. Subjective cosmetic and functional correlates of quality of life in women treated with breast-conserving surgical procedures and radiotherapy. *Cancer.* June 15, 2001;91(12):2273–2281.
3. Rabow MW, Hauser JM, Adams J. Supporting family caregivers at the end of life: "they don't know what they don't know." *JAMA.* January 28, 2004;291(4):483–491.
4. Berwick DM. A user's manual for the IOM's "Quality Chasm" report. *Health Aff (Millwood).* May–June 2002;21(3):80–90.
5. Reulen RC, Zeegers MP, Jenkinson C, et al. The use of the SF-36 questionnaire in adult survivors of childhood cancer: evaluation of data quality, score reliability, and scaling assumptions. *Health Qual Life Outcomes.* 2006;4:77.
6. Cella DF, Tulsky DS, Gray G, et al. The Functional Assessment of Cancer Therapy scale: development and validation of the general measure. *J Clin Oncol.* March 1993;11(3):570–579.
7. Schipper H, Clinch J, McMurray A, Levitt M. Measuring the quality of life of cancer patients: the Functional Living Index-Cancer: development and validation. *J Clin Oncol.* May 1984;2(5):472–483.
8. Osoba D, Zee B, Pater J, Warr D, Kaizer L, Latreille J. Psychometric properties and responsiveness of the EORTC quality of Life Questionnaire (QLQ-C30) in patients with breast, ovarian and lung cancer. *Qual Life Res.* October 1994;3(5):353–364.
9. Ganz PA, Schag CA, Lee JJ, Sim MS. The CARES: a generic measure of health-related quality of life for patients with cancer. *Qual Life Res.* February 1992;1(1):19–29.
10. Haley SM, McHorney CA, Ware JE, Jr. Evaluation of the MOS SF-36 physical functioning scale (PF-10): I. Unidimensionality and reproducibility of the Rasch item scale. *J Clin Epidemiol.* June 1994;47(6):671–684.
11. Fillenbaum GG, Smyer MA. The development, validity, and reliability of the OARS multidimensional functional assessment questionnaire. *J Gerontol.* July 1981;36(4):428–434.
12. Baecke JA, Burema J, Frijters JE. A short questionnaire for the measurement of habitual physical activity in epidemiological studies. *Am J Clin Nutr.* November 1982;36(5):936–942.
13. Godin G, Shephard RJ. A simple method to assess exercise behavior in the community. *Can J Appl Sport Sci.* September 1985;10(3):141–146.
14. Hudak PL, Amadio PC, Bombardier C. Development of an upper extremity outcome measure: the DASH (disabilities of the arm, shoulder and hand) [corrected]. The Upper Extremity Collaborative Group (UECG). *Am J Ind Med.* June 1996;29(6):602–608.
15. Granger CV HB, Keith RA, Zielesny M, Sherwin, FS. Advances in functional assessment for medical rehabilitation. *Top Geriatr Rehabil.* 1986;1:59–74.
16. Mahoney FI, Barthel DW. Functional evaluation: the Barthel index. *Md State Med J.* February 1965;14:61–65.
17. Lachs MS, Feinstein AR, Cooney LM, Jr., et al. A simple procedure for general screening for functional disability in elderly patients. *Ann Intern Med.* May 1, 1990;112(9):699–706.
18. Crooks V, Waller S, Smith T, Hahn TJ. The use of the Karnofsky Performance Scale in determining outcomes and risk in geriatric outpatients. *J Gerontol.* July 1991;46(4):M139–M144.
19. Conill C, Verger E, Salamero M. Performance status assessment in cancer patients. *Cancer.* April 15, 1990;65(8):1864–1866.
20. Guyatt GH, Sullivan MJ, Thompson PJ, et al. The 6-minute walk: a new measure of exercise capacity in patients with chronic heart failure. *Can Med Assoc J.* April 15, 1985;132(8):919–923.
21. Podsiadlo D, Richardson S. The timed "Up & Go": a test of basic functional mobility for frail elderly persons. *J Am Geriatr Soc.* February 1991;39(2):142–148.
22. Csuka M, McCarty DJ. Simple method for measurement of lower extremity muscle strength. *Am J Med.* January 1985;78(1):77–81.
23. Mathiowetz Volland G, Kashman N; Weber, K. Adult norms for the box and blocks test of manual dexterity. *Am J Occup Ther.* 1985;39:386–391.
24. Landy FJ. Stamp collecting versus science. *American Psychologist.* 1986;41:1183–1192.
25. Cheville AL. Troxel A.B.; Basford JR, Kornblith AB. Measuring function in cancer patients. *Arch Phys Med Rehabil.* In Press.

26. Haywood KL, Garratt AM, Fitzpatrick R. Quality of life in older people: a structured review of generic self-assessed health instruments. *Qual Life Res.* September 2005;14(7):1651–1668.

27. Survey USNH. Reporting of Hospitalization in the Health Interview Survey. *Health Statistics.* 1965; Series 3, No. 6.

28. Streiner DN, Norman GR. *Health Measurement Scales, a Practical Guide to Their Development and Use,* 2nd ed. New York: Oxford University Press; 1995.

29. Watson D, Pennebaker JW. Health complaints, stress, and distress: exploring the central role of negative affectivity. *Psychol Rev.* April 1989;96(2):234–254.

30. Massie MJ, Holland JC. Depression and the cancer patient. *J Clin Psychiatry.* July 1990;51(Suppl):12–17; discussion 18–19.

31. Steultjens MP, Roorda LD, Dekker J, Bijlsma JW. Responsiveness of observational and self-report methods for assessing disability in mobility in patients with osteoarthritis. *Arthritis Rheum.* February 2001;45(1):56–61.

32. Hollen PJ, Gralla RJ, Kris MG, Eberly SW, Cox C. Normative data and trends in quality of life from the Lung Cancer Symptom Scale (LCSS). *Support Care Cancer.* May 1999;7(3):140–148.

33. Fried LP, Young Y, Rubin G, Bandeen-Roche K. Self-reported preclinical disability identifies older women with early declines in performance and early disease. *J Clin Epidemiol.* September 2001;54(9):889–901.

34. Wicklund AH, Johnson N, Rademaker A, Weitner BB, Weintraub S. Profiles of decline in activities of daily living in non-Alzheimer dementia. *Alzheimer Dis Assoc Disord.* January–March 2007;21(1):8–13.

35. McCarthy EP, Phillips RS, Zhong Z, Drews RE, Lynn J. Dying with cancer: patients' function, symptoms, and care preferences as death approaches. *J Am Geriatr Soc.* May 2000;48(5 Suppl):S110–S121.

36. Lunney JR, Lynn J, Foley DJ, Lipson S, Guralnik JM. Patterns of functional decline at the end of life. *JAMA.* May 14, 2003;289(18):2387–2392.

37. Jette AM. Toward a common language for function, disability, and health. *Phys Ther.* May 2006;86(5):726–734.

38. Jette AM, Haley SM, Ni P. Comparison of functional status tools used in post-acute care. *Health Care Financ Rev.* Spring 2003;24(3):13–24.

39. Gardner W, Kelleher KJ, Pajer KA. Multidimensional adaptive testing for mental health problems in primary care. *Med Care.* September 2002;40(9):812–823.

40. McHorney CA, Haley SM, Ware JE, Jr. Evaluation of the MOS SF-36 Physical Functioning Scale (PF-10): II. Comparison of relative precision using Likert and Rasch scoring methods. *J Clin Epidemiol.* April 1997;50(4):451–461.

41. Hays RD, Morales LS, Reise SP. Item response theory and health outcomes measurement in the 21st century. *Med Care.* September 2000;38(9 Suppl):II28–II42.

42. Haley SM, Siebens H, Coster WJ, et al. Computerized adaptive testing for follow-up after discharge from inpatient rehabilitation: I. Activity outcomes. *Arch Phys Med Rehabil.* August 2006;87(8):1033–1042.

43. Haley SM, Fragala-Pinkham M, Ni P. Sensitivity of a computer adaptive assessment for measuring functional mobility changes in children enrolled in a community fitness programme. *Clin Rehabil.* July 2006;20(7):616–622.

44. Jette AM, Haley SM, Tao W, et al. Prospective evaluation of the AM-PAC-CAT in outpatient rehabilitation settings. *Phys Ther.* April 2007;87(4):385–398.

45. Saunders CM. *Cicely Saunders: Selected Writings 1958–2004.* New York: Oxford University Press; 2006.

46. Cummings S.D, Hulley S.R. *Designing Clinical Research.* Baltimore: Williams & Wilkins; 1988.

47. Hennekens CH Buring, J.E. *Epidemiology in Medicine.* First ed. Boston: Little, Brown and Company; 1987.

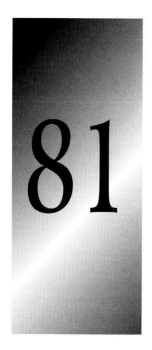

Research Funding Issues and Priorities in Cancer Rehabilitation

81

Beth Solomon
Cindy Pfalzer
Leighton Chan
Rebecca Parks

Despite the fact that cancer is one of the leading causes of morbidity and mortality (1) in the United States, there is strikingly little research in the area of cancer rehabilitation. Improved early detection and treatment has extended survival, making cancer a chronic disease much more amenable to rehabilitation interventions and strategies. In response to calls for increased quality of life (2–4), and contemporaneous with the rise of the hospice and palliative care movements, cancer rehabilitation programs were created and have been favorably received. There has been a dearth of research with respect to cancer rehabilitation, however (5,6). Cancer rehabilitation research capacity needs to be enhanced by increasing the numbers of cancer rehabilitation researchers, the number and quality of research facilities, and opportunities for funding (7).

A Pubmed search for the last 10 years reveals fewer than 500 publications related to rehabilitation and cancer (8). Likewise, a search of CRISP (a database that tracks all NIH funded grants) from 2005 to 2007, yields only 74 new or competing grants that focus on cancer rehabilitation research (9). Although crude, these numbers are disappointingly small, given the fact that more individuals are now surviving cancers and often face the long-term debilitating affects of the disease and its treatments (10).

The overall objective of any research effort in cancer is to make new discoveries, then translate findings into improvements into clinical care. One useful way to characterize the research process is to divide it into 5 phases (11):

- Phase 1—Basic research that leads towards an understanding of the pathophysiology of a disease or its treatment.
- Phase 2—Development of methods and the performance of pilot studies needed to do research in a particular area.
- Phase 3—Efficacy trials: evaluation of treatments under "ideal" scientific conditions.
- Phase 4—Effectiveness trials: evaluation of treatments under usual or "real life" conditions.
- Phase 5—Dissemination trials: once a treatment has been proven effective, to evaluate conditions which promote or impede its widespread use.

Unfortunately, the paucity of research in cancer rehabilitation extends throughout all five phases of this research process.

RESEARCH BY REHABILITATION PROFESSIONALS

Historically, rehabilitation professionals including physiatrists, physical therapists (PT), occupational therapists (OT), and speech language pathologists (SLP) have

---

KEY POINTS

- Cancer rehabilitation research capacity needs to be enhanced by increasing the numbers of cancer rehabilitation researchers, the number and quality of research facilities, and opportunities for funding.
- Cancer rehabilitation research could be better advanced by using the International Classification of Functioning, Disability, and Health (ICF) by the World Health Organization in 2001, standardization of outcome measures and formalization and published dissemination of intervention/treatment regimens.

- To enhance cancer rehabilitation research capacity, government and funding agencies and industry need to prioritize competition for limited rehabilitation research funding.
- Research begins with the generation of a clinical hypothesis, followed by appropriate literature reviews, assessment planning, and gathering and interpreting data. Given the changing continuum of oncology care, from diagnosis, treatment, recurrence, and late effects, significant challenges will occur even with the best research designs.

---

focused on the functional status of patients undergoing cancer treatments. Unfortunately, it has only been in recent years that large clinical investigations have used functional status to assess treatment outcomes.

Cancer special interest groups have been formed by the American Physical Therapy Association (APTA) and the American Academy of Physical Medicine and Rehabilitation (AAPMR); however, there have been no sections developed within the American Occupational Therapy Association (AOTA) and American Speech Language and Hearing Association (ASHA) or clinical specializations in these organizations. Within the last 20 years, rehabilitation specialists have developed cancer care programs in response to the needs of their own institutions' patient populations. When reviewing the literature regarding cancer rehabilitation research, one is struck by the preponderance of studies from outside the United States (12) and the lack of formal research ongoing or completed by specialists in rehabilitation of cancer patients within the United States. We speculate that this may be due to unified health care systems abroad and, possibly, the emphasis that other countries place on quality of life.

To advance the evolution of cancer rehabilitation for all specialties of PT, OT, SLP, and physiatry, concerted efforts must be made to progress from individual idiosyncratic local programs of care to utilization of conceptual frameworks for setting the cancer rehabilitation research agenda. The use of the International Classification of Functioning, Disability, and Health (ICF) by the World Health Organization in 2001 and the standardization of outcome measures and formalization and published dissemination of intervention/treatment regimens (Fig. 81.1), would advance the agenda.

The integrative ICF is structured around the following domains:

- Body functions and structure
- Activities (related to tasks and actions by an individual) and participation (involvement in a life situation)
- Additional information on environmental and personal factors including severity

Activities (eg, function) and participation (eg, disability) are viewed as complex interactions between the health condition of the individual and the contextual factors of the environment as well as personal factors. The view is of the person in his or her world and is produced by this combination of factors and domains. The ICF treats these domains as interactive and dynamic rather than linear or static. Based on the ICF, cancer rehabilitation can be defined as the health strategy that "aims to enable people with cancer experiencing or

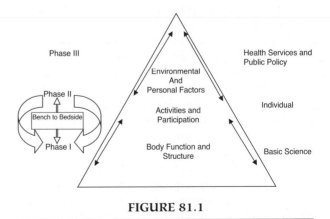

FIGURE 81.1

ICF construct for research.

likely to experience disability to achieve optimal function interacting with the environment" (13).

ICF AND CANCER REHABILITATION

Gerber et al. have proposed a framework for opportunities for rehabilitation interventions throughout the disease continuum that, when used in conjunction with the ICF, form a conceptual model for cancer rehabilitation research (Table 81.1). This continuum of care requires basic science, mechanistic research, translational and clinical research, and health services research at each of these points in the continuum of care.

Cheville and Tchou have discussed (1) the multidimensional and time-variable interventions used in rehabilitation that result in substantial variance; (2) that function is inherently multidimensional and difficult to accurately quantify even with the development of generic and disease specific instruments with reasonable statistical psychometric properties but lacking responsiveness to clinically meaningful change; and (3) that more variance is added by the multifactorial nature of rehabilitation outcomes (eg, function, return to work, community reintegration), and (4) that the sample size required to reject the null hypothesis and not create a type II error is directly proportional to variance in the primary outcome measure (14). This suggests that trials in cancer rehabilitation will be potentially limited by the large amount of variance in measures of function and other outcomes and interventions requiring large sample sizes that are costly studies and difficult to accrue at a single site. Multisite trials require more research capacity such as infrastructure and experienced research scientists, and are more costly to conduct. The statistical requirements for large sample sizes, limited generalizability, and deviance from the real-world clinical environment that characterize randomized clinical trials (RCT) have been outlined elsewhere (15). Large, prospective observational cohort studies that allow multivariate regression analyses are suggested as an alternative to the conventional gold standard RCT. Large databases permit analyses of the multifactorial interventions and outcomes characteristic of cancer rehabilitation. Additionally, several recent methodological evaluations found the results of such observational cohort studies comparable to those of RCTs with similar aims, thus offering a possible alternative to the RCT (16). Many research questions in cancer rehabilitation may not be answered with RCTs in a financially responsible manner. Additional barriers to rehabilitation arise from human, logistic, and financial sources. The scarcity of research, scientists, training programs, clinicians (17), physicians, and therapists specializing in cancer rehabilitation is also a barrier.

A basic question for cancer rehabilitation research to date is, "do we need a diagnosis specific functional assessment?" This can only be best answered with collection and analysis of functional outcome data specific to cancer type.

REHABILITATION RESEARCH QUESTIONS AND THE ICF

Analysis of the official websites of each of the rehabilitation professional organizations and associated foundations is instructive with regard to these organizations stated Research Priorities and Parameters of Practice. The organizations and respective foundations acknowledge that the research priorities and parameters are used to guide internal funding priorities and program development. The AOTA priorities, rooted in the International Classification of Function (ICF) (18) provide a scaffolding on which to build a possible future agenda for research in for the various rehabilitation specialties in cancer care. This easily can be adapted and applied to the other rehabilitation specialties as follows:

1. Are interventions effective in achieving targeted activity and participation outcomes and preventing/reducing secondary conditions?
2. To what extent does the intervention promote learning, adaptation, self-organization, adjustment to life situations, and self-determination across the life span?
3. Are environmental interventions that support activities effective in preventing impairment and promotion activity and participation at the individual, community, and societal levels?
4. Where, when, how, and at what level (Body Structure/Body Function, Activity, Participation, and Environment) should an intervention occur to maximize activity and participation, as well as cost-effectiveness of services?
5. What measures/measurement systems reflect the domain of activity and identify factors (body structure/body function, activity, participation, and environment) or document the impact of occupational therapy on these factors?
6. How do activity patterns and choices, both in everyday life and across the life span, influence the health and participation of individuals?
7. What is the impact of activity patterns and choices both in everyday life and across the life span, on society?

TABLE 81.1

Continuum of Care Model

CONTINUUM OF CARE FOR PATIENTS WITH CANCER	POSSIBLE SYMPTOMS AND IMPAIRED BODY STRUCTURE/ FUNCTION	FUNCTIONAL LIMITATIONS IN ACTIVITY AND PARTICIPATION	RESEARCH ISSUES TO ADDRESS
I. Staging/pretreatment	Anxiety, pain, functional loss	Daily routines, sleep, fatigue	Educate about functional impact of treatment(s), preserve function, pretreatment rehabilitation: ROM, ADL, strengthening, fit for mobility aids if needed
II. Primary treatment	Pain, anxiety, decreased mobility, wound and skin care, speech and swallowing deficits, decreased strength and fatigue	Daily routines, sleep, stamina, self-care, cosmesis, communication, eating/ nutrition	Evaluate effects of treatment, preserve and restore function through exercise, lymphedema management, ROM, increased activity, pain management, relaxation/sleep hygiene
III. After treatment	Pain, weakness, anxiety, depression, loss of mobility, edema, fatigue, deconditioning, weight gain	Sleep, fatigue, ADL, vocational and avocational concerns, cosmesis	Develop and support program to restore mobility and daily routines and to promote healthy lifestyle, educate patient about what to self-monitor, create maintenance program of exercise and edema management
IV. Recurrence	See II: Pain, weakness, anxiety, depression, fatigue, stamina, edema, bony instability, anorexia, possible central nervous system or other organ system involvement	Sleep, fatigue, disability, disruption of routines, cosmesis, vocational and avocational concerns	Educate patient about impact of recurrence and its effects on function and what to monitor in the context of new clinical status, supervise appropriate program to restore function and prevent decline (including orthotics, gait aids, adaptive equipment and aerobic exercise), assist patients in maintaining activity and QOL
V. End of life	Pain, fatigue, anorexia, fear, depression, spirituality	Decreased mobility and possible dependence in self-care, isolation/ withdrawal	Educate patient and family about energy conservation, transfer training with attention to body mechanics and assistive devices, manage pain and control symptoms, maintain independence and QOL, explore meaning and purpose of life/last wishes, legacy issues

Abbreviation: ROM, range of motion.
Source: From Ref. 17.

8. What are the conceptual models that explain the relationships among body structure/body function, activity, environment, and participation? What is the role of rehabilitation therapy within these models?

9. What factors contribute to effective partnerships between consumers and practitioners that foster and enhance participation of individuals with or at risk for disabling conditions?

10. What factors support professional practitioners' capacities to maximize the performance of the persons they serve?

Funding

Each of the rehabilitation national organizations fund various research endeavors. However, to our knowledge, few cancer rehabilitation research projects have been funded which may simply be an indicator of the lack of applications related to cancer rehabilitation. The APTA Foundation is currently funding the Clinical Research Network, its single largest project grant to date, moreover, the total awards granted by the Foundation equal approximately $12 million which has been leveraged into $75 million in additional funded research. During the 20-year period from 1979 to 1999, AOTF and AOTA jointly contributed a total of $2,460,179 to the profession's knowledge base, through grants awarded to members; establishment of three centers for Scholarship and Research; sponsorship of a series of bi-annual research symposia; and support for a new Center for Outcomes Research (CORE). The top three research categories receiving the largest portions of the funding were, in descending order of total dollar amounts awarded: Developmental Disabilities, Physical Disabilities, and Mental Health. The American Speech Language and Hearing Foundation has awarded almost $4 million to doctoral, post-doctoral researches, graduate students and leaders in the field supporting research and clinical recognition. In 2003, ASHA began a new randomized clinical trial assessing swallowing function and risks for aspiration in which a small cohort of patients were diagnosed with cancer. It appears that funding source opportunities are limited; however available for the eager scientist by our sister organizations and foundations.

Additional funding sources offered by the AAPMR, AOTA, ASHA and that APTA and their foundations are included in Table 81.2 (19–22).

TABLE 81.2
Organizations and Awards

APTA and APTA Foundation http://www.apta.org	AOTA and Foundation http://www.aotf.org/ http://www.aota.org	AAPMR and Foundation http://American Academy of Physical Medicine and Rehabilitation (AAPM&R)	ASHA and Foundation http://www.ashafoundation http://www.asha.org
Florence Kendall Doctoral Scholarships	Dissertation Research Grant Program of the Institute for the Study of Occupation and Health	ERF New Investigator Research Grants	Advancing Academic Research Careers http://www.aotf.org/
Promotion of Doctoral Studies (PODS) I & II Scholarships	Center for Outcomes Research and Education (CORE)	Musculoskeletal Research Grant	Minority Student Leadership Program (MSLP)
New Investigator Fellowship Training Initiative (NIFTI)	AOTF Research Grants Database	Medical Student Research Award	Students Preparing for Academic and Research Careers (SPARC)
Magistro Family Research Grants	North Coast Medical, Inc. (AOTF)		Clinical Research Grant-American Speech Language Foundation
Research Grant funded by the 2007 Pittsburgh Marquette Challenge	Progressus Therapy		New Investigators Research Grant
Legacy Endowment Fund Research Grant Recipient	Memorial scholarships in the name of prominent occupational therapy practitioners		Research Grant in Speech Science

To enhance cancer rehabilitation research capacity, government and funding agencies and industry need to prioritize competition for limited rehabilitation research funding. A list of federally funded cancer related rehabilitation research since 2004 demonstrates the breadth of currently funded research related to cancer rehabilitation (Table 81.3). However, compared to disease specific research funding this list indicates the relatively amount of funded research support. A current search using the NIH Active Funding Opportunities (RFAs & PAs) search feature yielded no results when searching for cancer rehabilitation and only 71 specific to rehabilitation in general. While the National Center for Medical Rehabilitation Research (23) is not on this list, NCMRR does provide active funding opportunities for rehabilitation research that can be related to cancer. NIH funding for rehabilitation research has remained approximately 300 million dollars per year over the last 5 years. Although somewhat large, the actual amount awarded to Physical Medicine and Rehabilitation Departments was approximately 27 million (11).

Frequently used research grant programs are listed in Table 81.4. It is important to note that NIH Institutes and Centers (ICs) may vary in the way they use activity codes; not all ICs accept applications for all types of grant programs as they often apply specialized eligibility criteria. Look closely at funding opportunity announcements (FOAs) to determine which ICs participate and the specifics of eligibility.

Cancer rehabilitation researchers will need to partner with national societies and foundations such as the American Cancer Society, Lance Armstrong Foundation and regional/state affiliates of national foundations such as Susan G. Komen Foundation to sponsor rehabilitation research. The National Comprehensive Cancer Network (NCCN) has a listing of its member institution at http://nccn.org/members/network.asp and many of these comprehensive cancer centers have their own affiliated foundation that provide research program/awards funding and funding for training programs (24). Selected foundations that have awards/programs directly related to cancer rehabilitation are listed in Table 81.5.

ETHICAL CONSIDERATIONS

In design of any research project, ethical considerations for the protection of human subjects are crucial. Concerns related to cancer rehabilitation research include (25):

1. Informed consent of the study subjects—This can be an issue, particularly in patients who are not cognitively intact. However, informed consent is the cornerstone of an ethically conducted research study.

2. Balancing patient safety with the potential benefits of new knowledge—In general, the benefits to society must outweigh the risks to the individual patient. This decision should not be made in isolation by an individual investigator, but should be supported by an Internal Review Board.

3. Insuring appropriate patient protections, including appropriate plans for patient recruitment, adverse events, and patient confidentiality. Cancer patients, many of whom are facing imminent death are particularly vulnerable. Even greater attention should be given to patient recruitment, which should not be coercive, and to minimizing risk, even in a terminally ill subject.

4. Researchers should to be in a state of "equipoise." That is, in any treatment trial, they need to be in doubt as to which treatment is better. If they are not in this state of "equipoise," then they cannot ethically randomize patients to one treatment over another. This may be a particular issue for many rehabilitation practitioners who have created standards of practice based on personal experiences and anecdotal evidence. They may not be able to make the transition to researcher.

CHALLENGES TO REHABILITATION RESEARCHERS

Both clinicians and researchers are faced with an impressive task on how best to conduct rehabilitation research in oncology. Unfortunately, there has been a lack of attention to functional status by oncologists either due to their lack of training, or ability to identify early functional changes of their patients, therefore prospective research within rehabilitation is limited.

Historically, research begins with the generation of a clinical hypothesis, followed by appropriate literature reviews, assessment planning, gathering, and interpreting data. Along the every changing continuum of oncology care, from diagnosis, treatment, recurrence, and late effects, the challenges are nearly endless even with the best research designs.

Hypothesis/Questions

Clinical researchers at large generally use a problem-based approach when asking the questions to be answered in the research. Although sometimes appropriate, this approach often fails address the personal

TABLE 81.3
Federally Funded Cancer Research

NIH/PHS ACTIVITY CODES/PROJECT AWARD NUMBER AND INSTITUTE	AUTHORS	TITLE	JOURNAL YEAR	VOLUME, PAGES
K22 CA87713-01/CA/NCI	Vallerand, A.H., et al.	Knowledge of and barriers to pain management in caregivers of cancer patients receiving homecare	*Cancer Nurs 2007*	30(1) 31–7
R01CA1048301A1/CA/NCI P50CA84719/CA/NCI	Graham, A.L. & D.B. Abrams	Reducing the cancer burden of lifestyle factors: opportunities and challenges of the Internet	*J Med Internet Res 2005*	7(3) e26
R01CA78955/CA/NCI	Mishel, M.H., et al.	Benefits from an uncertainty management intervention for African-American and Caucasian older long-term breast cancer survivors	*Psychooncology 2005*	14(11) 962–78
R01 DE 11255/DE/NIDCR C06 RR 14529-01/RR/NCRR	Garrett, N., et al.	Efficacy of conventional and implant-supported mandibular resection prostheses: study overview and treatment outcomes	*J Prosthet Dent 2006*	96(1) 13–24
R01DE11255/DE/NIDCR C06 RR-14529-01/RR/NCRR	Roumanas, E.D., et al.	Masticatory and swallowing threshold performances with conventional and implant-supported prostheses after mandibular fibula free-flap reconstruction	*J Prosthet Dent 2006*	96(4) 289–97
R21CA09736-1/CA/NCI	Main, D.S., et al.	A qualitative study of work and work return in cancer survivors	*Psychooncology 2005*	14(11) 992–1004
5P50CA089520-2/CA/NCI	Ornish, D., et al.	Intensive lifestyle changes may affect the progression of prostate cancer	*J Urol 2005*	174(3)1065–9
5U01-CA5572705/CA/NCI	Oeffinger, K.C., et al.	Health care of young adult survivors of childhood cancer: a report from the Childhood Cancer Survivor Study.	*Ann Fam Med 2004*	2(1) 61–70
91831 /PHS	Tercyak, K.P., et al.	Identifying, recruiting, and enrolling adolescent survivors of childhood cancer into a randomized controlled trial of health promotion: preliminary experiences in the Survivor Health and Resilience Education (SHARE) Program.	*J Pediatr Psychol 2006*	31(3) 252–61
91831 /PHS	Tercyak, K.P., et al.	Multiple behavioral risk factors among adolescent survivors of childhood cancer in the Survivor Health and Resilience Education (SHARE) program.	*Pediatr Blood Cancer 2006*	47(6) 825–30

(Continued)

TABLE 81.3
Federally Funded Cancer Research Continued

NIH/PHS ACTIVITY CODES/PROJECT AWARD NUMBER AND INSTITUTE	AUTHORS	TITLE	JOURNAL YEAR	VOLUME, PAGES
AG11268/AG / NIA CA106919/CA / NCI CA81191/CA / NCI CA92468/CA / NCI	Rao, A.V. & W. Demark-Wahne-fried	The older cancer survivor	*Crit Rev Oncol Hematol* 2006	60(2) 131–43
AG-02-004/AG / NIA R01CA60068/CA/ NCI	Chang, C.H., et al.	The SF-36 physical and mental health factors were confirmed in cancer and HIV/AIDS patients.	*J Clin Epidemiol* 2007	60(1) 68–72
AR52186/AR / NIAMS CA106919/CA / NCI CA81191/CA / NCI	Demark-Wahne-fried, W., B.M. Pinto, & E.R. Gritz	Promoting health and physical function among cancer survivors: potential for prevention and questions that remain	*J Clin Oncol,* 2006	24(32) 5125–31
CA13650/CA / NCI CA16116/CA / NCI CA23318/CA / NCI CA32102/CA / NCI CA49883/CA / NCI CA66636/CA / NCI	Eton, D.T., et al.	A combination of distribution- and anchor-based approaches determined minimally important differences (MIDs) for four endpoints in a breast cancer scale	*J Clin Epidemiol* 2004	57(9) 898–910
CA 75452/CA /NCI	Pinto, B.M., et al.	Home-based physical activity intervention for breast cancer patients	*J Clin Oncol* 2005	23(15)3577–87
K02AG20113/AG /NIA P30AG21342/AG /NIA R01AG19769/AG /NIA	Fried, T.R., et al.	Prospective study of health status preferences and changes in preferences over time in older adults	*Arch Intern Med* 2006	166(8)890–5
K05CA92395/CA /NCI K07CA87724/CA /NCI R01AG70818/AG /NIA R01CA57754/CA /NCI R01CA70818/CA /NCI	Lash, T.L., K. Clough-Gorr, & R.A. Silliman	Reduced rates of cancer-related worries and mortality associated with guideline surveillance after breast cancer therapy	*Breast Cancer Res Treat* 2005	89(1) 61–7
N01CN65064/CN /NCI	Bednarek, H.L. & C.J. Bradley	Work and retirement after cancer diagnosis	*Res Nurs Health* 2005	28(2) 126–35
N01CN65064/CN /NCI	Mellon, S., L.L. Northouse, & L.K. Weiss	A population-based study of the quality of life of cancer survivors and their family caregivers	*Cancer Nurs,* 2006	29(2)120–31
P20CA103676/CA/ NCI U01CA93324/CA / NCI	Ayanian, J.Z. & P.B. Jacobsen	Enhancing research on cancer survivors	*J Clin Oncol,* 2006	24(32) 5149–53
P20 / PHS	Hendrix, C. and C. Ray	Informal caregiver training on home care and cancer symptom management prior to hospital discharge: a feasibility study	*Oncol Nurs Forum, 2006*	33(4) 793–8
P30CA21765/CA / NCI	Hinds, P.S., et al.	End-of-life care preferences of pediatric patients with cancer	*J Clin Oncol,* 2005	23(36) 9146–54
P50CA92629/CA / NCI T32-82088 / PHS	Bianco, F.J., Jr., P.T. Scardino, and J.A. East-ham	Radical prostatectomy: long-term cancer control and recovery of sexual and urinary function ("trifecta").	*Urology, 2005*	66(5 Suppl)83–94

(Continued)

TABLE 81.3
Federally Funded Cancer Research Continued

NIH/PHS ACTIVITY CODES/PROJECT AWARD NUMBER AND INSTITUTE	AUTHORS	TITLE	JOURNAL YEAR	VOLUME, PAGES
R01CA63028/CA / NCI	Stanton, A.L., et al.	Outcomes from the Moving Beyond Cancer psychoeducational, randomized, controlled trial with breast cancer patients.	J Clin Oncol, 2005	23(25) 6009–18
R01CA78975/CA / NCI R03CA91577/CA / NCI	Bowman, K.F., J.H. Rose, and G.T. Deimling	Families of long-term cancer survivors: health maintenance advocacy and practice.	Psychooncology, 2005	14(12)1008–17
R01CA78940/CA / NCI	Campbell, B.H., et al.	Aspiration, weight loss, and quality of life in head and neck cancer survivors	Arch Otolaryngol Head Neck Surg, 2004	130(9)1100–3
R01CA79460/CA / NCI	Courneya, K.S., et al.	Exercise motivation and adherence in cancer survivors after participation in a randomized controlled trial: an attribution theory perspective.	Int J Behav Med, 2004	11(1) 8–17
R01CA01915/CA/ NCI T32NR07036/NR/ NINR	Hodgson, N.A. and C.W. Given	Determinants of functional recovery in older adults surgically treated for cancer	Cancer Nurs, 2004	27(1) 10–6
R01 CS82619 / PHS	Short, P.F., J.J. Vasey, and K. Tunceli	Employment pathways in a large cohort of adult cancer survivors	Cancer, 2005	103(6)1292–301
R03CA78972/CA/ NCI	Zebrack, B.J., et al.	Assessing the impact of cancer: development of a new instrument for long-term survivors	Psychooncology, 2006	15(5) 407–21
T32NR07088/NR/ NINR	Drake, D., et al.	Physical fitness training: outcomes for adult oncology patients	Clin Nurs Res, 2004	13(3) 245–64

Abbreviation: NCI, National Cancer Institute.
Source: From Refs. 33 and 34.

and environmental factors affecting each individual cancer patient. These individual do well and often become independent however still remain with functional impairments not identified in relation to their own participation in activities or their own environmental factors.

Recommendations to help clinical researcher in rehabilitation would included identifying the absolute functional questions for the population being studied, along with broadening the scope of secondary questions to include the changing continuum of cancer and patients personal factors. An example of this is often seen in the head and neck cancer population, when patients are faced with severe swallowing impairments associated with the acute effects of treatment. Swallowing tends to improve with intervention and time; however continued impairments are faced by persons in the late effect stages of the disease with diet limitations, embarrassments with eating in public, taste changes, xerostomia, and extended eating duration times (28,29). As clinical researchers, we need to be vigilant about not being satisfied with the fact that the patient is eating an oral diet when swallowing problems affect quality of life.

TABLE 81.4
Frequently Used Grant Research Programs

TYPE	DESCRIPTION	TYPE	DESCRIPTION
R01	NIH Research Project Grant Program (R01) • Used to support a discrete, specified, circumscribed research project • NIH's most commonly used grant program • No specific dollar limit unless specified in FOA • Advance permission required for $500K or more (direct costs) in any year • Generally awarded for 3 -5 years • All ICs utilize • See parent FOA at /grants/guide/pa-files/PA-07-070.html	R41/ R42	Small Business Technology Transfer (STTR) Intended to stimulate scientific and technological innovation through cooperative research/research and development (R/R&D) carried out between small business concerns (SBCs) and research institutions (RIs) Fosters technology transfer between SBCs and RIs Assists the small business and research communities in commercializing innovative technologies Three-phase structure: • I - Feasibility study to establish scientific/technical merit of the proposed R/R&D efforts (generally, 1 year; $100,000) • II - Full R/R&D efforts initiated in Phase I (generally 2 years; $750,000) • III- Commercialization stage (cannot use STTR funds) All ICs utilize except FIC See Parent FOA at http://grants.nih.gov/grants/guide/pa-files/PA-08-051.html

R03	NIH Small Grant Program (R03):
	• Provides limited funding for a short period of time to support a variety of types of projects, including: pilot or feasibility studies, collection of preliminary data, secondary analysis of existing data, small, self-contained research projects, development of new research technology, etc.
	• Limited to two years of funding
	• Direct costs generally up to $50,000 per year
	• Not renewable
	• Utilized by more than half of the NIH ICs
	• See parent FOA at /grants/guide/pa-files/PA-06-180.html
		R43/
		R44
			Small Business Innovative Research (SBIR)
			• Intended to stimulate technological innovation in the private sector by supporting research or research and development (R/R&D) for for-profit institutions for ideas that have potential for commercialization
			• Assists the small business research community in commercializing innovative technologies
			• Three-phase structure:
			  ○ I - Feasibility study to establish scientific/technical merit of the proposed R/R&D efforts (generally, 1 year; $100,000)
			  ○ II - Full research or R&D efforts initiated in Phase I (generally 2 years; $750,000)
			  ○ III- Commercialization stage (cannot use SBIR funds)
			• Multiple PD/PIs allowed.
			  ○ All ICs utilize except FIC
			  ○ See Parent FOA at http://grants.nih.gov/grants/guide/pa-files/PA-08-050.html

R13	NIH Support for Conferences and Scientific Meetings (R13 and U13) • Support for high quality conferences/scientific meetings that are relevant to NIH's scientific mission and to the public health • Requires advance permission from the funding IC • Foreign institutions are not eligible to apply • Award amounts vary and limits are set by individual ICs • Support for up to 5 years may be possible	R56	NIH High Priority, Short-Term Project Award (R56) • Will fund, for one or two years, high-priority new or competing renewal R01 applications with priority scores or percentiles that fall just outside the funding limits of participating NIH Institutes and Centers (IC). Investigators may not apply for R56 grants.

(Continued)

TABLE 81.4
Frequently Used Grant Research Programs Continued

TYPE	DESCRIPTION	TYPE	DESCRIPTION
R15	NIH Academic Research Enhancement Award (AREA) • Support small research projects in the biomedical and behavioral sciences conducted by students and faculty in health professional schools and other academic components that have not been major recipients of NIH research grant funds • Eligibility limited (see /grants/funding/area.htm) • Direct cost limited to $150,000 over entire project period • Project period limited to up to 3 years • All NIH ICs utilize except FIC an NCMHD • See parent FOA at /grants/guide/pa-files/PA-06-042.html	R21	NIH Exploratory/Developmental Research Grant Award (R21) • Encourages new, exploratory and developmental research projects by providing support for the early stages of project development. Sometimes used for pilot and feasibility studies. • Limited to up to two years of funding • Combined budget for direct costs for the two year project period usually may not exceed $275,000. • No preliminary data is generally required • Most ICs utilize • See /grants/guide/pa-files/PA-06-181.html
K99/R00	NIH Pathway to Independence (PI) Award (K99/R00) • Also see, New Investigators Program web page • Provides up to five years of support consisting of two phases ○ I - will provide 1–2 years of mentored support for highly promising, postdoctoral research scientists ○ II - up to 3 years of independent support contingent on securing an independent research position • Award recipients will be expected to compete successfully for independent R01 support from the NIH during the career transition award period • Eligible Principal Investigators include outstanding postdoctoral candidates who have terminal clinical or research doctorates who have no more than 5 years of postdoctoral research training • Foreign institutions are not eligible to apply • PI does not have to be a U.S. citizen	R34	NIH Clinical Trial Planning Grant (R34) Program • Designed to permit early peer review of the rationale for the proposed clinical trial and support development of essential elements of a clinical trial • Usually project period of one year, sometimes up to 3 • Usually, a budget of up to $100,000 direct costs, sometimes up to $450,000 • Used only by select ICs; no parent FOA
U01	Research Project Cooperative Agreement Supports discrete, specified, circumscribed projects to be performed by investigator(s) in an area representing their specific interests and competencies • Used when substantial programmatic involvement is anticipated between the awarding Institute and Center • One of many types of cooperative agreements • No specific dollar limit unless specified in FOA		National Institute of Arthritis and Musculoskeletal and Skin Diseases (NIAMS) (http://www.niams.nih.gov/) National Institute of Dental and Craniofacial Research (NIDCR), (http://www.nidcr.nih.gov/) National Institute of Nursing Research (NINR) (http://www.ninr.nih.gov) Public Health Service (PHS) (Non-Competing Grants) *NIH Research Grants (accessed 2/28/2008 http://grants.nih.gov/grants/funding/funding_program.htm)

TABLE 81.5
Selected Foundations With Cancer Research Awards

AWARD/PROGRAM	BRIEF AWARD/PROGRAM DESCRIPTION	AWARD/PROGRAM
American Cancer Society		http://www.cancer.org/docroot/RES/RES_5_1. asp?sitearea=RES
Research grants for independent investigators	Research scholar grants in basic, preclinical, clinical and epidemiology research	Support investigator-initiated research projects in basic, preclinical, clinical and epidemiologic research.
	Research scholar grants in cancer control: psychosocial and behavioral research	Support investigator-initiated research projects in psychosocial, behavioral, and cancer control research, including epidemiologic approaches to psychosocial and behavioral research.
	Research scholar grants in cancer control: Health services and health policy research	Support investigator-initiated research projects in health services and health policy outcomes research.
Mentored training and career development grants	Postdoctoral fellowships	This award is to support the training of researchers who have just received their doctorate to enable them to qualify for an independent career in cancer research (including basic, preclinical, clinical, psychosocial, behavioral, and epidemiologic research).
	Mentored research scholar grant in applied and clinical research	Support mentored research by full-time faculty, typically within the first four years of their appointment, with the goal of becoming independent investigators in clinical, cancer control and prevention, epidemiologic, psychosocial, behavioral, health services and health policy research.
Professors	Clinical research professor	a limited number of grants to established investigators in mid-career who have made seminal contributions that have changed the direction of clinical, psychosocial, behavioral, health policy or epidemiologic cancer research. Furthermore, it is expected that these investigators will continue to provide leadership in their research area.
Special initiatives	Research proposals directed at oor and underserved populations	Despite the steady overall decline in cancer incidence and mortality rates, the incidence of many cancers in poor and underserved populations is higher, and morbidity and mortality are often greater. The American Cancer Society is committed to reducing disparities and alleviating the disproportionate cancer burden borne by many underserved populations, and has designated this a high-priority area. The Extramural Grants Department of the Research Department has launched a special initiative to decrease disparities.
Lance Armstrong Foundation		**http://www.livestrong.org/site/c.khLXK1PxHmF/ b.2661021/k.A7DA/Grants Programs.htm**
Survivor-ship Centers		The LIVESTRONG Survivorship Center of Excellence Network is a collaborative effort of the LAF, cancer centers at leading medical institutions and their community affiliates to: • Provide essential direct survivorship services • Increase the effectiveness of survivorship care through research, the development of new interventions and sharing of best practices

(Continued)

TABLE 81.5

Selected Foundations With Cancer Research Awards Continued

	Through regular meetings, working groups and joint projects, the Network seeks to harness the expertise, experience, creativity and productivity of leading centers in an effort to significantly accelerate progress in the field of cancer survivorship.
Community program	Community program provides financial support and capacity-building to community-centered initiatives that address the physical, emotional and practical challenges of cancer survivorship. Award implementation and evolution grants to community, non-profit organizations to serve the needs of people living with cancer as identified by the *National Action Plan for Cancer Survivorship: Advancing Public Health Strategies.* Award grants in the areas of physical activity and nutrition; education and support for people living with cancer; and practical issues of survivorship. Each grant recipient completes a rigorous application process, and proposals are reviewed by a selection committee of cancer survivors and cancer community experts and advisors.
Research program	Fund cancer survivorship research that builds on the body of knowledge and services to improve quality of life for cancer survivors across physical, psychosocial and practical challenges. Fund community-based participatory research (CBPR), through which community members and researchers collaborate in a mutual learning process to research and solve survivorship issues identified by the community. Aiming to support research that is not readily fundable from traditional sources, award cancer survivorship research and CBPR grants to established investigators as well as young investigators in the early stages of their research careers. LAF funding attracts promising young investigators to the field of cancer survivorship and helps to ensure that these researchers have the opportunity to establish a foothold in the field of cancer survivorship research.
Susan G. Komen	**http://cms.komen.org/komen/GrantsProgram/index.htm**
Promise grants	Provide up to $1.5M annually over five years for integrated research programs that bring together laboratory and clinical investigators from different disciplines to work together to solve common causes of breast cancer mortality.
Investigator initiated research grants	Provide up to $600,000 over three years to stimulate exploration of new ideas and novel approaches in breast cancer research and clinical practice that will lead to reductions in breast cancer incidence and mortality within the next decade.
Career catalyst research grants	Provide unique opportunities for scientists in the early stages of their career to achieve research independence with an independent award of up to $450,000 over three years. CCR investigators lead a research project addressing an important question in breast cancer research and complete a self-defined career development plan with support from a mentor committee.

(Continued)

TABLE 81.5
Selected Foundations With Cancer Research Awards Continued

Susan G. Komen *Disparities research*	http://cms.komen.org/komen/GrantsProgram/index.htm A new RFA addressing one of our most important challenges in breast cancer, disparities in breast cancer screening, treatment, and mortality, is currently being designed. Will work to identify where research funding will have the greatest impact on breast cancer disparities and particularly, deaths from breast cancer among minority and underserved populations.
Training award program, Postdoctoral fellowships	Provides support for young investigators to explore important research questions and to pursue a career in breast cancer research. seek to attract pre-faculty scientists into breast cancer by providing up to $60,000 annually over three years. Fellows develop skills and expertise in one of two research tracks, basic and translational research leading to reductions in breast cancer incidence and mortality.
Community-based grants	Komen and their Domestic Affiliate Network fund non-duplicative, community-based grants that translate the findings from research into breast health education and seek to enhance the availability of breast cancer screening and treatment for the medically underserved.
Elsa U. Pardee Foundation	http://www.pardeefoundation.org/grants.aspx funds research to investigators in United States non-profit institutions proposing research directed toward identifying new treatments or cures for cancer. The Foundation particularly encourages grant applications for a one year period which will allow establishment of capabilities of new cancer researchers, or new cancer approaches by established cancer researchers. It is anticipated that this early stage funding by the Foundation may lead to subsequent and expanded support using government agency funding. Project relevance to cancer detection, treatment, or cure should be clearly identified.
William Bingham Foundation *Progams serving low-income breast cancer patients*	http://www.foundationcenter.org/grantmaker/bingham/procedures.html Makes grants to nonprofit organizations in Cleveland and other areas across the United States, is accepting applications for its 2008 funding priority, which is to assist organizations working to increase access to health care and services for low-income breast cancer patients, particularly in Cleveland, Ohio, and Washington, D.C. This focus is in effect only for 2008. Projects should seek to improve healthcare access through public education, diagnosis, treatment, and other means.
American-Italian Cancer Foundation *International cancer research opportunities*	http://www.aicfonline.org/ Funds Senior Scholar Consultancies for motivated scientists who are already conducting significant research and would benefit from cross training and/or research collaboration with other senior faculty at leading cancer institutions in the U.S. or Italy.

(Continued)

TABLE 81.5
Selected Foundations With Cancer Research Awards Continued

American-Italian Cancer Foundation		http://www.aicfonline.org/
		Applicants will be distinguished by their research productivity and should be working on an area where short-term, direct contact with a senior colleague in a host institution will make a significant difference in project outcomes. Faculty planning for a sabbatical from their parent institution may find this mechanism of support very useful for a productive extended visit to another institution.
Avon Products, Inc.		http://www.avoncompany.com/women/ Avon Hello Tomorrow Fund
		Every week for a year, commencing April 2007, the Hello Tomorrow Fund will award $5,000 to a U.S. individual to help realize a program, project, or idea to empower women in one of three areas: business development, community service, or awareness and outreach. Women and men are eligible to apply. Application submission and selection of winners will be organized in a quarterly cycle.
American Association for Cancer Research		http://www.aacr.org/home/scientists/research-funding ---training-grants.aspx
Research grants for independent investigators	Landon Foundation-AACR Innovator Award for International Collaboration	
Mentored grants and research fellowships	AACR Centennial predoctoral fellowships in cancer research	Provide full-time graduate students a rare opportunity to invest in their future cancer research careers. The grant terms are flexible, allowing applicants to tailor their grant funds to fit their individual research funding and salary needs. Grantees may also transfer their funds to a postdoctoral fellowship position, should they advance in their careers during grant term.
	AACR Centennial Postdoctoral Fellowships in Cancer Research	Provide $60,000 per year for up to three years to provide salary support and research funding for clinical and postdoctoral fellows in the 1st, 2nd or 3rd year of their fellowship status. In addition to financial flexibility these fellowships also provide career flexibility. Fellowship funds may be transferred to move with the grantee if the grantee's fellowship is completed during the grant term - a valuable commodity for a newly-independent investigator.
	Career Development Awards Fellows grants Research fellowships	
National Brain Tumor Foundation		
Research program	Epidemiology brain tumor research grant; grant amount = $50,000	Funds cutting edge research into new treatments, improving traditional treatments and enhancing the quality of life of all brain tumor patients. This grant will fund a research project focusing on the causes of brain tumors. Special consideration will be given to members of the Brain Tumor Epidemiology Consortium (BTEC).
	Caregiver/quality of life brain tumor research grant; grant amount = $15,000	Caregivers of brain tumor patients face unique challenges and stresses in caring for their loved one. Funding will be provided for research that has 2 components - qualitative/quantitative and interventional.

TABLE 81.6

Traditional Assessment Scales Compared to NIH Performance Scale

KARNOFSKY	EASTERN COOPERATIVE ONCOLOGY GROUP (ECOG)	NATIONAL INSTITUTES OF HEALTH REHABILITATION MEDICINE DEPARTMENT PERFORMANCE SCALE (NIH—RMDPS)
100—Normal no complaints, no evidence of disease.	**0**—Fully active, able to carry on all predisease performance without restriction.	**0**—Independent in Activities of Daily Living (ADLs), ambulation, speech, swallowing, work and recreational activities. No pain.
90—Able to carry on normal activity, minor signs or symptoms of disease. **80**—Normal activity with effort, some signs and symptoms of disease.	**1**—Restricted in physically strenuous activity but ambulatory and able to carry out a light sedentary nature, eg, light housework, office work.	**1**—Independent in ADLs community ambulator, speech, swallowing; able to perform light or sedentary work, reduce time spent in physical recreational activities; may begin experiencing mild pain and/or mild fatigue which is easily controlled.
70—Cares for self, unable to carry on normal activity or do active work. **60**—Requires occasional assistance, but is able to care for most of his/her needs.	**2**—Ambulatory and capable of all self care but unable to carry out any work activities. Up and about more than 50% of waking hours.	**2**—Independent in most ADLs (with or without adaptive equipment); Speech and swallowing independent with slight modifications (i.e. diet change); moderate pain and fatigue; engagement in passive leisure however not working full time or involved in physical recreation.
50—Requires considerable assistance and frequent medical care. **40**—Disabled, requires special care and assistance.	**3**—Capable of only limited self care, confined to bed or chair more than 50% of waking hours.	**3**—Requires assistance and adaptive equipment for most ADLs and mobility activities; may have moderate to severe difficulty with speech, and swallowing problems(alternate feeding device); moderate to severe pain and/or fatigue; enjoys quiet leisure activities.
30—Severely disabled, hospitalization indicated. Death not imminent. **20**—Very sick, hospitalization indicated. Death not imminent. **10**—Moribund fatal processes progressing rapidly.	**4**—completely disabled. Cannot carry on any self care. Totally confined to bed or chair.	**4**—Totally dependent in all ADLs and mobility activities. May require hospice care. May be unable to speak or understand intended messages; may be unable to swallow safely and may require total nutrition by alternate means; may require narcotics for pain control; may no longer participate in leisure activities.

Source: From Ref. 28.

Study Design

Rehabilitation researchers typically accrue their patients by referrals from larger medical treatment intervention studies. Often the homogeneity of the population groups is diminished by the time subjects are entered onto rehabilitation research protocols. The resulting population heterogeneity is theoretically not ideal but must be acknowledged and accepted if one is to engage in rehabilitation research at all. A common illustration is in the functional problems of patients who may have the same cancer medical diagnosis or same treatment; however the problems to be studied by rehabilitation are not necessarily the same. For example a group of patients with a common diagnosis of osteosarcoma may have widely divergent functional problems related to lower extremity amputation, chronic pain or difficulties with short term memory. This original homogenic group presented to rehabilitation with heterogeneous issues needing to be identified, studied and treated according to a research protocol. In anticipation of doing the research, the clinical researcher must engage in intensive study of how to identify and group the issues prior to embarking on any of the study.

Assessments

Deborah Franklin has stated the "optimal functional assessment tools for cancer have yet to be identified" (10). Use of the Karnofsky scale and other performance scales is common for specific medical research questions; however they fall short of providing sufficient information of many rehabilitation domains. The NIH Rehabilitation Medicine Department Performance scale was developed to capture patient's rehabilitation limitations and needs based on performance. Patients require only one functional limitation in an area to qualify for that specific performance category (Table 81.6). Often more than one rehabilitation domain needs to be assessed to gain an understanding of one's actual functional performance. This only underscores the need for continued interdisciplinary teamwork (28).

With the continued emphasis on performing research with oncology populations, rehabilitation researchers should consider utilizing Item Response Theory to evaluate outcome measures in their research domains. The Theory adopted as PROMIS (Patient Reported Outcome Information Systems) has been adopted by the National Institutes of Health's roadmap to help reduce the barriers in performing research. PROMIS has the goal to bring on new sciences such as Item Response Theory (IRT) and Computerized Adaptive Testing (CAT). IRT is the study of test and item scores based on assumptions concerning the mathematical relationships among questions asked of patients. Based on a mathematical probability model, IRT helps to predict how people will behave. With large study designs this theory may serve to be useful in oncology. It has a potential to reduce the amount of time patients spend filling out questionnaires by reducing the number of questionnaire items asked of patients based on their responses, which is especially important over the continuum of care. Additionally when combined with CAT, IRT can be applied to larger data banks for determining the outcome measures asked in research assessments creating a shorter dynamic approach (29).

An additional concern faced by rehabilitation researchers to determine timing when is the most appropriate time to assess an individual's performance. Clinically, this is typically a judgment call when one is demonstrating improvement or a change in functional status; however data collection times are often murky in the research domain and need stricter guidelines in the planning stages of the clinical research endeavor. This can be illustrated with the lymphedema populations as there is both a lack of standardized definition of upper and lower limb lymphedema and most studies lack a baseline measurement limb volume prior to treatment; therefore, underreporting of the prevalence of lymphedema is highly likely. Box et al. in 2002 is one of the few studies that demonstrates the effectiveness of early detection of lymphedema utilizing of utilizing baseline measures prior to medical treatment to enable early intervention (30).

Additionally best timing for therapeutic interventions has also been problematic on the continuum of cancer rehabilitation for clinical researchers. Knowing the best time to initiate treatment for optimal outcomes has been difficult to predict. Several trials of early physical therapy intervention have been conducted in the past with newer trials obtaining baseline measures prior to medical treatment and comparing two treatments to determine the best efficacy. In Australia, Box et al. showed in a randomized trial of 65 women with breast cancer that the physical therapy intervention group had greater functional recovery at one month was greater in those randomized to the control group (32). In Japan, 72 women with breast cancer were in groups approximately even between those that received modified radical mastectomy and those that received lumpectomy. The efficacy of the program was demonstrated by postoperative week four, when patients from both groups had restored the ROM of the arm on the affected side and all ADL items had become almost normal in approximately 90% of patients (31).

Common clinical intervention practices are often anecdotal and often little research is evident with evidence based practice for its efficacy. Additional therapeutic interventions in all rehabilitation domains need more rigorous study of their effectiveness with each modality and then applied to the oncology populations.

Data Analysis and Interpretation

As with many research efforts, cancer rehab research can generate an overwhelming amount of quantitative and/or qualitative data, this frequently challenges the researcher. Once statistical analysis is performed, translation to meaningful interpretation for possible clinical integration is the ultimate goal. This can be illustrated with previous head and neck cancer research conducted for pre-operative air insufflation testing for prediction of voice quality with secondary tracheoesophageal punctures prior to performing the actual procedure. The research results have now changed clinical practice with recommendations to utilize this assessment tool for prediction of speech quality during voice restoration for patients who have had laryngectomy (32).

CONCLUSIONS

Clinical research in rehabilitation is a well-accepted area of endeavor; however, the relative lack of oncology rehabilitation research is disappointing. The ultimate challenge at present is for rehabilitation specialties to further the development of oncology research, with emphasis on the cancer continuum. Additionally, the dynamic nature of the ICF mode has been overlooked (Fig. 81.2). So many of the research studies in rehabilitation have focused on the body and structure as well as the activity and participation domains, with strikingly little representation from the environmental and personal factors domains. Research projects in the future should consider how to slice through all ICF domains

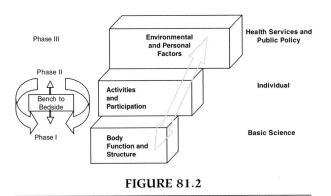

FIGURE 81.2

Ideal ICF construct for future cancer rehabilitation research.

from the outset (Table 81.7). A productive approach to this would be for a rehabilitation specialist to focus their hypothesis questions with primary, secondary and tertiary goals aligning with the ICF model's dimensions. This will have a more immediate impact on the state of practice and hence quality of rehabilitation care offered to patients.

As we have illustrated herein, the field of cancer research in rehabilitation is wide open, with numerous avenues to travel along the continuum of care through long-term survivorship. Additional future research is

imperative for all professionals to help determine the barriers to optimal rehabilitation for patients with cancer as well as test innovations in care delivery to improve overall outcomes. The time is right to start the desperately needed research in rehabilitation oncology and begin to address the rehabilitation issues with its comorbidities, psychosocial relationships, education to patient, family, and professional, and palliative care rehabilitation.

References

1. Accessed at http://www.cdc.gov/nchs/facts/icod.html.
2. Arzouman JM, Dudas S, Ferrans CE, Holm K. Quality of life of patients with sarcoma postchemotherapy. *Oncol Nurs Forum.* 1991;18:889–894.
3. Auchter RM SD, Adak S, Wagner H, Cella DF, Mehta MP. Quality of life assessment in advanced non-small-cell lung cancer patients undergoing an accelerated radiotherapy. regimen: Report of ECOG study 4593. *Int J Radiat Oncol Biol Phys.* 2001;50:1199–1206.
4. Axelsson B SP. Quality of life of cancer patients and their spouses in palliative home care. *Palliat Med.* 1998;12:29–39.
5. DeLisa J. A history of cancer rehabilitation. *Cancer.* 2001;92:970–974.
6. Whyte J. Training and retention of rehabilitation researchers. *Am J Phys Med Rehabil.* 2005;84(12):969–975.
7. Frontera WFJ, Jette A, Chan L, et al. Rehabilitation medicine summit: building research capacity. *Am J Phys Med Rehabil.* 2005;84:913–917.
8. Accessed at http://www.ncbi.nlm.nih.gov/sites/entrez/.
9. Accessed at http://crisp.cit.nih.gov. August 2008.

TABLE 81.7
Proposed Rehabilitation Research Domains for the Future

Research on limitations of current diagnostic testing or rehabilitation procedures for limitations in activity and participation in patients with cancer and ways to adapt technology to improve diagnosis and treatment of limitations in body structure and function, activity and participation.

Research on psychosocial factors, including impact of stigma, health beliefs, and body image on patient's with cancer decisions to seek rehabilitation services and subsequent health outcomes related to body structure and function, activity and participation.

Research on culturally appropriate patient/provider communication and rehabilitation in underserved/underrepresented minority groups with cancer.

Research focusing on the special needs of the elderly and/or medically disabled with cancer.

Research on patient or provider factors (including age, gender, ethnicity, type of cancer, or co-morbidities) leading to delayed rehabilitation in patients with cancer.

Research on the impact of modifications to the health care setting (including inpatient, outpatient, private practice office, home and hospice settings) on access to rehabilitation services, patient satisfaction with rehabilitation services, and health outcomes including body structure and function, activity and participation in patients with cancer.

Studies on the impact of modification of intervention procedures such as prescription of therapeutic exercise or mode of delivery in adults and/or children with cancer.

Research on the impact of improving rehabilitation provider knowledge, skills, and attitudes on body structure and function, activity and participation outcomes in patients with cancer.

Research on the interaction of type of cancer on the survivorship experience following primary treatment for cancer, including the capacity of patients to engage in self-management and the burden of care on family care-givers.

10. Franklin DJ. Cancer rehabilitation: challenges, approaches, and new directions. *Phys Med Rehabil Clin N Am.* 2007;18:899–924, viii.

11. Sussman S, Valente TW, Rohrbach LA, Skara S, Pentz MA. Translation in the health professions: converting science into action. *Eval Health Prof.* 2006;29:7–32.

12. Kealey P, McIntyre I. An evaluation of the domiciliary occupational therapy service in palliative cancer care in a community trust: a patient and carers perspective. *Eur J Cancer Care (Engl).* 2005;14:232–243.

13. Stucki G, Cieza A, Melvin J. The International Classification of Functioning, Disability and Health: A unifying model for a conceptual description of the rehabilitation strategy. *J Rehabil Med.* 2007;39:279–285.

14. Cheville AL. Current and future trends in Lymphedema management: implications for women's health. *Phys Med Rehabil Clin N Am.* 2007;18:539–553.

15. Horn SD, DeJong G, Ryser DK. Another look at observational studies in rehabilitation research: going beyond the holy grail of the randomized controlled trial. *Arch Phys Med Rehabil.* 2005;86:S8–S15.

16. Benson K, Hartz AJ. A comparison of observational studies and randomized, controlled trials. *N Engl J Med.* 2000;342:1878–1886.

17. Gerber LH, Vargo MM, Smith RG. Rehabilitation of the cancer patient. In: eds DeVita V, Hellman S, Rosenberg S, *Cancer: Principles and Practice of Oncology,* 7th ed. Philadelphia: Lippincott Williams and Wilkins; 2005:2719–2746.

18. Mayo NE, Poissant L, Ahmed S, et al. Incorporating the International Classification of Functioning, Disability, and Health (ICF) into an electronic health record to create indicators of function: proof of concept using the SF-12. *J Am Med Inform Assoc.* 2004;11:514–522.

19. Accessed at www.apta.com. August, 2008.

20. Accessed at www.asha.org. August, 2008.

21. Accessed at http://www.aapmr.org/. August, 2008.

22. Accessed at www.aota.org. August, 2008.

23. Accessed at www.nichd.nih.gov/about/org/ncmrr/. August, 2008.

24. Accessed at http://nccn.org/members/network.asp. August, 2008.

25. Accessed http://depts.washington.edu/bioethx/topics/resrch.html. August 2008.

26. List MA, Ritter-Sterr C, Lansky SB. A performance status scale for head and neck cancer patients. *Cancer.* 1990;66:564–569.

27. List MA, Bilir SP. Functional outcomes in head and neck cancer. *Semin Radiat Oncol.* 2004;14:178–189.

28. Solomon BI, Augustine E, Gerber L. New approaches to evaluation and intervention in the rehabilitation of cancer patients. In: *Recent Research Developments in Cancer.* Kerala, India: Transworld Research Network; 2002:553–568.

29. Accessed at http://www.nihpromis.org/default.aspx.

30. Box RC, Reul-Hirche H, Bullock-Saxton JE, Furnival C. Shoulder movement after breast cancer surgery: results of a randomized controlled study of postoperative physiotherapy. *Br Cancer Res Treat.* 2002;75:35–45.

31. Morimoto T, Tamura A, Ichihara T, et al. Evaluation of a new rehabilitation program for postoperative patients with breast cancer. *Nurs Health Sci.* 2003;5:275–282.

32. Lewin JS, Baugh RF, Baker SR. An objective method for prediction of tracheoesophageal speech production. *J Speech Hear Disord.* 1987;52:212–217.

33. Accessed at http://www.nia.nih.gov.

34. Accessed at http://www.ncrr.nih.gov/.

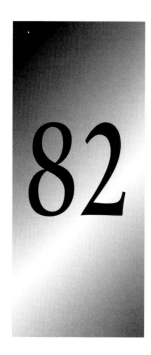

Public Policy Issues in Cancer Rehabilitation

Victoria Blinder
Madhu Mazumdar

The number of cancer survivors has tripled over the course of the last 30 years, and as a result issues pertaining to survivorship have come to the forefront of cancer research. Congress has enacted legislation to protect disabled persons, and many cancer patients and survivors qualify to receive these protections. They are protected from discrimination in the workplace under the Americans with Disabilities Act, and they may retain health care coverage when changing jobs under the Health Insurance Portability and Accountability Act. Many are also entitled to receive Medicare benefits, including inpatient and outpatient rehabilitation services. Multiple additional resources exist for cancer survivors provided by a variety of groups, including both governmental and nonprofit organizations. This chapter will focus on public policy regarding cancer rehabilitation and the resources available to patients and health care providers.

CANCER SURVIVORSHIP

Recent advances in oncology have improved long-term survival estimates, such that 67% of adults who are diagnosed with cancer are still living five years after diagnosis (1). The number of cancer survivors has, therefore, burgeoned over the course of the last several decades, and according to the National Cancer Institute (NCI), the number of people living with cancer in the United States increased from 3 to 10 million between

1971 and 2001 (2). As of 2003, cancer survivors represented approximately 3.6% of the United States population (3). This change in cancer demographics has resulted in the emergence of cancer survivorship as a promising research field, one that has continued to expand and blossom during the last decade. The growing awareness within the cancer community, among both patients and physicians, regarding the challenges facing cancer survivors has led to a surge in the investigation of issues such as return to work, the psychological burden of disease, and the interventions that are needed in order to facilitate the recovery of the patient with cancer and the transition to survivorship (4–9).

In 1996 the NCI, a division of the National Institutes of Health (NIH), established the Office of Cancer Survivorship (OCS) in recognition of the increasing number of cancer survivors and in order to help promote and support cancer survivorship research (10). According to the OCS, an individual is considered a cancer survivor from the time of diagnosis "through the balance of his or her life," regardless of the length of duration of this period (11). Friends, family members, and caregivers are included in this definition because they are also affected by the diagnosis. Since its inception, the OCS has distributed more than $28 million in research grants and currently funds more than 100 projects to investigate a broad range of issues, such as quality of life, disease and treatment-related cognitive deficits, vocational rehabilitation, exercise and weight loss, and the psychosocial effects of treatment (2,12).

KEY POINTS

- According to the National Cancer Institute (NCI), the number of people living with cancer in the United States increased from 3 to 10 million between 1971 and 2001.
- In 1996, the NCI, a division of the National Institutes of Health (NIH), established the Office of Cancer Survivorship (OCS) in recognition of the increasing number of cancer survivors and in order to help promote and support cancer survivorship research.
- Recent advances in oncology have improved long-term survival estimates, such that 67% of adults who are diagnosed with cancer are still living five years after diagnosis.
- According to the OCS, an individual is considered a cancer survivor from the time of diagnosis "through the balance of his or her life," regardless of the length of duration of this period.
- Title I of the Americans with Disabilities Act (ADA) of 1990 protects disabled persons from discrimination in the workplace.
- Cancer is generally considered a disability when the disease, its treatment, or the effects of either of these "substantially limits one or more of a person's major life activities," when it previously resulted in

- substantial limitations, or when it does not significantly alter a person's activities but an employer treats the individual as if it did so.
- The Health Insurance Portability and Accountability Act (HIPAA) is a federal law that protects health insurance coverage for employees and their families when they change or lose their jobs.
- Upon termination of employment, individuals are eligible for health insurance coverage under the Consolidated Omnibus Budget Reconciliation Act (COBRA) of 1986, which requires employers of at least 20 workers to allow these employees and their dependents to remain in the group plan for 18 months following job termination.
- Medicare is considered the "gold standard" of the insurance industry.
- Medicare's 75% rule may result in impaired access to inpatient rehabilitation facilities for cancer survivors.
- Memorial Sloan-Kettering Cancer Center, which has been at the forefront of survivorship planning, provides extensive resources for cancer survivors, regardless of whether or not they received their oncologic care at that institution.

Among the areas of particular emphasis in the OCS mission statement are health care disparities, economic outcomes (including work-related survivorship issues), optimization of follow-up care, and the development of study instruments to assess long-term quality of life and health outcomes (13). In addition to conducting and supporting research, the OCS seeks to educate professionals who work with cancer survivors and to communicate the results of research funded by the OCS to cancer survivors and their families through online resources and telephone education workshops. Despite the increased federal support for survivorship research, however, many areas of cancer survivorship remain unexplored. In particular, evidence-based guidelines for professionals providing follow-up care are needed in order to implement the products of research and develop appropriate interventions within this rapidly changing area of investigation.

In 2005, the Institute of Medicine published its groundbreaking report, *From Cancer Patient to Cancer Survivor: Lost in Transition* (2). In it, the Committee on Cancer Survivorship set forth various recommendations regarding the care of cancer survivors. They advocated for the inclusion of a comprehensive "Survivorship Care Plan," to be developed for each patient by the primary provider of oncologic care, and they emphasized the need for evidence-based guidelines for

the diagnosis and management of late effects of cancer and its treatment. The committee stressed the importance of congressional support for institutions providing care for these conditions. Employment concerns were paramount, and the committee cited not only the need to eliminate discrimination in the workplace, but also the importance of rehabilitation and return-to-work programs. The committee charged employers, health care providers, sponsors of support services, government agencies, and legal advocates with the task of supporting cancer survivors in their rehabilitation and reintegration. In their executive summary, committee members emphasized the need for improved education of patients and health care providers regarding the legal protections provided to cancer survivors. These are described in the section that follows.

LEGAL PROTECTIONS FOR CANCER PATIENTS AND SURVIVORS

Title I of the Americans with Disabilities Act (ADA) of 1990 protects disabled persons from discrimination in the workplace. Employers with at least 15 employees, including private businesses, state and local government agencies, labor unions, and employment agencies are prohibited from discriminating against qualified disabled individuals with respect to job applications, hiring, firing, advancement, compensation, job training, and other "terms, conditions, and privileges of employment" (14). The Rehabilitation Act exacts the same requirements of federal employers. According to the ADA, "An individual with a disability is a person who has a physical or mental impairment that substantially limits one or more major life activities, has a record of such an impairment, or is regarded as having such an impairment" (15). Most states also have additional laws to protect disabled persons from employment discrimination. Some of these include more expansive protections and/or provisions applicable to small-scale employers.

With respect to patients with cancer, the determination of whether or not an individual has a history of disability or is regarded as having a disability is made on a case-by-case basis (16). Cancer is generally considered a disability when the disease, its treatment, or the effects of either of these "substantially limits one or more of a person's major life activities," when it previously resulted in substantial limitations, or when it does not significantly alter a person's activities but an employer treats the individual as if it did so (16). The ADA prohibits employers from asking prospective or actual employees if they currently have or have previously suffered from cancer, and employees are not required to disclose this information unless they require special accommodations. Employers are permitted to ask questions or require employees to undergo a medical examination if they have reason to believe that a medical condition is affecting an individual's job performance, and they may likewise require employees who take a medical leave due to cancer to provide documentation or undergo a medical examination prior to returning to work. The ADA also requires employers to accommodate employees with disabilities unless such an accommodation would result in "undue hardship" for the employer. These accommodations include leave from work to attend doctor's appointments, undergo treatment, or recuperate from treatment; regular breaks or an area to rest or take medication; adjustments to the work schedule; permission to work at home; modification of office temperature; permission to use the work telephone to call physicians; redistribution of marginal tasks to other employees; and job reassignment (16).

Legal protection of employment-related health insurance benefits for cancer patients and survivors who are considering quitting or changing jobs varies between different states (8). The Health Insurance Portability and Accountability Act (HIPAA) is a federal law that protects health insurance coverage for employees and their families when they change or lose their jobs. HIPAA limits insurance companies' ability to exclude individuals based on preexisting conditions, prohibits group health plans from denying coverage or raising premiums based on an individual's past or current health status (or that of his or her family member), guarantees the legal right of some small employers and individuals who lose job-related insurance coverage to purchase new insurance, and guarantees that in general, employers and individuals who buy health insurance are able to renew their coverage regardless of any new health conditions that may develop (17). Although group health plans may refuse to cover the cost of treatment for preexisting conditions for a period of 12–18 months, this exclusion period can be reduced or eliminated if the individual had "creditable coverage" prior to enrollment. Such coverage includes most group or individual health insurance plans, Medicare, or Medicaid. Details regarding coverage of preexisting conditions, premiums, mandatory coverage of services, and requirements with respect to individuals with a history of cancer vary from state to state (8).

Upon termination of employment, individuals are eligible for health insurance coverage under the Consolidated Omnibus Budget Reconciliation Act (COBRA) of 1986, which requires employers of at least 20 workers to allow these employees and their dependents to remain in the group plan for 18 months following job termination (8,18). This period can be extended to 29 months for disabled employees, and serves to bridge the time gap between employment termination and Medicare enrollment (see below). Under COBRA, the former employee pays the full cost of the premium. In total, employees pay 102% of their premium price, including a 2% administrative fee. The premium may increase during the period of extension beyond 18 months.

Cancer patients and survivors who lose employment-related insurance may be eligible for Medicare or Medicaid. Medicare is an option for those who qualify for social security disability benefits, but the waiting period for enrollment is 29 months, during which the individual must find other means of insurance coverage, such as COBRA. Medicaid eligibility is based on income rather than disability and is available only to individuals whose earnings are below a certain limit. The program is administered by each state, and state governments determine the maximum income permitted for enrollment as well as other guidelines for eligibility and benefits (19).

MEDICARE AND CANCER REHABILITATION COVERAGE

Medicare is considered the "gold standard" of the insurance industry. Approximately 60% of cancer survivors are older than age 65, and 99% of these have health insurance through Medicare (2). As discussed above, cancer patients and survivors under age 65 may also be eligible for Medicare, making it the single largest health insurance provider for cancer survivors (2). Medicare covers inpatient rehabilitation services (including acute rehabilitation) in skilled nursing facilities, hospital units, freestanding rehabilitation centers, and long-term care hospitals, as well as outpatient rehabilitation at home and in the ambulatory clinic. Patients may also obtain durable medical equipment, prosthetics, orthotics, and supplies (DMEPOS) through Medicare. The next section focuses on the history of Medicare, the program's structure, and its coverage of rehabilitation.

Medicare was established in 1965 as a public health insurance administration for Americans aged 65 and older. In order to be eligible for Medicare, individuals must be citizens or permanent residents of the United States (19). In addition to the elderly, Medicare is available to those who are disabled and receive Social Security benefits, as well as to patients with end-stage renal disease. As discussed above, patients with cancer are not automatically eligible to receive Medicare benefits.

Medicare is divided into an inpatient insurance system and an outpatient or supplementary program. Medicare Part A covers inpatient hospital admissions, hospice, skilled nursing facilities, and some home health care services (20). Part B includes outpatient physicians' fees, laboratory tests, and other outpatient services (20). Although Medicare is a government agency, administered by the Centers for Medicare and Medicaid Services (CMS), most of its claims are processed by private contractors (20). Recent modifications have led to the creation of Medicare Part C or Medicare Advantage, which outsources insurance coverage to private carriers, and Medicare Part D, which includes the set of prescription drug plans that contract with Medicare.

In 1983, Medicare adopted the Prospective Payment System (PPS) as part of an attempt to improve the cost efficiency of the Medicare reimbursement system (21). Under PPS, hospitals would be reimbursed according to a payment schedule based on various diagnosis-related groupings (DRGs). Previously, there had been no incentive for physicians and hospital administrators to take cost efficiency into consideration when formulating a patient's plan of care. Any incentive had been in favor of increased spending, as hospitals were reimbursed in proportion to the costs accrued in caring for a patient. The use of DRGs to determine payment would, in theory, encourage physicians to be more economical when ordering tests or procedures. Reimbursement to hospitals would be determined by the DRG alone, regardless of the duration of the hospitalization or the number of tests ordered. If the fees incurred in the course of caring for a patient exceeded

the DRG-associated reimbursement, the hospital would not be reimbursed for the excess cost. Conversely, if the hospital spent less than the reimbursement schedule dictated in the course of caring for a patient, the institution would profit from the excess payment.

A system such as PPS would be difficult to apply to inpatient rehabilitation facilities (IRFs), however, since the range of services provided in this setting is different from the services provided in acute care hospitals and there is greater variability in the length of stay. Thus it was determined that IRFs would be reimbursed on a cost basis. The 75% Rule was established by Medicare to distinguish inpatient hospitals from IRFs. In order to qualify as an IRF, at least 75% of an institution's inpatients must be undergoing treatment for one or more of a list of ten conditions: stroke, spinal cord injury, congenital deformity, amputation, major multiple trauma, fracture of femur, brain injury, polyarthritis, neurological disorders, and burns (22). Using the 75% Rule as a guide, IRFs would continue to be reimbursed on a cost basis, while acute care hospitals adhered to the PPS system. However, in 1997, Congress initiated legislation to create a prospective payment system for IRFs as well, known as the IRF PPS. Under this system, which was implemented in 2002, reimbursement would be determined by a patient's assignment to one of 300 case-mix groups based on his or her characteristics, including a diagnosis requiring rehabilitation, the patient's functional and cognitive statuses, age, and comorbidities (22). Other factors would also be considered, such as regional wage adjustments, the proportion of low-income patients in the facility, whether or not the IRF was in a rural location, and whether or not it was considered a teaching facility.

Thus, Medicare continued to use the 75% Rule to determine whether a facility qualified to be an IRF, but the set of diagnoses used in this determination was not the same as the criteria dictating the payment schedule. Various groups, including the American Medical Rehabilitation Providers Association and the American Academy of Physical Medicine and Rehabilitation protested that the 75% Rule had become outdated in light of the alterations in the reimbursement system (23). They argued that the rule should be repealed or amended to include all of the diagnoses in the reimbursement schedule (except "Miscellaneous"). In 2002, the 75% Rule was temporarily suspended by CMS, when it was discovered that it was being inconsistently applied (22). Two years later, CMS redefined the inpatient rehabilitation facility criteria. Polyarthritis was replaced with three categories: osteoarthritis, rheumatoid arthritis, and joint replacement (bilateral, in patients aged 85 or older, or in those with body mass index of 50 or greater). In addition, systemic vasculidities was added to the list for a total of

13 diagnoses, known as the CMS-13 (22). A four-year transition period was planned to eventually achieve compliance with the 75% Rule. By July 2004, IRFs would be required to comply with the CMS-13 in 50% of their patients. One year later, a 60% rule would go into effect, followed by a 65% rule in 2007. Full compliance with the 75% Rule would be required by July 2008. Despite the expansion of the list of diagnoses from 10 to the CMS-13, it is likely that a large proportion of cancer patients will be excluded. Under the 75% Rule, patients with malignancies affecting the nervous system should have adequate access to rehabilitation, while those with solid and hematological malignancies lacking neurological involvement may not qualify. IRFs will have fewer incentives to accept large numbers of oncology patients due to a concern for noncompliance with the 75% Rule. It is not difficult to see how this may result in impaired access to inpatient rehabilitation facilities for cancer survivors.

Medicare also covers outpatient rehabilitation services, including outpatient physical therapy, occupational therapy, and speech-language pathology. Annual limits exist for these, unless they are provided in the outpatient department of a hospital (24). In 2006, these spending caps were $1,740 for physical therapy and speech-language pathology combined, and $1,740 for occupational therapy (24). Outpatient therapy provided in outpatient offices, comprehensive rehabilitation facilities, skilled nursing facilities, and at home, are subject to these limits, although patients may apply for exceptions and be granted additional funds.

DMEPOS are covered by Medicare under part B of the program. CMS is in the process of establishing a competitive bidding program for these, in which suppliers will be divided into Competitive Bidding Areas (CBAs) including ten of the largest Metropolitan Statistical Areas (MSAs) (25). Ten categories of devices will be chosen for this program, which is designed to decrease costs. Accreditation of the suppliers, already a CMS requirement, will be more rigorously implemented under this program, and will be based on new quality standards (26).

RESOURCES AVAILABLE TO PATIENTS AND PHYSICIANS

Despite the growing emphasis on cancer survivorship, relatively few comprehensive cancer rehabilitation programs have been developed to meet the complex and diverse needs of cancer survivors (8). Memorial Sloan-Kettering Cancer Center, which has been at the forefront of survivorship planning, provides extensive resources for cancer survivors, regardless of whether or not they received their oncologic care at that institution

(27). These include web-based information pages on survivorship issues including employment, emotional distress, sexual functioning, body image changes, fertility preservation, and cognitive changes. They also provide information on "managing ongoing and late effects of cancer and its treatment," including colostomy care, urinary incontinence, chronic pain, hearing loss, and physical therapy (28). The hospital has a comprehensive rehabilitation center, providing acute bedside rehabilitation and outpatient services that address a multitude of conditions related to cancer, including neuropathy, amputations, chronic pain, lymphedema, cognitive training, and energy conservation techniques.

Various nonprofit organizations also provide a range of services for cancer patients. The Lance Armstrong Foundation, CancerCare, and the American Cancer Society are only a few such groups. These groups are a source of financial and information resources for cancer patients during therapy and beyond. For example, through the Lance Armstrong Foundation's website, patients can obtain counseling and referrals to local services as well as assistance in addressing insurance and financial issues (29). Health care professionals can find information on survivorship, state-specific foundation-sponsored resources and efforts, and information to share with their patients. Through the Survivor*care* program, run jointly by CancerCare and the Lance Armstrong Foundation, patients can receive individualized support to help cope with their concerns. CancerCare, which was founded in 1944, provides individual help to approximately 91,000 people every year (30). The organization is a source of free information and support services to cancer patients and survivors, their families, and to health care providers. It sponsors educational programs, support groups, and individual counseling, which are available locally as well as online and by telephone. The group also provides financial assistance in addition to information about other sources of economic aid. The American Cancer Society and the National Cancer Institute also provide resources and information for cancer survivors. Grants to educators and researchers who mentor or employ a person with disability from cancer are also available. Table 82.1 lists various survivorship support organizations and their websites.

The Commission on Accreditation of Rehabilitation Facilities (CARF) is an international nonprofit organization that was founded in 1966, and provides information regarding a variety of rehabilitation services, such as facilities, durable medical equipment, career and job development, and counseling (31). Patients may request a regional list of providers for a particular service, or they may search specifically for various subcategories of services. The commission's

TABLE 82.1

Support for Cancer Survivors

The American Cancer Society	www.cancer.org
CancerCare	www.cancercare.org
Cancer Survivor's Project	www.cancersurvivorsproject.org
The Lance Armstrong Foundation	www.livestrong.org
The National Cancer Institute	www.cancer.gov
The National Coalition for Cancer Survivorship	www.canceradvocacy.org
People Living with Cancer	www.plwc.org

quality standards, which are updated annually, are based on recommendations from patients, rehabilitation providers, governmental organizations, and CARF funders. According to CARF, their accreditation helps assure patients that programs actively involve consumers in service planning, that they meet the CARF's consumer-oriented standards of performance, and that they focus on individualized goals and outcomes (32).

CONCLUSIONS

Cancer survivorship is a rapidly growing field of research, and the multiple facets of the care of cancer survivors are continuously evolving. Although the body of literature in this field has expanded dramatically over the course of last decade, a gap remains between the identification of survivorship issues and the development and implementation of appropriate interventions. Rehabilitation is an integral part of the transition to cancer survivorship for many patients, but its role in the care of the cancer survivor is not always clearly defined. Guidelines and benchmarks for adequate outcomes are needed, analogous to those used by oncologists in the delivery of acute cancer treatment, in order to ensure that all cancer survivors are assessed with respect to potential rehabilitation needs and that those who may benefit from this therapy are able to receive it. Cancer survivorship, including rehabilitation, must be recognized as an integral part of cancer care, and should be considered a component of the plan of care for each patient from the time of diagnosis. Finally, although a panoply of governmental and nonprofit resources are available to cancer survivors and health care providers, increased awareness is necessary in order to maximize

their reach. Treatment centers need to be the facilitators and advocates to ensure that each cancer patient is able to benefit from all that is available.

ACKNOWLEDGMENT

Dr. Mazumdar was partially suppoted by the following grants: UL1-RR024996, AHRQ RFA-HS-0514, NIGMS R25CA105012, NCI HHSN 26120062204C.

References

1. SEER Cancer Statistics Review, 1975–2004, National Cancer Institute. Bethesda, MD, http://seer.cancer.gov/csr/1975_2004/, based on November 2006 SEER data submission, posted to the SEER web site, 2007. (Accessed July 10, 2007, at http://seer.cancer.gov/csr/1975_2004/.)
2. Hewitt M, Greenfield S, Steovall E. *From Cancer Patient to Cancer Survivor: Lost in Transition.* Washington, DC: National Academies Press; 2006.
3. Estimated US Cancer Prevalence Counts: Who Are Our Cancer Survivors in the US? National Cancer Institute, 2007. (Accessed July 10, 2007, 2007, at http://dccps.nci.nih.gov/ocs/prevalence/index.html.)
4. Bouknight RR, Bradley CJ, Luo Z. Correlates of return to work for breast cancer survivors. *J Clin Oncol.* 2006;24(3):345–353.
5. Bradley CJ, Bednarek HL. Employment patterns of long-term cancer survivors. *Psychooncology.* 2002;11(3):188–198.
6. Maunsell E, Drolet M, Brisson J, Brisson C, Masse B, Deschenes L. Work situation after breast cancer: results from a population-based study. [see comment]. *J Natl Cancer Inst.* 2004;96(24):1813–1822.
7. Satariano WA, DeLorenze GN. The likelihood of returning to work after breast cancer.[see comment]. *Pub Health Rep.* 1996;111(3):236–241.
8. Short PF, Vargo MM. Responding to employment concerns of cancer survivors. *J Clin Oncol.* 2006;24(32):5138–5141.
9. Ganz PA, Coscarelli A, Fred C, Kahn B, Polinsky ML, Petersen L. Breast cancer survivors: psychosocial concerns and quality of life. *Breast Cancer Res Treat.* 1996;38(2):183–199.
10. About Cancer Survivorship Research: History. Office of Cancer Survivorship. National Cancer Institute. 2007. (Accessed July 10, 2007, at http://dccps.nci.nih.gov/ocs/history.html.)
11. Public Fact Sheet. Office of Cancer Survivorship. National Cancer Institute. 2007. (Accessed July 10, 2007, at http://dccps.nci.nih.gov/ocs/ocs_factsheet.pdf.)
12. Cancer Survivorship Research. Office of Cancer Survivorship. National Cancer Institute. 2007. (Accessed July 10, 2007, at http://dccps.nci.nih.gov/ocs/research-survivorship.html.)
13. Researchers Fact Sheets. Office of Cancer Survivorship. National Cancer Institute. 2007. (Accessed July 10, 2007, at http://cancercontrol.cancer.gov/ocs/researcher-factsheet.pdf.)
14. The Americans With Disabilities Act of 1990, Titles I and V. 1990. (Accessed July 10, 2007, at http://www.eeoc.gov/policy/ada.html.)
15. Disability Discrimination. The U.S. Equal Employment Opportunity Commission. 2007. (Accessed July 10, 2007, at http://www.eeoc.gov/types/ada.html.)
16. Questions and Answers about Cancer in the Workplace and the Americans with Disabilities Act (ADA). The U.S. Equal Employment Opportunity Commission. 2007. (Accessed July 10, 2007, at http://www.eeoc.gov/facts/cancer.html.)
17. What HIPAA Does and Does Not Do. Centers for Medicare and Medicaid Services. 2007. (Accessed July 10, 2007, at http://www.cms.hhs.gov/HealthInsReformforConsume/02_WhatHIPAADoesandDoesNotDo.asp#TopOfPage.)

18. An Employee's Guide to Health Benefits Under COBRA. The Consolidated Omnibus Budget Reconciliation Act of 1986. 2007. (Accessed July 10, 2007, at http://www.dol.gov/ebsa/pdf/cobraemployee.pdf.)

19. People with Medicare and Medicaid Center. Centers for Medicare and Medicaid Services. 2997. (Accessed July 10, 2007, at http://www.cms.hhs.gov/center/PeopleWithMedicareCenter.asp.)

20. Iglehart JK. The centers for medicare and medicaid services. *N Engl J Med.* 2001;345(26):1920–1924.

21. Patel K, Rushefsky ME. *Health Care Politics and Policy in America.* Armonk, New York: M.E. Sharpe; 1995.

22. Medicare Policy Advisory Commission. Report to the Congress: Medicare Payment Policy. 2006. (Retrieved from www.medpac.gov/publications/congressional_reports/mar06_ch04d.pdf))

23. ARN, AMRPA, AHA, FAH, AAN, AAPMR. Joint Position Statement Regarding the 75% Rule. Association of Rehabilitation Nurses, American Medical Rehabilitation Providers Association, Advancing Health in America, Federation of American Hospitals, American Academy of Neurology, American Academy of Physical Medicine and Rehabilitation. www.rehabnurse.org/docs/75rule.doc.

24. Medicare Limits on Therapy Services. 2006. (Accessed July 10, 2007, at http://www.medicare.gov/Publications/Pubs/pdf/10988.pdf.)

25. Competitive Acquisition for DMEPOS: Metropolitan statistical areas. 2007. (Accessed July 10, 2007, at http://www.cms.hhs.gov/CompetitiveAcqforDMEPOS/01b_MSAs.asp#TopOfPage.)

26. Competitive Acquisition for DMEPOS: New quality standards. 2007. (Accessed July 10, 2007, at http://www.cms.hhs.gov/CompetitiveAcqforDMEPOS/04_New_Quality_Standards.asp#TopOfPage.)

27. Memorial Sloan-Kettering Cancer Center: Survivorship. 2007. (Accessed July 10, 2007, at http://www.mskcc.org/mskcc/html/64233.cfm.)

28. Memorial Sloan-Kettering Cancer Center: Managing ongoing and late effects of cancer and treatment. 2007. (Accessed July 10, 2007, at http://www.mskcc.org/mskcc/html/65218.cfm.)

29. Livestrong Lance Armstrong Foundation: Cancer support. 2007. (Accessed July 10, 2007, at http://www.livestrong.org/site/c.khLXK1PxHmF/b.2662949/k.73BB/Get_OneonOne_Support.htm.)

30. Cancercare: Cancercare's mission. 2007. (Accessed July 10, 2007, at http://www.cancercare.org/about_us/.)

31. Commission on Accreditation of Rehabilitation Facilities: Who we are. 2007. (Accessed July 10, 2007, at http://www.carf.org/consumer.aspx?content=content/About/News/boilerplate.htm.)

32. Commission on Accreditation of Rehabilitation Facilities: CARF's mission, vision, core values, and purposes. 2007. (Accessed July 10, 2007, at http://www.carf.org/consumer.aspx?content=content/About/mission.htm.)

Health Maintenance and Screening in Cancer Survivors

Kevin C. Oeffinger

With recent advances in early detection, treatment, and supportive care, the number of cancer survivors in the United States increased from 3.0 million in 1971 to approximately 10.7 million individuals as of 2006 (1). Five-year survival rates now exceed 65% for adults with cancer and 80% for children and adolescents with cancer (2). This growing population of cancer survivors, expected to exceed 18 million by 2020, includes large groups of individuals diagnosed with breast cancer (22%), prostate cancers (18%), colorectal cancer (10%), and gynecologic (10%) malignancies (1). Pediatric cancer survivors represent less than 3% of all cancer survivors.

Success in curing cancer often comes with a cost in terms of physical and psychosocial health problems experienced by cancer survivors. Pediatric cancer survivors, due to the vulnerability of their developing organ systems, are particularly at risk to develop serious health problems as a consequence of their cancer therapy. It is estimated that by 30 years after the cancer diagnosis (eg, by age 40 for a patient treated at age 10), 73% of childhood cancer survivors will have a chronic physical condition, 42% with a severe, life-threatening, or disabling condition or death due to a chronic condition (3). Almost one in every two adult survivors of childhood cancer has at least one domain of their health status that is moderately to severely diminished, including limitations in activity, functional impairment, or symptoms of depression and anxiety (4). Adults, though in general less vulnerable to cancer therapy

than children, frequently experience health problems related to their cancer therapy. For example, women surviving breast cancer may experience weight gain and physical inactivity following their therapy. These two health outcomes in turn increase the risk for recurrence, cardiovascular disease, and diabetes (5–7). Other late effects experienced by breast cancer survivors include cognitive dysfunction (8,9), gonadal dysfunction, premature menopause and infertility (10,11), second malignant neoplasms (12–14), osteoporosis (15–17), anthracycline-related cardiomyopathy (18–22), body image changes and lymphedema (23,24), and psychosocial sequelae, including sexual dysfunction and fatigue (23–28). Many adults with cancer, particularly those who are older at diagnosis, have multiple comorbid health conditions that not only complicate cancer therapy but also increase their long-term risk (29,30). Importantly, while some serious problems occur during the cancer therapy or soon thereafter (long-term effects), the majority do not become clinically apparent until many years after the cancer is cured (late effects) (1,31,32).

Fortunately, the severity of many of the health outcomes experienced by cancer survivors can be either lessened or sometimes prevented by proactive and anticipatory survivor-focused health care. Highlighting this principle, the Institute of Medicine (IOM) released two seminal reports on cancer survivorship. In the 2003 report, *Childhood Cancer Survivorship: Improving Care and Quality of Life,*

KEY POINTS

- With recent advances in early detection, treatment, and supportive care, the number of cancer survivors in the United States increased from 3.0 million in 1971 to approximately 10.7 million individuals as of 2006.
- This success in curing cancer often comes with a cost in terms of physical and psychosocial health problems experienced by cancer survivors.
- Fortunately, the severity of many of the health outcomes experienced by cancer survivors can be either lessened or prevented by proactive and anticipatory survivor-focused health care.

- The National Comprehensive Cancer Network (NCCN) has developed the Clinical Practice Guidelines in Oncology, which provides recommendations for surveillance and/or follow-up applicable to 97% of patients with cancer.
- A key component of follow-up care is educating cancer survivors about the importance of their health behaviors.
- Longitudinal and targeted education and counseling is an integral aspect of risk-based health care.

the IOM strongly recommended lifelong follow-up health care for all childhood cancer survivors (32). This recommendation was echoed in the 2006 report focused on survivors of adult cancer, *From Cancer Patient to Cancer Survivor: Lost in Transition* (1). As described in these reports, the health care of cancer survivors should be based on their unique health risks following chemotherapy, surgery, and radiation. Content, intensity, and frequency of health care that addresses these risks vary from survivor to survivor. Risk-based health care refers to this conceptualization of lifelong health care that integrates the cancer and survivorship experience in the overall health care needs of the individual (33). Such care should include a systematic plan for lifelong screening, surveillance, and prevention that incorporates risks based on the previous cancer, cancer therapy, genetic predispositions, lifestyle behaviors, and comorbid health conditions. This includes surveillance for recurrent disease, screening for late effects and subsequent cancers, promotion of risk-reducing healthy lifestyles, and targeted counseling and education. In addition, some survivors will benefit from special services such as cognitive rehabilitation and genetic counseling.

Describing the content of risk-based health care by cancer group or treatment exposures is beyond the scope of this chapter. For further reading, several recent books (34–36) and journal reviews (37–39) have described survivor health care. *Establishing and Enhancing Services for Childhood Cancer Survivors: Long-Term Follow-Up Program Resource Guide*, developed by the Nursing Committee of the Children's Oncology Group (COG), is a tremendously rich resource that is intended to facilitate care of the long-term pediatric cancer survivors and can be downloaded from a public website, www.survivorshipguidelines.org. In the following sections, the key components of risk-based health care will be briefly described, including: surveillance for recurrence, screening for late effects and subsequent cancers,

promoting healthy lifestyles, educating and counseling cancer survivors, and using special services.

SURVEILLANCE FOR RECURRENCE

During the first few years after completion of therapy, the most important component of follow-up care is surveillance for recurrent disease. The National Comprehensive Cancer Network (NCCN) has developed the Clinical Practice Guidelines in Oncology, which provides recommendations for surveillance and/or follow-up applicable to 97% of patients with cancer (40). These include the frequency of follow-up visits and recommended labs and imaging studies (eg, mammogram). The guidelines were developed through an explicit review of the evidence integrated with expert medical judgment by multidisciplinary panels from NCCN member institutions, and continue to be updated on a regular basis.

SCREENING FOR LATE EFFECTS AND SUBSEQUENT CANCERS

In 2003, COG released the *COG Long-Term Follow-Up Guidelines for Survivors of Childhood, Adolescent, and Young Adult Cancers*. In preparation for the recommendations, an exhaustive review of the medical literature was completed and the quality of evidence of the association of late effects and cancer therapy was graded by the COG Late Effects Steering Committee; screening principles from the general population and other high-risk groups were applied (41). The guidelines can be found at www.survivorshipguidelines.org. For each chemotherapeutic agent, field of radiation, and type of surgery, and for special populations (eg, recipients of hematopoietic stem cell transplants), the following information is provided in a tabular format:

potential late effects, risk factors, highest risk groups, recommended periodic evaluation, health counseling information, up-to-date references, and the grade of evidence between the exposure and the late effect. The periodic evaluation includes pertinent aspects of the history and physical examination as well as recommended screening tests.

These guidelines are periodically updated by a multidisciplinary group that includes oncologists, primary care physicians, subspecialists of pediatric and adult medicine (eg, cardiologists, pulmonologists), surgeons, psychologists, and other experts in the field. A group from Baylor College of Medicine and Texas Children's Cancer Center, led by Poplack, Horowitz, and Fordis, has developed a web-based interactive and user-friendly format for these guidelines. This novel product, called *Passport for Care*, is being piloted among specialized long-term follow-up programs at cancer centers. Specifics of a patient's cancer and cancer therapy are entered into the system, using drop down menus, by a nurse, physician, or other trained individual. Then a set of individualized screening recommendations, based on the COG guidelines, are printed out and can be used by the clinician. With further development and refinement, the *Passport for Care* is intended to be used not only by specialized survivor clinics but also by primary care physicians or other clinicians following a cancer survivor. Ultimately, this tool can be used also in the care of survivors of adult cancer.

Evidence-based recommendations for screening of childhood cancer survivors have also been developed by several European groups, including the Scottish Intercollegiate Guidelines Network (SIGN) (42) and United Kingdom Children's Cancer Study Group Late Effects Group (43).

In contrast, the literature base of late effects following therapy for adult cancers has not yet evolved to the depth and breadth of that available for those following pediatric cancer (44). This gap was highlighted by the IOM, who called for further research in this area (1). Anticipating the growing body of evidence available, the American Society of Clinical Oncologists (ASCO) created a Cancer Survivorship Expert Panel to develop a set of screening recommendations for survivors of adult cancer. Recognizing the heterogeneity of therapeutic exposures used to cure adult cancers, this group decided to develop guidelines based upon affected organ systems, starting first with the heart and lungs. Because there was a lack of direct, high-quality evidence on the benefits and harms of screening for cardiac and pulmonary late effects, a set of evidence-based guidelines were not developed (45). The ASCO panel will soon review evidence regarding infertility/gonadal dysfunction and bone metabolism disorders associated with cancer therapy.

PROMOTING HEALTHY LIFESTYLES

A key component of follow-up care is educating cancer survivors about the importance of their health behaviors. Unhealthy behaviors and practices increase the risk of late effects among cancer survivors. For example, tobacco use increases lung cancer risk by more than 20-fold among Hodgkin lymphoma survivors who have been treated with mediastinal radiation (46,47). It is also anticipated that tobacco use among cancer survivors will increase risk of cardiovascular and pulmonary disease and other significant morbidities following chest radiation or chemotherapy that affects heart or lung function. Among women with breast cancer, obesity is associated with a twofold increased risk of cancer recurrence (48). Physical inactivity, which in the general population is associated with an increased risk of cardiovascular disease, diabetes mellitus, osteoporosis, and all-cause mortality, further modifies the risk faced by cancer survivors (6,49). Similarly, excessive alcohol intake, inadequate calcium intake, high-fat diets, and inadequate skin protection will increase the risk of various late effects or worsen comorbid health conditions.

In contrast, healthy lifestyles have been shown to improve outcomes of cancer survivors. Notably, Holmes and colleagues reported that physical activity following a breast cancer diagnosis appears to reduce the risk of death from this disease (7). Physical activity among cancer survivors has been shown to help with weight maintenance or loss, decrease levels of fatigue, and improved quality of life (6,50–52). Similarly, physical activity and adequate calcium intake are important practices to lessen the likelihood of developing osteoporosis following therapy that affects bone metabolism.

There is a common misperception that a cancer diagnosis motivates patients to alter their lifestyles and improve their dietary and exercise habits. However, this may not be the case, based upon a survey of prostate and breast cancer patients that noted 55% reported eating fewer than five fruits and vegetables daily, 42% indicated no routine exercise, and 20% currently smoked (53). Unhealthy diets, physical inactivity, and persistent smoking can continue to threaten the survival and quality of life for cancer survivors. This provides a "teachable moment" for medical care professionals, and an opportunity for patients to assume control of their lives as cancer survivors (53). The importance of general health promotion focused on lifestyle modifications, such as diet/nutrition, body weight, exercise, tobacco avoidance, and moderate use of alcohol, as well as maximizing rates of cancer screening, should be emphasized for cancer survivors as a method of empowerment and risk reduction (54–57).

EDUCATING AND COUNSELING CANCER SURVIVORS

Longitudinal and targeted education and counseling is an integral aspect of risk-based health care. It is imperative that the clinician spend time educating the patient and family members regarding the long-term implications of having survived cancer. Depending upon the cancer therapy, and modified by other risk factors such as genetic predispositions, lifestyle behaviors and practices, and comorbid health conditions, many cancer survivors have an increased risk of serious physical and psychological health problems. Discussing with survivors methods by which they can reduce risks and maximize their health, and addressing their concerns, fears, and sense of uncertainty is essential. In the following paragraphs, the importance of a treatment summary is described, followed by two important topics commonly addressed in a visit with a cancer survivor: fertility/gonadal function/sexuality and psychosocial issues.

Cancer Treatment Summary

The Institute of Medicine strongly recommends that all cancer survivors be provided a treatment summary that includes information regarding the cancer and cancer therapy (1,32). For the cancer, the key information includes the cancer type, stage at diagnosis if applicable, date of diagnosis, age at diagnosis, and date of completion of therapy. The cancer therapy should include a list of all surgeries, radiation field and dose, and chemotherapeutic agents. The cumulative dose of certain chemotherapeutic agents, such as doxorubicin (Adriamycin) or daunorubicin (DaunoXome) is important for individualizing screening recommendations. Lastly, a list of the primary (serious or common) potential late effects and associated screening recommendations can be quite helpful to cancer survivors.

For over two decades, the cancer treatment summary has been an integral component of educating childhood cancer survivors regarding the long-term risks associated with their cancer therapy (58). The COG Nursing and Late Effects Committees developed a standardized template for the treatment summary, provided as an appendix in the *IOM Workshop Summary, Implementing Cancer Survivorship Care Planning* (59). A template for both abbreviated and comprehensive treatment summaries can also be downloaded from the aforementioned *LTFU Program Resource Guide* (pp. 91–93) from the COG website, www.survivorshipguidelines.org. Several other templates to create treatment summaries for survivors of adult cancers are provided in the IOM Workshop Summary (59). The ASCO Cancer Survivorship Expert Panel is also in the process of developing and refining disease-specific treatment summary templates.

Fertility, Gonadal Function, and Sexuality

From the perspective of the survivor, alterations in gonadal function and the loss of fertility (or even the fear of impaired fertility) are perhaps the most life-altering sequelae of cancer, influencing a survivor's body image, sexuality, dating relationships, marriage patterns, and sense of well-being. Gonadal function is impacted by many different therapies, including chemotherapy with moderate to high dose alkylating agents; radiation to the pelvis, abdomen and brain; and pelvic surgery. Regardless of gender and age of the survivor, questions and concerns about fertility, premature gonadal failure, and sexuality are very common. It is imperative that the clinician provide both practical and accurate information, and offer other resources as needed. This topic is discussed in detail in four superb resource books (34–36,60). In addition, the Lance Armstrong Foundation has developed a very useful and user-friendly website, www.livestrong.org. This site provides some excellent and trustworthy information, including modules on female infertility, male infertility, and sexual dysfunction. ASCO has also published an excellent review of recommendations on fertility preservation in cancer patients (61).

Psychosocial Issues

The experience of being diagnosed and treated for cancer exerts considerable psychological strain on both the patient and the family. Despite this, many survivors report normal psychological health, and some even demonstrate psychological growth as a result of their cancer experience. However, on average, cancer survivors are more likely to experience chronic pain or fatigue than the general population (4,25,62). Hudson et al. reported that 17% of 9,535 young adult survivors of childhood cancer had depressive, somatic, or anxiety symptoms, and 10% reported moderate to extreme pain as a result of their cancer (4). Approximately one out of five young adult survivors of childhood cancer reports symptoms of posttraumatic stress disorder (PTSD), characterized by re-experiencing elements of their prior cancer experience or its associated emotions, avoidance of people or places that remind them of their previous cancer, and increased anxiety or arousal (63,64). Both parents and siblings of survivors may develop symptoms of PTSD, and thus, the primary care physician must extend the assessment of mental health to survivors' families (65,66). Posttraumatic stress symptoms and disorder are also common among adults diagnosed with cancer (67–69).

Importantly, some survivors demonstrate post-traumatic growth (PTG) and psychosocial thriving as a result of their cancer experience (70–72). Many rate themselves highly on their ability to cope as a result of their prior cancer, suggesting that this life-altering event promotes resiliency (73).

Clinicians must be sensitive to the concerns expressed by survivors who often worry about fertility and parenthood, obtaining health and life insurance, educational difficulties, job availability, and their risk for future health problems, including second cancer. In our experience, one of the most important components in delivering quality care to cancer survivors is having a psychologist as part of the team. In fact, screening for psychosocial problems, addressing fears and concerns, providing counseling, and managing psychological morbidity are some of the most important ways to maximize the health of a cancer survivor.

In addition, the Lance Armstrong Foundation website noted above, www.livestrong.org, provides very useful modules about emotional issues common to cancer survivors, including the following topics: body image, emotional effects of cancer, fear of recurrence, finding meaning, grief and loss, hope, living with uncertainty, sadness and depression, setting priorities, stress, communicating with your partner, dating and new relationships, and telling others you are a survivor. In addition, the website also provides an avenue for one-on-one peer support by telephone. Through this mechanism, counseling and referral to the local resources in the survivor's locale can be provided.

SPECIAL SERVICES

Some survivors will benefit from referral for special services. As described in this chapter, this includes cognitive and physical rehabilitation (74–77). Other special services that are occasionally needed include occupational and speech therapy, career counseling, peer support programs, and genetic testing and counseling (78–80). Developing a list of available special services can be helpful to the clinician following a cancer survivor.

CONCLUSIONS

In recent years, much has changed regarding our understanding of late effects and methods to maintain or improve the health of cancer survivors. In particular, the potential late effects following treatment of cancer in children and adolescents is reasonably well characterized, and the next generation of studies should be aimed at intervening to lower risk. In contrast, the frequency and severity of late effects following treatment of adult cancer is not as well characterized and research should be focused on gathering this information. Regardless, we now understand the uniqueness of the survivorship experience and the need for care that addresses a survivor's risks.

References

1. Hewitt M, Greenfield S, Stovall E. *From Cancer Patient to Cancer Survivor: Lost in Transition*. Washington DC: The National Academies Press; 2006.
2. Surveillance, Epidemiology, and End Results (SEER) Program. SEERStat Database: Incidence—SEER-9 regulations. Bethesda, Maryland:National Cancer Institute, Division of Cancer Control and Population Sciences, 2003. available at http://www.seer.cancer.gov
3. Oeffinger KC, Mertens AC, Sklar CA, et al. Chronic health conditions in adult survivors of childhood cancer. *N Engl J Med*. 2006;355:1572–182.
4. Hudson MM, Mertens AC, Yasui Y, et al. Health status of adult long-term survivors of childhood cancer: a report from the Childhood Cancer Survivor Study. *JAMA*. 2003;290: 1583–1592.
5. Chlebowski RT, Pettinger M, Stefanick ML, et al. Insulin, physical activity, and caloric intake in postmenopausal women: breast cancer implications. *J Clin Oncol*. 2004;22:4507–4513.
6. Herman DR, Ganz PA, Petersen L, et al. Obesity and cardiovascular risk factors in younger breast cancer survivors: The Cancer and Menopause Study (CAMS). *Breast Cancer Res Treat*. 2005;93:13–23.
7. Holmes MD, Chen WY, Feskanich D, et al. Physical activity and survival after breast cancer diagnosis. *JAMA*. 2005;293: 2479–2486.
8. Castellon SA, Ganz PA, Bower JE, et al. Neurocognitive performance in breast cancer survivors exposed to adjuvant chemotherapy and tamoxifen. *J Clin Exp Neuropsychol*. 2004;26:955–969.
9. McAllister TW, Ahles TA, Saykin AJ, et al. Cognitive effects of cytotoxic cancer chemotherapy: predisposing risk factors and potential treatments. *Curr Psychiatry Rep*. 2004;6:364–371.
10. Duffy CM, Allen SM, Clark MA. Discussions regarding reproductive health for young women with breast cancer undergoing chemotherapy. *J Clin Oncol*. 2005;23:766–773.
11. Ganz PA. Breast cancer, menopause, and long-term survivorship: critical issues for the 21st century. *Am J Med*. 2005;118: 136–141.
12. Hooning MJ, Aleman BM, van Rosmalen AJ, et al. Cause-specific mortality in long-term survivors of breast cancer: A 25-year follow-up study. *Int J Radiat Oncol Biol Phys*. 2006;64: 1081–1091.
13. Recht A, Edge SB, Solin LJ, et al. Postmastectomy radiotherapy: clinical practice guidelines of the American Society of Clinical Oncology. *J Clin Oncol*. 2001;19:1539–1569.
14. Roychoudhuri R, Evans H, Robinson D, et al. Radiation-induced malignancies following radiotherapy for breast cancer. *Br J Cancer*. 2004;91:868–872.
15. Chen Z, Maricic M, Bassford TL, et al. Fracture risk among breast cancer survivors: results from the Women's Health Initiative Observational Study. *Arch Intern Med*. 2005;165:552–558.
16. Chen Z, Maricic M, Pettinger M, et al. Osteoporosis and rate of bone loss among postmenopausal survivors of breast cancer. *Cancer*. 2005;104:1520–1530.
17. Chlebowski RT. Bone health in women with early-stage breast cancer. *Clin Breast Cancer*. 2005;5(Suppl):S35–S40.
18. Gianni L, Dombernowsky P, Sledge G, et al. Cardiac function following combination therapy with paclitaxel and doxorubicin: an analysis of 657 women with advanced breast cancer. *Ann Oncol*. 2001;12:1067–1073.

19. Meinardi MT, Van Der Graaf WT, Gietema JA, et al. Evaluation of long term cardiotoxicity after epirubicin containing adjuvant chemotherapy and locoregional radiotherapy for breast cancer using various detection techniques. *Heart*. 2002;88:81–82.

20. Meinardi MT, van Veldhuisen DJ, Gietema JA, et al. Prospective evaluation of early cardiac damage induced by epirubicin-containing adjuvant chemotherapy and locoregional radiotherapy in breast cancer patients. *J Clin Oncol*. 2001;19:2746–2753.

21. Shapiro CL, Hardenbergh PH, Gelman R, et al. Cardiac effects of adjuvant doxorubicin and radiation therapy in breast cancer patients. *J Clin Oncol*. 1998;16:3493–34501.

22. Zambetti M, Moliterni A, Materazzo C, et al. Long-term cardiac sequelae in operable breast cancer patients given adjuvant chemotherapy with or without doxorubicin and breast irradiation. *J Clin Oncol*. 2001;19:37–43.

23. Gotay CC, Muraoka MY. Quality of life in long-term survivors of adult-onset cancers. *J Natl Cancer Inst*. 1998;90:656–667.

24. Kornblith AB, Herndon JE, 2nd, Weiss RB, et al. Long-term adjustment of survivors of early-stage breast carcinoma, 20 years after adjuvant chemotherapy. *Cancer*. 2003;98:679–689.

25. Bower JE, Ganz PA, Desmond KA, et al. Fatigue in long-term breast carcinoma survivors: a longitudinal investigation. *Cancer*. 2006;106:751–758.

26. Bower JE, Ganz PA, Desmond KA, et al. Fatigue in breast cancer survivors: occurrence, correlates, and impact on quality of life. *J Clin Oncol*. 2000;18:743–753.

27. Deshields T, Tibbs T, Fan MY, et al. Differences in patterns of depression after treatment for breast cancer. *Psychooncology*. 2008;17(9):948–953.

28. Ganz PA, Rowland JH, Desmond K, et al. Life after breast cancer: understanding women's health-related quality of life and sexual functioning. *J Clin Oncol*. 1998;16:501–514.

29. Rowland JH, Yancik R. Cancer survivorship: the interface of aging, comorbidity, and quality care. *J Natl Cancer Inst*. 2006;98:504–505.

30. Yancik R, Ganz PA, Varricchio CG, et al. Perspectives on comorbidity and cancer in older patients: approaches to expand the knowledge base. *J Clin Oncol*. 2001;19:1147–1151.

31. Aziz NM, Rowland JH. Trends and advances in cancer survivorship research: challenge and opportunity. *Semin Radiat Oncol*. 2003;13:248–266.

32. Hewitt M, Weiner SL, Simone JV, eds. *Childhood Cancer Survivorship: Improving Care and Quality of Life*. Washington DC: The National Academies Press; 2003.

33. Oeffinger KC. Longitudinal risk-based health care for adult survivors of childhood cancer. *Curr Probl Cancer*. 2003;27:143–167.

34. Feuerstein M, ed. *Handbook of Cancer Survivorship*. New York, NY: Springer; 2007.

35. Ganz PA, ed. *Cancer Survivorship: Today and Tomorrow*. New York, NY: Springer; 2007.

36. Wallace WH, Green DM, eds. *Late Effects of Childhood Cancer*. London, UK: Arnold Publishers; 2004.

37. Bhatia S, Landier W. Evaluating survivors of pediatric cancer. *Cancer J*. 2005;11:340–354.

38. Ganz PA. Monitoring the physical health of cancer survivors: a survivorship-focused medical history. *J Clin Oncol*. 2006;24:5105–5111.

39. Oeffinger KC, Hudson MM. Long-term complications following childhood and adolescent cancer: foundations for providing risk-based health care for survivors. *CA Cancer J Clin*. 2004;54:208–236.

40. National Comprehensive Cancer Network: Welcome to the NCCN clinical practice guidelines in oncology. http://www.nccn.org/professionals/physician_gls/default.asp

41. Landier W, Bhatia S, Eshelman DA, et al. Development of risk-based guidelines for pediatric cancer survivors: the Children's Oncology Group long-term follow-up guidelines from the Children's Oncology Group late effects committee and nursing discipline. *J Clin Oncol*. 2004;22:4979–4990.

42. Scottish Intercollegiate Guidelines Network (SIGN). Long term follow up of survivors of childhood cancer. Guideline no. 76. Available at: www.sign.ac.uk/pdf/sign76.pdf

43. Skinner R, Wallace WH, Levitt G. Therapy based long-term follow up: a practice statement. United Kingdom Children's Cancer Study Group Late Effects Group. Available at: www.ukccsg.org

44. Earle CC. Cancer survivorship research and guidelines: maybe the cart should be beside the horse. *J Clin Oncol*. 2007;25:3800–3801.

45. Carver JR, Shapiro CL, Ng A, et al. American Society of Clinical Oncology clinical evidence review on the ongoing care of adult cancer survivors: cardiac and pulmonary late effects. *J Clin Oncol*. 2007;25:3991–4008.

46. Travis LB, Gilbert E. Lung cancer after Hodgkin lymphoma: the roles of chemotherapy, radiotherapy and tobacco use. *Radiat Res*. 2005;163:695–696.

47. Travis LB, Gospodarowicz M, Curtis RE, et al. Lung cancer following chemotherapy and radiotherapy for Hodgkin's disease. *J Natl Cancer Inst*. 2002;94:182–192.

48. Chlebowski RT, Aiello E, McTiernan A. Weight loss in breast cancer patient management. *J Clin Oncol*. 2002;20:1128–1143.

49. Oeffinger KC. Are survivors of acute lymphoblastic leukemia (ALL) at increased risk of cardiovascular disease? *Pediatr Blood Cancer*. 2008;50:462–467; discussion 468.

50. Bellizzi KM, Rowland JH, Jeffery DD, et al. Health behaviors of cancer survivors: examining opportunities for cancer control intervention. *J Clin Oncol*. 2005;23:8884–8893.

51. Irwin ML, Aiello EJ, McTiernan A, et al. Physical activity, body mass index, and mammographic density in postmenopausal breast cancer survivors. *J Clin Oncol*. 2007;25:1061–1066.

52. Schmitz KH, Holtzman J, Courneya KS, et al. Controlled physical activity trials in cancer survivors: a systematic review and meta-analysis. *Cancer Epidemiol Biomarkers Prev*. 2005;14:1588–1595.

53. Demark-Wahnefried W, Aziz NM, Rowland JH, et al. Riding the crest of the teachable moment: promoting long-term health after the diagnosis of cancer. *J Clin Oncol*. 2005;23:5814–5830.

54. Demark-Wahnefried W. Move onward, press forward, and take a deep breath: can lifestyle interventions improve the quality of life of women with breast cancer, and how can we be sure? *J Clin Oncol*. 2007;25:4344–4345.

55. Demark-Wahnefried W, Pinto BM, Gritz ER. Promoting health and physical function among cancer survivors: potential for prevention and questions that remain. *J Clin Oncol*. 2006;24:5125–5131.

56. Sunga AY, Eberl MM, Oeffinger KC, et al. Care of cancer survivors. *Am Fam Physician*. 2005;71:699–706.

57. Hudson MM, Oeffinger KC. Future health of survivors of adolescent and young adult cancer. In: Bleyer AW, Barr RD, eds. *Cancer in Adolescents and Young Adults*. New York, NY: Springer; 2007.

58. Aziz NM, Oeffinger KC, Brooks S, et al. Comprehensive long-term follow-up programs for pediatric cancer survivors. *Cancer*. 2006;107:841–848.

59. *Implementing Cancer Survivorship Care Planning: Workshop Summary*. Washington DC: The National Academies Press; 2006.

60. Bleyer AW, Barr RD, eds. *Cancer in Adolescents and Young Adults*. New York, NY: Springer; 2007.

61. Lee SJ, Schover LR, Partridge AH, et al. American Society of Clinical Oncology recommendations on fertility preservation in cancer patients. *J Clin Oncol*. 2006;24:2917–2931.

62. Ganz PA, Bower JE. Cancer related fatigue: a focus on breast cancer and Hodgkin's disease survivors. *Acta Oncol*. 2007;46:474–479.

63. Drotar D, Schwartz L, Palermo TM, et al. Factor structure of the child health questionnaire-parent form in pediatric populations. *J Pediatr Psychol*. 2006;31:127–138.

64. Rourke MT, Hobbie WL, Schwartz L, et al. Posttraumatic stress disorder (PTSD) in young adult survivors of childhood cancer. *Pediatr Blood Cancer.* 2007;49:177–182.

65. Kazak AE, Alderfer M, Rourke MT, et al. Posttraumatic stress disorder (PTSD) and posttraumatic stress symptoms (PTSS) in families of adolescent childhood cancer survivors. *J Pediatr Psychol.* 2004;29:211–219.

66. Kazak AE, Cant MC, Jensen MM, et al. Identifying psychosocial risk indicative of subsequent resource use in families of newly diagnosed pediatric oncology patients. *J Clin Oncol.* 2003;21:3220–3225.

67. Hegel MT, Moore CP, Collins ED, et al. Distress, psychiatric syndromes, and impairment of function in women with newly diagnosed breast cancer. *Cancer.* 2006;107:2924–2931.

68. Mehnert A, Koch U. Prevalence of acute and post-traumatic stress disorder and comorbid mental disorders in breast cancer patients during primary cancer care: a prospective study. *Psychooncology.* 2007;16:181–188.

69. Thornton AA, Perez MA. Posttraumatic growth in prostate cancer survivors and their partners. *Psychooncology.* 2006;15: 285–296.

70. Morrill EF, Brewer NT, O'Neill SC, et al. The interaction of post-traumatic growth and post-traumatic stress symptoms in predicting depressive symptoms and quality of life. *Psychooncology.* 2008;17(9):948–953.

71. Barakat LP, Alderfer MA, Kazak AE. Posttraumatic growth in adolescent survivors of cancer and their mothers and fathers. *J Pediatr Psychol.* 2006;31:413–419.

72. Parry C, Chesler MA. Thematic evidence of psychosocial thriving in childhood cancer survivors. *Qual Health Res.* 2005;15:1055–1073.

73. Zebrack BJ, Chesler MA. Quality of life in childhood cancer survivors. *Psychooncology.* 2002;11:132–141.

74. Gabanelli P. A rehabilitative approach to the patient with brain cancer. *Neurol Sci.* 2005;26(Suppl 1):S51–S52.

75. Fialka-Moser V, Crevenna R, Korpan M, et al. Cancer rehabilitation: particularly with aspects on physical impairments. *J Rehabil Med.* 2003;35:153–162.

76. Cole RP, Scialla SJ, Bednarz L. Functional recovery in cancer rehabilitation. *Arch Phys Med Rehabil.* 2000;81:623–627.

77. Stubblefield MD, Custodio CM, Franklin DJ. Cardiopulmonary rehabilitation and cancer rehabilitation. 3. Cancer rehabilitation. *Arch Phys Med Rehabil.* 2006;87:S65–S71.

78. Matthews BA, Baker F, Spillers RL. Oncology professionals and patient requests for cancer support services. *Support Care Cancer.* 2004;12:731–738.

79. Tesauro GM, Rowland JH, Lustig C. Survivorship resources for post-treatment cancer survivors. *Cancer Pract.* 2002;10: 277–283.

80. van Weert E, Hoekstra-Weebers J, Grol B, et al. A multidimensional cancer rehabilitation program for cancer survivors: effectiveness on health-related quality of life. *J Psychosom Res.* 2005;58:485–496.

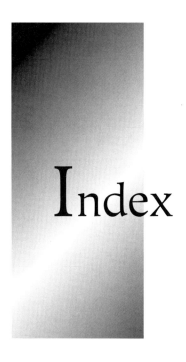

Index